THE MANAGEMENT OF PAIN

VOLUME

II

with collaboration of

John D. Loeser, M.D.

Professor of Neurological Surgery
Director, Multidisciplinary Pain Center
University of Washington
Chief, Division of Neurosurgery
Children's Orthopedic Hospital and Medical Center
Seattle, Washington

C. Richard Chapman, Ph.D.

Professor, Department of Anesthesiology,
 Psychiatry and Behavioral Sciences, and Psychology
Associate Director For Research, Multidisciplinary Pain Center
University of Washington
Director, Pain and Toxicity Research Program
Fred Hutchinson Cancer Research Center
Seattle, Washington

Wilbert E. Fordyce, Ph.D.

Professor Emeritus, Department of Rehabilitation Medicine
Senior Consultant in Clinical Psychology, Multidisciplinary Pain Center
University of Washington
Seattle, Washington

illustrations by

Marjorie Domenowske
Medical Illustrator

THE MANAGEMENT OF PAIN

SECOND EDITION

VOLUME

II

John J. Bonica, M.D., D.Sc., D. Med. Sc. (Hon.), F.F.A.R.C.S. (Hon.)

Professor and Chairman Emeritus
Department of Anesthesiology
Director Emeritus, Multidisciplinary Pain Center
University of Washington
Seattle, Washington
Founder and Honorary President
International Association for the Study of Pain

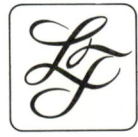

LEA & FEBIGER
Philadelphia • London
1990

Lea & Febiger
200 Chesterfield Parkway
Malvern, Pennsylvania   19355
U.S.A.
1-800-444-1785

Lea & Febiger (UK) Ltd.
145a Croydon Road
Beckenham, Kent BR3 3RB
U.K.

Library of Congress Cataloging-in-Publication Data

Bonica, John J., 1917–
 The management of pain.

 Rev. ed. of: The management of pain. 1953.
 Includes bibliographies and index.
 1. Pain—Treatment. I. Bonica, John J.,
1917–   Management of pain. II. Title.
[DNLM: 1. Pain—therapy. WL 104 B715m]
 RB127.B68   1989   616'.0472   88-8983
 ISBN 0-8121-1122-2

First Edition, 1953
  Reprinted 1954
Second Edition, 1990

The cover reproduction of the sculpture *Laocoonte* is used with the permission of Scala Istituto Fotografico Editoriale and Art Resource. The sculpture is housed at the Vatican, Museum Pio Clementino.

Reprints of chapters may be purchased from Lea & Febiger in quantities of 100 or more.

Printed in the United States of America

Print number: 5   4   3   2   1

This volume is dedicated to my children

Angela, Charlotte, Linda, and John

and to my grandchildren

Adrianna, Anna, Gianmarco, and William

in appreciation of their forbearance, sympathetic understanding, and the deprivation of my companionship during the long isolations necessary to the writing of this book and all other academic activities

PREFACE

The purpose of this textbook, like that of the first edition published in 1953, is to present a comprehensive discussion of the fundamental aspects of pain, of the various diseases and disorders in which pain is an important problem, and guidelines for managing patients with various acute painful disorders and chronic pain syndromes. Although a number of books and monographs on specific aspects of pain have been published during the past decade or so, none is complete enough to serve clinicians as a guide to the effective management of such a broad, multifaceted, and complex health problem as pain. It is necessary to consult several books in order to obtain information regarding the substrates, causes, pathophysiology, symptoms and signs, diagnosis, and treatment of pain and on the therapeutic modalities in current use and how to apply them appropriately. Unlike other major books on pain, which focus primarily or wholly on chronic pain, this book considers all acute painful disorders as well as virtually every chronic pain syndrome that has been described in the medical literature.

The book is intended to serve both as a textbook and as a complete reference work for practitioners of every field of medicine, because pain is universal and is the primary reason why patients seek the counsel of physicians and other care providers. It has been written for, and should be useful to, four groups of readers: (a) family physicians, dentists, and other caregivers, who are usually the first to see patients with pain; (b) specialists in internal medicine, neurology, neurosurgery, physiatry, psychology, psychiatry, and anesthesiology and others who have had no special training in clinical algology but who frequently encounter complex pain problems; (c) students of medicine, dentistry, nursing, and behavioral sciences and recently graduated physicians who are undertaking postgraduate training for specialization; and (d) clinical algologists. The first and second groups can use it as a reference source in helping to make or to confirm the correct diagnosis of complex pain problems and to deduce what therapy or combination of therapies should be carried out and what treatments should *not* be done. In many cases, therapy can and should be carried out by the patient's primary physician; in others the patient needs to be referred to a specialist with skills in a specific therapy, or more frequently to a multidisciplinary/interdisciplinary facility for diagnosis and therapy of pain. By providing appropriate guidelines, it is hoped that patients will be spared the risk of iatrogenic complications such as the development of chronic pain syndromes, drug toxicity, useless operations, and other ineffective therapies. Students and residents in specialty training will find useful the information on the basic aspects of pain as well as the clinical considerations of conditions encountered in their particular specialty. The clinical algologist will find indepth discussion of all aspects of complex chronic pain syndromes including guidelines to help in the differential diagnosis and the therapeutic modalities that can be used.

The book consists of five parts. The chapters in *Part I* contain basic scientific and clinical information. Chapter 1 is a historical overview of pain concepts and treatment, and Chapter 2 contains definitions and the taxonomy of pain published by the International Association for the Study of Pain (IASP). Section B (Chapters 3 through 5) presents an overview of the anatomic, physiologic, and biochemical substrates of pain and a discussion of the psychologic reactions to, and determinants of, pain. Section C is devoted to general considerations of various aspects of pain, including a chapter on applied anatomy especially relevant to the diagnosis and treatment of acute and chronic pain, followed by two chapters that consider the epidemiology, mechanisms, and effects of acute and chronic pain. The last chapter of Part I contains a brief discussion of the evolution and current status of multidisciplinary/interdisciplinary pain programs for research, education, training, and patient care. The material in this first part should prove especially useful to family physicians and to students and residents undertaking specialization.

Part II consists of 21 chapters on acute painful conditions and chronic pain syndromes that can involve different parts of the body. The information is intended to provide a general discussion that will minimize repetition of certain points regarding causes, pathophysiology, symptoms and signs, diagnosis, and therapy when considering a pain syndrome in a particular region of the body. For example, Section A contains chapters on pain of neuropathic origin such as peripheral nerve disorders, causalgia and other reflex sympathetic dystrophy, and central pain and other disorders, each of which can cause pain in several regions of the body. Thus, when considering neuropathy with neuralgia in the upper limb, chest, abdomen, or lower limb, the reader can refer to the general discussion in this part of the book and then turn to the appropriate chapter in Part IV. The last two chapters in Part II are devoted to special considerations of pain in infants, children, and the elderly.

The six chapters in *Part III* are devoted to the approaches and methods recommended for the assessment of patients with complex pain problems. Whereas diagnosis of causative factors is usually relatively simple in acute painful conditions such as injuries, burns, and visceral disease and in some chronic painful disorders such as arthritis and cancer, assessment of patients with complex chronic pain problems is necessarily comprehensive and time consuming.

Throughout this part as well as other parts of the book, emphasis is placed on an integrated approach to the evaluation and treatment of patients with pain.

Part IV deals with pain in the head, neck and upper limb, chest, abdomen, pelvis, and low back and lower limbs. Each section is introduced by a chapter that provides a brief overview of the anatomic and physiologic bases of painful conditions in that region, a summary of the most important points in evaluating patients with, for example, pain in the head, and a table summarizing the etiology and differential diagnosis of pain in the specific region. Subsequent chapters in Part IV deal with painful disorders and pain syndromes involving different body systems, such as the nervous system, musculoskeletal system, viscera, and vascular system. This classification of pain syndromes, according to regions and systems, was used in the first edition of this book and was considered to be one of the most important and practical contributions to the clinical management of pain. Moreover, this classification approach was adopted by the IASP as axes I and II of its classification. Many chapters in this part of the book discuss painful disorders not discussed at all in Part II, whereas others present material that complements the information contained in Part II.

Part V is devoted to discussion of all therapies currently used for the relief of pain. Each of the seven sections has chapters that describe specific therapeutic modalities for the symptomatic control of acute and chronic pain. The word symptomatic is intended to convey the fact that most of these therapies are not intended to eliminate the cause of the pain but rather to reduce or eliminate the pain per se. (Methods to eliminate the cause of pain, when this is possible, are discussed in various chapters of Part IV dealing with various diseases that cause acute or chronic pain.) The therapeutic modalities are presented in descending order of frequency and practicability of use by health professionals and according to whether they are invasive or noninvasive.

Each section is preceded by a brief historical perspective on the method or techniques, and in some sections, guidelines for their use. Each chapter includes such basic considerations as the pharmacologic, physiologic, psychologic, anatomic, or physical bases for the use of the procedure; its indications; a summary of the results obtained in its application to various painful disorders; and specific comments on side effects, complications, contraindications, and advantages and disadvantages of each procedure. Description of the technique of application varies according to the procedure: some simple techniques and procedures that can be done by family physicians or specialists—such as drug dosage or simple regional blocks, TENS, certain physical therapies, and certain psychologic techniques—are described in sufficient detail to permit either the generalist or the specialist to learn how to do and apply them.

Description of complicated regional anesthesia procedures and neurosurgical operations is brief and is not intended for physicians skilled in their application, nor is it intended to be used as the sole basis for learning and applying them. Rather, the primary objective is to provide readers who do not practice these procedures with information on what the procedure entails and its indications, advantages, disadvantages, and complications. This is in accordance with my long-held conviction that anyone managing patients in pain should be acquainted with all currently available therapeutic procedures, because only with such knowledge and broad perspective can the physician inform and guide the patient as to what therapy (or combination of therapies) is suitable for each particular pain problem.

The last section, composed of a single chapter, deals with multidisciplinary/multimodal therapies in the treatment of patients with complex chronic pain syndromes.

An attempt has been made to present a balanced view of how these modalities might be combined to achieve the best results in the management of patients with pain, particularly those with complex pain syndromes.

The book has been organized to minimize duplication of data and repetition of discussion of all aspects of painful disorders. For example, Chapters 7 and 8, devoted to an overview of epidemiology, mechanisms, and effects of acute and chronic pain, are intended to minimize repetition of these aspects in discussing the various acute and chronic pain disorders in Parts II and IV of the book. Similarly, the general discussions in Part II are intended to minimize repetition in Part IV. On the other hand, there is considerable repetition of some aspects of specific pain syndromes. Moreover, in discussing results obtained with each of the therapeutic modalities in Part V, there is duplication of data presented in various chapters in Parts II and IV. However, the data on results and complications presented in Part V are more comprehensive and include not only those experienced by the author(s) of each chapter, but a summary of data contained in the most important published reports. Repetitions, where they do exist, serve two purposes: to emphasize important issues and to minimize the need for readers to turn pages from one section to the other.

It is widely recognized that multiauthored books are often uneven in format and quality and frequently contain conflicting and contradictory information. These considerations prompted me to write virtually the entire first edition of the book. Subsequent reviewers emphasized its unity and described it as "encyclopedic," "monumental," and "a masterpiece," and it became known worldwide as "the bible of pain." These considerations would have suggested that I undertake the writing of the second edition alone. However, the recent vast advances in basic and clinical aspects of pain, the development of more sophisticated and highly specialized diagnostic and therapeutic modalities, my strong desire to publish the book in a reasonable time, and most importantly, my desire to produce a book that would reflect the multidimensional nature of pain and the multidisciplinary/interdisciplinary approach to its management compelled me to decide to have contributors.

To minimize the aforementioned disadvantages, I expanded hundreds of hours and exerted significant efforts during the four-year period required for the completion of the book. First, in the planning stage I developed a detailed outline of the book similar to, but larger than, the first edition and also developed uniform formats and outlines for chapters that would be in Parts II, IV, and V of the book. These were subsequently reviewed by my three collaborators: John D. Loeser, who assumed the responsibility of editing chapters dealing with neuropathic pain and neurosurgical operations, and C. Richard Chapman and Wilbert Fordyce, who had the task of reviewing chapters on pain of psychologic origin and the section on psychologic analgesic techniques. The outlines were sent to some four dozen authorities working in the field with the request to make suggestions for improving the organization of the volume. Subsequently I reviewed the responses and had semiweekly meetings with my three collaborators during the developmental stage of the book. In addition to considering the suggestions, they helped me in selecting contributors to the areas they were responsible for. Together with a letter of invitation, each prospective contributor was sent material that included a brief overview of the first edition, details of the objectives of the second edition, and description of the five parts. Once contributors accepted, they were sent copies of the aforementioned formats that were intended to be conducive to uniformity of chapters in the various parts of the book and were requested to submit a detailed outline of the chapter or chapter section they agreed to write. Once the outlines were received, I studied them carefully and reviewed the most current literature (books, review articles, etc.) on each specific subject to evaluate the proposed outline sent me and to make whatever revision I deemed important. I also enlisted the opinion of my collaborators. The revised outline was then returned to the author with a re-emphasis of the importance of adhering to the format and to the suggested size of the chapter. Each contributor was also requested to submit copies of illustrations to supplement the text. Some months later contributors sent in their initial drafts, which I reviewed and studied carefully. In some instances I enlisted the help of my collaborators in this review process. The chapters were then returned to the contributors, frequently with requests for deletion or addition of material, clarification or amplification of specific points, and revision of the format of both the text and tables. This process was repeated with subsequent drafts; consequently most chapters underwent at least three or four drafts, and some as many as six to eight drafts in order to make them comprehensive, up-to-date, and most important, uniform.

The many illustrations have been included to supplement the detailed description of the text and thus facilitate the task of the reader. Some of these have been taken from the first edition of this book and from other books I have written, many are new, and others are modifications of published figures. Mrs. Domenowske and I spent an immense amount of time and effort, not only to develop the new illustrations, but in modifying published figures rather than borrowing the original. This was done for the sake of uniformity of artistic style and because the modified illustration emphasizes important points relevant to the subject on hand not found in the original figure. A significant number of illustrations and data on anatomic structures in various chapters of Part IV are repeated in chapters in Part V. This repetition and the fact that the illustrations and the detailed description have been learned by physicians and can be found in textbooks of anatomy, orthopedics, anesthesia, neurosurgery, physical therapy, etc., might be considered by some as superfluous and unnecessary. However, I have included them to refresh the memory of physicians who have not retained the information, for health professionals who have not been taught such information, and most importantly to preclude the need for the reader to consult a number of other textbooks on reading this book. This is pursuant to my long-held philosophy expressed at the beginning of this preface that the comprehensive textbook should provide readers with a catholically thorough exposition of the subject.

Another aspect of the book intended to facilitate the task of a busy reader is that less relevant facts—material that has been included because of its academic importance, or for the sake of completeness, or for consumption by students and those who wish to delve deeper into the problem—are presented in small type. These can be skipped without losing continuity of thought. In this manner, completeness, detail, and thoroughness are not sacrificed and emphasis is laid on the practical aspects of the problem at hand. The references at the end of each chapter consist of the most important books or review articles containing more detailed exposition of subjects or citation of important publications on a particular subject.

Seattle, Washington   John. J. Bonica

ACKNOWLEDGMENTS

A book of this nature is made possible only by the contributions of many individuals. The information set forth in Chapters 3 and 4 and parts of other chapters represents the fruition of the efforts of many basic and clinical scientists who have spent untold time and efforts to solve the "puzzle of pain." In writing various chapters dealing with basic and clinical issues, I consulted numerous major textbooks on anatomy, neurophysiology, biochemistry, internal medicine, oncology, orthopedics, general surgery, neurosurgery, psychology, and psychiatry. Although these sources are cited in the introduction to each chapter, I wish to acknowledge the invaluable help I received from these books and thank their authors and publishers.

I wish to express my sincere appreciation and thanks to contributors to the two volumes for their cooperation, their patience, and the time spent in revising chapters and complying with my many requests. I am especially indebted to Dr. John D. Loeser, who not only contributed a significant number of chapters, but was extremely helpful in reviewing a number of early drafts of chapters and making editorial suggestions that helped me immensely. Drs. C. Richard Chapman and Wilbert Fordyce also contributed a number of chapters and helped in the editorial review process, particularly of chapters in Section B of Part II and in Part V. Andrew C.N. Chen provided immense help in reviewing the pain literature.

I owe special thanks and express deep appreciation to Drs. Ronald Dubner, Ken Casey, and Willie Dong, who carefully reviewed several drafts of Chapters 3 and 4 and made many valuable suggestions that improved and updated the information contained therein. I also thank the following colleagues who reviewed the page proofs of various other chapters: Drs. Peter Buckley, Stephen Butler, Felix Freund, Costantino Benedetti, and Terence Murphy. Mr. John F. Frlan, pharmacist, has provided advice and help pertaining to pharmaceutical issues.

I owe a great debt to Mrs. Marjorie Domenowske for the illustrations, most of which were developed after many hours of study of text and illustrations in other books, and for the many pleasant hours we spent together in developing the final copies. Mrs. Domenowske's superb artistic skill, patience, and cooperation greatly facilitated an arduous task. The expenses for the development of many of these illustrations were defrayed in part by three grants: one from the Breon/Winthrop Laboratories through the courtesy of the late Mr. Arthur Catalani and Mr. Joseph Scarlata, one from the Purdue Frederick Company through the courtesy of Drs. Robert Kaiko and Richard Sackler, and one from the Bristol-Myers Pharmaceutical Company through the courtesy of Dr. George Blewitt and Messrs. Harry Levine, Tom McCann, and Jon Weisberg. I also take this opportunity to express appreciation to the authors and publishers of illustrations that were used as a basis for development of new illustrations and of those that have been borrowed. In each case appropriate credit is given in the legend.

I wish to express immense appreciation to Dr. Thomas F. Hornbein, close friend and current Chairman of our Department of Anesthesiology for his encouragement in the development of this book, and for his sagacious foresight, immense interest, untiring efforts, and highly effective support of the Pain Center programs and for his vigorous leadership in the establishment of the John and Emma Bonica Endowed Chair for Anesthesiology and Pain Research.

It is difficult to express adequately my thanks and appreciation to my administrative secretary, Mrs. Donna Rowe, and transcription secretaries, Mrs. Eileen Holloway and Ms. Laura Hopkins, for their outstanding work and invaluable help. In addition to supervising the work of the other secretaries, Mrs. Rowe has been of inestimable value in coordinating all of the activities related to the book with the publisher and with all of the contributors, proofreading some of the text and doing many other tasks required for the development and publication of these two large volumes. Mrs. Kathleen A. Murray provided much appreciated help in some of the editorial aspects. I also wish to acknowledge the help given me by my children in secretarial assistance in my office at home. My special thanks are also due to Mr. Michael McIntosh of Health Sciences Photography for producing copies of original illustrations, to Mrs. Virginia Sheldon and Mrs. Hana Zeman of the Health Sciences Library in helping the secretarial staff in borrowing many major books, review articles, and reference lists, and to Dr. Jerry E. Prentiss and several librarians of the Straub Clinic and Hospital of Honolulu for their cooperation in researching and lending numerous major textbooks for consultation.

My sincerest thanks, appreciation, and gratitude are extended to Messrs. Carroll Cann, Tom Colaiezzi, and David Amundson of Lea & Febiger for their many courtesies, cooperation, remarkable help, and patience in the preparation and printing of this book.

John J. Boncia

CONTRIBUTORS

Tim A. Ahles, Ph.D.
Associate Professor of Psychiatry
Director, Behavioral Medicine Section
Dartmouth Medical School
Hanover, New Hampshire

Edward E. Almquist, M.D.
Clinical Professor of Orthopedics
University of Washington
Chief, Hand Surgery Service
Children's Orthopedic Hospital and Medical Center
Seattle, Washington

Julian S. Ansell, M.D.
Professor of Urology
University of Washington
Seattle, Washington

Joseph Barber, Ph.D.
Associate Clinical Professor of Psychiatry and Biobehavioral
  Sciences
University of California, Los Angeles
Consultant, Children's Hospital of Los Angeles
Los Angeles, California

Costantino Benedetti, M.D.
Associate Professor of Anesthesiology
Attending Physician/Algologist
Multidisciplinary Pain Center
University of Washington
Medical Director of Pain and Toxicity Research Program, Fred
  Hutchinson Cancer Research Center
Seattle, Washington

**Roger J. Berry, M.A., D.Phil., M.D., F.R.C.P.,
  F.R.C.R.(Hon.), F.A.C.R.**
Former Professor of Oncology
Middlesex Hospital Medical School
University of London
Director, Health and Safety and Environmental Protection
British Nuclear Fuels PLC
Risley, Warrington, Cheshire, England

Stanley J. Bigos, M.D.
Associate Professor of Orthopaedics
Director, Spine Resource Clinic
University of Washington
Seattle, Washington

Edward B. Blanchard, Ph.D.
Professor of Psychology
State University of New York at Albany
Co-Director, Center for Stress and Anxiety Disorders
Albany, New York

**John J. Bonica, M.D., D.Sc., D. Med. Sc.(Hon.),
  F.F.A.R.C.S.(Hon.)**
Professor and Chairman Emeritus, Department of
  Anesthesiology
Director Emeritus, Multidisciplinary Pain Center
University of Washington
Seattle, Washington
Founder and Honorary President
  International Association for the Study of Pain

Steven F. Brena, M.D.
Clinical Professor of Rehabilitation Medicine
Emory University
Atlanta, Georgia
Chairman, Pain Control and Rehabilitation Institute of Georgia
Decatur, Georgia

F. Peter Buckley, M.B., F.F.A.R.C.S.
Associate Professor of Anesthesiology
Attending Physician/Algologist
Multidisciplinary Pain Center
University of Washington
Seattle, Washington

Jeffrey A. Burgess, D.D.S., M.S.D.
Auxilliary Faculty, Department of Oral Medicine
Consultant, Multidisciplinary Pain Center
University of Washington
Seattle, Washington

Stephen H. Butler, M.D.
Associate Professor of Anesthesiology
Attending Physician/Algologist
Multidisciplinary Pain Center
University of Washington
Seattle, Washington

Margaret R. Byers, Ph.D.
Research Professor of Anesthesiology and Biological Structure
University of Washington
Seattle, Washington

René Cailliet, M.D.
Clinical Professor of Physical Medicine and Rehabilitation
University of Southern California
Los Angeles, California
Director of Rehabilitation Services
Santa Monica Hospital
Santa Monica, California

C. Richard Chapman, Ph.D.
Professor of Anesthesiology, Psychiatry and Behavioral
  Sciences, and Psychology
Associate Director for Research, Multidisciplinary Pain Center
University of Washington
Director, Pain and Toxicity Research Program
Fred Hutchinson Cancer Research Center
Seattle Washington

Charles W. Cummings, M.D.
Professor and Chairman, Department of Otolaryngology and
    Head and Neck Surgery
University of Washington
Seattle, Washington

Haile T. Debas, M.D.
Professor and Chairman, Department of Surgery
University of California, San Francisco
San Francisco, California

Antoine Depaulis, Ph.D.
Professor of Behavioral Neurophysiology and Biology
Center for Neurochemistry of the National Center for Scientific
    Research (CNRS)
Chief of Research, National Institute for Health and Medical
    Research (INSERM)
Strasbourg, France

Samuel F. Dworkin, D.D.S., Ph.D.
Professor of Psychiatry and Behavioral Sciences and Oral
    Medicine
Consultant, Multidisciplinary Pain Center
University of Washington
Seattle, Washington

Alice L. Eason, M.P.A., P.T.
Chief, Physical Therapy Service, Department of Rehabilitation
    Medicine
New York University
Physical Therapist, Goldwater Memorial Hospital
New York, New York

Margareta Eriksson, M.D., Ph.D.
Department of Neurophysiology
University of Lund
Lund, Sweden

Roseanne Filasky
Administrative Director and Senior Technical Instructor in
    Medical Thermography, Delaware Pain Clinic and
    Thermography Laboratory
Newark, Delaware

Wilbert E. Fordyce, Ph.D.
Professor Emeritus of Rehabilitation Medicine
Senior Consultant in Clinical Psychology
Multidisciplinary Pain Center
University of Washington
Seattle, Washington

Jonathan L. Franklin, M.D.
Formerly Chief Resident, Department of Orthopaedics
University of Washington
Seattle, Washington
Fellow in Sports Medicine, Salt Lake Knee and Sports Medicine
Salt Lake City, Utah

Peter R. Freund, M.D.
Associate Professor of Anesthesiology and Adjunct Associate
    Professor of Physiology and Biophysics
University of Washington
Chief of Anesthesiology and Operating Room Services
Veterans Administration Medical Center
Seattle, Washington

William F. Gee, M.D.
Assistant Clinical Professor of Urology
University of Kentucky
Consulting Urologist, Cardinal Hill Rehabilitation Hospital
Lexington, Kentucky

Phillip L. Gildenberg, M.D., Ph.D.
Clinical Professor of Neurosurgery
University of Texas
Houston, Texas

Bruce C. Gilliland, M.D.
Professor of Medicine and Laboratory Medicine
University of Washington
Director of Medical Education, Providence Medical Center
Seattle, Washington

C. Chan Gunn, M.A., M.D., F.I.C.A.E., F.A.A.A.
Director, Gunn Pain Clinic
Vancouver, British Columbia
Consultant Algologist, Multidisciplinary Pain Center
University of Washington
Seattle, Washington

Gay M. Guzinski, M.D.
Associate Professor of Obstetrics and Gynecology
Chief, Section of Benign Gynecology and Ambulatory
    Obstetrics and Gynecology
University of Maryland
Baltimore, Maryland

Karl E. Hammermeister, M.D.
Professor of Medicine
University of Colorado
Chief, Cardiology Section
Veterans Administration Medical Center
Denver, Colorado

Stephen W. Harkins, Ph.D.
Professor of Gerontology, Psychiatry, Psychology, and
    Biomedical Engineering
Medical College of Virginia
Virginia Commonwealth University
Richmond, Virginia

Josie Howard-Ruben, R.N., M.S.
Assistant Professor of Nursing
Rush Medical College of Rush University
Oncology Clinical Nurse Specialist
Rush-Presbyterian-St. Luke's Medical Center
Chicago, Illinois

Masayoshi Itoh, M.D., M.P.H.
Clinical Associate Professor of Rehabilitation Medicine
New York University
Associate Director, Department of Rehabilitation Medicine
Goldwater Memorial Hospital
New York, New York

Peter J. Jannetta, M.D.
Professor and Chairman, Neurological Surgery
University of Pittsburgh
Pittsburgh, Pennsylvania

Kaj H. Johansen, M.D., Ph.D.
Professor of Surgery
University of Washington
Chief, Vascular Surgery
Harborview Medical Center
Seattle, Washington

Robert E. Kalina, M.D.
Professor and Chairman, Department of Ophthalmology
University of Washington
Seattle, Washington

Jory N. Kaplan, M.D.
Clinical Assistant Professor of Otolaryngology
University of California at Irvine
Irvine, California

Michael B. Kimmey, M.D.
Assistant Professor of Medicine
Director of Therapeutic Endoscopy
University of Washington Medical Center
University of Washington
Seattle, Washington

Joseph Kwentus, M.D.
Medical Director and Director of Sleep Center
Modesto Psychiatric Center
Modesto, California

Joseph C. Langlois, M.D.
Clinical Faculty, Division of Dermatology
University of Washington
Department of Dermatology
Group Health Cooperative of Puget Sound
Seattle, Washington

William L. Lanzer, M.D.
Associate Professor of Orthopaedics
University of Washington
Seattle, Washington

Mathew H.M. Lee, M.D., M.P.H., F.A.C.P.
Professor and Acting Chairman, Department of Rehabilitation
Medicine
New York University
Director, Department of Rehabilitation Medicine
Goldwater Memorial Hospital
New York, New York

Pierre L. LeRoy, M.D., F.A.C.S., C.C.E.
Medical Director, Delaware Pain Clinic and Thermography
Laboratory
Newark, Delaware
Attending Physician, Section of Neurosurgery, St. Francis
Hospital and Medical Center of Delaware
Wilmington, Delaware

John C. Liebeskind, Ph.D.
Professor of Psychology and Anesthesiology
University of California, Los Angeles
Los Angeles, California

Frederick G. Lippert III, M.D.
Associate Professor of Orthopaedics
University of Washington
Chief of Orthopaedic Clinics
University of Washington Medical Center
University of Washington
Seattle, Washington

John D. Loeser, M.D.
Professor of Neurological Surgery
Director, Multidisciplinary Pain Center
University of Washington
Chief, Division of Neurosurgery
Children's Orthopedic Hospital and Medical Center
Seattle, Washington

John S. McDonald, M.D.
Professor and Chairman, Department of Anesthesiology
Ohio State University
Columbus, Ohio

Lora McGuire, R.N., M.S.
Instructor, Department of Nursing
Joliet Junior College
Joliet, Illinois
Complemental Faculty Member
Rush College of Nursing
Chicago, Illinois

Giuseppe Maggio, M.D.
Clinical Faculty, Department of Anesthesiology
University of Messina
Clinical Faculty, Department of Orthopedic Surgery and
Traumatology
University of Pisa
Director, EUMEDICA Center of Antalgic and Neurovegetative
Medicine
Lugano, Switzerland

Janet A. Marvin, R.N., M.N.
Associate Professor, Departments of Surgery and Physiological
Nursing
University of Washington
Associate Director, Burn Center
Harborview Medical Center
Seattle, Washington

Frederick A. Matsen III, M.D.
Professor and Chairman, Department of Orthopaedics
Chief of Orthopaedic Service
University of Washington Medical Center
University of Washington
Seattle, Washington

Amy M. Meacham, M.H.S., C.V.E.
Treatment Coordinator, Occupational Health Center
Georgia Baptist Medical Center
Vocational Evaluator, Emory Pain Control Center
Vocational Counselor and Evaluator, Pain Control and
Rehabilitation Institute of Georgia, Inc.
Atlanta, Georgia

**Harold Merskey, D.M., F.R.C.P., F.R.C.P.C.,
F.R.C.Psych., F.A.P.A.**
Professor of Psychiatry
University of Western Ontario
Director of Research
London Psychiatric Hospital
London, Ontario, Canada

Björn A. Meyerson, M.D., Ph.D.
Associate Professor and Acting Chairman, Department of
Neurosurgery
Karolinska Hospital
Stockholm, Sweden

Richard Monks, M.D., C.M., B.Sc., F.R.C.P.
Associate Professor of Psychiatry
McGill University
Senior Psychiatrist, Department of Psychiatry
Montreal General Hospital
Montreal, Québec, Canada

Guido Moricca, M.D.*
Formerly Chief of Anesthesia and Pain Service
National Cancer Institute Regina Elena
Rome, Italy

Michael W. Mulholland, M.D., Ph.D.
Assistant Professor of Surgery
University of Michigan
Ann Arbor, Michigan

* Deceased

Terence M. Murphy, M.B.Ch.B.
Professor of Anesthesiology
Attending Physician/Algologist, Multidisciplinary Pain Center
University of Washington
Seattle, Washington

Anne Naysmith, M.R.C.P.
Consultant in Palliative Medicine
Parkside Health Authority
London, England

Richard I. Newman, Jr., Ph.D.
Assistant Clinical Professor of Psychiatry
Oregon Health Sciences University
Co-Director, Northwest Pain Center
Portland, Oregon

George F. Odland, M.D.
Professor of Medicine and Biological Structure
Formerly Chief, Division of Dermatology
University of Washington
Seattle, Washington

George A. Ojemann, M.D.
Professor of Neurological Surgery
University of Washington
Director, Regional Epilepsy Center, Harborview Medical Center
Seattle, Washington

Jes Olesen, M.D.
Professor of Neurology
University of Copenhagen
Copenhagen, Denmark

James C. Orcutt, M.D., Ph.D.
Associate Professor of Ophthalmology
Adjunct Associate Professor of Otolaryngology, Head and
    Neck Surgery
University of Washington
Chief, Ophthalmology Section
Veterans Administration Medical Center
Seattle, Washington

Isacco Papo, M.D.
Chief, Division of Neurosurgery
Regional General Hospital
Ancona, Italy

Robert N. Pechnick, Ph.D.
Adjunct Assistant Professor of Pharmacology
University of California, Los Angeles
Los Angeles, California

**Issy Pilowsky, M.D., D.P.M., F.R.C.Psych.,
    F.R.A.C.P., F.R.A.N.Z.C.P.**
Professor and Chairman, Department of Psychiatry
University of Adelaide
Head, Department of Psychiatry and Attending Physician of
    Pain Clinic
Royal Adelaide Hospital
Adelaide, Australia

Charles E. Pope II, M.D.
Professor of Medicine
University of Washington
Chief, Gastroenterology
Veterans Administration Hospital
Seattle, Washington

Donald D. Price, Ph.D.
Professor of Anesthesiology and Director of Human Research
Medical College of Virginia
Virginia Commonwealth University
Richmond, Virginia

Paolo Procacci, M.D.
Professor of Systematic Medical Therapy
Director, Pain Center
University of Florence
Florence, Italy

L. Brian Ready, M.D., F.R.C.P.(C.)
Associate Professor of Anesthesiology
Attending Physician/Algologist and Chief of Acute Pain Service
Multidisciplinary Pain Center
University of Washington
Seattle, Washington

Joan M. Romano, Ph.D.
Assistant Professor of Psychiatry and Behavioral Sciences
Attending Psychologist, Multidisciplinary Pain Center
University of Washington
Seattle, Washington

Hubert L. Rosomoff, M.D., D.Med.Sc.
Professor and Chairman, Department of Neurological Surgery
University of Miami
Medical Director, University of Miami Comprehensive Pain
    and Rehabilitation Center
Chief, Neurological Surgery, Jackson Memorial Hospital
Miami, Florida

Armando Santoro, M.D.
Vice-Director, Department of Medical Oncology
National Cancer Institute
Milan, Italy

Joel L. Seres, M.D., F.A.C.S.
Associate Professor of Neurosurgery
Oregon Health Sciences University
Director, Northwest Pain Center
Portland, Oregon

Fred E. Silverstein, M.D.
Professor of Medicine
Chief of Gastrointestinal Endoscopy
University of Washington Medical Center
University of Washington
Seattle, Washington

Bengt, Sjölund, M.D., D.Med.Sc.
Associate Professor in Pain Research
Lund University
Lund, Sweden
Senior Consultant and Pain Director
Malmö General Hospital
Malmö, Sweden

Anders E. Sola, M.D., M.S.
Assistant Clinical Professor of Anesthesiology
Consultant Algologist, Multidisciplinary Pain Center
University of Washington
Seattle, Washington

Dan M. Spengler, M.D.
Professor and Chairman, Department of Othopaedics and
    Rehabilitation
Medical Director, Ability Assessment Center
Vanderbilt University
Nashville, Tennessee

Richard A. Sternbach, Ph.D.

Clinical Professor of Psychiatry
University of California, San Diego
San Diego, California
Program Director, Pain Treatment Center
Scripps Clinic and Research Foundation
La Jolla, California

Walter C. Stolov, M.D.

Professor and Chairman Department of Rehabilitation Medicine
University of Washington
Seattle, Washington

William H. Sweet, M.D., D.Sc.

Professor of Surgery Emeritus
Harvard Medical School
Senior Neurosurgeon
Massachusetts General Hospital
Boston, Massachusetts

Karen L. Syrjala, Ph.D.

Acting Assistant Professor of Psychiatry and Behavioral
  Sciences
University of Washington
Associate in Clinical Pain Research
Fred Hutchinson Cancer Research Center
Seattle, Washington

Ronald R. Tasker, M.D., F.R.C.S.(C.)

Professor of Surgery
University of Toronto
Head, Division of Neurosurgery
Toronto General Hospital
Toronto, Ontario, Canada

Carol C. Teitz, M.D.

Associate Professor of Orthopaedics
Acting Director, Division of Sports Medicine
University of Washington
Seattle, Washington

John M. Tew, Jr., M.D.

Professor and Chairman, Department of Neurosurgery
University of Cincinnati
Chief of Neurosurgery, University Hospital and Children's
  Hospital Medical Center
Chairman, Section of Neurosurgery, Good Samaritan Hospital
Cincinnati, Ohio

Edmond L. Truelove, D.D.S., M.S.D.

Associate Professor and Chairperson, Department of Oral
  Medicine
Consultant, Multidisciplinary Pain Center
University of Washington
Seattle, Washington

Eldon R. Tunks, M.D., F.R.C.P.(C.)

Professor of Psychiatry
McMaster University
Director, Pain Clinic
Chedoke-McMaster Hospitals
Hamilton, Ontario, Canada

Judith A. Turner, Ph.D.

Associate Professor of Psychiatry and Behavioral Sciences and
  Rehabilitation Medicine
Attending Psychologist and Assistant Director for Inpatient
  Services, Multidisciplinary Pain Center
University of Washington
Seattle, Washington

Robert G. Twycross, D.M., F.R.C.P.

Macmillan Clinical Reader in Palliative Medicine
University of Oxford
Consultant Physician, Sir Michael Sobell House, Churchill
  Hospital
Oxford, England

Donald C. Tyler, M.D.

Associate Professor of Anesthesiology and Pediatrics
University of Washington
Co-Director, Multidisciplinary Pain Program
Children's Orthopedic Hospital and Medical Center
Seattle, Washington

Harry van Loveren, M.D.

Associate Professor of Clinical Neurosurgery
University of Cincinnati Medical Center
Mayfield Neurological Institute
Cincinnati, Ohio

Vittorio Ventafridda, M.D.

Director, Pain Therapy and Palliative Care Service, National
  Cancer Institute
Director, WHO Collaborating Center for Cancer Pain Relief
Scientific Director, Floriani Foundation
Milan, Italy

Ernest P. Volinn, Ph.D.

Postdoctoral Research Associate, Department of Neurological
  Surgery
Consultant, Multidisciplinary Pain Center
University of Washington
Seattle, Washington

Nicholas G. Ward, M.D.

Associate Professor of Psychiatry and Behavioral Sciences
Director of Psychiatric Inpatient Services and Director of
  Psychopharmacology Clinic
University of Washington Medical Center
University of Washington
Seattle, Washington

Tony L. Yaksh, Ph.D.

Professor of Anesthesia and Adjunct Professor in
  Pharmacology
University of California, San Diego
La Jolla, California

Gai-Fu William Yang, M.D., R.P.T.

Coordinator, Howard A. Rusk Respiratory Rehabilitation
  Center
Goldwater Memorial Hospital
New York, New York

CONTENTS

VOLUME I

PART III · EVALUATION OF THE PATIENT WITH PAIN

PART IV · REGIONAL PAINS

SECTION A · PAIN IN THE HEAD

SECTION B · PAIN IN THE NECK, SHOULDER, AND UPPER EXTREMITIES

VOLUME II

SECTION C · PAIN IN THE CHEST

SECTION D · ABDOMINAL PAIN

SECTION E · PAIN IN THE PELVIS, PERINEUM, AND GENITALIA

SECTION F · PAIN IN THE LOW BACK, HIPS, AND LOWER EXTREMITIES

PART V · METHODS, PROCEDURES, AND TECHNIQUES FOR THE SYMPTOMATIC CONTROL OF PAIN

SECTION E · REGIONAL ANALGESIA/ANESTHESIA

SECTION F · ABLATIVE NEUROSURGICAL OPERATIONS

SECTION G · INTERDISCIPLINARY, MULTIMODAL PAIN MANAGEMENT PROGRAMS

53 · GENERAL CONSIDERATIONS OF PAIN IN THE CHEST

JOHN J. BONICA

THE chest is among the most common sites of pain, suffering, and disability encountered in clinical practice. The pain can be caused by disease of the thoracic viscera or by disorders of muscles, bones, and other pain-sensitive structures of the chest wall. It can also be projected from disease of the spinal cord or spinal nerves or referred from structures outside of the chest, or it can be a combination of two or more of these conditions. It is necessary for the clinician to have a thorough knowledge of the functional anatomy and physiology of the thorax and related structures to interpret the history properly and to carry out a meaningful general physical, neurologic, and orthopedic examination—prerequisites for making an accurate diagnosis and developing and implementing the most effective therapeutic strategy.

The first chapter of Section C, like other chapters that introduce the management of pain in various regions of the body, provides a concise discussion of these various considerations. The material is presented in four major sections: (A) Basic Considerations, including anatomy of the thorax and the muscles attached to it, a brief description of the thoracic spinal cord and thoracic spinal nerves, and a general description of the sympathetic and parasympathetic nerve supplies to the chest; (B) Innervation of the Thoracic Viscera; (C) History and Examination; and a table containing a summary of the characteristics of pain and other symptoms and signs in the chest that should help the clinician to make a differential diagnosis. Detailed information on pathophysiology as related to pain in the chest is given in subsequent chapters. Further discussions are found in relevant textbooks and reviews of anatomy and neuroanatomy (1–8).

A. BASIC CONSIDERATIONS

In this first section I discuss the clinically relevant aspects of the anatomy of the thoracic spine, chest, and abdominal wall, including a brief description of vertebrae, joints, ligaments, and muscles attached to these structures. (The muscles of the posterior chest are discussed with those of the lumbosacral spine in Chapter 70.) This is followed by a brief description of the thoracic spinal cord, spinal nerves, and the structures they supply in the chest and abdominal wall; these are presented here because the course of thoracic spinal nerves and the structures they supply (the chest and abdominal wall) are similar.

Anatomy of the Thorax

Skeletal Structures

Figure 53-1 depicts the skeletal parts of the thorax or chest, which form an osseocartilaginous cage that protects the principal organs of respiration and circulation (1). The thoracic cage extends inferiorly over the upper part of the abdomen and covers a portion of certain abdominal viscera. Its conical shape is a result of the fact that its superior or cervical inlet is of a lesser diameter than its inferior abdominal part. In transverse section the thorax appears to be kidney-shaped because of projection of the vertebral bodies into the cavity. The thoracic cage is formed by the ribs, with their costal cartilages attached anteriorly to the sternum (Fig. 53-1A) and posteriorly to the thoracic vertebrae of the spinal column (Fig. 53-1B).

The thorax is bounded posteriorly by the T12 vertebra and the posterior parts of the 12 ribs, anteriorly by the sternum and the costal cartilages, and laterally by the ribs. These are separated from each other by the 11 intercostal spaces, within which are located the intercostal muscles and membranes, nerves, and vessels. The superior opening of the thorax, formed by the T1 vertebra, the cranial margin of the sternum, and the first rib on each side, is broader from side to side than anteroposteriorly. The plane of the aperture slopes caudally from the spinal column down to the sternum, and its upper part lies 3 to 5 cm below the upper border of the body of the T1 vertebra. The inferior opening, or thoracic outlet, is formed posteriorly by the 12 thoracic vertebrae, laterally by the 11th and 12th ribs, and ventrally by the cartilages of the 7th to 10th ribs, which slope on each side to form the infrasternal angle of the xiphoid process.

The thorax of females differs from that of males in the following respects: its capacity is less; the sternum is shorter; the cranial margin of the sternum is on a level with the caudal part of the body of the T3 vertebra, whereas in the male it is on a level with the caudal part of the body of the T2 vertebra; and the upper ribs are more movable, permitting a greater expansion of the cephalad part of the thorax (1).

Thoracic Spine

The thoracic spine, composed of the 12 thoracic vertebrae, is concave anteriorly and articulates with the ribs, thus forming the supporting structure of the rib cage. Figure 53-2 depicts the anatomy and articulating surfaces of a typical thoracic vertebra, as well as its articulation with the head, neck, and proximal portion of the rib.

959

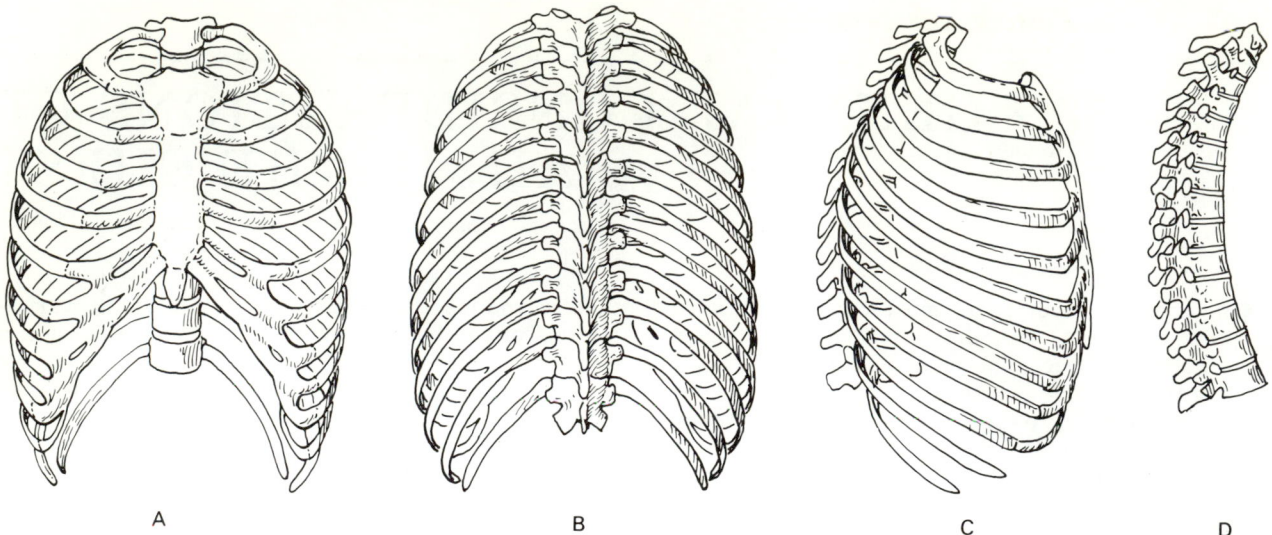

FIG. 53-1. Anatomy of the thoracic cage. **A.** Anterior view. Note that all 12 of the ribs articulate with their respective thoracic vertebrae, but only the first 7 attach directly to the sternum; the 8th and 9th ribs attach to the cartilages of the 7th rib on each side, while the 10th, 11th, and 12th pairs have no anterior articulation. **B.** Posterior view. Each rib articulates wtih its respective thoracic vertebra and, as the ribs encircle the trunk, they proceed in an inferolateral direction. **C.** Lateral view from the right side. Initially the ribs course in an anterolateral direction from the vertebral column and then proceed inferomedially to reach the costal cartilages and the sternum. **D.** View of the right side of the thoracic part of the vertebral column. Modified from Clemente, C.D.: Gray's Anatomy of the Human Body. 30th Ed. Philadelphia, Lea & Febiger, 1985, pp. 148–150.

The thoracic vertebrae are intermediate in size between the cervical and lumbar vertebrae, providing a gradual transition from the small cervical vertebrae cranially to the large lumbar vertebrae caudally. The body of a thoracic vertebra is larger posteriorly than anteriorly. The thoracic vertebrae are distinguished by the presence of costal facets on the side of the body for articulation of the heads of the ribs and by other articular facets in the transverse processes of the upper 10 thoracic vertebrae for articulation with the tubercles of the ribs. The T1 vertebra has an entire articular facet for the head of the first rib and a demifacet for the cranial half of the head of the second rib on each side of the vertebral body. The T2 to T8 vertebrae have similar demifacets, the T9 vertebra has only one demifacet above, and the T10, T11, and T12 vertebrae have one entire facet.

The pedicles of the thoracic vertebrae are directed dorsally and slightly cephalad from the transverse process; the inferior vertebral notches are large and extend more cephalad

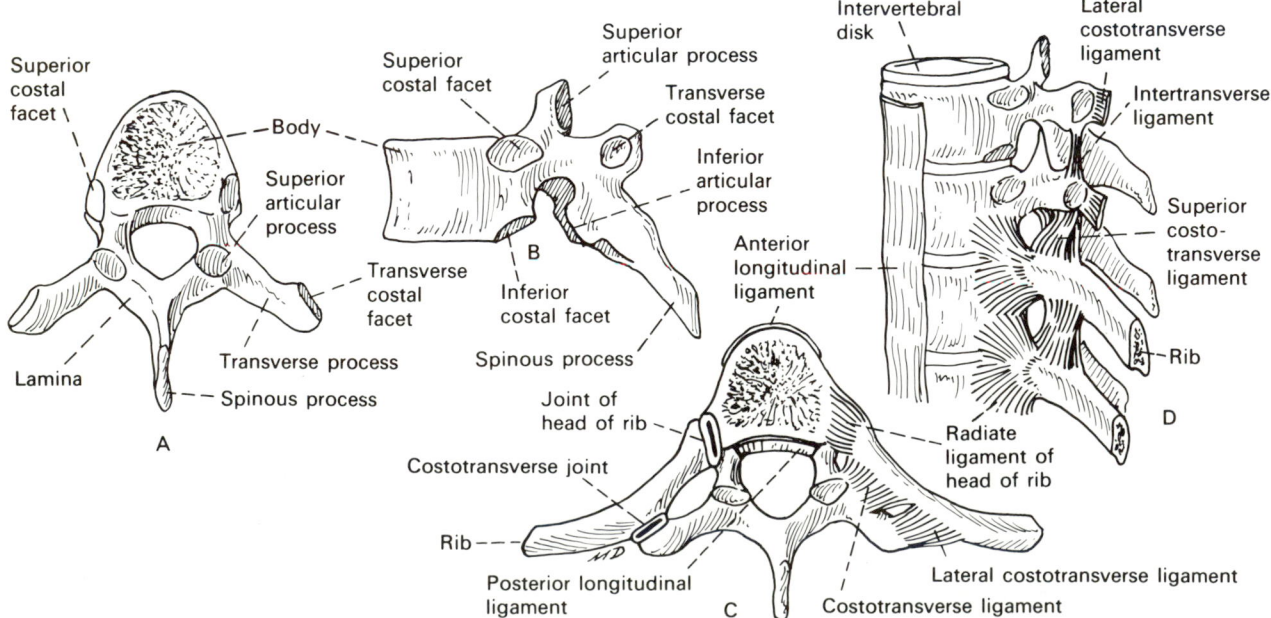

FIG. 53-2. Anatomy and articulations of the thoracic vertebrae. **A.** Superior view. **B.** Lateral view. The articular facets and the posteroinferior direction of the spinous processes are shown. **C.** Superior view. The synovial cavities of the joint of the head of the rib and the costotransverse joint are on the left, and the various ligaments are on the right. **D.** Lateral view of four thoracic vertebrae depicting the ligaments of the costovertebral joints.

than in any other region of the vertebral column, thus making the intervertebral foramina ample for the exit of the nerves. The laminae are broad, thick, and imbricated, with the one cephalad overlapping the next caudad like tiles on a roof. The spinous processes are long, triangular in coronal section, and directed obliquely caudally, and end in a tuberculated extremity. The spinous processes of the T5 to the T8 vertebrae are oblique and overlap to a greater degree than those of the upper and lower thoracic vertebrae.

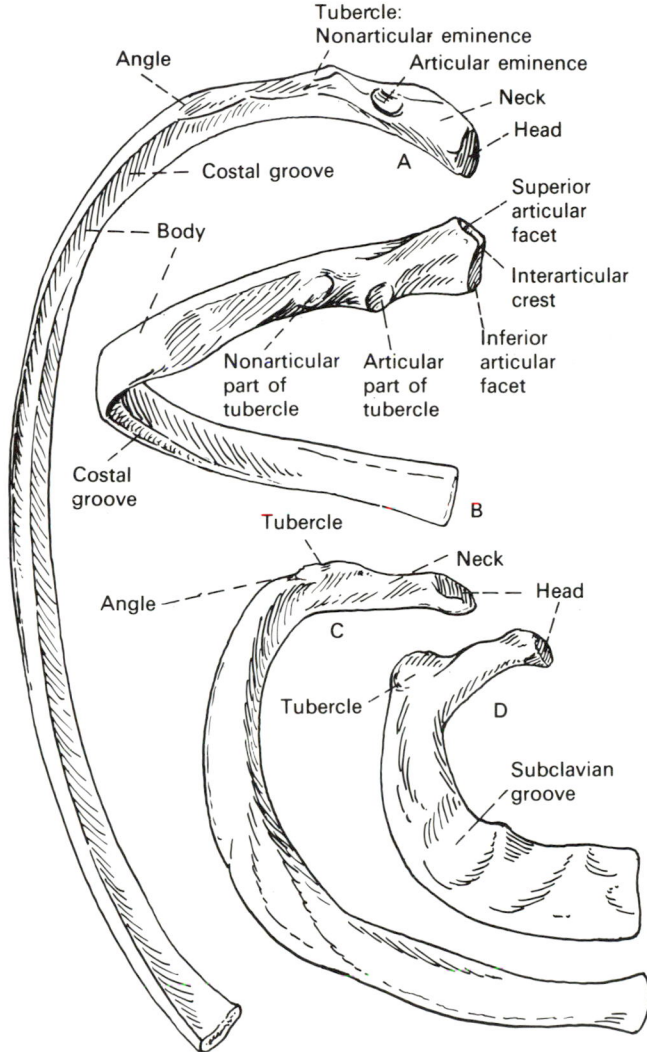

FIG. 53-3. Anatomy of the ribs. **A.** Inferior aspect of a typical central rib from the left side. The principal parts of the bone include the head, neck, tubercle (which possesses an articular eminence and a nonarticular eminence), and curved body of shaft. The costal groove contains the intercostal vessels and nerves. **B.** Typical central rib from the left side, viewed from behind. The vertebral extremity at the end of the head of the rib contains a large inferior facet for the numerically corresponding vertebra and a smaller facet for the adjacent vertebra above; the interarticular crest attaches to the intervertebral disk between the two facets. **C.** Right second rib, viewed from above. **D.** Right first rib, viewed from above; the subclavian groove below the head of the large tubercle is occupied by the subclavian artery and brachial plexus and the more anterior groove by the subclavian vein. Modified from Clemente, C.D.: Gray's Anatomy of the Human Body. 30th Ed. Philadelphia, Lea & Febiger, 1985, pp. 154–155.

Ribs

The ribs are flattened narrowed elastic arches of bone that form a large part of the thoracic skeleton. The first 7 of the 12 ribs are called true or vertebrosternal ribs; they connect dorsally with the vertebral column and ventrally with the sternum by means of costal cartilages. The remaining 5 pairs are "false" ribs and consist of two types; the 8th to 10th ribs have their cartilages attached to the cartilage of the rib above (vertebrochondral), while the 11th and 12th ribs are free at their anterior extremities and are therefore referred to as floating or vertebral ribs, because they do not attach to the sternum. Figure 53-3 depicts the anatomy of the typical central rib of the left side viewed from below and from the side, and shows the peculiar anatomy of the second and first ribs.

The *costal cartilages* are bars of hyaline cartilages that go along the ribs anteriorly and render the chest wall more elastic to accommodate, for example, the movements of respiration. The first seven pairs are connected to the sternum, the next three pairs articulate with the lower border of the cartilage of the preceding rib, and the last two pairs have pointed anterior extremities that end in the musculature of the abdominal wall.

Sternum

The sternum is an elongated flat bone that forms the middle portion of the anterior wall of the thorax and is composed of the manubrium, body, and xiphoid process. The upper portion of the manubrium articulates with the clavicle and the 1st and 2nd ribs. The body articulates with the cartilage of the 2nd to the 7th ribs, while the xiphoid process is a thin elongated structure that is cartilaginous in children but is more or less ossified proximally in adults (Figs. 53-1A and 53-5).

Joints and Ligaments

Joints and Ligaments of the Vertebral Column

The joints and ligaments of the thoracic portion of the vertebral column are similar to those discussed in Chapter 46 in relation to the cervical spine (1). These include the intervertebral disks and the anterior and posterior longitudinal ligaments (Fig. 53-2C, D). The intervertebral disks of the thoracic spine are nearly of uniform thickness, the anterior concavity of this part of the column is almost entirely a result of the shape of the vertebral bodies; as mentioned above, these are larger posteriorly than anteriorly. The intervertebral disks adhere to thin layers of hyaline cartilage that cover the superior and inferior surfaces of the vertebral bodies. Each disk is composed of an outer lamina of fibrous tissue called the annulus fibrosis and an inner core of a soft gelatinous and highly elastic substance called the nucleus pulposus.

The anterior longitudinal ligament, which extends from the occipital bone to the sacrum, is narrower but thicker in its passage over the anterior surface of the vertebral bodies than over the intervertebral disk. It consists of dense longitudinal fibers that adhere closely to the intervertebral disks and the prominent margins of the vertebrae but are not attached firmly to the middle parts of the body, where it is thick and fills the concavities of the anterior surfaces, thus giving the anterior aspect of the vertebral column a more even contour. This anterior aspect is composed of several layers of fibers that vary in length but are closely interlaced with each other. The most superficial fibers are the longest and extend across four or five vertebrae; a second subjacent set extends between two or three vertebrae and a third set, the shortest and deepest, reaches from one vertebra to the next.

The posterior longitudinal ligament extends from the axis to the sacrum and passes over the dorsal surface of the bodies of the vertebrae and the intervertebral disks. It is narrow and thick over the center of the bodies, from which it is separated by the basivertebral veins, and broadens over the intervertebral disks. It is composed of longitudinal fibers that are denser and more compact than those of the anterior ligaments.

JOINTS BETWEEN THE VERTEBRAL ARCHES. Joints between the articular processes of the thoracic (and other) vertebrae are plain or gliding joints enveloped by capsules lined by synovial membrane (Fig. 53-2B,C). The articular capsules are thin and loose and are attached to the margins of the articular processes of adjacent vertebrae. The ligamenta flava connect the laminae of adjacent vertebrae. Each ligamentum flavum consists of yellow elastic tissue attached to the anterior and inferior surfaces of the lamina above and to the posterior surface of the lamina below. The fibers of the ligamenta flava are almost perpendicular to the laminae to which they are attached. They are thin in the cervical region, thicker in the thoracic region, and thickest in the lumbar region. Their marked elasticity permits separation of the laminae during flexion of the vertebral column and also helps to preserve the upright posture (Fig. 53-4).

The interspinous ligaments are thin and membranous and interconnect adjoining spinous processes, extending from the root to the apex of each process. The supraspinous ligament is a strong fibrous cord that connects together the apices of the spinous processes from the C7 vertebra to the sacrum (Fig. 53-4). Fibrocartilage develops into ligament at its point of attachment to the tips of the spinous process and, in older persons, this can extend into the interspinous portions of the ligament. The intertransverse ligaments are interposed between the transverse processes, which in the thoracic region are rounded cords that are intimately connected with the deeper muscles of the back.

MOVEMENT. Normally the movements permitted in the vertebral column include flexion, extension, lateral flexion, circumduction, and rotation. In the thoracic region, however, notably in its upper part, all movements are limited to minimize interference with respiration (1). The almost complete absence of the upward inclination of the superior articular surfaces prohibits any marked flexion, whereas extension is checked by the contact of the inferior articular margins with the laminae and by the contact of the spinous processes with one another. The mechanism of the caudal end of the cervical spine limits extension and also serves to limit flexion of the thoracic region when the neck is extended. Rotation is free in the thoracic region; the position of the articular processes allows rotation around a vertical axis that passes through the bodies of the midthoracic vertebrae but is anterior to the vertebral bodies of the upper and lower thoracic vertebrae. The direction of the articular facets would allow free lateral flexion, but this movement is considerably limited by the resistance of the ribs and sternum.

Costovertebral Joints

The articulation of the ribs with the vertebral column can be divided into two sets, one connecting the heads of the ribs with the bodies of the vertebrae and the other uniting the necks and tubercles of the ribs with the transverse processes (1).

ARTICULATION OF THE HEADS OF THE RIBS. A series of plane or gliding joints are formed by the articulation of the heads of the typical ribs with the facets on the contiguous margin of the bodies of the thoracic vertebrae and with the intervertebral disks between them (Figs. 53-2C and D). Although the heads of the 2nd to 9th ribs each articulate by means of two facets, the articulation is considered to be a single joint because only one articular capsule is present, even with two synovial sacs. Figure 53-2C depicts two parts of this joint, the articular capsule and the radiate ligament. The radiate ligament connects the anterior part of the head of each rib with the sides of the bodies of two adjacent vertebrae and the intervertebral disks between them. The intra-articular ligament, situated in the interior of the joint, consists of a short flat band of fibers attached by one extremity to the crest separating the two articular facets on the head of the rib and by the other to the intervertebral disk. It divides the joint into two cavities, each of which is lined by a synovial membrane.

COSTOTRANSVERSE JOINTS. The articular surface on the tubercle of the upper ten ribs forms a plane or gliding joint

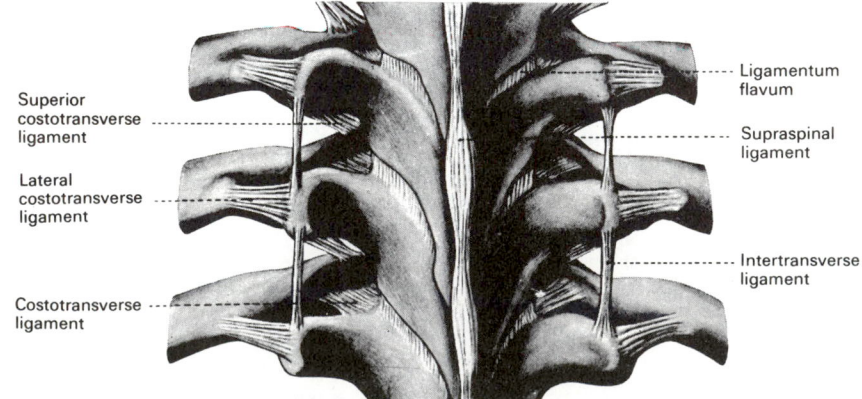

Superior costotransverse ligament

Lateral costotransverse ligament

Costotransverse ligament

Ligamentum flavum

Supraspinal ligament

Intertransverse ligament

FIG. 53-4. Posterior aspect of part of the thoracic spinal column showing the supraspinal, intertransverse, and costotransverse ligaments and the ligamentum flavum. From Clemente, C.D.: Gray's Anatomy of the Human Body. 30th Ed. Philadelphia, Lea & Febiger, 1985, p. 355.

with the articular facet on the adjacent transverse process of the corresponding vertebra (Fig. 53-2C and D). This articulation is missing in the 11th and 12th ribs. These joints include an articular capsule, which is a thin fibrous membrane attached to the circumference of the articular surface.

The superior costotransverse ligament is attached to the sharp crest of the superior border of the neck of the rib and passes obliquely upward and laterally to the lower border of the neck of the transverse process immediately above. It is composed of two layers; the anterior layer blends laterally with the internal intercostal membrane and is crossed by the intercostal nerves and vessels, while the posterior layer blends laterally with the external intercostal muscle. Its medial border is thickened and free and bounds an aperture that transmits the posterior division of the spinal nerves and posterior branches of the intercostal vessels.

The costotransverse ligament, sometimes called the ligament of the neck of the rib, consists of short strong fibers that connect the rough surfaces on the back of the neck of the rib with the anterior surface of the adjacent transverse process.

The lateral costotransverse ligament is a short, thick, and strong fasciculus. It passes obliquely from the apex of the transverse process of the vertebra to the rough and nonarticular portion of the tubercle of the corresponding rib.

MOVEMENT AT THE COSTOTRANSVERSE JOINTS. The heads of the ribs are so closely connected to the bodies of the vertebrae by the radiate and intra-articular ligaments that only slight gliding movements of the articular surfaces on one another can take place (1). Similarly, the strong ligaments binding the necks and tubercles of the ribs to the transverse process limit the movements of the costotransverse joints to a slight gliding motion. The joints at the head of the ribs and the costotransverse joints move simultaneously in the same direction, with total effect being that the neck of the rib moves as if on a single joint. The chief movement of the necks of the upper six ribs is one of rotation around their own long axes, with only slight upward and downward movements. Thus, backward rotation of the neck of the rib results in lowering of the anterior end of the rib, whereas forward rotation of the neck of the rib causes elevation of the anterior end. The necks of the 7th to the 10th ribs can move either upward, backward, and medialward, or downward, forward, and lateralward, thereby altering the shape of the rib cage with only a slight rotation accompanying these movements (1).

Articulation with the Sternum

STERNOCOSTAL JOINTS. The medial ends of the costal cartilages fit into the slight concavities along the lateral border of the sternum to form the sternocostal joints, which have an articular capsule and are strengthened by the radiate sternocostal ligaments, the intra-articular sternocostal ligaments, and the costal xiphoid ligaments (Fig. 53-5). These joints are supplied by the anterior perforating branches of the intercostal nerves. Sternocostal joints permit only a slight gliding movement.

INTERCHONDRAL AND COSTOCHONDRAL JOINTS. The contiguous borders between the 6th and 7th, 7th and 8th, 8th and 9th, and sometimes even those of the 9th and 10th costal cartilages, articulate with each other by small smooth oblong facets. Each joint is enclosed in a thin articular capsule lined by synovial membrane and strengthened laterally and medially by the fibrous interchondral ligaments (Fig. 53-5).

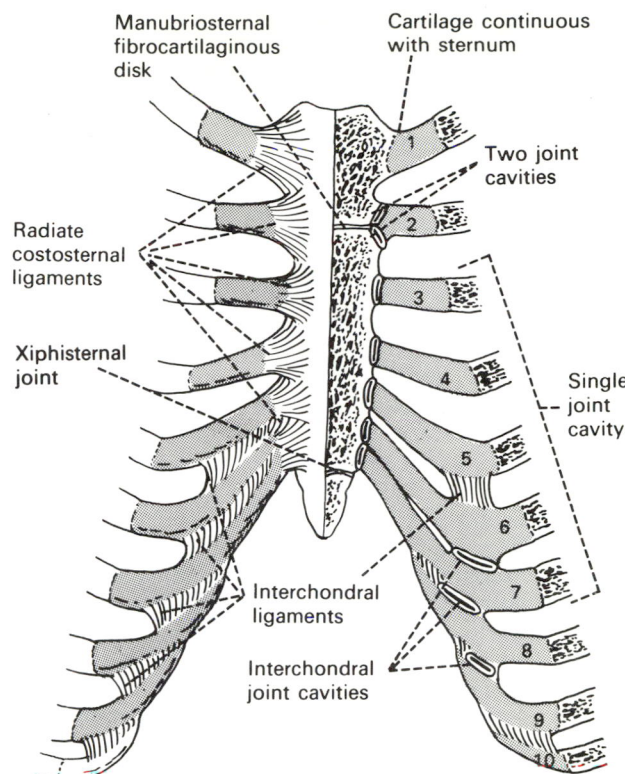

FIG. 53-5. Anterior view of the sternum and costal cartilages showing the sternocostal and interchondral articulations. On the left side of the sternum the synovial cavities are exposed by coronal section of the sternum and cartilages. Modified from Clemente, C.D.: Gray's Anatomy of the Human Body. 30th Ed. Philadelphia, Lea & Febiger, 1985, p. 356.

The lateral end of each costal cartilage is received into a slight depression of the sternal end of the rib. The cartilage and bone are bound together by the periosteum of the bone, which becomes continuous with the perichondrium of the cartilage.

Articulation of the Sternum

MANUBRIOSTERNAL AND XIPHISTERNAL JOINTS. The interior surface of the manubrium is united with the superior surface of the body of the sternum by a fibrocartilaginous disk, which is shaped to conform to the hyaline cartilage-covered bony surfaces. The lateral margins of this synthesis are contiguous with the second sternocostal joints. At this joint site, the manubrium and sternal body usually present a slight anteriorly projecting ridge called the sternal angle, which is palpable beneath the skin and serves as an important surface landmark for clinicians. The articulation between the xiphoid process and the inferior border of the sternal body is cartilaginous but, by 30 years of age, this joint has usually become ossified. The joint is secured laterally by radiating fibers of the sternocostal ligaments. Generally the 7th costal cartilage articulates with the sternum at the lateral margin of the xiphisternal junction (Fig. 53-5).

Muscles of the Thorax

The muscles considered in this section are primarily those attached to the ribs and concerned with movements, especially in relation to respiration. In addition, brief mention is made of the deep muscles of the back attached to the thoracic spine and ribs. The anterior muscles of the chest, including the pectoralis major, pectoralis minor, subclavius, and serratus anterior, were considered in the preceding section in connection with the shoulder.

Muscles of Respiration

The most important muscles that influence movement of the ribs and are concerned with respiration are listed in Table 6-2, which also presents their primary action and nerve supply. Only a brief description of these muscles is given below, particularly of the intercostal muscles, to provide a background for discussion of the position of the intercostal nerves. Before doing so, however, it is necessary to mention the fascia that covers the thoracic cage proper, composed of ribs and the intercostal muscles. The cage is covered internally and externally by thin layers of deep fascia. The outer layer essentially covers the external intercostal muscles while the inner layer, consisting of loose areolar tissue called the endothoracic fascia, lines the internal aspect of the thoracic cage. It covers the inner surface of the intercostal muscles and intervening ribs, along with the subcostal and transversus thoracis muscles and the diaphragm. It lies between the parietal pleura and the thoracic cage, which in the absence of adhesions can therefore be easily separated. Posteriorly, the endothoracic fascia continues over the bodies of the vertebrae and intervertebral disks. In this mediastinal region, certain structures such as the azygos and hemiazygos veins, the thoracic duct, the sympathetic chain, and the splanchnic nerves are partially or completely surrounded by the fascia. Superiorly, the endothoracic fascia extends over the apices of the lung where, somewhat thickened, it forms the suprapleural membrane, or Sibson's fascia. Inferiorly, it becomes thin over the superior surface of the diaphragm but is continuous with the internal investing fascia of the abdominal cavity, dorsal to the diaphragm at the lumbosacral arches and through the aortic hiatus (1).

INTERCOSTAL MUSCLES. The intercostal muscles are composed of three thin layers of muscular and tendinous fibers that occupy each of the intercostal spaces. The external intercostal muscles, 11 on each side, extend from the tubercles of the ribs posteriorly to the cartilages of the ribs anteriorly, where they each end as a thin fibrous sheet, the external intercostal membrane, which continues forward to the sternum (1). Each external intercostal muscle arises from the lower border of the rib above and is inserted into the upper border of the rib below. In the lowest two spaces the muscles extend to the ends of the cartilages, while in the uppermost two or three spaces they do not quite reach the ends of the ribs. These muscles are thicker than the internal intercostals; the fibers are directed obliquely inferolaterally on the posterior part of the thorax and inferolaterally and somewhat ventrally on the anterior aspect of the thorax (see Fig. 53-8).

The internal intercostal muscles, also 11 on each side, begin anteriorly at the sternum in the interspaces between the cartilage of two ribs and at the anterior extremities of the cartilages of the false ribs, and extend posteriorly as far as the angles of the ribs, where they continue to the vertebral column by thin aponeuroses, the internal intercostal membranes. Each muscle arises from the ridge on the inner surface of the rib above as well as from the corresponding costal cartilage, and inserts into the upper border of the rib below. These fibers are directed obliquely but pass in a direction perpendicular to that of the external intercostal muscles.

The innermost (intimi) intercostal muscles are frequently considered to be the deepest parts of the internal intercostal muscles. They are located deep to the intercostal nerves and vessels interposed between these structures and the parietal pleura (see Fig. 53-8, p. 968). They extend between the costal groove of the rib above to the inner lip of the upper margin of the rib below. The fibers generally course in the same direction as those of the internal intercostal muscles. The intimi intercostal muscles are not well developed and might be absent in the upper four or five interspaces.

The subcostal muscles consist of oblique muscular and aponeurotic fasciculi located on the inner surface of the posterior part of the chest. Usually they are well developed only in the lower part of the thorax (1). Each arises from the inner surface of one rib posteriorly near its angle and is inserted into the inner surface of the second or third rib below. Their fibers run in the same direction as those of the intimi intercostal muscles and, similarly, separate the intercostal nerves and vessels from the pleura (1) (Fig. 53-8).

The sternocostalis, or transversus thoracis muscles, are a thin plane of muscular and tendinous fibers situated on the inner surface of the anterior chest wall. They are situated deep to the intercostal nerves and vessels and deep to the internal mammary artery. They arise on each side from the caudal third of the inner surfaces of the body of the sternum, xiphoid process, and 2nd to 6th costal cartilages. The fibers fan out from the back of the body of the sternum and xiphoid process to the costal cartilages of the 2nd to 6th ribs; the upper fibers are ascending, while the lower fibers are horizontal and in continuity with the transversus abdominis muscle.

LEVATORES COSTARUM. The levatores costarum, 12 on each side, are located in the posterior surface of the thoracic cage. They consist of tendinous fleshy bundles that arise from the ends of the transverse process of the C7 and T1 to T11 vertebrae. The muscles pass obliquely inferolaterally like the fibers of the external intercostals in this posterior region. Each is inserted into the outer surface of the rib immediately below the vertebra from which it takes origin, between the tubercle and the angle. They elevate the ribs and bend the vertebral column laterally, rotating it slightly toward the opposite side. These muscles are also supplied by the intercostal nerves.

ACTION. All the intercostal muscles and levatores costarum are supplied by the intercostal nerves, which constitute the anterior division of the thoracic spinal nerves (see below). The external intercostal muscles raise the ribs during inspiration but can also be active during expiration (1-3). The action of the internal intercostal muscles varies; the anterior portion of the upper four or five intercostal muscles that interconnect the costal cartilages elevates the ribs during inspiration, whereas the more lateral and posterior of these muscles depress the ribs during expiration. The intimi intercostal muscles also depress the ribs, while the transversus thoracis muscles draw the ribs downward (2, 3). The levatores costarum elevate the ribs and then the vertebral column laterally and rotate it slightly to the opposite side.

DIAPHRAGM. The diaphragm is a dome-shaped musculofibrous septum that separates the thoracic cavity from the abdominal cavity. Its convex upper surface forms the floor of the thorax, while its concave inferior surface forms the roof of the abdomen. Its peripheral part consists of three groups of muscular fibers that originate from the circumference of the thoracic outlet and converge to be inserted into a central tendon. The sternal part of the muscular fibers arises from two fleshy slips from the dorsum of the xiphoid process, the costal part arises from the inner surface of the cartilages and from adjacent portions of the last six ribs on each side, interdigitating with the transversus abdominis muscle, and the lumbar part arises from two aponeurotic arches on each side (the medial and lateral arcuate ligaments) and from the lumbar vertebrae by two pillars, or crura. The most central portion of the diaphragm is innervated by the phrenic nerves, which arise from the two cervical plexuses (C3–C5), while its peripheral muscular fibers are supplied by the 6th to the 11th or 12th intercostal nerves.

Biomechanics of the Thorax

Through the action of the various muscles mentioned above, and of others, the thoracic cage either increases or decreases in size. Each rib possesses its own range of movements but, in combination, the ribs allow respiratory excursions of the thorax. Each rib can be regarded as a lever, the fulcrum of which is situated immediately lateral to the costotransverse joint so that the neck of the rib is depressed when the shaft of the rib is elevated, and vice versa (1). Because the arms of the lever are of different lengths, a slight movement at the vertebral end of the rib is greatly magnified at the anterior extremity.

The anterior ends of the rib lie at a more inferior plane than the posterior ends; thus, when the shaft of the rib is elevated, the anterior extremity is also thrust forward. Because the middle of the shaft of the rib lies at a plane inferior to one passing through the two extremities of the rib, the shaft is elevated at the same time as it is thrust forward from the median plane of the thorax (Fig. 53-6A). Moreover, each rib forms the segment of a curve that is greater than that of the rib immediately above it, and therefore the elevation of the rib also increases the transverse diameter of the thorax.

The first pair of ribs moves with the manubrium as a single piece, with the anterior portion being elevated by rotary movements of the necks of the ribs near the vertebral extremities. During normal quiet respiration the movement is virtually nonexistent. Movement of the second pair of ribs is also slight in normal respiration because their anterior extremities are fixed to the manubrium and are therefore prevented from moving upward. Elevation of the 3rd to the 6th ribs raises the thrust of their anterior extremities forward, with the greater part of the movement being affected by rotation of the rib neck (Fig. 53-6B).

The vertebrochondral ribs (8th–10th), along with the 7th rib, have movements that assist in enlarging the thorax for respiratory purposes but that also increase the upper abdominal space for viscera displaced by the action of the diaphragm (Fig. 53-6C). The costal cartilages of the 6th to 10th ribs articulate with one another so that each pushes up the costal cartilage above, with the final thrust being directed to pushing the lower end of the body of the sternum forward and upward. Slight rotation of the rib neck permits only a limited elevation of the anterior extremity. Elevation of the rib shaft is accompanied by an outward and backward movement that results in a considerable increase in the transverse diameter and a decrease in the median anteroposterior diameter of the lower chest and upper abdomen.

Even more important than the action of the ribs, and of the muscles that control their movements, is

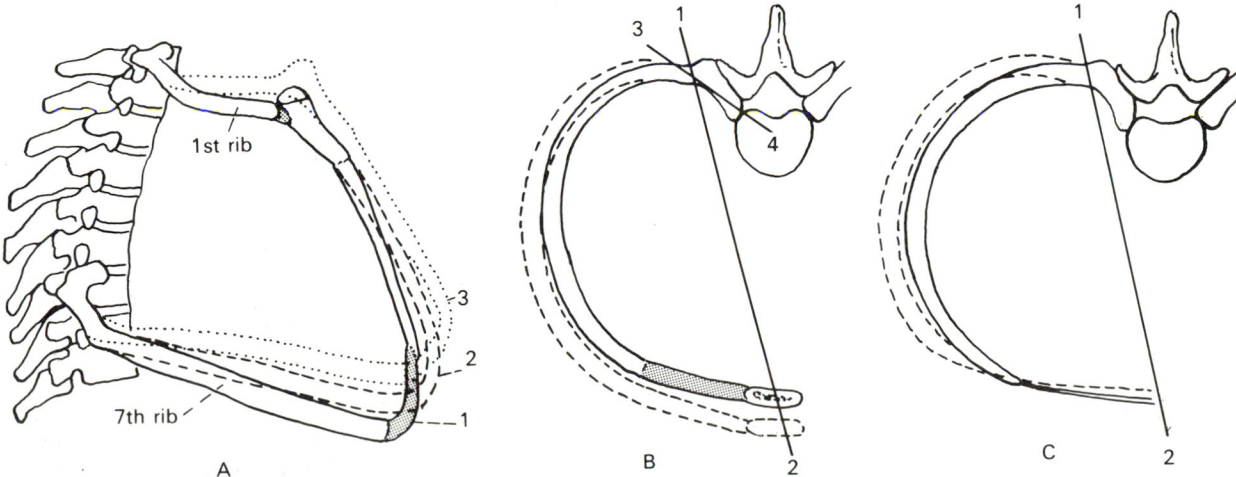

FIG. 53-6. Schematic depiction of the biomechanics of the thorax during respiration. *A.* Lateral view of the 1st and 7th ribs showing the movements of the sternum and ribs in ordinary expiration (*1*), quiet inspiration (*2*), and deep inspiration (*3*). *B.* Axes of movement (*1–2* and *3–4*) of the vertebrosternal rib. *C.* Axis of the movement (*1–2*) of the vertebrochondral rib. See text for more details. *Dotted lines,* position of rib during inspiration. Modified from Clemente, C.D.: Gray's Anatomy of the Human Body. 30th Ed. Philadelphia, Lea & Febiger, 1985, p. 365.

the action of the diaphragm. Acting from their attachment on the ribs and lumbar vertebrae, the muscle fibers of the diaphragm draw the central tendon downward and forward during inspiration. This tends both to increase the volume and decrease the pressure within the thoracic cavity and to decrease the volume and increase the pressure within the abdominal cavity.

All these structures take part in the respiratory cycle of inspiration and expiration, which is the result of the increase and decrease in the capacity of the thoracic cavity. Inspiration, the increase in the volume of the cavity, results from the muscular action of the descent of the diaphragm, which increases the vertical dimension of the thorax, and from the action of the muscles in the ribs, sternum, and vertebral column, which increases the transverse and anteroposterior dimensions of the thorax. Expiration, associated with a decrease in the volume of the thoracic cavity, is primarily a passive process because of the elastic recoil of the thoracic wall and of the tissues of the lungs

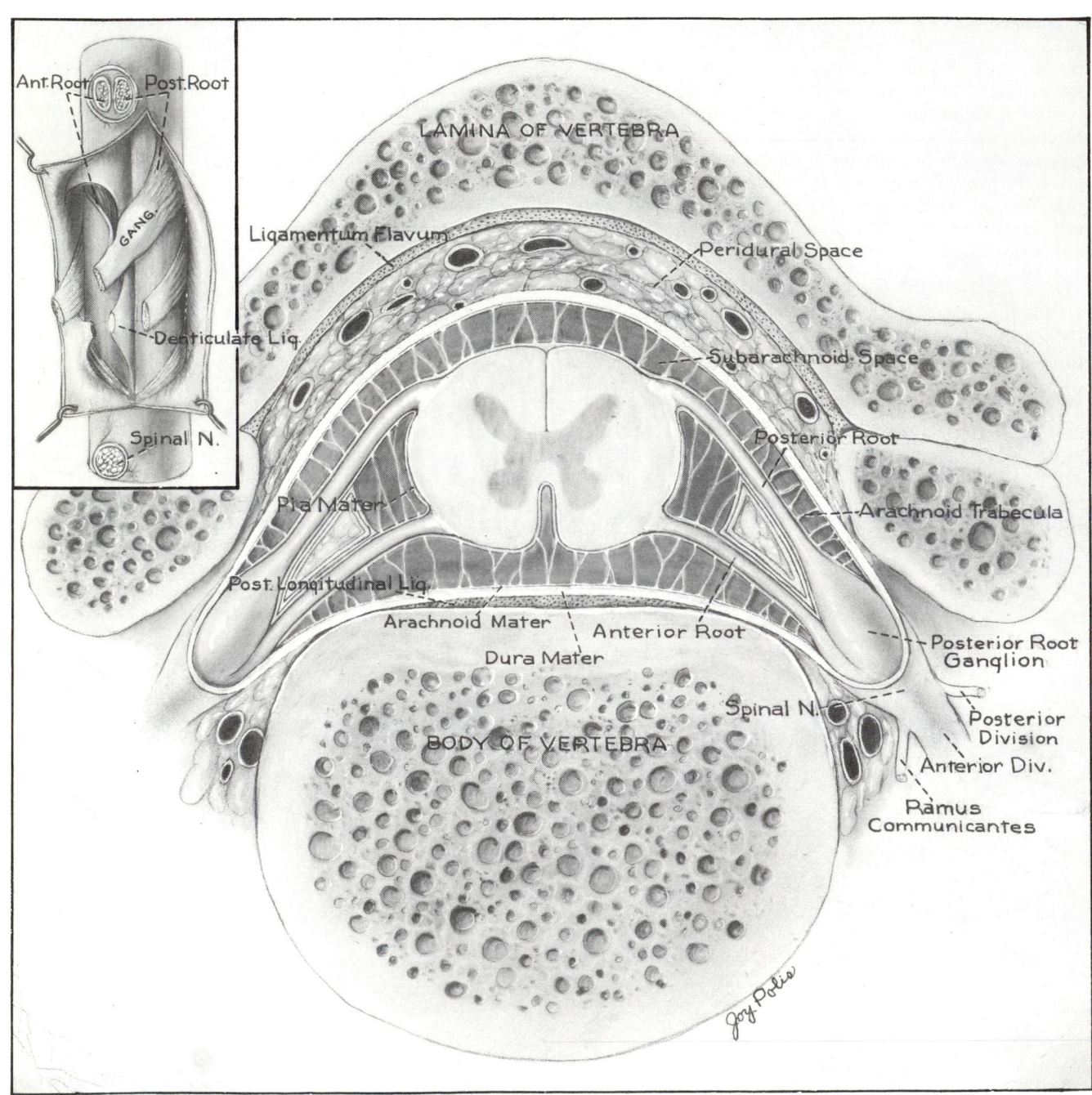

Fig. 53-7. Cross section of the thoracic spine showing detailed anatomy of the spinal cord and its meninges and the subarachnoid and epidural spaces. The section was taken between dentate ligaments (not shown). *Insert.* Attachment and coverings of the roots of spinal nerves.

966   *Pain in the Chest*

and bronchi. Thoracic volume can also decrease, however, as a result of the action of the abdominal muscles, which force the diaphragm upward by increasing the abdominal pressure, and by the action of certain muscles of the ribs and vertebral column, which actively contract the thoracic wall.

Neurologic Considerations

The canal of the thoracic portion of the spinal column in the adult contains more than two-thirds of the spinal cord. Although variations occur in most individuals, this portion of the canal contains the 2nd thoracic to the 1st sacral segments inclusively. As discussed in Chapter 46, the spinal cord only partially fills the spinal canal, its diameter being about half the diameter of the latter. Figure 53-7 shows the relationship of the spinal cord to the vertebral canal, and depicts the thoracic spine, the meninges, and the attachment of spinal nerves to the spinal cord. Because this was discussed in previous chapters, the remainder of this section describes the anatomy of the thoracic spinal nerves and the phrenic nerves because they supply motor fibers to the diaphragm and sensory fibers to the pericardium and other structures in the chest and abdomen.

Thoracic Spinal Nerves

The thoracic nerves consist of 12 pairs of somatic spinal nerves derived from homologous spinal cord segments located between the 7th cervical and 9th thoracic vertebrae (see Fig. 6-2). Generally, they retain their segmental relationship throughout their distribution by coursing below the corresponding rib to supply segments of muscles, skin, and other somatic structures of the thorax and abdomen. They also supply the parietal pleura and peritoneum.

Soon after they are formed within the spinal canal by the union of the anterior and posterior roots, the thoracic spinal nerves emerge below the corresponding vertebrae through the intervertebral foramen, and each divides into a posterior primary division and an anterior primary division (Fig. 53-8). Just before dividing, each of these nerves gives off a recurrent branch that returns through the foramen to supply the corresponding vertebra and its ligaments and a segment of the meninges covering the cord. Also before dividing, the formed thoracic spinal nerves are connected to the thoracic sympathetic chain by white rami communicantes, which contain myelinated preganglionic fibers and visceral afferents, and by gray rami communicantes, which contain unmyelinated postganglionic fibers.

The smaller posterior primary divisions diverge from their anterior counterparts and run posteriorly to supply the muscles and skin of the back through medial and lateral branches. In the upper six thoracic (and all cervical) segments the medial branches supply chiefly the skin and subcutaneous tissue, with the lateral branches almost entirely supplying muscles; in the lower thoracic (and lumbar and sacral) segments the reverse is true. The posterior division of each thoracic spinal nerve, often involved in painful conditions of the vertebrae and muscles, migrates within muscles caudally for a progressively greater distance before emerging from the muscle to supply the skin and subcutaneous tissue over the spinous process and the paravertebral region (Chapter 6 and Fig. 6-9). Thus, the cutaneous branch of the posterior division of the T6 nerve supplies the skin of the T9 to T10 dermatomes (posteriorly), the T10 nerve supplies the skin of the L2–L3 region, and the T12 nerve supplies that of the L5–S1 region (Table 6-1).

Each of the larger anterior primary divisions, after leaving the posterior primary division, proceeds laterally below the corresponding rib to become distributed to the parietes of the thorax and abdomen. The first 11 are situated between adjacent ribs and are therefore named the intercostal nerves, while the 12th nerve is called the subcostal nerve. The intercostal nerves are distributed chiefly to the parietes of the thorax and abdomen. They differ from other spinal nerves in that each pursues an independent course and, except for the 1st intercostal nerve, do not enter into the formation of plexuses.

The anterior primary division of the 1st thoracic nerve, after leaving the posterior primary division, divides into a larger superior branch and a smaller inferior branch. The superior branch runs in a superior and lateral direction across the neck of the 1st rib, leaves the thoracic cavity, and enters the interval between the anterior and middle scaleni muscles, where it joins the anterior primary division of the 8th cervical nerve to form the lower trunk of the brachial plexus. The inferior branch, which can be considered as the true 1st intercostal nerve, runs within the 1st intercostal space in the same fashion as other typical thoracic intercostal nerves. Usually it does not give off a lateral cutaneous branch, but sends a small branch to the intercostobrachial nerve.

Thoracic Intercostal Nerves

The anterior primary divisions of the 2nd through 6th thoracic nerves are often called the thoracic intercostal nerves because they supply the parietes of the chest. All these have a similar course and distribution and are therefore discussed as a group. After emerging through the intervertebral foramina they proceed laterally, each becoming situated for a short distance midway between the neck of the rib above and the neck of the rib below, lying between the pleura and the internal (posterior) intercostal membrane. About 3 cm lateral to the foramina they pierce the intercostal membrane and run obliquely across the interspace toward the angle of the rib above to enter the costal groove, where they come to lie below the intercostal vein and artery and between the innermost (intimi) intercostal muscles and the internal intercostal muscles (Fig. 53-8).

They continue their distal course between the two muscles as far as the junction between the ribs and costal cartilages, where they enter the interval between pleura and muscle. Proceeding within this interval they pass anteriorly to the internal mammary artery and the transverse thoracic muscle to within 1 to 2 cm of the lateral border of the sternum, where they pierce the internal intercostal muscle, the anterior intercostal membrane, and the pectoralis major to become the anterior cutaneous branches. Each of

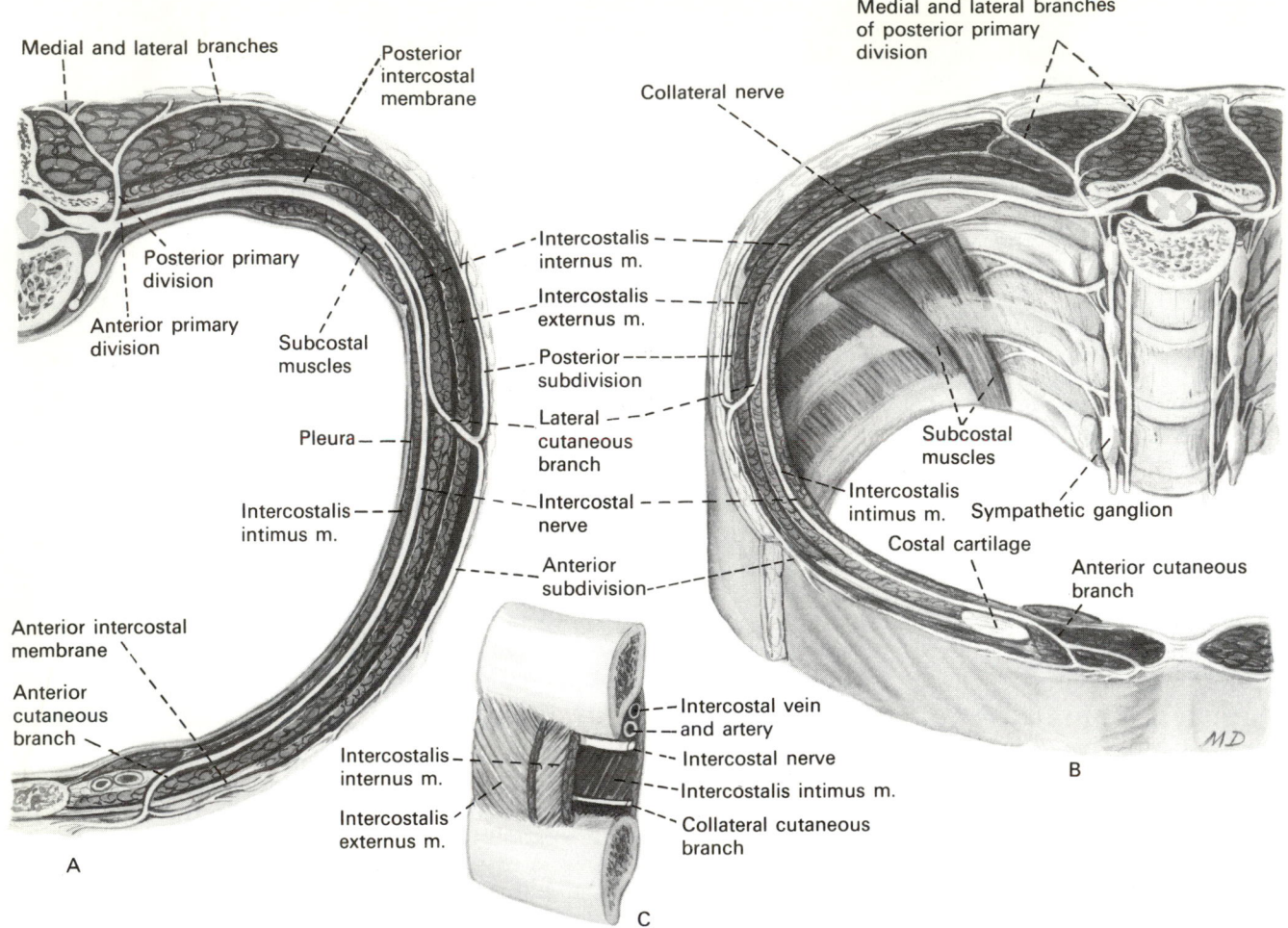

FIG. 53-8. A. Superior view of the intercostal space showing the various intercostal muscles and a thoracic spinal nerve dividing into posterior and anterior primary divisions, the latter becoming the intercostal nerve. **B.** Anterior view of the chest showing the relation of the intercostal nerves and their branches and the relation of the intercostal nerves to the sympathetic chain. **C.** Cut section of two adjacent ribs and the intercostal muscles showing the intercostal vessels and nerves. Note the direction of the fibers of the muscles. See text for details. Modified from Netter, F.H.: The CIBA Collection of Medical Illustrations. Vol. 7. Respiratory System. West Caldwell, NJ, CIBA Pharmaceutical, 1979, p. 11.

these branches supplies a segment of skin over the anterior chest and breast and sends filaments that overlap 2 cm beyond the midline to supply the skin of the opposite side. The anterior branch of the 1st intercostal is often absent, and that of the second frequently communicates with the medial supraclavicular nerves of the cervical plexus. The latter nerves supply the skin over the 1st, 2nd, and often the 3rd thoracic segments.

COLLATERAL AND LATERAL CUTANEOUS BRANCHES. At or near the neck of the rib, each intercostal nerve gives off a collateral branch and a lateral cutaneous branch (Figs. 53-8 and 53-9). The collateral branch runs along the lower border of the intercostal space and ends anteriorly as a separate cutaneous nerve or by rejoining the main nerve to supply the skin and other structures in the anterior chest.

The lateral cutaneous branch accompanies the main intercostal nerve as far as the midaxillary line before piercing the internal intercostal muscle and then runs obliquely through that muscle, the external intercostal muscle, and the serratus anterior muscle to reach the subcutaneous tissue, where it divides into anterior and posterior subdivisions. The anterior subdivisions run anteromedially to supply the skin of the lateral and anterior parts of the chest and breast; those of the 5th and 6th nerves also supply the cephalad digitations of the obliquus externus abdominis (Fig. 53-9). The posterior subdivisions supply the skin over the posterolateral and posterior parts of the chest that overlie the latissimus dorsi muscle and the scapular region.

The lateral cutaneous branch of the 2nd intercostal nerve, the intercostobrachial nerve, does not divide; it crosses the axilla to reach the medial side of the arm, where it pierces the deep fascia, communicates with branches of the medial and posterior brachial cutaneous nerves, and then proceeds to supply the skin of the upper half of the medial and posterior parts of the

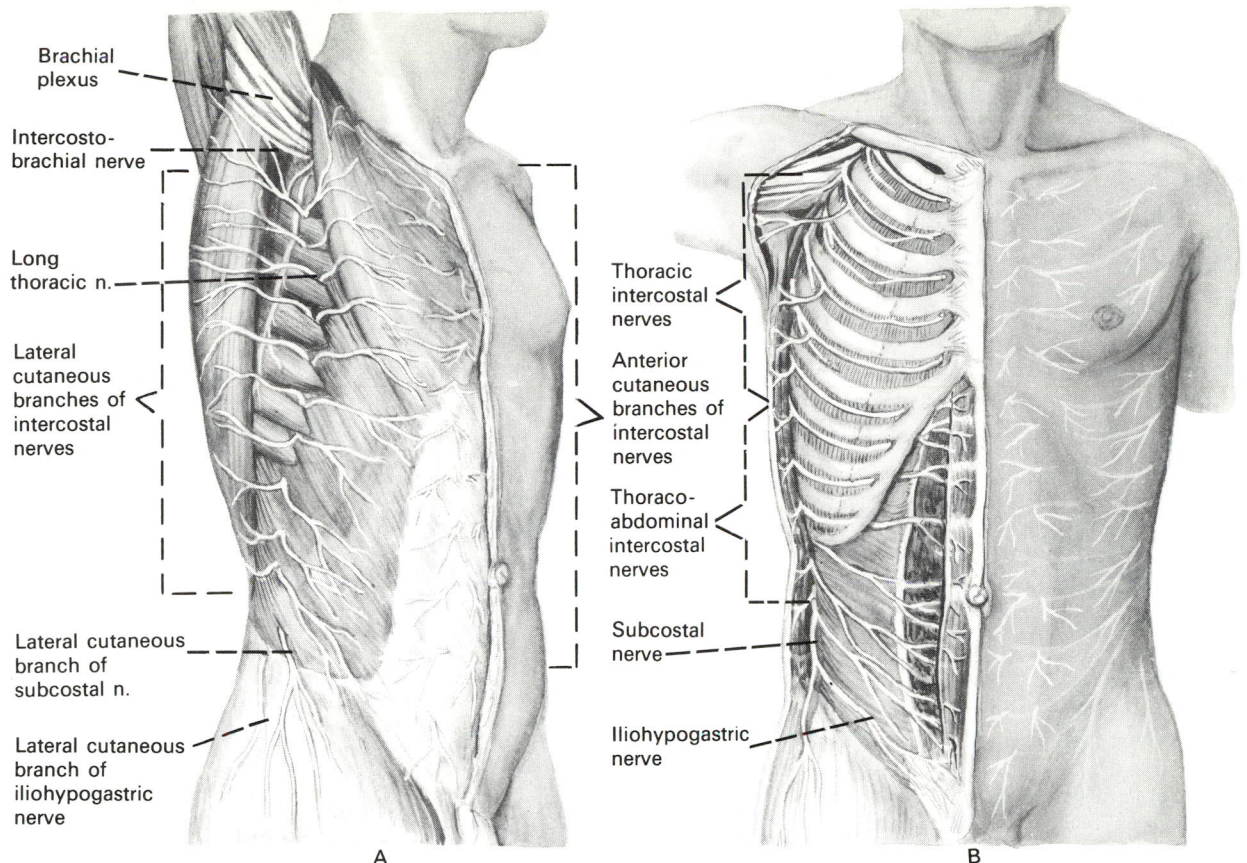

Brachial plexus

Intercosto-brachial nerve

Long thoracic n.

Lateral cutaneous branches of intercostal nerves

Lateral cutaneous branch of subcostal n.

Lateral cutaneous branch of iliohypogastric nerve

Thoracic intercostal nerves

Anterior cutaneous branches of intercostal nerves

Thoraco-abdominal intercostal nerves

Subcostal nerve

Iliohypogastric nerve

A

B

FIG. 53-9. Distribution of the intercostal nerves. **A.** Anterolateral view of the lateral cutaneous branches of the intercostal nerves emerging from the muscles and deep fascia and dividing into anterior and posterior subdivisions. Note especially the distribution of the lateral cutaneous branch of the 12th thoracic nerve, which supplies the anterior part of the gluteal region. The anterior cutaneous branches are also shown. **B.** Anterior view of the chest with the muscles removed on the right side to depict the location and distribution of the intercostal nerves. The anterior parts of the intercostal nerves enter the rectus abdominis muscle to provide motor branches to the muscle and then pass anteriorly through the muscle and its fascia to supply the cutaneous structures of the middle part of the abdominal wall.

arm. The anterior subdivision of the lateral cutaneous branch of the 3rd intercostal nerve often gives off a large filament that joins the intercostobrachial nerve to supply the axilla and upper medial aspect of the arm.

MUSCULAR BRANCH. The upper thoracic nerves give off numerous muscular branches to the intercostals, the subcostals, the levatores costarum, the serratus posterior superior, and the transversus thoracis muscles. At the anterior part of the thorax some of these muscular branches cross the costal cartilages from one intercostal space to another (1).

Thoracoabdominal Intercostal Nerves

The anterior primary division of the 7th to 11th nerves, often called the thoracoabdominal intercostal nerves, have the same course as those already described as far as the anterior end of the intercostal space. Here they run anteromedially to pass behind (posterior to) the costal cartilages and to enter the interval between the transversus abdominis and internal oblique muscles. They run medially within this interval as far as the semilunar line, where they perforate the posterior sheath of the rectus abdominis

muscle near its lateral margin. They then follow a medial course within the muscle, to which they give numerous filaments, and then abruptly turn anteriorly, piercing the anterior sheath of the rectus abdominis muscle to become the anterior cutaneous branches.

The anterior cutaneous branch of the 6th intercostal nerve supplies the skin over the xiphoid process, those of the 8th and 9th supply the skin between the xiphoid process and umbilicus, that of the 10th supplies the skin around the umbilicus, and that of the 11th supplies the skin just below the umbilicus.

The lateral cutaneous branches of these lower intercostals have similar subdivisions and distribution as the upper intercostals except that the anterior subdivisions supply the skin of the abdominal wall as far as the lateral margin of the rectus abdominis (linea semilunaris), while the posterior subdivisions supply the skin over the posterior part of the back as far as 4 to 5 cm from the midline (Fig. 53-9).

MUSCULAR BRANCHES. The thoracoabdominal intercostals give off muscular branches that supply the corresponding intercostals, the transversus abdominis, the external and internal oblique and rectus abdominis muscles, and the peripheral part of the diaphragm. The latter three also supply the serratus posterior inferior muscles.

TWELFTH THORACIC NERVE. The anterior primary division of the 12th thoracic nerve, the subcostal nerve, is much larger than the others. After emerging from its intervertebral foramen it gives off a branch that joins the 1st lumbar nerve and then passes laterally under the lateral lumbocostal arch in front of the quadratus lumborum to reach the transversus abdominis muscle, which it perforates to enter the interval between this and the internal oblique muscle. After this, its course and distribution are the same as those of the other lower intercostals, except that after perforating the muscles its lateral cutaneous branch does not divide but descends over the iliac crest to supply the skin of the anterior portion of the gluteal region as far as the greater trochanter. Its anterior cutaneous branch supplies a segment of skin about 3 to 4 cm above the pubis.

Phrenic Nerves

The phrenic nerves, generally considered to be the motor nerves of the diaphragm, also contain many sensory and sympathetic fibers. Each nerve is formed by a stout root from the anterior primary division of the C4 nerve, but is also augmented by fibers from the anterior division of the C3 and C5 nerves (Fig. 53-10). Each phrenic nerve receives gray rami communicantes from the superior and middle cervical sympathetic ganglia, and often from the vertebral ganglion and ansa subclavia. The three roots unite at the superolateral border of the anterior scalenus muscle. The nerve then passes downward on the anterior surface of that muscle, gradually crossing from its lateral to its medial side. It descends under cover of the sternocleidomastoid muscle and is crossed by the anterior belly of the omohyoid muscle and by the transverse cervical and suprascapular vessels. The nerve continues with the scalenus anterior between the subclavian vein and artery, and as it enters the thorax it crosses the origin of the internal thoracic artery and is joined by the pericardiophrenic branch of this artery. It then passes downward over the cupula of the pleura, and anterior to, the root of the lung, and along the lateral aspect of the pericardium between it and the mediastinal pleura until it reaches the diaphragm, where it divides into its terminal branches.

The right phrenic nerve is situated more deeply, is shorter, and runs more vertically downward than the left nerve. In the upper part of the thorax it is lateral to the right brachiocephalic vein and the superior vena cava. The left phrenic nerve is longer than the right because of the inclination of the heart toward the left and because of the more caudal position of the diaphragm on this side (Fig. 53-10). At the thoracic inlet the left nerve passes anterior to the subclavian artery behind the termination of the thoracic duct and proceeds downward between the left subclavian and left common carotid arteries. As it crosses the left side of the arch of the aorta it is lateral to the vagus nerve. It continues downward anterior to

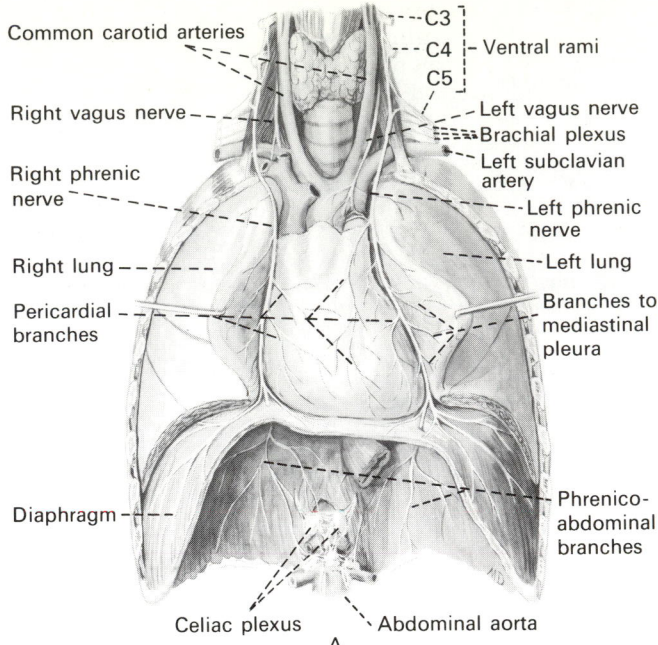

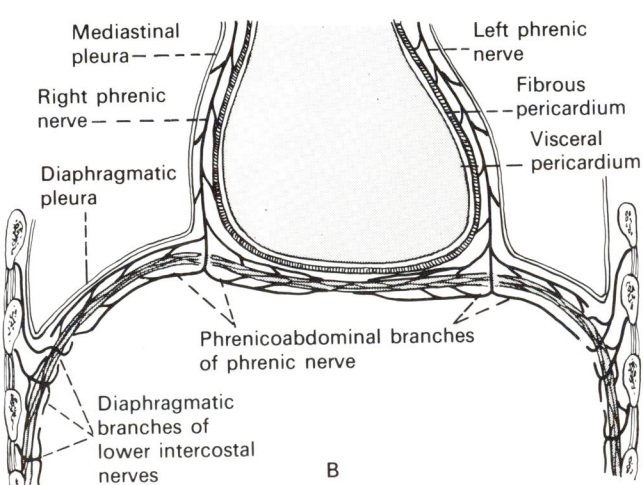

FIG. 53-10. Anatomy of the phrenic nerves. **A.** Anterior view of the chest with the lungs reflected to show the origin, course, and distribution of both phrenic nerves. **B.** Schematic depiction of the distribution of the motor and sensory fibers of the phrenic nerves. The sensory fibers contribute to the sensory innervation of the pericardium, the central portion of the superior and inferior surface of the diaphragm, and send branches to the inferior phrenic plexus (a subsidiary of the celiac plexus), through which the sensory nerves of the phrenic nerves supply a number of upper abdominal viscera. Modified from Netter, F.H.: The CIBA Collection of Medical Illustrations. Nervous System, Part I: Anatomy and Physiology. West Caldwell, NJ, CIBA Pharmaceutical, 1983, p. 114.

the root of the left lung and between the mediastinal pleura and fibrous pericardium covering the left surface of the heart to reach the diaphragm.

While passing through the thorax, both phrenic nerves supply nerve filaments to the fibrous pericardium, to the costal and mediastinal pleura over the apex of the lung, to the mediastinal pleura along its length, and to the central region of the diaphragmatic pleura. As previously mentioned, the sensory nerves to the margin of the diaphragm and to the corresponding areas of the overlying pleura and peritoneum are provided by lower intercostal nerves. The left phrenic nerve often sends a twig to the left pulmonary plexus and the right nerve supplies filaments to the inferior vena cava, with both nerves communicating with the superior thoracic splanchnic nerves.

The right phrenic nerve pierces the central tendon of the diaphragm through or near the orifice of the inferior vena cava, while the left nerve penetrates the diaphragm close to the anterior edge of its central tendon just lateral to the cardiac apex. Each nerve divides into three diverging phrenicoabdominal branches below the diaphragm. These supply the diaphragm from its inferior surface and also supply sensory fibers to most of the peritoneum covering the diaphragm except for marginal areas, which receive their nerve supply from the lower intercostal nerves. Sensory fibers also supply the coronary and falciform ligaments of the liver. On the right side a branch near the inferior vena cava communicates with the inferior phrenic plexus, a subsidiary of the celiac plexus, which accompanies the inferior phrenic arteries. A small phrenic ganglion is usually found at the point at which the filaments from the phrenic nerve join the phrenic plexus. Filaments from the inferior phrenic plexuses pass through the gastroesophageal junction, the cardiac end of the stomach, the porta hepatis, and the adrenal (suprarenal) plexuses.

Thoracic Sympathetic Nerves

The thoracic portion of the sympathetic trunk consists of a series of a paravertebral ganglia situated on each side of the thoracic vertebral column. Although it is usually stated that 1 ganglion is found on each side of each vertebra, with 12 ganglia in each of the two trunks, this occurs only rarely. In most cases the 1st ganglion fuses with the inferior cervical ganglion to form the stellate ganglion. According to Hovelacque (4), the 2nd thoracic can also take part occasionally in the formation of the stellate ganglion. In addition, fusion of 2 lower thoracic ganglia or of the 12th thoracic and 1st lumbar ganglia can occur, so that the number is reduced further. In most instances, therefore, 10, and not infrequently 11 ganglia, can be found in each of the thoracic sympathetic trunks (Fig. 53-11).

These ganglia vary greatly in size and shape. In most cases they are triangular or quadrangular and are 8 mm long and 3 mm wide. The 1st and 2nd ganglia are the largest and the 12th is next in size, whereas in the midportion of the trunk the ganglia can be so small as to be almost indistinguishable from the interganglionic cord.

As they emerge from the intervertebral foramina the spinal nerves pass posterior to the interganglionic cord. The pleura is immediately in front of and in close relation to the ganglia, separated from them by the thin endothoracic fascia.

Hovelacque (4) described the branches of the thoracic ganglia as internal and external. The external branches consist of one, two, sometimes three, and rarely four gray rami communicantes and one white

ramus communicans, which pass to the adjacent spinal nerves. The internal are vascular and visceral branches, with those of the upper four or five ganglia supplying the thoracic viscera and the thoracic aorta and its branches and those derived from the lower six or seven ganglia contributing to the formation of the splanchnic nerves. The thoracic visceral branches reach the viscera either directly or by first passing through the pulmonary, esophageal, and cardiac plexuses. The cardiac and pulmonary plexuses are described in the next section.

Splanchnic Nerves

The splanchnic nerves arise from the medial border of the lower seven ganglia and pass to the celiac plexus to effect a connection between this structure and the sympathetic trunk (5, 6). Usually three groups of these nerves are found on each side: the upper thoracic (greater) splanchnic nerves, the middle thoracic (lesser) splanchnic nerves, and the inferior thoracic (least) splanchnic nerves. DeSousa-Pereira (7) found a 4th splanchnic nerve in 4% of cases, and he called it the accessory splanchnic nerve.

SUPERIOR THORACIC SPLANCHNIC NERVE. The superior thoracic (greater) splanchnic nerve is formed by roots that arise from the midportion of the thoracic sympathetic chain. According to Hovelacque (4) it is usually formed by three roots, less frequently four, sometimes only two, and rarely five or six. This description of its formation, subsequently corroborated by the work of DeSousa-Pereira (7), who carefully dissected and studied the splanchnic nerves in 100 cadavers, is different from the usual textbook description, which states that it is most frequently formed by five or six roots. The roots are usually given off by the 7th, 8th, and 9th ganglia, each ganglion giving off only one filament. Sometimes, however, the uppermost root takes origin from the 6th or 5th ganglion, rarely the 4th or 3rd, while the lowest root originates from the 10th ganglion. In most cases the roots are given off by adjacent ganglia but in some cases are given off from a superior group and an inferior group, with two or three ganglia in between that do not contribute any fibers. These roots run inferiorly, anteriorly, and medially on the anterolateral aspect of the vertebral column and come together at the level of the 9th or 10th vertebra to form the superior thoracic splanchnic nerve. Near the origin of the formed nerve an enlargement called the splanchnic ganglion is usually found (70% of cases).

The superior thoracic (greater) splanchnic nerve is of considerable size, firm, and white. In its downward course it passes over the anterolateral aspect of the vertebrae, being separated at intervals from the vertebrae by the intercostal vessels and throughout its extent by the azygos vein on the right and by the hemiazygos vein and aorta on the left (Fig. 53-11). It is in close relation with the pleura, behind and medial to it. It passes through the diaphragm within the space that separates the internal from the external crura and enters the abdominal cavity. Its course within this cavity is short, never more than 2 cm (4), and is in an anteromedial and inferior direction. The nerve usually breaks up into its terminal branches, which spread out like a fan and terminate in one or more ipsilateral celiac ganglia (see Figs. 59-6 and 96-31).

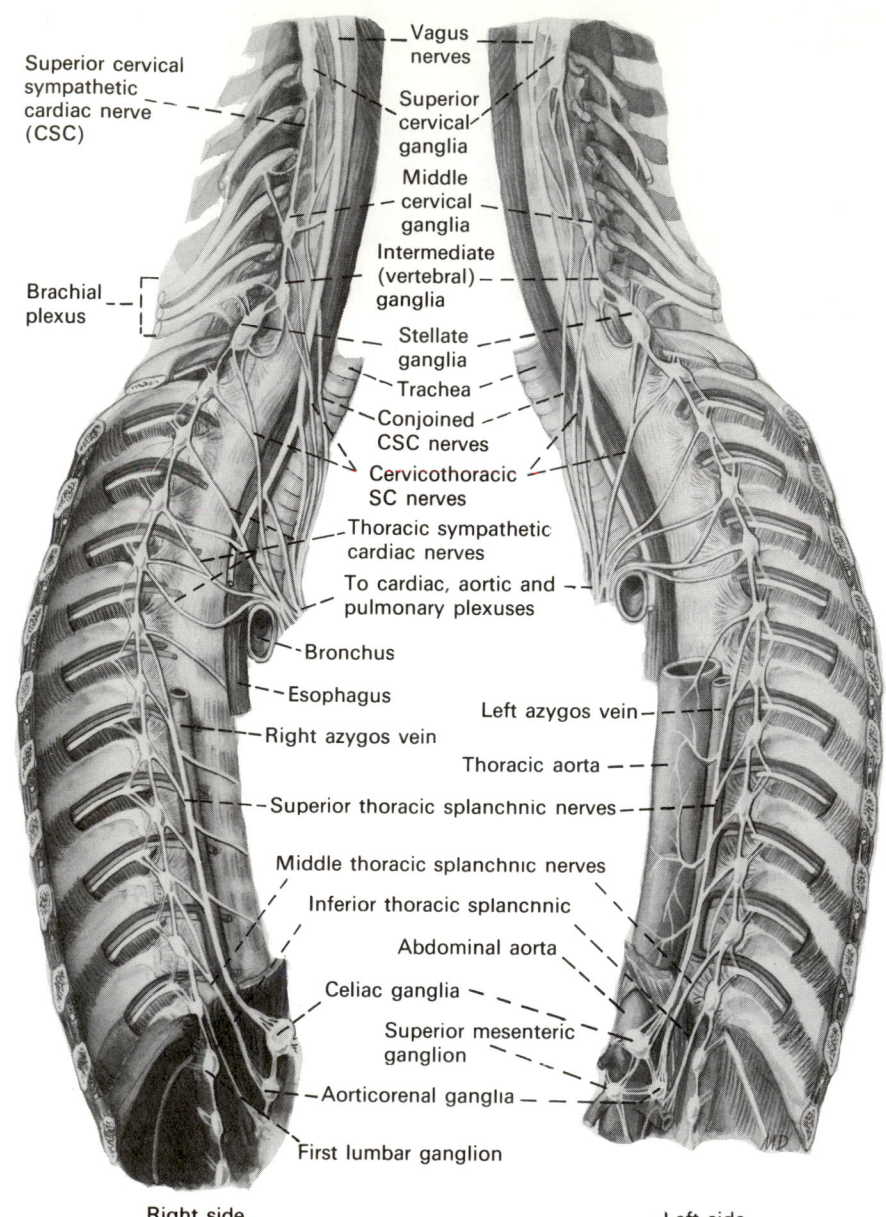

Superior cervical
sympathetic
cardiac nerve
(CSC)

Brachial
plexus

Vagus
nerves

Superior
cervical
ganglia

Middle
cervical
ganglia

Intermediate
(vertebral)
ganglia

Stellate
ganglia

Trachea

Conjoined
CSC nerves

Cervicothoracic
SC nerves

Thoracic sympathetic
cardiac nerves

To cardiac, aortic and
pulmonary plexuses

Bronchus

Esophagus

Right azygos vein

Left azygos vein

Thoracic aorta

Superior thoracic splanchnic nerves

Middle thoracic splanchnic nerves

Inferior thoracic splancnnic

Abdominal aorta

Celiac ganglia

Superior mesenteric
ganglion

Aorticorenal ganglia

First lumbar ganglion

Right side   Left side

Fig. 53-11. The cervical, thoracic, and upper lumbar sympathetic trunks and their branches. Note their relation to the vertebrae and ribs at various levels. CSC, cervical sympathetic cardiac; SC, sympathetic cardiac.

During its course the greater splanchnic nerve gives off fine collateral filaments that join the intercostal vessels, the azygos veins, and the aortic plexus and others going to the diaphragm and the spinal cord. In addition, some filaments join the lesser splanchnic nerve.

MIDDLE THORACIC (LESSER) SPLANCHNIC NERVE. The middle thoracic (lesser) splanchnic nerve is usually formed by two roots, sometimes by one or three, which arise from the lower portion of the thoracic chain. The roots are given off by the 10th and 11th ganglia, and rarely by the 12th ganglion (4). Soon after their origin these roots converge into one trunk, which descends inferiorly, anteriorly, and medially on

the anterolateral aspect of the vertebral column. It lies between the sympathetic chain, which is postero-lateral to it, and the greater splanchnic nerve, which is anteromedial to it. It leaves the thoracic cavity and enters the abdominal cavity by passing through the diaphragm lateral to and accompanied by the superior thoracic splanchnic nerve to terminate in the celiac or aorticorenal ganglion.

INFERIOR THORACIC (LEAST) SPLANCHNIC NERVE. The inferior thoracic (least) splanchnic nerve is usually formed by one root that arises from the 12th thoracic ganglion. This nerve is a fine cord that passes anteriorly, medially, and slightly inferiorly below the lesser splanchnic nerve. It perforates the diaphragm

972 *Pain in the Chest*

along with the other two splanchnic nerves to enter the abdominal cavity, where it proceeds toward and ends in the aorticorenal ganglion.

ACCESSORY SPLANCHNIC NERVE. The accessory splanchnic nerve, when present, arises from the 12th thoracic ganglion, has the same course as (but is independent of) the least splanchnic nerve, and ends in the aorticorenal ganglion.

B. INNERVATION OF THE THORACIC VISCERA

This section presents a detailed description of the anatomy of the nerves to the heart, the aorta, the lungs, and other visceral structures in the chest. More detailed reviews of these various aspects have been presented by Hovelacque (4), Kuntz (5), Mitchell (6), Miller (8), White and colleagues (9–11), Mizeres (12), and Hirsch and Borghard-Erdle (13).

Innervation of the Heart

The nerve supply of the heart is complex and, like other visceral organs, is composed of efferent and afferent sympathetic and parasympathetic efferent fibers (Fig. 53-12). Most of the nerves arise well above the cardiac level because the heart develops initially

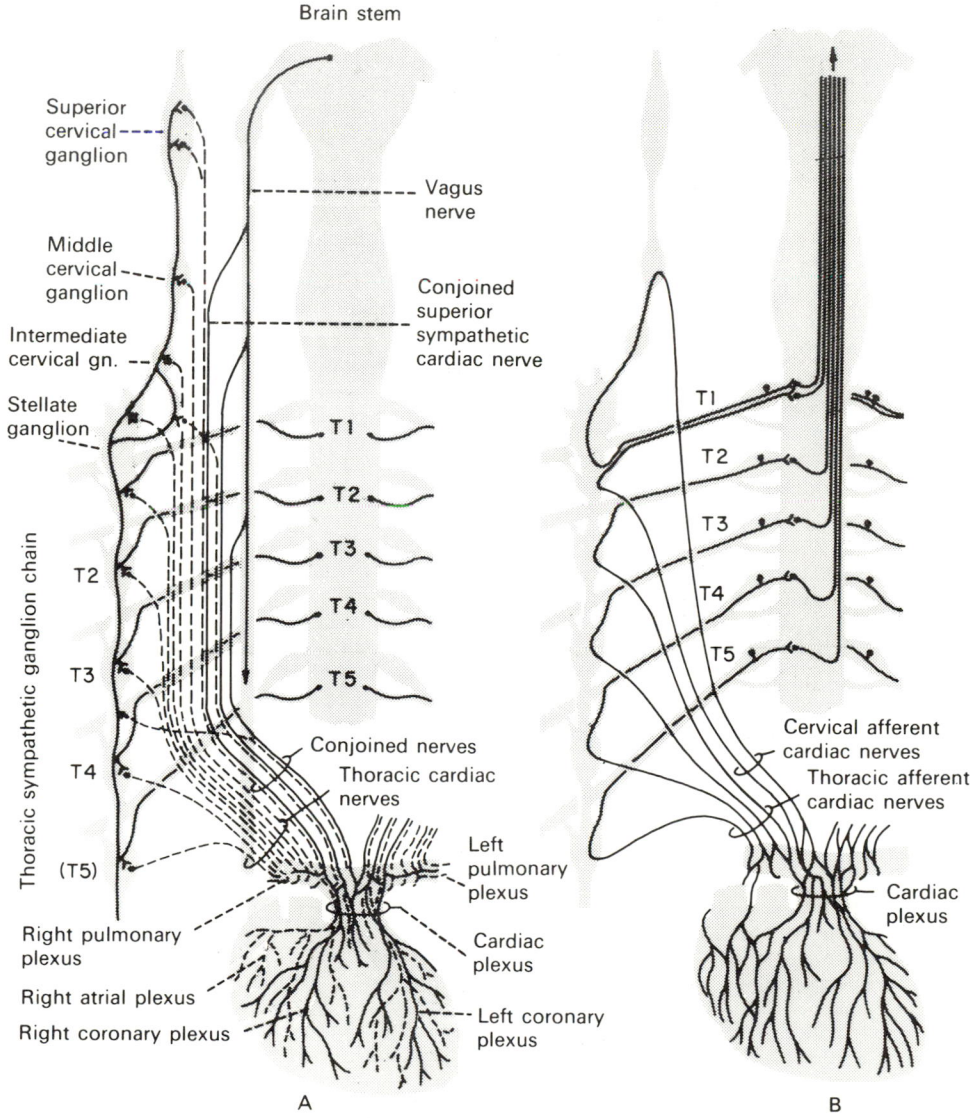

FIG. 53-12. Nerve supply of the heart. **A.** On the left is shown the sympathetic preganglionic fibers (*solid lines*), which have their cell bodies in the intermediolateral column of the T1 to T5 segments. These preganglionic axons synapse with cell bodies of postganglionic fibers (*dashed lines*), some of which join vagal fibers to form conjoint nerves. **B.** Sympathetic afferents. These transmit nociceptive information and have their cell bodies in the dorsal root ganglion. The proximal axons synapse with dorsal horn neurons whereas the distal axons pass through the white rami communicantes and thence through the sympathetic chain and the various cardiac sympathetic nerves that contribute to the cardiac plexus and its various subsidiary plexuses that supply the heart. No interruption or synapse of these fibers is found anywhere along their course. See text for details.

in the neck region and later migrates to the thorax (4). Efferent and afferent fibers are involved in important reflexes and are influenced in their activities by centrifugal and centripetal impulses from many parts of the body. This is not surprising considering the prime importance of the heart and major vessels in the body's physiologic economy, represented at every level in the nervous system (Chapter 6 reviews the central and peripheral portions of the autonomic nervous system). Here only those aspects relevant to the innervation of the heart are considered.

Sympathetic Nerves

The sympathetic nerves to the heart contain both efferent preganglionic and postganglionic fibers and afferent fibers. The sympathetic preganglionic cardiac fibers are the axons of cells located in the intermediolateral column of the spinal cord at the level of the T1 to the T4 or T5 spinal segments (in an undetermined percentage of individuals a cranial or caudal shift of one or even two segments might be present) (6). The representation is inverted, with the fibers destined for the ventricles arising above those destined for the atria (6). As emphasized below, these cells are influenced both by impulses coming from the heart and by impulses descending from the sympathetic centers in the hypothalamus, which in turn is influenced by higher centers of the brain as well as by impulses ascending from the neuraxis. These preganglionic myelinated axons leave the spinal cord via the ventral roots of the upper four or five thoracic spinal nerves and pass through the white rami communicantes to reach the paravertebral sympathetic chain. Some of these axons synapse with ganglionic cells in the ganglia that they enter, while most ascend in the trunk to end in the inferior, intermediate, middle, or superior cervical sympathetic ganglion.

The postganglionic axons have thin myelin sheaths, so thin that they appear to be unmyelinated when ordinary staining methods are used. The axons destined for the heart, aorta, and other large vessels pass through the superior, middle, and inferior cervical sympathetic cardiac nerves and the thoracic cardiac nerves. Like the parasympathetic nerves the sympathetic cardiac nerves vary in number, site of origin, size, and distribution. The following discussion is in accordance with the views of Hovelacque (4), Mitchell (6), and Mizeres (12) (Fig. 53-13).

SUPERIOR CERVICAL SYMPATHETIC CARDIAC NERVE. The superior cervical sympathetic cardiac nerve originates by one, two, or occasionally three rootlets from the lower and medial parts of the superior cervical sympathetic ganglion or can arise from any part of the upper cervical sympathetic chain, from its upper pole down through the level of the lower border of the C6 vertebra (5). The rootlets often unite, and soon thereafter often join with a corresponding cervical vagal branch to form a conjoined nerve that descends behind the common carotid sheath and its contents near the main sympathetic trunk and laterally through the trachea and esophagus. En route it communicates through slender filaments with the pharyngeal, laryngeal, carotid, and thyroid plexuses and with other cervical cardiac nerves. It then proceeds behind the homolateral subclavian artery at the root of the neck to reach the cardiac plexuses.

On the right side the nerve passes posterolateral to the innominate artery and aortic arch to end in the cardiac plexus. On the left side the nerve is in contact with the left side of the left common carotid artery and passes between this and the left subclavian artery or around the root of the latter vessel before curving downward across the left side of the arotic arch to the cardiac plexus. This nerve is often connected with the middle, or inferior, group of cardiac branches of the left vagus nerve somewhere between the root of the neck and the aortic arch, and always communicates with the middle and inferior cervical sympathetic cardiac nerves or with vagal branches. As described below, as these partially commingled nerves descend across the anterolateral side of the aortic arch they give off three to six filaments, which form the preaortic plexus.

MIDDLE CERVICAL SYMPATHETIC CARDIAC NERVE. The middle cervical sympathetic cardiac nerve originates by rootlets from the middle cervical ganglion or from the adjacent part of the sympathetic trunk and also receives rootlets contributed by the intermediate cervical (vertebral) sympathetic ganglion. Mitchell (6) stated that this is the largest of the sympathetic cardiac nerves. On the right side the nerve enters the thorax behind the subclavian and innominate arteries and reaches the cardiac plexus by passing between the tracheal bifurcation and aortic arch. On the left side it runs between the left common carotid and subclavian arteries or around the root of the latter and crosses the left side of the aortic arch to reach the cardiac plexus. Mitchell (6) and Mizeres (12) agreed that often this nerve cannot be distinguished as a complete and separate entity at the level of the aortic arch because of its intercommunication with other sympathetic and vagal cardiac branches. On both sides the nerve communicates with the thyroid, tracheal, esophageal, and aortic nerves and with filaments from the left recurrent laryngeal nerve. The nerve furnishes one or two filaments to the preaortic plexus.

INFERIOR CERVICAL SYMPATHETIC CARDIAC NERVES. The inferior cervical sympathetic cardiac nerves consist of a variable number of filaments arising from the stellate ganglion, the intermediate cervical (vertebral) sympathetic ganglion, and the ansa subclavia. When the inferior cervical and 1st thoracic ganglia are not fused into the stellate ganglion, the inferior cervical cardiac nerves arise from separate filaments from each ganglion. Their course is similar to that of the middle cervical sympathetic cardiac nerve. Mizeres (12) pointed out that, because these branches often arise from the sympathetic trunk at the level of the C7 and C8 and T1 vertebrae (which include the stellate ganglion, ansa subclavia, and vertebral or intermediate ganglion), they should be called the cervicothoracic cardiac sympathetic nerves. These nerves often fuse with the vagal branches to become conjoined nerves that pass caudad by coursing between the aorta and the bronchi to contribute to the cardiac and both pulmonary plexuses and to the plexus of the aortic arch, with some proceeding directly to the coronary plexuses. An inconstant communication exists between these nerves and the phrenic nerves.

THORACIC CARDIAC SYMPATHETIC NERVES. The cervical sympathetic cardiac nerves were recognized nearly 400 years ago by Fallopius (c. 1600 A.D.) and by many others thereafter. It was not until 1927, however, that the thoracic sympathetic cardiac nerves were identified. Their clinical importance was emphasized independently and simultaneously by Braeucker (14) and by Ionesco and Enachesco (15), although Mitchell (6) pointed out that they were noted in a calf by Weber (1815) and in humans by Swan (1830). Obviously these small anatomic structures are important clinically because they provide direct connection between the sympathetic trunk and the cardiac plexus. Usually three, four, or five rather slender branches on each side originate from the T2 to the T4 or T5 (rarely the T6) sympathetic ganglia, or from the interganglionic portion of the sympathetic trunk.

These nervelets pass anteriorly and medially; some enter the cardiac plexus directly or unite with neighboring filaments destined for the trachea, esophagus, aorta, or pulmonary structures, and then separate again as they appraoch the heart to contribute to the cardiac plexus. Mizeres (12) found that nervelets on the right side fuse immediately with at least one of the cervicothoracic cardiac sympathetic nerves and with one of the thoracic cardiac vagal nerves, and contribute directly to the right pulmonary and atrial plexuses. In contrast, on the left side, they do not fuse but proceed individually and send filaments into the plexus on the arch of the aorta, directly into the thoracic vagal trunk, and also to the left pulmonary and atrial plexuses.

Cardiac Branches of the Vagus Nerves

The vagus nerves that supply the heart and thoracic aorta have both preganglionic parasympathetic fibers and afferent fibers. The parasympathetic preganglionic fibers are contained in the vagus and in the cranial part of the accessory nerve that joins the vagus. The cell bodies of these preganglionic parasympathetic fibers are located in the dorsal motor nucleus of the vagus, which is an elongated structure that extends caudad to the upper cervical part of the spinal cord. These preganglionic axons course through each vagus nerve and through the cardiac vagal nerves on both sides to end in the terminal extrinsic ganglia in the cardiac plexus or in the small intrinsic cardiac ganglia in the subepicardial tissue of the heart and the myocardium. The finely myelinated preganglionic parasympathetic axons synapse with the cell bodies of the thinly myelinated or unmyelinated postganglionic fibers; these are short and, in contrast to the sympathetic postganglionic fibers, have a rather circumscribed distribution.

The vagal cardiac branches arise both in the neck and thorax and vary in size, number, and distribution. Nevertheless, it is generally agreed that these vagal cardiac nerves can be divided into three groups: the superior (referred to by Mizeres (12) as the cervical vagal cardiac nerves); the middle or cervicothoracic vagal cardiac nerves; and the lower or thoracic vagal cardiac nerves.

SUPERIOR (CERVICAL) VAGAL CARDIAC NERVES. The superior vagal cardiac nerves originate from any part of the cervical part of the vagus as far inferiorly as the lower border of the C6 vertebra (12). In some instances, two or three filaments arise just below the superior laryngeal nerve, while in others the vagus gives off only a single branch. In any case they soon coalesce to form a single nerve; as mentioned above, this invariably joins the superior cervical sympathetic cardiac nerve to form a conjoint nerve. The rootlets of the nerve itself often communicate with the pharyngeal and superior laryngeal nerves and occasionally with the carotid nerve. Mizeres (12) found that the right branch usually courses posteriorly to the aorta and enters the right pulmonary plexus, while the left branch descends anteriorly to the carotid sheath and arch of the aorta, contributing to its plexus and to the coronary plexuses. Occasionally both course anteriorly to the aortic arch.

MIDDLE (CERVICOTHORACIC) VAGAL CARDIAC NERVES. These nerves can consist of one, two, or three rootlets arising from the vagus in the lower half or third of the neck. They almost always communicate with the cervical sympathetic cardiac nerves and not infrequently course as conjoined nerves before reaching their destination. If these nerves remain separate they pass directly to the cardiac plexus, lying posterolaterally to the innominate artery and aortic arch on the right side and laterally to the left common carotid aortic arch on the left side. Mizeres (12) found that the right cervicothoracic vagal cardiac nerve usually arises by filaments from the right recurrent laryngeal nerve and from the vagal trunk at the level of the C7 and T1 vertebrae. Near their origin the filaments usually join the right cervical and cervicothoracic sympathetic cardiac nerves and course caudad as conjoined nerves posterolaterally to the innominate artery and aortic arch before reaching their destination, which is usually the right pulmonary plexus, a subsidiary of the cardiac plexus. The one or two left cervicothoracic vagal cardiac branches arise from the left vagal trunk at the level of the C7 and T1 vertebrae and usually course laterally to the left common carotid and subclavian arteries and then pass anteriorly to the arch of the aorta, contributing to the plexus on the arch and to the left atrial plexus.

INFERIOR (THORACIC) VAGAL CARDIAC NERVES. The two to four right thoracic vagal cardiac nerves arise from the thoracic vagal trunk between the level of the lower border of the T1 vertebra and the pulmonary hilus. They soon join the cervicothoracic or thoracic cardiac sympathetic nerves before coursing anteriorly to the right bronchus, where some filaments join the right pulmonary plexus and others proceed to the right atrial plexus. The left thoracic vagal cardiac branches arise from the left vagus at about the level of the origin of the left subclavian artery and run across the left side of the aortic arch to the cardiac plexus. Mizeres (12) found that in many instances one root arises from the left recurrent laryngeal nerve and another from the left vagal trunk just below it. Of the group of filaments that arise from the left recurrent laryngeal nerve, one group courses posteriorly to the arch of the aorta and joins the left atrial plexus directly while the other group courses anteriorly to join the left pulmonary plexus and proceeds in the fold of the left superior vena cava posteriorly to reach the left atrial plexus.

Afferent (Sensory) Fibers

The sensory fibers that supply the heart and great vessels pass centrally through the vagus nerves and the sympathetic nerves. Those associated with the vagus nerves have their cell bodies in the ganglion nodosum with the distal axons passing through the vagus and the cardiac vagal nerves to terminate in the heart, while the proximal axons enter the medulla to end in the nucleus of the tractus solitarius. The afferent fibers associated with the vagus that supply the heart carry impulses concerned with the subconscious reflex mechanisms that regulate cardiac action and blood pressure. Although some have suggested that some afferent fibers in the vagus convey all nociceptive impulses from the heart, clinical evidence does not support this notion (9–11, 16, 17). It has been shown that interruption of sympathetic afferents that pass into spinal cord segments T1 to T5 produce virtually complete relief of cardiac pain in the chest, arms, and neck, thus indicating they are the primary pathways for cardiac pain (9–11, 16, 17). Interruption of these sympathetic afferents may not relieve pain in the lower jaw, however, and does not eliminate the dyspnea and the feeling of constriction or tightness of the throat. It is possible that these sensations, which are the earliest and most frequent symptoms of myocardial ischemia in many patients, are transmitted by vagal afferents. Moreover, recent studies indicate that stimulation of the cardiac vagal afferents can activate cells in the brain stem; in turn, these cells produce descending modulating impulses that inhibit high-threshold and wide-dynamic-range cells of spinothalamic and other ascending systems at T1–T5 levels known to be involved in transmission of nociceptive ("pain") information to the brain (18–20). It has been suggested that this might be one of the mechanisms for the absence of pain in patients with silent myocardial infarction (18, 21) (see Chapter 54 for details).

The afferent fibers associated with the sympathetics, now commonly known as sympathetic afferents (22), are tonically active and not only mediate nociceptive impulses, but also mediate impulses involved in segmental and suprasegmental reflexes. These fibers are mainly excitatory in nature with positive-feedback characteristics and thus contribute to the neural regulation of circulatory functions (22). These sympathetic afferent fibers pass centrally through all the cardiac sympathetic nerves except those that arise from the superior cervical ganglia (Fig. 53-12B). The cell bodies of these sympathetic afferents are located in the posterior root ganglia of the upper four or five thoracic spinal nerves. Their central branches course to the spinal cord dorsal horn while their long peripheral branches pass distally through the upper four or five

thoracic white rami communicantes and through the upper four or five thoracic ganglia and the inferior, intermediate, and middle cervical sympathetic ganglia to reach the heart through the thoracic, cervicothoracic, and middle cervical sympathetic cardiac nerves. These peripheral branches travel uninterrupted in the ganglia or plexuses and terminate as typical sensory nerve endings in the pericardium, the walls of the heart, and the adventitial plexuses of the coronary arteries and the aorta. Many of these sensory fibers are of the A-delta and C categories, characteristic of nociceptive pathways (Chapter 54).

Cardiac Plexus

All vagal and sympathetic cardiac nerves and associated afferent fibers converge on the cardiac plexus, which is contained in the thoracic cavity (Figs. 53-13 and 53-14). Although it has generally been stated that the plexus lies between the concavity of the aortic arch and the tracheal bifurcation (1, 2–6). Mizeres (12), in his careful dissection of 36 cadavers of different ages, found that the cardiac plexus lies on the anterior and posterior walls of the pulmonary trunk at its bifurcation (Fig. 53-13). Moreover he, like Mitchell (6), believed that although the cardiac plexus is described as consisting of "superficial" and "deep" parts, this separation is an artifact created by dissection. The plexus, in its position on the adventitial wall of

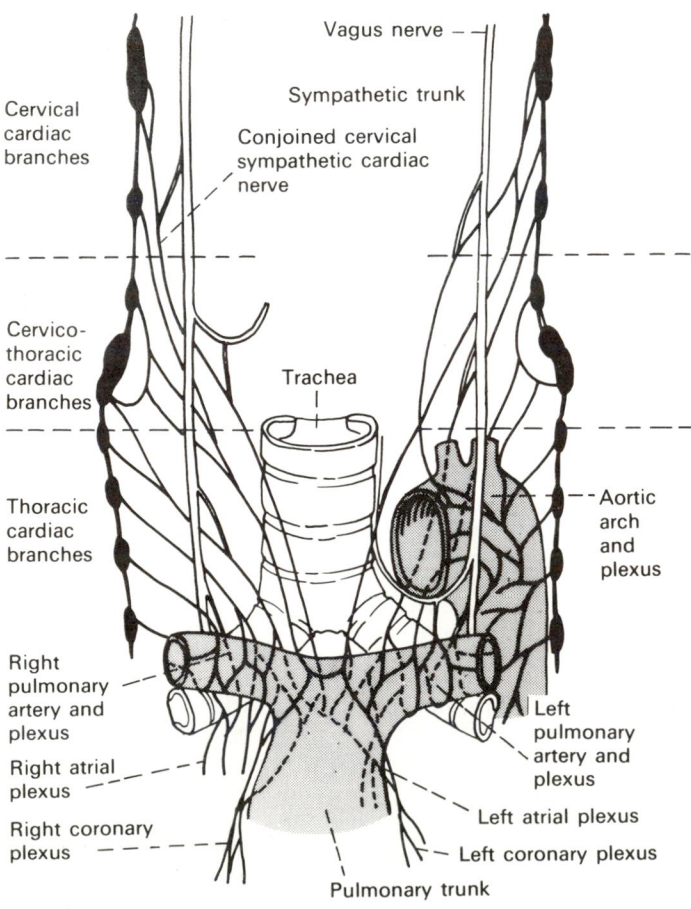

FIG. 53-13. The cardiac plexus and its subsidiary plexuses. See text for details. Modified from Mizeres, N.J.: The cardiac plexus of man. Am. J. Anat., *112*:143, 1963.

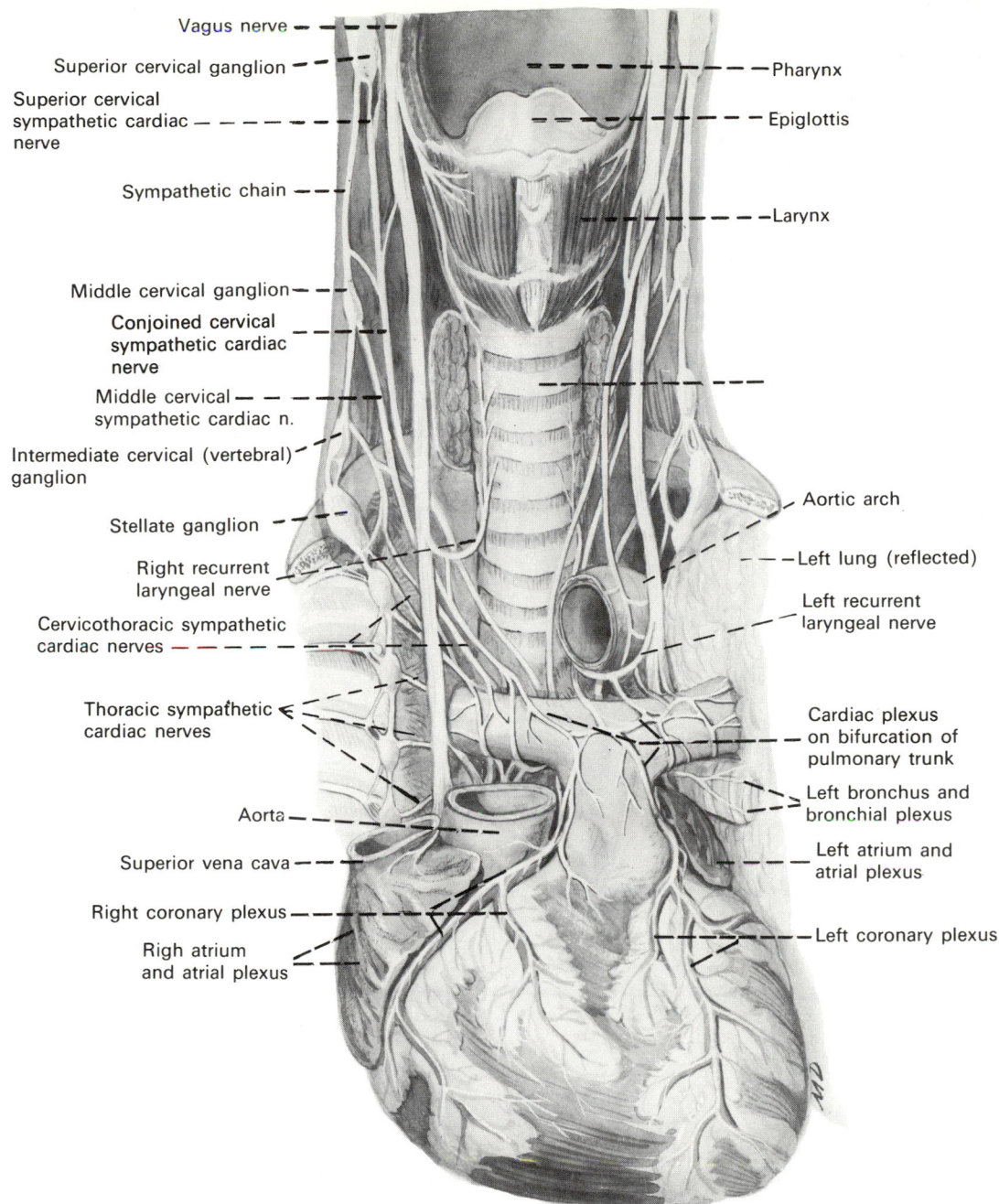

Vagus nerve

Superior cervical ganglion

Superior cervical
sympathetic cardiac
nerve

Sympathetic chain

Middle cervical ganglion

Conjoined cervical
sympathetic cardiac
nerve

Middle cervical
sympathetic cardiac n.

Intermediate cervical (vertebral)
ganglion

Stellate ganglion

Right recurrent
laryngeal nerve

Cervicothoracic sympathetic
cardiac nerves

Thoracic sympathetic
cardiac nerves

Aorta

Superior vena cava

Right coronary plexus

Righ atrium
and atrial plexus

Pharynx

Epiglottis

Larynx

Aortic arch

Left lung (reflected)

Left recurrent
laryngeal nerve

Cardiac plexus
on bifurcation of
pulmonary trunk

Left bronchus and
bronchial plexus

Left atrium and
atrial plexus

Left coronary plexus

FIG. 53-14. Anterior view of the chest depicting the anatomy of the nerves that contribute to the cardiac plexus and its subsidiary plexuses, including the coronary plexuses that follow the coronary vessels.

the pulmonary trunk, consists of the following subsidiary plexuses: the right and left pulmonary plexuses; the right and left coronary plexuses; the right and left atrial plexuses; and a plexus on the arch of the aorta. The pulmonary plexuses and the plexus on the arch of the aorta are discussed later in this chapter.

Coronary and Atrial Plexuses

The coronary plexuses are formed mainly by extensions of the right pulmonary plexus, with some contri-

bution from the left pulmonary plexus and from the plexus on the arch of the aorta. The coronary plexuses can also receive direct contributions from the cervical and thoracic cardiac branches, and usually send filaments into the anterior surfaces of the walls of both ventricles. Each coronary plexus follows its analogous artery and its branches, giving off subsidiary plexuses throughout the heart (Figs. 53-13 and 53-14).

The right atrial plexus is usually formed as an extension of the right pulmonary plexus, passing between the superior vena cava and aorta to end in the right atrium. The left atrial plexus is an extension of the left pulmonary plexus, coursing directly into the left posterior atrial wall and sending filaments into both posterior walls of the two ventricles. The plexus on the arch of the aorta sends filaments that course to the wall of the pulmonary arterial trunk, ending in both the left and right coronary plexuses. All these plexuses are interconnected.

Although sympathetic and vagal efferent and afferent fibers intermingle and lose their identities within the cardiac plexus a tendency toward subdivision into right and left halves exists, from which fibers are distributed to the heart along the two coronary arteries by the left and right coronary plexuses (5, 6). The right atrial and right coronary plexuses distribute mainly to the right atrium and ventricle, while the left plexuses are distributed to the corresponding parts of the heart on the left side.

The coronary nerves give off branches that ramify in the subepicardial tissues that overlie all the cavities of the heart. Whereas the larger branches of the nerves lie alongside the main coronary arteries, many of the smaller nerves run independently of vessels over the surface of the heart.

Several small extrinsic cardiac ganglia, in which a proportion of the vagal preganglionic fibers synapse with short postganglionic fibers, are present in the cardiac plexus. The largest is usually called the ganglion of Wrisberg, and is seldom more than 2 or 3 mm in diameter (6). Mizeres (12) found that this ganglion is not constant. The small intrinsic cardiac ganglia are located in the subepicardial tissue of the heart and, less commonly, in the myocardium.

Distribution of Nerves in the Heart

The heart is richly supplied with motor and sensory nerves containing myelinated and unmyelinated fibers derived from both sympathetic and vagus (parasympathetic) nerves. Hirsch and Borghard-Erdle (13) suggested that for purposes of orientation, the innervation of the heart can be categorized according to the distribution of the nerves to the several anatomic structures: the coronary arteries; the myocardial muscle tissue; the conducting system; and the supporting stroma, including the valves and their leaflets.

INNERVATION OF THE CORONARY ARTERIES. Coronary arteries and their branches have abundant motor and sensory nerves contributed by both sympathetic and parasympathetic nerves (5, 6). Indeed, it has been authoritatively stated that the coronary arteries in the heart have the richest nerve supply of all the arteries in the body (23). The following summary is based on the findings of Hirsch and Borghard-Erdle (13) in their studies of the human heart (except as otherwise noted). The adventitial fibrous tissue of the arteries has many large and small rounded nerve trunks containing myelinated and unmyelinated nerve fibers. These nerves accompany the arteries toward the endocardium and, at the arteriolar level, are diminutive round or flat structures. The thicker nerve trunks, which have vagal fibers, supply the adventitial and periadventitial fibrous tissue, while the thinner sympathetic nerves innervate the smooth muscle cells of the media of the coronary arteries to the level at which these contractile tissues disappear.

The coronary arterioles and precapillary blood vessels are supplied only by vagal fibers. At the precapillary level the vagal fibers have flat segments, but beyond this level they continue into or send terminal branches into the nearby myocardium, where they end either in a bulbous tip or in a brush-like terminus amidst the myocardial syncytium. These nerves have fine and slightly coarser fibrils that are in close continuity with the myocardial cells.

INNERVATION OF THE MYOCARDIUM. In addition to contributions by the coronary nerves, some large and small nerve trunks enter the myocardium directly and not in association with branches of the coronary arteries. These nerves divide dichotomously at considerable intervals in the heart muscle and some rather large ones reach the endocardium to divide further, being distributed in muscle tissue near the endocardial lining. After they have penetrated into the myocardium these nerves have scanty perineurium, and the fine nerve fibrils in them appear to extend directly into the contiguous myocardial cells. Motor end-plates resembling those of cell muscle have not been found in studies of the human heart (13).

The existence of sensory nerve endings in the heart was first suggested by Berkley (24) in 1894, and subsequently by others, who demonstrated that these sensory nerves are associated with both the vagus and sympathetic nerves to the heart (18). Early work by Wollard (23) and later by Nonidez (25), based on nerve degeneration following bilateral stellectomy, suggested that the largest proportion of cardiac sensory nerve endings are of vagal origin. Studies entailing the resection of the thoracic ganglia, however, showed that a significant proportion are associated with sympathetic nerves and are made up of myelinated and nonmyelinated afferents (26, 27).

In the heart the sensory fibers terminate as complex unencapsulated endings that are usually distinguished as either diffuse or compact (18, 25, 27, 28). The sensory nerve terminals exist in the subendocardial tissue as well as in the depth of the myocardium and around the coronary vessels. These sympathetic afferents innervate the same regions and layers of the heart as the vagal fibers. Moreover, the sympathetic afferents and endings frequently lie side by side with afferent fibers and endings of the vagus nerves (28).

INNERVATION OF THE CONDUCTING SYSTEM. Much evidence has shown that the sinoatrial node of Keith and Flack, the atrioventricular node of Tawara, and the atrioventricular bundle of His are abundantly supplied with nerve fibers and terminal networks around their constituent cells (5, 6, 13). Clusters of nerve cells are closely associated with these nerve bundles and plexuses, and belong to the intrinsic cardiac ganglia (5, 6, 13).

INNERVATION OF STROMA TISSUES. The fibrous tissues about the coronary arteries and their branches, down to the precapillary level, have a rich nerve supply that is mainly vagal. Nerve trunks extend throughout the myocardium, divide dichotomously, and split into compound terminal plexuses (13). The presence of myelinated fibers in nerves of supporting noncontractile tissues suggests that they are sensory fibers. Fibers in these nerves and their branches innervate the supporting stroma as well as form the endocardial plexus that extends into the leaflets of the valves.

Pericardium

The innervation of the pericardium varies according to its two major layers. The serous pericardium, which is composed of a single layer of mesothelial cells that covers the atria and the ventricles and extends beyond along the great vessel for 2 or 3 cm, is supplied by nerves derived from the cardiac, coronary, and epicardial plexuses containing sympathetic, parasympathetic, and afferent fibers. The serous layer that lines the inner surface of the fibrous pericardium, often called the parietal pericardium, together with the fibrous pericardium is supplied by sensory fibers derived from the phrenic nerves and the anterior parts of the thoracic intercostal nerves, and also receives sympathetic and vagal fibers through the cardiac plexus (6). Nociceptive information is transmitted by the sensory fibers principally in the phrenic nerves, by a few fibers from the intercostal nerves, and perhaps by sympathetic afferents.

Innervation of the Thoracic Aorta

The ascending aorta and arch of the aorta are supplied by both sympathetic and parasympathetic vagal fibers, many of which are afferent in nature and are distributed mainly in the adventitial plexus of the ascending aorta (4–6). Some vagal twigs enter the vessel directly, and others reach it through the cardiac plexus. The sympathetic fibers for the ascending aorta and the aortic arch arise from the stellate and upper thoracic ganglia and are often incorporated in the thoracic cardiac nerves, although occasionally separate filaments can be traced directly to the aorta (6). Aortic fibers in the thoracic cardiac sympathetic nerves pass to the cardiac and preaortic plexuses without interruption and reach the adjacent parts of the aorta in fine short branches (Fig. 53-15). The various aortic vagal and sympathetic filaments break up to form terminal plexuses in the walls of the aorta. The adventitial plexus is especially well marked around the ascending aorta, which is a special pressoreceptor area.

The small aortic arch body is a chemoreceptor structure similar to the carotid body, is usually located in the angle between the aortic arch and the ligamentum arteriosum and occasionally found at other points in the adventitia of the aortic arch. Additional small masses with similar morphologic characteristics sometimes exist in or adjacent to the adventitia of the ascending aorta or of the innominate artery.

Extensions from the aortic arch plexus continue along and supply the intrathoracic parts of the innominate, left common carotid, and left subclavian arteries.

The descending thoracic aorta is innervated by a variable number of direct filaments from the T4 and T5 sympathetic ganglia and from the superior thoracic (greater) splanchnic nerves or their rootlets of origin. Mitchell (6) pointed out that, in about 10% of individuals, on the right side and less often on the left side, a delicate para-aortic nerve is found lying along the posterolateral aspect of this part of the aorta and helps to supply it. This nerve interconnects the lowest thoracic cardiac nerve and the lower aortic and esophageal branches, and rarely extends above the level of the T4 or T5 vertebra.

Afferent fibers associated with both the vagus and sympathetic nerves supply the ascending aorta and arch of the aorta. White (11), White and associates (10, 17), Bonica (16), and others (29) suggested that the afferents that transmit nociceptive impulses from the ascending aorta and aortic arch, as well as from the descending aorta, pass through the neuraxis via sympathetic pathways. They produced symptomatic relief of the severe pain of aortic aneurysm by injecting the

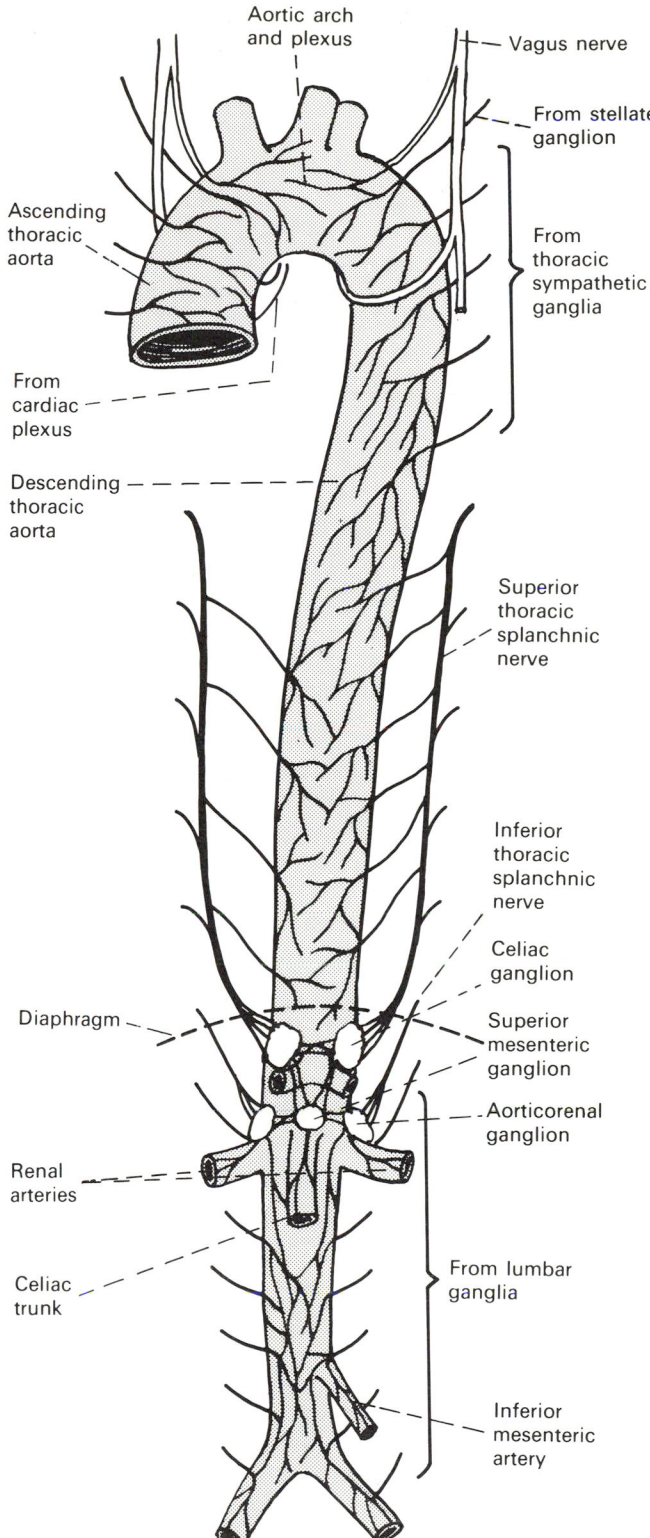

FIG. 53-15. Innervation of the thoracic aorta. See text for details.

upper thoracic sympathetic ganglia with a local anesthetic. Bonica (16) followed the diagnostic and prognostic injections with block of the sympathetic chain by alcohol. Injection of the ganglia on the right side is indicated for pain caused by aneurysm of the ascending aorta, but, if the arch or descending aorta is involved, the ganglia must be blocked on the left side or bilaterally to provide relief (16, 17, 29) (Chapter 94).

Reichert (personal communication, 1952) relieved severe pain from an aneurysm involving the lower part of the thoracic aorta by injecting the T2 to T6 ganglia with a local anesthetic. In one of White's patients, severe pain produced by a large aortic arch aneurysm that expanded upward into the thoracic inlet was referred to wide areas supplied by the cervical and intercostal nerves, suggesting it might be caused by pressure on neighboring structures, yet it was completely relieved by alcohol injection of the upper thoracic sympathetic ganglia (17).

The branches of the descending thoracic aorta, the most important of which are the bronchial, pericardial, mediastinal, esophageal, phrenic, posterior intercostal, and subcostal, all receive prolongations from a periarterial nerve plexus around the thoracic aorta. The bronchial arteries receive reinforcing filaments within the lungs. The esophageal arterial plexus is supplemented by twigs from the esophageal plexus, and branches of the phrenic nerves have been noted close to the pericardial and phrenic arteries, helping to innervate them. The posterior intercostal and subcostal arterial plexuses are also joined by small bundles of fibers from the adjacent intercostal and subcostal nerves, which contain a relatively high complement of sympathetic fibers, and from the thoracic splanchnic nerves at the points where the vessels pass behind them (5, 6).

Innervation of the Lungs

The lungs, including the trachea and bronchi, are innervated by both sympathetic and parasympathetic nerves, which contain efferent and afferent fibers. The nerves to the lungs reach the pulmonary vessels and lung tissue through the pulmonary plexuses. These are apart from filaments supplying the extrapulmonary parts of the bronchial arteries, which as noted above are extensions from the parent periaortic plexus surrounding the descending thoracic aorta.

Pulmonary Plexuses

The pulmonary plexuses are composed of larger vagal and smaller sympathetic contributions. The sympathetic pulmonary nerves are the axons of postganglionic sympathetic fibers that have already synapsed in sympathetic ganglia with preganglionic fibers. The cell bodies of the latter are located in the intermediolateral column of the spinal cord at the level of the T2 to T6 or T7 segments. The synapse with postganglionic fibers takes place in the T2 to T6 or T7 thoracic ganglia and occasionally in the stellate ganglion. The postganglionic fibers pass anteriorly and inferiorly and often merge with the thoracic cardiac, aortic, and esophageal branches and separate from them as they approach their destination. The sympathetic nerves, which also contain afferent nerves, run primarily to the posterior pulmonary plexus but also travel to the anterior pulmonary plexus (Fig. 53-16A). They unite with the corresponding branches of the vagus and are distributed along with them to the vessels, bronchi, and glands in the lungs.

The vagal pulmonary nerves contain both preganglionic and afferent fibers, the former originating in dorsal vagal nuclei and the latter having their cell bodies in the inferior vagal (nodose) ganglia. Just above the root of the lung each vagus nerve divides into smaller anterior and larger posterior parts, which embrace the lung root (Fig. 53-16B and C). Most of the pulmonary branches of the vagus derive from the larger part of the nerve lying behind the root of the lung but three or four branches are also given off before the main nerve splits, and smaller twigs are supplied by the smaller part of the nerve that passes anterior to the lung (4–6). The various branches form smaller anterior and larger posterior pulmonary plexuses. The nerves do *not* subdivide and reunite frequently, as shown in most illustrations, but rather they spring from the parent nerves almost perpendicularly and run straight outward anterior and posterior to the roots of each lung (6). They do divide as they enter the lung, however, and become dispersed around the vascular and bronchial structures. The posterior pulmonary branches are much more conspicuous than the anterior branches and receive direct or indirect contributions from the upper thoracic sympathetic ganglia.

The pulmonary plexuses always communicate with the cardiac, aortic, and esophageal plexuses, and the left anterior pulmonary plexus is often interconnected by delicate strands with the left phrenic nerve. The pulmonary plexuses proceed distally and, immediately after entering the lungs, the nerve filaments become partly segregated into groups that accompany the main bronchi and vessels and bronchial arteries. No plexus formation is noted around these structures, with the nerve bundles merely winding around them and giving off branches at irregular intervals. A plexus formation is well in evidence, though, by the level of the third-order bronchi and their accompanying vessels (6). Segregation between the perivascular and peribronchial nerves and plexuses is not at all complete; they are frequently interconnected by small bundles of fibers.

The supply to the various vessels within the lungs varies in richness: the small bronchial arteries have the best supply; the pulmonary arteries are less richly innervated; and the pulmonary veins have a poor supply limited to their extrapulmonary parts and large intrapulmonary branches (6). The larger bundles of pulmonary arterial nerve fibers are located on the side of the vessels facing the bronchi and can be traced to the extremities of these vessels, with some extending beyond them to the visceral pleura (6). The filaments passing through the bronchial arteries come from the adjacent extrachondral parts of the bronchial nerve plexus. Although some investigators have described rich nerve plexuses around the walls of the capillaries in the lung parenchyma (30), others could not confirm these findings (31).

Both myelinated and unmyelinated fibers have been found in the pulmonary nerves and plexuses. Some of these fibers have sensory receptors in the pulmonary blood vessels and are involved in reflex control of the pulmonary circulation, which apparently has vasoconstrictor and vasodilator fibers supplied by the sympathetic and parasympathetic efferent nerves, respectively.

The lung also has two types of receptors that probably have nociceptive function—the type J receptors with C afferents, and the "lung irritant receptors" with afferents in the A-delta range all running in the

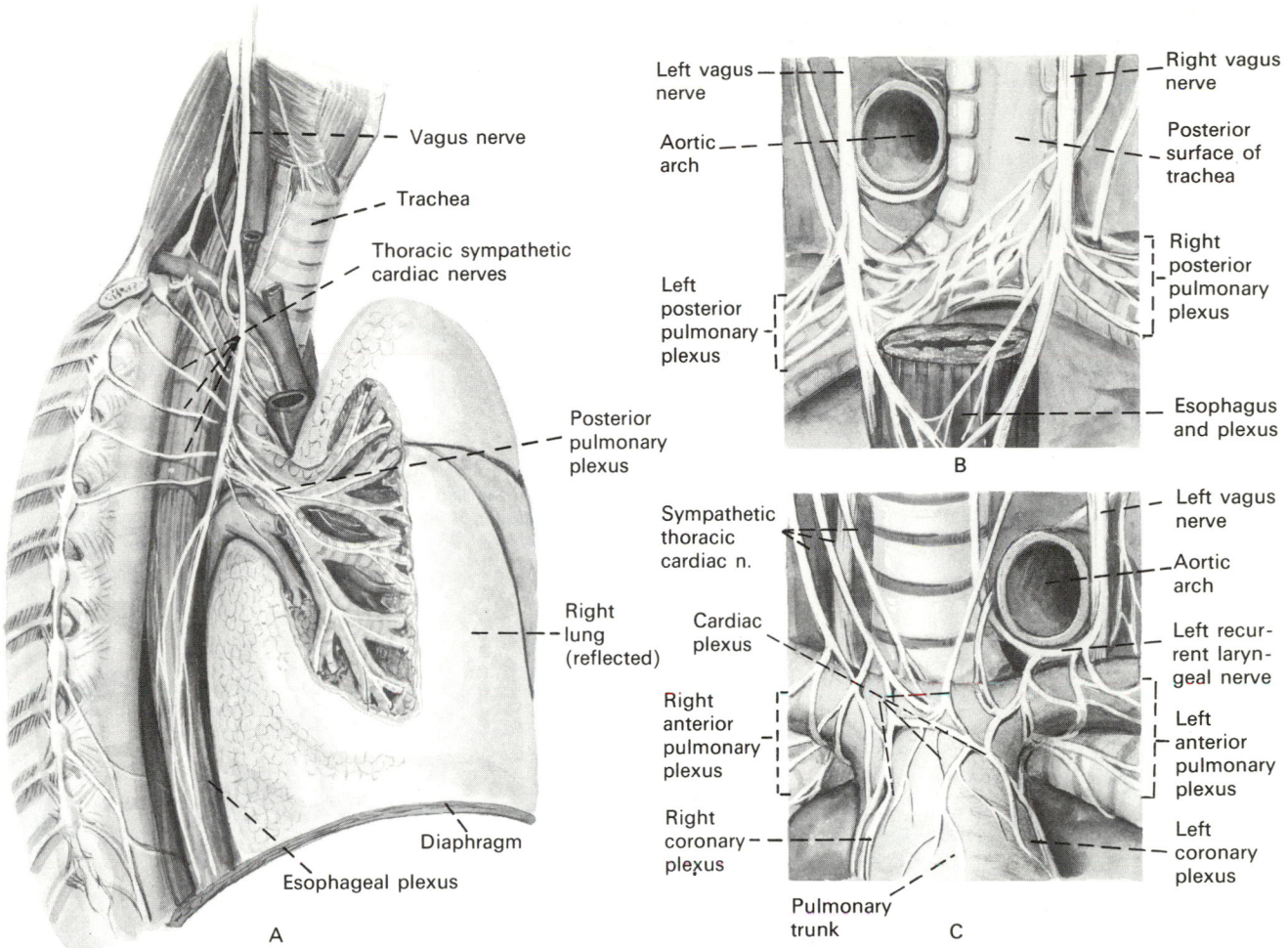

Fig. 53-16. Anatomy of the pulmonary plexuses and their distribution. **A.** Right parasagittal view showing origin, course, and termination of the nerves that contribute to the right pulmonary plexus. **B.** Posterior view. **C.** Anterior view of the trachea and two primary bronchi to show relation of the pulmonary plexus to these structures.

vagus nerves (32). The type J receptors are located in the interstitial space close to the capillaries whereas the lung irritant receptors are found in the epithelial lining of the lung and its airways. These are activated by various stimuli that produce mechanical distortion within the lung, such as pulmonary congestion, microembolism, atelectasis, pneumothorax, and chemical irritants. It is likely that this pain, caused by mechanical or chemical damage of the lung, is mediated by these A-delta and C fibers (32).

Larynx, Trachea, and Main Bronchi

Larynx

The nerves to the larynx are derived from the vagus nerve by way of the internal and external branches of the superior laryngeal nerve and by the recurrent laryngeal nerves. The internal laryngeal branch, which is sensory, enters the larynx by piercing the posterior part of the thyrohyoid membrane above the superior laryngeal vessels and divides into three branches. One is distributed to both surfaces of the epiglottis, a second to the aryepiglottic fold, and a third,

the largest, supplies the mucous membrane over the back of the larynx and communicates with a recurrent laryngeal nerve. The external laryngeal branch supplies the cricothyroid muscle. The recurrent nerve passes cephalad beneath the caudal border of the constrictor pharyngis inferior muscle immediately dorsal to the cricothyroid joint. It supplies all the muscles of the larynx except the cricothyroid. The sensory branches of the laryngeal nerves form subepithelial plexuses from which fibers end between cells that cover the mucous membrane. Fibers from the sympathetic nerves supply the blood vessels and glands of the larynx.

Trachea and Main Bronchi

The trachea and main bronchi are supplied by filaments from the vagus and the recurrent laryngeal nerves and by fibers from the sympathetic trunk. These filaments are distributed to the trachealis muscles and between the epithelial cells. As mentioned in Chapter 6, the sympathetic postganglionic nerve fibers produce relaxation of the trachealis muscles and increase the size of the trachea and bronchi, whereas the

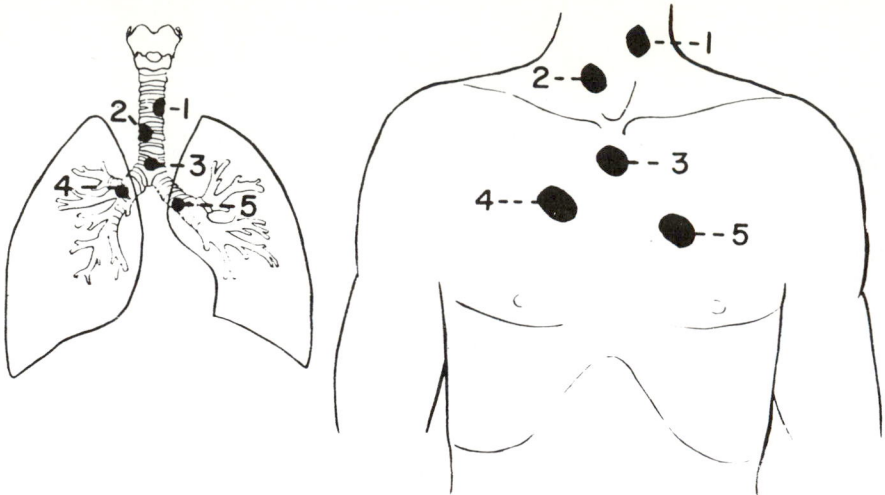

FIG. 53-17. Pain referred to the anterior chest wall from faradic stimulation of the mucous membrane of the tracheobronchial tree. The areas of pain are ipsilateral to the sites of stimulation. Modified from Morton, D.R., Klassen, K.P., Curtis C.M.: Clinical Physiology of Human Bronchi. I. Pain of tracheobronchial origin. Surgery, 28:669, 1950.

parasympathetic nerves have a bronchoconstrictor effect. Morton and colleagues (33) demonstrated that the sensory nerves that transmit nociceptive impulses are afferents of the vagus nerves and their branches. They carried out experiments in human volunteers in which electric stimulation of the tracheobronchial tree through a bronchoscope produced pain that was referred to the anterior chest or lower part of the neck (Fig. 53-17). They noted that points of the area of references were ipsilateral to the site of stimulation. Moreover, they demonstrated in patients with carcinoma that section of the vagus below the recurrent laryngeal nerve but above the pulmonary plexus abolished the pain on the side of vagotomy (34). In a few cases, following section of the one vagus nerve, pain of tracheobronchial origin was referred to the contralateral side, probably because of interconnection between nerves of each side.

Similar findings were reported by Teodori and Galletti (35). They noted that electrical stimulation of the normal mucosa produces little pain, but stimulation in patients with inflammation of the mucosa of the tracheobronchial tree produced pain in the anterior chest wall, even when the stimulus was applied to the posterior wall of the trachea and bronchi. When the stimulation was applied to the carina or at the beginning of the primary bronchi, painful sensation was localized in the parasternal region occupying the area between the 1st and the 5th intercostal spaces, whereas when the stimulation was applied more distally the pain extended as far as the 6th intercostal space. They also noted a decrease in electrical skin resistance limited to the T2 to T5 segments. In subjects with inflammation of the tracheobronchial mucosa, the stimulation was followed hours later by cutaneous hyperalgesia.

Pleura

The visceral pleura is supplied by sympathetic fibers that have a vasomotor function. It has afferent fibers, but these have no nociceptive function because the visceral pleura is insensitive to noxious stimuli and

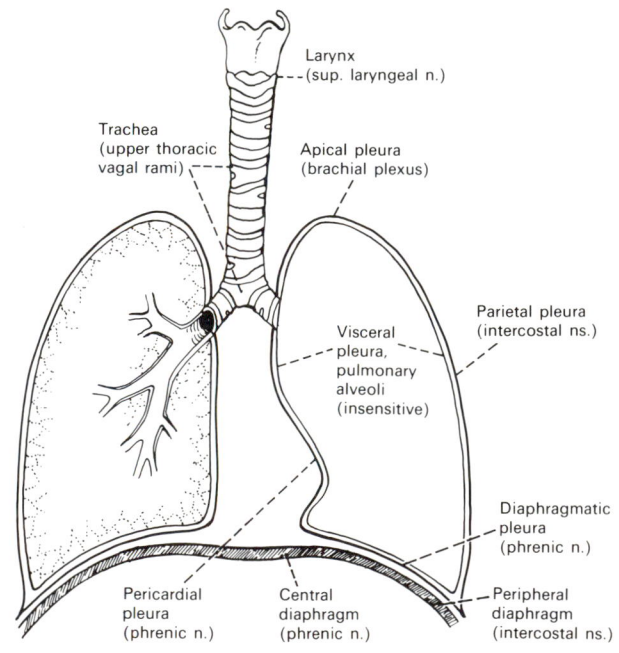

FIG. 53-18. Schematic of the sensory nerve supply to the tracheobronchial tree, parietal pleura, upper surface of the diaphragm, and the diaphragmatic pleura. From White, J.C.: Sensory innervation of the viscera: Studies on visceral afferent neurons in man based on neurosurgical procedures for the relief of intractable pain. In Pain. Edited by H.G. Wolff, H.S. Gasser, and J.C. Hinsey. Baltimore, Williams & Wilkins, 1943, pp. 373–390.

pain does not arise from disorders of the visceral pleura (36, 37). The visceral pleura also receives parasympathetic fibers through the pulmonary plexuses (32, 33).

The parietal pleura is supplied by the intercostal nerves on its lateral aspects, by the T1 spinal nerve on its apex, and by the phrenic nerves on the diaphragmatic surface (Fig. 53-18). In addition, the parietal pleura receives parasympathetic and sympathetic nerves through the pulmonary plexuses, and these nerves accompany the ramification of the bronchial arteries.

C. HISTORY AND EXAMINATION

A general consideration of the approach to diagnosing the specific cause(s) of pain in the chest is presented here. It is intended as a supplement to Chapter 31, which contains a detailed discussion of the evaluation of patients with pain. Comments made here are relevant to pain in the chest. Chapters 54 through 56 provide a more detailed discussion of diagnostic procedures for patients with pain of cardiac and aortic origin, pain of pulmonary origin, and pain of esophageal origin. This section and Table 53-1 are intended to help determine diagnostic possibilities, followed by a more detailed assessment of the probable cause(s) of pain in the chest.

In many instances the diagnosis of chest pain becomes relatively simple after the patient relates the story of the pain. Occasionally the cause is difficult to determine because so many lesions can cause similar pain. This is not surprising when one considers that the afferent nerves of the heart, aorta, esophagus, lungs, and upper chest wall have a common pathway in the spinal cord, and that visceral pain has somewhat similar qualities regardless of the organ affected (16, 38). The clinical application of this knowledge indicates that neither the location, quality, or area of reference of chest pain arising from these organs can denote the origin or nature of the underlying disorder with certainty. This information can only be obtained from a thorough history of the pain, particularly of the factors or circumstances that reproduce, aggravate, or relieve the pain, and from the history and character of the associated signs and symptoms.

Of course, the approach to the diagnosis of chest pain varies according to the circumstances in which patients are seen. Patients who present in acute distress require a vigorous investigation performed with dispatch, slanted initially either to establish or exclude life-threatening disease of the cardiorespiratory systems, such as myocardial infarction, large pulmonary embolism, and dissecting aneurysm of the aorta (38). The approach in such acute situations should be brisk; common sense dictates that in some circumstances (e.g., patients are in a state of collapse) immediate supportive treatment, such as clearing of the airway, adequate oxygenation, and maintenance of cardiac action and blood pressure, takes precedence over the formulation of an exact diagnosis.

With most patients who are seen in the physician's office or who present themselves at the emergency room, time can be taken to obtain an abbreviated history and physical examination and to perform a few tests, such as electrocardiography and chest radiography, before transferring patients to an intensive care unit. Patients with obvious acute myocardial infaction should be sent to a coronary care unit without delay, accompanied by someone who can perform cardiopulmonary resuscitation.

By contrast, with patients who come to the physician for consultation after having experienced chest pain that has dissipated, or who are in between episodes of recent pain, it is not necessary to hurry. The physician should take the time to carry out a detailed history and comprehensive physical examination supplemented by appropriate radiographic, electrocardiographic, and other laboratory tests and therapeutic trials. In such cases diagnosis can be made at the first visit or thereafter, when additional tests and trials have been done.

In assessing patients with chest pain, the following characteristics of the pain should be elicited through a detailed and meticulous history: speed of onset of the pain, the site, radiation, quality, and intensity of the pain, the temporal characteristics—that is, is the pain continuous or episodic and, if intermittent, what is the duration of each episode or attack? What time of day is it worse, and when is it better? What is the time-intensity curve and what is its relationship to meals and position of the body? Patients should be specifically asked to indicate the precise effect on pain of physical exertion, mental stress, breathing, coughing, straining, swallowing, defecation, urination, motion of the trunk, and motion of the neck (forward flexion, lateral flexion, extension, rotation). What effect does motion of the upper extremities, such as swinging of the arms, or lifting, have on the pain? How does walking influence the pain?

Perhaps the most important information to elicit is determination of those activities or factors that aggravate the pain, relieve the pain, and have no influence on the pain (16, 38). Thus, a history of sharp aggravation by breathing, coughing, or other respiratory movements usually indicates disorders of the pleura, pericardium, mediastinum, or chest wall. Similarly, the pain that regularly appears with rapid walking and vanishes in a few minutes on standing suggests a diagnosis of angina pectoris, although orthopedic disorders can also cause such chest pain.

Also important is obtaining a history of any *associated phenomena* such as the following: palpitation, dyspnea, coughing, expectoration, or hemoptysis, suggestive of lung disease; nausea, vomiting, distension, or abdominal tenderness, suggestive of gastrointestinal disease; dysphagia or odynophagia (pain on swallowing), suggestive of esophageal disorders. Following elucidation of the characteristics of the pain, the past medical and family histories and demographic data, a physical examination is carried out. Table 53-1 suggests the most important parts of such an examination.

The following points can help the clinician to determine the probable cause of pain and to make a tentative diagnosis. Bonica (16) and Levene and associates (38) have suggested that it is most practical to consider chest pain in several categories: (a) central chest pain caused by disease of viscera within the chest; (b) lateral pleuritic, musculoskeletal, or neurologic chest pain; (c) chest pain referred from disorders of structures outside the chest; and (d) chest pain primarily of psychologic origin.

Visceral (Central) Chest Pain

Structures producing central chest pain include the esophagus, the myocardium, the trachea and bronchi, the pericardium, the pulmonary arteries, and the aorta, in approximately that order of frequency (38). The following points in the history help to determine the causative factor.

TABLE 53-1. General Physical Examination for Chest Pain*

I. EXAMINATION OF THE CHEST
A. Observation
1. Posture—relation of shoulders, scapulae, clavicles, and costal margins
2. Shape and contour—normal, flattened, asymmetry, depression, prominences, pulsating tumors, other structural changes (specify)
3. Expansion—normal (inches), asymmetry
4. Skin—color, petechiae, prominent veins
5. Breasts—normal, tenderness, tumor

B. Palpation and percussion
1. Sternum—normal, pain and tenderness, local, referred, evidence of fracture
2. Cartilages—normal, pain and tenderness, prominences, depression, slip or dislocation
3. Ribs—normal, pain and tenderness, evidence of tumor, displacement, angulation, fracture
4. Spine—normal curves, kyphosis, scoliosis, flattening, prominences, gibbous
   a. Percussion—pain, tenderness, local, referred, paravertebral tenderness, site of pain radiation
5. Muscles—palpation for tenderness, trigger points

C. Neurologic examination
1. Sensations—pin scratch, pinprick, pinch; normal, hyperalgesia, allodynia, hyperpathia; local or segmental?
2. Muscle function—abduction, medial and lateral rotation of arms; anterior and lateral flexion and extension of neck; anterior and lateral flexion, extension, and rotation of spine

D. Examination of heart and lungs (respiratory rate and amplitude; pain on deep breathing, coughing)
1. Lungs
   a. Palpation—normal, fremitus, abnormal (specify)
   b. Percussion—normal, abnormal
   c. Auscultation—normal, abnormal (specify), friction sounds
2. Heart
   a. Point of maximum impulse (PMI) location, rate, rhythm, thrills, palpable friction rub, size
   b. Sounds—normal, abnormal (specify), friction

E. Examination of the diaphragm excursion—normal, abnormal; flutter; Litten's sign

F. Summary of findings

II. EXAMINATION OF THE ABDOMEN†
A. Observation
1. Shape and size—normal, pendulous, other
2. Skin—color, petechiae, dilated veins, striae, hernia (site), visible tumors
3. Diaphragmatic movements—normal, limited, singultus
4. Motion—forward bending, lateral flexion right and left, extension

B. Palpation
1. General palpation—normal, distension, ascites, fluid wave, bowel sounds
   a. Deep tenderness—local, diffuse
   b. Muscle spasm—local, diffuse, rigidity
2. Palpation of right hypochondrium
   a. Liver—normal, large, pain, tenderness, tumors
   b. Gallbladder—palpable, pain, tenderness
3. Palpation of left hypochondrium
   a. Spleen—normal, large, pain, tenderness
   b. Large bowel—normal, tumor?
4. Palpation of epigastrium—pain and tenderness (local, referred), tumor, palpating mass
5. Right and left flanks—pain, tenderness, kidney palpable, tumor, muscle spasm

C. Neurologic examination
1. Pinprick, pinscratch, pinch—normal, hyperesthesia, allodynia? segmental or local
2. Muscle function—muscle strength of abdominal wall
3. Abdominal reflexes—normal, hyperactive, decreased, absent

D. Summary of findings

*See Chapter 31 for a detailed description.
†Examination of the abdomen should always be carried out in any patient presenting with pain in the chest because the pain might be referred from an abdominal visceral disease.

History

SPEED OF ONSET. The sudden and severe onset of pain suggests dissecting aneurysm, ruptured esophagus, or pulmonary embolism. A less abrupt onset occurs with acute myocardial infarction, reflux esophagitis, and pneumothorax.

LOCATION AND RADIATION. Retrosternal chest pain with radiation to the jaw and arms suggests myocardial ischemia. Radiation of the pain to the back should suggest esophagitis, esophageal spasm or rupture, pancreatitis, or dissecting aortic aneurysm.

DURATION. Stable angina pectoris is characterized by short-lived pain, while the pain of unstable angina or myocardial infarction lasts longer, frequently much longer. Pain coming from other organs also lasts for minutes and hours.

AGGRAVATING FACTORS. Pain brought on by general body exertion, by emotional stress, or anger is considered to be caused by myocardial ischemia until proven otherwise. Exertion is a nonspecific stimulus, however, that can produce effects other than those on the cardiovascular system. For example, pain occurring with unaccustomed snow shoveling might be anginal but could also be caused by strain on the pectoral muscle or sternoclavicular joint. Pain after meals can either be esophageal or myocardial in origin, while pain after vomiting implicates the esophagus.

EFFECTS OF POSTURE. Pain that worsens on bending over, lying down, or stooping should suggest gastroesophageal reflux, pericarditis, or pancreatitis. Pain worsened by standing suggests a pneumothorax or emphysema. Pain made worse by deep breathing, coughing, sneezing, or laughing and relieved by quiet breathing suggests pleuritis (pneumonia, infarction, infectious process), or it can suggest fracture of the ribs, cartilages, sternum, or vertebra, or muscle strain.

PAIN-RELIEVING FACTORS. Pain relieved by antacids indicates an upper gastrointestinal pathophysiologic process. Nitroglycerin relieves the pain of stable angina completely, partially relieves the pain of unstable angina or esophageal spasm, but does not relieve the pain of myocardial infarction.

PRECEDING SYMPTOMS OF DISEASE. Preceding or concomitant symptoms should direct attention to various organs—heartburn to the esophagus, angina to the heart, alcohol abuse to the pancreas (38). Dyspnea should suggest left heart failure from myocardial infarction or right heart failure from massive pulmonary embolism. Recent postoperative immobilization or the use of contraceptive drugs should raise the suspicion of pulmonary embolism (38).

Physical Examination

Central chest pain associated with shock should suggest the following, in approximate order of frequency: acute myocardial infarction, massive pulmonary embolism, pericarditis or tamponade, dissecting aortic aneurysm, and acute pancreatitis (38).

Jugular venous distension implicates the cardiovascular system (myocardial infarction, pericardial tamponade, pulmonary embolism). Kussmaul's sign (distention of the jugular veins on inspiration) is seen in tamponade caused by pericarditis or mediastinal tumor.

Significant pulsus paradoxus (marked decrease in the pulse volume during inspiration) should immediately raise suspicion of pericardial tamponade unless airway obstruction is present.

Asymmetric pulses in a patient with central chest pain suggest dissecting aneurysm as the first consideration (38). Cardiac arrythmias and gallop rhythms are commonly seen in acute myocardial infarction. Moreover, the murmur of mitral regurgitation is heard in myocardial infarction, whereas the initial appearance of the murmur of aortic regurgitation is a clue to the presence of a dissecting aortic aneurysm.

Systemic hypertension is seen in both acute myocardial infarction and dissecting aneuryms, while subcutaneous emphysema indicates a ruptured viscus.

A pericardial friction rub occurring simultaneously with the onset of pain suggests a dissecting aortic aneurysm or acute pericarditis, whereas that beginning more than 24 hours after onset of pain suggests acute myocardial infarction.

Lateral Pleuritic, Orthopedic, and Neurologic Chest Pains

The most common structures that cause pain in the lateral chest wall are disorders of the chest wall, pleura, or thoracic spine.

History

Abrupt onset of lateral chest pain suggests a torn muscle, rib fracture, pulmonary embolism, or pneumothorax, in approximately that order (34). Aggravation of the pain by movement of the thorax during deep breathing or relief by immobilization suggests a rib fracture or torn muscle.

Purulent sputum accompanying the pain suggests bronchopulmonary infection, and bloody sputum suggests pulmonary embolism. Immobilization after recent operation and use of birth control pills can precede pulmonary embolism, whereas preceding symptoms of coryza or malaise suggest infection.

Segmental pain with vesicles suggests the onset of acute herpes zoster. Pain localized to the sternal region is usually caused by fracture of the sternum, chondritis, muscle strain, myofascial pain syndromes, mediastinal tumor, referred pain of herniated cervical disk, foreign body or carcinoma of the tracheobronchial tree, or diseases of the esophagus (retroesophageal esophagitis, carcinoma, ulcer). Less common causes are necrosis of the sternum, multiple myeloma, mediastinal tumors, mediastinitis, or mediastinal abscess.

Localized pain in the side of the chest is usually caused by muscle strain, myofascial syndromes, fractured ribs (trauma, carcinoma, osteoporosis), pleuritis, pneumonia, infarction, carcinoma, deep axillary abscess, diaphragmatic pleurisy, subphrenic abscess, and empyema. Less common causes include uncommon lesions of the ribs such as actinomycosis, myeloma, and periostitis, neurofibromata, epidemic pleurodynia, distension of the colon (left side), cholecystitis (right side), disseminated lupus erythematosus, and neurosis.

Pain localized in the back of the chest is usually caused by postural deformities, postural osteoarthritis, facet syndrome, and other disorders of the vertebral column, osteoporosis of the vertebrae or ribs, fracture of the vertebrae or ribs, displaced ribs, myofascial syndromes (particularly levator scapulae, latissimus dorsi, multifidi, rhomboids, and iliocostalis thoracis), fracture of the scapula, tuberculosis of the spine (Pott's disease), tumors of the vertebrae or posterior portion of the ribs, congenital disorders of the spine or thorax, osteomyelitis of the vertebrae, infectious arthritis, Kümmel's disease (traumatic spondylitis), osteitis deformans (Paget's disease), infectious vertebral epiphysitis (Scheuermann's disease), and herniated thoracic disk.

Physical Examination

Acute tenderness to palpation of the painful site strongly suggests that the lesion is in the chest wall, the site of tenderness indicating the diagnosis. Lumps suggest fractures, rib tumors, or inflamed costochondral or chondrosternal joints. In patients with rib fractures, mild compression of the ribs both in the lateral and anteroposterior planes produces intense pain.

Palpation of the muscles of the chest wall can reveal the presence of trigger areas indicative of myofascial pain syndromes. Tensing and stretching of each of the various muscles of the chest wall will cause pain if there has been an acute muscle strain or tear.

Palpation of the trachea can reveal deviation (to the opposite side) in pneumothorax. Percussion at the site of pain can produce acute tenderness if one or more underlying ribs are fractured. Dullness on percussion suggest consolidation of the lung or fluid in the pleural space. Hyper-resonance suggests pneumothorax.

Auscultation can reveal clicking of the ribs or the grating of rib fractures. A pleural rub suggests irritation caused by infection or embolism, whereas rales at the site of pain suggest underlying lung disease.

Pain from nerves and nerve roots is almost always lateralized and has a segmental pattern. The most common cause is herpes zoster, although spinal arthritis and disorders of the neuraxis can also cause segmental pain (neuralgia).

Chest Pain Referred from Extrathoracic Disorders

Pathology in Cervical Spine

Unilateral sharp or deep aching pain in the pectoral region associated with pain in the neck and upper limb is frequently caused by compression of lower cervical nerve roots by posterolateral herniation of a disk, by osteophyte fracture, or other pathologic process. Lesion of C8 on the left side produces angina-like pain in the left chest and medial arm, but the pain is unaffected by effort if the arm and neck are not moved. Pain is aggravated by ipsilateral neck flexion, head compression, cough, sneezing, and straining; it is relieved by head traction associated with sensory and reflex changes in the limb.

Pain in the upper anterior chest can be also caused by thoracic inlet syndromes, but pain that is most severe in the shoulder and limb, unaffected by effort but aggravated by extreme abduction of the arm is often associated with signs of vascular compression.

Pancoast's syndrome often causes pain in the scapular region and anterior chest, but the pain is most severe in the shoulder and in the medial aspect of the limb. The pain is associated with paresthesia, dysesthesia, hypesthesia, and weakness of the muscle supplied by the ulnar nerve. Fullness and tenderness may be noted in the medial supraclavicular and paravertebral regions.

Abdominal Disease

Gas entrapment syndrome produces abdominal pain with radiation to the lower chest. Gastric distension produces pain in the entire epigastrium and anterior and left lateral chest up to the xiphoid or the lower sternal region. Gas entrapment in the hepatic flexure produces pain in the right upper quadrant of the abdomen and right lateral anterior chest. Gas in the splenic flexure produces pain in the left upper abdominal quadrant and left anterior and lateral chest. Signs include abdominal distension, abdominal tympany, and positive radiographic evidence in the standing position.

Biliary colic produces pain in the epigastric or right subcostal regions, but the pain frequently extends to the back at the inferior angle of the scapula and sometimes into the low central anterior chest. Mild subcostal tenderness can be noted.

Biliary tract disease can provoke angina pectoris in patients with pre-existing coronary disease associated with T-wave changes. Cholecystitis is associated with nausea, vomiting, fever, jaundice, and a tender mass in the right upper quadrant of the abdomen.

Gastric ulcer located in the cardia (this is an uncommon site) is a frequent cause of laterally radiating pain in the central anterior and lower part of the chest. Gastric ulcer at other sites is not associated with chest pain. Duodenal ulcer can produce pain that radiates to the xiphoid, but chest pain is rare.

Some patients with acute pancreatitis complain only of chest pain that simulates the pain of myocardial infarction and often is associated with transient ECG abnormalities. The pain often radiates to the back; it is relieved by forward bending. It may be associated with diaphragmatic irritation resulting in pleuritic chest pain.

Distension or inflammation of the liver or spleen produces pleuritic pain in the chest and often in the shoulder. The pain is aggravated by breathing but is unaffected by effort. Subphrenic abscess produces inflammation of the diaphragm with consequent pleuritic pain on the side of the chest and/or shoulder. Usually there is sign of infection.

Chest Pain Primarily of Psychologic Origin

Anxiety, depression, hypochondriasis, and other psychologic factors can produce chest pain that is atypical in location, quality, and duration. Pain is usually in the left precordial or cardiac apical region. Chest pain does not always keep the patient from sleep, but it is present on awakening. Acute anxiety is usually associated with dyspnea, hyperventilation, palpitation, dizziness, perspiration, weakness, increased muscle tension, and diffuse chest tightness.

Chronic anxiety produces cardiac neurosis ("soldier's heart"), or neurocirculatory asthenia. The pain is usually dull and is felt at the cardiac apex; it can be associated with attacks of sharp pain. The pain varies in severity and location and is often related to physical activity. Patients complain of weakness, low energy level, dyspnea, and palpitation.

Pain can be caused by endogenous depression associated with signs of depressive illness, anorexia, weight loss, fatigue, low energy level, malaise, and insomnia.

A positive diagnosis of pain of psychologic origin is made by exclusion of disease of the heart and lungs and positive evidence acquired through psychologic tests.

Summary

Pain in the chest can be caused by various factors (see Table 53-2) and it is therefore most important for the physician to distinguish disorders that are not life-threatening from those that are serious. An incorrect diagnosis of a hazardous condition such as angina pectoris is likely to have harmful psychologic and economic consequences and can lead to unnecessary complex procedures such as coronary arteriography. Failure to recognise a serious disorder such as coronary artery disease or mediastinal tumor could result in a dangerous delay of much needed treatment. The situation must therefore be carefully assessed. (The most important points in examining a patient with chest pain are listed in Table 53-1.)

TABLE 53-2. Pain in the Chest: Summary of Differential Diagnosis

Etiology (Disease)	IASP Code Ref.*	Chapter No.	Important Diagnostic Features	
			Characteristics of the Pain	**Associated Symptoms and Signs**
I. PAIN CAUSED BY DISEASE OF THE HEART AND AORTA				
A. **Angina pectoris**, AP; (stable angina, SA; unstable angina, UA; variant angina, VA)	XVII-4	54	Mild, moderate, severe, or excruciating anterior chest pain felt predominantly retrosternally with radiation to parasternal region, left arm or right arm or both, epigastrium and, less frequently, to the interscapular region, neck, and lower jaw; discomfort felt as severe oppression or heaviness on the chest, a sense of constriction or band-like pressure, or a feeling of choking, strangling, or tight pressure on the neck; pain provoked by physical effort, severe emotional stress, or a large meal (except UA, which occurs at rest or with little or no provocation); lasts 2 to 5 minutes with SA, 15 to 30 minutes or longer with UA and VA; promptly relieved with nitroglycerin or discontinuation of effort	History of previous anginal attacks; can have normal ECG at rest but ST depression and other ECG changes during stress test; positive evidence with radionuclide stress testing and coronary arteriography; demonstration of coronary artery spasm in VA
B. **Acute myocardial infarction** (AMI)	XVII-5	54	Pain of same character, location, and reference as angina but of sudden onset, much more severe, and of longer duration (1 to 8 hours or more); little or no relief with nitroglycerin; intense pain often accompanied by strong alarm reaction and feeling of impending death	Frequently nausea, vomiting, and profuse sweating; many patients develop tenderness in pectoral muscle and deep muscle of interscapular region; some develop bradycardia and hypotension and others tachycardia and hypertension; ECG changes include Q-wave and ST-segment elevation and increased creatine kinase (CK) and other serum enzyme levels
C. **Aortic stenosis**	—	54	Dyspnea first symptom but angina occurs with severe aortic stenosis; chest pain occurs during physical exertion as a result of increased oxygen demand from increased myocardial mass and high ventricular systolic pressure	With severe disease exertional syncope is caused by decline in arterial pressure; left ventricular failure, palpitation, fatigue, weakness, peripheral cyanosis, narrow pulse pressure, and palpable systolic murmur; increased QRS-complex and ST- and T-wave alterations
D. **Aortic regurgitation**	—	54	Asymptomatic early in disease; dyspnea on exertion; pain late symptom of severe disease that can occur at rest as well as with exertion and persists longer than angina of coronary artery disease; some patients have neck and abdominal pain	Dyspnea on exertion, flushing, sweating, palpitation; increased fatigue progresses to orthopnea and eventually to paroxysmal nocturnal dyspnea; high-pitched crescendo dyastolic murmur along left sternal border
E. **Mitral valve prolapse**	—	54	Sharp, stabbing chest pain not provoked by exertion and unresponsive to nitroglycerin; more frequent in females	Cardiac arrhythmia produces palpitation and rarely dizziness, syncope, or even sudden death; midsystolic click and late systolic murmur
F. **Hypertrophic cardiomyopathy**	—	54	Most patients asymtomatic; symptomatic patients have dyspnea on exertion because of increased stiffness of left ventricular walls; typical angina pectoris with exertion	Atrial and ventricular arrhythmias produce palpitation, dizziness, and syncope; ECG shows QRS changes of left ventricular hypertrophy and abnormal Q wave

*See Table 2-2.

TABLE 53-2. (Cont.)

Etiology (Disease)	IASP Code Ref.*	Chapter No.	Important Diagnostic Features	
			Characteristics of the Pain	Associated Symptoms and Signs
G. Acute pericarditis	XVII-6	54	Severe, sharp chest pain; worse in supine position, partially relieved by sitting; markedly aggravated by deep breathing; pain usually retrosternal (central), radiates to the neck and trapezius ridge but not to the arms	Dyspnea occurs because of marked increase in pain with normal respiration; triphasic pericardial friction rub occurs with atrial systole, ventricular systole, and ventricular diastole, occasionally only biphasic; ECG initially shows ST-segment elevation and later T-wave flattening
H. Diseases of the thoracic aorta				
1. Dissecting aneurysm	—	54	Sudden, severe excruciating pain with maximal intensity at its onset; location of pain helps to localize dissection: ascending aortic dissection produces anterior chest pain in 65% of patients and posterior chest pain in 50%; dissection in descending thoracic aorta produces back pain in nearly all patients; radiation to the neck, throat, jaw, and abdomen in a small percentage of patients	Nausea, vomiting, diaphoresis, bradycardia and hypotension or tachycardia and hypertension; loss of one or more arterial pulses; sense of impending death, apprehension
2. Nondissecting aneurysm	XVII-7	53 96	Mild to severe continuous burning, aching pain with bouts of lancinating pain; radiation to the chest, shoulder and back caused by mechanical compression or injury of thoracic spinal nerves; erosion of bone causes boring, agonizing, intractable back pain	Dyspnea, cough, dysphagia, hoarseness; Horner's syndrome; pulsating mass; radiographic evidence
II. DISEASES OF THE RESPIRATORY SYSTEM				
A. Diseases of the tracheobronchial tree				
1. Acute tracheobronchitis (infectious; irritative; thermal injury)	—	55	Mild to moderate burning, aching pain in the retrosternal and parasternal regions; pain severe with thermal injury; associated with sore throat	Preceded by upper respiratory infection: coryza, malaise, chilliness, slight fever, back and muscle pain; with bronchitis, initially dry and nonproductive cough but later mucoid or mucopurulent; dyspnea might be present
2. Bronchiectasis	—	—	Mild to moderate aching pain in retrosternal and parasternal regions	Chronic cough and sputum production; with progression, cough becomes more productive, hemoptysis common, recurrent pneumonia frequent; wheezing, dyspnea in severe cases
B. Diseases of the pulmonary circulation				
1. Acute pulmonary hypertension	—	55	Severe crushing, gripping pain in the center of the chest simulating that of AMI, but does not radiate to arms or jaw and seldom to back	Usually decrease in arterial P_{O_2}; can have dyspnea, cyanosis, sweating
2. Chronic pulmonary hypertension (primary; secondary)	—	55	Pain in anterior chest, primarily retrosternal; radiation to neck; some patients have typical angina pectoris complicated by myocardial ischemia	Primary hypertension usually in females; dyspnea, easy fatigue, less frequently syncope; right ventricular hypertrophy can progress to failure

*See Table 2-2.

TABLE 53-2. (Cont.)

Etiology (Disease)	IASP Code Ref.*	Chapter No.	Important Diagnostic Features	
			Characteristics of the Pain	Associated Symptoms and Signs
3. Pulmonary embolism	—	55	With large embolus pain is sudden, severe, crushing, and of a visceral central type; simulates pain of myocardial infarction but does not radiate to the jaw or arms; lasts for minutes to several hours; small embolus produces localized severe pleuritic pain that is persistent and lasts a week or longer; aggravated by deep breathing or coughing	Feeling of impending death (angor animi), pressure on throat, desire to defecate; history of thrombi in leg, pelvis, occasionally in upper extremity; rarely, embiotic fluid or fat emboli; initially the large embolus usually produces pulmonary hypertension from increased pulmonary vascular resistance, leading to decreased cardic output, hypotension that can progress to shock, with sweating, tachypnea, dyspnea, arterial hypoxemia; hemoptysis, pleural friction rub with small embolus; radiography reveals wedge-shaped shadow
C. Diseases of the lungs				
1. Pneumonia	—	55	With lobar pneumonia patient develops pleuritis with moderate to severe pain in lateral chest or shoulder aggravated by deep breathing and coughing, (because of involvement of central diaphragmatic pleura); little or no pain with bronchopneumonia	Systemic symptoms and signs of infection: fever, cough, occasionally nausea, vomiting, malaise, and muscle pain; blood-streaked sputum, occasionally hemoptysis; rhonchi; percussion reveals dullness; radiographic evidence
2. Lung abscess	—	55	Typical pleuritic chest pain if abscess produces pleuritis; characteristics similar to those of lobar pneumonia (see above)	Malaise, anorexia, sputum-producing cough, sweats, severe prostration, and fever; putrid odor (anaerobic infection); fine moist rales
3. Atelectasis	—	—	Rapid occlusion with massive lung collapse causes moderate to severe pain on the affected side	Rapid collapse causes dyspnea, cyanosis, hypotension, tachycardia, fever, and shock; percussion, dullness or flatness; diminished or absent breath sounds; decreased chest excursion of affected side
D. Disorders of the pleura				
1. Pneumothorax (spontaneous)	—	55	Sudden moderate to severe stabbing, sharp pain felt across the chest or over abdomen or corresponding shoulder; can simulate pain of acute myocardial infarction or acute abdomen	Dyspnea, absent breath sounds; with large or tension pneumothorax tympany on percussion; decreased excursion of affected side; cardiac dullness and apex felt away from affected side; radiographic evidence
2. Pleuritis (pneumonitis; pulmonary infarct; pleural tumors; lung abscess; actinomycosis; coccidiomycosis; other infectious processes)	—	55	Localized, sharp, knife-like stabbing, piercing pain in various regions of the chest depending on the site of pathology (side, shoulder, epigastrium); markedly aggravated by deep breathing, coughing, laughing, movement of the chest; pain can be continuous with pleural carcinoma	Diagnostic pleural friction rub; history and systemic symptoms and signs of infection; chest signs (rales, rhonchi); radiographic evidence
3. Epidemic pleurodynia (Bornholm disease)	—	55	Severe paroxysmal sharp pain in side of chest wall, epigastrium, costovertebral region, and abdomen	Fever, headache; occasionally orchitis, encephalitis, and pericarditis occur during epidemic

*See Table 2-2.

TABLE 53-2. (Cont.)

Etiology (Disease)	IASP Code Ref.*	Chapter No.	Important Diagnostic Features	
			Characteristics of the Pain	Associated Symptoms and Signs
E. **Bronchogenic and metastatic carcinoma** (CA) of the lung, bronchial pleura (squamous cell CA; undifferentiated small or large cell adenocarcinoma, bronchoalveolar CA)	—	57	Location, quality, and severity of pain depend on location and type of spread: a. Endobronchial CA → sternal and parasternal pain b. Intrapulmonary CA → vague central (visceral) pain c. Pleural spread → sharp, stabbing, chest wall pain markedly aggravated by breathing, coughing, movement d. Mediastinal spread → neuropathy with segmental pain e. Pancoast's syndrome (brachial plexopathy) → pain in shoulder, scapula, medial arm	Weight loss; paraneoplastic syndromes; other signs and symptoms: a. Cough, hemoptysis b. Hypoxia, dyspnea, atelectasis c. Signs and symptoms of pleuritis (see above) d. Compression of superior vena cava → superior vena cava syndrome e. Horner's syndrome, hoarseness, weakness of all muscles supplied by the ulnar nerve

III. DISEASES OF THE ESOPHAGUS

A. **Esophagitis**				
1. Gastroesophageal reflux disease (GERD)	XIX-4	56	Retrosternal pain extends from suprasternal notch to xiphoid process; radiation to epigastrium, neck and back and, rarely, arms; simulates pain of myocardial ischemia; lasts seconds to many hours; aggravated by stooping or lifting, recumbency, citrus juices, exercise, heavy meal, coffee, alcohol, aspirin, tobacco, and obesity; relieved by antacids	Dysphagia, odynophagia, regurgitation, and occasionally aspiration; diagnosis helped by pH monitoring, acid perfusion test, and esophagoscopy
2. Acute and chronic esophagitis caused by infection or chemical agents	XIX-4	56	Corrosive agents: immediate, severe, burning pain in throat and behind the whole length of the sternum down to epigastrium, pain is constant with periodic increases in intensity produced by esophageal spasm; infection: pain appears gradually over a period of hours or days and is constant, mild to moderate, and burning in character; both are markedly aggravated by swallowing (odynophagia) and by citrus juices and other factors listed above for GERD	Infection: signs and symptoms of inflammation (e.g., fever, chills); chemical esophagitis: pharyngeal erythema; moniliasis; typical soft white patches in tongue, tonsil, and buccal mucosa; other associated symptoms as above (e.g., dysphagia, odynophagia)
B. **Esophageal motor disorders** (achalasia; diffuse spasm unclassified motor disorders)	XIX-3	56	Moderate to severe retrosternal pain; radiation to epigastrium and to back, neck, jaw, teeth, left arm, or both arms; aggravated by cold liquids, solids, and emotional stress; partially relieved by nitroglycerin; lasts seconds to many hours and can awaken patient from sleep; simulates pain of myocardial infarction	Dysphagia, odynophagia; diagnosis aided by manometry, scintigraphy, provocative tests (e.g., edrophonium or metacholine-induced esophageal spasm)
C. **Esophageal laceration and rupture** (Mallory-Weiss syndrome, MWS; Boerhaave's syndrome, BHS)	—	56	MWS: laceration of distal esophagus and proximal stomach during retching, vomiting, or hiccup causes pain in lower sternum and epigastrium; BHS: spontaneous rupture occurs during intense vomiting following a large meal and causes sudden, severe, excruciating crushing or tearing pain in lower retrosternal region and epigastrium, with radiation to the back	Dysphagia, odynophagia; rupture → mediastinitis → acute illness, epigastric tenderness, and later subcutaneous emphysema and left pleural effusion
D. **Carcinoma**	—	56	Moderate to severe retrosternal pain; radiation to epigastrium with lower lesions and to upper sternum with upper lesions; radiation to neck, interscapular region; pain continuous and aggravated by food ingestion	Dysphagia, odynophagia, weight loss; esophageal obstruction; radiographic, CT, and esophagoscopic evidence

*See Table 2-2.

TABLE 53-2. (Cont.)

Etiology (Disease)	IASP Code Ref.*	Chapter No.	Important Diagnostic Features	
			Characteristics of the Pain	Associated Symptoms and Signs
E. Paraesophageal hiatal hernia	XIX-2	56	Generally asymptomatic; might be feeling of epigastric fullness and lower retrosternal discomfort; with incarceration and strangulation, severe, excruciating epigastric and retrosternal pain	Possible massive gastrointestinal hemorrhage; radiographic and esophagoscopic evidence
IV. DISEASES OF THE MEDIASTINUM AND DIAPHRAGM				
A. Mediastinal disorders				
1. Spontaneous mediastinal emphysema	—	58	Sudden intense, violent, agonizing retrosternal or precordial pain; radiation to nape of neck and shoulder associated with pleural pain; persists for hours	Signs of emphysema: crunching sound in area of pain, decreased or obliterated cardiac dullness, pneumothorax, subcutaneous emphysema (crepitus); radiographic evidence
2. Acute or chronic mediastinitis	—	58	Continuous; mild to moderate; retrosternal, central; oppressive or burning, aching sensation; can be severe	Systemic signs of infection; history of esophageal rupture or other trauma
3. Neoplasms (anterior compartment, AC; superior compartment, SC; middle compartment, MC; posterior compartment, PC)	—	57	One-third of patients asymptomatic: remainder have chest pain, cough, dyspnea, and symptoms caused by compression or invasion of structures in mediastinum	MC: dysphagia, hoarseness; AC, SC: retrosternal and suprasternal discomfort, local chest pain from pressure on sternum; PC: neurogenic tumors, vague chest pain, cough, radicular pain from neuropathy, superior vena cava syndrome
B. Diseases of the diaphragm				
1. Diaphragmatic pleuritis	—	—	Sharp, stabbing "pleuritic" pain along the nape and shoulder and/or in the posterior and lateral parts of the lower chest and upper abdomen; aggravated by diaphragmatic motion	Signs and symptoms of pneumonitis or infectious processes with inflammation of diaphragmatic pleura
2. Acute primary diaphragmatitis (Hedblom's syndrome)	—	58	Moderate to severe pain in lower chest, upper abdomen, and shoulder	Chills and fever; muscle spasm of abdomen; decreased lung expansion on inspiration; radiographic evidence of flattened diaphragm
3. Diaphragmatic spasm	—	58	Precordial pain; radiation to shoulder	Dyspnea during sustained spasm of the diaphragm can cause occlusion of esophagus; some patients develop progressive dyspnea, pallor, sweating, hypotension and angor animi simulating that of AMI; occlusion of the esophagus causes dysphagia and odynophagia
4. Diaphragmatic flutter	—	58	Lower chest pain felt along the diaphragmatic attachment in the epigastrium, precordium; radiation to the shoulder and occasionally to the neck and arm	Dyspnea, palpatation; symptoms and signs of various causative factors (e.g., encephalitis, intoxication)

*See Table 2-2.

TABLE 53-2. (Cont.)

Etiology (Disease)	IASP Code Ref.*	Chapter No.	Important Diagnostic Features	
			Characteristics of the Pain	Associated Symptoms and Signs
V. PAIN OF NEUROPATHIC ORIGIN				
A. Lesions or diseases of the spinal cord (mylopathy)				
1. Intramedullary lesion (tumor; syringomyelia; trauma; multiple sclerosis, MS; abscess; hemorrhage)	I-6	14	Spontaneous, burning, diffuse, poorly localized pain; bouts of explosive pain; later radicular pain involving several segments, depending on the size of the lesion	Dissociation of sensation, loss of pain and temperature sensation, but little effect on proprioception; sensory changes often "spotty"; lower motor neuron signs; with MS spotty paresthesia, pain, symptoms and signs of other involved parts of CNS
2. Extramedullary lesion (primary or metastatic tumor; abscess; hemorrhage)	I-6	14, 57	Initially localized back pain but subsequently pain is radicular; aggravated by increase in CSF pressure, such as that caused by straining, sneezing, coughing	Paravertebral tenderness, paresthesia, followed by sensory loss, muscular weakness; lower motor neuron signs at level of lesion; increased deep reflexes; CSF changes early and marked; spinal cord compression with large lesion
3. Epidural spinal cord compression ESCC (primary or metastatic tumor; hemorrhage; posterior disk protrusion; abscess; hemorrhage)	—	57	Localized back pain at level of site of lesion in 95% of patients; bilateral radicular pain in segments affected by lesion in 55%; aggravated by neck flexion, straight leg raising, coughing, sneezing, Valsalva's maneuver	Back tenderness on deep palpation, fist pounding; no other early signs, but later muscle weakness ranging from mild degree to paraplegia; numbness and paresthesia in 50%; bladder and bowel dysfunction with low thoracic ESCC
B. Lesions of rootlets or roots of T1–T12 (radiculopathy)				
1. Herpes zoster (HZ)	I-1	13, 58	Continuous aching, itching, or burning pain, often with superimposed bouts of severe lancinating pain; hyperalgesia; aggravated by trunk motion, palpation of vesicles; persists until healing of rash (1 to 4 weeks)	Appearance of rash, later vesicles form and then crust; hyperalgesia and hyperesthesia of skin in affected segments; occasionally systemic symptoms of infection; mood and behavioral changes with unrelieved pain
2. Postherpetic neuralgia (PHN)	I-1	13	Severe, continuous, unrelenting burning pain, itching; accompanied by severe paroxysms of stabbing lancinating pain that persist long after acute phase	Hyperalgesia, hypesthesia, hyperpathia; scar in area of vesicles; reactive depression, sleep disturbances, anorexia, lassitude, constipation, decreased libido; high suicide rate among those with unrelieved PHN
3. Tabes dorsalis	I-6	14	Severe, sharp, lancinating, girdle-like (segmental) pain of brief duration with intervals of remission	History of syphilis; CSF evidence; other symptoms of CNS syphilis
4. Mechanical compression (tumor; disk protrusion; vertebral fracture; osteophyte; adhesive arachnoiditis)	—	58	Segmental sharp, burning pain; aggravated by cough, sneezing, straining, and movement of trunk	Hyperalgesia, hyperesthesia, hypesthesia, dysesthesia; radiographic evidence of pathology

*See Table 2-2.

TABLE 53-2. (Cont.)

Etiology (Disease)	IASP Code Ref.*	Chapter No.	Important Diagnostic Features	
			Characteristics of the Pain	Associated Symptoms and Signs
C. Diseases of formed thoracic spinal nerves (neuropathy)				
1. Vertebral compression (arthritis; metastatic or traumatic fracture; tumor of vertebrae; osteomyelitis)	—	58	Segmental neuralgia usually present: continuous burning or sharp pain affecting part or entire segment of nerve, associated with paroxysms of stabbing pain; compression of anterior root produces dull, aching, occasionally stabbing pain in part of affected segment; both aggravated by movement of thoracic spine; often worse at night	Paravertebral tenderness and segmental hyperalgesia, hyperesthesia, hypesthesia; radiographic evidence (CT scan)
2. Paravertebral compression (mediastinal tumors; aortic aneurysm; paravertebral abscess or adenopathy)	—	—	Continuous moderate to severe burning, aching segmental pain; aggravated by movement of spine; occasional bouts of lancinating pain	Paravertebral tenderness; segmental hyperalgesia, hypesthesia; radiographic evidence
3. Primary neurogenic tumors (neurofibroma; schwannoma; ganglioneuroma; neuroblastoma)	—	57	Possibly localized back pain and tenderness but usually continuous burning, aching pain; associated with lancinating pain in distribution of affected nerve	Sensory deficit (hypesthesia), paresthesia, dysesthesia; CT scan and radiographic evidence
4. Other neuropathies (systemic infection; alcoholism; avitaminosis; diabetes; metals)	—	—	Continuous or intermittent mild to moderate burning pain; associated with paroxysms of stabbing pain in one or more dermatomes	History of infection, alcoholism, nutrition deficiency, exposure to ingestion of metals; hyperesthesia, hyperalgesia, hypesthesia, paresthesia, dysesthesia; other signs and symptoms of primary disorder
D. Lesion or disease of the intercostal nerves—intercostal neuropathy (compression or irritation secondary to rib fracture; trauma; primary or metastatic tumor of ribs; pleuritis)	—	58	Superficial continuous burning pain in distribution of affected intercostal nerve; also, local pain with rib fracture or tumor, pleuritic pain with pleuritis	History of trauma or infection; paresthesia, hyperesthesia, dysesthesia, hypesthesia; superficial and deep tenderness; radiographic evidence; palpable tumor or fracture
VI. PAIN OF MUSCULOSKELETAL ORIGIN				
A. Lesions of the thoracic spine				
1. Fracture (trauma; neoplasm; osteoporosis; subluxation; dislocation)	—	58	Initially localized dull, aching pain, often referred to anterior part of chest; aggravated by motion, worse and throbbing at night; segmental pain with root compression	History of trauma; radiographic evidence; localized tenderness paravertebrally and over spinous processes; possibly segmental hyperalgesia, paresthesia
2. Metastatic or primary tumors	—	57	Intense aching, boring circumscribed pain; aggravated by motion and local pressure	Local tenderness or segmental hyperalgesia and hyperesthesia; CT scan and radiographic evidence

*See Table 2-2.

TABLE 53-2. (Cont.)

Etiology (Disease)	IASP Code Ref.*	Chapter No.	Important Diagnostic Features	
			Characteristics of the Pain	Associated Symptoms and Signs
3. Arthritis or deformity of spine	—	20, 58	Usually circumscribed aching pain in back and side; segmental pain with neuropathy	Signs of arthritis in other areas; deformity of spine evident; local tenderness; reflex muscle spasm; radiographic evidence
4. Ankylosing spondylitis	—	58, 90	Usually circumscribed dull aching pain in back; later paraspinal contractures develop with compression of nerve root, which causes segmental pain	Tenderness on deep palpation; radiographic evidence
5. Diffuse idiopathic skeletal hyperostosis	—	58	Mild to moderate localized, dull aching pain; aggravated by inactivity and cold	Tenderness and stiffness in thoracic spine; dorsal kyphosis; reduction of range of movement and in chest expansion; characteristic radiographic evidence
6. Inflammatory disease of vertebrae (osteomyelitis; actinomycosis; tuberculosis; syphilis; subperiosteal hematoma)	—	22, 58	Circumscribed, continuous, aching pain; moderate to severe; aggravated by pressure, often worse at night	Local and systemic symptoms and signs of inflammation; localized tenderness paravertebrally and over spinous process
7. Costovertebral joint arthritis	—	—	Localized deep aching pain similar to that arising from vertebral pathology; aggravated by movement; relieved by local infiltration of joint	Tenderness on deep palpation; radiographic evidence
8. Apophyseal facet syndrome	—	—	Moderate to severe, dull aching, localized pain and tenderness; aggravated by hyperextension; relieved by flexion of the spine	Tenderness; limitation of motion, flattening of normal kyphotic thoracic curve; paraspinal muscle spasm
B. Rib lesions				
1. Fracture or trauma (severe cough; osteoporosis; metastatic tumor)	—	58	Localized sharp pain at site of lesion; widespread chest pain with multiple rib fractures; pain aggravated by deep breathing, coughing, movement of thorax	History of accidental trauma or severe coughing; evidence of osteoporosis; exquisite tenderness on palpation of fracture site; radiographic evidence; with compound fracture can have pneumothorax and damage to lung, with respiratory symptoms and signs
2. Primary metastatic rib tumor (myeloma; chondrosarcoma; granuloma)	—	—	Mild to moderate or severe continuous unilateral dull, aching, chest pain; relatively localized but can also produce intercostal neuralgia	Palpable mass and tenderness to pressure; radiographic evidence
3. Other bone diseases (osteitis deformans; acromegaly; Paget's disease; osteoporosis; hyperostosis)	—	23, 58	Localized continuous aching pain; intercostal neuralgia if lesion irritates nerve	Evidence of disease elsewhere; tenderness on palpation; radiographic evidence
C. Disorders of the costal cartilages				
1. Costochondritis (anterior chest wall syndrome)	—	—	Unilateral or bilateral aching pain in lower anterior chest wall usually in region of cartilages of 3rd, 6th to 7th ribs; aggravated by deep breathing, coughing, palpation	No swelling of costochondral region; more frequent in younger than older people; development of anxiety and concern about heart disease if pain is on left side

*See Table 2-2.

TABLE 53-2. (Cont.)

Etiology (Disease)	IASP Code Ref.*	Chapter No.	Important Diagnostic Features	
			Characteristics of the Pain	Associated Symptoms and Signs
2. Tietze's syndrome	—	58	Localized moderate dull, aching pain in upper anterior chest in region of 2nd and perhaps 3rd costochondral junction; aggravated by palpation, movement of chest wall, coughing, respiratory infection; worse when lying down; recurs between intervals of remission	Palpable tender tumor-like swelling at site of costochondral joint; occurs mostly in people over 50; radiography not diagnostic; development of anxiety, fatigue, concern about heart disease
3. Slipping rib syndrome (rib tip syndrome; slipped cartilage)	XVII-10	58	Unilateral lower chest and upper abdominal localized aching or sharp pain; aggravated by hyperextension and raising of arms; relieved by forward bending to the affected side	Palpation produces tenderness and reveals upward curling of loosened end of cartilages of 8th, 9th and 10th ribs; hooking flexed finger under costal cartilage and exerting pressure anteriorly produces clicking noise
4. Fracture of cartilage or dislocation of costochondral joint	—	58	Sudden sharp pain from fracture or dislocation followed by continuous dull aching, burning discomfort in area of costal margin; reference to back	History of injury; tenderness on palpation; displaced cartilage is palpable and feels like lump
D. Lesions or disorders of the sternum				
1. Fracture of sternum	—	58	Localized pain in region of sternum, usually sharp initially but then continuous and aching; aggravated by deep breathing or palpation	History of blunt trauma to anterior chest; tenderness to palpation; leads to manubriosternal arthralgia
2. Rheumatoid arthritis or osteoarthritis	—	58	Continuous or intermittent pain localized to the angle of Louis; aggravated by deep breathing, coughing, sneezing, and yawning	Mild swelling of joint; exquisite tenderness to palpation; systemic arthritis present; radiographic evidence of arthropathy
3. Xiphoidalgia (hypersensitive xiphoid syndrome; xiphodynia)	—	57	Spontaneous deep aching or sharp pain varying in intensity from a slight to agonizing discomfort that simulates pain of myocardial infarction; aggravated by movements that act on xiphoid process (e.g., bending, stooping, turning) and by increase in intragastric pressure caused by a large meal; can be constant or recurs several times a day; lasts for minutes to several hours	Pressure on xiphoid process produces spontaneous pain that can radiate deep retrosternally and to the precordium, epigastrium, and across shoulder and back; persists for weeks or months but usually disappears spontaneously
4. Arthritis of sternoclavicular joint	—	—	Localized sharp or aching pain in region of joint; radiation to shoulder and upper chest	Joint swollen, tender on palpation; radiographic evidence
F. Muscle disorders				
1. Myofascial pain syndromes with trigger points (TPs)				
a. Anterior chest (major and minor, pectoralis; scaleni; sternalis; intercostals)	—	21, 58	Frequent cause of pain in anterior chest; pain is deep and aching; aggravated by activity; sternalis and pectoralis pain can simulate pain of angina pectoris; pain relieved by injection of TPs with local anesthetic	History of severe strain by heavy lifting; local tenderness, TPs present; unaffected by body activity
b. Lateral chest (serratus anterior; intercostals)	—	21, 58	Deep aching pain on the lateral aspect of the chest extending from the lower axilla to about the 7th to the 6th ribs; pain also in area near the inferior angle of the scapula; with intercostal syndrome site of pain varies with site of TPs; relief with TP injection	Localized tenderness and TP about the level of the 6th rib; pressure on trigger points produces spontaneous pain

*See Table 2-2.

TABLE 53-2. (Cont.)

Etiology (Disease)	IASP Code Ref.*	Chapter No.	Important Diagnostic Features	
			Characteristics of the Pain	Associated Symptoms and Signs
c. Posterior chest (rhomboidei; latissimus dorsi multifidi; serratus posterior superior; iliocostalis thoracis)	—	58	Deep aching pain in different parts of the back depending on the site of the TP and the muscles involved; aggravated by activity of muscles, unaffected by bodily activity	Localized tenderness and TPs
2. Acute muscle spasm	—	23	Sharp localized pain in area of the spastic muscle; some radiation to anterior and posterior chest; complete relief with infiltration of muscle	Palpation of spastic muscle; generalized tenderness
3. Muscle contractures	—	23, 90	Constant deep aching pain, often associated with early spondylosis	Possible localized tenderness of affected muscle or in an area of reference
4. Dermatomyositis and polymyositis	—	23	Rarely, a cause of chest pain; when present, pain aching and aggravated by palpation	Generalized weakness; elevated serum levels of skeletal muscle enzyme
VII. Pain of tegumentary origin (including the breast)				
A. Acute disorders				
1. Burns and other trauma	—	26	Sharp burning pain following burns, aching pain with trauma	History of injury or burn; emotional reactions
2. Postoperative pain	—	25	Fairly localized sharp, burning, aching pain primarily at the site of incision; can radiate to involve adjacent segments	Reflex muscle spasm, tenderness; hyperalgesia; tachycardia response; signs of neuroendocrine stress
3. Acute mastodynia (inflammatory)	—	—	Sharp, aching, burning pain in chest; radiation to axilla and inner arm; aggravated by movement of the breast	Extreme tenderness, tumefaction; evidence of infection
4. Deep axillary abscess	—	—	Sharp localized, diffuse dull, aching pain in axilla; radiation to anterior chest and medial arm	Tenderness, fluctuating mass; signs of infection
5. Acute dermatologic disorders (vesicles; furuncles; bullae; pustules; ulcers; erythema, cellulitis)	—	27	Aching, burning, itching pain localized to lesion	Possible evidence of local or systemic disease
B. Chronic disorders				
1. Postmastectomy syndrome 2. Post-thoracotomy syndrome	—	57	Sharp, burning, aching pain; accompanied by bouts of lancinating pain in distribution of the dermatomes supplied by the injured nerve or in part of the segment; aggravated by light touch of skin, palpation of neuroma, and emotional stress	Hyperesthesia, hyperalgesia, hypesthesia, paresthesia; neuroma often palpable; evidence of recurrent cancer by use of CT scan or other diagnostic procedures
3. Adiposis dolorosa (Dercum's disease)	—	27, 58	Enlarged painful fatty subcutaneous nodule most commonly in the chest and arms but can affect any part except the face; usually darting, shooting or stabbing pain; occurs spontaneously or provoked by palpation	Usually occurs in obese women; weakness, fatigue, emotional instability, occasional dementia

*See Table 2-2.

TABLE 53-2. (Cont.)

Etiology (Disease)	IASP Code Ref.*	Chapter No.	Important Diagnostic Features	
			Characteristics of the Pain	Associated Symptoms and Signs
4. Chronic mastalgia	—	58	Chronic persistent pain; cyclic in two-thirds of patients and continuous in the other third; deep, aching, diffuse pain over entire breast without palpable evidence of pathology; about 20% have spontaneous intermittent relief while others have relief at menopause or pregnancy or with use of oral contraceptives; those with noncyclic pain have pain that can persist for 2 to 3 years or for as long as 30 years	Psychologic tests usually reveal no abnormality; positive response to hormonal manipulation suggests a hormonal basis to the condition
5. Scleroderma (dermatomyositis; disseminating lupus erythematosus; polyarteritis nodosa)	—	—	Dull, aching, occasionally burning pain in the chest wall, usually in the area of the lesion; with scleroderma, chest pain can arise from skin, thoracic wall, or myocardial or esophageal lesions	Symptoms and signs of systemic disease; many types produce widespread visceral involvement
6. Other chronic dermatologic diseases	—	—	(See Chapter 27 for detailed discussion)	
7. Mondor's disease (phlebitis of anterolateral chest)	—	—	Rare condition manifested by thrombosis of superficial vein of thoracic wall that produces palpable painful cord within the skin; usually sharp and persistent; intensified by deep inspiration or flexion of the trunk	Presence of painful, tender, subcutaneous cord running obliquely across thorax in distribution of one or more superficial veins; lesion indolent after several weeks
C. Cancer of the breast	—	57	Early breast cancer not painful; in far advanced disease skin nodule eventually breaks down and formation also causes localized breast pain; metastasis to the pleura produces pleuritic pain; metastasis to the ribs causes localized pain and can be associated with segmental neuralgia; metastasis to the spine produces back pain and later can cause epidural spinal cord compression or plexopathy	Early: retracted nipple, bleeding, distorted areola or breast contour, skin dimpling (peau d'orange); later: axillary supraclavicular adenopathy; metastatic lesion demonstrated by radiography and CT scan

VIII. CHEST PAIN REFERRED FROM EXTRATHORACIC DISORDERS

A. Disorders of the cervical spine that cause neuropathy

1. Posterolateral protrusion of intervertebral disk (C7, C8) 2. Arthritis, osteophyte, fracture or other lesion that compresses root or nerve	—	48, 58	Pain in the neck, shoulder, medial aspect of the arm, and pectoral region of the chest; with left-sided lesion, pain can simulate that of myocardial ischemia but is differentiated by aggravation by lateral flexion and the Spurling test (Chapter 47); unaffected by activity if neck and arms not moved	Paravertebral and pectoral muscle tenderness; hyperalgesia, hyperesthesia, and paresthesia of the arm; decrease in reflexes and some muscle weakness in the upper limbs
3. Thoracic inlet syndromes (scalenus anticus syndrome; cervical rib or abnormal 1st rib; costoclavicular compression)	—	48, 58	Pain most prominent in the shoulder and upper limbs; radiation to the upper pectoral region; aggravated by severe arm abduction and walking with swinging arms; unaffected by activity if arms not moved	Supraclavicular (scaleni) tenderness and fullness; neurovascular signs and symptoms in the upper extremities; radiographic evidence of abnormal cervical rib

*See Table 2-2.

TABLE 53-2. (Cont.)

Etiology (Disease)	IASP Code Ref.*	Chapter No.	Important Diagnostic Features	
			Characteristics of the Pain	Associated Symptoms and Signs
4. Pancoast's syndrome	—	48, 58	Pain in shoulder, scapula, medial aspect of arm, and superior anterior chest; aggravated by extreme abduction of the arm and paravertebral pressure; unaffected by activity if neck and limbs are not moved	Signs and symptoms of plexopathy with paresthesia, dysesthesia, numbness in the medial aspects of the forearm and fourth and fifth fingers, also medial aspect of arm; marked weakness of muscles supplied by ulnar nerve; radiographic and CT scan evidence of lesion
B. Diseases of the abdominal viscera				
1. Gas entrapment syndromes (e.g., caused by aerophagia, excess production of gas in bowel)	—	—	Bloated sensation associated with pain in the epigastrium and central lower chest; if diaphragm irritated, pain also in shoulder; dull, aching pain worsens as day progresses; transiently relieved by belching; gas entrapment in hepatic flexure of colon produces discomfort in right upper quadrant and lower part of right chest, gas in splenic flexure causes pain in left upper quadrant and left lower chest	History of aerophagia, abdominal tympany; radiographic evidence
2. Peptic ulcer disease	—	60	Ulcer in cardia of stomach produces pain in the epigastrium and central lower anterior chest, ulcer in other locations not associated with chest pain; duodenal ulcer causes pain that radiates to xiphoid process but not higher	Peptic ulcer confirmed by radiography and endoscopy
3. Perforated ulcer	—	60	Sudden severe epigastric pain that can radiate to lower chest with severe hypotension → myocardial ischemia → anginal pain	History, physical signs (e.g., muscle spasm, shock, diaphoresis, hematemesis)
4. Biliary colic	—	61	Sudden moderate to severe epigastric pain; radiation to back; right subcostal region, and low central portion of right chest; rarely, pain confined only to chest mimicking that of MI, but no radiation to arm or jaw	Patient can have nausea but no vomiting; in distress but no fever; subcostal tenderness
5. Acute cholecystitis	—	61	Pain usually localized to right upper quadrant; lasts few days rather than a few hours; chest pain rare except in patients with coexisting coronary artery disease—in these patients, biliary pain provokes angina pectoris and ECG changes (low amplitude and inversion of T wave)	Nausea, vomiting, fever, jaundice, and tender right upper quadrant mass; abdominal muscle spasm
6. Acute pancreatitis	—	—	Sudden severe epigastric pain associated with retrosternal oppression; radiation to lower part of left side of chest; unaffected by effort; often provokes ECG changes similar to those of myocardial ischemia and infarction	Severe abdominal muscle spasm; often hypotension, hypoventilation, elevated blood amylase level
7. Subphrenic abscess	—	—	Pus from perforated viscus produces subdiaphragmatic abscess with inflammation of the diaphragm → pleuritic pain in the lower chest and often the shoulder; intrapleural rupture of amebic liver abscess → sudden severe chest pain	Dyspnea, fever, pleural effusion and, occasionally, hepatomegaly

*See Table 2-2.

TABLE 53-2. (Cont.)

Etiology (Disease)	IASP Code Ref.*	Chapter No.	Important Diagnostic Features	
			Characteristics of the Pain	Associated Symptoms and Signs
IX. CHEST PAIN PRIMARILY OF PSYCHOLOGIC ORIGIN				
A. Acute anxiety state	—	—	Sudden acute diffuse pain in chest in the precordial region near cardiac apex (not retrosternal); severe, sharp, stabbing pain or dull, heavy pressure experienced after effort, not during	Dyspnea (air hunger) leading to hyperventilation, tachycardia, dizziness, palpitations, perspiration, tremor, weakness, chest tightness; psychologic evaluation and testing reveal evidence of anxiety
B. Chronic anxiety (cardiac neurosis; soldier's heart; neurocirculatory asthenia; irritable heart; effort syndrome)	—	—	Pain usually at apex of the heart; felt as dull ache with or without attacks of sharp pain over same area; either of brief duration or continuous for hours and days; associated with fatigue rather than effort; responds poorly to all medication	Chronic anxiety and apprehension; severe dyspnea; respiratory distress both at rest and with exertion, sighing respirations; possible ECG changes; low energy level; psychologic evaluation and testing reveal psychopathology
C. Depression	—	—	Endogenous depression can cause atypical chest pain described as a heavy feeling or deep ache or tightness; possible radiation to left arm; usually worse in the morning, lessens as the day goes on	Feeling of overconcern with the heart; in primary affective disorder patient complains of feelings of depression, guilt, worthlessness, withdrawal, disinterest; occasional suicidal preoccupation, anorexia, weight loss, fatigue, low energy level, malaise, insomnia; psychologic evaluation and testing reveal psychopathology
D. Hypochondriasis	—	—	Precordial or apical pain; pain described by patient in minute detail regarding location, quality, and duration but does not fit pattern of any "organic" disease, and description of the pain changes from one visit to another	Feeling of overconcern with the heart; many other complaints (e.g., dysfunction of GI tract); may present different complaints at different visits. Psychologic evaluation and testing produces evidence of psychopathology
E. Operant pain (learned pain)	—	—	Initially patient has chest pain from disease of the heart or lungs that persists after healing because of reinforcing environmental factors. Develops chronic pain behavior and abnormal illness behavior	Progressive physical deterioration over time because of inactivity, muscle weakness, and other factors that cause pain and reinforce the behavior; psychologic evaluation and testing reveal psychopathology

*See Table 2-2.

REFERENCES

1. Clemente, C.D.: Gray's Anatomy of the Human Body. 30th Ed. Philadelphia, Lea & Febiger, 1985, pp. 147–158, 348–359, 475–482.
2. Lockhart, R.D., Hamilton, G.F., and Fyfe, F.W.: Anatomy of the Human Body. Philadelphia, J.B. Lippincott, 1959, pp. 176–177, 277–281.
3. Campbell, E.J.M., Agostoni, E., and Newsom-Davis, J.: The Respiratory Muscles: Mechanics and Neural Control. Philadelphia, W.B. Saunders, 1970.
4. Hovelacque, A.: Anatomie des Nerfs Craniens et Rachidiens et du Système Grand Sympathique chez l'Homme. Paris, G. Dion & Cie, 1927.
5. Kuntz, A.: Autonomic Nervous System. 4th Ed. Philadelphia, Lea & Febiger, 1953.
6. Mitchell, G.A.G.: Cardiovascular Innervation. London, E.S. Livingstone, 1956, pp. 196–238.
7. DeSousa-Pereira, A.: Blocking of the splanchnic nerves and the first lumbar sympathetic ganglion. Arch. Surg., 53:32, 1946.
8. Miller, H.R.: Angina Pectoris and Myocardial Infarction. New York, Grune & Stratton, 1950.
9. White, J.C., Garrey, W.E., and Atkins, J.A.: Cardiac innervation. Arch. Surg., 26:765, 1933.
10. White, J.C., and Bland, E.F.: Surgical relief of severe angina pectoris. Medicine, 27:1, 1948.
11. White, J.C.: Cardiac pain. Anatomic pathways and physiologic mechanisms. Circulation, 16:644, 1957.
12. Mizeres, N.J.: The cardiac plexus of man. Am. J. Anat., 112:141, 1963.
13. Hirsch, E.F., and Borghard-Erdle, A.M.: The innervation of the human heart. Arch. Pathol., 71:384, 1961.
14. Braeucker, W.: Der Brustteil des vegetativen Nervensystems und seine klinischchirurgische Bedeutung. Beitr. Klin. Tuberk., 66:1, 1927.

15. Ionesco, T., and Enachesco, M.: Nerfs cardiaques naissant de la chaine thoracicque du sympathique, au-dessous du ganglion stellaire. Les nerfs cardiaques thoraciques chez quelques mammiferes. Compt. Rend. Soc. Biol., (Paris), *97*:977, 1927.

16. Bonica, J.J.: The Management of Pain. 1st Ed. Philadelphia, Lea & Febiger, 1953.

17. White, J.C., and Sweet, W.H.: Pain and the Neurosurgeon. Springfield, Charles C Thomas, 1969.

18. Ammons, W.S., Blair, R.W., and Foreman, R.D.: Vagal afferent inhibition of primate T1–T5 spinothalamic neurons. J. Neurophysiol., *50*:926, 1983.

19. Ammons, W.S., Blair, R.W., and Foreman, R.D.: Raphe magnus inhibition of primate T1–T4 spinothalamic cells with cardiopulmonary visceral input. Pain, *20*:247, 1984.

20. Blair, R.W.: Noxious cardiac input onto neurons in medullary reticular formation. Brain Res., *326*:335, 1985.

21. Foreman, R.D.: Spinal substrates of visceral pain. In Spinal Afferent Processing. Edited by T.L. Yaksh. New York, Plenum Press, 1986, pp. 217–242.

22. Malliani, A.: Cardiovascular sympathetic afferent fibers. Rev. Physiol. Biochem. Pharmacol., *94*:11, 1982.

23. Wollard, H.H.: The innervation of the heart. J. Anat., *60*:345, 1926.

24. Berkley, H.J.: The intrinsic nerve supply of cardiac ventricles in certain vertebrates. Johns Hopkins Hosp. Rep., *4*:248, 1894.

25. Nonidez, J.F.: Studies on the innervation of the heart. II. Afferent nerve endings in the large arteries and veins. Am. J. Anat., *68*:151, 1941.

26. Nettleship, W.A.: Experimental studies on the afferent innervation of the cat's heart. J. Comp. Neurol., *64*:115, 1936.

27. Miller, M.R., and Kasahara, M.: Studies on the nerve endings in the heart. Am. J. Anat., *115*:217, 1964.

28. Khabarova, A.Y.: The Afferent Innervation of the Heart. New York, Consultants Bureau, 1963.

29. Rasmussen, T.B., and Farr, W.J.: Paravertebral injection of procaine for pain produced by aortic aneurysm. J. Neurosurg., *3*:267, 1946.

30. Ponzio, F.: Le terminazione nervose nel polmone. Anat. Anz., *28*:74, 1906.

31. Cookson, F.B.A.: The intrinsic arrangement of the nerve supplying the mammalian lung. B. Sc. Hons. Anat. Thesis. Manchester University, 1953.

32. Fillenz, M., and Widdicomb, J.C.: Receptors of the lung and airways. In Handbook of Sensory Physiology. Vol. 3 Pt. 1. Edited by E. Neil. Berlin, Springer-Verlag, 1972, pp. 81–112.

33. Morton, D.R., Klassen, K.P., and Curtis, G.M.: Clinical physiology of the human bronchi: I. Pain of tracheobronchial origin. Surgery, *28*:669, 1950.

34. Morton, D.R., Klassen, K.P., and Curtis, G.M.: The clinical physiology of the human bronchi: II. Effect of vagus section upon pain of tracheobronchial origin. Surgery, *30*:800, 1951.

35. Teodori, U., and Galletti, R.: Il Dolore Nelle Affezioni Degli Organi Interni del Torace. Rome, El Tozzi, 1962, pp. 183–233.

36. Capps, J.A.: An experimental and clinical study of pain in the pleura, pericardium and peritoneum. New York, Macmillan, 1932, pp. 1–67.

37. White, J.C.: Sensory innervation of the viscera: Studies on visceral afferent neurons in man based on neurosurgical procedures for the relief of intractable pain. In Pain. Edited by H.G. Wolff, H.S. Gasser, and J.C. Hinsey. Baltimore, Williams & Wilkins, 1943, pp. 373–390.

38. Levene, D.L. (Ed.): Chest Pain: An Integrated Diagnostic Approach. Philadelphia, Lea & Febiger, 1977.

54 · CARDIAC AND AORTIC PAIN

with contribution by
JOHN J. BONICA

MANY types of cardiac disease can produce pain in the chest, including coronary heart disease, valvular heart disease, pericardial disease, pulmonary hypertension, and aortic disease. Of these, coronary heart disease is clearly the most common cause of cardiac pain and is of the greatest public health importance. Coronary heart disease remains the leading cause of death in the United States despite a 30% drop in the mortality rate between 1972 and 1984 (1). Although sudden death accounts for about 50% of deaths caused by heart disease, sudden death in most patients is preceded by a recognizable cardiac pain or discomfort syndrome for a variable length of time. Moreover, because only a minority of heart disease deaths are the result of irreversible cardiac failure, most deaths are thought to be preventable. The recognition of a cardiac pain or discomfort syndrome is the single most powerful diagnostic tool available for the diagnosis of coronary heart disease. The pain of chronic coronary heart disease can generally be relieved by nonaddicting oral medications, with relatively few side effects. Thus, not only is cardiac pain easily treatable, but it is also important as a diagnostic tool in the recognition of coronary heart disease and the prevention of death.

Diseases of the thoracic aorta are much less common causes of chest pain, but when they do occur, a prompt, correct diagnosis and appropriate therapy are highly effective: if left untreated, most patients die. These various cardiovascular disorders are among the most important causes of severe pain that require effective management and therefore deserve detailed consideration.

This chapter contains a current and comprehensive overview of cardiac and aortic pain. The material is presented in five parts: A, Basic Considerations, which includes a historical review of the subject, the epidemiology of cardiac and aortic pain, and the characteristics, neurophysiology, and neuropathophysiology of cardiac pain; B, General Clinical Consideration of Coronary Heart Disease, including classification, etiology, pathophysiology, and general principles of diagnosis; C, Myocardial Ischemic Syndromes, in-cluding acute myocardial infarction, stable angina pectoris, unstable angina, sudden cardiac death, variant angina, and silent myocardial ischemia; D, Chest Pain from Other Cardiovascular Disease, including aortic stenosis and other valvular heart disease, hypertrophic cardiomyopathy, and acute pericarditis; and E, Diseases of the Thoracic Aorta, with emphasis on dissection of the thoracic aorta. Bonica contributed much of Section A, and the senior author developed the rest of the chapter. Major cardiology textbooks and recent articles provide more detailed consideration of both coronary heart disease and aortic dissection (2–9).

A. BASIC CONSIDERATIONS

Historical Overview of Cardiac Pain

The history of chest pain caused by disease of the heart goes back to the time of Hippocrates (8). In the book on the *morbus sacer*, as part of the Corpus Hippocraticum, specific reference is made to "palpation and piercing (pain) sensation felt in the breast and pain in the vertebral column" caused by "fluxions of humours in the heart" (8). In ancient Rome *angina* and *angor* were used by Celsus in his *De re Medicina* (30 A.D.) (10). A clear denomination of coronary pain is found in the work of Caelius Aurelianus, a Roman physician of the fifth century A.D. who used the term "*passio cardiaca propria*" to indicate pain of cardiac origin specifically. Like Celsus, he also used *angina* and *angor* to indicate acute disease characterized by a sense of choking and strangling (11). Although the condition was undoubtedly known throughout the Middle Ages, it wasn't until the Renaissance that the concept of "proper" heart pain re-emerged (8). Bartolomeo Castelli (12), in 1598, wrote that "*angor est nativi caloris cordis contractio, et centrum retractio, ad quam sequitur eiusdem cordis dolor, palpatatio et tristitia*" (angor is a contraction, and a retraction toward the center, of the natural heat of the heart, which is followed by heart pain, palpitation and anguish).

Some three decades later Girolamo Mercuriale, writing about diseases of the viscera, first used the term "cardialgia" to indicate heart pain (8). At the beginning of the eighteenth century, Bonet wrote in *Sepulechretum* that the *dolor pectoris* (chest pain) is a serious symptom and described the case of a patient with chest pain who died suddenly; on autopsy the coronary arteries were found to be occluded (13). During the ensuing seven decades, references to a relationship between recurrent heart pain and sudden death were by Lancisi (1707), Lieutaud (1759), Morgagni (1765), and Van Swieten (1768) (8).

Notwithstanding these precedents, credit for the first description of angina pectoris goes to William Heberden who, in 1768, presented a lecture titled "Some account of a disorder of the breast" before the Royal College of Physicians in London and published it 4 years later (14). Heberden's description is lucid, concise, and contains many important diagnostic clues used today:

There is a disorder of the breast marked with strong and peculiar symptoms, considerable for the kind of danger belonging to it, and not extremely rare, which deserves to be mentioned more at length. The seat of it, and sense of strangling, and anxiety with which it is attended, may make it not improperly to be called angina pectoris.

They who are afflicted with it, are seized while they are walking (more especially if it be uphill, and soon after eating), with a painful and most disagreeable sensation in the breast, which seems as if it would extinguish life, if it were to increase or continue; but the moment they stand still, all this uneasiness vanishes.

In all other respects, the patients are, at the beginning of this disorder, perfectly well, and in particular have no shortness of breath, from which it is totally different. The pain is sometimes situated in the upper part, sometimes in the middle, sometimes at the bottom of the os sterni, and more often inclined to the left than to the right side. It likewise very frequently extends from the breast to the middle of the left arm. The pulse is, at least sometimes, not disturbed by this pain, as I have had opportunities of observing by feeling the pulse during the paroxysm. Males are most liable to that disease, especially such as have past their fiftieth year.

After it has continued a year or more, it will not cease so instantaneously upon standing still; and it will come on not only when the persons are walking, but when they are lying down, especially if they lie on their left side, and oblige them to rise up out of their beds. In some inveterate cases, it has been brought on by the motion of a horse, or a carriage, and even by swallowing, coughing, going to stool, or speaking, or any disturbance of mind.

Such is the most unusual appearance of this disease; but some varieties may be met with. Some have been seized while they were standing still or sitting; also upon first waking out of sleep; and the pain sometimes reaches to the right arm, as well as to the left, and even down to the hands, but this is uncommon; in a very few instances the arm has at the same time been numbed and swelled. In one or two persons the pain has lasted some hours, or even days; but this has happened when the complaint has been of long standing, and thoroughly rooted in the constitution; once only the very first attack continued the whole night (14).

Heberden described the syndrome more diffusely in the *Commentari*, published two decades later (15). The term "angina" was used by Heberden not only to signify a sense of choking and strangling (according to Celsus), but also to indicate a terrible anxiety and anguish experienced by the patient (*angor animi*). In fact the word is derived from the Indo-European root *agh* which means "to choke, to oppress, to suffer." Although Heberden rightly deserves the recognition of being the first to describe the syndrome, it is not commonly recognized that he did not believe that angina originated in the heart, even though he implied this belief in the title of his monograph ". . . a disorder of the breast." Even in a later discussion, Heberden failed to associate angina pectoris with disease of the coronary arteries. This was surprising because toward the end of the eighteenth century, several British physicians strongly believed in a relationship between angina pectoris and myocardial ischemia. In 1772 Dr. John Wall, perhaps better known as an artist and founder of the Royal Worcester China Company, had a necropsy done on 1 of 13 persons with angina pectoris, who he had cared for and noted that he had aortic stenosis (16). Proudfit (7) has credited Wall for carrying out the first natural study of angina pectoris. Wall reported that 10 of his 13 patients with angina pectoris died suddenly, and he attributed this to disorders of the heart.

Early in 1786 Edward Jenner, who a decade later demonstrated the efficacy of vaccination for smallpox, carried out a necropsy on the body of a patient whom he had treated for angina pectoris and noted that the coronary arteries were so severely calcified that cutting through them produced an intense grating sound. Subsequently, after observing other necropsies in which "cartilaginous" obstruction of the coronary arteries was noted, he became convinced that coronary artery disease was the cause of angina pectoris:

. . . the importance of the coronary arteries and how much the heart must suffer from their not being able duly to perform their functions . . . it is possible that all the symptoms may arise from this one circumstance (17).

Dr. Caleb Parry, a close friend of Jenner, was familiar with Jenner's belief about angina pectoris. In the spring of 1788 he had a necropsy performed on the body of a patient who had suffered from angina for a number of years and also noted severe coronary artery disease. He reported this to the local medical society in July of that year. Using additional clinical material and Jenner's account of his experiences, as well as that of others, he published his monumental book on angina pectoris in 1799 (18). Parry wrote that

Though a quantity of blood may circulate through the arteries, sufficient to nourish the heart, as appears in some instances, from the size and firmness of the organ, yet there would probably be less than what is requisite for ready and vigorous action. Hence though a heart so diseased may be fit for the purposes of common circulation, during a state of bodily and mental tranquility, and of health otherwise good, yet when any unusual exertion is required, its powers may fail under the new and extraordinary demand (18).

A decade later Burns (19) emphasized the importance of Parry's contribution by stating that "the cause of this affection [angina pectoris] he had incontrovertibly proved to originate from some organic lesion of the nutrient vessels of the heart." This hypothesis was accepted by other English authors, including Johnstone (20) and Black (21).

In the early part of the nineteenth century, Home, Warren, Desportes, and others (see 8 for ref.) proposed that cardiac spasm was the cause of angina pectoris. They noted that, in some cases of angina pectoris, no coronary sclerosis was demonstrated, whereas in other cases severe coronary sclerosis observed at autopsy had not induced any anginal attack.

Despite all the efforts of these physicians, for over 150 years angina was not related to myocardial ischemia by "mainstream" physicians, including such stalwarts as Sir Clifford Allbutt, Regius Professor of Medicine at Cambridge University, and probably also Sir William Osler, his fellow Regius Professor at Oxford. Allbutt, in 1915, in his two-volume *Diseases of the Arteries Including Angina Pectoris* (22), stated that "angina pectoris is anything you please . . . a very popular sentiment." Allbutt and others attributed angina to disease of the aorta, perhaps distension. Beginning with Heberden, this discrepancy probably arose because the major cardiac diagnostic technique of that time, palpation of the pulse, generally revealed no abnormalities in patients with angina; this was Heberden's own observation during an anginal episode (14). Nine years after Allbutt's proposal, Wenckebach (23) stated a similar theory and postulated that the sudden distension of the aorta or distension of the coronary arteries proximal to the point of occlusion stimulated the nerve plexuses. In 1938 Martin and Gorham (24) were said to have proved the distension theory by their observation that pseudoaffective reactions could be induced experimentally in animals by stretching of coronary arteries without causing any change in blood flow.

At about the time that Allbutt was contesting the concept of myocardial ischemia, Herrick's (25) experiments provided strong support to the concept of a causal relationship between coronary insufficiency and cardiac pain. This was reaffirmed by Keefer and Resnik (26) in 1928 in their classic paper on angina pectoris, in which they stated that this symptom "was due to anoxemia of the myocardium . . . the attacks occur when the oxygen supply to the heart is inadequate to meet the oxygen demands of the heart." Further work in support of this theory was done by Sutton and Lueth (27) and White and co-workers (28), who carried out experiments on dogs that manifested pseudoaffective reactions (signs of pain) by repeated and intermittent occlusion of the orifices of coronary arteries. These painful reactions could be produced by occluding the orifices of the coronary arteries without causing distension; acute mechanical distension of the cavity of the left ventricle, the aortic ring, and the aortic arch produced no pain. At about the same time Wood and Wolferth (29) clearly demonstrated a causal relationship by observing electrocardiographic changes during angina; thus the concept of the ischemic origin of angina became widely accepted.

Epidemiology

Coronary Heart Disease

The American Heart Association (AHA) (1) estimated that in 1984, 12.8 million Americans had coronary heart disease, 2.1 million had rheumatic heart disease, and nearly 58 million had high blood pressure. It was further estimated that in 1984 over 440,000 Americans died of a heart attack and 350,000 of these died before they reached the hospital because the average victim waited 3 hours before deciding to get help. Other estimates have shown that among those aged 35–74 years, deaths from coronary heart disease approximately equal those from all other causes (30). The AHA also estimated that for 1986 as many as 1.5 million Americans had a heart attack, with about 540,000 deaths ensuing because of this.

Available data suggest that 5% of heart attacks occur in individuals under the age of 40 and 45% occur in those under the age of 65 (1). The AHA also estimated that in 1983 nearly 1.1 million years of potential life were lost by heart attack,* and 1.7 million deaths occurred from all types of heart disease. It is obvious that coronary heart disease is of epidemic proportions in the United States and other industrialized nations. Indeed, with the control of infectious diseases, coronary heart disease has become the most common cause of death in Western countries.

Fortunately, through various prophylactic and therapeutic measures between the years 1972 and 1984, deaths from coronary heart disease decreased by about 30% (1). This decrease in the mortality rate observed in the United States in the last 15 years has not been observed in a number of other Western countries, most notably Great Britain (31).

With the observation of an apparent decrease in the coronary heart disease mortality rate in Norway in World War II, it was hypothesized that a rich diet (which was austere in Norway during this period) might be a risk factor for coronary heart disease. Since then a number of studies have shown correlations between the coronary heart disease mortality rate and dietary fat or cholesterol intake (32), and a strong relationship between serum cholesterol level and coronary heart disease (33, 34). Despite numerous epidemiologic studies, however, the role of dietary fat intake in the genesis of coronary heart disease, and whether alteration in diet can reduce the risk of coronary heart disease, are still controversial.

Less disagreement exists in regard to the role of cigarette smoking and hypertension as risk factors for coronary heart disease. Cardiovascular mortality is 1.6 times as high among smokers as nonsmokers (35); the effect of cigarette smoking is dose-related and is most evident in younger men (33). The risk of a cardiovascular event returns to nearly that of a nonsmoker on cessation of smoking (36). A clear relationship also exists between hypertension and risk for coronary heart disease (33); some studies have shown a reduction in coronary deaths with control of hypertension (37, 38). Associations with risk for coronary heart disease have also been shown for habitual activity, personality traits, obesity, premature menopause, diabetes, oral contraceptive use, renal failure, and hyperuricemia. The strengths of these associations are much less, however, than those for the major reversible risk factors, smoking and hypertension. Furthermore, little evidence exists to indicate that alteration of these risk factors (if alterable) lowers the risk of coronary heart disease.

Aortic Disease

Of the two principal diseases of the thoracic aorta, chronic aneurysm and acute dissection, only dissecting aneurysms generally produce significant pain. In some patients, though, a large thoracic aortic aneurysm can produce severe excruciating pain in the side of the chest or back, either by irritating nerves or periosteum or other viscera (39). Aortic dissection is a relatively rare disease, with only about 2000 new cases annually in the United States (40). The initial presentation of acute dissection of the thoracic aorta is chest or back pain in over 90% of patients. Correct diagnosis and therapy (surgical in most cases) can achieve a 1-year survival rate of 70% or more (41); 90% of untreated cases die within 1 year—75% within the first month (42). The pain of aortic dissection often mimics that of coronary heart disease, esophageal disease, or musculoskeletal pain. Thus, correct diagnosis of dissection of the thoracic aorta is essential to the initiation of life-saving therapy; pain, although nonspecific in nature, is usually the first clue.

The major risk factor for dissection of the thoracic aorta is hypertension; 60 to 90% of patients with dissection have a history of hypertension (40, 43). Dissection occurs 10 to 20 times more frequently in patients with congenitally abnormal aortic valves (43). Patients with Marfan syndrome, a rare autosomal dominant genetic disease, also have a propensity for developing dissection of the thoracic aorta.

Impact of Disease and Pain on Patient, Family, and Society

As indicated previously, coronary heart disease has its major impact as the leading cause of death in most Western nations. Death from coronary heart disease frequently strikes during the most productive years, the fifth and sixth decades of life. Death is often sudden, leaving the family unprepared for the loss. In addition, angina and the sequelae of acute myocardial infarction, heart failure, and loss of functional capacity, are leading causes of disability and inability to work. Unfortunately, successful treatment of angina by either medical or surgical therapy seems to have little impact on the ability to work if the patient has been unemployed 3 months or more (44). The treatment of coronary heart disease consumes a large proportion of

---

*Years of potential life lost is an estimate based on deaths below age 65 by disease category.

American health care resources. Currently, the expenditure for coronary bypass surgery alone is over 4 billion dollars annually (about 200,000 operations yearly at a cost of $20,000 each) (4). The total cost of cardiovascular disease in 1987 was estimated by the AHA at over $85 billion dollars, a large portion being a result of coronary artery disease.

Aortic dissection has much less global impact because its incidence is less than 1% of that of coronary death. On the other hand, it occurs suddenly, often in otherwise healthy individuals (except for asymptomatic hypertension). Even with the best of modern surgical therapy, the acute mortality rate can be 30% or more. Other than those with Marfan syndrome, patients at risk for dissection cannot be prospectively identified because hypertension is too common to be a useful predictor. The surgical therapy of dissection and its complications is usually expensive both in terms of dollars and in terms of scarce resources—especially blood and intensive care beds. Fortunately, survivors of the acute treatment of dissection of the thoracic aorta can have relatively normal late survival (40) and may be able to lead relatively normal lives postoperatively.

Nature and Mechanisms of Cardiac Pain

The importance of understanding the nature and mechanisms involved in cardiac pain needs no elaboration. The nerve supply to the heart and other thoracic viscera is described in detail in Chapter 53. Here we discuss the nature and characteristics of cardiac pain, the neurophysiology, biochemical substates, and pathophysiologic mechanisms of pain originating in the heart, the physiologic and pathophysiologic effects of severe cardiac and thoracic aortic pain, and clinical implications of this information in regard to managing patients with cardiac pain.

Characteristics

The pains of stable angina pectoris, unstable angina, variant angina, and acute myocardial infarction all have a common denominator—myocardial ischemia. Thus, the pains of each of these conditions may have similar characteristics.

Cardiac pain is visceral in nature; that is, initially the pain is often vague, diffuse, poorly localized, and referred to varying anatomic areas. Patients often find it difficult to describe. Many patients refuse to use the word "pain" in describing angina pectoris, preferring instead to call it a discomfort, a tightness, a constricting feeling in the chest, "a band across the chest," "a weight on the center of the chest," or a strangling sensation. It was for this reason that Heberden chose the word "angina," which means strangling. Ischemic myocardial pain often carries with it the feeling of impending doom or death; Heberden used the Latin phrase *angor animi* to express this feeling of terror (15).

Patients often feel the need to stand absolutely motionless when they experience angina. Ischemic myocardial symptoms can also be described as paresthesia or a numbness or weakness, particularly in the arms. Some patients experience only dyspnea as a manifesta-

tion of their myocardial ischemia. Ischemic myocardial pain is commonly mistaken for pain of gastrointestinal origin because it can be epigastric in location, similar to the "heartburn" of esophagitis, and accompanied by an intense desire for eructation. It is not uncommon for patients suffering from angina pectoris to feel that they could obtain relief if only they could belch. The pain of acute myocardial infarction shares many of these characteristics, although usually it is more severe and of longer duration. Pain of myocardial ischemia is not pleuritic, and it is not exacerbated by deep breathing or coughing. It generally does not vary with position, as does the pain of acute pericarditis. The identification of precipitating factors, such as exercise or emotion, is an essential part of the diagnosis of stable angina pectoris (see below); unstable angina and variant angina, by definition, do not have recognizable external precipitating stimuli.

The visceral nature of cardiac pain provides a basis for its clinical differentiation from chest wall pain or pain from superficial structures. These differences in pain perception and in the stimuli required to evoke pain are summarized in Table 54-1. Pain from the skin can be localized precisely and is superficial and often sharp in nature. Pain from the chest wall (e.g., muscles, ribs, ligaments, parietal pleura) is intermediate in localization, depth, and sharpness (Chapter 7). Also, chest wall pain is often exacerbated by movement, such as with breathing or coughing.

Although ischemic myocardial pain can occur almost anywhere between the diaphragm and the mandible (Fig. 54-1), it is commonly felt in the anterior chest, retrosternally, with radiation to one or both arms, to the throat and mandible, or to all these areas. Less commonly the pain or discomfort is confined to the throat, arms, epigastrium, or even the interscapular region. Because of its visceral origin, ischemic myocardial pain or discomfort is generally referred to an area of substantial size—for example, size of the patient's fist or larger. Pain that is discretely confined to a small area on the chest or that can be localized by the patient with a single finger is usually not pain of myocardial ischemia but is chest wall pain. Indirect evidence has shown that the intensity and size of the area of true visceral and referred visceral pain are influenced to a

TABLE 54-1. Differences in Pain Perception from Heart, Chest Wall, and Skin

Structure	Effective Stimulus	Conscious Pain Perception
Skin	Discrete touch, pinprick, heat, cold	Precisely localized, superficial, burning, sharp
Chest wall	Deep pressure, movement	Intermediate in localization, aching, sharp or dull
Heart and thoracic viscera	Ischemia, distension, movement, muscle spasm	Vague, diffuse, deep, aching, usually dull

From Edmeads, J., and Billings, R.F.: Neurological and psychological aspects of chest pain. *In* Chest Pain: An Integrated Diagnostic Approach. Edited by D.L. Levene, et al. Philadelphia, Lea & Febiger, 1977.

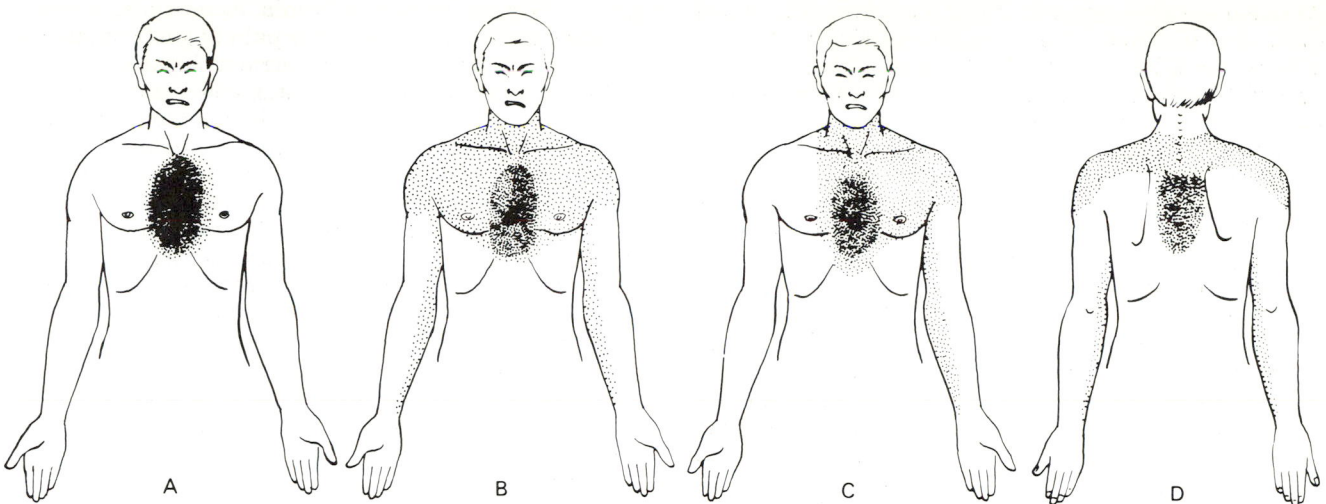

FIG. 54-1. Patterns of the pain produced by myocardial infarction and angina pectoris. The dark stippled area denotes the site of the most severe retrosternal pain while the lightly stippled area shows radiation of the pain. *A.* Initial phase of myocardial ischemic pain felt retrosternally, with some distribution to the anterior chest. Many patients also have a feeling of tightness of the throat and, indeed, in some patients this is the first symptom of myocardial ischemia. *B.* Distribution of the visceral and referred visceral pain to a wider part of the chest and to the medial aspects of the limbs and neck. *C.* Distribution reference to the anterior chest, left scapular region, and inner part of the left arm. *D.* Reference to scapular region posteriorly.

significant degree by the degree and size of the myocardial ischemia and myocardial necrosis. The greater the degree and area of myocardial ischemia the greater the nociceptive barrage into the neuraxis, with consequent spread of neuropathophysiology into the spinal cord and probably the brain stem and, consequently, the greater the spread and intensity of the pain. In addition to the pain, the patient develops hyperalgesia in the spinal segments involved.

In a study of 132 patients with severe chest pain admitted to the Coronary Care Unit of the Department of Medicine of the Karolinska Institute in Stockholm, Säwe (45) found that 51 patients had a proven diagnosis of acute myocardial infarction (AMI) and, in 81 patients, this diagnosis was excluded (he used this group as a "control"). He divided the chest into sections (Fig. 54-2) and carried out a careful assessment of the location of the pain by asking the patient to indicate its specific site. The following findings were reported: pain covering the mammary plane was indicated by 51% of AMI patients and 59% of those in the control group; 32% of AMI patients indicated pain above the mammary plane, as compared to 21%

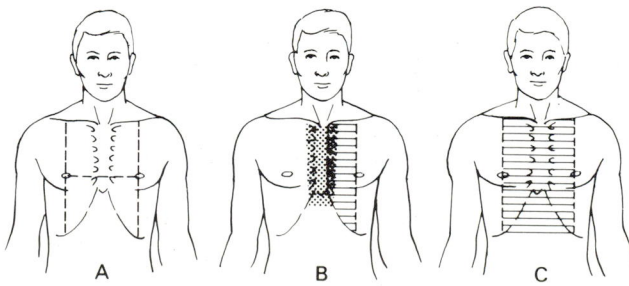

FIG. 54-2. Division of the chest into various sectors to which pain of myocardial ischemia can be referred. *A.* Mammary plane extending from the midclavicular line of one side to the other. *B.* Retrosternal and left parasternal areas. *C.* Pararetroparasternal area. Modified from Säwe, U.: Pain in acute myocardial infarction. Acta Med. Scand., *190*:79, 1971.

of controls; the pain was below the mammary plane in 27% of AMI patients and 20% of controls. Pain localized retrosternally was indicated by 12% of AMI patients and 16% of controls, whereas 35% of those in both groups indicated that the pain was outside the retrosternal area and that the pain extended from the right to the left midclavicular line. Statistical analysis revealed that none of these differences was significant, but a marked difference in the radiation of the pain was noted; 71% of AMI patients indicated radiation of pain to the neck as well as to the left or right arm or both as compared to 39% of patients without AMI, a highly significant difference. Radiation only to the neck was indicated by 7% of those in both groups. Radiation to the left arm alone was indicated by 29% of AMI patients versus 20% of controls ($p < 0.05$). Radiation of pain to both the left and right arms was present in 33% of AMI patients as compared to 12% of controls, possibly the most important difference between the two groups.

Ischemic myocardial pain generally lasts 5 to 15 minutes for stable, exertional angina, 15 to 30 minutes or longer for unstable angina and variant angina, and 1 to 8 hours or more for AMI. The pain of acute myocardial infarction is usually intense, often accompanied by a strong alarm reaction and a feeling of impending death, and not infrequently by nausea, vomiting, and profuse sweating. After a period of several hours, some AMI patients feel the pain to be localized more precisely, originating in the thoracic wall or upper limbs. Teodori and Galletti (46) considered this to be the second phase of AMI and reported that, among their patients, many experienced muscle tenderness in the pectoralis major, the deep muscles of the interscapular region, the muscles of the forearm, and less frequently the trapezius.

Fleeting pain lasting from a few seconds to a minute is almost certainly not pain of myocardial ischemia. Likewise, pain that persists for days is unlikely to be ischemic myocardial pain. Another differential diagnostic guideline is the response to rest or nitroglycerin. The prompt relief of pain or discomfort by rest or nitroglycerin is an important diagnostic characteristic of stable angina. Pain relief usually occurs within 2 to 5 minutes after taking sublingual nitroglycerin. Some patients might require a second nitroglycerin for complete relief, but the beginning of subsidence of the pain is still within 3 to 5 minutes. Pain that takes 15 minutes or longer to be relieved by rest or nitroglycerin either is not caused by myocardial ischemia or is a more severe form, such as unstable angina or AMI. Nitroglycerin is a somewhat unstable compound especially when exposed to heat or sunlight, and can lose its vasodilating potency. Use of old nitroglycerin is another reason for failure of prompt relief of angina. Many patients can recognize impotent nitroglycerin because it does not sting under the tongue or give a feeling of fullness in the head, as does the potent drug.

Somatic Components

It has long been known that ischemic myocardial pain must serve as a trigger for secondary musculoskeletal pain, which can be located in the anterior or posterior chest and is caused by spasm of the pectoralis or some of the posterior chest muscles, or by a combination of these. This phenomenon was initally pointed out to the senior author by an astute house officer who noted a high-frequency artifact in lead 1 (between the right and left arms) of the electrocardiogram of a patient with severe coronary artery disease who experienced persistent, intractable anterior chest pain. This patient, who had inoperable coronary artery disease, experienced considerable long-standing relief following training in biofeedback. This secondary pain, triggered initially by myocardial ischemia, can become the predominant pain syndrome, perpetuated by chronic anxiety. It can also explain some atypical features of the chest pain in patients with recognized and severe coronary artery disease, such as persistence for days, occurrence at rest without electrocardiographic changes, and failure to respond to antianginal therapy.

For nearly four decades, Bonica (39) and Rinzler and Travell (47), among others (see 39 for ref.) have stressed the importance of the somatic components of cardiac pain. They have explained the persistence of pain in the chest when painful visceral impulses are no longer present as follows. In addition to the visceral pain, a visceromotor reflex is set up following the initial insult to the myocardium or to the coronary vessels. This visceromotor reflex produces reflex spasm of the skeletal muscles in the reference zone in the same way that reflex spasm of abdominal musculature is produced by acute abdominal visceral disorders. The muscle spasm produces localized areas of tenderness in the chest muscles, called trigger points. Furthermore, this secondary muscle spasm acts as a new source of noxious stimuli, which produces pain and more muscle spasm (Chapters 7 and 21).

Thus, a vicious cycle of impulses is set up that can persist without further dependence on afferent impulses from the heart. These impulses are transmitted to and from the somatic structures by sustained facilitation of the noxious impulses by the closed self-exciting chains of the internuncial neurons in the central nervous system. Figure 54-3 depicts the sequential development of this somatic pain and the influence of blocking the somatic component for its relief.

Neuropathophysiology

During the past 25 years or so, the advent of sophisticated electrophysiologic techniques has permitted numerous studies that have greatly complemented and supplemented our knowledge of anatomy (Chapter 53). These studies, reviewed by Malliani (48), have led to a new understanding of the location and function of the sympathetic and vagal afferent nerves and of their roles in activating homeostatic reflex mechanisms, as well as contributing to the pathophysiologic states caused by cardiac disease.

Agostini and colleagues (49) demonstrated that the heart has a substantial afferent innervation of A-delta and C fibers from the vagus nerves. Others have shown

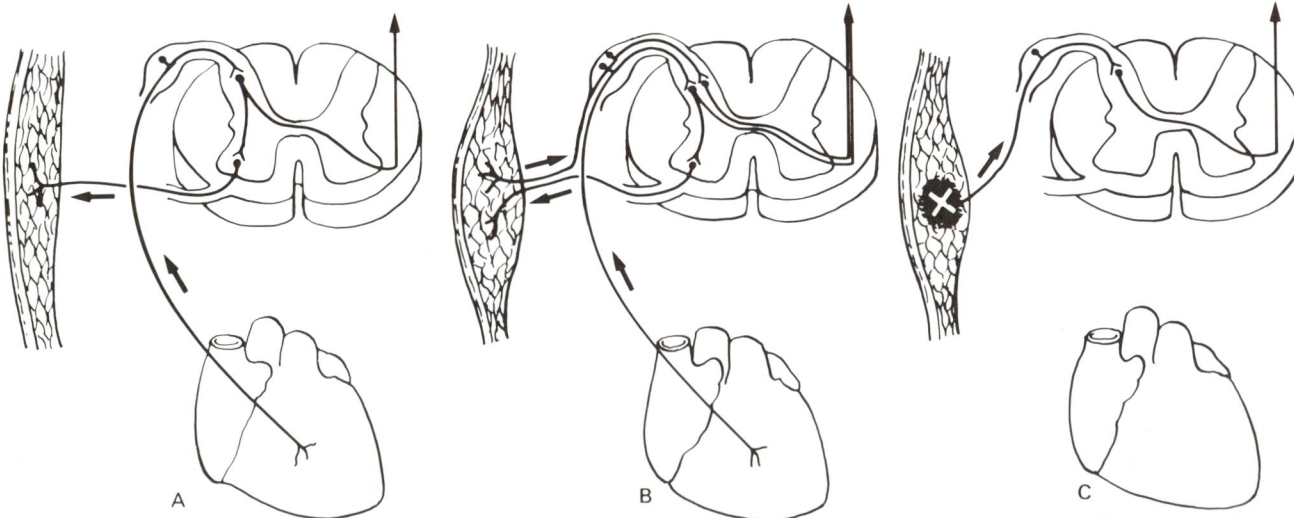

FIG. 54-3. Sequence of development of somatic components of cardiac pain. **A.** Nociceptive afferent input into dorsal horn causes efferent stimulation of muscles in the chest wall, which leads to muscle spasm. **B.** Muscle spasm acts as a new source of noxious input that produces trigger areas, and thus a vicious cycle develops. **C.** Nociceptive input from muscle continues after healing of the heart lesion. Injection of trigger areas with a local anesthetic eliminates the pain.

that many of these afferent fibers respond to brady-kinin and to ischemia, as well as to various mechanical stimuli (50, 51). As noted in Chapter 53, however, these are not involved in nociception, because cutting the vagi has no effect on responses to noxious stimuli (52). Clinical and laboratory evidence acquired since 1925 provides impressive testimony that nociceptive information is transmitted primarily by sympathetic afferents (28, 39, 53, 54), which are also involved in reflexes that control cardiovascular homeostasis. Vagal afferents may transmit information that provokes the tightness of the throat and a feeling of strangling during myocardial ischemia, and may also play a role in modulation of cardiac pain (see next section, Central Mechanisms).

Roughly equal numbers of myelinated A-delta and unmyelinated C fibers run in the cardiac sympathetic nerves; both types are spontaneously active when blood pressure and cardiac hemodynamics are normal (48, 55–57). Moreover, they manifest good response to blunt probing and mechanical deformation of the heart or surrounding structures. Some of these units have small receptive fields consisting of a single zone under 2 mm^2, while others have multiple zone fields that include the heart and adjacent structures (48, 56, 57). Most units have receptive fields located in the atria, ventricles, epicardium, coronary arteries and pericardium, aorta, pulmonary artery and veins, or visceral and parietal pleura (48, 56–61).

Single-unit recordings from white rami communicantes or dorsal roots of the thoracic sympathetics to the heart have shown that, during coronary occlusion, the activity of A-delta and C fibers increases significantly (48, 52, 61, 62). The responses of many A-delta units are slow (mean, 80 seconds), appear to depend on myocardial stretching, and have spontaneous active discharge that occurs in synchrony with cardiac rhythm (48, 57). Moreover, sympathetic afferent activity increases when the pressure within the heart increases (48, 57, 58). Responses of most C-fiber units are quicker, with a latency of 10 to 20 seconds following coronary occlusion, and the resulting irregular firing is unrelated to mechanical factors or to cardiac rhythm (48). Serotonin, histamine, bradykinin, and acids markedly excite both C and some A-delta sympathetic afferents (63–70), and the effects of bradykinin are markedly enhanced by prostaglandins (64, 71). These characteristics, observed by many (48, 52, 56, 58–70), have led to the proposal that most A-delta and a few C fibers are primarily mechanoreceptive in function and are concerned with the reflex regulation of circulation, while most C fibers and a few A-delta fibers are "nociceptors."

It has been suggested that cardiac pain is produced by the release of these humoral (algogenic) agents, from ischemic myocardial muscles, which sensitize or frankly activate the terminals of these sympathetic afferents (67, 68). Because bradykinin and prostaglandins are formed and released in heart muscles following ischemia (68–70), and because prostaglandins have been shown to potentiate the algogenic effects of bradykinin in other tissues (Chapter 4), it is thought that angina results from the excitation of afferent terminals by the joint release of prostaglandins and bradykinin (71). Serotonin, which could originate from

platelets accumulated and destroyed in the ischemic myocardium and histamine, has been shown to stimulate cardiac sympathetic afferents (66).

On the basis of these responses, many (52, 56, 58–64, 66, 72) have considered that most C and some A-delta fibers are specific cardiac nociceptor afferent units. This is based on animal studies that suggested two types of cardiac sympathetic afferents (72). One type is comprised of low-threshold A-delta or C fibers excited by abnormal bulging or stretching of the ventricular wall and consistently involved with cardiovascular reflexes that accompany cardiac failure. The second type is comprised of C-afferent fibers activated only by chemical substances released by ischemic myocardium and associated with pseudoaffective responses indicative of pain, but not activated by stimuli that do not evoke pain or nociceptive reflexes, even if these stimuli are abnormal and outside the physiologic range (72).

Among the early investigators were Brown and Malliani (73), who in 1971 noticed a recruitment of afferent sympathetic fibers during coronary occlusion, suggesting the existence of specific cardiac nociceptors. They later realized, however, that the results were obtained in animals with a transsected spinal cord and with a low baseline arterial pressure, so the hemodynamic factors were probably below the threshold for some mechanosensitive endings. These findings prompted Malliani and co-workers (48, 74) to review their earlier data and to carry out studies in conscious animals. As a result of those studies they now dispute the existence of specific cardiac nociceptors (48, 74). They base their contention on the fact that, to fulfill the criteria for a specific nociceptive function, afferent sympathetic fibers should normally be devoid of spontaneous impulse activity, unresponsive to physiologic hemodynamic events but conversely able to be excited during other stimulation, with possible pathophysiologic significance. They pointed out that all cardiac sympathetic afferents have some degree of mechanosensitivity that produces tonic impulse activity when the hemodynamic conditions are in the normal range, showing a clear response to normal hemodynamic stimuli.

Whereas Malliani and others noted that induction of coronary occlusion or administration of chemical substances suspected of involvement in the genesis of cardiac pain clearly excited the ventricular sympathetic afferent fibers, a recruitment of silent fibers was never seen in their studies. They explained the lack of background activity prior to stimulus seen by other authors (56, 58–64, 66) by suggesting that the hemodynamic condition of the experimental animals was so poor that the hemodynamic stimuli were below the threshold of mechanosensitive endings.

Extensive studies in conscious dogs have provided evidence to support this contention (see 48 for refs.). In the first study anesthetized dogs were instrumented with a pressure catheter covered by an inflatable rubber cylinder implanted in the thoracic aorta, which permitted stretching of the vessel without obstructing aortic blood flow. After the dogs had recovered from surgery the aortic diameter was increased nearly 10% by inflating the implanted cannula. This produced a significant increase in the mean aortic pressure without evoking any overt pain reaction.

In another study bradykinin was injected into a coronary artery 3 days after the animal had recovered from surgery and anesthesia, which produced a reflex rise in heart rate and arterial pressure together with a pain reaction characterized by vocalization, agitation, and struggling. Injection of the same or even larger dose 3 weeks after the surgery, however, produced a pressure response but no pain reaction. It was concluded that the early response was the result of interaction between trauma caused by the recent surgery and visceral stimulus, which disappeared as the animal recovered.

On the basis of these and other observations, Malliani and associates dispute the presence of specific nociceptors, thus casting into doubt the specificity theory in regard to cardiac pain. Indeed, the data also seem to detract from the "intensive theory" (Chapter 1). As a result, a modified version of the intensive theory was proposed as a working hypothesis: cardiac pain can result from the extreme excitation of a spatially restricted population of afferent sympathetic fibers: hence from an afferent code based on a peculiar spatiotemporal pattern. To cite Malliani (75), "More explicitly, an intense excitation of afferent sympathetic fibers would be more likely to reach the effectiveness of a nociceptive code when characterized by spatial heterogeneity. Thus, besides the extension and severity of ischemia, which would determine the background of the afferent excitation, further crucial stimulations of the sensory endings could occur in those regions where mechanical stretching is maximal or where an abnormal vasomotion takes place." Conversely, when the activation of the sympathetic afferent fibers is widely distributed, some central modulation can prevent pain perception. This would explain silent (nonpainful) myocardial infarction (see below).

Central Mechanisms

Myocardial ischemia, whether caused by atherosclerotic coronary artery disease or spasm of the artery, produces pain that initially is true visceral pain, felt deep in the chest and described as vague, poorly localized, and aching in character, and frequently radiating to sites outside of the chest, especially the inner aspects of the arms, neck, and occasionally the jaw. The mechanism of true visceral pain has not been precisely defined but it is probably a result of nociceptive impulses passing to the upper thoracic spinal cord, where they excite cell bodies of spinothalamic tract (STT) neurons and possibly the neurons of other ascending systems. Although STT cells that respond to visceral nociceptive impulses but not to cutaneous inputs have not been found, clinical evidence suggests that this is the mechanism for true visceral pain (72).

The mechanisms of "referred" visceral pain are discussed in Chapter 7. Some experimental studies concerning the neuropathophysiology of the referred pain produced by myocardial ischemia have been carried out. Foreman and associates (76–81), the foremost investigators in this field, have studied the effects of electrical stimulation of sympathetic afferents, the application of bradykinin into the heart, and noxious stimulation of the skin and muscle and of coronary artery occlusion (CAO) in monkeys. They noted that these all excited high-threshold (HT) and wide dynamic

range (WDR) spinothalamic neurons located primarily in laminae IV and V (68%), but also in laminae VII (24%) and I (8%) of the upper four or five thoracic segments. Of these STT cells, 64% were HT neurons, 26% were WDR neurons, and almost 10% were HT inhibitory neurons. Those in the latter category consisted of cells that were excited by pinch of the skin but inhibited by blowing hair on the skin (77). The following results were obtained: (a) these STT cells respond to A-delta and C, sympathetic afferents but not to A-beta afferents; (b) all the STT cells receive a convergent input from A-delta and C nociceptors in the skin and underlying muscles, as well as from the heart; and (c) the receptive fields of the cutaneous and muscle afferents are located in the ipsilateral upper anterior and lateral chest and in the medial and lateral aspects of the ipsilateral forelimb. In one study it was found that about 40% of STT cells received input from both A-delta and C sympathetic afferents, 50% received only A-delta fiber input, and 10% received only C fiber input (77).

These and other data support the "projection-convergence" theory of Ruch, which is responsible for cardiac pain being felt in the anterior chest and arms (see Chapter 7 for detailed discussion of this and other theories of referred pain). Moreover, it has been shown that neurons in the thalamic nuclei, where the axons of STT cells terminate (Chapter 3), respond to noxious cutaneous input and to noxious stimulation of the viscera. Viscerosomatic convergence has also been found in the somatosensory cortex (Chapter 7) (Fig. 54-4).

Other studies by Foreman and associates are also of great clinical importance. They compared excitation of

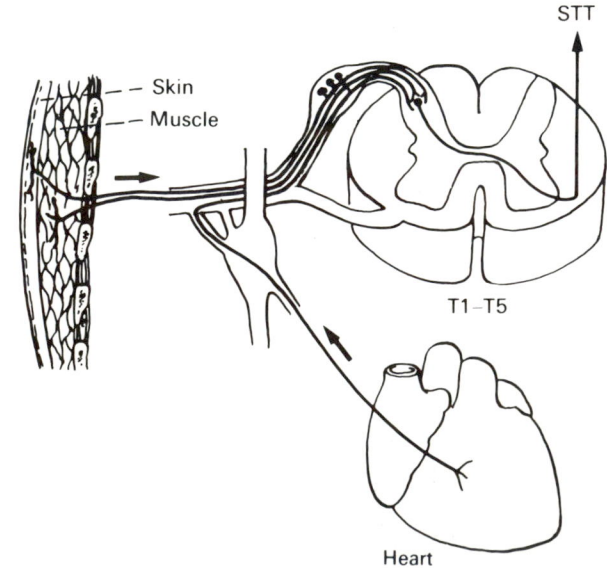

FIG. 54-4. Schematic depiction of the projection-convergence theory of Ruch to explain the mechanism of cardiac pain. Afferent sympathetic fibers from the heart, skin, and muscles converge on the same spinothalamic tract cell and the cell of spinoreticulothalamic tract that transmits the impulses to the lateral and medial thalamus respectively. Since the spinoreticulothalamic tract is a multisynaptic network, it mediates nociceptive impulses slowly and these are perceived as diffuse aching visceral pain. The spinothalamic tract cells project to the lateral thalamus that is concerned with the sensory discriminative function. (See Chapter 3 for details.)

STT neurons in T1 to T5 segments by electrical stimulation of the ansa subclavia and of the superior thoracic splanchnic nerve (78). Splanchnic stimulation excited 63 of 85 T1 to T5 STT neurons in 36 monkeys (78). All these STT neurons have somatic receptive fields and were electrically excited by stimulating the cardiopulmonary sympathetic afferents. STT cells in the more caudal segments and in deeper laminae were more responsive than cells in higher segments and in superficial laminae. This activity from splanchnic afferents stimulation reached T1 to T5 STT neurons by propriospinal pathways and by the sympathetic chain, which has afferents ending in the upper thoracic spinal segments. Distension of the gallbladder with saline solution to levels of 20 to 80 mm Hg excited STT cells in the T1 to T5 segments, with maximal responses obtained at 80 mm Hg; this caused an increase in cell activity from 13 ± 4 impulses/sec (control) to 24 ± 3 impulses/sec during distension (77) (Fig. 54-5). These results demonstrate that increased gallbladder pressure activates upper thoracic STT neurons, and might explain a number of clinical observations of chest pain resulting from gallbladder disease.

Ammons and associates demonstrated that electrical stimulation of the left thoracic vagus nerve caused inhibition of the spontaneous activity of 61% of STT cells in the T1 to T5 segments (79). Moreover, left thoracic vagal stimulation inhibited 100% of the STT cells that responded to noxious somatic stimulation (79). Stimulation of the cardiac vagal branch could produce responses similar to those of left thoracic vagal stimulation, but stimulation of the vagal fibers below the heart could not produce inhibition. Effects of vagal stimulation completely disappeared after the vagi were transsected in the cervical region. Vagal stimulation also inhibited the response of the STT cells to intracardiac injection of bradykinin (79). These results indicate that activation of descending pathways initiated by cardiac or cardiopulmonary vagal afferents is powerful enough to depress cell activity, even when the cell receives noxious input (79). It was also suggested that vagal inhibition of STT neurons was mediated by activation of descending systems that are part of the system for pain modulation (Chapter 4). Stimulation of the nucleus raphe magnus (NRM) inhibited all the STT cells in the upper thoracic segments that responded with an increased discharge to the intracardiac injection of bradykinin (80). It was postulated that the afferent vagal impulses that reach the nucleus of the tractus solitarius (NTS) activate efferent fibers that project to the medial reticular formation and the hypothalamus, which in turn causes stimulation of the NRM (81). It was speculated that this type of interaction explains the "silent" painless myocardial infarction or severe myocardial ischemia with no pain. Thus, under the proper conditions, myocardial ischemia can occur without pain because vagal input into the brain stem powerfully activates descending inhibitory pathways, which in turn reduce the responsiveness of STT cells to the excitatory effects of sympathetic afferent fibers.

These and other studies help to explain the mechanisms of referred pain to the chest, and even to the arms and neck. Possibly an intense afferent barrage produces stimulation of propriospinal fibers, which thus stimulates STT fibers in the cervical region.

It is difficult to elucidate the mechanisms of the spread of myocardial ischemic pain to the lower jaw and teeth. Davis and Pollock (82) suggested that nociceptive impulses that arose in the heart were transmitted by afferent fibers that coursed through the cervical sympathetic chain and from the superior cervical ganglion to the nucleus of cranial nerve V, presumably by the internal carotid nerve and plexus, which are known to communicate with the gasserian ganglion (and other cranial nerves). Clinical observations by White and Sweet (54, 83), however, somewhat disprove this theory; they found that the pain in the jaw and teeth persisted after resection of the superior cervical ganglion, as well as of the super-ficial cervical plexus. White and Sweet (83) reported a small percentage of their patients in whom surgical resection of the upper thoracic ganglia relieved the chest pain but did not relieve pain in the lower jaw. On the basis of this experience, and because others had reported relief of the jaw pain by injection of the mandibular nerve at the foramen ovale with a local anesthetic or alcohol, White and Sweet proposed another hypothesis. They suggested that activity of vagal afferents from the heart to the brain stem provokes some peripheral reflex mechanism that produces local pain in the trigeminal area. The vagi play no other role in the conduction of cardiac pain, but they probably transmit the sense of tightness in the throat and sense of oppression felt by some patients in the suprasternal region after complete sympathetic denervation of the heart. Thus, the sense of tightness, choking, and strangling,

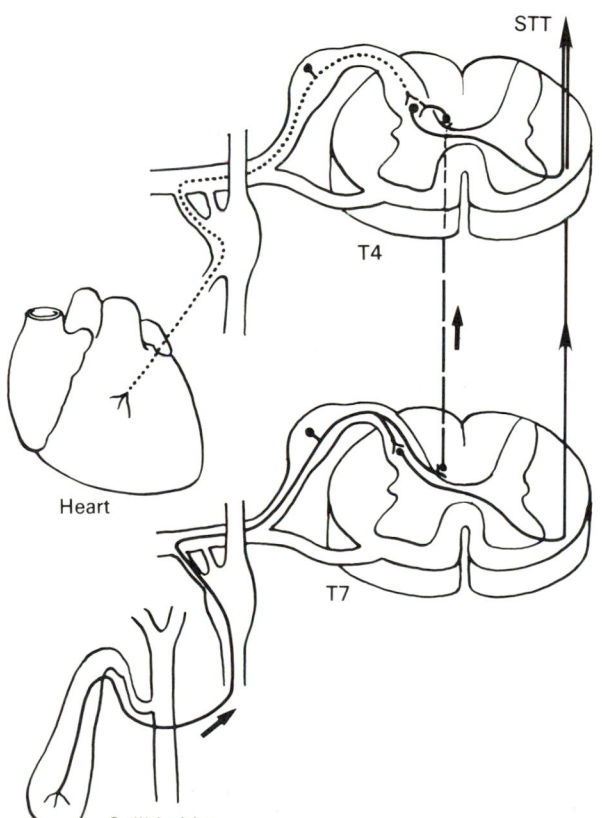

FIG. 54-5. Schematic depiction of the mechanism of pain caused by disease of the biliary tract, referred to the epigastrium and also to the chest. The impulses from the diseased gallbladder pass to the dorsal horn, where they stimulate spinothalamic tract cells of T6–T8. Some of the impulses also ascend through propriospinal fibers in the gray matter to stimulate the cells of the spinothalamic and other ascending tracts in the T5, T4, and higher segments of the thoracic spinal cord. (See text for details.)

which many patients experience as the earliest symptom of angina, might involve activity of afferents in the vagus.

Effects of Myocardial Ischemia and Pain

The pain of acute myocardial ischemia has the important biologic function of signaling to the patient that something is wrong and prompts the patient to limit activity and to seek medical counsel. Once it serves this function, however, it should be promptly relieved, because persistent severe pain and its associated reflex responses can aggravate the myocardial pathophysiology and produce widespread deleterious effects.

Tissue damage from myocardial ischemia and mechanical changes of the ventricles consequent to an acute infarct produce local biochemical changes and stimulate vagal and sympathetic afferents to produce pain and segmental and suprasegmental reflex responses (84). In addition to the excitation of these sympathetic afferents by the algogenic substances that excite and sensitize the sympathetic afferents directly, they can also be stimulated directly by physiologic motion of ischemic myocardium to produce a further increase in sympathetic reflex activity. Cardiac vagal afferents are mechanoreceptors that can also become sensitized after myocardial infarction and provoke abnormal reflexes.

Reflexes elicited by AMI involve afferents and efferents of both cardiac vagi and cardiac sympathetic nerves, which produce symptoms and signs characteristic of vagovagal and sympathosympathetic reflexes (48, 84). Under normal conditions these two extrinsic neurogenic controls of cardiac function have reciprocal neural organization, so that stimulation of sympathetic afferents not only elicits an increased action of sympathetic afferents but also, simultaneously, reduces the discharge of vagal efferents and vice versa. Under pathophysiologic conditions, however, this typical response is disturbed. Consequently, in most AMI patients, both systems are overactive. The one that predominates is determined by many interrelated factors, including the presence and intensity of pain and the size and location of the infarct; sympathetic overactivity predominates in cases of anterior infarction, while parasympathetic overactivity predominates in patients with inferior infarctions (84, 85).

An example of the potential danger of abnormal vagovagal reflexes is the Bezold-Jarisch reflex of severe bradycardia, atrioventricular block, peripheral vasodilation, and consequent severe hypotension. The concurrent sympathetic hyperactivity increases myocardial contractility and can be considered to be an important mechanism for opposing ventricular dilatation and cardiogenic shock. On the other hand, these potentially protective sympathetic reflexes can be detrimental by imposing a demand for increased oxygen consumption on the myocardium (84). Moreover, animal experimental evidence has shown that the alpha-adrenergic portion of the sympathetic nervous system can exert a vasoconstrictor effect on the coronary vessels, with a consequent decrease in both coronary blood flow and myocardial oxygen supply (86, 87). Although evidence in humans is limited, it was found that the vasoconstrictor tone can be augmented to the point of angina in patients with coronary artery disease (88). Laboratory and clinical evidence have also demonstrated the important role that sympathetic hyperactivity can play in the pathophysiology of myocardial infarction (89, 90) and fatal cardiac arrythmia (91, 92). In addition to the sympathosympathetic reflexes, stimulation of sympathetic afferents by mediation of nociceptive (pain) impulses can elicit widespread cardiac, vascular, and hormonal changes.

The afferent barrage of impulses to the neuraxis produces segmental, suprasegmental, and cortical responses (Chapter 7). *Segmental (spinal) reflexes* often can enhance nociception and produce alteration of ventilatory, circulatory, gastrointestinal, and urinary functions. Thus stimulation of somatomotor cells results in increased skeletal muscle tension, which decreases chest wall compliance and initiates a positive feedback loop that generates nociceptive impulses from the muscles. The segmental sympathosympathetic reflexes increase the heart rate and stroke volume and consequently, the cardiac workload and myocardial oxygen consumption, which might increase the risk of cardiac arrythmia. Moreover, if coronary constriction develops in vessels perfusing myocardial tissue adjacent to the affected myocardial muscle, it can make previously healthy myocardial tissue ischemic and previously ischemic tissue necrotic. In addition, sympathetic hyperactivity causes a decrease in gastrointestinal tone that can progress to ileus and a decrease in urinary function that reduces urinary output.

Suprasegmental reflex responses result from nociceptively induced stimulation of the medullary centers of ventilation and circulation, hypothalamic (predominantly sympathetic) centers, neuroendocrine function, and limbic structures. These responses consist of hyperventilation, increased neural sympathetic tone, and increased secretion of catecholamines and other catabolic hormones (e.g., cortisol, ACTH, glucagon), and a concomitant decrease in anabolic hormones (e.g., insulin, progesterone) (Chapter 7). This type of endocrine secretion, characteristic of the stress response, produces widespread metabolic effects, including increased levels of blood glucose, plasma cyclic AMP, free fatty acids, blood lactates, and ketones, as well as a generalized increase in metabolism and oxygen consumption. The endocrine and metabolic changes result in substrate transfer from storage to central organs and injured tissue, leading to a catabolic state and negative nitrogen balance. Moreover, the intense anxiety and fear that invariably develops in AMI patients, through cortical stimulation, greatly enhances the hypothalamic responses characteristic of stress, and can cause a cortically mediated increase in blood viscosity, clotting time, fibrinolysis, and platelet aggregation (Chapter 7).

Thus, it would seem obvious that segmental and suprasegmental sympathetic reflexes, anxiety, and psychologic stress greatly increase the workload of the heart and its oxygen consumption. Moreover, increased blood clotting times and possibly coronary vasoconstriction can further decrease blood flow in the already compromised arteriosclerotic coronary circulation and markedly increase the discrepancy between the oxygen supply and the oxygen demand, which may lead to further ischemia and possibly expanding the infarction. One or more of these responses can be a critical factor in causing the death of the patient. Therefore it is essential to relieve the pain, anxiety, and mental stress and decrease or eliminate the abnormal reflexes promptly and effectively. (See Chapter 94 for special techniques to achieve these objectives).

B. GENERAL CLINICAL CONSIDERATIONS OF CORONARY HEART DISEASE

Classification of Myocardial Ischemia Syndromes

Manifestations of myocardial ischemia can be classified according to clinical presentation, pathologic anatomy, and pathophysiology. I call these "syndromes" because often the pathophysiology is incompletely understood, especially in regard to sudden cardiac death (Table 54-2). The definitions in Table 54-2 are general statements designed to fit most cases; exceptions may occur.

Etiology and Pathophysiology of Coronary Artery Disease

Etiology

This discussion concentrates on atherosclerotic coronary artery disease because it accounts for 95% or more of patients with a myocardial ischemia syndrome caused by coronary artery disease. Myocardial ischemia can occur in the absence of anatomic coronary artery disease because of abnormal vasoreactivity (spasm) or of marked myocardial hypertrophy. The most common pathophysiologic substrate for myocardial ischemia in patients with normal coronary arteries is severe ventricular hypertrophy such that the myocardium outgrows its blood supply (e.g., aortic stenosis, severe hypertension, hypertrophic cardiomyopathy). Although the pathology is different the underlying biochemical mechanisms, symptoms, and electrocardiographic abnormalities are often similar to those of ischemia resulting from coronary artery disease. Similarly, not all coronary artery disease is caused by atherosclerosis. Coronary spasm, the causes of which are poorly understood, is discussed later in this chapter.

Syphilis can produce obstruction at the origins of the coronary arteries (Fig. 54-6) through extension of the aortitis to the coronary ostia; the myocardial ischemic syndrome is the same as if the obstruction were produced by atherosclerosis. Collagen vascular diseases can produce obstruction of the coronary arteries, usually smaller vessels, through an arteritis. Kawasaki's disease, a periarteritis-like disease of infants, can produce aneurysms of coronary arteries and other medium-sized arteries. Congenital anomalies of the coronary arteries can also produce myocardial ischemia; the most serious of these are the origin of a coronary artery from the pulmonary artery and the anomalous origin of the left coronary artery from the right coronary sinus with passage between the aorta and pulmonary artery.

Dissection of the aorta can produce acute occlusion of a coronary artery if the dissecting hematoma extends proximally to include the orifice of a coronary artery (see below). Acute coronary occlusion caused by embolism can occur with endocarditis or in patients with prosthetic aortic valves. Rarely, blunt chest trauma, such as with a steering wheel injury, can produce damage to a coronary artery, usually the left anterior descending artery. Rarely, coronary artery obstruction is caused by iatrogenic intimal damage by a catheter or cannula; this has been observed in coronary arteriography, coronary angioplasty, and aortic valve replacement, in which the coronary arteries are often perfused with a cannula.

Pathophysiology

Atherosclerosis involves the proliferation of smooth muscle cells, the deposition of cholesterol and other lipids, and the laying down of collagen just below the intima of medium-sized and large arteries. In large

TABLE 54-2. Classification of Myocardial Ischemia Syndromes

Syndrome	Clinical Presentation	Pathoanatomy	Pathophysiology
Stable angina	Exertional chest pain	Atherosclerotic coronary stenosis ≥50%	Provoked by increase in myocardial oxygen demand
Unstable angina	Chest pain at rest	Usually atherosclerotic coronary stenosis ≥90%; rarely, normal coronaries	Reduction in coronary blood flow by normal vasoreactivity, spasm, or partially occluding thrombus
Acute myocardial infarction			
Q-wave infarction	Severe unprovoked chest pain	Atherosclerotic coronary stenosis completely occluded by thrombus	Precipitating event unknown; possibly rupture of plaque, platelet aggregation, hemorrhage into plaque, or all three
Non-Q-wave infarction	Severe unprovoked chest pain	Atherosclerotic coronary stenosis ≥90%	Reduction in coronary blood flow by normal vasoreactivity, spasm, or partially occluding thrombus
Silent myocardial ischemia	Ischemic ST changes without pain	Uncertain; probably atherosclerotic coronary stenosis ≥50%	Defect in pain recognition versus subclinical ischemic episodes
Sudden cardiac death	Cardiac arrest	Atherosclerotic coronary disease plus myocardial damage from infarction	Unknown; possibly ventricular premature beats or ventricular tachycardia deteriorating to ventricular fibrillation

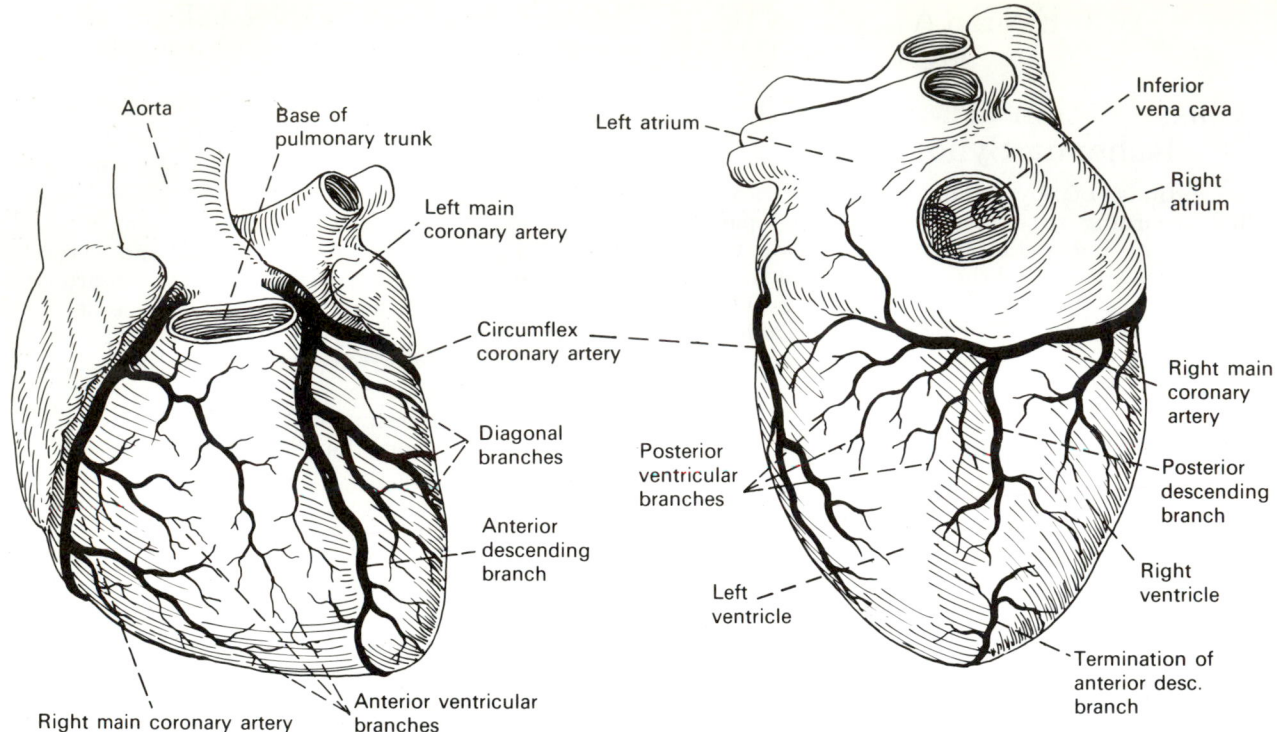

FIG. 54-6. Anatomy of the coronary arteries and their branches. **A.** Anterior view. **B.** A posterior diaphragmatic view.

arteries the atherosclerotic process can damage the media and result in the formation of aneurysms, as occurs commonly in the abdominal aorta. In medium-sized arteries the atherosclerotic process more commonly results in obstruction through the heaping up of the atheroma to impinge on the vessel lumen, as in the coronary and cerebral arteries. Development of atheroma probably begins in childhood and usually takes 30 to 50 years to progress to the stage at which clinical manifestations are produced.

The pathogenesis of atherosclerosis has been the subject of intense research activity for the past 40 years, but the basic pathophysiologic mechanisms are still largely speculative. Three hypotheses have been proposed: the response to injury hypothesis, proposed by Ross and Glomset (93); the monoclonal hypothesis of Benditt and Benditt (94), who proposed that the atheroma is essentially a benign tumor; and the lipogenic hypothesis, which emphasizes altered lipid metabolism. Presently the response to injury hypothesis seems best able to explain the available epidemiologic and biochemical data (Fig. 54-7). According to this theory, the endothelium is damaged by any of various noxious stimuli (e.g., mechanical forces, hyperlipidemia, homocysteine, immunologic factors, toxins, such as those from cigarette smoke, or viruses, resulting in abnormal permeability or even denudation (Fig. 54-7A). If the stimulus ceases, healing of the intima can occur (Fig. 54-7B and C). If the intimal injury is sufficiently severe or prolonged, however, transudation of lipids occurs together with migration of abnormal cells (smooth muscle cells and macrophages) into the subintimal region (Fig. 54-7 D and E). Platelets can adhere to the damaged intima and release a mitogenic

substance, platelet-derived growth factor, which stimulates proliferation of the smooth muscle cells in the atheroma. As the process continues collagen is laid down and cholesterol and its esters are taken up by cells in the lesion (Fig. 54-7F). This hypothesis is attractive because it takes into account the effects of most of the known risk factors but is not dependent on altered lipid metabolism, which is apparently normal in a substantial number of patients with coronary artery disease.

General Principles of Diagnosis
Importance of the History

The patient's history is the single most important diagnostic tool in the evaluation of coronary artery disease. The nature, frequency, and precipitating factors of the pain constitute the most useful information obtained from the history. In the vast majority of patients with angina pectoris the diagnosis can be made from the history alone, providing that proper history-taking skills are combined with a knowledge of the wide variation in symptoms that can occur. By its nature, ischemic myocardial pain is vague, diffuse, and ill-defined—hence, the "visceral nature." Many patients find it difficult to describe such vague symptoms; this is the setting in which directed yes or no questions can easily result in an incorrect data base. The importance of initiating the history taking with nondirected questions cannot be overemphasized. "Tell me about what brings you to see me today" or "Tell me about what troubles you," are examples of nondirected questions. The question "Do you have chest pain?"

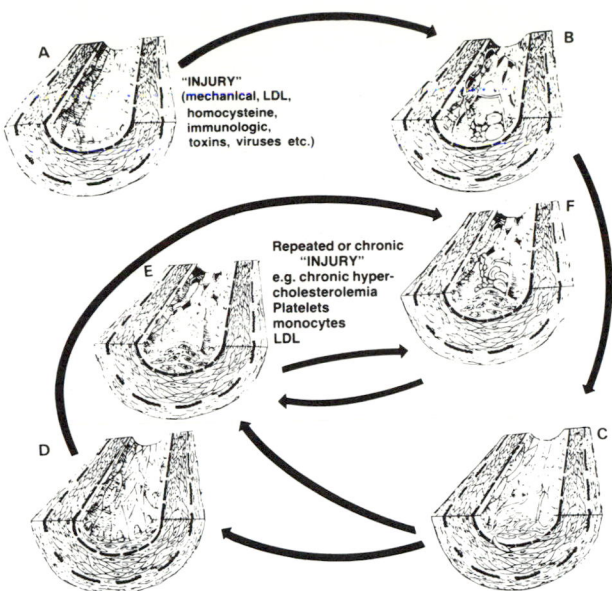

FIG. 54-7. Modified version of the response-to-injury hypothesis of atherosclerosis. A number of cyclic events can occur. **A–D.** In the outer or regression cycle, injury to the endothelium (**B**) is depicted by separations between endothelial cells or by frank desquamation of the endothelium in which both adherence of platelets and of monocytes or macrophages can occur. If platelet adherence occurs aggregation and release of platelet contents can also take place at such sites, whereas monocytes can go on to enter the tissue either at sites of desquamation or between endothelial cells. **C.** These interactions can be followed by migration of smooth muscle cells from the media into the intima, and by proliferation of these and possible pre-existing intimal smooth muscle cells in response to the released mitogens. **D.** End of the regression cycle. If the lesion is a single event and endothelial integrity is restored, the remnant of the proliferative response can simply be manifested as a somewhat thickened intima. **E.** If the intimal injury is sufficiently severe or prolonged, transudation of lipids occurs together with migration of abnormal cells (smooth muscle cells and macrophages) into the subintimal region. **F.** As the process continues, collagen is laid down and cholesterol and its esters are taken up by cells in the lesion. From Ross, R.: Atherosclerosis: A problem of the biology of arterial wall cells and their interactions with blood components. Arteriosclerosis, *1*:295, 1981.

invariably produces an affirmative response, because everyone has chest pain at one time or another.

It is useful to quantify the amount of exertion required to precipitate pain in patients with exertional angina. Even though the exertion required might vary within the same patient, a classification based on the level of precipitating activity is useful in assessing the severity of the disease, the patient's disability, the effects of therapy, and progression of the disease. The guidelines of the Canadian Cardiovascular Society for classifying angina are particularly useful because they were designed specifically for angina (95).

Class 1. Angina occurs only with strenuous or rapid or prolonged exertion at work or recreation. Ordinary physical activity such as walking or climbing stairs does not cause angina.

Class 2. Angina results in slight limitation of ordinary activity. It can be produced by walking or climbing stairs rapidly, walking uphill, walking or stair climbing after meals, exercise in cold or during emotional distress, or exercise in the first hours after awakening.

Class 3. Angina results in marked limitation of ordinary physical activity. It can be produced by walking one or two blocks on the level or climbing one flight of stairs in normal conditions and at a normal pace.

Class 4. Angina results in the inability to carry on any physical activity without discomfort. Angina can be present at rest.

Ischemic myocardial pain can be located anywhere between the diaphragm and mandible (Fig. 54-1); most often it is initially retrosternal (true visceral pain), but soon involves the anterior chest and radiates to both arms, neck, and occasionally the jaw.

Physical Examination

The physical examination is often overlooked as an important and useful diagnostic tool in patients with coronary heart disease because it is so often normal. Nevertheless, a careful physical examination is essential, even for the negative information it produces. Reversible risk factors for atherosclerosis can be detected by identifying hypertension, xanthomas of hyperlipidemia, or nicotine stains caused by cigarette smoking. The adequacy of myocardial function can be assessed by examining for evidence of congestive heart failure, such as elevated jugular venous pressure, pulmonary rales, gallop rhythm, cardiomegaly, and peripheral edema. Severe complications of AMI such as mitral regurgitation or ruptured interventricular septum are suspected by their murmurs. Noncoronary causes of myocardial ischemia, such as aortic valve disease or idiopathic hypertrophic subaortic stenosis, are usually detected easily on physical examination.

Routine Laboratory Studies

Routine laboratory studies are often normal, but still important, like the physical examination. Severe anemia must be excluded as a cause of angina. Diabetes as a risk factor for atherosclerosis needs to be identified and treated. Assessment of renal function is essential, particularly in patients being considered for coronary arteriography or coronary artery bypass surgery. The importance of measurement of serum lipid levels in patients with manifest coronary artery disease is still being debated because little evidence has been found to indicate that lowering serum lipid levels can reverse the atheroma once severe atherosclerosis has caused arterial obstruction. Certainly, patients with a strong family history or those with premature coronary artery disease should have a measurement of the fasting serum cholesterol level.

More sophisticated analyses for high- and low-density lipoproteins are primarily research tools at this time. Measurement of serum lipid levels during an acute event such as myocardial infarction or unstable angina is of little value because the stress of the event alters the lipid patterns. The serum enzymes creatine kinase and lactic dehydrogenase and their isoenzyme patterns are particularly useful in detecting myocardial necrosis and are discussed further below (see Acute Myocardial Infarction).

Resting Electrocardiogram

The resting ECG is a most cost-effective tool in the evaluation of coronary heart disease patients, providing that its limitations are recognized. It is frequently normal in patients with angina but no previous myocardial infarction. In the early phases of AMI it can also be normal or nonspecific. One of the more powerful noninvasive predictors of mortality in patients with coronary artery disease is ST-segment depression on the resting ECG (96), which can indicate ischemia under resting conditions. Increased QRS voltage and ST-segment or T-wave changes indicating left ventricular hypertrophy are also powerful predictors of survival (96). Finally, a number of studies have shown that ventricular arrhythmia in patients with coronary heart disease, particularly those with left ventricular dysfunction, is an indicator of increased risk of sudden cardiac death (96–98). The ECG is essential in the diagnosis of AMI and in the assessment of the arrhythmic complications of infarction (see Acute Myocardial Infarction, below).

Chest Roentgenogram

Most patients with coronary artery disease and preserved left ventricular function have normal cardiovascular structures on the chest roentgenogram. The primary value of the chest roentgenogram is in the assessment of heart failure. Important signs of heart failure are cardiomegaly, pleural effusions, redistribution of the pulmonary venous pattern to the upper lobes, and signs of interstitial edema and dilated lymphatics (Kerley's B lines). The physical examination is notoriously insensitive in detecting cardiac enlargement; although less sensitive than echocardiographic or angiographic techniques, the chest roentgenogram is a cost-effective way of assessing cardiac chamber enlargement. Furthermore, the heart size on the chest roentgenogram is an important prognostic indicator (99). In the absence of severe valvular regurgitation an inverse relationship between left ventricular size and ejection fraction (fraction of end-diastolic volume ejected with each beat) can be seen (100). Thus, significant left ventricular enlargement in the absence of valvular regurgitation is almost always associated with severe, chronic left ventricular dysfunction; the status of left ventricular systolic function is one of the two most powerful predictors of survival in patients with coronary artery disease (96).

Calcification of the coronary arteries is an uncommon finding on the chest roentgenogram but almost always indicates severe coronary atherosclerosis and often obstruction. Calcification seen in the region of the left ventricle can represent a calcified thrombus in a ventricular aneurysm. The chest roentgenogram is insensitive in the detection of left ventricular aneurysms, but deviation of the midportion of the left ventricular silhouette superiorly and to the left on the posteroanterior film can be a sign of an anterolateral aneurysm.

Special Tests

Exercise Stress Test

DIAGNOSTIC USEFULNESS. The exercise ECG is better called the exercise stress test because some of the more valuable information is derived not from the ECG but from other physiologic responses to exercise and the maximum exercise capacity. The exercise stress test has been the traditional noninvasive method for evaluating patients with chest pain syndromes, and has been used more recently as a useful indicator of subsequent risk following AMI. The exercise stress test is frequently misused, however, either because the wrong questions are asked about it or because attention is focused on the ECG and the other important data available are overlooked.

The value of the exercise stress test lies primarily in the diagnosis of the presence or absence of coronary artery disease and the assessment of prognosis in patients with known coronary artery disease. The stress test is also useful for assessing disability and evaluating the results of therapy. In males with a history of typical angina pectoris the probability is 90% that significant obstructive atherosclerotic coronary artery disease is present on coronary arteriography (101). In these patients the exercise test adds almost nothing to establishing a diagnosis of angina caused by atherosclerotic coronary artery disease.

The application of Bayes' theorem has been useful in deciding which patients are most likely to have the benefit of greater assuredness of diagnosis from the addition of exercise stress testing to the history, physical examination, and routine laboratory data, including the resting ECG (102). Patients whose pre-test probability of coronary artery disease is in the intermediate range benefit most diagnostically from the performance of the test; examples of such patients would be a middle-aged man with several risk factors for coronary heart disease and a chest pain syndrome not typical of angina pectoris and a premenopausal woman with typical angina pectoris. In both of these examples the probability of coronary artery disease causing the symptoms from the information given is in the range of 30 to 60%.

An exercise stress test with ST-segment depression $\geqslant 1$ mm significantly increases the probability of finding a significant coronary artery obstruction on angiography, whereas no significant ST-segment depression at maximal exercise significantly reduces this probability. In patients in whom the history and other data obtained prior to the exercise test provide a high degree of certainty regarding the diagnosis (i.e., the pretest probability of obstructive coronary artery disease is either extremely high or extremely low), exercise stress testing is not indicated for the sole purpose of establishing the diagnosis. For example, in the male with typical angina who has a pretest probability of obstructive coronary disease of >90%, a positive ST-segment response on exercise testing increases this probability only minimally, whereas a negative ST-segment response in no way excludes obstructive coronary artery disease.

ASSESSMENT OF PROGNOSIS. Exercise testing is also important for assessing the severity of disease, assessing prognosis, and evaluating the results of therapy. Many patients with angina whose diagnosis is clear from the history and resting ECG should have exercise stress testing to assess the severity of the disease, to provide an estimate of the likelihood of future cardiac events, and to aid in determining the need for coronary arteriography. Whereas the ST segment response to exertion is the most commonly used diagnostic criterion (usually depression ≥ 1 mm), the ST segment has more limited usefulness in the assessment of prognosis. In an analysis of patients in the Seattle Heart Watch Coronary Arteriography Registry, we found that the duration of exercise or maximal workload achieved, maximum heart rate, and maximum systolic blood pressure were the most powerful predictors of prognosis in patients with known coronary artery disease (96). In a multivariate analysis, the pressure-rate product (the product of maximal systolic pressure and maximal heart rate during exercise) included all the prognostic information available in the exercise test. In other studies marked ST-segment depression (≥ 2 mm) has been shown to be a useful prognostic indicator (2).

Radionuclide Imaging

Radionuclide imaging of the heart has been useful both in establishing the diagnosis and in assessing prognosis (103). Two techniques are in common clinical use: imaging of the myocardium with thallium-201 and imaging of the cardiac chambers, particularly the left and right ventricles, with technetium-99m tagged to red blood cells.

THALLIUM MYOCARDIAL IMAGING. Thallium is similar to potassium in that it is concentrated intracellularly; following IV injection it is taken up by viable cells, particularly myocardial cells. Areas of myocardium replaced by scar as a result of myocardial infarction do not take up thallium; similarly, viable cells whose metabolic functions have been disturbed by ischemia also do not take up thallium in a normal fashion. When the ischemia has been corrected, such as after an anginal episode, the cells once again take up thallium. These pathophysiologic principles are the basis of rest-exercise thallium myocardial imaging.

Patients are usually exercised with a standard treadmill protocol. At the time of development of angina or shortly before maximal exercise has been achieved, the thallium is injected through a peripheral vein. Imaging of the myocardium commences immediately with a standard gamma camera or with a tomographic system, such as single photon emission computed tomography (SPECT). If an area of myocardium was supplied by a significantly stenotic coronary artery, it becomes transiently ischemic because the restricted coronary flow cannot keep up with the increased metabolic demands; this area does not take up thallium and is visualized as a defect on the image obtained immediately on completion of exercise. With rest, however, normal metabolic function returns to this area of myocardium, allowing it to take up thallium once again. Over a period of several hours the thallium redistributes to the area that showed a defect on the early image; thus, an image obtained 3 or 4 hours after exercise shows normal uptake in the area of the defect on the early image. On the other hand, scar caused by myocardial infarction cannot take up thallium either on the early or late image. To summarize, a thallium defect seen both immediately following exercise and on the late redistribution image indicates myocardial infarction; a defect on the early image that becomes normal on the redistribution image indicates ischemic but viable myocardium.

TECHNETIUM BLOOD POOL IMAGING. Imaging of the blood pool in the cardiac chambers has proven to be a useful noninvasive technique for assessing ventricular function. This technique, sometimes known as multiple gated acquisition (MUGA), divides the cardiac cycle into 20 to 30 short segments, or gates. The image information from several hundred cardiac cycles is summed for each gate, reducing the noise caused by statistical variation in photon release. The resultant series of frames can be played back as a single cycle in a continuous loop or analyzed mathematically in various ways. Among the most useful data are the ejection fraction and the assessment of segmental wall motion. The ejection fraction, the proportion of the end-diastolic volume ejected with each beat, is easily calculated without having to make any geometric assumptions by subtracting the end-systolic counts from the end-diastolic counts and dividing by the end-diastolic counts. The ejection fraction measured at rest is one of the most useful measures of ventricular function because it is the most powerful predictor of survival in patients with coronary heart disease (96), and a resting ejection fraction of less than 0.30 correlates well with clinical congestive heart failure (100).

In subjects with normal cardiac function and normal coronary arteries, the left ventricular ejection fraction increases during exercise as the peripheral resistance decreases and the cardiac output increases. If exercise induces relative myocardial ischemia (as is the case in exertional angina), the involved myocardial segment cannot contract normally during exercise. Thus, blood pool imaging during exercise reveals the development of a segmental wall motion abnormality; also, the ejection fraction falls or fails to increase during exercise. Although the abnormal ejection fraction response to exercise is a sensitive indicator of coronary artery disease it is not specific. Other heart diseases, including valvular disease and hypertension, also show abnormal ejection fraction responses. The development of a new segmental wall motion abnormality during exercise, however, is relatively specific for localized ischemia.

Echocardiography

Imaging of the heart with ultrasound can also provide useful diagnostic and prognostic information regarding coronary heart disease. Two-dimensional echocardiography is much more useful than M-mode (motion mode) echocardiography because the latter can miss abnormal functioning segments. As with thallium and technetium imaging, wall motion abnormalities seen at rest usually represent either myocardial infarction or acute active ischemia. It is technically difficult to obtain echocardiographic images of the heart during exercise because of the increase in respiratory interference, but new wall motion abnormalities have been observed in patients with stress-induced ischemia. Additionally, echocardiography is particularly useful in diagnosing some complications of AMI. It presently is the best technique used clinically for the identification of left ventricular thrombi, with a sensitivity of about 90% (104). Rupture of the papillary muscle or of the interventricular septum, both catastrophic complications of AMI, can usually be diagnosed by echocardiography.

Computed Tomography and Magnetic Resonance Imaging

Computed tomography (CT scanning) has proven to be an exceptionally useful tool in the evaluation of pathology in organs with little or no motion. Because of the time required to acquire the images, however, the motion of the heart blurs the images obtained with conventional CT scanning. Experimental systems using multiple detectors and x-ray sources have been developed, but are expensive and expose the patient to substantial quantities of radiation.

Magnetic resonance imaging (MRI) can be used in a gated fashion as for radionuclide blood pool imaging; the images appear to be of excellent quality and are probably diagnostically useful. At present the expense and small number of MRI units available have limited the use of this procedure to investigational studies. Whether MRI will supplant the use of the much less expensive radionuclide and ultrasound imaging techniques in clinical practice is unclear at this time. Magnetic resonance spectroscopy is finding important research applications in the evaluation of metabolic function of the myocardium.

Cardiac Catheterization and Angiography

Selective coronary arteriography, introduced by Sones in 1959 (105) led to a totally new understanding of coronary anatomic pathology and made possible the development of the coronary artery bypass operation. In this procedure the coronary arteries are selectively cannulated, either with a single catheter, introduced through a brachial arteriotomy (Sones' technique), or with separate preformed catheters for the right and left coronary arteries, introduced percutaneously through the femoral artery in the groin (Judkins' technique). Injection of 3 to 10 ml of iodinated radiographic contrast material and filming the output phosphor of a radiographic image intensifier provide excellent definition of the coronary arteries. Roentgenographic and other equipment required for a modern adult cardiac catheterization laboratory is sophisticated and expensive (approximately $2,000,000). In skilled hands the risk of coronary arteriography is low, even in acutely ill patients such as those with AMI. Kennedy and associates reported on 53,581 patients undergoing cardiac catheterization and found a rate of significant complication of 1.8% (106) and a mortality rate of 0.14% (107). The risk of coronary arteriography is highest in the newborn, the elderly, the acutely ill, and those with severe left ventricular dysfunction.

Selective coronary arteriography is the only procedure currently available that accurately defines the location and severity of coronary arterial obstructions. As such it is an invaluable tool in the evaluation of patients with chest pain syndromes. It is an essential prerequisite to consideration of coronary revascularization. It is useful in patients whose chest pain syndrome cannot be diagnosed noninvasively. In addition, it provides much vital prognostic information, because prognosis is strongly related to the amount of myocardium placed in jeopardy by severe proximal coronary arterial stenoses. The following are some of the present indications for the use of coronary arteriography:

Angina
Patients with angina refractory to medical therapy who are being considered for coronary bypass surgery

Patients with medically controllable angina who exhibit evidence of high risk for coronary event on non-invasive testing:

ST-segment depression ≥ 2 mm

Drop or inadequate increase in blood pressure during exercise

Angina or ST-segment depression at low workload

Patients with angina or other evidence of coronary heart disease, who have high-risk occupation (e.g., airline pilots)

Patients with unstable angina who are otherwise acceptable candidates for coronary artery bypass surgery

Acute myocardial infarction
Patients with acute anterior myocardial infarction seen within 4 hours of onset of symptoms who might be candidates for streptokinase infusion

Patients experiencing spontaneous angina early following an acute myocardial infarction

Patients with angina or ST-segment depression on a low-level exercise test 7 to 10 days after an acute myocardial infarction

Other disorders
Patients over the age of 40 undergoing cardiac catheterization in consideration of valve replacement

Patients with incapacitating chest pain syndromes that cannot be diagnosed using noninvasive techniques

In the last few years coronary arteriography has formed the basis for a whole new specialty, interventional cardiology. Two interventions based on coronary arteriography technique are now in common use (intracoronary infusion of thrombolytic agents and percutaneous coronary transluminal angioplasty), and several other interventions are currently under development, including laser or mechanical removal of atheroma.

C. MYOCARDIAL ISCHEMIC SYNDROMES

Acute Myocardial Infarction (XVII-5)

Approximately 500,000 patients are hospitalized annually with AMI in the United States, and about 350,000 die before reaching the hospital (1). About 60% of deaths caused by AMI occur within 1 hour of onset of symptoms, mostly the result of malignant ventricular arrhythmias and ventricular fibrillation (see below, Sudden Cardiac Death). Many of these "electrical" deaths are preventable with effective antiarrhythmic therapy and defibrillation. The challenge has been to bring medical care to the patient quickly enough, or vice versa. Of patients hospitalized with AMI, about 15% die during hospitalization (most of left ventricular failure) and another 10% die in the first year after hospitalization of recurrent infarction or arrhythmia.

Pathophysiology

Acute myocardial infarction is irreversible myocardial cell death resulting from ischemia. AMI is classified into two types according to the ECG: Q-wave infarction (formerly known as transmural) and non-Q-wave infarction (formerly known as subendocardial). Further classification can be made according to location (Table 54-3), as determined from the ECG. Q-wave infarctions are most often (>80%) the result of total occlusion of a proximal coronary artery by a recent thrombus superimposed on a severe atherosclerotic lesion (108). In non-Q-wave infarctions the artery is usually still partially patent but severely obstructed by an atherosclerotic plaque, with or without superimposed thrombus.

TABLE 54-3. Classification, Pathophysiology, and Electrocardiographic Criteria of Acute Myocardial Infarction

Classification	Coronary Artery	Pathophysiology	Electrocardiographic Findings
Q-wave infarction			
Anterior	Left anterior descending	Complete thrombosis	Q waves in leads V_2 to V_4
Inferior	Right or posterior descending	Complete thrombosis	Q waves in leads II, III, aVF
Posterior	Circumflex	Complete thrombosis	Broad R waves in leads V_1 and V_2
Non-Q-wave infarction	Any	Severe stenosis	ST-segment depression, T-wave inversion, or both

The basic mechanisms leading up to the acute infarction are still controversial. For Q-wave infarctions two main theories have been proposed: (a) hemorrhage into a plaque, causing expansion of the plaque and further obstruction of the lumen; and (b) denuded or damaged endothelium over the plaque, leading to attachment of a platelet thrombus, which in turn leads to more thrombus formation and total occlusion of the artery. In a severely stenotic coronary artery a modest change in diameter from vasomotion or non-occlusive thrombus can result in a marked change in flow; this might be the mechanism of non-Q-wave infarctions.

The pain of AMI can be the result of the release of noxious pain-producing substances and of the abnormal mechanical action that occurs with myocardial segments that cannot shorten (see above, Basic Considerations). Cellular damage caused by the ischemia can result in the liberation of intracellular pain-producing (algogenic) substances such as potassium ions, lactic acid, serotonin, histamine, and bradykinin, all of which excite C-nociceptive afferents directly. The pain fibers can be sensitized by bradykinin (51, 64–66). The A-delta nociceptive afferents can also be stimulated directly by the nonphysiologic motion of the infarcting myocardium, having been sensitized by the algogenic substances (48, 59, 64). Finally, the cardiac vagal and sympathetic afferents can be sensitized by the release of algogenic substances caused by the abnormal motion of the myocardium, resulting in abnormal reflexes (50, 51, 75, 76). In anterior myocardial infarction sympathetic overactivity appears to dominate, while in inferior infarction it is vagal overactivity (84, 85). The latter contributes to the bradycardia, atrioventricular block, and peripheral vasodilation of inferior infarction responding to atropine (Bezold-Jarisch reflex) (84).

Symptoms and Signs

The clinical presentation is usually that of severe oppressive chest pain accompanied by diaphoresis and lasting from 20 minutes to several hours. Up to 50% of patients have a prodrome of intermittent angina-like pain lasting up to several days, but with onset at rest (i.e., unstable angina). The prodromal pain can be so mild or transient that patients do not seek medical attention. Even if they do, and are hospitalized for unstable angina, only about a 15% probability exists of progression to AMI. It is suspected that the pathophysiology might involve the transient closing and opening of the severely stenotic coronary artery, either by platelet plugs, vasomotion, or a combination of both.

The discomfort is sometimes epigastric, accompanied by a desire to belch, and often mistaken by both patient and physician for gastrointestinal upset. The pain can occasionally be interscapular, only in the arms, or only in the mandible. Data from the Framingham study, however, showed that AMI can be clinically silent in approximately 25% of patients, being recognized only on a subsequent ECG obtained for unrelated reasons (109). The reasons for the absence of pain in this large proportion of patients is unknown. It has been said that diabetics are more likely to have painless infarctions, but careful supporting epidemiologic evidence for this statement is lacking. Other commonly associated symptoms are dizziness and weakness from low cardiac output, marked diaphoresis from autonomic discharge, and palpitations or syncope from ventricular arrhythmia.

Despite relatively typical and severe symptoms in most cases, the average delay from onset of symptoms to arrival at a hospital is 1 to 3 hours in a number of studies (1); during this period the acutely ischemic myocardium is most unstable electrically and ventricular fibrillation is most likely to occur. Further patient and public education is needed to make at-risk patients knowledgeable of symptoms and aware of the danger of delay in seeking attention. Physicians must also be prepared to deal with false alarms in emergency rooms and some ultimately unnecessary hospital admissions.

The presenting physical signs can be surprisingly few. Either hypotension from low cardiac output or hypertension from sympathetic discharge can be present. Similarly, either bradycardia from vagal discharge (common in inferior infarction) or heart block or tachycardia from reduced stroke volume or sympathetic stimulation can be observed. In a minority of patients pulmonary congestion can be manifested by tachypnea, dyspnea, rales, or even frank pulmonary edema with frothy sputum. Examination of the heart is often normal; some patients, though, might have an S_3 gallop, a murmur of mitral regurgitation caused by papillary muscle dysfunction, or a precordial bulge reflecting dyskinetic myocardium (left ventricular wall moving outward with systole).

Diagnosis

ELECTROCARDIOGRAPHIC FINDINGS. Although the ECG is sometimes normal in the early phases of AMI, generally the ECG is the most useful, cost-effective diagnostic tool after the history in the initial phases of AMI. The classic electrocardiographic changes in myocardial infarction are shown in Table 54-3. An example of an acute anterior myocardial infarction with Q waves and ST-segment elevation in leads V_1 to V_4 is shown in Figure 54-8. Figure 54-9 shows an example of an old inferior myocardial infarction with Q waves in leads II, III, and aVF. The ST- and T-wave changes alone are not specific for AMI; these are the typical changes of a non-Q-wave-infarction but must be accompanied by serum enzyme level changes to make the definite diagnosis of infarction. The abnormal Q wave is relatively specific for myocardial infarction and a sign of dead or scarred myocardium that cannot generate an electrical field. The Q wave forms the basis for the diagnosis of a remote myocardial infarction from the ECG.

SERUM ENZYMES. The dying myocardial cell releases some of its enzymatic contents into the bloodstream; the detection of these enzymes in serum is diagnostically useful. Creatine kinase (CK) is usually detectable within a few hours of the onset of symptoms, peaks at 12 to 24 hours, and disappears within 48 to 72 hours. It is the most specific of the commonly used enzymes, but is also found in substantial quantities in skeletal muscle, vascular smooth muscle, and brain. The peak value of serum CK following an acute infarction correlates roughly with infarct size and with prognosis; more accurate estimates of infarct size can be obtained by estimating the area under the CK-time curve.

Serum lactate dehydrogenase (LDH) is also commonly used diagnostically; it is first detectable in serum 24 to 48 hours after onset of symptoms, peaks at 3 to 6 days, and shows elevated levels for as long as 8 to 14 days. It is this latter characteristic that makes determination of the serum LDH level useful diagnostically in patients who do not seek medical care for several days after the onset of symptoms. LDH is nonspecific for myocardial necrosis, however, being found in red blood cells, liver, kidney, and skeletal muscle. Analysis of the serum glutamic-oxaloacetic transaminase (SGOT) level, formerly a common diagnostic test, is presently of little diagnostic value because of its lack of specificity and its overlap with CK and LDH.

Separation into isoenzymes has greatly increased the specificity of both the CK and LDH assays. In fact, the finding of the MB isoenzyme of CK in serum is virtually specific for myocardial necrosis. Isoenzyme assays are expensive and overused, though, because the diagnosis is usually clear from the history, ECG, and standard enzyme determinations. Situations in which the CK isoenzyme assay would be particularly useful are out-of-hospital cardiac arrest (where high concentrations of skeletal muscle and liver enzymes are released as a result of the hypoxia and hypotension), alcoholism (liver and skeletal muscle enzymes are often present in the serum), and skeletal muscle trauma, including intramuscular injections, pericarditis, or a recent surgical procedure.

OTHER STUDIES. Imaging of the heart by ultrasound, radioisotopes, or magnetic resonance reveals abnormalities in AMI. They are not commonly used, however, because the diagnosis can almost always be made by the above procedures, and because these more expensive techniques can be nonspecific or unavail-

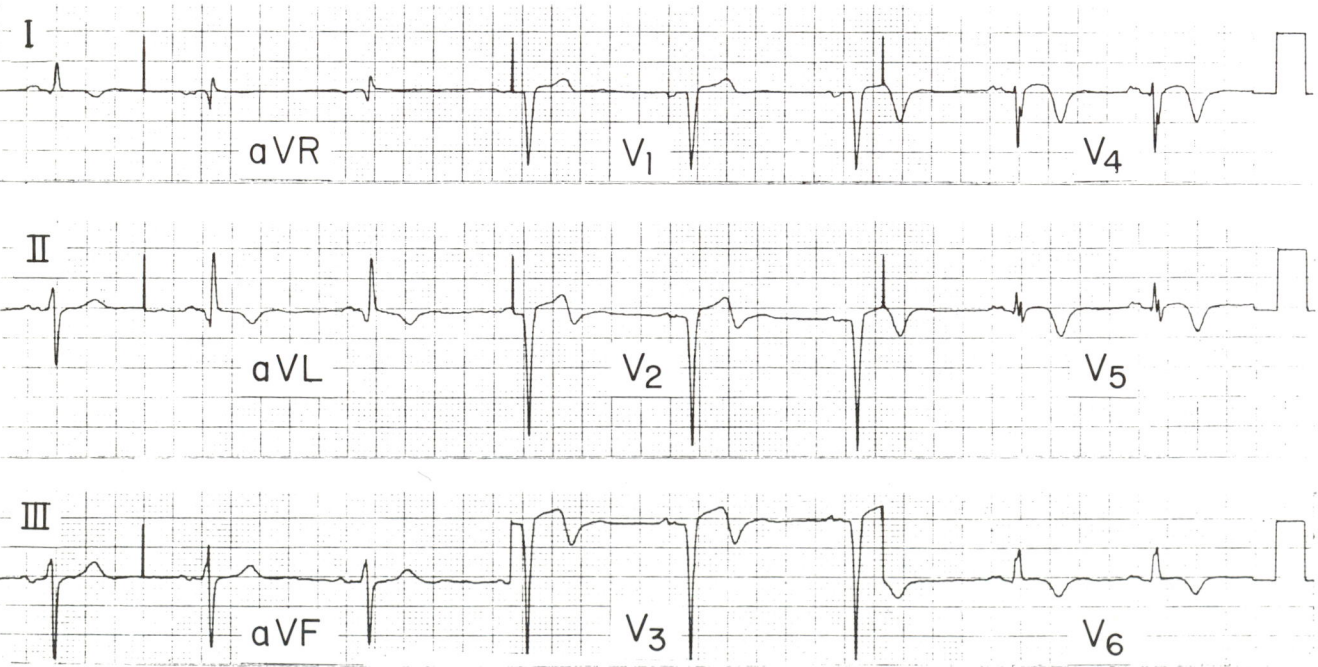

FIG. 54-8. ECG from a patient with recent anterior myocardial infarction showing Q waves in leads V_I to V_3, ST segment elevation in leads V_2 to V_5, and T-wave inversion in leads V_2 to V_6.

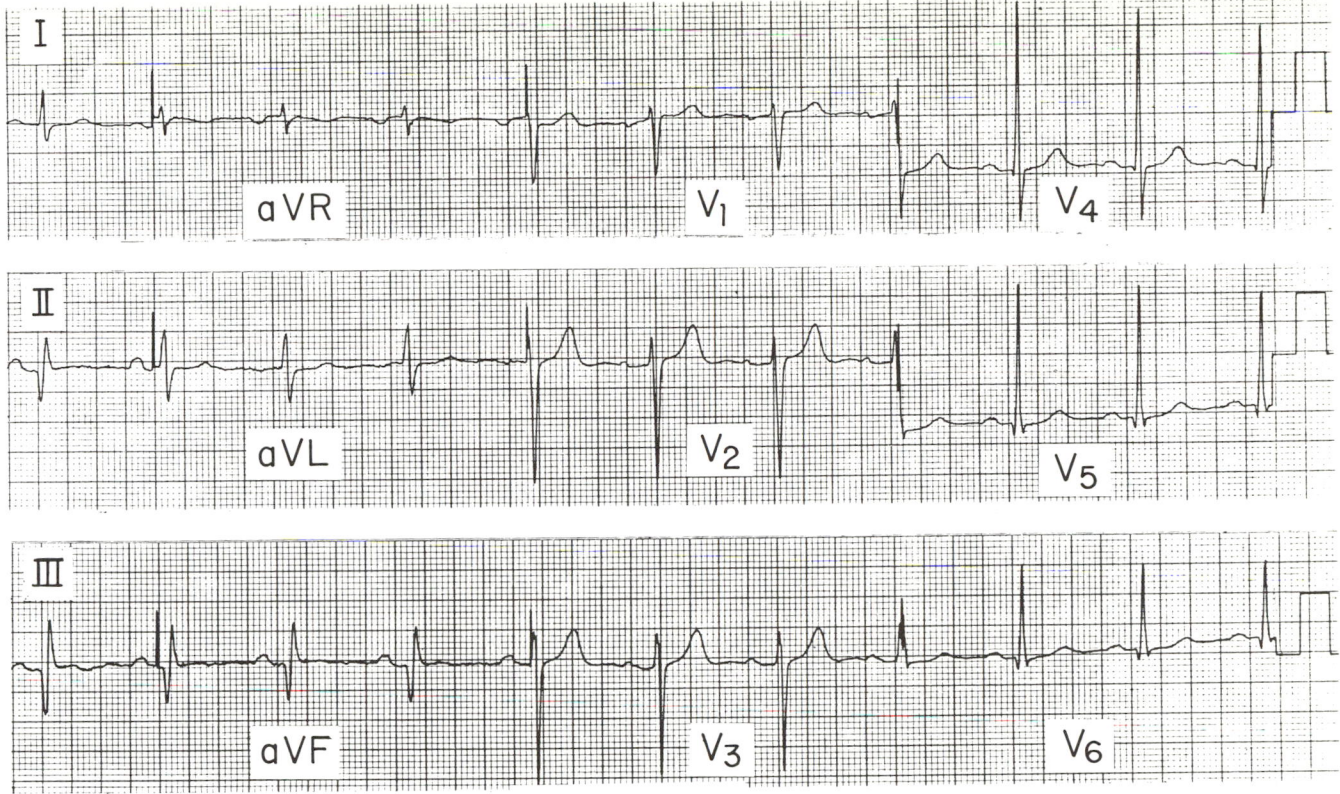

Fig. 54-9. ECG from a patient with an old inferior myocardial infarction showing Q waves in leads II, III, and aVF.

able, except in the research setting. Perhaps, the most useful is technetium-99m pyrophosphate scanning. This is the same radiopharmaceutical used for bone scans; the pyrophosphate complexes with calcium in the bone and carries with it the attached technetium-99m radionuclide. The mechanism of uptake by infarcting myocardial cells is presumably similar to that of uptake by bone. Infarcting myocardial cells collect large amounts of calcium in their mitochondria, to which the technetium-99m pyrophosphate complexes. This technique has its greatest use in patients with an atypical history and a pre-existing electrocardiographic abnormality that precludes a diagnosis (e.g., left bundle branch block or paced rhythm).

Differential Diagnosis

When a complete data base is available (history, ECG, and serum enzymes) the diagnosis is usually not difficult, but the pain is sometimes atypical or even absent in 25% of AMI patients. Other diseases that should be considered in the differential diagnosis are acute pericarditis, mitral valve prolapse, acute pulmonary embolism, aortic dissection (which can cause AMI by occluding the coronary ostium), stable angina, unstable angina, variant (Prinzmetal's) angina, costochondritis and other chest wall pain, esophageal spasm, biliary disease, cervical root compression, and psychosomatic pain. Acute pulmonary embolism can occasionally be particularly difficult to distinguish from AMI because it can produce visceral pain, acute decrease in cardiac output, an autonomic response to

this decrease, and electrocardiographic changes, all of which can resemble those of AMI. Table 54-4 lists some differentiating characteristics for these diagnoses.

Treatment

REPERFUSION. Treatment of AMI is rapidly evolving from a somewhat passive supportive role aimed primarily at prevention and treatment of lethal ventricular fibrillation to an aggressive interventional approach aimed at re-establishing myocardial perfusion and minimizing myocardial necrosis. The primary reasons for the evolution in treatment is the recognition once again (after having ignored for many years Herrick's (25) first description in 1912 of AMI as the result of "sudden obstruction of the coronary arteries") that AMI is most frequently the result of coronary thrombosis (108). Animal studies suggest that if perfusion is restored to acutely ischemic myocardium within 3 to 6 hours of coronary occlusion, some myocardium supplied by the occluded artery can be salvaged.

Three approaches have been tried in humans to restore myocardial blood flow promptly: emergent aortocoronary bypass surgery (ACBS), thrombolytic therapy (TT), and percutaneous transluminal coronary angioplasty (PTCA). Although bypass surgery can be performed in selected patients, and has acceptable morbidity and mortality rates, it has never been adequately scrutinized with a controlled clinical trial; moreover, it is expensive, and is extraordinarily demanding on acute care resources. TT and PTCA singly

TABLE 54-4. Differential Diagnosis of Acute Myocardial Infarction

Diagnosis	Pain Characteristics					
	Quality	Duration	Location	Provocation	Relief	Laboratory Findings
AMI	Visceral, severe	Hours	Thorax	None	Opiates, not Ntg*	ECG: Q waves, ST elevation and T inversion; serum enzyme levels increase
Stable angina	Visceral	Minutes	Thorax	Exercise, emotion	Rest, Ntg	ECG: ST depression; no enzyme level increase
Unstable angina	Visceral	Minutes to hours	Thorax	None	Ntg (sometimes)	ECG: ST depression; no enzyme level increase
Variant angina	Visceral	Minutes to hours	Thorax	None, smoking	Ntg (sometimes)	ECG: ST elevation; no enzyme level increase
Pericarditis	Sharp, positional, pleuritic	Days	Thorax	Motion	Anti-inflammatory agents	ECG: diffuse ST elevation; minimal enzyme level increase possible
Aortic dissection	Severe, sudden onset	Hours	Thorax back, abdomen	Acute motion sometimes	Opiates	Aortography: dissection Radiography: widened mediastinum lowered arterial pressure
Costochondritis	Localized, sharp	Days	Costo-chondral junction	Local pressure	Anti-inflammatory agents	All negative
Esophageal spasm	Visceral	Hours	Epigastrium	Swallowing, supine position	Antacids, Ntg (?)	Manometry: abnormal pressures Radiography: reflux
Cervical root compression	Sharp	Weeks to months	Arm, dermatomal	Neck motion	Difficult	Radiography: narrowing of ostial foramina

*Ntg, nitroglycerin.

and in combination are currently undergoing clinical evaluation in carefully designed randomized trials. In a well-designed randomized trial performed in university and community hospitals in the northwest, the intracoronary administration of streptokinase significantly reduced hospital mortality rates (110). The intracoronary administration of streptokinase is impractical for widespread use, however, because of the enormous demands it places on expensive cardiac catheterization resources 24 hours a day, 7 days a week.

Intravenous administration of thrombolytic agents, alone or in combination with antiplatelet agents, has been shown to significantly reduce the mortality of acute myocardial infarction. A randomized but unblinded trial in Italy with over 12,000 patients showed a statistically significant 18% reduction in mortality with intravenous streptokinase alone (111). Another recently completed trial with 17,000 patients—randomized, blinded, and placebo-controlled—has shown a dramatic 26% reduction in mortality with the combination of 1.5 million units of streptokinase intravenously and oral aspirin 160 mg daily (112). Statistically significant reduction in mortality was seen in the subgroup of patients treated as late as 12 to 24 hours after onset of symptoms. In the subgroup treated within 4 hours of onset of symptoms the reduction in mortality was 37%. Tissue plasminogen activator, a thrombin-specific thrombolytic agent, has been shown to be more effec-tive than streptokinase in re-establishing flow 90 minutes after intravenous administration in a very small (214 patients) randomized trial (113); bleeding complications were similar with the two agents. Tissue plasminogen activator is about 10 times as expensive as streptokinase, however, and has not been shown to reduce mortality because a placebo-controlled trial of appropriate size has not been performed. Large-scale trials to compare streptokinase and tissue plasminogen activator with mortality as an end point are in progress (Spring 1989).

A major unsolved problem following re-establishment of flow by thrombolysis, is that there is usually a severe residual atherosclerotic stenosis with presumably abnormal intima resulting in a substantial reocclusion rate following successful thrombolysis. Both coronary angioplasty and bypass surgery have been used in attempts to prevent reocclusion. A randomized trial comparing angioplasty performed immediately after reperfusion with tissue plasminogen activator with angioplasty performed electively 3 days later showed a higher mortality and complication rate in the early angioplasty group (114). However, there have been no randomized trials comparing survival in patients treated with thrombolytic therapy plus elective angioplasty versus thrombolytic therapy with no angioplasty. To summarize, the survival benefits of intracoronary intravenous streptokinase are well

Table 54-5. Determinants of Myocardial Oxygen Demand and Delivery

Myocardial Oxygen Demand	Myocardial Oxygen Delivery
Heart rate	Coronary blood flow
	Transcoronary pressure gradient
Contractility	Aortic diastolic pressure
	LV diastolic pressure
LV wall stress	Coronary vascular resistance
LV systolic pressure	
LV size (radius)	Oxygen extraction
	Arterial saturation
	Arterial-coronary sinus oxygen
	difference

established by randomized trials; there is further reduction in mortality with the concomitant administration of aspirin. The necessity for angioplasty in myocardial infarction patients not experiencing ongoing ischemia has not been established.

STANDARD THERAPY. Established (but not generally documented to be efficacious by clinical trials) forms of therapy for AMI include hospitalization in a coronary care unit with continuous electrocardiographic monitoring, treatment of pain with narcotic analgesics, administration of supplemental oxygen, and attempts to minimize myocardial oxygen demand through attention to the determinants of myocardial oxygen consumption (Table 54-5). Hypertension that persists after adequate pain and anxiety relief should be treated aggressively with parenteral antihypertensive agents such as intravenous nitroglycerin or nitroprusside. Tachycardia can be minimized by treating pain and anxiety. Morphine sulfate given intravenously in 2- to 4-mg increments is the preferred analgesic agent because of its potency, safety when given intravenously, lack of myocardial depressant effects, and generally minimal hemodynamic changes in the supine patient (115). Nitroglycerin has no analgesic properties; although it is effective in unstable angina, probably by relieving coronary spasm, it is generally ineffective in relieving the pain of AMI.

RISK ASSESSMENT. Patients with uncomplicated AMI are hospitalized for 7 to 10 days. Near the end of the hospitalization it has become accepted practice to perform a low-level exercise test to look for symptoms or signs of ischemia at a low workload. Provided that patients with severe left ventricular dysfunction or severe congestive heart failure or patients manifesting myocardial ischemia at rest or on minimal activity are excluded, the low-level exercise test can be performed safely. Some studies have shown a markedly increased risk for future coronary event in patients who exhibit ischemia in the form of angina or ST-segment depression on the low-level exercise test (116). Other studies, however, have suggested that other characteristics such as the ejection fraction or the occurrence of frequent ventricular ectopic beats are more powerful predictors of outcome (117). Nevertheless, it has become accepted practice to recommend coronary angiography in patients exhibiting symptoms of myocardial ischemia either spontaneously or on the low-level exercise test immediately following AMI. Such patients generally have multivessel coronary artery disease, but no well-controlled clinical trials in this subgroup of patients have been performed to demonstrate that coronary artery bypass surgery improves outcome compared to medical therapy.

BETA BLOCKADE. Three large well-done randomized trials have demonstrated that institution of a beta-adrenergic blocking agent prior to discharge for AMI reduces subsequent mortality significantly over the next several years (118–120). One study initiated beta blocker therapy with an intravenous drug (metoprolol) within hours after admission (118), while the other two studies (propanolol and timolol) began therapy 7 to 10 days after myocardial infarction (119, 120). In the metoprolol study, patients given intravenous metoprolol had less pain than those receiving placebo, but it is not clear whether the survival benefit seen in this study was dependent on the early administration of a beta-adrenergic blocking drug. Most physicians initiate oral therapy at 7 to 10 days because of fear of exacerbating congestive heart failure or inducing heart block.

ANTICOAGULATION. The use of anticoagulants following AMI is still subject to debate and investigation. One large randomized trial, the VA Cooperative Study, showed no difference in mortality rate between AMI patients anticoagulated for 30 days and the control group but a marked reduction in systemic embolization with anticoagulation was seen (121). Subsequent studies using two-dimensional echocardiography showed that intraventricular thrombus is predominantly seen only in patients with anterior myocardial infarction. Thus, it seems reasonable to anticoagulate patients with anterior myocardial infarction for about 1 month providing that no contraindications exist. Others would anticoagulate those patients in whom a thrombus can be detected by echocardiography; these patients are generally anticoagulated for 3 to 6 months.

Complications

VENTRICULAR ARRHYTHMIA. The most common complication of AMI is ventricular arrhythmia, which occurs in some form in over 90% of patients in the first 72 hours following onset of the infarction. Premature ventricular beats are almost universal; more complex forms such as couplets, triplets, and nonsustained ventricular tachycardia are also commonly seen early after myocardial infarction. Because of concern that these might deteriorate into ventricular fibrillation, they are usually treated with intravenous lidocaine, giving a 50- to 100-mg bolus initially followed by a drip of 1 to 4 mg/minute titrated to therapeutic blood levels of 2 to 4 μg/ml. Some recommend the prophylactic use of lidocaine in all patients with AMI based on the randomized trial of Lie and colleagues (122) showing a significant reduction in the incidence of ventricular fibrillation in the treated group. No difference in the mortality rate, however, was seen between the treated and control groups. Furthermore, acute infarction often cannot be distinguished from unstable angina for 24 to 48 hours after admission; this means treating many patients unnecessarily. Accelerated idioventricular rhythm also occurs relatively commonly in those with

AMI. It must be distinguished from ventricular tachycardia (on the basis of a rate between 50 and 110 beats/minute) because the former is generally benign and requires no treatment.

ATRIOVENTRICULAR BLOCK. Atrioventricular (A-V) conduction disturbances are relatively common and important complications of AMI. First-degree A-V block (PR interval >0.20 s) occurs in about 10% of patients and is almost always intranodal and benign. Progression to complete A-V block only occurs in the small proportion of patients in whom the first-degree A-V block is below the bundle of His; this is generally associated with a wide QRS caused by bifascicular block. Mobitz type I second-degree A-V block or Wenckebach block occurs in 4 to 10% of patients with AMI (usually inferior), is associated with a narrow QRS complex, is usually transient (up to 72 hours), is presumably caused by ischemia of the A-V node, rarely progresses to complete A-V block, and generally does not require pacing. Mobitz type II second-degree A-V block is rare in those with AMI (less than 1% of all cases), is caused by disease below the bundle of His, is associated with a wide QRS, often progresses to complete A-V block, is more often associated with anterior infarction, and generally requires pacing. When complete A-V block occurs in patients with inferior infarction, it is caused by relatively well-localized ischemia of the A-V node, the escape rhythm is most often nodal with a rate of 40 to 60 beats/minute, and generally well tolerated.

The mortality rate of acute inferior infarction complicated by complete A-V block (20 to 25%) is moderately increased over that of inferior infarction alone. This is in contrast to anterior infarction complicated by complete A-V block; then the block is a result of interruption of each of the three major fascicles below the bundle of His, meaning that the mass of infarcting myocardium is large. The escape rhythm is idioventricular, slow (<40 beats/minute), and subject to asystole. The mortality rate of anterior infarction complicated by complete A-V block is high (70 to 80%), mostly as a result of the extent of the infarction. Although some have argued that pacing does not improve the relatively benign prognosis of A-V block in inferior infarction, and nothing short of myocardial salvage can improve the disastrous prognosis of anterior infarction complicated by A-V block, temporary ventricular pacing is generally recommended for all AMI patients with complete A-V block.

CARDIOGENIC SHOCK. The other major complication of AMI is cardiogenic shock, which occurs in 10 to 15% of hospitalized AMI patients. Cardiogenic shock occurs when about 40% of the left ventricular myocardium has been destroyed by new and old infarction. Cardiogenic shock is defined as a cardiac output insufficient to meet the needs of vital organs despite an adequate intravascular volume and ventricular filling pressures. The hemodynamic findings in cardiogenic shock are hypotension (systolic pressure <80 mm Hg), left ventricular filling pressure ≥18 mm Hg, and cardiac index <1.8 L/minute/m². Peripheral manifestations of inadequate end-organ perfusion are oliguria, cool diaphoretic skin, and altered mental status.

When caused by left ventricular dysfunction, cardiogenic shock has a mortality rate of over 90% and is the most common cause of death in hospitalized AMI patients. It is essential to exclude hypovolemia when presented with a patient with signs of shock because it is easily treatable. Physical signs such as venous pressure and pulmonary rales and radiographic findings such as Kerley's B lines correlate poorly with left ventricular filling pressure, so nothing can substitute for direct invasive measurement of left and right ventricular filling pressures in patients with suspected cardiogenic shock. The Swan-Ganz catheter can generally be passed percutaneously through a vein (usually the internal jugular) at the bedside without fluoroscopic guidance through the right side of the heart to the pulmonary artery to measure the pulmonary artery wedge pressure, which is a good approximation of left atrial pressure and left ventricular diastolic pressure.

Another correctable cause of cardiogenic shock is right ventricular infarction, which often requires intravascular volume overexpansion to right atrial pressures ≥10 mm Hg to achieve an adequate cardiac output. Ventricular septal rupture and papillary muscle rupture each occur in 1 to 3% of hospitalized AMI patients and generally result in cardiogenic shock. These can be corrected surgically, although with a high operative mortality rate. When hypovolemia, right ventricular infarction, and rupture of the septum or papillary muscle have been excluded, acute left ventricular dysfunction involving 40% or more of the left ventricle is the likely cause of the cardiogenic shock. Temporary improvement in hemodynamic status can be obtained with the use of a mechanical support device such as the intra-aortic balloon; by inflating in diastole and deflating in systole this balloon can reduce left ventricular afterload and increase coronary perfusion pressure. The intra-aortic balloon alone, however, is rarely sufficient. In a few highly selected patients coronary angiography followed by coronary artery bypass surgery has been attempted, with a 30 to 40% survival rate (123).

Stable Angina Pectoris (XVII-4)

Briefly, angina pectoris can be defined as chest discomfort of a visceral nature precipitated by exertion or emotion and promptly relieved by rest or nitroglycerin. It is the most common symptomatic manifestation of stable coronary heart disease. Angina can occur in a stable pattern in many patients for a prolonged period of time (months to years). It differs from unstable angina in that a precipitating factor can generally be identified (usually exercise), and that relief occurs promptly with the removal of the precipitating factor or with the administration of sublingual nitroglycerin. The importance of angina pectoris is that it is often the most valuable clue to coronary artery disease, it is often disabling, and some patients with angina are at high risk for AMI or sudden cardiac death.

Pathophysiology

Stable angina pectoris occurs when the myocardial oxygen demand transiently exceeds the myocardial oxygen delivery because of an increase in a determinant of oxygen demand (see Table 54–5). The pathologic substrate in the vast majority of patients is a significant coronary artery obstruction caused by an atheromatous plaque. The clinical syndrome of angina pectoris can also occur in patients who have exertional coronary spasm despite anatomically normal coronary arteries, in patients with severe aortic valve disease (see below), in patients with hypertrophic cardiomyopathy, and in a small subset of patients without identifiable heart disease in whom the pathophysiology is unknown. It is generally believed that coronary blood flow and myocardial oxygen delivery are either unchanged or fail to increase sufficiently to meet the increased demands for myocardial oxygen delivery; an external factor (such as exercise-producing tachycardia) that increases myocardial oxygen demand is generally identifiable.

Symptoms and Diagnosis

Most patients can be diagnosed on the basis of the history alone (see above: General Principles of Diagnosis—Importance of the History). The most important information to elicit from the history regarding angina are the factors that precipitate the attack and what the patient does to relieve it. Typical precipitating factors are exertion and emotion. Isometric exertion, such as lifting over the head, is more likely to precipitate angina than isotonic exertion because of the marked increase in blood pressure that occurs with sustained isometric muscle contraction. Exertion performed after a large meal, during times of emotional distress, or on cold exposure is more likely to precipitate angina than exertion under other conditions. Angina tends to occur more frequently and with less provocation in the first hours after awakening. Stable angina is relieved within minutes by stopping exertion, alleviating the precipitating factor, or taking sublingual nitroglycerin. The response to nitroglycerin is one of the most useful clues from the history to the presence of coronary artery disease. In patients whose angina-like chest pain is promptly relieved by nitroglycerin, the probability of angiographically significant coronary artery disease is 0.90 (124). The time elapsed between taking nitroglycerin and the beginning of relief of the angina is a particularly vital part of the history. Relief occurring within minutes excludes a placebo or nonspecific effect of nitroglycerin. Although the pain of esophageal spasm can also be relieved by nitroglycerin, I have found this to be a rare phenomenon.

It is useful to quantify the amount of exertion required to precipitate exertion, although this is often variable within the same patient. The classification system of the Canadian Cardiovascular Society (95) is particularly useful because it was designed specifically for angina (see above, Importance of the History).

The nature and location of angina also provide useful diagnostic clues. Angina is diffuse and vague; many patients refuse to use the word "pain" in describing it, and correct the physician who uses it in questioning the patient. It is often described as a pressure sensation, a weight on the chest, or a constricting feeling in the chest and often in the neck. A clenched fist is often used by the patient to illustrate the constricting nature of the discomfort. Angina is not pleuritic and does not usually change with change in posture, as does pericardial pain. Angina is not fleeting; brief stabbing pains in the chest lasting only seconds are probably neuritic in origin. The duration of angina is generally 5 to 15 minutes. Although angina can occur almost anywhere between the diaphragm and mandible (Fig. 54-1) it is typically retrosternal with radiation into one or both arms, throat, and mandible. Occasionally it can occur only in the arms, only in the mandible, or only in the interscapular region. Sometimes the pain can occur in the epigastrium and might be mistaken for gastrointestinal pain by the physician or patient, such as esophagitis or peptic ulcer. Because of its visceral nature it generally encompasses a substantial area and is deep-seated; pain that is localized to a small area on the chest wall (e.g., less than 1 to 2 inches in diameter) or that is superficial is generally not angina. Pain localized by the patient with a single finger is not likely to be angina. Some characteristics of angina are summarized in Table 54-6.

PHYSICAL EXAMINATION. The physical examination is the least useful of the diagnostic tools, but some helpful information can be obtained. Often no cardiovascular abnormalities are detected. Particular attention to the major controllable determinants of myocardial oxygen consumption—heart rate and systolic pressure—is essential (see Table 54-5). Other causes of angina or angina-like pain, such as aortic valve disease, idiopathic hypertrophic subaortic stenosis, or mitral valve prolapse can be excluded by careful examination for the appropriate murmurs or midsystolic click (see below). Reproduction of the pain by firm palpation of the chest or by pressing on the ribs is useful in diagnosing chest wall pain. Costochondritis, a specific, but uncommon inflammation of the costochondral junction, is best diagnosed by eliciting exquisite pain with light pressure over the costochrondral junction about 1 to 2 inches lateral to the sternum. Symptoms and signs of congestive heart failure, such as elevated jugular venous pressure, pulmonary rales, or gallop rhythm, should be sought. Treatment of heart failure can also improve angina by lowering the left ventricular diastolic pressure, thereby improving the

TABLE 54-6. Diagnostic Clues of Angina Pectoris From the History

Definitely Angina	Possibly Angina	Not Angina
Precipitated by exertion or emotion	Pain at rest	Pleuritic or positional pain
Relieved within minutes by rest or nitroglycerin	Not promptly relieved by rest or nitroglycerin	Pain rarely or never relieved by nitroglycerin
Visceral or vague in nature	Dyspnea	Pain sharply localized to a small discrete area
Diffusely located	Well localized but to a substantial area	Brief, fleeting, stabbing pain
Worse in cold, after meals, or on arising	Not worse in cold, after meals, or on arising	Pain aggravated by palpation

perfusion gradient for coronary blood flow and reducing the wall stress (Table 54-6).

ROUTINE LABORATORY TESTS. The resting ECG is often normal. Q waves provide evidence of old myocardial infarction and thereby of coronary heart disease but do not necessarily help to identify the presenting chest pain. An ECG taken during an anginal episode is useful because it usually (but not always) shows ST-segment depression. The chest roentgenogram is useful to the extent that it permits assessment for cardiomegaly and evidence of congestive heart failure. Routine laboratory tests help to exclude severe anemia (hematocrit below 25%) as a precipitating factor for angina and to examine for risk factors of atherosclerotic heart disease such as diabetes or hyperlipidemia, but are of little direct value in determining whether the presenting complaints are the result of myocardial ischemia.

EXERCISE TESTING. The exercise stress ECG has been the traditional noninvasive diagnostic tool for the evaluation of angina pectoris, but it is commonly misused. The exercise test was discussed previously, but several points should be re-emphasized. The use of the exercise test should be considered in two principal categories: for diagnosis of the presence or absence of coronary artery disease; and for the assessment of prognosis in patients with known coronary artery disease. In males a history of typical angina pectoris indicates a 90% probability that significant atherosclerotic coronary artery obstruction will be present at coronary angiography (101); the exercise test adds almost nothing to the diagnosis in this situation. On the other hand, exercise testing is important for assessing severity of disease, prognosis, and response to therapy. Many patients whose diagnosis is clear from the history should therefore undergo exercise testing to determine if further diagnostic tests such as coronary arteriography are indicated or if coronary artery bypass grafting needs to be performed. Whereas the ST-segment response to exertion is the most commonly used diagnostic criterion (usually depression ≥ 1 mm), the ST-segment response has more limited usefulness in prognostication (96). The duration of exercise or maximum workload achieved and the maximum heart rate and blood pressure achieved are the most powerful prognostic indicators (96). Other useful prognostic indicators probably include marked ST-segment depression (≥ 2 mm) and exertional hypotension (a drop in blood pressure during exercise).

RADIONUCLIDE IMAGING. Radionuclide imaging of the heart has also been useful both in establishing the diagnosis and assessing prognosis (103). Two techniques are in common clinical use: imaging of the myocardium with thallium-201; and imaging of the cardiac chambers, particularly the left and right ventricles, with technetium-99m tagged to red blood cells (see above). They are most useful in patients whose baseline ECG precludes seeing diagnostic ST-segment changes with exercise testing (left ventricular hypertrophy with repolarization abnormalities and left bundle branch block). These tests are expensive and result in a small amount of radiation exposure; therefore they should not be used routinely.

CORONARY ARTERIOGRAPHY. Despite major advances in sophisticated noninvasive diagnostic procedures, coronary angiography is the only technique that can reliably determine the location, number, and severity of coronary artery obstructions. It can be performed with relatively low morbidity and mortality rates (0.1%), but it is expensive, uses ionizing radiation, and does carry a small risk. Generally accepted indications for coronary arteriography were presented previously (see above, Cardiac Catheterization and Angiography).

Treatment

MEDICAL THERAPY. Following diagnosis and assessment of risk for a major coronary event through noninvasive and invasive studies, if appropriate, the first step in therapy of stable angina should involve minimizing coronary artery disease risk factors and eliminating factors that aggravate angina. Cigarette smoking and hypertension are the two major controllable risk factors. Pipe and cigar smoking have also been associated with an increased risk of myocardial infarction or death, but to a lesser degree than cigarette smoking—probably because the dose is lower as a result of less inhalation of the pollutants. Weight reduction in obese patients, control of hyperglycemia in diabetics, correction of arterial hypoxemia in patients with pulmonary disease, control of tachycardia (particularly that caused by beta agonists used as bronchodilators), and a program of moderate isotonic exercise such as walking are also appropriate initial measures. Other medical conditions that aggravate angina, such as severe anemia, thyrotoxicosis, or congestive heart failure, should be diagnosed and treated.

Sublingual nitroglycerin (0.4 mg) has been the mainstay of treatment of symptomatic attacks ever since the first description of the response to amyl nitrate by Brunton in 1867 (125) and to nitroglycerin by Murrell in 1879 (126). Nitroglycerin can also be used prophylactically prior to performing exercise likely to precipitate angina, such as climbing stairs or sexual intercourse. If complete relief is not obtained by a single tablet, a second can be used in 5 to 10 minutes. Ischemic myocardial pain not responding to 3 nitroglycerin tablets within 15 to 20 minutes generally requires medical attention. Nitroglycerin is relatively unstable and loses its potency over several months, particularly if kept at room temperature. Patients can often tell when this occurs because the tablets no longer produce a stinging sensation under the tongue or give a feeling of fullness in the head. Most patients have headaches when initially taking any form of nitrate; tolerance to this side effect usually develops, but not to its angina-relieving properties.

The mechanism of action of nitroglycerin is still the subject of some debate. It probably both reduces myocardial oxygen demand through reducing left ventricular wall stress by decreasing afterload, and increases coronary blood flow to ischemic myocardium through dilation of the coronary stenoses (Table 54-7) (127). The duration of action of sublingual nitroglycerin is brief, usually 15 to 30 minutes; therefore, its use is not practical as a long-term prophylactic drug.

A number of long-acting nitrate preparations with mechanisms of action similar to that of sublingual nitroglycerin are available. Among the most commonly used are the oral organic nitrate, isosorbide

TABLE 54-7. Mechanism of Action of Antianginal Drugs

Determinant of Oxygen Supply-Demand Balance	Class of Drug		
	Nitrates	Beta Blocker	Calcium Channel Blocker
Myocardial oxygen demand			
Heart rate	Increases moderately	Decreases moderately	Variable, but usually little change
Contractility	No change	Decreases moderately	Variable degree of decrease
LV wall stress	Decreases moderately	No change unless CHF induced	Variable degree of decrease
Myocardial oxygen delivery			
Aortic systolic pressure	Decreases moderately	Decreases slightly	Decreases moderately
LV diastolic pressure	Decreases moderately	No change unless CHF induced	Variable, but usually no change
Coronary vascular resistance	Decreases moderately	No change or slightly increased	Decreases moderately
Arterial saturation	Decreases slightly	No change	No change

dinitrate, and various types of topical nitrates. Isosorbide can be begun at a dose of 10 mg tid and increased at 5- to 7-day intervals to 40 mg of the sustained-release form tid. Nitroglycerin ointment is probably the most effective nonparenteral form of nitroglycerin for patients with severe angina. It comes in tubes that supply a dose of 15 mg/inch. Doses of 7.5 mg (0.5 inch) to 30 mg (2 inches) applied to several square inches of nonhairy skin and covered with a plastic film up to qid are generally quite effective in relieving angina refractory to oral nitrates. There should be an 8- to 12-hour nitrate-free period each 24 hours to prevent development of tolerance. This form is particularly useful when applied just before sleep for patients having frequent nocturnal angina. Because the paste often soils underclothes, several pharmaceutical firms have developed sustained-release patches with the nitroglycerin impregnated in a polymer. Although these do result in sustained low blood levels, tolerance appears to develop rapidly; serious questions as to the efficacy of nitroglycerin patches are currently under investigation.

Beta-adrenergic blockers are highly effective in reducing the frequency of anginal attacks and in improving exercise tolerance in patients with stable exertional angina (128). Their primary mechanism of action is most likely the reduction of myocardial oxygen demand by decreasing resting and exercise heart rates and, to a lesser extent, systolic blood pressure (Table 54-7). The most common side effects are fatigue, mental depression, exacerbation of congestive heart failure in patients with severe left ventricular dysfunction, and bronchoconstriction. Beta-adrenergic blockers should be used cautiously or not at all in patients with a history of severe congestive heart failure or who have a left ventricular ejection fraction lower than 0.30. Nonselective beta-adrenergic blockers are also relatively contraindicated in patients with severe obstructive airway disease resulting in arterial desaturation or CO_2 retention. Beta-1 selective agents such as metoprolol have been developed to minimize bronchoconstriction, but in the larger doses often required for control of angina they lose their selectivity and can cause bronchospasm. Beta-adrenergic blockers are also relatively

contraindicated in patients with insulin-dependent diabetes because they block the sympathetic response to hypoglycemia, thereby prolonging the episode and impairing its recognition.

Calcium channel blockers are the most recently introduced drugs in the United States. These drugs cause vascular smooth muscle relaxation by blocking the calcium channel in the cell *membrane* and have proven to be highly effective in the treatment of angina (129). Although their mechanisms of action at the cellular or organ level are similar to those of the nitrates, their biochemical site of action is different; therefore these agents can be synergistic with nitrates in the treatment of angina. In contrast to nitrates these agents are also myocardial depressants, with verapamil being the most potent. Verapamil should be used cautiously or not at all in patients with severe congestive heart failure or left ventricular dysfunction. Nifedipine and diltiazem rarely cause serious congestive heart failure. Both verapamil and diltiazem slow A-V conduction and are relatively contraindicated in patients with advanced degrees of A-V block or sick sinus syndrome. Nifedipine commonly produces minor ankle edema that can usually be easily controlled with a diuretic. Because these are potent vasodilators, headache and orthostatic hypotension are common side effects, particularly when used in combination with large doses of nitrates.

The history is useful in choosing the first antianginal agent to initiate treatment. In patients whose angina is primarily exertional or is provoked by other stresses that increase myocardial oxygen demand, beta-adrenergic blocking agents are highly effective, as are the nitrates and calcium channel blockers. In patients with angina at rest, in whom the mechanism might be a spontaneous reduction in coronary blood flow caused by normal coronary vasoreactivity or spasm, nitrates or calcium channel blockers are probably preferable over beta-adrenergic blockers; the latter could theoretically exacerbate coronary spasm by leaving the alpha-constrictor tone unopposed. These three classes of antianginal drugs are useful in combination in patients with severe angina. Medical therapy is often not considered to be "maximal" unless the patient is receiving a drug from all three classes in therapeutic doses.

SURGICAL THERAPY. Various surgical procedures were tried for relief of severe angina in the middle decades of this century, but none were demonstrated to be more effective than a placebo or sham operation (130). With the description of the aortocoronary bypass operation by Favalaro in 1969, a truly effective way of improving myocardial blood flow at an acceptable risk was introduced (131). The operation is based on the angiographic observation that, in the earlier phases of symptomatic coronary artery disease, the atherosclerotic obstructions are in the proximal portions of the coronary arteries, leaving the distal portions of the vessels relatively free of disease. Direct surgical attack on the obstructive lesions (i.e., endarterectomy) did not work because of the small size of the arteries. The construction of a bypass conduit of saphenous vein from the ascending aorta to the coronary artery distal to the obstruction (Fig. 54-10) has been shown to be highly effective in relieving anginal symptoms and improving exercise tolerance. The operation, which requires the use of cardiopulmonary bypass to allow the delicate anastomoses to be made on the arrested heart, can now be performed with an operative mortality rate of about 2 to 3%. The probability of early graft patency is high (90%), as is the initial relief of symptoms (80%). As atherosclerosis progresses in the native coronary

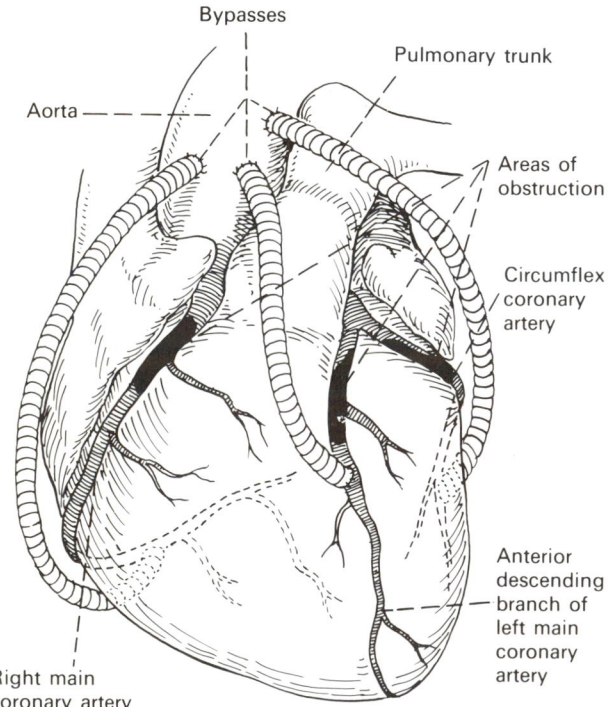

Bypasses

Pulmonary trunk

Aorta

Areas of obstruction

Circumflex coronary artery

Anterior descending branch of left main coronary artery

Right main coronary artery

FIG. 54-10. Triple coronary aortic bypass on patient ELB carried out by Dr. R. Anderson in two stages 9 years apart. The bypasses to the left anterior descending branch of the left coronary and the one to the posterior part of the circumflex coronary artery were carried out in 1974, and the bypass to the posterior descending branch of the right coronary was carried out in 1983. Angiogram done in 1988 revealed that all three vessels remained patent, but the native vessels were severely obstructed as follows: left main coronary artery 80%, left anterior descending artery 100%, circumflex artery 90%, right coronary artery 100%. The names of the branches of the arteries have been omitted for the sake of clarity. See Figure 54-6 for details. Courtesy of Dr. R. Riggins.

arteries and develops in the saphenous veins, however, symptoms return at a rate of 3 to 4%/year so that by 5 years after surgery about 30% of operated patients are again symptomatic (4). The internal thoracic artery is now frequently used as the bypass conduit to coronary arteries on the anterior surface of the heart because it does not appear to develop atherosclerotic obstruction, resulting in better late patency rates.

Whereas the beneficial symptomatic results of coronary bypass surgery in patients who are severely limited by angina preoperatively are quite clear, the effect of surgery on survival has been more controversial. With the publication of three large randomized trials comparing survival or surgically and medically treated patients (132–134), it is now accepted that survival is improved with surgical therapy in patients with significant obstruction of the left main coronary artery (132) and in patients with three-vessel coronary artery disease and left ventricular dysfunction (134). No study has shown improved survival in patients with single-vessel coronary artery disease. A European randomized trial showed substantially improved survival in symptomatic patients with three-vessel disease and normal left ventricular function (133). The Coronary Artery Surgery Study conducted in the United States and Canada, however, showed no survival benefit for minimally symptomatic patients with three-vessel disease and normal left ventricular function (134). Although neither the VA Cooperative Study nor the Coronory Artery Surgery Study showed improved survival in patients with two-vessel disease, some data from the European study suggest that, if one of the two involved vessels is the anterior descending coronary artery, survival might be prolonged with surgery (133). These and other data relating to the effects of coronary artery bypass surgery on survival have been reviewed in greater detail by the senior author (4, 135).

The indications for coronary bypass surgery can be considered in two categories, relief of symptoms and prolongation of life:

Generally accepted indications
Relief of symptoms—patients meeting all the following criteria:
　　Unacceptable angina despite adequate medical therapy
　　One or more major coronary vessels obstructed and bypassable
　　Age, general condition, and left ventricular function make risk of surgery reasonable
　Prolongation of survival
　　Patients with left main coronary obstruction ≥50%
　　Patients with three-vessel disease and left ventricular dysfunction
Possible indications
　Patients with three-vessel disease and normal left ventricular function (for prolongation of survival)
　Patients with two-vessel disease, one of which is the anterior descending coronary artery (for prolongation of survival)
　Patients requiring valve replacement who also have coronary artery disease
　Patients in cardiogenic shock caused by AMI

Patients who are significantly limited by angina despite adequate medical therapy, with one or more coronary arteries that could be bypassed, and whose left ventricular function and general medical condition make the risk of surgery acceptable, should be offered surgery for relief of symptoms. Patients who have 50% or more obstruction of the left main coronary artery or who have three-vessel disease and moderate left ventricular dysfunction and are at a reasonable risk for surgery should be offered bypass surgery for prolongation of survival.

OTHER THERAPIES. In selected patients *percutaneous transluminal coronary angioplasty* (PTCA) provides effective revascularization without a surgical procedure. This catheterization procedure, developed by Gruntzig in the late 1970s (136), consists of passing a flexible guide wire across the coronary artery stenosis and following with a balloon catheter over the guide wire. The balloon is inflated and the stenosis is dilated. In skilled hands the procedure promptly relieves the obstruction in about 90% of attempts but a small risk of occluding the artery or damaging it is involved, so that emergency surgery is required in 2 to 4% of patients. The procedure seems to be most effective in patients with limited coronary artery disease involving one or at most two vessels. A major unresolved problem is the recurrence of the stenosis in about 30% of patients within 6 months of the procedure.

Because of the likelihood that ischemic myocardial pain can serve as the "trigger" for secondary skeletal muscle spasm, it seems logical that forms of therapy directed at relieving this secondary pain will prove beneficial. Chapter 58 describes several myofascial pain syndromes with trigger points (TPs) that frequently develop in the anterior chest in these patients and contribute to the patients' discomfort. Although not well described in the cardiologic literature, there is much evidence that injections of the TPs promptly relieve the pain (see Chapter 58 for references). Biofeedback, meditation, or other forms of relaxation may also prove beneficial.

Depression is common in patients with serious heart disease. Depressed patients are likely to magnify somatic symptoms or be unable to take effective steps in their own care. Thus, identification and treatment of depression can serve to improve angina.

Much has been said about the potentially lethal side effects of tricyclic antidepressants and of phenothiazines in patients with heart disease. Specifically, it was debated whether ventricular arrhythmias might be aggravated by these drugs. Little or no sound epidemiologic evidence has been found to indicate that these drugs precipitate sudden cardiac death. To the contrary, it now appears that imipramine might be an effective antiarrhythmic agent.

Nerve interruption procedures, such as upper thoracic sympathectomy, were used for the treatment of intractable angina, with almost complete relief of chest pain in most patients (39, 54, 82). These procedures are rarely done now since the advent of effective long-acting antianginal medications and revascularization procedures. In patients in whom these therapies do not provide adequate relief of severe pain, however, a prognostic sympathetic block with a long-acting local anesthetic should be carried out under sedation. If this provides good pain relief, a sympathectomy should be considered in patients who can tolerate the surgery or a neurolytic block of the upper sympathetic chain should be done with alcohol or phenol in high risk patients (39, 82) (Chapter 97).

Unstable Angina (XVII-4)

Unstable angina can be defined as angina occuring at rest or with little or no provocation. Previously, patients with new-onset angina and patients with a crescendo pattern to their exertional angina were included with those in the unstable angina group, but these two subgroups probably have a different pathophysiology and a different prognosis.

Pathophysiology

Patients with unstable angina generally have a severe stenosis ($\geqslant 90\%$ in one or more major coronary arteries, but the vessel is still patent. The angina occurs without any change in the determinants of myocardial oxygen demand, and therefore must be the result of a reduction in coronary blood flow caused by an increase in coronary vascular resistance (Table 54-5). The increase in resistance is thought to occur primarily at the severe atherosclerotic stenosis because of partial occlusion by a platelet thrombus, by an increase in vasomotor tone producing a small reduction in lumen area that can effect a large increase in resistance, or by a combination of both these mechanisms. Rarely, an unstable angina pattern can occur in patients with arteriographically normal coronary arteries; in these patients coronary spasm must be the primary mechanism.

Diagnosis

HISTORY. As with stable angina, the history provides most of the diagnostic information required. The pain is similar to that of stable exertional angina; within the same patient, the nature and location of the pain is usually the same as that experienced with exercise. The major difference is that the pain comes on at rest with no change in heart rate or blood pressure preceding the onset of pain. The pain can be more severe than that of the exertional pain and can last 30 minutes or longer. In a patient without previous objective evidence of coronary heart disease, such as prior myocardial infarction or typical exertional angina, the presenting complaint of chest pain at rest can be difficult to distinguish from noncardiac pain on the basis of the history alone. The pain is often less responsive to sublingual nitroglycerin than exertional angina.

PHYSICAL EXAMINATION. As in stable angina, the physical examination is often unrevealing. Nevertheless, evidence of congestive heart failure, aortic valve disease, uncontrolled hypertension, tachycardia, fever, severe anemia, and marked anxiety should be sought.

ELECTROCARDIOGRAPHY. Most patients with unstable angina have transient ST-segment depression or elevation or T-wave inversion with the anginal episode. The absence of electrocardiographic changes with the pain, however, does not exclude the diagnosis.

LABORATORY STUDIES. Frequently, unstable angina can only be differentiated from a non-Q-wave infarction by the absence of an increase in serum enzyme levels. The pain pattern and electrocardiographic changes alone do not distinguish unstable angina from a non-Q-wave infarction. Thallium myocardial imaging during an episode of unstable angina reveals a perfusion deficit that returns to normal following relief of pain. This observation forms the basis for the understanding of the pathophysiology (i.e., transient reduction in coronary flow), but thallium imaging is generally not required to establish the diagnosis. Exercise testing is generally contraindicated in patients having chest pain at rest; in patients in whom immediate coronary arteriography is not appropriate, exercise testing, if required, can be performed after a period of stability of several days to weeks.

CORONARY ARTERIOGRAPHY. In most patients whose age and general medical condition make them potential candidates for coronary bypass surgery, coronary arteriography should be performed during the same hospital admission for two reasons. First, the incidence of severe coronary artery disease requiring surgery for prolongation of survival (e.g., left main coronary artery obstruction or three-vessel disease) is higher in patients with unstable angina than in those with other manifestations of coronary heart disease. Second, failure of medical therapy resulting in readmission for recurrent unstable angina or myocardial infarction has been relatively common.

Treatment

Patients with unstable angina should be admitted to the hospital and placed at bed rest in a quiet, anxiety-free environment. If arterial hypoxemia is present oxygen should be administered. Factors that increase myocardial oxygen demand or coronary artery resistance should be vigorously treated; the most important of these are hypertension and cigarette smoking.

MEDICAL THERAPY. Nitrates are the primary mode of medical therapy. If oral or topical nitrates are unsuccessful in providing prompt relief of pain, nitroglycerin should be given intravenously starting at $10 \mu g$/minute, increasing by $10 \mu g$/minute every 10 minutes until the initial rate of $50 \mu m$/minute is achieved. If the pain persists or recurs, nitroglycerin can be titrated upward to a maximal dose of $300 \mu m$/minute providing that the systolic arterial blood pressure does not fall below approximately 100 mm Hg. Calcium channel blockers are useful adjuncts to therapy. The initiation of beta-adrenergic blockers in unstable angina is more controversial because of the possibility of increasing coronary vascular resistance, but little or no evidence has been found to show a deleterious effect of these drugs in unstable angina aside from the usual side effects discussed for stable angina. If the patient has been on a beta-adrenergic blocker at the time of admission it should be continued unless congestive heart failure or marked bradycardia is present. Sudden withdrawal of beta-adrenergic blockers has been associated with a rebound phenomenon, resulting in more severe angina or myocardial infarction.

Two randomized trials have shown a marked beneficial effect of aspirin in the prevention of myocardial infarction and death over the subsequent several months (137, 138). Many surgeons believe, however, that aspirin increases the risk of bleeding at the time of surgery. If the patient is not a surgical candidate, aspirin should be instituted at a dose of 300 mg/day. If the patient is a potential surgical candidate coronary arteriography might be performed first, and a decision regarding medical versus surgical therapy made on the basis of coronary anatomy and clinical status.

SURGICAL THERAPY. Coronary bypass surgery is the therapy of choice for patients with graftable coronary arteries whose angina cannot be controlled by oral or topical antianginal agents, or both, and for those in whom surgery prolongs life (see above, Stable Angina: Surgical Therapy). The intra-aortic balloon is highly effective for the temporary control of pain and can probably prevent infarction until coronary arteriography and surgery can be performed for those patients whose angina cannot be controlled by intravenous nitroglycerin. The mechanism whereby the intra-aortic balloon affords myocardial protection involves augmentation of diastolic aortic pressure, increasing coronary flow, and reducing systolic pressure, thus reducing myocardial oxygen demand.

Sudden Cardiac Death

Epidemiology

Sudden cardiac death can be defined as unexpected death occurring without symptoms or preceded by symptoms of no more than 1 hour's duration. The incidence of sudden cardiac death in the United States is approximately 440,000 annually, 80% of which are caused by coronary artery disease (1). Conversely, of all deaths from coronary artery disease, one-half to two-thirds are sudden. There is a strong male predominance, with an average age of approximately 60 years. In 75% of patients dying suddenly, some clinical manifestation of heart disease was present prior to the episode—most commonly, angina or previous myocardial infarction. In 20 to 25% of cases, however, sudden death is the first manifestation of heart disease. Because atherosclerotic coronary artery disease is the most common cause of sudden cardiac death, the risk factors for coronary heart disease are also associated with sudden death, particularly smoking, hypertension, and hyperlipidemia. In patients with heart disease, frequent or complex ventricular ectopy such as nonsustained ventricular tachycardia were shown to be associated with an increased risk for sudden death (97). If associated ventricular dysfunction is present the risk of sudden death becomes substantial, as high as 25% in a 2-year period (139), but asymptomatic, complex ventricular ectopy appears to carry little risk of sudden death in patients without demonstrable heart disease.

Pathophysiology

Almost all patients in whom an ECG was recorded during sudden cardiac death have had ventricular fibrillation, often triggered by premature ventricular beats or ventricular tachycardia. Studies in patients resuscitated from out-of-hospital sudden cardiac death in Seattle showed that only about one-third had myocardial necrosis; in other words, sudden death is purely the result of electrical instability in about two-thirds of patients (140). Preventive measures would offer the most hope for those in this latter group.

The mechanism by which patients with coronary heart disease progress from their stable, nonacutely ill state to ventricular fibrillation and sudden death is unknown. Currently the mechanism and prevention of sudden death are areas of intense investigation. It has been widely speculated that the autonomic nervous system might play a major role in triggering sudden death. For example, the sudden release of catecholamines from sympathetic nerve fibers to the heart can alter the membrane characteristics of myocardial cells, thus setting up the opportunity for re-entry leading to ventricular tachycardia and fibrillation. A second possible mechanism is that the catecholamine release makes myocardial cells relatively ischemic by increasing their oxygen demand at a time when oxygen delivery cannot be increased because of coronary artery obstruction. A third possibility is that alterations in autonomic tone result in vasomotor changes in the coronary arteries. If such vasospasm occurs at the site of an atherosclerotic stenosis, small changes in diameter at the stenosis can result in critical changes in flow. Finally, some studies have shown that myocardial infarction interrupts sympathetic innervation to the myocardium distal to the infarction. This sets the stage for an imbalance in autonomic impulses reaching different portions of the heart, which in turn increases electrical instability.

A large variety of cardiovascular diseases comprise the underlying pathologic substrate in the 25% of patients in whom atherosclerotic coronary artery disease does not seem to be causative of sudden cardiac death. These include aortic stenosis and, less commonly, other forms of valvular heart disease, hypertrophic cardiomyopathy (both obstructive and nonobstructive), dilated cardiomyopathy, congenital anomalies of the coronary arteries, other forms of complex congenital heart disease, primary pulmonary hypertension, Marfan's syndrome, and dissecting hematoma of the aorta. It is rare that a careful autopsy does not reveal a significant cardiovascular lesion in patients dying suddenly.

Diagnosis

The diagnosis of the acute event is not difficult but is nevertheless important because institution of cardiopulmonary resuscitation in someone temporarily unconscious from a vasovagal faint, seizure, or transient cerebral ischemia can result in injury such as broken ribs, separated costochondral cartilages, or even pneumothorax. Because forward cardiac output has totally ceased, patients are pallid, often ashen in appearance, and diaphoretic. They are nearly always completely flaccid, with no or agonal respirations. Seizure movements are rare and always brief because of the total cerebral ischemia. The most important physical sign is the absence of any detectable pulses; the femoral, carotid, and temporal arteries are usually the most reliable and accessible. An ECG is not always available but usually shows ventricular fibrillation initially. Asystole is generally a late finding and indicates a poor prognosis.

The identification of patients at risk for sudden cardiac death has been the subject of intense research for several decades. Left ventricular dysfunction and congestive heart failure are among the most powerful predictors of sudden death (96, 141, 142). Myocardial ischemia manifested by angina, painless ST-segment changes, and angiographic findings of the extent of coronary artery disease are also a powerful predictor (96, 142). Among patients with angiographically proven coronary artery disease, those who continue to smoke have almost twice the risk of sudden cardiac death as those who quit (143). In patients with structural heart disease, the frequent occurrence of premature ventricular depolarizations or complex ventricular arrhythmia (e.g., multiform beats, couplets, nonsustained ventricular tachycardia) is also a powerful predictor of sudden death (97, 139, 141).

Treatment

Treatment should be considered in two areas: resuscitation from the acute event and prevention of ventricular fibrillation. Most episodes occur outside the hospital, far from any medical care facility. It has been known for many years that primary ventricular fibrillation (i.e., that occuring as the result of electrical instability and not cardiogenic shock) in the intensive care unit could be easily treated by prompt defibrillation; patients experiencing such an event often had a relatively good prognosis on leaving the hospital. Beginning in the early 1970s the intensive care unit experience was transferred to the community setting by the development of "mobile coronary care units." The system developed in Seattle by Cobb and associates has been extraordinarily successful and has served as a model for those in many other communities (140). They reasoned that one or several mobile coronary care units (as had been tried in other communities earlier) could not arrive at the scene of sudden death within 4 minutes of onset (the time at which irreversible cerebral damage begins) and be cost-effective. Instead, they developed a tiered response. The first tier consists of the general public trained in cardiopulmonary resuscitation (CPR). The second tier is the fire department, most of whose members have received an intermediate level of training and can administer CPR but no drugs or defibrillation. The final tier is the mobile coronary care unit, staffed by highly trained and skilled paramedics who are capable of tracheal intubation, drug administration under a physician's orders by radio, and cardiac defibrillation. The first tier, the general public trained in CPR, has proven to be a particularly vital link in the success of this system. Over 50% of adults in Seattle have received CPR training, generally through the fire department. The long-term survival rate for patients with out-of-hospital ventricular fibrillation is almost twice as high for victims in whom cardiopulmonary resuscitation was initiated by a bystander than if it were initiated by the firemen, because of the faster response time of the bystander. Presently, about 30% of victims of out-of-hospital ventricular fibrillation survive to hospital discharge, most in their previous state of health (140, 144). Permanent cerebral dysfunction from anoxia has been surprisingly uncommon.

Even with this highly successful and innovative system in Seattle, now being used in many other communities, two-thirds of patients experiencing out-of-hospital ventricular fibrillation are not long-term survivors. Thus, prevention is vital. Unfortunately, it is not known how to identify patients at risk, sensitively and specifically, nor is it known how to prevent episodes of lethal electrical instability. Many therapeutic procedures shown to prolong survival in patients with angina or following a myocardial infarction (see above) are effective by reducing the incidence of sudden death. Beta-adrenergic blockers administered for several years following acute myocardial infarction prolong survival by reducing sudden death and recurrent infarction (118–120). Coronary bypass surgery prolongs survival in certain subsets of patients with severe coronary artery disease by preventing sudden death (142, 145). These studies, however, represent only a small proportion of those at risk for sudden death. Because two-thirds of patients with sudden cardiac death appear to have "pure" electrical instability, often occurring in the setting of asymptomatic, complex, or frequent ventricular ectopic beats, the role of antiarrhythmic agents needs to be considered. This is an area of active investigation, but no controlled clinical trials have shown prolonged survival with treatment by an antiarrhythmic agent.

Variant Angina

Clinical Description and Pathophysiology

Variant angina, or Prinzmetal's angina, was described by Prinzmetal as angina at rest accompanied by ST-segment elevation in the absence of exertional angina (146). He postulated that it might be caused by transient narrowing as the result of changes in the vasomotor tone of proximal coronary artery stenoses. Subsequent angiographic investigation of patients fitting this definition has shown findings that vary from normal coronary arteries to severe atherosclerotic coronary artery disease; thus, it is not a single disease entity, with the latter group overlapping with unstable angina patients. Nevertheless, it appears that a small group of patients has predominantly unprovoked, at-rest angina with dramatic ST-segment changes and sometimes malignant ventricular arrhythmias. Many patients are premenopausal women who smoke cigarettes. Anginal attacks are most frequent in the morning hours, with marked variability over time in the disease activity. The mechanism of the coronary spasm is unknown, although in about 25% of patients evidence has been found of a more generalized vasospastic syndrome such as Raynaud's phenomenon or migraine headaches.

Diagnosis

The diagnosis is best made by demonstrating marked ST-segment shifts during episodes of unprovoked angina in a patient who otherwise has normal exercise tolerance. Coronary arteriography during an anginal episode usually shows spasm in the coronary artery predicted by the electrocardiographic ST-segment changes. Because anginal episodes occur unpredictably, however, such an episode might not occur spontaneously during coronary arteriography. Ergonovine maleate, an ergot alkaloid, has been used to provoke coronary spasm during coronary arteriography; a good relationship between provokable spasm and the clinical syndrome seems to exist.

Treatment

Both nitrates and calcium channel blockers are generally effective in these patients, either separately or in combination. Of course, cessation of smoking should be advised. The prognosis in patients with angiographically normal coronary arteries is good although, rarely, acute myocardial infarction can occur.

Silent Myocardial Ischemia

Silent myocardial ischemia is the occurrence of unprovoked ST-segment shifts consistent with myocardial ischemia, but without pain or other discomfort. It is best detected on ambulatory electrocardiographic monitoring. Many patients with more typical exertional angina also have episodes of silent myocardial ischemia; some patients have no symptoms whatever. Most patients with silent ischemia probably have significant atherosclerotic coronary artery disease. It is unknown whether this represents relatively small areas of ischemic myocardium that do not reach the pain threshold, or whether these patients have a defect in visceral pain perception (147, 148)

A possible mechanism (see above, Basic Considerations) is that intense cardiac vagal stimulation activates centers in the brain stem involved with descending modulating (inhibiting systems), which impair the transmission of nociceptive impulses in the dorsal horn to the spinothalamic tract and other ascending "pain" systems (78). The clinical and prognostic significance of silent myocardial ischemia is unknown at this time. Because by definition no symptoms are found, the only reason for treatment would be to prevent myocardial infarction and improve prognosis. The relation of silent ischemia to sudden death or subsequent myocardial infarction is unclear, so, treatment at this time might be premature.

D. CHEST PAIN FROM OTHER CARDIOVASCULAR DISEASE

Aortic Stenosis

Pathophysiology

Aortic stenosis in the adult has three causes. The most common cause of severe isolated aortic stenosis is a congenitally abnormal valve. The valve might have been originally bicuspid, one of the most common congenital cardiac anomalies, or might have had three unequal-sized cusps. The valve functions with little or no hemodynamic derangement for the first three or four decades of life. The abnormal anatomy predisposes to fibrotic thickening and deposition of calcium, however, until the valve becomes severely stenotic in middle life. This is a disease predominantly of males. A second pathologic picture is seen in the elderly, in whom gradual wear and tear produces thickening of three originally normal cusps. This process is a common cause of systolic ejection murmurs and mildly thickened leaflets seen on echocardiography in the elderly, but most often does not result in the severe stenosis that requires valve replacement. The third pathologic picture is that created by the late sequelae of rheumatic fever. The inflammatory process of rheumatic fever produces thickening and shortening of the leaflets with commissural fusion; this usually results in the hemodynamic findings of mixed stenosis and regurgitation. In almost all cases the mitral valve is also affected by the rheumatic process.

The thickening and calcification of the aortic valve leaflets produce obstruction to ejection of blood from the left ventricle. The left ventricle hypertrophies (increases its wall thicknesses) in response to this "pressure overload" and can only maintain a normal stroke volume by markedly increasing the intraventricular systolic pressure from the normal 120 mm Hg to (frequently) over 200 mm Hg. The normal aortic valve produces no measurable pressure gradient between the left ventricle and aorta; in severe aortic stenosis this pressure gradient can be as high as 100 mm Hg (Figure 54-11). The left ventricle might be able to compensate for this marked pressure overload for many years, but eventually myocardial failure develops. The left ventricle increases its preload (filling pressure) to maintain the falling stroke volume. With increasing preload comes ventricular dilatation and a falling ejection fraction. The rising diastolic pressure required to maintain cardiac output results in pulmonary venous hypertension, decreased pulmonary compliance, and the sensation of dyspnea. Once the full syndrome of congestive heart failure ensues prognosis of untreated aortic stenosis is guarded; 50% of such patients die within 2 years if the valve is not replaced.

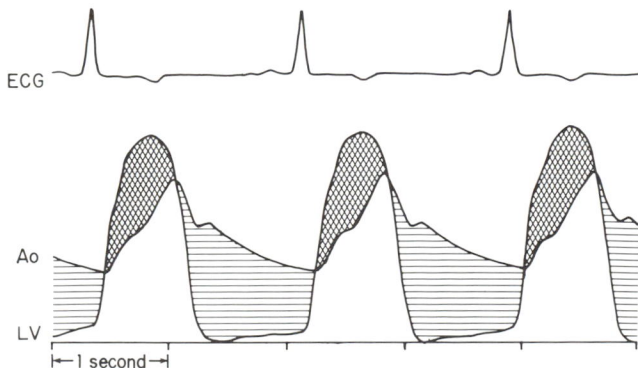

FIG. 54-11. ECG and pressure recordings from a patient with moderately severe aortic stenosis (calculated valve area = 1.0 cm²). The cross-hatched area indicates the pressure gradient between the aorta (Ao) and the left ventricle (LV); normally, no gradient is measurable. The area marked by horizontal lines represents the diastolic pressure gradient across the coronary bed—that is, the head of pressure driving blood through the coronary arteries. Because of the low aortic diastolic and increased left ventricular diastolic pressures, this driving gradient is reduced.

Symptoms and Signs

The most common symptom in aortic stenosis is dyspnea. This results from the increased left ventricular diastolic pressure producing pulmonary venous hypertension, which in turn results in transudation of fluid into the pulmonary interstitium. This transudation reduces pulmonary compliance and impairs oxygen transport, with both resulting in the symptom of dyspnea.

Angina is a relatively common symptom in patients with severe aortic stenosis. The pathophysiology is similar to that of angina caused by atherosclerotic coronary artery disease in that it is the result of myocardial ischemia. It differs in that significant coronary artery disease is present in 50% or less of adult patients with aortic stenosis. In patients without obstructive coronary artery disease the myocardial ischemia is the result of increased oxygen demand caused by the high left ventricular wall stress resulting from the high left ventricular systolic pressures required to overcome the obstructed valve. The impaired coronary blood flow is caused by the reduced driving pressure across the coronary bed as a result of the elevated left ventricular diastolic pressure and reduced aortic diastolic pressure (Table 54-5, Fig. 54-11). Finally, the myocardial fiber hypertrophy can exceed the capillary growth. Even in patients with obstructive coronary artery disease similar pathophysiology of angina may pertain, because aortic valve replacement alone usually relieves the angina.

Diagnosis

The most common clinical presentation is that of a relatively asymptomatic middle-aged male with a systolic ejection murmur and possibly evidence of left ventricular hypertrophy on the ECG. Although the symptoms of angina, congestive heart failure, and syncope were emphasized in the past, the most common early symptom is dyspnea on exertion. If the diagnosis is delayed until congestive heart failure has developed, irreversible myocardial failure can also have occurred. In other words, aortic stenosis must be diagnosed and treated before left ventricular dilatation and heart failure occur. Because the anginal pain of aortic stenosis is the result of myocardial ischemia, it shares many characteristics with that of angina caused by obstructive coronary artery disease. It is vague, diffuse, retrosternal, often exertional, and promptly relieved by rest. Although it can be promptly relieved by nitroglycerin, the administration of nitroglycerin might present some risk to patients with left ventricular outflow obstruction. The drop in peripheral resistance cannot be compensated for by increased left ventricular ejection; hence, the arterial pressure can fall precipitously and produce dizziness or syncope.

PHYSICAL EXAMINATION. Physical signs are useful in determining that aortic valve disease is present, but are less useful in assessing the severity of the stenosis. The characteristic finding is a systolic ejection murmur in the aortic area, with radiation to both carotid arteries. Often, however, the ejection murmur is clearly heard, or even is loudest, at the apex. In severe stenosis the peripheral pulses can have reduced amplitude and slowed upstroke—pulsus parvus et tardus. Abnormal peripheral pulses are often modulated by the compliance of the vascular system, however, and have not been consistently useful in judging severity. The left ventricular impulse is often sustained, a sign of hypertrophy, but is in the normal location if dilatation has not occurred. A thrill palpable over the upper sternum is uncommon but, when present, usually indicates severe stenosis. Because the thickened calcified leaflets are relatively immobile they do not make a sound when closing, so splitting of the second sound is not heard in adults with aortic stenosis. Similarly, a systolic ejection click is almost never heard in adults but is often present in children with aortic stenosis, in whom it is caused by the valve snapping upward at the onset of ejection.

ELECTROCARDIOGRAM AND CHEST ROENTGENOGRAM. The ECG provides important clues to the presence of left ventricular hypertrophy, which in the absence of systemic hypertension often means significant stenosis. The chest roentgenogram is generally of little help in assessing the severity of the stenosis. It is useful in evaluating for the presence of left ventricular dilatation and pulmonary vascular congestion, both signs of myocardial failure. Rarely, evidence of calcification can be seen on the chest roentgenogram but, because calcification is universally present in adults with significant stenosis, more sensitive techniques for detecting the calcification must be used, such as fluoroscopy. The absence of valve calcification in the adult means that the stenosis is not severe; obviously this is not the case in children with congenital aortic stenosis.

ECHOCARDIOGRAM. M-mode and two-dimensional echocardiograms provide useful anatomic information, but cannot provide precise indications of the severity of the stenosis. The severely thickened, immobile leaflets can be seen, but the anatomic derangement correlates poorly with the physiologic derangement. The one useful finding is that a leaflet opening of 15 mm or more on the M-mode echocardiogram reliably excludes significant stenosis. More recently, the measurement of blood velocity by the Doppler principle has proven to be useful in the noninvasive assessment of the severity of aortic stenosis (149). To maintain a normal stroke volume the blood passing through the narrowed aortic orifice must do so at an increased velocity. Using the Bernoulli equation relating pressure drop across a stenosis to change in velocity, the instantaneous aortic valve gradient can be reliably estimated from blood velocity in the aortic root measured by Doppler ultrasound (149).

CARDIAC CATHETERIZATION. Cardiac catheterization has been useful in defining the severity of aortic stenosis, assessing ventricular function, and determining whether associated coronary artery disease is present. Now, with accurate ultrasound techniques for quantitating the severity of aortic stenosis and radionuclide or echocardiographic techniques for assessing ventricular function, some younger patients can undergo valve replacement without prior cardiac catheterization. Cardiac catheterization is still the preferred definitive diagnostic study in older patients with a substantial risk of concomitant coronary artery disease (over the age of 40), however, because it is the only reliable technique for identifying and localizing coronary artery obstructions.

Treatment

The primary therapeutic issue in aortic stenosis patients is the timing of valve replacement. Medical therapy has little to offer in symptomatic patients other than minimizing the risks of valve replacement by optimizing hemodynamic status. Certainly, all patients with angina, syncope, or congestive heart failure caused by aortic stenosis should be offered valve replacement if their general medical condition makes the risk of surgery acceptable and allows a meaningful life following valve replacement. In patients with symptomatic aortic stenosis cardiac catheterization usually shows a mean aortic valve gradient of 40 mm Hg or more and an estimated valve orifice area of 1.0 cm^2 or less. It is still controversial whether asymptomatic patients with severe aortic stenosis should also be offered valve replacement.

Aortic valve replacement can be accomplished with an operative mortality rate of 5 to 10%. Reparative procedures on the aortic valve have been tried but are not effective, either because of failure to relieve the stenosis or because of rapid recurrence of the stenosis. Two types of prosthetic valves are currently in common use, the totally prosthetic mechanical valve and the bioprosthetic valve (150, 151). The mechanical valves are either of the tilting disk or ball-in-a-cage variety. The bioprosthetic valve is a porcine aortic valve mounted on a stent for easier placement in the recipient. Because the porcine valve is avascular and perhaps because of its sterilization and treatment with glutaraldehyde, it is nonantigenic. Nevertheless, it is a nonliving biologic structure; the stresses imposed by millions of openings and closings under pressure result in gradual disintegration of the collagen and elastic fibers in the valve. Thus, biologic valves are expected to have a finite life-span, perhaps in the range of 10 years. On the other hand, they are relatively nonthrombogenic and generally do not require anticoagulation, with its attendant risk of bleeding. Mechanical prostheses are durable but are thrombogenic and require permanent anticoagulation with warfarin. Two randomized trials comparing outcome of patients undergoing valve replacement with a mechanical prosthesis with bioprosthesis have shown no difference in survival (150, 151). One trial (initiated by the senior author) has shown fewer valve-related complications in patients receiving the bioprosthesis, because of fewer clinically significant bleeds.

Prognosis

Patients with aortic stenosis who are asymptomatic and maintain normal exercise tolerance probably have a good prognosis. On the other hand, the prognosis changes precipitously with the onset of symptoms; 25% die in the first year and 50% within 2 years of the onset of symptoms. The prognosis is worst if the symptoms are those of congestive heart failure, with nearly all patients dying within 2 years. Unfortunately, although valve replacement improves prognosis in patients with congestive heart failure caused by aortic stenosis, the prognosis is worse than in aortic stenosis patients without heart failure undergoing valve replacement.

Aortic Regurgitation

Pathophysiology

Aortic regurgitation has many causes; some of the more common are a congenitally bicuspid valve, rheumatic heart disease, endocarditis, many connective tissue disorders, and collagen vascular diseases. To compensate for the loss of a portion of left ventricular ejection back into the left ventricle, the left ventricle increases its stroke volume by dilating to as much as five times its normal volume.

Rarely, patients with pure aortic regurgitation and no coronary artery disease experience angina pectoris. The pathophysiology is analogous to that presented for aortic stenosis. The marked left ventricular dilatation that represents the compensation for significant chronic volume overload results in increased left ventricular wall stress. Although left ventricular systolic pressures are usually normal, the increased radius of the left ventricle results in increased wall stress (and, thereby, the increased myocardial oxygen demand) according to the LaPlace relationship. Coronary blood flow can be impaired both by a low aortic diastolic pressure from the low-resistance runoff back into the left ventricle and by an increased left ventricular diastolic pressure.

Symptoms and Signs

Aortic regurgitation can be asymptomatic for many years, even if it is severe. Like aortic stenosis, the most common symptom is dyspnea on exertion. Late in the course of the disease the full picture of congestive heart failure can be seen—including marked fatigue, orthopnea, paroxysmal nocturnal dyspnea, and edema.

Diagnosis

The diagnosis is usually easily made from the physical examination, which reveals the typical diastolic, decrescendo, high-pitched murmur at the left sternal border, wide pulse pressure, bounding peripheral pulses, and a displaced cardiac impulse caused by the left ventricular dilatation. Echocardiography and Doppler ultrasound are useful in confirming the diagnosis and in assessing left ventricular size and function and the severity of the regurgitation. Cardiac catheterization is helpful in assessing coronary artery disease, quantitating the severity of the regurgitation, evaluating for other valve involvement, and assessing left ventricular function.

Treatment

Patients with severe symptomatic aortic regurgitation should undergo valve replacement. Controversy persists regarding the timing of valve replacement in patients with significant regurgitation but few or no symptoms.

Mitral Valve Prolapse

Chest pain is frequently associated with mitral valve prolapse, although the exact pathogenesis of chest pain is unclear. Mitral valve prolapse is one of the most frequent cardiovascular abnormalities, occurring in 5 to 10% of females and in 1 to 2% of males. In the milder forms the distinction from normal is often unclear. The full syndrome consists of typical auscultatory findings of a midsystolic click and late systolic murmur, atypical chest pain, and arrhythmias (152, 153).

Etiology and Pathophysiology

Although there are multiple causes, the common denominator appears to be a mitral apparatus that is too large; thus, as the ventricle becomes smaller with systolic ejection, the mitral leaflets prolapse into the left atrium. The chordae are too long, and the mitral leaflets large and redundant. Histologic examination of the leaflets reveals a loose myxomatous material in the leaflets. Haphazard arrangement and disruption of the collagen can be seen on electron microscopy. Although mitral valve prolapse can be seen in those with known connective tissue disorders such as Marfan's and Ehlers-Danlos syndromes, most patients with prolapse do not have another identifiable connective tissue disorder. Nevertheless, it is thought that mitral valve prolapse can be a specific genetic syndrome because it is inherited in many patients, often with a characteristic body habitus including pectus excavatum and an asthenic appearance.

In early systole the valve might be competent; as the ventricle becomes smaller and the valve prolapses, regurgitation occurs and produces the late systolic murmur. The systolic click occurs at the time of prolapse, usually in midsystole, and is thought to be caused by the snapping of the leaflets as they become taut at the full extent of the prolapse.

Symptoms and Signs

Mitral valve prolapse should be considered in the differential diagnosis of most types of chest pain, especially if the pain is not typical of angina and the patient is female. The pain often is sharp, stabbing, and nonexertional. It usually does not respond to nitroglycerin. The pathophysiology of the pain is unknown. Some have attributed it to abnormal tension on the papillary muscles, but proof is lacking.

Palpitations from the cardiac arrhythmias associated with this syndrome are also common. Rarely, the arrhythmias can produce alterations in cardiac output resulting in dizziness, syncope, or even sudden cardiac death (154).

Diagnosis

The diagnosis can be made from the physical examination alone if the typical findings of midsystolic click and late systolic murmur are present. Only a portion of the classic findings can be present; however, the physical signs are dynamic, varying greatly with the hemodynamic state. Some patients can have a pansystolic murmur indistinguishable from that of other forms of mitral regurgitation. Thus, echocardiography has become the diagnostic tool of choice, because the prolapsing leaflets can generally be seen on either the M-mode or two-dimensional study (Fig. 54-12). Cardiac catheterization is rarely required unless the mitral

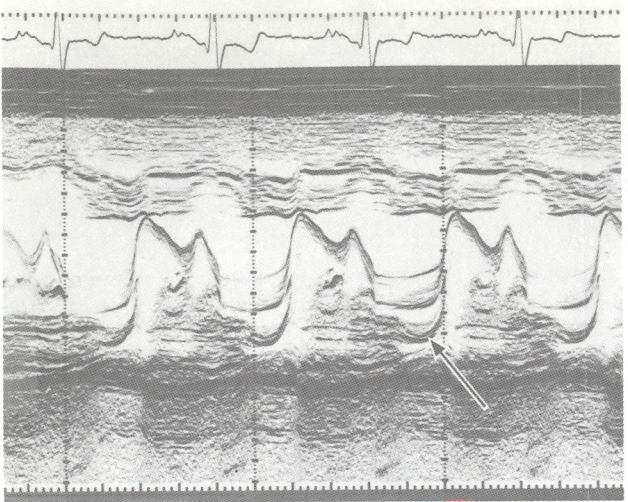

FIG. 54-12. M-mode echocardiogram of the mitral valve in a patient with severe mitral valve prolapse. A portion of the posterior leaflet (arrow) has begun to move posteriorly (i.e., prolapses) in midsystole. The normal motion is gradual anterior motion throughout systole.

regurgitation is severe enough to lead to consideration of mitral valve replacement or repair.

If the patient has palpitations or symptoms of transient cerebral ischemia, evaluation for arrhythmias should be done. The 24-hour ambulatory ECG is the most useful tool, although sometimes the arrhythmias can be identified on the resting or exercise ECG. The full range of arrhythmias from atrial or ventricular premature beats to supraventricular and ventricular tachycardias has been observed.

Treatment

Most patients require no treatment. Patients who have mitral regurgitation should receive endocarditis prophylaxis for dental and other procedures in which bacteremia is likely to occur. If symptomatic arrhythmias are present, antiarrhythmic therapy should be initiated. The identification of an effective agent often requires trial and error with repetitive ambulatory electrocardiographic monitoring. Beta-adrenergic blockers can be effective for both the arrhythmias and chest pain.

Rarely, the mitral regurgitation is severe enough to require mitral valve replacement.

Hypertrophic Cardiomyopathy

Hypertrophic cardiomyopathy is a relatively rare, genetically transmitted disease. Chest pain is a frequent symptom in patients with hypertrophic cardiomyopathy, although dyspnea is probably the most common symptom. The major significance of this disorder is that death may occur suddenly. It is a relatively common cause of sudden cardiac death in young people (155).

Pathophysiology

Hypertrophic cardiomyopathy is a disease of unknown cause characterized by marked hypertrophy of the left ventricular wall without dilatation of the chamber. Systolic function of the ventricle is preserved or even supernormal in the earlier stages of the disease. The dyspnea and exercise intolerance are the result of diastolic dysfunction secondary to abnormal ventricular compliance caused by the massive hypertrophy of the ventricular walls. Some patients have disproportionate hypertrophy of the interventricular septum (asymmetric septal hypertrophy, ASH) that, together with the anterior leaflet of the mitral valve may result in obstruction to systolic outflow from the left ventricle. This subset of patients with hypertrophic cardiomyopathy is known as idiopathic hypertrophic subaortic stenosis (IHSS) in the United States and as hypertrophic obstructive cardiomyopathy (HOCM) in Britain.

Diagnosis

Most patients with hypertrophic cardiomyopathy are asymptomatic. The diagnosis can be suspected by a family history of sudden cardiac death or hypertrophic cardiomyopathy, by an ECG showing unexplained left ventricular hypertrophy, or by the murmur in those patients with the obstructive variety of the disease.

The most common symptom among symptomatic patients is dyspnea on exertion. The chest pain is anginal in character and is usually the result of myocardial ischemia. Although the epicardial coronary arteries are typically large and free of obstructive disease, an imbalance exists between myocardial oxygen demand and supply (Table 54-5). Patients with the obstructive variety have increased left ventricular wall stress because of the high systolic pressures. Coronary blood flow can be impaired because of the high diastolic pressure in the left ventricle. Also, the marked myocardial fiber hypertrophy outstrips capillary growth. Both atrial and ventricular arrhythmias are relatively common and can produce palpitations, dizziness, or even syncope.

The ECG is nearly always abnormal, most commonly showing the QRS voltage and repolarization abnormalities of left ventricular hypertrophy. Also, abnormal Q-waves, which are sometimes confused with myocardial infarction, are seen in 30 to 50% of patients.

The diagnostic procedure of choice is the echocardiogram. The increased left ventricular wall thicknesses and normal chamber size are usually easily identified. In patients with the obstructive variety, the systolic anterior motion of the anterior mitral valve leaflet is characteristic.

Treatment

No specific therapy is required for asymptomatic patients. Echocardiography of family members and genetic counseling, however, should be recommended for all patients with this disorder. Beta-adrenergic blockade with propranolol has been the primary mode of therapy in symptomatic patients (156). It is relatively beneficial in relieving the angina, but not the dyspnea. It is effective through several possible mechanisms: (a) slowing the heart rate and reducing myocardial oxygen demand, as in coronary artery disease; (b) reducing the left ventricular outflow gradient in patients with the obstructive variety; and (c) controlling the arrhythmias. For a selected group of patients with persistent symptoms despite maximal doses of propranolol and a persistent left ventricular outflow gradient, resection of a portion of the disproportionately hypertrophied septum has resulted in symptomatic improvement (157). No form of therapy has been clearly shown to reduce the risk of sudden cardiac death.

Acute Pericarditis (XVII-6)

Acute pericarditis is caused by inflammation of the pericardium and produces a characteristic pain syndrome, pericardial friction rub, and electrocardiographic changes. Other forms of pericarditis such as subacute effusive pericarditis and constrictive pericarditis are not discussed here, because these usually do not produce pain but cause hemodynamic abnormalities.

Pericarditis occurs more frequently than recognized clinically. Evidence of previous pericardial inflammation has been found in 2 to 6% of autopsies, whereas acute pericarditis accounts for only about 0.1% of hospital admissions.

Pathophysiology

Pathologic examination reveals acute inflammatory cells within both the visceral and parietal pericardium. The inflammation can invade the myocardium beneath the visceral pericardium, which probably accounts for the characteristic electrocardiographic changes (see below). Fibrin becomes deposited on the pericardium, giving it a shaggy, reddened appearance; an accompanying pericardial effusion may be present. Most cases of acute pericarditis heal, leaving little in the way of residual changes except for a few clinically insignificant adhesions between the visceral and parietal pericardium. In a few cases, however, acute pericarditis leaves marked fibrotic changes in both layers of adherent pericardium, resulting in constriction of the heart.

The following are some common causes of acute pericarditis:

a. Idiopathic
b. Infection: viral; pyogenic bacteria
c. Immunologic disorders: acute rheumatic fever; rheumatoid arthritis; systemic lupus erythematous; scleroderma; postmyocardial infarction (Dressler's syndrome; postpericardiotomy syndrome
d. Acute myocardial infarction
e. Drugs: procainamide; hydralazine; isoniazid

It is thought that viral infection (particularly Coxsackie B and echovirus type 8) accounts for a large percentage of cases of acute pericarditis, although documentation of viral infection is often not possible. Uremia and drugs (procainamide and hydralazine) are other common causes of acute pericarditis. Bacterial infection is a rare but potentially lethal form of acute pericarditis that requires immediate diagnosis and treatment with drainage and antibiotics (158).

Symptoms and Signs

Acute pericarditis characteristically produces severe sharp chest pain that worsens in the supine position and is partially relieved by sitting. It is often markedly exacerbated by deep breathing, leading to confusion with pleuritis (which can accompany acute pericarditis). Some patients experience a pulsating nature to the pain with each heartbeat. The pain is more often retrosternal but can radiate to the anterior neck, the mandible, and the trapezius ridge (159). Patients can be dyspneic because of the marked increase in severity of the pain with normal respiration.

Diagnosis

The diagnosis can generally be made by the history of typical positional pain, as described above, the physical signs, and the ECG.

PHYSICAL EXAMINATION. The prime physical sign is the pericardial friction rub. Since the time of Laennec the rub has been described as sounding like creaking leather. Typically, three separate components to the rub have been noted: systole, rapid ventricular filling in early diastole, and atrial contraction. Often only one or two components are present, however, with the systolic component usually being the last to disappear. In its complete form the rub is easily distinguishable from cardiac murmurs but, if only the systolic component is present, this distinction is often unclear. The rub often changes with position; to exclude a pericardial friction rub the patient must be examined in multiple positions, including on hands and knees.

ELECTROCARDIOGRAM. The typical electrocardiographic finding is ST-segment elevation in most leads. Later, T-wave flattening, inversion, or both can develop. New Q-waves never develop—this is a feature that distinguishes acute pericarditis from an acute Q-wave myocardial infarction. The distinction from non-Q-wave infarction is much more difficult, however, and requires the identification of the rub, no or minimal changes in cardiac enzyme levels, and a rapid response to anti-inflammatory agents. ST-segment elevation is, of course, nonspecific; in addition to occurring in the early stages of AMI, ST-segment elevation can be a normal variant known as early repolarization, a sign of a ventricular aneurysm, or a sign of coronary artery spasm.

OTHER STUDIES. The chest roentgenogram is of relatively little value. If an accompanying pericardial effusion is present, the cardiac silhouette can be enlarged. Levels of cardiac enzymes, creatine kinase and lactate dehydrogenase, are most commonly within the normal range, but occasionally minor elevations with positive isoenzymes can be found. The echocardiogram, although commonly ordered, provides little specific information. Whereas the echocardiogram is the best diagnostic tool available for pericardial effusion, effusion is often absent in acute pericarditis.

Treatment

The pain of acute pericarditis usually promptly responds to institution of anti-inflammatory agents. If the pain is mild, aspirin, 650 mg tid or qid, can be adequate. For more severe cases a nonsteroidal anti-inflammatory agent should be tried; indomethacin, 25 to 75 mg tid or qid, seems to be highly effective in most cases. In fact, the pain relief can be dramatic and rapid, within 4 to 8 hours. If no relief has been obtained in 24 to 48 hours, prednisone should be started at a dose of 60 to

80 mg daily in divided doses; this can usually be tapered and stopped after about 2 weeks of therapy. The response to anti-inflammatory agents is so characteristic that failure to respond to the above regimen should lead to questioning of the diagnosis. If the pain is severe, narcotic analgesic agents should be used until relief is obtained with anti-inflammatory agents.

In a minority of patients acute pericarditis can recur weeks or months after completion of the initial course of therapy, requiring repeat treatment. In a few patients pericardiectomy might be required to control the pain of multiple recurrence and avoid the side effects of sustained prednisone therapy. In most patients the pericarditis heals without recurrence or late sequelae. A few patients, however, develop chronic constrictive pericarditis.

E. DISEASES OF THE THORACIC AORTA

The major diseases involving the thoracic aorta are dissecting hematoma, thoracic aortic aneurysms, false aneurysm of the aorta, annuloaortic ectasia, Takayasu's arteritis, and giant cell arteritis. Of these, dissecting hematoma is of the greatest significance clinically, and the only one in which pain is the primary presenting complaint.

Dissection of the Thoracic Aorta (XVII-7)

This fortunately rare disease begins with an intimal tear followed by progressive formation of a plane within the media of the aorta by extravasating blood. Untreated, it is lethal in most patients because of rupture of the aorta. In a large autopsy series 21% died within 24 hours of onset of symptoms, 37% by 48 hours, and 74% within 2 weeks (160). It is the most common clinical catastrophe involving the aorta, far exceeding rupture of the abdominal aorta. Initially it is neither a true aneurysm (thinning and dilatation of the wall of the aorta involving all layers) nor a false aneurysm (the aneurysmal wall being only the adventitial layer); therefore, the terms "dissecting hematoma" or "aortic dissection" are preferable to "dissecting aneurysm."

The first clear description was by Morgagni, who in 1769 described the autopsy of a case with an intimal tear in the ascending aorta and rupture into the pericardial space (161). In 1760 King George II of England died suddenly while at stool. The autopsy revealed an intimal tear and a pericardial space distended with blood.

Dissection of the aorta occurs in all adult age groups, but has its greatest incidence in middle age and older. Other than a history of hypertension, patients are often completely healthy right up to the acute event, which in a few cases seems to have been precipitated by abrupt motion such as swinging a golf club. Males predominate over females by a ratio of 2 or 3:1. The most common associated risk factor is hypertension. The incidence of aortic dissection appears to be increased in pregnant females and in patients with congenitally bicuspid aortic valves, Marfan's syndrome, or Ehlers-Danlos syndrome.

Pathogenesis

CYSTIC MEDIAL NECROSIS. Some difference of opinion exists regarding the primacy of cystic medial necrosis in the pathogenesis of aortic dissection. It is agreed that cystic medial necrosis is seen in the unaffected aortic wall of most patients dying of aortic dissection; both elastic and collagen fibers degenerate, with cystic spaces within media. Although a similar pathologic picture is seen in patients with Marfan's syndrome, an autosomal dominant connective tissue disorder susceptible to aortic dissection, an inherited biochemical defect cannot be identified in most patients with dissection. The cystic medial necrosis can be the result of excessive mechanical stress and strain, because it increases in frequency in patients with systemic hypertension or hypertension of the ascending aorta caused by coarctation of the aorta. This observation is the source of the controversy of the role of cystic medial necrosis because it seems to occur with equal frequency in hypertensives without dissection as in patients with dissection, most of whom have also had hypertension (162). Nevertheless many authorities believe that the weakening of the media of the aorta through degeneration of elastic and collagen is an important factor in the pathogenesis of dissection of the aorta (163, 164).

INTIMAL TEAR. A tear of the intima of the aorta can be identified in most but not all autopsied cases of aortic dissection; this tear can also frequently be seen by aortography. It is now generally thought that this tear is the initial event in the dissection. Previously, some suggested that the dissection began with bleeding within the media because of rupture of the vasa vasorum; the intimal tear would then be a secondary event, releasing the medial bleeding into the lumen of the aorta. The vasa vasorum supply primarily the outer third of the media and adventitia, while the dissection begins in the inner half of the aortic wall (163). The intimal tear is seen twice as frequently in the ascending aorta, where the hydrodynamic forces of left ventricular ejection are the greatest, than elsewhere in the aorta. Thus, it is thought that abnormal stress and strain play a role in the initiation of the intimal tear, as well as in the development of cystic medial necrosis and the propagation of the dissection itself. The hemodynamic variables that seem to be important are the rate of rise of aortic pressure (dP/dT), the systolic pressure, and the pulse pressure (systolic pressure minus diastolic pressure). The stress within the wall of the aorta is a function of both the intraluminal pressure and the radius (the LaPlace relationship). Thus, for a given aortic pressure, the stress in the wall of the aorta is greater in a dilated aorta than in a nondilated one. Similarly, the increased stroke volume and decreased vascular resistance of pregnancy, resulting in a widened pulse pressure and increased aortic dP/dT, might be why dissection appears with increased frequency in pregnant women.

PROPAGATION OF THE DISSECTION. Once the intimal tear allows intraluminal blood access to the media of the aorta, the hydrostatic forces of each heartbeat

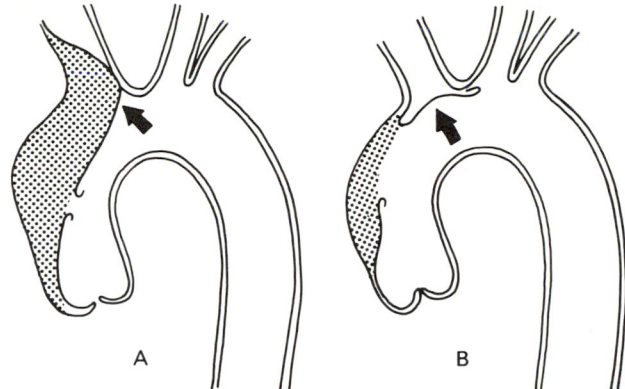

FIG. 54-13. Mechanism of occlusion of branch vessels in aortic dissection. *A*. Dissection blocks brachiocephalic artery with loss of pulse and no blood pressure in the right upper limb. *B*. Part of a lining of the aorta blocks the vessels. Modified from Slater, E.E.: Aortic dissection: Presentation and diagnosis. *In* Aortic Dissection. Edited by R.M. Doroghazi and E.E. Slater. New York, McGraw-Hill, 1983, p. 65.

result in further tearing and separation of the media. The dissection can extend as far distally as the iliac arteries and proximally to the aortic valve cusps and ostia of the coronary arteries. Although the term "dissecting hematoma" is commonly used, this does not imply that the blood dissecting between the layers of media is clotted. Rather, a second lumen to the aorta is formed, known as a "false lumen," which can be detected angiographically and by CT scanning. Sometimes the false lumen can rejoin the true lumen distally through a second tear in the intima; this can relieve some of the pressure in the false lumen and slow or stop the dissecting process.

As the dissection passes the orifice of a side branch of the aorta, the displaced intima can result in obstruction of that branch (Fig. 54-13). Thus, loss of distal limb pulses or occlusion of a coronary artery resulting in myocardial infarction is frequently seen in aortic dissection. Also, the blood supply to other vital organs such as the kidney and bowel can be disrupted by this process. If the dissection extends to the aortic valve, the support of the valve leaflets can be altered so that aortic regurgitation ensues (Fig. 54-14).

Although the interruption of blood supply to vital organs can be devastating the usual cause of death is external rupture, either into the pleural space or the pericardial space.

Symptoms and Signs

PAIN. Pain, which is usually excruciating, is a presenting symptom in over 90% of patients with dissection and the predominant presenting symptom in over 75% (165). The pain is usually maximal in intensity at its onset in contrast to the pain of myocardial ischemia or infarction, which often waxes and wanes. The pain is sometimes described as a tearing or ripping sensation. The pain can migrate from an anterior retrosternal location to posterior or back pain as the dissection propagates. The location of the pain is of some value in localizing the dissection (165) (Table 54-8). Two-thirds of patients with dissection in the ascending aorta have anterior chest pain, compared to only 27% of patients with dissection in the descending thoracic aorta. Nearly all (94%) patients with dissection in the descending thoracic aorta have pain in the back, but 50% of patients with dissection in the ascending aorta also have back pain.

OTHER SYMPTOMS AND SIGNS. Commonly associated with the pain are symptoms and signs of autonomic nervous system hyperactivity such as diaphoresis, bradycardia or tachycardia, apprehension, nausea, and vomiting. Other presenting symptoms are syncope, stroke, paraplegia from interruption of the spinal arteries, pulse loss with resultant limb ischemia, and congestive heart failure from aortic regurgitation. In the large series from Massachusetts General Hospital, only 8 of 124 patients had no pain: 4 presented with congestive heart failure, 2 with stroke, and 2 with an abnormal chest roentgenogram (165).

Hypertension, sometimes severe, is commonly present—more frequently with dissection of the descending thoracic aorta than the ascending. In one series 60% of patients with dissection of the descending aorta had a diastolic pressure exceeding 120 mm Hg, and in 42% it exceeded 140 mm Hg (166). Conversely, up to 20% of patients with ascending aortic dissection can be hypotensive.

Loss of one or more arterial pulses is common, having been reported in 50% of patients with dissection involving the ascending aorta and in 16% of those with dissection of the descending thoracic aorta (166). This sign is particularly useful if the state of the pulses has been carefully recorded previously.

FIG. 54-14. Three potential mechanisms for the development of aortic regurgitation in aortic dissection. *A*. A circumferential hematoma widens the aortic root and separates the aortic cusps. *B*. Displacement of one cusp substantially below the level of the others by asymmetric pressure of the dissecting aneurysm. *C*. Actual destruction of the annular leaflet support leading to a flail cusp. Modified from Slater, E.E.: Aortic dissection: Presentation and diagnosis. *In* Aortic Dissection. Edited by R.M. Doroghazi and E.E. Slater. New York, McGraw-Hill, 1983, p. 65.

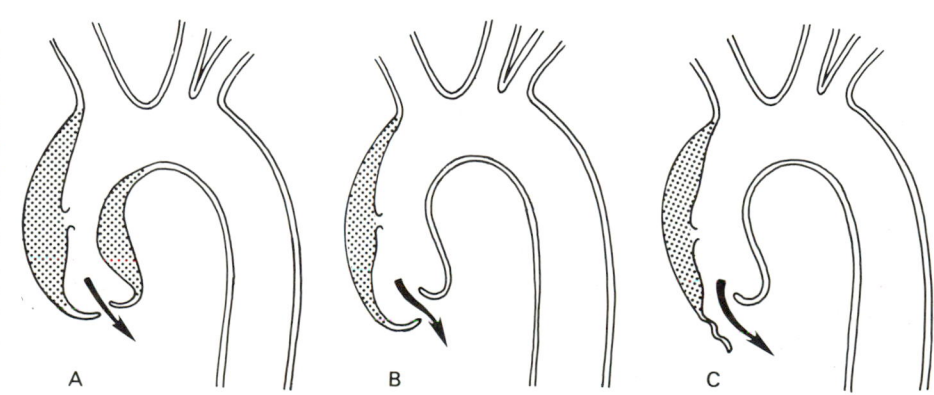

TABLE 54-8. Relationship of Site of Pain to Location of Dissection

Site of Pain	Site of Dissection (% of Total)	
	Proximal*	Distal†
Major Pain		
Chest, anterior	65	27
Chest, posterior	10	57
Chest, both anterior and posterior	9	12
Neck and throat	9	0
Abdomen	6	3
Suprapubic	0	1
Any Pain		
Anterior only	50	6
Posterior only	10	36
Anterior and posterior	40	57
Any pain in back	50	94
Jaw and throat	26	10
Low back pain	13	21

*47 cases.
†69 cases.
Adapted from Slater, E.E., and De Sanctis, R.W.: The clinical recognition of dissecting aortic aneurysm. Am. J. Med., *60*:625, 1976.

One-half to two-thirds of patients with dissection of the ascending aorta develop the high-pitched decrescendo murmur of aortic regurgitation. It has been reported to be commonly heard along the right sternal border in contrast to the more common types of aortic regurgitation, which are best heard along the left sternal border. The other well-known signs of severe aortic regurgitation (e.g., bounding peripheral pulses, wide pulse pressure, left ventricular heave) however, might not be present early in the course of dissection because not enough time has passed for left ventricular dilatation and increased stroke output to occur.

Although rupture of the dissection into the pericardial space is usually promptly fatal and is the most common cause of death from dissection, a few patients can have a limited leak into the pericardium. These patients can exhibit a pericardial rub or hypotension and pulsus paradoxus from pericardial tamponade.

About 20% of patients have neurologic deficits on presentation. Hemiparesis with or without change in consciousness occurs most commonly in patients with dissection of the ascending aorta, while neurologic compromise of the lower extremities (e.g., paraparesis) is seen more commonly with dissection of the descending thoracic aorta.

Diagnosis

The definitive diagnosis of aortic dissection is based on demonstration of the separation of the aorta into true and false lumens. Aortography by selective injection of radiographic contrast material into the ascending aorta accurately distinguishes aortic dissection from other types of aortic aneurysms (167), and is still the diagnostic procedure of choice in most centers. Some controversy exists as to the necessity of establishing the exact site of the intimal tear and the full extent of the dissection, because the decision to undertake surgical therapy and the planning of the surgical approach requires knowledge only of whether or not the ascending aorta is involved (40). Nevertheless, because aortic dissection is such a devastating disease, and still has a substantial surgical mortality rate, as much diagnostic information as possible should be obtained within the constraints of time and safety. Aortography is commonly performed with a catheter passed percutaneously from the femoral artery under continuous pressure monitoring and fluoroscopic guidance. The fear that the passage of the catheter might further damage the fragile aorta, leading to rupture, has not been borne out. The use of a guide wire with a flexible tip or of a looped catheter provides protection against aortic damage. Filming can be performed either directly onto large radiographic film or by cine filming of the output phosphor of an image intensifier. In either case, filming should be done in at least two planes for optimal demonstration of the lesion. Some have claimed that cine filming is more effective in demonstrating the site of the intimal tear because the intimal flap can be seen in motion.

CT scanning with intravenous administration of contrast material appears to accurately distinguish aortic dissection with its true and false lumens from a fusiform aneurysm (168). Many surgeons, however, do not accept this noninvasive procedure as the sole diagnostic procedure before undertaking surgical repair. Because time is of the essence, most centers perform aortography as the sole diagnostic procedure.

The decision to undertake aortography is generally based on the history of the typical tearing, excruciating pain, and a widened thoracic aorta seen on the chest roentgenogram. An abnormal width to the ascending aorta or mediastinum is seen in 85% or more of patients with aortic dissection; a previous chest roentgenogram showing a normal mediastinum is particularly helpful. If the arch of the aorta is involved by the dissection and if calcium is present, the radiographically visible calcium can be separated from the aorta-lung interface by 1 cm or more. This is because the calcification occurs in the intima; this sign is almost diagnostic of dissection.

Dissection can also be diagnosed with echocardiography. Because only the first few centimeters of the ascending aorta are imaged well, however, this procedure has limited sensitivity and is not used as the definitive procedure. The major value of cardiac ultrasonography is in the evaluation for pericardial effusion and the confirmation of aortic insufficiency by the use of Doppler ultrasonography. Other diagnostic procedures are of secondary importance, but aid in the assessment of complications of dissection of the aorta. The mild leukocytosis sometimes seen is probably related to stress. The lactate dehydrogenase level can be elevated if red cells passing through the false lumen are hemolyzed or if myocardial necrosis has occurred. Evidence of myocardial damage should be sought on the ECG and by evidence of elevation of the serum creatine kinase level. Falling urine output and an increasing serum creatinine level can indicate occlusion of a renal artery by the dissection.

Treatment

The first effective therapy, resection, and replacement of the ascending aorta was reported by DeBakey and colleagues in 1955 (169). Although their patients had a relatively low operation mortality rate—21%—these results were not initially duplicated elsewhere. Thus, Wheat and associates introduced the concept that reducing aortic pressure and the dP/dT would limit the dissection and provide an effective means of nonsurgical therapy (170). This was based on the observation that reserpine reduced the mortality rate in turkeys, which are susceptible to aortic dissection. The initial experience of Wheat and colleagues in a small series of patients was favorable, although subsequent follow-up indicated continuing mortality.

MEDICAL THERAPY. Present therapy consists of medical therapy aimed at reducing pressure and dP/dT in all patients and early surgical resection in some subgroups. If the history and chest roentgenogram are strongly suggestive of dissection, antihypertensive therapy should be started even before the definitive diagnosis has been made with aortography. Intravenous nitroprusside or trimethaphan are given to lower the mean arterial pressure to 55 to 70 mm Hg or the systolic pressure to 100 to 120 mm Hg. Beta-adrenergic blockade is also essential; propranolol is given 1 mg intravenously every 5 minutes until the resting heart rate is 60 to 80 beats/minute for a maximal total initial dose of 0.15 mg/kg.

SURGICAL THERAPY. The indications and results of surgery are highly dependent on the type and acuity of the dissection. Many classifications have been proposed, but the Stanford classification proposed by Daily and co-workers in 1970 is the simplest, and is now widely used (171). An aortic dissection is classified as type A if the ascending aorta is involved, regardless of where the intimal tear is and whether the descending aorta is also involved; type B dissections are limited to the descending thoracic aorta. An acute dissection is one diagnosed within 2 weeks of onset of symptoms; a chronic dissection is diagnosed after 2 weeks or longer.

Surgery is recommended for all acute type A dissections provided that the status of other organ systems does not impose an excessive surgical mortality and provides the possibility of satisfactory quality of life. The surgery consists of resection of the ascending aorta from just above the sinus of Valsalva to the origin of the innominate artery, followed by replacement with a Dacron prosthesis. The false lumen is obliterated while making the distal anastomosis if the dissection extends beyond, as it often does. No attempt is made to resect all the involved aorta if the dissection involves the arch or the descending aorta. If coronary occlusion or significant aortic regurgitation has occurred, however, the aortic valve is also replaced and the coronary arteries are reattached to the aortic prosthesis. The operative mortality rate for 24 consecutive patients operated at Stanford between 1976 and 1981 was only 8% (40).

Surgery is recommended for chronic type A dissections if a complication, such as aortic regurgitation, exists that causes heart failure or an expanding aneurysm. The operative procedure is similar to that for acute type A dissections, with an operative mortality rate of 13% in 16 patients operated at Stanford (40).

The role of surgery in acute type B dissections is controversial. Because some centers have reported a high operative mortality rate and a significant incidence of paraplegia from interruption of spinal arterial supply, medical therapy has been recommended unless a complication ensued, however, such as uncontrollable dissection or an expanding aneurysm. Miller suggested, however, that the high operative mortality rate was the result of waiting for a life-threatening complication to occur, and reported only a 13% (1 of 8) operative mortality rate by operating promptly on all acute type B dissections at Stanford between 1976 and 1981 (40). In chronic type B dissections surgery is usually withheld until complications develop. The surgical procedure involves replacement of a relatively short segment of the descending thoracic aorta by a left lateral thoracotomy, obliterating the false lumen at both the distal and proximal anastomoses in the process.

REFERENCES

1. American Heart Association: 1987 Heart Facts. New York, American Heart Association, 1986.
2. Braunwald, E. (ed.): Heart Disease: A Textbook of Cardiovascular Medicine. Philadelphia, W.B. Saunders, 1984.
3. Hurst, J.W., et al. (eds.): The Heart, Arteries and Veins. New York, McGraw-Hill, 1985.
4. Hammermeister, K.E. (ed.): Coronary Bypass Surgery: The Late Results. New York, Praeger, 1983.
5. Dillard, D.H., and Miller, D.W.: Atlas of Cardiac Surgery. New York, Macmillan, 1983.
6. Pruit, R.D.: Historical vignette: Symptoms, signs, signals, and shadows. The pathophysiology of angina pectoris—a historical perspective. Mayo Clin. Proc., 58:394, 1983.
7. Proudfit, W.L.: Origin of concept of ischemic heart disease. Br. Heart J., 50:209, 1983.
8. Procacci, P., and Maresca, M.: Historical considerations of cardiac pain. Pain, 22:325, 1985.
9. Doroghazi, R.M., and Slater, E.E. (eds.): Aortic Dissection. New York, McGraw-Hill, 1983.
10. Celsus, A.C.: De medicina libri octo. Ad fidem optimorum librorum denuo recensuit, adnotatione critica indicibusque instruxit C. Daremberg, Lipsiae, B.B. Teubneri, 1891.
11. Caelius, A.: De Morbis Acutis et Chronicis. Amsterdam, Wetsteniana, 1722.
12. Castelli, B.: Lexicon Medicum Graeco-Latinum ex Hippocrate et Galeno Desumptum. Brae, Mesanae, 1598.
13. Bonet, T.: Selpulchretum sive Anatomia Practica ex Cadaveribus Morbo Denatis. Geneva, Cramer et Perachon, 1700.
14. Heberden, W.: Some account of a disorder of the breast. Med. Trans. R. Coll. Physicians (Lond.), 2:59, 1772.
15. Heberden, W.: Commentaries on the History and Cure of Diseases. London, Payne, 1802.
16. Wall, J.: A letter from Dr. Wall to Dr. Heberden, on the same subject (angina pectoris). Med. Trans. R. Coll. Physicians (Lond.), 3:12, 1785.
17. Baron, J.: The Life of Edward Jenner, M.D. London, Henry Colburn, 1838.
18. Parry, C.H.: An Inquiry into the Symptoms and Causes of the Syncope Anginosa, Commonly Called Angina Pectoris. (With Jenner's letter to Parry.) London, Cadell and Davis, 1799.
19. Burns, A.: Observations on Some of the Most Frequent and Important Diseases of the Heart. Edinburgh, Bryce, 1809.
20. Johnstone, J.: Case of angina pectoris from an unexpected disease in the heart. Mem. Med. Soc. (Lond.), 1:376, 1787.
21. Black, S.: Angina Pectoris, Clinical and Pathological Reports. London, Longman, 1819.
22. Allbutt, C.: Diseases of the Arteries Including Angina Pectoris, Vol. 2. London, Macmillan, 1915, pp. 350–426.
23. Wenckebach, K.F.: Angina pectoris and the possibilities of its surgical relief. Br. Med. J., 1:809, 1924.
24. Gorham, L.W., and Martin, S.J.: Coronary occlusion with and without pain. Arch. Intern. Med., 62:821, 1938.
25. Herrick, J.B.: Sudden obstruction of the coronary arteries. JAMA, 59:2015, 1912.
26. Keefer, C.S., and Resnik, W.H.: Angina pectoris, a syndrome caused by anoxemia of the myocardium. Arch. Intern. Med., 41:469, 1928.

27. Sutton, D.C., and Lueth, H.C.: Pain. Experimental production of pain on excitation of the heart and great vessels. Arch. Intern. Med., *45*:827, 1930.
28. White, J.C., Garrey, W.E., and Atkins, J.A.: Cardiac innervation. Arch. Surg., *26*:765, 1933.
29. Wood, F.C., and Wolferth, C.C.: Angina pectoris: The clinical and electrocardiographic phenomena of the attack and their comparison with the effects of experimental temporary coronary occlusion. Arch. Intern. Med., *47*:339, 1931.
30. Levy, R.I.: Declining mortality in coronary heart disease. Arteriosclerosis, *1*:312, 1981.
31. Dwyer, T., and Netzel, B.S.: A comparison of trends of coronary heart disease mortality in Australia, U.S.A. and England and Wales with reference to three major risk factors—hypertension, cigarette smoking and diet. Int. J. Epidiomol., *9*:65, 1980.
32. Keys, A.: Coronary heart disease in seven countries. Circulation, *41*(Suppl. I):1, 1970.
33. Kannel, W.B., McGee, D., and Gordon, T.: A general cardiovascular risk profile: The Framingham Study. Am. J. Cardiol., *38*:46, 1976.
34. Glueck, C.J., Mattson, F., and Bierman, E.L.: Sounding boards: Diet and coronary heart disease: Another view. N. Engl. J. Med., *298*:1471, 1978.
35. Feinlieb, M., and Williams, R.R.: Relative risks of myocardial infarction, cardiovascular disease and peripheral vascular disease by type of smoking. Proceedings of the Third World Conference on Smoking and Health, Vol. 1. 1976, p. 243.
36. Gordon, T., Kannel, W.B., and McGee, D.: Death and coronary attacks in men after giving up cigarette smoking. A report from the Framingham Study. Lancet, *2*:1345, 1974.
37. Berglund, G., et al.: Coronary heart disease after treatment of hypertension. Lancet, *1*:1, 1978.
38. Hypertension Detection and Followup Program Cooperative Group: Five-year findings of the Hypertension Detection and Followup Program: I. Reduction in mortality of persons with high blood pressure, including mild hypertension. JAMA, *242*:2562, 1979.
39. Bonica, J.J.: The Management of Pain. Philadelphia, Lea & Febiger, 1953, pp. 1310–1361.
40. Miller, D.C.: Surgical management of aortic dissections: Indications, perioperative management and long-term results. *In* Aortic Dissection. Edited by R.M. Doroghazi and E.E. Slater. New York, McGraw-Hill, 1983, pp. 193–243.
41. Anagnostopoulos, C.E., Prabhakar, M.J.S., and Kittle, C.F.: Aortic dissection and dissecting aneurysms. Am. J. Cardiol., *30*:263, 1972.
42. Wheat, M.W., Jr.: Acute dissecting aneurysms of the aorta: Diagnosis and treatment—1979. Am. Heart J., *99*:373, 1980.
43. Larson, E.W. and Edward, W.D.: Risk factors for aortic dissection: A necropsy study of 161 cases. Am. J. Cardiol., *53*:849, 1984.
44. Hammermeister, K.E., et al.: Effect of surgical versus medical therapy on return to work in patients with coronary artery disease. Am. J. Cardiol., *44*:105, 1979.
45. Säwe, U.: Pain in acute myocardial infarction. Acta Med. Scand., *190*:79, 1971.
46. Teodori, U., and Galletti, R.: Il Dolore nelle affezione degli organi interni del Torace. Rome, El Tozzi, 1962, pp. 183–233.
47. Rinzler, S.H., and Travell, J.: Therapy directed at the somatic component of cardiac pain. Am. Heart J., *35*:248, 1948.
48. Malliani, A.: Cardiovascular sympathetic afferent fibers. Rev. Physiol. Biochem. Pharmacol., *94*:11, 1982.
49. Agostini, E., et al.: Functional and histological studies of the vagus nerve and its branches to the heart, lung, and abdominal viscera in the cat. J. Physiol., *135*:182, 1975.
50. Thoren, P.: Role of cardiac vagal C-fibers in cardiovascular control. Rev. Physiol. Biochem. Pharmacol. *86*:1, 1979.
51. Kaufman, M.P., et al.: Stimulation by bradykinin of afferent vagal C-fibers with chemosensitive endings in the heart and aorta of the dog. Circ. Res., *46*:476, 1980.
52. Brown, A.M.: Excitation of afferent cardiac sympathetic nerve fibres during myocardial ischemia. J. Physiol. (Lond.), *190*:35, 1967.
53. Mandl, F.: Die Wirkung der paravertebralen Injektion bein "Angina pectoris." Arch. Klin. Chir., *136*:495, 1925.
54. White, J.C.: Cardiac pain. Anatomic pathways and physiologic mechanisms. Circulation, *16*:644, 1957.
55. Oldefield, B.J., and McLachlan, E.M.: Localization of sensory neurons traversing the stellate ganglion of the cat. J. Comp. Neurol., *182*:915, 1978.
56. Coleridge, H.M., and Coleridge, J.C.G.: Cardiovascular afferents involved in regulation of peripheral vessels. Ann. Rev. Physiol., *42*:413, 1980.
57. Mallinani, A., et al.: Nervous activity of afferent cardiac sympathetic fibres with atrial and ventricular endings. J. Physiol. (Lond.), *229*:457, 1973.
58. Ueda, H., Uchida, Y., and Kamisaka, K.: Distribution and responses of the cardiac sympathetic receptors to mechanically induced circulatory changes. Jpn. Heart J., *10*:70, 1969.
59. Uchida, Y., et al.: Mechanosensitivity of afferent cardiac sympathetic fibers. Am. J. Physiol., *226*:1088, 1974.
60. Casati, R., et al.: Afferent sympathetic unmyelinated fibres with left ventricular endings in cats. J. Physiol. (Lond.), *292*:135, 1979.
61. Uchida, Y.: Afferent aortic nerve fibers with their pathways in cardiac sympathetic nerves. Am. J. Physiol., *228*:990, 1975.
62. Uchida Y., and Murao, S: Excitation of afferent cardiac sympathetic nerve fibers during coronary occlusion. Am. J. Physiol., *226*:1094, 1974.
63. Uchida, Y., and Murao, S.: Potassium-induced excitation of afferent cardiac sympathetic nerve fibers. Am. J. Physiol., *226*:603, 1974.
64. Baker, D.G., et al.: Search for a cardiac nociceptor: Stimulation by bradykinin of sympathetic afferent nerve endings in the heart of the cat. J. Physiol. (Lond.), *306*:519, 1980.
65. Lombardi, F., et al.: Effects of intracoronary administration of bradykinin on the impulse activity of afferent sympathetic unmyelinated fibers with left ventricular endings in the cat. Circ. Res., *48*:69, 1981.
66. Nishi, K., et al.: Activation of afferent cardiac sympathetic nerve fibers of the cat by pain producing substances and by noxious heat. Pflugers Arch., *372*:53, 1977.
67. Burch, G.E., and DePasquale, N.P.: Bradykinin. Am. Heart J., *65*:116, 1963.
68. Kimura, E., et al.: Changes in bradykinin level in coronary sinus blood at the experimental occlusion of a coronary artery. Am. Heart J., *85*:635, 1973.
69. Block, A.R., et al.: Anoxia-induced release of prostaglandins in rabbit-isolated hearts. Circ. Res., *36*:34, 1975.
70. Wennmalm, A., Chanh, P.H., and Junstad, M.: Hypoxia causes prostaglandin release from perfused rabbit hearts. Acta Physiol. Scand., *91*:133, 1974.
71. Staszewska-Barczaka, J., Ferreira, S.H., and Vane, J.R.: Excitatory nociceptive cardiac reflex elicited by bradykinin and potentiated by prostaglandins and myocardial ischemia. Cardiovasc. Res., *10*:314, 1976.
72. Cervero, F.: Mechanisms of visceral pain. *In* Persistent Pain: Modern Methods of Treatment, Vol. 4. Edited by S. Lipton and J. Miles. New York, Grune & Stratton, 1983, pp. 1–19.
73. Brown, A.M., and Malliani, A.: Spinal sympathetic reflexes initiated by coronary receptors. J. Physiol. (Lond.), *212*:685, 1971.
74. Malliani, A., Pagani, M., and Lombardi, F.: Visceral versus somatic mechanisms. *In* Textbook of Pain. Edited by P.D. Wall and R. Melzack. Edinburgh, Churchill Livingstone, 1984, pp. 100–109.
75. Malliani, A.: The elusive link between transient myocardial ischemia and pain. Circulation, *73*:203, 1986.
76. Foreman, R.D.: Spinal substrates of visceral pain. *In* Spinal Afferent Processing. Edited by T.L. Yaksh. New York, Plenum Press, 1986, pp. 217–242.
77. Blair, R.W., Weber, R.N., and Foreman, R.D.: Characteristics of primate spinothalamic tract neurons receiving viscerosomatic convergent inputs in T3–T5 segments. J. Neurophysiol., *46*:797, 1981.
78. Ammons, W.S., Blair, R.W., and Foreman, R.D.: Greater splanchnic excitation of primate T1–T5 spinothalamic neurons. J. Neurophysiol., *51*:592, 1984.
79. Ammons, W.S., Blair, R.W., and Foreman, R.D.: Vagal afferent inhibition of primate T1–T5 spinothalamic neurons. J. Neurophysiol., *50*:926, 1983.
80. Ammons, W.S., Blair, R.W., and Foreman, R.D.: Raphe magnus inhibition of primate T1–T4 spinothalamic cells with cardiopulmonary visceral input. Pain, *20*:247, 1984.
81. Blair, R.W.: Noxious cardiac input onto neurons in medullary reticular formation. Brain Res., *326*:335, 1985.
82. Davis, L., and Pollock, L.J.: The role of the sympathetic nervous system in the production of pain in the head. Arch. Neurol. Psychiatry, *27*:282, 1982.
83. White, J.C., and Sweet, W.H.: Pain and the Neurosurgeon. Springfield, IL, Charles C Thomas, 1969, pp. 530–533.
84. Zanchetti, A., and Malliani, A.: Neural and psychological factors in coronary disease. Acta Cardiol., *20*(Suppl.):69, 1974.

85. Webb, S.W., Adgey, A.A.J., and Pantridge, J.F.: Autonomic disturbance at onset of acute myocardial infarction. Br. Med. J., *3*:89, 1972.
86. Feigl, E.O.: Sympathetic control of the coronary circulation. Circ. Res., *20*:262, 1967.
87. Feigl, E.O.: Control of myocardial oxygen tension by sympathetic coronary vasoconstriction in the dog. Circ. Res., *37*:88, 1975.
88. Mudge, G.H., et al.: Reflex increase in coronary vascular resistance in patients with ischemic heart disease. N. Engl. J. Med., *295*:1333, 1976.
89. Khan, M.I., et al.: Early arrhythmias following experimental coronary occlusion in conscious dogs and their modification by beta-adrenoceptor blocking drugs. Am. Heart J., *86*:347, 1973.
90. Mueller, H.S., et al.: Propranolol in the treatment of acute myocardial infarction. Circulation, *49*:1078, 1974.
91. Kliks, B.R., Burgess, M.J., and Abildskov, J.A.: Influence of sympathetic tone on ventricular fibrillation threshold during experimental coronary occlusion. Am. J. Cardiol., *36*:45, 1975.
92. Schaal, S.F., et al.: Protective effect of cardiac denervation against arrhythmias of myocardial infarction. Cardiovasc. Res., *3*:241, 1969.
93. Ross, R., and Glomset, J.A.: The pathogenesis of atherosclerosis. N. Engl. J. Med. *295*:369, 420, 1976.
94. Benditt, E.P., and Benditt, J.M.: Evidence for a monoclonal origin of human atherosclerotic plaques. Proc. Natl. Acad. Sci. U.S.A., *70*:1753, 1973.
95. Campeau, L.: Letter to the Editor: Grading of angina pectoris. Circulation, *54*:522, 1976.
96. Hammermeister, K.E., DeRouen, T.A., and Dodge, H.T.: Variables predictive of survival in patients with coronary disease. Selection by univariate and multivariate analyses from the clinical, electrocardiographic, exercise, arteriographic and quantitative angiographic evaluation. Circulation, *59*:421, 1979.
97. Ruberman, W., et al.: Ventricular premature complexes and sudden death after myocardial infarction. Circulation, *64*:297, 1981.
98. Califf, R.M., et al.: Prognostic implications of ventricular arrhythmias during 24-hour ambulatory monitoring in patients undergoing cardiac catheterization for coronary artery disease. Am J. Cardiol., *50*:23, 1982.
99. Hammermeister, K.E., et al.: Relationship of cardiothoracic ratio and plain film heart volume to late survival. Circulation, *59*:89, 1979.
100. Hamilton, G.W., Murray, J.A., and Kennedy, J.W.: Quantitative angiography in ischemic heart disease. Circulation, *45*:1065, 1972.
101. Weiner, D.A., et al.: Correlations among history of angina, ST segment response and prevalence of coronary artery disease in the Coronary Artery Surgery Study (CASS). N. Engl. J. Med., *301*:230, 1979.
102. Hamilton, G.W., et al.: Myocardial imaging with 201-thallium: An analysis of clinical usefulness based on Bayes theorem. Semin. Nucl. Med., *8*:358, 1978.
103. Beller, G.A.: Radionuclide techniques in the evaluation of the patient with chest pain. Mod. Conc. Cardiovasc. Dis. *50*:43, 1981.
104. Stratton, J.R., et al.: Detection of left ventricular thrombus by two-dimensional echocardiography: Sensitivity, specificity, and causes of uncertainty. Circulation, *66*:156, 1982.
105. Sones, F.M., Jr., et al.: Cine-coronary arteriography (Abstr.). Circulation, *20*:773, 1959.
106. Kennedy, J.W., and the Registry Committee of the Society for Cardiac Angiography: Complications associated with cardiac catheterization and angiography. Cathet. Cardiovasc. Diagn., *8*:5, 1982.
107. Kennedy, J.W. and the Registry Committee of the Society for Cardiac Angiography: Mortality related to cardiac catheterization and angiography. Cathet. Cardiovasc. Diagn., *8*:323, 1982.
108. DeWood, M.A., et al.: Prevalance of total coronary occlusion during the early hours of transmural myocardial infarction. N. Engl. J. Med., *303*:897, 1980.
109. Margolis, J.R., et al.: Clinical features of unrecognized myocardial infarction—silent and symptomatic. Eighteen year follow-up: The Framingham Study. Am. J. Cardiol., *32*:1, 1973.
110. Kennedy, J.W., et al.: Western Washington randomized trial of intracoronary streptokinase in acute myocardial infarction. N. Engl. J. Med., *300*:1477, 1983.
111. Gruppo Italiano Per Lo Studio Della Streptochinasi Nell' infarto Myocardico (Gissi): Effectiveness of intravenous thrombolytic treatment in acute myocardial infarction. Lancet, *1*:397, 1986.
112. ISIS-2 (Second International Study of Infarct Survival) Collaborative Group. Randomized trial of intravenous streptokinase, oral aspirin, both or neither among 17,187 cases of suspected acute myocardial infarction: ISIS-2. Lancet, II: 349, 1988.
113. TIMI Study Group: The thrombolysis in myocardial infarction (TIMI) trial: Phase I findings. N. Engl. J. Med., *312*:932, 1985.
114. Topol E.J. et al.: A randomized trial of immediate versus delayed elective angioplasty after intravenous tissue plasminogen activator in acute myocardial infarction. N. Engl. J. Med., *317*:581, 1987.
115. Thomas, M., et al.: Haemodynamic effects of morphine in patients with acute myocardial infarction. Br. Heart J., *27*:863, 1965.
116. Theroux, P., et al.: Prognostic value of exercise testing soon after myocardial infarction. N. Engl. J. Med., *301*:341, 1979.
117. Bigger, J.T., et al., and the Multicenter Post-Infarction Research Group: The relationships among ventricular arrhythmias, left ventricular dysfunction, and mortality in the 2 years after myocardial infarction. Circulation, *69*:250, 1984.
118. Hjalmarson, A., et al.: The Goteborg metoprolol trial. Effects on mortality and morbidity in acute myocardial infarction. Circulation, *67* (Suppl. I):26, 1983.
119. The Norwegian Multicenter Study Group: Timolol-induced reduction in mortality and reinfarction in patients surviving acute myocardial infarction. N. Engl. J. Med., *304*:801, 1981.
120. Beta Blocker Heart Attack Study Group: The beta-blocker heart attack trial. JAMA, *246*:2073, 1981.
121. Anticoagulants in acute myocardial infarction: Results of a cooperative clinical trial. JAMA, *225*:724, 1973.
122. Lie, K.I., et al.: Lidocaine in the prevention of primary ventricular fibrillation. A double-blind randomized study of 212 consecutive patients. N. Engl. J. Med., *291*:1324, 1974.
123. Mundth, E.D.: Surgical treatment of cardiogenic shock and of acute mechanical complications following myocardial infarction. Cardiovasc. Clin., 8241, 1977.
124. Horwitz, L.D., Herman, M.V., and Gorlin, R.: Clinical response to nitroglycerin as a diagnostic test for coronary artery disease. Am. J. Cardiol., *29*:149, 1972.
125. Brunton, T.L.: Use of nitrate of amyl in angina pectoris. Lancet, *2*:97, 1867.
126. Murrell, W.: Nitro-glycerine as a remedy for angina pectoris. Lancet, *1*:80, 151, 225, 1879.
127. Abrams, J.: Current concepts: Nitroglycerin and long-acting nitrates. N. Engl. J. Med., *302*:1234, 1980.
128. Frishman, W.H.: Beta-adrenoreceptor antagonists: New drugs and new indications. N. Engl. J. Med., *305*:500, 1981.
129. Krikler, D.M., and Rowland, E.: Clinical value of calcium antagonists in treatment of cardiovascular disorders. J. Am. Coll. Cardiol., *1*:355, 1983.
130. Cobb, L.A., et al.: An evaluation of internal-mammary-artery ligation by a double-blind technique. N. Engl. J. Med., *260*:115–118, 1959.
131. Favalaro, R.G.: Saphenous vein graft in the surgical treatment of coronary artery disease. Operative technique. J. Thorac. Cardiovasc. Surg., *58*:178, 1969.
132. Takaro, T., et al.: The VA Cooperative randomized study of surgery for coronary arterial occlusive disease. II. Subgroup with significant left main lesions. Circulation, *54*(Suppl. III):107, 1976.
133. European Coronary Surgery Study Group: Prospective randomized study of coronary artery bypass surgery in stable angina pectoris. Lancet, *2*:491, 1980.
134. CASS Principal Investigators and their Associates: Coronary Artery Surgery Study (CASS). A randomized trial of coronary bypass surgery. Survival data. Circulation, *68*:939, 1983.
135. Hammermeister, K.E.: The effect of coronary bypass surgery on survival. Prog. Cardiovasc. Dis., *15*:297, 1983.
136. Gruntzig, A.: Transluminal dilatation of coronary artery stenosis. Lancet, *1*:263, 1978.
137. Lewis, H.D., Jr., et al.: Protective effects of aspirin against acute myocardial infarction and death in men with unstable angina. Results of a Veterans Administration Cooperative Study. N. Engl. J. Med., *309*:396, 1983.
138. Cairns, J.A., et al.: Aspirin, sulfinpyrazone, or both in unstable angina. Results of a Canadian multicenter trial. N. Engl. J. Med., *313*:1369, 1985.

139. Mukharji, J., et al., and the MILIS Study Group: Risk factors for sudden death after acute myocardial infarction: Two-year follow-up. Am. J. Cardiol., *54*:31, 1984.

140. Cobb, L.A., Werner, J.A., and Trobaugh, G.R.: Sudden cardiac death: I. A decade's experience with out-of-hospital resuscitation. Mod. Conc. Cardiovasc. Dis., *49*:31, 1980.

141. Bigger, J.T.: Relation between left ventricular dysfunction and ventricular arrhythmias after myocardial infarction. Am. J. Cardiol., *57*:8B, 1986.

142. Holmes, D.R., et al., and Participants in the Coronary Artery Surgery Study: The effect of medical and surgical treatment on subsequent sudden cardiac death in patients with coronary artery disease: A report from the Coronary Artery Surgery Study. Circulation, *73*:1254, 1986.

143. Vlietstra, R.E., et al.: Effect of cigarette smoking on survival of patients with angiographically documented coronary artery disease. Report from the CASS registry. JAMA, *255*:1023, 1986.

144. Baum, R.S., Alvarez, H., III, and Cobb, L.A.: Survival after resuscitation from out-of-hospital ventricular fibrillation. Circulation, *50*:1231, 1974.

145. Hammermeister, K.E., et al.: Effect of aortocoronary saphenous vein bypass grafting on death and sudden death: Comparison of nonrandomized medically and surgically treated cohorts with comparable coronary disease and left ventricular function. Am. J. Cardiol., *39*:925, 1977.

146. Prinzmetal, M., et al.: Angina pectoris. I. A variant form of angina pectoris. Am. J. Med., *27*:375, 1959.

147. Cohn, P.F.: Silent myocardial ischemia in patients with a defective anginal warning system. Am. J. Cardiol, *45*:697, 1980.

148. Droste, C., and Roskamm, H.: Experimental pain measurement in patients with asymptomatic myocardial ischemia. J. Am. Coll. Cardiol, *1*:940, 1983.

149. Currie, P.J., et al.: Continuous-wave Doppler echocardiographic assessment of severity of calcific aortic stenosis: A simultaneous Doppler-catheter correlative study in 100 adult patients. Circulation, *71*:1162, 1985.

150. Bloomfield, P., et al.: A prospective evaluation of the Björk-Shiley, Hancock, and Carpentier-Edwards heart valve prostheses. Circulation, *73*:1213, 1986.

151. Hammermeister, K.E., et al.—Participants in the VA Cooperative Study on Valvular Heart Disease: Comparison of outcome after valve replacement with a bioprosthetic valve versus a mechanical prosthesis. J. Am. Coll. Cardiol. *10*:719, 1987.

152. Jersaty, R.M.: Mitral Valve Prolapse. New York, Raven Press, 1979, p. 251.

153. Perloff, J.K.: Evolving concepts of mitral valve prolapse. N. Engl. J. Med., *307*:369, 1982.

154. Ritchie, J.L., Hammermeister, K.E., and Kennedy, J.W.: Refractory ventricular tachycardia and fibrillation in a patient with prolapsing mitral leaflet syndrome. Successful control with overdrive pacing. Am. J. Cardiol., *37*:314, 1976.

155. Maron, B.J., et al.: Sudden death in young athletes. Circulation, *62*:218, 1980.

156. Cohen, L.S., and Braunwald, E.: Amelioration of angina pectoris in idiopathic hypertrophic subaortic stenosis with beta-adrenergic blockade. Circulation, *35*:847, 1967.

157. Maron, B.J., et al.: Long-term clinical course and symptomatic status of patients after operation for hypertrophic subaortic stenosis. Circulation, *57*:1205, 1978.

158. Hammermeister, K.E., and Belcher, H.V.: Acute streptococcal pericarditis: Report of a case treated with pericardiectomy. Md. State Med. J., *20*:50, 1971.

159. Dunn, M., and Rinkenberger, R.L.: Clinical aspects of acute pericarditis. Cardiovasc. Clin., 7:131, 1976.

160. Hirst, A.E., Jr., Johns, V.J. Jr., and Kime, S.W., Jr.: Dissecting aneurysm of the aorta. A review of 505 cases. Medicine, *37*:217, 1958.

161. Morgagni, J.B.: The Seats and Causes of Diseases Investigated by Anatomy, Vol. 1. Translated by B. Alexander. London, A. Miller, T. Cadele, 1769, pp. 8089–8090.

162. Schlatmann, T.J.M., and Becker, A.E.: Pathogenesis of dissecting aneurysm of the aorta. Comparative histopathologic study of significance of medial changes. Am. J. Cardiol., *39*:21, 1977.

163. Wheat, M.W.: Pathogenesis of aortic dissection. *In* Aortic Dissection. Edited by R.M. Doroghazi and E.E. Slater. New York, McGraw-Hill, 1983, pp. 55–60.

164. Slater, E.E., and De Sanctis, R.W.: Diseases of the Aorta. *In* Heart Disease: A Textbook of Cardiovascular Medicine. 2nd Ed. Edited by E. Braunwald. Philadelphia, W.B. Saunders, 1984, pp. 1540–1571.

165. Slater, E. E., and De Sanctis, R.W.: The clinical recognition of dissecting aortic aneurysm. Am. J. Med., *60*:625, 1976.

166. Lindsay, J., Jr., and Hurst, J.W.: Clinical features and prognosis in dissecting aneurysm of the aorta: A reappraisal. Circulation, *35*:880, 1967.

167. Dinsmore, R.E., Willerson, J.T., and Buckley, M.J.: Dissecting aneurysm of the aorta. Aortographic features affecting prognosis. Diagn. Radiol., *105*:567, 1969.

168. Godwin, J.D., et al.: Evaluation of dissections and aneurysms of the thoracic aorta by conventional and dynamic CT scanning. Radiology, *136*:125, 1980.

169. DeBakey, M.E., Cooley, D.A., and Creech, O., Jr.: Surgical considerations of dissecting aneurysm of the aorta. Ann. Surg., *142*:586, 1955.

170. Wheat, M.W., Jr., et al.: Treatment of dissecting aneurysms of the aorta without surgery. J. Thorac. Cardiovasc. Surg., *50*:364, 1965.

171. Daily, P.O., et al.: Management of acute aortic dissections. Ann. Thorac. Surg., *10*:237, 1970.

55 · PAINFUL DISORDERS OF THE RESPIRATORY SYSTEM

JOHN J. BONICA

THIS chapter includes discussion of painful disorders of the trachea, bronchi, lungs, and pleura. Because the primary focus of this book is on pain, disorders involving these structures that do not produce pain, such as respiratory distress syndrome, asthma, and other nonpainful ventilatory disorders, are not considered here. Moreover, because disorders of the upper airway (nose and mouth, pharynx and larynx) are discussed in Chapters 38 and 43, they are not considered here. The information is presented in five parts: A, Basic Considerations; B, Painful Disorders of the Tracheobronchial Tree; C, Pain Caused by Diseases of the Lung; D, Disorders of the Pulmonary Circulation; and E, Chest Pain Caused by Disorders of the Pleura. As with most other chapters in the book, only key references are included. More detailed discussion can be found elsewhere (1–2).

A. BASIC CONSIDERATIONS

Anatomic and Neurologic Aspects

This section contains a summary of the anatomy of the trachea, bronchi, lungs, and pleura, and is presented as a review. This supplements the information in Chapter 53 (pp. 980–982). More detailed discussion can be found elsewhere (3–6).

Anatomy of the Trachea, Bronchi, and Lungs

Trachea and Bronchi

The trachea is a cartilaginous membranous tube that extends from the larynx on a level with the C6 vertebra to the upper border of the T5 vertebra, where it divides into the right main bronchus and the left main bronchus. The trachea is nearly but not quite symmetric, and is flattened posteriorly. It is about 11 cm (10 to 12 cm) long and its diameter from side to side ranges from 2 to 2.5 cm, being always greater in the male than in the female. The trachea is smaller, more deeply placed, and more movable in the child than in the adult (3, 6).

The right main bronchus is wider, shorter, and less abrupt in its divergence from the trachea than the left main bronchus. It is usually about 2.5 cm long but, in a study of about 20 cadavers, Bonica and Hall (7) found that the right main stem bronchus varied from 0.3 to 2.5 cm long. The left bronchus is smaller in caliber, but longer than the right bronchus, usually being about 5 cm long. Each main bronchus gives off secondary bronchi, one for each lobe of the lung, which in turn give off tertiary bronchi for each lobule of the lung. Figure 55-1 depicts the anatomy of the tracheobronchial tree.

Lungs and Pleura

The two lungs and the parietal pleura are shown in Figure 55-2. Each lung is invested by two layers of serus membrane, the pulmonary or visceral pleura and the parietal pleura. The visceral pleura covers the surface of each lung and dips into the fissures between its lobes. The parietal pleura lines the inner surface of the chest wall, covering the diaphragm, and is reflected over structures occupying the middle of the thorax. The two layers are contiguous with each other and on and below the root of the lung; normally they are in actual contact with each other, with a small amount of liquid in the potential pleural space permitting movement of the two layers without friction (see below, Section E).

When the lung collapses, or when air or fluid collects between the two layers, the cavity becomes apparent. The right and left pleural sacs are entirely separate from each other: between them are the thoracic viscera, except the lungs (Fig. 54-2A). The parietal pleura sacs touch each other only for a short distance anteriorly behind the upper part of the body of the sternum. In the center of the chest cavity the two pleural sacs are separated by the mediastinum.

Different portions of the parietal pleura have special names to indicate their position: the costal pleura lines the inner surface of the ribs and the intercostal muscles; the diaphragmatic pleura covers the convex (superior) surface of the diaphragm; the mediastinal pleura covers the medial aspects of the lungs and is in contact with other thoracic viscera; and the cupula of the pleura (cervical pleura) arises in the neck and overlies the apex of the lung.

Neurophysiology

Trachea, Bronchi, and Lungs

Chapter 53 contains a description of the nerve supply to the tracheobronchial tree, the pulmonary vessels, the lungs, and the pleura. Figures 55-3 and 55-4 are reproduced here from Chapter 53 for the convenience of the reader. Figure 55-5 is a schematic depiction of the segmental nerve supply to the lungs.

The tracheobronchial tree receives contributions from the vagus, which contains preganglionic parasympathetic and afferent fibers, and also from the sympathetic postganglionic fibers derived from the T2 to the T6 or T7 sympathetic ganglia and occasionally the stellate or middle cervical ganglia. The trachea receives some vagal afferent and efferent fibers through the recurrent laryngeal nerve, which is frequently joined by fibers from the middle cervical sympathetic ganglion. The lower part of the trachea receives vagal fibers directly from the vagus nerves and postganglionic sympathetic fibers from the stellate and T1 ganglia.

The two bronchial trees and the pulmonary vessels derive their nerve supply from a larger posterior pulmonary plexus and a smaller anterior pulmonary plexus located at the beginning of each pulmonary artery on each side (4). Each pulmonary plexus contains vagal efferent and afferent fibers, as well as sympathetic efferent and afferent fibers, which leave the root of the lung and proceed distally. Immediately after

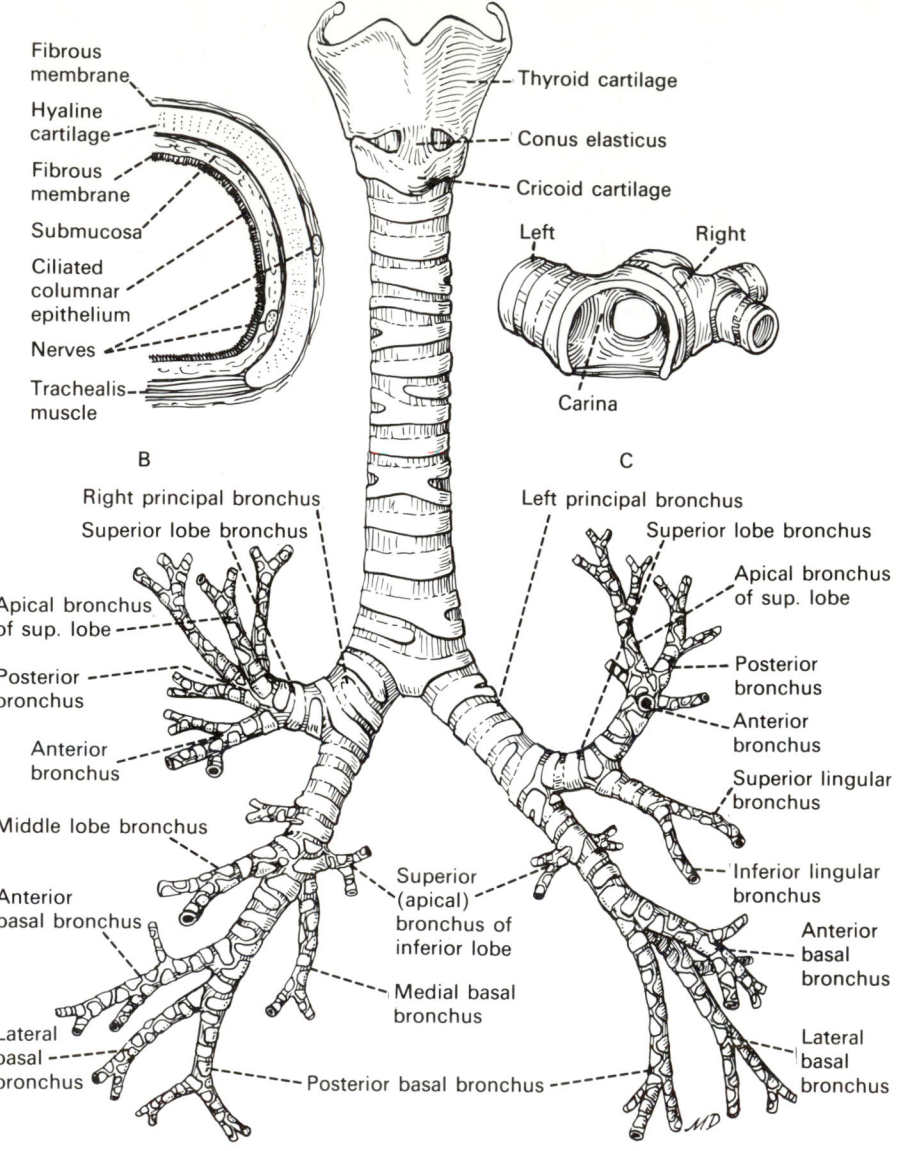

FIG. 55-1. Anatomy of the tracheobronchial tree. *A.* Anterior view of the trachea and primary and secondary bronchi and tertiary bronchial tubes. The right main stem bronchus makes an angle of about 20° with the midsagittal plane, whereas the left main stem bronchus makes an angle of 45°. *B.* Cross section of the adult trachea showing the nerves that supply the submucosa and mucosa. *C.* Bifurcation of the trachea viewed from above. The interior shows the carina as it would be seen through a bronchoscope. Modified from Clemente, C.D.: Gray's Anatomy of the Human Body. 30th Ed. Philadelphia, Lea & Febiger, 1985.

entering the lungs the nerve filaments become partially segregated into groups that accompany the main bronchi, the pulmonary vessels, and the bronchial arteries. At the level of the main bronchi is a subepithelial plexus, located between cartilaginous plates and the bronchial musculature, and a deep plexus, located between cartilaginous plates in the submucous and mucous membranes.

From the walls of the smaller bronchi the two plexuses blend into a single plexus that can be traced as far as the respiratory bronchioles, but nerve fibers running either singly or in small bundles continue still further into the walls of the atria (4). Afferent fibers extend distally as far as the proximal end of the alveolar duct (Fig. 55-6).

The nerve supply to the various vessels within the lungs varies in richness: the small bronchial arteries have the best supply, the pulmonary arteries are less richly innervated, and the pulmonary veins have a poor supply, limited to their extrapulmonary parts and the large intrapulmonary branches (5). The larger bundles of the pulmonary arteriolar nerve fibers are located on the side of the vessels, facing the bronchi, and can be traced to the extremities of these vessels; some extend beyond them to the visceral pleura. Filaments passing through the bronchial arteries come from the adjacent extrachondrial parts of the bronchial nerve plexus.

Both myelinated and unmyelinated fibers have been found in pulmonary nerves and plexuses. Many of these have sensory receptors in the pulmonary blood vessels and are involved in the reflex control of the pulmonary circulation, with vasoconstrictor and vasodilator fibers supplied by the sympathetic and parasympathetic efferent nerves, respectively. The lungs have two types of receptors that probably have nociceptive function: type J receptors of C afferents and "lung irritant" receptors with afferents in the

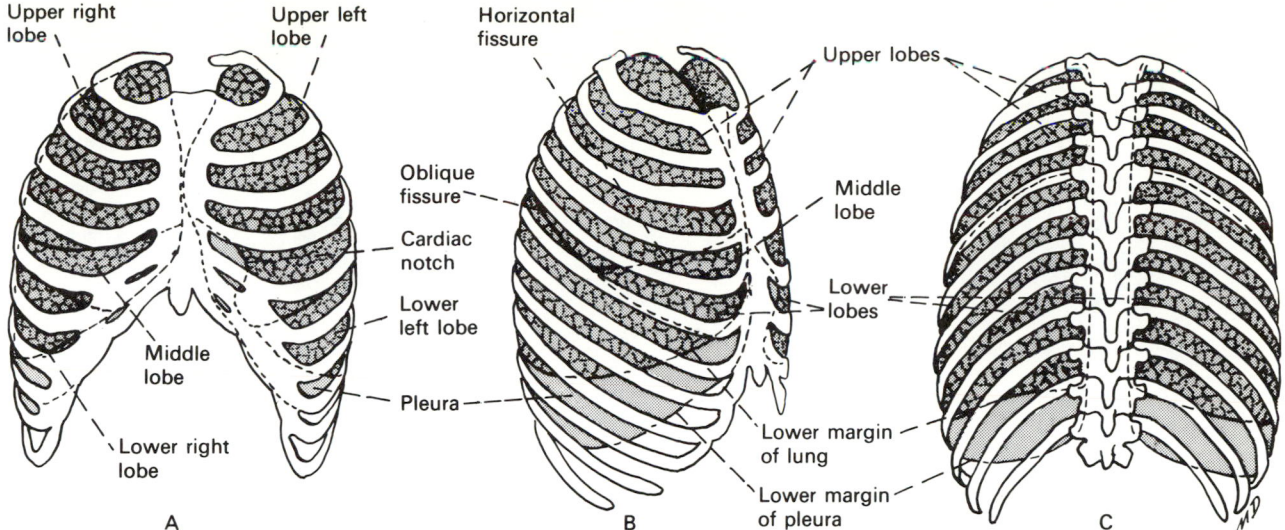

Upper right lobe
Upper left lobe
Horizontal fissure
Upper lobes
Middle lobe
Oblique fissure
Cardiac notch
Lower left lobe
Middle lobe
Lower lobes
Pleura
Lower right lobe
Lower margin of lung
Lower margin of pleura
A
B
C

FIG. 55-2. Anterior (*A*), lateral (*B*), and posterior (*C*) views of the thorax showing the relationship of the pleurae and lungs to the chest wall. The pleura from each side approaches the other behind the midportion of the manubrium. The extension of the caudal portion of the pleurae is seen in *B* and *C*.

A-delta range, all running in the vagus nerves (4, 8). The type J receptors are located within the interstitial space, close to the capillaries, whereas the lung irritant receptors are found in the epithelial lining of the lung and its airways. These receptors are activated by various stimuli that produce mechanical distortion within the lung such as pulmonary congestion, microembolism, atelectasis, and pneumothorax, and

biochemical irritants. Pain caused by mechanical or chemical damage of the lung is probably mediated by these A-delta and C fibers. The sympathetic afferents might have a role in the transmission of nociceptive impulses, and are involved in reflex control of the circulation and of the tracheobronchial tree.

The sensory nerves that transmit nociceptive impulses from the trachea and bronchi are afferents of

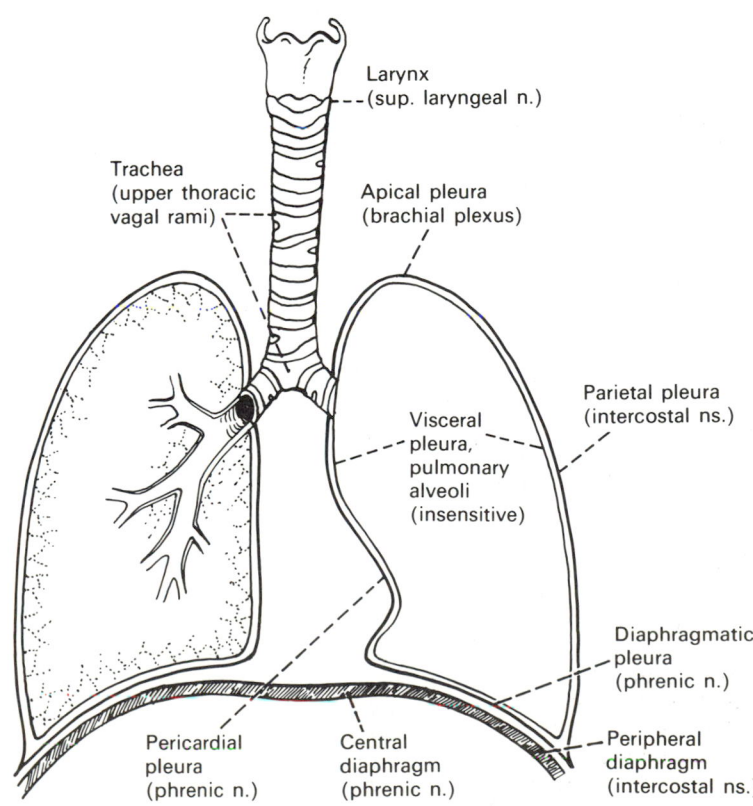

Larynx (sup. laryngeal n.)
Trachea (upper thoracic vagal rami)
Apical pleura (brachial plexus)
Visceral pleura, pulmonary alveoli (insensitive)
Parietal pleura (intercostal ns.)
Diaphragmatic pleura (phrenic n.)
Pericardial pleura (phrenic n.)
Central diaphragm (phrenic n.)
Peripheral diaphragm (intercostal ns.)

FIG. 55-3. Schematic representation of the sensory nerve supply to the tracheobronchial tree, parietal pleura, and upper surface of the diaphragm, as well as to the diaphragmatic pleura. Modified from White, J.C.: Sensory innervation of the viscera. *In* Pain Res. Publ. Ass. Nerv. Ment. Dis. Vol. 23. Edited by H.G. Wolff, H.S. Gasser, and J.C. Hinsey. Baltimore, Williams & Wilkins, 1943, Fig. 97, p. 377.

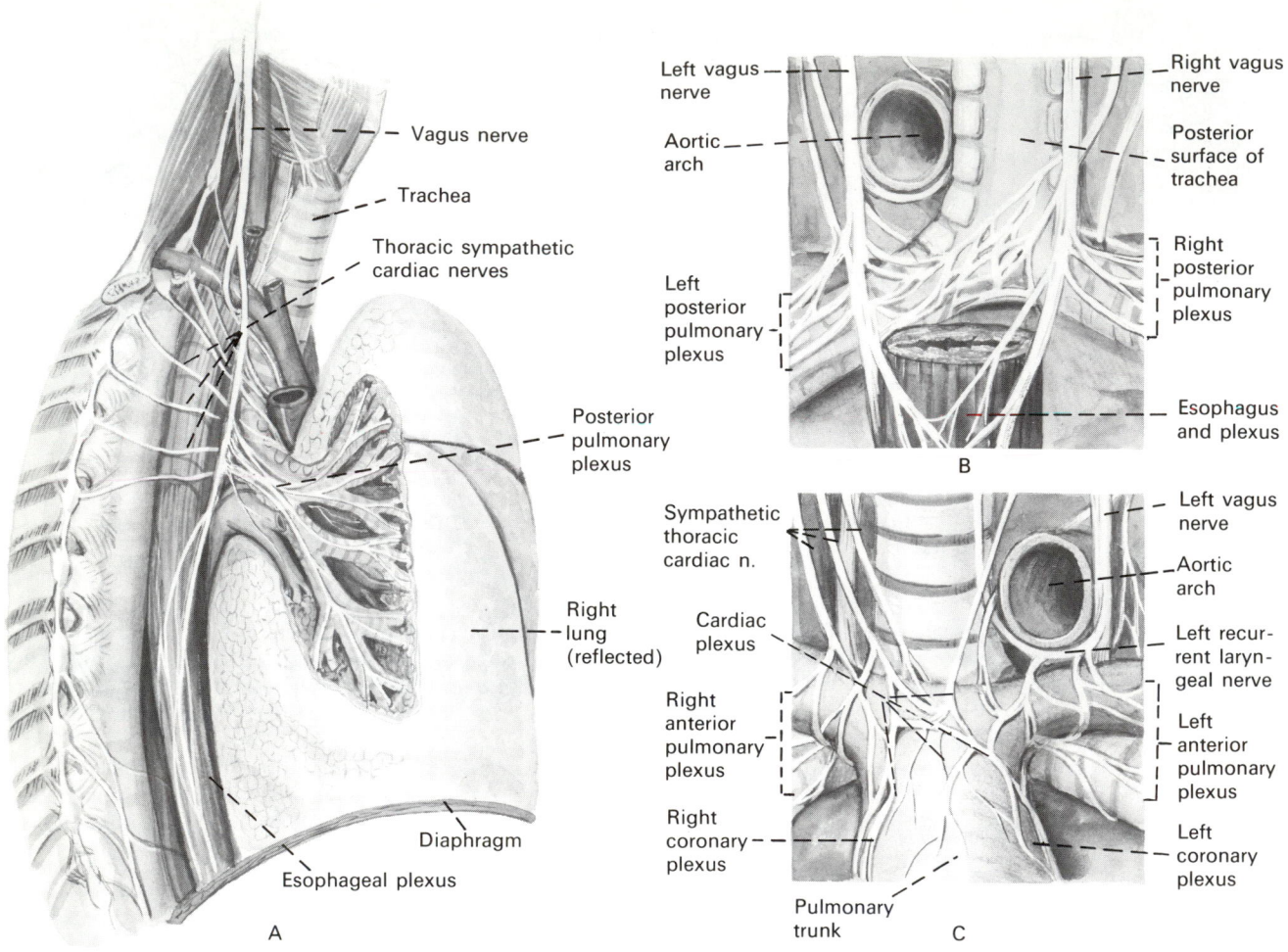

FIG. 55-4. Anatomy of the pulmonary plexuses and their distribution. **A.** Right parasagittal view showing origin, course, and termination of the nerves that contribute to the right pulmonary plexus. **B, C.** Posterior and anterior views of the trachea and two primary bronchi to show the relation of the pulmonary plexus to these structures. Developed from data in Mitchell, G.A.G.: Cardiovascular Innervation. London, E.S. Livingstone, 1956, pp. 196–238, and Netter, F.H.: The CIBA Collection of Medical Illustrations. Vol. 7. The Respiratory System. West Caldwell, New Jersey. CIBA Pharmaceuticals, 1979, p. 28.

the vagus nerves and their branches (Chapter 53; also see Fig. 53-17). It appears that each side of the tracheobronchial tree derives its sensory supply from the ipsilateral vagus nerves because, when the mucous membrane of the tree is noxiously stimulated, the area of pain reference is ipsilateral to the site of stimulation. Section of the vagus nerve below the recurrent laryngeal nerve but above the pulmonary plexus has been found to abolish the pain caused by carcinoma.

Pleura

The visceral pleura is supplied by sympathetic fibers that have a vasomotor function; these have afferent fibers that apparently have no nociceptive function because noxious stimulation of the visceral pleura does not result in pain. As previously mentioned, the visceral pleura also receives parasympathetic fibers through the pulmonary plexuses. In contrast, the parietal pleura is richly supplied by nerves containing sensory fibers that carry nociceptive information. The costal pleura is supplied by the intercostal nerves. The cupula of the pleura (cervical pleura) is supplied by the first thoracic spinal nerve, while the mediastinal pleura and diaphragmatic pleura are supplied by sensory fibers contributed by the phrenic nerves (see Fig. 53-8).

Evaluation of the Patient

Evaluation of patients who present with pain in the chest suspected of being caused by disease of the tracheobronchial tree, lung, or pleura requires a detailed history, physical examination and, frequently, chest roentgenograms. The history and physical examination should be carried out as discussed in Chapters 31 and 53. Pulmonary function tests, arterial blood gas analysis, chemical and microbiologic tests, or special studies such as endoscopy, biopsy, or radionuclide scanning might also be necessary. Because disorders of

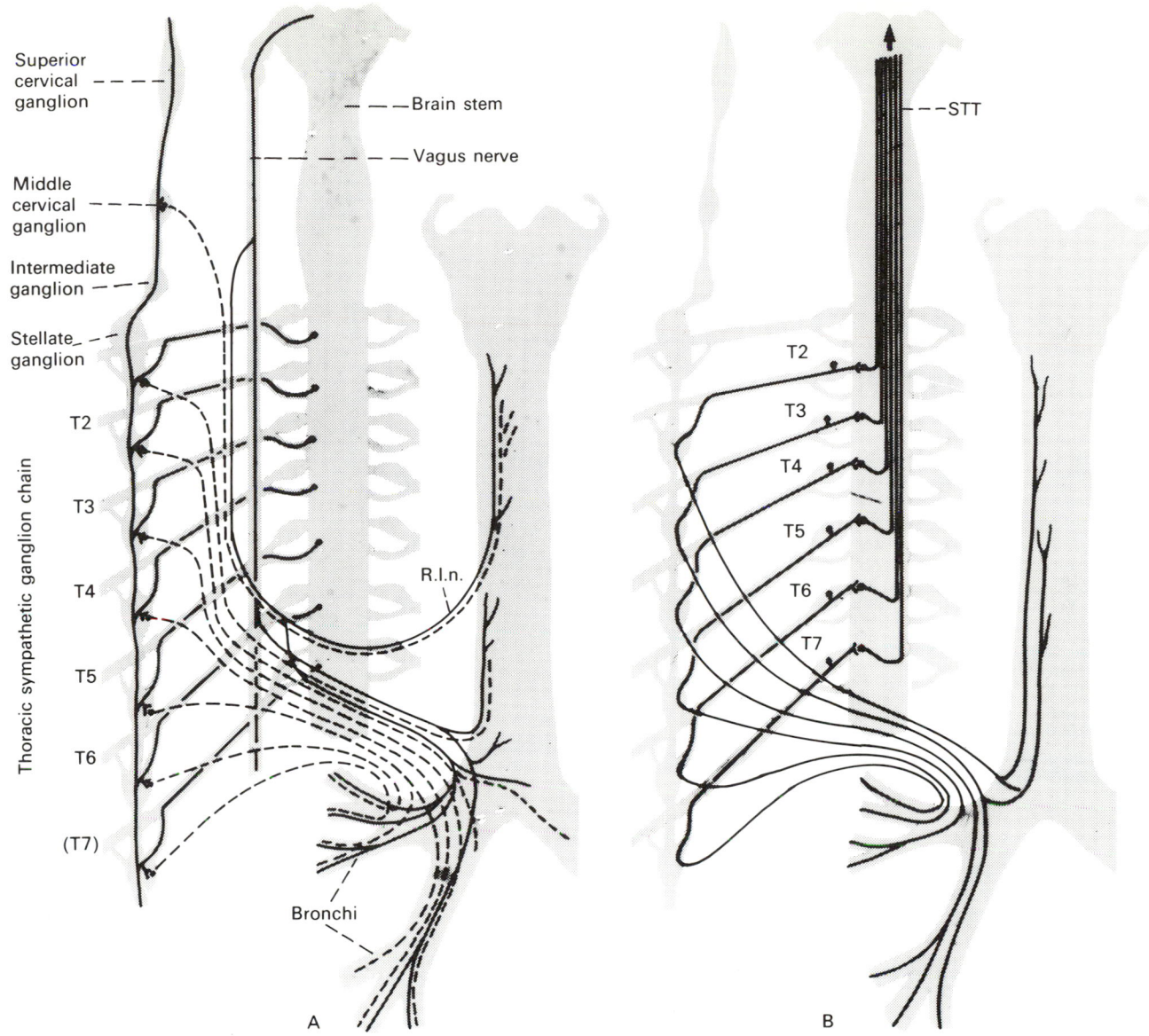

FIG. 55-5. *A.* Schematic representation of the segments of the spinal cord and sympathetic chain that provide sympathetic efferent and afferent nerves and of the vagal nerves that supply parasympathetic efferent and afferent fibers to the tracheobronchial tree, the lungs, and their blood vessels. Preganglionic sympathetic and parasympathetic fibers are shown as solid lines, and postganglionic sympathetic fibers are shown as dashed lines. R.I.n = recurrent laryngeal nerve. *B.* The sympathetic afferents with their cell bodies in the dorsal root ganglia, their proximal branches synapsing in the dorsal horn of the spinal cord and the distal branches accompanying the sympathetic nerves. Both sympathetics and afferents pass through the white rami communicantes, the thoracic sympathetic chain, the thoracic cardiac and aortic nerves, and the esophageal nerves and then proceed to their destination.

the respiratory system are frequently a manifestation of the systemic process, attention must be focused not only on the chest but also on the comprehensive evaluation of the patient's entire health status.

History taking provides essential information and initiates the physician's understanding of the patient as a person, the patient's environment, and the type and place of work, as well as the patient's expectations and fears. As discussed in Chapter 31, data should include past and present history, information on previous illnesses, medications, and other therapies, a family history, and history of the occupation; if warranted, information should be obtained about exposure to such hazards as asbestos, coal,

silica, beryllium, iron oxide, tin oxide, cotton dust, titanium, silver, and nitrogen dioxide (9).

Obviously, much time should be devoted to obtaining a detailed description of the presenting chest pain and other major respiratory symptoms such as cough, dyspnea, wheeze, and hemoptysis. The most important respiratory system disorders that produce pain include inflammation of the tracheobronchial tree or of the pleura, as in pneumonia, pulmonary thromboembolism, tuberculosis, and malignancy. Pleuritic pain is usually localized to one side of the chest and is related to movements of the thorax and to respiration. Lesions confined to the pulmonary parenchyma do not produce pain except as previously

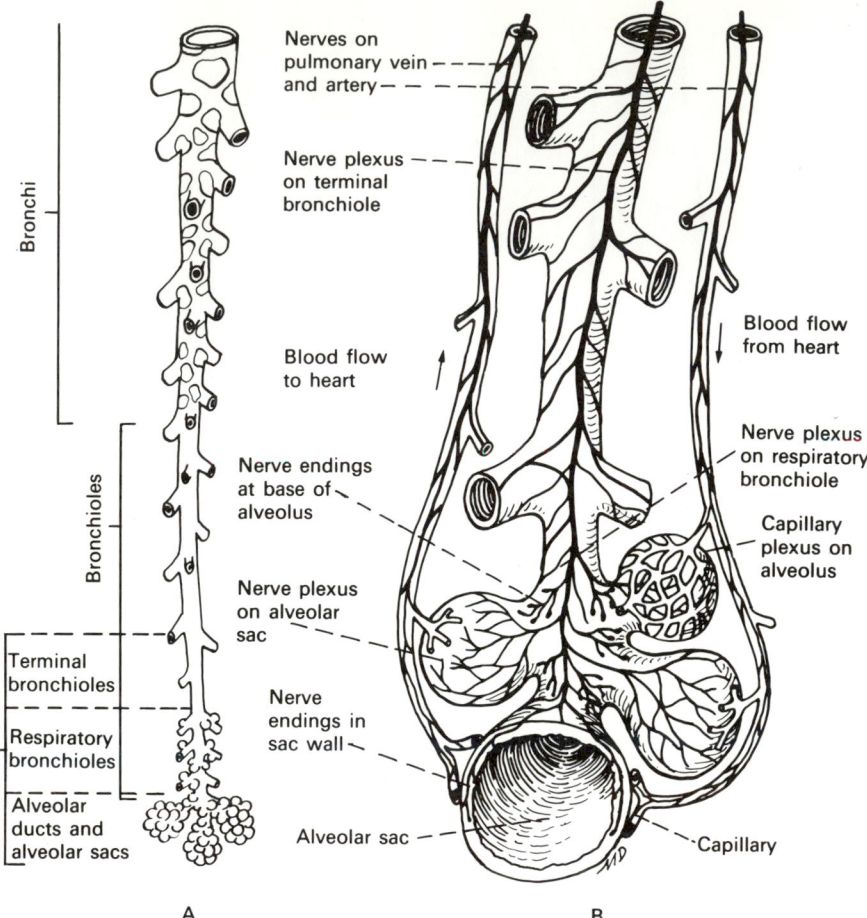

FIG. 55-6. **A,** Anatomy of the distal part of a tertiary bronchus and of the bronchioles, alveolar ducts, and alveolar sacs. **B.** Nerve supply to the terminal portion of the pulmonary artery, the pulmonary vein, and respiratory bronchioles, all of which contribute to the nerve supply of the alveolar ducts and alveolar sacs. The number of alveolar sacs has been greatly reduced for the sake of clarity. Note the nerve endings within the wall of the alveolar sac that has been cut. **A** and part of **B** modified from Netter, F.H: The CIBA Collection of Medical Illustrations. Vol. 7. The Respiratory System. West Caldwell, New Jersey. CIBA Pharmaceuticals, 1979, p. 28. Distal part of **B** was developed from data of Fillenz, M., and Widdicombe, J.G.: Receptors of the lungs and air-ways. *In* Handbook of Sensory Physiology. Vol. 3/1. Edited by E. Neil. Berlin, Springer-Verlag, 1972, pp. 81–112.

mentioned, when pathophysiologic processes stimulate the J or the lung irritant receptors. Detailed information must be obtained about the various characteristics of the pain, including the speed of onset, location, radiation, intensity, duration, and factors that aggravate and relieve the pain (10, 11) (Chapter 53). A detailed history and a comprehensive physical examination, carried out along the lines summarized in Table 53-1, together with a review of Chapter 53C, permit a presumptive diagnosis. Important diagnostic points (see Table 53-2) should also help the physician to make a differential diagnosis among pain caused by respiratory disorders, pain of the chest wall resulting from orthopedic or neurologic problems, and pain referred to the chest from diseases of the abdominal viscera or from neck and upper limb disorders.

Epidemiology

Acute respiratory disorders afflict more Americans than any other group of acute conditions. The 1986 estimates published by the National Center of Health Statistics (NCHS), based on the National Health Interview Survey (NHIS), indicated that, of a total of 448.6 million acute conditions, 228.8 million (51%) involved the respiratory system (12) (Table 55-1).* Because the survey excluded those conditions that did *not* involve restricted activity or medical attention, the ac-

*The numbers do not reflect the numbers of patients afflicted but the total number of acute conditions estimated in the survey. Some people had more than one acute condition.

tual figure is even larger. The next most frequent group of acute conditions included about 65 million injuries and 54 million infectious and parasitic diseases. As noted in Table 55-1, these respiratory disorders caused 795 million days of restricted activity, 405 million days of bed disability, and nearly 148 million days lost from work among those 18 years of age or older who were fully employed. If the work days lost by those under 18 years of age who were fully employed and those partially employed are added, as well as days lost from being unable to do housework, it is obvious that the total loss of days of productivity are probably more than 80 million days.

Table 55-1 lists the percentage of acute conditions that were medically attended (12). As might be expected the highest percentage of medical attention was obtained for upper respiratory infections, acute bronchitis, and pneumonia. The number of physician visits for each condition (last column) was computed by multiplying the total number for each condition by its percentage. The total was nearly 89 million visits. Available data about hospitalization for acute respiratory conditions were found in an NCHS publication (13) containing data for 1983 and extrapolated to the 1986 population. These calculations revealed that 1.1 million patients were hospitalized for acute upper respiratory infections for a total of 3.7 million hospital days and 960,000 patients were hospitalized for pneumonia for a total of 4.5 million days. Using the mean figures for the cost of each hospital day, the cost of physicians' visits, and the median income it can be suggested that acute respiratory disorders cost the American people about 18 billion dollars in 1986.

In regard to chronic respiratory conditions, the only information for a few "selected" disorders is available: chronic

Table 55-1. Incidence and Impact of Acute Respiratory Disorders (Numbers in Millions)

Conditions	Total Number	Restricted Activity (Days)	Bed Disability (Days)	Work Loss (Days)	Attended by Physicians	
					Percentage of Conditions	Total Physician Visits
Common cold	63.4	184.8	62.6	23.3	35.2	22.3
Other upper respiratory infections	21.8	52.0	25.3	7.4	69.0	15.0
Influenza	130.5	461.9	260.6	100.8	30.9	40.3
Acute bronchitis	6.3	37.8	15.9	6.6	82.3	5.2
Pneumonia	2.6	39.9	29.7	5.4	96.2	2.5
Other acute respiratory conditions	4.2	18.9	11.2	4.4	84.0	3.5
All:	228.8	795.3	465.3	147.9	38.8	88.8

bronchitis, 11.4 million; asthma, 10 million; emphysema, 2 million; chronic sinusitis, 34.4 million; and other chronic respiratory conditions, 26.1 million (12). This does not include data on neoplasms (presented in Chapter 57). No figures are available about the number of restricted activity days, bed disability days, and days of lost work, but it is likely that the numbers are significantly larger because of the chronicity of these disorders. Data relevant to this chapter were obtained from the National Ambulatory Medical Care Survey (NAMCS) and include the number of visits to physicians for "new pain" and for "chronic pain" (pain of 3 months or longer duration) (14, 15). Management of the pain was the primary reason for the patient's visit to the physician. During the 2-year period from January 1, 1980 to December 31, 1981, 6.5 million visits were for new chest pain and 6.8 million were for chronic chest pain. After the principal diagnosis was determined the new pain considered to be a result of respiratory diseases accounted for 5.5 million visits and chronic pain prompted 4.4 million visits during the 2-year period. Extrapolating to the 1986 population (1 year) suggests 3 million visits for new pain and about 2.3 million visits for chronic pain caused by respiratory disorders.

B. PAINFUL DISORDERS OF THE TRACHEOBRONCHIAL TREE

Acute Tracheobronchitis

Acute inflammation of the upper respiratory tract causes mild to moderate pain, which is perceived as soreness and irritability of the airway. The patient can also experience retrosternal burning or soreness, often associated with a sore throat or laryngeal irritation. The condition is generally self-limiting, with eventual complete healing and return of function. Although often mild, bronchitis can be serious in debilitated patients and in those with chronic lung or heart disease. Pneumonia is a critical complication (16).

Etiology

Acute bronchitis can be caused by an infectious process or by various irritants. An acute infectious process, most prevalent in winter, is often part of an acute upper respiratory infection. Not infrequently this develops after a common cold or other viral infection of the nasopharynx, throat, or tracheobronchial tree, and is often complicated by a secondary bacterial infection. Exposure to air pollutants and possibly chilling, fatigue, or malnutrition are predisposing or contributing factors (11). Recurrent attacks often complicate chronic bronchopulmonary disease, which impair bronchial clearance mechanisms. Repeated infections can be associated with chronic sinusitis, bronchiectasis, or bronchopulmonary allergy.

Various irritating gases can also cause inflammation of the tracheobronchial tree. Acute irritative bronchitis can also be caused by various mineral and vegetable dusts and by fumes from strong acids, ammonia, certain volatile organic solvents, chlorine, hydrogen sulfide, sulfur dioxide, or chlorine. During a temperature inversion, polluted air can settle over an area and highly irritant gases such as sulfur dioxide and nitrogen peroxide can increase in concentration until clinical symptoms result (11). Inhalation of extremely hot air produces a burning in the upper airway that is exceedingly painful and slow to heal (16). When associated with inhalation of soot and burning particles, such a burn can be rapidly fatal.

Pathophysiology

Acute infectious tracheobronchitis initially causes hyperemia of the mucous membranes followed by desquamation, edema, leukocytic infiltration of the submucosa, and production of a sticky or mucopurulent exudate. The protective function of the bronchial cilia, phagocytes, and lymphatics is disturbed, and bacteria can invade the normally sterile bronchi and cause accumulation of cellular debris and mucopurulent exudate. Coughing, although distressing, is essential to eliminate bronchial secretion. Airway obstruction can result from edema of the bronchial walls retained secretions, and, in some cases, spasm of the bronchial muscles. Burning of the upper airways from inhalation of hot air, if not fatal, causes the patient to cough up eschar before recovering. The healing process is prolonged and difficult.

Symptoms and Signs

Acute infectious bronchitis is often preceded by symptoms of upper respiratory infection: coryza, malaise, chilliness, slight fever, back and muscle pain, and sore throat (16). The onset of tracheobronchitis is signaled by a cough that is initially dry and nonproductive but raises small amounts of viscid sputum for a few hours a day, and then becomes more abundant and mucopurulent. At this time patients can feel retrosternal irritation and discomfort or frank pain. In severe or complicated cases, fever up to 38.3° or 38.9° C (101° or 102° F) can be present for 2 to 5 days, after which a few symptoms subside while the cough can continue for several weeks. Some patients continue to cough and some bring up abundant mucoid or mucopurulent sputum. Dyspnea, which is secondary to the underlying obstruction, can be experienced.

Auscultation in patients with uncomplicated acute bronchitis reveals scattered high- or low-pitched rhonchi, occasional crackling or moist rales, or both at the base of the lungs. Wheezing after coughing is commonly noted. Patients with acute irritative bronchitis usually have a dry nonproductive cough but, with invasion of bacteria, patients develop the same symptoms and signs as those of acute infectious bronchitis.

Patients who manifest persistent fever are likely to be developing bronchopneumonia, which produces persistent localized signs of consolidation. This and other serious complications are usually seen only in patients with underlying chronic respiratory disorders and, in such patients, acute bronchitis can lead to severe blood gas abnormalities.

Diagnosis

Diagnosis is easily made through a detailed history and physical examination. If the symptoms and signs are serious and persist, a chest roentgenogram should be taken to rule out other diseases or complicating pneumonia. When serious underlying chronic respiratory disease is present, arterial blood gases should be monitored at frequent intervals. Gram-staining should be done to determine the infective organism in those who do not respond to antibiotic therapy.

Treatment

Treatment consists of rest until pain subsides, fluids in amounts of 3 to 4 L/day during the febrile course, and the administration of nonsteroidal anti-inflammatory drugs (NSAIDs) to reduce the fever and relieve the muscle pain that most of these patients have. NSAIDs should be given in sufficient doses to provide effective analgesia and achieve an antipyritic effect. For example, aspirin in doses of 600 mg q4h should be given but, if this does not provide effective relief, the dose should be increased to 1000 mg q4h. Of course, in patients who are allergic to aspirin, other NSAIDs should be used. In any case patients should be monitored closely for any adverse side effects (Chapter 78). If the patient has a severe cough that continues to produce muscle pain and interferes with sleep, codeine in doses of 32 to 64 mg should be added to NSAIDs. Care should be taken if patients also have chronic obstructive pulmonary disease (COPD). Other measures include steam inhalation or a vaporizer for coughing and bronchodilators for wheezing.

In patients in whom the high fever persists and who have purulent sputum, or in those who have a concomitant COPD, antibiotics should be given (16). Oral tetracycline or ampicillin 250 mg q6h is adequate for most patients. Smear and sputum cultures are indicated if symptoms persist or recur, or in those with unusually severe disease, and then the most appropriate antibiotic chosen.

Bronchiectasis

Bronchiectasis is an irreversible focal dilation of the bronchioles, usually accompanied by infection. Although pain is not the most severe symptom, many patients experience some retrosternal and general chest pain (17, 18).

Etiology and Pathophysiology

Acquired bronchiectasis results from direct bronchial wall destruction after infection, inhalation of bronchial chemicals, and immunologic reaction of vascular abnormalities that interfere with bronchial nutrition, or from mechanical alterations secondary to atelectasis or loss of parenchymal volume that lead to bronchial dilation and secondary infection. Conditions commonly leading to bronchiectasis include the following: (a) severe pneumonia (especially complicating measles, pertussis, or certain adenovirus infections in children); (b) necrotizing infection at any age caused by Klebsiella, staphylococci, influenza virus, fungi, microbacteria, and perhaps Mycoplasma; and (c) bronchial obstruction from any cause such as foreign bodies, enlarged lymph nodes, mucous infection, or lung cancer. Other miscellaneous factors can also produce bronchiectasis.

Bronchiectasis can be unilateral or bilateral and is most common in the lower lobes, but the right middle lobe or a portion of the left upper lobe can also be involved. Examination reveals extensive inflammatory destruction, chronic inflammation, increased mucus, and loss of cilia.

Symptoms and Signs

Although patients might be completely asymptomatic, chronic cough and sputum production are the most characteristic and common symptoms; these usually begin insidiously following a respiratory infection and tend to worsen gradually over a period of years (17–19). As the condition progresses the cough eventually becomes more productive, occurring with typical regularity in the morning on arising, late in the afternoon, and on retiring, but many patients are affected with cough during intervening hours. Concurrent pneumonia and hemoptysis are common, and the latter can be the first and only symptom. Physical findings are not specific, but persistent rales occur over the affected part of the lungs. Pulmonary functional and hemodynamic changes depend on the extent of the accompanying pathologic changes, such as diffuse chronic bronchitis, pulmonary emphysema, or pulmonary fibrosis, and can include reduction in lung volumes and air flow rates, ventilation or perfusion defects, hypoxemia and, in severe cases, pulmonary hypertension.

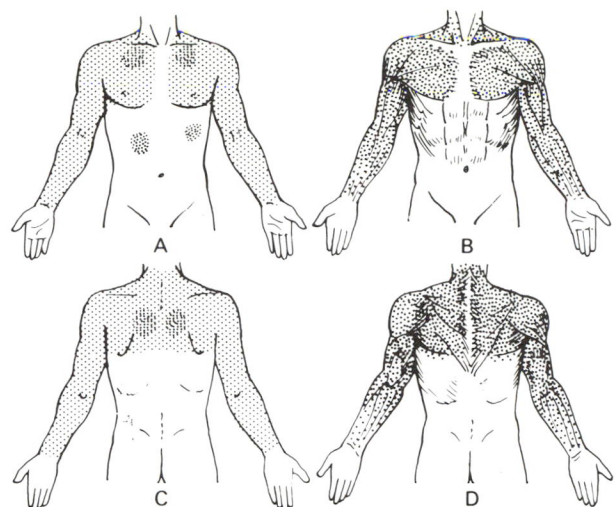

FIG. 55-7. Distribution of pain and of cutaneous and deep hyperalgesia in patients with bilateral bronchiectasis. **A, B.** Anterior views of distribution of the pain, indicated by heavy stipples and of the cutaneous hyperalgesia, indicated by the cross-hatched areas. **C, D.** Posterior views showing the distribution of deep hyperalgesia involving muscles of the chest. Modified from Teodori, U., and Galletti, R.: Il Dolor Nelle Affezioni Degli Organi Interni del Torace. Rome, El Tozzi, 1962, p. 262.

Pain is not a common symptom but it can occur and produces significant discomfort, particularly in patients in whom the bronchiectasis is associated with osteoarthritis—so-called rheumatic bronchiectasis. Such patients have pain not only in the chest but also in the limbs. A number of cases were reported (20) in which the patients with bronchiectasis had pain in the chest and in the arms that was moderate and poorly localized. Teodori and Galletti (20) studied 18 patients with bronchiectasis and found that 10 patients had deep marked diffuse pain of variable location: in 3 of these the pain was in the shoulders and arms, in 2 the pain was located in the interscapular region, in 2 it was located in the scapular region and anterior chest, in 1 it was limited to the interscapular vertebral region, in 1 it was limited to the shoulder, and in 1 it was diffuse over the entire chest. All the patients manifested cutaneous hyperalgesia that was located in two areas: one area involved the anterior chest below the clavicles, extending between the anterior axillary line and the peristernal region between the 1st to 3rd ribs, while the second area involved the interscapular vertebral region posteriorly between the medial aspect of the two scapulae and between the 3rd and 6th ribs. Of the 18 patients, 12 had deep hyperalgesia involving the muscles of the chest. Figure 55-7 depicts the most frequent sites of the pain, cutaneous hyperalgesia, and deep hyperalgesia. It was concluded that the pain was a referred phenomenon from stimulation of the tracheobronchial tree, while the cutaneous and deep hyperalgesia were caused by viscercutaneous reflexes (20).

Diagnosis

Diagnosis of bronchiectasis is made through a history and physical examination and by symptoms and signs, as described above. Standard chest radiographs can show increased bronchovascular markings, areas of honeycombing, or cystic areas with or without fluid levels, but often the radiographs are normal. A CT scan of the chest can provide other confirmatory evidence but bronchography is necessary to confirm the diagnosis and extent of the lesions, especially if surgery is being contemplated (17, 18).

Treatment

Treatment consists of appropriate antibiotics, drugs, and physical therapy to promote bronchial drainage. The flora in the sputum are usually mixed gram-positive and gram-negative microorganisms, and anaerobes commonly inhabit the bronchiectatic cysts. A broad-spectrum antibiotic such as ampicillin or tetracycline in doses of 250 to 500 mg orally q6h is continued until the sputum is nonpurulent and less voluminous, usually for 1 to 2 weeks. The combination of trimethoprim, 120 mg, and sulfamethoxazole, 600 mg, orally q12h for 14 days has also been successful in reducing bronchiolar volume and eliminating pathogens (17). Antibiotics should be repeated at the first sign of returning infection; if it recurs frequently prolonged chemoprophylaxis with ampicillin or tetracycline can be tried but is generally disappointing. If bronchopneumonia or serious respiratory infection occurs, a parenteral antibiotic guided by gram-stained cultures and sensitivity studies is indicated.

The mild to moderate pain that is usually present in a number of patients should be managed with nonsteroidal NSAIDs in moderate to high doses (650 to 1000 mg aspirin q4h). If these are not effective and the patient has a persistent cough, moderate doses of codeine can be added to the NSAIDs. If physical examination reveals the presence of myofascial syndrome, trigger points should be injected with a local anesthetic and other therapy should be carried out (Chapters 21 and 57).

C. PAIN CAUSED BY DISEASES OF THE LUNG

Lung tissue is generally considered to be insensitive to noxious stimuli but, under certain pathophysiologic conditions, the J receptors in the interstitial space near the capillaries, the lung irritant receptors in the epithelial lining of the lung and its airways, or both types of receptors, are excited by stimuli that produce mechanical distortion within the lung tissue, such as pulmonary congestion. In addition, infectious diseases such as pneumonia or lung abscess can extend to produce inflammation of the pleura and cause pleuritic pain. Disorders of the pulmonary circulation such as pulmonary hypertension and pulmonary embolism can also be a source of chest pain.

Pulmonary Infections

Pneumonia

Pneumonia is defined as an inflammation in the lung parenchyma in the portion distal to the terminal bronchioles, and comprised of the respiratory bronchioles, alveolar ducts, alveolar sacs and alveoli, and interstitial tissues (21, 22). In lobar pneumonia the infection is confined to an entire lobe, in segmental or lobular pneumonia it is confined to a segment of the lobe, in bronchopneumonia it is confined to alveoli contiguous to the bronchi, and in interstitial pneumonia it is confined to the interstitial tissues. These distinctions are generally based on roentgenographic evidence.

Etiology and Epidemiology

The most common causes of pneumonia in adults are bacteria—Streptococcus pneumonia, Staphylococcus aureus, Hemophilus influenzae, Klebsiella pneumoniae, and other gram-negative bacilli. In addition, Mycoplasma pneumoniae, a bacteria-like organism, can cause pneumonia, especially in older children and young adults. Various other types of bacteria can also cause specific types of pneumonia.

Predisposing factors include respiratory viral infection, alcoholism, age extremes, debility, immunosuppressive disorders and therapy, compromised consciousness, dysphagia, and exposure to transmissible agents (21). The usual mechanism is either inhalation of droplets small enough to reach the alveoli or aspiration of secretions from the upper airways. Other mechanisms include hematogenous dissemination or through the lymphatics or directly from contiguous infection. An important contributing factor is postoperative or post-traumatic decrease in chest wall and pulmonary compliance with consequent hypoventilation, impairment of the cough reflex, bronchiolar spasm, and dehydration. All these cause retention of bronchial secretions, which lead to segmental atelectasis and in turn to lung infection.

Another unusual but important cause of pneumonia is aspiration of gastric contents (Mendelson's syndrome), which causes chemical pneumonitis with serious lung pathophysiology. This disorder is the most frequent cause of anesthetic morbidity and mortality among patients who receive general anesthesia (23).

Other contributing factors are weakness from malnutrition or neuromuscular diseases, thoracic deformities such as severe kyphoscoliosis, or severe lung disease that prevents the full inspiration and brisk expiration necessary to generate an effective cough (22).

In the United States over 2 million people develop pneumonia annually and, of these, 40,000 to 60,000 die (21). Pneumonia is the most common lethal infection and ranks sixth among all disease categories as cause of death; it is the most frequently occurring fatal hospital-acquired infection. In developing countries, lower respiratory tract infections are usually either major causes of death or rank second only to diarrhea. Despite this impressive prevalence, few infections have causative agents that are so difficult to identify. In 30 to 50% of patients no pathogen is identifiable, despite a clinical impression of bacterial pneumonia (21).

Pathophysiology

The earliest stage of pneumonia is congestion characterized by extensive serous exudation, vascular engorgement, and rapid bacterial proliferation. The next phase is called "red hepatization," reflecting the liver-like appearance of the consolidated lung or lobule. The air spaces are full of polymorphonuclear cells, with vascular congestion; extravasation of red blood cells provides the basis for the reddish discoloration on gross examination (21). The parenchyma can be intact but the usual air-containing spaces change into a solid organ with a dense inflammatory response—hence the term "hepatization." The next stage is gray hepatization, in which accumulation of fibrin is associated with inflammatory white and red blood cells in various stages of disintegration, and the alveolar spaces are packed with an inflammatory exudate. The final stage is resolution characterized by resorption of the exudate.

Symptoms and Signs

The major symptoms of pneumonia occur in varying combinations of cough, fever, chest pain, dyspnea, and the production of sputum, which can be mucoid, purulent, or even bloody. In some patients extrapulmonary features such as confusion or disorientation are prominent features. Occasionally, in elderly, alcoholic, or neutropenic patients, respiratory symptoms and signs are absent altogether.

Chest pain occurs predominantly in lobar pneumonia that involves the peripheral lung tissues, frequently sparing the airways (11). The inflammation involves the pleura early and thus pleuritic pain is an initial symptom. The onset of pain is fairly rapid, occurring over a few hours. Most sufferers seem to awake in the early morning with pain. Pleurisy is frequent with pneumonococcal lobar pneumonia, occurs not infrequently with Klebsiella pneumonia, but is noted infrequently in mycoplasmal and viral pneumonias. Because the pleura is unaffected in bronchopneumonia pneumonia and interstitial pneumonia, pain is not a prominent symptom.

The common physical findings are fever, tachycardia, and tachypnea, and patients with severe hypoxemia appear cyanotic. Chest examination usually reveals a decreased respiratory excursion on the affected side because of the pleuritic pain and dullness to percussion from pneumonic consolidation or an accompanying pleural effusion (22). Among the earliest auscultatory findings is the presence of high-pitched end-inspiratory crackles originating from fluid-filled alveoli, which are often increased and heard only after coughing. Consolidated lung surrounding a patent bronchus produces bronchial breath sounds. Examination of the skin with a pinprick or pinch reveals cutaneous hyperalgesia in the same segments supplying the pleura. If the diaphragmatic pleura is involved, the hyperalgesia is found in dermatomes C3 to C5 and perhaps in T9, T10, and T11 (see Chapter 53 for details of innervation of the pleura).

Patients with lower lobe involvement also have hyperalgesia of the chest, whereas if the pneumonia involves the upper lobes, the hyperalgesia is present in T2 to T5 or T6. In addition, pinch reveals deep hyperalgesia and increased muscle tension. Both the cutaneous and deep types of hyperalgesia are present on the side ipsilateral to the pneumonia (20).

Diagnosis

A presumptive diagnosis is usually made through a detailed history, physical examination, and roentgenographic studies, which invariably show the pulmonary infiltrate. Culture and gram-staining of appropriate specimens and a complete red cell count are helpful. For definitive diagnosis it is necessary to demonstrate the pathogen in pleural fluid, blood, or lung or transtracheal aspirate (21).

Treatment

GENERAL THERAPY. Treatment of patients with pneumonia includes general measures such as rest, fluids, and antibacterial agents specific for the bacterial pathogen. Patients with pneumonococcal pneumonia should be treated with penicillin G or V in doses of 250 to 500 mg orally q6h (21). Alternative oral regimens include tetracycline, erythromycin, or cephalexin 500 mg q6h, or clindamycin 300 mg q6h. For parenteral therapy, procaine penicillin 600,000 U IM q12h, or aqueous penicillin G 500,000 to 1,000,000 U q4h or q6h is the preferred regimen. Alternative parenteral agents are cephalosporins, erythromycin, or clindamycin. The recommended therapy for staphylococcal pneumonia is a penicillinase-resistant penicillin such as oxacillin or nafcillin, 2 g IV q4h or q6h. Other important alternative derivatives are cephalosporins such as cephalothin or cefamandole, 2 g IV q4h or q6h. Other types of pneumonia require appropriate antimicrobial agents.

PAIN THERAPY. The treatment of pain associated with pneumonia depends on its severity. Patients with mild pain should be given NSAIDs in the medium range of dosages listed in Chapter 78. For moderate pain it might be necessary to give high doses (e.g., 1000 mg of aspirin) together with 64 to 128 mg of codeine. Because the pain is severe in many of these patients it is necessary to combine NSAIDs with morphine or other potent narcotics. A highly effective way of providing good pain relief with potent narcotics is by the use of patient-controlled analgesia (Chapter 78).

In patients with severe excruciating pain that is not adequately relieved by systemic analgesics, serious consideration should be given to having an anesthesiologist carry out posterior intercostal block of the segment involved with pain using a long-acting local anesthetic, such as bupivacaine. To obviate the minimal discomfort from the needle punctures, I usually give patients a bolus of 150 mg of thiopental sodium to produce amnesia (not anesthesia) for 3 to 5 minutes, during which time the needles are inserted. This procedure provides complete pain relief for 8 to 12 hours and also eliminates the reflex segmental and suprasegmental responses described in Chapter 7.

An alternate technique for managing severe pain is the use of epidural opioid analgesia, which is achieved by placing a catheter in the lower thoracic epidural space and injecting appropriate doses of a narcotic. Although this is not as effective in blocking nociceptive impulses as the use of local anesthetic, it usually provides excellent pain relief and has the advantage over the use of intercostal block of involving only one

puncture. Because the pain only lasts 3 or 4 days with effective antibiotic therapy, all these therapeutic procedures to manage pain are practical, and are associated with only minimal adverse side effects.

Lung Abscess

Lung abscess consists of a localized pus-containing cavity resulting from necrosis of lung tissue and surrounding pneumonitis. It can be a cause of chest pain, especially if the inflammation extends to the parietal pleura.

Etiology and Pathophysiology

Lung abscesses are usually caused by aspiration of infected material from an upper airway when a patient is unconscious or obtunded from alcoholism, central nervous system disease, general anesthesia, or excessive sedation. Lung abscesses are usually produced by anerobes and are not infrequently associated with periodontal disease. Sometimes multiple organisms act synergistically. Bacteria cultured from a lung abscess include the common pyogenic bacteria and nasopharyngeal flora, particularly anaerobes and, less often, aerobic bacteria and fungi. Bronchogenic carcinoma is an occasional cause of lung abscess in persons over the age of 55 (21).

A single abscess is most common, but multiple abscesses that are usually unilateral, also occur, and can develop simultaneously or spread from a single focus (21). In abscesses caused by aspiration the superior segment of the lower lobe and the posterior segment of the upper lobe are most frequently affected. The solitary abscess consequent to bronchial obstruction or an infected embolus starts as necrosis over the major portion of the involved bronchopulmonary segment, with its base adjacent to the chest wall and the pleural space; the affected part is often obliterated by inflammatory adhesions. Abscesses as a result of hematogenous spread are frequently caused by Staphylococcus aureus, and can occur in multiple sites in noncontiguous parts of the lung (21, 22).

An abscess usually ruptures into a bronchus and its contents expectorated into the air- and fluid-filled cavity. With adequate drainage the walls usually collapse and contract, eventually obliterating the cavity. If drainage is inadequate the abscess becomes fibrotic and rigid, and healing does not occur. Occasionally an abscess ruptures into a pleural cavity, resulting in empyema and not infrequently in a bronchopleural fistula.

Symptoms and Signs

Symptoms can develop acutely or are insidious. Early symptoms are often those of pneumonia, characterized by malaise, anorexia, sputum-producing cough, and fever. Unless the abscess is completely walled off the sputum is purulent and is frequently blood-streaked. About 60% of patients with abscess caused by anaerobic bacteria develop a putrid odor discernible at some distance from the patient (21). Some patients manifest severe prostration and a temperature of 39° to 40° C.

Chest pain occurs invariably with pleural involvement. Teodori and Galletti (20) carefully studied the

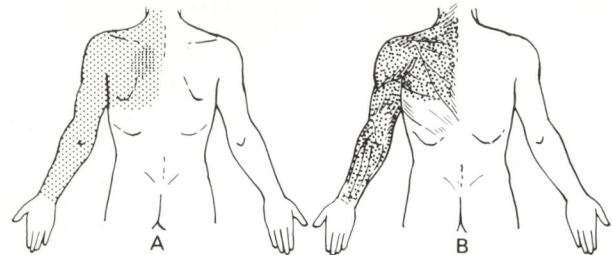

Fig. 55-8. Distribution of pain and of cutaneous hyperalgesia in patients with an abscess in the left lung. *A, B.* Posterior views showing the distribution of the pain, indicated by heavy stipples, and of the cutaneous hyperalgesia, indicated by the cross-hatched areas. Modified from Teodori, U., and Galletti, R.: Il Dolore Nelle Affezioni Degli Organi Interni del Torace. Rome, El Tozzi, 1962, p. 72.

location, quality, and intensity of pain in 15 patients with lung abscess. They noted that all but 2 patients had pain that was dull and aching in character, and it was mild in 2, moderate in 8, and severe in 3. Pain caused by abscess in the superior lobe was usually referred to the ipsilateral scapula, pain from the midportion of the lung was usually referred to the ipsilateral shoulder and arm and mammary region, while pain that involved the lower part of the lung was usually referred to the shoulders bilaterally. In the latter case it is likely that the diaphragmatic pleura was involved in the inflammatory reaction. Pain was continuous in 8 of the patients, and occurred at intervals during the day in the rest. All the patients had cutaneous hypergesia, and 12 had deep muscular hyperalgesia. Figure 55-8 shows the distribution of spontaneous pain and the cutaneous hyperalgesia in one patient who had unilateral pain.

Physical signs of lung abscess include a small area of dullness indicating localized pneumonic consolidation, suppressed rather than bronchial breath sounds, and fine or medium moist rales.

Diagnosis

The presumptive diagnosis can be made through a history and physical examination that reveals the aforementioned signs (9). Chest roentgenography initially shows a segmental or lobar consolidation that becomes globular as it distends with pus. Following a rupture into a bronchus, a cavity with a fluid level appears on the film. Failure of an area of pneumonia to resolve should always suggest abscess formation, bronchial neoplasm, or both. The patient should be followed with roentgenography at 1- to 2-week intervals in search of central areas of diminished density. The sputum should be examined by smear and cultured for bacteria, including mycobacteria. If anaerobes are suspected as the causative agents, a specimen of bronchial secretion should be acquired by transtracheal aspiration and not through the mouth, which contains anaerobic organisms that could contaminate the sputum.

Treatment

Prompt and complete healing of a lung abscess depends on adequate antibiotic treatment and drainage; most patients recover without surgical intervention. As soon as the sputum and blood have been collected for culture and sensitivity testing, antibiotic therapy should be initiated promptly (21, 22). The drug of choice is usually penicillin G 1.2 million U (750 mg) orally qid or 10 to 12 million U IV daily (22). If no clinical response is seen in 4 to 7 days and a specific pathogen has not been located, clindamycin 600 mg IV qid or tid should replace the penicillin. Treatment should be continued until the pneumonitis has resolved and the cavity has disappeared or stabilized on serial roentgenograms. Postural drainage can be a helpful adjunct but can also cause spillage to other bronchi, with extension of the process or acute obstruction. If the patient is weak or paralyzed tracheostomy and suction should be considered. Rarely, bronchoscopic aspiration might be required for tenacious sputum. Pulmonary resection is the procedure of choice for an abscess resistant to medical therapy, particularly if bronchogenic carcinoma is suspected. Management of the chest pain associated with the lung abscess is similar to that described above for pneumonia.

D. DISORDERS OF THE PULMONARY CIRCULATION

Pulmonary Arterial Hypertension

Acute pulmonary hypertension is a common cause of severe pain, often in the center of the chest, which is crushing or gripping in quality and is easily confused with the pain of acute myocardial infarction (11). In contrast to the pain of myocardial infarction, however, the pain of acute pulmonary arterial hypertension does not radiate to the jaw or to the arms, and seldom to the back.

Etiology and Pathophysiology

Davies (11) suggested that the pain is produced by acute dilatation of the main pulmonary artery or its major branches because acute distension of a large blood vessel anywhere in the body can cause pain, and this is also true of pulmonary arteries. The fall in Pa_{O_2} is a potent cause of rapid small pulmonary arterial constriction, leading to a rise in pulmonary arterial pressure with consequent distension of the larger vessels, which in turn causes pain. Davies believed that pain can occur in a previously healthy patient with an acute rise in pressure or in a patient with chronic pulmonary hypertension when an extra load raises pressure still further.

The cause of chronic primary pulmonary hypertension is unknown but some possible factors have been suggested. Because pathologic examination in some patients with chronic primary pulmonary hypertension revealed minimal or no changes in the pulmonary vessels, it has been suggested that a neurohumoral vasoconstrictor mechanism is involved (24, 25). Support for this view is provided by the observation that the pulmonary vascular resistance can be acutely reduced in some patients with this disease by intrapulmonary injection of vasodilators or by breathing oxygen (26). The occurrence of the disease in young women has prompted the suggestion that unrecognized thromboemboli or amniotic fluid emboli during pregnancy might play a role. Oral contraceptives might be a contributing factor. The association and occurrence of Raynaud's disease or scleroderma, disseminated lupus erythematosus, rheumatoid arthritis, and dermomyocitis have led to the speculation that primary pulmonary hypertension might represent a form of collagen vascular disease (24).

On pathologic examination of patients with chronic primary pulmonary hypertension the findings are usually confined to the right side of the heart and lungs, with the right atrium often enlarged and right ventricle hypertrophy. Frequently the large pulmonary arteries exhibit atherosclerotic plaques. The small pulmonary arteries (30 to 300 μm in diameter) exhibit muscular hypertrophy and intimal hyperplasia, sometimes with fibrosis (24).

With the development of severe pulmonary vascular disease, abnormal elevation of pulmonary arterial pressure occurs, often to a striking degree, and the pulmonary arterial pressure can be equal to that of the systemic arterial pressure. In many patients the mean right atrial pressure is increased and the a wave in the right atrium is markedly elevated, which is an indication of the forceful atrial contraction necessary to fill the hypertrophied right ventricle. Interestingly, pulmonary arterial wedge pressure is normal, the cardiac output is normal or reduced, and no intracardiac shunts are detected (24). Mild systemic arterial oxygen desaturation is quite common, even in the absence of heart failure, and might be a result of shunting within the lungs. Pulmonary function is generally normal, although hyperventilation is often present, resulting in hypocapnia and a decrease in serum bicarbonate concentration.

Symptoms and Signs

Patients with acute pulmonary hypertension have severe central chest pain located retrosternally, often associated with anxiety and sense of impending death (11). As previously mentioned, unlike myocardial infarction pain, it does not radiate to the arms or jaw. Patients with chronic primary pulmonary hypertension relate a history of relatively recent onset of symptoms consisting of exertional dyspnea, weakness, and fatigue; 50 to 60% have angina-type chest pain (24, 25, 27). Hoarseness caused by compression of the left recurrent laryngeal nerve by the enlarged pulmonary artery occurs in about 6 to 8% of patients (28).

Patients with acute pulmonary arterial hypertension can be in shock if the pain is severe. Cyanosis is usually present with both acute and chronic pulmonary hypertension. The jugular pulse shows a prominent a wave, a right ventricular heave is present and a pulse can be felt in the region of the main pulmonary artery. An ejection click can be audible at the pulmonic area. The pulmonary closure sound is markedly accentuated and often palpable, and the second heart sound is narrowly split (24). An atrial valve sound is heard at the lower left sternal border and, in some patients, an ejection murmur at the pulmonic area or the early diastolic murmur of pulmonic regurgitation is heard. Chest roentgenograms can show cardiac enlargement of the right ventricle and right atrial prominence, with marked dilatation of the pulmonary artery segments.

Diagnosis

Ross (24) emphasized that it is imperative that the diagnosis of primary (chronic) pulmonary hypertension not be made until potentially treatable causes of elevated pulmonary arterial pressure have been excluded. This requires not only a thorough history but a complete physical examination and special tests, including pulmonary function tests, cardiac catheterization, angiography, and radioactive lung scanning studies.

Treatment

Acute pulmonary hypertension is usually treated by eliminating the causative factor. Inhalation of high concentrations of oxygen is effective in decreasing the pulmonary arterial pressure and, consequently, the pain. If this is ineffective intrapulmonary injection of vasodilator should be considered (28).

In patients with chronic primary pulmonary hypertension, Ross (24) indicated that the downward course is progressive in many patients, despite treatment, and therapy must be palliative. Right-sided heart failure should be treated with cardiotonic and diuretic regimens. Because no hypocapnia is present the hypoxemia that can occur with heart failure can be treated safely with oxygen therapy. It has been noted that, in some patients, pharmacologic therapy can produce clinical and hemodynamic improvement (25–28). Four groups of drugs have been found to be useful: (a) direct vascular smooth muscle relaxants, such as nitroprusside, diazoxide, and hydralazine; (b) beta agonists, such as sublingual isoproterenol and oral terbutaline; (c) alpha-adrenergic blockers, such as phentolamine and phenoxybenzamine; and (d) calcium blockers, such as nifedipine and verapamil. In some patients stable hemodynamic effects from orally administered drugs such as diazoxide or hydralazine have been sustained for many months, with clinical improvement manifested by relief of dyspnea and pain and by a reduction in the number of episodes of syncope (24, 28). Prior to instituting long-term therapy, measurements of the acute responses of the pulmonary artery pressure, pulmonary vascular resistance, cardiac output, and arterial pressure are indicated to aid in prognosis.

The management of pain depends on the severity and duration. In patients with severe and excruciating central pain caused by acute pulmonary hypertension, cessation of the severe exertion or elimination of the causative factor, such as giving oxygen to patients who have pain at high altitudes, is usually sufficient. If the severe excruciating pain persists after a reasonable trial period, intravenous narcotics should be administered. In patients with chronic pulmonary hypertension the pain is usually not as severe and can be managed with NSAIDs given alone or in combination with codeine.

Pulmonary Embolism*

Acute pulmonary embolism is a relatively common event, particularly in hospitalized, acutely ill patients (29, 30). The incidence of symptomatic pulmonary embolism in the United States has been estimated at 650,000 annually (30). Evidence of pulmonary emboli

---

*Some of the information in this section was contributed by Dr. K.H. Hammermeister, senior author of Chapter 54.

can be found in 60% of autopsies, most of which are probably clinically insignificant (31). Even these data underestimate the incidence, because emboli in many patients resolve without a trace and are not found on postmortem examination. Acute pulmonary embolism might be the most common cause of acute pulmonary disease in hospitalized patients (32, 33) and is one of the most common causes of sudden unexpected death in this population (34).

Etiology

The pulmonary embolus can consist of thrombus, air, amniotic fluid, fat, or bone marrow (35). Available data indicate, however, that 95% of pulmonary emboli arise from thrombi forming in the leg or pelvic veins (36). Thrombi occur in the right cardiac chambers or other veins and account for most of the remaining 5% of pulmonary emboli. Amniotic fluid, fat, or bone marrow emboli represent less than 1% of all cases of pulmonary embolism (29). The most significant risk factor for the formation of thrombus and subsequent pulmonary embolism is venous stasis, such as that which occurs postoperatively, with prolonged periods of bed rest, with low cardiac output from any cause, and with prolonged immobility during lengthy travel.

Other predisposing factors include the use of oral contraceptives, pregnancy, obesity, malignancy, COPD, hematologic disorders (e.g., polycythemia vera), vascular injuries from minor trauma, and prolonged immobilization of patients with chronic disease states (36–38). Several studies have shown that patients undergoing hip surgery with general anesthesia have a significantly greater incidence of thromboembolism than those undergoing the same surgery with regional anesthesia (39, 40).

Once released into the venous circulation, emboli are distributed to both lungs in 65% of cases, to the right lung in 20%, and to the left lung in 15% (36). The lower lobes are involved four times more often than the upper lobes.

Pathophysiology

Most of the consequences of pulmonary embolism can be explained by obstruction of the pulmonary vasculature to produce hypoxemia, acute pulmonary hypertension, right ventricular failure, and reduced cardiac output or cardiogenic shock. Symptomatic pulmonary embolism is associated with obstruction of approximately 30% or more of the segments of the pulmonary arterial tree (41). Acute obstruction of the right or left main pulmonary artery with a balloon, however, produced relatively few hemodynamic changes or symptoms (42). Therefore, it is generally thought that the acute pulmonary embolism leads to the release of humoral substances such as serotonin, prostaglandins, and histamine, resulting in constriction of the pulmonary arterial bed (29, 43). The combined effect of the mechanical obstruction by thrombus and vasoconstriction leads to unperfused but ventilated alveoli (V:Q mismatch), resulting in the arterial hypoxemia that is almost universal. Hypoxemia, in turn, can increase the pulmonary vasoconstriction. Pulmonary vascular resistance, pulmonary arterial pressure, right ventricular systolic and diastolic pressures, and right atrial pressure are increased, while the cardiac index is decreased. If pulmonary vascular resistance increases acutely to the extent that the right ventricle cannot generate sufficient pressure to maintain cardiac output, arterial hypotension results, and this can progress to shock. In patients without preexisting cardiopulmonary disease this only occurs after massive embolization involving at least 50% and usually 75% of the pulmonary vascular bed (29).

Symptoms and Signs

The most common symptoms of pulmonary embolism are chest pain, dyspnea, and tachypnea (44). The frequency of these and other symptoms and signs reported by 327 patients in two large clinical trials of thrombolytic therapy for pulmonary embolism (44, 45) are shown in Table 55-2. The chest pain was pleuritic in over 75% of patients. The pleurisy is often caused by pulmonary infarction, which produces inflammation on the pleural surfaces, a pleural rub, and pleuritic pain. The pleuritic pain is a relatively late finding, because it can take several days for pulmonary infarction and pleural inflammation to develop. The pleuritic pain is characteristically severe and persistent, lasting several days longer than that of pneumonia, for example (11). Indeed, the persistence of pleuritic pain for more than 7 days in an acutely ill patient should suggest pulmonary embolism (Fig. 55-9).

Patients with large pulmonary emboli usually experience a severe, visceral, retrosternal (deep) crushing pain at the time of the embolism, similar to that of myocardial ischemia except that the pain does not radiate. This is thought to be caused by sudden distension of the pulmonary artery, right ventricle, or both, or even by right ventricular ischemia resulting in sudden increase in wall stress and myocardial oxygen demand. When this type of pain occurs together with T-wave or ST-segment changes, distinction from unstable angina or acute myocardial infarction can be difficult. The classic triad of hemoptysis, pleuritic chest pain, and a pleural rub is uncommon (29).

In patients with massive pulmonary artery obstruction consequent marked increase in pulmonary artery pressure can cause right ventricular failure, with resultant distension of cervical veins and other signs of right ventricular failure. In such patients auscultation reveals a right ventricular heave and a right ventricular presystolic and protodiastolic gallop. Cyanosis is usual with massive pulmonary embolism, but not with a lesser degree of obstruction. Examination of the lungs is usually normal in the absence of pulmonary infarct. Wheezing is sometimes heard, particularly if underlying bronchopulmonary or cardiac disease is present.

Tachypnea, often with dyspnea, almost always occurs after an embolic episode; it appears to be of reflex origin, most likely caused by stimulation of juxtacapillary receptors in the alveolar membrane by swelling of the alveolar interstitial space (44, 45). This stimulation increases vagal afferent activity that in turn stimulates medullary respiration, with consequent alveolar hyperventilation manifested by a lower Pa_{CO_2}.

TABLE 55-2. Symptoms and Signs in 327 Patients with Acute Pulmonary Embolism

Symptoms and Signs	All Patients n = 327 (%)	Patients with Massive Emboli n = 197 (%)	Patients with Submassive Emboli n = 130 (%)
Symptoms			
Chest pain	88	85	82
Dyspnea	84	85	82
Apprehension	59	65	50
Cough	53	53	52
Hemoptysis	30	23	40
Diaphoresis	27	29	23
Syncope	13	20	4
Signs			
Tachypnea (resp. >16/min)	92	95	87
Rales	58	57	60
Increased pulmonic 2nd sound	53	58	45
Tachycardia (pulse >100/min)	44	48	38
Fever (temp. >37.8° C)	43	43	42
Gallop	34	39	25
Diaphoresis	36	42	27
Phlebitis	32	36	26
Edema	24	23	25
Murmur	23	27	16
Cyanosis	19	25	9

From Bell, W.R., Simon, T.L., and DeMets, D.L.: The clinical features of submassive and massive pulmonary emboli. Am. J. Med., *62*:355, 1977.

Diagnosis

All the symptoms, signs, and routine laboratory data in acute pulmonary embolism are nonspecific; their usefulness lies in leading to a suspicion of the diagnosis. The diagnosis rests on establishing a defect in pulmonary artery perfusion that cannot be explained by coexisting lung disease. The "gold standard" for the diagnosis of pulmonary embolism is the pulmonary arteriogram (29). The passage of a catheter to the main pulmonary artery and performance of the angiogram can be performed by a trained angiographer, with minimal risk (approximately 0.2% mortality rate). The use of perfusion imaging to guide the angiographer in performing subselective angiography with small doses of contrast material reduces this risk even further. The identification of filling defects within the pulmonary arteries or abruptly terminated arteries establishes the diagnosis of pulmonary embolism. Thrombi lyse over a period of 7 to 10 days; therefore, pulmonary angiography (and radionuclide imaging) are most sensitive in the first few days after onset of symptoms.

Pulmonary angiography is performed in only a minority of patients with suspected pulmonary embolism because of greater confidence in the use of radionuclide ventilation perfusion scintigraphy (29). When first introduced this technique involved only perfusion imaging using radionuclide-tagged macroaggregated albumin, which was embolized to the pulmonary arterioles. Because many pulmonary diseases—most particularly COPD and pneumonia—also result in abnormal pulmonary artery perfusion, this technique was sensitive but nonspecific. With the addition of simultaneous ventilation scanning and better diagnostic criteria, however, the sensitivity and specificity of the procedure have improved to the point that it is the primary diagnostic tool for most patients with suspected pulmonary embolism. Ventilation usually remains normal in most segments of lung with pulmonary emboli, at least until infarction occurs; ventilation is abnormal in those with COPD and pneumonia.

Electrocardiographic changes in acute pulmonary embolism are nonspecific and do not aid in differentiating from other causes of chest pain and acute dyspnea. The typical electrocardiographic pattern of right heart strain (right axis deviation of the QRS wave and T-wave inversion in the right precordial leads) is seen in only about 19% of patients with pulmonary embolism. T-wave inversion and ST-segment shifts that might suggest myocardial ischemia are seen in 30 to 40% of patients (46).

The chest roentgenogram is similarly nonspecific. The most common finding is no acute change, because

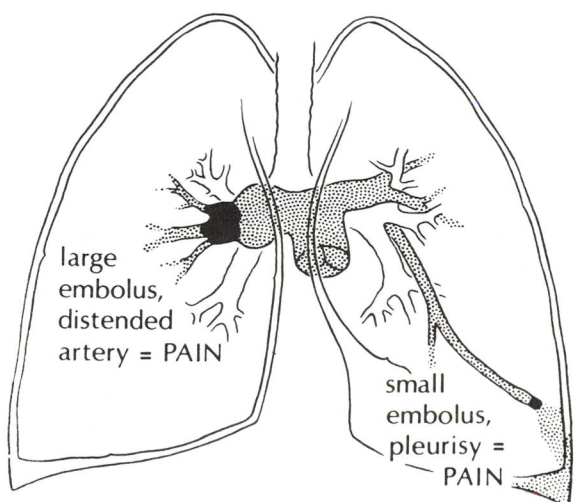

FIG. 55-9. The origin of pain in pulmonary embolism. From Levene, D.L. (ed.): Chest Pain: An Integrated Diagnostic Approach. Philadelphia, Lea & Febiger, 1977, p. 77.

Painful Disorders of the Respiratory System **1057**

most pulmonary emboli do not cause pulmonary infiltrates. The classic pleural-based wedge-shaped infiltrate is uncommon. When pre-existing pulmonary infiltrates are present the diagnosis becomes more difficult because the ventilation perfusion scan is less reliable. These are patients in whom pulmonary angiography might be necessary if establishment of the diagnosis is required.

The serum lactic dehydrogenase level might be increased with pulmonary infarction, but this is of little diagnostic value because it is nonspecific and insensitive for pulmonary embolism.

Treatment

PROPHYLAXIS. The most important aspect of treatment is prevention. Early ambulation following surgery or acute myocardial infarction is thought to be effective. Alternatively (or in combination with early ambulation), a number of studies have shown that low-dose heparin (5000 U bid) is highly effective in preventing venous thrombosis, pulmonary embolism, or both (47), except in patients undergoing hip replacement or prostatic surgery (48). With the use of these prophylactic measures, it is generally believed that the incidence of clinically significant pulmonary embolism has decreased substantially over the past decade. As previously mentioned, several studies have shown that patients undergoing hip replacement operations under regional anesthesia have significantly less incidence of thromboembolism than those managed with general anesthesia (39–40).

GENERAL THERAPY. Treatment of the acute event is primarily aimed at preventing further pulmonary embolism, supporting the circulation, and administering oxygen until the natural lytic processes result in dissolution of the emboli. If the diagnosis is strongly suspected and no significant contraindication to anticoagulation is present, therapy with heparin should be started even before the diagnosis is definitely established with ventilation perfusion scanning, pulmonary angiography, or both (29). Heparin can be given as a 10,000-U loading dose followed by continuous IV infusion of 1000 U/hour or by a dose sufficient to prolong the partial thromboplastin time twofold. Oral anticoagulation with warfarin is then instituted for a period of 6 weeks to 6 months. If no prior embolism has occurred and the inciting cause has resolved (e.g., recent surgery), it seems to be of little benefit to continue anticoagulation therapy beyond 6 weeks (49). A few patients with recurrent pulmonary embolism and persisting risk factors might need to remain on chronic anticoagulation indefinitely.

Thrombolytic therapy has been carefully studied (46); the administration of urokinase or streptokinase results in more rapid lysis of the emboli and restoration of normal hemodynamics, but produces no decrease in the mortality rate. Presently, thrombolytic therapy is reserved for patients with massive emboli with marked hemodynamic compromise. Pulmonary embolectomy using cardiopulmonary bypass has also been used in patients in cardiogenic shock from pulmonary emboli, but carries a high operative mortality rate (50); it is rarely used at present. If pulmonary embolism recurs while patients are adequately anticoagulated with heparin or warfarin, interruption of the inferior vena cava by direct ligation or by the percutaneous placement of an umbrella should be considered. Caval interruption is thought to be only a temporary prophylaxis, because sizable collateral channels develop around the site of interruption (29).

PAIN THERAPY. The management of the pain associated with pulmonary embolism depends on the rate of onset, severity, duration, and quality. The patient who experiences sudden, severe crushing central pain caused by a large pulmonary obstruction should be given morphine or another potent narcotic intravenously slowly. The initial dose of 4 to 5 mg diluted in 5 ml of saline solution is injected slowly over a period of 2 or 3 minutes. This should produce some relief in 5 minutes and good relief in 10 to 15 minutes. If the patient still experiences severe pain a second dose of 5 mg should be administered and the patient monitored closely. Usually the second dose provides ample pain relief but, if it does not within 15 to 20 minutes of the injection, a third dose should be given; following this the patient can be managed with a continuous infusion of opioids or patient-controlled analgesia, if available.

An even more effective alternative is the use of a cervicothoracic sympathetic block with a long-lasting local anesthetic, provided, of course, that a physician expert in its administration is available in the hospital. This procedure produces complete pain relief ipsilateral to the injection within 5 to 8 minutes of injection, and the pain relief will last for 6 to 10 hours. Leriche and colleagues (51) were the first to suggest the use of this procedure in the treatment of pulmonary embolism; they believed that it not only relieved pain by blocking afferent impulses from the lungs but also interrupted efferent impulses taking part in the production of sympathetic reflex mechanisms thought to be involved in the pathophysiology. More recent data did not substantiate this claim but suggested that reflexes involved in the pathophysiology are mediated primarily by the vagus nerves (52). Nevertheless, the procedure is effective in relieving the central type of pain (53). Moreover, because it blocks some of the sympathetic afferent input to the neuraxis, it should decrease the segmental and suprasegmental reflex responses that are invariably associated with severe pain and nociceptive input (Chapter 7). Another relatively new procedure for relief of the pain is the use of intraspinal narcotics.

Patients who develop pleuritic pain can usually be relieved with NSAIDs combined with a potent narcotic agent given orally or parenterally. If the patient has experienced severe pleuritic pain unrelieved by systemic analgesics, however, a posterior intercostal block with bupivacaine should be considered (Chapter 94). The procedure is carried out in the manner described for the pleurisy of pneumonia.

In several major medicine and cardiology textbooks reviewed during the writing of this section, the treatment was exclusively focused on prevention and treatment with anticoagulant and thrombolytic therapies (29, 30). The management of pain was not discussed; from the viewpoint of the patient, this is an important issue. The lack of discussion of pain management in textbooks of medicine and surgery continues to surprise and concern me.

E. CHEST PAIN CAUSED BY DISORDERS OF THE PLEURA

The most important disorders of the pleura that produce chest pain are either of inflammatory origin, as in pleuritis, or from mechanical distortion, as in pneumothorax.

Pleuritis

Inflammation of the pleura can occur with underlying pulmonary diseases including pneumonia, lung abscess, pulmonary infarct caused by an embolus, and neoplasm (54). As discussed above, the pleuritis is associated with localized chest pain and needs no further comment. Pleural pain in the absence of physical and radiographic findings or underlying disease suggests the diagnosis of epidemic pleurodynia, infection of the pleura, or a connective tissue disorder such as systemic lupus erythematosis.

Pleurodynia. Pleurodynia, also known as Bornholm disease and epidemic myalgia, is characterized by malaise, sore throat, and anorexia, followed by increased debility, fever, and sudden onset of muscle, pleuritic, and abdominal pain (55). The pain is sharp, severe, and paroxysmal over the lower ribs or substernal area. It is markedly aggravated by moving, breathing, coughing, sneezing, and hiccuping, and can be referred to the shoulders, neck, scapula, or chest. In about 50% of patients pain and spasm of the anterior abdominal muscles occur in combination with chest pain. Many patients complain of cutaneous hyperalgesia, hyperesthesia, and paresthesia in the area of the pain.

This condition usually occurs as an epidemic and lasts 3 to 7 days, but relapses can occur (55, 56). Coxsackieviruses B were isolated from the striated muscle of patients with pleurodynia during an epidemic (56). Occasionally the pleuritis is accompanied by pleural effusion, and the virus has been isolated from the pleural fluid. Bornholm disease can occur in those of any age but is most common in children and young adults. Early in the course of the illness meningitis, myocarditis, or hepatitis can ensue. Liver biopsy in patients with complicating jaundice show some acute partial triaditis and intense clouding and swelling of central zone hepatocytes. A late complication is orchitis, occurring in 3 to 5% of patients with pleurodynia during relapse (56).

Treatment

Treatment of pleuritis is directed toward the underlying disease and relief of pain. In patients with mild to moderate pain, NSAIDs given alone or in combination with codeine in optimal doses usually suffice. For more severe pain, potent narcotics with NSAIDs should be tried. As I pointed out in the first edition of this book and in the preceding pages, however, systemic analgesics even in optimal doses do not completely relieve the pain associated with deep breathing and coughing, thus preventing the patient from bringing up secretions. In such patients serious consideration should be given to the use of posterior intercostal blocks or segmental epidural analgesia with long-lasting anesthetic agents such as bupivacaine. Intraspinal opioids, although not quite as effective, are a

good alternative. These procedures require the skill of a clinical anesthesiologist, available in most medical centers.

Occasionally acute pleuritis leads to chronic adhesive pleuritis as a sequelae of empyema, hemothorax, or tuberculosis. Adhesive pleuritis is characterized by marked thickening of the pleura, which can interfere with pulmonary function. Under these circumstances the thickened pleura encases the lung and "traps" it so that the lung behaves as if it were small and stiff, despite having intrinsically normal mechanical processes. If symptoms such as dyspnea are severe, surgical removal of the thickened pleura (decortication) might be indicated (54).

Pleural Effusion

Although not usually painful, pleural effusion is discussed briefly here for the sake of completeness. The visceral and parietal pleurae form a continuous membrane that encloses a potential space that normally contains only a small amount of liquid. This liquid is dynamic and, as with all movements of liquid between vascular and extravascular compartments, the principle of Starling's equation applies (54). Under normal circumstances the liquid is filtered out of the parietal pleura, which is supplied by systemic capillaries at a mean pressure of 30 cm H_2O; most of this is taken up at the visceral pleura, supplied by the pulmonary circulation with a mean capillary pressure of 11 cm H_2O. For the removal of macromolecules plus some liquid, there are in addition lymphatic stomata in the diaphragmatic and vascular portions of the parietal pleura.

An abnormal accumulation of liquid, designated as pleural effusion, occurs with changes in hydrostatic and oncotic forces (transudation) or with an alteration in membrane permeability (exudation), such as with inflammation or neoplastic involvement. The finding of pleural effusion in the absence of parenchymal disease suggests primary tuberculosis, subdiaphragmatic abscess, mesoepithelioma, or primary bacterial infection of the pleural space. Many pleural effusions are asymptomatic, but patients can complain of dyspnea, pleuritic chest pain, or a dull uncomfortable sensation in the chest (54). Physical signs include deviation of the trachea to the contralateral side, dullness on percussion, and diminished breath sounds over the affected side.

Empyema is the presence of infected liquid or frank pus in the pleural space and is usually a complication of pneumonia, abscess from the lung, or diaphragmatic or esophageal perforation. Chest pain, fever, cough, night sweats, and weight loss are common complaints.

Treatment of symptomatic pleural effusion or empyema includes adequate drainage of the pleural space, antimicrobial therapy, and the control of pain as discussed in previous sections.

Pneumothorax

In pneumothorax a collection of gas in the pleural space occurs that results in complete or partial collapse of a lobe or entire lung. When air enters the pleural space, pleural pressure in the affected hemithorax tends to approach atmospheric pressure, thus eliminating the normal negative pressure that keeps the lung expanded (54, 57). The less negative the pleural pressure, the greater the degree of lung collapse. The normal elastic recoil of the unaffected lung causes a shift of the mediastinum from the affected to the unaffected side. If pressure inside the pneumothorax increases above atmospheric pressure, as with a one-way leak into the pleural space ("ball valve leak"), or when a pneumothorax occurs as a complication of positive pressure ventilation, a tension pneumothorax is present. Under these circumstances the affected lung is compressed, the mediastinum is further shifted toward the unaffected side, and cardiac output can be severely compromised because of the positive intrathoracic pressure that decreases venous return to the heart.

Tension pneumothorax is a medical emergency (54, 57). A pneumothorax can occur spontaneously or can be secondary to underlying lung disease, chest trauma, mechanical ventilation, or perforated esophagus. Spontaneous pneumothorax most commonly occurs in previously healthy adults between 20 and 40 years of age (54). In many of these patients air leaks into the pleural space as a result of rupture of small blebs on the surface of the visceral pleura. The cause of the blebs is unclear, but they tend to be located around the apex of the lung.

Symptoms and Signs

Spontaneous pneumothorax usually manifests itself by sudden chest pain of pleuritic type, localized to one side and associated in most cases with a sensation of dyspnea. The most helpful feature of the pain is its sudden onset, so that often patients can describe their activities at the moment it appeared (11, 54, 57). The severity of pain and degree of dyspnea at onset are not indicative of the size of the pneumothorax. Usually both pain and dyspnea disappear within 2 to 3 hours following a small pneumothorax in healthy people. Persistence of dyspnea and pain that increases in severity suggest a large pneumothorax, and perhaps intrapleural hemorrhage.

The sudden change in volume of the lungs with shift of the mediastinum is likely to cause a visceral-type deep central pain, retrosternal pressure, or heaviness, but this usually does not persist and is overshadowed by the pleuritic pain.

Physical examination reveals tachypnea, asymmetric expansion of the chest on the affected side (because of outward recoil of the chest wall as the lung collapses), mediastinal shift with deviation of the trachea, cardiac dullness and apex beat away from the pneumothorax, hyper-resonance to percussion, and diminished breath sounds over the affected side (54, 57). Chest roentgenograms reveal a visible visceral pleural edge with no lung markings between this edge and the chest wall (54). It is important to take the chest roentgenograms with the patient in the upright position because, in a supine posture, upward movement of air with approximation of the visceral and parietal pleura can obscure the presence of a pneumothorax.

Treatment

Treatment depends on the size of the pneumothorax. A small pneumothorax is best managed by reassuring the patient and close observation because the air leak has usually sealed by the time the patient presents to the physician. The pain is generally managed easily with systemic analgesics given orally. Large pneumothoraces are usually accompanied by moderate to severe pain that requires therapy in the form of evacuation of air and the use of a combination of a NSAID and a narcotic. It is best to achieve aspiration of air with closed thoracostomy tube drainage (54, 57). Spontaneous tension pneumothorax is unusual but, if present, should be treated as an emergency by immediate aspiration through a wide-bore needle placed in the pleural space at the level of the 2nd intercostal space anteriorly in the midclavicular region.

REFERENCES

1. Fishman, A.P. (ed.): Pulmonary Diseases and Disorders. New York, McGraw-Hill, 1980.
2. Snider, G.L. (ed.): Clinical Pulmonary Medicine. Boston, Little, Brown & Co., 1981.
3. Clemente, C.D.: Gray's Anatomy of the Human Body. 30th Ed. Philadelphia, Lea & Febiger, 1985, pp. 1377–1401.
4. Kuntz, A.: Autonomic Nervous System. 4th Ed. Philadelphia, Lea & Febiger, 1953, pp. 184–206.
5. Mitchell, G.A.G.: Cardiovascular Innervation. London, E. & S. Livingstone, 1956, pp. 196–238.
6. Netter, F.H.: The CIBA Collection of Medical Illustrations. The Respiratory System. West Caldwell, NJ, CIBA Pharmaceuticals, 1979, p. 28.
7. Bonica, J.J., and Hall, W.M.: Endobronchial anesthesia for intrathoracic surgery. Anesthesiology, 12:344, 1951.
8. Fillenz, M., and Widdicombe, J.G.: Receptors of the lungs and air-ways. In Handbook of Sensory Physiology, Vol. 3/1. Edited by E. Neil. Berlin, Springer-Verlag, 1972, pp. 81–112.
9. Braunwald, E.: Approach to the patient with disease of the respiratory system. In Harrison's Principles of Internal Medicine. 10th Ed. Edited by R. G. Petersdorf et al. New York, McGraw-Hill, 1983, pp. 1498–1500.
10. Levene, D.L. et al. (eds.): Chest Pain: An Integrated Diagnostic Approach. Philadelphia, Lea & Febiger, 1977.
11. Davies, G.M.: The lung in chest pain. In Chest Pain: An Integrated Diagnostic Approach. Edited by D.L. Levene et al. Philadelphia, Lea & Febiger, 1977, pp. 71–87.
12. National Center for Health Statistics: Current Estimates from the National Health Interview Survey: United States 1986. DHHS Publ. No. 87-1592. Hyattsville, MD, National Center for Health Statistics, 1987.
13. National Center for Health Statistics: Health United States 1985. DHHS Publ. No. 81-1232. Hyattsville, MD, National Center for Health Statistics, 1985.
14. Knapp, D.A., and Koch, H.: The management of new pain in office-based ambulatory care: National Ambulatory Medical Care Survey 1980–1981. National Center for Health Statistics Advance Data, 97:1, 1984.
15. Koch, H.: The management of chronic pain in office-based ambulatory care: National Ambulatory Medical Care Survey. National Center for Health Statistics Advance Data, 123:1–12, 1986.
16. Burrows, B.: Acute bronchitis. In The Merck Manual of Diagnosis and Therapy. 15th Ed. Edited by R. Berkow. Rahway, NJ, Merck, Sharp & Dohme Research Laboratories, 1987, pp. 634–636.
17. Murray, J.F.: Bronchiectasis and broncholithiasis. In Harrison's Principles of Internal Medicine. 10th Ed. Edited by R.G. Petersdorf et al. New York, McGraw-Hill, 1983, pp. 1539–1542.
18. Davies, A.L.: Bronchiectasis. In Pulmonary Diseases and Disorders. Edited by A.P. Fishman. New York, McGraw-Hill, 1980, pp. 1209–1219.
19. Davies, A.L.: Bronchiectasis. In The Merck Manual of Diagnosis and Therapy. 15th Ed. Edited by R. Berkow. Rahway, NJ, Merck, Sharp & Dohme Research Laboratories, 1987, pp. 643–646.
20 Teodori, U., and Galletti, R.: Il Dolore Nelle Affezioni Degli Organi Interni Del Torace. Rome, L. Tozzi, 1962, pp. 183–233.
21. Bartlett, J.G.: Pneumonia and lung abscess. In The Merck Manual of Diagnosis and Therapy. 15th Ed. Edited by R. Berkow. Rahway, NJ, Merck, Sharp & Dohme Research Laboraties, 1987, pp. 657–674.
22. Hirschmann, J.V., and Murray, J.F.: Pneumonia and lung abscess. In Harrison's Principles of Internal Medicine. 11th

Ed. Edited by E. Braunwald et al. New York, McGraw-Hill, 1987, pp. 1085–1082.

23. Bonica, J.J.: Principles and Practice of Obstetric Analgesia and Anesthesia. Philadelphia, F.A. Davis, 1967, pp. 673–688.

24. Ross, J., Jr.: Primary pulmonary hypertension. *In* Harrison's Principles of Internal Medicine. 10th Ed. Edited by R.G. Petersdorf et al. New York, McGraw-Hill, 1983, pp. 1559–1561.

25. Grossman, W., Alpert, J.S., and Braunwald, E.: Pulmonary hypertension. *In* Heart Disease: A Textbook of Cardiovascular Medicine. 2nd Ed. Edited by E. Braunwald. Philadelphia, W.B. Saunders, 1984, pp. 823–848.

26. Lupi-Herrera, E. et al.: The role of hydralazine therapy for pulmonary arterial hypertension of unknown cause. Circulation, *65*:645, 1982.

27. Voelkel, N., and Reeves, J.T.: Primary pulmonary hypertension. *In* Pulmonary Vascular Diseases, Vol. 14. Edited by K.M. Moser. New York, Marcel Dekker, 1979, pp. 573–628.

28. Camerini, F. et al.: Primary pulmonary hypertension: The effects of nifedipine. Br. Heart J., *44*:352, 1980.

29. Moser, K.M.: Pulmonary thromboembolism. *In* Harrison's Principles of Internal Medicine. 10th Ed. Edited by R.G. Petersdorf. New York, McGraw-Hill, 1983, pp. 1561–1567.

30. McFadden, E.R., Jr., and Braunwald, E.: Cor pulmonale and pulmonary thromboembolism. *In* Heart Disease: A Textbook of Cardiovascular Medicine. 2nd Ed. Edited by E. Braunwald. Philadelphia, W.B. Saunders, 1984, pp. 1572–1604.

31. Bell, W.R., and Simon, T.L.: Current status of pulmonary thromboembolic disease: Pathophysiology, diagnosis, prevention, and treatment. Am. Heart J., *103*:239, 1983.

32. Freiman, D.G., Suyemoto, J., and Wessler, S.: Frequency of pulmonary thromboembolism in man. N. Engl. J. Med., *272*:1278, 1965.

33. Israel, H.L., and Goldstein, F.: The varied clinical manifestations of pulmonary embolism. Ann. Intern. Med., *47*:202, 1957.

34. McIntyre, K.M., and Levine, H.J.: Cardiac arrest and resuscitation. *In* Emergency Medical Management. Edited by S. Spitzer, W.W. Oaks, and J. Moyer. New York, Grune & Stratton, 1971, p.4.

35. Fishman, A.P.: Pulmonary thromboembolism. Pathophysiology and clinical features. *In* Pulmonary Diseases and Disorders. Edited by A.P. Fishman. New York, McGraw-Hill, 1980, p. 809.

36. Sharma, G.V.R.K. et al: Deep venous thrombosis as a diagnosis clue to pulmonary embolism. Am. J. Cardiol, *33*:170, 1974.

37. Havig, O.: Deep vein thrombosis and pulmonary embolism. Acta Chir. Scand. (Suppl.), *42*:478, 1977.

38. Alexander, J.K.: Pulmonary embolism. *In* The Merck Manual of Diagnosis and Therapy. 15th Ed. Edited by R. Berkow. Rahway, NJ, Merck, Sharp & Dohme Research Laboratories, 1987, pp. 649–657.

39. Modig, J., Malmberg, P., and Karlstrom, G.: Effect of epidural vs. general anesthesia on calf blood flow. Acta Anesthesiol. Scand., *24*:350, 1980.

40. Modig, J.: Thromboembolism and blood loss. Continuous epidural block vs. general anesthesia with controlled ventilation. Reg. Anaesth. *7*:S84, 1982.

41. McIntyre, K.M., and Sasahara, A.A.: Hemodynamic response to pulmonary embolism in patients free of prior cardiopulmonary disease. Am. J. Cardiol., *28*:228, 1971.

42. Brandfonbrenner, M. et al.: Effects of occlusion of one pulmonary artery on pulmonary circulation in man. Fed. Proc., *17*:19, 1958.

43. Halmajay, D.F., Starzecki, B., and Horner, G.J.: Humoral transmission of cardiorespiratory changes in experimental lung embolism. Circ. Res., *14*:546, 1964.

44. Bell, W.R., Simon, T.L., and DeMets, L.L.: The clinical features of submassive and massive pulmonary emboli. Am. J. Med., *62*:335, 1977.

45. Stein, P.D., Willis, P.W., and DeMets, D.L.: History and physical examination in acute pulmonary embolism in patients without preexisting cardiac pulmonary disease. Am. J. Cardiol., *47*:218, 1981.

46. National Cooperative Study. The urokinase-pulmonary embolism trial. Circulation, *47* (Suppl. II):1, 1973.

47. Kakkar, U.V., Corrigan, T.P., and Fossard, D.P.: Prevention of fatal postoperative embolism by low-dose heparin: An international multicenter trial. Lancet, *2*:45, 1975.

48. Evarts, M., and Alfide, J.: Thromboembolism after total hip reconstruction: Failure of low doses of heparin in prevention. JAMA, *225*:515, 1973.

49. O'Sullivan, E.F.: Duration of anticoagulant therapy in venous thromboembolism. Med. J. Aust., *2*:1104, 1972.

50. Alpert, J.S. et al.: Treatment of massive pulmonary embolism: The role of pulmonary embolectomy. Am. Heart J., *89*:413, 1975.

51. Leriche, R., Fontaine, R., and Friedmann, L.: L'infiltration Stellaire est elle Justifiée dans l'embolie Pulmonaire du Point de Vue Physiologique et Anatomo-pathologique? J. Chir., *50*:737, 1937.

52. Widdicombe, J.G.: Reflex mechanisms in pulmonary thromboembolism. *In* Pulmonary Thromboembolism. Edited by K.M. Moser and M. Stein. Chicago, Year Book Medical Publishers, 1973, pp. 178–193.

53. Bonica, J.J.: The Management of Pain. Philadelphia, Lea & Febiger, 1953, pp. 1344–1348.

54. Ingram, R.H., Jr.: Diseases of the pleura, mediastinum, and diaphragm. *In* Harrison's Principles of Internal Medicine. 10th Ed. Edited by R.G. Petersdorf et al. New York, McGraw-Hill, 1983, pp. 1580–1586.

55. Lerner, A.M.: Enteric viruses. *In* Harrison's Principles of Internal Medicine. 10th Ed. Edited by R.G. Petersdorf et al. New York, McGraw-Hill, 1983, pp. 1125–1132.

56. Bain, H.W. et al.: Epidemic pleurodynia (Bornholm's disease) due to coxsackie B5 virus: The interrelationship of pleurodynia, benign pericarditis and aspectic meningitis. Pediatrics, *27*:889, 1961.

57. Snider, G.L.: Pleural disorders; pneumothorax. *In* The Merck Manual of Diagnosis and Therapy. 15th Ed. Edited by R. Berkow. Rahway, NJ, Merck, Sharp & Dohme Research Laboratories, 1987, pp. 703–705.

56 · CHEST PAIN OF ESOPHAGEAL ORIGIN

CHARLES POPE *and* JOHN J. BONICA

ALTHOUGH the esophagus normally transports solids and liquids to the stomach without pain or discomfort, it can develop discomfort that is clearly of esophageal origin as well as pain that is indistinguishable from the chest pain of myocardial ischemia. Because of the fear of coronary artery disease, such pain can lead to anxiety, multiple workups, and expensive hospitalizations. Failure to consider the esophagus as a potential source of chest pain can lead to repeat hospitalization and unnecessary invasive diagnostic procedures.

Pain of esophageal origin is not uncommon; in one study, it accounted for the pain in as many as 20% of an unselected group of patients evaluated for chest pain at a local hospital (1). Tibbling (2) conducted a survey of the frequency of esophageal disorders and angina pectoris among an urban Swedish male and female population selected at random. She reported that the frequency of esophageal disorders was 5.7% among those who were 25 years old and 30% among those who were 55 years old. The frequency of angina pectoris using the Rose questionnaire (3) (employed in field surveys to diagnose ischemic heart disease) was 5% and 13%, respectively, for the two ages. When a cardiologist took the history among the group of 55-year-olds with angina pectoris (according to the questionnaire), he found definite angina in 4.2%, suspected angina in 4.2%, and no angina in 5.5%. Thus, correct diagnosis of chest pain of esophageal origin not only reassures the patient but allows proper therapy to be undertaken.

Two main types of disorders generate pain in the esophagus: disorders of the esophageal mucosa via diverse processes, and failure of coordinated muscular function (motor disorders). The factors that produce mucosal disease are usually easily identified, whereas esophageal pain of muscular origin is both hard to identify and to understand. In this chapter disease processes involving the mucosa and the esophageal muscle are discussed separately. Mucosal disease can be either acute or chronic, whereas problems involving the muscle tend to produce pain that often persists for months or years. Some etiologic factors in these two types of disorders are discussed, although it should be recognized that many of the factors that produce esophageal pain remain unknown. Diagnostic tools are reviewed with an understanding that some of the tests are specific but not very sensitive in establishing pain of esophageal origin. Correct diagnosis is often essential in choosing optional therapeutic maneuvers. Some forms of esophageal pain respond promptly to therapy; others remain extremely recalcitrant.

The information is presented in five sections: A, basic considerations including the anatomy and physiology of the esophagus; B, esophageal mucosal disorders; C, esophageal motor disorders; D, cancer of the esophagus; and E, other painful disorders of the esophagus. More detailed information can be found in reports by Pope (4–6), Brand (7), and the monograph by Areskog and Tibbling (8).

A. BASIC CONSIDERATIONS

Anatomy of the Esophagus

General Structure

The esophagus is a tube consisting of striated muscle in the upper one-third and smooth muscle in the remainder of the organ. It is approximately 30 to 35 cm long, 3.0 cm in lateral diameter, and 1.9 cm in anterior-posterior diameter (Fig. 56-1). It begins at the cricopharyngeus muscle, which effectively separates the lumen of the esophagus from that of the hypopharynx. It passes through the mediastinum, traverses the hiatus of the diaphragm, and ends in the lower esophageal sphincter muscle, which separates the esophageal lumen from the gastric lumen. Careful dissections in human cadavers show a thickening of the circular, but not the longitudinal, muscle in the lower esophageal sphincter zone as well as an unusual distribution of the circular muscle fibers. The esophagus is lined with stratified squamous epithelium, which is lubricated by specialized mucous glands located in the submucosal layer. The esophagus contains no serosal layer, which accounts for difficulties encountered by surgeons making anastomoses in the esophagus.

Blood Supply

The arterial supply to the cervical esophagus comes from the terminal branches of the inferior thyroid artery. The thoracic portion is supplied by branches of the thoracic aorta and from the bronchial arteries. The lowest portion of the thoracic and the abdominal part of the esophagus receives its arterial supply from the left gastric branch of the celiac artery and from the inferior phrenic branch of the abdominal aorta (Fig. 56-1).

The venous drainage of the cervical esophagus is into the inferior thyroid vein, which empties into the brachiocephalic veins. The thoracic esophagus is drained through the periesophageal plexus, which empties into the azygos system. The lowest part of the thoracic and the abdominal esophagus drains into the gastric veins which, in turn, empty into the portal vein.

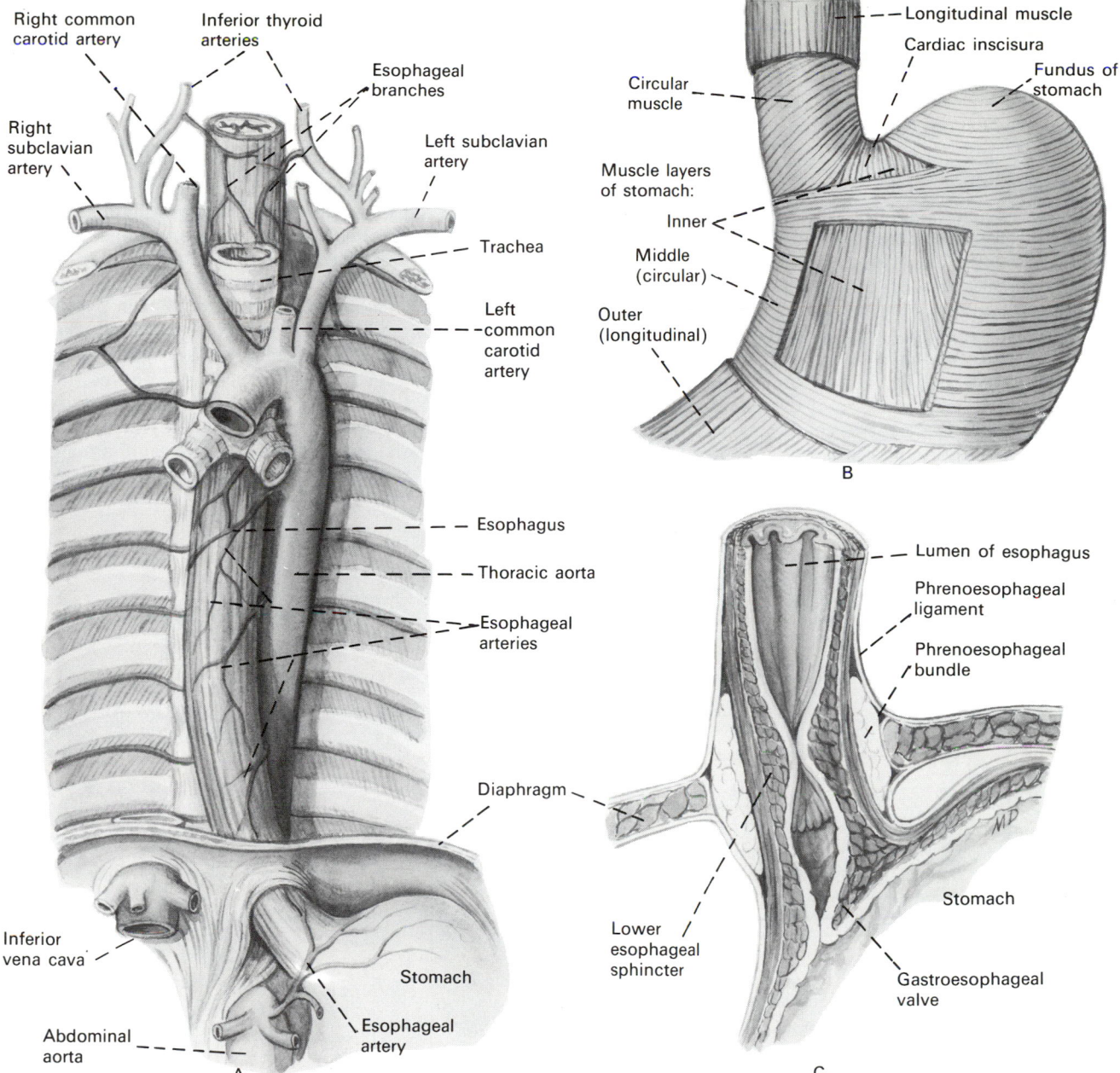

FIG. 56-1. Anatomy of the esophagus. **A.** Relationship of the esophagus (except the uppermost part which has been resected) to the lower trachea, the proximal bronchi, and the aorta and its arterial blood supply. **B.** Lower esophagus and upper stomach showing the direction of the longitudinal and circular muscle fibers of the lower esophagus and the upper part of the stomach. **C.** Coronal section depicting the component parts of the gastroesophageal junction and the component parts of the antireflux barrier including the lower esophageal sphincter (LES) made up of thick circular musculature. The phrenoesophageal ligament arises from the circumference of the hiatus as an extension of the inferior fascia of the diaphragm and breaks up into an ascending and descending leaf; the former passes cephalad for several centimeters above the hiatus where it is inserted circumferentially into the adventitia of the esophagus, while the descending leaf passes downward and is inserted around the cardia deep to the peritoneum. Within the cavity, thus formed by the phrenoesophageal ligament and below the diaphragmatic hiatus, lies a ring of dense fibroareolar and fatty tissue which together with the ligament make up the phrenoesophageal bundle. Also the gastroesophageal valve is created by the acute angle of His and consists of a flat lateral leaf approximating against the mucosa of the lesser curvature of the stomach. *A* and *B* modified from Netter, F.H.: The CIBA Collection of Medical Illustrations. Vol. 3: Digestive System: Part I, Upper Digestive Tract. Caldwell, NJ, CIBA Pharmaceutical Co., 1959, pp. 38–41. *C* was developed from data in Hill, L.D., Thor, K., and Mercer, D.: Surgery for hiatal hernia and esophagitis. *In* The Esophagus: Medical and Surgical Management. Edited by L.D. Hill. Philadelphia, W.B. Saunders, 1988, p. 98.

Nerve Supply

The esophagus is supplied by sympathetic nerves and the vagus nerves, which contain both afferents and efferents and which convey impulses to and from the mucous coat, glands, blood vessels, and the smooth and striated muscles of this viscus. The following information is derived from the first edition of this book (9) and from the works by Kuntz (10) and Netter (11).

Vagus Nerves

The vagus nerves supply general visceral efferents, visceral afferents, and somatic efferents to the esophagus (Fig. 56-2). The general visceral efferents are parasympathetic fibers, arising from cell bodies in the dorsal nucleus of the vagus, whose axons pass peripherally to supply the nonstriated muscle and glands of the esophagus (10, 11). Visceral afferent fibers arise from cell bodies in the superior (jugular) and inferior (nodose) ganglia of the vagus whose proximal axons end in the tractus solitarius, while the distal axons supply the mucous membrane of the esophagus. The somatic efferent fibers arise from cell bodies in the nucleus ambiguus and supply the striated muscles of the pharynx and the upper part of the esophagus. From the neck down, the branches of the vagus nerves communicate with sympathetic fibers derived from the paravertebral sympathetic chain to form dense plexuses.

In the neck, the esophagus receives fibers from the recurrent laryngeal nerve, which passes cephalad on each side in a groove between the esophagus and the trachea and gives parallel branches that enter the wall of the cervical portion of the esophagus. In general, these branches neither cross the median plane nor enter a plexus formation (10). The cervical portion of the esophagus also receives (inconstant) branches directly from the vagus. In the thorax, the part of the esophagus in the superior mediastinum receives filaments from the left recurrent laryngeal nerve and from both vagus nerves. Both vagus nerves descend posterior to the roots of the lung and below these structures they break up into two to four branches, which become closely opposed to the esophagus in the posterior mediastinum (11). The branches from the

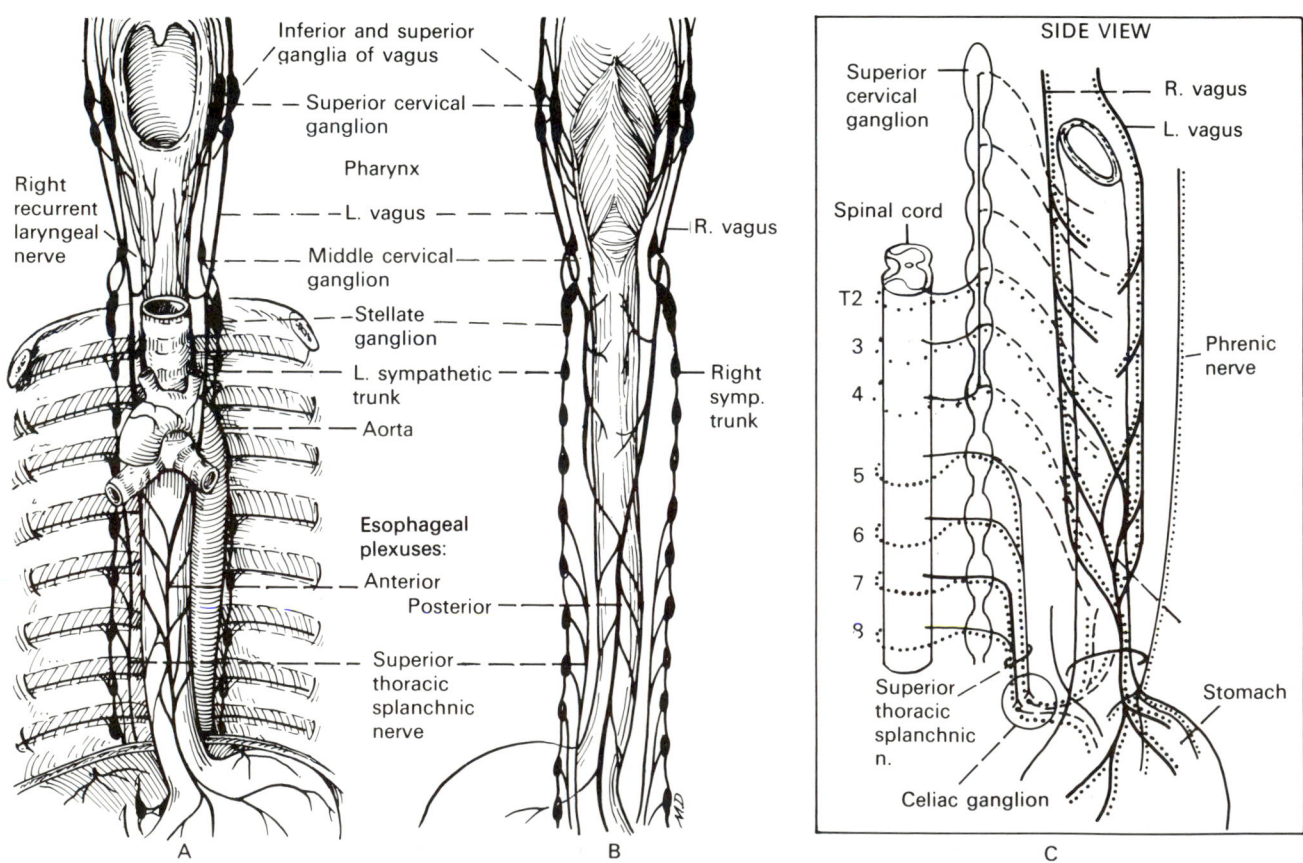

FIG. 56-2. Nerve supply of the esophagus. **A.** Anterior view showing the relationship of the esophagus posterior to the larynx, trachea, beginning of the main bronchi, and aorta. Note the transition from the thoracic to the abdominal aorta through the esophageal hiatus. The nerve supply is provided by the vagus, the paravertegral sympathetic chain, and the phrenic nerve. **B.** Posterior view of the esophagus showing the relationship of the vagus nerve and the sympathetic trunks. **C.** Schematic illustration of a side view of the esophagus showing the nerve supply. The solid lines in the vagus and the sympathetic system indicate preganglionic fibers; the dashed lines in the sympathetic system indicate postganglionic fibers; and the dotted lines indicate sensory nerve supply. Note that the dotted lines indicating pathways from T2–T4 are staggered to suggest that these may be uncertain. On the right side is the phrenic nerve, which ends in the inferior surface of the diaphragm as the phrenic plexus; this probably contributes sensation to the lower esophagus and part of the stomach. Modified from Netter, F.H.: The CIBA Collection of Medical Illustrations. Vol. 3: Digestive System; Part I, Upper Digestive Tract. Caldwell, NJ, CIBA Pharmaceutical Co., 1959.

right vagus incline posteriorly and those from the left vagus anteriorly (Fig. 56-2). These branches divide and reunite to form an open-meshed esophageal plexus containing small ganglia. At a variable distance above the esophageal hiatus in the diaphragm, the meshes of the esophageal plexuses become reconstituted into one or, less often, two or more vagal trunks, which are located anterior and posterior to the lowest part of the esophagus, lying on the surface or partially embedded in its wall (10). Offshoots from the esophageal plexus and from the anterior and posterior vagal nerve trunks sink into the esophageal wall. Within the wall, the parasympathetic preganglionic fibers synapse with cell bodies of the short postganglionic neurons; the afferent fibers pass through the muscular wall to end in the submucosa and mucosa of the esophagus.

Sympathetic Nerve Supply

The sympathetic supply to the esophagus originates in the intermediolateral column of the spinal cord where the cell bodies of preganglionic neurons are located in spinal segments T2 to T8 (Fig. 56-2C). The axons of these fibers pass from the spinal cord through the anterior nerve roots of the analogous spinal nerves and thence pass as the white rami communicantes to reach the paravertebral sympathetic chain.

As noted in Table 6-6 and Figure 56-2, those sympathetic fibers destined to supply the cervical portion of the esophagus originate in spinal cord segments T2 to T4 and, after reaching the paravertebral chain, ascend and synapse with postganglionic fibers in all of the cervical sympathetic ganglia. Postganglionic fibers pass to contribute to the pharyngeal plexus and also join the recurrent laryngeal nerve to supply the uppermost part of the esophagus.

The thoracic portion of the esophagus (except the lowermost part) receives sympathetic fibers that originate in spinal cord segments T3 to T6. After passing to the sympathetic chain, they ascend to the stellate and the uppermost thoracic sympathetic ganglia where they synapse with postganglionic neurons. Some of the axons of postganglionic neurons pass directly from the stellate ganglia or ansae subclaviae to the esophagus, others pass via the thoracic cardiac nerves, and still others pass directly from the sympathetic chain to the esophagus.

The sympathetic fibers that supply the lowermost thoracic and the abdominal portion of the esophagus originate in T5 to T8 (and often T9) spinal segments; after passing through the sympathetic chain, they become part of the superior thoracic (greater) splanchnic nerves and synapse in the celiac ganglia. Postganglionic fibers become part of the plexuses that surround the left gastric and inferior phrenic arteries and pass to supply the lowermost part of the thoracic and the abdominal portion of the esophagus.

Sensory Nerves

Sensory nerves that supply the esophagus are derived from afferents associated with both the vagus and sympathetic nerves. The cervical and upper thoracic parts of the esophagus are primarily supplied by afferents associated with the vagus, although there is some evidence that afferents associated with the sym-

pathetics contribute to transmission of nociceptive information from these parts of the esophagus. The lower part of the thoracic esophagus and the abdominal esophagus are supplied by afferents that accompany primarily the sympathetic nerves, although those that accompany the vagus nerve may also be involved. The abdominal portion of the esophagus also receives afferent fibers from the phrenic plexuses that lie on the inferior surface of the diaphragm. These phrenic afferent fibers enter the spinal cord at C3, C4, and C5. The endings of all the phrenic afferent fibers supply and penetrate the muscular coats and also supply the submucosa and mucosa.

Intrinsic Innervation

The esophagus, like the rest of the gastrointestinal tract, contains intrinsic innervation effected through enteric plexuses. These are composed of numerous groups of ganglion cells interconnected by a network of fibers, which lie between the layers of the muscular coats (Auerbach's plexus) and in the submucosa (Meissner's plexus). These enteric plexuses contain postganglionic sympathetic and pre- and postganglionic parasympathetic fibers, afferent fibers, and the intrinsic ganglia cells and their processes. The afferent fibers from the esophagus (as well as the stomach and duodenum) are carried to the brain stem and spinal cord through the vagal and sympathetic nerves supplying these parts, but they form no synaptic connection with the ganglion cells in the enteric plexuses (10).

Sites of Pain Reference

As with pain in other viscera, the pain due to diseases of the esophagus is referred to the parietes, primarily in the front but also in the back, depending on the site and type of the noxious stimuli. During the past eight decades, numerous investigators have attempted to determine the area of pain reference by mechanical distension of the esophagus with a balloon or by electrical or chemical stimulation. Jones (12) carried out one of the more extensive studies in 29 normal subjects in which he distended the esophagus at different levels. He noted that moderate distension produced substernal pain experienced at the level of the balloon (Fig. 56-3). Thus, pain arising from the upper esophagus was felt in the midline over the upper portion of the manubrium, while that produced at the cardiac end of the esophagus was felt at the level of the xiphoid cartilage. The same observations had been previously reported by Payne and Poulton (13), who suggested that pain is due to distension and deformation of nerve endings in the esophageal wall. They noted that pain was diminished by peristaltic contraction that reduced the distension, whereas if the peristaltic wave did not relieve the contraction, the pain became worse, resulting in severe paroxysmal cramping pain.

Teodori and Galletti (14), in studies using an esophageal balloon, determined not only the site of pain but also electric skin resistance. They reported that rapid inflation of the balloon with 30 to 50 ml of air produced moderate to severe pain, the site of which

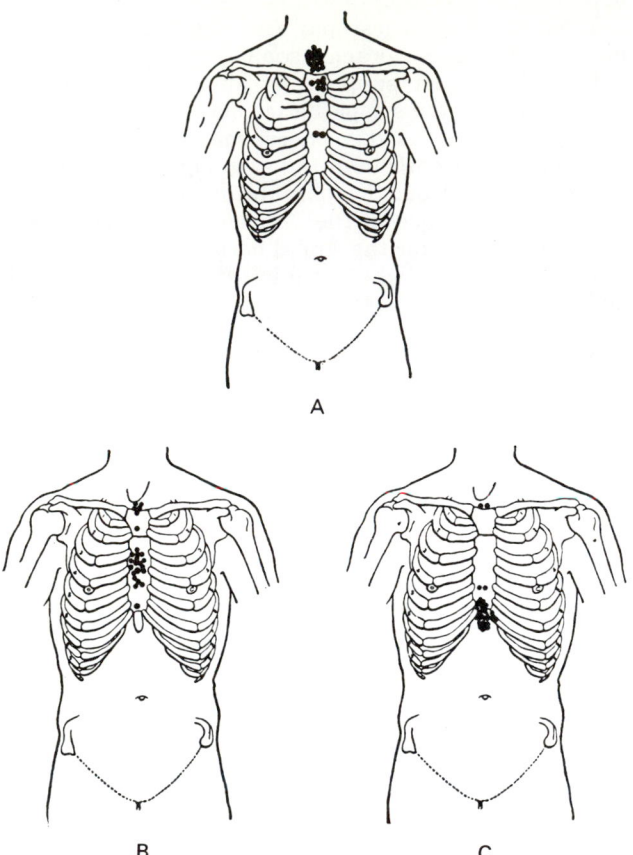

Fig. 56-3. Sites of referred pain from inflation of a balloon in the upper (**A**), middle (**B**), and lower (**C**) esophagus. Each dot represents one subject. Compare with Figures 56-4 and 56-6. From Jones, C.M.: Digestive Tract Pain. New York, Macmillan, 1938, p. 11.

depended on the level of the distension. Distension in the upper third of the esophagus produced pain referred to the area of the manubrium and upper part of the sternum without producing any pain in the back. In contrast, stimulation of the lower third of the esophagus produced pain in the xiphoid process and the epigastric area and posteriorly in the midline at

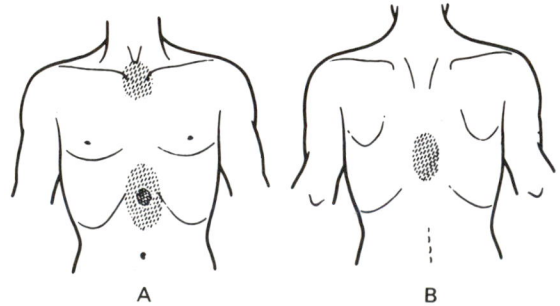

Fig. 56-4. A. Anterior view showing reference of pain caused by inflation of the upper third and lower third of the esophagus. **B.** Posterior view showing reference of pain in the back from mechanical stimulation of the lower esophagus. From Teodori, U., and Galletti, R.: Il Dolore Nelle Affezioni Degli Organi Interni del Torace. Rome, L. Pozzi, 1962, pp. 169–178.

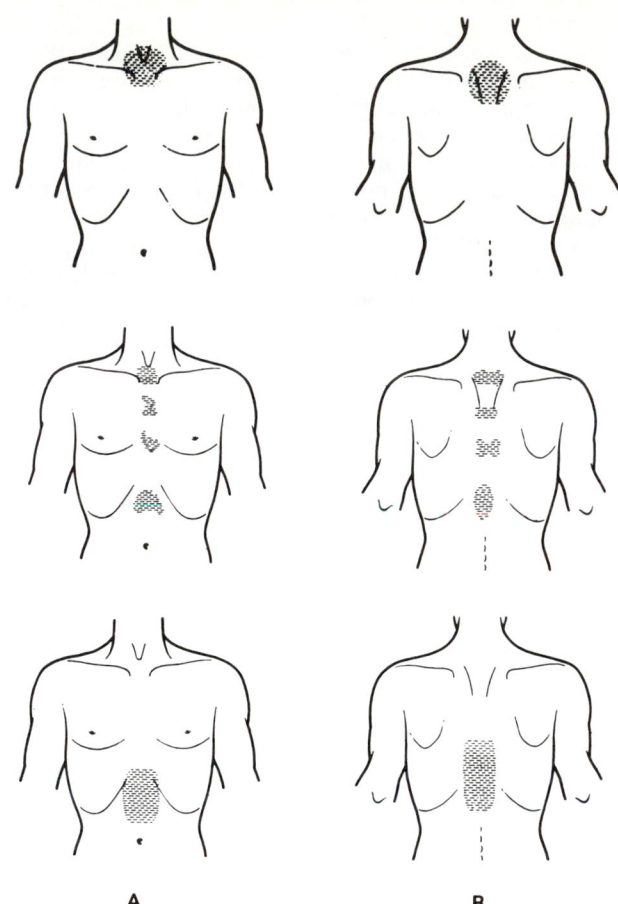

Fig. 56-5. Zones in which there was a reduction in the cutaneous electrical resistance (RCER) consequent to mechanical stimulation of the esophagus with an inflated balloon that produced pain in the anterior (**A**) and posterior (**B**) portion of the chest. The top panel shows the areas of RCER from stimulation of the upper third of the esophagus. Posteriorly the area of the pain overlies the midline and paravertebral region at the level of the 7th cervical to the 1st thoracic vertebrae inclusive. The middle panel shows the area of RCER from stimulation of the middle third of the esophagus. Note the variability. The bottom panel shows the area of RCER from stimulation of the lower third of the esophagus. Posteriorly this area overlies the paravertebral region at the level of the 6th to the 11th thoracic vertebrae. From Teodori, U., and Galletti, R.: Il Dolore Nelle Affezioni Degli Organi Interni del Torace. Rome, L. Pozzi, 1962, pp. 169–178.

the level of the 6th to 7th thoracic vertebrae (Fig. 56-4). They noted that referred pain produced by stimulation of the middle third of the esophagus usually was less intense and more variable in location. In some subjects the pain was felt in both the manubrium and xiphoid process, in others in one or the other, and in still others in the retrosternal region. Interestingly, the areas of decreased electric resistance were consistently in approximately the same sites as the areas of referred pain (Fig. 56-5). Cutaneous hyperalgesia developed in most subjects in the epigastric region and in the skin overlying the lower portion of the sternocleidomastoid muscles bilaterally.

Physiology of the Esophagus

The action of the upper esophageal sphincter (cricopharyngeus and some circular esophageal muscles) is closely correlated with the constrictor muscles of the pharynx and is under direct nerve control of cranial nerves IX and X through the pharyngeal plexus and the external laryngeal and recurrent laryngeal nerves. The upper esophageal sphincter (UES) relaxes as the bolus is propelled toward it by the tongue and the pharyngeal muscles, and then it closes immediately after passage. A stripping wave originates at the UES and travels down the esophagus at a velocity of 3 to 4 cm/s. A luminal pressure of 80 to 130 mm Hg is developed by the circular muscle during peristalsis, and the wave lasts 4 to 6 seconds.

The lower esophageal sphincter (LES) usually develops a normal intraluminal pressure of 15 to 30 mm Hg. This pressure falls to the gastric level on initiation of deglutition and remains low until the peristaltic wave reaches the region, whereupon the elevated resting pressure is restored. The LES and other components make up the gastroesophageal (GE) junction, which is a highly efficient and complex mechanism that allows for swallowing of a bolus and yet maintains a resting pressure that prevents reflux of gastric contents. The GE junction distinguishes between gas and liquid, permits belching and vomiting, and prevents continuous bathing of the esophageal mucosa by gastric juice. When reflux, belching, or vomiting occurs in normal individuals, the esophagus clears the gastric juice rapidly and efficiently. Disturbance in the body of the esophagus or impairment of the function of the LES and other components, which normally act as the "antireflux barrier," leads to heartburn, chest pain, and other symptoms discussed in the sections that follow.

B. ESOPHAGEAL MUCOSAL DISORDERS

The most common cause of chest pain due to disorders of the esophageal mucosa is GE reflux. Other causes of chest pain include infectious and systemic disease, physical agents, and trauma. Most of the following discussion is devoted to GE reflux. This is followed by brief sections on the other causes of chest pain due to mucosal disorders.

Gastroesophageal Reflux Disease (XIX-5)

Etiology and Pathophysiology

The most common mucosal disorder leading to chest pain results from reflux of gastric and duodenal contents (gastroesophageal reflux disease, GERD). Some esophageal reflux is present in all persons, but when the mucosa is exposed to a strong concentration of gastric acid and pepsin or to a combination of gastric acid and bile salts for a sufficiently long time, histologic changes of the esophagus occur and pain can result. The squamous epithelium of the esophagus affected by reflux shows an increased number of basal cells and elongation of the dermal pegs (15). In addition, there are increased spaces between the basal cells of the mucosa. These changes can be demonstrated in patients shown to have reflux and symptoms whose mucosa appears grossly normal to the endoscopist.

More severe forms of esophageal damage due to refluxed material lead to microulcers. These are very thin, shallow ulcers, which usually occur on top of the esophageal folds and usually cannot be demonstrated by normal radiographic techniques. Finally, in a very few subjects, severe reflux leads to a penetrating deep esophageal ulcer, which is easily seen radiologically and is often associated with severe constant esophageal pain.

Numerous factors can lead to prolonged reflux and subsequent esophageal damage. The lower esophageal sphincter, a specialized bundle of muscle between the esophagus and stomach, can have poor intrinsic tone or relax inappropriately, allowing gastric contents to reach the esophagus. Cigarette smoking, use of alcohol, obesity, and pregnancy all can lead to or intensify reflux and esophageal damage (16, 17). Further information on GE reflux is presented in a review by Richter and Castell (18).

Once the mucosa has been breached by reflux disease or trauma, pain can be caused by inflammation and by increased permeability of the mucosa, which permits luminal contents to reach the underlying lamina propria and nerve endings. When hyperosmotic solutions such as fruit juices are imbibed, burning or discomfort can result. Most of the esophageal pain and distress caused by mucosal disease is not accompanied by esophageal motor abnormalities, although a transition from a normal motor pattern to an abnormal one during reflux associated with pain has occasionally been noted.

Symptoms and Signs

The most common from of discomfort produced by mucosal irritation is *heartburn*. Most patients describe the discomfort as "burning," "heat," or "hot feeling," although some use the same terms as those suffering from esophageal motor disorders or coronary artery disease. The heartburn is diffuse, extending from the substernal notch to the epigastrium (Fig. 56-6). The heartburn is usually relieved, albeit transiently, by ingestion of antacids. Angina-like pain from mucosal irritation usually responds less readily to antacids (19).

Several other types of chest pain of esophageal mucosal origin can be distinguished. When the discomfort is related to bolus ingestion, the discomfort is termed *odynophagia*. Odynophagia occurs only during the passage of a bolus, usually a solid one, down the esophagus. It is more common when the mucosa is

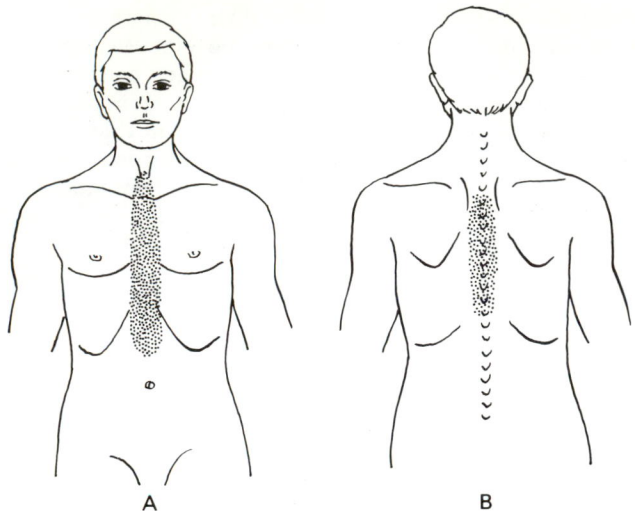

FIG. 56-6. Anterior (*A*) and posterior (*B*) sites of pain of esophageal mucosal origin. The patient experiences retrosternal pain extending from the suprasternal notch to the epigastrium, which has a burning, stabbing quality. Compare with Figures 56-3 and 56-4. The more extensive pattern of the pain in patients with GE reflux suggests that nociceptive input is coming from the mucosa of the entire esophagus.

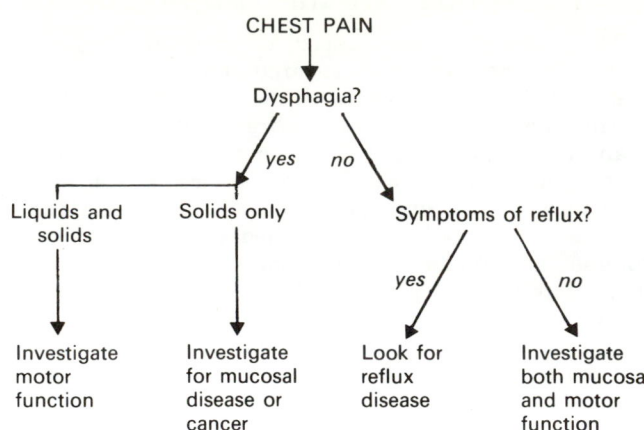

FIG. 56-7. Flow chart for diagnosis of chest pain of esophageal origin.

affected by a viral infection or a burn due to a retained tablet than in GERD. A very mild variant of odynophagia may occur in patients with GERD, but this is not necessarily perceived as pain. In this stituation, the patient is aware of the location of a bolus as it moves down the esophagus, although the bolus does not necessarily hesitate or stick on the way down the esophagus. Other symptoms that accompany mucosal disorders are regurgitation of acid or bile into the pharynx and even the mouth on bending or at night, and laryngeal stridor when refluxed material irritates the vocal cords.

Another point to determine is whether *dysphagia* is present. Although dysphagia does not necessarily occur at the time of chest pain, many patients with dysphagia have pain of esophageal origin. It is often necessary to pursue the possibility of dysphagia with some diligence. Words such as "does the food stick, hesitate, or pause" must be used in addition to merely asking patients whether they have trouble swallowing. Many patients consider mild dysphagia to be a normal phenomenon, or they assume they have simply eaten too large a bolus. When dysphagia is present, however, the physician should focus increased diagnostic emphasis on the esophagus, as this condition is common in both mucosal disease and motor disorders of the esophagus.

Diagnosis

A flow chart for diagnostic investigation of chest pain of esophageal origin is presented in Figure 56-7. First, the physician should determine whether the mucosa of the esophagus is sensitive, thus producing esophageal pain. If dysphagia is not present and if the patient has suffered regurgitation of gastric contents, then it is likely that the mucosa is involved and its acid sensitivity should be investigated. Conversely, if

dysphagia, especially for liquids as well as solids, is a prominent part of the history, then the initial investigations might be directed at the function of the esophageal muscle. Important characteristics that help in the differential diagnosis of these two esophageal conditions and other causes of chest pain are listed in Table 56-1.

MUCOSAL SENSITIVITY. The most effective way to demonstrate whether chest pain is coming from the esophageal mucosa is to determine the effect of contact of the mucosa with a stimulating agent, which can be either the patient's own refluxed juice or an exogenous stimulus.

Endogenous stimulation is determined by short-term or long-term pH monitoring. In this technique, an indwelling pH probe records bursts of reflux. If the patient's pain occurs soon after an episode of reflux is recorded, then the conclusion is that the chest pain is due to mucosal sensitivity to refluxed material. At the present time, prolonged pH monitoring is not available to most patients in the United States. Development of practical systems for long-term pH monitoring would allow many more patients to be observed during their ordinary working activity and during events in their life that are associated with pain. Although long-term pH monitoring is in its infancy, this technique promises to be quite useful in the differential diagnosis of chest pain (20).

If short-term or long-term pH-monitoring facilities are not available, the acid perfusion test (21) can be used to determine whether chest pain is of esophageal origin. This relatively simple test, which involves placing a nasogastric tube high in the esophagus and then first dripping in saline and then 0.1 N hydrochloric acid, can be performed in any physician's office. Although 0.1 N hydrochloric acid is used for convenience, sensitive mucosa will respond to other solutions such as bile salts or even materials of high osmotic activity. If the patient's symptoms occur readily during the acid perfusion and vanish relatively rapidly after perfusion with saline, then an esophageal origin of the pain is likely. Some workers

TABLE 56-1. Differential Diagnosis of Chest Pain

| Disorder | Characteristics of Pain | | | Aggravating Factors | Associated Symptoms | Special Diagnostic Tests |
	Intensity	Distribution (Radiation)	Duration			
Esophageal mucosa	Mild to severe	Substernal; radiates to epigastrium, neck, and back, rarely to arms	10 sec to many hours	Exercise Citrus juices Stooping or lifting Recumbency	Dysphagia Regurgitation Aspiration	pH monitoring Acid perfusion Esophagoscopy Response to antacids
Esophageal motor disorders	Mild to severe	Substernal; radiates to epigastrium, back, neck, jaw, teeth, left arm, or both arms	10 sec to many hours	Cold liquids Emotional stress (??)	Dysphagia	Manometry Scintigraphy Provocation tests
Esophageal cancer	Moderate to severe	Substernal; radiates to epigastrium, neck, interscapular region	Constant	Food ingestion	Dysphagia Weight loss Esophageal obstruction	Radiography Esophagoscopy CT scan
Coronary artery disease	Mild to severe	Substernal, jaw, neck, teeth, arm(s)	5 sec to 5 min	Exercise Emotion Cold exposure	Congestive heart failure	ECG Stress test Thallium scan Coronary angiography Ergonovine stimulation
Thoracic outlet syndrome	Mild to severe	Substernal; radiates always to affected arm	5 min to hours	Lifting suitcases Driving a car Use of arms overhead	None	Adson's maneuver Nerve conduction velocities
Thoracic spine disease	Mild to moderate	Substernal; radiates to back	5 min to hours	Twisting Poor posture	None	Pressure over T4 or T5 spinous process
Pancreatic biliary disease	Mild to severe	Subxiphoid, interscapular	30 min to hours	Eating Alcohol	Jaundice Nausea and vomiting	Ultrasound ERCP*
Pulmonary diseases (embolism pleurisy cancer)	Moderate to severe	Substernal; left or right chest	5 min to constant	Breathing	Hemoptysis Weight loss Pleurisy	Chest film Bronchoscopy V/Q scan

*Endoscopic retrograde cholangiopancreatography.

have disputed the sensitivity and specificity of this examination, but it is the best technique presently available to demonstrate mucosal sensitivity.

Interpreting the results of the acid perfusion test is not always easy. Some patients with both chest pain and heartburn will develop heartburn during the test, but not necessarily chest pain. Even when acid perfusion is continued to the point that heartburn becomes very uncomfortable, chest pain is not often produced. Another problem in interpretation of this test is the production of a different set of symptoms. Although this may be interesting, it should be scored as an indeterminate test. Only onset during perfusion of the symptoms that are troubling the patient should be rated as a positive test.

In a series of patients undergoing antireflux operations and complaining of chest pain, acid perfusion reproduced the pain in over 90% (19). Although many of these patients complained of radiation of pain to the back, arms, or ears, acid perfusion was less successful in reproducing these components of the pain syndrome. In a series of nonsurgical patients being evaluated for chest pain, acid reproduction of the pain occurred in only 10% (22).

DIRECT EVALUATION. Direct evaluation of the state of the mucosa by radiography or endoscopy is of little benefit. Radiographic investigation of the mucosa, even with double-contrast studies, is not sensitive enough to pick up mucosal erosions. Endoscopy of patients with mucosal disease often shows a normal-appearing mucosa, which is interpreted as uninvolved (even though the mucosa is in fact acid sensitive), or reveals erosions that are present but are not, in fact, the cause of chest pain. Other items that can be demonstrated by endoscopy or by radiographic studies such as the presence or absence of reflux or hiatal herniation are much less important in the evaluation of chest pain. Demonstration of hiatal herniation, for instance, does not establish the esophagus or hiatal hernia as the cause of chest pain. Grave clinical mistakes can be made if a surgical approach is taken against a hiatal hernia in a patient with chest pain when in fact the hernia is not the cause of the pain.

If the clinical history points to a specific cause of pain, then endoscopy might be a useful diagnostic procedure. One might see a circumscribed ulcer with an alarming-looking necrotic base. Fungal stains of biopsies and scrapings from this area will be negative.

Both physician and patient can be assured that such a lesion will heal without scarring.

Treatment

As is true in most other areas in medicine, specific diagnosis of chest pain of esophageal origin aids in the selection of treatment. Unfortunately, as emphasized in the last section, this diagnosis sometimes is extremely difficult to make, and occasionally a therapeutic trial must be instituted not only to confirm the diagnosis but also to aid the patient to cope with chest pain. Nonspecific therapy, of course, can also be given if specific therapy is not effective.

REMOVAL OF CAUSE OF PAIN. When the cause of pain is due to mucosal sensitivity, efforts should be made to strengthen the mucosa so it will no longer be sensitive. The most common situation involves the treatment of esophageal reflux. Table 56-2 lists the currently accepted methods for treating this condition. The first line of attack is to decrease nocturnal reflux by elevating the patient's head. This is best done by placing 6- to 8-in. blocks under the legs at the head of the bed. Elevation of the head with pillows is not as effective, as there is a tendency for the patient to roll off the pillows during the night. Elevation decreases the exposure time of the esophageal mucosa to reflux material (23). Other prophylactic measures include avoidance of citrus fruit juices, reduction of fat in the diet, and strict avoidance of alcohol and smoking; both alcohol and smoking have been shown to decrease LES pressure. Weight loss of as little as 10 lb can relieve all symptoms in some patients. Although many patients find these recommendations difficult to follow, they should be encouraged to comply because these measures often reduce or eliminate symptoms.

For compliant patients in whom these prophylactic measures prove ineffective, active pharmacologic therapy, also listed in Table 56-2, is used. Antacids are useful for intermittent attacks of heartburn. Since these agents leave the stomach rapidly, hourly ingestion is mandatory for intensive therapy. Agents used for this purpose include liquid aluminum hydroxide–magnesium hydroxide and proprietary tablets containing calcium carbonate, dihydroxyaluminum sodium carbonate, or sodium bicarbonate. Both cimetidine (Tagamet) and ranitidine (Zantac) are histamine H2-receptor antagonists and thus decrease both daytime and nocturnal basal acid secretions and secretions stimulated by food (24). Both agents can be effective when ordinary antacids are not.

TABLE 56-2. Treatment of Esophageal Reflux

Prophylactic Therapy	Pharmacologic Therapy
Elevation of head of bed by 6–8 inches No bedtime snacks Cessation of alcohol and smoking	Antacid Therapy Antacids: 30 ml q3h pc and hs Cimetidine: 300 mq qid Ranitidine: 150 mg bid Drugs to Strengthen LES Bethanechol: 10–25 mg qid Metoclopramide: 10 mg qid

Two drugs have been used to strengthen the LES pharmacologically. Farrell et al. (25) reported that bethanechol (Urecholine), a cholinergic agent, increased LES pressure in both normal subjects and those with reflux and significantly reduced both reflux symptoms and antacid use (25). In our experience, however, this drug helps some, but not all, persons with reflux symptoms. Metoclopramide (Reglan) stimulates smooth muscle contraction and has been shown to strengthen the LES, increase LES pressure, decrease pH probe–proven reflux after a protein meal, and reduce the symptoms of reflux (26, 27). For maximum benefit with pharmacologic therapy, the patient should be under the care of a gastroenterologist with special interest and experience in management of reflux esophagitis.

The pharmacologic treatment of chest pain due to reflux is difficult. Nevertheless, in spite of our clinical impression that medical therapy is not as effective in chest pain of esophageal origin as desired, it is uncommon for us to recommend antireflux surgery solely on the basis of chest pain.

NONSPECIFIC CONTROL OF PAIN. Occasionally, just the interest of the physician in the patient and the demonstration by manometry or other techniques that there is an esophageal cause of chest pain can be beneficial. For patients who have been told that they have a life-threatening illness (myocardial ischemia), knowledge that their chest pain is not associated with the possibility of sudden death often is reassuring and allows them to undergo discomfort even though specific therapeutic efforts may not relieve their symptoms.

Patients svverely compromised by esophageal pain present the physician with a serious dilemma. Most physicians are quite correctly reluctant to embark on long-term use of narcotics to control esophageal pain, but for intermittent episodes of pain that do not respond to therapeutic modalities, the use of morphine or meperidine (Demerol) can be of benefit. One always has to be concerned about the possibility of having the patient develop physical dependence or psychologic dependence (addiction). Generally, efforts should be made to identify the specific cause of esophageal pain and then to correct this if possible.

Infections, Systemic Disease, and Chemical Injuries (XIX-4)

Etiology and Pathophysiology

The mucosa of the esophagus can be damaged by infections, certain systemic illnesses, and some chemical agents. Any of these can produce heartburn or other forms of chest pain, odynophagia, and dysphagia.

INFECTIONS. Infectious agents such as Candida albicans (28), herpes simplex virus (29), and cytomegalic virus can affect not only immunocompromised hosts but also normal individuals. Factors that allow colonization of these pathogens are not well understood. They tend to produce acute self-limited illnesses which include esophagitis with very striking clinical manifestations.

SYSTEMIC DISEASE. Several systemic disorders also produce esophagitis with consequent odynophagia, dysphagia, and, occasionally, heartburn. Esophagitis associated with mucocutaneous disease occurs in epidermolysis bullosa (30) and pemphigoid (31), the former occurring more frequently than the latter. Epidermolysis bullosa can occur as a simple form in which the bullae heal without scarring, but in the dystrophic form, bullae come in crops and progress from tense fluid-filled bullae to exuding ulcers, which occur initially; eventually scarring and stricture formation develop. Pemphigoid occurs relatively late in life and is not associated with extensive scarring of the skin or esophagus.

Another important systemic disease, which can cause both gastroesophageal reflux and esophagitis, is scleroderma, also known as progressive systemic sclerosis. The esophagus is involved in over 50% of the cases (32) of this connective tissue disorder, which is characterized by progressive fibrosis of the skin and a variety of internal organs. The cause of this disease is unknown, but its pathophysiology involves a markedly weakened LES with consequent severe impairment of peristalsis leading to gross esophageal reflux and prolonged contact between irritants and the esophageal mucosa. Stricture formation is a frequent complication.

CHEMICAL INJURIES. Chemical agents can also produce acute mucosal damage in the esophagus. The accidental or purposeful (in attempted suicide) ingestion of caustic compounds (e.g., lye, drain cleaners, and detergents) can produce serious damage to squamous epithelium and even dissolve fat and cause muscle necrosis. Less-damaging chemical agents include certain capsules that can lodge in the esophagus and produce localized mucosal burn. Medication such as doxycycline and aspirin have been implicated in such burns (33).

Symptoms and Signs

Most of the infections, systemic disorders, and chemical agents mentioned in the previous section produce mucosal irritation with consequent heartburn, odynophagia, and dysphagia. The severity of symptoms varies depending on the degree of injury to the mucosa, submucosa, and muscle. Patients who have one of the mucocutaneous disorders with esophageal involvement will describe dysphagia and odynophagia in addition to the manifestations in the skin, nails, and occasionally teeth. Those with epidermolysis bullosa develop scarring and stricture formation and have severe dysphagia and odynophagia. Patients who have scleroderma experience chest pain, which is due to reflux esophagitis. Pain tends to be more prominent than that seen in "ordinary" reflux esophagitis because the pathology is much more severe and extensive.

Most patients who ingest caustic substances promptly complain of intense pain in the mouth and chest, are unable to swallow saliva or any other material, appear to be in considerable distress with tachycardia, and usually will spit out large amounts of frothy mucus. If damage has been severe, the patient may retch and vomit, bringing up quantities of blood

and esophageal tissues. Physical examination during the acute phase will show evidence of oropharyngeal burns with white membranes and edema of the soft palate and uvula. Usually, the acute distress of the episode fades in 3 to 4 days, and the patient will be able to ingest fluid and solid material. This period of improvement is then followed by renewed symptoms of dysphagia secondary to stricture formation.

Diagnosis

Diagnosis of these various conditions is made by thorough history, physical examination, and, when indicated, laboratory and instrumentation studies. Patients with viral illness or yeast infection of the esophagus experience pain and odynophagia. Endoscopy is helpful in confirming the presence of mucosal ulceration and allows specimens to be taken for a specific diagnosis, which may affect the therapeutic strategy to be followed. Diagnosis of scleroderma in patients with symptoms of reflux esophagitis is facilitated by the presence of typical changes in the skin and Raynaud's phenomenon (32). When these are inconspicuous, cinesophagography and esophageal motility studies can be used to reveal marked reduction in the amplitude of smooth muscle contractions, which may be peristaltic or nonperistaltic.

The onset of chest pain immediately following ingestion of a capsule, accompanied by simultaneous odynophagia, is adequate information for a diagnosis, but if symptoms persist more than 3 days or are increasing, then endoscopy is warranted. One might see a circumscribed ulcer with an alarming-looking necrotic base.

The history and characteristics of oropharyngeal burns usually establish diagnosis of ingestion of caustic agents, but the extent of an injury must be ascertained in order to plan further therapy. Esophagoscopy within the first 24 hours of caustic ingestion is essential for delineating the extent of esophageal injury and therefore determining what needs to be done. Radiographic studies after a barium swallow occasionally show evidence of segmental spasm, but mucosal injury cannot always be demonstrated by this method.

Treatment

INFECTIONS. Treatment of mucosal disorders due to infection or physical agents is much more likely to be successful than treatment of "ordinary" gastrointestinal reflux esophagitis. If diagnostic studies have shown infection of the mucosa with yeast or herpes virus, then the specific therapies listed in Table 56-3 are indicated. No treatment is presently available for esophageal infection due to cytomegalic virus.

SYSTEMIC DISEASE. Steroid therapy occasionally helps in the management of the bullous phase of epidermolysis bullosa. An initial oral dosage of 75 to 80 mg of prednisone per day is recommended; after the desired effects have been obtained, the dosage is tapered to between 10 and 20 mg steroid per day. If scarring and contraction of the esophagus become so marked as to interfere with nutrition, a colonic interposition should be considered. Currently, no effective treatment exists for the motor dysfunction caused by

TABLE 56-3. Treatment of Esophageal Infection

Pathogen	Treatment
Candida albicans	Nystatin: 50,000 u q4h
	Ketoconazole: 200–600 mg tid
	Chlortrimazole
Herpes simplex virus	Acyclovir
Cytomegalic virus	No therapy available at present; topical anesthesia for pain relief

scleroderma. Reflux esophagitis and its complications should be treated aggressively as described in the preceding sections.

CHEMICAL INJURIES. Treatment of patients who have incurred a caustic burn varies according to the liquid ingested and the degree of injury. Patients who have ingested liquid lye should undergo emergency esophagogastrectomy (33, 34). Damage by other caustics can be treated at a more leisurely pace. Large doses of steroids have been shown to decrease the incidence of stricture significantly, to 8 to 10% (35, 36). Typical doses are 200 mg parenteral hydrocortisone every 6 hours for 3 weeks or prednisone given in an initial dose of 80 mg/day and then tapering to 20 mg/day until esophageal healing takes place. In severe cases, steroid therapy may continue as long as 3 to 5 months. Steroid therapy is best accompanied by antimicrobial therapy (e.g., 250 mg tetracycline four times a day or 500 mg ampicillin four times a day).

Introduction of a nasogastric tube or a larger plastic tube to serve as a splint (34) also can help prevent stricture formation. Although such a tube maintains an open lumen, it also serves as an irritating factor, which may enhance scar formation. If such a tube is used, suction should be applied so that the gastric acid cannot use the indwelling tube as a wick, thus further compounding the problem of esophageal tissue healing.

Bougienage, another means to prevent stricture formation, can be used in patients who have superficially damaged esophagus, but in those who have sustained severe damage it carries the risk of esophageal perforation. Generally, this treatment should not be started until 5 or 6 days after the injury. Because no evidence exists that routine bougienage is helpful, it probably should be withheld unless radiologic evidence shows a compromised esophageal lumen is present.

Late treatment of caustic ingestion is focused on maintenance of an adequate esophageal lumen. If the stricture that forms is limited, dilatation by weighted mercury bougies should be adequate to open and maintain the esophageal lumen. If the stricture is severe or there are multiple strictures, esophageal interposition with a colon transplant should be considered, although some patients develop recurrent stricture where the colon is anastomosed to the damaged cervical esophagus.

C. ESOPHAGEAL MOTOR DISORDERS (XIX-3)

Etiology and Pathophysiology

Normally, the muscle of the esophagus, both striated and smooth, is in a state of rest with only the upper and lower esophageal sphincters continuously contracted. When a person swallows, a peristaltic wave begins in the top of the esophagus and sweeps down to the lower esophageal sphincter; this muscular activity is not perceived by the normal person. In patients with esophageal motor abnormalities, however, persistaltic waves are felt as a sensation of pressure or pain and rarely as a burning sensation. The most common type of motor abnormality associated with chest discomfort consists of peristaltic waves of very high amplitude and long duration, which often have a very low rate of propagation (Fig. 56-8). Not every swallow produces such a wave, but the waves with the highest amplitude and duration often are correlated with the greatest intensity of discomfort.

A much less common motor disorder that can produce pain is diffuse spasm of the esophagus. In this, the entire esophagus is clamped down and subject to simultaneous repetitive contractions and localized areas of spasm, usually in the lower end of the esophagus (Fig. 56-9). Very rarely, peristaltic waves that appear normal in terms of amplitude and velocity can be associated with pain. This association can only be discovered by simultaneous monitoring of symptoms and intraluminal measurements of muscle activities. Before the advent of modern diagnostic methods, many of these conditions were lumped under the label

"cardiospasm." We prefer to either discard this term or restrict its use to patients with achalasia.

The actual mechanism of pain production in esophageal motor disorders has not been elucidated. When high-amplitude waves are present, some have suggested that muscle tension receptors in the esophageal body respond to the increased tension by producing nociceptive impulses that are conveyed to the central nervous system. Such "pain" receptors, however, have not been histologically described. The histology of the muscle and myoneural network in most patients with painful motor abnormalities

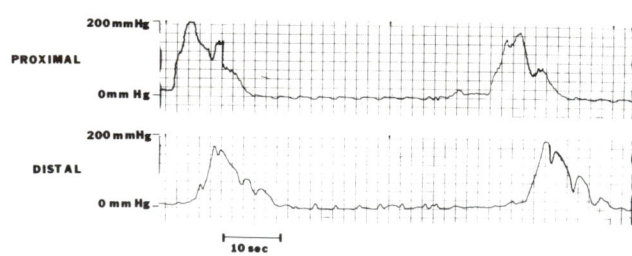

FIG. 56-8. Manometric record of high-amplitude peristaltic contraction. Tracings obtained for two tips 5 cm apart show waves of very high amplitudes (175 to 200 mmHg compared with normal values of 60 to 100 mmHg), long duration (14 to 16 sec compared with normal value of less than 6 sec), and slow velocity of propagation (50 to 60 cm/sec compared with a normal value of 4 cm/sec). Pain can be present throughout the duration of such waves.

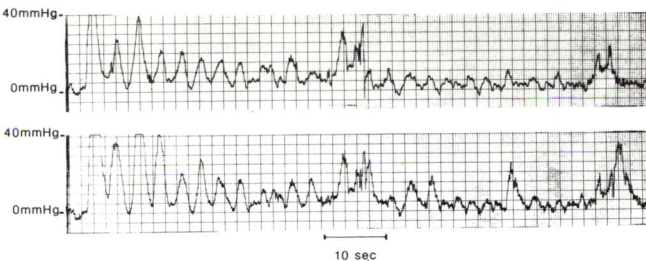

FIG. 56-9. Manometric record of diffuse spasm of the esophagus. Note elevation of the baseline pressure on the left side of the tracings with superimposed simultaneous contractors. The baseline pressure returns to normal in the center of the tracings. A peristaltic contraction is recorded on the far right portion of the tracings. Pain, if present, would be experienced during the period of baseline elevation.

appears to be normal. Another possibility is that the muscle of the esophagus becomes ischemic during prolonged periods of contraction. Since it is not possible at the present time to measure esophageal muscular blood flow with any accuracy, obtaining evidence for this theory is difficult.

Symptoms and Signs

ESOPHAGEAL COLIC. Pain of esophageal origin that mimics myocardial ischemia is called esophageal colic to distinguish it from heartburn, which also can be quite severe. Esophageal colic is usually described by the patient in terms of a pressure—a boring or aching sensation—and can range in intensity from a feeling of slight constriction to a life-threatening intense pressure associated with diaphoresis, a gray color, and a feeling of impending death. Esophageal colic is usually felt substernally but sometimes is felt only in the neck or the epigastric area (Fig. 56-10). Radiation through to the back is a clinical clue that the chest pain under consideration might be of esophageal origin. Radiation into the neck, jaw, teeth, and shoulder is common. Occasionally pain radiates to the left arm or both arms as it does in myocardial ischemia. It is uncommon for esophageal pain to radiate to the abdomen and legs.

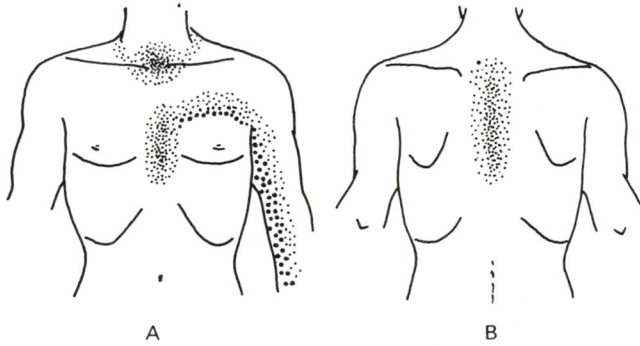

FIG. 56-10. Area of pain reference from esophageal colic. The pain is usually felt substernally, but it can be felt also in the neck or the epigastric area (A) and almost always in the back (B). Radiation occurs into the neck, jaw, teeth, and shoulder and occasionally to the left or both arms.

The duration of esophageal colic can be from a few seconds to many hours. Most commonly it will come in short bursts of 5 to 10 min. Esophageal colic can mimic pain due to coronary artery disease not only in terms of location and intensity but also in the factors that aggravate or relieve it. An exercise-related component to the pain is present in over half of the patients whose pain is later determined to be of esophageal origin. Unlike coronary artery pain, however, the effect of exercise tends to be quite variable in terms of the amount of exertion required to bring on an attack. Sometimes esophageal colic can be triggered by the ingestion of cold or less commonly very warm beverages. Esophageal colic occasionally is related to the ingestion of food, but this is relatively uncommon and the patient does not correlate the onset of pain with eating.

An attack of esophageal colic can occur during moments of emotional tension, but the relationship between pain and stress seems to be less well marked than in the case of pain due to myocardial ischemia. Although population studies suggest that people with chest discomfort of esophageal origin are more likely to have associated psychiatric disturbances (37), clinicians rarely see cases of stress causing chest pain of esophageal origin.

DYSPHAGIA. As in the case of mucosal disease, the presence of dysphagia is a useful clue to esophageal motor disorders, although the dysphagia need not be temporally associated with the chest pain. Patients undergoing an attack of esophageal colic usually are not interested in food intake. If a history of inability to swallow water during an attack of chest pain is obtained, then a motor disorder is likely. In motor disorders, dysphagia can be produced by either solid or liquid bolus ingestion, whereas dysphagia associated with mucosal disease tends to manifest itself only with a solid bolus.

Diagnosis

MANOMETRIC EVALUATION. To implicate a motor disorder of the esophagus as the cause of chest pain, it is necessary not only to demonstrate the presence of a motor disorder but also to correlate it temporally with the occurrence of chest pain. At the present time, manometric examination of the esophagus is the best way to establish that chest pain is due to motor disorder. A discussion of the techniques necessary for this type of examination is beyond the scope of this chapter, but is available in Weihrauch's textbook (38). Current techniques employ an intraluminal catheter assembly, which is attached to appropriate recording instruments. Most laboratories involved in this type of investigation do only short-term monitoring (maximum of 1 to 2 hours). Long-term monitoring of esophageal motor activity is still in the preliminary stages, although several groups around the world are involved in fabricating and testing long-term methods of measuring esophageal motor function.

The most common manometric abnormality associated with pain is the intermittent occurrence of high-amplitude, long-duration, and occasionally low-velocity waves. These waves have been termed "super-squeeze" (39) or "the nutcracker esophagus" (40). A patient undergoing an attack during manometric evaluation will complain of a baseline of constant esophageal pain on top of which are superimposed periods of increased discomfort. These increases in discomfort can be exactly correlated with the pressure waves being observed. Usually, patients do not associate chest pain with the act of swallowing. This is because there is often a lag time between swallowing and the occurrence of pain, especially when the propagation velocity of the wave causing discomfort is quite low.

During manometric monitoring, the manometrist can tell the patient when an attack is coming, how long it will last, and the intensity of each wave by viewing the tracing emerging from the recorder. When the pain can be predicted based on the manometric tracing, then the diagnosis of chest pain of esophageal origin is firmly established. Occasionally, large waves of high amplitude and long duration can be observed at times when the patient is not symptomatic. In this situation, the pain might be due to esophageal motor abnormalities, but the diagnosis is not conclusive. Giant waves are rarely seen in totally asymptomatic patients but can be seen in individuals whose primary and only complaint is dysphagia.

Classic diffuse spasm, characterized by the presence of elevated baseline pressure in multiple leads following a swallow and accompanied by rhythmic, simultaneous contractions of the esophagus, is an uncommon pattern. Often the elevation of the baseline is not marked, and it is difficult to understand why minor elevations of esophageal pressure are accompanied by severe chest pain. As in the case of the high-amplitude, long-duration waves, diffuse spasm abnormalities can be correlated with episodes of chest pain when present. Although many physicians believe that spasm is quite a common abnormality, manometric demonstration of this disorder is difficult in many patients.

Other less well characterized manometric abnormalities, which are usually lumped under the title of nonspecific motor disorders (NSMD), are also associated with chest pain. For example, some patients have no peristaltic waves but develop simultaneous contractions in response to a swallow. The contractions can be either single, resembling a peristaltic wave, or multiple, in which case the tracing momentarily resembles that seen in patients with esophageal spasm. Pain is usually experienced only during episodes of multiple esophageal contractions. Less-dramatic abnormalities can also be associated with chest pain. A few individuals have normal peristaltic waves interspersed with simultaneous contractions; only the simultaneous waves are associated with chest discomfort. Such patients usually have fleeting episodes of chest pain.

In all of these motor abnormalities, the clinical situation must be correlated with manometric recordings of the esophagus. This requires an alert technician or physician. The chance of patients experiencing chest pain during a short recording session is limited; indeed, chest pain occurs in only 10 to 15% of all patients undergoing short-term manometric evaluation. Thus this type of examination has low sensitivity but high specificity. When long-term pressure monitors are available, they will incorporate a method for the patient to indicate when chest pain is present. The physician will then simply have to review the tracing and try to correlate periods of chest pain with the manometric changes.

RADIOGRAPHY. Other techniques for studying esophageal motility have been less helpful than manometry in determining the cause of chest pain due to motor abnormality of the esophagus. Radiography can occasionally be helpful. For instance, if the patient has chest pain during the time he or she is swallowing barium and abnormal contractions of the esophagus can be demonstrated, then the diagnosis is established. Since the radiologist only follows the progress of two or three mouthfuls of barium, however, it is unusual to see the patient during the middle of an attack. If the chest pain attack is of prolonged duration, and a barium swallow can be arranged during this time, then radiographic examination has more utility. Perfectly normal function of the transport of barium during an attack of chest pain would seem to make at least diffuse spasm unlikely. Since the roentgenographic equivalent of high-amplitude, long-duration waves is not known, normal transport of barium might be seen during prolonged high-amplitude wave contractions.

SCINTIGRAPHY. The newer scintigraphic methods for evaluating motor activity in the esophagus share many of the benefits and deficiencies of the barium swallow. These studies, which are performed by ingesting a bolus of radioactive technetium–sulfur colloid and recording the progress of the bolus on a gamma camera, provide sensitive measures of esophageal motor function (41). Unlike manometry, in which many swallows can be evaluated over several hours if necessary, the total time of esophageal monitoring with a radioactive swallow is very brief indeed. As in the case of both manometry and radiography, scintigraphic demonstration of an abnormal motor pattern during an asymptomatic period proves the presence of a motor disorder, but does not definitely establish the motor disorder as the cause of the pain.

PROVOCATIVE TESTS. Since it is so difficult to catch the esophagus misbehaving manometrically, some have tried to provoke the esophagus into abnormal motility in order to see whether chest pain is produced. If the history indicates that chest pain follows the ingestion of ice cold liquids, it is logical to try to provoke an attack with a swallow of ice water. Although prolonged swallows of ice water will produce an aperistaltic esophagus and pain by a different mechanism (42), one or two swallows of ice water can serve as a useful provocative test for motor disorders if the patient has previously noticed a sensitivity to extremes of temperature.

In the experience of the senior author the infusion of acid as a provoking agent has been of very little benefit. Often when chest pain is produced by acid infusion, concomitant monitoring of muscle activity shows no change and certainly no production of spasm. However, a few patients have been observed in whom normal peristaltic waves were replaced by high-amplitude long-duration contractions associated with

TABLE 56-4. Pharmacologic Stimulation of Abnormal Motor Activity

Agent	Dose
Edrophonium (Tensilon)	100 µg/kg, IV
Pentagastrin	6 µg/kg, IV
Bethanechol (Urecholine)	40 µg/kg, subcutaneous
Ergonovine	0.5 mg/kg, IV

chest pain during acid infusion. In this situation the therapeutic endeavors should, of course, be addressed to the control of esophageal reflux.

Several pharmacologic agents (Table 56-4) have been used to stimulate the esophagus (43). Clinical experience suggests that, edrophonium (Tensilon) is the most useful agent. The advantages of edrophonium are that it can be given intravenously and that it has a short duration of action. Therefore, provocation of a positive response will be limited in time. The use of this agent, unfortunately, uncovers only 10 to 15% of individuals whose chest pain is due to a motor disorder not diagnosed by other methods. The actual sensitivity of this stimulus as well as any other has never been established by experimentation. In order to do so, it would be necessary to take patients with chest pain known to be from the esophagus and stimulate them. Such patients are understandably reluctant to undergo such testing!

Ergonovine has also been used to provoke abnormal esophageal motor activity (44, 45). This agent has been used to stimulate both coronary artery spasm and esophageal spasm. Unfortunately, its use is not without side effects. Death has been reported during its use even under maximally controlled situations in the coronary catheterization laboratory. Therefore, this agent should never be used except under very precise cardiovascular monitoring.

No one agent currently available is likely to prove to be a universal stimulant of abnormal esophageal motor activity. The search will continue for a compound that is safe and well tolerated and has high sensitivity. Various studies are in progress to attempt to find the best agent and dosage to produce safe stimulation of the esophageal muscle.

Treatment

No uniformly effective forms of medical therapy for esophageal motor disorders are available at the present time. Drugs commonly used to treat esophageal motor disorders are listed in Table 56-5.

NITRATES. Nitroglycerin can be effective, since it

TABLE 56-5. Treatment of Esophageal Motor Disorders

Agent	Dose
Nitroglycerin	0/4 mg prn
Isosorbide	10 mg qid
Hydralazine	50–200 mg qd
Nifedipine	50–30 mg qid
Diltiazem	60–90 mg qid

can be taken soon after the onset of pain. Approximately 50% of the patients with an esophageal cause for chest pain will respond to nitroglycerin. If there is a response to nitroglycerin sublingually, then more long-acting forms such as isosorbide or nitropaste can be employed (46), although no large series of successes with this form of therapy have been reported. There may also be a selection bias in the patients referred for esophageal testing. Thus, if a patient responds to nitroglycerin, that patient may be assumed to have coronary artery disease when esophageal spasm may be the cause of the pain. Consequently, the patient may assume that a life-threatening illness is present when in fact the esophagus is the causative factor. On the other hand, failure of nitroglycerin therapy may cause referral for esophageal investigation. Therefore, the true prevalence of patients with esophageal pain that respond to sublingual nitroglycerin probably is underestimated.

CALCIUM-BLOCKING AGENTS. Theurapeutic response to calcium channel blocking drugs, such as nifedipine, diltiazem, and verapamil, seems to occur in some patients with esophageal pain but not in all. Open trials that suggest benefit of these agents have been conducted but no double-blind studies, which must be undertaken to determine if calcium blockers are really of benefit. At the present state of knowledge, it would seem worthwhile to at least test the esophagus manometrically before embarking on a course of these expensive drugs, which have significant side effects.

DILATATION. There has been some interest in the use of dilatation of the esophagus either with bougies or with balloon dilators. Again, with very little data available, it would seem worthwhile before embarking on a surgical course of therapy to try dilatation at least in patients with concomitantly high lower esophageal sphincter pressures (47).

SURGICAL THERAPY. Surgical therapy has been used in the treatment of chest pain of esophageal motor origin, but reported use of this therapy is limited (48). The most common operation is a long myotomy. If a high pressure in the lower esophageal sphincter accompanies the abnormality in the body of the esophagus, myotomy is usually carried on through the area of the lower esophageal sphincter. Long-term results of this type of therapy are few. In the experience of the senior author it has been of benefit only in highly selected patients. Before considering a surgical approach, the physician should first have established that the chest pain is of muscular origin. This can only be done by getting the patient in an attack and showing by manometric recordings that the motor abnormality occurs at the same time as the patient's pain.

Manometric results can also be used to determine the extent of the myotomy. If the surgery is effective, pain relief results even though the patient may suffer some postoperative reflux. Several patients have experienced initial relief after myotomy but subsequent return of chest pain. One unfortunate individual who underwent two myotomies and an esophageal replacement, still has chest pain, presumably still of esophageal origin. It would seem reasonable not to proceed to a surgical solution for this type of difficulty until all medical forms of therapy have been exhausted.

D. CANCER OF THE ESOPHAGUS

Epidemiology and Etiology

Cancer of the esophagus is one of the most unpleasant malignancies of the gastrointestinal tract, and its clinical manifestations and resistance to therapy seem to be increasing worldwide. It approaches epidemic proportions in the Transkei region of Capetown Province of South Africa (49), the Caspian region of Iran, the Northern Province of China, and that part of the USSR near the Caspian region (50). In these areas, the incidence rates per 100,000 people have been estimated to be 246, 140, 130, and 60, respectively (49, 50). In contrast, in the United States the rate per 100,000 population was reported in 1975 to be about 6 for males and 1.6 for females (51). Estimates by the American Cancer Society suggest that in the United States there were 9700 new cases of cancer of the esophagus (6800 in men and 2900 in women) and 8800 deaths (6400 men and 2400 women) in 1987 (52). The high ratio of deaths to new cases indicates that cancer of the esophagus often is incurable.

In North America, black males who smoke cigarettes and abuse alcohol seem to be at highest risk with an incidence over four times that of white males (51). Comparison between the white and black population reveals that the incidence rates have been 4 among white males, 1.2 among white females, 16 among black males, and 4 among black females. Other etiologic factors play a role among the general population worldwide. Chronic irritation of the esophageal mucosa may be one of the predisposing factors leading to carcinoma. For example, the incidence in patients with lye strictures and ionized radiation is estimated to be higher than in age- and sex-matched controls (53). Irritation from long-term stasis and untreated achalasia has also been incriminated (54). Another type of irritation is chronic and persistent reflux. There appears to be a particularly relevant relation between reflux (Barrett's) epithelium and adenocarcinoma of the esophagus (54).

Clinical association between esophageal cancer and Plummer–Vinson syndrome also exists (55). For example, in those countries that have a high incidence of esophageal carcinoma, the use of very hot tea is a common custom. Studies in human volunteers showed that the ingestion of extremely hot beverages can raise intraesophageal temperature to a level at which tissue damage can be expected (56).

Pathology

More than 90% of malignant esophageal tumors are squamous cell carcinomas, which arise from the squamous cell epithelium lining the lumen of the esophagus. Variants of squamous cell carcinoma include spindle cell carcinoma, pseudosarcoma and carcinosarcoma, and verrucous carcinoma.

Adenocarcinoma of the esophagus also seems to be on the increase, although this type represents only about 3 to 5% of all esophageal cancers (54). Originally thought to be a cancer invading the esophagus from the stomach or occurring in the esophageal glands, it is now clear that this malignancy often arises from columnar (Barrett's) epithelium.

Symptoms and Signs

Pain as a presenting manifestation of carcinoma tends to be overshadowed by dysphagia, weight loss, and symptoms of esophageal obstruction. Although mentioned in passing in many articles, exact estimates of the incidence of pain due to esophageal cancer are rare in the modern literature. In a series of 153 cases in the United States, chest pain was experienced by only 17 (11%), bony metastatic pain by another 7 (4%), and pain in the throat or neck by 20 (13%) (57). In a South African series of 206 patients, 36 (17.5%) presented with retrosternal pain, 10 (5%) had interscapular pain, and 27 (13%) had epigastric discomfort (58).

Pain of esophageal carcinoma is usually felt in the retrosternal region and often radiates to the back. It is steady and can be quite intense, thus presenting a problem in patient management. The presence of pain usually signals mediastinal, bony, or visceral involvement and is a poor prognostic sign.

Diagnosis

A careful double-contrast examination of the esophagus is the least invasive and most productive method of investigation. Any suspicious area seen in the examination or the presence of unrelenting chest pain in a patient with multiple risk factors for carcinoma of the esophagus and/or dysphagia should suggest the need for endoscopy. Through the endoscope, target biopsies or brushings of a suspicious lesion can be made.

Computerized tomography scanning seems to be the most accurate method of defining the extent of extraesophageal and mediastinal involvement, and it has almost supplanted mediastinoscopy. Other invasive methods of evaluation such as lymphangiography and diagnostic pneumomediastinography have also been abandoned.

Treatment

No agreement exists about the best method for treating esophageal carcinoma, either for cure or for palliation (54). Luminal patency can be restored by surgery (either bypass or resection), by radiation therapy, by dilatation of the tumor, by intubation with a stent, or by local debulking of the tumor with a laser or a heater probe. Pain, which usually signals inoperability, is best managed by appropriate use of narcotics, nerve blocks, and other therapeutic modalities discussed in Chapter 24.

E. OTHER PAINFUL DISORDERS OF THE ESOPHAGUS

This section contains a very brief discussion of two other esophageal conditions that cause pain: laceration and perforation of the esophagus and hiatus hernia.

Lacerations and Perforations

Etiology and Pathophysiology

Esophageal laceration, intramural dissection, and perforation occur as a result of trauma. The most common form of trauma is mucosal laceration during the act of vomiting (Mallory-Weiss syndrome) (6). Several causes of actual perforation or rupture of the esophagus are known. A marked increase in esophageal pressure (up to 250 to 300 mm Hg) associated with very forceful vomiting or retching after a large meal, which presumably occurs because the upper esophageal sphincter does not relax during the vomiting (6), can result in spontaneous rupture (Boerhaave's syndrome). External trauma to the body, usually in the form of high-speed automobile accidents, also can result in transection or perforation of the esophagus. Diseases of the esophagus, such as a corrosive ingestion, peptic ulcer, neoplasm, and esophagomalacia, can progress to a perforation of the esophagus. Finally, instrumentation of the esophagus can cause iatrogenic damage.

The site of perforation is variable and depends on the cause. Spontaneous perforation due to high intraesophageal pressure consequent to forceful vomiting occurs at the weakest point, which is in the posterolateral aspect of the esophagus. Iatrogenic perforation usually occurs in the pharynx and in the lower esophagus. With rupture there is leakage of contents into the mediastinum.

Symptoms and Signs

Patients with esophageal mucosal laceration experience little pain but invariably vomit bright red blood. Instrumental laceration or perforation usually is accompanied by relatively mild symptoms and is free of complications.

Spontaneous rupture of the esophagus often causes sudden severe pain, described as tearing or crushing, much like that of dissecting aortic aneurysm. If the rupture is high, the pain is in the upper part of the sternal region, whereas if the rupture is lower, the pain is located in the restrosternal and epigastric area, often radiating to the thoracic spine. Swallowing is frequently painful. The patient becomes dyspneic, cyanotic, and diaphoretic and appears gravely ill. Examination reveals a pale, sweaty patient with tachycardia and not infrequently signs of shock. The pain often mimics myocardial infarction, pancreatitis, or a ruptured abdominal viscus.

Vomiting in patients with spontaneous rupture of the esophagus usually deposits gastric contents into the mediastinum, which causes severe mediastinal complications. In addition, free air enters the mediastinum and spreads to neighboring structures and causes palpable subcutaneous emphysema in the neck, mediastinal cracking sounds on auscultation, and

pneumothorax. This may be followed by pleural effusion and hydropneumothorax, which, if severe, causes shock. With time, secondary infection supervenes, and mediastinal abscess and pleuropulmonary suppurative complications develop.

Diagnosis

Diagnosis of mucosal laceration rests on suspicion and demonstration of the tear at endoscopy. Diagnosis of rupture is suggested by the history and physical findings. Plain upright chest radiography often demonstrates air in the mediastinum, widening of the mediastinum, and left pleural effusion. Confirmation of the presence of a tear, as well as its localization, is provided by radiologic contrast examination. Esophageal perforation must be differentiated from perforation of the stomach due to a penetrating ulcer in which case there is free air under the diaphragm but pleural effusion and mediastinal air are absent. The presence of the latter as well as subcutaneous emphysema helps to differentiate esophageal perforation from acute pancreatitis and dissecting aortic aneurysm.

Treatment

Treatment of mucosal tears consists of watchful waiting, as most patients stop bleeding spontaneously. Vasopressin, balloon tamponade or angiographic embolization is used if bleeding persists (6). If surgery is necessary, preoperative endoscopy should be done to localize the lesion or lesions and thus facilitate the surgical repair (6). Iatrogenic perforation of the cervical esophagus can also be managed medically with intravenous nourishment and antibiotics; if the patient shows signs of continuing infection or leak, limited drainage can be done through a supraclavicular incision (59).

Perforation in the midthoracic or lower esophagus is best treated by immediate thoracotomy and repair of the lesion and drainage (60, 61). If significant time elapses between perforation and surgery, the muscle around the site of perforation becomes inflamed and necrotic, impairing the ability of sutures to hold the tissues (6). In such cases, the tear should be repaired primarily by buttressing the incision with pleura or by gastric patch or by esophageal diversion (62). Another approach that involves less surgery is to drain the area with a small thoracotomy and then cauterize the perforation through an endoscope with sodium hydroxide until the perforation heals (63). If perforation occurs proximal to a pre-existing esophageal pathologic process (e.g., stricture, cancer, or achalasia), the coexisting disorder must be treated at the same time by resection in the case of a tumor or stricture or by myotomy in the case of achalasia (54). In patients with terminal carcinoma, surgical repair may not be feasible. Extensive corrosive damage may require esophageal diversion and subsequent excision.

Methods to control the pain depend on its severity. Obviously, oral medication cannot be used. Patients experiencing severe pain should be given an intitial dose of a narcotic as an intravenous bolus, followed by either intramuscularly administered narcotics or intravenous analgesia, either in repeated doses or with continuous infusion. In patients requiring surgery, these techniques can be used preoperatively and postoperatively to control pain due to the residual effects of the initial lesion and that due to the surgical procedure. In medical centers where the technique is available, patient-controlled analgesia is highly effective. Another highly effective technique is continuous segmental epidural analgesia with local anesthetics limited to those segments where the pain is referred. This technique produces virtually complete relief of severe or excruciating pain and diminishes or completely eliminates the reflex skeletal muscle spasm and the severe neuroendocrine response inherent in the intense nociceptive input associated with rupture of the esophagus (see Chapters 7 and 94 for details). In patients requiring surgery, the preoperative analgesia can be used as a complement to general endotracheal anesthesia for the operation and can then be continued for the control of postoperative pain. Obviously, epidural analgesia in the upper thoracic and lower cervical region requires great skill and experience on the part of the anesthesiologist.

Hiatus Hernia

Although hiatus hernia usually is considered in connection with reflux esophagitis, it is discussed here to re-emphasize certain points made in Section B (Esophageal Mucosal Disorders) and also because its therapy remains a controversial issue. The two types of hiatus hernia that occur differ significantly in terms of diagnosis and therapy. In *sliding hiatus hernia*, the GE junction and a portion of the stomach are above the diaphragm with one side of the stomach covered by peritoneum. In *paraesophageal hiatus hernia*, the GE junction remains fixed in its normal location but a portion of the stomach is adjacent to the esophagus (Fig. 56-11).

Sliding Hiatus Hernia

In the past, sliding hiatus hernia was considered a synonym for gastroesophageal reflux disease. This mechanistic and simplistic belief misled clinicians into attaching a multitude of symptoms to a common radiologic finding. Although sliding hiatus hernia can be demonstrated in more than 40% of the population, most patients are asymptomatic. Pope (4) stated that if sliding hiatus hernia and reflux esophagitis are viewed as synonymous, two possibly serious errors may occur. If a patient whose nonspecific symptoms led to an upper gastrointestinal radiographic series shows a pouch at the lower end of the esophagus and if all of the patient's symptoms are attributed to this pouch, it is likely that the patient will be operated on for repair of the hernia but the symptoms will remain. Conversely, a patient with severe symptoms of reflux in whom a pouch at the lower end of the esophagus is not demonstrated by radiography may be ignored or mistreated.

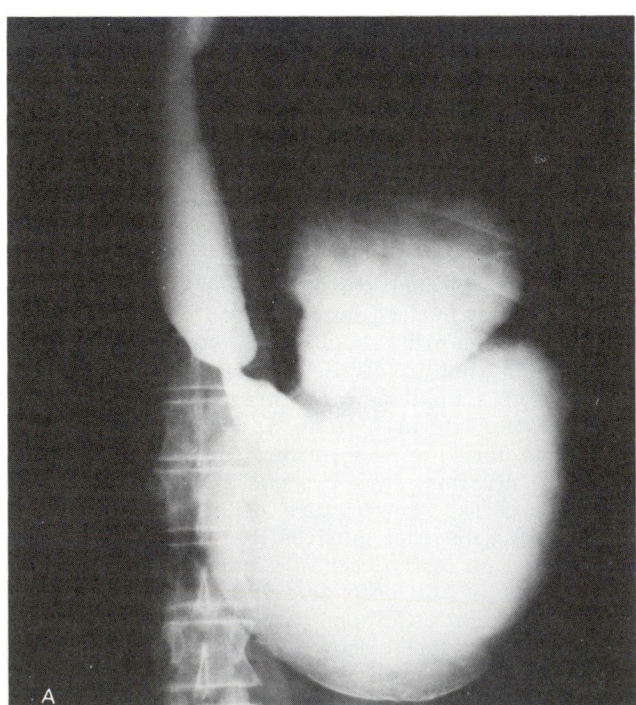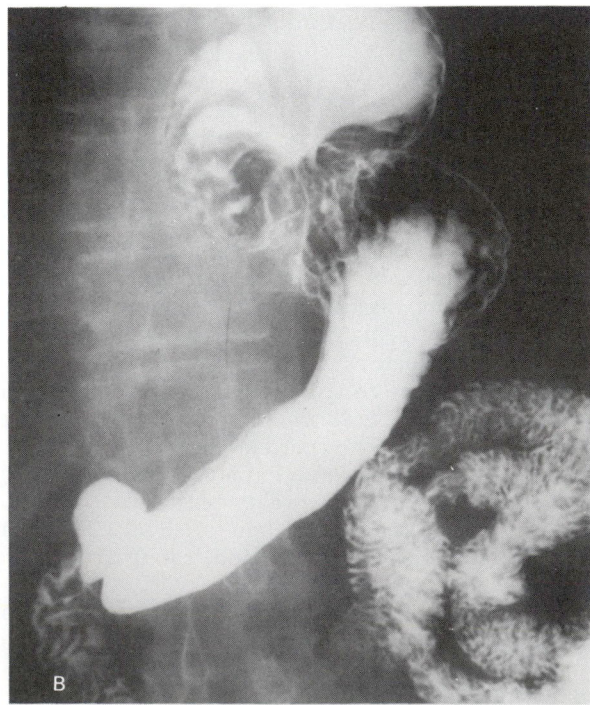

FIG. 56-11. *A.* Paraesophageal hernia. Note that the esophagogastric junction is located well down in the abdomen and that the fundus rises into the chest. *B.* Large hiatus hernia. The impression of the diaphragm is seen in the midfundal region. The gastroesophageal junction is located high in the mediastinum. Radiographs courtesy of C.A. Rohrmann, M.D.

Another related problem is that to determine whether a sliding hiatus hernia is present or not requires knowing precisely the location of the junction of the esophagus and stomach as well as the relationship between this junction and the esophageal hiatus. Pope (4) presented impressive evidence that this is difficult or impossible, even with the use of the latest radiographic techniques, intraluminal manometry, and even the flexible gastroscope. Thus the question of how often esophageal reflux is caused by sliding hiatus hernia remains difficult to resolve. Since hiatus hernia is not an illness but an anatomic condition, the main thrust of the physician's activities is to focus on the diagnosis and effective treatment of reflux, not hiatus hernia (Fig. 56-11).

Treatment

The conservative medical treatment of reflux esophagitis, whether or not it is associated with a sliding hiatus hernia, was discussed in Section B and need not be repeated here. However, because surgical therapy was not discussed in that section, it is considered here.

Surgical therapy for patients with sliding hiatus hernia associated with reflux esophagitis remains a controversial issue, but it is used much less frequently than in earlier years. In one referral medical center, of nearly 35,000 patients who underwent upper gastrointestinal radiographic series, hiatus hernia was revealed in over 7300, but only 90 were subjected to surgery (64). On the basis of his broad experience, Pope (4) concluded that surgical therapy should be considered only for patients who develop such complications of reflux as stricture formation, significant bleeding from ulceration, and pulmonary aspiration. Intractability of symptoms despite effective medical management, which probably is the most common indication for surgery, is one of the most difficult to define and remains the "gray area" in the field. Although the use of the diagnostic tests mentioned in Section B may be of help, the eventual decision to operate will be a clinical one made by the surgeon on the basis of information from the patient and consultation with the referring physician (4).

Earlier surgical techniques were directed toward the anatomic obliteration of the hernia, but clinical experience showed that most patients continued to experience reflux symptoms and its complications after such operations. More recent techniques have concentrated on enhancing the complex mechanisms of the GE junction. With some procedures, this is achieved by invaginating the esophagus on itself by creating a gastric wrap-around with or without fixation. But even these procedures often failed and were associated with some complications. More recently, Hill et al. (65) suggested that in addition to strengthening the lower esophageal sphincter, the operative procedure should also consider the role of the GE valve, esophageal clearance, and posterior fixation of the esophagus, each of which also contributes to the antireflux barrier.

The GE valve, created by the acute angle of His, is a flat lateral leaf that approximates against the mucosa of the lesser curvature of the stomach (Fig. 56-1C). Increase in intragastric pressure pushes the valve medially, thus occluding the lumen and preventing reflux. Hill et al. (65) demonstrated in cadavers that there is a measurable pressure gradient across the GE junction, which requires from 7 to 15 cm of water pressure in the stomach before reflux occurs. Conversely, if the fundus of the stomach is depressed to about 45°, the angle of His becomes obtuse, thus eliminating the valve and converting the osteum of the esophagus into a funnel, allowing free reflux and elimination of the gradient.

Another factor of importance is esophageal clearance. In the normal individual, reflux produces an instantaneous and powerful peristaltic wave that rapidly cleanses the lower esophagus of reflux material. A direct correlation between the duration of exposure to acid reflux and severity of objective esophagitis has been demonstrated (16). Other studies have revealed that more than 40% of patients with GE reflux have delayed esophageal clearance, which persists even after correction of the reflux and relief of symptoms (see 65 for references). The third factor emphasized by Hill et al. (65) is posterior fixation. Normally, the GE junction is anchored within the abdomen, usually at the level just above the median arcuate ligament, so that the esophagus has a fulcrum from which it can generate powerful peristaltic waves. When this anchoring is lost, the esophagus loses its ability to generate forceful peristaltic waves. Hill et al. (65) stressed that the posterior attachment of the GE junction, by the dorsal mesentery to the preaortic fascia, is a key to the integrity of the entire antireflux barrier. In patients with hiatus hernia and GE reflux, the function of one or more of the components of the GE junction is impaired or completely lost.

The Hill operation, called *gastroesophageal restoration* (GER) by its developers, is intended to improve the function of the various components of the GE junction. Hill et al. (65) insist that the procedure is a posterior gastropexy, in which the phrenoesophageal bundles are imbricated together, and is not a fundoplication because there is actually no wrap of stomach around the lower esophagus. The GER procedure depends on augmentation of the intrinsic sphincter and its special features. By placing tension on the collar sling musculature, the repair automatically accentuates the valve of His and anchors the GE junction posterior to its normal primary attachment—the preaortic fascia. In contrast to some other operations, with the GER procedure no sutures into the esophagus are used because the esophagus has no serosa and no strength and if sutures are placed deeply there is a risk of fistula formation. Intraoperative manometry is used to measure the pressure in the GE junction during the operation, thus objectively determining whether an adequate repair had been created (Fig. 56-12).

Hill et al. (65) carefully selected patients by comprehensive preoperative evaluation of the following: the function of the LES, the presence of reflux, the

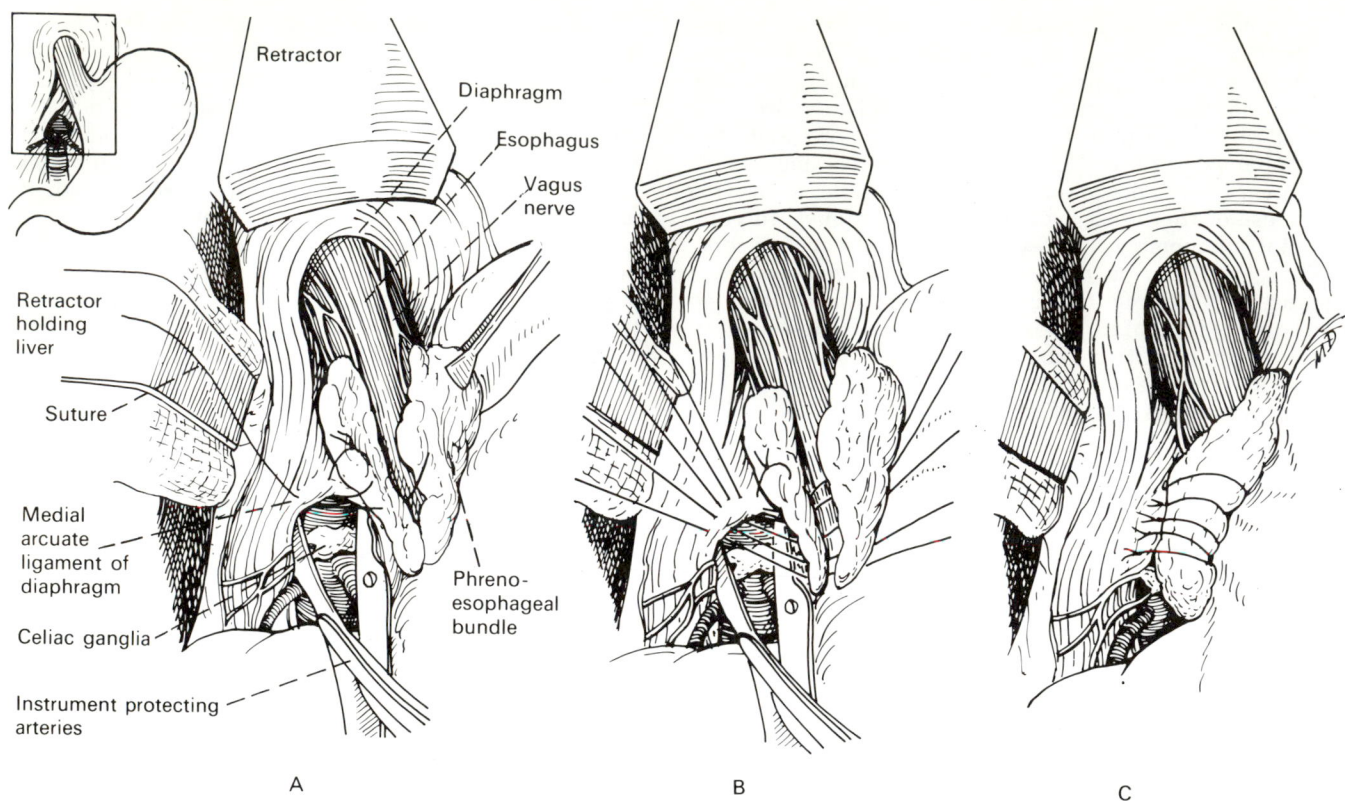

Retractor

Diaphragm

Esophagus

Vagus nerve

Retractor holding liver

Suture

Medial arcuate ligament of diaphragm

Celiac ganglia

Instrument protecting arteries

Phreno-esophageal bundle

A   B   C

FIG. 56-12. The final stages of the Hill operation. These stages are achieved after very careful exploration of the upper abdomen, especially the pylorus; precise and gentle dissection and maneuvers to avoid damage to the celiac artery, the celiac ganglia, and the vagus nerves; and dissection of the preaortic fascia. The stomach is rotated in a clockwise direction to expose its posterior part, thereby displaying the anterior and posterior phrenoesophageal bundles. **A.** Five strong nonabsorbable sutures are placed in the anterior and posterior phrenoesophageal bundles (care taken not to injure the vagus nerve); subsequently, the sutures are passed through the preaortic fascia and the medial arcuate ligament. **B.** After the sutures are in place, a single knot is placed through the top three sutures, which are clamped with a hemostat. Measurements of the barrier pressure are then made; if it is above 55 mmHg, the sutures are loosened; if it is below 30 mmHg, they are tightened. After the proper pressure is obtained, all five sutures are tied and a final pressure measurement is made. **C.** The repair is complete. In addition to strenghtening the lower esophageal sphincter, the operation can be easily palpated through the wall of the stomach. This operation accentuates the valve of His and anchors the GE junction posteriorly to its normal primary attachment—the preaortic fascia. Modified from Hill, L.D., Thor, K., and Mercer, D.: Surgery for hiatal hernia and esophagitis. *In* The Esophagus: Medical and Surgical Management. Edited by L.D. Hill. Philadelphia, W.B. Saunders, 1988, pp. 101–103.

level of gastric acid, determination of whether the patient has esophagitis or Barrett's esophagus, and exclusion of neoplasm. Although intractability to medical management is the most common indication for the surgery, the second most important indication is objective evidence of serious esophagitis using Pope's criteria. About 15% of patients were operated on for stricture and ulceration; others were selected for surgery because of bleeding, respiratory complications, very large sliding hiatus hernia, and severe inflammation of the esophagus demonstrated both by biopsy and by endoscopy. The results obtained in more than 1300 patients operated on during the past quarter century have been excellent or good in some 95% of the patients, with a failure and recurrence rate of 1.5 to 5% and a complication and mortality rate of 0.2% (65).

Paraesophageal Hiatus Hernia

The much less common paraesophageal hiatus

hernia is quite a different problem in regard to diagnosis and therapy. Radiography will usually demonstrate that the GE junction is below the diaphragm and reflux is not a clinical problem. Patients present with a feeling of fullness and discomfort in the epigastrium and lower chest. Complications, which are not infrequent, include strangulation, infarction, and ulceration of the herniated stomach. Patients with strangulation or infarction present with severe acute chest pain, dyspnea and other symptoms that simulate myocardial infarction, ruptured aortic aneurysm, and other serious visceral disorders.

Because of the possibility of these severe complications, some authorities recommend surgical reduction of all paraesophageal hiatus hernia when discovered (66). Certainly, when patients present with severe pain due to strangulation, infarction, or ulceration with severe bleeding, emergency surgery is mandatory.

SUMMARY

Chest pain of esophageal origin can be due to mucosal disease, dysfunction of the muscles of the esophagus, esophageal carcinoma, and laceration or rupture of the esophagus. Arriving at a correct diagnosis and differentiating pain of esophageal origin from other causes of chest pain frequently is difficult. Table 56-1 lists the signs, symptoms, and tests that help to make a differential diagnosis. A logical diagnostic flow chart is shown in Figure 56-7, which highlights the decision points in determining the sequential tests to employ.

REFERENCES

1. Davies, J.A., Jones, D.B., and Rhodes, J.: Esophageal angina as the cause of chest pain. JAMA, 248:2274, 1982.
2. Tibbling, L.: Oesophageal dysfunction and angina pectoris in a Swedish population selected at random. Acta Med. Scand. 644(Suppl.):71, 1981.
3. Rose, G.A.: The diagnosis of ischaemic heart pain and intermittent claudication in field surveys. Bull. WHO, 27:645, 1962.
4. Pope, C.E., II: Gastroesophageal reflux disease. In Gastrointestinal Disease. 3rd Ed. Edited by M.H. Sleisenger and J.S. Fordtran. Philadelphia, W.B. Saunders, 1983, pp. 449–476.
5. Pope, C.E., II: Motor disorders. In Gastrointestinal Disease. 3rd Ed. Edited by M.H. Sleisenger and J.S. Fordtran. Philadelphia, W.B. Saunders, 1983, pp. 424–448.
6. Pope, C.E., II: Involvement of the esophagus by infections, systemic illnesses and physical agents. In Gastrointestinal Disease. 3rd Ed. Edited by M.H. Sleisenger and J.S. Fordtran. Philadelphia, W.B. Saunders, 1983, pp. 495–504.
7. Brand, D.L.: Chest pain of esophageal origin. In Diseases of the Esophagus. Edited by S. Cohen. New York, Churchill Livingstone, 1982.
8. Areskog, N., and Tibbling, L. (eds.): Differential diagnostic aspects of chest pain. Acta Med. Scand. 544(Suppl.), 1981.
9. Bonica, J.J.: The Management of Pain. Philadelphia, Lea & Febiger, 1953, pp. 1369–1372.
10. Kuntz, A.: The Autonomic Nervous System. 4th Ed. Philadelphia, Lea & Febiger, 1953, pp. 207, 208.
11. Netter, F.H.: The CIBA Collection of Medical Illustrations. Vol. 3: Digestive System; Part I, Upper Digestive Tract. Caldwell, NJ, CIBA Pharmaceutical Co., 1959, pp. 44, 45.
12. Jones, C.M.: Digestive Tract Pain. New York, MacMillan, 1938.
13. Payne, W.W., and Poulton, E.P.: Experiments on visceral sensations. J. Physiol., 63:217, 1927.
14. Teodori, U., and Galletti, R.: Il Dolore Nelle Affezioni Degli Organi Interni del Torace. Rome, L. Pozzi, 1962, pp. 169–178.
15. Ismail-Beigi, F., Horton, P.F., and Pope, C.E.; II: Histologic consequences of gastroesophageal reflux in man. Gastroenterology, 58:163, 1970.
16. Pope, C.E., II: Pathophysiology and diagnosis of reflux esophagitis. Gastroenterology, 70:445, 1976.
17. Doddes, W.S., et al.: Pathogenesis of reflux esophagitis. Gastroenterology, 81: 376, 1981.
18. Richter, J.E., and Castell, D.O.: Gastroesophageal reflux. Ann. Intern. Med., 97:93, 1982.
19. Henderson, R.D., and Marryatt, G.: Characteristics of chest pain. Acta Med. Scand. 641(Suppl.):49, 1982.
20. Branicki, F.J., et al.: Ambulatory monitoring of oesophageal pH in reflux oesophagitis using a portable radiotelemetry system. Gut, 23:992, 1982.
21. Bernstein, L.M., and Baker, L.A.: A clinical test for esophagitis. Gastroenterology, 24:760, 1958.
22. Brand, D.L., Ilves, R., and Pope, C.E., II: Evaluation of esophageal function in patients with central chest pain. Acta Med. Scand. 641(Suppl.):53, 1981.
23. Johnson, L.F., and DeMeester, T.R.: Evaluation of elevation of the head of the bed, bethanechol, and antacid foam tablets on gastroesophageal reflux. Dig. Dis. Sci., 26:673, 1981.
24. Fiasse, R., et al.: Controlled trial of cimetidine in reflux esophagitis. Dig. Dis. Sci., 25:750, 1980.
25. Farrell, R.L., Roling, G.T., and Castell, D.O.: Cholinergic therapy of chronic heartburn. Ann. Intern. Med., 80:573, 1974.
26. Behar, J., and Biancani, P.: Effect of oral metoclopramide on gastroesophageal reflux in the post-cibal state. Gastroenterology, 70:331, 1976.
27. McCallum, R.W., et al.: A controlled trial of metoclopramide in symptomatic gastroesophageal reflux. N. Engl. J. Med., 296:354, 1977.
28. Eras, P., Goldstein, M.J., and Sherlock, P.: Candida infection of the gastrointestinal tract. Medicine, 51:367, 1972.
29. Fishbein, P.G., et al.: Herpes simplex esophatitis. Dig. Dis. Sci., 24:540, 1979.
30. Orlando, R.C., et al.: Epidermolysis bullosa: Gastrointestinal manifestations. Ann. Intern. Med., 81:203, 1974.
31. Foroozan, P., et al.: Loss and regeneration of the esophageal mucosa in pemphigoid. Gastroenterology, 52:548, 1967.
32. Gilliland, B.C., and Mannik, M.: Progressive systemic sclerosis (diffuse scleroderma). In Harrison's Principles and Practice of Internal Medicine. 10th Ed. Edited by R.G. Petersdorf. New York, McGraw-Hill, 1983, pp. 2002–2006.
33. Ritter, F.N., et al.: The rationale of emergency esophagogastrectomy in the treatment of liquid caustic burns of the esophagus and stomach. Ann. Otol., 80:513, 1971.
34. Ray, J.F., et al.: The natural history of liquid lye ingestion. Arch. Surg., 109:436, 1974.
35. Balasegaram, M.: Early management of corrosive burns of the oesophagus. Br. J. Surg., 62:444, 1975.
36. Cardona, J.C., and Daly, J.F.: Current management of corrosive esophagitis. Ann. Otol., 80:521, 1971.
37. Clouse, R.E., and Lustman, P.J.: Psychiatric illness and contraction abnormalities of the esophagus. N. Engl. J. Med., 390:1337, 1983.
38. Weihrauch, T.R.: Esophageal Manometry. Baltimore, Urban & Schwarzenberg, 1981.
39. Brand, D.L., Martin, D., and Pope, C.E., II: Esophageal manometrics in patients with angina-like chest pain. Am. J. Dig. Dis., 22:300, 1977.
40. Benjamin, S.B., Gerhardt, D.C., and Castell, D.O.: High amplitude, peristaltic esophageal contractions associated with chest pain and/or dysphagia. Gastroenterology, 77:478, 1979.
41. Russell, C.O.H., et al.: Radionuclide transmit: A sensitive screening test for esophageal dysfunction. Gastroenterology, 80:887, 1981.
42. Meyer, G.W., and Castell, D.O.: Human esophageal response during chest pain induced by swallowing cold liquids. JAMA, 246:2057, 1981.
43. Benjamin, S., et al.: Prospective manometric evaluation with pharmacologic provocation of patients with suspected esophageal motility dysfunction. Gastroenterology, 84:893, 1983.
44. London, R., et al.: Provocation of esophageal pain by ergonovine or edrophonium. Gastroenterology, 81:10, 1981.
45. Eastwood, G.L., et al.: Use of ergonovine to identify esophageal spasm in patients with chest pain. Ann. Intern. Med., 94:768, 1981.
46. Swamy, N.: Esophageal spasm: Clinical and manometric response to nitroglycerin and long-acting nitrates. Gastroenterology, 72:23, 1977.
47. Ebert, E.C., et al.: Pneumatic dilatation in patients with symptomatic diffuse esophageal spasm and lower esophageal sphincter dysfunction. Dig. Dis. Sci., 28:481, 1983.
48. Leonardi, H.K., et al.: Diffuse spasm of the esophagus. J. Thorac. Cardiovasc. Surg., 74:736, 1977.
49. Gilder, S.S.B.: Carcinoma of the esophagus. Ann. Intern. Med., 87:494, 1977.
50. Kmet, J., and Mahboubi, E.: Esophageal cancer in the Caspian Littoral of Iran. Science, 175:846, 1972.
51. Cutler, S.J., and Young, J.L.: Third national cancer survey: Incidence data. Natl. Cancer Inst. Monogr., 41:1, 1975.
52. Cancer Facts and Figures: 1987. New York, American Cancer Society, 1988.
53. Lansing, P.B., Ferrante, W.A., and Ochsner, J.L.: Carcinoma of the esophagus at the site of lye stricture. Am. J. Surg., 118:108, 1969.

54. Pope, C.E., II: Tumors of the esophagus. *In* Gastrointestinal Disease. 3rd Ed. Edited by M.H. Sleisenger and J.S. Fordtran. Philadelphia, W.B. Saunders, 1983, pp. 479–490.

55. Wynder, E.L., et al.: Environmental factors in cancer of upper alimentary tract: Swedish study with special reference to Plummer-Vinson (Paterson-Kelly) syndromes. Cancer, *10*:470, 1957.

56. DeJong, U.W., et al.: The relationship between the ingestion of hot coffee and intraoesophageal temperature. Gut, *13*:24, 1972.

57. Takita, H., et al.: Squamous cell carcinoma of the esophagus: A study of 153 cases. J. Surg. Oncol., *9*:547, 1977.

58. Stein, D.: Early and late symptomatology of carcinoma of the esophagus. *In* Carcinoma of the Esophagus. Edited by W. Silber. Rotterdam, A.A. Balkema, 1978, pp. 151–155.

59. Bombeck, C.T., Boyd, D.R., and Nyhus, L.M.: Esophageal trauma. Surg. Clin. North Am., *52*:219, 1972.

60. Janssen, C.W.: Perforation of the intrathoracic oesophagus. Scand. J. Thorac. Cardiovasc. Surg., *10*:189, 1976.

61. Sandrasagra, F.A., English, T.A.H., and Milstein, B.B.: The management and prognosis of oesophageal perforation. Br. J. Surg., *65*:629, 1978.

62. Finley, R.I., et al.: The management of nonmalignant intrathoracic esophageal perforations. Ann. Thorac. Surg., *30*:575, 1980.

63. Gunning, A.J., and Kingsworth, A.: Treatment of chronic oesophageal perforations with special reference to an endoscopic method. Br. J. Surg., *66*:226, 1979.

64. Polk, H.C., and Zeppa, R.: Hiatal hernia and esophagitis: A survey of indications for operation and technique and results of fundoplication. Ann. Surg., *173*:775, 1971.

65. Hill, L.D., Thor, K., and Mercer, D.: Surgery for hiatal hernia and esophagitis. *In* The Esophagus: Medical and Surgical Management. Edited by L.D. Hill. Philadelphia, W.B. Saunders, 1988. 98, 101–103.

66. Hill, L.D.: Incarcerated paraesophageal hernia: A surgical emergency. Am. J. Surg., *126*:286, 1973.

57 · CHEST PAIN RELATED TO CANCER

JOHN J. BONICA

IN this chapter I discuss malignant and some benign neoplasms that arise from various structures in the chest as well as metastatic lesions that cause chest pain. The material is presented in two major parts: A, Basic Considerations of cancer of the lungs, including the tracheobronchial tree and pleura, neoplasms of the mediastinum, and cancer of the breast; and B, Management of Cancer-Related Chest Pain. Part A includes a brief discussion of the epidemiology, etiology, pathology, symptoms and signs, diagnosis, and treatment of the various tumors. Part B supplements the information contained in Chapter 24 but provides greater detail about the control of pain for various specific cancers. More detailed discussion of the various aspects of the basic considerations can be found in major oncology textbooks (1–4).

A. BASIC CONSIDERATIONS

Cancer of the Lung

Epidemiology

Cancer that involves the tracheobronchial tree and lung tissue and pleura is the most frequently occurring type of cancer in most western countries. The American Cancer Society estimated that in 1987 150,000 new cases of primary cancer of the lung afflicted 99,000 males and 51,000 females and it was the cause of death in 136,000 persons, including 92,000 males and 44,000 females (5) (Table 57-1). Many of those who developed cancer in 1987 died in the same year. Age-adjusted lung cancer is the leading cause of cancer deaths in males from age 35 on, and the second leading cause of cancer deaths in females ages 35 to 74. In 1987 lung cancer caused about 22% of all male deaths and about 8% of all female deaths but, among the cancer population, cancer of the lung accounted for 36% of all male and 20% of all female cancer deaths. Most cases for both sexes occur at a median age of about 35 years, with a peak at age 55 to 56 for each sex. The incidence is increasing every year and, unless a drastic change is seen (i.e., elimination of smoking by all Americans), this progressive increase will cause the age-adjusted lung cancer death rate for both sexes to double every 15 years (5).

At diagnosis only 20% of patients with lung cancer have local disease, 25% have spread to regional lymph nodes, and 55% have spread to distant sites (6). Unfortunately, even in those patients with supposedly localized disease, the overall 5-year survival rate is only 30% for males and 15% for females, a survival rate that has not changed significantly over the past 20 years. Studies of age-adjusted death rates per 1,000 population for selected sites in 48 countries reveal that cancer of the lung is also a major health problem that afflicts a high percentage of those in the adult population. Indeed, these data reveal that among males in 20 countries the death rate is 60/100,000 or higher compared with 70/100,000 in the United States. Obviously, primary carcinoma of the lung is a major health problem with a generally grim prognosis. Equally important from the viewpoint of this book is that many of these patients have severe intractable pain that is difficult to manage.

Much of the information in the following discussion was obtained from Minna (6), Minna and colleagues (7), DeCaro and Benfield (8), and other sources (9–12).

Etiology

Most lung cancers are associated with and probably caused by cigarette smoking—benzo[a]pyrene is a major carcinogen in tobacco smoke (6, 7). A dose-response relationship exists between the lung cancer death rate and the total amount of cigarettes smoked, usually expressed in "cigarette pack/year" (6). Comparison of the incidence of lung cancer between nonsmokers and smokers reveals that the risk is increased 60- to 70-fold for the man smoking two packs a day for 20 years compared to the nonsmoker. Conversely, the chances of developing lung cancer decreases with cessation of smoking, but is not likely to decrease to the nonsmoker level. As shown in Figure 57-1, in 1965, lung cancer in women began to go up strongly; the age-adjusted death rate is expected to increase from about 5/100,000 in 1965 to about 28/100,000 by the year 2000 (6) only as a result of the increase in cigarette smoking among women. Pipe smoking does not appear to be related to lung cancer.

Other suggested lung cancer carcinogens include ionizing radiation, uranium ore, asbestos, halochromates, metallic iron and iron oxide, nickel, beryllium, and arsenic (6, 10). Radiation and haloether exposure are particularly associated with the development of small cell and epidermoid lung cancers. These environmental pollutants apparently enhance the carcinogenic effects of smoking.

Pathology

PULMONARY LUNG TUMORS. The histologic classification of primary lung neoplasms recommended by the World Health Organization in 1977 (Table 57-2) is used most widely (6, 7). The first four major cell groups comprise 95% of all primary lung neoplasms and, of these, epidermoid (squamous cell) carcinoma is the most common histologic type in males, while adenocarcinoma is the most common type in females (6, 10). The influence of smoking is re-emphasized by the fact that 95% of patients with lung cancer of all histologic types are cigarette smokers while the rare

TABLE 57-1. 1987 Estimates of New Cases and Deaths from Lung and Breast Cancer

Parameter	Lung Cancer	Breast Cancer
New Cases		
Male	99,000	900*
Female	51,000	130,000*
Total	150,000	130,900*
Deaths		
Male	92,000	300
Female	44,000	41,000
Total	136,000	41,300

*Invasive cancer only.
From American Cancer Society: Cancer Facts and Figures—1987. New York, American Cancer Society, 1987.

TABLE 57-2. World Health Organization (WHO) Classification of Malignant Pleuropulmonary Neoplasms

Classification	Type of Neoplasm
I	Epidermoid carcinoma
II	Small cell carcinoma (including fusiform, polygonal, lymphocyte-like, and others)
III	Adenocarcinoma (including acinar, papillary, and bronchioloalveolar)
IV	Large cell carcinoma (including solid tumors with and without mucin and giant cell and clear cell tumors)
V	Combined epidermoid and adenocarcinomas
VI	Carcinoid tumors
VII	Bronchial gland tumors (including cylindromas and mucoepidermoid tumors)
VIII	Papillary tumors of the surface epithelium
IX	"Mixed" tumors and carcinosarcomas
X	Sarcomas
XI	Unclassified
XII	Mesotheliomas (including localized and diffuse)
XIII	Melanomas

From Kreyberg, L.: Histologic typing of lung tumors. *In* International Classification of Tumors No. 1. Edited by L. Kreyberg. Geneva, World Health Organization, 1967, pp. 19–26.

nonsmoking patient who develops lung cancer usually has adenocarcinoma (6, 7, 10, 11).

The various cell types have different natural histories and responses to therapy; thus, a correct histologic diagnosis is the first step in the determination of correct treatment. Treatment decisions are made on the basis of whether the neoplasm can be histologically classified as a small cell lung cancer (SCLC, or "oat cell" cancer) or one of the non-small cell cancers, which include epidermoid carcinoma, adenocarcinoma, large cell carcinoma, bronchioloalveolar carcinoma, and mixed versions of these (6–11) (Table 57-3). Small cell carcinoma, which accounts for 25% of all cases of lung cancer, has the highest incidence of distant metastasis, the lowest incidence of surgical resectability, and the least likelihood of 5-year survival.

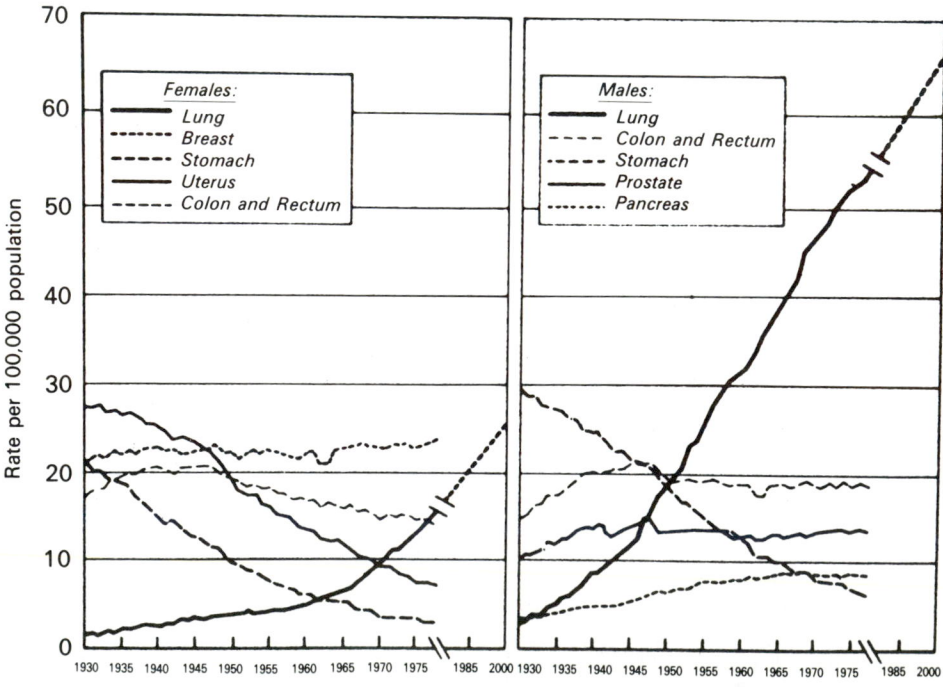

FIG. 57-1. Age-adjusted cancer death rates in the United States for lung cancer and cancer of other selected sites with theoretical projections for lung cancer mortality to the year 2000. From Minna, J.D., et al.: Cancer of the lung. *In* Principles and Practice of Oncology. 2nd Ed. Edited by V.T. DeVita, S. Hellman, and S.A. Rosenberg. Philadelphia, J.B. Lippincott, 1985, p. 508.

TABLE 57-3. Incidence, Frequency of Metastases, and Surgical Resectability of the Major Lung Cancer Histologic Types

Cell Type	Incidence in Autopsy Series (%)	Necropsy Frequency of Distant Metastases When Clinically Localized (%)*	Resectability Rate (AJC† Study) (%)	5-year Survival Rate After Curative Section (%)
Non-small cell carcinoma:				
Epidermoid	33	17	60	37
Adenocarcinoma	25	40	38	27
Large cell carcinoma	16	14	38	27
Small cell carcinoma	25	63	11	<1

*Determined from autopsy studies of patients dying of causes other than cancer within 30 days following an apparent curative surgical resection.
†AJC, American Joint Committee Study for Cancer Staging and End Results Reporting indicating percentage of cases thought to undergo a curative resection.
From Minna, J.D.: Neoplasms of the lung. *In* Harrison's Principles of Internal Medicine. 11th Ed. Edited by E. Braunwald et al. New York, McGraw-Hill, 1987, p. 1116.

Epidermoid (squamous cell) carcinoma grows centrally toward the main-stem bronchus and locally invades underlying bronchial cartilage, adjoining lung parenchyma, and lymph nodes (7, 8). The bronchial mucosa usually presents evidence of squamous metaplasia, dysplasia, or frank intraepithelial neoplasia. Small cell carcinoma also usually presents as a central mass with submucosal infiltrates in the early phase of the disease. Obstruction of the bronchial lumina by extrinsic compression or endobronchial tumor occurs in the advanced stage (7). Most adenocarcinomas are peripheral in location, unrelated to bronchi except by contiguous growth or lymph node metastasis. They usually present as firm localized subpleural masses and tend to invade the overlying pleura. Similarly, large cell carcinoma often presents as peripheral subpleural large lesions, usually unrelated to the bronchi except by contiguous growth, and have a tendency to invade the pulmonary parenchyma and the overlying pleura. Epidermoid and large cell cancers cavitate in 20 to 30% of cases (6). Bronchioloalveolar carcinoma can present either as a single mass, a diffuse multinodular lesion, or a fluffy infiltrate.

NEOPLASMS OF THE TRACHEOBRONCHIAL TREE. Primary tracheal and bronchial tumors, which represent 1% of all neoplasms of the respiratory tract (6–8), always express themselves intraluminally and are diagnosed by bronchoscopic biopsy. Benign tracheal tumors include papillomas and hemangiomas and the rarer tumors, such as lipomas, fibromas, neurofibromas, chemodectomas, and granular cell myoblastoma (8). These benign neoplasms can present as obstructing tumors that might cause respiratory difficulties. Tracheal cancers include exothytic or ulcerating squamous carcinoma, adenoid cystic carcinoma (cylindroma), mucoepidermoid carcinoma, chondroma, carcinoid sarcoma, and other rare tumors (8).

PLEURAL TUMORS. With pleural tumors, the mesothelial cells of the pleura can assume bizarre shapes transiently as part of an inflammatory or non-neoplastic disease. Mesotheliomas can be benign, stimulating fibromas that arise from the visceral or parietal pleura, or malignant, with the diffuse infiltration of the visceral and parietal pleura encapsulating the lungs (8). Diagnosis of pleural malignancy can be made through cells found in pleural effusion, but a large sample is usually needed to help differentiate metastatic adenocarcinoma from primary pleural mesothelioma (8).

METASTATIC PULMONARY TUMORS. The lungs are frequently the site of metastatic disease from primary cancer outside the lung. Approximately 30% of patients with malignancies have pulmonary metastasis at some time during the clinical course of their disease (15). Almost 20% of patients dying of pulmonary metastasis have no other detectable focus of disease. Pulmonary metastasis represents a major and often the only site of occurrence in a number of childhood tumors, including Wilms' tumor and Ewing's sarcoma,

and might be the only site of failure of testicular tumors as well as of small and soft tissue sarcomas (15). Most sarcomas and some carcinomas tend to metastasize in children by the hematogenous route, while most carcinomas spread by way of the lymphatics. The hematogenous spread of most tumors is to the lung, because the venous blood return of most organs is to the right side of the heart and from there to the pulmonary capillary bed (15). This includes tumors of the head and neck, lungs, kidneys, and testes, myelomas originating from the skin, osteochondrosarcomas, and liver and endocrine tumors (15). Organs drained by the systemic venous system give rise to 84% of cases of solitary metastasis (15).

Symptoms and Signs

Lung cancer usually begins with cytologic changes of atypia in the bronchial epithelial cells, progressing to carcinoma in situ, and eventually to frank invasion (6, 7). These changes usually occur before symptoms or signs have developed and are only seen in cytologic studies of sputum, bronchial washings, and biopsies (6, 7). At the onset of local tumor growth and invasion, lung cancer can produce signs and symptoms as well as positive chest radiographic findings, which can arise from local tumor growth, invasion of adjacent structures, regional growth (from metastasis to peribronchial hilar, mediastinal, and supraclavicular nodes), lymphatic spread, or growth in distant metastatic sites from hematogenous dissemination. Symptoms and signs can also result from a remote effect of the tumor (6, 7), usually from peptide hormone secretion by the tumor that produces a paraneoplastic syndrome (6, 7). Several reports indicated that only 5 to 15% of patients are detected while asymptomatic, usually on a routine chest radiograph, while the vast majority of patients present with some sign or symptom (13, 14).

The following are common signs and symptoms of lung cancer, as reported by Cohen (16):

Symptoms secondary to central or endobronchial growth of the primary tumor:
   Cough
   Hemoptysis
   Wheeze and stridor
   Dyspnea from obstruction
   Pneumonitis from obstruction (fever, productive cough)

Symptoms secondary to peripheral growth of the primary tumor:

Pain from pleural or chest wall involvement

Cough

Dyspnea on a restrictive basis

Lung abcess syndrome from tumor cavitation

Symptoms related to regional spread of the tumor in the thorax by contiguity or by metastasis to regional lymph nodes:

Tracheal obstruction

Esophageal compression with dysphagia

Recurrent laryngeal nerve paralysis with hoarseness

Phrenic nerve paralysis with hemidiaphragm elevation and dyspnea

Sympathetic nerve paralysis with Horner's syndrome

Eighth cervical and first thoracic nerves with ulnar pain and Pancoast's syndrome

Superior vena cava syndrome from vascular obstruction

Pericardial and cardiac extension with resultant tamponade, arrhythmia, or cardiac failure

Lymphatic obstruction with pleural effusion

Lymphangitic spread through lungs with hypoxemia and dyspnea

Signs and symptoms secondary to the central or endobronchial growth of primary tumor include cough, hemoptysis, wheeze, striated dyspnea, and pneumonitis from obstruction. Signs and symptoms secondary to the peripheral growth of primary tumor include pain from pleural or chest wall involvement, cough, dyspnea on a restrictive basis, and symptoms of lung abscess resulting from tumor cavitation. Tumors of the apex of the lung that usually grow by local extension to involve the C8 and T1 (and occasionally the C7 and T2) spinal nerves and often the sympathetic chain produce Pancoast's or superior pulmonary sulcus tumor syndrome. (See below, Section B).

INTRATHORACIC SPREAD. Intrathoracic spread of lung cancer, either by direct extension or by lymphatic metastasis, produces regional disease symptoms in the thorax. Tracheal obstruction and irritation can be associated with retrosternal and anterior chest wall pain, as well as with cough and hemoptysis (6, 7). Entrapment of the recurrent laryngeal nerve produces paralysis and hoarseness and, because of the longer intrathoracic course of the left nerve, these symptoms more commonly occur on the left side than on the right side. Involvement of the phrenic nerve can lead to paralysis and elevation of the hemidiaphragm, with resulting dyspnea.

Compression of the esophagus by the tumor can lead to dysphagia, odynophagia and, not infrequently, deep visceral pain caused by the involvement of sensory nerves to the esophagus. Also, dysphagia of both solids and liquids can result with recurrent laryngeal nerve paralysis; because this nerve supplies part of the cricoid musculature and proximal esophagus it can cause aspiration of gastric contents. Compression of the thin-walled low-pressure system of the superior vena cava by a right-sided tumor or large lymph nodes in the mediastinum, produces the superior vena cava syndrome (see below).

Metastasis to the heart occurs in 15 to 35% of patients with lung cancer (15). Tumor extension into the pericardium and heart can produce pericardial tamponade or congestive heart failure. Other problems of regional spread include lymphatic obstruction, with resulting pleural effusion, and lymphangiectatic spread to the lungs, with production of hypoxemia and dyspnea. Bronchioalveolar carcinoma can spread transbronchially with consequent tumor growing along the multiple alveolar surfaces and resulting in impairment of oxygen transfer, respiratory insufficiency, dyspnea, hypoxemia, and production of large amounts of sputum (6, 7). Some of these patients have deep, retrosternal, diffuse visceral-type pain.

EXTRATHORACIC METASTATIC DISEASE. Extrathoracic metastatic disease is found on autopsy in 25 to 55% of patients with epidermoid carcinoma, in 50 to 80% of patients with adenocarcinoma and large cell carcinoma, and in 74 to 95% of patients with small cell cancer (12, 17). Autopsy studies revealed lung cancer metastasis in almost every organ system. In addition to the pleura, diaphragm, pericardium, and myocardium, the most frequent sites of metastasis are the liver, adrenals, bone, central nervous system, meninges, gastrointestinal tract, esophagus, and thyroid gland. These produce common clinical problems, which include neurologic deficit from brain metastasis, pain from bone metastasis and pathologic fracture, biochemical liver dysfunction, anorexia, and biliary obstruction with pain. Some patients with metastasis to the lymph nodes in the supraclavicular region, and occasionally in the axilla and groin, have pain and ulceration. Extension of the tumor into the spinal cord frequently causes spinal cord compression, with consequent neurologic signs and symptoms.

PARANEOPLASTIC SYNDROMES. Paraneoplastic syndromes, which are remote effects of cancer, are common in patients with lung cancer and can be the initial finding or the first sign of occurrence of the lung cancer (7). In addition, a paraneoplastic syndrome can mimic metastatic disease and, unless detected, might lead to inappropriate palliative rather than curative treatment. The paraneoplastic syndrome is often relieved by successful treatment of the tumor, so this can be the basis for correcting such a syndrome (7).

Diagnosis

It is essential to screen high-risk individuals (those over 45 years old, smoking 40 or more cigarettes daily) for lung cancer. Minna (6) reported that screening with sputum cytology tests and chest radiographs done at 4-month intervals showed a prevalence rate of lung cancer in asymptomatic patients of 4 to 8 cases/1000 persons; with follow-up screening, 4 new cases of lung cancer/1000 persons followed each year were found. Minna (6) reported that these cancers can be detected 72% of the time by radiography, 20% by cytology, and 6% by both methods. About 90% of screened patients who develop lung cancer are asymptomatic, and 62% have resectable lung cancer (6). In view of the poor prognosis of lung cancer, such screening programs should be expanded to try to salvage as many of these patients as possible.

ESTABLISHING TISSUE DIAGNOSIS. Once signs and symptoms or diagnostic studies suggest that lung cancer is present, it is necessary to establish a tissue diagnosis of malignancy to determine the histologic cell type and to stage the patient for appropriate treatment (7). In patients who have a solitary pulmonary nodule or some other local lesion tissue diagnosis is made by definitive surgical resection, while in larger lesions tumor tissue or tumor cells in washings are obtained through a fiberoptic bronchoscopy with bronchial biopsy. Other techniques for obtaining lung tissue include mediastinal node biopsy through a mediastinoscope, percutaneous biopsy of a large supraclavicular lymph node, soft tissue mass, or lytic bone lesion, bone marrow biopsy, and cytologic examination of pleural fluid or needle biopsy of the involved pleura (6). A transthoracic fine-needle aspiration biopsy or transbronchial forcep biopsy can be used for high-risk patients or for those who are determined to be unresectable.

STAGING FOR LUNG CANCER. The next step in the diagnostic and prognostic process is staging of the patient with lung cancer. A detailed description of cancer staging is beyond the scope of this chapter, and Table 57-4 is included only for completeness. Lung cancer staging consists of anatomic staging, determination of the location and size of the tumor, and physiologic staging, consisting of assessment of the patient's ability to withstand various anticancer therapies. The TNM staging system listed in Table 57-4 is used for anatomic staging of the tumor. For staging of non-small cell lung cancer, the TNM factors are combined to form three different groups, stages I, II, and III.

GENERAL DIAGNOSTIC PROCEDURES. All lung cancer patients should have a complete history and physical examination, with evaluation of all other medical problems and determination of performance status and weight loss. It is especially important to examine the ear, nose, and throat carefully because of the frequent occurrence of secondary cancers in these areas (6). Chest radiographs and CT scans should be obtained, and tomography for special diagnostic problems should be done. A complete laboratory workup, including electrocardiography, pulmonary function studies, and measurement of blood gases, is frequently indicated. If signs and symptoms suggest tumor involvement of other organs, appropriate radionuclide studies are indicated. These and other procedures for making a correct diagnosis and determining proper staging of the patient have been discussed in detail by Minna and associates (6, 7) and by DeCaro and Benfield (8).

Treatment

TRACHEAL TUMORS. Tracheal tumors can be treated by local excision (6, 8). For primary cancers of the trachea, which are most often of the adenocystic or mucoepidermoid type and have a propensity to spread submucosally and by local extension, wide excision of the neoplasm is required. It is usually possible to resect six to eight tracheal rings (or sometimes more) and to re-establish a primary anastomosis by immobilization of the entire pulmonary hilum and use of the laryngeal release procedure. Although tracheal prostheses have been used, they are of limited value

TABLE 57-4. TNM Classification of Lung Cancer

Classification	Characteristics
Primary Tumor*	
TX	Occult cancer: only evidence in bronchial washings cytologically
T1	Less than 3 cm surrounded by lung or visceral pleura, and without bronchoscopic invasion proximal to a lobar bronchus
T2	Tumor more than 3 cm; or tumor with atelectasis or pneumonitis extending to hilum but less than entire lung, within a lobar bronchus, and more than 2 cm distal to carina; no pleural effusion
T3	Tumor of any size with extension into parietal pleura, chest wall, diaphragm, mediastinum; less than 2 cm from carina; or atelectasis, pneumonitis of entire lung; pleural effusion with or without malignant cells
Regional lymph nodes†	
N0	Negative hilar and mediastinal nodes
N1	Positive ipsilateral hilar nodes
N2	Positive mediastinal nodes (also scored when vocal cord paralysis, superior vena cava obstruction, and tracheal or epsophageal compression are present, all of which strongly indicate mediastinal node invasion)
Distant metastasis‡	
M0	No known distant metastasis
M1	Distant metastasis present with site specified (e.g., brain)
Stage grouping	
Occult carcinoma	TX, N0, M0
Stage I	T1, N0, M0; T1, N1, M0; T2, N0, M0
Stage II	T2, N1, M0
Stage III	T3 with any N or M; N2 with any T or M; M1 with any T or N

*T, tumor size.
†N, regional nodal involvement.
‡M, Absence or presence of distant metastasis.
From Minna, J.D.: Neoplasms of the lung. *In* Harrison's Principles of Internal Medicine. 11th Ed. Edited by E. Braunwald et al. New York, McGraw-Hill, 1987, p. 1118.

(8). Therefore, a bronchoplastic procedure with primary anastomoses of autogenous tissue is the approach of choice in the treatment of tracheal cancers. Following appropriate surgical resection, 95% of patients with bronchial adenoma survived 5 years, but this decreased to 70% if regional lymph nodes were involved (6).

LUNG TUMORS. It was previously thought that *small cell lung carcinoma* (SCLC) should not be resected because of poor results, but evidence now exists to show that resection of T1, N0, M0 lesions (Table 57-4), combined with adequate chemotherapy, radiation therapy, or both can offer a 5-year survival to more than 25% of patients (18, 19). Many patients with more advanced disease have a good response to cyclophosphamide, methotrexate, adriamycin, and hemibody radiation. The percentage of disease-free patients 2 years after initiation of treatment, however, has remained at 7 to 30%; few if any patients with proven SCLC have survived for 5 years (18).

In patients with *non-small cell lung cancer* in stages I and II (localized disease) who can tolerate operation, the treatment of choice is pulmonary resection (6). Resection should also be considered in rare patients with stage III cancer of favorable age, cardiopulmonary function, and anatomy. In general, conservative resection that often encompasses all known tumor has a survival rate equal to that obtained with the use of more extensive procedures. Thus, lobectomy is preferred to pneumonectomy, while wedge resection and segmental resections are reserved for patients with poor pulmonary reserve and small peripheral lesions. Approximately 43% of all lung cancer patients undergo thoracotomy and, of these, 77% have a definitive resection, 12% have a palliative procedure with no disease left behind, and 12% are only explored for disease extent (6).

Minna (6) reported that the incidence of long-term survivors following definitive surgical therapy is remarkably similar for major medical centers performing lung cancer surgery in the United States. Approximately 30% of all patients resected for cure survive 5 years, and 15% survive 10 years. The 5-year survival rates for different histologic types are as follows: squamous cell (epidermoid carcinoma), 33%; adenocarcinoma, 26%; large cell carcinoma, 28%; and bronchioalveolar carcinoma, 51%. For those with small cell carcinoma, however, the survival rate is less than 1%.

Of patients who turn out to have *unresectable disseminated non-small cell cancer*, 70% have a poor prognosis. Minna (6) reported that the median survival for patients with performance status scores at 0 (asymptomatic) is 34 weeks; for those with 1 (symptomatic, fully ambulatory) it is 25 weeks; for those with a score of 2 (in bed less than 50% of the time) it is 17 weeks; for those with a score of 3 (in bed more than 50% of the time) it is 8 weeks; and for those with a score of 4 (bedridden all the time) it is only 4 weeks. Such patients should be managed appropriately with medical therapy, analgesics, and radiotherapy.

Patients whose primary tumors cause symptoms such as bronchial obstruction and pneumonitis, hemoptysis, or upper airway or superior vena cava obstruction should usually have radiotherapy to the primary tumor. Prophylactic treatment should be carried out in asymptomatic patients in whom follow-up is uncertain to prevent major symptoms from developing, but, if the patient can be followed closely, deferring treatment until symptoms appear is appropriate (6). Usually a course of radiation therapy of 30,000 to 40,000 mGy (3000 to 4000 rad) over 2 to 4 weeks is applied to the tumor. Radiation therapy relieves intrathoracic symptoms of hemoptysis in 85% of patients, superior vena cava (SVC) syndrome in 80%, dyspnea in 60%, cough in 60%, atelectasis in 23%, and vocal cord paralysis in 6% (6).

Other symptoms of metastatic disease treated by radiotherapy include cardiac tamponade, painful bone metastasis (in which relief occurs in about 65% of cases), brain metastasis, spinal cord compression, and brachial plexus involvement. As mentioned in Chapter 24, with brain and spinal cord compression, dexamethasone administered in a daily dose of 25 to 100 mg, qid, can also be given and then rapidly tapered to the lowest dosage that relieves neurologic symptoms.

Anticancer chemotherapy is not yet standard therapy for non-small cell lung cancer except in those centers in which clinical trials are being carried out. Trials to date have shown that, in patients given the most active single drug, 10 to 20% have objective tumor shrinkage while the figure increases to 30 to 40% with combination chemotherapy (6). Unfortunately, a complete clinical regression of tumor occurs in less than 5% of patients. Those patients with tumor who respond to chemotherapy have a median survival of about 30 to 40 weeks, whereas for those that do not respond to chemotherapy it is 10 to 20 weeks (6).

Pulmonary metastatic disease is usually considered to be incurable, with two exceptions. The first is development of a solitary pulmonary shadow seen on a chest radiograph in a patient known to have an extrathoracic neoplasm (6). This can represent metastasis or a new primary lung tumor. Because the natural history of lung cancer is worse than for most other primary tumors, it is best to approach the single pulmonary nodule in the patient with a known extrathoracic tumor as though the nodule were a primary lung cancer, especially if the patient is over 35 years old and a smoker (6). The second exception is multiple pulmonary nodules that are resected for cure. Resection is usually recommended if, after careful staging, the patient can tolerate the contemplated pulmonary resection, the primary tumor has been definitely and successfully treated, and all known metastatic disease can be encompassed by the projected pulmonary resection. Primary tumors with pulmonary metastases that have been successfully resected for cure include osteogenic sarcoma, and colorectal, uterine cervix or corpus tumor; head and neck, breast, testis, bladder, and kidney tumors. The 5-year survival rate in carefully selected patients is between 20 and 30% (6).

Neoplasms of the Mediastinum

Various benign and malignant tumors (and cysts) occur with considerable frequency in the mediastinum. Although one-third to one-half of these tumors are asymptomatic and are found on routine chest radiography, the remainder of mediastinal neoplasms produce chest pain or a feeling of tightness, dyspnea, hoarseness, general malaise, anorexia and weight loss, and other symptoms and signs secondary to displacement or compression of the adjacent mediastinal structures (20, 21). The symptoms and signs are partly related to the size of the tumor and its location. Figure 57-2 depicts the boundaries and compartments of the mediastinum.

Epidemiology and Pathology

The most common mediastinal masses in adults are metastatic carcinomas, lymphomas, and thymomas; other neoplasms include germ cell, neurogenic, and mesenchymal tumors. Table 57-5 lists the relative incidence of mediastinal tumors and cysts found by Sabiston and colleagues (22, 23) among 1881 adults and 354 children. One-fourth of the masses were malignant, whereas in children the overall incidence of malignancy was estimated at 50%. Figure 57-3 indicates the most common sites of these tumors in various

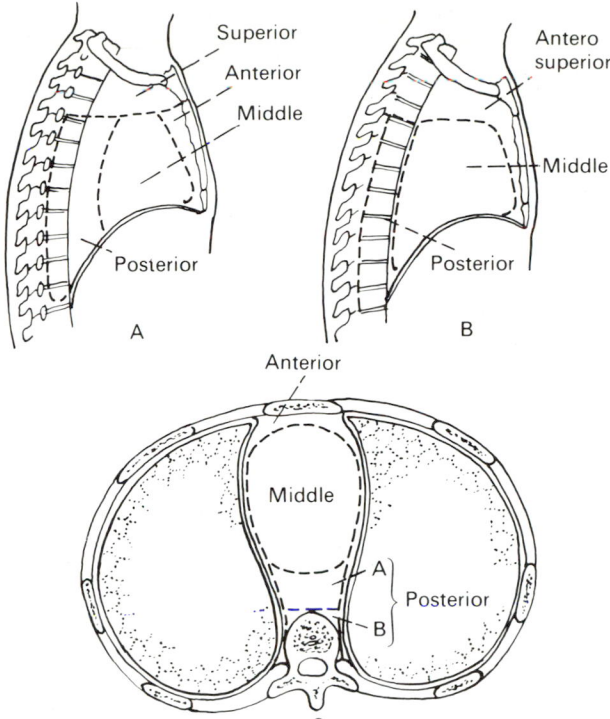

FIG. 57-2. *A* and *B.* Two different classifications of the compartments of the mediastinum. *C.* Cross section showing the compartment including the posterior compartment as classified in *A* and *B*.

TABLE 57-5. Relative Incidence of Mediastinal Tumors and Cysts

Type	All Patients (%)	Children (%)
Thymomas	21	—
Neurogenic tumors	20	38
Lymphomas	12	19
Germ cell neoplasms	11	12
Mesenchymal tumors	7	10
Endocrine tumors	6	—
Primary carcinoma	3	4
Cysts	19	17

From Hammon, J.W., Jr., and Sabiston, D.C., Jr.: The mediastinum. *In* Thoracic Surgery. Edited by H.E. Ellis and H.S. Goldsmith. Hagerstown MD, Harper & Row, 1979.

compartments of the mediastinum. Neurogenic tumors are the most common primary mediastinal neoplasms and are found almost exclusively in the posterior mediastinum near the paravertebral gutter. Most of these neoplasms are benign, including neurofibromas, schwannomas, and ganglioneuromas. The most common tumors in the superior, anterior, and middle mediastinum are lymphomas and metastatic carcinoma. The presence of numerous lymph nodes in the mediastinum leads to frequent metastasis.

Symptoms and Signs

The symptoms and signs of mediastinal tumors are as follows (20):

Nonspecific:
    Chest discomfort—fullness, tightness, pain
    Anorexia
    Weight loss
    Malaise
Secondary to compression or displacement of adjacent mediastinal structures:
    Tracheobronchial compression—cough, wheezing, stridor, dyspnea, recurrent respiratory infections
    Esophageal compression—dysphagia
    Superior vena cava syndrome
    Horner's syndrome
    Vocal cord paralysis—dysphonia
    Pulmonic stenosis—murmurs
    Cardiac tamponade or arrhythmias
Secondary to endocrine function:
    Cushing's disease
    Gynecomastia
    Hypertension
    Hypoglycemia
Systemic syndromes:
    Thymoma—myasthenia gravis, red cell aplasia, hypogammaglobulinemia, autoimmune diseases
    Carcinoid of thymus—multiple endocrine abnormalities (type I), Cushing's syndrome
    Neurofibroma—osteoarthritis
    Lymphoma—alcohol-induced pain, fever
    Teratoma—hypoglycemia, insulin-producing tumor

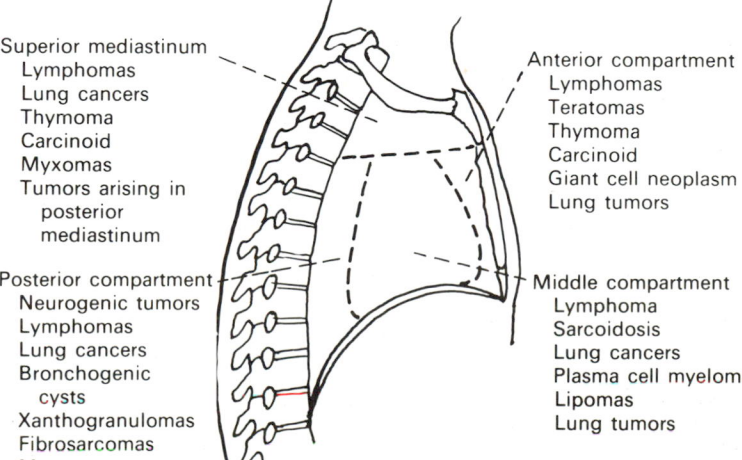

FIG. 57-3. Locations of the most frequently occurring mediastinal neoplasms.

As mentioned, pain, tightness, or fullness in the chest occur frequently and are often associated with anorexia, weight loss, and malaise. Other symptoms and signs are secondary to compression of the displacement of the tracheobronchial tree, esophagus, sympathetic chain, recurrent laryngeal nerve, or heart. In addition, various systemic syndromes, can occur caused by thymomas, carcinoids of the thymus, new fibromas, lymphomas, and teratomas (20).

Diagnosis

Investigation of the mediastinal mass begins with posteroanterior and lateral chest radiographs. In addition, it might be necessary to obtain oblique views, do a contrast study of the esophagus, and perform a CT scan to define the anatomic location and borders of the neoplasm more clearly. The anatomic location and site of the lesion are of diagnostic importance and can help to determine other procedures that are necessary to reach definitive diagnosis (24). CT scanning of the chest with injection of contrast material into a peripheral vein or angiography of the pulmonary circulation or aorta might be needed to distinguish vascular from nonvascular lesions, a differentiation of special importance if biopsy of the mass is being considered. Another use of CT scanning is detection of a cystic lesion, which strongly indicates that a mass is benign.

Mediastinoscopy with biopsy is useful in the diagnosis of mediastinal masses if metastatic carcinoma, lymphoma, or sarcoidosis are suspected (24). In the absence of palpable nodes, scalene node biopsy is useful in patients thought to have lymphoma or metastatic carcinoma. Bronchoscopy and esophagoscopy should be performed whenever the radiographic abnormality could be caused by a lung or esophageal tumor in any way. The frequency of lung cancer requires that this diagnosis be considered in patients who are 40 years of age and over, with a history of smoking (20, 24).

Treatment

The treatment of the various neoplasms varies according to histologic type. The treatment of metastatic lung tumors has been discussed in the preceding section. Complete resection of the tumor is the treatment of choice for all types of thymoma. Complete resection of a well-encapsulated benign thymoma is curative (21). On the other hand, neither external radiation therapy nor surgery used alone is sufficient to control malignant thymomas. Radiation therapy should be added to the surgical treatment whether tumor removal has been accomplished. Martini and associates (21) have recommended colloidal radioactive phosphorus (^{32}P) instillation if pleural involvement by seeding or malignant effusion is found to control both effusion and superficial pleural seeding.

Surgical resection is the treatment of choice for neurogenic tumors. Differentiation between a benign and malignant neurogenic tumor is based on its growth, appearance at surgery, and histologic examination of the resected specimen. Benign tumors are generally well encapsulated and easily removed in their entirety. If malignant tumors are suspected by the presence of infiltration and erosion of the sur-

rounding structures, whether soft tissue or bone, a complete resection should be done whenever possible to encompass all involved tissues. In addition, it might be necessary to do a partial resection of ribs and vertebral bodies. When resection is incomplete, radiation therapy is also given either internally or externally, to the tumor bed.

Treatment of a germ cell tumor depends on whether it is benign or malignant. Benign (adult) teratomas are easily excised, and this is curative. Treatment of seminomas (germinomas) of the mediastinum is by surgery and radiation therapy consisting of 2000 to 3000 rad over 2 to 3 weeks applied to the mediastinum as well as to the supraclavicular, infraclavicular, and low cervical lymph nodes (20). Nonseminomatous and mixed germ cell tumors are treated by resection of the tumor as much as possible, followed by combination chemotherapy.

Mesenchymal tumors are also treated by surgical section. Section of lipomas, fibromas, myxomas, and encapsulated leiomyomas and leiomyosarcomas in curative. Complete excision of fibrosarcomas or liposarcomas is usually not possible because of invasion of surrounding tissues. Repeated surgical excision and radiation in patients with liposarcomas might extend survival, but fibrosarcomas are not sensitive to radiation therapy or chemotherapy and the prognosis is dismal (21).

Superior Vena Cava Syndrome

The superior vena cava (SVC) syndrome is an acute or subacute oncologic emergency with typical clinical features that require prompt action (25). The incidence of SVC syndrome has been reported to vary from 3 to 8% in patients with carcinoma of the lung and malignant lymphomas (24–26). Approximately 75 to 80% of cases of SVC syndrome are caused by bronchogenic carcinoma, and lymphomas account for almost all remaining cases (24–26). Rarely, the syndrome occurs with fibrosing mediastinitis and by retrosternal thyroid and aortic aneurysms.

Pathophysiology

The pathophysiology of SVC syndrome is related to obstruction of venous drainage in the upper part of the thorax. Increased venous pressure leads to dilation and distension of collateral veins, facial plethora, conjunctival edema with or without proptosis, and various central nervous system (CNS) symptoms, such as moderate to severe headache, visual disturbances, and altered states of consciousness (27). The CNS effects are ascribed to increased intracranial pressure secondary to SVC obstruction.

The vulnerability of the SVC to compression from mediastinal lesions is related to the thinness of the vessel walls and to the low venous pressure (25, 28). The SVC is located in a tight compartment of the anterior-superior mediastinum behind the rigid sternum, adjacent to the right main stem bronchus and completely encircled by chains of lymph nodes that drain all the structures of the right thoracic cavity and the lower part of the left cavity. Anterior to the SVC lie the right anterior mediastinal nodes and posterior to it lie the right lateral or paratracheal nodes.

The azygos vein, the main auxiliary vessel to the SVC, is also threatened by enlarged paratracheal nodes. In some patients the SVC syndrome is associated with spinal cord compression, which occurs because of the proximity of these structures (25).

Perez and co-workers (27) studied 84 patients with SVC syndrome and noted that it was caused by bronchogenic carcinoma in 80% of patients, by lymphomas in 17%, and by other cancers in about 3%. Of the cases caused by lung cancer, small cell undifferentiated cancer was responsible in 46%, epidermoid carcinoma in 25%, large cell carcinoma in 15%, adenocarcinoma in 12%, and other malignant lesions in 3%.

Symptoms and Signs

In the analysis of their 84 patients, Perez and colleagues (27) noted vein distension in the thorax in 67%, vein distension in the neck in 59%, edema of the face in 56%, tachypnea in 40%, plectora of the face in 19%, cyanosis in 15%, and edema of the upper extremity in 10%. Chest pain occurred in 20% of patients, as did cough and dysphagia. Many patients also experienced severe intractable head pain caused by the marked increase in intracranial pressure, which was not relieved by potent opioids.

Diagnosis

The clinical diagnosis of SVC syndrome is usually apparent without the use of extensive diagnostic tests (25). Chest films show a mass in the right side of the superior mediastinum, pulmonary lesions of hilar adenopathy, or both. Mediastinal tomography can further delineate the mass and show obstruction of the tracheobronchial tree, but should not be pursued at the expense of prompt treatment of the condition. Venography might be contraindicated because interruption of the integrity of the vessel wall in the presence of increased intraluminal pressure can result in excessive bleeding from the puncture site (25). Invasive diagnostic procedures such as bronchoscopy, esophagoscopy, mediastinoscopy, scalene node biopsy, and exploratory thoracotomy are needed to establish a histopathologic diagnosis of the extent of the disease. Such studies can only be pursued, however, if abnormal tissues are superficial and readily accessible or if the syndrome is stable, slowly progressive, or has been found relatively early in its clinical stage. If the SVC syndrome presents as an oncologic emergency, such investigations should be deferred and immediate therapy carried out to alleviate the symptoms. Once this is done, a diagnostic biopsy procedure can be performed. Perez and associates (27) noted that a 100% positive diagnosis could be established in 19 patients who had thoracotomy and biopsy and in 4 patients who had pleural effusion and in whom pleural fluid cytology was done. They noted that sputum cytology, bronchoscopy, bronchial washing, and biopsy of palpable supraclavicular nodes yielded the correct diagnosis in about 70% of patients.

Treatment

The SVC syndrome can be treated by radiation therapy, chemotherapy, surgery, and medical measures, including anticoagulation (25). High-dose radiation consisting of two to four large initial fractions of 300 to 400 rad followed by additional daily doses of 180 to 200 rad, up to a total dose of 3000 to 3500 rad, produced improvement within 15 days in 70% of patients, compared to 50% of patients treated with the conventional radiation dosage of 180 to 200 rad/day (25). With such treatment complete symptomatic relief is produced, including resolution of dyspnea, facial edema, and neck vein distension in 75% of patients with malignant lymphoma, compared to 20% of patients with bronchogenic carcinoma.

Chemotherapy has been used in connection with radiation therapy; in cases in which radiation tolerance of the mediastinum has been reached, it has been used as a primary therapeutic procedure. Primary chemotherapy as the sole form of treatment is especially indicated in those with SVC syndrome resulting from small cell carcinoma of the lung (25). Direct surgical intervention with a bypass graft of the SVC obstruction has the advantage of rapid removal of the obstruction and has an ancillary benefit with tissue diagnosis, but the mortality rate is considerable, with a high incidence of complications, including hemorrhage. Medical measures, including anticoagulation with fibrinolytic drugs as a complement to radiotherapy, have been found to produce more rapid clinical improvement and prolong survival than therapy without them (25). Steroids are of limited efficacy and can be used in the presence of respiratory complications. Patients with increased intracranial pressure associated with severe headache should be given large IV doses of dexamethasone (Decadron) and methylprednisolone (Medrol) followed by 50 g of mannitol given IV either as a bolus or in a 20% sterile water solution.

Cancer of the Breast

Epidemiology

Cancer of the breast causes more deaths among American women than any other malignancy. The American Cancer Society estimated 130,000 new cases of breast cancer in women and 900 in men in 1987, about a 6% increase over the previous year (5) (Table 57-1). It has been estimated that about 1 out of 10 women will develop breast cancer some time during her life (29). It was also estimated that in 1987 breast cancer killed 41,000 women and 300 men, thus making breast cancer second only to lung cancer as the foremost cause of cancer deaths in American women.

The mortality from breast cancer is about five times as high in North America and northern Europe as in many Asian and African countries, with seven European and South American countries having intermediate rates. Rates among American blacks are a little different from those among white women (5).

Etiology

The principal risk factors for breast cancer include menstrual and reproductive history, family history, and history of benign breast disease (29–31). Except for a plateau at age 50, the risk of breast cancer increases with the patient's age. Moreover, early menstruation, late menopause (after 55), and irregularity in menstrual cycle all appear to be factors that increase a woman's chances of developing breast cancer.

Castration, either by surgery or radiotherapy prior to the age of 35, is associated with a reduction of risk to one-third of that experienced by women undergoing a natural menopause (32). Women who bear their first child before the age of 18 have one-third the risk of those who bear their first child after the age of 30.

Women who have a first-degree relative with breast cancer have a risk two to three times greater than those in the general female population (33). Women whose female relatives were premenopausal when they developed breast cancer, particularly if it was bilateral, are at greatest risk.

A history of benign chronic breast conditions, particularly those associated with epithelial hyperplasia, increases the risk as much as fourfold. This increase appears to last at least 30 years after the diagnosis of benign disease (34).

Other risk factors include high animal fat intake, obesity, exposure of the breast to ionizing radiation, and the intake of exogenous estrogens for the relief of menopausal symptoms (29, 30). Other factors that have been suggested but not proven include the use of reserpine to control hypertension and hair dyes and other chemicals frequently used by women.

Pathology

HISTOLOGIC CONSIDERATIONS. The most common forms of breast cancer include infiltrating duct-NOS (not otherwise specified), medullary, lobular invasive, and colloid or mucinous tumors (29, 30). These histologic types are generally seen in their pure form, but can also appear in combination. Rare histologic types of breast cancer include tubular, adenocystic, papillary, and carcinosarcoma tumors. Although tumors can arise from any of the three anatomic units of the female breast (i.e., small, medium, and large ducts), carcinoma of the breast most frequently arises in a large duct. Hellman and associates (29) suggested that no distinct histologic structure can be distinguished; such infiltrating duct carcinomas, which comprise 70 to 75% of breast tumors, have been designated as NOS.

Medullary carcinomas comprise about 6% of all breast cancers and, unlike intraductal carcinoma, are of a large size but are not likely to infiltrate. Another slow-growing invasive carcinoma that becomes large and bulky is colloid carcinoma, a mucin-producing tumor that comprises about 3% of breast cancers.

Lobular carcinoma, which makes up about 5% of breast cancers, arises in the small end ducts and can either be invasive or noninvasive. In the noninvasive type, carcinoma in situ, the anaplastic cells are contained within the lubules, whereas in the invasive form the tumor extends beyond the lobule or end ducts from which it arises (30).

Two special manifestations of breast cancer are Paget's disease, seen in 1 to 4% of all patients with breast cancer, and inflammatory breast cancer. In Paget's disease the nipple epithelium contains nests of tumor cells, but the tumor can either be intraductal or of the invasive duct type. Inflammatory breast cancer is characterized clinically by skin redness and warmth and a visible erysipeloid margin on the underlying breast.

An important breast tumor characteristic is multicentricity indicating that microscopic foci of invasive and noninvasive tumors can be detected in about 13% of patients in quadrants of the breast other than that in which the primary lesion was diagnosed; therefore, such tumors are regarded as independent cancers (30). Hellman and associates (29) noted that the clinical significance of such lesions is unclear because it is unusual for multiple cancers in a single breast to become clinically overt or for bilateral cancers to occur synchronously. This issue should be resolved after the long-term follow-up of women who are currently undergoing clinical trials of segmental resection of the breast with or without radiation. Obviously, if segmental mastectomy proves equally as effective in terms of curability, it should be cosmetically more acceptable and therefore preferable.

METASTATIC SPREAD. The most common routes of breast cancer metastasis are the axillary, internal mammary, supraclavicular, and intercostal regional lymph nodes. Breast cancer can metastasize to various organs. In two studies of autopsies (35, 36) it was suggested that the most common sites of metastasis are the following: liver and lungs, involved in 60 to 70% of cases; bones, 45 to 70%; pleura and adrenals, 30 to 50%; and kidneys, spleen, pancreas, ovaries, uterus, brain, and thyroid, 15 to 25%. Less common sites are the heart, diaphragm, pericardium, intestines, peritoneum, and skin.

Metastases to the skeleton are frequently associated with local pain or neuropathic pain, or with both. Metastasis to the rib can cause local or intercostal neuralgia while metastasis to the vertebral column is likely to produce brachial or lumbosacral plexopathy and epidural cord compression, all of which can result in severe intractable pain. Table 57-6 lists the sites of skeletal metastasis from breast cancer in studies done by Lenz and Freid (37), Galasko (38), and Schider (39). In one study, Greenberg and colleagues (40) found that in 43 patients with metastasis to the base of the skull, cancer of the breast was the primary tumor in 17. Another study by Greenberg and associates (41) in regard to the incidence of epidural spinal cord compression (ESCC) found that cancer of the breast was the primary tumor that produced ESCC in 14% of cases in the cervical region, in 79% of cases in the thoracic region, and in 7% of cases in the lumbosacral region (see below, Management of Cancer-Related Chest Pain).

Symptoms and Signs

The symptoms and signs associated with breast cancer are determined by the size of the cancer and by the site of metastasis. Tumors smaller than 2 cm in diameter are generally associated with the most favorable outcome and rarely cause pain or other symptoms. Larger tumors can be associated with a dull aching pain that is localized to the chest in the region of the breast and is probably caused by compression or irritation of nociceptive nerve endings in the underlying soft tissue. Metastasis to regional lymph nodes occurs in 38% of patients with lesions that are 1 cm or smaller whereas it occurs in 70% of patients with lesions that are 5.5 cm or larger (30). A correlation exists between increased tumor size and the presence of four or more positive axillary lymph nodes involved in the tumor. Generally, small regional lymph nodes that are involved do not produce pain or other symptoms. If they are large they can cause localized pain in the axilla and, if the intercostobrachial nerve or one or more of the major nerves to the upper limb is compressed or irritated, patients experience burning,

TABLE 57-6. Sites of Skeletal Metastasis from Breast Cancer

Parameter	Source		
	Lenz and Freid (37)	Galasko (38)	Schider (39)
Number of patients	81*	100 (no. of bones involved)†	50‡
Site of metastasis (% of total patients studied)			
Ribs	40	35 (134)	62
Pelvis	63	57 (85)	66
Skull	35	12	44
Femur	55	24 (34)	44
Humerus	27	8 (9)	14
Clavicle and scapula		3 (3)	10
Vertebrae:			
Cervical		18 (37)	26
Thoracic		42 (142)	72
Lumbar		41 (101)	68

*Studied by radiography and autopsy.
†Studied by scintigraphy in 100 early and late breast cancers.
‡Studied by scintigraphy in 50 advanced breast cancers.

aching pain accompanied by bouts of lancinating pain. Patients who neglect seeing a physician can present with necrosis and ulceration of the skin and deeper tissues of the breast associated with a severe burning aching pain that is predominantly in the affected region, but that can radiate to the anterior chest and axilla.

Metastases to bones and various viscera are associated with pain and other symptoms and signs, depending on the site. Of particular importance are metastasis to the ribs, which produces localized chest pain frequently associated with intercostal neuralgia, and metastasis to the vertebral column, which often produces pain localized in the back or signs of ESCC, with consequent back and radicular pain. Radicular pain also occurs with metastatic fracture and sudden compression of the spinal nerve. Invasion of the brachial plexus results in metastatic brachial plexopathy. These and other pain syndromes are discussed in more detail in the second section of this chapter.

Diagnosis

SCREENING. Because the earlier clinical stages of breast cancer have a more favorable outcome, the National Cancer Institute, the American Cancer Society, and other agencies have placed major emphasis on developing methods for screening large populations for cancer. In approximately 90% of cases, the breast mass is found by the patient herself during deliberate or accidental self-examination. In the remaining 10% the tumor is found during examination by a physician or by mass screening. The value of mass screening was demonstrated by a study carried out by the Health Insurance Plan (HIP) of New York. The screening included both mammography and physical examination in 62,000 patients (42). A 9-year follow-up period showed a 30% reduction in the mortality rate for women 50 years or older who had been screened compared to those in a control group. Although some concern has been expressed about the risk of exposing large numbers of women to ionizing radiation, high-quality mammography can now be performed that exposes the patient to a radiation dose no greater than 0.01 Gy. Currently it is recommended that mammography be done annually for women over 50 years of age and for women from 40 to 49 years old who are considered at high risk, defined as anyone who has had prior breast cancer or a mother or sibling with the disease.

MEDICAL HISTORY AND PHYSICAL EXAMINATION. Once breast tumor is suspected or indicated, a complete medical history and thorough physical examination followed by biopsy or needle aspiration should be carried out (30). It is most important to elicit information about when the patient first noted pain and mass in the breast and about breast and axillary symptoms, such as discharge from the nipple, nipple or skin retraction, axillary mass or pain, and arm swelling (30). The medical history should elicit information about the following: prior breast disease, including prior biopsy; details of the reproductive history, such as age of onset of menses and frequency, duration, and regularity of menstrual periods; age at first pregnancy and number of pregnancies, children, and abortions; history of breast feeding; age at onset of menopause; history of hormone use, including birth control pills; if the patient has any other signs and symptoms, particularly those related to possible metastasis, the family history should be obtained for information about the diagnosis and death of family members with breast cancer.

The physical examination should include the following: careful evaluation of the breast mass, including size, location, shape, consistency, and fixation to skin, pectoral muscle, or chest wall; skin changes such as erythema, edema, dimpling, and satellite nodules; and nipple changes, such as retraction, discoloration, thickening, reddening, and erosion. Examination of the axillary lymph nodes should determine the number, location, size, fixation to other nodes or underlying structures, and whether infraclavicular fullness, supraclavicular nodes, or areas of swelling are present.

In 75% of patients in whom a tumor is detected the lesions are benign. About 75% of the other 25% of patients present with a hard circumscribed mass in the breast. If the mass is fixed to the skin or deep muscle, or if edema of the skin or retraction of the nipple is present, cancer is almost a certainty (30). In 45% of

TABLE 57-7. Breast Cancer Clinical Stages and Prognosis

Stage	American Joint Committee Staging	Approximate Frequency of Stage at Presentation (%)	Approximate 5-Year Survival (%)
I	Primary tumor <2 cm; nodes, if palpable, not felt to contain metastases; no distant metastases	55–70	80
II	Primary tumor >2 cm and <5 cm; nodes, if palpable, not fixed; no distant metastases evident	20–25	65
III	Tumor >5 cm or fixed to chest wall or skin invasion present; supraclavicular nodes palpable; no distant metastases evident	10	40
IV	Distant metastases	10	10

From Henney, J.E., and DeVita, V.T., Jr.: Breast cancer. *In* Harrison's Principles of Internal Medicine. 11th Ed. Edited by E. Braunwald et al. New York, McGraw-Hill, 1987, p. 1568.

patients breast cancer presents in the upper outer quadrant of the breast, in 25% it is in the central or subareolar portion of the breast, in 15% it is in the upper inner quadrant, and in 5% it is in the lower inner quadrant (30). A mobile mass with well-defined margins in a woman under 30 years old is likely to be a benign fibroadenoma. Table 57-7 lists the clinical staging and prognosis of patients with breast cancer.

OTHER TESTS. In addition to the physical examination it is necessary to perform posteroanterior and lateral radiography of the chest, a complete blood count, and liver chemistry tests. Although a radionuclide scan is a sensitive test for the detection of early bone metastasis, its diagnostic value in asymptomatic patients with early breast cancer is small (29, 30). Similarly, a positive pretreatment liver scan is even less accurate in regard to diagnosis than a bone scan. Hellman and associates (29) emphasized that a positive bone or liver scan does not necessarily establish metastatic disease. On the other hand, brain and CT scanning of the head are both sensitive tests for detecting early metastatic involvement.

Treatment

STAGE I AND STAGE II BREAST CANCER. Until a decade or so ago radical mastectomy, entailing the removal of the breast, the pectoralis major, and minor muscles, and the ipsilateral axillary lymph nodes, and the ipsilateral supraclavicular and mediastinal lymph chains in medial lesions was considered to be the only treatment for breast cancer. Many clinical trials have shown, however, that breast cancer is localized only briefly and then disseminates simultaneously into the circulatory and lymphatic channels early in its course. Consequently, the current method of therapy involves removal of the primary site of tumor with the minimum disfigurement necessary to obtain local control and control of the microscopic foci of disease with adjuvant therapies (29, 30).

Results of clinical trials have shown that various other surgical approaches produce survival rates similar to those in patients treated with radical mastectomy while obtaining a more acceptable cosmetic result. These include the following: *modified radical mastectomy*, in which the pectoralis muscles are spared but the axillary dissection is done en bloc; *total simple mastectomy*, in which both the pectoralis muscles and axillary nodes are spared; *segmental mastectomy and tylectomy*, which entail removal of the primary tumor and a minimal amount of surrounding tissues to preserve most of the breast (both are appropriate for women who have lesions smaller than 2 cm located in the periphery of the breast); and *quadrantectomy*, which involves the removal of the breast quadrant in which the lesion is located together with the overlying skin and the fascia of the pectoralis major (also done in women who have lesions smaller than 2 cm).

Adjuvant therapies for stages I and II breast cancer include postoperative radiation therapy and chemotherapy. Postoperative radiation therapy can reduce the overall local regional recurrence rate to less than 5% but does not increase the overall survival rate (29, 30). Patients who have received adjuvant chemotherapy have a similar incidence of local regional recurrence but the additional benefit of longer survival (30).

DISSEMINATING BREAST CANCER. Although only about 10% of patients have stage IV breast cancer, about one-third to one-half of all breast cancer patients treated with surgery or radiation alone eventually experience a recurrence of the disease that becomes widespread. It is necessary to assess the size, location, and rate of progression of the cancer and the status of the estrogen receptor (ER) protein to select the optimum method of therapy. Hormone manipulation therapy aims to abolish estrogen or estrogen precursors; it includes the use of antiestrogens, castration, adrenalectomy or hypophysectomy, estrogen, and androgens. An antiestrogen such as tamoxifen 10 mg bid is considered the drug of choice, and produces a good response in 60% of patients who are ER-positive, except in those with hepatic metastasis who respond poorly (29, 30). Castration should be considered in premenopausal women who relapse after having had a good response to tamoxifen and who have no evidence of hepatic metastasis or lymphatic spread to the lungs (30). About 50% of ER-positive women respond to this therapy. Adrenalectomy or hypophysectomy should be considered for premenopausal patients who have a recurrence of the cancer after having responded to antiestrogen, or castration, or both. About 50% of patients who were previously hormone-sensitive respond to such treatment.

Patients who have failed or exhausted prior hormonal manipulation or who are ER-negative, and those with visceral disease that is progressing rapidly, should be considered for chemotherapy. Although single-agent chemotherapy produces a partial response in 20 to 40% of patients, best results are achieved with combination chemotherapy (30). This and other therapeutic procedures have been discussed in detail by Hellman and co-workers (29) and by others (30, 43). The efficacy of surgical therapy, hormonal manipulation, and chemotherapy for relieving pain is shown in Tables 24-7, 24-8, and 24-9.

B. MANAGEMENT OF CANCER-RELATED CHEST PAIN

In Chapter 24 data are presented to show that cancer of the tracheobronchial tree and lung is associated with pain in 35 to 60% (mean 50%) of patients with early and intermediate stages of the disease, and pain occurs in about 60 to 85% of patients with advanced or terminal cancer. Table 24-4 lists data from six reports indicating a 73% incidence (mean) of pain among patients with advanced or terminal lung cancer. Using these figures along with the 1987 estimates from the American Cancer Society (5) suggests that 103,000 of the approximately 206,000 patients in the prevalence group (new and old cases) had pain, and about 99,000 of the 136,000 who died (and therefore were in the advanced or terminal stage of the disease) had pain; in over 70% of these the pain was moderate to severe.

Neoplasms of the mediastinum produce retrosternal chest pain in only a small percentage of the patients, but those few who develop the SVC syndrome experience moderate to severe headache. Early cancer of the breast also produces only moderate pain in a small percentage of patients but, as shown in Table 24-3, advancing breast cancer causes pain in 56 to 100% of patients, with a mean of 74%. Using these figures with the 1987 estimates by the American Cancer Society (5) suggests that between 50,000 and 60,000 of those in the prevalence group (new and old cases) had mild to moderate pain and 30,000 of those in the advanced and terminal stages had moderate to severe pain.

General Principles

The initial approach to the treatment of pain caused by cancer of the lungs, mediastinum, or breast involves the use of oncologic therapies discussed above, including surgery, radiation therapy, chemotherapy, and hormone therapy. Their value in regard to curing patients and eliminating the cause of pain have also been discussed. Their efficacy as palliative measures, particularly for relieving pain, are listed in Tables 24-9, 24-10, and 24-11.

During the course of either curative or palliative anticancer therapy the patient's pain should be managed effectively but this is usually not done, because many oncologists believe that the pain is an important criterion for monitoring and assessing the usefulness of the oncologic therapy. Although this point has validity it is not necessary for patients to suffer severe pain because sufficient amounts of analgesics can be given to provide good but not complete pain relief. With proper titration of the analgesics, patients can have a sustained degree of mild pain that disappears completely when the oncologic therapy has been successfully completed.

In patients in whom oncologic therapy fails to relieve the pain, effective pain control should be carried out by using the various pharmacologic, psychologic, physical, chemical, and neurosurgical techniques discussed in Chapter 24. Proper selection of the therapy or, more frequently, combination of therapies, requires a thorough evaluation of the pain and of the physical, psychologic, and psychosocial status of the patient, as well as of the personnel and therapeutic procedures available. Because cancer of the lungs, trachea, bronchi and breast produce various pain syndromes that have different characteristics and are caused by different pathophysiologic mechanisms, the management of specific pain syndromes is discussed separately.

Pain Syndromes

In the first edition of this book I discussed a number of pain syndromes caused by cancer of the lung, mediastinum, and breast (44). These included the following: superior pulmonary sulcus tumor (Pancoast's) syndrome; the costopleural syndrome; the tracheothoracic syndrome (pain in the chest produced by cancer of the trachea and main stem bronchi); peripheral pain syndromes caused by metastatic lesions in the bones and other organs; headache and other head pain caused by compression of the superior vena cava in the chest; and a visceral type of pain syndrome. In addition, I mentioned the occurrence of chronic pain following thoracotomy and mastectomy and that associated with metastatic and postradiation brachial plexopathy.

About 25 years later, Turnbull (45) reported on the incidence of some of these syndromes among 280 patients admitted to the Cancer Control Agency of British Columbia (formerly the B.C. Cancer Institute) for palliative treatment of the pain after being considered incurable. These patients were in two groups; one group, studied in 1960, consisted of 100 consecutive patients with lung cancer who were only studied when first seen, when the diagnosis of incurable cancer was established. Turnbull studied the pattern of pain and related this to the clinical evidence and to autopsy findings, which prompted him to conclude that six syndromes were possible: (a) no pain; (b) substernal pain syndrome; (c) deep lateral pain syndrome; (d) brachial pain syndrome; (e) costplural pain syndrome; and (f) peripheral pain syndrome. At the initial visit 71% had one of the five pain syndromes while 29% had no pain. Because the data did not provide information regarding pain during treatment and before death, a second survey of 180 consecutive patients was initiated in 1970. In this group 32 patients (18%) developed new pain during the treatment, 81 patients (45%) had persistent pain when treatment of the disease ended, and 117 (65%) had persistent pain during their last 2 months of life.

In 1981 an international symposium on the superior pulmonary sulcus syndrome was held in Italy to discuss the symptoms and signs and treatment of this condition (46). Kanner and associates (47) analyzed the incidence of pain and other symptoms and signs and reviewed the most pertinent literature. (See below, Pancoast's Syndrome).

In 1987 Watson and Evans (48) reported on the largest number of patients to date (221) with intractable pain associated with lung cancer. In this retrospective study they examined the natural history, classification, clinical and pathologic features, and results of treatment of intractable pain of these patients, who had been referred to their pain clinic for relief. In 189 patients (86%) the pain was related to cancer, in 11 (5%) the pain was related to cancer treatment (post-thoracotomy neuralgia), in 9 (4%) no obvious pathologic cause for the pain was seen, and in 12 (5.4%) the pain was unrelated to cancer. Of the 189 patients in whom the intractable pain was related to cancer, the pain was caused by skeletal metastasis in 64 (34%), the pain was part of Pancoast's syndrome in 50 (31%), the pain was caused by invasion of soft tissue in ribs and the chest wall in 26 (14%), the pain was caused by intra-abdominal metastasis to the liver, adrenal, or retroperitoneal space in 19 (10%), and the pain was a result of metastasis to other structures, including the cerebrum, epidural space, esophagus, and SVC compression in 22 (11.6%). Additional information on these patients is discussed below for each specific syndrome.

Foley, Posner, and associates (41, 49–52) have also studied pain syndromes in the chest and upper limbs caused by metastasis from lung and breast (and other cancers) and by cancer therapy. These include plexopathy resulting from cancer and radiation therapy (49), epidural spinal cord compression (41), the postmastectomy syndrome (50), the post-thoracotomy syndrome, and other syndromes listed in Table 24-7 and discussed elsewhere (52).

Most published reports on chest pain caused by cancer of the lung and breast pertain to persistent or intractable pain in patients with advanced disease. Little information is available about pain characteristics such as site, quality, intensity, duration, and response to therapy in the early stages of disease. This is not surprising because, as mentioned above, most patients have advanced disease by the time lung cancer is diagnosed. Although only 10% of patients with breast cancer have negative signs with stage III and another 10% with stage IV, some 50 to 65% eventually have recurrence of the disease, including metastasis to various organs (see above).

The following discussion of various specific pain syndromes is based on the aforementioned reports, review of other published reports, and personal experience during the past 45 years. The following syndromes are discussed in order of their listing:

a. Superior pulmonary sulcus (Pancoast's) syndrome
b. Other cancer-related brachial plexus syndromes
c. Costopleural syndrome
d. Pain syndromes caused by vertebral metastasis
e. Postmastectomy pain syndrome
f. Post-thoracotomy syndrome
g. Epidural spinal cord compression (ESCC)

Although the superior pulmonary sulcus (Pancoast's) syndrome and metastatic and postradiation plexopathy produce pain predominantly in one or both of the upper limbs and less in the upper chest, they are considered here in detail because cancer of the lung and breast are the most common causes of these syndromes. The costopleural syndrome and the pain syndrome resulting from vertebral metastasis are frequent causes of pain in the chest, and the latter can also cause metastatic brachial plexopathy. Because the diagnostic procedures and therapy for controlling pain in the first four syndromes listed are similar, they are discussed after the epidemiology, pathology, and symptoms and signs have been described for each condition separately.

Superior Pulmonary Sulcus (Pancoast's) Syndrome (IX-12)

Historical Overview

The symptoms and signs of cancer of the superior pulmonary sulcus have probably been known since ancient times, but the first report published in the English literature was by E.S. Hare in 1838 (53). I have reviewed the literature and found that, during the ensuing 80 years, other writers, including Colby of Montreal, Schmidt of Vienna, Ricaldoni of Italy, and Freeman of the United States, mentioned that lesions of the apex of the lung produce pain in the shoulder and inside the arm (see 46).

In 1924, H.K. Pancoast, an American radiologist, called attention to the importance of careful radiologic investigation of "apical chest tumors" by reporting on three patients whose chest radiographs showed a homogeneous density at the apex of the lung, with destruction of the upper two or three ribs and with pain in the shoulder and arm associated with wasting of the hand muscles, a contracted pupil, and drooping of the eyelid (54). Pancoast suggested that the tumor was separate from the lung and it was subsequently called Pancoast's tumor. Eight years later Pancoast published his classic paper, Superior Pulmonary Sulcus Tumor, in which he reported on four additional patients who had similar symptoms and signs and clinical findings (55). In this report Pancoast defined such tumors as always occurring "at a definite location at the thoracic inlet" and characterized clinically by "pain around the shoulder and down the inner side of the arm and often the ulnar side of the forearm, loss of power and wasting of the muscles of the hand, Horner's syndrome, and signs mainly of dullness in the apex of the chest." Pancoast postulated that it arose from extrapulmonary structures such as embryonic epithelial rests of branchial clefts that formed an abnormal sulcus in the apex of the lung, hence the name "superior pulmonary sulcus tumor." Subsequently, the symptoms and signs became known as Pancoast's syndrome, or superior pulmonary sulcus syndrome.

During the ensuing decades others reported the same symptoms and signs and central features caused by primary carcinoma of the lung, metastatic pulmonary tumors, and other types of neoplasm, while still others reported the syndrome associated with tuberculosis, pulmonary abscess, laryngeal and branchial cleft tumors, myeloma, trauma, cervical rib, and neoplasms of the cervical sympathetic ganglia. Notwithstanding these reports, which have caused confusion among nononcologic practitioners, Paulson (56), an outstanding American authority on the subject, stressed that, in many cases, the superior pulmonary sulcus syndrome is caused by bronchogenic carcinoma of the apex of the lung.

Epidemiology and Pathology

Berrino (57) carried out an epidemiologic survey of Pancoast's tumor and reviewed two dozen reports. The data revealed that Pancoast's syndrome is found in 3 to 5% of patients with pulmonary tumors, suggesting that in 1987 between 6000 and 10,000 patients in the United States with lung cancer had Pancoast's tumor. Berrino also found that histologic types of pulmonary carcinoma were associated with Pancoast's syndrome, as follows: epidermoid (squamous cell) carcinoma, 48%; adenocarcinoma, 22%; anaplastic carcinoma with large cells, 19%; and microcytoma, mixed tumors, and other rare tumors, 11%. Data from 11 reports indicated that the male:female ratio was 9:1 and the mean age at the time of diagnosis was between 54 and 58 years.

Kanner and associates (47) reported that, of 962 patients with lung cancer, 30 (3%) had tumor of the superior pulmonary sulcus. In this group of 30 patients the male:female ratio was 23:7 and the mean age was 56 years. All the patients had primary carcinoma of the lung; 12 of them had adenocarcinoma, 10 had epidermoid (squamous cell) carcinoma, 4 had poorly differentiated carcinoma, 1 had small cell carcinoma, 1 had mixed cell carcinoma, and 2 were unclassified.

Symptoms and Signs

Table 57-8 summarizes data on the incidence of the various symptoms and signs of Pancoast's tumor (47, 48, 55). Of the 688 patients, 90 to 100% had severe intractable pain. In Pancoast's tumor it begins as a moderate to severe, deep, aching pain felt in the shoulder, scapula, medial aspect of the forearm and hand and, less frequently, the medial upper arm. Figure 57-4

depicts the distribution of pain in the 58 patients studied by Watson and Evans (48); as noted, it was common for the pain to occur at a single site in the chest or arm (65% of patients) and, in those in the group with more than one site, the combination of scapular and shoulder pain was most frequent.

The pain is caused by compression and infiltration of the lower part of the brachial plexus and eventually becomes severe or excruciating and neuralgic in quality, often associated with lancinating pain—symptoms of deafferentation pain. Although a few reports suggested that pain occurs in less than 50% of patients, most published reports indicated that 80 to 100% of patients had pain, which occurs early (47). Thus, Watson and Evans (48) reported that, in their 58 patients, the median interval between the diagnosis and pain onset was 0. It is generally agreed that persistent or recurrent pain is a harbinger of progressive disease.

Pancoast (54) reported that Horner's syndrome was present in all of his patients, but subsequent published reports indicated that the incidence varies from 35 to 90% (47, 58). I believe that a mean of 45 to 60% approximates the actual incidence. Some clinicians have reported that, in the early phases of disease, patients manifest the opposite of Horner's syndrome (mydriasis and hyperhydrosis), presumably because of irritation of the uppermost thoracic and lower cervical parts of the sympathetic chain. As the tumor enlarges and expands medially, the chain is first compressed and later destroyed with a Horner's syndrome that becomes permanent.

Because the superior pulmonary sulcus is directly below (subjacent) to the lower trunk of the brachial plexus, as the tumor grows it first irritates and then compresses the lower trunk and its C8 and T1 roots and, in some patients, the C7 and T2 roots are also involved. The latter explains the distribution of pain in the axilla and upper part of the medial aspect of the arm, which is supplied by the intercostobrachial nerve.

In addition to the pain, sensory disturbances such as paresthesia, dysesthesia, and hyperpathia and motor deficits are present, with consequent atrophy of those muscles supplied by the ulnar nerve. The muscles involved are the flexor carpi ulnaris, flexor digitorum profundus, muscles of the hypothenar group, adductor pollicis, flexor pollicis brevis, third and fourth

TABLE 57-8. Signs and Symptoms of Pancoast's Tumors in Percentage of Total Patients Studied

Parameter	Source		
	Berrino (57)	**Kanner et al. (47)**	**Watson and Evans (48)**
Number of patients assessed	600	30	58
Symptoms and signs (in % of total patients studied)			
Pain	90	93	100
Horner's syndrome	62	40	58
Brachial plexopathy	65	17 (75)†	40
Spinal cord compression	NS*	20	5
Vocal cord paralysis	NS	3	10
Bone invasion	45	7	NS
Cough, hemoptysis	24	3	NS

*NS, not stated.
†17% at presentation, but 75% eventually developed plexopathy.

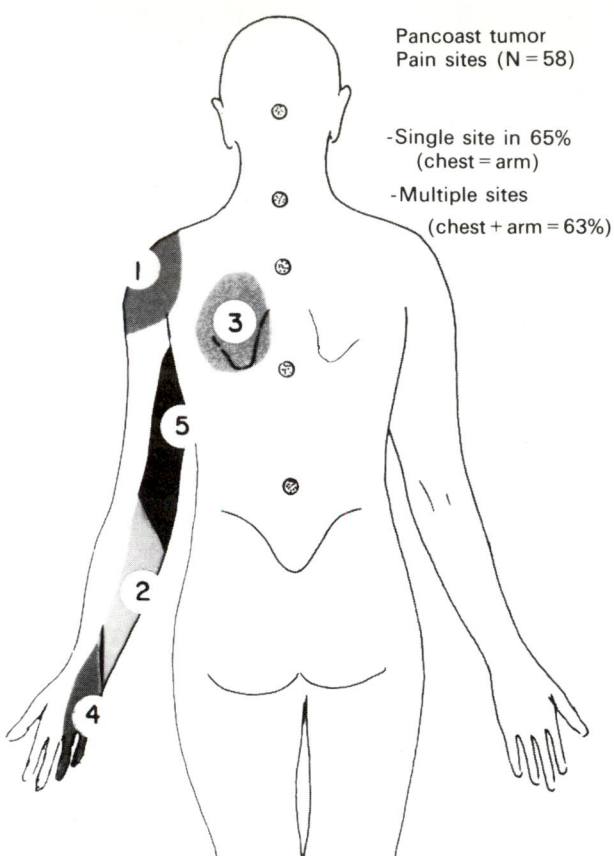

FIG. 57-4. Sites of pain in Pancoast's syndrome in order of frequency. Of 58 patients, 28 (49%) had pain in the shoulder, 24 (41%) in the medial forearm, 23 (40%) in the scapula, 9 (15.5%) in the fourth and fifth fingers, and 4 (7%) in the medial part of the upper arm. From Watson, P.N., and Evans, R.J.: Intractable pain with lung cancer. Pain, *29*:163, 1987.

Pancoast tumor
Pain sites (N = 58)

-Single site in 65%
 (chest = arm)
-Multiple sites
 (chest + arm = 63%)

lumbricales, and all the interossei, both palmar and dorsal, with consequent atrophy of much of the hand. The incidence of brachial plexus involvement noted at time of presentation varies. When the patient presents early the incidence can be low; in most patients, however, a delay of 6 to 12 months or longer occurs before diagnosis (47, 48, 59, 60), so between 65 and 90% of patients have clinical evidence of brachial plexus involvement when they are first seen. Moreover, 5 to 10% have compression of the recurrent laryngeal nerve with consequent hoarseness and, less frequently, cough.

Epidural spinal cord compression (ESCC) occurred in 25% of patients studied, and this more commonly occurred late in the course of the disease (56–58). Kanner and associates (47) found that 1 patient had ESCC at the time of presentation, whereas another 5 developed the condition 2 to 12 months after presentation and after initial therapy for the tumor. The low incidence of definable bony metastatic disease found by Kanner and colleagues (47) and by Galasko (61) suggests that ESCC occurs from tumor growth through the intervertebral foramina along the nerve roots without involvement of bone. This contrasts with the common presentation of ESCC with metastatic vertebral body disease (see below, Epidural Spinal Cord Compression).

Brachial Plexopathy From Other Causes (X-4)

Epidemiology and Pathology

In addition to lung cancer, brachial plexopathy can be caused by metastatic lesions from the breast and other primary tumors or can result from radiation therapy (49, 52). Pain is the most common presenting symptom, with its distribution and neurologic involvement dependent on the site of tumor infiltration. In patients with carcinoma of the breast, tumor infiltration of the brachial plexus can occur with the first symptoms appearing as pain in the shoulder, biceps region, elbow, or hand. Patients who develop tumor infiltration in the supraclavicular region experience burning pain and dysesthesia in the index finger and thumb, indicating involvement of the upper portion of the brachial plexus. A significant number of patients who undergo radiation therapy develop brachial plexopathy that produces pain and other symptoms and signs that make it difficult to differentiate it from tumor infiltration flexopathy (Chapter 24).

Kori and colleagues (49) studied 100 patients with well-documented brachial plexopathy; in 78 patients it was caused by metastatic tumor and in the other 22 it was a result of radiation therapy. These patients were studied to determine whether any differences in symptoms and signs would help to differentiate tumor infiltration from radiation fibrosis. Of the 78 patients who had metastatic lesions 44 had never received radiation therapy to the plexus (group IA), while the other 34 had previously received radiation therapy (group IB). The diagnosis of metastatic plexopathy in these groups was accepted if the following criteria were met: (a) surgical exploration of the plexus revealed tumor; (b) multiple metastases were demonstrated in adjacent lung, clavicle, or vertebral body; and (c) evidence of new and widespread metastatic disease was found. The diagnosis of radiation injury was made if the following criteria were met: (a) surgical exploration of the plexus failed to reveal tumor; (b) follow-up for several years failed to show evidence of tumor recurrence; or (c) radiation had been administered in the absence of any tumor because of incorrect diagnosis (49).

In patients in whom plexopathy was caused by tumor infiltration, in 54 (69%) the primary tumor was in the lung or breast. Of the other 24 patients with other primary tumors, in 16 (20%) the tumors had metastasized to the upper lobe of the corresponding lung before spreading to the plexus, and in 3 the ipsilateral axillary lymph nodes were involved. Tumor metastasis involved the plexus mainly by lymphatic spread of the disease, with tumor most commonly situated in the area drained by the lateral group of the axillary lymph nodes (49–52). Table 57-9 lists the three most important histologic types of primary tumors involved in these patients.

TABLE 57-9. Histology and Symptoms and Signs of Brachial Plexopathy

(Figures in percent of total patients in each group.)

Parameter	Group		
	I: Metastatic		II: Postradiation
	IA	IB	
Total number of patients	44	34	22
Histologic type tumor			
Lung	32	44	14
Breast	30	35	59
Lymphoma	7	9	14
Other	31	12	13
Symptoms			
Pain	75	89	18
Dysesthesia	25	6	55
Weakness of arm	0	6	27
Signs			
Edema of arm	0	0	40
Horner's syndrome	53	56	14
Lymphedema	13	15	73
ESCC	(Both groups: 56)		0
Part of plexus involved			
Upper trunk (C5–C6)	0	9	77
Lower trunk (C8, T1)	75	68	0
Entire plexus (C5–T1)	25	23	23

*ESCC, epidural cord compression.
From Kori, S., Foley, K.M., and Posner, J.B.: Brachial plexus lesions in patients with cancer: Clinical findings in 100 cases. Neurology, *31*:45, 1981.

Symptoms and Signs

The symptoms and signs found by Kori and associates (49) are summarized in Table 57-9. Pain was the most common presenting symptom in those in group I. Pain was of moderate to severe intensity, beginning in the shoulder girdle and radiating to the elbow, medial aspect of the arm, and fourth and fifth fingers, indicating involvement of the lower part of the brachial plexus caused by Pancoast's tumor. In some patients the pain was localized in the posterior aspect of the arm or elbow, while others complained of a burning or freezing sensation and hypersensitivity of the skin along the outer aspects of the hand, suggesting involvement of the upper part of the brachial plexus. About 15% of patients had paresthesia in the ulnar distribution, while others had paresthesia in the distribution of the median nerve. Pain was the first symptom in 89% of those in group IB, preceding other symptoms or neurologic signs, and a correct diagnosis was not made for up to 9 months. In 2 patients in group IB pain was the only symptom of tumor recurrence, and diagnosis was established by exploration and biopsy.

In contrast to this high incidence of pain in patients with metastatic lesions, only 18% of postradiation plexopathy patients presented with pain. Although 65% had some pain later pain was never a major symptom in 35%. The pain had different characteristics in these patients: some patients complained of aching in the shoulder or hand and this symptom was difficult to separate from other more common presenting symptoms, which included paresthesia of the entire hand, swelling and heaviness of the arm, and proximal weakness of the arm. Paresthesia often started in the thumb and forefinger, later extending throughout the rest of the hand. Significant differences in these symptoms were seen between those in the metastatic and postradiation groups.

Significant differences in motor and neurologic signs were also found. Whereas 75% of group I patients had focal weakness, atrophy, or sensory changes in the distribution of the C8 and T1 roots, no group II patients had neurologic findings restricted to these nerves. Similarly, no group IA patients and only 9% of group IB patients had signs limited to the C5 and C6 roots, whereas 77% of the 22 group II patients had involvement of these two roots. Thus, the lower trunk of the brachial plexus is most often involved by metastatic disease while the upper trunk is damaged by radiation therapy. The incidence of involvement of the entire brachial plexus (C5–T1) was similar in all three groups, about 25% for each group.

Significant differences were also found between those in the metastatic group and in the postradiation plexopathy group in regard to the incidence of Horner's syndrome, lymphedema and swelling of the ipsilateral limb, and development of epidural deposits. Epidural deposits were found in 25 (56%) of 45 group I patients in whom myelography was performed, whereas this diagnostic test revealed no epidural deposits in 4 patients with radiation plexopathy. Of the 25 patients with epidural deposits, the epidural disease was consequent to lung cancer in 19 (76%). All 25 patients had Horner's syndrome and 14 (56%) had signs implicating the entire plexus that differed from the lower trunk signs in other group I patients. Moreover, of these 25 patients, vertebral body metastasis was present in 12 (48%), pyramidal tract signs in 10 (40%), and pain localized in vertebrae in 14 (56%). In 4 patients with no clinical signs of epidural tumor this lesion was found by myelography and, in 2 additional patients without clinical signs, ESCC was found at autopsy.

Costopleural Syndrome

The costopleural syndrome is caused by tumor invasion of the pleura, soft tissue and ribs of the chest wall, and frequently the intercostal nerves. This is the most frequently occurring syndrome that develops in patients with cancer of the lung, and can occur early in the disease. Metastasis to the pleura and chest wall occurs in about 50 to 60% of patients with epidermoid and small cell carcinoma and in 75 to 85% of patients with adenocarcinoma and large cell carcinoma (17). Turnbull (45) reported that this syndrome was present in less than 20% of patients when first seen but was found in nearly 22% of 280 patients seen during their last 2 months of life. Of 189 patients with pain caused by lung cancer managed by Watson and Evans (48), 58 (31%) had this syndrome. Of 101 patients seen by Deely (60), costopleural pain secondary to apical and other lung tumors was experienced by about 50% of patients.

The costopleural syndrome is infrequent in patients with primary mediastinal neoplasm. Metastasis from breast cancer to the pleura, however, occurs in 35 to 50% of patients (35, 36). Lenz and Freid (37) reported metastasis to the ribs in 40% of 81 patients studied by radiography and autopsy. In one series of 100 patients with breast cancer (50 early, 50 advanced), radionuclide bone scans revealed skeletal lesions in 24% of patients with early disease and in 84% of those with advanced disease (39). A total of 134 metastases were found in the ribs of 35 patients (38). In advanced breast cancer the ribs were involved in 62% of patients (see Table 57-6). Regardless of the primary tumor, metastasis to the pleura and chest wall produces pain that can have different characteristics, depending on the tissue involved.

THE PLEURA. Involvement of the pleura produces pleuritic irritation that causes a sharp aching or burning pain, localized in the chest wall anterolaterally or posteriorly and overlying the pathologic process (Fig. 57-5). If the process involves the diaphragmatic pleura, the patient experiences a well-localized sharp or aching pain in the shoulder and ridge of the trapezius if the lesion is limited to the central portion of the diaphragmatic pleura, which is supplied by sensory fibers of the phrenic nerves. In most instances, however, the lesion also involves the pleura overlying the muscular part of the diaphragm, which is supplied by the lower intercostal nerves (Chapter 53), so the patient also experiences referred pain in the upper lumbar region of the back and in the upper two-thirds of the abdomen. This pain is dull and aching in character, and is usually not as sharp and well localized as the pain caused by irritation of the costal pleura. Pain is usually associated with cutaneous hyperalgesia and deep tenderness and is not infrequently accompanied by increased tension or spasm of the muscles supplied by the same segments that supply the involved pleura.

Tumor involvement of the cupula of the pleura, which is supplied by the T1 and T2 nerves, usually produces pain in the upper interscapular or vertebral area and in the medial aspect of the arm. This part of

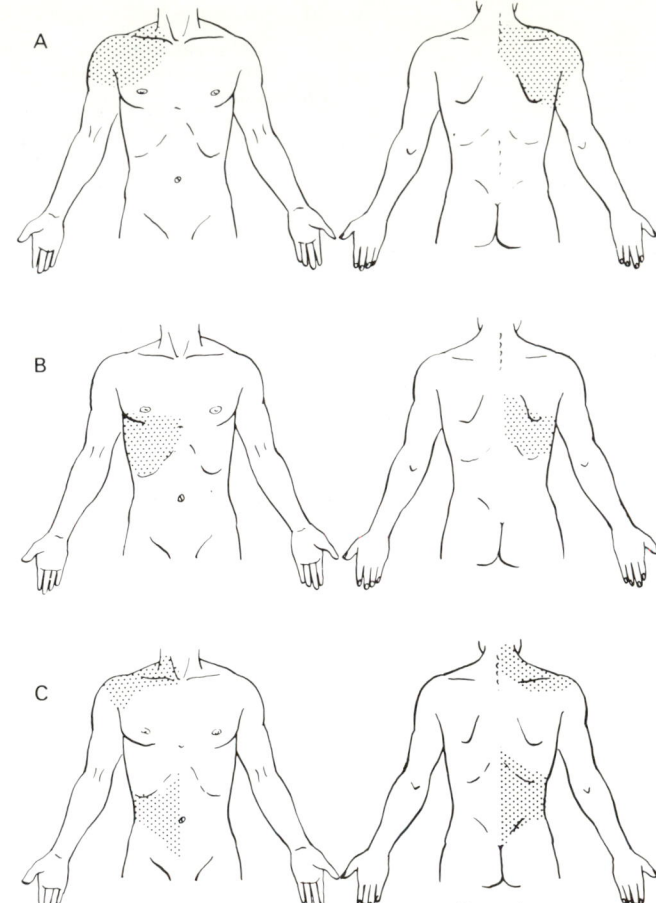

FIG. 57-5. Sites of pain in various costopleural syndromes. **A.** Pain pattern from pathology in the right upper part of the thoracic cage, or apical parietal pleura. **B.** Pain pattern of the right middle part of the chest and parietal pleura. **C.** Pain pattern from irritation of the right portion of the diaphragmatic pleura producing pain in the shoulder, outer abdomen, and back (parts supplied by the phrenic nerves and the lower thoracoabdominal intercostal nerves, respectively. See text for details.

the pleura is invariably involved in the superior pulmonary sulcus syndrome and by metastasis from breast cancer.

Involvement of the mediastinal pleura produces pain felt deep in the central portion of the chest and also in the shoulder and trapezius region as a result of nociceptive impulses transmitted by the phrenic nerves. The pain caused by pleural involvement is markedly aggravated by deep breathing, coughing, and other maneuvers that cause movement of the pleura against the endothoracic fascia or visceral pleura.

SOFT TISSUE AND RIBS. If the endothoracic fascia and the fascia over the intercostal muscles and ribs are involved in the pathologic process, patients also experience well-localized sharp pain, cutaneous hyperalgesia, and deep tenderness. Deely (60) found radiographic evidence of metastasis to the ribs only in 44% of 101 patients, only the vertebrae in 4%, and to both vertebrae and ribs in 3%. Not infrequently metastatic lesions from the lungs involve the lower ribs, in which case patients have sharp localized pain that is markedly aggravated by deep breathing or movement of the chest. Point pressure on the affected rib(s) causes excruciating pain.

INTERCOSTAL NEUROPATHY. Metastatic lesions to the ribs often produce compression, irritation, or damage of one or more intercostal nerves, or direct invasion of the nerves can occur. In these situations pain is the earliest symptom, with progressive sensory loss distal to the site of compression or infiltration. These patients experience a continuous severe, burning, aching pain associated with bouts of lancinating pain that is unilateral and segmental in distribution. Posterior expansion of the pulmonary tumor can result in tumor compression and eventually infiltration and damage of the spinal nerves as they exit through the intervertebral foramina deep to the internal intercostal membrane. These patients can develop neuralgia characterized by a burning aching pain associated with bouts of lancinating pain, dysesthesia, hyperesthesia, and paresthesia along the distribution of the affected nerves.

Pain Syndromes Caused by Vertebral Metastasis

Pain in the chest is a frequent symptom of a metastatic lesion of the thoracic vertebrae from primary tumors in the lung, breast, prostate and, less frequently, the kidney, lymphoma, and other sites. Indeed, the vertebral column is the most common site of bone metastasis from primary tumors involving various structures. In Galasko's (38) study of 100 patients with breast cancer, the thoracic spine was the most common site of vertebral column involvement, involving 42 patients with 142 lesions, the lumbar spine was affected in 41 patients with 101 lesions, and the cervical spine was the site of metastasis in 18 patients with 37 lesions. Of 50 patients with advanced breast cancer, metastases were found in the thoracic spine in 72% of patients, in the lumbar spine in 68%, and in the cervical spine in 26% (38). Lenz and Freid (37) found vertebral metastasis in 59% of 81 breast cancer patients (Table 57-9). Watson and Evans (48) found that, of 189 patients with cancer-related severe intractable pain caused by lung neoplasm, 64 patients (34%) had metastases in 164 sites, including 53 in the thoracic spine and 21 in the lumbar spine but only 2 in the cervical spine (Fig. 57-6).

Galasko (61) and Posner (62) noted that the reason for the high incidence of vertebral involvement in patients with cancer of the lung, breast, and prostate is the peculiar anatomy of the vertebral venous (Batson's) plexus. Batson's plexus is an intercommunicating system of thin-walled veins with no intraluminal pressure and is valveless, so that free movement is possible in either a cranial or caudal direction. Studies done in humans have shown that the plexus can be easily filled when dye is injected into mammary, pleural, or prostatic veins (61). Thus, cancer of the breast, lung, and pelvic organs has a potential connection with the spine, which is therefore easily invaded by primary tumors in these organs. Moreover, with every act of straining, coughing, or lifting, blood is squeezed out of the thoracic abdominal cavity into the vertebral venous plexus. Studies in experimental

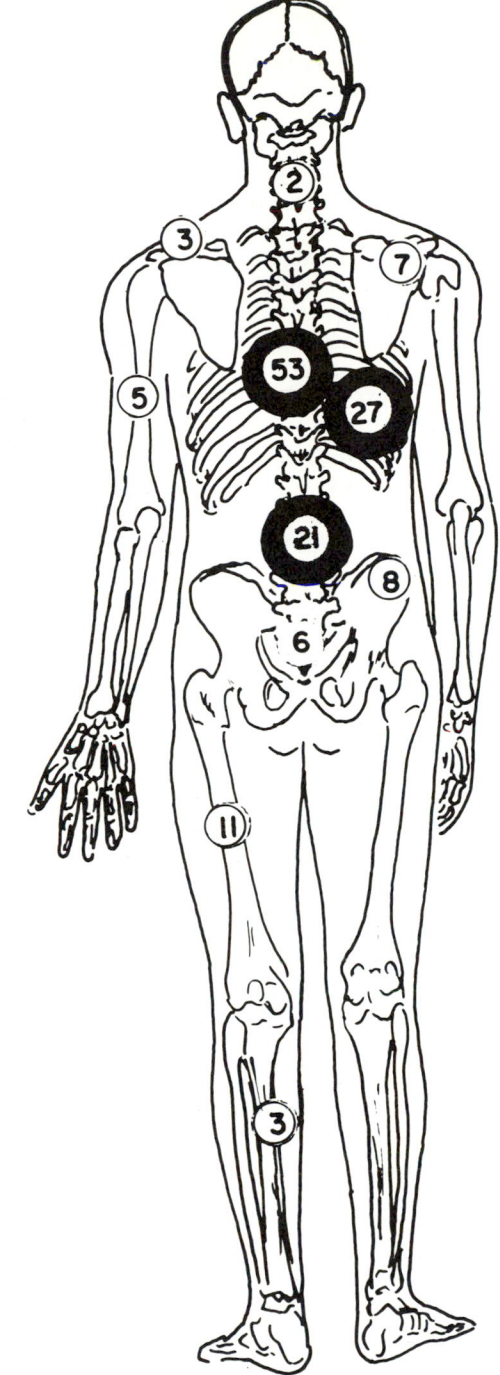

FIG. 57-6. Sites of intractable pain caused by skeletal metastasis in 64 patients consequent to lung cancer. The circles contain the number of metastases at various sites. The most frequently involved regions of the 101 painful sites were the thoracic vertebrae, the ribs, and the lumbar vertebrae. The sites indicated do not relate to lateralization. From Watson, P.N., and Evans, R.J.: Intractable pain with lung cancer. Pain, *29*:163, 1987.

animals (rats and rabbits) demonstrated that tumor cells injected into the tail or femoral vein while the intra-abdominal pressure was briefly elevated were found to lodge in the vertebral veins rather than in the systemic arterioles, indicating that they pass directly into the vertebral venous system (62). In addition to the hematogenous spread of primary tumors, the spine and the soft tissue structures it contains can be affected by metastasis to lymph nodes and other structures in the paravertebral space that then invade bone secondarily.

Growth of metastatic disease either in the bone or surrounding structures, if unchecked, eventually affects neural structures, including nerve roots and spinal cord or cauda equina. In most cases, particularly cancer of the breast, lung, or prostate, the vertebral body or other bony structure of the spine is affected first. Nerve roots and the spinal cord can be secondarily compressed, either by tumor growing into the epidural space or intervertebral foramina or by fracture or collapse of the vertebra, thus causing a combination of tumor in bone to impinge on the epidural space. Posner (62) indicated that, less frequently, tumor in the paravertebral space can grow through the intervertebral foramina and compress first the spinal nerve roots and subsequently the spinal cord.

Symptoms and Signs

Almost all patients with vertebral metastasis experience local or radicular pain, or both, depending on the predominant pathophysiologic process. Patients with metastasis that involves a vertebra have localized pain and tenderness to palpation. Patients with predominantly involvement of the spinal nerve roots have radicular pain, whereas those with spinal cord compression can have radicular pain and funicular pain as a result of compression of the long tracts of the spinal cord. In addition, some patients have reflex spasm of the paraspinal muscles, which becomes a new source of nociceptive input and pain. Because of the clinical importance of ESCC, because the lesion can produce not only pain in the chest but also in other parts of the body, and because treatment of its pain is somewhat different than for that caused by local vertebral lesions, it is discussed separately in the last section of this chapter.

Diagnostic Procedures

This section contains a brief discussion of special procedures to be used to help diagnose the four pain syndromes discussed above. Although each syndrome requires individual consideration, all four have common clinical characteristics that require a similar diagnostic approach. Obviously a thorough physical and neurologic examination is essential.

In patients with superior pulmonary sulcus (Pancoast's) syndrome and other types of metastatic plexopathy, the shoulder and arm pain is frequently mistaken for cervical arthritis, shoulder bursitis, cervical outlet syndrome, or peripheral neuropathy. Consequently patients are referred to an orthopedic surgeon or neurologist who proceeds to treat these conditions. Martini (63) stated that the vast majority of patients lose from 6 to 12 months while being investigated by orthopedists, neurologists, neurosurgeons, and chiropractors. A late diagnosis is finally made when Horner's syndrome develops. In the study by Kanner and associates (47), 27 of 28 patients had been treated for osteoarthritis or bursitis for up to 12 months (mean, 5 months) before the tumor was diagnosed. Other reports cited by Kanner and

colleagues (47) indicated that some patients went as long as 48 months before diagnosis. As noted in the last section of this chapter, vertebral metastasis can also cause back and chest pain without other signs of ESCC, and thus can be mistaken for and treated as arthritis or as some other nonmalignant musculoskeletal problem, with consequent delay of correct diagnosis.

In attempting to diagnose superior pulmonary sulcus syndrome and other types of plexopathy and chest pain caused by cancer, and to aid in the differential diagnosis, it is necessary to carry out various radiographic techniques, including sophisticated imaging procedures, in addition to a detailed history and complete physical examination. In all these patients plain radiographs and bone scans, if negative, do not rule out metastatic disease. Paulson (56) suggested that, in patients who have the characteristic pain and neurologic signs of Pancoast's tumor, and in whom radiographs are negative, one can usually prove the presence of tumor by planography, thereafter proceeding to the use of CT scanning limited to that region. Needle biopsy is necessary to make the histologic diagnosis. In some patients, it might be necessary to carry out surgical exploration of the plexus but this can be difficult. A negative result does not rule out the presence of metastatic disease but does prove helpful in demonstrating the pathology of radiation fibrosis.

To differentiate metastatic from radiation plexopathy, it is important to know the exact radiation dose of patients who have received radiation therapy. Kori and co-workers (49) analyzed the radiation history of cancer patients with brachial plexus lesions and concluded that, if more than 6000 rad were given and if neurologic symptoms appeared within a year, the cause was radiation fibrosis consequent to radiation therapy. If the radiation therapy dose was less than 6000 rad, and symptoms appeared after 1 year, it could have been radiation fibrosis or recurrence of tumor (49).

Foley (52) stated that the advent of CT scanning has dramatically reduced the need to perform surgical exploration of the brachial plexus and, when exploration is necessary, the CT scan is used to direct the surgeon to the appropriate site for needle biopsy and exploration. Foley believes that CT scan of the brachial plexus provides the best two-dimensional view of tumor infiltration and detects bony changes earlier than standard radiographs. The CT scan is a useful guide for surgical exploration of the brachial plexus but does not differentiate tumor infiltration from radiation fibrosis. Careful study of the CT scan, however, reveals other differences, as shown in Table 57-10, which also contains the results of other diagnostic procedures that help to differentiate between these two conditions.

In patients with costopleural syndrome and in those with pain caused by vertebral metastasis, radiographs often provide positive evidence of the metastasis, but this occurs late in the disease. Again, the CT scan permits much earlier detection of bony changes than can be determined with standard radiographs. Magnetic resonance imaging (MRI) also shows promise for providing not only identification of the present metastasis to the spine but also the site and degree of spinal

TABLE 57-10. Results of Diagnostic Tests in Patients with Breast Cancer

Diagnostic Procedure	No. (%) of Total Patients Studied	
	Metastatic Plexopathy	Radiation Plexopathy
CT scan		
Abnormal	41/46 (89)	4/5 (80)
Circumscribed soft tissue mass	40/41 (98)	0/4 (0)

Diffuse soft tissue
    infiltration with loss
    of tissue planes
	5/41 (12)	4/4 (100)

Paravertebral soft tissue extension	19/41 (46)	0/4 (0)
Bony erosion	13/41 (32)	0/4 (0)
Epidural extension	0/41 (0)	0/1 (0)
Other tests		
Radionuclide bone scan	4/32 (13)	0/3 (0)
Myelography (epidural mass)	6/35 (17)	0/0 (0)
Cervical spine radiography	4/39 (10)	0/0 (0)
Chest radiography (apical mass)	10/46 (22)	1/5 (20)*

*Radiation pneumonitis.
From Foley, K. Overview of cancer pain and brachial and lumbar plexopathy. In Management of Cancer Pain. Edited by K. Foley. New York, Memorial Sloan-Kettering Cancer Center, 1985.

cord compression, if present, and might thus obviate the need for myelography. Prior to carrying out therapies to control pain, of course, a clear diagnosis of the syndrome, its cause, and the histologic type of tumor involved should be established.

Management of the Pain

This discussion applies to the management of pain of the four previously described syndromes. Much of the discussion is focused on the superior pulmonary sulcus syndrome, however, not only because of the intensity and frequency of pain and the difficulty in relieving it, but also because more information is available for the symptomatic relief of this condition than for the other syndromes. Obviously, the initial phase of symptomatic pain control is to carry out additional cancer therapy in the form of further surgical resection of the lesion, radiation therapy, chemotherapy, or a combination of these.

Most studies indicate that anticancer therapy, whether surgical or radiation therapy for the superior pulmonary sulcus syndrome, provides some pain relief in 55 to 80% of patients (47, 55, 58). Kanner and colleagues (47) reported on initial pain relief in 23 of 28 patients presenting with pain and, of this group, 2 patients obtained initial relief with surgery, 15 patients were relieved by radiation therapy, and 6 patients derived no relief. Of 17 patients, 4 obtained permanent relief and survived longer than 36 months without recurrence of pain or tumor. In the other 13 of these patients pain returned with evidence of tumor progression, with 11 showing signs of increased brachial plexopathy, ESCC, or both, and 2 showing evidence of bone metastasis. Of the 101 patients referred to Deely (60), 80 patients were given radiation therapy for pain control. Of this group, 55 (68%) obtained partial or complete relief so that their symptoms could be fairly well controlled by mild analgesics. This group included 82% of those with pleural involvement only, 70% of those with bone involvement only, and 75% of those with metastasis elsewhere, but only 11% of those with Pancoast's syndrome. The pain relief lasted among those who survived a short period of time. In 25 patients (32%) of the treated group radiation therapy was ineffective; many of these patients required cordotomy, tractotomy, or neurolytic blockage.

Watson and Evans (48) evaluated the efficacy of radiation therapy in 105 of their patients presenting with severe and intractable pain caused by lung cancer. Good relief was obtained by 28% of 50 patients with Pancoast's tumor, by 49% of 37 patients with skeletal metastasis, and by 44% of 18 patients with metastasis elsewhere. Overall, 40 patients (38%) achieved good pain relief, with a median duration of 1 month.

Obviously, in patients in whom anticancer therapy provides no relief or who have recurrence of the pain that is not amenable to further palliative measures, it is essential to treat the pain symptomatically with pharmacologic therapy, neurostimulating techniques, neurosurgical procedures, neurolytic nerve blocks, or a combination of these, always complemented with psychologic analgesia. It is essential to study the mechanism of the pain to select the optimal therapy or, more frequently, the combination of therapies.

In patients with superior pulmonary sulcus syndrome, metastatic plexopathy, or bone involvement, pain is caused by peripheral (noceptive) mechanisms or peripheral-central (deafferentation) mechanisms. Nociceptive pain is usually localized and continuous and increases with time, and is caused by tumor invasion of the nearby vertebrae, the cupula of the pleura, and other soft tissue. Deafferentation pain is caused by compression, infiltration, and destruction of the involved spinal nerves, which produces burning pain with allodynia, hyperalgesia, hyperesthesia, dysesthesia, and hyperpathia, with a segmental distribution. In patients with costopleural syndrome with pain localized in the pleural rib the pain is predominantly caused by a peripheral mechanism but, if intercostal nerves are involved, deafferentation pain plays a predominant role in the patients' discomfort.

Although the following discussion of symptomatic pain control is mainly relevant to the treatment of those with superior pulmonary sulcus syndrome, it is also applicable to patients who have brachial plexopathy caused by metastasis from other primary tumors. Moreover, many of these procedures are also effective in relieving pain associated with the costopleural and vertebral metastasis syndromes.

PHARMACOLOGIC THERAPY. Pharmacologic therapy in the form of nonsteroidal anti-inflammatory drugs (NSAIDs) alone or combined with codeine should be used as a first choice in patients who have mild to moderate pain caused by any of the four syndromes described above. These drugs should also be used for the relief of severe pain caused by involvement of bone, myofascial structures and tendons, serous membranes, and periosteum. Tricyclic antidepressants are especially indicated in patients with deafferentation pain. De Conno and associates (64) reported that the administration of 50 to 100 mg of amtriptyline at night with 2 to 3 mg of fluphenazine (an anxiolytic drug) during the day proved effective in 50 to 85% of patients with deafferentation pain. They found these drugs to be especially useful in increasing the number of hours of sleep, an important benefit that suggests less pain during the night. Potent narcotics should be used in patients with severe pain who are in the advanced phase of the disease and have a short life expectancy. As emphasized in Chapter 24, morphine or methadone, given in recommended doses, is usually preferred. Slow-release morphine is particularly useful.

De Conno and co-workers (64) reported the results of pharmacologic therapy and percutaneous cordotomy (see below) in 19 patients with severe pain caused by Pancoast's syndrome (Fig. 57-7). NSAIDs combined with weak narcotics such as codeine were more effective than therapy with NSAID alone. These drugs were effective for about 7 to 10 days, after which the pain progressively returned to its former intensity. A cordotomy was then done that produced complete pain relief for about 5 weeks, after which analgesia began to fade. At this time the patients began to experience mild to moderate pain that was effectively relieved with the resumption of pharmacologic therapy. Oral morphine given to 14 patients with Pancoast's syndrome produced a rapid decrease of pain with an average intensity of 8.1 on the visual analogue scale at the start of treatment to an average of 0.8 at 60 days after the onset of treatment (Fig. 57-8). It is now well established that pharmacologic therapy is an important part of a multimodal therapeutic program that provides effective relief in 70 to 80% of patients.

NEUROSURGICAL PROCEDURES. *Cervical percutaneous cordotomy* has been widely used for the relief of cancer pain below the clavicle in many medical centers throughout the world (see Chapters 24 and 98A for details). Ventafridda and colleagues (65) collected data from 18 neurosurgical centers in which this procedure was used for the treatment of Pancoast's syndrome. Effective pain relief was obtained in 79% of 336 patients promptly after the procedure, but this was reduced to 50% at 3 months' follow-up. One group that studied 130 patients (the largest series) reported that

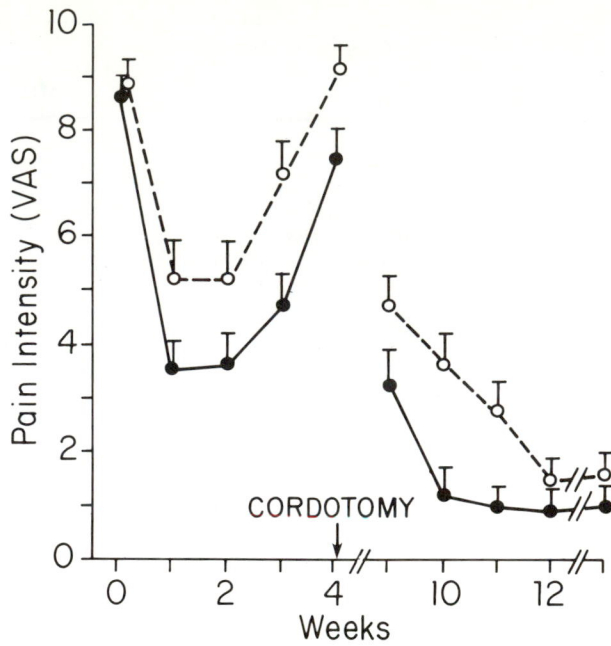

FIG. 57-7. Time course of analgesia observed in two groups of patients. One group (nine patients) was managed with nonsteroidal anti-inflammatory drugs (NSAIDs) combined with mild opioids (solid lines) or with NSAIDs alone (broken lines) during 4 weeks, which was considered to be the control period before percutaneous cervical cordotomy was done. The operation provided highly effective analgesia but this began to fade 5 weeks later, at which time pharmacologic therapy was restarted and provided good pain relief. See text for details. From DeConno, F., Sjanzerla, E., and Ventafridda, V.: Analgesic drugs. *In* Advances in Pain Research and Therapy, Vol. 4. Edited by J.J. Bonica et al. New York, Raven Press, 1982, p. 130.

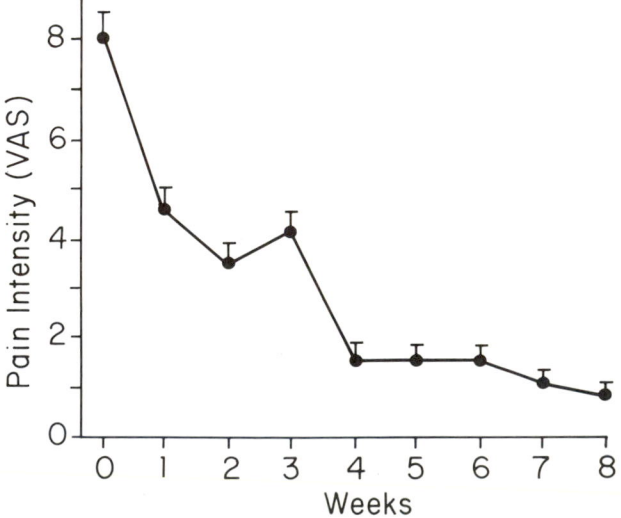

FIG. 57-8. Time course of analgesia in 14 patients with Pancoast's syndrome on oral morphine administered during 8-week follow-up. From DeConno, F., Sjanzerla, E., and Ventafridda, V.: Analgesic drugs. *In* Advances in Pain Research and Therapy, Vol. 4. Edited by J.J. Bonica et al. New York, Raven Press, 1982, p. 131.

pain relief occurred in 83% of patients, however, and persisted at 3 months' follow-up, and several other groups noted persistence of 100% pain relief at 3 months' follow-up (65).

Ventafridda and associates (65) analyzed 33 of their own patients with Pancoast's syndrome who underwent cervical percutaneous cordotomy. All the 33 patients experienced pain relief after the operation, but this decreased to 80% during the first 4 weeks, to 60% at 8 weeks, and to 47% at 12 weeks. They emphasized that, although the patients were not completely relieved of the pain, most had adequate analgesia achieved with supplementary analgesic drugs but usually required smaller doses than those needed before the procedure. About 46% of patients had recurrence of pain caused by the phenomenon of fading in one-third of the patients and by the development of contralateral pain in the other two-thirds. Moreover, at 1 month after the procedure, the number of hours of sleep increased significantly; this was maintained for the ensuing 5 months, indicating a decrease or elimination of nociceptive input at night. Despite the fact that these patients were debilitated, with no increase in physical performance, their quality of life was improved. Side effects included a 10 to 20% decrease in forced expiratory volume, transient hypotension in 30% of patients, and transient weakness of the contralateral lower limb in 25%. It was concluded that, despite these side effects and the phenomenon of fading, percutaneous cordotomy is useful and should be carried out before beginning a prolonged treatment with strong opioids (65).

Watson and Evans (48) carried out percutaneous cervical cordotomy in 32 patients with severe pain caused by lung cancer that was not relieved by "maximally" tolerated doses of narcotics, and noted good pain relief in 24 patients (75%), which lasted a median of 3 months. The efficacy of this procedure varied according to the site and cause of the pain. The best results were obtained in patients with unilateral pain from skeletal spread and chest wall disease, and the least satisfactory results were seen in patients with Pancoast's syndrome. Thus, of 6 patients with chest wall syndrome, 5 (83%) obtained good pain relief for 6 months, and, of 10 patients with skeletal metastasis, 9 (90%) obtained relief for 3 months. Of 16 patients with Pancoast's syndrome, 10 (63%) obtained good relief that lasted only 2 months; 9 of these patients (28%) had a total of 13 complications, the most common being ipsilateral leg weakness in 6 (19%) of the patients, but this was transient in 3 patients. All required a permanent urinary catheter, 1 suffered significant postcordotomy dysesthesia, and 1 patient had respiratory arrest that resulted in death.

From these and other data it is obvious that percutaneous cervical cordotomy provides effective pain relief for a longer period of time in a high percentage of patients who have unilateral chest or back pain, than in those with Pancoast's syndrome. This is probably because, in such cases, the pain involves spinal cord segments below T2; by making a slightly deeper lesion, analgesia of the entire chest wall and thoracic spine is provided, and the fading phenomenon is less likely to occur. In contrast, in patients who have metastatic

upper brachial (C5–C7) plexopathy, percutaneous cervical cordotomy is less likely to provide effective relief because the incidence of the fading phenomenon is likely to be even greater than in patients with Pancoast's syndrome.

Open cervical cordotomy reports were reviewed by Pagni (66). Of 99 patients who underwent this procedure, 44% derived effective pain relief for several months or until the time of their death, while another 15% had partial relief. This group had a 17% mortality rate, and late failures occurred in 5%. Pagni (66) concluded that the relatively high failure rate (56%) and the return of pain in 5% was a result of the fact that the level of analgesia, which was initially at C3–C4, dropped after a few weeks below the level of pain; also, some patients developed pain in the midline or contralaterally.

Spinothalamic tracototomy in the brain stem is another neurosurgical operation that has attempted to obtain a higher level of analgesia and thus improve the incidence of effective pain relief in patients with Pancoast's syndrome or metastatic plexopathy. The procedure has been done at the bulbar and mesencephalic levels by open operation. Although both types have proven effective they have been abandoned because of the high operative mortality rate, high incidence of complications, and production of dysesthesia.

This technique has been replaced by *stereotactic mesencephalotomy*, which can be performed in high-risk patients with minimal operative morbidity and complications. Pagni (66) found that, of 46 patients with Pancoast's syndrome, 34 (74%) obtained good pain relief and 4% partial relief, with a mortality rate of 4%. This procedure is also effective in patients with costopleural or vertebral metastatic pain syndromes.

Posterior spinal rhizotomy for the treatment of Pancoast's syndrome entails section of the posterior rootlets of C4 to T4–T7 inclusively, and thus requires an extensive laminectomy that is not tolerated by patients with advanced disease. Moreover, a significant percentage of patients develops dysesthesia and other deafferentation phenomena. Richardson (67), among others, has reported the use of percutaneous radiographically controlled radiofrequency coagulation of nerve roots at the neural foramen in patients with unilateral pain caused by cancer of the chest, with good results. Prior to carrying out the procedure diagnostic and prognostic blocks are used to determine the segments involved. Richardson (67) believed that these procedures can be useful in patients who have post-thoracotomy pain syndrome (see below).

Dorsal root entry zone (DREZ) lesions, described in Chapter 98, can prove highly effective in relieving the severe excruciating pain associated with Pancoast's syndrome or other brachial plexopathy. Theoretically this procedure should provide good pain relief without injuring motor tracts and producing weakness of the lower limb, as is the case with cordotomy. The procedure does require a laminectomy and is therefore limited to patients who are in fairly good physical condition and who are expected to live 3 to 5 months or longer.

Stereotactic thalamotomy is another procedure that has been used to relieve severe cancer-related pain in the chest and upper limb and, indeed, in the entire half of the body. The procedure is done under local anesthesia and involves minimal morbidity and mortality rates. Pagni (66) cited several reports indicating favorable results for patients with Pancoast's syndrome and other metastatic plexopathy, as well as for severe unilateral chest pain. The major disadvantage of the procedure is that the pain relief does not last longer than 6 to 12 months. (A detailed description of this procedure is given in Chapter 99.)

At the international symposium on superior pulmonary sulcus syndrome, Sweet and colleagues (68) reported on the use of a supracallosal anterior cingulate lesion (*cingulotomy*) in patients with severe excruciating cancer pain associated with a significant degree of psychologic distress. He emphasized that he has obtained excellent results with lesions placed more posteriorly than the classical operation. Unfortunately, most of these and the other neurosurgical procedures mentioned above require a great deal of skill and experience, and are not available to many patients with severe cancer pain.

NEUROSTIMULATION TECHNIQUES. Transcutaneous electrical nerve stimulation (TENS), spinal cord stimulation (SCS), and deep brain stimulation (DBS) are newer procedures that are used in the treatment of cancer pain and other chronic pain syndromes. Richardson (67), who was among the first to use stimulation of the periventricular gray, reported good results in a relatively small number of patients with Pancoast's syndrome and other cancer-related pain in the chest. The advantage of this procedure is that it can be carried out under local anesthesia and thus does not produce a central nervous system lesion, which has the potential complication of neural destruction. The stimulation is under patients' control so that it can be used as needed, and it controls both bilateral and unilateral pain.

NERVE BLOCKS. Neural blockade using anesthetic or neurolytic agents is also important in managing patients with Pancoast's syndrome, metastatic plexopathy, costopleural syndrome, and pain caused by vertebral metastasis. Blocks with a long-acting local anesthetic, such as bupivacaine, can be used as diagnostic and prognostic procedures prior to attempting prolonged interruption of neural pathways and can also be used to provide temporary relief in patients with severe or excruciating pain. For example, in patients with unilateral chest pain, posterior intercostal nerve block of the affected segments provides relief for 6 to 12 hours and, in patients with excruciating pain, it can be done on a daily basis for 5 to 7 days. To obviate the discomfort associated with the needle punctures I usually have someone inject 150 to 200 mg of thiopental IV just prior to insertion of the needle. This amount produces amnesia for 3 to 6 minutes, which is long enough to insert the needles and inject the solution. In patients with bilateral chest pain it is best to carry out a continuous segmental epidural block for 4 to 6 days, achieved either with a continuous infusion or repeated "top-up" injection. If either of these procedures produces good pain relief, serious consideration should be given to subarachnoid neurolysis (see below).

Another effective method of providing pain relief in patients with severe cancer pain is intraspinal opioid analgesia. This technique is likely to provide better pain relief in patients with pleuritic pain but is not likely to be as effective in patients with deafferentation pain.

Neurolytic blockade should be considered in patients who are poor risks and in whom pharmacologic therapy does not provide complete pain relief. Subarachnoid neurolysis is the most frequently used and the most effective procedure. I have used subarachnol alcohol in 21 patients with Pancoast's syndrome and of these, 11 (52%) had good pain relief, 4 (19%) had partial relief, and 6 (29%) had no relief. The pain relief lasted from 5 weeks to 2 months until the death of the patient. In most patients a second and, in some, a third injection of alcohol was necessary to obtain effective analgesia. In those in whom partial or no relief was obtained tumor invasion of the epidural space had occurred.

I have also used the technique in patients with severe pain associated with costopleural syndrome and with pain caused by metastatic lesions of the thoracic vertebrae with even better results. Subarachnoid neurolysis produces the best results in the thoracic region (Chapter 96). Although it is likely that the drug diffuses to involve the anterior roots, no major respiratory difficulty is usually encountered. On the other hand, about 20 to 30% of patients with pain in the upper limb caused by Pancoast's syndrome experience transient (and some even prolonged) muscle weakness, paresthesia, and other sensory disturbances in the affected upper limb.

Ventafridda and Martino (69) carried out 132 subarachnoid blocks using either alcohol or phenol in glycerin in 89 patients with pain in the C7–T5 region and obtained good results in 42 (47%) of the patients. They reported that good pain relief was obtained in 71% of those with chest wall pain, in 44% of those with lung and chest wall involvement, and in 56% of those with tumor involvement of the upper lung and brachial plexus. Surprisingly, the mean duration of analgesia ranged from 16 to 21 days, a much shorter period than that reported by most other clinicians. They noted complications of muscle weakness and dysesthesia, which lasted a few weeks.

Swerdlow (70) reported the results of subarachnoid neurolysis using phenol or chlorocresol in 20 patients and using subarachnoid alcohol in 4 others. Of those treated with phenol or chlorocresol, 11 obtained moderate to good pain relief until their death, which occurred in 2 weeks in 3, in less than 2 weeks in 4, and in 3 or more weeks in 4. Of the 4 patients managed with subarachnoid alcohol, 2 obtained moderate or good relief for 2 months while the other 2 obtained only transient relief. Swerdlow (70) reviewed the results of 5 other reports, which indicated that relief of pain of Pancoast's syndrome occurred in 30 to 50% of patients. In another report, Swerdlow (71) indicated better results in patients with cancer pain in the chest.

Other blocks that can be used include cervicothoracic sympathetic blocks, which should be tried in patients who complain of severe burning pain in the chest or upper limb. The block should be carried out with a long-acting local anesthetic on three or four occasions. If this produces good relief of the burning pain a neurolytic block using 5 to 7% phenol, should be considered, which produces blockade for several weeks.

It has always been my belief that neurolytic blockade of nerves to the limbs should be avoided because it produces an almost useless limb. In patients with excruciating pain in the upper limb caused by plexopathy, in whom oncologic therapy is no longer effective, and who have a short life expectancy, however, paravertebral block of the involved roots of the brachial plexus should be tried. If three or more prognostic blocks with a local anesthetic produce good pain relief serious consideration should be given to injection of 50% alcohol into the nerve, provided, of course, that the effects and complications are discussed with the patient in advance and the patient has decided that the paralysis is preferable to the severe pain. An alternative is injection of the brachial plexus with 2% aqueous phenol. This should be preceded by a block of the brachial plexus with a long-lasting local anesthetic to obviate the severe pain that can occur from the use of the neurolytic agent.

HYPOPHYSECTOMY. Hypophysectomy should be considered in patients with severe excruciating diffuse (bilateral) pain, especially in those in whom the chest pain is caused by breast or prostate carcinoma. The destruction of the pituitary can be achieved by a surgical transnasal or transfrontal approach, by radiofrequency coagulation of the pituitary, or by injection of alcohol into or near the gland. Richardson (67) and Moricca (72) and others (see Chapter 96) have reported effective pain relief in 50 to 70% of patients with severe chest pain.

Other Cancer-Related Chest Pain Syndromes

Postmastectomy Pain Syndrome (XXII-11-13)

Postmastectomy pain syndrome consists of persistent pain in the anterior chest, axilla, and medial and posterior parts of the arm that follows any surgical procedure on the breast. It can occur after a relatively simple operation such as the lumpectomy but occurs more frequently following radical mastectomy and axillary node dissection. Granek and associates (50) have reported an incidence of 4 to 6% following breast surgery, with the time of onset varying from 2 weeks to 6 months after operation.

Etiology and Pathophysiology

The postmastectomy pain syndrome develops consequent to damage of the intercostobrachial nerve, which is the lateral cutaneous branch of the second intercostal nerve. The anterior subdivision of the lateral cutaneous branch of the 3rd intercostal nerve often sends a branch to join the intercostobrachial nerve (Chapter 53). These nerves pass from the intercostal space by penetrating the internal and external intercostal muscles proceeding from there to the floor of the axilla and to the medial and posterior aspects of the upper arm. During radical mastectomy or extensive dissection of the axilla these nerves can be injured, producing a neuropathy with consequent neuralgia or, if the nerve(s) is sectioned, resulting in neuromata.

In addition, a radical mastectomy can damage the lateral cutaneous branches of the 4th and 5th nerves and, if the dissection approaches the midline of the anterior chest, the anterior cutaneous branches of these nerves can also be damaged. The neuropathophysiologic mechanisms of neuroma are discussed in detail in Chapters 8 and 10. Why neuromata produce pain in only 5 to 10% of those who sustain nerve injury is not known. Foley and associates (50, 52, 73) noted that the postmastectomy syndrome occurs more frequently in patients who have postoperative complications, such as wound infection or fluid retention, which presumably put patients at risk for local fibrosis in and about the nerve.

Symptoms and Signs

The postmastectomy pain syndrome is characterized by a tight, constricting, burning pain in the anterior part of the chest, the axilla, and the medial and posterior aspects of the arm. The pain is often associated with bouts of lancinating pain, paresthesia, and dysesthesia, and often hyperpathia, hypesthesia, and hyperesthesia in the distribution of the injured nerves. The pain and other symptoms are exacerbated by movement of the arm and relieved by immobilization, causing patients to posture the arm in a flexed position close to the chest wall. The tendency to keep the arm immobilized is enhanced by the development of lymphedema of the limb because of impairment of venous return. Then, unless patients are given effective pain relief and become involved in an active postoperative rehabilitation program, these factors result in the development of frozen shoulder (Chapter 50). Some patients develop reflex sympathetic dystrophy (RSD) involving the affected limb, frequently in the form of the "shoulder-arm" syndrome (Chapters 11 and 52).

Many of these patients have such intense hyperesthesia and allodynia that contact with undergarments becomes uncomfortable and palpation of the skin markedly aggravates the pain and other symptoms. Moreover, palpation of the neuroma causes a lancinating electric shock sensation.

Diagnosis

The diagnosis is usually clear-cut and is based on the detailed description of the pain, history of the mastectomy, presence of sensory disturbances, and identification of neuroma. These symptoms and signs should clearly distinguish it from brachial plexopathy caused by metastasis of the primary tumor to the brachial plexus. Posterior intercostal block of the affected segments performed by a skilled operator helps to differentiate the postmastectomy syndrome from brachial plexopathy. If neuroma can be identified, injection with a local anesthetic can provide dramatic pain relief, thus helping in the differential diagnosis.

Treatment

Good pain relief and aggressive physical therapy and active motion of the arm not only help to prevent a frozen shoulder but also to eliminate the pain of muscle movement caused by disuse atrophy. The first step in pain control is prescription of a nonopioid analgesic in combination with a tricyclic antidepressant, such as amitriptyline. The use of TENS can help the pain control strategy (see Chapter 92).

In patients in whom these therapies are ineffective, and who experience severe pain, a series of diagnostic and prognostic posterior intercostal blocks should be carried out with a long-acting local anesthetic to help in developing future strategies. An alternative is continuous segmental epidural block with local anesthetic, provided only three or four segments are needed to provide relief. Another alternative is epidural opioid analgesia. These procedures usually provide good pain relief in patients experiencing excruciating pain. Consideration should be given to neuroablative procedures, such as DREZ lesions or spinal rhizotomy. Obviously, because these procedures entail extensive laminectomy, they should only be considered in patients who are in good physical condition and who have a good prognosis.

Post-Thoracotomy Syndrome (XVII-14)

The post-thoracotomy syndrome is characterized by moderate to severe pain in the distribution of one or more intercostal nerves, which persists beyond the usual course of postoperative pain.

Etiology and Pathophysiology

Almost all patients who undergo thoracotomy for nonmalignant or malignant lesions have postoperative pain in the distribution of the incision, associated with some sensory loss. In most patients the pain ceases after 6 to 10 days (Chapter 25). In a small percentage of patients who undergo thoracotomy for nonmalignant disease, however, the pain persists for weeks and months and usually involves injury or section of one or more of the intercostal nerves. As for postmastectomy syndrome, injury of the nerve results in fibrosis neuropathy with consequent neuralgia, and with section of the nerve a neuroma results. In a significant percentage of patients who undergo thoracotomy for cancer therapy the persistent pain is caused by infection or recurrence of the neoplasm.

Kanner and co-workers (51) prospectively followed for 5 months 126 cancer patients who had thoracotomies at the Memorial Sloan-Kettering Cancer Center (MSKCC) to define the pattern of the pain. Of this group, 9 patients were lost to follow-up. The remaining 117 patients were separated into three groups based on the evolution and pattern of pain. In the first group, consisting of 79 patients, the pain was reduced or disappeared in 31 patients at 1 month, in 33 patients at 2 months, and in the remaining 15 patients during the follow-up period. Pain recurred in 13 of these patients though, because of recurrence of the tumor locally or in the pleura, chest wall, bone, or other site. In the second group, consisting of 20 patients, the pain persisted and increased in intensity during the follow-up

period. In this group the increasing pain was a result of local recurrence in 10, of pleura, chest wall, or spine recurrence in 6, of infection in 2, of widespread disease in 1, and of SVC syndrome in another. The third group, consisting of 18 of the 117 patients (15%) who were followed up, had stable or decreasing pain that resolved over time and did not represent a difficult management problem. In a total of 33 of the 117 patients (28%) followed prospectively, the postoperative pain remained because of persistent or recurrent tumor or infection. At the time of surgery 31 of these patients had evidence of pleural or chest wall involvement or residual disease, and therefore represented a high-risk group of patients for tumor recurrence. Kanner and colleagues (51) concluded that persistent or recurrent pain in the distribution of the thoracotomy scar in patients with cancer is most commonly associated with recurrent tumor, while in a small percentage it is caused by traumatic neuroma at the site of the thoracotomy scar.

Symptoms and Signs

The characteristics of the pain depend on the underlying pathophysiologic mechanism. Patients in whom persistent pain is caused by recurrent cancer can present with a costopleural syndrome, vertebral tumor metastasis, or ESCC. These types of pain are usually moderate to severe in intensity. The pain can be localized to the chest wall or can have a segmental (radicular) distribution. It can be associated with paresthesia, dysesthesia, and other sensory changes and, in those with ESCC, pyramidal signs can be present (see below). In the small percentage of patients in whom the persistence of pain is a result of traumatic neuroma the pain is usually of a burning aching quality associated with bouts of lancinating pain. Palpation of the chest wall can reveal hyperesthesia and allodynia. Some of these patients also develop RSD in the ipsilateral upper limb with consequent burning aching pain and other symptoms and signs of RSD. Like postmastectomy pain, the patient can develop a frozen shoulder unless the pain is relieved.

Diagnosis

Diagnosis of the pain presents no problem but, to determine the cause of the pain, a thorough history and physical examination are required. Because in most patients the pain is caused by recurrence of the cancer, other diagnostic procedures must be carried out. Chest radiographs are insufficient for evaluating recurrent disease and a CT scan through the chest with bone and soft tissue windows is the diagnostic procedure of choice. Kanner and associates (51) believed that CT scanning is also necessary prior to consideration of intercostal nerve blocks for the managment of the pain. If a neuroma is present injection of the lesion with local anesthetic provides dramatic pain relief; Kanner and colleagues (51) noted that this would indicate that the neuroma is the probable cause of the pain.

Management of the Pain

In patients in whom the pain is caused by recurrent or residual tumor anticancer therapy is to be carried out, which depends on the type of cancer and on the specific antitumor therapies that are available. During the oncologic therapy it is absolutely essential to relieve any pain and to carry out early and active mobilization of the arm by physical therapy. Pain relief can be obtained with nonopioid and opioid analgesics, occasionally combined with steroids. In patients with bouts of lancinating pain, amitryptiline should be given trial. If pharmacologic therapy does not produce complete pain relief, prognostic or therapeutic nerve blocks should be considered, provided someone skilled in these techniques is available. In patients with unilateral pain, posterior intercostal block using a long-acting local anesthetic is repeated daily for 4 to 6 days. This can produce a reduction in the intensity of the pain, which can then be managed with analgesics. In patients with bilateral pain whose CT scan reveals no epidural tumor deposits, segmental epidural block with local anesthetic or with opioids should be tried. Cervicothoracic sympathetic block can be helpful for some patients with severe burning pain. Patients with pain caused by a neuropathy can be given a trial on analgesics but, if these do not relieve severe pain, a neurosurgical operation or neurolytic block should be considered (see Chapters 94, 97, and 98).

Epidural Spinal Cord Compression

A significant percentage of patients with cancer have metastasis to the spinal cord, nerve roots, or both. Indeed, this is the second most common neurologic complication of systemic cancer, occurring in 5 to 10% of cancer patients. Although spinal metastasis usually occurs in those with advanced disease (72, 74) it can occur any time during the illness. In as many as 8% of patients with spinal involvement it is the first manifestation of the underlying malignancy (74). ESCC is considered here because it occurs most frequently in the thoracic spine and thus produces pain and other symptoms and signs in the chest and abdomen. It can also occur in the cervical or lumbosacral region, however, and produce pain in the neck and upper limb or pelvis and lower limb, respectively. The discussion in this section is based primarily on work done by Posner and associates (41, 62, 74, 75), who are among the leading authorities on this problem.

Etiology and Pathophysiology

Spinal cord damage can result either from compression by tumor in the epidural space or by direct invasion of the spinal cord parenchyma. Figure 57-9 depicts the pathophysiology of myelopathy caused by metastatic cancers. The tumor can arise in, or metastasize hematogenously to, the substance of the spinal cord, or it can be extraparenchymal but intradural. Much more common is metastatic ESCC, in which the tumor reaches the epidural space and compresses the spinal cord in one of two ways. In most cases a metastasis to the vertebral body later spreads to the epidural space. Less common, particularly in patients with lymphomas and neuroblastomas, is a paravertebral tumor that grows into the spinal canal through the intervertebral foramina. Table 57-11 lists the sites of primary tumor in 318 patients, and Table 57-12 lists the primary tumor and location of spinal cord compression

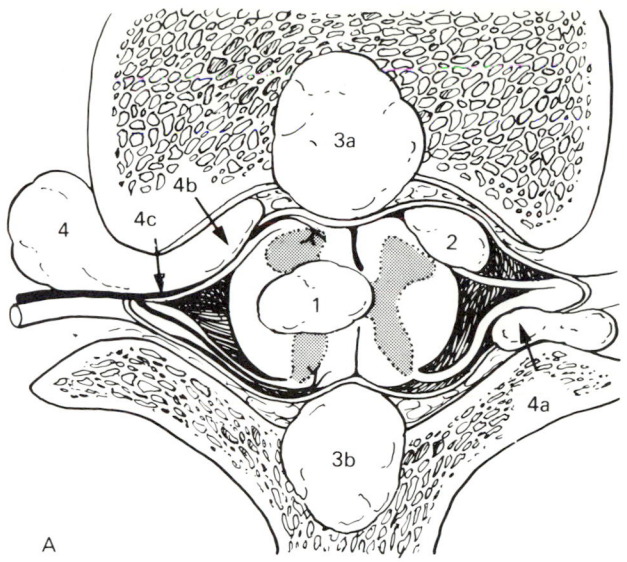

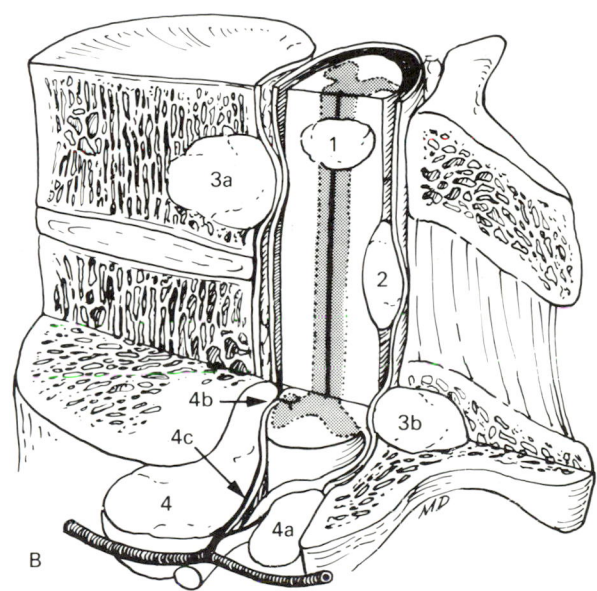

FIG. 57-9. Pathophysiology of myelopathy caused by neoplasms. *A* shows a cross section of the vertebral column at the mid-thoracic region depicting the spinal cord and the type of tumors that invade it. *B* is a sagittal section showing the right part of the vertebra and spinal cord and also a cross section to give the viewer a perspective of the pathways of the neoplasms that cause myelopathy. 1. The tumor can arise in or metastasize hematogenously to the substance of the spinal cord (intramedullary). 2. The tumor can be extraparenchymal but intradural. 3. The tumor can be extradural, extending either from the vertebral body (3a) or from the spinous process (3b), and cause symptoms by compressing the spinal cord. 4. The tumor can originate in or spread to the paravertebral space and produce symptoms either by invading the nerve roots (4a) or by invading the epidural or subdural space through the intervertebral foramen (4b) or by compressing radicular arteries (4c) to cause spinal cord ischemia. Modified from del Regato, G.A.: Pathways of metastatic spread of malignant tumors. Seminars in Oncology, 4:33, 1977.

in 130 patients studied by Posner and associates (41, 62, 74, 75).

Posner (62) stated that the exact cause of neurologic symptoms with spinal cord or chronic compression has

TABLE 57-11. Primary Tumor Causing Epidural Cord Compression in 318 Patients*

Primary Tumor	No.	(%)
Breast	69	(21.7)
Lung	41	(12.9)
Prostate	33	(10.4)
Lymphoma	28	(8.8)
Sarcoma	26	(8.2)
Kidney	20	(6.3)
Head and neck	19	(6.0)
Gastrointestinal	15	(4.7)
Melanoma	13	(4.1)
Myeloma	10	(3.1)
Female reproductive	9	(2.8)
Embryonal cell carcinoma	7	(2.2)
Neuroblastoma	6	(1.9)
Miscellaneous	15	(4.7)

*In 7 patients (2.2%) the primary tumor was unknown.
From Posner, J.B.: Back pain and epidural spinal cord compression. *In* Management of Cancer Pain. Edited by K.M. Foley. New York, Memorial Sloan-Kettering Cancer Center, 1985.

TABLE 57-13. Symptoms and Signs of Epidural Spinal Cord Compression in 130 Patients

Symptoms and Signs	First Symptom or Sign No. (%)		Symptom or Sign at Diagnosis No. (%)	
Pain	125	(96)	125	(96)
Weakness	2	(1.5)	99	(76)
Autonomic dysfunction	0	(0)	75	(57)
Sensory loss	0	(0)	66	(51)
Ataxia	2	(1.5)	4	(3)
Herpes zoster	0	(0)	3	(2.3)
Flexor spasm	0	(0)	2	(1.5)

From Gilbert, R.W., Kim, J.H., and Posner, J.B.: Epidural spinal cord compression from metastatic tumor: Diagnosis and treatment. Ann. Neurol., *3*:40, 1978.

not been firmly established. In most instances dysfunction probably results from compression of neural tissues. Animal experiments have demonstrated several stages, depending on the degree of compression (76). Axonal swelling and mild edema of the white matter occur early but, as the tumor increases in size, it produces more compression and more edema in the white matter resulting from breakdown of the blood-spinal cord barrier (76, 77). Gray matter is preserved until late; prolonged compression, however, produces necrosis of both the gray and white matter (77). Posner (62) noted that some authorities believe that the early stages of edema are caused by venous stasis and later changes are caused by arteriolar compression from the tumor. In rare instances the spinal cord signs can result from compression of radicular arteries as they pass through the intervertebral foramina.

Symptoms and Signs

Pain is the first symptom of ESCC in about 90% of patients. In their study of 130 consecutive patients with ESCC, Posner and co-workers (75) noted pain in 125 patients (96%) (Table 57-13). They also noted that

the pain occurs days or weeks before other neurologic symptoms and signs appear. The pain begins as localized discomfort in the back near the midline and is frequently accompanied by referred or radicular pain. The back pain is usually dull, aching, constant, and progressive in nature and is exacerbated by lying down, straining, neck flexion, or straight leg raising, and is partially relieved by sitting or standing. Invariably local tenderness to percussion of the spinous process of the affected vertebrae is present. When root compression is the primary problem only radicular pain might be present; this is usually unilateral if the lesion is in the cervical or lumbosacral spine and bilateral if the lesion is in the thoracic spine. ESCC does not produce pain in a small percentage of patients.

In patients in whom diagnosis is not made early and treatment is not instituted, neurologic signs develop, so that by the time of diagnosis 75% of patients have weakness and about 50% have some sensory loss, autonomic dysfunction, or both (Table 57-13). The small percentage of patients without pain presents either with weakness or occasionally with ataxia, which is probably caused by compression of the spinocerebellar pathways. Posner (62) noted that ataxia in the absence of pain with sensory loss can lead the physician to believe that the disorder is in the cerebellum or that the patient is hysterical, rather than having ESCC.

TABLE 57-12. Sites of Spinal Cord Compression by Metastatic Tumor in 130 Patients

Primary Tumor	Cervical Spine No. (%)		Thoracic Spine No. (%)		Lumbosacral Spine No. (%)		Total No. (%)	
Breast	4	(14)	22	(79)	2	(7)	28	(21.5)
Lung	8	(38)	12	(57)	1	(5)	21	(16.2)
Prostate	2	(14)	12	(57)	2	(14)	14	(10.8)
Kidney	1	(8)	9	(25)	2	(17)	12	(9.2)
Lymphoma	1	(13)	5	(63)	2	(25)	8	(6.0)
Myeloma	1	(13)	5	(63)	2	(29)	7	(5.4)
Melanoma	1	(14)	4	(57)	2	(29)	5	(3.8)
GI	0	(0)	2	(40)	3	(60)	5	(3.8)
Others	2	(7)	20	(74)	5	(19)	27	(20.8)
All:	20	(15)	89	(68)	21	(16)	130	(100)

From Gilbert, R.W., Kim, J.H., and Posner, J.B.: Epidural spinal cord compression from metastatic tumor: Diagnosis and treatment. Ann. Neurol., *3*:40, 1978.

Diagnosis

Once neurologic signs of ESCC have developed diagnosis is not difficult, and the site of the lesion can be localized on the basis of these signs. Posner (62) emphasized that the diagnostic challenge is identification of those patients with spine metastasis, with or without spinal cord compression, when pain is the only symptom. In such cases, and when the patient is not known to have cancer, the condition can be wrongly diagnosed and treated as an orthopedic musculoskeletal problem. In such cases pain in the thoracic region, which is exacerbated on assuming the recumbent position and that is progressive and unremitting despite rest, should suggest a structural lesion, so appropriate radiographs and CT scans should be obtained.

Portenoy and colleagues (78) developed the algorithm depicted in Figure 57-10 to help in the diagnosis of patients known or suspected of having cancer

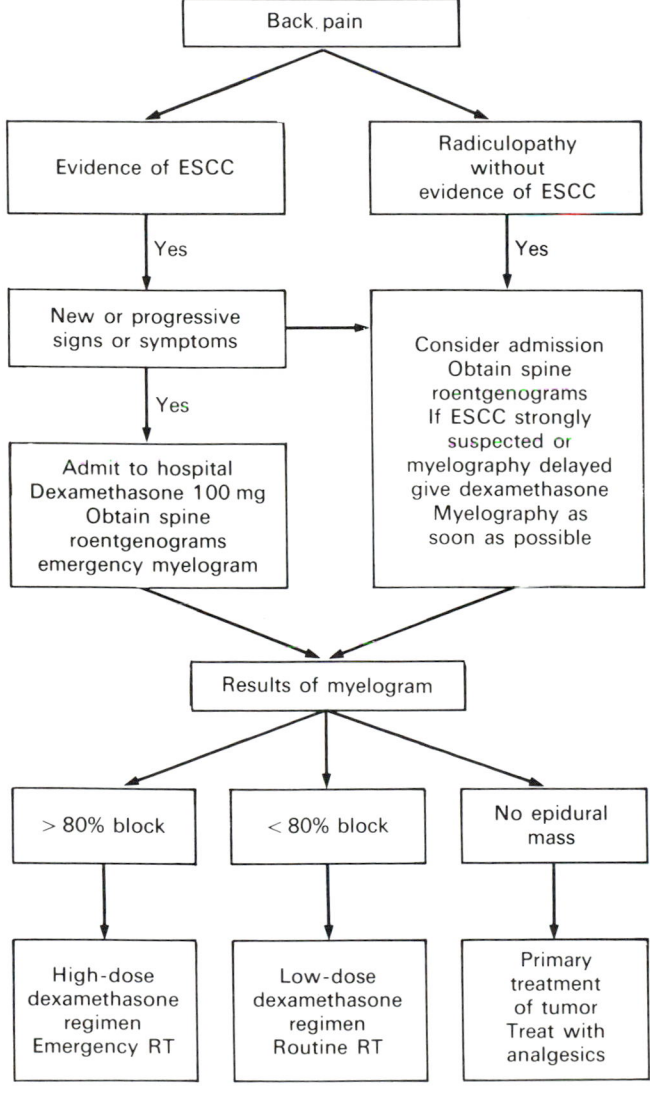

FIG. 57-10. Algorithm for the diagnosis and treatment of epidural spinal cord compression (ESCC). Modified from Portenoy, R.K., Lipton, R.B., and Foley, K.M.: Back pain in the cancer patient: An algorithm for evaluation and management. Neurology, *37*:134, 1987.

who present with back pain. If the physical examination reveals no neurologic signs, plain radiography of the spine is the first step. Posner (62) suggested that MRI might become the diagnostic test of choice because it identifies not only the presence of metastasis to the spine but also the site and degree of spinal cord compression, thus obviating the need for myelography. Presently, however, the evidence is too meager to define clearly the role of MRI in the evaluation of these patients.

Plain radiographs identify spinal cord involvement in 85% of patients with ESCC (62). Although CT and radionuclide bone scanning are more sensitive tests, the former can only cover a small portion of the spine while the latter is less specific than plain radiographs. On the other hand, CT scanning is useful in identifying paravertebral lesions that can invade the spinal canal through the intervertebral foramina. In patients with back pain but no neurologic signs, in whom plain radiographs and CT scans of the area are negative, the likelihood of ESCC is small. In patients with positive plain radiographs and back pain (high-risk patients) but with no neurologic signs the likelihood of ESCC is as high as 20% (78, 79). Myelography, when used to define the presence of ESCC and its actual extent, can identify the presence of asymptomatic epidural lesions and allow sampling through the spinal fluid to identify the concomitant presence of leptomeningeal metastasis.

Treatment

Several therapeutic procedures are available for treatment of spinal metastasis and ESCC. The goals of treatment are to retain or regain ambulation and to control pain.

Medical therapy involves the use of corticosteroids such as IV dexamethasone 100 mg, followed by 100 mg/day in divided doses, to relieve pain and improve other symptoms and signs by reducing the vasogenic edema in the spinal cord. The initial 100-mg dose usually reduces the intense pain associated with ESCC dramatically, and sometimes either stabilizes or improves the neurologic dysfunction (62). Tapering is begun within 48 to 70 hours of introducing high doses of steroids but, if the pain worsens, the steroid dose should be increased. Intravenous steroids occasionally produce a transient itching or burning sensation in the anogenital region that can be quite intense but that does not disturb patients if they are forewarned.

Radiation therapy has become the mainstay of treatment for ESCC because most patients present at a late stage of their cancer and are not surgical candidates. Tumors that are highly radiosensitive, such as lymphomas, respond better than those that are less radiosensitive, such as renal tumors. It has been suggested that most patients who are ambulatory before treatment is started retain ambulation as a result of radiation therapy (62, 74). Posner and associates (41, 62, 74, 75) noted that 50% of those who are paraparetic retain ambulation while only about 3 to 5% of paraplegic patients respond. Fortunately, pain is relieved in about 75% of the patients.

Surgical approaches to patients with ESCC include decompressive laminectomy and vertebral body resection. Posner (62, 74) noted that, because in most instances the tumor lies anterior rather than posterior to the spinal cord, the surgeon often cannot identify or remove much of the tumor even though the spinal cord can be decompressed. Several studies have compared the effects of laminectomy combined with radiation therapy to those of radiation therapy alone, and have demonstrated no significant differences in motor performance, sphincter function, and pain relief after either therapy (62, 74, 75). Moreover, in patients with vertebral collapse and subluxation, laminectomy increases the instability of the spine and sometimes leads to worsening of the symptoms (62, 74).

Vertebral body resection with stabilization of the spine by one of several mechanical devices might be a better procedure. Because most of the tumors are within the vertebral body, such resection decompresses the spinal cord by removing the tumor and, at the same time, stabilizes the spine so that postoperative instability is not a problem. Posner (62) cited several reports suggesting that in suitable patients vertebral body resection can be superior to either laminectomy or radiation therapy.

REFERENCES

1. DeVita, V.T., Jr., Hellman, S., and Rosenberg, S.A. (eds.): Cancer: Principles and Practice of Oncology. 2nd Ed. Philadelphia, J.B. Lippincott, 1985.
2. Moossa, A.R., Robson, M.C., and Schimpff, S.C. (eds.): Comprehensive Textbook of Oncology. Baltimore, Williams & Wilkins, 1986.
3. Becker, F. (ed.): Cancer: A Comprehensive Treatise. 2nd Ed. New York, Plenum Press, 1982.
4. Holland, J.F., and Frei, E., III (eds.): Cancer Medicine. Philadelphia, Lea & Febiger, 1982.
5. American Cancer Society: 1987 Cancer Facts and Figures. New York, American Cancer Society, 1987.
6. Minna, J.D.: Neoplasm of the lung. In Harrison's Principles of Internal Medicine. 11th Ed. Edited by E. Braunwald et al. New York, McGraw-Hill, 1987, pp. 1115–1123.
7. Minna, J.D., Higgins, G.A., and Glatstein, E.J.: Cancer of the lung. In Cancer: Principles and Practice of Oncology. 2nd Ed. Edited by V.T. DeVita, S. Hellman, and S.A. Rosenberg. Philadelphia, J.B. Lippincott, 1985, pp. 507–597.
8. DeCaro, L.F., and Benfield, J.R.: Respiratory tract neoplasm. In Comprehensive Textbook of Oncology. Edited by A.R. Moossa, M.C. Robson, and S.C. Schimpff. Baltimore, Williams & Wilkins, 1986, pp. 723–743.
9. Cohen, M.H.: Diagnosis, staging and therapy. In Pathogenesis and Therapy of Lung Cancer. Edited by C.C. Harris. New York, Marcel Dekker, 1978, pp. 653–700.
10. Selawry, O.S., and Hansen, H.H.: Lung cancer. In Cancer Medicine. Edited by J.F. Holland and E. Frei. Philadelphia, Lea & Febiger, 1973, pp. 1473–1518.
11. Straus, M.J.: Lung Cancer: Clinical Diagnosis and Treatment. New York, Grune & Stratton, 1977.
12. Kreyberg L.: Histologic typing of lung tumors. In International Classification of Tumors No. 1. Edited by L. Kreyberg. Geneva, World Health Organization, 1967, pp. 19–26.
13. Matthews, M.J., and Gordon, P.R.: Morphology of pulmonary and pleural malignancies. In Lung Cancer: Clinical Diagnosis and Treatment. Edited by M.J. Straus. New York, Grune & Stratton, 1977, pp. 49–69.
14. Yesner, R., Gerstl, B., and Auerbach, O.: Application of the World Health Organization classification of lung carcinoma to biopsy material. Ann. Thorac. Surg., 1:33, 1965.
15. Ultmann, J.E., Phillips, T.L., and Flye, M.W.: Treatment of metastatic cancer to the lung. In Cancer: Principles and Practice of Oncology. Edited by V.T. DeVita, S. Hellman, and S.A. Rosenberg. Philadelphia, J.B. Lippincott, 1982, pp. 1539–1552.
16. Cohen, M.H.: Signs and symptoms of bronchogenic carcinoma. In Lung Cancer: Clinical Diagnosis and Treatment. Edited by M.J. Straus. New York, Grune & Stratton, 1977, pp. 85–94.
17. Strauss, B.L., et al.: Cardiac metastasis in lung cancer. Chest, 71:607, 1977.
18. Shores, D.F., and Paneth, M.: Survival after small cell carcinoma of the bronchus. Thorax, 35:819, 1980.
19. Li, W., et al: Unpredictable course of small cell undifferentiated carcinoma of the bronchus. J. Thorac. Cardiovasc. Surg., 81:34, 1981.
20. Roesenberg, J.C.: Neoplasm of the mediastinum. In Cancer: Principles and Practice of Oncology. 2nd Ed. Edited by V.T. DeVita, Jr., S. Hellman, and S.A. Rosenberg. Philadelphia, J.B. Lippincott, 1985, pp. 599–620.
21. Martini, N., et al.: Tumors of mediastinum. In Comprehensive Textbook of Oncology. Edited by A.R. Moossa, M.C. Robson, and S.C. Schimpff. Baltimore, Williams & Wilkins, 1986, pp. 703–722.
22. Silverman, N.A., and Sabiston, D.C., Jr.: Primary tumors and cysts of the mediastinum. In Current Problems in Cancer. Vol. 11. Edited by R.C. Hickey et al. Chicago, Year Book Medical Publishers, 1977, pp. 1–55.
23. Hammon, J.W., Jr., and Sabiston, D.C., Jr.: The mediastinum. In Thoracic Surgery. Edited by H.E. Ellis and H.S. Goldsmith. Hagerstown, MD, Harper & Row, 1979, pp. 135–147.
24. Ingram, R.H., Jr.: Disease of the pleura, mediastinum and diaphragm. In Harrison's Principles of Internal Medicine. 10th Ed. Edited by R.G. Petersdorf et al. New York, McGraw-Hill, 1983, pp. 1584–1585.
25. Caravell, S.C., and Goodman, R.L.: Superior vena caval syndrome. In Cancer: Principles and Practice of Oncology. Edited by V.T. DeVita Jr., S. Hellman, and S.A. Rosenberg. Philadelphia, J.B. Lippincott, 1982, pp. 1582–1586.
26. Schechter, M.M.: The superior vena cava syndrome. Am. J. Med. Sci., 227:46, 1954.
27. Perez, C.A., Presant, C.A., and Amburg, A.L.: Management of superior vena cava syndrome. Semin. Oncol., 5:123, 1978.
28. Roswit, B., Kaplan, G., and Jacobson, H.G.: The superior vena cava obstruction in bronchogenic carcinoma. Radiology, 61:722, 1953.
29. Hellman, S., et al.: Cancer of the breast. In Cancer: Principles and Practice of Oncology. Edited by V.T. DeVita Jr., S. Hellman, and S.A. Rosenberg. Philadelphia, J.B. Lippincott, 1982, pp. 914–970.
30. Henney, J.E., and DeVita, V.T., Jr.: Breast cancer. In Harrison's Principles of Internal Medicine. 11th Ed. Edited by E. Braunwald et al. New York, McGraw-Hill, 1987, pp. 1567–1574.
31. Cuschieri, A.: Tumors of the breast: An overview. In Comprehensive Textbook of Oncology. Edited by A.R. Moossa, M.C. Robson, and S.C. Schimpff. Baltimore, Williams & Wilkins, 1986, pp. 959–967.
32. Smith, P.G., Doll, R.: Late effects of x-irradiation in patients treated for metropathia haemorrhagica. Br. J. Radiol., 49:224, 1976.
33. Petrakis, N.L.: Genetic factors in the etiology of breast cancer. Cancer, 39:2709, 1977.
34. Monson, R.R., et al.: Chronic mastitis and carcinoma of the breast. Lancet, 2:224, 1976.
35. Warren, S., and Witman, E.M.: Studies on tumor metastases: The distribution of metastases in cancer of the breast. Surg. Gynecol. Obstet., 57:81, 1937.
36. Haagensen, C.D.: Diseases of the Breast. 2nd Ed. Philadelphia, W.B. Saunders, 1971.
37. Lenz, M., and Freid, J.R.: Metastases to skeleton, brain and spinal cord from cancer of the breast and effect of radiotherapy. Ann. Surg., 93:278, 1931.
38. Galasko, C.S.B.: Skeletal metastases and mammary cancer. Ann. R. Coll. Surg. Engl., 50:3, 1972.
39. Schider, F.: An Atlas of Anatomy for Artists. 3rd Ed. New York, Dover Publications, 1957, p. 58.
40. Greenberg, J.S., et al.: Metastasis to the base of the skull: Clinical findings in 43 patients. Neurology, 31:530, 1981.
41. Greenberg, J.S., Kim, J.H., and Posner, J.B.: Epidural spinal cord compression from metastatic tumor: Results with a new treatment protocol. Ann. Neurol., 8:361, 1980.
42. Shapiro, S.: Evidence on screening for breast cancer from a randomized trial. Cancer, 39:2772, 1977.
43. Margolese, R.: Primary breast cancer treatment—surgical and adjuvant chemotherapy. In Comprehensive Textbook

of Oncology. Edited by A.R. Moossa, M.C. Robson, and S.C. Schimpff. Baltimore, Williams & Wilkins, 1986, pp. 968–978.

44. Bonica, J.J.: The Management of Pain. 1st Ed. Philadelphia, Lea & Febiger, 1953.
45. Turnbull, F.: The nature of pain that may accompany cancer of the lung. Pain, 7:371, 1979.
46. Bonica, J.J., Ventafridda, V., and Pagni, C.A. (eds): International symposium on the superior pulmonary sulcus syndrome. In Advances in Pain Research and Therapy. Vol. 4. New York, Raven Press, 1982.
47. Kanner, R.M., Martini, N., and Foley, K.M.: Incidence of pain and other clinical manifestations of superior pulmonary sulcus tumor (Pancoast's tumor). In Advances in Pain Research and Therapy, Vol. 4. Edited by J.J. Bonica, V. Ventafridda, and C.A. Pagni. New York, Raven Press, 1982, pp. 27–38.
48. Watson, P.N., and Evans, R.J.: Intractable pain with lung cancer. Pain, 29:163, 1987.
49. Kori, S., Foley, K.M., and Posner, J.B.: Brachial plexus lesions in patients with cancer: Clinical findings in 100 cases. Neurology, 31:45, 1981.
50. Granek, I., Ashikari, R., and Foley, K.M.: Postmastectomy pain syndrome: Clinical and anatomic correlates. Proc. Am. Soc. Clin. Oncol. 3:122, 1983.
51. Kanner, R., Martini, N., and Foley, K.M.: Nature and incidence of postthoracotomy pain. Proc. Am. Soc. Clin. Oncol., 1:152, 1982.
52. Foley, K.M.: Overview of cancer pain and brachial and lumbosacral plexopathy. In Management of Cancer Pain. Edited by K.M. Foley. New York, Memorial Sloan-Kettering Cancer Center, 1985, pp. 25–50.
53. Hare, E.S.: Tumor involving certain nerves. Lond. Med. Gaz., 23:16, 1838.
54. Pancoast, H.K.: Importance of careful roentgen-ray investigation of apical chest tumors. JAMA, 83:1407, 1924.
55. Pancoast, H.K.: Superior pulmonary sulcus tumor. JAMA, 99:1391, 1932.
56. Paulson, D.L.: Combined preoperative irradiation and extended resection for carcinoma in the superior pulmonary sulcus. In Advances in Pain Research and Therapy, Vol. 4. Edited by J.J. Bonica, V. Ventafridda, and C.A. Pagni. New York, Raven Press, 1982, pp. 47–64.
57. Berrino, F.: Epidemiology of superior pulmonary sulcus syndrome (Pancoast syndrome). In Advances in Pain Research and Therapy, Vol. 4. Edited by J.J. Bonica, V. Ventafridda, and C.A. Pagni. New York, Raven Press, 1982, pp. 15–22.
58. Hepper, N.G.G., et al.: Thoracic inlet tumors. Ann. Intern. Med., 64:979, 1966.
59. Miller, J.I., Mansour, K.A., and Hatcher, C.R.: Carcinoma of the superior pulmonary sulcus. Ann. Thorac. Surg., 28:44, 1979.
60. Deeley, T.J.: Radiation therapy. In Advances in Pain Research and Therapy, Vol. 4. Edited by J.J. Bonica, V. Ventafridda, and C.A. Pagni. New York, Raven Press, 1982, pp. 87–112.
61. Galasko, C.S.B.: The anatomy and pathways of skeletal metastases. In Bone Metastasis. Edited by L. Weiss and H.A. Gilbert. Boston, G.K. Hall, 1981, pp. 49–63.
62. Posner, J.B.: Back pain and epidural spinal cord compression. Med. Clin. North Am., 71:185, 1987.
63. Martini, N.: General clinical manifestations of superior

pulmonary sulcus carcinoma. In Advances in Pain Research and Therapy, Vol. 4. Edited by J.J. Bonica, V. Ventafridda, and C.A. Pagni. New York, Raven Press, 1982, pp. 23–26.
64. De Conno, F., Spanzerla, E., and Ventafridda, V.: Analgesic drugs. In Advances in Pain Research and Therapy, Vol. 4. Edited by J.J. Bonica, V. Ventafridda, and C.A. Pagni. New York, Raven Press, 1982, pp. 125–132.
65. Ventafridda, V., De Conno, F., and Fochi, C.: Cervical percutaneous cordotomy. In Advances in Pain Research and Therapy, Vol. 4. Edited by J.J. Bonica, V. Ventafridda, and C.A. Pagni. New York, Raven Press, 1982, pp. 185–198.
66. Pagni, C.A.: Neurosurgical treatment: Status of the problem. In Advances in Pain Research and Therapy, Vol. 4. Edited by J.J. Bonica, V. Ventafridda, and C.A. Pagni. New York, Raven Press, 1982, pp. 165–183.
67. Richardson, D.E.: Role of neurosurgery and pain involving the chest and brachial plexus. In Advances in Pain Research and Therapy, Vol. 2. Edited by J.J. Bonica, and V. Ventafridda. New York, Raven Press, 1979, pp. 577–586.
68. Sweet, W.H., Poletti, C.E., and Umansky, F.: Neurosurgical techniques to control the pain of superior pulmonary sulcus and other tumors in this region. In Advances in Pain Research and Therapy, Vol. 4. Edited by J.J. Bonica, V. Ventafridda, and C.A. Pagni. New York, Raven Press, 1982, pp. 211–233.
69. Ventafridda, V., and Martino, G.: Clinical evaluation of subarachnoid neurolytic blocks in intractable cancer pain. In Advances in Pain Research and Therapy, Vol. 1. Edited by J.J. Bonica and D. Albe-Fessard. New York, Raven Press, 1976, pp. 699–703.
70. Swerdlow, M.: Spinal and peripheral neurolysis for managing Pancoast syndrome. In Advances in Pain Research and Therapy, Vol. 4. Edited by J.J. Bonica, V. Ventafridda, and C.A. Pagni. New York, Raven Press, 1982, pp. 135–144.
71. Swerdlow, M.: Role of nerve blocks and pain involving the chest and brachial plexus. In Advances in Pain Research and Therapy, Vol. 2. Edited by J.J. Bonica and V. Ventafridda. New York, Raven Press, 1979, pp. 567–576.
72. Moricca, G.: Chemical hypophysectomy for cancer pain. In Advances in Neurology, Vol. 4: International Symposium on Pain. Edited by J.J. Bonica. New York, Raven Press, 1974, pp. 707–714.
73. Kanner, R.: Postsurgical pain syndromes. In Management of Cancer Pain. Edited by K.M. Foley. New York, Memorial Sloan-Kettering Cancer Center, 1985, pp. 65–69.
74. Posner, J.B.: Back pain and epidural spinal cord compression. In Management of Cancer Pain. Edited by K.M. Foley. New York, Memorial Sloan-Kettering Cancer Center, 1985, pp. 51–59.
75. Gilbert, R.W., Kim, J.H., and Posner, J.B.: Epidural spinal cord compression from metastatic tumor. Ann. Neurol., 3:183, 1978.
76. Kato, A., Ushio, Y., and Hayakawa, T.: Circulatory disturbance of the spinal cord with epidural neoplasm in rats. J. Neurosurg., 63:260, 1985.
77. Ushio, Y., et al: Experimental spinal cord compression by epidural neoplasms. Neurology, 27:422, 1977.
78. Portenoy, R.K., Lipton, R.B., and Foley, K.M.: Back pain in the cancer patient: An algorithm for evaluation and management. Neurology, 37:134, 1987.
79. Rodichok, L.D., et al: Early diagnosis of spinal epidural metastases. Am. J. Med., 70:1181, 1981.

58 • CHEST PAIN CAUSED BY OTHER DISORDERS

JOHN J. BONICA

with contributions by
ANDERS F. SOLA

THIS chapter contains a discussion of pain in the chest caused by various disorders not considered in the preceding chapters. The material is presented in five major sections: A, Pain of Neuropathic Origin; B, Pain Primarily of Musculoskeletal Origin; C, Pain of Tegumentary Origin; D, Referred Pain Caused by Extrathoracic Disorders; E, Relation of Chest Pain and Psychologic Factors (Table 58-1). Because of the high frequency of occurrence of the first two categories of pain, it is essential to have a thorough knowledge of the anatomy and biomechanics of the thoracic cage, as discussed in Chapter 53. Moreover, because the pathologic processes in the first two categories also produce pain in the abdomen, they are described in detail in this chapter and are only mentioned in Chapter 64 in the sections dealing with abdominal pain of neuropathic and musculoskeletal origin. Sola contributed some information on the subsection of myofascial pain syndromes.

A. PAIN OF NEUROPATHIC ORIGIN

Pain in the anterior, lateral, and posterior parts of the chest can be caused by lesions or diseases of the upper six segments of the thoracic spinal cord, by pathologic processes that affect the rootlets, roots, or short formed nerve trunks of the upper six spinal nerves, or by lesions or diseases that are limited to the anterior primary division of these nerves, referred to as the thoracic intercostal nerves (Table 58-2.) If the pathologic process affects the lower six segments of the spinal cord or the rootlets, roots, or formed nerve, the pain is distributed in the affected segments of the abdomen, lower thoracic and lumbar spines, and paraspinal regions. Diseases or lesions of the thoracoabdominal intercostal nerves produce pain that is experienced in the anterior abdominal wall and the lateral aspect of the trunk, depending on the site of the pathologic process.

Before describing the various pain syndromes caused by neuropathic pathology, definitions are given because they help to indicate the site of the lesion. As noted below, the symptoms and signs and their distribution vary according to the site of the pathologic process. Lesions or diseases that affect the spinal cord produce symptoms and signs of a *myelopathy*; pathologic processes involving the roots or rootlets of the thoracic spinal nerves produce a *radiculopathy* with segmental pain (radiculalgia) and other signs and symptoms that are limited to the segment(s). When the pathologic process involves the short formed nerve trunk of the thoracic spinal nerve before it divides into the anterior primary division and posterior primary division the condition is known as a *thoracic spinal neuropathy*, whereas if the pathologic process involves part of or the entire anterior primary division it is known as an *intercostal neuropathy*. In rare instances only branches of the primary division are involved and the term "peripheral neuropathy" can be used. A similar term can be used when the posterior primary division alone is involved in the pathologic process.

Thoracic Myelopathy

Contrary to general belief, disorders of the spinal cord are common causes of pain in the chest as well as in the abdomen and back. The lesion or disease can be intrinsic within the spinal cord, extramedullary but within the meninges, located in the epidural space, or a combination of these.

Intrinsic and Extramedullary Spinal Cord Lesions

As noted in Table 58-2, intrinsic spinal cord lesions or diseases include primary tumors, metastatic neoplasms, syringomyelia, trauma, multiple sclerosis, hemorrhage, infarct, and abscess. Approximately 50% of spinal cord tumors originate in the thoracic portion (1). Neurofibromas and meningiomas each account for about 25% of intraspinal neoplasms, intramedullary sarcomas and extramedullary hemangioendotheliomas each account for about 10% of spinal cord tumors, and other types account for the remaining 20%.

Primary spinal cord tumors and syringomyelia tend to arise in the center of the cord and to spread centrifugally. Thus, in contrast to nerve root tumors, these usually produce compelling evidence of spinal cord damage long before involvement of the dorsal root entry zones produces circumferential chest pain.

Multiple sclerosis (Charcot's disease, disseminated sclerosis, insular sclerosis) is a degenerative disease of the central nervous system that produces sporadic patches throughout the spinal cord, brain stem, and brain. Pathologically it is characterized by circumscribed areas of demyelinization. As the acute lesions subside the glia proliferates and forms scars.

Symptoms and Signs

Spinal cord tumors produce pain that is often varied and difficult to describe because at times it can appear to be caused by a visceral disease or an infectious

TABLE 58-1. Chest Pain Caused by Other Neuropathic, Musculoskeletal, and Other Disorders

I. PAIN PRIMARILY OF NEUROPATHIC ORIGIN
A. **Disease of the spinal cord** (myelopathy)
B. **Lesions of the rootlets or roots of thoracic spinal nerves** (radiculopathy)
C. **Lesions of the formed spinal nerves** (neuropathy)
D. **Lesions of the intercostal nerves** (intercostal neuropathy)
E. **Disorders of the peripheral branches of spinal nerves** (peripheral neuropathy)

II. PAIN PRIMARILY OF MUSCULOSKELETAL ORIGIN
A. **Lesions or disease of bones**
  1. Disease or lesions of the thoracic vertebrae
  2. Disease or lesions of the ribs
  3. Diseases or disorders of the costal cartilages
  4. Disease or disorders of the sternum
  5. Disease of the sternoclavicular joint
B. **Disorders of muscles**
  1. Myofascial pain syndromes
  2. Chest pain caused by other disorders of muscles

III. DISEASES OF TEGUMENTARY ORIGIN
A. **Burns and other trauma**
B. **Cicatrices**
C. **Postoperative pain syndromes**
D. **Mastodynia**
E. **Deep axillary abscess**
F. **Adiposis dolorosa**
G. **Phlebitis of the anterolateral chest**
H. **Other dermatologic painful disorders**

IV. CHEST PAIN CAUSED BY EXTRATHORACIC DISEASES
A. **Disorders of the cervical spine and shoulder**
  1. Intervertebral disk disease
  2. Thoracic outlet syndromes
B. **Abdominal diseases**
  1. Gas entrapment syndromes
  2. Disorders of the gastrointestinal tract
  3. Disease of the biliary tract
  4. Disease of the pancreas
  5. Other abdominal visceral disease
C. **Diseases of the diaphragm**
  1. Acute primary diaphragmatis
  2. Subphrenic abscess
  3. Diaphragmatic flutter

V. CHEST PAIN PRIMARILY OF PSYCHOLOGIC ORIGIN
A. **Abnormal emotional reactions to visceral disease**
B. **Anxiety syndrome**
C. **Depression syndrome**
D. **Conversion reaction**
E. **Hypochondriasis**
F. **Psychiatric syndromes**

TABLE 58-2. Chest Pain Primarily of Neuropathic Origin

I. DISEASES OF THE SPINAL CORD (MYELOPATHY)
A. **Intrinsic spinal cord diseases:** primary tumors, metastatic tumors, syringomyelia, trauma, multiple sclerosis, infarction, abscess
B. **Extramedullary intrathecal disorders**
  1. Primary tumors: meningioma, neurofibroma
  2. Metastatic tumors
C. **Epidural spinal cord compression**
  1. Primarily caused by vertebral pathology
  2. Metastatic neoplasm from breast, lung, prostate
  3. Epidural abscess
  4. Hematoma
  5. Adhesive arachnoiditis

II. DISEASES OF THE ROOTLETS AND ROOTS OF SPINAL NERVES (radiculopathy)
A. **Infection and inflammation**
  1. Herpes zoster
  2. Syphilis (tabes dorsalis)
  3. Meningitis
  4. Systemic infection
  5. Tuberculosis
  6. Other infectious diseases
B. **Mechanical compression or injury**
  1. Osteoarthritis
  2. Other arthritides
  3. Ruptured intervertebral disk
  4. Fracture of vertebra
  5. Abscess or tumor of the vertebra
  6. Paget's disease of the spine

III. DISEASES OF THE FORMED THORACIC SPINAL NERVES (thoracic neuropathy)
A. **Vertebral compression** (same as II-B)
B. **Paravertebral compression**
  1. Paravertebral adenopathy
  2. Mediastinal tumors
  3. Paravertebral abscess
  4. Aortic aneurysm
C. **Primary nerve tumors**
  1. Neurofibroma
  2. Schwannoma
D. **Systemic infection, neuropathy**
E. **Other neuritides**
  1. Alcoholism
  2. Avitaminosis
  3. Intoxication by heavy metals, food, amoebae
  4. Vitamin metabolic disorders and others

IV. DISORDERS OF THE INTERCOSTAL NERVES (intercostal neuralgia)
A. **Compression or injury secondary to fracture or tumors of ribs**
B. **External trauma** (e.g., stab wounds)
C. **Postinfectious intercostal neuropathy**
D. **Postoperative neuropathy**
  1. Postmastectomy syndrome
  2. Post-thoracotomy syndrome

---

process of the spinal cord. The pain can be constant or intermittent, occurs at rest, and is relieved by exercise (2). It frequently awakens the patient for a few hours at a time and forces the patient to walk the floor or sleep in an unusual position, often sitting up. The pain recurs in an identical thoracic distribution each time it occurs. The constant pain is usually associated with bouts of lancinating pain and is aggravated by coughing, sneezing, or straining. Associated motor or sensory deficits are frequent signs of these lesions. With significant compression of the spinal cord a typical Brown-Sequard syndrome can develop, with spastic paralysis of the muscles below and on the ipsilateral side of the lesion and loss of pain and temperature sensibility

on the contralateral side. Compression of posterior columns of the spinal cord results in a decrease in deep sensibility, position sense, vibratory sense, and ataxia below the level of the lesion.

Syringomyelia and multiple sclerosis can cause pain in the chest but frequently the patient feels a zone of numbness around the chest or abdomen, depending on the site of the lesion. Common physical signs of the disease are weakness of the lower limbs, visual changes (e.g., reduction of the visual field, scotomata, nystagmus, pallor of the optic disk), tremor, ataxia, reflex changes, loss of vibratory and positional sensibilities, mental aberrations, and impaired sphincter tone.

Diagnosis

A complete physical and neurologic examination usually demonstrates sensory and motor deficits in the lower part of the body. Finding the level below which sensation is impaired is extremely helpful. Examination of the cerebrospinal fluid (CSF) reveals increased protein levels and other findings that support the diagnosis. Radiographs alone might not show evidence of the lesion unless the vertebrae are involved. Computerized tomography is helpful, and myelography can localize the lesion. Magnetic resonance imaging (MRI) can localize the lesion without myelography.

Treatment

Treatment is usually by radiation therapy if the lesion is radiosensitive; if not, neurosurgical excision of the tumor is necessary. The results of therapy are improved by early ambulation and exercise. During the evaluation of the patient it is essential to control the pain with systemic analgesics (Chapter 24).

Epidural Lesions

Epidural lesions invariably produce epidural spinal cord compression (ESCC) (Chapter 57). In addition to the metastatic neoplasms mentioned, ESCC can be caused by giant cell tumor, myeloma, osteogenic sarcoma of the vertebra, osteochondroma, epidural abscess, infection of the vertebra or intravertebral space, Paget's disease, and epidural hematoma. As indicated in Table 57-11, metastatic lesions that produce ESCC originate primarily in the lung, prostate, and breast but can also arise from other primary tumors.

Pain is the first and most frequent symptom of ESCC, occurring in over 95% of patients even before other symptoms and signs develop. Initially the pain can be localized to the thoracic spine at the level of the lesion and is associated with tenderness on palpation of spinous process and the paravertebral region. Later signs and symptoms of sensory and motor deficits and reflex changes develop.

The diagnosis and treatment of epidural spinal cord compression are discussed in detail in Chapter 57.

Radiculopathy and Neuropathy (Segmental Neuralgia)

Radiculopathy of sensory (dorsal) rootlets or roots and neuropathy of the short formed thoracic spinal nerves before they divide into the primary anterior and posterior divisions produce radiculalgia and segmental neuralgia, respectively. The pain is usually continuous, has a sharp burning or constricting quality, and is often accompanied by bouts of brief stabbing or lancinating pain. The pain is felt in the skin and subcutaneous tissue of part of or the entire segmental distribution of the affected nerve(s). The pain is often worse at night (perhaps because of spinal sagging) and is aggravated by movements of the thoracic spine, as in twisting and bending. It is increased by changes in intraspinal pressure, as with coughing, sneezing, and straining. Hyperesthesia, hyperalgesia, and hyper-

pathia of the affected segments can accompany the pain. Because of the extensive overlapping of adjacent spinal nerves it is possible that no demonstrable sensory deficit can be noted if only one or two nerves are affected, but a careful examiner might elicit hypalgesia to pinprick and other stimuli in the affected dermatomes (3). If several contiguous roots are involved segmental hypesthesia can be defined in the dermatome or dermatomes that are in the middle of the band of hyperalgesia.

Diagnosis at this point is often extremely difficult. It hinges on recognition of the characteristics of radicular pain and on painstaking examination of the patient for minimal sensory deficits in the thoracic dermatomes. Many patients have tenderness to fist pounding of the affected vertebrae. A comprehensive radiologic investigation is essential. As noted by Edmeads (3), the dimension of the diagnostic problem is indicated by the fact that 10% of all patients with thoracic nerve root compression undergo surgery for nonexistent disease of the abdominal and thoracic viscera.

In patients in whom the lesion enlarges, the adjacent spinal cord is compressed and results in symptoms and signs of cord compression, including weak spastic hyper-reflexic lower limbs, impaired sensation below the level of the lesion, and sphincteric disturbances. These symptoms and signs of spinal cord involvement facilitate diagnosis. Plain radiography of the spine, CT scanning, and myelography might be necessary to define the location and extent of the lesion. Magnetic resonance imaging (MRI) provides this type of information without myelography and can even suggest the nature of the problem (4).

Because most conditions listed in Table 58-2 that produce radiculopathy and neuropathy are discussed elsewhere in this book, my comments here are limited to a brief discussion of conditions that are considered to be especially significant in regard to the production of chest and abdominal wall pain. These include herpes zoster, herniation of a thoracic intervertebral disk, neurogenic tumors, and traumatic fracture of a vertebra.

Herpes Zoster (XVII-1)

Acute herpes zoster (HZ) and postherpetic neuralgia (PHN) are discussed in detail in Chapter 13. HZ is briefly considered here because it involves the thoracic region in 50% of patients (5, 6) and is the source of severe pain in the chest or lower back and abdomen.

Etiology

Acute HZ is caused by the varicella zoster virus (VZV). Its incidence increases with age and is higher in patients with cancer, especially hematologic or raticuloendothelial malignancies, and in other immunocompromised patients, including those receiving immunosuppressive drugs. Portenoy and colleagues (7) indicated that patients with acquired immune deficiency syndrome (AIDS) are also likely to be at increased risk. Use of corticosteroids has been reported to increase the severity of primary varicella-zoster infection and to augment the risk of dissemination during HZ in patients with underlying diseases that compromise immune function.

Pathophysiology

Acute varicella begins as an oral or respiratory infection with consequent viremia in which the skin is seeded with the virus. Retrograde axonal transport carries the virus from the skin to the dorsal root ganglion cells, in which a latent phase occurs. Acute HZ is the result of a dynamic interaction between the viral genome and the neuron in which it is latent in the host immune system. Clinical HZ occurs by the spread of reactivated virus within the ganglia and by orthograde axonal transport to the skin.

The pathology of acute HZ was first elucidated by Head and Campbell (8) in their classic investigation. It is characterized by an acute inflammatory process involving chiefly the dorsal root ganglion cells and various degrees of degeneration involving the corresponding sensory nerves, posterior roots or rootlets, posterior horn cells, and occasionally anterior horns of the involved segments. Lymphocytic infiltration usually occurs, followed by hemorrhagic necrosis of the ganglion cells. As the mononeuropathy extends peripherally from the dorsal root ganglia myelin breakdown and axonal degeneration occur and the number of cutaneous nerve fibers around the lesion in the skin is diminished.

Symptoms and Signs

Pain, itching, tingling, or a feeling of formication are the first and most important symptoms of HZ, typically preceding the appearance of a rash by several days to a week or longer (Fig. 58-1). In some patients the pain is felt concurrently with the rash while in others it begins after the rash. The pain is felt in the distribution of one or more contiguous thoracic dermatomes and, unless an underlying immunodeficient state is present, it is almost unilateral, seldom involving more than four contiguous thoracic segments. The pain is sharp, severe, superficial, and burning in quality, with superimposed bouts of severe stabbing or lancinating pain that can occur spontaneously or can be precipitated by emotional stress or by touching or moving the involved area. The affected dermatome becomes hyperalgesic and hyperesthetic, frequently with exquisite tenderness around the vesicles that can worsen as ulceration and secondary infection occur. Patients with HZ in the thoracic dermatomes commonly splint the region and have reflex muscle spasm and secondary musculoskeletal pain as a result. If the pain cannot be relieved by the initial treatment patients can exhibit mood changes and prominent alterations in behavior, including diminished appetite, sleep disruption, and increased social isolation that might evolve into a pattern of abnormal illness behavior and depression (7).

Diagnosis

A diagnosis of HZ should be suspected even in the pre-eruptive stage when a patient complains of

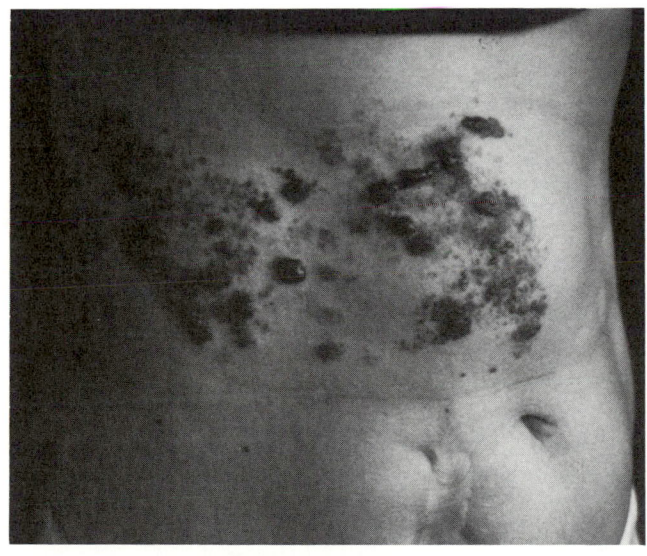
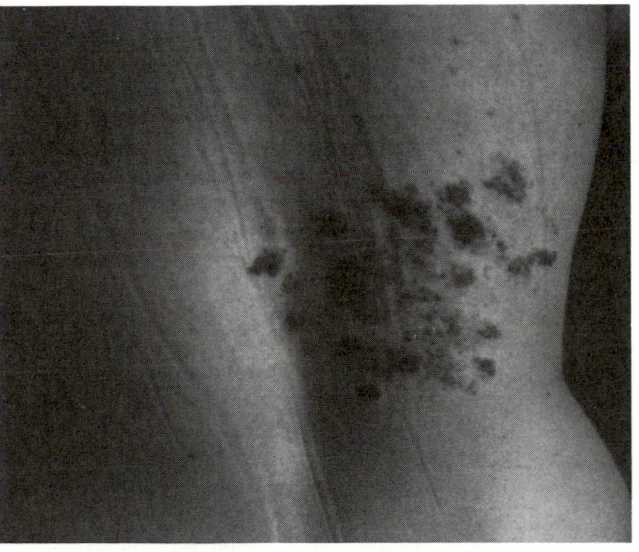

A   B

FIG. 58-1. Photographs of a 40-year-old woman with full-blown vesicles of herpes zoster involving the 8th and 9th right thoracic nerves. Because of her age she was treated by a dermatologist conservatively with systemic analgesics and corticosteroids, with little pain relief. The patient continued to have moderate to severe pain and, 1 week after these photographs were taken the lesions extended to involve the 7th and 10th right thoracic nerves. Acyclovir was prescribed 3 weeks after onset but did not relieve the pain, which remained severe. Continuous segmental epidural analgesia was then induced, extending from T6 to T10. This produced prompt relief of pain and was continued for 6 days, after which mild burning pain persisted for another week. By the 10th week after onset the cutaneous ulcerations dried up and the patient was relatively free of pain. Three weeks later, however, she began to experience mild to moderate burning pain associated with bouts of lancinating pain that lasted 1 to 3 days and occurred at 3- to 6-week intervals. *A.* Anterior distribution of the initial vesicles. *B.* Posterior distribution. The vesicles in the posterior region are opposite L1 to L3 as a result of the natural migration of the posterior division of each spinal nerve. (See Chapter 6 for details on this issue.)

peculiar burning aching pain in a segmental distribution. A correlation between the severity and duration of the pain and consequent emotional reactions seems to exist as well as an increased incidence of postherpetic neuralgia, so it is essential to initiate analgesia and antiviral therapy as soon as possible.

Treatment

In Chapter 13 the many types of therapy that have been used for HZ and for PHN are noted. Based on experience in managing nearly 200 patients for over 30 years and on a review of recent literature, I am firmly convinced that HZ should be treated with a combination of antiviral drugs and segmental epidural analgesia or somatic and sympathetic block of the involved nerves achieved with a local anesthetic to provide immediate and complete relief of pain. Controlled studies have provided evidence that repeated intramuscular injection of interferon or acyclovir, given soon after disease onset, shortens the duration of the rash and diminishes the pain and dissemination of disease (9, 10). Vidarabine also improved healing and reduced dissemination, resulting in a more rapid resolution of the pain. Although the efficacy of antiviral therapy in preventing PHN has not been demonstrated conclusively, such an effect has been suggested (9).

Combining antiviral therapy with sympathetic and somatic nerve blocks has the advantage of producing prompt relief of severe pain and significantly reducing the duration and degree of skin eruption. Moreover, it has been found to reduce the incidence of PHN in about 30% of patients. To achieve these benefits it is essential to administer the block as soon as the initial symptoms (e.g., pain, itching) or sign of erythema develop and to continue the therapy for 5 to 7 days. When done by skilled personnel, paravertebral block using the paralaminar approach, with injection of 5 ml of 0.5% bupivacaine daily, is effective in blocking both the somatic nerves and the sympathetic chain. If multiple segments are involved I usually prefer to obviate discomfort from needle punctures by giving patients 150 mg of thiopental IV; this dose produces amnesia for 3 to 5 minutes, during which time the punctures are done without subsequent recall by the patient. An alternative and somewhat easier technique is production of a segmental epidural block, also with a dilute solution of bupivacaine. This technique has the advantage of involving only one puncture and, by using the appropriate amount, two or more segments can be blocked. In patients who experience severe excruciating pain, the production of continuous segmental epidural analgesia by giving repeated doses or by using an infusion pump should be considered (Chapter 94). This procedure can be carried out on an outpatient basis, and the patient should be monitored for several hours to determine the efficacy of analgesia and sympathetic blockade and to detect any arterial hypotension from the vasomotor block or other adverse reactions. If the condition involves only two to four segments, and the patient is normovolemic, the procedure entails almost no risk of clinically significant arterial hypotension. For continuous blockade, it is best to have the patient in the hospital for continuous monitoring of the system and the patient.

Neural blockade has the relative disadvantage of requiring someone skilled in such techniques and of carrying out the procedure in an outpatient clinic. Notwithstanding these disadvantages, I am convinced that they are highly effective, not only in providing prompt pain relief but also in reducing the duration and degree of the cutaneous eruptions and decreasing the incidence of PHN. I am so convinced of the efficacy of the procedure that I have had neural blockade as the sole treatment for my own case of HZ and for that of my wife and one of my siblings. Neural blockade was initiated the same day that the first symptom (pain) or sign (rash) occurred and was repeated daily for 1 week. In each case the response was similar to that of 85% of patients whom I have treated with this procedure: immediate relief of pain, the number and size of vesicles were markedly reduced, and complete healing occurred within 6 to 10 days. At the time of this writing 6 to 9 years after treatment (carried out when all of the patients were in their early 60s), none have developed PHN. This is in contrast to the experience of one of my daughters who, because of her age (40 years), was treated conservatively with systemic analgesics consisting of non-steroidal anti-inflammatory drugs, codeine, and corticosteroids. She continued to have moderate to severe pain; after 1 week the skin lesions had extended from two to four segments that developed large blebs and on the third week began to ulcerate, markedly aggravating her pain. The administration of acyclovir on the third week had no effect on the pain. Indeed, the pain intensity increased to such a degree as to prompt me to initiate a continuous segmental epidural block to provide her with pain relief and rest for a period of 6 days, after which the pain gradually diminished in intensity. The cutaneous ulcerations finally dried up on the tenth week. Since the thoracic attack (which occurred 2 years prior to this writing), and despite her relative youth, she has experienced bouts of mild to moderate burning pain associated with lancinating pain at intervals of 3 to 6 weeks.

The aforementioned four cases are anecdotal reports but the results are similar to those I have observed in patients managed with neural blockade, as well as the results reported by many others. Because many of these are cited in Chapter 94 I only mention results reported by Colding (11, 12), who carried out two large uncontrolled studies in which patients were managed with paravertebral somatic and sympathetic blocks for HZ below the head and with cervicothoracic (stellate) block for trigeminal HZ. One to four blocks usually provided relief in 85 to 90% of patients treated within 2 weeks of onset but the success rate dropped to 40% in patients treated 2 weeks or more after onset. The incidence of PHN was lower than that reported in an epidemiologic survey of untreated patients, suggesting that neural blockade is effective in reducing the incidence of this serious complication of HZ. Similar results have been noted by myself and others, as discussed in more detail in Chapter 94. The management of PHN is discussed in Chapter 13.

Ruptured Intervertebral Disk

Extrusion of a thoracic intravertebral disk, with a consequent radiculopathy and the symptoms and signs associated with it, was formerly considered as uncommon or rare but is now being recognized with increasing frequency (13). Although the incidence of herniated disk in the thoracic region is lower than in the cervical and lumbar regions, it requires early diagnosis and appropriate therapy to prevent or halt dysfunction of the spinal cord, either directly by compression of the cord or indirectly by interruption of its vascular supply.

Etiology and Pathophysiology

The causative factor can be sudden severe trauma, either immediate or a remote or minor accident, such as falling from a sitting position, that can go unrecognized. People in middle age or older are predisposed, especially those with a pre-existing spinal deformity such as scoliosis or degenerative changes. The herniation can occur at any level of the thoracic spine but occurs most frequently in its lower half.

Changes in the disk annulus and adjacent ligaments initially produce back pain that can be present for weeks or months before actual protrusion into the intervertebral foramina or spinal canal occurs. Such protrusions are usually posterolateral, compressing a nerve root and producing unilateral radicular chest pain or radicular pain in the abdomen (the lower thoracic dermatomes). Further protrusion posterolaterally or protrusion posteriorly compresses the spinal cord. A midline disk protrusion is especially critical, not so much because the dura-arachnoid is compressed but because of compression of the anterior median longitudinal artery, which is an end artery that produces ischemia of several segments of the spinal cord when compressed. As Turek (13) emphasized, that portion of the spinal cord lying within the spinal canal and extending from vertebral segments T4 to about T9 is the "critical zone" of the spinal cord. This is because it is the narrowest zone of the spinal canal corresponding to the part of the spinal cord that possesses the least amount of vascular supply (14). Therefore, the spinal cord can be compromised by two factors, by compression or by interruption of the vascular supply, resulting in ischemia that produces edema and central necrosis.

Symptoms and Signs

The patient usually presents with a history of antecedent trauma, often of an insignificant degree, so that the onset can be sudden but more commonly is insidious. A vague poorly localized aching pain in the back is the most common initial symptom but later the patient can have unilateral or bilateral radicular pain that extends girdle-like around the chest wall or radiates to the abdomen; with low (T7–T12) lesions it can involve the groin. Typically the pain is intensified by neck flexion or by increasing CSF pressure by coughing, sneezing, or straining and is usually relieved by recumbency. Subjective numbness and paresthesia, such as coldness and a burning sensation, are early and outstanding symptoms.

With spinal cord compression the patient can experience back pain and, with a low lesion, pain in the groin and lower limbs, weakness, and heaviness of the legs. If not promptly and effectively treated it progresses to paraplegia, often associated with sphincter weakness. Physical findings of upper motor neuron lesions include clonus, hyperactive deep reflexes, spasticity, and the Babinski response. The degree of sensory deficit is highly variable and is noted at least several dermatomes below the level of disk protrusion.

Diagnosis

In its early stage the clinical picture of disk protrusion varies greatly, so a high degree of suspicion is essential. In patients who have unilateral or bilateral radicular pain that is aggravated by coughing, sneezing, or straining, however, a presumptive diagnosis of herniated disk should be made. In patients with low-grade steady encroachment on the spinal canal the condition is often misdiagnosed as multiple sclerosis or arteriosclerotic myelopathy. On the other hand, acute protrusion of the disk that produces sudden compression of the spinal cord and a severe neurologic deficit usually alerts the physician to a threatening situation that requires prompt therapy. The diagnosis is made by CT, which can be carried out in conjunction with myelography. MRI localizes and defines the lesion without myelography.

Treatment

Patients who have a posterolateral herniation of the thoracic disk that produces symptoms and signs only of a radiculopathy should be treated conservatively by bed rest, systemic analgesics for the management of pain, and traction. If the patient is experiencing severe pain and manifests intense reflex muscle spasm a continuous segmental epidural block should be considered because it provides complete pain relief and elimination of the reflex muscle spasm. The catheter is inserted through a needle placed two or three vertebral levels below the disk. The catheter is then advanced 3 or 4 cm, placing it just below the level of the disk. Injection of 4 to 6 ml of 2% lidocaine or 0.5% bupivacaine is usually sufficient to produce a band of analgesia that extends two to three segments above and below the disk.

In patients who have beginning signs of spinal cord compression it is essential to prevent irreversible damage to the spinal cord by surgical removal of the protruded disk. Attempts to remove the disk from the anterior portion of the spinal canal through a posterior approach entails the risk of additional damage to the cord. Turek (13) has recommended an anterolateral approach by removal of the rib and transverse process, or by the transthoracic approach.

Neurogenic Tumors

In Chapter 57 benign and malignant tumors that arise from the thoracic spinal nerves and frequently occupy the posterior mediastinum in the paravertebral gutter were discussed briefly. These include such benign tumors as neurofibromas, schwannomas, and ganglioneuromas. Malignant neoplasms of the thoracic spinal nerves such as neurofibrosarcomas or neurogenic sarcomas can originate from a previously existing neurofibroma but ordinarily present signs of malignant growth from the time of onset.

Thoracic neurofibromas are nodular outgrowths of nerves that can attain a great size by expanding and displacing the soft intrathoracic structures, especially the lung. They can assume a dumbbell shape, with the smaller part within the spinal canal and the larger expansion in the posterior mediastinum (15). The tumor can compress the superior vena cava to produce the superior vena cava syndrome or can compress the tracheobronchial tree or esophagus.

Symptoms and Signs

Pain is a common symptom that arises in some cases from the compression of a neighboring structure such as the esophagus or tracheobronchial tree or as a neuropathic pain arising from involvement of the nerve itself. Patients with benign neurogenic tumors usually complain of pain in the chest wall at the site of the tumor, with radiation of pain along the course of the involved nerve (16). The pain is often continuous and severe and, according to Wehrmacher (2) the pain is frequently of long duration before help is sought. By the time patients are seen by a physician, considerable local tenderness or pressure has occurred at the site of the tumor. Sensory disturbances are unusual signs of benign tumors because these displace rather than invade the nerve trunk of origin. Sensory changes are common with malignant tumors, however, which destroy nerve fibers by infiltration and local pressure.

Diagnosis

In addition to the history, including details of the characteristics of the pain and laboratory examination, radiographs of the chest are needed. When a neurogenic tumor is present the radiograph reveals a certain shadow adjacent to the chest wall. With multiple projections or tomographic studies the separation from the underlying structure can usually be demonstrated. The tumor can erode the vertebra or rib but erosion is more apt to result from malignant than from benign growth (2).

Treatment

Treatment of these tumors is usually by surgical excision, which is easily done with benign tumors because they can be peeled away from the nerve trunk of origin. In contrast, malignant tumors that invade the surrounding tissue require radical surgical excision. The prognosis with benign tumors is good but, with neurogenic sarcomas, the prognosis is poor, either because the tumor cannot be excised completely or the patient dies from progressive cachexia. Radiation therapy has little effect on these tumors and is of no use in management except as a palliative measure during the terminal stage.

Vertebral Fractures (XVII-9)

A crushed fracture of the vertebral body can cause sudden severe compression of nerve roots as they pass through the intervertebral foramina, thus producing unilateral or bilateral radicular pain. Vertebral fractures seldom produce cord compression. Underlying bone pathology should be sought in patients who develop vertebral fractures without severe trauma. Osteoporosis is noted most frequently, although metastatic cancer to the vertebra is also a factor.

Patients who present with mild to moderate pain should be managed conservatively with systemic analgesics, bed rest, and physical therapy. In patients with severe unilateral radicular pain and intense reflex muscle spasms, paravertebral nerve blocks should be given consideration. For patients with bilateral radicular pain and other symptoms and signs of radiculopathy, a segmental epidural block provides the advantages of bilateral analgesia with only one needle puncture. Neural blockade not only provides complete pain relief but also relieves reflex muscle spasm, which in many cases adds to the nociceptive input through feedback loops. In a surprisingly and significantly high percentage of patients, the duration of pain relief and the elimination of reflex muscle spasms far outlast the pharmacologic effects of the drug. Obviously, if the pathologic process is severe, surgical intervention is necessary.

Other Causes of Radiculopathy and Neuropathy (XVII-3)

Thoracic nerve roots can be compressed by marked scoliosis of the spine or by such rare lesions as angiomas, tuberculomas, and epidural abscesses. Regardless of the nature of the lesion the current history of local back pain, associated with the radicular pain with or without evidence of spinal cord compression, should suggest the probability of neurologic disease and the need for comprehensive evaluation.

The thoracic spinal nerves can also be damaged by a wide variety of toxins, infections, and circulatory and metabolic disorders. Although many such causes of painful neuropathy exist, they infrequently involve the thoracic spinal nerves to produce chest or abdominal pain. Even when they do, the nerves to the limb are almost always involved, so the differential diagnosis of chest pain should not be difficult.

Intercostal and Peripheral Neuropathy

One or more intercostal nerves can be injured by compression, trauma, stab wound, or infection or in the course of thoracic surgery or mastectomy. The latter two conditions are discussed in detail in Chapter 57. The following brief discussion of traumatic intercostal neuropathy is included here for completeness; a more detailed discussion is given in Chapter 10.

The intercostal nerves, in their positions immediately inferior to each rib, are vulnerable to rib trauma. Fracture of a rib can cause injury to the subjacent nerve that is followed by a sharp superficial burning pain in its distribution. The pain can be aggravated by respirations or movements of the rib cage that mimic those of pleurisy. Because of significant overlap not much sensory deficit is found unless several nerves are involved. Even when only one nerve is injured, however, a thin segment of subtle hyperalgesia and hyperesthesia is produced. Palpation usually elicits superficial and deep tenderness, particularly over the site of the rib fracture. If the fracture becomes displaced it can lacerate the pleura and might even damage the lung, with additional symptoms and signs being produced.

When the history and physical examination reveal evidence of chest wall trauma the diagnosis is easily made. When the trauma has been forgotten by the patient and no features such as rib tenderness or irregularity are found, however, the diagnosis can be extremely difficult. In such cases an appropriately located fractured line or rib callus on chest radiography can aid in diagnosis.

Mild to moderate intercostal neuralgia can be managed with systemic analgesics consisting of nonsteroidal inflammatory drugs (NSAIDs) and weak opioids. In patients who have severe intercostal neuralgia the best relief is achieved by producing a posterior intercostal block with a long-acting local anesthetic, such as 0.25 to 0.5% bupivacaine (see Chapter 94 for more details).

B. PAIN PRIMARILY OF MUSCULOSKELETAL ORIGIN

Table 58-3 lists the most important musculoskeletal disorders that produce pain in the chest. As noted previously, disorders of the lower thoracic vertebrae and the spinal cord contained therein can produce pain in the low back and abdomen. Because many of the conditions listed in Table 58-3 are discussed in detail elsewhere in this book, they are only mentioned briefly here. Other conditions that are especially relevant to pain in the chest are discussed in more detail in the following sections.

Disorders of the Thoracic Spine

Many disorders of the thoracic portion of the vertebral column, including simple fracture or minor subluxation or dislocation, arthritis, osteomyelitis, metabolic disorders, acromegaly, and Paget's disease, frequently produce only localized pain in the back (13). When these conditions produce compression or irritation of the thoracic spinal nerve a radiculopathy or neuropathy is associated with the condition (see above, Pain of Neuropathic Origin).

The localized pain in the back caused by vertebral lesions is produced by stimulation of nociceptive endings in periosteum, ligaments, and joints secondary to inflammation, compression, or local biochemical changes. Back pain can also be produced by the associated reflex spasm of the paravertebral muscles. Fist pounding palpation or deep finger palpation of the spinous processes and the paravertebral region aggravate the pain and elicit superficial and local tenderness. Pain is also aggravated by movements of the spine. When the vertebral bodies are affected the pain tends to worsen at night and is throbbing in character. Stiffness is usually associated with this pain, as is pain in the spastic paraspinal muscles.

The diagnosis of localized back pain is based on the history, the characteristics of the pain, and physical, neurologic, roentgenographic, and laboratory examinations. Treatment should be directed toward elimination of the cause. Therapy of arthritis is discussed in detail in Chapter 20. Acute and chronic osteomyelitis are discussed in Chapter 23, as are the metabolic bone disorders that might cause localized back pain. Pain caused by primary and metastatic tumors of the spine are considered above (see Neurogenic Tumors). The following brief discussion of three disorders that involve the thoracic spine is included for the sake of completeness.

Postural Deformities

Postural kyphosis, or rounded shoulders, and lateral scoliosis can be the result of congenital deformities or acquired structural defects secondary to disease, trauma, a shortened lower extremity, or poor posture.

The most satisfactory and efficient treatment consists of rectifying the muscle imbalance by strengthening with exercise. If scoliosis is caused by a short lower limb a shoe lift is essential. Mild pain can be well controlled by NSAIDs alone or in combination with codeine (Chapter 78). If the patient has severe pain associated with excessive muscle spasm, local infiltration of the muscle or paravertebral block of the

TABLE 58-3. Chest Pain Primarily of Musculoskeletal Origin

I. DISORDERS OF THE UPPER THORACIC SPINE
  A. **Fracture, dislocation, subluxation**
  B. **Arthritis**
    1. Osteoarthritis
    2. Rheumatoid arthritis
    3. Acute pyogenic arthritis
    4. Traumatic arthritis
    5. Ankylosing spondylitis
    6. Interarticular facet syndrome
    7. Costovertebral arthritis
    8. Diffuse idiopathic skeletal hyperostosis
  C. **Infection**
    1. Acute osteomyelitis
    2. Chronic osteomyelitis
    3. Syphilis
    4. Tuberculosis
    5. Brucella infection
  D. **Metabolic disorders**
    1. Osteoporosis
    2. Osteomalacia
    3. Acromegaly
  E. **Postural deformities**
  F. **Osteitis ossificans** (Paget's disease of the spine)
  G. **Tumors**
    1. Primary
    2. Metastatic

II. LESIONS OR DISEASES OF THE RIBS
  A. **Fractures**
  B. **Primary tumors**
  C. **Metastatic tumors**
  D. **Osteitis deformans**
  E. **Acromegaly**
  F. **Slipping rib syndrome**
  G. **Costovertebral arthritis**

III. DISEASES OF THE COSTAL CARTILAGES
  A. **Costochondritis**
  B. **Tietze's syndrome**
  C. **Costochondral dislocation**
  D. **Traumatic chondritis**

IV. DISEASES OF THE STERNUM
  A. **Sternoclavicular arthritis**
  B. **Manubriosternal arthritis**
  C. **Manubriosternal dislocation**
  D. **Fracture of the sternum**
  E. **Osteomyelitis**
  F. **Neoplasm**

V. DISORDERS OF MUSCLES
  A. **Myofascial syndromes**
  B. **Chest pain from other muscle disorders**

affected segments provides highly effective pain relief and permits more effective physical therapy. Daily injections with a long-acting local anesthetic done just prior to the active exercise and physical therapy produce good results.

Ankylosing Spondylitis

Spondylitis is an arthritic condition of the intervertebral joints, including the costovertebral, costotransverse, and thoracic apophyseal joints, that is usually of a degenerative or rheumatoid type and that can cause moderate aching pain in the back aggravated by movements and limitation of chest expansion (17). As discussed in Chapter 90 many patients with even mild spondylosis develop a subtle radiculopathy, which in turn produces muscle spasm and later contractures that cause localized pain by squeezing intramuscular nociceptors. When paraspinal contractures compress nerve roots they can create a vicious circle of pain → contraction → pain. Sustained contraction can lead to degeneration and secondary pain in activity-stressed parts of the body.

Treatment aims at releasing the contractions, promoting healing, and removing the source of nerve irritation. The treatment of choice is penetration of the motor point with acupuncture needles (Chapter 90). Infiltration of the spastic muscle with a dilute solution of local anesthetic has also been used (see Chapters 21 to 23).

Costovertebral Arthritis

Arthritis of the costovertebral and costotransverse joints is associated with osteoarthritis and ankylosing spondylitis and rarely with other arthritides (18). It is an uncommon cause of thoracic back pain. The pain is often increased by deep breathing, coughing, or chest compression (18, 19). The anatomic characteristics and increased mobility of the 1st, 11th, and 12th costovertebral joints account for the high frequency of occurrence of degenerative arthritis in these joints. Arthritis of the 1st costovertebral joint is a rare cause of thoracic outlet syndrome.

Arthritis in these two joints causes localized back pain and tenderness elicited by deep pressure or fist pounding. The pain is usually localized, deep and aching in character, and continuous.

A presumptive diagnosis is made on the characteristics of the pain and by the presence of arthritis in other joints and is confirmed by radiographic demonstration of joint space narrowing, subchondral bony sclerosis, and marginal osteophytes or intra-articular loose bodies (19).

Treatment is symptomatic, involving the use of systemic analgesics and physical therapy (Chapter 20). Intra-articular injection of a local anesthetic and corticosteroid compound is indicated in refractory cases (Chapter 94).

Diffuse Idiopathic Skeletal Hyperostosis

Diffuse idiopathic skeletal hyperostosis (DISH), also known as Forestier's disease (20), is a relatively common disorder of middle-aged and elderly individuals, particularly men (21). The predominant symptom of the condition is pain and stiffness in the thoracolumbar spine. The pain is generally mild to moderate and dull and aching in character, and does not radiate, but is aggravated by inactivity and exposure to cold and dampness. Physical findings in the thoracic spine include a slight increase in dorsal kyphosis, minimal reduction in the range of movement and chest expansion and, frequently, local tenderness.

The diagnosis requires, in addition to a history and physical examination, radiographic studies that show spinal hyperostosis, particularly in the thoracic region, resulting in linear ossification and bridging osteophytosis (21). Radiographic features include flowing, undulating, anterior ossification of four or more contiguous thoracic vertebrae, radiolucency between the deposited bone and the underlying vertebral bodies, and relative preservation of the intervertebral disk height. The absence of sacroiliitis, true syndesmophytes, and apophyseal joint ankylosis distinguishes this condition from ankylosing spondylitis (18).

Treatment is symptomatic, involving the use of salicylates or other NSAIDs, physical therapy consisting of application of heat, and exercise programs to strengthen the back muscles.

Apophyseal Facet Syndrome

The apophyseal facet syndrome results from excessive and rapid muscular movement in an unguarded position such as sudden rotation of the trunk, working with the hands extended over the head, or lifting with the body in a twisted position. Such trauma can cause excessive stress and strain on the apophyseal joints and their ligaments, causing the latter to pull the joint surface so tightly together that they tend to "bind" or "lock" on one another (22). This results in loss of function of the joint and often in pain that can vary in degree from persistent annoying discomfort to total disability. In the event of tearing of the ligaments, the facets subluxate on one another and cause even greater restriction and pain (13).

Symptoms and Signs

The chief symptom is decrease or total loss of mobility of that portion of the back accompanied by pain that usually involves the side and even the anterior part of the chest. The pain is aggravated by all movements, especially hyperextension, and is reduced by flexion. If the "locking" is high in the thoracic spine the patient can move the neck in a guarded position. If more than one vertebra is involved a flattening of the normal kyphotic thoracic curve is noted (22). A tender painful spasm is sometimes present in the erector spinae muscle just above and below the site of the lock.

Diagnosis

The diagnosis is based on the history and physical findings. Roentgenograms of the spine are necessary to exclude other disorders. Careful study of the radiograph sometimes shows slight rotation of the vertebral and occasionally what Mennell (22) labeled as "localized curve," which is a definite narrowing of the intervertebral disk on one side or an alteration in the general line thrown by the shadow of the articular or spinous processes. Oblique views of the spine show subluxation of the facet, if present.

Treatment

Treatment consists of relief of pain by infiltration of the facet, application of heat, and active physical therapy, including exercise. The exercises, which should be done under the supervision of a physical therapist, are intended to strengthen the abdominal muscles and to stretch and strengthen the erector spinae muscles.

Chest Pain Caused by Disorders of the Ribs

Fractures

Fractures of one or more ribs constitute one of the most common causes of acute pain in the chest of musculoskeletal origin. Fractures are commonly encountered in industrial medical practice and in most cases result from trauma. Fractures can also occur during a severe paroxysm of coughing—so called "tussive fracture" of the ribs—a condition that was first described in 1773 by Gooch (23) and redescribed in the medical literature periodically since then (24). Spontaneous fracture of the ribs can also occur in patients with severe osteoporosis or metastatic cancer involving one or more ribs.

Pathophysiology

The pathophysiology and symptoms and signs vary according to the severity of the injury, the type of fracture, whether adjacent structures are involved, and resulting complications. In most cases the fracture is partial or complete. Marked displacement and overriding of the fragment occur only with violent trauma associated with crush injuries. Fractures often involve several ribs or multiple fractures of the same rib. Stress or insufficiency fractures involving the ribs occur in patients with rheumatoid arthritis, osteoporosis, osteomalacia, and Paget's disease of bone (18, 25, 26). Patients with long-standing deforming rheumatoid arthritis who have stiff shoulders can also have rib erosions involving the outer aspect of the 2nd to 6th ribs near their angles (25). The erosions are usually painless and are thought to be a result of pressure from the scapula on the ribs and of the development of bursa between them.

Symptoms and Signs

Single fractures produce a localized sharp aching pain that is aggravated by deep breathing, coughing, and other movements that involve the thoracic cage. Palpation of the site of fracture with the finger elicits severe tenderness, and voluntary splinting of the chest is often present.

Fracture with displacement produces severe and often intolerable pain that prevents adequate breathing, coughing, and even slight chest movements. Such fractures traumatize the adjacent soft tissue and not infrequently penetrate the thoracic cavity to tear the pleura and rupture the lung, resulting in pneumothorax or hemopneumothorax. Even if the lung is not injured, damage to the adjacent nerves, vessels, and muscles initiates reflex mechanisms that result in skeletal muscle spasm, vasospasm, and decreased chest wall compliance. These together with the pain produce severe splinting of the thoracic wall, suppression of cough, and inadequate pulmonary ventilation—factors that predispose to atelectasis, hypoxemia, and perhaps pneumonitis.

Diagnosis

Diagnosis is usually not difficult and is based on the history of trauma or bouts of severe coughing, on the symptoms and signs, and on radiographic evidence. In the absence of radiographic evidence the site of the lesion can be determined by gently palpating the chest, having the patient breathe deeply, or both. Application of gentle pressure with one hand over the sternum and the other over the back is a helpful diagnostic maneuver.

Treatment

Treatment of simple fractures consists of relieving the pain and immobilizing the chest with adhesive tape to obtain prompt alignment of bone fragments. The tape should not be applied so tightly as to impair adequate ventilation. Displaced fractures require bed rest and pain control, whereas multiple rib fractures that cause instability of ventilation require pain control and assisted or controlled ventilation with an endotracheal tube or tracheostomy.

Effective relief of the chest pain is crucial to a favorable outcome. Although potent opioids given by mouth or intramuscularly have been used for many years, the suppression of cough that follows their administration leaves much to be desired. Even if given with the greatest care, it is difficult to maintain the precise balance between sufficient analgesia on the one hand and avoidance of respiratory depression and suppression of cough on the other. During the past 30 years or so the value of various forms of nerve blocks has been amply demonstrated. These procedures not only completely relieve the pain and the voluntary splinting but also interrupt reflex mechanisms, thus eliminating muscle spasm, vasospasm, and decrease in chest wall compliance. Following nerve block the patient can breathe deeply and cough without discomfort (the results of many studies are summarized in Chapter 94).

Infiltration of local anesthetic directly at the fracture site is a simple method that produces good pain relief but has several disadvantages. The skin area immediately over the fracture can be contused or infected, or both, and therefore might be an unfavorable site for the introduction of a needle. Moreover, the duration of pain relief is usually short, about 3 to 4 hours.

Posterior intercostal nerve block achieved by injection of a long-acting local anesthetic such as 0.5% bupivacaine produces complete pain relief for 6 to 10 hours. It should be done twice daily, early in the morning and in the evening. During the period of analgesia the patient is encouraged to cough and expectorate productively and to ventilate deeply.

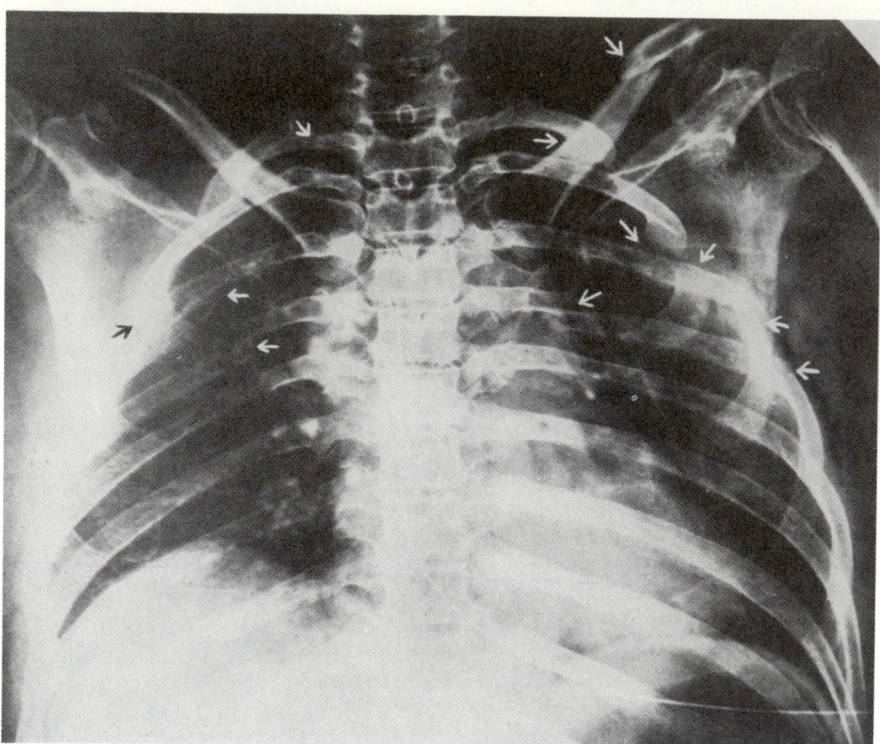

FIG. 58-2. Roentgenogram showing multiple fractures of the upper four ribs sustained in an automobile accident by a 56-year-old nurse. Promptly after the accident she entered the hospital complaining of severe pain and inability to breathe, cough, or move without aggravating the pain. The respirations were shallow, at a rate of 60/minute, the pulse was 120/minute, and the blood pressure was 90/60. The pain was initially treated with 15 mg of morphine IM and, although this produced some relief, the patient was unable to cough effectively. Following consultation with her physician a continuous segmental epidural analgesia was initiated by inserting a catheter percutaneously into the epidural space and advancing it to the level of the T3 vertebra. Injection of 6 to 8 ml of 0.1% tetracaine produced a band of analgesia extending from the C8 to T5 vertebrae. Within 10 minutes the patient was completely relieved and the pulse and respiratory rates decreased gradually to 90 and 28/minute, respectively. The block was continued for 7 days until trial without block for 30 hours indicated that it was no longer necessary. From Bonica, J.J.: The Management of Pain. Philadelphia, Lea & Febiger, 1953, p. 1171.

Continuous segmental epidural analgesia is particularly suitable in the management of multiple rib fractures, in which it offers significant advantages over the use of intercostal or even paravertebral block. It has the advantage of producing a region of analgesia that covers all painful areas; this effect can be made continuous by giving "top-up" injections or by continuous infusion. Figure 58-2 shows the use of an epidural catheter to provide continuous segmental analgesia of the upper portion of the chest. The disadvantage of epidural analgesia with local anesthetic is that it produces vasomotor blockade and thus, in patients who are hypovolemic or who are otherwise in a high-risk group it is relatively contraindicated.

Epidural opioid analgesia is now considered to be the method of choice for managing patients with chest pain caused by fractured ribs. Although the number of cases reported to date is small, it is likely that this procedure is being used worldwide with increasing frequency. The technique is described in detail in Chapter 95.

Rib Trauma Without Fracture

Trauma to the rib cage without fracture is also a common cause of chest wall pain that is aggravated by deep breathing and movement. Usually point tenderness occurs at the site of trauma and a local swelling can be present. (Fig. 58-3).

The significance of metastasis from carcinoma of the lung, breast, prostate, thyroid, and kidney as a cause of costopleural pain is discussed in Chapter 57. These lesions often present either as a painful rib swelling or as a pathologic fracture. Primary neoplasms and tumor-like conditions are rare and include osteochon-droma, multiple exostoses, chondrosarcoma, multiple myeloma, and eosinophilic granuloma (18).

Slipping Rib Syndrome (XVII-10)

The slipping rib syndrome was first described by Davies-Colley (27) in 1922, and has been frequently reported as a cause of chest pain since then (28–30). It is characterized by pain at the lower costal margin associated with an increasing mobility of the anterior end of the costal cartilage, most often that of the 10th rib and occasionally that of the 8th and 9th ribs. This syndrome has been called by various names, including slipping rib, clicking rib, rib gliding, rib-tip syndrome, slipping rib cartilage, displaced ribs, and nerve nipping at the intercostal margin (see 2 and 18 for references).

Etiology and Pathophysiology

The syndrome is thought to be traumatic in origin because many patients, when questioned, recall past injury to the affected side. The injury causes separation of the costal cartilages. Figure 53-5 shows that the upper seven ribs articulate directly with the sternum by their respective cartilages but the cartilages of the 8th, 9th, and 10th ribs articulate with the cartilage above by endochondral synovial membrane, which is surrounded by fibrous tissue. Structurally this is the weakest point in the chest and so is particularly vulnerable to trauma. Following separation the loosened end of the cartilage curls upward; this automatically slips up and down during respiration or it can slip anteriorly and posteriorly over the border of the upper cartilage, with a click and pain that are diagnostic

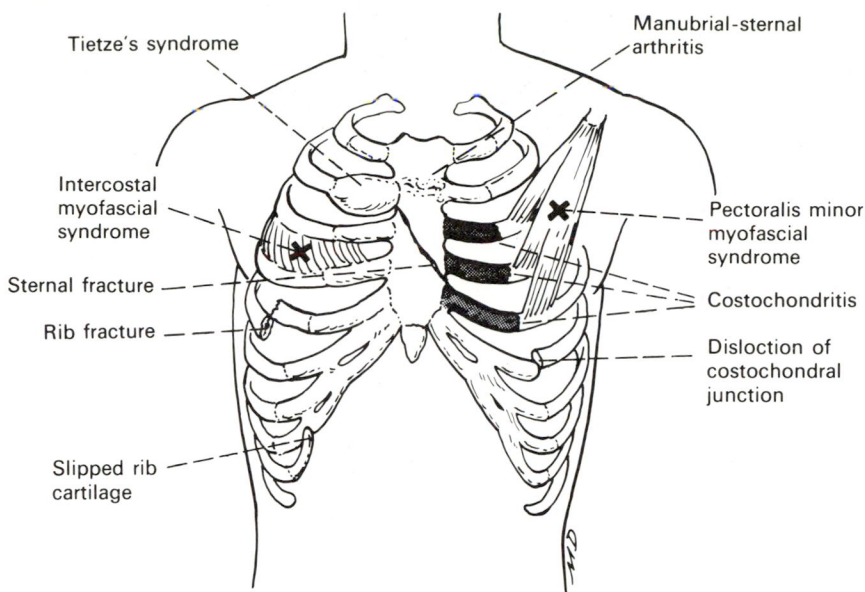

FIG. 58-3. Schematic diagram of the chest showing some of the most important musculoskeletal disorders that cause chest pain.

(27–30). This slipping of cartilage can traumatize the perichondrium of the cartilage above as well as the intercostal nerve.

Symptoms and Signs

Several types of pain can be associated with this syndrome. The pain is often sharp and stabbing and is localized to the upper quadrant or to the epigastric area. The pain is aggravated by hyperextension of the rib cage caused by raising the arms. In the acute phase the pain causes the patient to bend forward and to the side to relieve the tension on the abdominal muscles, which are attached to the costal margins. Occasionally the pain is dull, aching, or burning, located below the costal margin and radiating to the back. The involved costal cartilage is tender and moves more freely than normal.

The symptoms are readily confused with pain originating from abdominal viscera, with many reports of needless laparotomies performed to diagnose what seemed to be visceral pain (30). Often hyperesthesia can be demonstrated along the course of the intercostal nerve, possibly with spasm of the associated intercostal muscles. To confuse the clinical picture further, the patient might react to the pain with nausea and vomiting. The persistence of the distress and the inability of the physician to make a correct diagnosis can cause mental anguish in the patient, with possible ensuing depression.

Diagnosis

The diagnosis can be made only by acumen and by bearing this condition in mind. No associated laboratory findings can be found, which should cause one to think of chest wall syndromes in the diagnosis of abdominal pain. The rib margin is radiologically normal and fluoroscopy is not helpful. Holmes (29) described the pathognomonic test, which involves "hooking" the curled fingers of the examiner under the inferior rib margin and pulling anteriorly. This maneuver produces a clicking noise as the detached cartilage slides over the rib cartilage above and aggravates the pain. Because the condition is almost always unilateral, performing the hooking maneuver on the contralateral side should not produce a similar pain (30). The diagnosis can be confirmed by infiltrating the space between the detached cartilage and rib with 5 ml of 0.5% lidocaine, waiting about 10 minutes, and repeating the maneuver, at which time it should prove painless.

Treatment

Conservative treatment consists of reassurance of the patient and administration of systemic nonopioid analgesics to relieve the pain. I have obtained prolonged pain relief by repeated injection of 0.1% tetracaine or 0.25% bupivacaine combined with a corticosteroid. In patients for whom repeated injections do not produce prolonged relief, surgical resection of the rib margin produces permanent relief (28, 30).

Tietze's Syndrome

Tietze's syndrome, first described by Tietze in 1921 (31), consists of a nonspecific, benign, self-limiting, nonsuppurative painful swelling of the costal cartilages, most often the 2nd and occasionally the 3rd. The condition is often confused with costochondritis, another clinical syndrome associated with pain and tenderness of the costochondral junctions, that occurs much more frequently than Tietze's syndrome.

Etiology and Pathophysiology

True Tietze's syndrome is a relatively rare condition affecting young people (including children), with a predilection for those in their second and third decades and of either gender. The causes are unknown but respiratory straining, such as severe cough, heavy manual work, and deficient nutrition, have been suggested as causative factors (2). Motulsky and Rohn (32) suggested that coughing and sudden movements produce small tears (microtrauma) in the inconstant intra-articular sternocostal ligaments. Clinically, respiratory disease and rheumatic conditions often precede the onset of chest pain (33). No occupational, racial, or geographic disposition has been noted, although clustering of cases has been reported (33).

The disorder has a predilection for the 2nd and 3rd costochondral junctions (31–34). The 2nd alone is involved in 60% of patients (35). The chondrosternal, manubriosternal, sternoclavicular, and xiphisternal articulations are affected less frequently. Lesions are unilateral and single in more than 80% of patients (36). The swelling can progress to an irregular mass that obliterates the adjacent intercostal spaces.

Symptoms and Signs

Pain of variable intensity in the anterior chest wall is the predominant symptom. It is usually localized to the involved synchondrosis but can radiate widely over the anterior chest wall, occasionally to the shoulder and neck. In some patients the pain is similar to that produced by a heavy weight pressing on the chest but in others it is a vague soreness or tightness. The pain is aggravated by coughing, deep breathing, and lying prone. The affected costal cartilage(s) is tender and swollen but the overlying skin shows no alteration and moves freely over the overlying tender bulbous or fusiform swelling. Heat and erythema are absent, and no constitutional disturbances are noted.

The disorder runs a self-limited course of remissions and exacerbations (31–34, 36). The pain can cease spontaneously within 2 to 3 weeks but not infrequently it lasts months, and the residual swelling can persist for much longer, months or even several years (2).

Diagnosis

The diagnosis is made by a careful history and thorough examination of the chest and by exclusion of other conditions affecting the costal cartilages, such as rheumatoid arthritis, pyogenic arthritis, tumors, and relapsing polychondritis (37). No characteristic radiographic features are found, and calcification of costal cartilages is not characteristic of this syndrome. Abnormal accumulation of radionuclide of the involved costochondral joint has been reported (35) but similar findings are seen in patients with costochondritis and thus this is not helpful in the differential diagnosis. Laboratory and other tests are used to exclude other conditions but are not helpful in diagnosing this syndrome.

Treatment

One of the most important parts of management of patients with Tietze's syndrome is reassurance about the benign character of the disorder to allay fears and apprehension about cardiac disease. Local application of heat and the use of salicylates or other NSAIDs provide relief of mild to moderate pain. In patients who have severe and persistent pain, local infiltration of the involved costal cartilages with a long-lasting local anesthetic such as bupivacaine, alone or in combination with steroid, provides effective relief, often for many hours or even days. Block of the intercostal nerves done 1.5 to 2 inches proximal to the costochondral joint of the affected level is likely to produce even longer lasting pain relief and is indicated if other measures are not effective.

Anterior Chest Wall Syndrome (Costochondritis)

The anterior chest wall syndrome, or costochondritis, is a relatively frequent cause of anterior chest pain, both as a primary condition and in combination with coronary heart disease. The condition is recognized under various other labels, including chest wall syndrome, costosternal syndrome, and costosternal chondrodynia (2, 18, 38–42). In addition to the fact that it is a frequent cause of anterior chest pain, it is important because its pain simulates cardiac pain and thus causes great concern in the patient and confusion in the clinician. This is particularly true in patients who have this syndrome associated with a type of heart disease that can produce angina pectoris, such as coronary artery disease, hypertrophic cardiomyopathy, mitral valve prolapse, or aortic valve disease.

Etiology and Pathophysiology

The pathogenesis of costochondritis, or its relationship to Tietze's syndrome, is unknown. A traumatic cause has been proposed but pathologic abnormalities have not been described (2, 43). The condition has been observed in association with myofascial pain syndromes and with cervical osteoarthritis (18).

Symptoms and Signs

Costochondritis is characterized by pain of the anterior chest wall that can radiate widely. Palpation of the affected portions of the thoracic cage elicits local tenderness at multiple sites and also reproduces radiation of the pain as previously described by the patient. In contrast to Tietze's syndrome, in which only one level is involved in 80% of patients, multiple sites are present in 90% of patients with costochondritis (Table 58-4). The 2nd to 5th costal cartilages are most frequently affected (39, 40). Usually the pain and tenderness are located more easily than with Tietze's syndrome and, in contrast to Tietze's syndrome, no local swelling is present. The condition occurs more frequently in women (a ratio of 3:1) and at a later age in life (two-thirds of patients are over the age of 40). Respiratory symptoms occur only in about 12% of patients with costochondritis, as compared to about 85% of those with Tietze's syndrome. Movement of the chest and body can frequently aggravate the pain.

Inflammation of the upper costal cartilages can cause intense chest pain that often is mistaken for that of cardiac disease, and the patient is referred to a cardiologist (40, 41). When the condition involves the lower costal cartilages the pain is in the upper abdomen, and such patients are frequently referred to a gastroenterologist (43).

The importance of this condition in causing chest or abdominal pain in adolescents was emphasized by

TABLE 58-4. Tietze's Syndrome and Costochondritis

Feature	Tietze's Syndrome	Costochondritis
Frequency	Rare	More common
Age group most commonly affected	<40 years	≥40 years
Number of sites affected	One in 80%	More than one in 90%
Costochondral junctions most commonly involved	2nd (occasionally 3rd)	2nd to 5th
Local swelling	Present	Absent
Associated conditions	Respiratory tract infections	Cervical strain syndrome, coronary heart disease, myofascial syndrome

Modified from Fam, A.G., and Smythe, H.A.: Musculoskeletal chest wall pain. Can. Med. Assoc. J. *133*:379, 1985.

Brown (44). In a study of 100 patients in an adolescent outpatient clinic who complained of chest or upper abdominal pain, 79 were found to have only tender costal cartilages. In this group the pain was usually located in the anterior chest but, in a number of patients, it radiated to the back and abdomen. The condition was more often unilateral than bilateral, affecting the left side more often than the right side. The left 4th sternocostal cartilage was most frequently involved. A simple program of mild analgesic and reassurance was sufficient treatment for all patients.

Diagnosis

Because this syndrome is often confused with pain of cardiac or abdominal origin, it is essential to carry out a comprehensive history and physical examination including a complete neurologic and musculoskeletal evaluation. Epstein and associates (43) carefully studied 12 patients with severe and often incapacitating chest pain that was believed to be cardiac in origin but that on subsequent evaluation was shown to be the anterior chest wall syndrome. Several maneuvers were found to be helpful in establishing the diagnosis, including a noninvasive test to differentiate it from cardiac disease. A maneuver was considered to be positive for chest wall syndrome if it precipitated pain similar in quality and location to the spontaneous pain. Part of the examination required the application of firm steady pressure to the sternum and to the left and right parasternal junctions, the intercostal spaces, the ribs, the inframammary area, and the entire pectoralis major muscle, including its insertion. Another maneuver, the "horizontal flexion test," consisted of having the arm flexed across the anterior chest and applying steady prolonged traction in a horizontal direction while at the same time, the patient's head was rotated as far as possible toward the ipsilateral shoulder (43). Another test, the "crowing rooster maneuver," consisted of having the patient extend the neck as much as possible by looking toward the ceiling while the clinician, standing behind the patient, exerted traction on the posteriorly extended arms. Epstein and co-workers (43) also used radionuclide cineangiographic studies performed both at rest and during symptom-limited bicycle exercise performed in the supine position, which allowed visualization of regional heart wall motion abnormalities as well as calculation of the left ventricular ejection fraction.

Of the 12 patients, 11 had exertional chest pain, all experienced pain at rest, and 8 had episodes of pain that awakened them from sleep (43). One patient with isolated chest wall syndrome described what was considered to be classic angina pectoris. All patients had chest wall tenderness, the location of which is shown in Figure 58-4. The most common site of tenderness was the left parasternal region (7 of 12 patients), followed by the inframammary region, (5 of 12), the left pectoral muscles, including their insertions (4 of 12), and the sternum (3 of 12). Of the 12 patients, 11 had a positive horizontal flexion test and 4 had a positive "crowing rooster" test. All patients with the chest wall syndrome had a normal ejection fraction and normal regional wall motion, both at rest and during exercise. Epstein and colleagues (43) concluded that the radionuclide cineangiographic test, which is

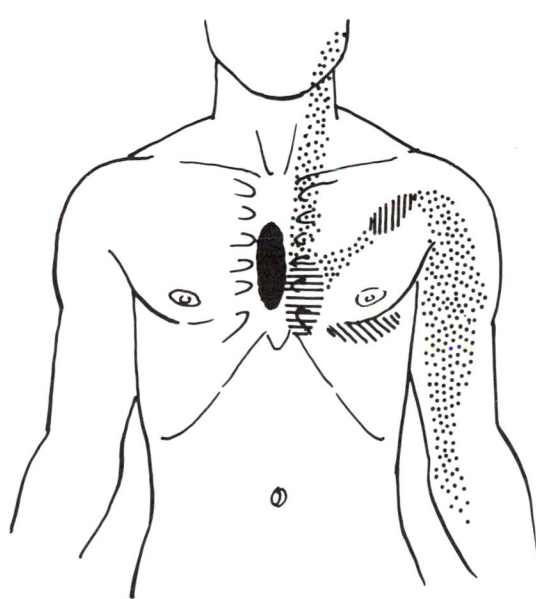

FIG. 58-4. Pattern of pain in patients with anterior chest wall syndrome showing the regions in the anterior chest in which spontaneous pain was most frequently experienced and where tenderness could be elicited. The black and striped areas represent primary sites of pain and of tenderness and the stippled areas represent radiation of the pain. Modified from Epstein, S.E., Gerber, L.H., and Borer, J.S.: Chest wall syndrome: A common cause of unexplained cardiac pain. JAMA, *241*:2793, 1979.

invariably positive in patients with coronary artery disease, is a sensitive method for differentiating between anterior chest wall syndrome and cardiac pathology.

In patients who have the chest wall syndrome in association with organic heart disease, the characteristics of the pain and tenderness also help in differentiating between the two conditions. In most patients with anterior chest wall syndrome the pain is localized mainly in the precordium or the left parasternal region, usually at the level of the left 3rd or 4th intercostal space, and often radiating superiorly toward the left shoulder and down the left arm—characteristics that differ from the pain of myocardial ischemia. Moreover, the pain usually occurs at rest and lasts for many minutes to hours, which also distinguishes it from pain of cardiac origin. In the relatively small percentage of patients in whom the pain is indistinguishable from that of typical angina pectoris caused by coronary disease, careful questioning often discloses that the pain has atypical precipitating features that are more closely related to postural changes and to stresses imposed on chest wall structures than to physical exertion per se. Although the prompt pain-relieving effect of nitroglycerin is usually considered good evidence that the pain is a result of myocardial ischemia, some patients with chest wall pain and no evidence of any organic heart disease have reported relief after taking sublingual nitrate.

The most critical finding establishing the diagnosis of chest wall syndrome is the detection of chest wall tenderness on physical examination, which is present in all patients. Tenderness located in the region of origin of spontaneous pain, particularly when the quality of the pain evoked by the physician reproduces the spontaneous pain, together with a negative radionuclide test, provides the strongest evidence of chest wall syndrome.

A highly reliable and effective differential diagnostic procedure that can be carried out in such patients is producing intercostal block at the posterior axillary line. This provides complete relief of pain from chest wall pathology but has little or no effect on cardiac pain because the nociceptive pathways from the heart are in the sympathetic afferents located in the paravertebral region.

Treatment

Treatment of costochondritis, or chest wall syndrome, consists of reassurance of the patient, the use of NSAIDs, alone or in combination with codeine, the application of heat, and other physical therapeutic measures. Perhaps the most important of these is reassuring the patient that the pain is of benign origin, thus helping to avoid the emotional and financial burdens often associated with an erroneous diagnosis of organic heart disease. Epstein and associates (43) reported that many of their patients had been admitted to coronary care units many times because of the suspicion of acute myocardial infarction. Other patients manifested chronic anxiety, largely because they believed that the chest pain was a harbinger of imminent death. Contributing to their anxiety were the fears generated by well-meaning physicians, who

often misdiagnosed coronary artery disease. The reassurance that can be provided by a diagnosis of an annoying but non-life-threatening condition can often in itself lead to dramatic symptomatic improvement and rehabilitation. In patients with anterior chest wall syndrome who have severe pain, intercostal block at the posterior axillary line provides complete relief for 6 to 10 hours (see Chapter 94). This procedure can also be used to demonstrate to the patient that the disease is in the anterior chest wall by explaining the difference in the nerve supplies to the chest wall and the heart.

Tumors of the Costal Cartilages

Tumors of the costal cartilages are rare; when they occur, however, they usually attract notice by their growth rather than by obscure chest pain. They should be distinguished from tuberculosis or fungus abscess, gumma, malunited fractures, deformities, and Tietze's syndrome. When a tumor mass can be felt diagnosis is rarely difficult. Pain can be a heavy, chronic, boring distress but can be pleuritic and referred along the course of the intercostal nerve. Treatment is usually by surgical excision.

Costochondral Dislocation

Dislocation at the costochondral junction, secondary to trauma, causes pain in the injured part of the chest. It is frequently seen in patients under 30 years of age. The pain can be continuous, dull, aching, and burning, with discomfort localized to an area of the costal margin and occasionally referred to the back, or it can have the sharp and lancinating character of radicular pain. Occasionally the pain is more disabling than that associated with a simple fracture of the rib. Local tenderness is invariably present. Palpation of the area can reveal a tumor mass that probably represents the accumulation of excess cartilaginous material at the point of injury.

Treatment consists of reduction of the dislocation and subsequent pain relief. If the condition is of recent origin it can be reduced by manipulation after the region has been anesthetized by local infiltration of the site of dislocation or, more effectively, by block of the intercostal nerves above and below the site of dislocation. The site of injection can be the anterior axillary line or the midclavicular line (Chapter 94).

Pain Caused by Pathology of the Sternum and Its Articulation

Trauma and Arthritis of the Sternoclavicular Joint

Pain arising from the sternoclavicular joint can radiate to the anterior chest wall and thereby simulate pain of cardiopulmonary origin. The major causes of sternoclavicular joint arthritis include osteoarthritis, rheumatoid arthritis, ankylosing spondylitis, psoriatic arthritis, and infection (18, 45). Pain in the sternoclavicular joint can also result from traumatic subluxation or dislocation (Chapter 50) or from tumor metastases.

The pain is aggravated by shrugging the shoulder and is associated with severe tenderness on palpation of the joint. Local swelling and crepitus are usually present.

Treatment of these conditions is discussed in detail in Chapters 20 and 50. The pain is usually controlled with NSAIDs alone or in combination with modest doses of codeine. Except for those patients who have an infectious process, injection of the joint with local anesthetic and corticosteroid provides good relief that can last several days or even longer.

Sternoclavicular Hyperostosis

Sternoclavicular hyperostosis is a recently recognized syndrome that is manifested by bilateral chronic painful swelling of the clavicles, sternum, and first ribs (46). Radiologic abnomalities include hyperostosis, widening and increased bone density of the clavicles and sternum, ossification of the 1st costal cartilage, and sternoclavicular synostosis (46). Skeletal scintigraphy demonstrates increased activity in the involved bones. Histologic examination shows ossifying periostitis associated with general hyperostosis. The cause of this condition is unknown, although a relation to pustular psoriasis and psoriatic arthritis has been suggested (47). Laboratory values are normal except for occasional elevation of the erythrocyte sedimentation rate and hypergammaglobulinemia.

The condition follows a relapsing course. Bone enlargement and extension of the inflammatory process can lead to occlusion of the subclavian vein or can cause a thoracic outlet syndrome (46).

The diagnosis is based on radiographic and scintigraphic findings. This condition can be distinguished from Paget's disease of bone by the characteristic symmetric involvement of the clavicles, sternum, and upper ribs, the presence of sternoclavicular synostosis, and a finding of normal serum alkaline phosphatase and urinary hydroxyproline levels (18).

Treatment is symptomatic and consists of the use of anti-inflammatory drugs, including indomethacin and corticosteroids. Radiotherapy can be beneficial in severe cases (18).

Manubriosternal Arthritis

Arthritis of the manubriosternal joint can cause localized pain in the upper sternal region. The pain occurs in those with ankylosing spondylitis, rheumatoid arthritis, or psoriatic arthritis, and is rarely caused by infection (48, 49). The resulting pain is either localized to the joint or radiates widely along the upper ribs to the shoulders, mimicking the pain of angina. The pain can either be constant or intermittent and is sometimes periodic (2). It is aggravated by motion of the chest and deep breathing, particularly when the movements are intensified as in deep inspiration, coughing, sneezing, and yawning. The pain is often associated with localized tenderness and swelling of the joint.

The diagnosis should include identification of the pathologic process. Treatment of these various arthritides is discussed in detail in Chapter 20. The pain is usually well controlled with NSAIDs used alone or in combination with modest doses of codeine. In patients with severe pain who do not have infection of the joint, infiltration with a local anesthetic and corticosteroids produces good pain relief for several days or longer.

Trauma to Sternum

Blunt injury to the sternum can cause strain or even partial subluxation of the manubriosternal joint. At the time of or soon after injury the patient experiences sharp pain localized to the area of the angle of Louis. Pain can also radiate into a broader area. Simple joint sprain can be managed conservatively with systemic analgesics and the application of heat. If the patient has severe pain local infiltration of the joint with a long-lasting anesthetic and steroid produces effective relief. If the displacement is sufficient to require surgical intervention, it is best done with regional analgesia achieved by blocking the intercostal nerves at the midclavicular line at the level of the 2nd and 3rd ribs.

Xiphoidalgia Syndrome

Xiphoidalgia syndrome is characterized by spontaneous pain in the anterior chest associated with distinct discomfort and tenderness of the xiphoid process of the sternum (2). This relatively rare condition is also known by various other names, including painful xiphoid syndrome, hypersensitive xiphoid, and xiphoid cartilage syndrome. Lipkin and colleagues (50) quoted a study of 24 patients with this syndrome associated with tender xiphoid and, as a control study, they examined 200 consecutive unselected ward patients. Among those in the control group, 6 were found to have a tender xiphoid process, and 4 of these complained of chest pains strongly suggestive of this syndrome.

Etiology and Pathophysiology

Little is known about the cause and pathophysiology of the xiphoid syndrome. The disorder generally occurs without the presence of known disease but has been observed concurrently in patients with coronary artery disease, intestinal disease, arthritis, and neurologic and metabolic disorders, and is likely to be confused with some of these when it occurs independently (2). Because the xiphoid process receives its nerve supply from the phrenic nerves and the T4 to T7 intercostal nerves, pathology in this structure produces widespread pain.

Symptoms and Signs

The xiphoidalgia syndrome is characterized by intermittent low substernal or epigastric pain that can radiate to the precordium or abdomen, simulating the pain of cardiac and abdominal disease, respectively. The xiphoid cartilage is tender, and pressure duplicates the pain and its radiation. Lipkin and colleagues (50) described the spontaneous pain as "a deep slightly nauseating ache, somewhat like that experienced after a blow in the celiac plexus." The intensity varies considerably from an annoying, slight, aching discomfort to an agonizing pain, which the patient might believe arises from cardiac disease or an abdominal disorder (2).

The pain can be precipitated or aggravated by movement that acts on the xiphoid, such as bending, stooping and turning, particularly after a full meal, which itself increases the pressure behind the xiphoid process (2). Usually it is not precipitated by exertion, but careful questioning might be necessary to determine whether a particular movement rather than exercise itself has brought on the pain. The pain of this condition generally does not subside immediately after the aggravating motion has ceased, as do many other types of chest pain. The frequency of pain is variable but can occur several times a day. Its duration varies from minutes to several hours but it usually lasts for an appreciable time after it is provoked. In addition to reproducing the spontaneous pain and its radiation, deep pressure can cause the pain to be felt deep in the chest (retrosternal), shoulder, and back.

Diagnosis and Treatment

The diagnosis of xiphoidalgia syndrome is made on the basis of the characteristics of the pain and tenderness and on the exclusion of other causes of pain in this region. The disorder ordinarily persists for weeks or months but usually disappears spontaneously without special treatment (2). Mild to moderate pain and tenderness are effectively controlled with nonopioid systemic analgesics. If these prove ineffective in patients with severe pain, injection of a long-lasting local anesthetic and a steroid into the xiphosternal joint usually provides effective relief for hours and sometimes days. In patients in whom these conservative measures fail to relieve severe pain surgical resection should be considered, but this is rarely necessary (2).

Chest Pain Caused by Myofascial Pain Syndromes

Myofascial pain syndrome (MPS) with trigger points (TPs) are among the most common causes of pain in the anterior and posterior chest. MPSs are characterized by local and referred pain, muscle spasm, tenderness, stiffness, limitation of motion and, occasionally, autonomic dysfunction. Although most of these syndromes develop gradually, they can develop rather suddenly in some patients; symptoms and signs can be mistaken by the patient as being caused by heart disease, thus resulting in great concern, anxiety, and apprehension (51–53). Unless the physician keeps these conditions in mind when consulting with the patients who present with chest pain, the rapid onset of pain, especially in the anterior chest, can mislead the physician into making a wrong diagnosis and proceeding with highly sophisticated and costly laboratory tests. Although the causes, symptoms and signs, and therapy are described in detail in Chapter 21, they are summarized here briefly before describing specific syndromes.

General Considerations

Etiology and Pathophysiology

Myofascial pain in the chest is usually the result of a specific traumatic event in the form of unusual stress of the affected muscle, or it can result from repetitive or continuous stress during work or certain athletic exercises. In some patients MPS in the chest can result from poor posture, degenerative disease of the thoracic spine, or emotional stress, which through psychophysiologic mechanisms can cause tension in the affected chest muscles. These in turn produce abnormal muscle sensitivity secondary to sympathetic hyperactivity and reflex spasm, which become a new source of nociceptive input.

Symptoms and Signs

The pain of myofascial syndromes in the chest can vary from a slight ache to severe, unrelenting, and disabling discomfort. The pain can either be sharp or dull and, because it is often referred, it can mislead the patient and clinician to suspect disorders of the thoracic viscera.

In the absence of specific clinical findings in patients complaining of pain in the chest, the muscles should be carefully examined for hyperactive TPs. The clinician must also remember that TPs are likely to be activated as a secondary cause of pain in association with any injury or strain, and that failure to diagnose and treat hyperactive points intensifies the pain, thus delaying healing and making rehabilitation more difficult.

Diagnosis

Screening for myofascial syndromes should include a complete history and thorough physical examination, as discussed in Chapter 21. To identify TPs in specific muscles it is necessary to palpate the suspected muscle or muscles systematically with a finger or blunt object and to compare the particular muscle with the contralateral muscle.

The patient should be positioned for examination so that the muscles of the chest as well as those of the shoulder and upper back can be examined both in relaxed and stretched positions. The entire surface of the suspected muscle or muscles should be systematically palpated for masses, tightness, and ropiness, as well as for the hypersensitive TP.

Treatment

In approaching treatment of a chest MPS, it is important to understand that regional findings are likely to be associated with one or more predictable patterns of MPS, as discussed below. Treatment of hyperactive points in the chest without identification and treatment of dominant points can have limited success or can intensify myofascial activity in the dominant areas (usually the low back and hip regions).

The need for a comprehensive treatment approach is emphasized in Chapter 21, in which such a program is discussed in detail. We prefer penetration and injection of TPs. For this purpose a short (2.5 cm) and fine (27- or 30-gauge) needle is adequate for TPs in most chest muscles. For each TP we use 1 to 2 ml of 0.5% procaine or lidocaine or 0.125 to 0.25% bupivacaine. When the trigger point is penetrated the tight muscle can actually be felt to "grab" the needle and, after injection, the muscle is felt to relax, releasing the needle dramatically.

Following injection the patient is maintained in a comfortable position with warm moist packs applied to the treatment area for approximately 10 minutes. Treated muscles should be guarded against overuse for several days because they are highly susceptible to reactivation of the TPs.

Specific Myofascial Pain Syndromes

The most important MPSs with TPs that produce pain in the chest are listed in Table 58-5, according to the predominant location of the pain. As noted below, the site of pain produced by each of these syndromes overlaps the sites of other syndromes. Thus, it can be seen that the levator scapulae and trapezius muscles

TABLE 58-5. Myofascial Syndromes Causing Chest Pain

Location of Pain	Muscle Involved
Anterior chest	Sternalis; pectoralis major; pectoralis minor; scaleni muscle; sternocleidomastoid (sternal head); subclavius; iliocostalis cervicis
Upper thoracic back	Levator scapulae; trapezius multifidi
Midthoracic back	Latissimus dorsi; rhomboid; serratus posterior superior; trapezius serratus anterior
Low thoracic back	Serratus posterior inferior; iliocostalis thoracis multifidi

frequently cause pain in back of the chest with spillover to the shoulder but, because the most intense pain is found in the neck, they are discussed in Chapter 47. Similarly, although the scaleni, subscapularis, and teres major muscles can cause localized pain over the scapula, the predominant pain is located in the shoulder and is therefore discussed in Chapter 52. In the illustrations of myofascial syndromes included in this chapter (and elsewhere), the black area represents an "essential" zone, indicating that the pain is felt most intensely in this area and by most or all patients, while the stippled area represents the "spillover" zone, indicating that the pain referred to this region is milder and is experienced only by some patients.

Pectoralis Major Muscle Syndrome

Pain in the anterior part of the shoulder caused by TPs in the clavicular section of the pectoralis major muscle is described in Chapter 52. In this section we describe various pain syndromes caused by TPs in the intermediate sternal section of the pectoralis major, pain caused by TPs in the lateral free margin of the

muscle, and pain in the anterior chest caused by TPs in the parasternal region of the muscle.

Figure 58-5 depicts the patterns of referred pain and the site of the trigger points. As indicated, the solid black shows the essential areas of referred pain, whereas the stippled area shows the spillover pain areas (51–53). Activation of TPs in the intermediate sternal section of the pectoralis muscles produces intense pain in the anterior chest, with occasional spillover into the medial aspect of the arm and occasionally the forearm. TPs located in the lateral free margin of the muscle can cause pain and tenderness in the breast associated with hypersensitivity of the nipple and intolerance to wearing of clothing. In women the pain can be attributed to pathology within the breast and might be a source of severe anxiety and apprehension about the significance of the pain. TPs in the parasternal region of the pectoralis muscles cause pain in the parasternal region, which is a common site of pain produced by coronary artery disease.

The development and persistence of TPs in these various parts of the pectoralis major muscle can be initiated and reactivated in many ways, some of which are mentioned in Chapter 52. A frequent cause is excessive strain caused by heavy lifting, especially when reaching up in front, by overuse of the arm in abduction, by a repeated circle of movements, such as changing the tire of an automobile, or by sustaining lifting in a fixed position, such as with the use of a power saw (53). Contributing factors include high levels of anxiety, exposure of fatigued muscle to cold air, and prolonged round-shouldered posture that causes sutained shortening of the pectoral muscles.

Travell and Rinzler (54) long ago emphasized the relationship between acute myocardial infarction and the development of TPs in the pectoralis major and minor muscles. As indicated in Chapter 54, pain in acute myocardial infarction is commonly referred to

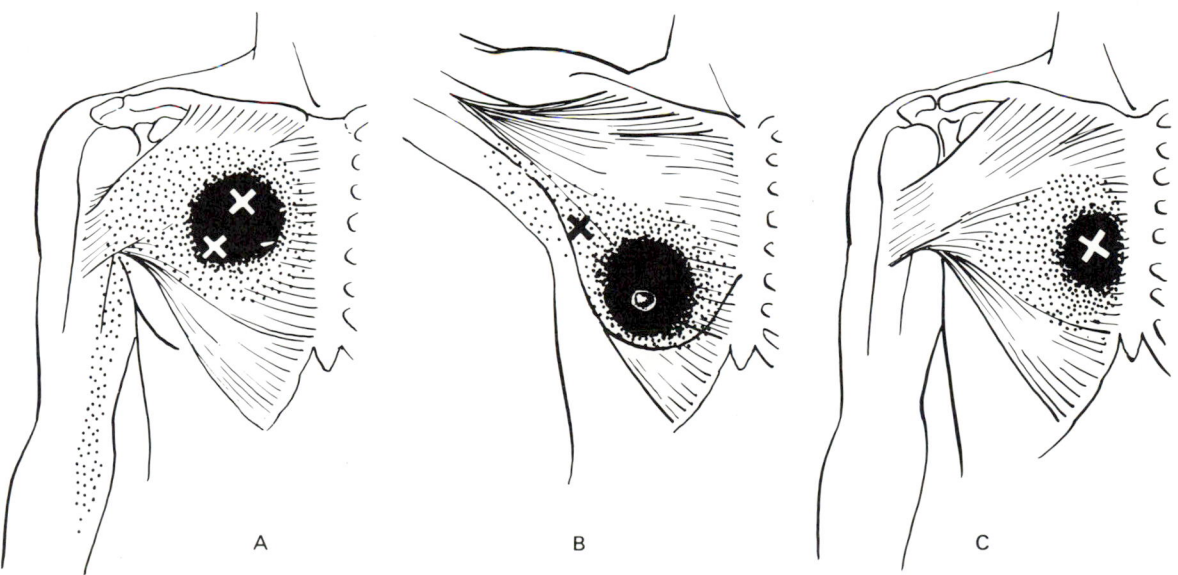

FIG. 58-5. Patterns of pain provoked by trigger points in different parts of the right pectoralis major muscle. **A.** Pattern provoked by trigger points (X) in the intermediate sternal section of the muscle. **B.** Pain and trigger points in the lateral margin of the muscle. **C.** Trigger point (X) in the medial margin of the muscle. The black area depicts the essential zone of pain while the stippled area shows the spillover zone.

sternal and parasternal regions in the area where the medial portions of the pectoralis major and minor muscles are attached. Injury to heart muscle initiates a viscerosomatic process that activates TPs in the pectoral and other anterior chest muscles. Following recovery from acute infarction, these self-perpetuating TPs tend to persist in the chest wall and to continue to cause chest pain (51, 54–57). The somatic component of cardiac pain that persists long after the acute attack is of great clinical relevance because it can cause continued anxiety and apprehension in the patient and might be confusing to the physician (Chapter 54).

Diagnosis of active myofascial TPs in the pectoralis muscles should be suspected in all patients who present with anterior chest pain. The location of the TP is ascertained by careful and systematic palpation of every square centimeter of the anterior chest, particularly the sternal, costal, and clavicular section of the muscles. Palpation of the TPs usually causes a strong local twitch response and markedly aggravates spontaneous pain or reproduces latent pain. The diagnosis of the syndrome is confirmed by the dramatic relief that follows the injection of the TP with small amounts of local anesthetics, as described above.

Relief of chest pain with therapy does not exclude cardiac disease because, in some patients, cardiac pain can be relieved by application of vapocoolant spray or by infiltration of local anesthetics subcutaneously into areas of referred cardiac pain (51, 54–58). Adding to the diagnostic challenge is the fact that many patients with myofascial syndromes obtain good pain relief by the use of nitroglycerin or nitrates. Moreover, it is well known that noncardiac pain can induce transient T-wave changes in the electrocardiogram (59). It is therefore essential to exclude heart disease as the cause of chest pain by appropriate tests of cardiac function as suggested in Chapter 54 and by Epstein and colleagues (43) in connection with anterior chest wall syndrome. For effective treatment of the pectoral muscle syndrome, needle penetration and injection of local anesthesia, as described above and in Chapter 21, is effective in relieving the pain and permitting stretch of the muscle. It is best when using vapocoolant spray to have the patient seated, abducting and flexing the arm at the shoulder and applying the vapocoolant spray cephalad over the stretched muscle (see Chapter 21). In addition patients should be made to carry out measures to correct poor posture and poor standing, to avoid mechanical overload of the muscle, and to exercise the muscle appropriately.

Sternalis Muscle Syndrome

The sternalis muscle is a frequent site of TPs that cause pain over the entire sternal and retrosternal regions. The pain can extend to the ipsilateral upper pectoral area, the front of the shoulder, and the medial aspect of the arm (51–53) (Fig. 58-6). This pattern closely mimics that of the retrosternal pain of myocardial infarction or angina pectoris and consequently produces anxiety and apprehension in patients who develop this syndrome. Fortunately, this syndrome can be differentiated from cardiac pain by the fact that movement does not aggravate myofascial pain. Some patients have trigger points in both the sternalis and

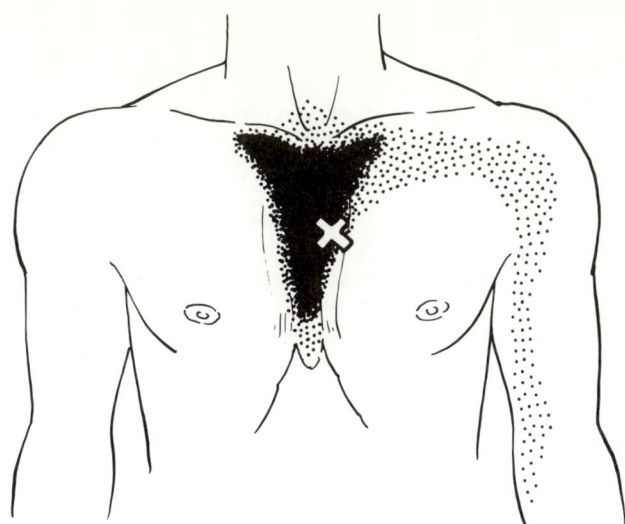

FIG. 58-6. Pattern of pain and trigger point (X) in the sternalis muscle. See text for details.

pectoralis muscles on the same side, or bilaterally (53–57).

Developments and persistence of TPs in the sternalis can be caused by direct trauma to the costosternal area but they are most frequently activated in patients with acute myocardial infarction (55–59). TPs in the sternalis that are activated by such episodes of myocardial ischemia are likely to persist long after healing.

The TPs are located by systematic palpation against the underlying sternum and costal cartilage. Although the TPs can appear anywhere in the muscle, including the midline, they are most likely to occur to the left of the midline at the midsternal level (53, 57).

When multiple areas of localized tenderness are found over the costochondral junction, with or without the area of pain, it is necessary to differentiate MPS from costochondritis, Tietze's syndrome, and other anterior chest well pain syndromes. The diagnosis of MPS is facilitated if dramatic relief of the wide area of pain is obtained by injection of the TPs with a small amount of local anesthetic. In contrast to other myofascial syndromes, the sternalis syndrome is not amenable to stretch and spray because the sternalis cannot be stretched.

Anterior Chest Pain From Other Myofascial Syndromes

Pain in the anterior portion of the chest can also be caused by TPs in the pectoralis minor, scaleni, sternal head of the sternocleidomastoid, and subclavius muscles. Because the first two syndromes mainly produce pain in the shoulders and upper limbs, with some spillover to the anterior chest, they are discussed in Chapter 52. The most prominent sites of pain caused by TPs in the sternocleidomastoid are the head and neck (Chapter 40). TPs in the sternal head of the muscle and TPs in the subclavius produce only a small area of pain in the region of the sternoclavicular joint and the intraclavicular area, respectively. They are not sufficiently important to be considered here. TPs in the serratus posterior superior muscle produce pain in the posterior aspect of the shoulder, as well as over the scapular region (Chapter 52). The following syndromes produce pain predominantly in the lateral and posterior parts of the thorax.

Serratus Anterior Muscle Syndrome

TPs in the serratus anterior muscles are usually located in the subcutaneous portion of the muscle in the midaxillary line, at about the level of the 5th or 6th rib (Fig. 58-7A). The essential zone of the pain pattern is located in and around the area of the TP on the lateral aspect of the chest (Fig. 58-7B) and is medial to the inferior angle of the scapula (Fig. 58-7C) (51–55). In a small number of patients the spillover zone can extend to the medial aspect of the upper limb. Moreover, in some patients, TPs in this muscle contribute to abnormal breast sensitivity in addition to the TPs in the pectoralis major muscle.

TPs in the serratus anterior muscle are developed and sustained by muscle strain during excessively fast or prolonged running, pushups, lifting heavy weights overhead, or severe coughing caused by respiratory disease (51–53). Contributing factors can be anxiety and other psychologic problems. The TPs are located by careful systematic point pressure over the muscle.

For injection of the trigger area, except for obese patients, only short needles should be used to minimize the risk of missing the muscle, passing through the intercostal space, and puncturing the lung. It is best to place the 2nd and 3rd fingers of one hand over the intercostal space above and below the level of the TP (to protect the space and prevent intercostal puncture) and, with the other hand to penetrate the TP

with the needle. Usually 2 to 3 ml of local anesthetic solution is sufficient. To use stretch and spray it is best to have patients lying on their unaffected side, retracting their arm to cause full retraction of the scapula. The spray is directed first posteriorly and then anteriorly to cover the muscle and its entire pain pattern (53). Corrective measures include reduction or elimination of overuse of the muscle and appropriate self-stretch exercises.

Intercostal Myofascial Syndrome

Intercostal muscles are frequently involved with painful TPs as a result of trauma, excessive coughing, or chest surgery (Fig. 58-8). Intercostal nerve blocks can only relieve these painful syndromes temporarily. The TP is located by carefully examining the involved intercostal spaces with the fingers. Once located, these trigger points should be injected with a long-acting anesthetic using a 30-gauge needle. Great care must be taken so that the patient does not flinch on injection.

Thoracic Paraspinal Muscle Syndromes

The paraspinal muscles consist of a superficial group of long-fibered longitudinal muscles collectively known as the erector spinae; these are comprised of the longissimus thoracis, iliocostalis thoracis, and a deep group of short diagonal muscles—including the semispinalis, multifidus, and rotators at successively deeper levels (53). Figure 58-9 depicts the referred pain patterns provoked by TPs in the iliocostalis thoracis and multifidus thoracis. These all produce pain in the posterior part of the chest.

TPs are activated and sustained either by a sudden overload, as when lifting objects with the back twisted and flexed, or by a sustained overload, as when stooping or when the back muscles are maintained in a fully shortened (hyperlordotic) position (53). In addition to the pattern of pain, the patient has restricted range of

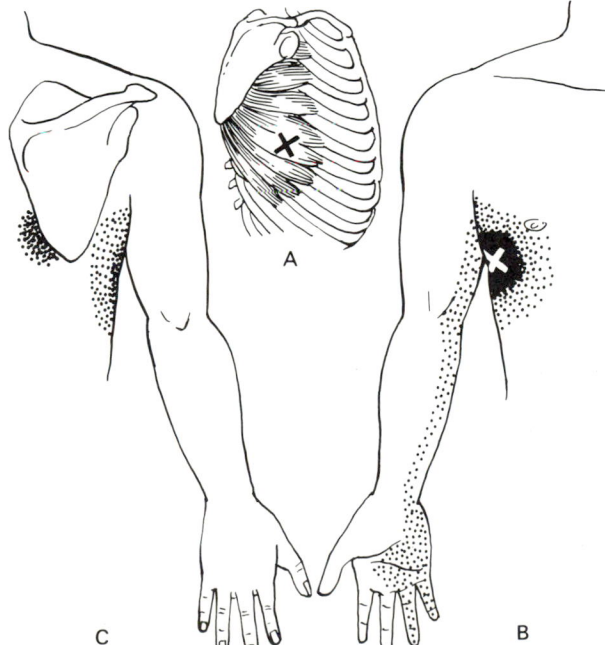

FIG. 58-7. Areas of pain and sites of trigger points (X) of the serratus anterior myofascial syndrome. **A.** Site of TP. **B.** Anterior view showing pain pattern. **C.** Posterior view showing spillover zone. See text for details.

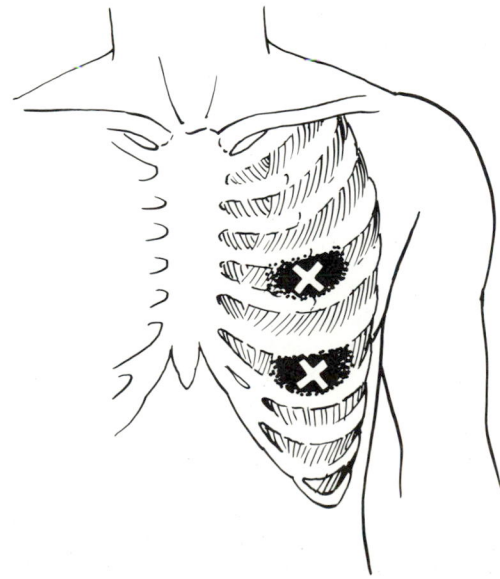

FIG. 58-8. Pattern of referred pain provoked by trigger points (X) in the intercostal muscles. This is a frequent cause of anterior chest pain.

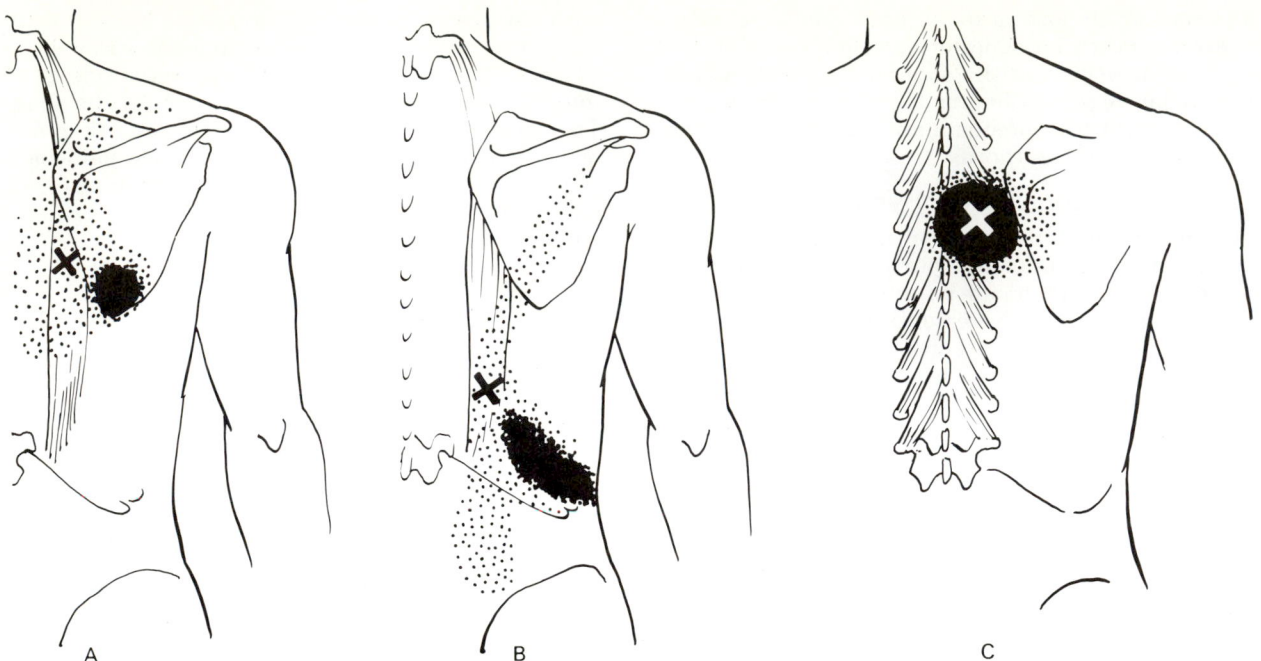

FIG. 58-9. Pain patterns with their corresponding trigger points (X) in the iliocostalis and multifidus thoracis muscles. **A.** Trigger point in the iliocostalis muscle just medial to the medial edge of the scapula. **B.** Trigger point in the lower portion of the iliocostalis thoracis. **C.** Posterior chest pain pattern provoked by trigger point in the upper part of the multifidus thoracis muscle.

back motion and spasm or tightness of the muscles. The TPs are located by systematic finger point palpation, covering the entire area in which the TP is suspected to be located on the basis of the pain pattern. Pressure over the TPs elicits the characteristic referred pain pattern. In many patients TPs produce reflex spasms, which develop into tense bands in the paraspinal muscles; these entrap the posterior primary divisions of the thoracic nerves and thus produce additional pain.

Treatment consists of penetration of the TPs and injection of a local anesthetic solution. In patients who are obese, muscular, or both, penetration of the deeper muscles requires a 5-cm 25- or 22-gauge needle. The stretch-and-spray technique for the long fiber erector spinae muscles is accomplished by flexing the spine of the seated patient while a jet stream of vapocoolant is applied with a downward parallel sweep. Successively deeper muscle layers require progressively more spinal rotation, with the patient's face turned toward the affected side and the vapocoolant sprayed diagonally. Corrective measures include compensation for body asymmetries, modification of daily activities to reduce stress on the back muscles, and graduated stretch and strengthening exercises (53).

Latissimus Dorsi Muscle Syndrome

The latissimus dorsi muscle is a frequently overlooked myofascial cause of midback pain. The TPs are usually located in the axillary portion of the muscle in the posterior axillary fold. Figure 58-10 shows the location of the TPs and the area of the pain pattern, which is generally concentrated in the region of the inferior angle of the scapula but occasionally has spillover to the back of the shoulder and down the

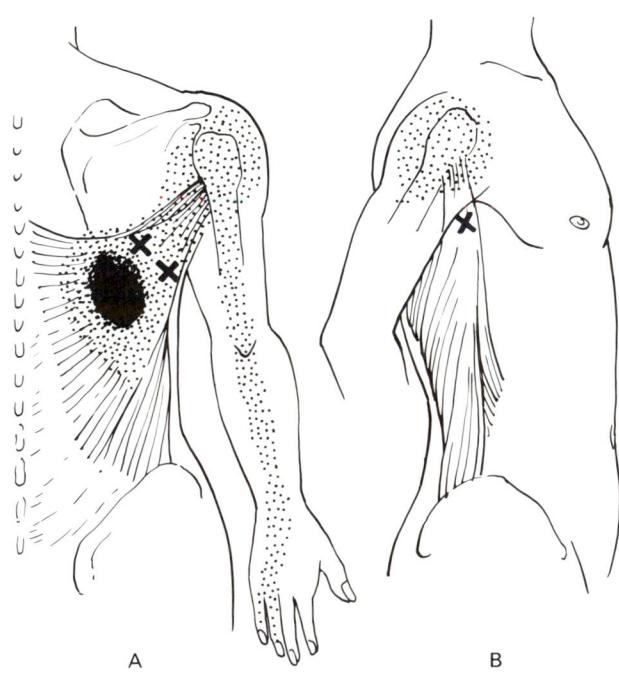

FIG. 58-10. Pain in the posterior part of the chest with spillover into the shoulder and arm caused by trigger points (X) in the right latissimus dorsi muscle. **A.** Posterior view. **B.** Lateral view.

medial aspect of the arm (53). The trigger area usually develops as a result of repetitive reaching forward and upward, either to manipulate some large object or to pull something down. In addition to the pain the patient might have minimal restriction of the range of motion.

The trigger point is located by pincer palpation of the posterior axillary fold at approximately the mid-scapular level. Injection and penetration of the TP are performed by grasping the muscle fibers within the posterior axillary fold in a pincer grip to inject them. Stretch and spray of the muscle is done from the iliac crest upward over the entire muscle and is continued over the referred pain pattern. Corrective measures should include avoidance of overloading the muscle, application of hot packs to the area, and having the patient perform progressive stretching exercises regularly.

Rhomboidei Muscle Syndromes

Pain referred from TPs in the rhomboidei major and minor muscles concentrates in the interval between the vertebral border of the scapula and the spinous processes (51, 54). Figure 58-11 depicts the composite referred pain pattern and the site of the TPs in the right rhomboidei muscles. TPs in the muscles are activated by prolonged leaning forward and working in a round-shouldered position, by overload caused by prominence of the scapula over the convex side in upper thoracic scoliosis, and by prolonged holding of the arm in abduction at 90° (53).

TPs in the middle transverse fibers of the trapezius muscle produce a referred pain pattern located in the paraspinal region opposite to the spinous processes of T1 to T3 or T4, just above the site of the rhomboid pain pattern.

The TPs are located by systematic palpation of the muscles between the medial border of the scapula and the spinous processes. Having the patient cross the arms anteriorly causes the scapula to retract and places the muscles under tension. Injection and penetration of the trigger point should be carried out with care, using a short needle to avoid accidental penetration of the pleura and lung. The risk can be almost eliminated by placing the 2nd and 3rd fingers over the intercostal space above and below the site of the TP, as described above. Stretch and spray requires protraction of the scapula with upper rotation of the

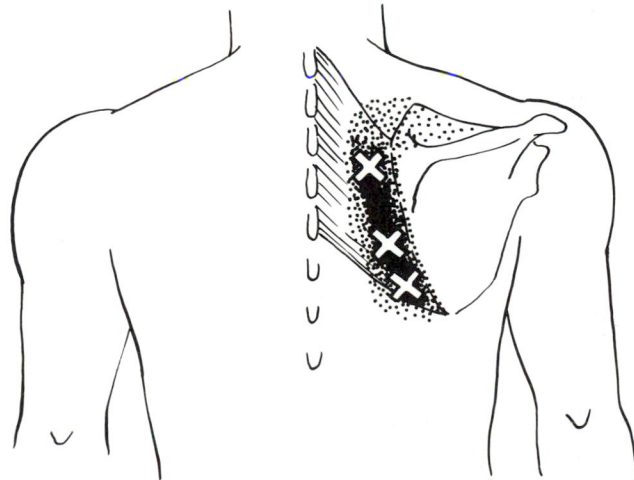

FIG. 58-11. Posterior chest pain caused by trigger points in the rhomboid muscles.

glenoid fossa to place the muscles in full stretch (53). The spray is applied in a caudad direction parallel to the muscle fibers. Corrective measures include inactivation of pectoral muscle TPs, correction of functional scoliosis, and strengthening exercises.

Other Painful Muscular Disorders

Traumatic Muscle Strain

Trauma to muscles of the chest can cause injury to muscle fibers throughout the entire muscle. The trauma might be in the form of repeated stress or excessive muscular activity, such as lifting, painting a ceiling, chopping wood, coughing, or exercising untrained muscles. These are the same causative factors that produce myofascial syndromes with TPs; in some patients, however, widespread "strained" muscles are produced with consequent pain and tenderness over the entire muscle. The pain is usually made worse by maneuvers that tense or stretch the muscle. Careful examination of the muscle does not reveal any localized tender or trigger points but indicates generalized tenderness over the entire muscle.

The diagnosis of traumatic pectoral and other chest muscle pain is made from the history and physical findings. Treatment consists of reassurance, local application of heat, use of systemic analgesics, rest of the injured muscles, and avoidance of repeating the activities responsible for the pain. In patients who have severe pain, infiltration of a dilute solution of a long-acting local anesthetic (e.g., 0.1% bupivacaine) throughout the muscle produces prompt pain relief.

Precordial Catch Syndrome

The precordial catch syndrome, also called the chest wall twinge syndrome, is a rare, benign, self-limited disorder of unknown cause, characterized by episodes of brief, sharp, stabbing precordial pain (18, 60, 61). The condition usually occurs in young healthy individuals and is not associated with major trauma. The sharp stabbing pains, referred to as "catches" or "stitches" of pain, are felt in the anterior chest wall, usually in the left parasternal area or near the cardiac apex and last from 30 seconds to 3 minutes. Some patients report the onset of pain while slouching or bending over. The pain is aggravated by deep breathing and is usually relieved by shallow respiration, moderate activity, or assuming a correct posture. No local tenderness is associated, such as that which occurs with other pain syndromes of the chest wall.

The cause of this condition is unknown, although intercostal muscle spasm from faulty posture or a pleuritic origin of pain has been postulated (60). Treatment consists of reassurance and correction of any postural abnormality. Because the pain is short-lived and unpredictable, analgesics are not usually indicated.

Precordial Migraine

Although casually mentioned by Tissot in 1788, with a number of case reports published from 1900 to 1940, it was Fitz-Hugh (62) who, in 1940, described the syndrome of precordial angina in detail. He reported that, among 88 patients suffering from migraine, 27%

described a recurring precordial pain that he considered to be a migraine equivalent, and he called it precordial migraine. Briggs and Bellomo (63) 2 years later reported that, among 684 migraine patients, 158 (23%) had precordial discomfort and 37 had anginal pain associated with palpitations and tachycardia. More recently Leon-Sotomayor (64) studied 12 migraine patients who had, between and during their attacks, paroxysmal chest pain associated with spells of tremulousness, weakness, tachycardia, or high-frequency bitemporoparietal spikes on the EEG. Ergotamine aggravated the symptoms while glycerol trinitrate or propranolol alleviated them. Saibil and Edmeads (65) cited other reports and stated that the chest pain is alleged to be caused by vascular changes in the thoracic viscera, muscles of the chest wall, or both, and the situation is said to be analogous to abdominal migraine. In managing these patients it is important to avoid ergotamine because it could precipitate myocardial ischemia.

Chest Pain Caused by Diseases of the Mediastinum and Diaphragm

A number of rather rare disorders of the mediastinum and diaphragm can cause chest pain and deserve brief mention in this section.

Diseases of the Mediastinum

In addition to tumors (Chapter 57), two disorders of the mediastinum can cause chest pain and should be considered in the differential diagnosis. These are mediastinal emphysema and mediastinitis.

Mediastinal Emphysema

Air within the planes of the mediastinum can appear spontaneously or can be secondary to chest trauma, perforation of the esophagus, trachea, or bronchus, spread from fascial planes of the nasopharynx, or dissection from the retroperitoneal space. When pneumomediastinum occurs with no apparent cause, it is referred to as spontaneous mediastinal emphysema or spontaneous pneumomediastinum. Air is thought to dissect from the alveoli to the interstitial space into the vascular adventitia and into the hilum, from which it moves into the mediastinum, neck, or retroperitoneal space.

If the volume of air reaching the mediastinum is small the resulting pain can be severe while other physiologic disturbances might be minimal. Occasionally the condition is self-limited, with spontaneous recovery. When great volumes of air accumulate, as in what Wehrmacher (2) called malignant mediastinal emphysema, profound physiologic disturbances result. Because of compression of the great vessels returning venous blood to the heart this causes circulatory shock, impaired exchange of oxygen and carbon dioxide between the alveoli and the blood, and cardiovascular collapse that can progress to death if the increased mediastinal pressure is not promptly relieved.

Spontaneous pneumothorax produces rather sudden onset of pain in the absence of effort while the patient is quietly standing, sitting, or lying. The pain usually begins beneath the sternum and sometimes radiates to the back, neck, or shoulders, but rarely to the arms. Physical examination can reveal subcutaneous crepitus in the upper body and a crunching sound synchronous with the heart beat is often heard over the precordium (Hamman's sign). Fever and mild leukocytosis are common with uncomplicated mediastinal emphysema.

A radiograph of the chest in a patient with spontaneous mediastinal emphysema demonstrates air in the mediastinum and usually a small pneumothorax. Mediastinal air is much more difficult to demonstrate than pneumothorax and is usually best seen along the pleural line parallel to the left heart border on films made during full expiration (2).

Therapy for the benign type of mediastinal emphysema is purely symptomatic but, for malignant emphysema, surgical drainage of the mediastinum is essential to release the entrapped air. Oxygen therapy might be necessary to relieve dyspnea and cyanosis. The pain is controlled with appropriate systemic analgesics and sedatives administered carefully and appropriate monitoring of the patient is essential to detect any adverse side effects.

Mediastinitis

Acute mediastinitis occurs as an extension from a mediastinal lymphadenitis secondary to pulmonary or pleural infections, from inflamed neighboring structures, or from rupture of the esophagus or trachea. The infection can be nonsuppurative, phlegmonous, or suppurative, and an abscess can result. A rather peculiar chronic cicatrizing mediastinitis of uncertain origin that manifests extensive fibrosis with retraction and displacement of various mediastinal structures was cited by Wehrmacher (2).

The usual symptoms of acute mediastinitis are those referrable to the underlying infection. As discussed in Chapter 56, rupture of the esophagus usually produces severe, excruciating, retrosternal pain simulating that of acute myocardial infarction. The esophageal perforation is a surgical emergency and should be suspected if pain increases and is aggravated by swallowing or fever.

With other causes of mediastinitis the chest pain can be overshadowed by other manifestations of the causative factor. Treatment varies according to the cause of mediastinitis but invariably requires antibacterial therapy. The management of the pain depends on its severity. Mild to moderate pain can be adequately controlled with NSAIDs combined with codeine or some other mild opioid. Severe pain requires potent opioids that should be injected intravenously as soon as the diagnosis is made and analgesia is then maintained, either with intramuscular injections at regular intervals or, preferably, with patient-controlled analgesia (see Chapter 78).

Disorders of the Diaphragm

The diaphragm can be the site of inflammatory diseases, tumors, hemorrhage, edema, and degeneration. In Chapter 55 the various causes of pleuritis involving the diaphragmatic pleura are discussed, including viral infection (pleurodynia) and other infectious processes involving the thoracic viscera. In Chapter 56 diaphragmatic hernia is discussed. Many causes of diaphragmatic peritonitis are discussed in detail in Chapters 61, 62, and 64. Here the discussion is limited to three conditions: acute primary diaphragmatitis, sustained diaphragmatic spasm, and diaphragmatic flutter.

Acute Primary Diaphragmatitis

Acute primary diaphragmatitis, also known as Heddron's syndrome, is manifested by moderate to severe pain in the lower chest, upper abdomen, and shoulder. The cause of this condition is unknown, but some (2) have suggested that it can follow chilling or acute nasopharyngeal infection and is attributed to a primary myositis of the diaphragm, bearing no relationship to lesions of the pleura, lungs, or subphrenic organs.

Clinically the pain limits the respiratory effort beyond a fixed depth, invariably with spasm of the abdominal muscle below the costal margin associated with pain in the upper quadrants but no deep tenderness. The costal margins flare and remain relatively immobile; fluoroscopy shows the diaphragm to be immobilized in midposition during the acute phase. As the myositis subsides and the muscles are replaced by fibrous tissue, flattening of the diaphragm persists.

The symptoms usually subside within 1 or 2 weeks, but can recur during inclement weather (2). Treatment of this condition is symptomatic and should include encouragement, reassurance, and effective pain control with systemic analgesics.

Sustained Spasm of the Diaphragm (XVII-8)

Rare cases of persistent contraction of the diaphragm have been reported as a cause of chest pain (2). In each instance, a characteristic disorder of diaphragmatic function was demonstrable by fluoroscopic observation: inspiration became jerky and the excursion of the diaphragm during inspiration was exceeded, so that during expiration the structure assume a progressively lower position. When the state of contracture of the diaphragm was such that adequate respiratory excursions were no longer possible dyspnea was experienced, with the feeling of inability to take a breath. During the attacks of sustained diaphragmatic contractions the patient experienced pain in the pericordium or elsewhere in the chest, with radiation to the shoulder. In some patients the attacks were accompanied by pallor, sweating, hypotension, and angor animi, simulating that of acute myocardial infarction. In others a diaphragmatic spasm caused occlusion of the esophagus, with consequent dysphasia and odynophagia.

Such patients require a thorough workup to exclude severe thoracic visceral disorders. Because the attack is provoked by emotional conflicts in many patients, psychologic management is especially important. If patients have severe dyspnea, oxygen can be helpful. Pain can usually be adequately relieved with systemic analgesics. In patients who have severe contraction, unilateral or bilateral phrenic nerve blocks might be necessary to relieve the spasm.

Diaphragmatic Flutter

Diaphragmatic flutter is a rare but disturbing cause of chest pain that usually escapes recognition for a long time. The cause of the condition is frequently unknown but some have reported it to be precipitated by excitement, emotional tension, severe cough, pressure on the upper abdomen, exercise, and sneezing (2). Wehrmacher (2) mentioned that symptoms can be suppressed at times by deep inspiration, swallowing, or supraclavicular pressure, and can cease during a period of natural sleep.

The patient has pain in the chest, shortness of breath, and palpitations. The pain occurs along the diaphragmatic attachment, in the epigastrium, and over the precordium, and radiates into the neck, shoulder, and down the arm. Clock-like sounds and plethysmographic oscillation at the base of the lung as visualized by fluoroscopy establish the rapid movement of the diaphragm.

Management should be conservative for patients in whom the condition does not cause significant emotional or physiologic disturbances. In those in whom the condition persists and causes severe emotional and physiologic disturbances several prognostic blocks of the phrenic nerve should be carried out to determine what effect they might have on the condition. This is best achieved by injecting 5 to 10 ml of local anesthetic on the anterior surface of the scalenus anticus (Fig. 94-7). The block should be attempted on one side and later on the other and, if the condition of the patient warrants, a bilateral block can be carried out to determine its efficacy. If the patient has no respiratory difficulties following the block a continuous infusion block might be considered.

C. CHEST PAIN OF TEGUMENTARY ORIGIN

A number of the disorders of the skin can cause pain in the chest (Table 58-1). These include burns, (Chapter 26) and various pain syndromes of dermatologic origin (Chapter 27). In this section I mention several rather rare conditions usually not considered in the differential diagnosis of pain in this region.

Idiopathic Chronic Mastalgia

Chronic mastalgia is characterized by chronic severe pain felt in the entire breast that persists for years without a demonstrable pathologic process, hence the term "idiopathic mastalgia." This condition has remained a controversial subject since the early report by Atkins (66). Although many clinicians believe that the condition has a psychologic basis, tests reveal no emotional or psychologic abnormality (67) and the condition responds to hormonal manipulation (68, 69).

Based on reports and follow-up studies done for 2 to 7 years on 258 patients with severe idiopathic mastalgia seen at the Welsh National School of Medicine in

Cardiff, Wisbey and colleagues (70) reported that, in about two-thirds of patients, the pain was cyclical and predominantly premenstrual and, in about 27%, it was continuous throughout the month. Among those in the cyclic pain group, the age of onset of the syndrome was before or during the third decade, while in those with continuous pain the age of onset was the fourth decade or later. Without treatment the pain persisted for many years, especially among those women with cyclic pain who began to have the syndrome before the age of 20 years. Some of those with noncyclic pain had pain for only 2 to 4 years, while others had pain for as long as 30 years.

Among the 174 patients with cyclic pain, 104 (60%) had complete or substantial relief of the pain. Of this group of 104 patients, in 81 (78%) the pain relief was related to menopause, the use of contraceptives, or pregnancy, while in 23 (22%) relief occurred spontaneously. Among the 67 patients with noncyclic pain, 32 (48%) experienced relief, and of this group, in 16 (50%), relief occurred spontaneously while in 8 (25%) relief occurred with breast operation, in 6 (19%) relief was related to menopause, and in 2 (6%) it was related to intake of contraceptive pills.

Wisbey and associates (70) concluded that the persistent cyclic mastalgia should prompt consideration of specific hormonal therapy now that new drugs with proven efficacy are available, such as bromocriptine and danazol (64, 65). Management remains difficult for those with noncyclic pain; menopause and contraceptives relieve only 10 to 15% of patients. Patients with localized pain might be considered for excision biopsy and those with retroareolar pain associated with signs of periductal mastitis can be treated with ductal excision, but a satisfactory result cannot be guaranteed.

Adiposis Dolorosa

In 1892 Dercum reported a new syndrome characterized by pain in areas with a fatty swelling and proposed that it be named adiposis dolorosa (71). The condition is characterized by painful circumscribed adipose deposits in subcutaneous tissues of various regions of the body and extremities (72). Lesions vary in size from 0.5 to 5 cm in diameter. Pain and paresthesia can occur spontaneously or result from pressure. The condition most frequently occurs in women (ratio of women to men, 30:1) who are usually obese. The syndrome is associated with weakness, fatigue, emotional instability, and occasional dementia, and rarely begins until after menopause (72). Although studies in the early part of the century suggested that the condition was caused by abnormalities of the pituitary and other endocrine glands, this has not been substantiated by modern endocrinologic assessment.

Treatment is frequently unsatisfactory, although Atkinson (73) reported that intravenous lidocaine was effective in providing relief to two patients (Chapter 94).

Mondor's Disease

Mondor's disease is a form of cord phlebitis of the anterior lateral chest that is usually caused by thrombosis of the superficial vein of the thoracic wall. It is characterized by a palpable painful cord within the skin (2, 74, 75). This condition is usually not well known by practicing physicians and can provoke considerable anxiety until its benign character is recognized. Although either sex can be afflicted, most patients reported to date have been women (2).

The initial inflammatory phase is characterized by the rather sudden appearance of a painful, tender, subcutaneous cord running somewhat obliquely across the thorax in the distribution of one or more of the superficial subcutaneous veins. The cord can be linear or Y-shaped, corresponding to the linear or branching course of the affected vein. During the inflammatory phase the lesion can grow as if a worm were crawling beneath the skin (2). After the initial inflammatory phase, usually lasting several weeks, an indolent phase follows with little or no discomfort and only the palpable cord, extending like a urethral catheter beneath the skin, remains as evidence of the disorder.

Laboratory studies are of little value although the eosinophils in the peripheral blood might be slightly increased. Biopsy usually reveals a white indurated cord that macroscopically appears as a small-caliber vessel.

The most important feature in the management of this disorder is its recognition so that the patient can be spared unnecessary anxiety and apprehension. The disease is self-limited and requires nothing more than symptomatic relief of the pain with systemic analgesics.

D. REFERRED CHEST PAIN CAUSED BY EXTRATHORACIC DISORDERS

Throughout this section on chest pain, it has been noted that chest pain can be caused by diseases or lesions in structures outside of the thoracic cavity. These include disorders of the neck, herniated cervical disk, thoracic inlet syndromes, and disorders of the abdominal viscera. Because each of these conditions is discussed in detail elsewhere, only brief comments relevant to chest pain are made here.

Disorders of Cervical Nerve Roots

Cervical Disk Disease (IX-1)

Pain in the anterior upper part of the chest can be caused by herniation of the intervertebral disk of the lower part of the cervical spine. The pectoral muscles and fascia are supplied by the lateral and medial pectoral nerves with the former derived from C5 to C7 and the latter derived from C8 and T1. Compression of any of these roots can cause pain referred to the pectoral region, even though the compression lesion is in the neck. Posterolateral herniation of a degenerated cervical intervertebral disk causes anterior chest pain that is deep, aching, steady, and, at times, severe. The pectoral muscles can be tender when they are the seat of the referred pain. The pain is aggravated by lateral flexion to the affected side and by coughing, sneezing, and straining. Unless these and other features are kept in mind, the pain can be confused with that of myocardial ischemia.

The diagnosis is based on history and physical examination, with emphasis on detection of changes in affected muscles in the neck and the limbs and on examination of passive and active motion of neck muscles. Patients with referred pain from cervical disk disease almost always have referred pain in the shoulder and upper limb. The diagnosis and therapy of this condition are discussed in Chapter 48.

Thoracic Outlet Syndrome (IX-13)

Various types of thoracic outlet syndromes are discussed in Chapter 48. In addition to producing neuropathic pain in the distribution of the major nerves to the upper limb, pain can also be referred to the chest. Chest and left arm pain produced by left-sided thoracic outlet syndrome can simulate cardiac pain, but many features are associated that indicate the correct diagnosis. Symptoms and signs, diagnosis, and treatment of these disorders are considered in detail in Chapter 48.

Disorders of Abdominal Viscera

Gas Entrapment Syndromes

Gas entrapment syndromes occur as a result of gaseous distension of a portion of the gastrointestinal tract. The pain is caused by tension on the wall of the hollow viscus. If the viscus is adjacent to the diaphragm, chest pain frequently results. Pain caused by gastric distension is felt in the epigastrium and in the lower part of the anterior chest. Gas in the hepatic flexure of the colon causes pain in the right hypo-

chondrium and in the right side of the lower chest. If the gas is in the splenic flexure, the pain is felt in the left hypochondrium and left side of the chest. These conditions are discussed in detail in Chapter 64.

Biliary Tract Disease

Biliary tract disease includes biliary colic, acute and chronic cholecystitis, and choledocholithiasis. All these conditions are frequent causes of pain in the epigastrium or right hypochondrium, and the pain frequently extends into the lower part of the chest. In patients with biliary colic the pain is usually in the epigastrium or right subcostal region and not infrequently extends into the lower central anterior chest. Rarely, pain is confined to the chest, mimicking that of myocardial ischemia. The pain frequently radiates to the back, particularly to the inferior angle of the right scapula and, less frequently, is referred to the right shoulder. The mechanism of this type of referred chest pain is discussed in Chapter 54.

The pain of acute cholecystitis is similar to that of biliary colic except that it is usually localized to the right upper quadrant and lasts a few days.

Acute Pancreatitis

Some patients with acute pancreatitis complain only of chest pain that simulates that of myocardial infarction. This type of presentation is complicated by the fact that acute pancreatitis can cause transient electrocardiographic abnormalities, which might include the entire spectrum of changes seen in myocardial ischemia and infarction. Obviously a careful differential diagnosis is essential.

Other Abdominal Visceral Diseases (XIX-1-8)

Other abdominal disorders that can cause pain that is extended or referred to the lower part of the chest include peptic ulcer disease, tumors of the gastric cardia, subphrenic abscess, amebic liver abscess, and various other conditions discussed in the next section (Section E).

E. RELATIONSHIPS BETWEEN CHEST PAIN AND PSYCHOLOGIC FACTORS

In this section I first re-emphasize some important psychologic reactions to chest pain caused by pathologic processes and then discuss pain primarily resulting from psychologic mechanisms. This subject is presented last in this chapter not because it is the least important but because psychologic and emotional factors are the most frequent causes of chest pain, or are frequent concomitants of chest pain associated with heart disease or other thoracic visceral and somatic disorders. Emotional "stress" is a significant contributing factor in the development of coronary artery disease and some of its complications, but a detailed discussion is beyond the scope of this chapter. Evidence from animal experiments and human studies indicates that emotional factors are important

in producing psychophysiologic responses that aggravate coronary artery disease and that can precipitate cardiac arrhythmia, possibly ending in sudden death. A recent summary of the most important of these studies has been presented by Buell and Elliot (76).

Emotional Reactions to Organic Chest Pain

Patients with sudden acute chest pain, regardless of the cause, experience varying degrees of anxiety, apprehension, and fear, depending on their interpretation of the cause of pain. Those who believe that they are experiencing a heart attack become extremely frightened of possible impending death. Many patients who have acute myocardial infarction (AMI) pass through reactions of denial, anxiety, depression, and finally acceptance (77). In AMI patients anxiety and apprehension provoke a marked increase in general neural sympathetic tone and produce an increase in the neuroendocrine response to stress that can aggravate the existing pathophysiology and prove deleterious to the patient (Chapter 54). It is therefore essential to relieve the pain and also the associated anxiety and apprehension promptly to minimize or prevent these serious psychophysiologic responses.

Patients with persistent angina pectoris frequently develop reactive depression as a consequence of the limitation imposed by the illness, which is seen as a threat affecting the patient's life-style, self-image, status, family relationships, and security (77). As emphasized in Chapter 8, persistent chronic pain is frequently associated with reactive depression, regardless of the causative factor. The depression frequently aggravates the physical disability and, if it remains untreated it sets up a vicious circle that produces progressive physical and psychologic deterioration. Reactive depression is an even greater problem in patients with chronic cancer-related chest pain, not only because of the significance of the pain but also because of the progressive physical and psychologic deterioration that these patients undergo (Chapters 24 and 57).

Chest pain caused by nonmalignant musculoskeletal or neuropathic disorders provokes a great deal of anxiety and apprehension until patients have been reassured about the "benign" nature of the painful condition. In most patients reassurance about the nonthreatening nature of the pain decreases or eliminates the depression. On the other hand, some patients in whom moderate to severe pain persists because its cause remains unknown or because the pain remains unrelieved as a result of ineffective therapy are also likely to develop reactive depression if the pain is intense enough to affect work and life-style.

These examples are mentioned to emphasize that, in addition to assessing the patient to diagnose the primary cause, it is also important to assess the emotional reactions to, and psychologic impact on, the patient's pain and pathologic process. Obviously, in addition to treating the pain and underlying disorder, aggressively it is also essential to assess emotional reactions and to treat these aggressively.

Chest Pain Primarily Resulting From Psychologic Mechanisms

Although precise epidemiologic data are not available it has been suggested that, in patients with chest pain with no evidence of coronary or other types of heart disease or diseases of the esophagus, the pain is frequently a result of psychologic mechanisms. The most common causes of such pain are anxiety disorders, affective disorders, operant mechanisms, psychophysiologic factors, and somatoform disorders. Pain caused by each of these mechanisms, together with a listing of their diagnostic criteria as contained in the

Diagnostic and Statistical Manual (DSM-IIIR) of the American Psychiatric Association (78), is discussed in Section C of Part II of this book (Chapters 15 to 19 inclusive). In this section comments are limited to those relevant to chest pain caused by one or more of these psychologic mechanisms. The characteristics of the pain and other signs and symptoms are discussed first for each of these mechanisms and then the diagnostic procedures and therapy for all these factors are considered.

Anxiety Disorders

Anxiety disorders, which were formerly lumped together under the term of "anxiety neurosis," are now recognized as a number of relatively distinct clinical syndromes according to diagnostic criteria in the DSM-IIIR (78). They are classified into two major groups: (a) *anxiety disorders*, comprised of panic disorder, generalized anxiety state, obsessive-compulsive disorder, and post-traumatic stress disorder; and (b) *phobic disorders*, comprised of agoraphobia, social phobia, and simple phobia. Of these, the panic disorder, characterized by a sudden acute attack of anxiety, fear, and apprehension, and the generalized anxiety disorder, characterized by a persistent chronic anxiety state, have chest pain as a prominent symptom.

Acute Anxiety Attack

An acute anxiety attack usually begins as a sudden unexpected sense of terror, a feeling of apprehension, which increases in severity, leads to dyspnea, and is associated with a sense of choking or smothering, palpitations, and chest pains that are often so severe patients believe that they are having a heart attack or dying. Dyspnea, or a feeling of air hunger, can produce the hyperventilation syndrome, which is characterized by a marked increase in ventilation that produces severe respiratory alkalosis with a consequent marked decrease in the CO_2 tension in arterial blood and cerebral tissue that leads to marked cerebral vasoconstriction and hypoxia. As a result of these changes patients experience tachycardia, sweating, tremor, dizziness, and increased muscle tension, which can be accompanied by a diffuse chest tightness and paresthesia, a feeling of tingling in the hands, feet, face, or throat—feelings that cause patients to conclude that their initial fears are substantiated and they are suffering from a fatal heart attack (77).

The chest pain associated with an acute anxiety attack can occur even without hyperventilation and is described by patients as a severe, sharp, precordial pain or pain in the left inframammary region (Fig. 58-12). The pain can be diffuse in the chest but is rarely retrosternal. The pain does not occur during physical effort but can develop after the effort has ceased. After the acute pain subsides patients can continue to have a dull ache or mild pain that persists for some time. The chest pain can become the patients' focus of concern and the complaint that brings them to the physician or emergency room.

An acute anxiety attack usually lasts for a few minutes, rarely for more than 30 minutes. Following the attack the patient can feel fatigued and exhausted. As the attacks recur, some of the symptoms mentioned

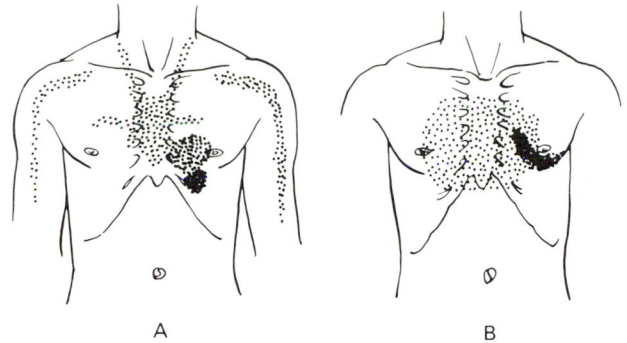

Fig. 58-12. Patterns of pain provoked by psychologic factors. **A.** Pattern of pains in a patient who has true angina (light stipple) coexisting with psychologic pain usually felt at the cardiac apex or over the area where the patient thinks the heart lies (heavy stipple). **B.** Pattern of pain in acute anxiety felt diffusely throughout the chest or precordially. In patients with conversion pain, it is usually also felt precordially at the cardiac apex or along an operative scar if one is present.

above become the focus of the patient's attention. Frequently this is comprised of the sensation of palpitations, dyspnea, and chest pain, which can become recurrent complaints.

The clinical importance of chest pain caused by an acute anxiety attack cannot be overemphasized. Hurst, a world authority on heart disease, stated that "The most common cause of chest pain is not related to cardiovascular disease, but is associated with anxiety" (79). Moreover, because acute anxiety is accompanied by elevated plasma catecholamine levels, it is a common precipitant of angina. Indeed, in patients who have some degree of coronary artery disease, myocardial infarction can occur during periods of sustained anxiety (77). It is therefore obvious that early diagnosis and treatment of the anxiety attack are critically important and are crucial in the prevention of chronicity.

Chronic Anxiety State

In patients with chronic anxiety chest pain various other symptoms and signs are present in a common pattern that has been called the syndrome of "cardiac neurosis," in which cardiovascular, respiratory, and nervous symptoms are prominent features in the absence of an explanatory diagnosis. This syndrome has been known for over a century—in 1871 Da Costa referred to it as "irritable heart syndrome" (80). Since then this condition has undergone many name changes, including soldier's heart (81), Da Costa's syndrome (82), effort syndrome (83), neurocirculatory asthenia (84), and vasoregulatory asthenia (85).

Patients with this syndrome complain of a moderate to severe shortness of breath, usually described as an inability to fill the lungs, palpitations, chest pain, nervousness, anxiety, fatigue and generalized weakness, and low energy level. Among the most important precipitating or aggravating factors are emotion-provoking situations, illness, hard physical labor, pregnancy, and military service (77). Billings (77) theorized that this syndrome tends to develop in patients who have problems relating to dependency needs and

who are attempting to function in a situation that is taxing their coping ability. Under this stress anxiety and concern about the heart can develop, and one symptom is precordial pain. This concern might be aggravated by the physician's uncertainty about the diagnosis and by the performance of unnecessary and repeated tests that refocus patients' attention on their heart.

Pain felt at the cardiac apex is often described as a dull ache, with or without attacks of sharper pain also felt in the same area, because that is where the patient thinks cardiac pain should be experienced (77) (Fig. 58-12). The patient might relate the pain to physical exertion but it usually occurs after the physical exertion has ceased and is associated with fatigue rather than effort. The shortness of breath, usually described as an inability to fill the lungs, is a prominent symptom, as are generalized weakness and low energy levels. Other manifestations of anxiety can be present but are not prominent.

Many clinical and experimental laboratory studies have been done on patients with this disorder but their results have not generally been helpful in delineating a clinical picture useful for making a diagnosis (76). Standard blood chemistry findings are unremarkable and no characteristic electrocardiographic pattern for this syndrome has been found. Some studies have revealed abnormalities in oxygen consumption, blood lactate levels, and palmar sweat during psychologic testing, muscular work, or application of painful stimuli (76). Exercises tend to cause an abnormal rise in blood lactate levels and administration of lactate to such patients has induced anxiety attacks in the vast majority (86). Diminished work capacity is reflected by a lower maximal oxygen consumption than normal and by a narrow arteriovenous oxygen difference (85).

This condition tends to persist for years, with periods of exacerbation and remission. A number of patients can recover entirely and some show improvement (76, 77). The prognosis for disappearance of symptoms is poor if a serious psychiatric background and a long history of symptoms are present and the syndrome appears after relatively brief and minor physical strain (77).

Depression

Many depressed patients complain of pains for which no physical basis can be found. Although these might not be the presenting complaints, some patients who are depressed from any cause describe a heavy feeling or deep ache in the chest. The chest pain is usually precordial, is described as an ache or tightness, possibly radiates into the left arm, and is associated with overconcern about the heart. This overconcern can be so marked that patients neglect or deny the other psychologic or physiologic symptoms. Like other symptoms of depression chest pain is usually worse in the morning, is present on awakening or soon after, and lessens as the day goes on. It is not particularly affected by physical activity (see Chapter 18).

Conversion Reactions (XVIII-3)

Conversion is an unconscious mechanism used to repress the anxiety resulting from intrapsychic conflict and is usually related to dependency needs, sexual feelings, or aggressive drives. Repression converts the psychic conflict into physical symptoms, which reflect both the unconscious drive and the inhibiting mechanisms.

Conversion pain, when located in the chest, presents difficult diagnostic problems. The usual location of pain in the chest is in the region of the heart; concern about the heart is usually present but not to the same degree as that seen in cardiac neurosis (77). The psychodynamics of conversion pain are discussed in Chapter 18.

Some characteristics of the pain and of the reaction to the pain can help in arriving at the correct diagnosis of conversion pain. Whereas a patient with an organic basis of pain is more likely to accept the suggestion that the pain is psychologic in origin, the patient with conversion pain resists the idea vehemently. In conversion pain syndromes the patient might show *la belle indifférence*. The patient is usually overconcerned about the pain, demanding further investigation or relief, but indifference is demonstrated by lack of concern about the affect of the pain on life-style. Moreover, conversion pain varies in location from examination to examination. It is incompletely relieved by an analgesic, tranquilizer, or placebo, and does not awaken the patient from sleep. The pain is usually described in a dramatic way and is associated with overreaction and a self-protective behavior.

Hypochondriasis (I-16)

Hypochondriac patients tend to worry particularly about their heart, lungs, brain, gastrointestinal tract, and sexual organs. Chest pain is frequent and, if associated with worry about the heart, the pain is usually precordial, initially felt over the apex (Fig. 58-12). The pain is described in minute specific detail with respect to location, quality, and duration, but it does not fit any of the pain patterns discussed in this section and, of course, no abnormal physical findings are seen. Description of the character of the pain changes from one visit to another. Complaints of chest pain also occur in patients worrying about lung disease, particularly cancer. Unlike the pain that is associated with carcinoma of the lung, the hypochondriac pain is likely to vary in intensity and location and is described as sharp or stabbing.

Operant (Learned) Chest Pain

Some patients who have acute chest pain caused by an acute pathologic process develop chronic pain behavior as a consequence of reinforcing environmental factors. In such pain patients the pain behavior persists far beyond the course of the acute disease process, and can be associated with progressive physical deterioration and disability. The theoretic underpinnings of this type of pain are described in detail in Chapter 16.

Diagnostic Procedures

The assessment of psychologic factors is not easy when a patient first presents at the physician's office or in the emergency room. In general, the diagnosis of chest pain primarily of psychologic origin should be made not only by the systematic exclusion of organic pathology but by the finding of positive psychologic factors using various psychometric and psychologic tests. Because of the potential seriousness of a physical cause of the chest pain, a complete and thorough history, a physical examination, and full investigative procedures are essential prerequisites to the diagnosis. When pain primarily of psychologic origin is suspected the examination and investigation should be done in a reassuring way to avoid undue concern in the patient.

During the initial evaluation of a patient with chest pain, certain factors should alert the physician in a general way to the possibility that the pain is wholly a result of psychologic or emotional factors, or perhaps is a psychologic concomitant of organic pain. The following points suggested by Billings (77) can be used as indications that the patient's complaint are primarily of psychologic origin:

a. The pain is usually located in the precordial region at the apex of the heart and is rarely central (Fig. 58-12).

b. Description of the pain is atypical and stated in dramatic terms, such as "tearing pain through the chest wall" or "stabbing pain like a knife cutting through the heart." Thus, it does not fit an organic syndrome nor does it follow a physiologic pattern.

c. The distribution is not anatomically explicable and the development of the pain involves events that are not physiologically related.

d. Often more than one system is involved or several different pain patterns are noted on different occasions.

e. "Psychogenic" pain does not awaken patients from sleep but can be present on awakening or soon thereafter.

f. In most patients an emotional precipitant usually precedes the development of acute pain, and patients manifest symptoms and signs of anxiety, depression, or other neurotic patterns.

g. In contrast with pain of "organic" origin, which responds consistently to appropriate analgesics or other forms of therapy, pain primarily of psychologic origin is more likely to show a variable response on different occasions.

Billings (77) emphasized that, although all these might indicate diagnosis of pain primarily of psychologic origin, each has limitations and should be considered only as suggestive. They must be complemented by the use of well-established psychologic tests, such as the Minnesota Multiphasic Personal Inventory (MMPI) and others (Chapter 33). Levene (87) emphasized that it is dangerous to diagnose a psychologic cause for chest pain (or pain in any other location) if, after careful and extensive interviews and psychologic tests, no accompanying psychologic or psychiatric disorders or secondary gain can be positively identified.

In most instances patients with acute or chronic chest pain have undergone various diagnostic tests to rule out coronary artery disease and other cardiovascular problems, respiratory disorders, and cancer. Stress electrocardiography, radionuclear stress testing, and coronary arteriography are considered the standards for defining coronary artery stenosis and other cardiac problems. About 20 to 30% of those who undergo these tests have normal coronary arteries or only minimal insignificant coronary stenosis at catheterization and have normal heart function (88, 89). The prognosis of those in this group with normal arteries in terms of morbidity and mortality is excellent (88, 90, 91). Frequently, however, their functional status does not improve (90, 91). One study showed that, 16 months after catheterization, about 50% of those with normal arteries were limited by chest pain and were unable to work (90). A significant percentage of patients who have chest pain without coronary disease have esophageal disorders as the cause, but in many the chest pain has a psychologic or psychiatric basis.

This has been shown by a number of reports of patients with persistent chest pain and negative evidence of coronary artery disease in whom psychologic testing demonstrated a psychologic basis for their pain. Bass and Wade (92) found that two-thirds of patients with chest pain and normal coronary angiograms had predominant psychiatric rather than cardiac disorders, and concluded that the patients' chest pain represented somatic manifestation of anxiety.

Using the hospital anxiety and depression scale, Channer and colleagues (93) measured anxiety and depression in 87 consecutive patients (65 males, 22 females) with chest pain before diagnostic exercise treadmill testing. Chest pain was assessed as typical or atypical of angina by an independent observer. A positive exercise test was found in 50 patients (58%), and in 37 patients the test was negative. Patients with negative tests had significantly higher scores for anxiety and higher depression scores than those with positive tests. Among the patients who had negative tests, 27 (73%) had atypical pain as compared with 6 (12%) who had positive tests. Depressed patients walked for a significantly shorter time than those who were not depressed. By using discriminant analysis, it was found that the probability of a negative exercise test in males who were both anxious and depressed with atypical chest pain was 97% and in females it was 99%.

Wielgosz and colleagues (90) used the MMPI and demonstrated that the strongest predictor for continued chest pain in patients who had normal coronaries or stenosis less than 75% was a high score for hypochondriasis. In another study, Costa and associates (94) noted that high scores for neuroticism as determined by the Cornell Medical Index were related not to coronary heart disease but to expressions of anger, fear, and severity of pain. Wielgosz and Earp (95) reported the development of a new scale consisting of six variables that elicit information about the patients' views concerning cause, history, future, kinship, admission, and disability; these factors were combined into a single scale called the "Self-Label of Coronary Vulnerability." It was demonstrated that this variable was strongly associated with continued unimproved chest pain in patients with normal coronary arteries.

Treatment

Treatment of patients who have acute or persistent chest pain primarily of psychologic origin should be tailored according to the primary psychologic disorder involved. In patients with an acute anxiety attack, reassurance, relaxation techniques, anxiolytic drugs, sedatives, tranquilizers, and time reduce anxiety.

In patients with chronic anxiety, winning and retaining their confidence and providing reassurance are the most important therapeutic measures. In addition to obtaining a detailed history and physical examination, it is important to demonstrate a complete understanding of, and an interest in, patients' symptoms. Reassurance should not stop with the exclusion of organic heart disease but should include an emphasis on a good prognosis for life expectancy and a low incidence of disability. Precipitating factors should be identified, explained, and dealt with in terms of patients' life style, attitudes, and emotional reactions. Buell and Elliot (76) cited studies indicating that intensive psychotherapy or psychoanalysis appear to have no better result than simple reassurance, appropriate drug therapy for acute episodes, and advice about aggravating factors. In patients who manifest tachycardia, beta-adrenergic blocking agents can be used to reduce heart rate (96).

Billings (77) suggested that, if the evaluation indicates there is a secondary gain factor, such as avoidance of an unpleasant situation, maintenance of a distorted family or marital relationship, or seeking of a disability pension, treatment is difficult because these reactions are often fixed and held onto tenaciously by the patient. Although granting of a disability pension might be effective, attempts to remove secondary gain factors more often result not in improvement but in an elaboration of symptoms.

Patients who complain of chest pain caused by endogenous depression require specialized psychologic or psychiatric care (Chapter 86). Patients whose chest pain is caused by operant mechanisms are treated by contingency management (Chapter 81). As part of the contingency management, a multimodal approach to these patients is needed (Chapter 100).

REFERENCES

1. Rasmussen, T.B., Kernohan, J.W., and Adson, A.W.: Pathologic classification with surgical consideration of intraspinal tumors. Ann. Surg., *111*:513, 1940.
2. Wehrmacher, W.H.: Pain in the Chest. Springfield, IL, Charles C Thomas, 1964, pp. 71–99.
3. Edmeads, J.: Pain arising from thoracic nerves, nerve roots and spinal cord. In Chest Pain. An Integrated Diagnostic Approach. Edited by D.L. Levene. Philadelphia, Lea & Febiger, 1977, pp. 107–117.
4. Posner, J.B.: Back pain and epidural spinal cord compression. Med. Clin. North Am. *71*:185, 1987.
5. Burgoon, C.F., Burgoon, J.S., and Baldridge, G.D.: The natural history of herpes zoster. JAMA, *164*:265, 1957.
6. Mazur, N., and Dolin, R. Herpes zoster at the NIH: A 20-year history. Am. J. Med., *65*:738, 1978.
7. Portenoy, R.K., Duma, C., and Foley, K.M.: Acute herpetic and postherpetic neuralgia: Clinical review and current management. Ann. Neurol., *20*:651, 1986.
8. Head, H., and Campbell, A.W.: The pathology of herpes zoster and its bearing on sensory localization. Brain, *23*:335, 1900.
9. Merigan, T., et al.: Human leukocyte interferon for the treatment of herpes zoster in patients with cancer. N. Engl. J. Med., *298*:981, 1978.

10. Peterslund, N.A., et al.: Acyclovir in herpes zoster. Lancet, 2:827, 1981.
11. Colding, A.: The effect of sympathetic blocks on herpes zoster. Acta Anaesthesiol. Scand., 13:133, 1969.
12. Colding, A.: Organization of pain clinic: Treatment of herpes zoster. Proc. R. Soc. Lond. [Biol.], 66:541, 1973.
13. Turek, S.L.: Orthopaedics: Principles and Their Application. 4th Ed. Philadelphia, J.B. Lippincott, 1984, pp. 1519–1521.
14. Arseni, C., and Nash, F.: Protrusion of thoracic intervertebral discs. Acta Neurochir., 11:3, 1963.
15. Heuer, G.J.: The so-called hourglass tumors of the spine. Arch. Surg., 18:935, 1929.
16. Hochberg, L.A., and Rivkin, L.M.: Benign neurogenic tumors of the chest wall. Ann. Surg., 138:104, 1953.
17. Good, A.D.: The chest pain of ankylosing spondylitis. Its place in the differential diagnosis of heart pain. Ann. Intern. Med., 58:926, 1963.
18. Fam, A.G., and Smythe, H.A.: Musculoskeletal chest wall pain. Can. Med. Assoc. J., 133:379, 1985.
19. Nathan, H., et al.: The costovertebral joints; Anatomical-clinical observations in arthritis. Arthritis Rheum., 7:228, 1964.
20. Forestier, J., and Lagier, R.: Ankylosing hyperostosis of the spine. Clin. Orthop., 74:65, 1971.
21. Resnick, D., et al.: Diffuse idiopathic skeletal hyperostosis (DISH) (ankylosing hyperostosis of Forestier and Rotes-Querol). Semin. Arthritis Rheum., 7:153, 1978.
22. Mennell, J.: The Science and Art of Joint Manipulation. New York, Blakiston, 1952.
23. Gooch, B.: Medical and Chirurgical Observation. London, Robinson, 1773.
24. Fam, A.G., et al.: Stress fractures in rheumatoid arthritis. J. Rheumatol., 10:722, 1983.
25. Anderson, I.F., Corrigan, A.B., and Champion, G.D.: Rib erosions in rheumatoid arthritis. Ann. Rheum. Dis., 31:16, 1972.
26. Daffner, R.H.: Stress fractures: Current concepts. Skeletal Radiol., 2:221, 1978.
27. Davies-Colley, R.: Slipping rib. Br. Med. J., 1:432, 1922.
28. Bonica, J.J.: The Management of Pain. 1st Ed. Philadelphia, Lea & Febiger, 1953, pp. 1164–1176.
29. Holmes, J.F.: A study of the slipping rib-cartilage syndrome. N. Engl. J. Med., 224:928, 1941.
30. Heinz, G.J., and Zavala, D.C.: Slipping rib syndrome. Diagnosis using the "hooking maneuver." JAMA, 237:794, 1977.
31. Tietze, A.: Über eine eigenartige Haufung von Fallen mit Dystrophie der Rippenknorpel. Berl. Klin. Wochenschr., 58:829, 1921.
32. Motulsky, A., and Rohn, R.J.: Tietze's syndrome: Cause of chest pain and chest wall swelling. JAMA, 152:504, 1953.
33. Gill, G.V.: Epidemic of Tietze's syndrome. Br. Med. J., 2:499, 1977.
34. Levey, G.S., and Calabro, J.J.: Tietze's syndrome: Report of two cases and review of the literature. Arthritis Rheum., 5:261, 1962.
35. Sain, A.K.: Bone scan in Tietze's syndrome. Clin. Nucl. Med., 3:470, 1978.
36. Calabro, J.J., and Marchesano, J.N.: Tietze's syndrome: Report of a case with juvenile onset. J. Pediatr., 68:985, 1966.
37. Kayser, H.L.: Tietze's syndrome: A review of the literature. Am. J. Med., 21:982, 1956.
38. Wehrmacher, W.H.: The painful anterior chest wall syndromes. Med. Clin. North Am., 38:111, 1958.
39. Calabro, J.J., et al.: Classification of anterior chest wall syndromes. JAMA, 243:1420, 1980.
40. Carabasi, R.J., Christian, J.J., and Brindley, H.H.: Costosternal chondrodynia: A variant of Tietze's syndrome? Dis. Chest, 41:559, 1962.
41. Wolf, E., and Stern, S.: Costosternal syndrome: Its frequency and importance in differential diagnosis of coronary heart disease. Arch. Intern. Med., 136:189, 1976.
42. Scobie, B.A.: Costochondral pain in gastroenterologic practice. N. Engl. J. Med., 295:1261, 1975.
43. Epstein, S.E., Gerber, L.H., and Borer, J.S.: Chest wall syndrome: A common cause of unexplained cardiac pain. JAMA, 241:2793, 1979.
44. Brown, R.T.: Costochondritis in adolescence. J. Adolesc. Health Care, 1:198, 1981.
45. Reuler, J.B., Girard D.E., and Nardone, D.A.: Sternoclavicular joint involvement in ankylosing spondylitis. South Med. J., 71:1480, 1978.
46. Resnick, D., Vint, V., and Poteshman, N.L.: Sterno-costoclavicular hyperostosis. J. Bone Joint Surg., 63:1329, 1981.
47. Fallet, G.H., Arroyo, J., and Vischer, T.L.: Sternocostoclavicular hyperostosis: Case report with a 31-year follow-up. Arthritis Rheum., 26:784, 1983.
48. Parker, V.S., et al.: The sternomanubrial joint (SMJ) in rheumatic diseases. Arthritis Rheum. 24 (Suppl. 108):S75, 1981.
49. Sebes, J.I., and Salazar, J.E.: The manubriosternal joint in rheumatoid arthritis. A.J.R., 140:117, 1983.
50. Lipkin, M., Fulton, L.R., and Wolfson, E.A.: Xiphoidalgia syndrome. N. Engl. J. Med., 253:609, 1955.
51. Bonica, J.J.: Management of myofascial pain syndrome in general practice. JAMA, 164:732, 1957.
52. Sola, A.E.: Myofascial trigger point therapy. Resident Staff Physician, 27:38, 1981.
53. Travell, J.G., and Simons, D.J.: Myofascial Pain and Dysfunction: The Trigger Point Manual. Baltimore, Williams & Wilkins, 1983, pp. 576–640.
54. Travell, J.G., and Rinzler, S.H.: Pain syndromes of the chest muscles: Resemblance of effort angina and myocardial infarction and relief by local block. Can. Med. Assoc. J., 59:333, 1948.
55. Travell, J.G., and Rinzler, S.H.: Relief of cardiac pain by local block of somatic trigger areas. Proc. Soc. Exp. Biol. Med., 63:480, 1946.
56. Rabzkerm S.H., and Travell, J.G.: Therapy directed at the somatic component of cardiac pain. Am. Heart J., 35:248, 1948.
57. Travell, J.G.: Early relief of chest pain by ethyl chloride spray in acute coronary thrombosis. Circulation, 3:120, 1951.
58. Lindgren, I.: Cutaneous precordial anaesthesia in angina pectoris and coronary occlusion (an experimental study). Nord. Med. Cardiologia, 11:207, 1946.
59. Gold, H., Kwip, N.T., and Modell, W.: The effect of extra cardiac pain on the heart. In Pain (Proceedings of Association for Research in Nervous and Mental Disease). Vol. 23. Edited by H.G. Wolff. Baltimore, Williams & Wilkins, 1943, pp. 345–351.
60. Sparrow, M.J., and Bird, E.L.: "Precordial catch": A benign syndrome of chest pain in young persons. N.Z. Med. J., 88:325, 1978.
61. Miller, A.J., and Texidor, T.A.: "Precordial catch," a neglected syndrome of precordial pain. JAMA, 159:1364, 1955.
62. Fitz-Hugh, T.: Precordial migraine: An important form of "angina innocens." Int. Clin., 3:141, 1940.
63. Briggs, J.F., and Bellomo, J.: Precordial migraine. Dis. Chest, 21:635, 1952.
64. Leon-Sotomayor, L.A.: Cardiac migraine: Report of twelve cases. Angiology, 25:161, 1974.
65. Saibil, F.B., and Edmeads, J.: Chest pain arising from extrathoracic structures. In Chest Pain: An Integrated Diagnostic Approach. Edited by D.L. Levene. Philadelphia, Lea & Febiger, 1977, p. 130.
66. Atkins, H.J.B.: Treatment of chronic mastitis. Lancet, 1:707, 1938.
67. Preece, P.E., Mansel, R.E., and Hughes, L.E.: Mastalgia: Psychoneurosis or organic disease? Br. Med. J., 1:29, 1978.
68. Mansel, R.E., Preece, P.E., and Hughes, L.E.: A double-blind trial of the prolactin inhibitor bromocriptine in painful nodular benign breast disease. Br. J. Surg., 65:724, 1978.
69. Mansel, R.E., Wisbey, J.R., and Hughes, L.E.: Controlled trial of the antigonadotropin danazol in painful nodular benign breast disease. Lancet, 2:928, 1982.
70. Wisbey, J.R., et al.: Natural history of breast pain. Lancet, 2:672, 1983.
71. Dercum, F.X.: Three cases of a hitherto unclassified infection resembling in its grosser aspects obesity, but associated with special nervous syptoms: Adiposis dolorosa. Am. J. Med. Sci., 104:521, 1892.
72. Foster, D.W.: Lipodystrophies and other rare disorders of adipose tissue. In Harrison's principles of Internal Medicine. 11th Ed. Edited by E. Braunwald et al. New York, McGraw-Hill, 1987, p. 1680.
73. Atkinson, R.L.: Intravenous lidocaine for the treatment of intractable pain of adiposis dolorosa. Int. J. Obes., 6:351, 1982.
74. Mondor, H.: Phlebite en cordon de la paroi thoracique. Mem. Acad. Chir., 70:96, 1944.
75. Lunn, G.M., and Potter, J.M.: Mondor's disease (subcutaneous phlebitis of the breast region). Br. Med. J. 1:1074, 1954.

76. Buell, J.C., and Elliot, R.S.: The heart and emotional stress. *In* The Heart, Arteries and Veins. 6th Ed. Edited by J.W. Hurst et al. New York, McGraw-Hill, 1986, pp. 1520–1530.
77. Billings, R.F.: Chest pain related to emotional disorders. *In* Chest pain: An Integrated Diagnostic Approach. Edited by D.L. Levene. Philadelphia, Lea & Febiger, 1977, pp. 133–150.
78. American Psychiatric Association: Diagnostic and Statistical Manual of Mental Disorders. 3rd Ed. Revised. Washington, DC, American Psychiatric Association, 1987.
79. Hurst, J.W., et al: Atherosclerotic coronary heart disease: Recognition, prognosis, and treatment in the heart. *In* The Heart, Arteries and Veins. 6th Ed. Edited by J.W. Hurst et al. New York, McGraw-Hill, 1986, pp. 907–908.
80. Da Costa, J.M.: On irritable heart: A clinical study of a form of functional cardiac disorder and its consequences. Am. J. Med. Sci., *61*:2, 1871.
81. Lewis, T.: The Soldier's Heart and the Effort Syndrome. New York, Hoeber, 1919.
82. Vaisrub, S.: Da Costa syndrome revisited. JAMA, *232*:164, 1975.
83. Soley, M.H., and Shock, N.W.: The etiology of the effort syndrome. Am. J. Med. Sci., *196*:840, 1938.
84. Wheeler, E.B., et al.: Neurocirculatory asthenia (anxiety neurosis, effort syndrome, neurasthenia): A 20-year follow-up study of 173 patients. JAMA, *142*:878, 1950.
85. Holmgren, A., et al.: Lung physical working capacity in suspected heart cases due to inadequate adjustment of peripheral blood flow. (Vasoregulatory asthenia.) Acta Med. Scand., *159*:413, 1957.
86. Cohen, M.E., Consolazio, F.C., and Johnson, R.A.: Blood lactate response during moderate exercise in neurocirculatory asthenia, anxiety neurosis or effort syndrome. J. Clin. Invest., *26*:339, 1947.
87. Levene, D.L.: Chest Pain: An Integrated Diagnostic Approach. Philadelphia, Lea & Febiger, 1977.
88. Ockene, I.S., et al.: Unexplained chest pain in patients with normal coronary arteriograms: A follow-up study of functional status. N. Engl. J. Med., *303*:1249, 1980.
89. DeCaestecker, J.S., et al.: The oesophagus as a cause of recurrent chest pain: Which patients should be investigated and which tests should be used? Lancet, *2*:1143, 1985.
90. Wielgosz, A.T., et al.: Unimproved chest pain in patients with minimal or no coronary disease: A behavioral phenomenon. Am. Heart J., *108*:67, 1984.
91. Pamelia F.X., et al.: Prognosis with chest pain and normal thallium-201 exercise scintigrams. Am. J. Cardiol., *55*:920, 1985.
92. Bass, C., and Wade, C.: Chest pain with normal coronary arteries: A comparative study of psychiatric and social morbidity. Psychol. Med. *14*:51, 1984.
93. Channer, K.S., et al.: Anxiety and depression in patients with chest pain referred for exercise testing. Lancet, *2*:820, 1985.
94. Costa, P.T., et al.: The relation of chest pain symptoms to angiographic findings of coronary artery stenosis and neuroticism. Psychosom. Med., *47*:285, 1985.
95. Wielgosz, A.T., and Earp, J.: Perceived vulnerability to serious heart disease and persistent pain in patients with minimal or no coronary disease. Psychosom. Med., *48*:118, 1986.
96. Wolf, E., Braun, K., and Stern, S.: Effects of beta-receptor blocking agents propranolol and practolol on SP-T changes in neurocirculatory asthenia. Br. Heart J., *36*:872, 1974.

59 · GENERAL CONSIDERATIONS OF ABDOMINAL PAIN

JOHN J. BONICA

THE abdomen is one of the most frequent sites of regional acute pain and various chronic pain syndromes caused by disorders of the abdominal viscera or referred by diseases of the thoracic viscera. Abdominal pain can also represent neuropathic pain caused by disease of the spinal cord or of the lower six thoracic nerves. Injury or disease of muscles and the fascia and other somatic structures that are part of the abdomen can also cause abdominal pain. This chapter, like others that introduce pain in various body regions, is intended to provide information on the anatomic, neurologic, and pathophysiologic bases of pain in the abdomen and a general approach to its diagnosis. Although the pelvis is considered to be part of the abdominal cavity, the various pain syndromes in this region are discussed separately in Section F (Part IV) to emphasize their importance and also because pain in the pelvis is often related to diseases of the perineum and external genitalia.

The information in this chapter is presented in four major sections: A, Basic Considerations, including an overview of the most common causes of pain in the abdomen and their mechanisms, and a brief discussion of the epidemiology of abdominal pain; B, Anatomy and Neurologic Aspects of the abdomen and viscera contained therein, including anatomy of the muscles of the abdomen, a brief description of the peritoneum, the nerve supply to these structures, and a general description of the autonomic and afferent nerve supplies to the abdominal viscera; C, Summary of Evaluation of the Patient and Differential Diagnosis of patients presenting with abdominal pain; and D, a table that presents all possible causes of abdominal pain, the characteristics of the pain, and other symptoms and signs that should help to make a differential diagnosis. The subsequent five chapters are more detailed and present specific information on these various aspects as they pertain to the disease of each viscus.

A. BASIC CONSIDERATIONS

Classification of Abdominal Pain

Pain in the abdomen is usually caused by disorders of the viscera contained within the abdominal cavity, including the pelvic viscera. Referred pain to the abdomen from diseases of the chest is the next common cause and often is a source of difficulty in differential diagnosis because the lower thoracic cavity and the abdomen, other than the pelvis, can be considered as one neurologic unit because the somatic and visceral nerve supplies of both regions have a common segmental distribution in the spinal cord. To be more specific, the lower half of the thoracic parietal pleura, the periphery of the diaphragmatic pleura, and about the upper 85% of the abdominal wall are supplied by the lower six or seven thoracic (and the first lumbar) somatic spinal nerves. Moreover, the proximal ends of the afferent nerves, which mediate nociceptive and other sensory impulses from the abdominal viscera (except the pelvis), synapse in the same spinal cord segments as the somatic spinal nerves. It is not surprising, therefore, that lesions of these various structures produce pain with similar localization in the trunk. These neuroanatomic and neurophysiologic factors also explain the common features of pain in the chest and abdomen caused by neuropathic disorders. The same neurologic lesions of the spinal cord or of the lower six or seven thoracic and first lumbar spinal nerves or their roots frequently produce a similar type of pain in the lower chest or the abdominal wall, depending on the level of the lesion. Less common

causes of abdominal pain are disorders of muscles and certain systemic diseases.

Abdominal Visceral Disease

The characteristics and mechanisms of pain caused by abdominal visceral disease are discussed in detail in Chapter 7. To briefly recapitulate, cutting and tearing or crushing of the viscera does not result in pain or in other perceptible sensation (1). Tension or stretching of the walls of hollow viscera, traction or stretching of the peritoneum, and increased tension caused by rapid stretching of the capsule of solid viscera constitute "the adequate stimulus" for visceral pain, specifically the following (2–5): (a) spasm of the smooth muscle of a hollow viscus; (b) sudden abnormal distension, stretching, or tearing of any part of the gastrointestinal tract (including the biliary ducts) or of the genitourinary system (including the ureters, urinary bladder, and uterus); (c) contraction of a hollow viscus under isometric conditions (i.e., the outlet of the viscus is obstructed); (d) rapid abnormal stretching of the capsule of such solid organs as the liver, spleen, or kidney; (e) traction, compression, or twisting of the mesentery, parietal peritoneum, ligaments, or blood vessels; (f) rapidly developing ischemia of the viscera; and (g) inflammation and necrosis of the pancreas or other viscera.

Inflammation, whether of bacterial or chemical origin, or ischemia of a hollowed viscus liberates algogenic (pain producing) substances such as bradykinin, serotonin, histamine, and prostaglandins that stimulate and sensitize nerve endings and thus lower their threshold for the adequate stimulus to activate sensory nerve endings. Thus, whereas pinching the wall of the healthy gastric mucosa or applying faradic stimulation or chemical irritants to it produces no pain, such procedures do produce pain of considerable intensity when done to inflamed, congested, and edematous gastric mucosa (5). Severe ischemia has a similar effect by increasing the concentration of these algogenic substances in the region of nerve endings.

Pain in the abdomen can be separated into two types according to the origin of the nociceptive impulses, visceral pain and parietal (somatic) pain. Based on localization, either type can be felt in or near the structure from which it arises or can be felt at a region that is removed from the structure that is the seat of noxious stimuli. Thus, four types of pain are associated with visceral disease: (a) unreferred or true visceral pain; (b) referred visceral pain; (c) unreferred or local parietal pain; and (d) referred parietal pain.

UNREFERRED VISCERAL PAIN. Unreferred or true visceral pain is dull, poorly localized in the epigastrium, periumbilical region, or lower midabdomen, and usually felt around the midline because with few exceptions the abdominal organs are supplied with afferents bilaterally. Exceptions to this are the kidneys, ureters, cecum, ascending colon, and descending and sigmoid colon, which have unilateral innervation. The poor localization of the pain occurs because innervation of most viscera is multisegmental and the viscera contain fewer nerve endings than the skin. The quality of the pain is usually gnawing, cramping, and associated with nausea, sweating, vomiting, perspiration, and pallor. When the nociceptive input is intense the pain is referred to the skin and deeper somatic tissue.

On the basis of the lack of evidence for a sensory channel specifically concerned with the transmission of visceral sensory impulses and the considerable amount of experimental data on viscerosomatic convergence in the central nervous system, Cervero and Tattersall (6) dispute this century-old classic concept of true visceral pain.

REFERRED VISCERAL PAIN. Referred visceral pain is somewhat more localized than true visceral pain. It is located in the dermatomes and myotomes that are supplied by the same spinal cord segments as the affected viscus and is the result of the convergence-projection mechanism (Chapter 7). Thus, distension of the intestine with a balloon causes a vague, aching, poorly localized discomfort at first but, with greater distension, the pain is referred to the abdominal wall and back (7).

UNREFERRED PARIETAL PAIN. Parietal pain is considered to be unreferred or local when the inflammation of the parietal peritoneum produces pain localized in the body wall directly over the site of the inflammation, such as the localized pain in acute appendicitis produced by inflammatory involvement of the parietal peritoneum at McBurney's point. The pain results from stimulation of nociceptive fibers in the parietal peritoneum in the right lower quadrant.

REFERRED PARIETAL PAIN. Referred parietal pain is characterized by pain felt in an area that is remote from the site of nociceptive stimulation. A typical example is the pain felt in the shoulder when the parietal peritoneum of the middle portion of the diaphragm is inflamed and stimulated.

Pain of Neuropathic Origin

Lesions of the spinal cord, such as primary or metastatic tumors, or spinal cord compression cause pain in the abdomen when the lesion involves one or more of the lower six thoracic segments of the spinal cord. The pain can be dull, aching, and not well localized or radicular, depending on the lesion. Compression or inflammation of the rootlets and roots of the lower six or seven thoracic nerves, such as in herpes zoster, tabes dorsalis, or compression from vertebral tumors or herniated disks, produces sharp, burning, segmental pain in the abdomen and is associated with hyperalgesia, hyperesthesia, and other sensory disturbances. Intercostal neuropathy produced by mechanical or inflammatory processes can also cause pain in the anterior abdomen.

Pain Caused by Musculoskeletal Disorders

In addition to producing radiculopathy or neuropathy with segmental pain, disorders of the lower thoracic spine can cause local or regional pain in the back or occasionally referred to the side of the trunk. Fracture or dislocation of the lower ribs or their cartilages causes localized pain on the side of the injury. Fracture or slippage of the cartilages causes sharp localized epigastric pain that is aggravated by movement and pressure. Myofascial pain syndromes involving muscles of the abdomen are much less frequent causes of pain from the abdomen than from other parts of the body. Trauma with hemorrhage to the anterior abdominal wall can cause localized pain. In all these conditions the pain is fairly well localized and sharp and is associated with tenderness. Postoperative pain is a source of moderate to severe discomfort, especially following operation in the upper abdomen. This type of pain is markedly aggravated by movement, coughing, and straining and is often associated with reflex muscle spasm and other segmental and suprasegmental responses (Chapter 25).

Other Causes of Abdominal Pain

Various systemic, toxic, allergic, hematologic, and endocrine disturbances can cause episodes of severe, deep abdominal pain that can simulate that of visceral disease. The pain of porphyria or lead colic is usually difficult to distinguish from that of intestinal obstruction because severe hyperperistalsis is a prominent feature of both (8). The pain of uremia or diabetes is nonspecific and the pain and tenderness frequently shift in location and intensity. Black widow spider bites produce pain and rigidity of abdominal muscles and of back muscles, an area not frequently involved in disease of intra-abdominal origin.

Disease of intra-abdominal arteries and veins can cause severe, diffuse pain as in embolism or thrombosis of the superior mesenteric artery or rupture of abdominal aortic aneurysm, or it can cause mild continuous diffuse pain for 2 or 3 days before vascular collapse or evidence of peritoneal inflammation appears (8). The early, seemingly insignificant, discomfort is caused by hyperperistalsis rather than by peritoneal inflammation. The absence of tenderness and rigidity and the presence of continuous diffuse pain in a patient likely to have vascular disease is characteristic of occlusion of the superior mesenteric artery (8).

Pain primarily caused by psychologic or emotional factors varies enormously in type, location, and other characteristics, usually has no relation to meals, and is often accentuated during the night; nausea and vomiting are rarely observed and no reflex spasm of abdominal muscles is seen. Frequently, the site of the pain varies from visit to visit.

Table 59-1 presents the most common causes of abdominal pain. (A more detailed listing is given below in Table 59-6, which contains the important diagnostic features of each condition.)

Epidemiology

The precise incidence and prevalence of abdominal pain are not known, but data from the 1986 National Health Interview Survey (9) suggest that nearly 15 million Americans suffered acute disorders of the digestive system and about 2 million had acute disorders of the kidney and ureters in 1986. These conditions resulted in over 105 million days of restricted activity, about 44 million days of bed disability, and about 25 million days of lost work. In addition, over 30 million people were listed as having "selected chronic digestive conditions," including 4.5 million patients with ulcers, nearly 3 million patients with gastritis or duodenitis, 2.5 million patients with enteritis or colitis, 5.3 million patients with frequent recurrent periods of pain caused by indigestion, and over 1.6 million patients with spastic colon associated with abdominal pain.

The 1986 National Hospital Discharge Survey (10) indicated that about 5.8 million patients were hospitalized for digestive and kidney diseases in 1986, resulting in nearly 38 million days of hospitalization. Moreover, about 6.7 million operations were performed to diagnose and treat digestive and renal disorders (Table 59-2).

The 1987 estimates of the American Cancer Society (11) included 224,000 new cases of cancer of the digestive organs and 22,000 new cases of cancer of the kidney and ureters, while the total deaths from each group of cancers were 125,000 and 9400, respectively (Table 59-3). The total of new cases and deaths from cancer of the digestive system is the highest of any organ system or cancer site.

Computations based on the incidence of pain with these various abdominal and renal conditions, and data on the incidence of cancer pain with various types of cancers (Chapter 24), suggest that in 1986 about 20% of Americans had abdominal pain that required medical attention. The Nuprin Pain Report suggested that these numbers underestimate the actual figures and noted that, in 1985, 46% of Americans had abdominal ("stomach") pain (12).

TABLE 59-1. Major Causes of Abdominal Pain

I. INTRA-ABDOMINAL DISEASE
  A. Parietal peritoneal inflammation
    1. Generalized peritonitis
       a. Primary bacterial infection (e.g., pneumococcal, streptococcal, enteric bacillus)
       b. Bacterial contamination (e.g., perforated appendix, pelvic inflammatory disease, ruptured hepatic abscess)
       c. Chemical peritonitis (e.g., perforated ulcer, pancreatitis, ruptured ovarian cyst, rupture of follicle)
    2. Localized peritonitis (e.g., acute appendicitis, cholecystitis, peptic ulcer, colitis, regional enteritis, abdominal abscess, Meckel's diverticulitis, pancreatitis, gastroenteritis, hepatitis)
    3. Distension or traction of mesentery (e.g., tumor)
  B. Mechanical obstruction of hollow viscus that leads to increased tension stretching
    1. Obstruction of small or large intestine (e.g., tumor, adhesions, hernia, volvulus, intussusception)
    2. Obstruction of biliary system (e.g., gallstones, strictures, tumors)
    3. Obstruction of ureter (e.g., calculi, external tumors, kinking)
    4. Obstruction of uterus (e.g., tumor, childbirth)
  C. Rapid distension of capsule of solid viscus that leads to increased tension or stretching
    1. Capsule of liver (e.g., hepatitis—toxic or viral, rapidly growing tumor, common duct obstruction)
    2. Capsule of spleen (e.g., acute splenomegaly, hemorrhage, abscess, cyst, tumor)
    3. Capsule of kidney (e.g., pyelonephritis, hemorrhage, abscess, ureteral obstruction)
  D. Acute ischemia
    1. Mesenteric embolism or thrombosis
    2. Splenic embolism or thrombosis
    3. Hepatic infarction or toxemia
    4. Rapid torsion of gallbladder, spleen, ovarian cyst, testicle, appendix
    5. Vascular rupture
    6. Sickle cell anemia

II. EXTRA-ABDOMINAL DISEASE
  A. Thoracic visceral disease
    1. Pneumonia, pulmonary embolism, pneumothorax
    2. Acute myocardial infarction, myocarditis, angina pectoris
    3. Esophageal rupture, esophageal spasm
  B. Neuropathic and musculoskeletal disorders
    1. Diseases of the spinal cord (e.g., tumor tabes dorsalis, spinal cord compression)
    2. Infectious or mechanical radiculopathy (e.g., herpes zoster, postherpetic neuralgia, compression by disorders of the spine)
    3. Fracture of lower ribs leading to neuropathy and neuralgia
    4. Fracture or dislocation of the lower costal cartilages
    5. Myofascial pain syndromes, trauma to abdominal muscles, polymyositis

III. METABOLIC DISORDERS AND TOXINS OR POISONS
  A. Exogenous causes
    1. Spider bite (e.g., black widow)
    2. Lead and other heavy metal poisoning
  B. Endogenous causes
    1. Uremia
    2. Porphyria
    3. Diabetes mellitus
    4. Allergic diseases

IV. ABDOMINAL PAIN PRIMARILY OF PSYCHOLOGIC ORIGIN
  A. Irritable bowel syndrome
  B. Anxiety states
  C. Depression
  D. Hypochondriasis
  E. Operant abdominal pain

TABLE 59-2. Hospitalizations and Operations Performed for Digestive and Renal Diseases in 1986

| Disease | Inpatient Discharges | | | Operations | |
	Number of Patients (in Thousands)	Average Length of Stay (Days)	Total Hospital Days (in Thousands)	Type	Total (in Thousands)
Digestive tract				Digestive Tract	
Peptic ulcer	295	7.1	2,095	Endoscopy	642
Gastritis or duodenitis	196	4.5	882	Gastrectomy	293
Appendicitis	250	4.9	1,225	Appendectomy	275
Inguinal hernia	304	3.0	912	Cholecystectomy	502
Enteritis or colitis	429	4.8	2,059	Repair of inguinal hernia	329
Cholelithiasis	494	6.9	3,409	Division of adhesions	325
Other disorders	2,047	4.2	8,775	Hemorrhoidectomy	114
				Other	3,248
Subtotal:	3,732	6.1	27,765		
				Subtotal:	5,728
Renal or ureteral				Renal or ureteral	984
Calculi	331	3.6	1,192		
Other	1,703	5.2	8,856		
Subtotal:	2,034	4.9	10,048		
All:	5,766	6.5	37,813	All:	6,712

National Center for Health Statistics: Advanced Data 1986 Summary: National Hospital Discharge Survey. Hyattsville, MD, National Center for Health Statistics, 1987, Publ. No. 145.

TABLE 59-3. Estimates of New Cancer Cases of the Digestive and Renal Systems and Cancer Deaths in 1987

| Site | Estimated New Cases | | | Estimated Deaths | | |
	Male	Female	Total	Male	Female	Total
Digestive organs						
Esophagus	6,800	2,900	9,700	6,400	2,400	8,800
Stomach	15,000	9,600	24,600	8,300	5,900	14,200
Small intestine	1,300	1,200	2,500	400	400	800
Large intestine	47,000	55,000	102,000	25,000	27,000	52,000
Rectum	23,000	20,000	43,000	4,100	3,900	8,000
Liver and biliary passages	7,100	6,900	14,000	5,300	5,300	10,600
Pancreas	13,000	13,200	26,200	12,300	12,000	24,300
Other cancers	2,800	1,200	4,000	600	600	1,200
Subtotal:	114,400	110,000	224,000	62,400	57,500	125,200
Kidney	13,800	8,000	21,900	5,700	3,700	9,400

American Cancer Society: Cancer Facts and Figures, 1987. New York, American Cancer Society, 1987.

B. ANATOMIC AND NEUROLOGIC ASPECTS

Anatomy of the Abdomen

The abdomen, the region of the trunk below the diaphragm, is composed of an upper part, the abdomen proper, and a lower part, the lesser pelvis (13, 14). The anatomy of the pelvis is described in Chapter 65. The abdomen is largely bounded by muscles and its shape and size can thus be altered under different conditions, such as varying degrees of distension of the hollow organs contained therein and the different phases of respiration. Moreover, the tone of the muscles is important in maintaining the abdominal (and pelvic) viscera in position.

The abdomen proper is bounded anteriorly by the rectus abdominis muscles, the pyramidalis, and the aponeurotic parts of three muscles—the external oblique, internal oblique, and transversus abdominis. It is bounded at its sides by the fleshy parts of these three muscles and by the iliac muscles and iliac bones and posteriorly by the lumbar part of the vertebral column, the crura of the diaphragm, the psoas and quadratus lumborum muscles, and the posterior part of the iliac bones. Superiorly it is bounded by the diaphragm and inferiorly by the superior aperture of the lesser pelvis. Because of the dome shape of the diaphragm a considerable part of the abdominal cavity extends superiorly and is inside the framework of the thorax. The abdomen proper contains the greater part of the gastrointestinal tract as well as the liver, pancreas, spleen, kidneys, part of the ureters,

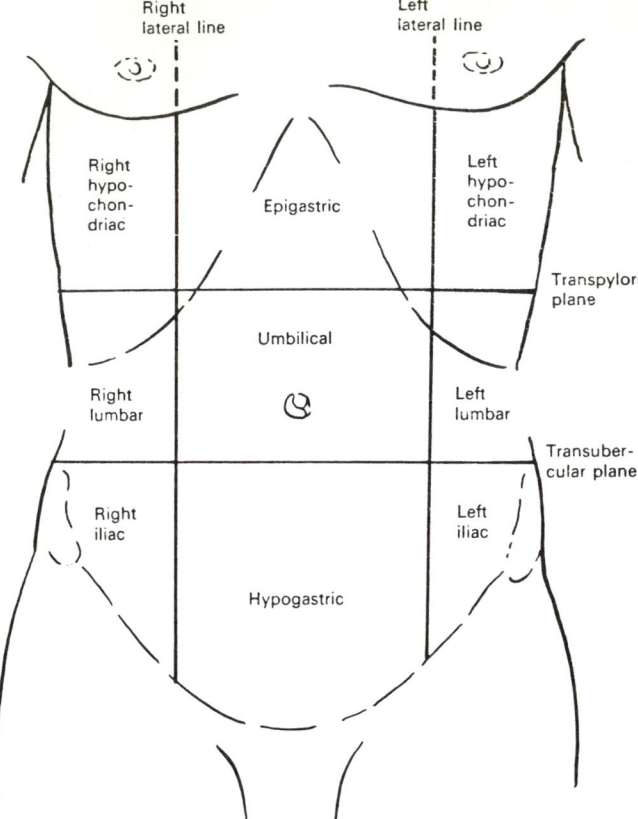

FIG. 59-1. Regions of the abdominal wall. The wall is divided into nine regions by four imaginary lines, of which two pass horizontally around the body and two vertically. The upper horizontal line or plane, also called the transpyloric plane, is at a level midway between the suprasternal notch and the symphysis pubis, intersects the front of the body of the 1st lumbar vertebra near its lower border, and meets the costal margin at the tip of the 9th costal cartilage. The lower transtubercular plane is at the level of the top of the crests of the iliac bones and intersects the front of the body of the 5th lumbar vertebra near its upper border. The vertical lines, one on each side of the body, descend from the cartilages of the 8th rib to the center of the inguinal ligament.

supra-adrenal glands, and numerous blood vessels, lymph vessels, lymph nodes, and nerves.

For purposes of location of the viscera, especially in clinical practice, the abdomen is divided into nine regions by imaginary planes. Two horizontal and two sagittal planes pass through the cavity, with the edges of each plane being indicated by lines projected onto the surface of the body (Fig. 59-1). Figure 59-2 depicts the relationship of various abdominal viscera and other structures to the dermatomes and to the ribs.

Muscles

The muscles of the abdomen are conveniently divided into an anterolateral group and a posterior group. The anterolateral group consists of four large flat muscular sheets that form the anterior abdominal wall, including the internal and external oblique, the transversus and rectus abdominis, and two smaller elements, the cremaster and pyramidalis, which are involved in the suspension of the testes and in the

tensing of the midline tendinous raphe of the abdominal wall. The posterior muscles of the abdomen include the psoas major and minor, the iliacus, and the fasciae covering them, as well as the quadratus lumborum muscle. The superior part of the abdomen is composed of the inferior surface of the diaphragm, which although discussed briefly in connection with the chest is considered in some detail here; the other muscles are then described briefly.

Diaphragm

Figure 59-3 depicts the inferior surface of the diaphragm with the various nerves and some of the major vessels, but without any of the other structures. This dome-shaped musculofibrous sheet, which separates the thoracic from the abdominal cavities, consists of the central tendon, which consists of a thin but strong aponeurosis of closely interwoven fibers situated near the center of the dome, and the peripheral part, which consists of muscular fibers that are attached to the circumference of the thoracic outlet and converge into the central tendon (13, 14).

The musculofibers are grouped into three portions: the sternal part, arising from two fleshy slips from the back of the xiphoid process; the costal part, arising from the internal surface of the cartilage and from adjacent parts of the lower six ribs on each side and interdigitating with the transversus abdominis muscle; and the lumbar part, arising from two aponeurotic arches, from the medial and lateral arcuate ligaments, and from the lumbar vertebrae by two pillars, or crura.

The diaphragm has three large openings—the aortic, esophageal, and vena caval—and a number of smaller ones that transmit the superior and middle splanchnic nerves. The aortic aperture is the lowest and most posterior of the large openings and is situated at the level of the lower border of the T10 vertebra and the thoracolumbar intervertebral disk, slightly to the left of the median plane. In addition to being an opening for the passage of the aorta, the aortic aperture also transmits the thoracic duct and occasionally the azygos and hemiazygos veins.

The esophageal aperture is an elliptic opening in the muscular part of the diaphragm at the level of the T10 vertebra that is formed by the splitting of the medial fibers of the right crus (14). In addition to transmitting the esophagus it allows the passage of the vagal and sympathetic nerves that surround the lower esophagus and then proceed to the stomach, the esophageal branches of the left gastric vessels, and some lymphatics. The fascia on the inferior surface of the diaphragm, which is continuous with the transversalis fascia and is rich in elastic fibers, extends upward into the opening in a conical fashion to be attached to the wall of the esophagus about 2 cm above the gastroesophageal junction, with some of the elastic fibers penetrating to the submucosa of the esophagus. This fascial extension, often called the phrenoesophageal ligament, is an important structure in the treatment of esophageal reflux (Figure 56-12). The vena caval aperture is the highest of the three large openings and is situated at about the level of the disk between the T8 and T9 vertebrae. It transmits the inferior vena cava and some branches of the right phrenic nerve, which is the major motor nerve supply to the diaphragm, and also contains some sensory fibers (Chapter 53).

Anterolateral Muscles

The anterolateral group of muscles of the abdomen are covered by a fascia that is divisible into two

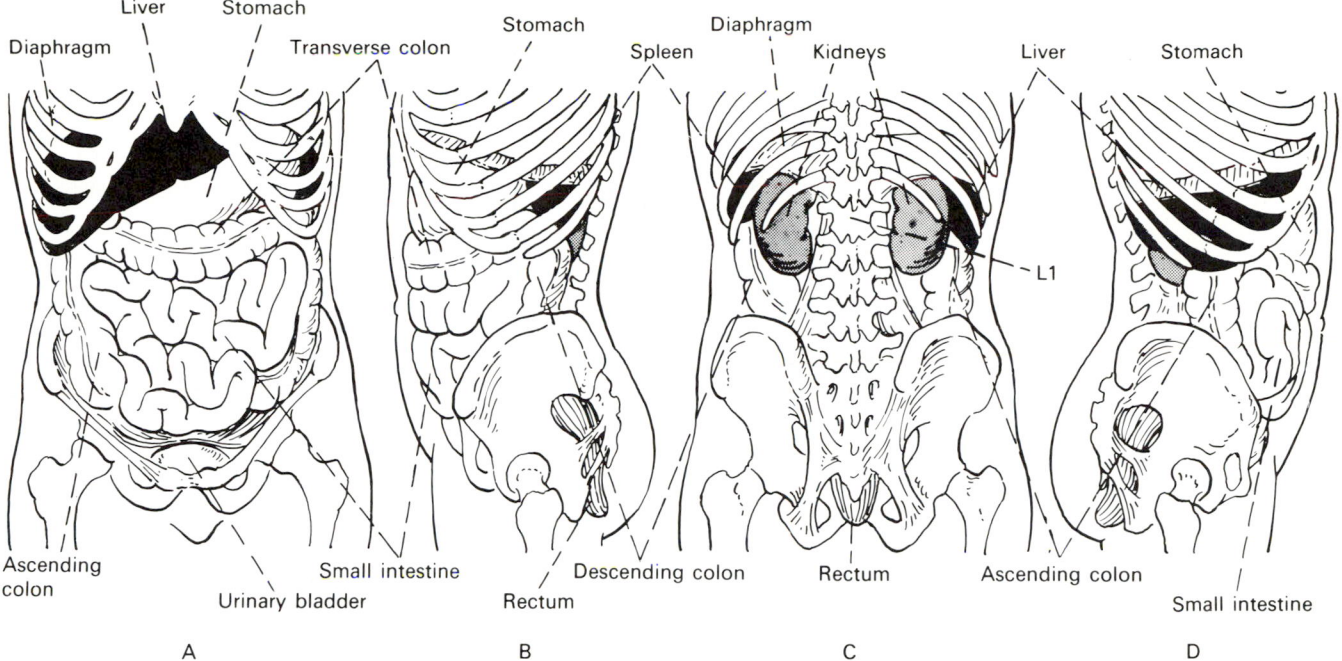

Fig. 59-2. Abdominal viscera shown in their normal relationship in the skeleton. **A.** Anterior view. **B.** View from the left side. **C.** View from the back. **D.** View from the right side. Modified from Clemente, C.D. (ed.): Gray's Anatomy of the Human Body, 30th Ed. Philadelphia, Lea & Febiger, 1985.

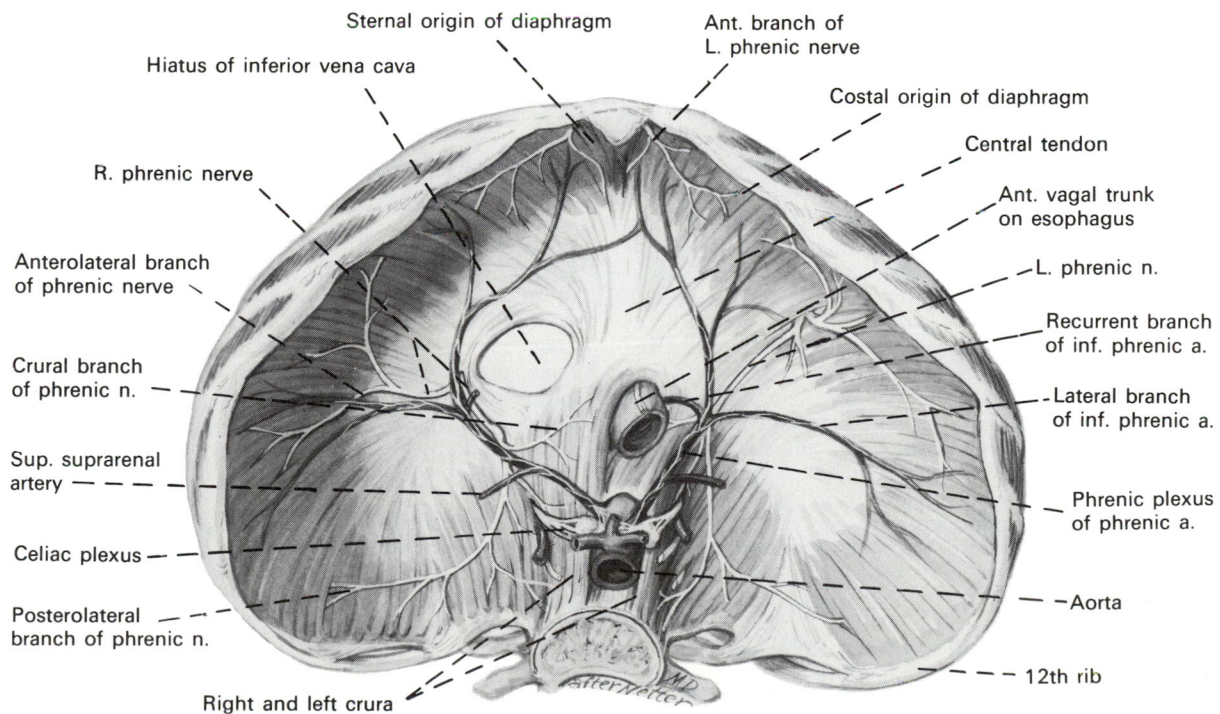

Fig. 59-3. Abdominal surface of the diaphragm depicting the phrenic nerves and arteries and the phrenic plexus, as well as the major openings. See text for details. Modified from Netter, F.H.: The CIBA Collection of Medical Illustrations, Vol. 2, Digestive System. Part III, Lower Digestive Tract. Summit, NJ, CIBA, 1979, p. 21.

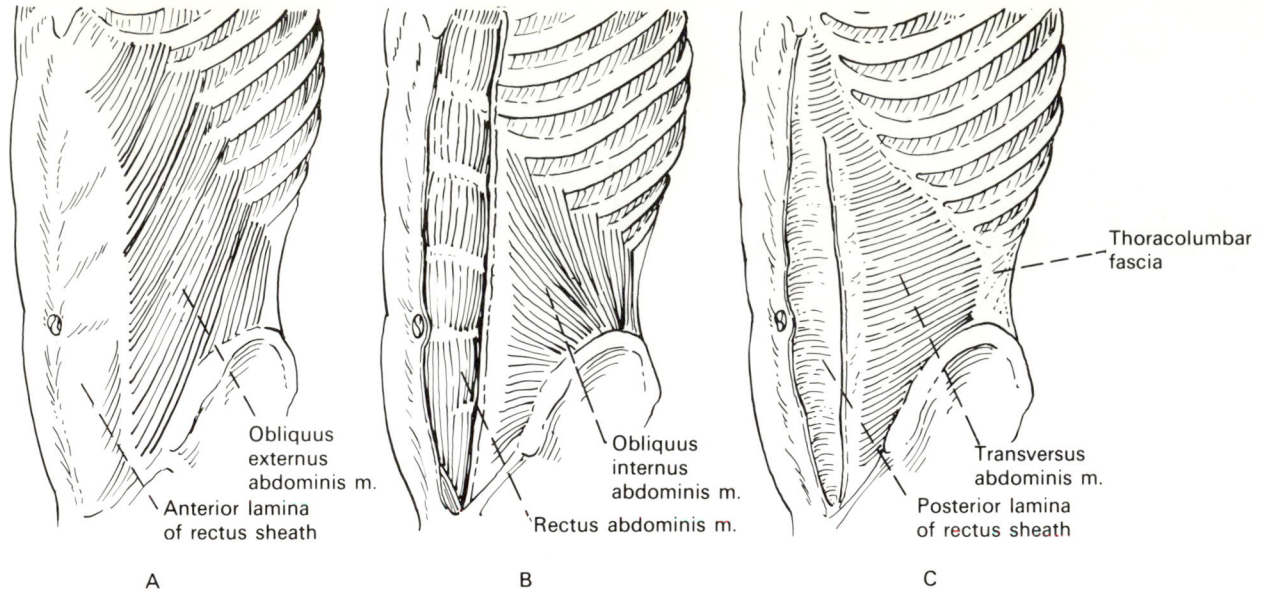

Thoracolumbar fascia

Obliquus externus abdominis m.

Anterior lamina of rectus sheath

Obliquus internus abdominis m.

Rectus abdominis m.

Transversus abdominis m.

Posterior lamina of rectus sheath

A B C

FIG. 59-4. Muscles and fascia of the abdominal wall. *A.* Obliquus externus abdominis and anterior lamina of the rectus sheath; *B.* Rectus abdominis and obliquus internus abdominis. *C.* Transversus abdominis, thoracolumbar fascia, and posterior lamina of the rectus sheath.

layers, between which are superficial vessels, nerves, and superficial inguinal lymph nodes. The superficial layer of the fascia is thick, is areolar in texture, and contains a varying quantity of fat in its meshes. Below it passes over the inguinal ligament and is continuous with the superficial fascia of the thigh. The deep layer of the fascia is more membranous than the superficial, contains elastic fibers, and is loosely connected by areolar tissue to the aponeurosis of the external oblique muscle except in the medial plane, where it adheres intimately to the linea alba and to the symphysis pubis (Fig. 59-4).

OBLIQUUS EXTERNUS ABDOMINIS. The obliquus externus abdominis muscle, the largest and most superficial of the three flat muscles, arises by eight fleshy slips from the external surfaces and inferior borders of the lower eight ribs; these slips interdigitate with the serratus anterior and latissimus dorsi (Fig. 59-4A). The fibers diverge from these attachments as they pass into their insertion: those from the lower two ribs pass inferiorly to become attached to the outer lip of the iliac crest, whereas the middle and upper fibers are directed inferiorly and anteriorly, end in an aponeurosis that is a strong tendinous sheath and whose fibers are directed downward and medially. In the medial plane its fibers end in the linea alba, which is a tendinous raphe that stretches from the xiphoid process to the symphysis pubis. At the raphe it is continuous with the aponeurosis of the opposite muscle and together these two cover the anterior part of the abdomen. The margin of the aponeurosis between the anterior superior iliac spine and the pubic tubercle is a thick band formed and then turned on itself to present a grooved upper surface. This is the inguinal, or Poupart's, ligament.

OBLIQUUS INTERNUS ABDOMINIS. The obliquus internus abdominis muscle is internal to and is thinner and less bulky than the obliquus externus muscle. It arises by muscular fibers from the lateral two-thirds of the grooved upper surface of the inguinal ligament, from the anterior two-thirds of the intermediate line of the iliac crest, and from the thoracolumbar fascia (Fig. 59-4B). The posterior fibers pass cepha-

lad and laterally to the inferior border of the lower three or four ribs and are continuous with the internal intercostal muscles. The fibers from the inguinal ligament arch across the spermatic cord in the male and the round ligament of the uterus in the female, become tendinous, and attach to the corresponding part of the aponeurosis of the transversus abdominis muscle to the crest in the medial part of the pecten ossis pubis, forming the conjoint tendon or falx inguinalis. The rest of the fibers pass anteriorly and anterosuperiorly, ending in an aponeurosis that gradually broadens from below upward. In its upper two-thirds this aponeurosis splits at the lateral border of the rectus abdominis into two layers, which pass around it and reunite in the linea alba that they help to form.

TRANSVERSUS ABDOMINIS. The transversus abdominis is the innermost of the flat muscles of the abdominal wall and is internal to the obliquus internus abdominis. It arises from the lateral third of the inguinal ligament, the anterior two-thirds of the inner lip of the iliac crest and thoracolumbar fascia between the iliac crest and the 12th rib, and the internal aspects of the lower six costal cartilages, where it interdigitates with the diaphragm (Fig. 59-4C). The muscle fibers pass anteriorly and end in its aponeurosis. The lower fibers of the aponeurosis pass inferiorly and medially, together with those of the aponeurosis of the internal oblique, to the crest and pecten of the pubis; these contribute to the falx inguinalis while the rest pass horizontally over the aponeurosis toward the medial plane and blend with the linea alba.

RECTUS ABDOMINIS. The rectus abdominis muscle is a long, thick, rather narrow muscle that extends along the whole length of the front of the abdomen and is separated from its counterpart by the linea alba. It arises by two tendons, a lateral and larger tendon attached to the crest of the pubis and a medial tendon that interlaces with the larger one and becomes connected with ligamentous fibers of the symphysis pubis (Fig. 59-4B). Superiorly each muscle is inserted by three fascicles of unequal size to the 5th, 6th, and 7th costal cartilages. The muscle fibers of the rectus are interrupted by three fibrous bands called tendinous intersections. The rectus abdominis is enclosed in the rectus sheath,

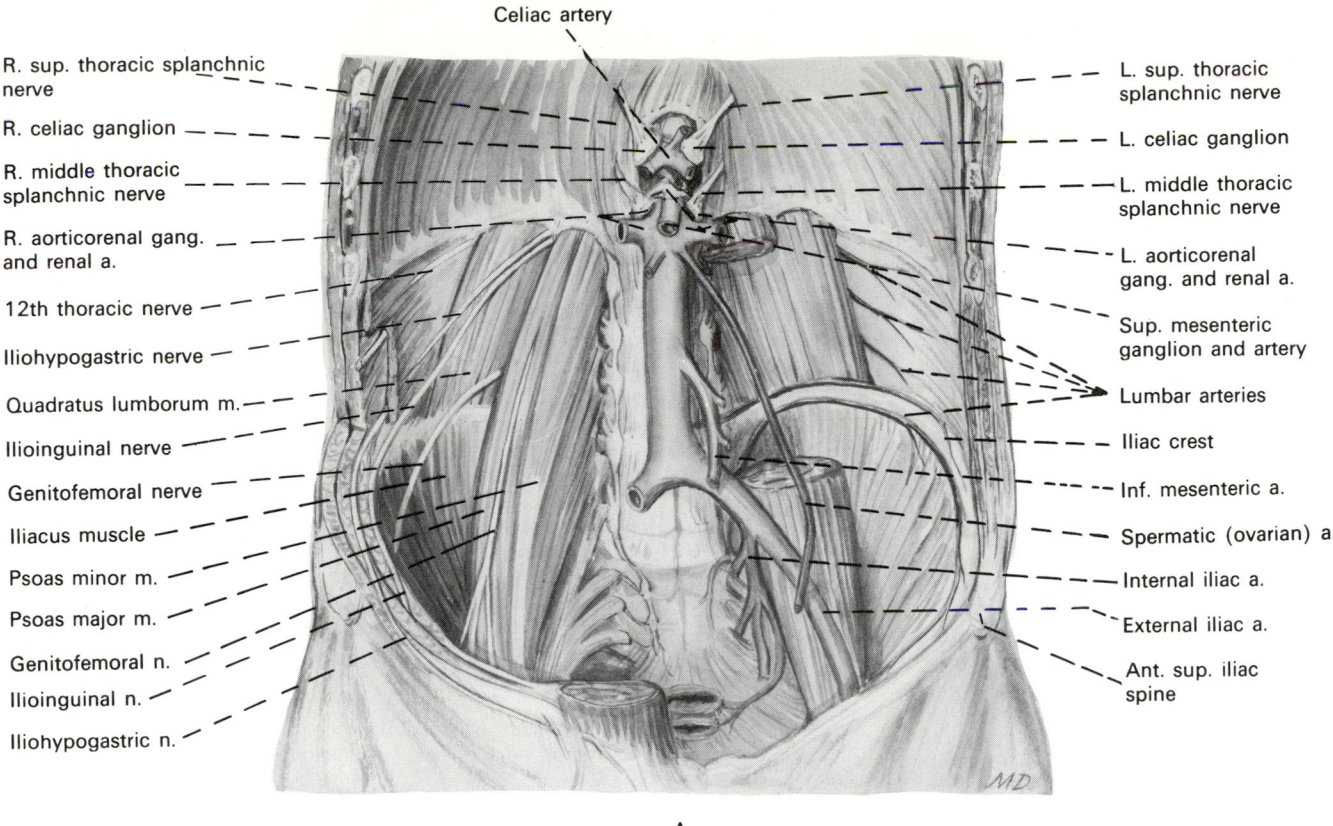

Celiac artery

R. sup. thoracic splanchnic nerve

R. celiac ganglion

R. middle thoracic splanchnic nerve

R. aorticorenal gang. and renal a.

12th thoracic nerve

Iliohypogastric nerve

Quadratus lumborum m.

Ilioinguinal nerve

Genitofemoral nerve

Iliacus muscle

Psoas minor m.

Psoas major m.

Genitofemoral n.

Ilioinguinal n.

Iliohypogastric n.

L. sup. thoracic splanchnic nerve

L. celiac ganglion

L. middle thoracic splanchnic nerve

L. aorticorenal gang. and renal a.

Sup. mesenteric ganglion and artery

Lumbar arteries

Iliac crest

Inf. mesenteric a.

Spermatic (ovarian) a.

Internal iliac a.

External iliac a.

Ant. sup. iliac spine

A

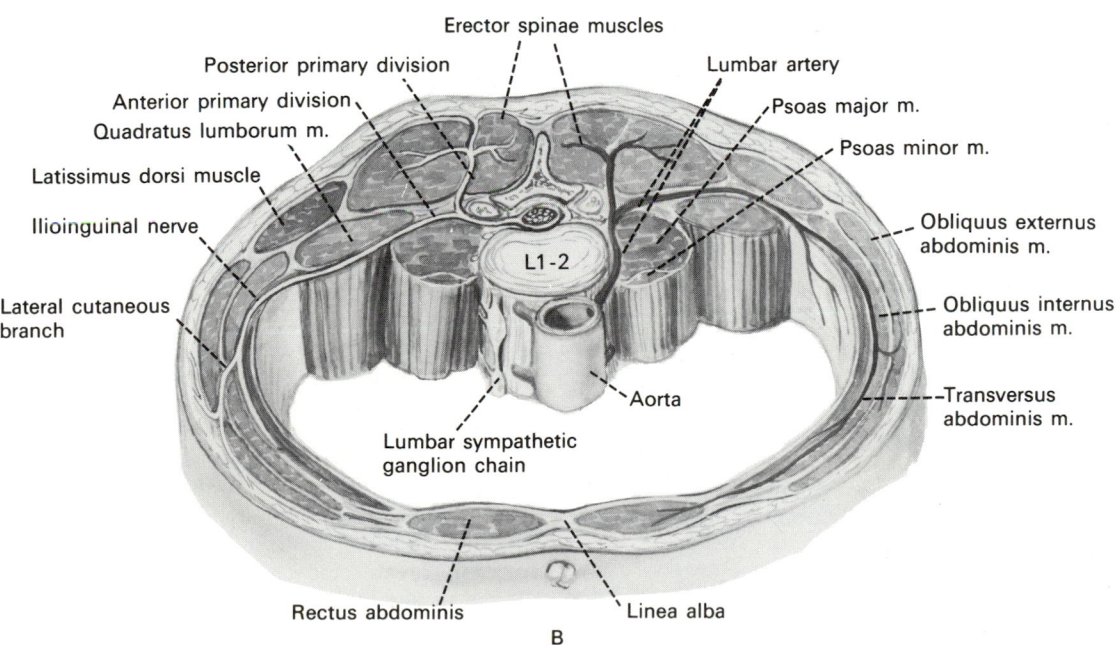

Erector spinae muscles

Posterior primary division

Anterior primary division

Quadratus lumborum m.

Latissimus dorsi muscle

Ilioinguinal nerve

Lateral cutaneous branch

Lumbar artery

Psoas major m.

Psoas minor m.

L1-2

Obliquus externus abdominis m.

Obliquus internus abdominis m.

Transversus abdominis m.

Aorta

Lumbar sympathetic ganglion chain

Rectus abdominis

Linea alba

B

FIG. 59-5. *A.* Posterior wall of the abdomen showing the blood vessels on the right and the lumbar nerves on the left, as well as the muscles that make up the posterior boundary of the abdomen proper. *B.* Cross section of the trunk depicting the anterior and posterior abdominal muscles and course of the lumbar artery (right) and the 1st lumbar nerve on the left. *A* Modified from Netter, F.H.: The CIBA Collection of Medical Illustrations, Vol. 3, Digestive System. Part II, Lower Digestive Tract. Summit, NJ, CIBA, 1979, pp. 35, 43.

which is the aponeurosis of the oblique and transverse muscles. Figure 59-5 depicts a transverse section through the anterior and posterior abdominal walls showing the termination of the abdominal muscles and the fascia that covers them.

Only the quadratus lumborum is described here because the other, posterior muscles of the abdomen are muscles of the lower limb and are described in Chapter 70. The quadratus lumborum is an irregularly quadrilateral-shaped muscle that is broader inferiorly (Fig. 59-5). It arises below by aponeurotic fibers of the iliolumbar ligament and by the adjacent portion of the iliac crest for about 5 cm, while above it is inserted into the medial half of the lower border of the last rib and to the apices of the transverse processes of the upper four lumbar vertebrae by four small tendons. Anterior to the quadratus lumborum are the colon, kidney, psoas major and minor, and diaphragm.

Peritoneum

The peritoneum is the largest and most complexly arranged serous membrane of the body. In the male it consists of a closed sac; part of this lines the abdominal wall and the remainder is reflected over viscera. In the female the lateral ends of the uterine tube open into the peritoneal cavity. The part that lines the abdominal wall is called the parietal peritoneum while that reflected over the viscera is the visceral peritoneum. The free surface of the membrane is covered with a layer of flattened mesothelium and is kept moist and smooth by a thin film of serous fluid, so that the viscera can glide unrestricted over each other on the wall of the cavity.

A fairly large amount of areolar connective tissue intervenes between the parietal peritoneum and the abdominal wall, blending with the fascia lining. This structure, known as the extraperitoneal tissue, varies in quantity and contains a varying amount of fat in different regions. The areolar connective tissue is loosely connected to parietal peritoneum in the abdominal wall but is dense in adherence on the inferior surface of the diaphragm and behind the linea alba. It is especially loosely arranged in some places to allow alteration in size of certain organs, such as the urinary bladder. The extraperitoneal tissue is usually heavily laden with fat on the posterior abdominal wall in relation to the kidney. The visceral peritoneum, on the other hand, is firmly united to the viscera that it covers and cannot be easily stripped off. Indeed, the connective tissue layer, the subserous fascia of the visceral peritoneum, is directly continuous with the fibrous tissue stroma of the viscera. The parietal and visceral layers of the peritoneum are in actual contact, the peritoneal cavity being the potential space between them. The peritoneal cavity consists of a main region, called the greater sac, and a diverticulum from this called the omental bursa, or lesser sac. The neck or communication between the greater and lesser sacs is the epiploic foramen, or foramen of Winslow (13).

Omenta

LESSER OMENTUM. The lesser omentum is the fold of peritoneum that extends to the liver from the lesser curvature of the stomach and the beginning of the duodenum. It is continuous with the two layers that cover the anterosuperior and posteroinferior surfaces of the stomach and about the first 2 cm of the duodenum. A portion of the lesser omentum that extends between the liver and stomach is known as the hepatogastric ligament, and that between the liver and duodenum is known as the hepatoduodenal ligament.

GREATER OMENTUM. The greater omentum is the largest peritoneal fold. It consists of a double sheet folded on itself so that it is made up of four layers. The two layers that descend from the stomach and the beginning of the duodenum pass downward in front of the small intestine for a variable distance. They then turn on themselves and ascend as far as the anterosuperior aspect of the transverse colon. They adhere to but are separable from the peritoneum on the upper surface of the transverse colon and the upper layer of the transverse mesocolon.

Mesenteries

The peritoneal fold, collectively known as the mesenteries, includes the mesentery of the small intestine, called the mesentery proper, and the mesoappendix, the transverse mesocolon, and the sigmoid mesocolon. The mesentery of the small intestine is a broad, variably shaped fold of peritoneum that connects the convolutions of the jejunum and ileum to the posterior abdominal wall. The part attached to the posterior wall of the abdomen is called the root of the mesentery. The mesoappendix is a triangular fold of peritoneum around the vermiform appendix that is attached to the back of the lower end of the mesentery close to the ileocecal junction. Its layers include the blood vessels, nerves, and lymph vessels of the appendix, together with a lymph node. The transverse mesocolon is a broad fold that connects the transverse colon to the posterior abdominal wall. Its two layers pass from the anterior surface of the head and the anterior border of the body of the pancreas to the posterior surface of the transverse colon. The sigmoid mesocolon is a fold of peritoneum that attaches the sigmoid to the pelvic wall. These structures are important because they contain blood vessels, nerves, and lymph vessels and, when stretched, provoke nociceptive impulses.

Vessels and Nerves

The parietal and visceral layers of the peritoneum are developed from the somatopleural and splanchnopleural layers of the lateral plate mesoderm, respectively. Correlated with their embryologic origin is the fact that the parietal peritoneum derives its nerve supply from the spinal nerves, which also supply the muscles and skin of the parietes (the same applies to its arterial supply and to drainage of the venous systems). The visceral peritoneum, which is considered to be an integral part of the viscera themselves, derives its nerve supply from the autonomic nerves supplying the viscera. The difference in the sensibility of the two layers of the peritoneum is thus correlated with the different innervation. In conscious patients pain can be elicited by noxious stimuli applied to the parietal peritoneum, but these stimuli are ineffective when applied to the visceral peritoneum or to the viscera themselves. The region of the gastrointestinal tract that is insensible to stimuli that are normally painful when applied to the skin and other than somatic structures extends from about the middle of the esophagus down to the junction of the endodermal and extradermal parts of the anal canal. Conversely, tension or stretch applied to the viscera or the visceral peritoneum, such as overdistension of the hollow viscera or traction of the mesentery that stretches the nerve plexus in the walls of the organs or the nerves in the mesentery, produces pain. Other effective stimuli are spasm or contraction of the visceral muscle, particularly under isometric conditions, ischemia, and inflammation, which lowers the threshold of nerve endings.

The somatic nerve supply of the parietal peritoneum also supplies the corresponding segmental area of the skin and trunk muscles, and noxious stimuli applied to these structures produce pain and reflex muscle contraction or spasm. The parietal peritoneum of the undersurface of the diaphragm is supplied centrally by both phrenic nerves and peripherally by the lower six intercostal and subcostal nerves, so that inflammation or irritation of the peripheral part of the diaphragmatic peritoneum causes pain, tenderness, and muscular rigidity in the distribution of the lower intercostal nerves whereas stimulation of the central portion produces pain in the distribution of the cutaneous branches of the C3 to C5 nerves (neck and shoulder regions) (Chapter 53 and Fig. 53-9 describe the thoracoabdominal intercostal nerves in more detail).

Autonomic and Sensory Nerve Supply to the Abdominal Viscera

This section presents a general overview of the anatomy of the parasympathetic, sympathetic, and afferent (sensory) nerves to the viscera of the abdomen proper. The information that follows is an extension of the description of the nerves to the thoracic viscera of the abdomen, which includes a discussion of the origin and course of the thoracic splanchnic nerves (see also Fig. 53-11). The nerves to the pelvic viscera and the nerves to the structures of the pelvis are described in Chapter 65.

Figures 59-6 to 59-13 (see below) depict the anatomy of the parasympathetic, sympathetic, and sensory nerves that supply the viscera in the abdomen proper. The parasympathetic efferent (motor) and afferent (sensory) fibers are contributed by branches of the vagus nerves and by the sacral splanchnic nerves (nervi erigentes). The sympathetic supply is provided by thoracic and lumbar splanchnic nerves. Below I describe the course and distribution of the vagus nerves, splanchnic nerves, and celiac and subsidiary plexuses.

Vagus Nerves

The vagus nerves supply parasympathetic preganglionic fibers and sensory nerves to the viscera of the abdomen proper, except the left half of the transverse colon and the descending colon, which are supplied by the sacral parasympathetic nerves. As discussed in Chapters 6 and 53, the cell bodies of the parasympathetic preganglionic fibers are located in the motor nucleus of the vagus in the brain stem while the cell bodies of the sensory nerves are located in the inferior (nodose) ganglion, with the proximal processes entering the medulla and the distal processes incorporated into the vagus nerves. The two vagus nerves pass vertically from the base of the skull down the neck within the carotid sheath until they reach the root of the neck. The further course of the nerve differs on the two sides of the body.

Right Vagus Nerve

On the right side the vagus descends posteriorly to the internal jugular vein. It crosses the first part of the subclavian artery, enters the thorax, and descends through the superior mediastinum, lying posterior to the right brachio-

cephalic vein. It then passes to the right of the trachea posteromedially to the superior vena cava and medially to the pleura and lung, passing posteriorly to the right principal bronchus to reach the posterior aspect of the root of the right lung, where it breaks up into posterior pulmonary branches that unite with filaments from the thoracic sympathetic nerves to form the right posterior pulmonary plexus. From the lower part of the posterior pulmonary plexus two or three branches descend on the posterior aspect of the esophagus and, with a branch from the left vagus, form the posterior esophageal plexus.

From the posterior esophageal plexus a trunk is formed that continues posteriorly to the esophagus to enter the abdomen through the esophageal opening in the diaphragm. This is *the posterior vagal trunk*, which contains fibers from both vagus nerves. In the abdomen the posterior vagal trunk divides into a small gastric branch, which supplies the posteroinferior surface of the stomach with the exception of the pyloric canal, and a large celiac branch, which ends chiefly in the celiac plexus but also sends fibers directly to the splenic, hepatic, renal, suprarenal, and superior mesenteric plexuses.

Left Vagus Nerve

The left vagus nerve enters the thorax between the left common carotid and left subclavian arteries, posterior to the left brachiocephalic vein, and then descends through the superior mediastinum and crosses the left side of the aortic arch to pass behind the root of the left lung, where it divides into posterior pulmonary branches that unite with the sympathetic fibers and form the left posterior pulmonary plexus. Two branches descend from this left posterior pulmonary plexus in front of the esophagus where they form the anterior esophageal plexus with a twig from the right posterior pulmonary plexus.

From the anterior esophageal plexus a trunk containing fibers from both vagus nerves continues in front of the esophagus, enters the abdomen through the esophageal opening of the diaphragm, and becomes the anterior vagal trunk. In the abdomen *the anterior vagal trunk* sends branches to the cardiac antrum and then divides into right and left branches. The fibers of the left group follow the lesser curvature of the stomach and supply the anterosuperior surface of this viscus. The right group consists of three main branches. One proceeds between the layers of the lesser omentum toward the porta hepatis. Here it divides into an upper branch that enters the porta hepatis and a lower branch that chiefly supplies the pyloric canal, pylorus, superior and descending parts of the duodenum, and the head of the pancreas. The second branch is distributed to the anterosuperior surface of the body of the stomach, and the third branch follows the lesser curvature of the stomach as far as the angular notch.

Sympathetic Nerves

The viscera of the abdomen proper are supplied by sympathetic efferent (motor nerves) whose cell bodies are located in the T5 to L2 spinal cord segments and whose axons pass through the anterior nerve roots, short formed nerves, and white rami communicantes to reach the sympathetic chain. These axons pass through the chain without synapsing and pass through the splanchnic nerves to end in the three prevertebral ganglia—the celiac, aorticorenal, and inferior mesenteric ganglia—where they synapse with cell bodies of postganglionic neurons (Chapter 6). The axons of the postganglionic neurons, together with axons of preganglionic parasympathetic fibers and afferent fibers, comprise the celiac plexuses and then proceed as subsidiary plexuses that supply the various abdominal viscera. Although the origin and course of the thoracic splanchnic nerves are described in Chapter 53 and depicted in Figure 53-11, a brief discussion of their course and origin, their contribution to the celiac and subsidiary plexuses, the origin and course of the lumbar splanchnic nerves, and the anatomy of the celiac plexus and its subsidiary plexuses is presented here.

Superior Thoracic Splanchnic Nerve

The superior thoracic splanchnic nerve, consisting mainly of myelinated preganglionic sympathetic and afferent fibers, is formed by three or four roots that are given off by the T5 or T6 to the T9 or T10 ganglia inclusively. These roots run inferiorly, anteriorly, and medially on the anterolateral aspect of the vertebral column and come together at the level of the 9th or 10th vertebra to form the nerve. Near the origin of the formed nerve is usually found (70% of cases) an enlargement called the splanchnic ganglion of Lobstein (14). Its downward course in the thorax is described in Chapter 53 (Fig. 53-8). It passes through the diaphragm within the space that separates the internal from the external crus and enters the abdominal cavity. In the abdomen it has a short course in an anteromedial and inferior direction before it breaks up into its terminal branches, which spread out like a fan and terminate in the celiac ganglia; some also terminate in the ipsilateral aorticorenal ganglion. In its course it gives off fine collateral filaments that join the esophageal and aortic plexuses, intercostal vessels, azygos veins, and aortic plexus. Some filaments supply the diaphragm and contents of the spinal canal and some filaments join the middle thoracic splanchnic nerve.

Middle Thoracic Splanchnic Nerve

The middle thoracic splanchnic nerve is usually formed by two roots that arise from the 10th and 11th ganglia and soon thereafter converge into one trunk that descends inferiorly, anteriorly, and medially on the anterolateral aspect of the vertebal column. This then passes through the diaphragm accompanied by the superior thoracic splanchnic nerve to terminate in the ipsilateral aorticorenal ganglion, although some fibers can terminate in the celiac ganglia, and one or two filaments pass to the renal plexus, or superior mesenteric plexus.

Inferior Thoracic Splanchnic Nerve

The inferior thoracic splanchnic nerve is usually formed by one fine root that arises from the last thoracic ganglion and then passes anteriorly, medially, and a little inferiorly below the middle thoracic splanchnic nerve. It perforates the diaphragm along with the other two thoracic splanchnic nerves to enter the abdominal cavity, where it proceeds to and ends in the posterior renal ganglion and the adjacent part of the renal plexus.

Lumbar Splanchnic Nerves

The lumbar splanchnic nerves, usually four, arise from the lumbar portion of the paravertebral sympa-thetic chain and pass anteriorly to join the celiac intermesenteric (abdominal aortic) and superior hypogastric plexuses. The L1 splanchnic nerve arises from the uppermost lumbar ganglion and joins the celiac, renal, and intermesenteric (aortic) plexuses (Fig. 59-6). The L2 splanchnic nerve arises from the 2nd (and sometimes 3rd) ganglia and joins the lower part of the aortic plexus. The L3 splanchnic nerve arises as two or three stouter roots from the 2nd, 3rd, or 4th ganglia and passes in front of the common iliac vessels to join the superior hypogastric plexus. The lowest (usually the L4) splanchnic nerve arises from the lowest lumbar ganglion and passes posterior to the common iliac vessels to join the lower part of the superior hypogastric plexus or the hypogastric nerve. On one or both sides it supplies twigs to the aorta, inferior vena cava, and common iliac artery and communicates with the gonadal (spermatic or ovarian) and ureteral plexuses.

Celiac Plexus and Subsidiary Plexuses

The celiac plexus, also called the solar plexus and sometimes the epigastric plexus, is the largest prevertebral plexus. It is composed of two or more large aggregates of ganglion cells, the right and left celiac ganglia, a number of smaller ganglia, and a dense network of parasympathetic and sympathetic efferent and afferent fibers that enmesh these ganglia (Fig. 59-6). The plexus is situated in the epigastrium just anterior to the crura of the diaphragm and the body of the first lumbar vertebra, surrounding the celiac artery and the root of the superior mesenteric artery. The entire plexus lies posterior to the stomach and the omental bursa. The right half of the plexus lies behind the upper part of the head of the pancreas, the small part of the duodenum, the lower end of the portal vein, and the inferior vena cava. The left half is also covered by the pancreas and splenic vessels. In the midline the plexus rests anterior to the beginning of the abdominal aorta. The phrenic arteries are superior and the renal vessels inferior to the plexus while the suprarenal vessels often pass through interstices in the plexus (14–17).

The celiac plexus and ganglia are joined by the superior and middle thoracic splanchnic nerves of both sides, which contain sympathetic preganglionic and afferent fibers, and also by branches of the vagus nerves, composed of preganglionic parasympathetic and afferent fibers as well as sensory fibers from the phrenic nerves. Many of these fibers cross from one side to the other to form a dense network. Numerous secondary or subsidiary plexuses are derived from the celiac plexus; these follow the branches of the celiac artery and also surround neighboring arteries.

The celiac plexus occupies an area about 3 cm in length and 4 cm wide. In the transverse plane it occupies the region between the two adrenal glands and extends beyond the lateral borders of the aorta on both sides. In the longitudinal plane it occupies the area delineated by the celiac artery above and the renal arteries below. It is thus situated in front of the entire L1 vertebra and often even the upper portion of the L2 vertebra. The plexus lies in loose areolar tissue, which is rich in fat.

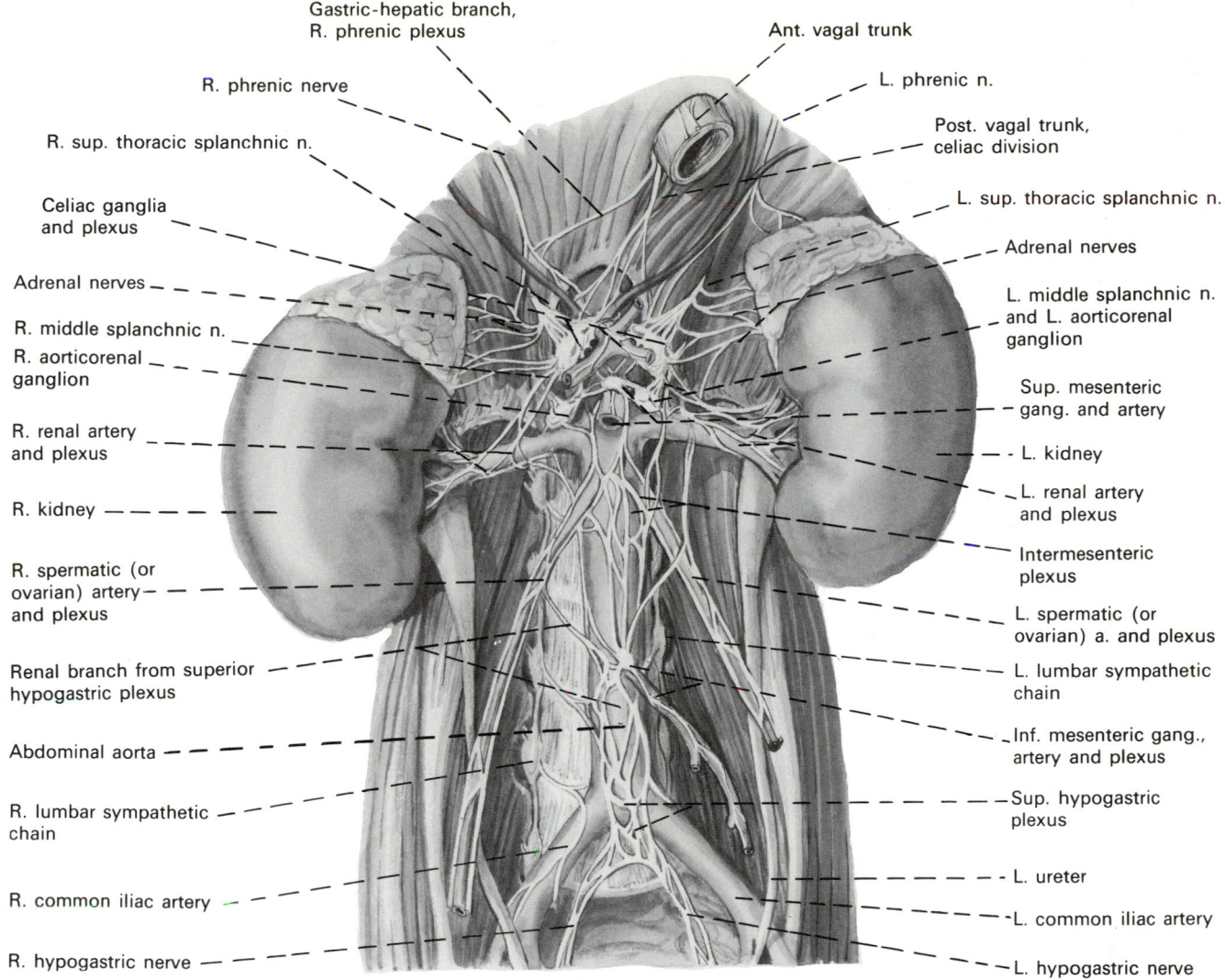

FIG. 59-6. Anterior view of the abdomen showing the celiac plexuses and the ganglia as well as the subsidiary plexuses, including the phrenic, suprarenal, renal, testicular, and superior and inferior mesenteric plexuses. Modified from Mitchell, G.A.G.: Cardiovascular Innervation. Edinburgh, E.S. Livingstone, 1956, p. 258.

Prevertebral Ganglia

The ganglia associated with the celiac plexus and its subsidiary plexuses are, according to the classic description, in three pairs—the celiac, the aorticorenal, and the superior mesenteric. According to Hovelacque (18), however, such a description, although serving the purpose of simplicity, is merely schematic, because the actual number and shape of the ganglia are variable (Fig. 59-6).

CELIAC GANGLIA. The celiac ganglia, usually described as two large masses, semilunar in shape and located on each side of the origin of the celiac artery, in reality vary in number, shape, and size (18). In most cases their surfaces are irregular and reddish gray in color, and they are flattened anteroposteriorly. Sometimes they are semilunar in shape with the concavity facing superomedially or inferolaterally, whereas at other times they are quadrilateral or stellate in shape. Frequently one or both are divided into several small portions that are scattered around the celiac axis.

Because of the variability in size and shape it is difficult to give exact measurements. On average the celiac ganglia collectively are 20 to 25 mm by 10 to 15 mm and 3 to 5 mm in thickness (14, 16). The distance separating them also varies, ranging from 6 or 7 mm up to as much as 20 to 25 mm. The ganglia receive the terminations of the ipsilateral superior and middle thoracic splanchnic nerves that synapse with cell bodies of postganglionic neurons contained within the ganglia. The celiac ganglia are covered by a dense network of fibers that cross from one side to the other, some passing anteriorly to the celiac artery and others passing posteriorly to it.

AORTICORENAL GANGLIA. The aorticorenal ganglia can be regarded as the detached lower and outer portions of the celiac ganglia to which they are almost always united by one or more bands containing nerve fibers and ganglion cells (16). They are intermediate in size between the celiac and superior mesenteric ganglia and are fusiform or irregular in shape. Usually

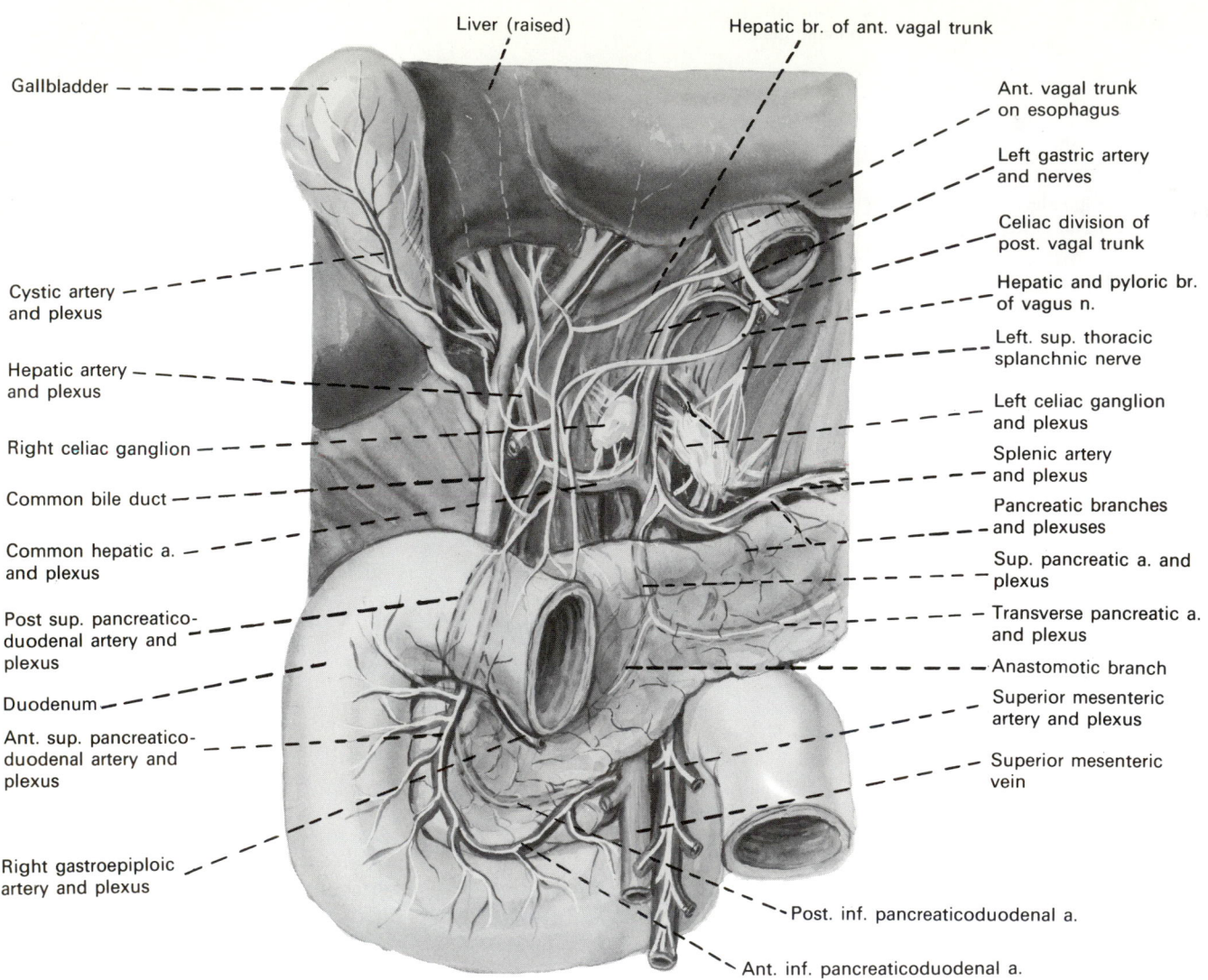

Gallbladder

Liver (raised)

Hepatic br. of ant. vagal trunk

Ant. vagal trunk
on esophagus

Left gastric artery
and nerves

Celiac division of
post. vagal trunk

Cystic artery
and plexus

Hepatic and pyloric br.
of vagus n.

Hepatic artery
and plexus

Left. sup. thoracic
splanchnic nerve

Right celiac ganglion

Left celiac ganglion
and plexus

Splenic artery
and plexus

Common bile duct

Pancreatic branches
and plexuses

Common hepatic a.
and plexus

Sup. pancreatic a. and
plexus

Post sup. pancreatico-
duodenal artery and
plexus

Transverse pancreatic a.
and plexus

Anastomotic branch

Duodenum

Superior mesenteric
artery and plexus

Ant. sup. pancreatico-
duodenal artery and
plexus

Superior mesenteric
vein

Right gastroepiploic
artery and plexus

Post. inf. pancreaticoduodenal a.

Ant. inf. pancreaticoduodenal a.

FIG. 59-7. Hepatic plexus and its various subsidiary plexuses. See text for details.

they are situated above the origin of the renal arteries, although sometimes they are anterior or anterosuperior to the arteries. Each ganglion receives fibers from the middle and inferior thoracic splanchnic nerves. The two aorticorenal ganglia are often connected by fibers that cross in front of the aorta.

SUPERIOR MESENTERIC GANGLION. The superior mesenteric ganglion is a small irregular mass about 5 mm in diameter that lies on the anterior surface of the aorta just above, or occasionally below, the origin of the superior mesenteric artery.

Secondary (Subsidiary) Plexuses

The secondary plexuses arising from or connected with the celiac plexus include the phrenic, gastric, hepatic, splenic, adrenal, renal, superior mesenteric, intermesenteric (abdominal aortic), spermatic (ovarian), and inferior mesenteric plexuses.

PHRENIC PLEXUS. The phrenic plexus arises from the upper part of the celiac plexus and from some sensory filaments contributed by the phrenic nerves (see Fig. 59-3). Both sets of nerves accompany the

phrenic arteries to become distributed to the diaphragm and send a few filaments to the suprarenal glands by way of the suprarenal plexus (Fig. 56-6). On the right side the plexus closely accompanies the phrenic artery. In addition, the left plexus sends some filaments to the esophagus, while the right plexus sends filaments to the inferior vena cava and to the hepatic plexus. At the point of junction of the right phrenic plexus with the phrenic nerve is a small mass called the phrenic ganglion (Chapter 53). Because this plexus contains sensory fibers that pass to the phrenic nerves and into the spinal cord at the C3 to C5 level, it has special clinical importance in regard to referred pain caused by disease in the upper abdomen.

HEPATIC PLEXUS. The hepatic plexus, the largest of the subsidiary plexuses, receives fibers directly from the left and right vagus nerves that do not traverse the celiac plexus and also receives sensory fibers from the right phrenic nerve (Fig. 59-7). The plexus accompanies the hepatic artery, portal vein, and their branches into the liver; in the liver the nerves are confined to the vicinity of blood vessels. Branches from the hepatic plexus form tertiary plexuses that accompany all the branches of the hepatic artery, including the right gastric, gastroduodenal, and cystic arteries.

The right gastric plexus is reinforced by filaments from the pyloric branches of the vagal trunks and supplies sympathetic, parasympathetic, and sensory fibers to the upper parts of the anterior and posterior surfaces of the stomach and also the pylorus (Fig. 59-8).

The gastroduodenal plexus accompanies the gastroduodenal artery and its branches, the right gastroepiploic and superior pancreaticoduodenal arteries. Branches from the gastroduodenal plexus pass to the pylorus and superior part of the duodenum, while many of the nerves that pass with the right gastroepiploic artery supply the right part of the stomach and its greater curvature.

The superior pancreaticoduodenal plexus supplies the descending part of the duodenum, head of the pancreas, and lower part of the bile duct. Fibers passing to the gallbladder arise from the cystic plexus, with some branches also passing to the bile ducts. These various plexuses contain both afferent and efferent sympathetic and parasympathetic fibers that supply the liver, gallbladder, stomach, duodenum, and pancreas. The functions of the sympathetic and parasympathetic fibers in these structures are presented in Table 59-4 (below). The sensory fibers associated with the vagus probably constitute the afferent limb of subconscious reflexes, while the sympathetic afferents mediate nociceptive and other sensory impulses.

LEFT GASTRIC PLEXUS. The left gastric plexus is derived from the celiac plexus and from both vagal trunks that pass directly to it. It accompanies the left gastric artery along the lesser curvature of the stomach (Fig. 59-8B). The plexus supplies fibers to the stomach and to the abdominal portion of the esophagus through the subsidiary plexuses that accompany the two or three esophageal branches of the left gastric artery. The gastric sympathetic nerves are motor to the pyloric sphincter but are inhibitory to the muscular coat of the stomach.

SPLENIC PLEXUS. The splenic plexus is formed by branches from the celiac plexus, left celiac ganglia, and posterior vagal trunk. It accompanies the splenic, pancreatic, short gastric, and left gastroepiploic arteries (Fig. 59-9). The small plexus around the left gastric or left gastroepiploic artery communicates

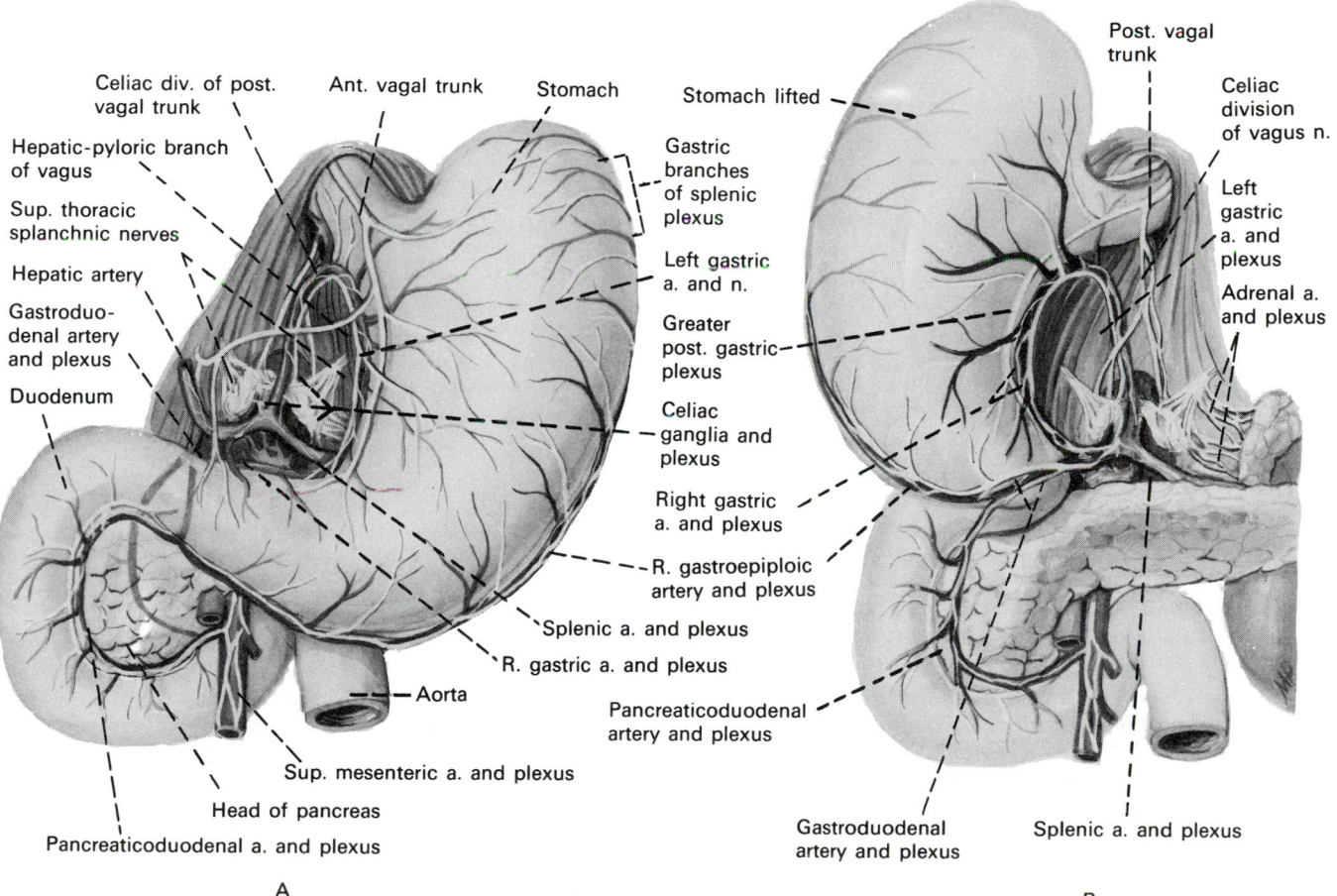

FIG. 59-8. Autonomic nerve supply to the stomach and duodenum. *A.* Anterior view showing the anterior vagal trunk and its direct contribution to the hepatic plexus and the celiac plexus, which gives off the left gastric plexus that meets with the right gastric plexus; all of these supply the lesser curvature of the stomach. The gastroduodenal plexus supplies the duodeum and head of the pancreas; the greater curvature of the stomach is supplied by the right gastroepiploic plexus and gastric branches of the splenic plexus. *B.* The stomach has been shifted to the right to show the celiac gastric, right gastroepiploic, and other nerves that supply the stomach. Modified from Mitchell, G.A.G.: Cardiovascular Innervation. Edinburgh, E.S. Livingstone, 1956, p. 242.

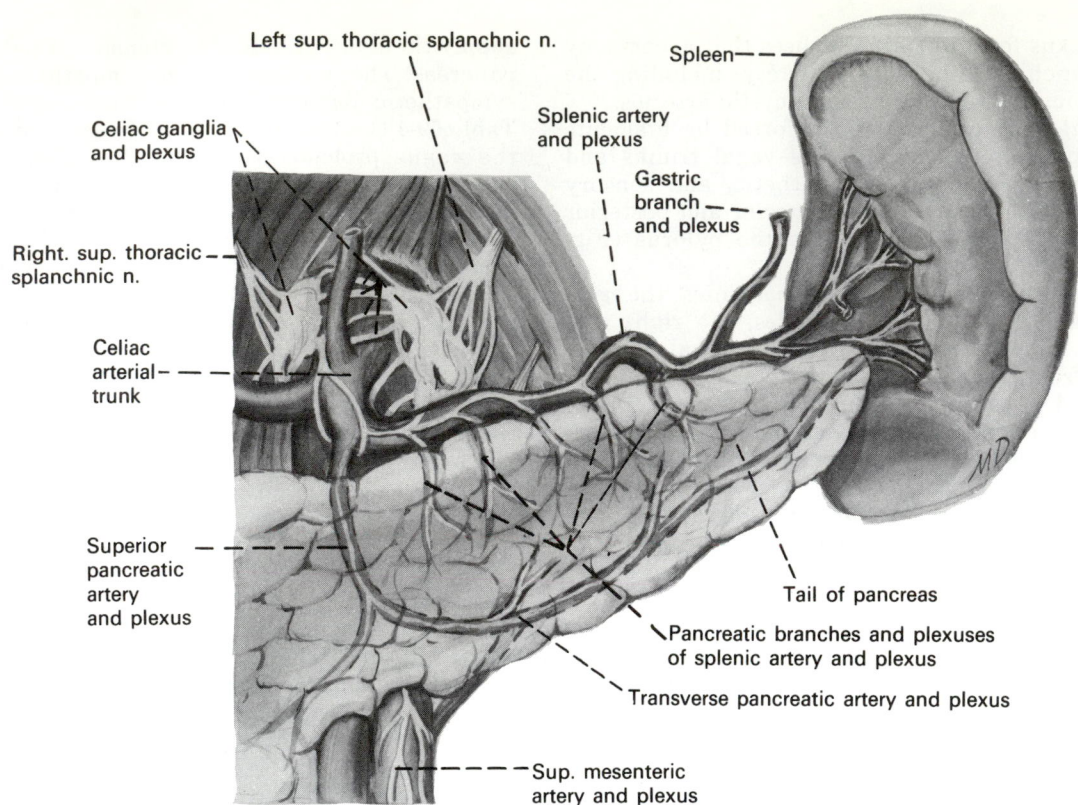

Fig. 59-9. Splenic plexus. Note its origin and distribution to the pancreas, spleen, and stomach. Modified from Mitchell, G.A.G.: Cardiovascular Innervation. Edinburgh, E.S. Livingstone, 1956, p. 249.

with gastric branches of the posterior vagal trunk and with gastroesophageal branches of the left phrenic plexus that run to the gastroesophageal junction (16, 17). The plexus around the pancreatic branch supplies the pancreas. The fibers that terminate in the spleen are principally, if not wholly, sympathetic efferents and afferents, with the efferents terminating on blood vessels and unstriated muscle of the splenic capsule and trabeculae (14–16). The sympathetic afferents convey nociceptive impulses provoked by rapid distension of the splenic capsule.

The subsidiary plexus that surrounds the pancreatic branches of the splenic artery supplies the neck, body, and tail of the pancreas. The subsidiary plexus that surrounds the short gastric branches of the splenic artery is distributed to the fundus of the stomach while the plexus around the posterior gastric branch contributes fibers to the fundus and posterior wall of the stomach. The subsidiary plexus surrounding the left gastroepiploic branch contributes fibers to the upper third of the greater curvature of the stomach. The plexuses that continue along the omental branches of the left gastroepiploic artery, and those of the right gastroepiploic artery supply nerve fibers to the greater omentum.

SUPRARENAL PLEXUSES. The suprarenal plexuses are formed by branches from the celiac plexus, celiac ganglia, phrenic plexus, and ipsilateral superior thoracic splanchnic nerves (Fig. 59-6). The plexuses supply the suprarenal glands, which, relative to their size, have a larger autonomic nerve supply than any other

organ (16). Most of the nerve fibers are preganglionic sympathetic fibers that terminate and synapse with the large chromaffin cells, the pheochromocytes, which are analogous with postganglionic sympathetic neurons. The suprarenal plexuses also have parasympathetic preganglionic fibers and afferent fibers (15).

RENAL PLEXUSES. The renal plexuses are formed by filaments from the ipsilateral celiac ganglion, celiac plexus, aorticorenal ganglion, inferior thoracic splanchnic nerve, L1 splanchnic nerve, aortic plexus, and superior hypogastric plexus (14–18) (Fig. 59-6; also see Fig. 63-2). Collections of nerve cells (ganglia) are found in each plexus, with the largest, the renal ganglion, usually lying posteriorly or posterosuperiorly to the commencement of the renal artery. The plexus continues into the kidney around the branches of the renal artery to supply the vessels and renal glomeruli and tubules, particularly the tubules in the cortex of the kidney (19). Most fibers of this plexus are sympathetic efferents that have vasomotor function and sympathetic afferents that transmit nociceptive information. The plexus also has parasympathetic preganglionic fibers that synapse in small ganglia in the hilum of the kidney, but not within its parenchyma (16, 17). The renal plexus gives off fibers that contribute to the upper third of the ureteric plexus that supplies the ureter and also contributes to the testicular or ovarian plexuses. The middle third of the ureteral plexus is derived from the superior hypogastric plexus and hypogastric nerve, while the lower part is derived from the hypogastric nerve and inferior

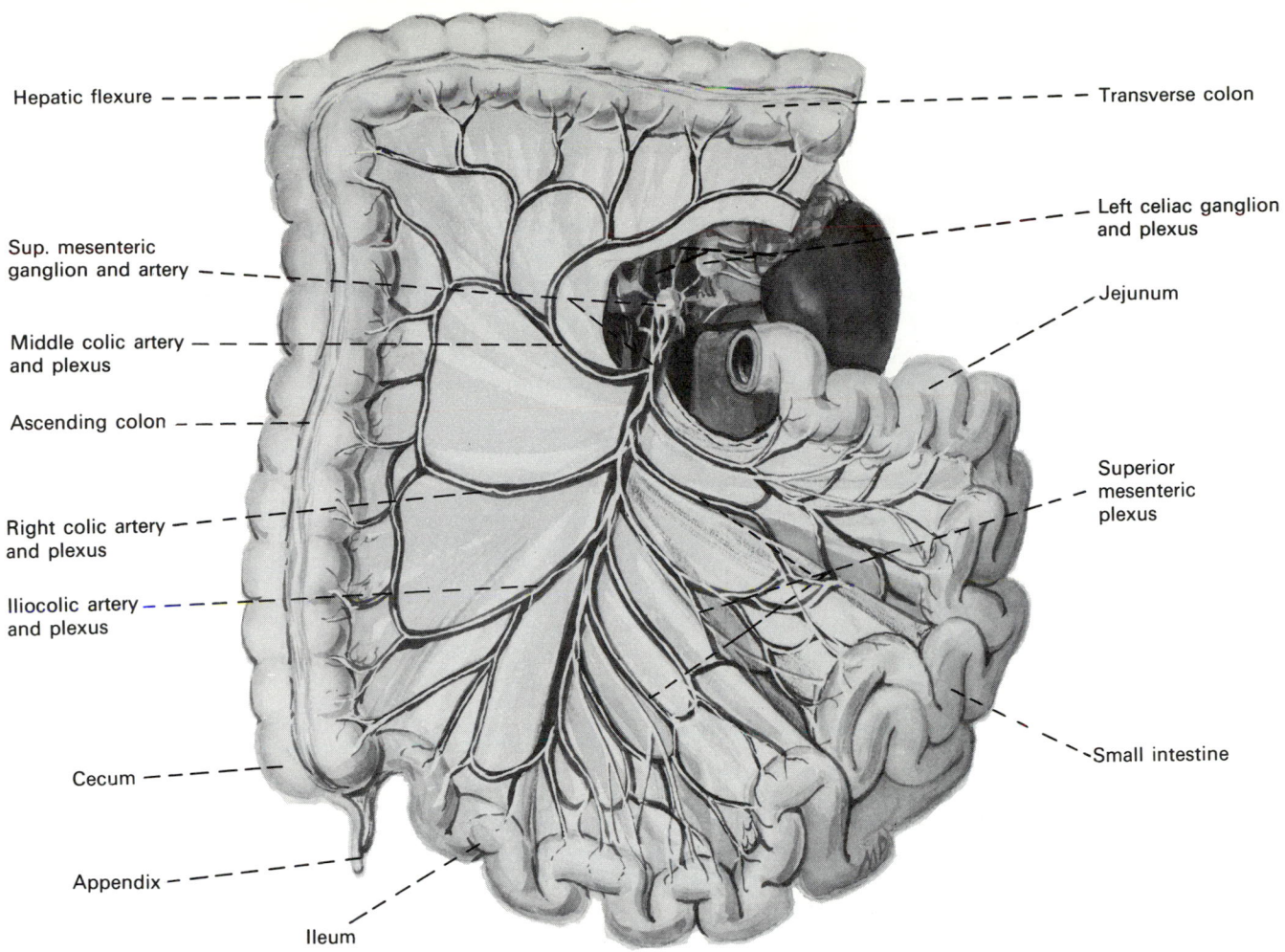

Hepatic flexure

Sup. mesenteric ganglion and artery

Middle colic artery and plexus

Ascending colon

Right colic artery and plexus

Iliocolic artery and plexus

Cecum

Appendix

Ileum

Transverse colon

Left celiac ganglion and plexus

Jejunum

Superior mesenteric plexus

Small intestine

FIG. 59-10. Superior mesenteric plexus. Modified from Mitchell, G.A.G.: Cardiovascular Innervation. Edinburgh, E.S. Livingstone, 1956, p. 251.

hypogastric plexus (these are discussed in detail in Chapter 62, and the testicular and ovarian plexuses are discussed in Chapter 65, which introduces the section on pain in the pelvis).

SUPERIOR MESENTERIC PLEXUS. The superior mesenteric plexus is a continuation of the lower part of the celiac plexus but also receives fibers directly from the posterior vagal trunk and from the celiac and aorticorenal ganglia of both sides. The superior mesenteric ganglion is often incorporated into the origin of the plexus (Fig. 59-10; also see Fig. 60-8). The plexus surrounds the superior mesenteric artery, accompanying it into the mesentery, and divides into a number of secondary plexuses that are distributed to all structures supplied by the artery. These include the following: (a) the pancreaticoduodenal plexus, which contributes to the nerve supply of the pancreas; (b) the jejunal and ileal plexuses, which supply the small intestine; and (c) the ileocolic, right colic, and middle colic plexuses, which supply the corresponding parts of the large intestine. The sympathetic efferent fibers decrease motility, relax the sphincters, and inhibit secretions of the intestine, while the parasympathetic fibers have opposite effects. The parasympathetic afferents have a subconscious reflex function while

the sympathetic afferents participate in the reflexes but also convey nociceptive information (Table 59-4).

ABDOMINAL AORTIC PLEXUS. The abdominal aortic plexus, also known as the intermesenteric plexus, is formed by fibers contributed by the celiac plexus and ganglia and by the L1 and L2 splanchnic nerves (Fig. 59-6). The plexus is situated on the anterior and lateral parts of the aorta between the origins of the superior and inferior mesenteric arteries. It is continuous above with the celiac plexus and celiac and aorticorenal ganglia and below with the superior hypogastric plexus. Fibers derived from this plexus contribute to the formation of the adrenal, renal, spermatic, inferior mesenteric, iliac, and superior hypogastric plexuses and also supply the inferior vena cava.

INFERIOR MESENTERIC PLEXUS. The inferior mesenteric plexus is derived chiefly from the aortic plexus but also receives fibers from the L2 and L3 splanchnic nerves (Fig. 59-11). Below the origin of the artery the plexus is connected by oblique bundles with the superior hypogastric plexus and with parasympathetic fibers from the sacral splanchnic nerve (16, 17). Usually the parasympathetic supply to the distal colon and its vessels runs in fine long nerves that arise on

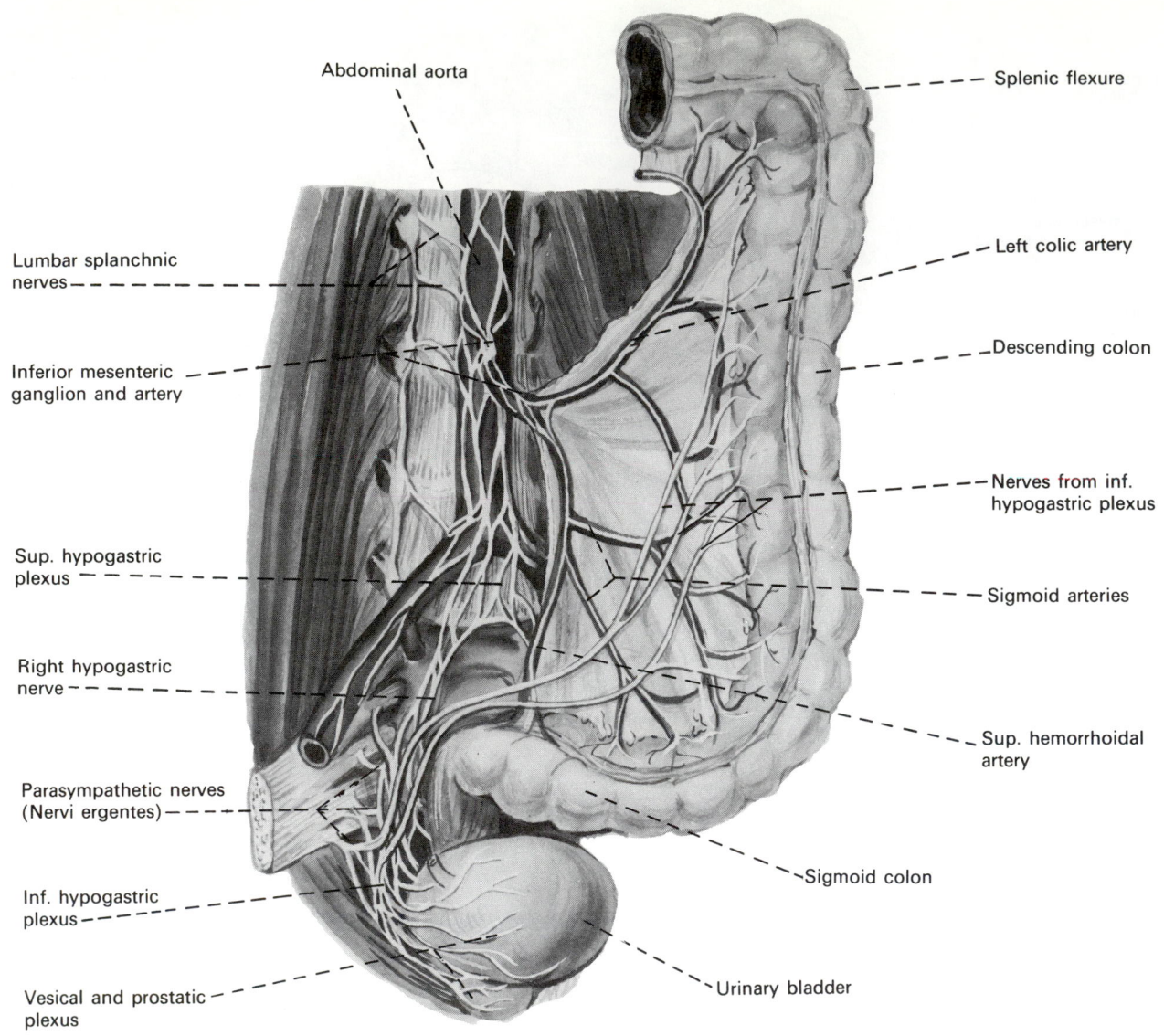

Abdominal aorta

Lumbar splanchnic nerves

Inferior mesenteric ganglion and artery

Sup. hypogastric plexus

Right hypogastric nerve

Parasympathetic nerves (Nervi ergentes)

Inf. hypogastric plexus

Vesical and prostatic plexus

Splenic flexure

Left colic artery

Descending colon

Nerves from inf. hypogastric plexus

Sigmoid arteries

Sup. hemorrhoidal artery

Sigmoid colon

Urinary bladder

FIG. 59-11. Inferior mesenteric plexus. Modified from Mitchell, G.A.G.: Cardiovascular Innervation. Edinburgh, E.S. Livingstone, 1956, p. 245.

each side by several rootlets from the inferior hypogastric (pelvic) plexus and hypogastric nerves or as direct offshoots from the sacral splanchnic nerves (nervi erigentes), passing upward to join the inferior mesenteric plexus (for a more detailed description of these nerves see Chapter 65). The plexus surrounds the inferior mesenteric artery and then forms a subsidiary plexus. Near its beginning at the origin of the artery the inferior mesenteric ganglion, or a number of small discrete ganglia, is found. Through its subsidiary plexuses around the superior and inferior left colic arteries it supplies the left part of the transverse colon and the descending colon, and through the superior rectal plexus it supplies the sigmoid colon.

Superior and Inferior Hypogastric Plexuses

The superior hypogastric plexus, considered to be a continuation of the abdominal aortic plexus with

contributions from other parts, the hypogastric nerve, and the inferior hypogastric plexuses are discussed in Chapter 65 because they contribute sympathetic, parasympathetic, and afferent nerves to the pelvic viscera. Illustrations depicting the nerve supply for each of the major organs within the abdomen proper are presented in the respective chapters.

Intrinsic (Enteric) Nervous System

The gastrointestinal tract is supplied by the extrinsic nerves mentioned above and also by an intrinsic nervous system consisting of cell bodies and short axons. Two major and three minor networks or plexuses of neurons and their axons form the intrinsic nervous system (20–22). The two main ganglionated plexuses are the myenteric (Auerbach's) plexus and the submucous (Meissner's) plexus (Fig. 59-12).

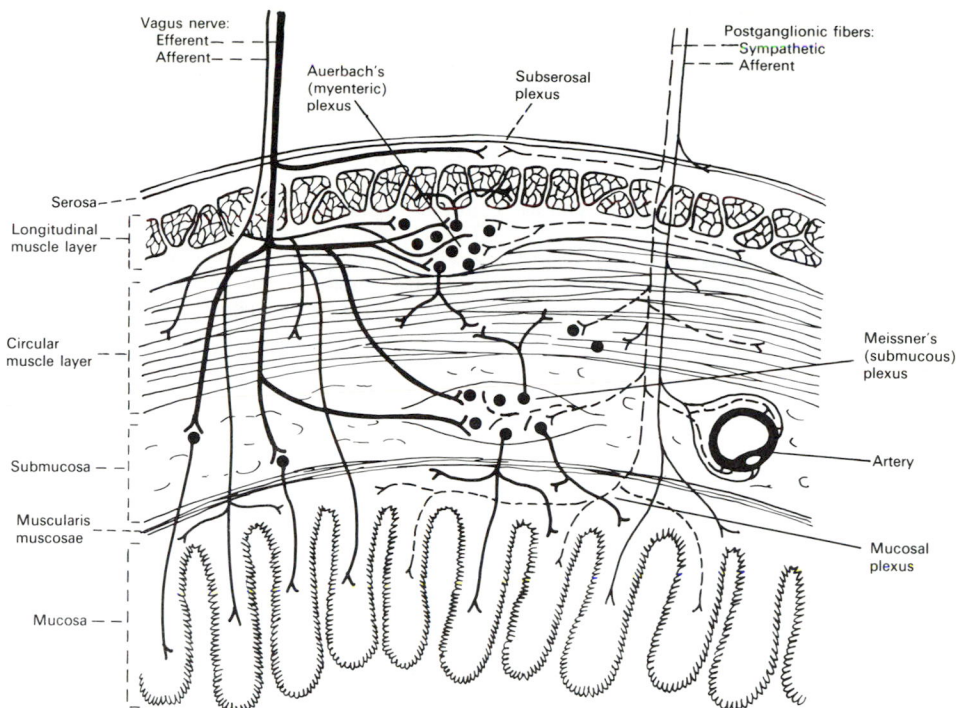

Fig. 59-12. Arrangement of nerve cells and nerve fibers in the intramural plexuses in the intestine. The axonal endings of the parasympathetic preganglionic neurons synapse in the wall of the intestine, whereas the axonal endings of postganglionic sympathetic neurons are largely distributed to the intramural ganglia and the blood vessels. Modified from Kuntz, A.: Autonomic Nervous System. 4th Ed. Philadelphia, Lea & Febiger, 1953, p. 215.

Auerbach's plexus lies between the longitudinal and circular muscle layers and consists of three plexiform networks (20, 21). The primary network is a coarse structure consisting of large bundles of unmyelinated fibers that link various ganglia. Although its meshes vary within relatively wide limits in regard to size and form, they exhibit primarily a longitudinal arrangement (20). The secondary plexus is intimately connected with the primary one but is made up of more slender bundles of nerve fibers, with few neurons interspersed. This secondary plexus is, in turn, continuous with the tertiary plexus and lies in intimate contact with the circular muscle. Nerve fibers extend from this plexus into the muscles that terminate in relation to muscle cells.

The submucous, or Meissner's, plexus consists of a meshwork of relatively slender fiber bundles, with small ganglia located at nodal points (20). It is not confined to a definitively limited zone in the submucous layer; some fiber bundles lie near the circle of muscle layer and others lie close to the muscularis mucosae. Mechanical separation of the mucosa and submucosa from the outer muscular layer usually effectively removes the submucous from the circular muscle layer.

In addition to these two main plexuses are three variably developed plexuses (22): (a) the subserosal plexus, situated beneath the serosa and consisting of bundles of nerve fiber with few ganglia; (b) the deep myenteric plexus, situated within the circular muscle coat, similar in structure to the tertiary network of Auerbach to which it is continuous, and also connected with the adjacent submucous plexus; and (c) the mucous plexuses, which are widely distributed and are further named according to their positions in the mucosa—namely, subglandular, intraglandular, and intravillous mucous plexuses. These plexuses usually contain no neurons and are mere extensions of submucous plexuses.

Auerbach's plexus is associated with smooth musculature

of the gut from the esophagus to the internal anal sphincter, including the biliary tract, and is also present in the striated muscle of the upper esophageal pharynx (21). The function of Auerbach's plexus in the striated muscle is not known, but it might innervate the muscularis mucosae, glands, and blood vessels (22). The density of ganglia in the myenteric plexus varies in different parts of the gut (23). In the esophagus the ganglia are scantier than in the stomach, small bowel, or colon. In the colon the greatest concentration of neurons occurs in relation to the tenia. Few ganglia are found in the distal 2- to 3-cm segment of the rectum. This should be borne in mind to avoid making a wrong diagnosis of Hirschsprung's disease (24).

The ganglia in the submucous plexus are more abundant in the small bowel than in other parts of the gut. No ganglia are in the submucous plexus in the esophagus or in the anal canal distal to the pectinate line. During development the enteric ganglia first appear in the proximal gut wall and then migrate caudally toward the anus.

Enteric nerves are of three types (25). Type I cells have numerous thick dendrites and a single slender axon that enters one of the fasciculi to reach the target cells. These neurons are thought to have a motor function. Type II cells have long smooth dendrites that arise from the mucosa and are thought to be sensory neurons. Type III cells have dendrites of intermediate length that terminate in the same or neighboring ganglia; they might serve as interneurons or integrating neurons. It is thought that the submucous plexus contains only type II (sensory) neurons.

Electrophysiologic studies have found several distinct types of enteric neurons (26, 27): (a) neurons that respond to sensory stimuli; (b) neurons that generate patterned outputs of spontaneously discharged action potential; and (c) neurons that show temporal coupling of firing with other neurons, suggestive of synaptic interaction between neurons. These results suggest that the enteric nervous system is capable of intrinsic integration and is involved in local reflex mechanisms (20).

The axons from the efferent intramural neurons are distributed to various effector cells, including the smooth muscle cells, secretory cells, absorptive cells, and endocrine cells. The axons branch and rebranch as they proceed to their target cells, and as they come into contact with the target cells, they end in a swelling that contains vesicles of neurotransmitters and they make synaptic contacts with the effector cells.

The intrinsic nervous system has contacts with the endings of axons of postganglionic sympathetic and parasympathetic neurons and afferent fibers that connect the intrinsic system with the central nervous system. This makes possible independent function by the intrinsic system; also, however, it can influence and be influenced by the extrinsic nervous system, which of course is under the influence of the central nervous system.

The gastrointestinal tract is rich in various cells that contain hormones and transmitter substances (22, 28, 29). A number of hormones are found together in the gut and in the brain, including gastrin, somatostatin, substance P, vasoactive intestinal polypeptide (VIP), and gastrin-releasing peptide (GRP). The gut also contains various chromaffin cells, particularly enterochromaffin cells. Some of these have a common origin in the neural crest and are included in a series of APUD (amine precursor uptake and decarboxylation) cells that share the common property of synthesizing and storing amines such as dopamine, histamine, and serotonin. These cells are probably innervated by the intrinsic autonomic nerves and thus might also influence the function of the intramural system, which appears to play a key role in the neuroendocrine regulation of the function of the gastrointestinal tract (22).

Summary of Neurologic Function

Parasympathetic and Sympathetic Nerves

The roles of the parasympathetic and sympathetic nerves are summarized in Table 59-4.

Afferent (Sensory) Innervation

The afferent fibers associated with the parasympathetic and sympathetic nerves are widely distributed throughout the gastrointestinal tract and other viscera in the abdomen. About 90% of fibers in the vagus are afferents, and of these 80 to 90% are amyelinated fibers (30). The rest are myelinated afferents of which the majority are A-delta and a smaller percentage are A-beta fibers. Recent studies in cat have shown that each superior thoracic splanchnic nerve contains 3000 to 3500 afferent fibers, which are less than 20% of the total numbers of fibers in this nerve (the remainder are preganglionic fibers) (6, 30, 31). The majority of these afferent fibers (2000 to 3000) are unmyelinated (C) fibers, 250 to 400 are A-delta, and about 20 to 350 are A-beta fibers. The middle and inferior thoracic splanchnic nerves contain another 1000 to 2000 afferents, the lumbar splanchnic nerves contain about 4600, and the sacral parasympathetic inervation contains about 7300 afferents. Thus it appears that a total of 22,000 to 25,000 spinal afferents (associated with splanchnic nerves and the sacral parasympathetics) are responsible for signal afferent information from the abdominal and pelvic viscera of the cat.

Afferent fibers convey information about mechanical, chemical, thermal, and osmotic changes, which are transduced into impulses that are transmitted to integrating neurons in the neuraxis. In the neuraxis they are subjected to

TABLE 59-4. Physiologic Responses to Autonomic Stimulation

Structures or Organs	Sympathetic Stimulation	Adrenergic Receptors	Parasympathetic Stimulation
Stomach			
Motility	Decreased	α, β	Increased
Sphincters	Contracted	α	Relaxed
Secretion	Inhibited	α	Increased
Liver	Glycogenolysis Gluconeogenesis	β	
Gallbladder and biliary ducts	Relaxed	β	Contracted
Pancreas	Vasoconstriction		
Insulin secretion	Reduced	α	Increased secretion
Spleen	Contraction of capsule	α	
Intestines			
Motility	Decreased	α, β	Increased
Sphincters	Relaxed	β	Contracted
Secretion	Decreased	α	Increased
Suprarenal glands	Secretion of 80% E, 20% NE*	α	
Kidneys	Arteriolar construction	α	Controls glomerular secretion
Ureters: tone and motility	Decreased	α	Increased

*E, epinephrine; NE, norepinephrine.

modulating influences and are transmitted either to efferent neurons at segmental levels or to the brain stem to provide information to the hypothalamus, the limbic system, the thalamic nuclei, and finally the cortex (see Chapter 3).

Under physiologic conditions, these afferent fibers are involved in the regulation of visceral functions, in sensations, and in various spinal and supraspinal reflexes.

The mechanoreceptors consist of two types, those with a slowly adapting response able to detect static and dynamic events and those with a rapidly adapting response able to detect dynamic events only (32, 33).

Slowly adapting mechanoreceptors have been shown to exist in the walls of the esophagus, stomach, and intestine, are "in series" with muscle fibers, and act as tension receptors rather than length receptors (34). They are stimulated by balloon distension and by spontaneous or drug-induced muscle contraction. These receptors lie in the muscle layer, and those in the stomach are of two types: receptors with a low tension threshold that excite gastric centers in the neuraxis and cause reflex gastric activity, and those with a higher threshold that have inhibitory effects (34). It has been speculated that low-tension-threshold receptors help to set the level of smooth muscle contraction in the quiescent stomach, and when the stomach starts to contract, input from these receptors controls the timing and force of contraction. When the contraction becomes strong it can be inhibited by the high-threshold mechanoreceptors. The slowly adapting tension receptors also signal sensations of gastric distension and can mediate hunger pains resulting from gastric contraction in an empty stomach (22, 34).

Rapidly acting mechanoreceptors are those that give an "on" and an "off" response when a steady mechanical stimulus is applied and later removed, but give no response while the stimulus is held steady. Rapidly adapting receptors have been found in the mesentery and include pacinian corpuscles beneath the serosa of the small intestine (e.g., movement receptors) and receptors in the muscularis mucosa of the intestine (muscularis mucosa receptors) and in the mucosa (mucosal receptors). The rapidly adapting receptors serve various functions. Mesenteric pacinian corpuscles located at the root of the mesentery and next to the branches of the mesenteric arteries stabilize blood flow through the splanchnic bed. The movement receptors located beneath the submucosa signal distortion of the intestine and the dynamic phase of inflation or deflation of an intraluminal balloon. The muscularis mucosa receptors are thought to act as the flow receptors while some mucosal receptors are sensitive to tactile stimulation. The transitional epithelium in the anal canal possesses sensitive receptors that can distinguish between gas and liquid (33). They serve to let the flatus pass while retaining the feces.

Chemoreceptors can be activated by a chemical substance that acts as a stimulus either by its structural configuration or by its physical characteristics. Most of the chemoreceptors in the gastrointestinal tract, such as acid receptors and osmoreceptors, are activated by the physical characteristics of chemical substances (32, 33, 35). Acid receptors have been described in the gastric mucosa and duodenal mucosa and osmoreceptors have been identified in the duodenal mucosa (22, 32).

In Chapters 3 and 7, mention is made of Cervero's experiments on the biliary duct of the ferret in which he found low-threshold and high-threshold fibers and concluded that the high-threshold biliary afferents probably have a nociceptive function (36). Jänig and Morrison, however, in a recent comprehensive review (37), concluded that no evidence exists for a population of high-threshold afferents that would qualify as visceral nociceptors. Their analysis of an immense number of data on the functional and morphologic properties of spinal afferent neurons supplying the abdominal viscera led them to conclude that these neurons are functionally homogeneous, that is, that the same population of afferents encodes various events that give rise to non-noxious and noxious sensations, a number of reflexes, and to the regulation of viscera.

Most of the available data dispute both concepts and suggest that visceral sensory receptors encode nociceptive events by peripheral recruitment of receptors showing a wide range of threshold (summation). While this interpretation denies the existence of two distinct and separate populations of sensory receptors (nociceptive and non-nociceptive), it also does not support a notionally single population of afferent fibers with a narrow range of excitability threshold as claimed by Jänig and Morrison. Instead, it is based on the existence of different kinds of afferent fibers whose thresholds form a continuum ranging from anoxious to noxious levels. Thus, as the stimulus intensity increases, more and more of these receptors will be activated and pain will be felt by a process of central summation (38).

C. SUMMARY OF EVALUATION OF THE PATIENT

This section presents a general approach to the assessment of patients with abdominal pain. Each of the subsequent five chapters contains a more detailed description of the evaluation of patients presenting with disease suspected to involve specific organs. Obviously, other than in patients who are hemorrhaging and require urgent operative intervention, it is essential to obtain a detailed history and carry out a comprehensive physical examination, including a neurologic and orthopedic evaluation as discussed in Chapter 31 and summarized in Table 53-1. In many cases it is also necessary to obtain laboratory data, including a complete blood count and urinalysis and, in specific cases, roentgenographic studies to detect free air.

History

As emphasized in Chapter 31 and elsewhere in this book, an orderly, systematic, and painstakingly detailed history is the most important aspect of the patient's assessment, and often the correct diagnosis can be made on the basis of the information obtained. Particularly important is inclusion of information about the rapidity of onset of the pain, its quality, intensity, duration, and temporal characteristics, and factors that relieve and aggravate it. If the pain has been present for several days before the patient seeks a physician's counsel, it is important to ascertain whether any of its features have changed and what time of the day the pain is better and what time it is worse. The patient should be asked specifically what effects the following activities or functions have on the pain: eating, swallowing, belching, deep breathing, coughing, straining, release of flatus, defecation, urination, lateral or forward flexion of the trunk or other movements, and supine and prone positions. Specific information should be obtained about associated symptoms and signs or phenomena such as nausea, vomiting, dyspnea, hematemesis, hemoptysis, melena, and the presence of weakness or numbness in various parts of the body. Details about the history of the pain are presented below.

Physical Examination

The physical examination should begin with a simple critical inspection of the patient regarding the facies, color, degree of hydration, respiratory movements, and the various other parts of the examination listed in Table 53-1, beginning with the abdomen and then the chest. In regard to the examination, Silen (8) emphasized that the amount of information to be gleaned from the physical examination is directly proportional to the gentleness and thoroughness of the examiner. In a patient suspected of having peritonitis, one should avoid palpating deeply and eliciting rebound tenderness because this markedly aggravates the pain and increases reflex muscle spasm. The same information can be obtained by gentle percussion of the abdomen (rebound tenderness on a miniature scale, a maneuver that can be far more precise and localizing). Asking the patient to cough elicits true rebound tenderness without the need for placing a hand on the abdomen. Moreover, the brusque illustration of rebound tenderness startles and induces protective spasm in a nervous or worried patient in whom true rebound tenderness is not present. It is especially important to carry out a rectal (and vaginal, if appropriate) examination in every patient with abdominal pain. Similarly, it is essential to examine the chest and spine to exclude referred abdominal pain caused by disorders in these structures.

Laboratory Studies

The results of the laboratory examination, including a complete blood count, should be integrated with the information obtained from the history and physical examination. The urinalysis is helpful in providing some indication of the state of hydration and in ruling out severe renal disease, diabetes, and urinary infection. Determination of blood urea nitrogen, blood sugar, and serum bilirubin levels can also be helpful. Silen (8) emphasized that the serum amylase determination is overrated in helping to reach a diagnosis of acute pancreatitis because many other conditions, such as perforated ulcer, strangulating intestinal obstruction, and acute cholecystitis, can be associated with a marked increase in its value.

Plain and upright or lateral decubitus roentgenograms are useful in helping to reach a diagnosis of intestinal obstruction, perforated ulcer, and various other conditions that can be associated with pneumoperitoneum. Other specialized tests can be used in connection with disease of the gastrointestinal tract, liver, gallbladder, and kidney (Chapters 60, 61, and 62).

Key Points to the Differential Diagnosis

The following points given here, as in Chapter 53, can help the physician in making a differential diagnosis. These include the various characteristics and location of the pain at the time of onset and during the interval between onset and the time the patient is being evaluated, as well as at the time of evaluation, its relation to other bodily functions, and associated signs and symptoms. Much of the information contained in this section is taken from the first edition of this book (39), from material by Currie (40) and others (41, 42), and from material contained in the next five chapters.

Characteristics of Pain at Onset

Site of the Pain

The patient should be asked to point to the site of pain when the pain began. It is important to determine, if the pain was in the midline, whether it was located in the epigastrium, periumbilical area, or hypogastric region and, if it was felt on the side, whether it was in the upper or lower part of the side. The conditions that produce pain in these regions are listed below.

Time Course and Circumstances

Sudden severe pain that occurs instantaneously is a sign of perforated ulcer, rupture of an abscess or hematoma, rupture of the esophagus, rupture of ectopic pregnancy, rupture of infarct of an abdominal organ, heart, or lung, spontaneous pneumothorax, ruptured or dissecting aortic aneurysm, or ruptured spleen. Table 59-5 lists these and other conditions according to the rate or time course of onset (39).

A clear statement of what the patient was doing at the time of onset of the pain is important (40). Did the pain follow an injury or intake of food, fluids, or alcoholic beverages? Did the pain occur while doing heavy work or carrying out a special movement? An injury to the upper abdomen, or to the lower chest and left flank, followed by sudden pain, should suggest rupture of the spleen. Pain that follows drinking alcohol should suggest pancreatitis, gastritis, peptic ulcer, or esophagitis. Sudden epigastric and lower chest pain that occurs with severe vomiting immediately after a large meal suggests perforation of the esophagus. If the pain developed during sleep and awakens the patient it is usually of organic rather than of psychologic origin. (It is rare for pain of psychologic origin to awaken the patient.) Pain following endoscopic examination of any part of the gastrointestinal tract should immediately raise the suspicion of injury and possible perforation. Cramps followed by diarrhea are expected after a laxative but cramps without diarrhea might indicate an obstruction (40). Sudden pain

TABLE 59-5. Classification of Abdominal Pain According to the Rate of Onset

Sudden Onset (Instantaneous)	Rapid (in Minutes)		Gradual (in Hours)
Rupture of the esophagus	Acute pancreatitis		Chronic cholecystitis
Perforated gastric or duodenal ulcer	Acute cholecystitis	Less common than gradual onset	Pyelonephritis or pyelitis
Ruptured spleen	Acute appendicitis		Chronic pancreatitis
Splenic embolism or infarction	Biliary colic		Duodenal or gastric ulcer
Rupture of abscess	Ureteral colic		Gastritis
Rupture of hematoma	Renal colic		Ulcerated colitis
Acute hemorrhagic pancreatitis	Strangulation of viscus (torsion)		Regional enteritis
Ruptured aortic aneurysm			Crohn's disease
Mesenteric embolism	Torsion of ovarian cyst		Meckel's diverticulitis
Rupture of kidney		can be sudden	Sigmoid diverticulitis
Perforation of the appendix	Torsion of pedunculated tumor		Mesenteric lymphadenitis
Ruptured uterus			Ectopic pregnancy before rupture
Ruptured ovarian follicle	Ectopic pregnancy		Cystitis
Infarct of abdominal organ	Acute diverticulitis		Salpingitis
Acute myocardial infarction	Small bowel obstruction		Prostatis
Pulmonary embolism	Porphyria		Urinary retention
Tabetic crisis	Arachnidism		Mesenteric cyst
Ruptured ectopic pregnancy	Sickle cell anemia		Small bowel tumor or infarct
	Lead poisoning		
	Toxic or metabolic disease		
	Pneumonitis with pleurisy		
	Angina pectoris		

Modified from Way, L.E.: Abdominal pain and the acute abdomen. *In* Gastrointestinal Disease: Physiology, Diagnosis, Management. 3rd Ed. Edited by M.H. Sleisenger and J.S. Fordtran. Philadelphia, W.B. Saunders, 1984, pp. 394–410.

caused by straining, such as coughing, sneezing, or bearing down, suggests a neuropathic process if the pain is segmental or renewed enlargement of an abdominal aneurysm if the pain does not have a segmental distribution.

Quality

Sharp pain suggests pain of superficial cutaneous and somatic structural origin or pain that is being produced by a neuropathic lesion, such as radiculopathy of herpes zoster or that caused by compression of one or more of the lower seven thoracic spinal nerves. Segmental burning pain felt in the abdominal wall and lower part of the chest can be a result of postherpetic neuralgia or chronic neuropathic lesions of the spinal cord. Burning epigastric pain suggests peptic ulcer, gastritis, or esophagitis. Severe tearing abdominal pain suggests a dissecting aneurysm, while pain of the same quality in the anal region during defecation is caused by an anal fissure. Poorly localized, diffuse, "sickening" abdominal pain, difficult for the patient to describe, suggests abdominal visceral disease.

Intensity and Rate of Onset

The intensity or severity of the pain depends partly on the rate of change and the intensity of the stimuli. If the rate of change is slow, little or no pain is felt even though a pathologic process has progressed to a marked degree, whereas if the rate of change is rapid the pain is intense. Therefore, severe pain occurs with sudden obstruction of hollow organs, abrupt impairment of blood supply, chemical peritonitis caused by a ruptured viscus or hemorrhage, or acute inflammation. Moderate pain occurs with localized or chronic inflammatory disease and with progressive chronic obstruction by tumors or gradual enlargement of the liver, spleen, or kidney, with a consequent progressive increase in tension on the capsule. It is critically important to evaluate the patient's assessment of the intensity or severity of the pain within the framework of the psychologic evaluation of the patient, as well as noting the specific manner (e.g., facial expression, pallor, frowning, clenched jaws, body position, movements) and the type of words the patient uses.

Time of Day or Month

Information should be obtained about the time of day and perhaps month that the pain is aggravated or relieved. Peptic ulcer pain, especially that caused by duodenal ulcer, tends to occur several hours after breakfast, at midmorning coffee time, just before lunch, several hours after lunch, immediately before supper, a few hours after supper, and during the night (40). Pain that awakens the patient at night is more frequently seen with duodenal ulcer disease. The pain of peptic ulcer rarely begins before breakfast, which is in contrast to the pain of irritable colon that usually starts early in the morning.

Back pain, especially if it causes the patient to awaken, is significant and usually indicates organic disease. Currie (40) attributed this to the fact that sleep allows increased autonomic activity so that the pain of peptic ulcer and cramping pain can be bothersome at night. Burning retrosternal pain, felt when the patient first lies down, is typical of heartburn caused by esophageal reflux. The constant pain of an infiltrating tumor can also be more distressing to the patient once the distractions of the day cease. Pain of primarily psychologic origin rarely awakens the patient but, if such a patient has insomnia, it can produce troublesome discomfort at night (40).

Lower abdominal pain occurring 2 weeks before expected menstruation can be caused by bleeding at ovulation. The problem is not likely to occur in women who take contraceptive pills because these generally suppress ovulation and consequently pain from such bleeding is unlikely to occur. Currie (40) stated that a venereal infection can become established more readily during menstruation than at other times, and therefore acute salpingitis associated with lower abdominal pain occurs more frequently soon after menstruation than at other times in the menstrual cycle.

Characteristics of the Pain Since Onset and at Present Time

Any change in location, quality, intensity, and duration of the pain during the interval between onset and the time the patient is being evaluated is important in deciding on the diagnosis. In most diseases of the gastrointestinal tract the initial pain is true visceral pain and is felt as a poorly localized, diffuse, sickening pain in the midline. Spread of the infection and inflammation to the parietal peritoneum causes more localized and rather a sharp burning pain in one region of the abdomen. The classic example is the steady or cramping periumbilical pain with acute appendicitis that changes to a well-localized pain at McBurney's point in the right lower quadrant of the abdomen. Similarly, biliary colic initially produces pain usually in the midline but, when this is complicated by acute cholecystitis, the patient begins to have pain in the right upper quadrant and often in the inferior angle of the right scapula (referred parietal pain). If the pathologic process worsens, empyema, gangrene, and perforation with diffuse peritonitis produce diffuse parietal pain and referred parietal pain in the right shoulder and trapezius region.

Steady visceral pain suggests increasing distension or ischemia, whereas cramping pain indicates exaggerated intestinal activity. Most patients with visceral pain are likely to experience change with time and therefore require repeated evaluation. This is especially true of patients with an undiagnosed abdominal pain because of possible changes in the quality and location of the pain and with probable changes in abdominal physical signs, any of which can help in the diagnosis (40). With each examination it is important to assess the location, quality, intensity, and temporal characteristics of the pain, as well as determining factors that make the pain worse or better. These include such factors as the type and amount of food intake, changes in bodily functions and, most importantly, the associated symptoms and · signs. These factors are discussed first and then I focus on the most common causes of pain in different regions of the abdomen.

Temporal Features

Acute continuous pain is encountered with peritonitis secondary to a ruptured viscus, impairment of blood supply, hemorrhage into the abdominal cavity, and to an increase in the tension of the supporting elements of organs (capsules, ligaments, or mesentery). Intermittent or colicky pain is usually caused by intermittent and recurrent disturbances of the function of a hollow viscus. This can be produced by the following: (a) intrinsic lesions, such as tumors, stones, intussusception, segmental enteritis or extrinsic factors, such as hernias, tumors, bands, or torsion; (b) metabolic ileus, which can either be spastic (e.g., lead intoxication, porphyria, uremia, diabetes, arachnidism, endocrine disorders) or mesenteric embolism or thrombosis, hypoxemia secondary to pneumonia, or potassium and sodium deficit. Constant chronic pain suggests a progressively developing or static lesion such as cancer. Constant pain felt in different parts of the abdomen usually implies a functional or emotional disorder rather than a progressive disease such as neoplasm.

Aggravating and Relieving Factors

FOOD OR FLUID INTAKE. The type, quality, and quantity of food eaten aggravate various pathophysiologic processes and consequently the intensity, character, and duration of the pain. Appealing and tasty foods, including sweets and such irritants as hot and cold foods, spices, acids, and alcoholic beverages, increase gastric acidity and thus aggravate the pain of peptic ulcer, gastritis, and reflux esophagitis (40). Food roughage is also said to increase the pain of peptic ulcer. Peptic ulcer pain becomes worse several hours after eating when gastric acid is unbuffered because food has left the stomach. Intake of fatty food delays gastric emptying and thus delays the onset of the peptic ulcer pain that occurs after meals. Fatty foods stimulate the gallbladder to contract and can precipitate or aggravate biliary colic. Protein stimulates pancreatic secretion so that foods rich in protein can exacerbate the pain of pancreatitis. Food or alcoholic beverages tend to aggravate pancreatitis regardless of its cause. Lactose contained in dairy products causes bloating, cramps, and diarrhea in lactase-deficient individuals. Aerophagia, or air swallowing, can cause gastric distension with consequent abdominal distress within a few minutes of eating. Because eating stimulates the gastrocolic reflex that produces stimulation of the lower intestine, pain that might exist in the lower bowel is intensified by eating.

RELIEVING FACTORS. Factors that relieve abdominal pain are often opposite to those that aggravate it, although some exceptions to this rule have been noted (40). Fasting does not relieve but rather aggravates the pain of peptic ulcer; this can be relieved by bland, soft, nonstimulating foods. Peptic ulcer pain is best controlled by food ingestion and antacid medication. The time that it takes for the medication to relieve burning pain is of significant diagnostic importance (40). Immediate relief on swallowing a liquid antacid localizes the site of irritation to the esophagus, whereas in patients with gastric or stomal ulcer relief occurs within 10 to 15 minutes, and that of duodenal ulcer takes 7 to 15 minutes (40). Avoiding fatty foods does not relieve biliary colic but might prevent some attacks.

Avoiding large meals or food altogether affords some relief in patients with painful lower intestinal disorders. The partial small bowel obstruction in Crohn's disease improves with starvation. Avoidance of lactose-containing dairy products can relieve abdominal bloating, cramps, and diarrhea. Similarly, belching relieves the distress of early postprandial pain caused by air swallowing. Pain from lesions of the lower bowel is relieved by a bowel movement, and urgent defecation followed by relief of periumbilical visceral pain occurs frequently in patients with regional ileitis. Unplugging a colonic obstruction by enemas or intubating a sigmoid volvulus produces immediate relief with passage of flatus and liquid feces. Temporary relief of abdominal pain might not indicate improvement but can be followed by worsening of the patient's condition. Frequent examples are the temporary relief of local pain consequent to rupture of an empyema of the appendix or gallbladder or to rupture of an acute paracolic abscess or other intra-abdominal abscess into the peritoneal cavity.

RELATION TO OTHER BODILY FUNCTIONS. Pain intensified by movement of the diaphragm suggests thoracic visceral disease, diaphragmatic disease, or subphrenic abscess or disease of the upper abdominal viscera. Pain aggravated by factors such as movement of the trunk, coughing, or sneezing suggests a radiculopathy or neuropathy caused by tumor or compression in the spine. Pain made worse by the supine position and improved by forward bending suggests acute pancreatitis or cancer of the pancreas. Recumbency, straining, or stooping aggravates the pain of esophageal reflux disease, whereas standing or forward bending relieves it. Back pain or upper abdominal pain that appears while the patient is standing an hour or so after drinking fluids, and is relieved soon after lying down, suggests poor drainage from the renal pelvis. Pain made worse by contraction of abdominal muscles suggests myofascial pain syndromes or trauma with hemorrhage into the muscle.

Associated Symptoms and Signs

SYMPTOMS. The time relation of nausea, vomiting, diarrhea, and obstipation is an important point to aid the differential diagnosis between abdominal visceral disease and extra-abdominal causes of pain (39–42). Vomiting without nausea suggests central nervous system disease (4). In patients with abdominal visceral disease, nausea and vomiting are usually accompanied by autonomic reactions such as sweating, pallor, palpipation, weakness, and fainting. Fainting alone can indicate the presence of severe pain. Other than diseases of the central nervous system, vomiting is preceded by anorexia and nausea. Nausea and vomiting occur readily in children with gastroenteritis, in alcoholics, and in adults with peptic ulcer disease. Pyloric obstruction, with which the stomach is greatly distended, causes vomiting of large volumes. The large vomitus can contain recognizable vegetable matter eaten several meals prior to the vomiting but does not contain bile if the pylorus is completely occluded, whereas the presence of bile indicates that the pylorus and biliary ducts are open.

Early and frequent vomiting occurs with small bowel obstruction. Toxic vomiting complicates pancreatitis, gastritic, peritonitis with advanced ileus, and high small bowel obstruction.

SIGNS. The presence of hyperalgesia or hyperesthesia that has a segmental distribution is of diagnostic value because it suggests a neuropathic origin of the pain. Marked localized tenderness to palpation indicates inflammation of visceral disease and, because it usually occurs directly over the involved organ, its diagnostic value is obvious. Reflex spasm of the abdominal muscles occurs with neuropathic and musculoskeletal disorders as well as with intra-abdominal visceral disease but, in the latter, the spasm is more marked and is aggravated by deep pressure. In acute abdominal conditions, such as appendicitis, cholecystitis, and acute pancreatitis, spasm of the rectus muscle occurs over the involved structure. It is important to differentiate between voluntary and involuntary (reflex) spasm. The presence of distension indicates obstruction of the gastrointestinal tract (see Table 59-1 for causes). An abdominal mass associated with the pain is of course diagnostically significant because it could be the direct or indirect cause of the pain.

Location and Distribution

The location and distribution of pain at the time of assessment are important diagnostic characteristics. Segmental pain suggests radiculopathy or neuropathy whereas pain that does not conform to dermatomal or peripheral nerve distribution is either visceral or musculoskeletal in origin. Abdominal visceral diseases have relatively specific areas of pain reference. For example, the pain of hepatic or biliary disease is in the epigastrium or right hypochondrium with radiation to the right posterior chest, lumbar region, and scapula. It is obviously important to know the possible causes of pain in the various regions of the abdomen (see Fig. 59-1).

GENERALIZED ABDOMINAL PAIN. Generalized abdominal pain occurs with acute or chronic peritonitis caused by bacteria, tuberculosis, fungal infection, parasitic disease, granulomatous peritonitis, widespread neoplasm of the peritoneum such as primary mesothelioma, secondary carcinomatosis, vasculitis, Henoch-Schönlein purpura, eosinophilic peritonitis, Whipple's disease, and sclerosing peritonitis, as well as with acute intestinal obstruction, gastroenterocolitis, chronic ulcerative colitis, dysentery, epidural spinal cord compression, acute rheumatic fever, brucellosis, typhoid fever, sickle cell anemia, lead poisoning, and other generalized processes that cause metabolic disturbances of the gastrointestinal tract. Psychologic and environmental factors are often primary causes of pain in the abdomen, especially in children and women. This pain can be generalized or frequently can be in the periumbilical region (Chapter 63).

PAIN IN THE EPIGASTRIUM. Pain in the epigastrium is produced mainly by lesions of the stomach, gallbladder, duodenum, pancreas, liver, lower esophagus, heart, lungs, and certain nervous system

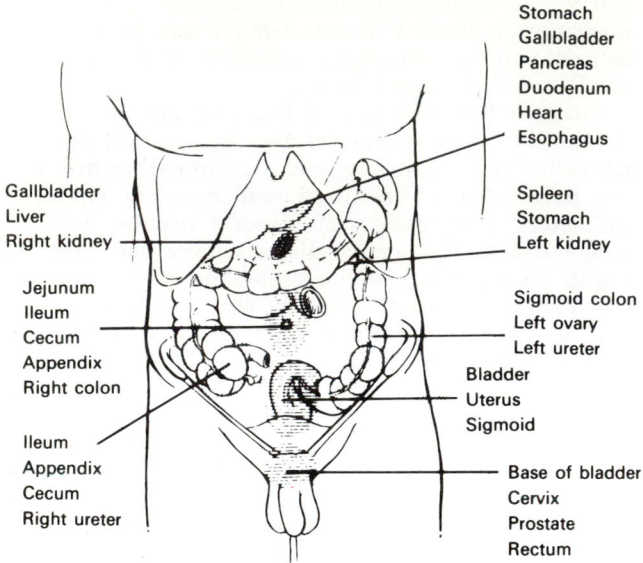

FIG. 59-13. Abdominal pain according to site. Visceral pain occurs mostly in the midline, epigastric, periumbilical, and hypogastric regions. Parietal pain occurs because of involvement of the parietal peritoneum that causes reference to the right and left lateral regions. From Currie, D.J.: Abdominal Pain. New York, McGraw-Hill, 1979, p. 188.

disorders (Fig. 59-13). The most important include chronic peptic ulcer, perforated ulcer, acute gastritis, pylorospasm, gastric carcinoma, acute and chronic pancreatitis (early), cholecystitis with lithiasis (early), perforation of the lower esophagus, chemical or bacterial esophagitis, myocardial infarction, pericarditis, congestive heart failure, and epigastric hernia. Less common causes include ulcer of the lower esophagus, aneurysm of the abdominal aorta, primary or metastatic tumors of the lower thoracic spinal cord, gastric crisis (tabes dorsalis), diaphragmatic hernia, acute hepatitis, diabetic acidosis, myofascial syndromes, pleurisy, and pericarditis.

PAIN IN THE RIGHT HYPOCHONDRIAC REGION.
Pain in the right hypochondriac region is usually produced by diseases of the liver, gallbladder, and hepatic flexure of the colon, by diseases of the right chest or right hemidiaphragm, and by disorders of the nervous system, muscle, and bone. The most important diseases include acute and chronic cholecystitis, biliary colic, cancer of the liver or gallbladder, abscess of the liver or pancreas, acute or chronic hepatitis, right hemidiaphragmatic pleurisy, subphrenic abscess, duodenal ulcer, right segmental or intercostal neuralgia, postcholecystectomy syndrome, right-sided slipped costal cartilage, pneumonia, and pleurisy. Less common causes include tender postoperative or post-traumatic scar, gas entrapment at the hepatic flexure of the colon, carcinoma of the hepatic flexure of the colon, and carcinoma of the bile ducts.

PAIN IN THE LEFT HYPOCHONDRIAC REGION. Pain in the left hypochondriac region is usually caused by disease of the spleen, splenic flexure of the colon,

lesion of the left chest, cancer of the tail of the pancreas, and neurologic and musculoskeletal disorders. The most common are embolism or thrombosis of the splenic vessels, splenic infarction, splenic abscess, splenomegaly, colitis, carcinoma of the splenic flexure of the colon, ruptured spleen, left-sided pneumonia, pleurisy, segmental or intercostal neuralgia, gas entrapment syndrome in splenic flexure of the colon, left-sided slipped costal cartilage, diaphragmatic hernia, pericarditis, and angina pectoris. Less common causes include contusion of the spleen, perisplenitis, abscess of the spleen, tuberculosis or amyloid disease of the spleen, congestion of the spleen, and neoplasm of the cardia of the stomach.

PAIN IN THE RIGHT OR LEFT LUMBAR REGIONS.
Pain in the right or left lumbar (lateral) region is caused by disease of the kidney, ureters, head or tail of the pancreas, and colon. The most common causes include carbuncle or furuncle of the kidney, perinephritic abscess, pyelitis, pyelonephritis, renal abscess, tuberculosis of the kidney, tumor of the kidney, postnephrectomy pain syndrome, and segmental or intercostal neuralgia of one or more of the T8 to T11 nerves resulting from mechanical compression by tumors or vertebral disease.

PAIN IN THE PERIUMBILICAL REGION. Pain in the periumbilical region is usually a result of disease of the small intestine, appendix, cecum, body of the pancreas or of neurologic or musculoskeletal disorders. The most common causes are acute intestinal obstruction, acute diverticulitis, chronic intestinal obstruction, Meckel's diverticulitis, embolism of the superior mesenteric artery, metabolic ileus, enterocolitis, regional enteritis, umbilical hernia, tabes dorsalis, bilateral segmental (T9–T11) neuralgia, myofascial syndromes, and postoperative scars. Periumbilical pain in children and in women is frequently caused by psychologic and environmental factors. Less common causes include peptic ulcer, cholelithiasis, epithelioma of the umbilicus, pancreatic calculi, omphalitis, omental cyst or carcinoma, aneurysm of the abdominal aorta, tumors of the spinal cord, and segmental or intercostal neuralgia.

PAIN IN THE RIGHT ILIAC REGION. Pain in the right iliac region of the abdomen is usually caused by disorders of the appendix, small intestine, cecum, right kidney and ureter, and right uterine tube or ovary or by neurologic or musculoskeletal disorders. The most important include acute appendicitis, acute salpingitis, ruptured ectopic pregnancy, chronic salpingitis, oophoritis, twisted ovarian cyst, ruptured graafian follicle, acute oophoritis, Meckel's diverticulitis, renal colic (see Table 59-6-IV for causes), acute pyelitis, carcinoma of the cecum, inguinal hernia, Crohn's disease, iliac adenitis, acute epididymitis, right psoas or midabdominal abscess, segmental neuralgia of T12 to L1 nerves, and postoperative scar. Less common causes include inguinal adenitis, ileocecal adenitis, sarcoma of the ilium, suppurative periostitis of the ilium, strangulated retroperitoneal hernia, sigmoid volvulus, and aneurysm of the iliac artery.

PAIN IN THE LEFT ILIAC REGION. Pain in the left iliac region is usually caused by disease of the sigmoid colon, left urinary tract, and internal genitalia (female) or by neurologic or musculoskeletal disorders. The most common causes include acute salpingitis, chronic salpingo-oophoritis, ectopic pregnancy, twisted ovarian cyst, ruptured graafian follicle, acute oophoritis, ulcerative colitis, midabdominal or psoas abscess, acute diverticulitis, carcinoma of the sigmoid colon, sigmoid volvulus, intussusception (children), intestinal obstruction, fecal impaction, inguinal hernia, acute epididymitis, left lower ureteral calculus, radiation of pain from disease of the kidney and pelvis, segmental neuralgia (e.g., herpes zoster, herniated disk, spinal tumor), segmental neuralgia of lower thoracic nerves (e.g., vertebral disease, osteoarthritis, tumors, deformity), iliohypogastric and ilioinguinal neuralgia (e.g., retroperitoneal tumor, infections), lumbar myofascial syndrome, left psoas abscess, and postoperative scar. Less common causes include disease of the hip and sacroiliac joints, aneurysm of the left iliac artery, strangulated retroperitoneal hernia, rectal polyp, and cyst of the canal of Nuck.

PAIN IN THE HYPOGASTRIC REGION. Pain in the hypogastric region is usually caused by urinary bladder, internal genitalia, and intestinal diseases or by neurologic or musculoskeletal disorders. The most common causes include acute cystitis, urinary bladder distension, prostatitis, seminal vesiculitis, hypertrophy of the prostate, calculi in the urinary bladder, carcinoma of the urinary bladder, ulcer of the urinary bladder, various diseases of female genitalia (including dysmenorrhea, acute salpingitis, ruptured ectopic pregnancy, acute or chronic endometritis, retrodisplacement of the uterus, carcinoma of the uterus, pelvic peritonitis, and prolapse of the uterus), acute diverticulitis, volvulus, intussusception, chronic colitis, rupture of the urinary bladder, tumors of the rectosigmoid, Meckel's diverticulum, chronic constipation, regional enteritis, various neuralgias (see above), myofascial syndromes, and occasionally postoperative scar.

TABLE 59-6. Summary of Etiology and Differential Diagnoses of Abdominal Pain

Etiology (Disease)	IASP Code Reference*	Chapter No.	Important Diagnostic Features	
			Characteristics of the Pain	Associated Symptoms and Signs
I. PAIN CAUSED BY DISEASE OF THE GI TRACT				
A. Esophagus 1. Rupture 2. Esophagitis 3. Motor disorders 4. Carcinoma	—	56	Pain usually retrosternal, with radiation to the epigastrium, but can be sufficiently severe to confuse the diagnosis; pain usually aggravated by swallowing	Dysphagia early sign; odynophagia, anorexia, and age of patient (cancer); radiographic and esophagoscopic evidence
			See Section III of Table 53-2 for detailed summary	See Section III of Table 53-2 for summary
B. Stomach and duodenum	—	60		
1. Gastritis				
a. Acute erosive			Mild to moderate aching, burning intermittent pain in epigastrium in 10% of patients; relieved by antacids and meals	Bleeding, nausea and vomiting, anorexia but no weight loss
b. Chronic erosive			Mild to moderate to severe, dull, aching intermittent pain in epigastrium associated with a feeling of fullness; relieved by meals in 50% of patients	Nausea, vomiting, anorexia, weight loss; endoscopic and radiographic evidence
c. Hypertrophic gastropathy			Aching, burning pain of variable intensity, slow in onset, variable duration; meals occasionally relieve the pain	Bleeding (occasionally massive), nausea, vomiting, anorexia, weight loss, edema; radiographic and histologic evidence
d. Nonulcer dyspepsia			Aching burning pain in epigastrium in 50% of patients, back pain in 25%; associated with fullness; pain mild to moderate, slow in onset, intermittent duration; pain relieved by antacids in 50% and meals in 25%	Little or no incidence of bleeding, nausea, vomiting, anorexia, or weight loss; sometimes patient has clinical depression; exclude ulcers by radiography and endoscopy

*See Table 2-2 (p. 22) for code.

TABLE 59-6. (Cont.)

Etiology (Disease)	IASP Code Reference*	Chapter No.	Important Diagnostic Features	
			Characteristics of the Pain	Associated Symptoms and Signs
2. Peptic ulcer				
a. Gastric ulcer (GU)	XXI–4	60	Gnawing, burning, aching epigastric pain with radiation to the back and right upper quadrant (RUQ) with DU; pain gradual in onset, moderate to severe with GU and mild to moderate with DU; pain intermittent during day; none in the morning, but pain 1 to 2 hours after each meal; often awakens patients; pain relieved by food or antacid in 50% of patients with DU and less so in those with GU; periodic pain becomes more frequent, more severe, and lasts longer until pain-free periods disappear	Nausea, vomiting, anorexia, more severe with GU than DU; also heartburn, bloating, belching; can have mild iron deficiency anemia and elevated ESR; bleeding can produce hematemesis or melena; radiographic and endoscopic evidence
b. Duodenal ulcer (DU)	XXI–5	60		
c. Penetrating ulcer (into pancreas, omentum, or biliary system)			Severe continuous epigastric pain with radiation to back; back pain dull, deep, and constant; with irritation of retroperitoneal tissue leads to radicular pain; pain only partially or not relieved by food and antacid therapy	Nausea, vomiting, anorexia; can have hematemesis or melena; severe spasm of paraspinal muscles in lower thoracic region and abdominal muscles
d. Perforation of ulcer	—	60	Sudden severe continuous pain that begins in epigastrium but quickly spreads to involve entire abdomen as peritonitis ensues; pain is markedly aggravated by movement so that patient lies immobile; frequently pain in the shoulder; occasionally ulcer perforates and partially seals, leading to rapid spillage of duodenal contents to right paracolic gutter that produces pain in right lower quadrant (RLQ)	Severe tenderness and muscle spasm with board-like rigidity of abdomen; irritation of central portion of diaphragmatic peritoneum produces rapid shallow breathing with hypoxemia; possible signs of shock; ulcer history; radiography shows free air in peritoneal cavity
3. Postgastrectomy pain syndromes				
a. Gastric pouch too small			Steady moderate to severe midepigastric pain appearing soon after the start of a meal and subsiding shortly thereafter	Many patients have diarrhea, vasomotor phenomena, vomiting, weight loss, anemia, metabolic bone disease; some might develop obstruction of the gastric outlet, which causes pain as well as frequent vomiting; rarely, patients develop volvulus, intussusception, or internal hernia that causes small bowel obstruction with consequent abdominal pain
b. Afferent loop syndrome			Severe continuous burning pain in right upper abdomen similar to ulcer pain; exacerbated by eating; not relieved by antacid but by vomiting of bile	
c. Dumping syndrome			Crampy periumbilical pain 20 to 60 minutes after eating associated with flushing, sweating, lightheadedness	
d. Reflux alkaline syndrome			Upper abdominal pain accompanied by distal gastritis	

*See Table 2-2 (p. 22) for code.

TABLE 59-6. (Cont.)

Etiology (Disease)	IASP Code Reference*	Chapter No.	Important Diagnostic Features	
			Characteristics of the Pain	Associated Symptoms and Signs
4. Gastric neoplasm (e.g., adenocarcinoma, lymphoma, leimyosarcoma)	XXI-6	60	Early gastric cancer can be asymptomatic; patient then develops vague epigastric pain similar to pain of gastric ulcer; later local invasion causes pancreatitis, gastrocolic fistula, and severe continuous abdominal and back pain	Weight loss, anorexia, vomiting, occult or overt GI bleeding, anemia, palpable epigastric mass; laboratory and radiographic evidence
5. Other gastric diseases				
a. Volvulus			Severe upper abdominal steady pain	Nausea, vomiting, shock
b. Paraesophageal hiatus hernia		56	Severe pain in left chest and epigastrium	Nausea, vomiting, shock; radiographic evidence
c. Phlegmonous gastritis			Severe upper abdominal pain caused by infection of gastric wall	Signs of peritonitis, fever, purulent ascitic fluid, nausea, vomiting; normal serum amylase level
d. Pyloric stenosis and pylorospasm			Colicky pain in epigastrium radiating to both sides and to back; relieved by vomiting	Occurs 2 to 3 hours after meals; rhythmic; endoscopic evidence
e. Gastric granuloma			Variable degree of epigastric pain, usually mild	Leukocytosis; disease can cause pyloric obstruction not responsive to corticosteroids; endoscopic evidence
C. Intestines				
1. Acute appendicitis		60	Most frequent cause of acute severe abdominal pain that requires surgery; initially pain in periumbilical region (visceral pain); usually cramping or colicky but occasionally steady; later replaced by right lower quadrant, steady continuous parietal pain	Anorexia, nausea, occasionally vomiting after onset of pain; exquisite local tenderness, percussion tenderness, and rebound tenderness; hyperalgesia and muscle spasm and rigidity; fever, tachycardia, leukocytosis, perspiration
2. Infectious enterocolitis	—	60	Intermittent cramping or colicky abdominal pain in periumbilical region or right in the hypogastrium	Pain often preceded by nausea and vomiting and followed by watery, bloody, or mucoid diarrhea; fever can be present; hyperactive peristaltic noises coinciding with cramps
3. Postradiation enterocolitis		60	Pain mild to moderate or severe; mid and lower abdominal cramping pain months to years after radiation therapy; periumbilical cramping pain suggests presence of partial small or large bowel obstruction caused by stricture formation	Nausea, vomiting, and diarrhea can occur with treatment, later associated with tenesmus indicating rectal and lower colonic mucosal involvement; a significant obstruction present leading to progressive abdominal distension, nausea, and vomiting; rectal bleeding, malabsorption, fistula formation
4. Diverticulitis	XXI-12	60	Pain generally moderate, steady or cramping; in the left and right lower quadrants; sometimes radiates to the back	Nausea, vomiting, diarrhea, or constipation or mucus in stool; lower abdominal tenderness, but no rigidity or rebound tenderness; leukocytosis with left shift; usually in patients 60 years or older; sigmoid colon felt as firm tender cord in left lower quadrant

*See Table 2-2 (p. 22) for code.

TABLE 59-6. (Cont.)

Etiology (Disease)	IASP Code Reference*	Chapter No.	Important Diagnostic Features	
			Characteristics of the Pain	Associated Symptoms and Signs
5. Crohn's disease	XX-1–9	60	Pain located in area of inflammation but most frequent in RLQ; continuous, occasionally radiating to right upper thigh and causing patient to limp; usually not associated with bowel movements but exacerbated by eating; severe cramping periumbilical pain often superimposed on continuous pain and relieved by bowel movement	Signs of partial obstruction: nausea, vomiting, diarrhea, bloody stool, fever, weight loss, rectal involvement causes sensation of urgency to tenesmus; also perianal pain caused by fistula, fissures, or abscess
6. Ulcerative colitis	—	60	Moderate cramping pain in LLQ; pain relieved by defecation	Diarrhea, hematochezia (passage of bloody stools); occasional perianal pain caused by fissures
7. Acute intestinal obstruction				
a. Small bowel obstruction (adhesion and bands; strangulated hernia; intussusception; volvulus)	—	60	Crampy periumbilical pain with intervals of 5 minutes between attacks; later, pain is continuous and persistent	Distension, bilious vomiting, visible peristalsis at first; diarrhea with necrosis, exquisite local tenderness
b. Large bowel obstruction (tumors, strictures; extrinsic compression—tumors; fecal impaction)			Pain in infraumbilical or hypogastric region in midline or on either side; occurs after onset of distension	More severe distension than in small bowel obstruction with pain and vomiting occurring later; patient might continue to pass feces but ceases to pass flatus; radiography shows dilated bowel filled with air and fluid; barium enema useful in defining site of obstruction
c. Neurogenic obstruction (postoperative trauma, infection, metabolic drugs)			Usually generalized mild to moderate pain, continuous	Distension, nausea, vomiting, absent bowel sounds; when severe causes push on diaphragm, leading to respiratory insufficiency, dyspnea, tachypnea, hypopnea, hypoxemia
8. Carcinoma	XX-1–13	60	Painless until tumor produces obstruction or compression of adjacent structures, leading to continuous dull aching pain or paroxysmal colicky pain in LUQ (splenic flexure), left iliac region and over sacrum (sigmoid colon), or right lower quadrant (ascending colon); with perforation acute abdominal pain and signs of peritonitis	Caused by obstruction; pain synchronous with constipation or emesis relieved by evacuation; occult blood alternating diarrhea and constipation; radiographic evidence
9. Irritable bowel syndrome	XXI-11	60, 65	Cramping or aching pain below level of umbilicus; relieved by bowel movement or passing of flatus; lasts from a few minutes to hours and is usually recurrent; can be in epigastrium and frequently shifts to various sites	Distension, nausea, vomiting, diarrhea alternating with constipation, mucus in stool, excessive flatus; symptoms and signs of emotional stress.
10. Intestinal ischemia	XX-1–8	64	See Section IX, below	

*See Table 2-2 (p. 22) for code.

TABLE 59-6. (Cont.)

Etiology (Disease)	IASP Code Reference*	Chapter No.	Important Diagnostic Features	
			Characteristics of the Pain	Associated Symptoms and Signs
11. Other intestinal lesions				
a. Regional ileitis		64	Pain in right lower quadrant simulating that of appendicitis	Tenderness and hyperalgesia, neuralgia of iliohypogastric and ilioinguinal nerves
b. Dysentary (amebic, bacillary)			Sudden, diffuse abdominal pain with tenesmus and extreme tenderness	Frequent stools with blood and mucus, vomiting, tachycardia, variable temperature; laboratory evidence
c. Typhoid			Acute abdominal pain, often simulating that of appendicitis	Fever, splenomegaly, neutrophilic leukopenia; positive blood culture
d. Tuberculosis, actinomycosis, other mycotic diseases			Chronic, dull pain in right lower quadrant with occasional paroxysm of colicky pain	History and signs and symptoms of disease; radiographic evidence
II. DISEASES OF THE GALLBLADDER	XXI–2	61		
A. Cholelithiasis (biliary colic)			Sudden, severe, constant, poorly localized pain in the midepigastrium; later moves to RUQ with radiation to right shoulder and scapula; severe pain persists for 1 to 8 hours, subsiding gradually or rapidly followed by residual mild ache or soreness in RUQ that persists for 24 hours or more	Anorexia, nausea, vomiting; no inflammation; little or no RUQ tenderness or guarding
B. Acute cholecystitis		61	Usually well-localized pain in RUQ, with radiation to interscapular area, inferior angle of right scapula, and shoulder regions; pain aggravated by deep inspiration or cough during subcostal palpation of RUQ (Murphy's sign); also aggravated by light blow to right subcostal area	Anorexia, nausea, vomiting, mild leukocytosis, fever; localized rebound tenderness, severe muscle spasm in RUQ; often abdominal distension and hypoactive bowel sounds from paralytic ileus; mild increase in serum bilirubin, alkaline phosphatase, and amylase levels
C. Empyema of gallbladder		61	Severe RUQ pain with radiation to interscapular region, inferior angle of scapula, and right shoulder; aggravated by deep inspiration or cough and Murphy's sign	Same as acute cholecystitis, but more severe; high fever; marked leukocytosis and often prostration
D. Postcholecystectomy syndrome (incorrect diagnosis, unrecognized disease, malignancy, remnant structures, biliary dyskinesia)	XXI-3	61	Pain in RUQ; often develops after a short initial pain-free period following cholecystectomy; pain similar to gallbladder pain, can be colicky, dull or intense, lasting all day, possibly continuing for months or years; usually absent at night; aggravated by eating	History of cholecystectomy, nausea, occasional vomiting; tenderness in RUQ; laboratory studies normal
E. Carcinoma		61	Mild to moderate or severe unremitting RUQ pain; aggravated by deep pressure	Anorexia, weight loss, jaundice, palpable RUQ mass

*See Table 2-2 (p. 22) for code.

TABLE 59-6. (Cont.)

Etiology (Disease)	IASP Code Reference*	Chapter No.	Important Diagnostic Features	
			Characteristics of the Pain	Associated Symptoms and Signs
III. DISEASES OF THE LIVER	—	61		
A. Acute hepatitis (viral or bacterial infection)			Early, little or no pain but later mild to moderate or severe dull aching pain in right upper abdomen caused by hepatic enlargement and stretching of capsule; often radiation to right shoulder and scapula	Anorexia, fatigue, nonspecific systemic complaints; jaundice; hepatomegaly; palpable and tender
B. Abscess (pyogenic, amebic)		61	Constant dull aching moderate to severe pain in RUQ; radiation to right shoulder and scapula	Large tender liver; systemic signs of sepsis, fever, chills, rigor, tachycardia; malaise, anorexia, weight loss, nausea
C. Gonococcal perihepatitis (Fitz-Hugh-Curtis syndrome)		61	Sudden RUQ pain; radiation to right shoulder; aggravated by deep inspiration	Fever, tenderness and rebound tenderness in RUQ; usually presence of pelvic infection
D. Carcinoma				
1. Primary tumor (hepatocellular CA, hepatoma)			Insidious onset of mild to moderate pain in RUQ or epigastrium described as pressure, fullness, or heaviness; with hepatoma, sudden acute RUQ pain	Hepatic mass, weight loss, ascites with carcinoma; fever and jaundice mimicking those of cholecystitis with hepatoma; hemorrhagic phenomena frequent; associated with apparent neoplastic syndrome (polycythemia, hypoglycemia, thrombocytosis, hypercalcemia)
2. Metastatic tumors		61	Asymptomatic in 15 to 20% of patients; rest have constant dull aching pain localized to epigastrium with hemorrhage into necrotic tumor, sudden acute RUQ pain	Anorexia, weight loss, fatigue, fever, epigastric fullness; jaundice and ascites uncommon until advanced stage
E. Other disorders (Echinococcus cyst; choledochus cyst— cyst of common bile duct; passive congestion; aneurysm of hepatic artery; hepatomegaly from any cause)			Feeling of dull, aching pain and pressure in RUQ; pain continuous with congestion	Radiographic evidence (cyst); palpable tumor (aneurysm); jaundice, hepatomegaly; positive liver dysfunction tests
IV. DISEASES OF THE PANCREAS	XXI-7	61		
A. Acute pancreatitis			Abdominal pain major symptom of disease; can vary from mild intolerable discomfort to severe constant and excruciating pain that is steady and boring in character; located in epigastrium and periumbilical region; radiation to back, chest, flanks, and lower abdomen; persists for hours to days; aggravated by recumbency; relieved by sitting or standing with trunk flexed	Nausea, vomiting, abdominal distension caused by gastrointestinal hypomotility, chemical peritonitis, fever, tachycardia, hypotension, often shock; severe reflex muscle spasm, tachypnea, hypopnea, hypercapnea, hypoxemia may lead to respiratory insufficiency and death; elevated serum amylase level in 65% of patients; radiographic evidence

*See Table 2-2 (p. 22) for code.

TABLE 59-6. (Cont.)

Etiology (Disease)	IASP Code Reference*	Chapter No.	Important Diagnostic Features	
			Characteristics of the Pain	Associated Symptoms and Signs
B. Chronic pancreatitis		61	Pain central feature of disease; in 50% of patients it is constant gnawing, mild to severe, but never subsides; usually felt in epigastrium with radiation to back; aggravated by eating; in some patients pain is maximal in right or left upper quadrants or in the back or diffuse throughout upper abdomen; can be referred to anterior chest or flank; aggravated by alcohol and ingestion of heavy meals; other 50% of patients experience severe episodes of epigastric pain with pain-free intervals between; can last for days to weeks; constant pain associated with alcoholic chronic pancreatitis, intermittent pain more common with nonalcoholic pancreatitis; often pain so severe it requires frequent use of narcotics, leading to physical dependence	Weight loss, abnormal stools, other signs and symptoms of malabsorption; mild abdominal tenderness and fever; evidence of endocrine insufficiency
C. Carcinoma	XXI-7	61	Pain hallmark symptom of pancreatic cancer; usually begins as mild epigastric discomfort that rapidly becomes more severe, gnawing, relentless, and visceral in character; radiation to back in about 25% of patients.	Anorexia, weight loss, nausea, vomiting, weakness, palpable abdominal mass in 20% of patients; jaundice frequent
D. Occlusion of pancreatic duct (tumors, calculi or inflammation)			Colicky deep-seated epigastric pain, often excruciating; radiating along the left costal margin to the left side of the back; promptly relieved by relief of obstruction	Colic accompanied by vomiting, exhaustion, high amylase level, glycosuria, hyperglycemia, fatty stools; radiographic evidence; swelling of parotid glands
E. Other diseases of pancreas (cysts, aseptic necrosis due to arterial thrombosis)			Deep-seated pain in epigastrium or back with cysts; dull aching pain in epigastrium; radiating to front of chest and shoulder with aseptic necrosis	Palpable mass (cysts); signs of some tenderness in left hypochondriac region
V. DISEASES OF THE SPLEEN	—	64		
A. Perisplenitis			Acute continuous pain in left hypochondriac region	Tenderness in region of spleen
B. Splenomegaly (infections, hematologic or metabolic disorders, abscess)			Constant dull aching pain in left hypochondriac region caused by massive splenomegaly	Tenderness, sense of tension, palpable mass
C. Splenic abscess			Moderate to severe pain in left hypochondriac region, lower chest, and flank; can radiate to left shoulder	Leukocytosis; palpable mass with radiographic evidence of mass; gas in abscess; displacement of colon, kidney, and stomach; elevation of left hemidiaphragm

*See Table 2-2 (p. 22) for code.

TABLE 59-6. (Cont.)

Etiology (Disease)	IASP Code Reference*	Chapter No.	Important Diagnostic Features	
			Characteristics of the Pain	Associated Symptoms and Signs
D. Splenic infarction			Sudden violent pain in left hypochondriac and splenic regions; sudden severe pain in left hypochondriac region, often radiating to shoulder	Splinting of left diaphragm, tenderness, and guarding in LLQ; friction rub in splenic area
E. Splenic rupture (traumatic or iatrogenic)			Sudden severe LUQ pain with radiation to left scapular region	Severe reflex spasm with abdominal guarding and rigidity; evidence of internal hemorrhage, shock, and anemia
F. Other disorders (tumor, cyst, Banti's syndrome)			Mild to moderate pain in left LUQ from splenomegaly	Palpable mass, tumor or cyst, with latter containing fluid seen on CT scan
VI. DISEASES OF THE KIDNEY AND URETERS	—	63		
A. Congenital	—	63		
1. Polycystic kidney disease			Hematuria initial symptom in young males; chronic intermittent dull bilateral flank pain; aggravated by hyperextension of spine	Palpable mass; uremia and hypertension in patients over 40 years; typical ultrasound findings
2. Simple (solitary) cyst			Chronic, dull, intermittent unilateral flank or back pain	Solitary renal mass; clear fluid on cyst puncture
3. Calyceal diverticulum			Most patients asymptomatic, but chronic dull intermittent flank pain in others	Stones trapped in diverticula; typical urographic findings
4. Horseshoe kidney			Dull intermittent abdominal pain; worsens with hyperextension of spine	Can have obstructive lesion; typical urographic findings
5. Vesicoureteral reflux			Renal pain or colic before, during, or immediately after voiding	Typical cystographic findings
B. Acquired vascular disease	—	63		
1. Renal vein thrombosis			Acute flank pain or chronic flank ache	Urography shows nonfunction; venography shows occluded renal vein; proteinurea
2. Renal artery occlusion			Sudden severe prostating abdominal and flank pain	Usually develops shock; reflex muscle spasm; arteriography shows occlusion of main renal artery
3. Renal artery aneurysm			Mild flank pain from compression; if aneurysm ruptures severe abdominal and flank pain can result	Ring-like calcification in renal hilus; occlusion of renal artery on arteriogram; shock with rupture
4. Hypertensive renal vascular disease			Headache and other symptoms with severe hypertension	Hypertension, stenosis of renal artery and vein; other signs and symptoms of hypertension
C. Renal infection	—	63		
1. Acute pyelonephritis			Acute continuous aching pain in flank over affected kidney	Severe flank tenderness; pyuria, fever, leukocytosis, malaise, chills
2. Renal carbuncle			Vague intermittent back pain aggravated by movement of spine	Weight loss, spiking fever; CT scan shows intrarenal mass; kidney nonmotile (fixed to surrounding structures)
3. Renal abscess			Sudden severe continuous flank pain; radiation to the back	Flank tenderness, chills, fever with medullary abscess, pyuria but not with cortical abscess; microscopic hematuria

*See Table 2-2 (p. 22) for code.

TABLE 59-6. (Cont.)

Etiology (Disease)	IASP Code Reference*	Chapter No.	Important Diagnostic Features	
			Characteristics of the Pain	Associated Symptoms and Signs
4. Perinephritic abscess (rupture or renal abscess into perinephritic space)			Dull persistent unilateral flank pain	Flank or abdominal mass and tenderness, fever, leukocytosis, pyuria, dysuria; CT scan shows extrarenal collection; kidney nonmotile
5. Pyelonephrosis			Dull unilateral flank pain of late onset; aggravated by palpation of flank or abdomen	Fever, malaise; signs of sepsis; urography shows delay or nonfunction secondary to obstruction of ureter
6. Tuberculosis			Usually painless; can have dull flank pain or colic	Typical findings on excretory urography
7. Renal echinococcus			Acute ureteral colic secondary to passage of cyst through ureter	Histologic diagnosis
D. Obstruction	—	63		
1. Renal and ureteral calculus			Acute colic and flank pain of sudden onset; radiating to gonadal and inguinal regions, unrelieved by position change; patient moves about frantically seeking relief	Flank and abdominal tenderness, hyperesthesia, allodynia, retraction of testicle; nausea, vomiting; microscopic hematuria; urography shows calculus
2. Noncalculus obstruction			Usually painless; can have dull ache in flank	Typical findings on excretory urography
3. Acute intermittent hydronephrosis			Intermittent bouts of acute colic; aggravated by high fluid intake	Urography shows partial obstruction of ureteropelvic junction
4. Blood clot obstruction (clots from trauma, polycystic kidney, carcinoma)			Acute severe colic and flank pain; similar characteristics to those of calculus	Tenderness and spasm of flank and abdominal muscles; clots in urine
5. Papillary necrosis (sloughed renal papilla)			Acute moderate to severe colic and flank pain; continuous; unrelieved by position change	Flank tenderness; urography shows typical findings
6. Retroperitoneal fibrosis (compression and medial displacement of ureters, usually bilateral)			Vague, continuous dull aching flank and low back pain; compression or irritation of lumbar nerves produces radicular pain in thigh and low back	Mild flank tenderness; can have spasm of paraspinal muscles
7. Ovarian vein syndrome (obstruction of ureter by aberrant ovarian vein)			Severe, continuous flank and abdominal pain occurs prepartum or 2 to 6 weeks postpartum; relieved by bypassing obstruction	Flank tenderness, fever, chills, nausea and vomiting, pyuria; urography shows obstruction at S1 level
8. Fraley's syndrome (infundibular stenosis)			Intermittent moderate to severe flank pain, right or left side; relieved by lying down	Flank tenderness; urography shows typical findings
E. Neoplasm	—	63		
1. Renal cell CA			Triad or flank pain; pain prominent in 35 to 45% of patients	Hypertension, weight loss, hematuria, palpable mass; radiographic evidence
2. Metastatic renal cell CA			Pain caused by metastasis (e.g., to bones, nerves)	Weight loss, cachexia; radiographic evidence of metastasis
3. Sarcoma			Flank pain radiating to inguinal region caused by stretching of capsule; radicular pain from pressure of spinal nerves	Palpable mass, weight loss; radiographic evidence

*See Table 2-2 (p. 22) for code.

TABLE 59-6. (Cont.)

Etiology (Disease)	IASP Code Reference*	Chapter No.	Important Diagnostic Features	
			Characteristics of the Pain	Associated Symptoms and Signs
4. Carcinoma of the renal pelvis			Pain caused by obstruction of ureter or ureteropelvic junction by tumor; pain localized to psoas, quadratus lumborum, and back muscles	Palpable flank mass, urinary frequency, dysuria; radiographic evidence
F. Idiopathic nephralgia	—	63	Lesion nondemonstrable; long history of "renal" pain with radiation to right ipsilateral flank and lower quadrant; aggravated by physical activity, emotional stress, menstruation	Absence of pathophysiologic or psychologic abnormality
VII. INTRA-ABDOMINAL VASCULAR DISEASES	—	64		
A. Enlarging or ruptured intra-abdominal aneurysm (aortic, iliac, visceral artery)			Steady excruciating pain (sudden in case of rupture); initially epigastric with radiation to back, flank, groin, or upper thigh, especially on left side	Tenderness over pulsatile mass; nausea and vomiting, hypotension, and shock; deviation of ureters on pyelography; erosion of lumbar vertebral bodies; calcifications in aneurysm wall on plain abdominal films
B. Acute mesenteric occlusion (embolus or thrombus; "nonocclusive mesenteric ischemia")	XXI–8	64	Initially colicky epigastric pain, then becoming steady and diffuse; not relieved by vomiting or evacuation of bowels; with more gradual thrombosis or nonocclusive variant pain is steady, boring, ill-localized	Initially pain out of proportion to physical findings, then vomiting, hyperperistalsis, melena, distension; with perforation, ileus, leukocytosis, acidosis, shock, peritonitis; history of abdominal angina, atrial fibrillation, widespread atherosclerosis; patients with nonocclusive mesenteric ischemia frequently aged; volume-depleted, hemoconcentrated, on digitalis, with chronic heart failure
C. Chronic mesenteric insufficiency (multiple visceral arterial stenoses; "celiac compression" syndrome	XXI–8	64	Recurrent attacks of colicky midabdominal pain, poorly localized; usually postprandial; lasts minutes to hours	Substantial weight loss, abdominal bruits, other evidence of severe atherosclerosis; at least two visceral arteries occluded or stenotic on arteriography
D. Vasculitis (polyarteritis nodosa, lupus erythematosus, Henoch-Schönlein purpura)			Sudden severe pain of acute infarction with large vessel involvement; mild to moderate pain with small vessel involvement	With large vessel involvement, symptoms and signs similar to those of acute ischemia; with small vessels, variable degrees of obstruction and bleeding; plain radiographs show "thumbprinting" caused by localized edema, hemorrhage, ulceration
VIII. DISEASES OF THE PERITONEUM AND MESENTERY	—	64		
A. Diseases of peritoneum 1. Acute generalized peritonitis (bacterial, chemical)			Severe diffuse persistent continuous pain in entire abdomen, usually worse in periumbilical region; onset insidious with bacterial infection, sudden and intense with chemical irritation; markedly aggravated by motion; relieved by being on one side with hips flexed	Extreme generalized tenderness with rebound tenderness referred to the point of pressure; severe abdominal muscle spasm; abdomen unyielding; rapid ileus, nausea, vomiting, distension, tympany with rigidity, fever, tachycardia, prostration; fast shallow breathing leads to hypoxemia

*See Table 2-2 (p. 22) for code.

TABLE 59-6. (Cont.)

Etiology (Disease)	IASP Code Reference*	Chapter No.	Important Diagnostic Features	
			Characteristics of the Pain	Associated Symptoms and Signs
2. Granulomatous peritonitis			Mild to moderate abdominal pain; usually localized to region of granulomatous inflammatory reaction	Abdominal tenderness, fever, nausea, vomiting, distension, small bowel obstruction in 25% of patients
3. Familial paroxysmal peritonitis (familial Mediterranean fever)	XXII-1	64	Recurring episodes of peritonitis produce localized or diffuse, moderate to severe, abdominal pain	Sudden onset of fever, exquisite abdominal tenderness with marked rebound tenderness, leukocytosis; symptoms and signs subside after 6 to 12 hours, patients well in 24 to 48 hours; attacks recur at irregular and unpredictable intervals
4. Neoplasm a. Mesothelioma			Abdominal pain	Anorexia, nausea, vomiting, constipation, weight loss; abdominal mass
b. Carcinomatosis			Diffuse abdominal pain	Ascites, weight loss, nausea and vomiting less frequent
B. Diseases of the mesentery	—	64		
1. Mesenteric inflammatory disease			Recurrent episodes of cramping abdominal pain; localized or diffuse	Weight loss, nausea, vomiting, low-grade fever
2. Mesenteric tumors			Moderate diffuse abdominal pain	Abdominal mass, weight loss
3. Torsion of the omentum			Sudden or rapid severe abdominal pain in RLQ (80%) or RUQ (10%)	Tenderness, guarding, ileus, nausea, vomiting; abdominal mass; leukocytosis
C. Diseases of the diaphragm		64		
1. Herniation (Bochdalek hernia)			Vague intermittent abdominal pain (50%), chest pain (25%) with incarceration of intestine; severe acute sharp retrosternal pain radiating to LUQ or back	Dyspnea; symptoms and signs of cardiovascular dysfunction caused by compression of heart and great vessel
2. Rupture (trauma)			Severe epigastric and chest pain caused by herniation of abdominal viscera	Nausea, vomiting, cramps, dyspnea, bowel obstruction with strangulation
3. Tumors and cysts			Mild to moderate upper abdominal pain; predominantly in epigastrium	Radiographic evidence shows irregularity of diaphragm or large mass
IX. OTHER INTRA-ABDOMINAL DISEASES				
A. Intra-abdominal abscesses	—	64		
1. Subphrenic (postoperative)			Pain in the lower anterior and lateral chest, occasionally in epigastrium with radiation to shoulder and occasionally to interscapular region	Nonproductive cough, dyspnea; rales, rhonchi, or friction rub; localized tenderness, abdominal distension, hypoactive bowel sounds; elevated or immobile hemidiaphragm
2. Hepatic and subhepatic abscesses			Moderate to severe pain in RUQ; associated with pleuritic chest pain	Chills, nausea, vomiting, anorexia, weight loss, weakness; hepatomegaly with hepatic abscess; radiographic evidence of atelectasis, pneumonia, pleural effusion, elevated right hemidiaphragm; abnormal liver function tests

*See Table 2-2 (p. 22) for code.

TABLE 59-6. (Cont.)

Etiology (Disease)	IASP Code Reference*	Chapter No.	Important Diagnostic Features	
			Characteristics of the Pain	Associated Symptoms and Signs
3. Pancreatic abscess (in site of pancreatic necrosis)			Periumbilical or right-sided abdominal pain; mild to moderate or severe; occurs 10 to 21 days after acute pancreatitis	Abdominal tenderness, nausea, vomiting, persistent ileus, fever, leukocytosis; palpable mass in 50% of patients; radiographs can show left pleural effusion, atelectasis, or pneumonia
4. Midabdominal abscesses			Abdominal pain in RLQ, LLQ, or periumbilical region	Tenderness, signs of paralytic ileus
5. Anterior retroperitoneal abscess			Moderate to severe abdominal or flank pain; radiation to the hip, thigh, or knee from psoas muscle involvement; aggravated by extension of hip	Fever, nausea, vomiting, abdominal and flank tenderness; palpable mass
B. Neurogenic intestinal obstruction (adynamic ileus)	—	64	Cramping abdominal pain; continuous or intermittent	Distension, vomiting, absence of bowel sounds; evidence of intestinal obstruction
C. Gas entrapment syndromes	—	64		
1. Gastric entrapment syndrome			Pain in midanterior abdomen and chest or right upper quadrant or left upper quadrant, depending on site of distension; pain dull, constant, becomes worse as day progresses; aggravated at mealtime; with splenic flexure pain radiates to left shoulder	Abdominal tympany; plain films reveal excess gas
2. Hepatic flexure syndrome				
3. Splenic flexure syndrome				
D. Abdominal migraine	XXII-2	64	Recurrent bouts of periumbilical pain associated with headaches; attacks last less than 6 hours	Nausea, vomiting, headache, pallor, perspiration, bradycardia, fever, occasional diarrhea

X. ABDOMINAL PAIN ASSOCIATED WITH SYSTEMIC DISORDERS

Etiology (Disease)	IASP Code Reference*	Chapter No.	Characteristics of the Pain	Associated Symptoms and Signs
A. Hematologic disorders	—	64		
1. Sickle cell anemia			Recurrent episodes of severe, diffuse colicky pain (abdominal crises) simulating those of acute abdomen	Vomiting, diarrhea, constipation; laboratory evidence
2. Acute hemolytic crises			Sudden onset of moderate to severe pain in abdomen, back, or limbs; severe abdominal pain	Abdominal muscle spasm, rigidity, hypertension, profound prostration, shock, pallor, jaundice, tachycardia, other symptoms of severe anemia
3. Chronic hemolytic anemias			Occurrence of abdominal crises manifested by severe acute abdominal pain	Anemia, jaundice, splenomegaly, muscular spasm and rigidity
B. Metabolic disorders				
1. Acute intermittent porphyria (hereditary porphyria, variegated porphyria)	XXII-3, 4, 5	64	Recurrent acute attacks of severe abdominal pain precipitated by various drugs and environmental factors; pain can be moderate but frequently is severe; cramping or colicky; localized in one lower quadrant or periumbilical region; more frequently diffuse through the abdomen; radiates to back or loins	Low-grade fever, mild leukocytosis, tachycardia, hypertension, postural hypotension, sweating; can have evidence of peripheral neuropathy

*See Table 2-2 (p. 22) for code.

TABLE 59-6. (Cont.)

Etiology (Disease)	IASP Code Reference*	Chapter No.	Important Diagnostic Features	
			Characteristics of the Pain	Associated Symptoms and Signs
C. Systemic toxic disorders 1. Lead and other heavy metal poisoning 2. Food poisoning 3. Uremia	—	64	Generalized moderate to severe paroxysmal colicky abdominal pain; worse in umbilical region; associated with gastrointestinal spasm and abdominal tenderness	Nausea, vomiting, diarrhea, abdominal tenderness, fever, leukocytosis; other signs of disorder (lead line in gums, basophils, stippling in RBC, lead in urine); history of exposure to heavy metals, ingestion of food
D. Biologic factors 1. Spider bite	—	64	Severe excruciating waves of cramping abdominal pain; begins 10 to 20 minutes after bite, persists for hours or days	Abdomen boardlike; labored breathing, nausea, vomiting, headache, sweating, salivation, hyperactive reflexes, twitching, tremor, paresthesia
2. Allergy to food			Sudden acute colicky pain with mild tenderness	History of ingestion of food or administration of drugs; other signs of allergy
E. Endocrine disturbances			Moderate to severe abdominal colicky pain caused by spasm of gastrointestinal and biliary tracts	History and other signs of hyperthyroidism, adrenal insufficiency, Simmond's pituitary cachexia
XI. EXTRA-ABDOMINAL DISORDERS				
A. Thoracic visceral disease 1. Acute myocardial infarction 2. Pericarditis 3. Pulmonary embolism 4. Pneumonia 5. Pleuritis	—	54, 55	Pain most intense in chest (retrosternal or lateral chest); radiation to epigastrium, RUQ or LUQ; pleuritic pain aggravated by deep breathing	Nausea, vomiting, tachycardia or bradycardia; pericardial friction rub; ECG changes; dyspnea, fever; signs of lung consolidation; see Table 53-2, Sections I and II
B. Pelvic diseases 1. Gynecologic disorders	—	67	See Table 65-1, Section I	
a. Acute disorders (pregnancy, infection, ectopic pregnancy, torsion of adnexa) b. Recurrent pain, chronic pain			Mild to moderate or severe suprapubic and low back pain; radiation to inguinal region and medial thigh; intermittent or cramping pain from uterine contractions; torsion of ovaries or tubes; rupture of cyst or ectopic pregnancy leads to sudden severe pain	Rectal or cervical tenderness on palpation; spasm of lower abdominal muscles, suprapubic tenderness; signs of infection; vaginal bleeding
2. Urinary bladder and prostatic disorders	—	68	Suprapubic pain; radiation to back and upper lumbar region; prostatic disease caused deep pelvic and perineal pain	Urgency, frequency, dysuria, tenesmus, fever, other signs of sepsis with infection
C. Abdominal pain of neuropathic origin 1. Lesion of brain or brain stem	—	14	Burning aching pain in half of trunk and extremities	Hyperesthesia, hyperpathia, and other neurologic manifestations
2. Lesion of the spinal cord (lower thoracic part)	—	14	Pain initially localized to back, later radicular pain radiates to abdominal wall	Same as above
3. Lesion of roots or trunk of spinal nerves (T5–L1)	XX-2	10, 13, 58	Segmental pain in one or more dermatomes of abdomen, flank, and back	Hyperalgesia, hyperesthesia, hypesthesia, other neurologic evidence
4. Intercostal neuropathy			Segmental pain in anterior abdomen and lateral chest	Neuropathic manifestations

*See Table 2-2 (p. 22) for code.

TABLE 59-6. (Cont.)

Etiology (Disease)	IASP Code Reference*	Chapter No.	Important Diagnostic Features	
			Characteristics of the Pain	Associated Symptoms and Signs
5. Abdominal cutaneous nerve entrapment syndrome	XX-5	58	Intermittent pain in region of rectus abdominis muscle or segmental neuralgia; provoked by increase in intra-abdominal pressure and twisting of trunk; relieved by injection of local anesthetic into painful area	Fingertip tenderness over lateral edge of rectus with herniation of neurovascular bundle, feels like pea-sized mass
D. Abdominal Pain of musculoskeletal origin				
1. 12th rib syndrome		64	Unilateral chronic persistent flank pain (simulate renal disease); aggravated by lateral flexion to affected side and extension; relieved by forward flexion	Tenderness over affected rib; manipulation of rib reproduces patient's pain; no radiographic findings
2. Slipping rib syndrome	XVII-10	64	Unilateral lower chest and upper abdominal pain; aggravated by extension	Palpation produces tenderness and reveals upward curling of loosened cartilage
3. Xiphoidalgia		64	Aching or sharp pain in region of xiphoid process; radiation to epigastrium and lower chest	Pressure produces pain and tenderness over xiphoid process
4. Myofascial pain syndrome with trigger points			Dull aching or sharp pain in any part of the abdominal wall	Location of trigger point reproduces or aggravates pain; can have visceral dysfunction caused by somatovisceral reflex
5. Hematoma in muscles (trauma)		64	Mild to severe pain localized to area of injury	Palpable mass, tenderness
E. Abdominal Pain of tegumentary origin				
1. Painful scars	—	64	Aching burning pain; associated with bouts of lancinating pain in region of scar	Pressure on scar reproduces lancinating pain, tenderness, palpation of neuroma
2. Dermatologic disorders	—	27	Continuous aching burning pain in region of skin lesion	Usually lesion also in other parts of the body
3. Postburn scars	—	26	Dull aching burning pain in region of scar	Evidence of burns elsewhere in the body
4. Postoperative pain	—	25	Acute sharp aching pain in site of incision; associated with deep vague visceral pain	Usually muscle spasm, hyperalgesia, hyperesthesia; tenderness; ileus with distension, hypoventilation leading to hypoxemia
XII. ABDOMINAL PAIN OF PSYCHOLOGIC ORIGIN				
A. Somatoform (psychophysiologic)				
1. Peptic ulcer 2. Ulcerative colitis 3. Crohn's disease		50, 60	Pain of variable intensity and location depending on the disease. See IB, C above	See IB, C above for summary
B. Learned pain		16, 63	Pain of variable intensity and location that persists after abdominal visceral disease has been cured	Abnormal illness behavior develops consequent to organic pathology through environmental factors
C. Delusional or hallucinatory pain	XXIII-2	19	Persistent abdominal pain of variable intensity and site. In manic depressive, schizophrenic, or other psychosis	No physical or laboratory findings or pathologic lesions. Symptoms of psychosis. Very rare; less than 2% of patients with chronic pain
D. Hysterical or hypochondriacal	XXIII-3	19	Continuous abdominal pain described in sensory terms; fluctuates in intensity; does not awaken patient from sleep; usually lasts more than 6 months; attributable to thought processes	No physical or laboratory findings of pathologic lesions. The depressive complaint and resentment frequent. Loss of function (paralysis, anesthesia) without physical basis

*See Table 2-2 (p. 22) for code.

TABLE 59-6. (Cont.)

Etiology (Disease)	IASP Code Reference*	Chapter No.	Important Diagnostic Features	
			Characteristics of the Pain	Associated Symptoms and Signs
E. Depression		18	Patients with major depression may complain of persistent pain in abdomen. Pain of variable intensity and site. More frequent in women than in men	Depressed mood, decrease of interest or pleasure, sleep disturbance, decrease in appetite, fatigue, decrease in self-esteem, no organic pathology, not superimposed on schizophrenia or delusional or psychotic disorders

See Table 2-2 (p. 22) for code.

REFERENCES

1. Lennander, K.G.: Über die sensibilitat der Bauchloehle ünd uber lokale und allgemeine Anasthesie bei Bruch und Bachoperationen, Zentralbl. Physiol., 28:209, 1901.
2. Hurst, A.F.: On the sensibility of the alimentary canal in health and disease. Lancet, 1:1051, 1911.
3. Bonica, J.J.: The Management of Pain. Philadelphia, Lea & Febiger, 1953, pp. 109–120.
4. Procacci, P., Zoppi, M., and Maresca, M.: Experimental pain in man. Pain, 6:123, 1979.
5. Wolf, S., and Wolff, H.G.: Pain arising from the stomach and mechanisms underlying gastric symptoms. In Pain-Proceedings, Research Nervous Mental Disease. Vol. 23. Edited by H.G. Wolff. Baltimore, Williams & Wilkins, 1943, pp. 289–294.
6. Cervero, F., and Tattersall, J.E.H.: Somatic and visceral sensory integration in the thoracic spinal cord. In Visceral Sensation. Edited by F. Cervero and J.E.H. Morrison. Amsterdam, Elsevier, 1986. pp. 189–205.
7. Jones, C.M.: Digestive Tract Pain. New York, Macmillan, 1939.
8. Silen, W.: Abdominal pain. In Harrison's Principles of Internal Medicine. 10th Ed. Edited by R.G. Petersdorf, et al. New York, McGraw-Hill, 1983, pp. 31–35.
9. National Center for Health Statistics: Current Estimates From the National Health Interview Survey. United States, 1986. Hyattsville, MD, National Center for Health Statistics, 1987, DHHS Publ. No. (PHS) 87-1592.
10. National Center for Health Statistics: Advanced Data 1986 Summary: National Hospital Discharge Survey. Hyattsville, MD, National Center for Health Statistics, 1987, Publ. No. 145.
11. American Cancer Society: Cancer Facts and Figures, 1987. New York, American Cancer Society, 1987.
12. Taylor, H.S.: The Nuprin Pain Report. New York, Lou Harris Associates, 1985.
13. Clemente, C.D. (ed.): Gray's Anatomy of the Human Body. 30th Ed. Philadelphia, Lea & Febiger, 1985, pp. 483–498, 1450–1489.
14. Williams, P.L., and Warwick, R. (eds.): Gray's Anatomy. 36th Br. Ed. Philadelphia, W.B. Saunders, 1980.
15. Netter, F.H.: The CIBA Collection of Medical Illustrations, Vol. 3: Digestive System. Part II, Lower Digestive Tract. Summit, NJ, CIBA, 1979.
16. Mitchell, G.A.G.: Anatomy of the Autonomic Nervous System. London, Livingstone, 1953.
17. Mitchell, G.A.G.: Cardiovascular Innervation. Edinburgh, Livingstone, 1956.
18. Hovelacque, A.: Anatomie des Nerfs Crainiens et Rachidiens et du Système Grand Sympathique chez l'Homme. Paris, G. Doin, 1927.
19. Norvell, J.E.: The aorticorenal ganglion and its role in renal innervation. J. Comp. Neurol., 133:101, 1969.
20. Kuntz, A.: Autonomic Nervous System. 4th Ed. Philadelphia, Lea & Febiger, 1953, pp. 207–260.
21. Schoefield, G.C.: Anatomy of muscular and neural tissues in the alimentary canal. In Handbook of Physiology, Vol. 4, Sec. 6. Edited by C.F. Code. Washington DC, American Physiological Society, 1968, pp. 1579–1628.
22. Goyal, R.K.: Neurology of the gut. In Gastrointestinal Disease: Pathophysiology, Diagnosis, Management. 3rd Ed. Edited by M.H. Sleisenger and J.S. Fordtran. Philadelphia, W.B. Saunders, 1983, pp. 97–114.
23. Gabella, G.: Structure of the Autonomic Nervous System. London, Chapman & Hall, 1976.
24. Weinberg, A.G.: Hirschsprung's disease: A pathologist's view. Perspect. Pediatr. Pathol., 2:207, 1975.
25. Dogiel, A.S.: Zwei arten sympathischer Nervenzellen. Ant. Anz: 11:679, 1986.
26. Wood, J.D.: Neurophysiology of Auerbach's plexus and control of intestinal motility. Physiol. Rev., 55:307, 1975.
27. Burnstock, G.: Structure of smooth muscle and its innervation. In Smooth Muscle. Edited by E. Bulbring et al. Baltimore, Williams & Wilkins, 1970, pp. 1–69.
28. Wilbourn, R.B., et al.: The APUD cells of the alimentary tract in health and disease. Med. Clin. North Am., 58:1359, 1974.
29. Paintal, A.S.: Action of drugs on sensory nerve endings. Ann. Rev. Pharmacol., 11:231, 1971.
30. Andrews, P.L.R.: Vagal afferent innervation of the gastrointestinal tract. In Visceral Sensation. Edited by F. Cervero and J.E.H. Morrison. Amsterdam, Elsevier, 1986, pp. 65–86.
31. Kuo, B.C., et al.: A wide field electronic microscopic analysis of the fiber constituents of the major splanchnic nerve in the cat. J. Comp. Neurol., 210:49, 1982.
32. Leek, B.F.: Abdominal visceral receptors. In Handbook of Sensory Physiology, Vol. 3. Edited by E. Neil. New York, Springer-Verlag, 1972, 113–160.
33. Sharma, K.N.: Receptor mechanisms in the alimentary tract: Their excitation and functions. In Handbook of Physiology, Vol. 1, Sec. 6. Edited by C.F. Code. Washington, DC, American Physiological Society, 1967, 225–237.
34. Iggo, A., and Leek, B.F.: Sensory receptors in the ruminant stomach and their reflex effects. In Physiology of Digestion and Metabolism in the Ruminant. Edited by A.T. Phillipson. Newcastle-upon-Tyne, Oriel Press, 1970, pp. 23–34.
35. Thomas, J.E., and Baldwin, M.V.: Pathways and mechanisms of regulation of gastric motility. In Handbook of Physiology, Vol. 4, Sec. 6. Edited by C.F. Code. Washington, DC, American Physiological Society, 1968, 1937–1964.
36. Cervero, F.: Afferent activity evoked by natural stimulation of the biliary system in the ferret. Pain, 13:137, 1982.
37. Janig, W., and Morrison, J.F.B.: Functional properties of spinal visceral afferents supplying abdominal and pelvic organs with special emphasis on visceral nociception. In Visceral Sensation. Edited by F. Cervero and J.E.H. Morrison. Amsterdam, Elsevier, 1986, pp. 87–114.
38. Cervero, F.: Visceral Pain. In Proc. Fifth World Congress on Pain. Edited by R. Dubner, G.F. Gebhart, and M.R. Bond. Amsterdam, Elsevier, 1988, pp. 216–226.
39. Bonica, J.J.: The Management of Pain. Philadelphia, Lea & Febiger, 1953, pp. 730–743.
40. Currie, D.J.: Abdominal Pain. New York, McGraw-Hill, 1979, pp. 77–96, 124–194.
41. Way, L.W.: Abdominal pain in the acute abdomen. In Gastrointestinal Disease: Pathophysiology, Diagnosis, Management. 3rd Ed. Edited by M.H. Sleisenger and J.S. Fordtran. Philadelphia, W.B. Saunders, 1983, pp. 207–221.
42. Mellinkoff, S.M.: The Differential Diagnosis of Abdominal Pain. New York, McGraw-Hill, 1959.

60 · DISEASES OF THE GASTROINTESTINAL TRACT

MICHAEL B. KIMMEY *and* FRED E. SILVERSTEIN

with contributions by
JOHN J. BONICA

PAIN is an important and common symptom of gastrointestinal tract disease. It can be the first indication of a new pathologic process, or it can signify a change in a known condition. The recognition of the pain pattern and its significance is crucial to the early diagnosis and treatment of these problems. The relief of pain is frequently of diagnostic importance and is often the best indicator of successful treatment.

Abdominal pain is a common complaint. One survey of over a million adults selected randomly from the United States population found current complaints of "stomach pain" in 13% and "pain in lower abdomen" in 11% of men and in 17% of women who responded to the questionnaire (1). Because abdominal pain caused by diseases of the gastrointestinal tract can be mimicked by painful conditions of other abdominal and extra-abdominal structures, the evaluation of this symptom often requires physicians to use the full breadth of their medical knowledge.

A patient with abdominal pain of gastrointestinal origin can be completely disabled by this symptom. This disability involves all aspects of the patient's life, including bodily functions, employment, and family relations. These problems can be continuous, as in a patient with unresectable cancer or, more commonly, can be intermittent, as in inflammatory bowel disease or irritable bowel syndrome. The complex interaction between the course of inflammatory bowel disease and psychologic factors is a good example of the importance of the patient's family and social environment (2). Recurrent pain can cause the disruption of employment or family structure; psychosocial influences can affect the activity of the inflammatory bowel disease.

Painful gastrointestinal diseases have a large economic impact as well. For example, irritable bowel syndrome is a leading cause of absence from work, and is the basis of extensive use of diagnostic facilities; drugs for peptic ulcer disease, such as the H_2 receptor blockers, are among the most widely prescribed prescription medications.

In this chapter the diagnostic and therapeutic principles outlined above are applied to painful diseases of the gastrointestinal tract. The information is presented in four sections: A, General Considerations of Diagnosis and Management; B, Diseases of the Stomach and Duodenum; C, Diseases of the Small and Large Intestines; and D, Diseases of the Anus and Rectum. The beginning of each section contains a brief discussion and illustrations of the anatomy and nerve supply of each specific viscus, contributed in part by Bonica. A more detailed discussion of these disorders has been presented by Sleisenger and Fordtran (3).

A. GENERAL CONSIDERATIONS OF DIAGNOSIS AND MANAGEMENT

Patient Evaluation

The management of abdominal pain caused by gastrointestinal disease is based on accurate diagnosis. The history, physical examination, and use of selected laboratory tests and procedures usually yield the correct diagnosis and a list of differential diagnoses, and help to determine further management. The severity and acuteness of pain often determines the pace of further diagnostic testing. This chapter does not discuss extraintestinal or extra-abdominal causes of abdominal pain because they are reviewed elsewhere (4–6) and are presented in other chapters.

History

The character and location of the pain often help to suggest the mechanism of the pain. The location, intensity, rate of onset, quality, duration, frequency, time of day, and relationship to factors that increase or decrease the pain should be determined for each pain described by the patient. The sudden onset of severe pain that does not diminish, for example, is characteristic of a perforated viscus, embolism, torsion, or hemorrhage. Crampy intermittent pain is commonly caused by small intestinal disease, but biliary tract, urinary system, and fallopian tube problems can also cause crampy pain. Pain severity can be a misleading feature because of individual differences in pain perception. Nonetheless, the most severe pains of abdominal origin are caused by intestinal infarction, perforated ulcer, dissecting aortic aneurysm, and ureterolithiasis. Associated symptoms are also useful in diagnosis. Upper gastrointestinal symptoms of nausea, vomiting, anorexia, and bleeding should be sought. Useful lower digestive tract symptoms include diarrhea, constipation, flatulence, and bleeding, as well as stool color and caliber. A review of urinary and gynecologic symptoms should also be obtained. Other systemic symptoms such as weight loss are also helpful.

Physical Examination

Physical examination of the patient with abdominal pain often determines the immediate management course. General examination can reveal signs of increased autonomic activity that are associated with visceral pain, such as flushing, diaphoresis, tachycardia, and mydriasis. Body posture can suggest certain diagnoses. Patients with intestinal, renal, or biliary colic move frequently in an attempt to decrease the pain, often in a writhing fashion; on the other hand, patients with peritonitis lie quietly on their back, usually with knees and hips flexed to reduce pain. Abdominal examination must be thorough and include inspection, auscultation, palpation, percussion, and rectal examination. Signs of peritonitis on examination dictate a more expedient evaluation, usually culminating in surgical exploration of the abdomen.

Laboratory Evaluation

Laboratory evaluation should be directed by the diagnoses suggested by the history and physical examination. Hematocrit, white blood count, and urinalysis are useful and inexpensive tests that are obtained on most patients with abdominal pain. Serum liver function tests (e.g., bilirubin, alanine aminotransferase, alkaline phosphatase), creatinine, and amylase can be useful for excluding diseases of the liver, bile ducts, kidney, and pancreas. Abdominal roentgenograms are useful in the acute setting in patients with moderate or severe abdominal tenderness, after abdominal trauma, and when the clinician suspects bowel obstruction, ischemia, perforation, or renal and biliary calculi (7).

Contrast radiography and fiberoptic endoscopy of the gastrointestinal tract are complementary in the diagnosis of diseases of the stomach, proximal small intestine, and colon (8–11). The choice of test depends on the clinical situation and on local availability and expertise. A recent study comparing upper endoscopy and the double-contrast barium meal in patients with upper gastrointestinal symptoms found endoscopy to be particularly useful in patients who were unable or unwilling to cooperate with the maneuvers required for a radiologic examination (8). Several studies have suggested that endoscopy is more specific and sensitive than roentgenography. Diagnosis of small intestinal disease depends on radiographic examination without the advantages of endoscopic observation. Plain abdominal radiographs, contrast examinations, arteriography, ultrasound, and CT scanning are useful in the diagnosis and management of intestinal causes of abdominal pain (12, 13).

Pathophysiology

Understanding the mechanism of gastrointestinal tract pain is diagnostically useful. Most pain from the gut begins with stimulation of visceral pain receptors. Relatively little is known about the anatomy and physiology of gut pain receptors (4, 14). Mucosal and serosal inflammation, traction on the mesentery, rapid luminal distension, ischemia, and forceful smooth muscle contraction under isometric conditions (i.e., with obstruction distal to the contraction) are known stimulants of these "pain" receptors (14). These receptors are endings of the A-delta and C afferent nerve fibers that accompany the sympathetic nerves from the stomach and small and large intestine, which pass through the celiac plexus and subsidiary plexuses, the splanchnic nerves, the sympathetic chain, and the white rami communicantes and have their cell bodies in dorsal root ganglia of spinal nerves. Pain fibers from the rectum accompany the parasympathetic fibers to the dorsal root ganglia of the S2 to S4 spinal nerves. Central nervous system pathways for visceral afferent (nociceptive) fibers are similar to those of somatic afferent nerves. Cortical areas receiving visceral pain sensations are intermixed with those receiving somatic pain input (Chapter 3).

The characteristics of visceral pain have been described in previous chapters. Visceral pain caused by distension, inflammation, or ischemia of the gut can be a continuous aching or gnawing, or can be of a burning character (15, 16). An intermittent cramping sensation is produced when a strong smooth muscle contraction is the source of pain. Forceful gut contraction can be a result of increased peristalsis without obstruction, as in gastroenteritis, or it can be stimulated by distal mechanical obstruction. Visceral pain is generally poorly localized, is often described as deep within the abdomen, and can be associated with signs of autonomic overactivity. This type of pain is most commonly felt in the midline because most areas of the gut have bilateral spinal connections. Some normal subjects and many patients with the irritable bowel syndrome, however, have lateralizing pain in response to luminal distension (17).

Gastrointestinal diseases cause somatic pain when they involve the parietal peritoneum or the anus. Peritoneal irritation can either be localized or diffuse. When an inflamed organ such as the appendix or a colonic diverticulum touches the peritoneum, a well-localized and usually severe somatic pain is felt by the patient. A perforated ulcer, on the other hand, causes a generalized peritonitis with diffuse severe abdominal pain. Either of these pains is usually aggravated by any movement of the patient. The anal canal is also innervated by somatic nerves, so inflammatory and infiltrating diseases in this area produce a severe localized pain.

Treatment

Management of gastrointestinal pain involves both treatment of the underlying disorder causing the pain and the use of nonspecific pain-relieving measures. Specific treatment of the underlying disease usually leads to improvement of symptoms, which is often the best indicator of successful therapy. On the other hand, use of nonspecific measures such as systemic analgesics and nerve blocks is also an important part of the therapeutic approach to patients with abdominal pain. Nonspecific pain relief is indicated in situations in which specific corrective therapy is not available, such as patients with advanced gastric or colon cancer. Nonspecific pain control measures should also be used for patients with benign disease while they are awaiting specific therapy.

Pain relief is an important part of patient management during therapy for gastrointestinal disease. The selection of nonspecific analgesic measures depends on the severity of pain and on the nature of the underlying disease. Simple measures such as the application of heat or a change in diet are effective in some situations. Potent narcotic analgesics are required in other circumstances. Caution must be exercised, however, in the use of potent analgesics before a diagnosis or specific diagnostic plan is made. Pain might be the only symptom of a significant underlying disease; masking pain could thus delay diagnosis and definitive therapy (18).

Complete pain relief should be a management priority in patients awaiting surgical treatment. The use of adequate quantities of narcotic analgesics to relieve pain should not be deterred by concerns of respiratory depression and addiction. Pain is a powerful respiratory stimulant, and the short-term use of narcotics does not cause psychologic or physical dependence. Pain that is not relieved by parenteral narcotic analgesics can often be managed with subarachnoid or epidural narcotics. Splanchnic and celiac plexus blocks with long-acting local anesthetic agents are also useful in the management of intractable pain while patients are awaiting specific therapy.

B. DISEASES OF THE STOMACH AND DUODENUM

Basic Considerations

Anatomy

An understanding of the anatomy and embryology of the stomach and duodenum is useful in the diagnosis and management of painful diseases of these organs. (Fig. 60-1). The stomach is fixed proximally at its attachment to the distal esophagus, where the esophagus penetrates the diaphragm. This esophagogastric junction is just to the left of midline at the level of the T10 vertebra. The stomach has a variable shape but lies predominantly in the left upper quadrant. The distal end of the stomach crosses the midline at approximately the level of the L1 vertebra and is separated from the duodenum by a band of connective tissue and muscle fibers, which constitute the pyloric sphincter.

The portion of the duodenum proximal to the papilla of Vater originates from the embryonic foregut. The distal duodenum is derived from the midgut and passes posterior and to the left of the midline to become the jejunum at the ligament of Treitz.

Nerve Supply

As in the rest of the gastrointestinal tract, pain receptors in the stomach and duodenum are stimulated by distension, traction, and direct pressure generated by contraction of the muscles of these structures. Local inflammation and ischemia lower the receptor's threshold to nociceptive stimuli. These nociceptive stimuli are transmitted through afferent pathways that accompany the visceral sympathetic fibers through the celiac plexus, the greater splanchnic nerves, the paravertebral sympathetic chain, and the white rami communicantes, and have their cell bodies in dorsal root ganglia of spinal nerves, which in turn transmit the impulse to the dorsal horn of the spinal cord. Nociceptive impulses from the stomach and proximal portion of the duodenum are transmitted primarily through the T6 to T9 roots inclusively, although in some individuals the T5 or T10 root (or both) is also involved (16). Nociceptive impulses from the distal portion of the duodenum are transmitted to the spinal cord through the T8 to T10 spinal nerves, although T11 and, rarely, T12 can also be involved. The nerve supply of the stomach and duodenum is illustrated in Figure 60-2. (Also see Fig. 59-8, page 1159.)

Characteristics of the Pain

Visceral pain originating in the stomach is usually felt in the midepigastric area (15). Gastric diseases that involve the overlying parietal peritoneum can cause pain in the left upper quadrant alone or can be combined with epigastric pain. Diseases of the duodenal bulb cause visceral pain that is usually felt in the epigastrium but occasionally also in the right upper quadrant. Diseases of the distal duodenum cause pain that is usually felt in the periumbilical region.

Clinical Considerations

Anatomic Abnormalities

Most congenital abnormalities of the stomach and duodenum present in infancy or early childhood with symptoms of gastric outlet obstruction. Epigastric pain that is exacerbated by eating and relieved by vomiting is characteristic. Hypertrophic pyloric stenosis is most commonly seen in infants, but can rarely be found in adults who present with vomiting, epigastric pain, and weight loss. Partial or complete duodenal obstruction caused by webs or atresia, malrotation, or an annular

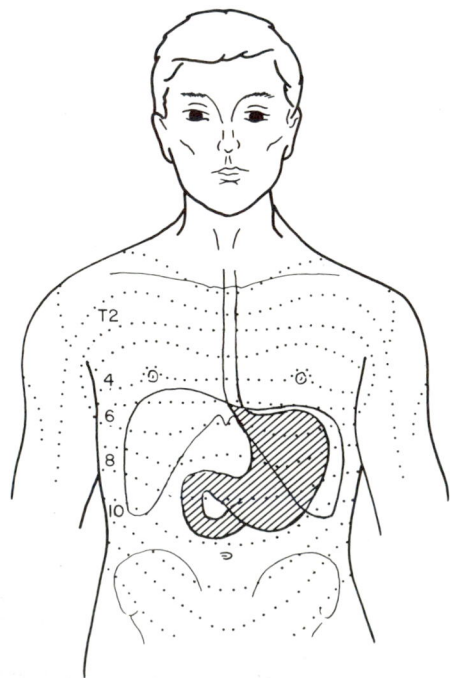

FIG. 60-1. Location of the stomach and duodenum in relationship to the diaphragm and the dermatomes.

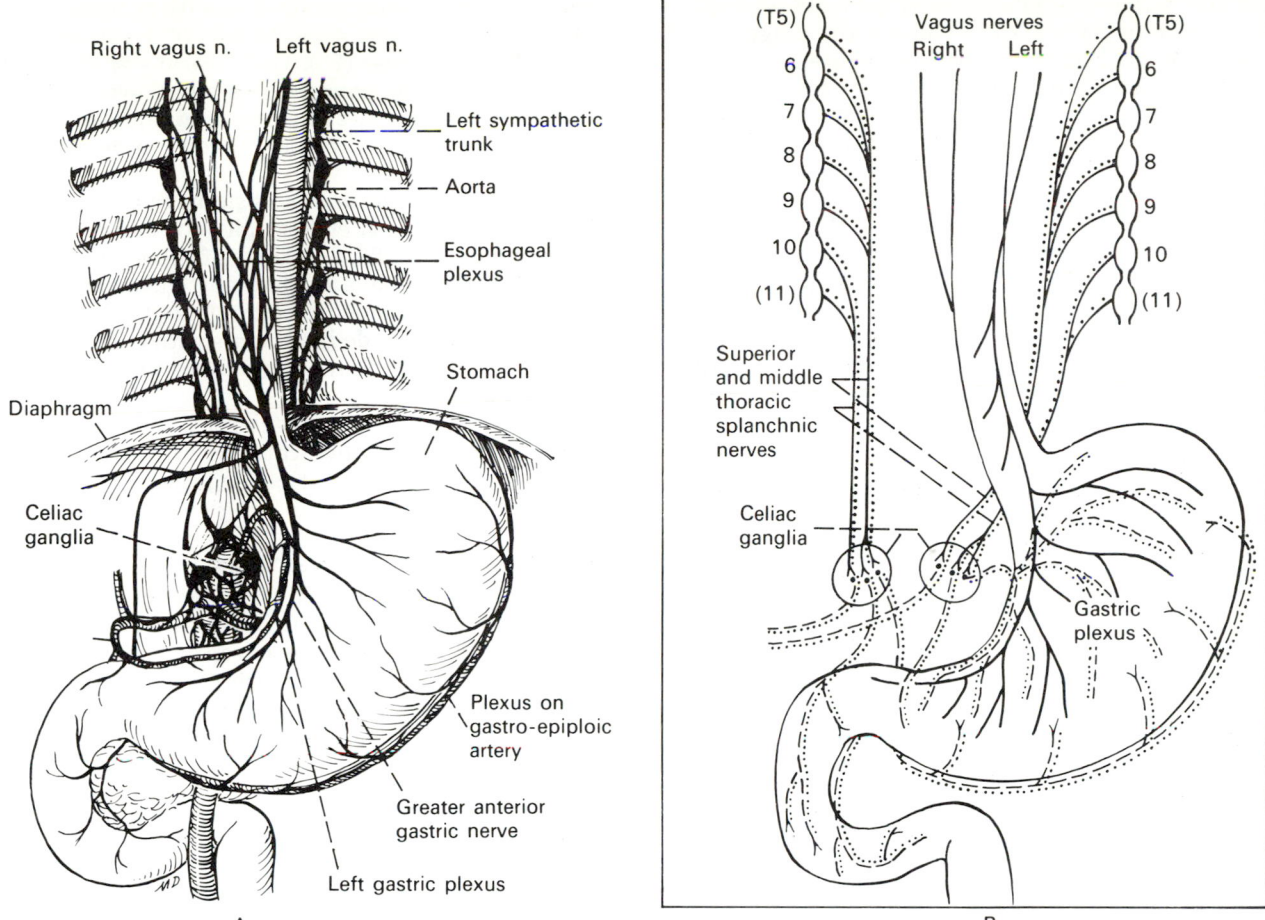

FIG. 60-2. Innervation of the stomach and duodenum. *A.* Relationship of the vagus nerves and the thoracic sympathetic chain and their distribution to the lower esophagus and to the stomach and duodenum. As noted, both vagus nerves continue from the esophagus to the stomach, where the anterior vagus trunk passes along the lesser curvature of the stomach, supplying the anterior surface of this viscus as far as the pylorus. The posterior vagus gives off branches that are distributed to the posterior part of the stomach. Both nerves give off one branch that is greater than the others, and hence are called the greater anterior gastric nerve and greater posterior gastric nerves, respectively. The various gastric branches can be traced for some distance before they sink into the muscle coat, where they synapse with postganglionic parasympathetic neurons. The vagus nerves also give off celiac branches that pass along the left gastric artery and reach the celiac plexus, where they intermingle with sympathetic fibers. Vagal fibers from the celiac branches are distributed to the pylorus and duodenum. Both vagi have afferent fibers that transmit sensory information, except nociception. The sympathetic preganglionic fibers derive from the paravertebral sympathetic chain, pass peripheralward as the superior (greater) thoracic splanchnic nerves, and end in the celiac ganglia, where they synapse with postganglionic neurons. The axons of the latter pass to the stomach and duodenum along the side of the various branches of the celiac and superior mesenteric arteries, around which they form plexuses. These arterial plexuses are comprised mainly of sympathetic efferent and afferent (nociceptive) fibers but also contain some parasympathetic fibers, which, as mentioned above, reach the celiac plexus by way of the celiac branches of the two vagal trunks. The celiac plexus breaks up into subsidiary plexuses that follow the various arteries to the stomach and duodenum to supply these structures. *B.* Innervation of the stomach and duodenum by the vagus nerves and by the segmental sympathetic and sensory nerve supplies. The solid lines for the vagus and sympathetic nerves indicate preganglionic fibers, the dashed lines indicated postganglionic fibers, and dotted lines indicate the nociceptive pathways. The parenthesis for T5 and T11 indicates that these are inconstant segments. Frequently the celiac ganglia are composed of more than two, as shown here. (See Chapter 59 for more details of the origin and relation of these nerve pathways.) Modified from Netter, F.H.: Innervation of the stomach and duodenum. *In* The CIBA Collection of Medical Illustrations, Vol. 3: Digestive System, Pt. 2, The Digestive Tract. West Caldwell, NJ, CIBA Pharmaceutical Co., 1959, pp. 64, 65, and Bonica, J.J.: The Management of Pain. First Ed. Philadelphia, Lea & Febiger, 1953, pp. 395, 397.

pancreas can also present with similar symptoms (19). Treatment by surgical correction of the underlying abnormality is usually successful in these conditions (20).

Gastric diverticula are found on radiographic and endoscopic evaluation of the stomach in less than 0.3% of these examinations. Less than half of these patients have symptoms of epigastric pain that in some is relieved and in others exacerbated by meals. Epigastric fullness and nausea are also common (21). Treatment is rarely indicated unless hemorrhage occurs, in which case surgical resection might be necessary.

Paraesophageal hiatal hernias are caused by a diaphragmatic defect adjacent to the esophagogastric junction, which allows herniation of large portions of the stomach into the thorax. Patients with this disorder often complain of epigastric fullness or mild discomfort. The most feared complication of this anatomic defect is acute gastric volvulus caused by rotation of the stomach on its longitudinal axis (22). Patients with acute gastric volvulus usually present with epigastric pain and forceful vomiting. This diagnosis should be suspected when these symptoms are present and there is difficulty in passing a nasogastric tube. Radiographic contrast examination should confirm the diagnosis of a paraesophageal hiatal hernia and acute gastric volvulus, if present. Emergency surgery is required in the latter situation. Some surgeons recommend elective surgery in all cases of paraesophageal hernia to prevent the development of a volvulus (20, 22).

Gastritis, Duodenitis, and Nonulcer Dyspepsia

Gastritis is a common finding in the general population, but its significance as a cause of abdominal pain is difficult to determine. Symptoms do not always correlate with the histologic and endoscopic findings that are used to define the diagnosis. Serious semantic differences exist in this category of stomach abnormalities. A distinction is made in the following discussion between the erosive and nonerosive forms of gastritis because these can usually be separated by both endoscopic and histologic differences (23). Infectious causes and hypertrophic gastropathy are discussed because these diagnoses can be made on clinical grounds. Patients with upper abdominal symptoms and no histologic or endoscopic evidence of gastritis should be considered to be in the category of nonulcer dyspepsia.

Duodenitis is either an endoscopic diagnosis, characterized by erythema and friability of the duodenal bulb, or a histologic diagnosis made on duodenal biopsies.

Duodenitis does not correlate well with symptoms (24). Duodenitis can in some cases be part of the spectrum of duodenal ulcer disease (25). The clinical significance of duodenitis without symptoms is unknown. Patients with upper abdominal symptoms and endoscopic evidence of duodenitis are considered to be in the category of nonulcer dyspepsia.

Patients with *nonulcer dyspepsia* have upper abdominal symptoms without endoscopic or radiographic evidence of ulceration (26, 27). Some of these patients can have gastritis or duodenitis, but most have normal gastric and duodenal mucosa. Nonulcer dyspepsia is a common diagnosis made in patients with chronic upper abdominal pain, particularly in those under 40 years old (26, 27).

The inter-relationship of gastritis, duodenitis, and nonulcer dyspepsia is illustrated in Figure 60-3. Characteristics of these diagnostic categories are compared in Table 60-1.

Etiology and Pathophysiology

EROSIVE GASTRITIS. Erosive gastritis is seen in association with stressful illnesses such as burns, intracranial diseases, trauma, sepsis, and ingestion of certain drugs, especially aspirin and other nonsteroidal anti-inflammatory agents (NSAIDs) (28). Acute gastric ulcers can be associated. Several pathogenic mechanisms are probably involved in this

TABLE 60-1. Characteristics of Gastritis and Nonulcer Dyspepsia

Condition	Etiology and Pathophysiology	Symptoms					
		Pain					
		Incidence (%)	Site	Quality	Intensity	Rate of Onset	Duration
Acute erosive gastritis	Stressful illness (burns, trauma, sepsis, shock); aspirin and NSAID use	10	Epigastrium	Aching, burning	Mild to moderate	Slow	Intermittent
Chronic erosive gastritis	Hypersensitivity (IgE staining plasma cells in gastric mucosa)	70	Epigastrium	Aching, fullness	Mild to moderate	Slow	Intermittent
Nonerosive gastritis	Infection with Campylobacter pylori; also seen with pernicious anemia and postgastrectomy	Most patients are asymptomatic; small subset with atrophic mucosa develop Vitamin B$_{12}$					
Hypertrophic gastropathy	Unknown cause; large gastric folds with loss of protein through mucosa	75	Epigastrium	Aching, burning	Variable	Slow	Variable
Nonulcer dyspepsia	Acid hypersecretion; motility disturbance sensitivity to distensions; unknown factors	50	Epigastrium; 25%, have back pain	Aching, burning, fullness	Mild	Slow	Intermittent

disorder, including acid production, decreased mucosal blood flow, and alterations in other mucosal defenses, such as surface mucus and local tissue prostaglandin levels. Chronic erosive or varioliform gastritis is rare and can have a hypersensitivity basis, because large quantities of IgE-containing plasma cells are frequently found in the gastric mucosa (29).

NONEROSIVE GASTRITIS. Nonerosive gastritis is a histologic finding that correlates poorly with symptoms and endoscopic findings. This type of gastritis is seen in mucosa surrounding gastric ulcers and has been associated with the presence of a bacterium, Campylobacter pylori, on the mucosal surface (30). Nonerosive gastritis is also seen in patients with pernicious anemia and in patients after gastrectomy. Hypertrophic gastropathy (Menetrier's disease) is a type of nonerosive gastritis of unknown cause characterized by large gastric folds with loss of protein through the gastric mucosa (31). In addition, other bacteria, fungi, and viruses have been associated with the development of gastritis.

NONULCER DYSPEPSIA. Nonulcer dyspepsia is a syndrome of multiple causes (26, 32). One cause of this illness is acid hypersecretion, as in some patients with duodenal ulcer disease. A minority of patients with nonulcer dyspepsia eventually develop a duodenal ulcer. Other possible factors contributing to this syndrome include altered gastric motility and increased sensitivity to gastric distension (32). Some patients with nonulcer dyspepsia have an underlying depression (33).

Symptoms and Signs

Upper gastrointestinal hemorrhage and abdominal pain are the most frequent symptoms in patients with erosive gastritis. Bleeding is the predominant finding in stress-associated gastritis. In the absence of perforation, epigastric pain is present in less than 10% of patients. Pain is more commonly reported when erosive gastritis is caused by aspirin and other NSAIDs than when caused by stress. When pain is present with drug-induced erosive gastritis it is usually epigastric, and is frequently relieved by meals and antacids (34).

Patients with chronic or varioliform erosive gastritis frequently have upper abdominal symptoms (29). Approximately 70% of patients have epigastric pain. Half of these patients obtain relief of pain by eating. Anorexia, nausea, vomiting, and weight loss occur in patients with chronic erosive gastritis.

Most patients with nonerosive gastritis are asymptomatic. A minority of the subset with atrophic mucosa can develop neurologic symptoms caused by vitamin B_{12} deficiency. Paresthesias, loss of sensation, and dementia can be the only complaints because abdominal pain does not occur in this disease. Symptoms of anemia can also be present with vitamin B_{12} deficiency.

and Signs

| Pain Relief | | Other Symptoms | | | | | Diagnosis |
Antacids	Meals	Bleeding	Nausea, Vomiting	Anorexia	Weight Loss	Other	
Yes	Yes	+	+	+	−		Endoscopy and clinical setting
	50% have relief with meals	−	+ +	+ +	+ +	−	Endoscopy or radiology
deficiency that produces neurologic symptoms, paresthesia, hypesthesia, dementia, and symptoms of anemia							Histology, culture for Campylobacter pylori
	Occasional relief with meals	± (occasionally massive)	+ +	+ +	+ +	Edema	Radiology, histology
50%	25%	−	±	±	−	Sometimes clinical depression	Clinical; exclude ulcers on roentgenography or endoscopy

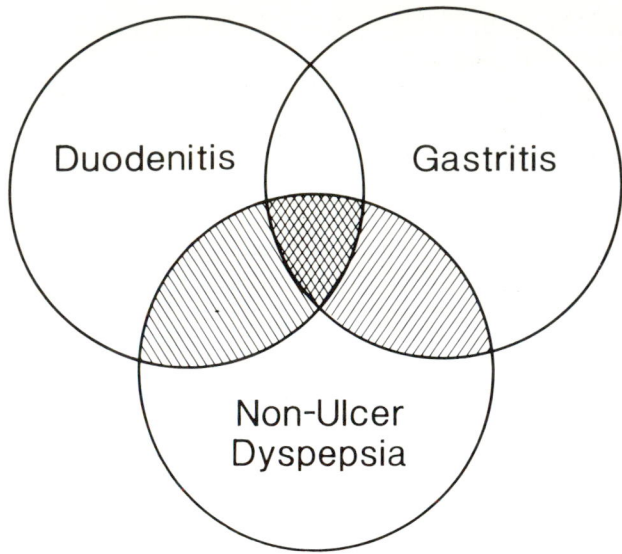

FIG. 60-3. Graphic depiction of the relationship among gastritis, duodenitis, and nonulcer dyspepsias.

Approximately 75% of patients with hypertrophic gastropathy have abdominal pain. This pain is usually epigastric and is occasionally relieved by meals (31). Anorexia, weight loss, and peripheral edema are frequent associated symptoms. Most patients have a long history of abdominal pain before the diagnosis of hypertrophic gastropathy is made.

Over 50% of patients with nonulcer dyspepsia report epigastric pain. In 25% of patients the pain radiates to the back. Episodic pain of longer than 3 years' duration is described by over 90% of patients. Most report no relation of pain to meals but approximately 25% describe some relief with antacids. Nausea is present in most patients whereas weight loss, nocturnal pain, and a change in bowel pattern are uncommon. Symptoms of depression or psychologic tension are frequent. Nonulcer dyspepsia does not cause upper gastrointestinal bleeding.

Diagnosis

The diagnosis of gastritis and nonulcer dyspepsia are usually considered in patients with upper abdominal pain. It is difficult to distinguish among gastric ulcer, duodenal ulcer, and nonulcer dyspepsia by symptoms alone. A therapeutic trial of antacids or an H_2-receptor antagonist can be the most cost-effective approach to this problem. Further diagnostic studies with roentgenography or endoscopy might only be indicated if symptoms persist, increase, or change. Further workup is mandatory in patients whose symptoms suggest complications of peptic ulcer disease. If a diagnostic procedure is required, upper endoscopy is a more sensitive technique for detecting erosive gastritis than radiography. High-quality air contrast barium radiography, however, usually excludes significant gastric and duodenal ulcerations and a gastric mass (8). Endoscopic mucosal biopsy is required for the diagnosis of nonerosive gastritis (23). The presence of this histologic finding, however, is not clinically significant and does not affect management.

Other diagnostic tests might be required in patients with atypical symptoms or if diagnosis is unclear after an endoscopy or roentgenography. Patients with low serum albumin levels, and large folds on radiographic or endoscopic examination, can require a surgical full-thickness gastric biopsy to diagnose hypertrophic gastropathy. Dyspeptic symptoms can be similar to those caused by cholecystitis. If symptoms are persistent and troublesome, abdominal ultrasonography should be used to look for gallstones.

Treatment

The objectives of therapy of acute and chronic erosive gastritis are pain relief and the prevention of complications. Antacids and cimetidine have been shown to prevent the development of acute erosive gastritis and ulceration in patients with serious underlying disease if the intragastric pH is kept above 3.5. Use of these agents to treat erosions is less successful but is generally attempted. Patients with erosive gastritis caused by aspirin and other NSAIDs should stop taking these drugs if possible. When this type of medication must be continued, enteric-coated aspirin can be less harmful to the gastric mucosa (34). Cimetidine (Tagamet), 1 g/day, and sodium chromoglycate, 200 mg/day, have been reported to be effective in the treatment of chronic erosive and varioliform gastritis (35).

Patients with hypertrophic gastropathy can do well for years without therapy (31). If pain or hypoalbuminemia from gastric protein loss is disabling, relief can be obtained with gastrectomy. Patients with infectious gastritis should be treated with specific antimicrobial agents whenever possible.

The treatment of nonulcer dyspepsia is not well defined and is frequently unsuccessful. Therapy must be individualized and directed toward the patient's most troublesome symptoms (36). Cimetidine (Tagamet), 1 g/day, can decrease pain in some patients with nonulcer dyspepsia, but a controlled trial has failed to show significant benefit over the use of placebo (37). Antacids and sucralfate (Carafate) are also frequently tried. Metoclopramide (Reglan), 10 mg before each meal, can enhance gastric emptying and benefit patients with early satiety. Tricyclic antidepressant medication is useful in patients with chronic pain who have symptoms of depression. Nonulcer dyspepsia can be chronic and is not associated with decreased longevity. Therefore, any treatment attempted should be monitored and stopped if side effects occur. Systemic analgesics are never indicated for treatment of this category of gastric disorders.

Peptic Ulcer Disease (XXI-4, 5)*

Ulceration of the stomach and duodenum constitutes one of the most important diseases of the gastrointestinal tract. Because it results in significant pain and a high morbidity rate, it is a leading cause of health care expenditures. It was estimated that in 1975 four million people in the United States had ulcers, with a resulting cost of medical care and time lost from work of approximately 2.7 billion dollars. New diagnostic and therapeutic techniques have contributed to this expense but have also dramatically changed the management of

*IASP code ref.—see Chapter 2.

TABLE 60-2. Characteristics of Gastric Ulcer, Duodenal Ulcer, and Non-Ulcer Dyspepsia

Characteristic	Condition		
	Gastric Ulcer	Duodenal Ulcer	Nonulcer Dyspepsia
Etiology			
Hyperacidity	±	+ +	±
Impaired mucosal defense	+ +	+	−
Stress	+ +	+	±
Aspirin/NSAIDs	+ +	+	±
Tumor	<5%	Rare	−
Symptomatology			
Pain			
Incidence	75%	75%	50%
Site	Epigastrium	Epigastrium RUQ	Epigastrium
Radiation to back	25%	25%	25%
Intensity			
Severe	+ +	+	±
Mild/moderate	+	+	+ +
Rate of onset	Gradual	Gradual	Gradual
Quality	Burning, aching	Burning, aching	Burning, aching
Nocturnal	+	+ +	±
Pain Relief			
Antacids	+	+ +	+
Foods	±	+ +	±
Other Symptoms			
Nausea/vomiting	+ +	+	+
Anorexia	+ +	+	+
Heartburn	+	+ +	+
Bloating/belching	+	+	+

patients with ulcers over the last 10 years. Gastric and duodenal ulcers are considered together here because of similarities in symptoms, diagnostic approaches, and therapies. These two types of ulcer disease are compared to nonulcer dyspepsia in Table 60-2.

Etiology and Pathophysiology

An ulcer is a localized loss of the normal gastric or duodenal mucosa. Granulation tissue and inflammatory exudate are found in the base of an ulcer, overlying the submucosal layer of the gastrointestinal wall (Fig. 60-4). Ulcers are formed because of an imbalance between aggressive factors such as acid and defensive factors that usually protect against mucosal damage (38). The role of gastric acid in the pathogenesis of peptic ulcer disease is widely appreciated. Excessive acid can be present in absolute terms, as in the Zollinger-Ellison syndrome, in which a gastrin-producing tumor causes a marked increase in gastric acid production, or the acid might only be increased relative to the ability of the gastric or duodenal mucosa to protect itself. Acid is clearly linked to duodenal ulcer production, and is also an important factor in the development of gastric ulcers. If no acid is present no gastric ulcer is formed although most patients with gastric ulcer have acid secretory rates that are normal or less than normal. Interestingly, intragastric infusion of acid reproduces ulcer pain in only a minority of duodenal ulcer patients (39).

Factors other than acid are also involved in the pathogenesis of gastric and duodenal ulcers. Psychologic and genetic factors have been implicated in the development of ulcers (40). In addition, the importance of local mechanisms in protecting both the gastric and duodenal mucosa from the harmful effects of acid and pepsin is now better appreciated. Regional blood flow, mucus and bicarbonate production, and local prostaglandins are probably all important in this mucosal defense (38).

Environmental influences can also be involved in the pathogenesis of peptic ulcers. Ingestion of aspirin and NSAIDs has been associated with the development of both gastric and duodenal ulcers (28). Smoking has been linked epidemiologically to the development of duodenal ulcers and is responsible for an increased rate of ulcer relapse after therapy is stopped (41, 42).

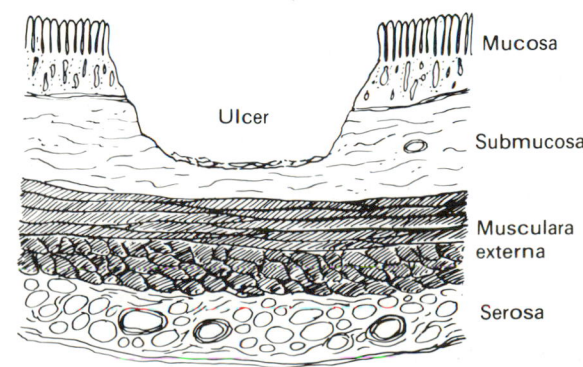

FIG. 60-4. Schematic diagram of a peptic ulcer.

Symptoms and Signs

Symptoms alone do not differentiate reliably among the diagnoses of duodenal ulcer, gastric ulcer, and nonulcer dyspepsia. Only minor differences in symptoms are seen in patients with these problems (26, 27) (Table 60-2). In all these diseases pain is most often felt in the epigastrium, although right upper quadrant pain is seen in some patients with duodenal ulcer and left upper quadrant pain can be seen with gastric ulcer (Fig. 60-5). The pain is variously described as gnawing or burning, and a sense of fullness is common. Radiation of pain to the back occurs in 20 to 30% of patients. Pain relief by food or antacid is described by half of patients with a duodenal ulcer and by less of those with gastric ulcer and nonulcer dyspepsia. Pain that awakens the patients at night is more frequently seen with duodenal ulcer disease. Nausea, vomiting, heartburn, and anorexia are reported in a significant number of patients with these diseases. Although patients with gastric ulcer tend to be older and patients with nonulcer dyspepsia have milder degrees of pain, these findings do not help to distinguish among these diagnoses in an individual patient. Patients with ulcers associated with NSAID consumption are often asymptomatic until they present with a complication (43).

Symptoms also correlate imperfectly with ulcer healing (44). Patients who become asymptomatic can still have an ulcer crater approximately 15% of the time. Furthermore, two-thirds of patients who are still symp-tomatic after a 6-week course of antacid therapy are found to have healing of their ulcer at endoscopy.

Bleeding, perforation, penetration, obstruction, and intractable pain are the most common complications of peptic ulcer disease. Gastrointestinal bleeding, presenting either as melena or hematemesis, complicates peptic ulcer disease in 10 to 20% of patients. Bleeding can be associated with pain or it can be the first and only manifestation of the ulcer. Approximately 5% of patients with ulcers experience perforation.

Perforation presents with the sudden onset of severe epigastric pain that quickly spreads to involve the entire abdomen as peritonitis ensues. If a duodenal ulcer perforates and partially seals it can present as right lower quadrant pain because of the accumulation of gastric contents in the right paracolic gutter.

Penetration of a duodenal or gastric ulcer into the pancreas, adjacent omentum, or hepatobiliary system is usually suspected if the patient has severe continuous pain that resists medical therapy. Radiation of pain to the back occurs in over half of patients with posterior penetration. Somatic pain with a radicular quality is also frequently described in this situation, probably because of inflammation of retroperitoneal structures.

Gastric outlet obstruction should be suspected in patients with ulcers who develop frequent vomiting, particularly if the vomiting occurs at night or if the emesis contains food residue eaten several hours earlier. Patients who develop pyloric obstruction frequently have a long history of ulcer pain that has recently changed character. With the onset of obstruction, pain can become more continuous and be relieved by vomiting. Intractable pain can be caused by penetration or by inadequate therapeutic regimen.

Symptoms follow surgery for peptic ulcer disease in 10 to 50% of patients, depending on the type of operation and the population studied (45). Abdominal pain, diarrhea, vasomotor phenomena, vomiting, weight loss, anemia, and metabolic bone disease are the most commonly encountered problems. Abdominal pain caused by alkaline reflux gastritis is usually a continuous burning pain, often similar to the initial ulcer pain, and frequently exacerbated by eating. Antacids do not relieve the pain. Vomiting of bitter bile-stained material is frequently described. Crampy or steady epigastric pain occurring 30 to 60 minutes after eating and associated with flushing, diaphoresis, and lightheadedness is referred to as the "dumping" syndrome. Other considerations in the patient with chronic postoperative pain are recurrent ulceration, obstruction of the gastric outlet, and malfunction of the afferent loop in a patient with a Billroth II anastomosis.

Diagnosis

Physical findings and laboratory tests are often not specific for peptic ulcer disease. For example, epigastric tenderness is found just as frequently in patients with ulcers as in those without ulcers (46). The serum amylase level is normal in patients with peptic ulcer disease but is elevated if the ulcer has penetrated into the pancreas. The serum gastrin level should be measured in patients with multiple ulcers, recurrent ulcers, or when ulcers are present in the distal duodenum, or are refractory to medical or surgical therapy, because

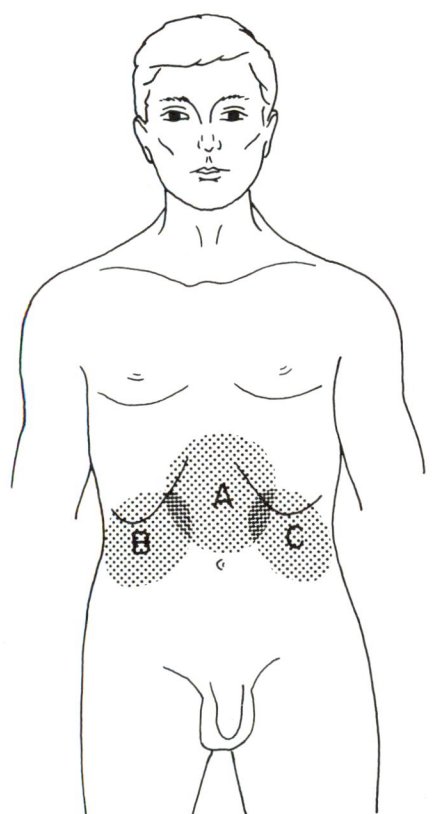

FIG. 60-5. Locations of referred pain from peptic ulcer. Most commonly, the pain is referred to the epigastrium (**A**). In some patients the pain of duodenal ulcer is referred to the right upper quadrant (**B**) or left upper quadrant in patients with gastric ulcer (**C**).

this picture suggests Zollinger-Ellison syndrome (ZES).*

Demonstration of an ulcer requires radiographic contrast examination or endoscopy. Contrast examinations are less expensive but endoscopy is more sensitive and has the capability of biopsy. Patients generally prefer roentgenography. The choice of tests often depends on the quality and local availability of these two procedures.

Patients with gastric ulcers should have follow-up roentgenography or endoscopy to document complete healing because a gastric cancer can present as a benign-appearing ulcer. Many think that all gastric ulcers should be examined endoscopically, with six to eight biopsies of the rim and brush cytology taken. Nonhealing gastric ulcers and those ulcers that have a suspicious appearance on initial examination should be re-examined and rebiopsied to exclude malignancy.

Postgastrectomy syndromes should be considered in all patients with upper abdominal pain and a history of gastric surgery. A diagnosis of dumping or alkaline reflux gastritis is often based on the characteristic clinical presentation. Recurrent ulceration is best detected by endoscopy because postsurgical changes make radiographic findings difficult to interpret. On the other hand, gastric and afferent loop obstruction are best demonstrated radiographically.

Treatment

MEDICAL THERAPY. The mainstay of therapy for both gastric and duodenal ulcers has been acid neutralization. Antacids have been shown to heal 80 to 90% of both gastric and duodenal ulcers in 6 to 12 weeks (47, 48). Liquid antacid preparations should be taken 1 hour after each meal and at bedtime in a dose of 15 to 30 mL. Combinations of magnesium and aluminum hydroxides are best tolerated. If diarrhea occurs, one of these preparations should be alternated with an antacid containing only aluminum hydroxide. Exclusive use of calcium carbonate should probably be avoided because of rebound acid hypersecretion. The H_2-receptor antagonists cimetidine (Tagamet) and ranitidine (Zantac) are alternatives to antacids because they are equally effective (47, 49). The recommended dose of cimetidine is 400 mg twice daily. Alternatively, ranitidine should be taken twice daily in a dose of 150 mg. Confusion, particularly in the elderly, bone marrow suppression, gynecomastia, and azoospermia are infrequently reported side effects of cimetidine. Ranitidine is associated with fewer of these side effects, but experience with the use of this drug is not as extensive as that with cimetidine, and side effects do occur with ranitidine (49). Both drugs generally are effective and well tolerated.

Agents that bind to ulcers have also been shown to promote healing. Sucralfate (Carafate) is the only one of these drugs presently available in the United States. Given in a dose of 1 g qid, sucralfate is as effective as cimetidine for healing duodenal ulcers (42, 50). Constipation is an infrequent side effect of sucralfate. Sucralfate should not be taken at the same time as other medications to avoid interference with absorption of the other drugs.

Aspirin, other NSAIDs, and alcohol should be avoided by patients with ulcers. Other dietary limitations are not associated with improved healing. Patients should be encouraged not to smoke, because smoking impairs ulcer healing (42). Avoidance of unnecessary stress is always commendable, but too much emphasis on this aspect cannot be recommended on the basis of available information concerning the effects of stress on ulcer formation and healing.

Patients with the ZES should have resection of the gastrin-producing tumor if it is found and has not spread (51). Acid secretion and ulcer pain can be controlled with cimetidine when surgical resection is not possible. Cimetidine dosages 2.5 to 5 g/day might be required. Anticholinergic drugs such as propantheline bromide (Pro-Banthine), 15 mg qid, or glycopyrrolate (Robinul), 1 mg qid, in addition to cimetidine might be required if cimetidine alone is ineffective. Total gastrectomy should be reserved for patients with ZES who have continued ulceration despite maximum medical therapy.

SURGICAL THERAPY. Surgery for peptic ulcer disease is most often recommended for patients who have persistent pain despite maximum medical management. Other indications for surgery include persistent bleeding, obstruction, penetration, and perforation. Parietal cell vagotomy by a surgeon experienced in this procedure is the operation of choice for intractable pain. Dumping, diarrhea, and alkaline reflux gastritis are all less frequent with this operation, although recurrent ulcers are more common than with other ulcer surgery and occur in 5 to 10% of patients. Vagotomy with pyloroplasty, and vagotomy with antrectomy and either gastroduodenostomy or gastrojejunostomy, are alternative ulcer operations. Repeat surgery might be needed for complications of severe alkaline reflux gastritis or for obstruction of surgical anastomoses.

All patients with ulcer pain should be managed with the medical and surgical treatments outlined above. Antacids, and acetaminophen if necessary, generally provide sufficient pain relief during the healing phase. Narcotic analgesics or anesthetic blocks should be used in patients with severe pain caused by perforation or penetration after diagnosis has been made and surgery is planned. Patients should not be left in pain while awaiting surgery.

Neoplasms of the Stomach

Gastric cancer is a leading cause of cancer deaths worldwide. Adenocarcinoma accounts for over 80% of malignant gastric neoplasms, lymphoma and leiomyosarcoma making up the remainder. Although the incidence of gastric cancer is decreasing in the United States, this malignancy remains a cause of upper abdominal pain and a therapeutic challenge to physicians (see Table 59-3, p. 1149 for 1987 estimates used). A monograph on most aspects of gastric neoplasms is available (52).

Etiology and Pathophysiology

Both environmental and genetic factors have significant roles in the pathogenesis of gastric cancer.

---

*ZES is characterized by the presence of upper gastrointestinal ulcer, marked increase in secretion of gastrin, and a non-beta islet cell tumor of the pancreas, known as a gastrinoma.

Dietary salt and nitrates have been linked epidemiologically to gastric cancer. An increased incidence of gastric cancer occurs in patients with pernicious anemia, chronic atrophic gastritis, and large adenomatous gastric polyps (52).

Symptoms and Signs

Patients with early gastric cancer can be asymptomatic or can have vague epigastric pain or a sensation of fullness. Pain can be similar to the pain of gastric ulcer. Weight loss, anorexia, vomiting and occult or overt gastrointestinal bleeding can be present. Local invasion can cause pancreatitis, gastrocolic fistulas, or severe continuous abdominal or back pain. Metastases from gastric cancer can be responsible for ascites, pleural effusions, or jaundice. Physical examination reveals an epigastric mass, enlarged liver, or ascites, or enlarged supraclavicular, axillary, or umbilical lymph nodes (52).

Diagnosis

A combination of diagnostic procedures is used in the detection of gastric cancer. Upper gastrointestinal roentgenography can reveal a mass or suspicious ulcer. Gastroscopy provides direct visualization and an opportunity to biopsy an ulcer or mass lesion and to brush it for cytology. Biopsies and brushings for cytology should be taken of gastric ulcers and of any irregular-appearing mucosas. Diffuse carcinomatous involvement of the stomach wall ("linitus plastica") and lymphoma sometimes requires an open surgical biopsy for diagnosis. CT scanning is currently the most useful nonsurgical method for determining the degrees of local extension and for detection of metastatic spread.

Treatment

CANCER THERAPY. Treatment of gastric cancer usually includes surgery and chemotherapy (53). Patients who have no evidence of spread of the neoplasm outside the stomach should have a subtotal gastrectomy and lymph node dissection. Palliative surgery is also indicated for luminal obstruction and hemorrhage. Adjuvant chemotherapy with 5-fluorouracil and nitrosourea compounds has been shown to lengthen survival of patients who have undergone potentially curative surgery (54). Patients with locally advanced or metastatic disease can benefit from chemotherapy using combinations of the above compounds with adriamycin and mitomycin C. Radiotherapy has not been useful in the treatment of locally advanced gastric cancer, but can relieve pain caused by metastases to bone.

PAIN THERAPY. The treatment of severe pain in patients with advanced inoperable gastric cancer is a significant problem and challenge, and is discussed in detail in Chapter 24. Both visceral and somatic pain mechanisms are usually involved because of abdominal wall or retroperitoneal invasion. For such patients available therapies include narcotic analgesics, orally or parenterally, intraspinal narcotics, block of the splanchnic nerves or celiac plexus alone or combined with intracostal block, neurostimulation techniques, and ablative neurosurgical operations. Two or more of these techniques are frequently used to provide relief.

Pain can be controlled in most patients with maximum life expectancy of less than 3 months by appropriate use of narcotic analgesics PO. In patients with mild to moderate pain, NSAIDs are used initially and, if necessary, can be combined with codeine or more potent narcotics such as morphine. Regularly scheduled oral administration of a pain cocktail containing methadone is often effective. A dose of 10 mg every 8 hours is prescribed initially but must then be titrated to the patient's needs. The addition of hydroxyzine (25 to 50 mg/ 6 h) or prochlorperazine to the cocktail is useful for the treatment of nausea and vomiting, which is frequent in these patients. Moreover, hydroxyzine potentiates the analgesic action of narcotics. Intraspinal narcotics are increasingly being used and are effective in many of these advanced cancer patients.

Neurolytic blocks are used for the management of a subset of patients with advanced gastric cancer associated with severe pain. This therapy is usually reserved for situations in which the overall condition of the patient is fairly good and the pain is localized and severe. Significant pain relief has been reported in over 90% of patients with gastric cancer who have had bilateral celiac plexus block with 50% alcohol solution (55) (Chapter 96). Pain relief often lasts for months following this procedure. Recurrent pain sometimes responds to repeated injections but, when these fail, extension of the cancer to the peritoneum or abdominal wall is likely. This requires neurolytic blocks of the involved intracostal nerves. Neurolytic blocks are often combined with pharmacologic therapy or psychologic techniques or both.

Neurostimulation techniques that can be used in patients with severe pain caused by stomach cancer include dorsal column stimulation or deep brain stimulation (Chapter 93).

Neurosurgical procedures are sometimes used for the treatment of severe intractable pain in patients with advanced gastric cancer (56). These procedures should be used when life expectancy is greater than 3 months and when pharmacologic therapy is not effective or is associated with unacceptable side effects (see Chapters 24, 98, and 99 for more detailed discussions of these techniques).

C. DISEASES OF THE SMALL AND LARGE INTESTINES

Basic Considerations

Anatomy

The small intestine begins at the distal end of the stomach, the pyloroduodenal junction, and ends as it joins the colon at the ileocecal valve. The proximal 10 inches of small bowel comprises the duodenum (this was discussed above, with the stomach, because of similarities in the clinical presentation of diseases of these two organs). The remainder of the small intestine, suspended on its mesentery, is approximately 10 feet long and occupies most of the abdomen (see Fig. 60-6).

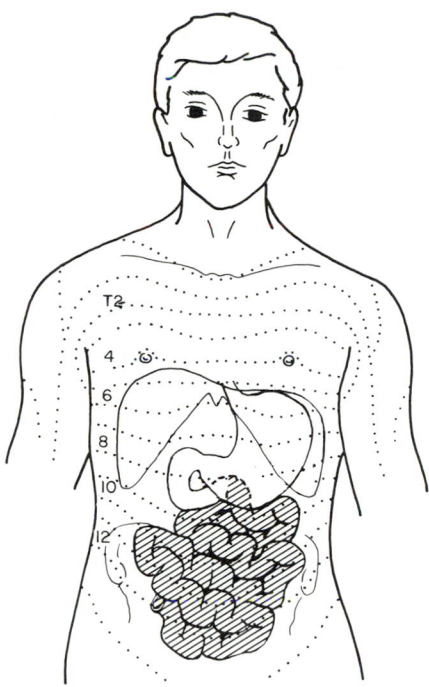

FIG. 60-6. Location of the small intestine in relationship to the dermatomes.

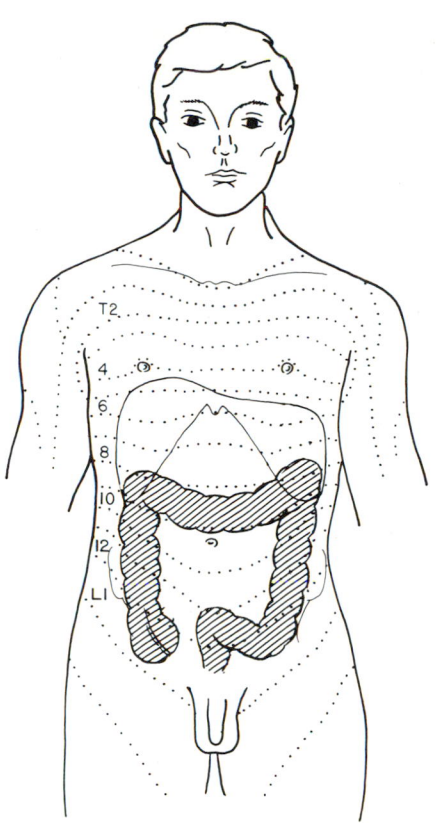

FIG. 60-7. Location of the large intestine in relationship to the diaphragm and the dermatomes.

The large intestine, or colon, begins at the ileocecal valve and ends at the anus. The cecum is the most proximal aspect of the colon and usually lies in the right lower quadrant. The ascending and descending portions of the colon do not have a mesentery and are relatively fixed in the retroperitoneum. The transverse colon has a mesentery and can form variable-sized loops across the midabdominal cavity. The sigmoid colon also has a mesentery and can stretch to a great length, particularly in the elderly. The rectum, which is fixed in the retroperitoneum, forms the most distal 12 to 15 cm of large intestine. Some disease processes of the distal rectum are clinically similar to anal diseases (see below). The position of the small and large intestines within the abdomen are shown in Figures 60-6 and 60-7.

The embryologic development of the intestine accounts for some of the abnormalities encountered clinically. During normal fetal development the small bowel is transiently occluded by proliferating epithelial cells. Defective recanalization can result in the formation of gut duplications, cysts, and webs, which all can cause problems subsequently. Another embryologic remnant that might be clinically relevant later in life is a Meckel's diverticulum, which forms at the junction of the primitive gut and the vitelline duct. This diverticulum often contains gastric mucosa and can cause abdominal pain and intestinal bleeding.

Nerve Supply

Visceral sensation, including pain from the jejunum and ileum, is carried by sympathetic afferent nerves through the least and lesser splanchnic nerves, and from there through the superior mesenteric and part of the celiac plexuses to enter the spinal cord at the T8 to T12 levels (Fig. 60-8). Sensation from the cecum,

ascending colon, and right half of the transverse colon is carried by sympathetic afferent fibers that pass through the least and lesser splanchnic nerves, and from these through the inferior mesenteric and superior mesenteric plexuses to enter the spinal cord at the T10 to L2 levels. Pain sensation from the left half of the transverse colon and from the descending colon and rectum is mediated by afferent fibers; some of these accompany sympathetic fibers to the lower thoracic and lumbar sympathetic trunks and others course with the parasympathetic nerves through the pelvic plexus and pelvic nerves (nervi erigentes) and then enter the spinal cord at the S2 to S4 levels (Figs. 60-8 and 60-9). In a few persons afferent sensation can also be carried by the vagus nerve because midgut visceral pain can be felt after spinal cord transection above T1 as well as after bilateral splanchnic nerve resection (18).

Characteristics of the Pain

Pain from the small intestine is usually felt as a periumbilical cramp or colic. This pain can be triggered by luminal distension or by excessive motor activity. In patients with functional abdominal pain, experiments with balloon distension of the jejunum and ileum produced pain that was felt in various quadrants of the abdomen by different patients (15, 57, 58). Steady visceral pain can be caused by intestinal distension or ischemia. Inflammatory and infiltrative processes that extend to the parietal peritoneum can cause localized somatic pain from the involved area of peritoneum. Traction on the root of the mesentery can cause a

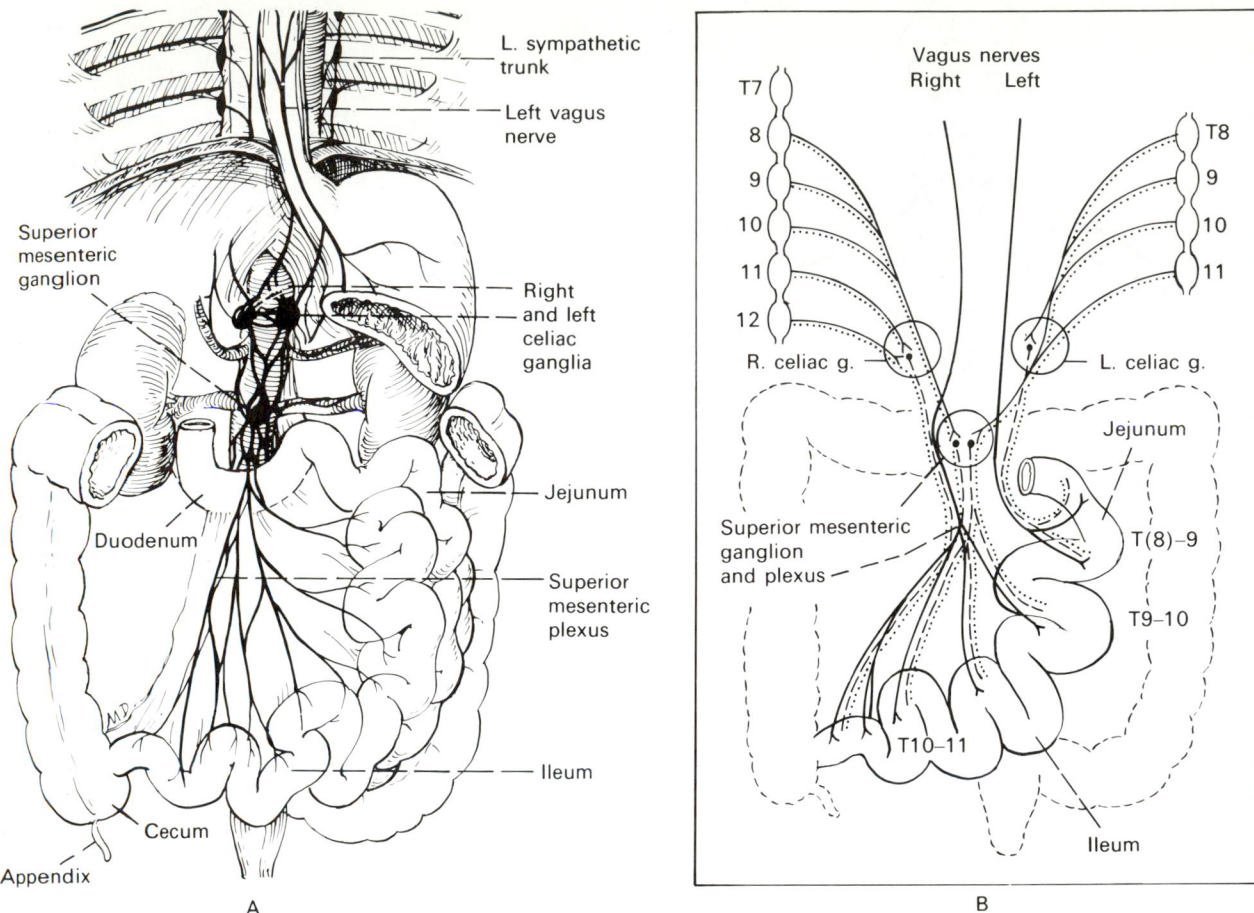

FIG. 60-8. Innervation of the small intestine. **A.** Relationship of the vagus nerves, sympathetic trunk, celiac ganglia, superior mesenteric ganglion, and superior mesenteric plexus supplying the small intestine. **B.** Schematic depiction of the nerve supply to the small intestine. The vagus nerves supply the small intestine with parasympathetic preganglionic fibers, which end in the wall of the gut and synapse with short postganglionic fibers. These also contain sensory fibers that convey sensations other than nociception. The small intestine received sympathetic supplies through preganglionic sympathetic fibers (*solid lines*) derived from T8 to T12 on the right and T8 to T11 on the left. These synapse in the celiac and superior mesenteric ganglia with postganglionic fibers (*dashed lines*). Sensory fibers, which transmit nociceptive information (*dotted lines*), follow the sympathetic nerves and enter the spinal cord at T8 to T12 on the right and T8 to T11 on the left. The segments that supply sympathetic and sensory fibers to different parts of the small intestine are indicated by numbers. The segments in parentheses in the sympathetic chain are inconstant. (For more detailed information of the origin and course of these nerve pathways, see Chapter 59.) Modified from Netter, F.H.: Innervation of the small intestine. *In* The CIBA Collection of Medical Illustrations, Vol. 3, Digestive System, P. 2, Lower Digestive Tract, Summit, NJ, CIBA Pharmaceutical Co., 1979, pp. 76–79, and Bonica, J.J.: Management of Pain. 1st Ed. Philadelphia, Lea & Febiger, 1953, pp. 395, 397.

similar type of somatic pain but usually produces a periumbilical visceral type of pain (59) (Fig. 60-10).

Distension of the ascending and right half of the transverse colon generally causes periumbilical pain, although a significant number of patients also have suprapubic pain. Because the right colon is fixed to the retroperitoneum, severe distension causes right-sided pain, similar to that of infiltrating and inflammatory processes. Stimulation of somatic nerves in the underlying peritoneum is the probable mechanism of this type of pain.

Distension of the left half of the transverse colon and descending colon usually produces pain in the midline below the umbilicus and in the suprapubic region. Severe distension causes left-sided pain localized over the region of distension. Sigmoid colon lesions that involve the overlying peritoneum can cause right lower

quadrant, suprapubic, or left lower quadrant pain because of the long mesentery from which the sigmoid colon is suspended, which enables it to touch a wide area of abdominal wall. The common positions of referred pain from the small and large intestines are shown in Figure 60-10.

Clinical Considerations

Anatomic Abnormalities

Etiology and Pathophysiology

Most congenital anatomic derangements of the intestine that cause abdominal pain do so by producing luminal obstruction. Incomplete canalization of the gut lumen or in utero ischemia can cause atresia or stenosis of any part of the intestine. Failure of the intestine

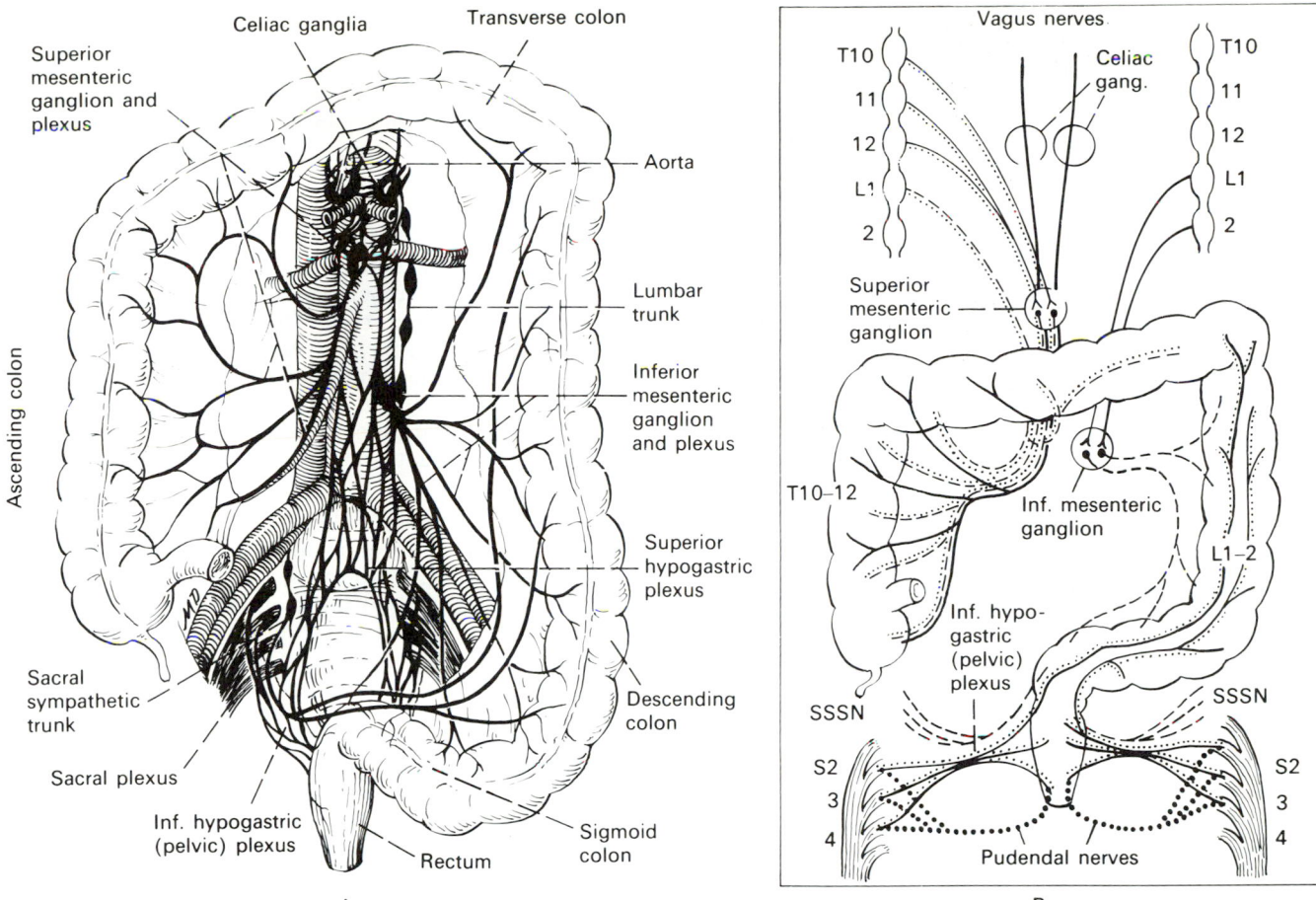

FIG. 60-9. Innervation of the large intestine. **A.** Anatomic relationship of the nerves supplying various parts of the colon and rectum. **B.** Schematic depiction of the innervation by the vagus, sympathetic, and sensory fibers. The right and transverse colon up to the splenic flexure is supplied by preganglionic parasympathetic fibers of the vagus nerves, which synapse in the wall of the viscus with short postganglionic fibers. The sympathetic supply is through preganglionic fibers derived from T10 to T12 (*solid lines*), which synapse with postganglionic fibers (*dashed lines*) in the superior mesenteric ganglion. This portion of the gut also receives postganglionic fibers derived from the L1 ganglion. This part of the colon is supplied by sensory (nociceptive) fibers that accompany the sympathetic nerves and enter the spinal cord at T10 to L1 inclusively. The descending colon receives preganglionic sympathetic fibers from L1 to L2, which synapse in the inferior mesenteric ganglion with the postganglionic fibers that supply the viscus as far as the sigmoid colon. Postganglionic sympathic fibers to the rest of the colon from the rectosigmoid junction and rectum are derived from sacral sympathetic splanchnic nerves (SSSN), which are derived from the sacral portion of the sympathetic chain. The descending colon is supplied with parasympathetic preganglionic fibers, which originate in spinal cord segments S2, S3, and S4 and pass through the inferior hypogastric (pelvic plexus) and from there to the colon and rectum, where they end in the wall of the viscus and synapse with short postganglionic fibers. The sensory fibers that conduct nociceptive impulses accompany the parasympathetic nerves and enter the spinal cord in the S2, S3, and S4 segments. Sensory supply to the rectum is through the pudendal nerve. (See Chapter 59 for a more detailed description of the origin and course of these nerve pathways.) Modified from Netter, F.H.: Innervation of the small intestine. *In* The CIBA Collection of Medical Illustrations, Vol. 3, Digestive System, P. 2, Lower Digestive Tract. Summit, NJ, CIBA Pharmaceutical Co., 1979, pp. 76–79, and Bonica, J.J.: The Management of Pain, 1st Ed. Philadelphia, Lea & Febiger, 1953, pp. 395, 397.

to rotate on its mesentery when it re-enters the abdomen in the second trimester can result in malrotation of various portions of the bowel. Malrotation can be present without any symptoms. Pain is produced by this anomaly only if intestinal obstruction results from internal herniation or formation of a volvulus. Meckel's diverticula are embryologic remnants of the connection of the vitelline duct and terminal ileum. Intestinal obstruction can be induced by these diverticula either by formation of a volvulus or by intussusception. An ulcer can occur in the diverticulum if ectopic gastric mucosa is present.

Symptoms and Signs

Symptoms caused by anatomic abnormalities of the gut are similar to those produced by other causes of intestinal obstruction (see below, Intestinal Obstruction). Most congenital abnormalities present in infancy or early childhool. Occasionally, symptoms of these disorders first appear in adults. Therefore, these anomalies should be considered in the differential diagnosis of abdominal pain in adults as well as in children.

Continuous burning or aching abdominal pain can also be caused by anatomic defects. Intestinal

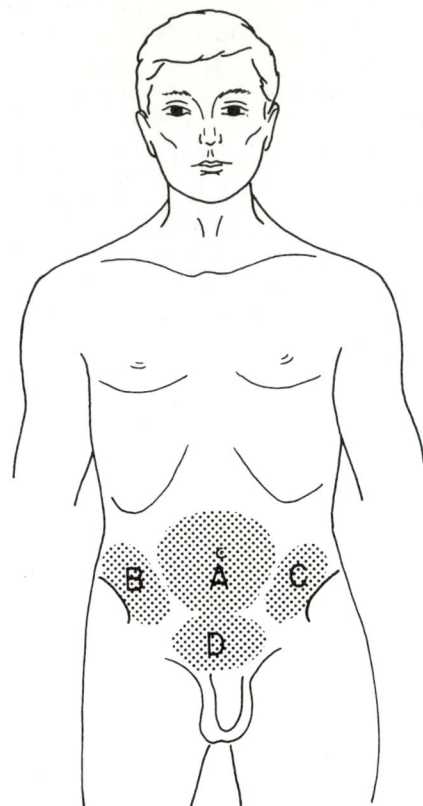

FIG. 60-10. Sites of referred pain from diseases of the small and large intestine. Periumbilical pain (**A**) is caused by distension or disease of the ascending and right half of the colon, but a significant number of patients also have suprapubic pain (**D**). Pain in the right lower quadrant (**B**) is caused by severe distension or disease of the appendix and small intestine, as well as of the beginning of the ascending colon. Pain in the left lower quadrant (**C**) is caused by disease of the descending or sigmoid colon.

duplications usually occur in the ileum and can contain acid-producing gastric mucosa. This can lead to local intestinal ulceration that causes pain directly or after perforation of the gut wall. Ectopic gastric mucosa is also responsible for the pain associated with a Meckel's diverticulum, which is often postprandial. The mucosal ulceration can cause lower gastrointestinal bleeding (60). Inflammation of a Meckel's diverticulum can cause right lower quadrant pain that mimics that of appendicitis.

Diagnosis and Treatment

Most cases of congenital intestinal anomalies are first detected when laparotomy is performed for the relief of intestinal obstruction. Surgical resection of the area of stenosis or duplication is curative. Areas of internal herniation should be reduced and repaired. Meckel's diverticula should be resected.

Patients with less severe symptoms can have their anatomic abnormality diagnosed prior to laparotomy, usually by radiographic contrast examination. Many of these anomalies are asymptomatic and therefore the challenge is to be certain that the symptoms are actually caused by the anomaly and not by another condition.

Appendicitis

Appendicitis is the most common cause of acute severe abdominal pain that requires surgery. Approximately 10% of the population develops appendicitis at some time (61). Although appendicitis can occur in the very young and the elderly, the peak incidence is in the second and third decades of life.

Etiology and Pathophysiology

More than half of appendicitis cases are caused by obstruction of the appendiceal lumen by fecaliths, calculi, or other material. This blockage leads to swelling, mucosal ischemia, and bacterial invasion. Other pathogenic mechanisms can be involved but are largely unknown. Within 24 to 36 hours after luminal obstruction, perforation can occur, leading to peritonitis and abscess formation.

Symptoms and Signs

Patients with acute appendicitis have moderate to severe pain that begins in the epigastric or periumbilical region (6, 62). This initial pain is of a visceral type and is caused by luminal obstruction and distension of the appendix. Pain is most often steady, but some patients have cramping or colicky pain. Movement does not seem to affect this initial pain. The pain generally increases in severity over several hours and then can subside before localizing in the right lower quadrant.

When inflammation extends to the appendiceal serosa, stimulation of overlying parietal peritoneal somatic nerves results in well-localized right lower quadrant pain. This pain is usually severe, continuous, and exacerbated by bodily movement and coughing. Vomiting and defecation do not affect the quality or severity of this pain.

Most patients with appendicitis have anorexia, nausea, and vomiting. A useful diagnostic feature is that nausea and emesis follow the onset of pain. Diarrhea is reported by less than 25% of patients. Some patients report a sensation of constipation.

Diagnosis and Treatment

Diagnosis and treatment of appendicitis requires laparotomy when symptoms, physical examination, and laboratory findings suggest the diagnosis. Physical examination reveals a temperature of over 38° C in 50% of patients. Rebound tenderness and involuntary guarding, usually in the right lower quadrant, are common findings. Tenderness on rectal examination is frequently present. Peripheral leukocytosis is seen in over 90% of patients. An appendiceal fecalith is seen on plain abdominal roentgenography in less than 10% of patients. Other laboratory findings are nonspecific. Laparotomy must be done early in the course of the illness to prevent the significantly increased morbidity and mortality rates associated with perforation.

The physican must also be aware of atypical presentations of acute appendicitis caused by unusual locations of the appendix (6). Inflammation of a retrocecal appendix causes less severe pain that can remain poorly localized and not cause discrete localized abdominal tenderness. Ureteral irritation can lead to urinary frequency and pyuria. An appendix that hangs down over the pelvic brim can cause severe pain that localizes to the low midline or left abdomen after beginning in the periumbilical region. Rectal and pelvic tenderness are more commonly seen in those in this group.

Many diseases that simulate acute appendicitis can sometimes only be excluded by laparotomy. Infectious gastroenteritis, lymphadenitis, ureterolithiasis and, in women, salpingitis, ruptured ovarian cysts, and ruptured ectopic pregnancy, must be considered in the differential diagnosis. Intravenous urography, culdocentesis, and laparoscopy obviate the need for laparotomy in some patients.

Once the decision has been made to perform exploratory laparotomy in a patient with presumed appendicitis, all efforts should be made to relieve the abdominal pain. Parenteral narcotics and segmental epidural analgesic blocks are useful in this situation.

Infectious Enterocolitis

Infections of the small and large intestines are a common cause of self-limited abdominal pain. Infectious enterocolitis should be suspected in any person who develops diarrhea and abdominal cramping.

Etiology and Pathophysiology

Infectious agents that cause enterocolitis include bacteria, protozoans, and viruses. These organisms produce intestinal dysfunction and pain by mucosal invasion, toxin production, or both (63). Specific organisms are considered below (see Diagnosis and Treatment).

Symptoms and Signs

Symptoms of infectious enterocolitis are similar for all organisms that cause this problem. Abdominal cramps are usually intermittent and can be localized to the periumbilical region or lower in the hypogastrium. Rectal urgency is frequent when the rectum is involved. Diarrhea can be watery, bloody, or mucoid; associated symptoms of nausea, vomiting, and fever can be present.

Diagnosis and Treatment

Identification of the causative infectious organism depends on using the known epidemiologic associations to determine appropriate culture media and other laboratory tests. A specific diagnosis is critical to direct appropriate treatment of enterocolitis. Invasive infections are most commonly caused by bacteria and typically cause severe pain and bloody diarrhea. The presence of fecal leukocytes suggests the presence of invasive organisms, but both false positive and false negative test results are common. Stool cultures are the only reliable way of determining the specific organism involved (64).

INVASIVE ORGANISMS. Campylobacter jejuni is the most common cause of invasive infections. Campylobacter enterocolitis is treated with erythromycin, 500 mg qid for 7 days, if symptoms are persistent, but usually the disease remits spontaneously. Some cases have been associated with household pets, but the source of infection in most patients is unknown. Salmonella and Shigella can cause a similar clinical illness, sometimes associated with eating contaminated foods. Antimicrobial therapy of these infections is usually unnecessary but might be warranted in selected instances.

FOODBORNE ORGANISMS. Foodborne organisms cause enterocolitis that is usually self-limited and requires no treatment. Staphylococcus aureus, Bacillus cereus, and Clostridium perfringens often produce severe abdominal pains and watery diarrhea, which begin several hours after eating contaminated food and last less than 24 hours. S. aureus and B. cereus infections are frequently associated with severe vomiting.

TRAVELER'S DIARRHEA. Travelers to developing countries with tropical climates can develop enterocolitis (65). Contaminated food and water are responsible for transmitting the organism. In addition to the bacterial pathogens mentioned above, the protozoan organisms Entamoeba histolytica and Giardia lamblia should also be considered in this setting. Diagnosis depends on finding characteristic cysts and trophozoites in the stool of infected patients. Diarrhea and abdominal cramping usually persist for 2 to 7 days. Treatment of traveler's diarrhea includes nonspecific agents to reduce diarrhea (see below) and empiric antibiotics such as trimethoprim-sulfamethoxazole (Septra, Bactrim), one double-strength tablet bid. Use of other specific antimicrobial agents requires recovery of a pathogenic agent from the stool.

ANTIBOTIC-ASSOCIATED COLITIS. Patients who develop abdominal cramping and diarrhea, and who have been on antibiotics in the previous 6 weeks, should be suspected of having pseudomembranous colitis (66). This condition has been associated with the use of nearly all antibiotics, but cephalosporins, ampicillin, and clindamycin are most frequently implicated. Overgrowth of the toxin-producing organism Clostridium difficile causes this syndrome by destruction of the colonic epithelium. Diagnosis depends on identifying characteristic pseudomembranes on the rectal mucosa at sigmoidoscopy and by detecting the presence of the C. difficile organism and cytotoxin in the patient's stool. Treatment with oral vancomycin (Vancocin), 500 mg qid for 7 days, or metronidazole (Flagyl), 250 mg tid for 7 days, is usually curative. A severe colitis can result from this syndrome, producing a serious life-threatening situation.

SUPPORTIVE THERAPY. Supportive therapy for the patient with abdominal cramping and diarrhea caused by an infectious agent is important. Maintenance of hydration with liquids and oral electrolyte solutions is important. Cramping and diarrhea can often be reduced by using bismuth subsalicylate (Pepto-Bismol) in a dose of 30 ml each half hour, up to 8 ounces, or until diarrhea and cramps subside. Antiperistaltic agents such as diphenoxylate, loperamide, and codeine reduce the severity of diarrhea but should be used cautiously in patients with a fever or bloody diarrhea because of the risk of increasing the severity and prolonging the illness.

Radiation Enterocolitis

Etiology and Pathophysiology

Patients undergoing abdominal or pelvic irradiation for the treatment of neoplasia can develop intestinal complications. These can occur while the radiation is being administered, immediately after completion of treatment, or many months or years after treatment has been discontinued. Most patients so affected have recieved a total radiation dose of over 4000 rad (67). Patients undergoing recent radiation therapy have symptoms produced by mucosal edema and ulceration. Late symptoms after abdominal radiation are usually caused by partial small bowel obstruction from radiation-induced intestinal fibrosis. Diarrhea, when present, is caused by malabsorption, fistulas, or bacterial overgrowth.

Symptoms and Signs

Patients can have gastrointestinal symptoms while undergoing a course of radiation treatment. Nausea, vomiting, and diarrhea can occur, beginning at the end of the first week of treatment. A sensation of incomplete rectal evacuation and tenesmus indicates rectal and lower colonic mucosal involvement. Increased mucus and blood can be present in the stool. Mid- and lower abdominal cramping are present with significant small intestine involvement.

Abdominal symptoms can present months to years after radiation therapy has been completed. Symptoms of proctitis, including rectal burning, urgency, and mucoid diarrhea, are most frequent. Decreased stool caliber often indicates the presence of a rectal stricture. Periumbilical cramping pain suggests the presence of partial small or large bowel obstruction caused by stricture formation. If significant obstruction is present, progressive abdominal distension, nausea, and vomiting occur. Rectal bleeding, malabsorption, fistula formation, and perforation can also be late manifestations of radiation injury (68).

Diagnosis

The diagnosis of radiation enterocolitis should be considered in patients with abdominal pain who have a history of undergoing abdominal radiation therapy. The presence of the clinical syndrome described above is usually sufficient for diagnosis if other causes of pain are excluded. Proctosigmoidoscopy should be done to exclude other diseases, such as colonic cancer. Typical mucosal changes of radiation proctitis, including friability, ulceration, and telangiectasias, can be seen. Infectious enterocolitis needs to be ruled out using stool cultures, particularly in recently treated and potentially immunosuppressed patients with diarrhea. The diagnosis of partial mechanical intestinal obstruction is best made by plain abdominal roentgenography and contrast radiography.

Treatment

Treatment of radiation enterocolitis is directed at the patient's most distressing symptoms. Pain associated with ongoing radiation can respond to a decrease either in radiation dose or frequency of treatments. Stool bulking agents such as psyllium (Metamucil), 1 to 2 tablespoons daily, anticholinergic drugs such as propantheline (Pro-Banthine), 15 mg qid, and antiperistaltic drugs such as loperamide (Imodium), 2 mg qid, can also be helpful in reducing diarrhea and cramping. Rectal symptoms can respond to warm sitz baths and topical 2% lidocaine (Xylocaine) ointment. Diarrhea and pain in patients with a history of remote radiation treatment can sometimes be reduced by sulfasalazine (Azulfidine), 500 mg qid. Surgery can be hazardous in the patient with radiation enterocolitis because of a reduced vascular supply that results in impaired wound healing. Laparotomy is required, however, if tight strictures, complete obstruction, or symptomatic fistulas are present.

Diverticulitis

Etiology and Pathophysiology

Herniation of a small piece of intestinal mucosa and submucosa through the muscular wall of the bowel forms a diverticulum. These diverticula can be caused by increased colonic intraluminal pressure from chronic constipation. Diverticula are frequent in populations whose diets contain low quantities of fiber. Approximately 50% of people in the United States develop colonic diverticula by the ninth decade of life (69). The diverticula are usually multiple and are most frequently found on the left side of the colon. Diverticula rarely cause abdominal pain unless they become inflamed; this condition is called diverticulitis, and occurs at some time in about 10 to 20% of patients with diverticula (69).

Symptoms and Signs

Most patients with diverticulitis are over the age of 60 and complain of lower abdominal pain and fever. The pain is generally of moderate severity, can be either steady or cramping, and is frequently associated with nausea, vomiting, and a change in bowel habit (i.e., diarrhea, constipation, or mucus in the stool). Although diverticula are most commonly seen in the left colon, pain is frequent in the right as well as the left lower quadrants, possibly because of a redundant sigmoid colon that loops to the right of midline in many of these patients. Pain sometimes radiates to the back. Fever is usually present, and a peripheral leukocytosis with left shift is seen in most patients. Lower abdominal tenderness is a frequent finding, but significant rigidity and rebound tenderness are unusual. The sigmoid colon can sometimes be felt as a firm, tender cord in the left lower quadrant.

Diagnosis

The clinical diagnosis of diverticulitis can be made without difficulty in most cases. Gentle proctosigmoidoscopy with minimal air insufflation is useful in excluding other mass lesions, such as carcinoma, and diffuse mucosal diseases, such as inflammatory bowel disease and infectious colitis. Ischemic colitis must be considered in this group of patients, particularly when abdominal tenderness and pain are extreme and when antibiotic therapy has little effect. Radiographic contrast examination is best delayed until patients have clinically improved. Barium enemas have been reported to cause perforation when performed in patients with acute diverticulitis. The presence of diverticula can be confirmed and areas of luminal narrowing safely defined when the radiographic examination is performed after the fever and pain have subsided.

Treatment

Most patients with diverticulitis respond to medical treatment with broad-spectrum antibiotics, correction of fluid and electrolyte losses, and general supportive care. Severely ill patients should initially be given nothing by mouth and then should be advanced slowly to a low-residue diet as symptoms improve. Use of parenteral narcotics is best avoided whenever possible to lessen the risk of masking a diverticular perforation or some other process, such as colonic ischemia. Surgical drainage is necessary when fever does not respond to antibiotics or when radiography shows abscess formation. If the colonic obstruction does not resolve, surgical decompression with a colostomy might be necessary. Later, when the area of diverticulitis is less inflamed, the segment can be resected as part of a two- or three-stage surgical procedure. Resection of strictured bowel might be required for diagnosis and treatment when carcinoma cannot be ruled out by endoscopic biopsies.

Crohn's Disease (XXI-9)

Crohn's disease is a frequent cause of both acute and chronic abdominal pain, particularly in young people. Crohn's disease is an idiopathic inflammatory disease of the intestine. Either the small or large intestine, or both, is involved with a transmural inflammatory process. Areas of normal mucosa, referred to as skip areas, can be present between the inflamed regions of bowel.

Etiology and Pathophysiology

The cause of Crohn's disease is unknown, although numerous pathogenic mechanisms have been postulated (70). One or all of the mechanisms could be involved in a given patient. Abnormalities in both antibody-mediated and cell-mediated immunities have been reported. The importance of these immune systems might lie in their determining individual susceptibility rather than causing disease directly. Infectious agents, including bacteria and viruses, have been postulated to cause inflammatory bowel disease, and might also be responsible for some exacerbations of disease activity. Psychologic factors are certainly important in the course of inflammatory bowel disease, and have been proposed by some to be involved in disease pathogenesis.

Symptoms and Signs

Pain in patients with Crohn's disease is caused by either obstruction or inflammation (71). Inflammatory pain can be found anywhere in the abdomen, depending on location of the area of inflammation. Right lower quadrant pain is most frequent because of the common involvement of the terminal ileum and cecum. This pain is a continuous ache and occasionally radiates to the right upper thigh. It can be severe enough to cause the patient to limp. The pain is not necessarily associated with bowel movements but can be exacerbated by eating. Often superimposed on this continuous aching discomfort is a more severe crampy pain, which is located in the periumbilical region and is often relieved by bowel movements. This type of pain is usually a sign of partial intestinal obstruction induced by the inflam-matory process, and can be associated with nausea and vomiting. Diarrhea, which can be bloody, fever, and weight loss are other frequent symptoms.

Symptoms of anal and rectal involvement can also be prominent in patients with Crohn's disease (70). Rectal involvement causes a sensation of urgency or tenesmus, a feeling of rectal irritation or discomfort that makes the patient feel that a bowel movement is about to occur; in fact, only a small amount of diarrhea might be present, or no stool at all. Perianal pain caused by fistula, fissure, or abscess is found in about half of patients with Crohn's disease at some time in their illness. Severe pain localized to the anus and perianal area, accompanying or following bowel movements, is characteristic of these complications (these anorectal problems are discussed in more detail below).

Patients with Crohn's disease can also have symptoms caused by extraintestinal complications (72). These problems are most common during periods of active inflammation and often respond to medical or surgical treatment of the bowel disease. Arthritis is seen in approximately 25% of patients with Crohn's colitis but is less frequent when Crohn's disease is limited to the small bowel. A few large joints or multiple smaller joints can be affected. Skin involvement in the form of erythema nodosum, pyoderma gangrenosum, and other rashes is also seen in patients with colonic inflammation. Conjunctivitis, uveitis, and oral aphthous ulcerations are seen in 5 to 10% of patients with colitis. Liver disease, including pericholangitis, fatty liver, and, less commonly, sclerosing cholangitis, is also seen in patients with Crohn's disease.

Diagnosis

The diagnosis of Crohn's disease is usually made by a suggestive history and physical examination, with the aid of radiographic contrast examinations, endoscopy, and endoscopic biopsies. Small intestinal involvement is best detected with barium radiography. Colonic involvement can be defined by both roentgenography and colonoscopy. Rectal mucosal biopsies taken through the sigmoidoscope are also helpful. It is sometimes difficult to distinguish between Crohn's disease limited to the colon and ulcerative colitis.

Patients presenting with complaints of abdominal pain and diarrhea must have infectious enterocolitis ruled out by appropriate cultures and serologic tests. Campylobacter, Shigella, and Amoeba can all cause a clinical picture similar to that of Crohn's colitis. Pseudomembranous colitis should be considered in all patients who have been taking antibiotics. Yersinia can also cause right lower quadrant pain and diarrhea that mimics Crohn's disease.

Appendicitis, ischemic enterocolitis, and intestinal malignancy should also be considered in patients thought to have inflammatory bowel disease. Patients who have an abrupt onset of ileitis are frequently operated on for presumed appendicitis. Appendectomy should not be done in these patients if the cecum is grossly involved with Crohn's disease at the time of surgery because enterocutaneous fistulas could form at the appendectomy site. Intestinal ischemia should be considered in elderly patients with intestinal inflammatory disease, especially in patients with a history of other atherosclerotic cardiovascular diseases. Colonic cancer and small intestinal lymphoma must be ruled out when a mass is present on radiographic studies of the intestine.

Treatment

Treatment of the patient with Crohn's disease involves a multidisciplinary approach. The gastroenterologist, surgeon, psychologist, and nutritionist all have valuable roles, but it is crucial that the patient maintain close contact with one physician. The emotional support, provided by a trusted and concerned physician, is invaluable over the long course of illness (70). The role of stressful life events in the exacerbation of inflammatory bowel disease is well recognized, and underlines the role of the primary physician for major psychologic support. Formal psychotherapy is indicated in selected patients with prominent psychologic problems.

Pain is best controlled by appropriate management of the underlying inflammatory disease (73). Systemic corticosteroids such as prednisone in a dose of 1 mg/kg are useful in treating acute exacerbations of Crohn's disease. These drugs must be used cautiously and should be tapered rapidly because of their long-term side effects and the difficulty some patients have in discontinuing the medication. Systemic cortiscosteroids do not prevent relapses of Crohn's disease and therefore long-term use is discouraged. Hydrocortisone enemas are useful in the treatment of rectal and left colonic inflammations. This can be particularly helpful in reducing the troublesome symptom of tenesmus. Sulfasalazine (Azulfidine) in a dosage of 2 to 4 g/day is useful in treating flares of Crohn's colitis but probably does not prevent relapse in the patient with quiescent disease. 6-Mercaptopurine and azathioprine can prevent relapse and decrease steroid requirements in patients with Crohn's disease (73). Metronidazole (Flagyl) in a dosage of 15 to 20 mg/kg/day is frequently helpful in patients with perineal disease (74).

Narcotic analgesics should be used judiciously in the management of patients with inflammatory bowel disease. The decreased intestinal motility associated with the use of these agents can precipitate toxic megacolon in patients undergoing severe attacks of Crohn's colitis. Paradoxically, narcotics can increase pain in some patients by increasing intestinal spasm. Nevertheless, the less potent narcotics are helpful in managing the chronic diarrhea and cramping. Four to eight tablets daily of codeine, loperamide (Imodium), or diphenoxylate with atropine (Lomotil) are commonly used. Anticholinergic drugs such as propantheline (Pro-Banthine), 15 mg qid, and dicyclomine (Bentyl), 20 mg qid, also relieve intestinal cramping in some patients.

Dietary manipulation can benefit some patients with inflammatory bowel disease. Patients with significant obstructive symptoms can obtain relief by eating low-residue foods. Many patients with Crohn's disease are lactose-intolerant; a trial of eliminating dairy products from the diet can decrease pain and diarrhea. Other dietary manipulations should aim at providing adequate amounts of protein and calories.

Resective surgery should be avoided whenever possible because the disease can recur in previously uninvolved segments of bowel. Nevertheless, significant intestinal obstruction and unhealed fistulas remain a common indication for surgery in this disease. Surgery is also indicated for the drainage of abscesses and for repair of intestinal perforation. Massive intestinal hemorrhage and toxic dilatation of the colon unresponsive to medical therapy are other rare indications for surgery in Crohn's disease.

Ulcerative Colitis

Etiology and Pathophysiology

Ulcerative colitis is another common type of idiopathic inflammatory bowel disease. Inflammation is limited to the mucosal surface of the colon, beginning at the anus and extending proximally for variable distances. Unlike Crohn's disease, the inflammatory process does not involve the small intestine and does not skip over areas of normal colonic mucosa. Like Crohn's disease, the cause is unknown; the same pathogenetic factors discussed in the previous section might also be involved in ulcerative colitis.

Symptoms and Signs

Most patients with ulcerative colitis have some combination of abdominal pain, diarrhea, and hematochezia during active flares of the disease. Bloody diarrhea is a more common complaint than pain (70). Pain is usually not as severe as that seen in some patients with Crohn's disease. Pain is usually located in the left lower quadrant of the abdomen, is cramping in character, and is generally accompanied by an urge to defecate, which often relieves the pain. A minority of patients have a fulminant onset of ulcerative colitis, known as toxic megacolon. In this situation the colon distends to a large diameter and can produce severe diffuse abdominal pain and fever.

Perianal pain is not as common in ulcerative colitis as it is in Crohn's disease. Patients with ulcerative colitis can suffer from anal fissures that cause pain during bowel movements, but perianal fistulas are not part of this disease.

Diarrhea is often a prominent symptom. Stools can be soft but formed, watery, full of mucus, or frankly bloody. Diarrhea can be present, with or without abdominal pain. Stools can be as frequent as every half hour and often awaken the patient at night.

Extraintestinal manifestations of ulcerative colitis are similar to those seen in Crohn's disease (72). Joint, skin, eye, and liver involvement can be indistinguishable from that seen in Crohn's disease.

Diagnosis

The diagnosis of ulcerative colitis is usually made when sigmoidoscopy is performed to investigate diarrhea and abdominal pain. The rectal mucosa is red, friable, and sometimes ulcerated in patients with active disease. Crohn's disease, infectious colitis, and ischemic colitis can give a similar clinical and sigmoidoscopic appearance and should be considered as other diagnostic possibilities. Stool cultures and serology for amebiasis should always be done in this setting to rule out an infectious cause. Rectal mucosal biopsies can sometimes help to distinguish among infectious colitis, Crohn's colitis, and ulcerative colitis.

Patients with ulcerative colitis have an increased risk for the development of colon carcinoma. Patients with disease that has involved the entire colon for longer than 10 years are at highest risk. Those with a change in the character of their diarrhea or abdominal pain should be investigated for this complication. Colonoscopy with multiple biopsies is the procedure of choice for detecting colon cancer or dysplasia in patients with ulcerative colitis.

Treatment

The same multidisciplinary approach used in the management of patients with Crohn's disease should be followed for patients with ulcerative colitis. Medical, surgical, psychologic, and nutritional therapies all have roles in the management of patients with this disease. The specific treatment selected depends on the severity, extent, and duration of the disease.

Pain in patients with ulcerative colitis is best managed by controlling the colonic inflammation. Sulfasalazine (Azulfidine), in a dosage of 2 to 4 g/day PO, is usually effective in inducing remission and preventing relapse in patients with mild to moderate disease. About 25% of patients taking this drug have nausea, epigastric pain, or headache; these side effects can be reduced by lowering the dose of azulfidine.

Corticosteroids are effective in controlling colonic inflammation and the resultant abdominal pain and diarrhea. Patients with disease limited to the rectum and descending colon often benefit from the daily administration of hydrocortisone enemas (Cortenema) or hydrocortisone suppositories. These preparations are especially helpful in patients with rectal urgency and tenesmus. More severe and diffuse colonic disease usually requires systemic steroids. Prednisone, 40 to 60 mg/day, rapidly controls the symptoms of pain and diarrhea in most patients. Because disease relapse is not prevented by systemic steroids, however, these drugs should be tapered rapidly and discontinued whenever possible.

Antiperistaltic drugs are useful in decreasing the frequency of diarrhea in patients with ulcerative colitis. Diphenoxylate with atropine (Lomotil) and loperamide (Imodium) are the most frequently used agents. A dosage of four to eight tablets/day is commonly used. These drugs can also decrease some of the lower abdominal cramping pain associated with bowel movements. Opiates should not be used in patients with severe disease because they have been associated with the development of toxic megacolon (75).

Colectomy is indicated in patients with ulcerative colitis for intractable disease and for specific complications. Colectomy is life-saving in patients with toxic megacolon unresponsive to medical management. Others with continued abdominal pain and bloody diarrhea that is only controlled by high-dose corticosteroids should also be offered surgery. Total protocolectomy cures ulcerative colitis and prevents the sequelae of long-term corticosteroid use in these patients. Colectomy is also indicated to prevent the development of carcinoma when mucosal biopsies show dysplasia in patients with long-standing disease.

Several surgical procedures are available to patients with ulcerative colitis; protocolectomy with ileostomy, subtotal colectomy with ileorectal anastomosis, and proctocolectomy with ileoanal anastomosis and ileal reservoir are currently used operations. The choice of operation depends on the medical condition and preference of the patient and the experience of the surgeon.

Intestinal Obstruction

Etiology and Pathophysiology

Mechanical or nonmechanical obstruction to the normal passage of intestinal contents from the stomach to the anus is another common cause of abdominal pain (6). Interruption of the luminal pathway can be a result of several different mechanisms, all of which produce the symptoms of abdominal pain, distension, vomiting, and failure to pass flatus. The causes and mechanisms of intestinal obstruction are listed in Table 60-3. In adults, adhesions most commonly cause mechanical small bowel obstruction, and cancer is the most frequent cause of large bowel obstruction. Nonmechanical obstruction of the intestine is caused by abnormal intestinal motor function, which can be either a primary intestinal abnormality, as in primary intestinal pseudo-obstruction (76) or, more commonly, secondary to other problems.

Symptoms and Signs

Abdominal pain resulting from intestinal obstruction is usually caused by intestinal distension proximal to the area of obstruction. Crampy periumbilical pain is characteristic of small bowel obstruction. The interval between cramps is about 5 minutes when the blockage is proximal and longer with more distal obstruction. Abdominal distension is usually present, except with the most proximal obstructions. Vomiting is bilious with upper intestinal obstruction and becomes darker and even feculent as the area of blockage is increasingly distal. Patients with colonic obstruction usually have more distension, pain and vomiting occurring later. The pain caused by large bowel obstruction is often infraumbilical, in the midline or on either side. Patients might continue to pass feces after the onset of

TABLE 60-3. Causes of Intestinal Obstruction

Mechanical Obstruction	Nonmechanical Obstruction
Luminal contents	Pseudo-obstruction
Foreign bodies	Primary
Gallstones	Secondary: drugs,
Bezoars	endocrinopathy, systemic
Feces	illness
Intrinsic lesions	Paralytic ileus
Neoplasms	Surgery
Strictures	Trauma
Atresia	Infection
Extrinsic compression	Metabolic
Neoplasms	
Adhesions	
Abscess	
Intussusception	
Volvulus	
Herniation	

obstruction because of preserved colonic motility, but they cease to pass flatus. Patients with nonmechanical obstruction generally have less severe pain than those with mechanical obstruction. Further diagnostic tests are required to distinguish between those in the two groups.

Diagnosis

Physical examination of the obstructed patient is important for diagnosis and for determining management. Measurement of the orthostatic blood pressure and assessment of mucous membranes help to guide fluid resuscitation. These patients are usually dehydrated. Bowel sounds are generally decreased, possibly with high-pitched rushes, but these findings are neither sensitive nor specific for obstruction. Although abdominal distension with mild diffuse or periumbilical tenderness is often present, marked localized or rebound tenderness and fever should raise the suspicion that intestinal infarction or perforation has complicated the obstruction.

Plain abdominal roentgenography is the single most useful test in the diagnosis of intestinal obstruction. Dilated bowel, filled with air and fluid, is seen except with early or extremely proximal intestinal obstruction. The location and appearance of dilated bowel help both to localize the obstruction and to determine whether a mechanical or nonmechanical mechanism is involved. Elevated peripheral white blood cell counts increase the suspicion of perforation or strangulation. Whereas radiographic contrast examinations help to localize the point of obstruction, they are best used when the patient has been decompressed, especially with small bowel obstruction. Barium enemas are useful in defining a colonic obstruction and can even be therapeutic if a volvulus or intussuception is present.

Treatment

The management of the patient with intestinal obstruction includes general supportive care, treatment of the underlying abnormalities, and avoidance of complications. Initially, dehydration should be corrected with intravenous fluids, and the bowel decompressed with nasogastric suction. When clinical findings and plain films suggest complete mechanical obstruction, early laparotomy both defines the cause of obstruction and allows intestinal diversion or definitive correction of the abnormality. Parenteral narcotics are indicated for relief of pain while the patient is awaiting surgery. The major complications of intestinal obstruction are perforation and strangulation or infarction. Both problems carry high morbidity and mortality rates, require immediate surgery, and could be masked by analgesic use. Therefore, analgesics should be withheld in this situation if the diagnosis is unclear and if surgical intervention is not yet planned. Significant pain relief is often obtained by bowel decompression alone.

Treatment of nonmechanical obstruction involves supportive care and correction of any underlying abnormalities. Surgery is rarely indicated. Paralytic ileus secondary to the postoperative state, infections, and electrolyte imbalance usually resolves with time and treatment of the causative factors. Supportive care with nasogastric suction and fluid therapy is helpful in

episodes of primary intestinal pseudo-obstruction because the episodes are recurrent, and no effective definitive therapy is available (76).

Intestinal Neoplasms (XXI-13)

Etiology and Pathophysiology

Benign and malignant neoplasms of the colon, including polyps and cancers, are common. Colon cancer is the third most common cause of cancer deaths in the United States and is the most common type of gastrointestinal cancer. Most carcinomas of the colon are thought to begin as small growths of neoplastic tissue, known as adenomatous polyps. These polyps have an increasing degree of malignant potential with increasing size (77). Other types of polyps, with little or no malignant potential, are also commonly found in the colon, including hamartomatous and hyperplastic polyps. Neoplasms of the large intestine other than adenocarcinoma are rare; these include carcinoid tumors, lymphomas, and leiomyomas. The cause of the tumors is unknown, but both genetic and dietary factors are probably involved. Certain patients have conditions that place them at high risk of developing colon cancer, such as ulcerative colitis, familial polyposis syndromes, and a family history of colon cancer (Table 58-3, p. 1149).

Tumors of the small intestine are uncommon. Adenocarcinoma, lymphoma, carcinoma, and leiomyosarcoma all occur in the small bowel but overall account for less than 5% of all intestinal neoplasms.

Symptoms and Signs

Most neoplasms of the intestine are painless until they produce luminal obstruction or extend to adjacent structures (78). When obstruction is present the cancer is often unresectable; the tumor must reach a large size before it causes obstruction. Occasionally, a small polyp presents with pain caused by intussusception. The characteristics of pain caused by intestinal obstruction and intussusception are similar to those described in the preceding section. Locally advanced carcinomas can cause abdominal pain by erosion into adjacent organs, such as the retroperitoneum and sacrum. Carcinomas can perforate and cause acute abdominal pain and signs of peritonitis. Other symptoms of neoplasms include bleeding, which is often occult, and changes in bowel habits, such as constipation. A reduction in stool caliber is often noted if the tumor is in the rectum or distal colon. Metastatic colon cancer frequently causes profound inanition, weight loss, and pain.

Diagnosis

Selection of diagnostic tests to detect intestinal cancer is based on the patient's clinical presentation. Patients with pain caused by complete intestinal obstruction usually require laparotomy, both for diagnosis and for treatment of the obstruction. Intermittent abdominal pain caused by partial bowel obstruction should be investigated by contrast radiography. Upper gastrointestinal roentgenography with a small bowel follow-through examination can detect small intestinal mass lesions, but laparotomy is sometimes required for diagnosis of these lesions. If symptoms or plain abdominal films suggest the presence of large bowel obstruction, rigid or flexible sigmoidoscopy followed by a barium enema should delineate the level of obstruction. Colonoscopy is necessary to biopsy mass lesions detected by roentgenography and can also reveal small polyps or cancers missed by radiography (10, 79).

Patients with gross or occult blood in their stools, or a change in stool character and frequency, should have rigid or flexible sigmoidoscopy followed by a double-contrast barium enema to exclude the presence of a colon cancer. If fecal occult blood is still unexplained by these tests, a full colonoscopy is indicated because polyps and small cancers can be missed by roentgenography. Blood tests (e.g., the level of carcinoembryonic antigen) can be useful in following patients with a history of resected colon cancer to monitor for recurrence.

Treatment

Treatment of intestinal neoplasms involves several types of therapy, including surgery, radiation therapy, and chemotherapy. Polyps can usually be removed by colonoscopy, but colectomy is needed if an invasive carcinoma is present (10). Surgical resection provides the best chance for cure of colon cancer; prognosis is directly related to the degree of invasion and spread. Radiation therapy decreases pain caused by spinal metastases and advanced pelvic tumors (78). Chemotherapy does not increase survival rates for colon cancer but can be useful in certain cases. Hepatic arterial infusion of 5-fluorouracil can decrease the size of liver metastases and thus decrease right upper quadrant pain caused by distension of the liver capsule, but survival might not be prolonged by this procedure (80). This therapy should be utilized in patients with symptomatic liver metasteses who are in otherwise good condition; implantable infusion pumps are available that allow for long-term outpatient therapy (80).

Treatment of pain in patients with advanced colorectal cancer is a challenging problem that often requires multiple medical disciplines. Many of these patients can be managed with narcotic analgesics, using the principles outlined in Chapters 24 and 78. When narcotics are not well tolerated or are ineffective, other procedures should be attempted. Upper abdominal pain can be relieved by celiac plexus block with alcohol (55). Because pain is more commonly seen in the lower abdomen and pelvis in these patients, however, subarachnoid injection of alcohol to interrupt the affected segments can be used; epidural administration of morphine or some other narcotic is an alternative to neurosurgical procedures in patients with intractable lower abdominal, pelvic, and sacral pain caused by colorectal cancer (81, 82). Such treatment is sometimes successful, but tolerance to the narcotic can develop (82). Subcutaneous reservoirs are available to facilitate simple daily injections at home, but these measures do not relieve severe pain. If life expectancy is greater than 3 months, neurosurgical intervention can be useful (56). Detailed discussions of these aspects of managing cancer pain can be found in Chapters 24, 96, and 98.

Irritable Bowel Syndrome (XXI-11)

Etiology and Pathophysiology

Irritable bowel syndrome is a frequent cause of abdominal pain in the general population and is the most common diagnosis among patients referred to gastroenterologists (83). The cause of this disorder is unknown but most likely is multifactorial and related to altered intestinal motility (84, 85). Emotional stress is often associated with exacerbations of the irritable bowel syndrome and has been shown to alter intestinal motility (84). Patients with this disorder also perceive pain produced by small and large intestinal distension in more diverse abdominal and extra-abdominal sites than do normal people (17, 57). Irritable bowel syndrome is twice as common in females than males, most often begins in the third or fourth decade of life, and commonly recurs for the lifetime of the patient.

Symptoms and Signs

Most patients with irritable bowel syndrome have abdominal pain, a cramping or aching pain below the level of the umbilicus that is relieved by a bowel movement or by passing flatus (86). Pain lasts from a few minutes to hours and is usually recurrent. Some patients with irritable bowel syndrome have predominantly epigastric pain and are part of those in the nonulcer dyspepsia spectrum (36).

Alteration of bowel habits occurs in 90% of patients with irritable bowel syndrome. Constipation, diarrhea, or alternating episodes of constipation and diarrhea can occur. Individual patients often have a typical pattern of bowel evacuation that is constant over their lifetime. Stools are often loose with an episode of pain, but the pain is usually relieved by the bowel movement (86). Abdominal distension, mucus in stools, nausea, vomiting, and excessive flatus are frequent associated symptoms. Symptoms are recurrent and are often associated with stressful life events.

Diagnosis

Diagnosis of irritable bowel syndrome requires recognition of the positive clinical features outlined above, as well as exclusion of other known causes of the patient's symptoms (86). Lactose intolerance, giardiasis, inflammatory bowel disease, and intestinal obstruction should be considered in patients with recurrent abdominal pain and altered bowel habits. A trial lactose-free diet, examination of stool for blood, ova, and parasites, sigmoidoscopy, and barium enema examinations are usually needed to exclude these possibilities. Patients who have blood in their stool, fever, weight loss, progressive symptoms, nocturnal pain, or nocturnal diarrhea are more likely to have an illness other than irritable bowel syndrome; those in this group should have a more thorough investigation for other causes of their symptoms.

Treatment

No cure is available for irritable bowel syndrome, but patients can be helped in several ways. The concerned and supportive physician can do much to relieve patients' concerns about their symptoms. The importance of a supportive role is illustrated by the beneficial effects of placebo in reducing pain in these patients (87). Stress management techniques can also be useful in decreasing the frequency of symptoms. Tricyclic antidepressants such as trimipramine (Surmontil), 50 mg PO at bedtime, have been shown to reduce abdominal pain and nausea significantly more than placebo in patients with irritable bowel syndrome (87).

Other medical therapies for irritable bowel syndrome can benefit individuals, but controlled trials have not proven their efficacy in large groups of patients. A high-fiber diet is usually helpful in reducing constipation, but abdominal pain might not be relieved. Diphen-oxylate with atropine (Lomotil) or loperamide (Imodium), one or two tablets in the morning and evening, can be used in severe exacerbations of diarrhea, but chronic use should be avoided. Anticholinergic agents such as dicyclomine (Bentyl), 10 to 20 mg, and propantheline (Pro-Banthine), 15 to 30 mg given before meals, can decrease abdominal pain that is induced by eating. Narcotic analgesics for pain in this syndrome are contraindicated because of the risk of psychologic and physical dependence. Reassurance that symptoms usually resolve with time and that the patients' longevity is not decreased in irritable bowel syndrome are critical to successful long-term management.

D. DISEASES OF THE ANUS AND RECTUM

Basic Considerations

Anatomy

The rectum constitutes the distal 12 to 15 cm of the large intestine, beginning at approximately the level of the S3 vertebra. Many diseases of the rectum are part of the spectrum of other colonic diseases, and have been considered in the previous section, (e.g., carcinoma, inflammatory bowel disease, and various obstructive lesions). Other disease processes involving the rectum produce symptoms that are similar to those of anal disease and are included here to facilitate clinical recognition. The terminal 3 cm of the rectum pass through the anal canal, which is comprised of an internal sphincter of smooth muscle and an external sphincter of striated muscle. The rectum is lined with columnar mucosa as far distally as the pectinate line, which is about 2 cm inside the anal verge.

Nerve Supply

Sensory innervation of the rectum is through visceral afferent nerves that course with parasympathetic nerves by way of the pelvic splanchnic nerves and the pelvic plexus to enter the spinal cord at the S2 to S4 levels (see Fig. 60-9). Rapid distension, inflammation, and infiltration of the rectum produce a sensation of aching in the region of the rectum or a poorly localized deep central pelvic pain. Patients with rectal diseases also often report a dull or aching pain in the region of the midsacrum (88).

The anal canal distal to the pectinate line is covered with stratified squamous epithelium and is innervated by somatic sensory nerves. These nerve fibers are carried by the inferior hemorrhoidal nerve and synapse in the dorsal root ganglion at the S2 to S4 levels. Unlike other parts of the rectum and intestine, the anal canal is sensitive to cold, heat, and touch. Pain from the anus is well localized and often severe. The pain is usually continuous and can be of a burning, throbbing, or aching nature (88).

Clinical Considerations

Anatomic Abnormalities

Anal stenosis and atresia with fistula formation to other perineal structures are common congenital defects caused by incomplete development of the hindgut. They are generally diagnosed by inspection in early infancy and thus are not considered further here.

Hirschsprung's disease, or congenital megacolon, is caused by the absence of the intramural neural plexuses of a segment of the colon and results in dilatation of the bowel proximal to the abnormal segment (88). Over two-thirds of cases involve only the rectum and distal sigmoid colon. Most patients present in infancy with abdominal distension and vomiting, suggesting intestinal obstruction. If the problem remains undetected until later in childhood, constipation, failure to gain weight, and diffuse abdominal pain can result. The diagnosis is usually suspected when a dilated colon is seen on plain abdominal radiographs or with barium enema. Diagnostic confirmation requires the demonstration of the absence of intramural nerve plexuses by rectal biopsy. Surgical resection of the rectosigmoid usually corrects the problem.

Foreign Bodies

Numerous types of foreign bodies have been known to be introduced into the rectum, causing local pain and irritation. Perforations and lacerations can also occur, resulting in severe pain and sometimes peritonitis. Blood or mucus might be seen in the stool. Some homosexual men practice fisting, in which the hand and forearm are introduced into the rectum (89). The diagnosis is usually suspected from the patient's history. The presence of foreign bodies and the extent of mucosal damage can usually be assessed by sigmoidoscopy. Most foreign objects in the rectum can be removed through the sigmoidoscope, although anesthesia is usually required for this procedure. Laparotomy is required for foreign bodies that cannot be removed endoscopically and for intestinal perforation.

Hemorrhoids

Etiology and Pathophysiology

Hemorrhoids are dilated blood vessels of the anal canal. They are classified as internal if above the pectinate line and external if below the pectinate line. Several theories have been proposed to explain the formation of hemorrhoids (90). Increased venous pressure in the pelvis, high anal sphincter tone, low-residue diets with resulting hard stool, and prolonged straining with defecation can all contribute to hemorrhoid pathogenesis.

Symptoms and Signs

Internal hemorrhoids are usually painless and cause symptoms either by bleeding or by prolapsing into the anal canal (90). Most patients with internal hemorrhoids reveal a history of anal discomfort at some time, although this might only be a mild irritation. If prolapsed hemorrhoids become incarcerated and thrombose, however, intense pain can be produced. The pain is localized to the anal area and is made worse by bowel movements, sitting, and walking. Hemorrhoidal bleeding is usually bright red and painless and can be seen on the surface of the stool, on the toilet tissue, or in the toilet bowl.

External hemorrhoids are usually asymptomatic. They are frequently seen in young people as small perianal bluish masses covered with normal perianal skin. These hemorrhoids can be painful if they thrombose or rupture into the surrounding skin, causing traction on adjacent nerves. This usually follows an episode of constipation and straining with defecation. The patient presents with well-localized perianal pain that is continuous and exacerbated by sitting and defection. External hemorrhoids usually do not cause rectal bleeding.

Diagnosis

Hemorrhoids are usually diagnosed by inspection of the anus, and by use of simple maneuvers. Internal hemorrhoids can be seen at anoscopy, but the best way to detect them is with a stress test. The patient is asked to sit on the toilet and strain as one would during defecation. After 30 seconds, and while the patient continues to strain, the examiner inspects the anal region by placing a hand-held mirror under the patient's buttocks. Internal hemorrhoids are visualized as bluish structures that protrude from the anus. Incarcerated internal hemorrhoids can be seen directly without patient straining as erythematous masses in the anal canal, covered with pink rectal mucosa. These lesions are tender and might not easily reduce back into the rectum. Thrombosed external hemorrhoids are bluish masses outside the anus that are covered with normal perianal skin, and are usually tender to palpation.

Patients with anorectal pain or bleeding should have nonhemorrhoidal causes of the symptoms ruled out. Infectious proctitis, inflammatory bowel disease, anorectal neoplasms, and anal fissures should be considered in these patients. Sigmoidoscopy usually excludes these problems in patients under the age of 35. If pain or bleeding persists after treatment, and in older patients, a barium enema or colonoscopy should be performed to exclude lesions in more proximal areas of the colon (90). Care must be taken so that bleeding caused by a colon cancer above the area of sigmoidoscopy is not incorrectly attributed to hemorrhoids. Often barium enema roentgenography or colonoscopy is necessary to resolve this question.

Treatment

Most patients with mild bleeding and discomfort caused by hemorrhoids can be managed medically. An increase in dietary fiber is often sufficient to soften stools, resulting in decreased straining with defecation. Topical application of ointments containing local anesthetics such as 2.5% lidocaine (Xylocaine) or 1% pramoxime (Tronolane) can be soothing to patients with thrombosed external hemorrhoids. Hydrocortisone ointment 1% is also sometimes helpful for this condition. Warm water baths can decrease painful spasms of the anal sphincter.

Surgical therapy of hemorrhoids should be used in patients with persistent pain, bleeding, and prolapse. Rubber band ligation is a simple outpatient procedure that is quite effective in patients with internal hemorrhoids that are reducible and not too large (91). This ligation is more efficacious and has fewer complications than cryosurgery or injection of sclerosing solutions. Surgical resection of hemorrhoids is the treatment of choice for large and unreducible prolapsing hemorrhoids. Incarcerated hemorrhoids can usually be reduced after 1% lidocaine is injected around the anus and under the protruding hemorrhoid. Pain usually subsides within several days. Early surgical hemorrhoidectomy should be performed if thrombosis or gangrene is present (92). Patients with persistent pain, despite medical treatment of thrombosed external hemorrhoids, should have the associated clot excised. A single elliptic incision after injection of a local anesthetic such as 1% lidocaine allows clot evacuation. The procedure is safe, effective, and well tolerated.

Proctitis

Etiology and Pathophysiology

Inflammation of the anus and rectum has both infectious and noninfectious causes. Infectious proctitis is seen most frequently in homosexual men in whom frequent and widespread anogenital and orogenital contact is common (89). Infectious causes of proctitis are listed in Table 60-4. Inflammatory bowel disease limited to the rectum, trauma from foreign bodies and anal intercourse, radiation therapy, and allergies to lubricants and enemas are noninfectious causes of proctitis.

Symptoms and Signs

Bleeding, mucous or purulent discharge, pain, burning, and rectal urgency are the chief symptoms produced by anorectal inflammation; these symptoms are similar for all causes of proctitis. Diarrhea can be present if inflammation extends to more proximal areas of the colon (Table 60-4). Pain is often increased by bowel movements and by wearing tight clothing. The most severe pain occurs when inflammation is present distal to the pectinate line.

TABLE 60-4. Causes and Symptoms and Signs of Infectious Proctitis

Symptoms and Signs	Causative Organism
Pain and anal discharge	Neisseria gonorrhoeae Herpesvirus hominis Treponema pallidum Chlamydia trachomatis
Pain and diarrhea	Entamoeba histolytica Campylobacter jejuni Shigella species Chlamydia trachomatis

Diagnosis

Specific diagnosis of the cause of proctitis is important for directing therapy and determining prognosis. Sigmoidoscopy usually reveals erythematous and friable rectal mucosa, with or without ulcerations, and areas of adherent purulent material. Herpes simplex infections can show characteristic grouped vesicles. Cultures for bacterial, chlamydial, and herpes organisms should be obtained from swabs obtained at sigmoidoscopy. Rectal ulcers should be swabbed for dark-field microscopic examination, and a serum serologic test for syphilis should be obtained if the patient has a history of anal intercourse. Rectal biopsies should be obtained when symptoms are persistent and cultures are negative to rule out inflammatory bowel disease.

Treatment

Treatment of proctitis is directed at the specific cause as well as symptomatic relief. Antibiotic therapy should be based on the results of appropriate cultures. Treatment of inflammatory bowel disease has been discussed above. Sitz baths, warm compresses applied to the perianal region, and local analgesic ointments such as 2.5% lidocaine (Xylocaine) can provide some relief. If maceration is present all lubricants and ointments should be avoided and the area kept as dry as possible. Oral narcotic analgesics are sometimes necessary in severe cases. Persistent pain and bleeding caused by radiation proctitis can require surgical resection of the involved bowel (68, 88).

Anorectal Abscess

Etiology and Pathophysiology

Localized abscesses are common in the perianal and anorectal areas. These infections can arise in pre-existing tears, fissures, or thrombosed hemorrhoids, or can be seen in systemic illnesses such as Crohn's disease, ulcerative colitis, and leukemia (88, 93). An underlying cause, however, often cannot be found. Abscesses can be superficial and in the perianal region, or they can be deep, in any of several potential spaces around the rectum.

Symptoms and Signs

Perianal abscesses, the most common type of anorectal abscess, present as painful localized masses. Pain is usually throbbing and constant until the abscess bursts.

Symptoms of deep anorectal abscesses are often not as well defined as those of the more superficial lesions. An aching sensation in the rectum, or poorly defined lower abdominal and pelvic pain, can be present. Fever is common in these deep perirectal infections.

Diagnosis

Physical examination in patients with anorectal abscesses usually reveals the diagnosis. Superficial abscesses are easily recognized by the presence of a red, tender, localized swelling near the anus. Deeper abscesses are detected by an exquisitely tender area of rectum found on digital examination. If deeper abscesses have burst into the rectal lumen, a purulent discharge is present. Peripheral leukocytosis is common, especially with deeper abscesses. Anorectal abscesses are distinguished from pilonidal, Bartholin's, and periurethral abscesses by their anatomic relationships to other perineal structures.

Treatment

Treatment of all anorectal abscesses centers around surgical drainage (88, 93). It is not necessary to wait for fluctuance before carrying out incision and drainage. Antibiotics are useful when cellulitis is present around the abscess. The patient should have a follow-up examination for the detection of complications, such as fistula formation.

Anal Fissures

Etiology and Pathophysiology

Fissures of the anus are one of the most frequently seen painful anal conditions. These superficial tears of the anal epithelium are localized to the posterior midline of the anus in over 90% of cases (88). Most commonly found in young adults with a recent history of constipation, fissures are probably formed by a tearing force associated with the passage of a large firm stool (90). Most fissures heal spontaneously within a few weeks. Chronic fissures, which are less likely to heal, occur in patients with high internal anal sphincter pressures. Other chronic fissures are seen in patients with Crohn's disease, ulcerative colitis, carcinoma, syphilis, and tuberculosis.

Symptoms and Signs

Most patients can relate the acute onset of pain caused by a fissure to defecation. Pain is localized to the anal area. The pain is continuous but is exacerbated by sitting and further defecation. Secondary constipation often occurs because of the fear of provoking pain with further bowel movements. A small amount of rectal bleeding and discharge can be present.

Diagnosis

The diagnosis of an anal fissure can usually be made by physical examination. Inspection of the anus often reveals an edematous skin tag adjacent to the distal aspect of the fissure. Rectal examination, with the examiner's smallest finger lubricated with 2% lidocaine (Xylocaine) jelly, confirms the localized indurated anal wall and excludes associated mass lesions. Anoscopy and sigmoidoscopy must usually be postponed until the fissure has healed, but should eventually be done to exclude other rectal lesions.

Treatment

Treatment of anal fissures involves local analgesics and stool softeners to avoid pain and recurrent tears (90, 94). Orally administered mineral oil or bulk agents such as psyllium usually loosen the stool, which facilitates stool passage and results in decreased straining. After the fissure has healed, additional fiber in the diet in the form of bran is often all that is needed to prevent recurrence. Local application of a lubricant containing a local anesthetic is helpful before bowel movements. This is best applied into the anal canal with the patient's little finger. Surgical resection or lateral subcutaneous spincterotomy is usually required to treat chronic idiopathic fissures (95).

Anorectal Neoplasms (XXVIII-1)

Etiology and Pathophysiology

Neoplasms of the anal canal and perianal region account for less than 5% of lower gastrointestinal malignancies (78). Approximately 50% of the neoplasms that present as anal masses are adenocarcinomas of the rectum, with distal growth through the anal canal. Most of the remainder are epidermoid carcinomas of the anal canal. Melanomas, basal cell carcinomas, and cloacogenic carcinomas are other rare neoplasms of this region (88) (see Table 59-3, p. 1149 for 1987 estimates).

Anal epidermoid carcinomas are associated with the presence of benign anorectal disorders, although the exact role of these conditions in the pathogenesis of the carcinoma is unknown. Over 50% of patients with these cancers have a history of hemorrhoids, fistulas, fissures, leukoplakia, abscesses, or anal warts (96).

Symptoms and Signs

Neoplasms of the anus and distal rectum present with symptoms different from those of more proximal colorectal cancers. These tumors are first detected either as an anal mass, because of bleeding or mucous discharge, or because of painful defecation. Continuous localized pain unassociated with defecation can also occur. Narrowing of stool caliber is often noted. Symptoms of large bowel obstruction can be seen with advanced cases. Weight loss and inguinal adenopathy usually indicate the presence of metastases.

Diagnosis

The diagnosis of an anorectal neoplasm is usually obvious after visual inspection of the anus and a gentle rectal examination. Any firm or indurated lesion of the anal canal should be suspected as being neoplastic. These mass lesions can be biopsied through the anoscope to obtain a histologic diagnosis. If the patient can tolerate the procedure, the proximal extent of the tumor should be assessed by sigmoidoscopy.

Treatment

Therapy of anorectal neoplasms can involve radiotherapy, surgery, or chemotherapy. Radiotherapy, either alone or prior to surgical excision, has been effective in about 75% of patients with anal epidermoid carcinomas (78, 97). Preoperative radiation therapy can also increase survival in some patients with adenocarcinomas of the rectum (98). Abdominoperineal resection is the operative treatment of choice for rectal and large anal cancers. Wide local excision should be reserved for anal tumors smaller than 4 cm^2 (78). Combined radiotherapy and chemotherapy using 5-fluorouracil and nitrosoureas in patients with rectal adenocarcinoma that has extended through the bowel wall decreases the incidence of recurrent disease but does not change overall survival (99). Chemotherapy has not been effective in the treatment of metastatic cancers of the anus and rectum.

Palliative treatment of anorectal neoplasms involves multiple therapeutic procedures. Radiation therapy of unresectable rectal cancers relieves symptoms of pain, bleeding, and discharge in about 75% of patients, (78, 100). Narcotic analgesics should be used liberally during radiation therapy and in patients with pain unresponsive to radiation. The use of intra-arterial chemotherapy, chronic intrathecal morphine administration, and ablative neurosurgical procedures in patients with intractable pain caused by anorectal neoplasms is similar to the use of these treatments for intestinal neoplasms. Pain management in patients with advanced cancer remains a challenging problem (Chapter 24).

REFERENCES

1. Hammond, E.C.: Some preliminary findings on physical complaints from a prospective study of 1,064,004 men and women. Am. J. Public Health, 54:11, 1964.
2. Whitehead, W.E., and Schuster, M.M.: Inflammatory bowel diseases. In Gastrointestinal Disorders—Behavioral and Physiological Basis for Treatment. Orlando, Academic Press, 1985, pp. 125–154.
3. Sleisenger, M.H., and Fordtran, J.S. (eds.): Gastrointestinal Disease. 3rd Ed. Philadelphia, W.B. Saunders, 1983.
4. Curie, D.J.: Abdominal Pain. New York, McGraw-Hill, 1979.
5. Kimmey, M.: Abdominal pain. In Blue Book of Medical Diagnosis. Edited by R.O. Cummins and M.S. Eisenberg. Philadelphia, W.B. Saunders, 1986, pp. 434–442.
6. Silen, W.: Cope's Early Diagnosis of the Acute Abdomen. 16th Ed. New York, Oxford University Press, 1983.
7. Eisenberg, R.L., et al.: Evaluation of plain abdominal radiographs in the diagnosis of abdominal pain. Ann. Intern. Med., 97:257, 1982.
8. Dooley, C.P.: Double-contrast barium meal and upper gastrointestinal endoscopy, a comparative study. Ann. Intern. Med., 101:538, 1984.
9. Silverstein, F.E., and Tytgat, G.N.J.: Atlas of Gastrointestinal Endoscopy. Philadelphia, W.B. Saunders, 1987.
10. Hunt, R.H., and Waye, J.D.: Colonoscopy: Techniques, Clinical Practice, and Colour Atlas. London, Chapman and Hall, 1981.
11. Eisenberg, R.L.: Gastrointestinal Radiology. Philadelphia, J.B. Lippincott, 1983.
12. Moss, A.A., Gamsu, G., and Genant, H.K.: Computed Tomography of the Body. Philadelphia, W.B. Saunders, 1983.
13. Goldberg, B.B.: Abdominal Ultrasonography. 2nd Ed. New York, John Wiley & Sons, 1984.
14. Morrison, J.F.B.: The afferent innervation of the gastrointestinal tract. In Nerves and the Gut. Edited by F.P. Brooks and P.W. Evers. Thorofare, NJ, Charles B. Slack, 1977, pp. 297–322.
15. Jones, C.: Digestive Tract Pain: Diagnosis and Treatment. New York, MacMillan, 1939.
16. Hansen, K., and Schliack, H.: Segmental Innervation. Georg Thieme Verlag, Stuttgart, 1962.
17. Swarbick, E.T., et al.: Site of pain from the irritable bowel. Lancet, 2:443, 1980.
18. Bingham, J.R., Ingelfinger, F.J., and Smithwick, R.H.: The effects of sympathectomy on abdominal pain in man. Gastroenterology, 15:18, 1950.
19. Silverberg, M., and Daum, F.: Textbook of Pediatric Gastroenterology. 2nd Ed. Chicago, Year Book Medical, 1988.
20. Filston, H.C.: Surgical Problems in Children. Recognition and Referral. St. Louis, C.V. Mosby, 1982.
21. Palmer, E.: Gastric diverticulosis. Am. Fam. Physician, 7:114, 1973.
22. Babb, R., Peck, O., and Jamplis, R.: Gastric volvulus and obstruction in paraesophageal hiatal hernia. Am. J. Dig. Dis., 17:119, 1972.
23. Sauerbruch, T., et al.: Endoscopy in the diagnosis of gastritis: Diagnostic value of endoscopic criteria in relation to histological diagnosis. Endoscopy, 16:101, 1984.

24. Kreuning, J., et al.: Gastric and duodenal mucosa in "healthy" individuals—an endoscopic and histopathological study of 50 volunteers. J. Clin. Pathol., *31*:69, 1978.
25. Thomson, W.O., et al.: Is duodenitis a dyspeptic myth? Lancet, *1*:1197, 1977.
26. Horrocks, J.C., and DeDombal, F.T.: Clinical presentation of patients with "dyspepsia." Gut, *19*:19, 1978.
27. Mollman, K.M., et al.: A diagnostic study of patients with upper abdominal pain. Scand. J. Gastroenterol., *10*:805, 1975.
28. Silvoso, G.R., et al.: Incidence of gastric lesions in patients with rheumatic disease on chronic aspirin therapy. Ann. Intern. Med., *91*:517, 1979.
29. Lambert, R., et al.: Diffuse varioliform gastritis. Digestion, *17*:159, 1968.
30. Dooley, C.P., and Cohen, H.: The clinical significance of Campylobacter pylori. Ann. Intern. Med., *108*:70, 1988.
31. Scharschmidt, B.F.: The natural history of hypertrophic gastropathy (Menetrier's disease). Am. J. Med., *63*:644, 1977.
32. Thompson, W.G.: The Irritable Gut. Baltimore, University Park Press, 1979.
33. Gomez, J., and Dally, P.: Psychologically mediated abdominal pain in surgical and medical outpatient clinics. Br. Med. J., *1*:1451, 1977.
34. Hoftiezer, J.W., et al.: Comparison of the effects of regular and enteric-coated aspirin on gastroduodenal mucosa of man. Lancet, *2*:609, 1980.
35. Andre, C., et al.: Randomized placebo-controlled double-blind trial of two dosages of sodium chromoglycate in treatment of varioliform gastritis: Comparison with cimetidine. Gut, *23*:348, 1982.
36. Thompson, W.G.: Functional diseases of the upper gastrointestinal tract. *In* Current Therapy in Gastroenterology and Liver Diseases 1984–1985. Edited by T.M. Bayless. Philadelphia, B.C. Decker, 1984, pp. 99–102.
37. Nyren, O., et al.: Absence of therapeutic benefit from antacids or cimetidine in non-ulcer dyspepsia. N. Engl. J. Med., *314*:339, 1986.
38. Flemstrom, G., and Turnberg, L.A.: Gastroduodenal defense mechanisms. Clin. Gastroenterol., *13*:327, 1984.
39. Harrison, A., et al.: Most patients with active symptomatic duodenal ulcers fail to develop ulcer-type pain in response to gastroduodenal acidification. J. Clin. Gastroenterol., *4*:105, 1982.
40. Peters, M.N., and Richardson, C.T.: Stressful life events, acid hypersecretion, and ulcer disease. Gastroenterology, *84*:114, 1983.
41. Sontag, S., et al.: Cimetidine, cigarette smoking, and recurrence of duodenal ulcer. N. Engl. J. Med., *311*:689, 1984.
42. Lam, S.K., et al.: Sucralfate overcomes adverse effect of cigarette smoking on duodenal ulcer healing and prolongs subsequent remission. Gastroenterology, *92*:1193, 1987.
43. Armstrong, C.P., and Blower, A.L.: Non-steroidal anti-inflammatory drugs and life threatening complications of peptic ulceration. Gut, *28*:527, 1987.
44. Ippoliti, A., et al.: Recurrent ulcer after successful treatment with cimetidine or antacid. Gastroenterology, *85*:875, 1983.
45. Kennedy, T.: The failures of gastric surgery. Brit. J. Surg., *68*:677, 1981.
46. Priebe, W.M., et al.: Is epigastric tenderness a sign of peptic ulcer disease? Gastroenterology, *82*:16, 1982.
47. Isenberg, J.I., et al.: Healing of benign gastric ulcer with low dose antacid or cimetidine. N. Engl. J. Med., *308*:1319, 1983.
48. Peterson, W.L., et al.: Healing of duodenal ulcer with an antacid regimen. N. Engl. J. Med., *297*:341, 1977.
49. McCarthy, D.M.: Editorial: Ranitidine or cimetidine? Ann. Intern. Med., *99*:551, 1983.
50. Martin, F., et al.: Comparison of the healing capacities of sucralfate and cimetidine in the short-term treatment of duodenal ulcer: A double-blind randomized trial. Gastroenterology, *82*:401, 1982.
51. Malegelada, J.R., et al.: Medical and surgical options in the management of patients with gastrinoma. Gastroenterology, *84*:1524, 1983.
52. Herfarth, C., and Schlag, P. (eds.): Gastric Cancer. Berlin, Springer-Verlag, 1979.
53. Friedman, M., Ogawa, M., and Kisner, D. (eds.): Diagnosis and Treatment of Upper Gastrointestinal Tumors. Amsterdam, Excerpta Medica, 1981.
54. Gastrointestinal Tumor Study Group: Controlled trial of adjuvant chemotherapy following curative resection for gastric cancer. Cancer, *49*:1116, 1982.
55. Thompson, G.E., et al.: Abdominal pain and alcohol celiac plexus nerve block. Anesth. Analg., *56*:1, 1977.
56. Loeser, J.D.: Role of neurosurgery in visceral and perineal pain. *In* Advances in Pain Research and Therapy, Vol. 2. Edited by J.J. Bonica and V. Ventafridda. New York, Raven Press, 1979, pp. 607–614.
57. Moriarity, K.J., and Dawson, A.M.: Functional abdominal pain: Further evidence that whole gut is affected. Br. Med. J., *284*:1670, 1982.
58. Kingham, J.G.C., and Dawson, A.M.: Origin of chronic right upper quadrant pain. Gut, *26*:783, 1985.
59. Doran, F.S.A.: Observations on referred pain from the posterior abdominal wall and pelvis. Br. J. Surg., *49*:376, 1962.
60. Wansbrough, R.M., et al.: Meckel's diverticulum: A 42-year review of 273 cases at the Hospital for Sick Children, Toronto. Can. J. Surg., *1*:15, 1957.
61. Ashley, D.J.B.: Observations on the epidemiology of appendicitis. Gut, *8*:533, 1967.
62. Staniland, R., Ditchburn, J., and de Dombal, F.T.: Clinical presentation of acute abdomen: A study of 600 patients. Br. Med. J., *3*:393, 1972.
63. Plotkin, G.R., Kluge, R.M., and Waldman, R.H.: Gastroenteritis: Etiology, pathophysiology, and clinical manifestations. Medicine, *58*:95, 1979.
64. Blaser, M.D., et al.: Campylobacter enteritis in the United States. Ann. Intern. Med., *98*:360, 1983.
65. Gorbach, S.L.: Traveler's diarrhea. N. Engl. J. Med., *307*:881, 1982.
66. George, W.L., Rolfe, R.D., and Finegold, S.M.: Treatment of antimicrobial agent-induced colitis and diarrhea. Gastroenterology, *79*:366, 1980.
67. Novak, J.M., et al.: Effects of radiation on the human gastrointestinal tract. J. Clin. Gastroenterol., *1*:9, 1979.
68. Galland, R.B., and Spencer, J.: The natural history of clinically established radiation enteritis. Lancet, *1*:1257, 1985.
69. Almy, T.P., and Howell, D.A.: Diverticular disease of the colon. N. Engl. J. Med., *302*:324, 1980.
70. Kirsner, J.B., and Shorter, R.G., (eds.): Inflammatory Bowel Disease. 2nd Ed. Philadelphia, Lea & Febiger, 1980.
71. Mekhjian, H.S., et al.: Clinical features and natural history of Crohn's disease. Gastroenterology, *77*:898, 1979.
72. Greenstein, A.J., Janowitz, H.D., and Sachar, D.B.: The extraintestinal complications of Crohn's disease and ulcerative colitis: A study of 700 patients. Medicine, *55*:401, 1976.
73. Korelitz, B.I.: Therapy of inflammatory bowel disease including use of immunosuppressive agents. Clin. Gastroenterol., *9*:331, 1980.
74. Brandt, L.J., et al.: Metronidazole therapy for perineal Crohn's disease: A follow-up study. Gastroenterology, *83*:383, 1982.
75. Garrett, J.M., Sauer, W.G., and Moertel, C.G.: Colonic motility in ulcerative colitis after opiate administration. Gastroenterology, *53*:93, 1967.
76. Schuffler, M.D., et al.: Chronic intestinal pseudo-obstruction: A report of 27 cases and review of the literature. Medicine, *60*:173, 1981.
77. Morson, B.C.: Genesis of colorectal cancer. Clin. Gastroenterol., *5*:505, 1976.
78. Spratt, J.S.: Neoplasms of the Colon, Rectum, and Anus. Philadelphia, W.B. Saunders, 1984.
79. Winawer, S.J., et al.: Colonoscopic biopsy and cytology in the diagnosis of colon cancer. Cancer, *42*:2849, 1978.
80. Weiss, G.R., et al.: Long-term hepatic arterial infusion of 5-fluorodeoxyuridine for liver metastases using an implantable infusion pump. J. Clin. Oncol., *1*:337, 1983.
81. Cobb, C.A., French, B.N., and Smith, K.A.: Intrathecal morphine for pelvic and sacral pain caused by cancer. Surg. Neurol., *22*:63, 1984.
82. Greenberg, H.S., et al.: Benefit from and tolerance to continuous intrathecal infusion of morphine for intractable cancer pain. J. Neurosurg., *57*:360, 1982.
83. Switz, D.M.: What the gastroenterologist does all day. Gastroenterology, *70*:1048, 1976.
84. Wangle, A.G., and Deller, D.J.: Intestinal motility in man: III. Mechanisms of constipation and diarrhea with particular reference to the irritable colon syndrome. Gastroenterology, *48*:69, 1965.
85. Sullivan, M.A., Cohen, S., and Snape, W.J.: Colonic myoelectrical activity in irritable-bowel syndrome. N. Engl. J. Med., *298*:878, 1978.
86. Manning, A.P., et al.: Towards positive diagnosis of the irritable bowel. Br. Med. J., *2*:653, 1978.

87. Myren, J., et al.: A double-blind study of the effect of trimipramine in patients with the irritable bowel syndrome. Scand. J. Gastroenterol., *19*:835, 1984.
88. Goligher, J.C.: Surgery of the Anus, Rectum, and Colon. 5th Ed. London, Balliere Tindall, 1984.
89. Owen, W.F.: Sexually transmitted diseases and traumatic problems in homosexual men. Ann. Intern. Med., *92*:805, 1980.
90. Lieberman, D.A.: Common anorectal disorders. Ann. Intern. Med., *101*:837, 1984.
91. Murie, J.A., Sim, A.J., and MacKenzie, I.: Rubber band ligation versus haemorrhoidectomy for prolapsing haemorrhoids: A long-term prospective clinical trial. Br. J. Surg., *69*:536, 1982.
92. Mazier, W.P.: Emergency hemorrhoidectomy: A worthwhile procedure. Dis. Colon Rectum, *16*:200, 1973.
93. MacLeod, J.H.: A Method of Proctology. Hagerstown, MD, Harper & Row, 1979.
94. Gough, M.J., and Lewis, A.: The conservative treatment of fissure-in-ano. Br. J. Surg., *70*:175, 1983.
95. Jensen, S.L.: Lateral subcutaneous sphincterotomy versus anal dilatation in the treatment of fissure in ano in outpatients: A prospective randomized study. Brit. Med. J., *289*:528, 1984.
96. Beahrs, O.H., and Wilson, S.M.: Carcinoma of the anus. Ann. Surg., *184*:422, 1976.
97. Green, J.P., et al.: Anal carcinoma: Current therapeutic concepts. Am. J. Surg., *140*:151, 1980.
98. Higgins, G.A., and Roswit, B.: The role of radiotherapy in the surgical treatment of large bowel cancer. Prog. Clin. Cancer, *7*:71, 1981.
99. Gastrointestinal Tumor Study Group: Prolongation of the disease-free interval in surgically treated rectal carcinoma. N. Engl. J. Med., *312*:1465, 1985.
100. Uradaneta-Lafer, N., Kligerman, M.M., and Knowlton, A.H.: Evaluation of palliation in rectal carcinoma. Radiology, *104*:673, 1972.

61 · DISEASES OF THE LIVER, BILIARY SYSTEM, AND PANCREAS

MICHAEL W. MULHOLLAND *and* HAILE T. DEBAS

with contributions by
JOHN J. BONICA

PAIN is a frequent concomitant of diseases of the liver, biliary system, and pancreas. Pain is important both as a diagnostic symptom to be interpreted and as a clinical management problem. Because of the high frequency of hepatobiliary and pancreatic disease in clinical practice, familiarity with hepatic, biliary, and pancreatic pain syndromes is essential.

In this chapter, pain syndromes associated with hepatic disorders (A), biliary disorders (B), and pancreatic disorders (C), are discussed separately. The causes and pathophysiology of primary disease processes involving each of these organ systems are discussed. Painful symptoms are examined from the viewpoint of underlying disease mechanisms. An outline of essential diagnostic tests is provided. Discussion of treatment options focuses on therapy of primary disease processes and on palliation of accompanying organic pain. Path-ologic processes are examined to determine mechanisms of pain production as a guide to rational pain management. Bonica contributed to the description and illustration of the nerve supply of these organs and the illustrations of the pain patterns.

A. LIVER

Basic Considerations

In humans, branches of both vagus nerves and branches of splanchnic nerves innervate the liver (1). Two separate, but intercommunicating plexuses are formed by the sympathetic and parasympathetic nerve fibers (Figs. 61-1 and 61-2). An interior plexus composed of parasympathetic fibers from the anterior vagus and of sympathetic fibers from the celiac ganglion surrounds the hepatic artery. The posterior plexus is located behind the bile duct and portal vein, and is derived from the posterior vagus and right celiac ganglion. Hepatic nerves enter the liver in association with blood vessels and bile ducts and parallel these structures as they arborize within the liver parenchyma.

Hepatic pain is not transmitted by the vagi, although the liver receives a substantial vagal innervation and approximtely 90% of vagal fibers are primary afferents. Vagotomy does not eliminate the perception of hepatic pain. Hepatic pain is believed to be transmitted to the central nervous system by afferent sympathetic fibers. In the cat, approximately 50% of visceral sympathetic fibers are afferent (2).

Clinical experience has attributed hepatic pain to stretch of the liver capsule by parenchymal swelling. The rate of hepatic enlargement can be the important variable in the production of pain; gradual hepatic enlargement is often painless. Morphologic evidence suggests that hepatic nerves might also be sensitive to changes in hepatic venous pressure (3). Nerve fibrils have been demonstrated in humans in association with intimal endothelial cells of hepatic veins that are structurally similar to known sensory nerves (4).

Hepatic inflammatory processes can produce well-localized somatic pain if the parietal peritoneum is involved. Sharp, intense, upper abdominal or lower thoracic discomfort is characteristic. Typically, inspiration intensifies such pain. Referred hepatic pain is usually noted in the right shoulder and scapular areas (Fig. 61-3).

Clinical Considerations

Viral Infection

Symptoms and Signs

Acute viral hepatitis is frequently accompanied by hepatic enlargement and pain. During the early prodromal stage of the illness, pain is usually absent and

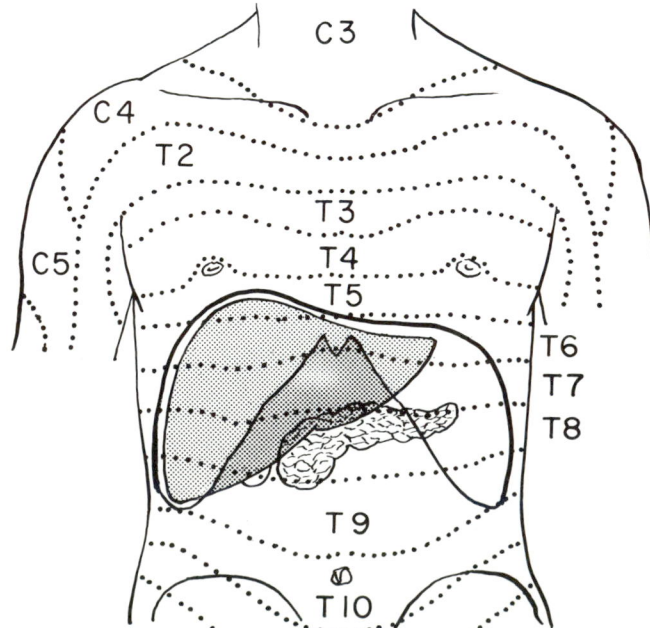

FIG. 61-1. Schematic depiction of the position of the liver and pancreas in relation to body wall and dermatomes. The liver extends from T5 to T9 while the pancreas is located within T7 to T9.

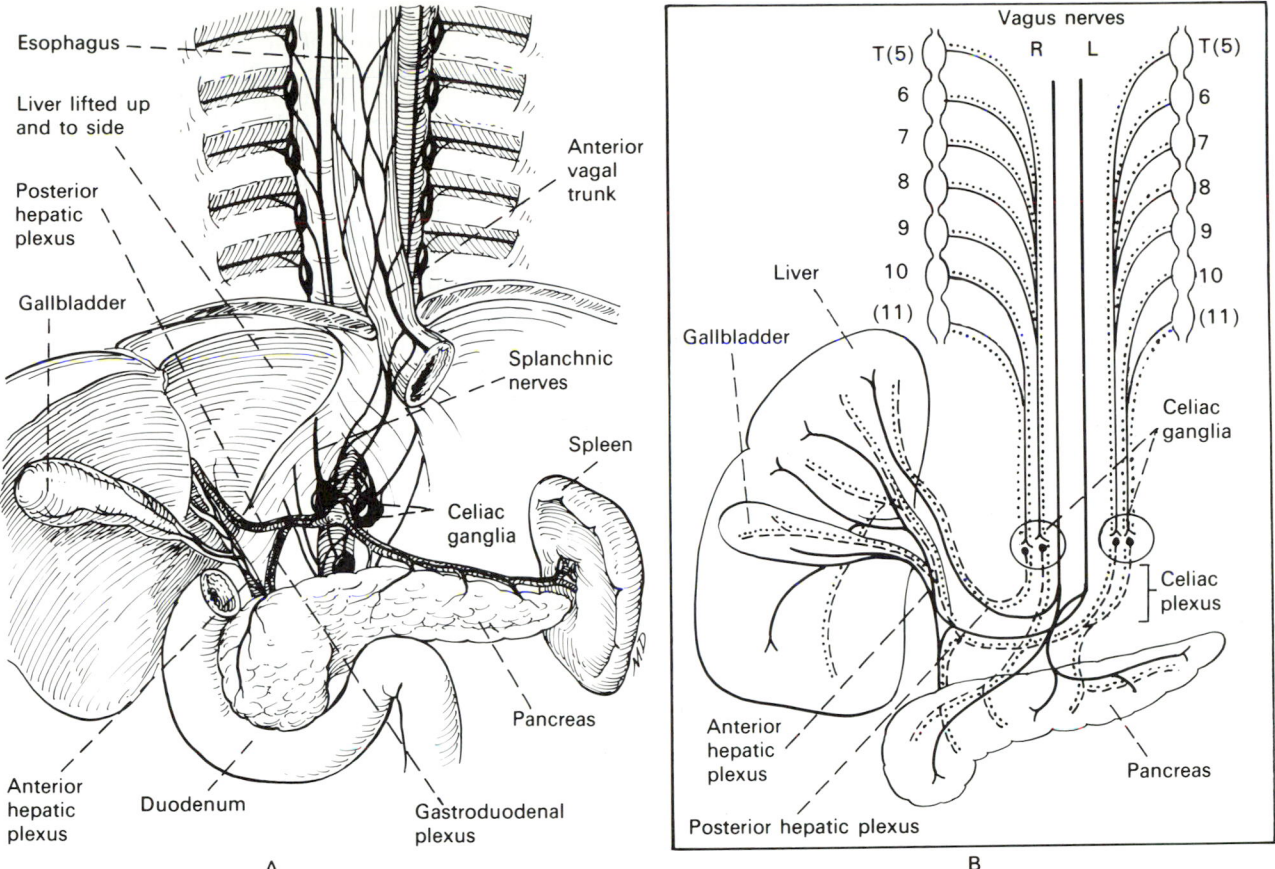

FIG. 61-2. Anatomy of nerve supply to the liver, biliary system, and pancreas. **A.** Relationship of the vagus and sympathetic nerves contributing to the celiac plexus and the subsidiary plexuses which follow vessels supplying the viscera. **B.** Schematic depiction of the course and distribution of two vagal nerves consisting primarily of preganglionic fibers, which synapse in the wall of the viscera with short postganglionic fibers (*not shown*). Preganglionic sympathetic fibers passing primarily from T6 to T9 (but also possibly from T5, T10, and T11) pass through the superior and middle thoracic splanchnic nerves to the celiac ganglia, where they synapse with postganglionic fibers (*dashed lines*). Segments in parentheses in the sympathetic chain are variable. The afferent fibers are shown by the dotted lines. See text for details.

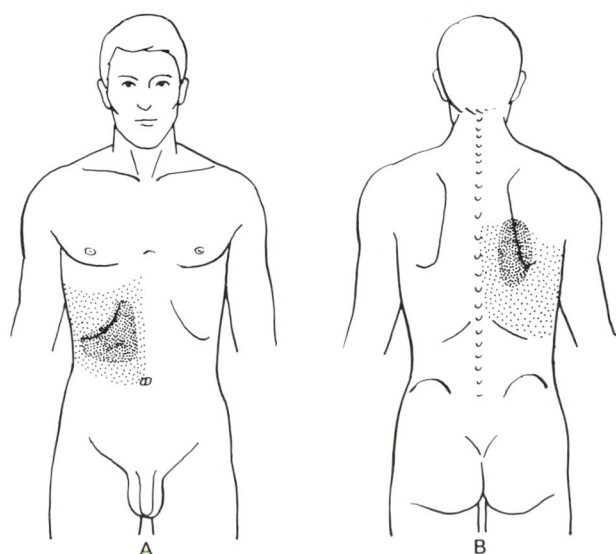

FIG. 61-3. Areas of referred hepatic pain in the anterior (**A**) and posterior (**B**) regions of the body. The heavy stipple indicates the area of pain reference while the light stipple indicates the extensive cutaneous hyperalgesia often associated with the pain.

physical findings are minimal. Fatigue, anorexia, nonspecific constitutional complaints, and arthralgias predominate. By the time jaundice appears, over half of affected patients are symptomatic with hepatic pain. The discomfort is often described as a dull, heavy, unpleasant sensation, localized to the right upper abdomen. Hepatomegaly is common; the liver edge is usually smooth and tender to palpation.

Diagnosis

In the presence of appropriate symptoms, acute viral hepatitis can be diagnosed by determination of progressively elevated serum transaminase levels. The serum alkaline phosphatase levels can be normal or moderately elevated. Increases in the serum bilirubin level are variable. Assays to detect circulating viral antigens should be performed to characterize the disease further.

Treatment

Treatment of uncomplicated acute viral hepatitis is supportive, consisting of nutritional care, pain relief, and avoidance of hepatotoxic drugs or agents. The accompanying hepatic discomfort is usually not a difficult management problem, but caution should be exercised in the administration of sedatives or analgesics; agents with significant hepatic metabolic effects should be avoided.

Bacterial Infection

Symptoms and Signs

Hepatic abscess should be suspected when hepatic pain is present in a patient with systemic sepsis. The most frequent localizing symptom is a constant dull pain in the right upper quadrant of the abdomen, present in 50 to 90% of such patients (5–7). Radiation of pain to the right shoulder and scapula is common. Most patients with hepatic abscess have a large, tender liver on physical examination. Jaundice is unusual, occurring in only 10% of patients (5). Ascites is rare. Systemic signs of sepsis predominate. Fevers, chills, rigor, and tachycardia are usually present. Malaise, anorexia, weight loss, and nausea are frequent, nonspecific complaints.

Pathophysiology

Bacterial infection of the liver usually manifests as a parenchymal abscess. Hepatic abscesses can develop following bacterial contamination from several routes—by direct extension from an adjacent suppurative process, by portal venous bacteremia from a distant septic focus, and through the biliary system during ascending cholangitis. In 20% of hepatic abscesses, the source cannot be determined after thorough clinical and pathologic evaluation (cryptogenic abscess) (6). The microbiology of hepatic abscesses reflects their common association with other gastrointestinal inflammatory diseases. Enteric organisms are recovered from cultures of the abscess in 80% of cases. Escherichea coli and Klebsiella species are discovered in greater than 50% of hepatic abscesses; anaerobic bacteria are frequent copathogens. Multimicrobial abscesses are common.

Diagnosis

Radiologic evaluation is essential to diagnose hepatic abscesses, to define the disease process anatomically, and to detect other foci of intraperitoneal sepsis. Ultrasonography is essential to rule out biliary tract disease. It is also a useful screening procedure for locating hepatic masses and to differentiate solid and cystic processes (7). CT scanning, however, currently provides the most detailed and accurate anatomic information for hepatic abscesses. In most cases, CT scanning should be employed in planning definitive therapy (8). Optimistic reports have also been published using [99]technetium and [111]indium radionuclide scans to diagnose hepatic sepsis (9).

Treatment

The treatment of hepatic abscesses requires long-term (6-week) antibiotic therapy and drainage of the abscess. Antibiotic therapy is usually started prior to detection of the abscess because most patients have signs of systemic sepsis. The choice of antibiotic should reflect the polymicrobial enteric flora commonly associated with hepatic abscess; broad coverage of aerobic gram-negative organisms and anaerobes should be achieved. Percutaneous catheter drainage of hepatic abscesses is often successful, especially if the infection is solitary and not associated with other intraperitoneal pathology. Operative therapy of accompanying foci of infection (e.g., suppurative cholangitis), however, is frequently required. Treatment of the pain associated with hepatic infection depends on successful treatment of the abscess. Chronic pain syndromes have not been associated with parenchymal hepatic infection.

Gonococcal Perihepatitis

Pathophysiology

Gonococcal perihepatitis, described in women as a cause of right upper quadrant pain, is known as the Fitz-Hugh-Curtis syndrome. The gonococcal organism is transmitted venereally and has an affinity for the urogenital epithelium. Ascending infection presumably enters the peritoneal cavity through the fallopian tubes and reaches the perihepatic space through the right paracolic gutter. Pelvic infection might not be clinically obvious. Chlamydia can also cause the syndrome in women in the presence or absence of gonococci.

Symptoms and Signs

Acute gonococcal perihepatitis begins as sudden right upper quadrant pain with radiation to the right shoulder. Inspiration intensifies the pain. Fever, tenderness, and rebound are common. Acute gonococcal perihepatitis can be suspected when these symptoms are present in sexually active women with clinical evidence of pelvic inflammatory disease or gonococcal organisms demonstrated on cervical culture.

Treatment

Treatment of acute gonococcal perihepatitis requires antibiotic therapy appropriate for treatment of the underlying pelvic inflammatory disease. Painful symptoms should resolve promptly (10).

Chronic or incompletely treated perihepatitis has been reported to result in formation of adhesions from the liver to the surrounding parietal peritoneum. A chronic upper abdominal pain syndrome can result from traction of such adhesions on the parietal peritoneum. Peritoneoscopy can be used to identify this process. Lysis of offending adhesions should eliminate the pain (11).

Neoplastic Disease

Involvement of the liver by primary and metastatic neoplasms remains a great challenge to those interested in the treatment of pain. The magnitude of this problem can be appreciated by considering that 20 to 25% of cancer deaths in the United States are caused by primary or metastatic hepatic cancers. Results of a study by Jaffe and colleagues (12) suggested that metastatic replacement of the liver is the aspect of visceral cancers that most directly contributes to mortality. In most reports the mean survival of patients with symptomatic liver tumors was less than 1 year. Because cure of primary or metastatic hepatic tumors is rarely achieved, palliation, including palliation of painful symptoms, is a major clinical goal.

Primary hepatic tumors cause approximately 1% of cancer deaths in the United States and other developed countries. In parts of Africa and Asia, however, hepatocellular carcinomas cause up to 20 to 40% of cancer-related deaths. Hepatomas frequently develop in the setting of pre-existing severe liver disease. More than 50% of patients who develop hepatocellular carcinoma have histologic evidence of cirrhosis. Approximately 5% of patients with alcoholic cirrhosis in the United States develop hepatocellular carcinoma. The frequency is even greater in individuals with postnecrotic cirrhosis (10%), untreated hemochromatosis (20%), or cirrhosis caused by alpha-1-antitrypsin deficiency. Because of the high absolute number of patients with alcoholism, the majority of patients in most reported series have Laennec's cirrhosis typical of alcohol abuse (13).

Symptoms and Signs

Most authors, while emphasizing that symptoms caused by hepatoma are vague and nonspecific, have reported that pain is a prominent symptom when patients first seek medical attention. Ihde and associates (14) noted that more than 70% of hepatoma patients have right upper quadrant or epigastric pain of a chronic nature, most commonly associated with a hepatic mass, weight loss, or ascites. The pain is frequently described as an epigastric pressure, fullness, or heaviness. The onset of symptoms is usually insidious. A second relatively common presentation, noted in 8% of patients with hepatoma, consists of acute right upper quadrant pain, fever, and jaundice, mimicking that of acute cholecystitis.

Because hepatocellular carcinomas tend to develop in patients with hepatic functional impairment, systemic symptoms can be prominent and rapidly progressive. Cachexia and wasting, development of jaundice or worsening of pre-existing jaundice, and intractable ascites are common. Hemorrhagic phenomena are frequent. Hemorrhage, including gastrointestinal bleeding from varices and hemoperitoneum caused by intraperitoneal rupture of tumors, is a proximate cause of death in 50% of hepatocellular cancer patients. Hepatomas are among the tumors most frequently associated with paraneoplastic syndromes. Secondary paraneoplastic syndromes include polycythemia, thrombocytosis, hypoglycemia, hypercalcemia, and production of ectopic adrenocorticotropic hormones.

Treatment

Curative therapy is not currently available for the large majority of patients. On the basis of physical examination and noninvasive tests, two-thirds of patients with hepatocellular carcinoma are clearly unresectable when they first come to medical attention, and only one in three of the patients who undergo laparotomy can have potentially curative hepatic resection. Thus, at present, only 10% of all patients with hepatocellular carcinoma are potentially curable. The response of hepatocellular carcinoma to intravenous single-agent and multiagent chemotherapy has been unimpressive. Response rates of 25% or less have been reported, with no significant increase in survival time (15). The continuous infusion of chemotherapeutic agents into the hepatic artery has recently been described for the treatment of hepatomas (16). Initial results suggest a modest improvement in palliation compared to those obtained with intravenous chemotherapy (17). Pain during therapy is controlled with nonsteroidal anti-inflammatory drugs and potent narcotics. In hospitals in which qualified personnel are available, severe pain can be temporarily relieved with segmental epidural analgesia (Chapter 94) or intraspinal narcotics (Chapter 95). See Chapter 24 for a comprehensive summary of the management of cancer pain.

Hepatic Adenoma

Diagnosis

In a woman of child-bearing age, who has been taking birth control pills and presents with chronic right upper quadrant pain, the diagnosis of hepatic adenoma should be seriously considered. Biliary tract disease is first excluded by ultrasonography, which can also show the presence of a solid tumor in the liver. If the ultrasonography is negative, CT scanning or peritoneoscopic examination of the liver surface might be required. These adenomas are highly vascular and should not be biopsied to avoid life-threatening hemorrhage.

Treatment

The first step in treatment is to stop the birth control tablets. If the tumor is larger than 6 to 8 cm in diameter or pain is not rapidly relieved, surgical excision is necessary. Pain rapidly resolves after excision. In patients for whom discontinuation of birth control medication and follow-up is decided on, gradual resolution of pain and tumor regression should occur. Otherwise, surgical excision should be considered.

Hepatic adenomas can also present acutely, either with severe right upper quadrant pain or with spontaneous hemorrhage into the peritoneal cavity. Emergency surgery is indicated in these situations.

Metastatic Tumors

Metastatic tumors occur with 20 to 30 times the frequency of primary hepatic cancers. Hepatic metastatic disease is a particular problem for cancers drained by the portal venous system, being 7 times more likely to occur than tumors arising outside the portal bed (18). In a series of 8455 autopsies reported from the Roswell Park Cancer Center, 39% of adult patients with solid tumors had hepatic involvement (18).

Symptoms and Signs

Many patients with hepatic metastases are asymptomatic. Asymptomatic hepatic metastases are discovered in 15 to 20% of patients with colorectal carcinoma during staging of the cancers before operation or during laparotomy. Most patients with hepatic metastases are symptomatic, however, with pain as a prominent complaint. The pain associated with hepatic metastases is usually constant, dull, and localized to the epigastrium. Accompanying anorexia, weight loss, fatigue, fever, and epigastric fullness are common. Occasionally, acute episodes of right upper quadrant pain can herald hemorrhage into a hepatic metastasis or tumor necrosis. Unlike primary hepatomas, jaundice and ascites are uncommon until the advanced stages of hepatic metastatic disease. When jaundice occurs as an initial finding, malignant biliary obstruction by enlarged nodes in the porta hepatis or by direct growth of biliary or pancreatic carcinomas is the usual finding. Death occurs as a result of liver failure from progressive replacement of the liver parenchyma.

Prognosis

The survival pattern in cases of hepatic metastasis depends on patients' functional status, the extent of hepatic replacement by the metastatic tumor, and the presence or absence of an extrahepatic tumor. A prospective study of 101 patients with colorectal cancer reported no survivors after 4 years for patients with multiple or widespread hepatic metastases. Only 16% of those with solitary hepatic metastases lived for 5 years (19). Survival is markedly decreased in patients who are nutritionally debilitated when metastases are discovered, or if extrahepatic tumor is also present.

Treatment

Selected patients with metastatic hepatic neoplasms (primarily colorectal cancers) can be candidates for curative surgery. They must meet rigorous criteria: control of the primary cancer; absence of extrahepatic metastases; adequate functional hepatic reserve; and confinement of disease to one hepatic lobe. Fewer than 10% of all patients with hepatic metastases fulfill these criteria, and only 30% of potential candidates for surgical excision have resectable disease at the time of exploration. Approximately 25% of patients who undergo resection survive for 5 years postoperatively (20). Response to systemic chemotherapy depends on the site of the primary neoplasm, the extent of hepatic involvement, and the route of administration. Long-term palliation is occasionally possible (21).

Because cure of hepatic neoplasms is uncommon, symptomatic palliation is of cardinal importance. Measures to control the secondary manifestations of hepatic dysfunction are important therapeutic adjuncts. Relief of ascites by pharmacologic or mechanical means, treatment of the pruritis accompanying biliary obstruction, and attention to nutrition are examples of measures that make palliation of pain much more effective.

A commitment should be made to maintain patients with hepatic neoplasms on oral medications for as long as possible. It is generally possible and practical to maintain most patients with hepatic tumors on oral opioids and nonopioids plus adjuvants until the last few days of their lives (22). Sedation, the major adverse side effect, must be monitored but is generally not debilitating. Most patients remain ambulatory and can retain some independence. A discussion of specific agents, routes of administration, and dosage schedules is found in Chapter 24. If large doses of oral opioids are ineffective in relieving severe pain, intraspinal opioids should be given a trial. In patients with severe excruciating pain unaffected by the aforementioned procedures, a celiac plexus block with alcohol should be considered if a physician skilled in its administration is available.

B. BILIARY SYSTEM

Basic Considerations

In humans, the biliary system is supplied by sympathetic afferent fibers originating from the T6 through T10 dermatomes (Fig. 61-2). Although sympathetic afferent innervation of the biliary system is bilateral, most fibers transmitting visceral pain traverse the right splanchnic nerves. The gallbladder and bile ducts receive extensive parasympathetic innervation, both through the hepatic branches of the left vagus and the celiac division of the posterior vagus. Visceral biliary pain, however, is not transmitted by afferent vagal fibers. Vagotomy does not alter the perception of biliary pain.

Visceral pain fibers in the biliary system are primarily sensitive to distension of the gallbladder or bile ducts and to forceful muscular contraction of the gallbladder in the presence of distal ductal obstruction (see Chapter 3 for details). Distension of the gallbladder or common bile duct most often causes pain when the distension occurs acutely; gradual enlargement usually does not cause painful symptoms. In humans, experimental dilatation of these structures causes an intense crampy pain in the epigastrium or right upper quadrant (23). The pain can be referred to the back at the level of the right scapula (Fig. 61-4). Active contraction of the gallbladder accompanying complete or nearly complete duct obstruction causes the pain of biliary colic. Colic is initiated when gallbladder contraction is stimulated by the hormone cholecystokinin. Cholecystokinin release, in turn, is stimulated by intraduodenal fats (24) or amino acids (25). Biliary visceral pain is usually not dramatic if the obstruction develops gradually within the common bile ducts, perhaps because of the capacity afforded by the extrahepatic and intrahepatic biliary systems.

Inflammatory disease of the gallbladder can cause stimulation of the afferent nerve fibers of the parietal peritoneum, which is experienced as somatic pain. Nerve fibers that are activated by stimulation of the parietal peritoneum are distributed in the areolar conective tissue beneath the parietal mesothelium. These myelinated fibers are organized in dermatomes; biliary inflammation generally stimulates somatic afferents that reach the spinal cord through the 6th to 9th intercostal nerves corresponding to dermatomes T6 through T9. Somatic pain associated with biliary disease is intense, easily described, and well localized to the right upper quadrant. When present, somatic pain tends to obscure accompanying visceral pain.

Clinical Considerations

Gallstones (XXI-2)

Calculous biliary tract disease is a major problem in the United States. Approximately 12% of adults in this country are prone to the development of symptomatic

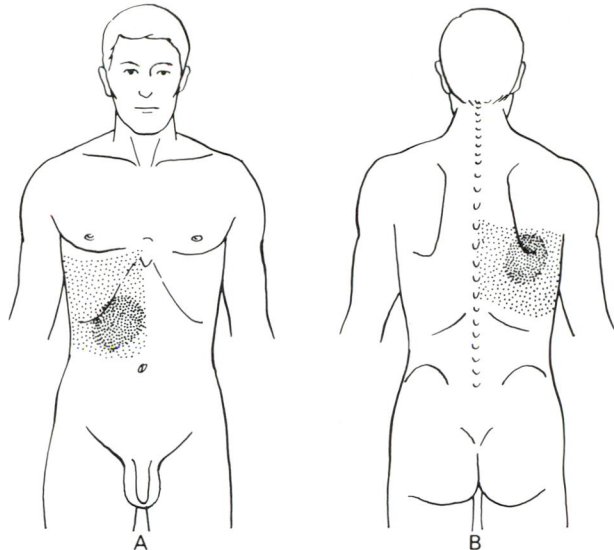

FIG. 61-4. Areas of referred biliary pain in the anterior (**A**) and posterior (**B**) regions of the body. The heavy stipple indicates the area of pain reference while the light stipple indicates the extensive cutaneous hyperalgesia often associated with the pain.

gallstones; more than 500,000 biliary tract operations are performed each year (26). Of those with symptoms from biliary calculi, 60 to 75% have colic as their initial symptom.

Symptoms and Signs

An episode of biliary colic usually begins with poorly localized pain in the midepigastrium. The pain can eventually move to the right upper quadrant. The discomfort is constant and surprisingly intense. Symptoms can persist for 4 to 8 hours before gradually abating. Accompanying anorexia, nausea, and vomiting magnify the unpleasant visceral sensations. Somatic pain is absent unless obstruction is complicated by inflammation. Referral of biliary visceral pain to the scapular area is frequently observed. Right upper quadrant tenderness and guarding are usually absent, as are systemic signs of inflammation.

The completeness of obstruction and the promptness of relief of obstruction probably determine whether gallbladder inflammation will occur to complicate biliary colic. In most people (90%) the obstruction relents and inflammatory changes are minimal and nonprogressive. If obstruction is not relieved, continued distension can result in the progressive inflammation of the gallbladder wall that characterizes acute cholecystitis.

Pain associated with acute cholecystitis is usually well localized by history and physical examination to the right upper quadrant. Somatic pain can be present if the inflammatory process is in contact with the parietal peritoneum. Referred pain to the right shoulder can also be noted. Localized tenderness is noted in the right upper quadrant on physical examination. Gentle deep palpation heightens the discomfort. In one-third of patients a palpable mass representing gallbladder and adherent omentum and bowel is noted. Low-grade fever (less than 101° F) is common but does not reliably distinguish biliary colic and acute cholecystitis.

Diagnosis

Mild to moderate cases of acute cholecystitis are accompanied by modest leukocytosis, about 12,000 white blood cells per mm^3. Serum bilirubin values are reported to be elevated in 20% of patients with acute cholecystitis (usually lower than 4 mg/100 ml). Serum alkaline phosphatase and serum amylase levels can also be modestly and nonspecifically elevated.

Ultrasonography has become the method of choice for demonstrating the presence of gallstones within the gallbladder. Using modern equipment and a real-time technique, several authors have reported that gallstones can be detected with sensitivity and specificity of diagnosis that exceed 90% (27). The presence of acute cholecystic inflammation can be implied by the sonographic presence of a thickened gallbladder wall or pericholecystic edema. Occasionally, radionuclide scanning of the biliary system can be useful in demonstrating cystic duct obstruction (28). Alternative examinations, such as oral cholecystography, endoscopic retrograde cholangiopancreatography (ERCP), and percutaneous transhepatic cholangiography have limited usefulness in uncomplicated cases.

Treatment

Cholecystectomy is the recommended treatment for biliary colic and for acute or chronic cholecystitis. In the presence of gallstones, the typical visceral pain associated with biliary tract disease is permanently relieved in 95% of patients (29). Nonspecific dyspeptic symptoms associated with definite gallbladder calculi are relieved in 75% of patients.

Postcholecystectomy Pain (XXI-3)

In certain patients, cholecystectomy can be one of the most effective operations employed for relief of pain. Nonetheless, approximately 5 to 20% of patients continue to have abdominal pain that is severe enough to prompt medical evaluation after surgery (30). These patients represent difficult diagnostic and therapeutic problems. They are frequently evaluated and cared for by physicians interested in chronic pain.

Pathophysiology

Several factors have been identified that place patients at increased risk of post-cholecystectomy pain. Those individuals who have a functioning gallbladder identified preoperatively by oral cholecystography have a significantly higher incidence of postoperative distress than those with nonfunctioning gallbladders. Those who have non-inflamed gallbladders or gallbladders without calculi have a high incidence of postcholecystectomy pain. In addition, the risk of developing postoperative symptoms increases the longer the symptoms were present preoperatively.

Possible causes of postcholecystectomy pain can be separated into four general categories: incorrect preoperative diagnosis, unrecognized accompanying hepatobiliary disease, incomplete cholecystectomy, and papillary obstruction (Table 61-1).

TABLE 61-1. Causes of Postcholecystectomy Pain Syndromes

General Category	Histopathologic Diagnosis	Method of Investigation
Incorrect preoperative diagnosis	Peptic ulcer	Upper gastrointestinal GI endoscopy
	Pancreatitis	Serum amylase determination, ultrasonography
	Functional bowel disorders	Barium, enema, colonoscopy
Unrecognized hepatobiliary disease	Retained common duct stone; biliary stricture; neoplasms	ERCP*
Incomplete cholecystectomy	Gallbladder remnant; cyst duct remnant	ERCP
Papillary obstruction	Sphincter of Oddi stenosis; ampulla of Vater dyskinesia	ERCP and biliary manometry

*Endoscopic retrograde cholangiopancreatography.

INCORRECT DIAGNOSIS. In patients with persistent abdominal pain after cholecystectomy, the possibility of an incorrect preoperative diagnosis must always be considered. Unrecognized peptic ulcer, pancreatitis, and functional bowel disorders are the disturbances most frequently misidentified as calculous biliary disease. The possibility of incorrect diagnosis is greatest for those patients who are found to have noninflamed or acalculous gallbladders at the time of operation. Patients with persistent symptoms following cholecystectomy should be evaluated for these possibilities (and others) using appropriate endoscopic, radiologic, and laboratory tests.

UNRECOGNIZED DISEASES. The second general category of disorders that cause persistent pain following operation includes co-existent unrecognized hepatobiliary disorders originating in a portion of the biliary system separate from the gallbladder. The most frequent pathologic entities identified in this category are retained common bile duct stones, postoperative biliary strictures, and unrecognized biliary or pancreatic neoplasms.

Retained stones constitute the most common cause of recurrent biliary-type pain following cholecystectomy. Residual common bile duct stones have been reported in approximately 2% of patients following cholecystectomy (31), and calculi are found in 80% of patients who undergo secondary biliary operations following cholecystectomy (30). Retained bile duct stones should be suspected in patients with biliary pain and biochemical evidence of cholestasis or pancreatitis. A history of previously performed common bile duct exploration should heighten suspicion, because this maneuver is associated with a five-to-tenfold increase in the risk of retained or recurrent stones. ERCP is the preferred method for demonstrating suspected common duct stones. Endoscopy also provides the options of therapeutic papillotomy and endoscopically guided stone extraction (32). If endoscopic stone removal is not possible or successful, reoperation might be recommended, often with formation of a biliary-enteric anastomosis to prevent recurrence (33).

Postoperative biliary strictures are second in frequency to retained biliary stones as causes for post-cholecystectomy pain caused by residual hepatobiliary disease. In more than 90% of patients, biliary stricture results from iatrogenic injury to the extrahepatic bile ducts during cholecystectomy (34). In most of the remaining patients, ductal obstruction occurs because of cicatrization of the intrapancreatic common bile duct as a result of pancreatitis. Clinical symptoms can appear months to years postoperatively. Typical biliary-type pain and laboratory evidence of cholestasis are common findings. Endoscopic cholangiography is essential for identifying the injury and for defining the extent of damage anatomically. Postoperative biliary strictures have been treated by operative repair (35), stenting (36), and balloon dilation (37), and by combinations of these techniques. Experience, familiarity with available options, and clinical judgment dictate the most appropriate approach for individual patients.

MALIGNANCY. Because symptoms caused by biliary, periampullary, and pancreatic malignancies can sometimes mimic pain from calculous biliary disease, these cancers, if not recognized at operation, can cause persistent postoperative distress. The treatment of pain resulting from retained biliary stones or biliary strictures consists of treating the residual disease. Restoration of anatomic and functional normality results in relief of pain. Treatment of malignancy-associated pain is covered later in this chapter.

REMNANT STRUCTURES. Two frequently cited causes of persistent symptoms after cholecystectomy are remnants of gallbladder or remnant cystic ducts (38). A cystic duct remnant is defined as a residual ductal structure demonstrated by cholangiography to be larger than 1 cm. Such remnants have been hypothesized to cause symptoms by harboring residual calculi, by allowing new stones to form in an area of relative stagnation, and by continued chronic inflammation. The causal relationship of cystic duct remnants to symptoms has been difficult to prove. Several large studies have shown that most patients with cystic duct remnants are asymptomatic, and that symptomatic patients generally have other possible explanations for their pain (usually residual common duct stones) (39).

The best treatment for the retained cystic duct syndrome, of course, is prevention. The routine use of operative cholangiography for detecting long cystic ducts permits removal at the first operation. Operative removal of a cystic duct remnant by a second laparotomy can be recommended if residual calculi are demonstrated by postoperative cholangiography. The reported results do not support removal of cystic duct remnants in the absence of demonstrable calculi if pain relief is the therapeutic objective (40).

FUNCTIONAL DISORDERS. The last general category of causes of postcholecystectomy pain includes functional disorders of biliary emptying. Two different mechanisms have been suggested to account for biliary pain and apparent biliary obstruction. In one group, the continued presence of chronic inflammation of the ampulla of Vater has been postulated to result in fibrosis and fixed stenosis of the ampulla. Sphincter of Oddi dyskinesia has been suggested in the absence of inflammation, with spasm of the sphincter raising intraductal pressure and impeding emptying.

These two mechanisms are the basis for the "postcholecystectomy syndrome," a nonspecific and poorly defined term. Biliary dyskinesia is a preferable appellation, but this term is best reserved for clinical situations in which typical biliary-type pain, biochemical evidence of cholestasis, and cholangiographic and manometric evidence of papillary dysfunction exist in the absence of one of the previously described causes of postoperative symptoms.

Diagnosis

Biliary dyskinesia is a diagnosis of exclusion. ERCP is the preferred method of radiologic investigation. Biliary manometry is confirmatory. Diagnostic manometry employs single-lumen or multilumen perfused catheters positioned across the sphincter of Oddi and recording pressures in the common bile duct, the sphincter, and the duodenum. In humans, common bile duct pressure is about 10 mm Hg above duodenal pressure (41, 42). In turn, the sphincter of Oddi basal pressure is 5 to 10 mm Hg greater than the common bile duct pressure. Phasic high-pressure contractions occur periodically within the sphincter at a rate of 4 to 6/minute. These contractions appear to be peristaltic, moving in antegrade fashion from the common bile duct to the duodenum. Intravenous infusion of cholecystokinin decreases the basal sphincter of Oddi pressure as well as the frequency and amplitude of phasic contractions (43). The effects of morphine are opposite to those of cholecystokinin; morphine increases resting sphincter pressure and increases the frequency of phasic contractions (44).

It has been suggested that a subset of patients with pain after cholecystectomy have identifiable manometric abnormalities and demonstrable obstruction to ductal emptying. In affected patients, manometrically measured basal sphincter of Oddi pressure is elevated to about twice control values (45). In addition, in those

TABLE 61-2. Distinguishing Features of Biliary Dyskinesia

Feature	Findings Characteristic of Biliary Dyskinesia
Associated hepatobiliary disease	Absence of retained or recurrent biliary stones, biliary stricture, neoplasms; transient elevation of alkaline phosphatase and parenchymal liver enzyme levels with symptomatic episodes
Cholangiographic results	Mild to moderate dilatation of extrahepatic bile ducts; delayed emptying of cholangiographic contrast medium
Biliary manometry	Increased basal sphincter pressure; retrograde propagation of phasic pressure waves; paradoxic response to cholecystokinin
Response to therapy	Symptomatic improvement after sphincterotomy in 85% of patients

patients with suspected biliary dyskinesia, propagation of phasic pressure waves is frequently retrograde, in an antiperistaltic direction. Furthermore, provocative testing with cholecystokinin infusion suggests that some patients with this disorder respond to the hormone not with the expected ampullary relaxation, but with a paradoxic increase in sphincter pressure (46). The functional significance of manometric abnormalities is confirmed by observing delayed emptying either of endoscopically injected radiographic contrast medium or hepatically excreted radionuclide (47).

Only those patients with manometric abnormalities and documented delayed biliary emptying, in whom other pathophysiologic processes have been excluded, should be considered to have biliary dyskinesia (Table 61-2). It is not currently possible to distinguish between fixed fibrotic stenosis and spasm; elements of each can be present in any one patient.

Treatment

Endoscopically performed sphincterotomy is currently the recommended treatment for patients with suspected biliary dyskinesia who meet the above criteria. Symptomatic improvement has been reported in 85% of patients treated in this fashion (47). Less invasive forms of therapy might be possible for mildly symptomatic individuals. Nitrates relax the sphincter of Oddi and can prove helpful if sphincteric spasm is present (48). Narcotics, particularly morphine, should not be used in these patients because of their known contractile effects on the sphincter of Oddi. Patients with severe persistent pain should be considered for surgical chemical splanchnicectomy after several prognostic blocks have indicated that interruption of these nociceptive pathways provides complete pain relief (Chapters 94 and 97).

C. PANCREAS

Basic Considerations

The pancreas is subject to a number of disease processes, both inflammatory and neoplastic, in which pain is a major clinical feature. Patients with pancreatic disorders constitute a large proportion of those seen by physicians interested in pain control. The location of the pancreas in the retroperitoneum of the upper abdomen, its anatomic relationships to surrounding organs, and its complex physiologic functions present difficulties in the diagnosis and management of pancreatic pain syndromes. An understanding of pancreatic pathophysiology is essential to all physicians caring for such patients.

The pancreas is a roughly triangular organ that lies transversely in the upper retroperitoneum between the duodenum on the right and the spleen on the left. The pancreas is related anteriorly to the pylorus, stomach, gastrocolic omentum, and liver. Inferiorly, the pancreas is in contact with the transverse portion of the duodenum, the jejunum, and the transverse mesocolon. The transverse colon can also form a portion of the inferior border.

The pancreas receives both sympathetic and parasympathetic innervation. Sympathetic innervation is derived from the upper thoracic splanchnic nerve, which is composed of preganglionic fibers from the T5 through T10 spinal segments (Fig. 61-2). Additional pancreatic sympathetic fibers travel in the lesser splanchnic nerve, and are derived from the T9 through T11 segments. Before reaching the pancreas, fibers from the upper and middle thoracic splanchnic nerves traverse the celiac plexus and ganglion. The cell bodies of efferent nerves to the pancreas are in the celiac ganglion. Cell bodies of afferent pancreatic sympathetic nerves are located in dorsal root ganglia. Sympathetic afferent connections with the central nervous system are bilateral; some afferent fibers cross the midline on traversing the celiac ganglion.

Parasympathetic innervation of the pancreas is derived from the celiac division of the posterior vagal trunk. The cell bodies of afferent vagal fibers are located in the nucleus ambiguus of the medulla of the brain. Efferent vagal fibers are dendrites of neurons with cell bodies in the dorsal motor nucleus. Both efferent and afferent parasympathetic fibers pass through the celiac ganglion. Neither type of parasympathetic nerve fiber synapses within this ganglion.

Pancreatic visceral pain is usually sensed as a severe constant discomfort localized to the upper midabdomen. Although intensely unpleasant and often intractable, pancreatic pain is often difficult to describe. "Stabbing," "burning," and "boring" are commonly used adjectives. Radiation of pancreatic pain to the back in the area of the lower thoracic spine is common (Fig. 61-5). Because the pancreas does not contact the somatically innervated parietal peritoneum, somatic pain is not associated with pancreatic disorders unless peripancreatic inflammatory complications extend beyond the lesser sac.

Vagal afferents do not appear to mediate pancreatic pain. Vagotomy alone is ineffective in the relief of pancreatic pain (49). Sympathetic afferents have been shown to transmit painful impulses from the pancreas. The use of sympathectomy in the treatment of pancreatic pain is discussed in Chapter 97.

Clinical Considerations

Acute Pancreatitis

Acute pancreatitis is one of the most common causes of acute abdominal pain requiring hospitalization. The disorder can vary in its clinical presentation, ranging from a transient mildly symptomatic illness to a rapidly fatal abdominal catastrophe. Acute pancreatitis has proven difficult to diagnose reliably and to treat specifically. Palliation of the pain that accompanies acute pancreatic inflammation remains a major clinical challenge.

Etiology and Pathophysiology

Although the pathogenesis of acute pancreatitis in most cases is not definitely established, a number of factors are clearly associated with this disease (Table 61-3). Chronic alcohol abuse is the most common metabolic cause of acute pancreatitis. Histologic evidence of antecedent pancreatitis has been reported in up to 45% of alcoholics in autopsy studies (50), but acute pancreatitis is recognized in fewer than 10% of such patients premortem. Individuals who develop acute alcoholic pancreatitis have abused alcohol for an average of 11 to 18 years before becoming symptomatic (51), with the mean ethanol consumption in these patients approximating 150 g/day. The triggering mechanism that initiates an episode of acute pancreatitis in the midst of chronic heavy alcohol intake is not known. The acute toxicity of ethanol for pancreatic acinar cells is believed to be the pathogenetic factor. Ethanol

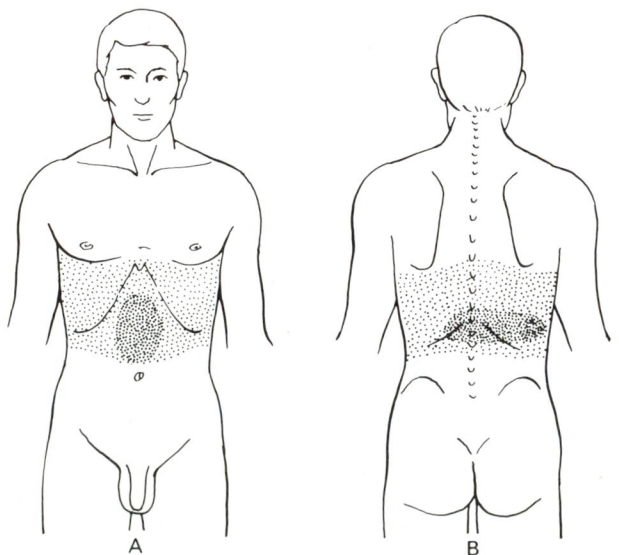

FIG. 61-5. Areas of referred pancreatic pain in the anterior (*A*) and posterior (*B*) regions of the body. The heavy stipple indicates the pain reference while the light stipple indicates the extensive cutaneous hyperalgesia often associated with the pain.

TABLE 61-3. Causative Factors in Acute Pancreatitis

Factor	Examples
Metabolic	Alcohol, hyperlipoproteinemia, hypercalcemia
Mechanical	Gallstones, post-traumatic, postoperative, after pancreatography
Vascular	Shock, cardiopulmonary bypass, polyarteritis nodosa
Drugs	Steroids, azathioprine, thiazide, estrogens, tetracycline, furosemide
Miscellaneous	Familial, viral infections, idiopathic

and its primary metabolite, acetaldehyde, have been shown to be toxic to pancreatic acinar cells. Cellular damage is postulated to occur by altering cellular membrane fluidity and composition (52), reducing mitochondrial protein synthesis (53), and enhancing abnormal amylase, trypsinogen, and chymotrypsinogen secretion (54).

Acute pancreatitis has been reported in patients with both familial and acquired forms of hypertriglyceridemia (55). Individuals with Frederickson type I hyperlipoproteinemia have a 30% risk of developing clinical pancreatitis. Pancreatitis occurs in 15% of those with type IV disease and in approximately 40% of those with type V hyperlipoproteinemia. A severe form of pancreatitis has been noted in association with the chylomicronemia syndrome (56).

Pancreatitis has been reported in association with hypercalcemia caused by hyperparathyroidism (57), multiple myeloma, and intravenous administration of calcium (58). Pancreatitis has been most clearly related to hyperparathyroidism that is long-standing and symptomatic. Acute pancreatic necrosis has been reported during hyperparathyroid crisis.

Gallstones are recognized in more than 50% of nonalcoholic patients with acute pancreatitis. It seems likely that passage of a gallstone through the ampulla of Vater is responsible for initiating pancreatitis in these patients. Gallstones can be retrieved from the stool of 85 to 95% of patients recovering from gallstone pancreatitis (59). In patients who underwent laparotomy within 48 hours of the onset of biliary pancreatitis, gallstones were reported to be present in the ampulla of Vater in 75% (60). In some patients, but not all, the anatomic structure of the ampulla of Vater can be a factor in the induction of gallstone pancreatitis by permitting transient obstruction of the pancreatic duct or obstruction of a common pancreatic-biliary channel. Mechanical disruption of primary or secondary pancreatic ducts by trauma, operative complications, or forceful ductal injection during pancreatography can also result in pancreatitis.

Many drugs have been reported to cause acute pancreatitis. Corticosteroids, thiazide diuretics, and estrogens have been implicated most frequently. Less common causes of pancreatic inflammatory disease include vasculitis, viral infections (Coxsackie and mumps viruses), and familial pancreatitis.

Although a number of associations with acute pancreatitis have been clearly identified as causative factors, the mechanism of injury is not known in most cases. The pancreas responds to a spectrum of injuries in a stereotyped fashion. The essential pathogenetic feature of this response is the extravasation of activated pancreatic enzymes into pancreatic and peripancreatic tissues. Tissue necrosis, edema, and local and systemic inflammatory reactions result from this extravasation.

Symptoms and Signs

Abdominal pain is the hallmark symptom in patients with pancreatic inflammation. The abdominal pain begins acutely and usually increases gradually over several hours before reaching maximum intensity. The pain is most severe in the upper abdomen with penetration through to the back, often radiating to the chest and flanks. The pain of acute pancreatitis usually persists without relenting for hours to days. It is often aggravated by recumbency. If abdominal pain fluctuates markedly in intensity or ceases for periods of time, acute pancreatitis should be suspected. The rapid onset of symptoms and the severity of pain associated with acute pancreatitis can mimic those of other acute inflammatory processes such as gangrenous cholecystitis, perforated peptic ulcer, and intestinal ischemia. Nausea and vomiting are nearly constant accompanying symptoms in acute pancreatitis. Vomiting does not relieve the pain and is not progressive. Fever, tachycardia, and evidence of dehydration are present in most patients.

Acute pancreatitis usually results in intense nociceptive input that not only produces severe pain but also reflex responses that are usually inherent in serious tissue damage (Chapter 7). Many patients develop severe reflex skeletal muscle spasm of the abdominal and lower chest walls, with a consequent marked decrease in chest wall compliance. Moreover, visceral reflexes also produce a decrease or inhibition of gastrointestinal tone with varying degrees of ileus, and also reflex bronchiolar constriction. The pain and reflex responses markedly impair ventilation, which frequently becomes rapid and shallow and produces hypercapnia and hypoxemia caused by increased physiologic shunting (61). As a result, the arterial oxygen tension (Pa_{O_2}) falls steadily. In one series, 40% of patients with acute pancreatitis developed a Pa_{O_2} of less than 60 mm Hg while breathing room air some time during the first week of the ileus (62). Unless aggressively treated, this results in respiratory failure and death (J.J. Bonica, personal communication, 1988).

Diagnosis

Acute pancreatitis is a clinical diagnosis, suspected in susceptible individuals with acute abdominal pain and confirmed by appropriate laboratory and radiologic investigations. The diagnosis can be subtle. Pancreatic symptoms can be deceptive. In a recent report from a teaching institution, experienced clinicians correctly diagnosed severe pancreatitis in only 35% of patients at the time of admission (63). After 24 hours of hospitalization, 73% of patients had the disease correctly identified as pancreatitis. Even after 48 hours of hospitalization, however, only 83% of patients with severe acute pancreatitis had been diagnosed correctly.

Diagnostic confusion might be a result of the frequently nonspecific nature of pancreatic symptoms and of difficulties in physical examination. In addition, commonly used laboratory examinations, although sensitive, are relatively nonspecific. A serum amylase determination is the most useful indicator of pancreatic inflammation. Unfortunately, hyperamylasemia can persist for only 24 to 48 hours after the initiation of pancreatitis, and the degree of hyperamylasemia might not correlate with the severity of pancreatic damage. Only 65% of patients with elevated serum amylase levels have pancreatitis. Normal serum amylase values are found in 10 to 15% of patients with acute pancreatitis. Urinary amylase measurements do not improve diagnostic capabilities, and the calculation of the urinary amylase:creatinine clearance ratio is generally not helpful.

Radiographic studies are often useful for evaluating the pancreas and supporting the clinical diagnosis of pancreatitis. In the setting of acute pancreatitis, CT scanning and ultrasonography have largely replaced other radiologic procedures in evaluation of the pancreas. These methods can provide useful anatomic information about the pancreatic gland, biliary system, and surrounding organs.

Newer CT scanners, with improved resolution and faster scanning times, have become the preferred technology in most patients. CT scanning has been reported to demonstrate pancreatic abnormalities in 90% of patients with acute pancreatitis (64). The most common finding on CT examination is diffuse enlargement of the gland. The most frequent complication of acute pancreatitis detected by CT scanning is an extrapancreatic fluid collection. Pancreatic pseudocysts and pancreatic abscesses that occur frequently as sequelae of acute pancreatitis are readily identified by CT scanning.

Ultrasonography is only slightly less effective than CT scanning for demonstrating pancreatic edema, phlegmons, and pseudocysts. Because of the absence of ionizing radiation, ultrasound is a superior procedure to use for pregnant women. Ultrasound is also well suited to young children who might not be cooperative. Although CT scanning is superior to ultrasound in providing anatomic information about the pancreas, ultrasound is more sensitive for detecting biliary calculi as a cause for pancreatitis.

Treatment

The clinical management of patients with acute pancreatitis combines measures to control the pancreatic inflammatory process with efforts to minimize pain and discomfort. The therapy of pancreatitis can be considered to have three phases: efforts to resuscitate and support the patient during the initial illness; attempts to limit pancreatic inflammation and abort development of complications; and measures to treat complications that do occur. Physicians treating patients with acute pancreatitis must be aware that the process evolves, often unpredictably, over a period of time; therapeutic objectives must thus be re-evaluated periodically. Relief of painful symptoms is a prime aspect of therapy throughout the course of the illness.

Patients with acute pancreatitis are at greatest risk of dying during the initial few days of the illness.

Shock, respiratory failure, and hemorrhage are the main causes of mortality during this phase of the disease. Vigorous patient support has proven effective in preventing death during the early phase of acute pancreatitis. Maintenance of tissue perfusion by the appropriate restoration of intravascular volume is crucial. Respiratory support, prophylaxis against gastric stress ulceration, and appropriate transfusion have been shown to be effective measures in these patients. Intravenous nutritional supplementation is also essential and should be instituted early.

Numerous therapeutic measures and agents have been investigated in attempts to limit pancreatic inflammation and to prevent complications. Most proposed therapies have been empiric and based on an incomplete understanding of the pathophysiology of pancreatitis. Not surprisingly, most of the proposed therapies have not been found to be efficacious when subjected to controlled trials. The following are proposed measures for limiting pancreatic inflammation and preventing complications: (a) nasogastric suction; (b) hypothermia; (c) pancreatic irradiation; (d) steroids; (e) enzyme inhibitors (e.g., Trasylol); (f) early biliary operations; and (g) drugs (e.g., anticholinergics, cimetidine, glucagon, calcitonin, antibiotics). Nasogastric suctioning prevents the accumulation of fluid and air in the gastrointestinal tract and treats the ileus that occurs with pancreatitis, but nasogastric suctioning has not been shown to result in a more rapid symptomatic or biochemical resolution of the pancreatic inflammatory process (66). Pancreatic inflammation is not positively influenced by steroid administration, trypsin inhibitors (67), or various other drugs, from anticholinergics to cimetidine [68]. Unfortunately, the administration of antibiotics prophylactically does not prevent the occurrence of pancreatic abscess or infection of peripancreatic phlegmons (69). Because food normally increases pancreatic secretion, fasting has been employed to minimize pancreatic stimulation. Withholding food is logical and is usually effective in promoting pancreatic quiescence.

Because the passage of common bile duct stones is so frequently associated with the initiation of pancreatitis, it has been postulated that the length of the period of ampullary obstruction and the completeness of obstruction determine the severity of the resultant pancreatitis. Early biliary operation with disimpaction of the offending stone has been proposed as a means of limiting pancreatic inflammation. In a controlled trial of early operation reported by Stone and colleagues, no amelioration of pancreatic inflammation was noted (70). Because of the lack of positive effect on the pancreatic inflammatory process, and because of the increased risk of infecting a sterile pancreatic phlegmon by operative manipulations, laparotomy during the early phase of acute pancreatitis is to be discouraged. An important exception to this recommendation exists for patients in whom serious coexistent pathology cannot be excluded. Positive evidence of acute pancreatitis does not exclude the presence of concomitant duodenal perforation, mesenteric infarction, or gangrenous cholecystitis.

Management of the pain associated with acute pancreatitis is an important aspect of patient care. Because of the severity of pancreatic symptoms, narcotic analgesia is the usual method of providing relief. Before narcotics are employed, however, certainty of diagnosis is important. Relief of abdominal pain could remove an important diagnostic clue of some other nonpancreatic disease that might be mimicked by pancreatitis.

Morphine should be avoided in patients with pancreatitis because of its contractile actions on the sphincter of Oddi. Meperidine (Demerol) also produces spasm of the biliary tract but its spasmogenic effect is less than that caused by morphine, and thus is the preferred parenteral systemic analgesic for pancreatic pain. Epidural opioids produce better pain relief with less spasmogenic effects. Bonica (personal communication, 1988) has pointed out, however, that none of the procedures completely relieves the severe pain of the reflex muscle spasm and of the massive neuroendocrine catabolic response. Segmental epidural (T5 to T10) analgesia with a dilute solution of local anesthetic relieves pain, markedly improves ventilation, and decreases or eliminates the reflex muscle spasm and neuroendocrine response. Of course, hypovolemia should be treated before this procedure is initiated to minimize the hypotension caused by vasomotor blockade (Chapters 7 and 94).

Chronic Pancreatitis

Chronic pancreatitis is a distinct clinical entity frequently encountered by those caring for patients with chronic pain. Chronic pancreatitis differs markedly from acute pancreatitis in pathogenesis, sequelae, and response to treatment. Numerous experimental studies in animals and clinical observations in humans suggest that, for most patients, chronic pancreatitis does not evolve from recurrent episodes of acute pancreatitis with progressive, additive inflammatory changes. Most investigators agree that the mechanisms of injury for the two disease processes are fundamentally different. Support for this view has been provided by Sarles et al. (71), who noted that the average age of onset for chronic pancreatitis is 38 years whearas the average age of onset for acute pancreatitis is 51 years.

Etiology and Pathophysiology

Although numerous causative factors have been associated with chronic pancreatitis, pathogenic mechanisms are largely unknown. Therapy continues to be empiric and limited to management of symptoms, side effects, and complications of the disease. For most patients chronic abdominal pain is the most prominent symptom and the most difficult complication of chronic pancreatitis to treat.

In the United States, the cause of chronic pancreatitis in 80 to 90% of patients is alcoholism (72). For most of the remaining patients the cause is not known, and the disease is labeled "idiopathic" chronic pancreatitis. Biliary calculi, so common as a cause of acute pancreatitis, are rarely a factor in the development of chronic pancreatitis.

The histologic changes that characterize chronic pancreatitis usually develop in the setting of prolonged periods of excessive alcohol intake. Chronic alcohol ingestion, by mechanisms that are incompletely understood, causes sustained secretion of protein by pancreatic acinar cells. Increased secretion of protein, without a proportionate increase in secretion of pancreatic water and bicarbonate, has been postulated to cause precipitation of protein within the pancreatic ducts. Obstruction of primary and secondary pancreatic ducts by the precipitate can cause the damage to pancreatic acini, with the accompanying inflammation and fibrosis that typify chronic pancreatitis. Persistent ductal obstruction and lobular destruction result in the progressive loss of pancreatic exocrine tissue that characterizes chronic pancreatitis histologically. Although the islets of Langerhans are not initially involved in the inflammatory process, gradual loss of endocrine tissue occurs as well.

Symptoms and Signs

Pain is the central feature of chronic pancreatitis. Virtually 100% of patients suffer from chronic abdominal pain. Approximately 50% of patients with chronic pancreatitis experience a constant, gnawing epigastric pain. The pain can vary in intensity but never subsides completely. The discomfort frequently radiates to the back. Pain is frequently worsened by eating and weight loss is a prominent accompaniment. Narcotic addiction is frequent. Steady employment is rarely achieved. In a second group of patients, severe attacks of epigastric pain are episodic, with the affected individual pain-free between attacks. Painful episodes might or might not be associated with signs of acute pancreatitis superimposed on chronic pancreatitis. The pain from episodic attacks can last for days to weeks. Constant pain is most frequently associated with alcoholic chronic pancreatitis, whereas intermittent pain is more common with nonalcoholic pancreatitis.

In addition to various pain syndromes, most patients with chronic pancreatitis have evidence of endocrine insufficiency. Of patients with chronic pancreatitis, 15% are insulin-dependent; most non-insulin-dependent patients have abnormally low basal insulin levels and abnormal glucose tolerance tests (73). Even when insulin dependence does occur, the patients have some circulating endogenous insulin and are not prone to diabetic ketosis. Nonetheless, the chronic complications of diabetes mellitus are significant causes of death in patients with chronic pancreatitis.

Exocrine insufficiency is detectable in approximately 50% of patients when they seek medical attention and occurs with increasing frequency over time. The repetitive cycles of tissue destruction result in a significant reduction in the ability of the pancreas to secrete amylase, lipase, and proteolytic enzymes. Steatorrhea and malabsorption result and contribute to chronic weight loss.

The natural history of chronic pancreatitis is not known with certainty. Most reported series have been retrospective and confounded by including patients undergoing pancreatic operations or patients with significant accompanying illnesses. A prospective report suggested that only 20% of patients with chronic pancreatitis die from causes directly related to pancreatitis or its complications (74). Malignancies, cardiovascular diseases, and severe infections were common nonpancreatic causes of death.

Diagnosis

Chronic pancreatitis should be suspected in all individuals with intractable abdominal pain. Chronic pancreatitis is a clinical diagnosis, based on appropriate signs and symptoms in susceptible individuals. Determination of serum enzyme values is usually of little value; serum amylase and serum lipase levels are infrequently elevated in patients with chronic abdominal pain and are nonspecific in their interpretation. Findings of endocrine or exocrine insufficiency strengthen the clinical impression.

CT scanning and endoscopic pancreatography have improved the diagnostic evaluation of chronic pancreatitis in recent years. Approximately 50% of patients with chronic pancreatitis have ductal abnormalities that can be demonstrated by these techniques (75). In these patients, pseudocysts or strictures, obstructions or stones in the pancreatic duct, or alternating areas of dilatation and narrowing are demonstrated. In the other half, normal biliary and pancreatic ducts are demonstrated. Ductal abnormalities constitute strong positive evidence for chronic pancreatitis. Pancreatic calcification is pathognomonic.

Treatment

The treatment of chronic pancreatitis consists of three aspects: abstinence from alcohol; support for endocrine and exocrine insufficiency; and palliation of painful symptoms. Management of endocrine insufficiency usually requires administration of insulin, whereas support for exocrine insufficiency can be accomplished by oral administration of pancreatic enzyme preparations. When patient compliance is good, management of endocrine and exocrine disturbances is readily achieved; it is not discussed further here.

MEDICAL THERAPY. For most patients with chronic pancreatitis in whom pain is severe, medical therapy is not successful and surgical intervention becomes necessary. Simple nonoperative measures, such as manipulations of diet, have not been shown to ameliorate pancreatic pain in a controlled clinical trial. Pharmacologic attempts to suppress pancreatic secretion have also been largely unsuccessful. Anticholinergic drugs have been demonstrated experimentally to decrease pancreatic secretion, but administration of atropine-like drugs to patients has not reduced pancreatic pain. Cimetidine, a potent inhibitor of gastric acid secretin, has been employed to decrease stimulation of the pancreas by secretin released by introduodenal acid. Cimetidine, however, does not relieve pancreatic symptoms. In most instances, the medical management of chronic pancreatic pain relies on the use of narcotic analgesics. The long-term commitment to such analgesics required by patients with chronic pancreatitis often leads to physical dependence. Data reported by Ammann and co-workers (76) suggest that medically treated patients experience abdominal pain for a mean of greater than 5 years before pancreatic dysfunction becomes so severe that pain is relieved. The nihilistic approach of waiting until the disease "burns out" is not to be encouraged.

Various procedures to ablate afferent nerves from the pancreas have been employed in attempts to palliate pancreatic pain. Dramatic temporary relief of pain from acute pancreatitis can be obtained by injecting solutions of lidocaine or bupivacaine into the splanchnic nerves or the left celiac ganglion (77). Positive results in patients with acute pancreatitis have encouraged many investigators to extend these techniques to patients with chronic pancreatitis. Neural ablation may be achieved by several operative or nonoperative methods. One nonoperative approach involves the use of celiac plexus block with alcohol after prognostic blocks have produced effective pain relief (Chapter 94). In patients who are undergoing operative pancreatic procedures, alcohol can be injected into the celiac ganglia directly at the time of laparotomy. Destruction of the celiac ganglia has also been accomplished by resection. The ganglia can be removed by a posterior incision through the twelfth rib below the diaphragm.

A prospective controlled study of splanchnicectomy for relief of chronic pancreatic pain has not been performed. Retrospective clinical series by proponents of the procedure claimed that permanent pain control is achieved in greater than 90% of patients (78). These initial encouraging results, however, have not been reproduced by most other surgical investigators. A definitive statement of the usefulness of neural ablative procedures in treatment of chronic pancreatitis cannot be made. A more complete discussion may be found in Chapters 96 and 97.

SURGICAL THERAPY. The use of endoscopic retrograde cannulation of the pancreas, ultrasonography, and CT scanning, has improved the ability to assess the structural changes associated with chronic pancreatitis and its complications. Two major patterns have been recognized. Some patients, both alcoholic and nonalcoholic, have enlarged major pancreatic ducts alternating with segmental areas of narrowing. The ectatic ducts are often associated with intraductal stones and calcification. This form of structural abnormality has been termed "large duct" or "obstructive" disease. Many physicians have interpreted these changes as resulting from pancreatic ductal hypertension caused by blockage of the flow of pancreatic secretions. Such an assumption has yet to be supported by endoscopic measurements or by direct ductal pressure recordings. An alternative explanation is that the structural changes are a result of atrophy of pancreatic parenchyma and periductal scarring.

A second form of pancreatitis has been termed "small duct disease." In these patients, pancreatography demonstrates chronic calcifying pancreatitis, in which major pancreatic ducts are not enlarged. Proteinaceous plugs can be seen in terminal ductules and acini. Atrophy and dilatation of the fine aborizations of the pancreatic ductal system can be present.

The surgical treatment of chronic pancreatitis is based on two assumptions about the functional significance of these structural abnormalities. The first assumption is that pancreatic ductal obstruction is the cause of pain in large duct disease and that decompression of the pancreatic duct by operative manipulations relieves pain. The second assumption is that ductal hypertension is absent in small duct disease. Periductal or perineural inflammation is assumed to cause the chronic abdominal pain in patients with nondilated ducts. For these patients, pancreatic resection has been proposed to remove the source of chronic inflammatory stimuli.

Operative therapy in chronic pancreatitis is effective in reducing pain, but should not be undertaken for the purpose of improving endocrine or exocrine function. Glucose intolerance and fat malabsorption are not improved by operations for chronic pancreatitis (79).

Longitudinal pancreaticojejunostomy has become the standard surgical approach for patients in whom pancreatography demonstrates dilated pancreatic ducts or alternating areas of dilatation and stricture. As currently performed, the procedure decompresses the entire pancreatic duct by creating a side-to-side anastomosis between the opened pancreatic duct and a Roux-en-Y limb of jejunum (Fig. 61-6). The pancreatic duct should be 8 mm in diameter or larger for this procedure to be appropriate. The gland is left in situ. The main pancreatic duct is filleted along its

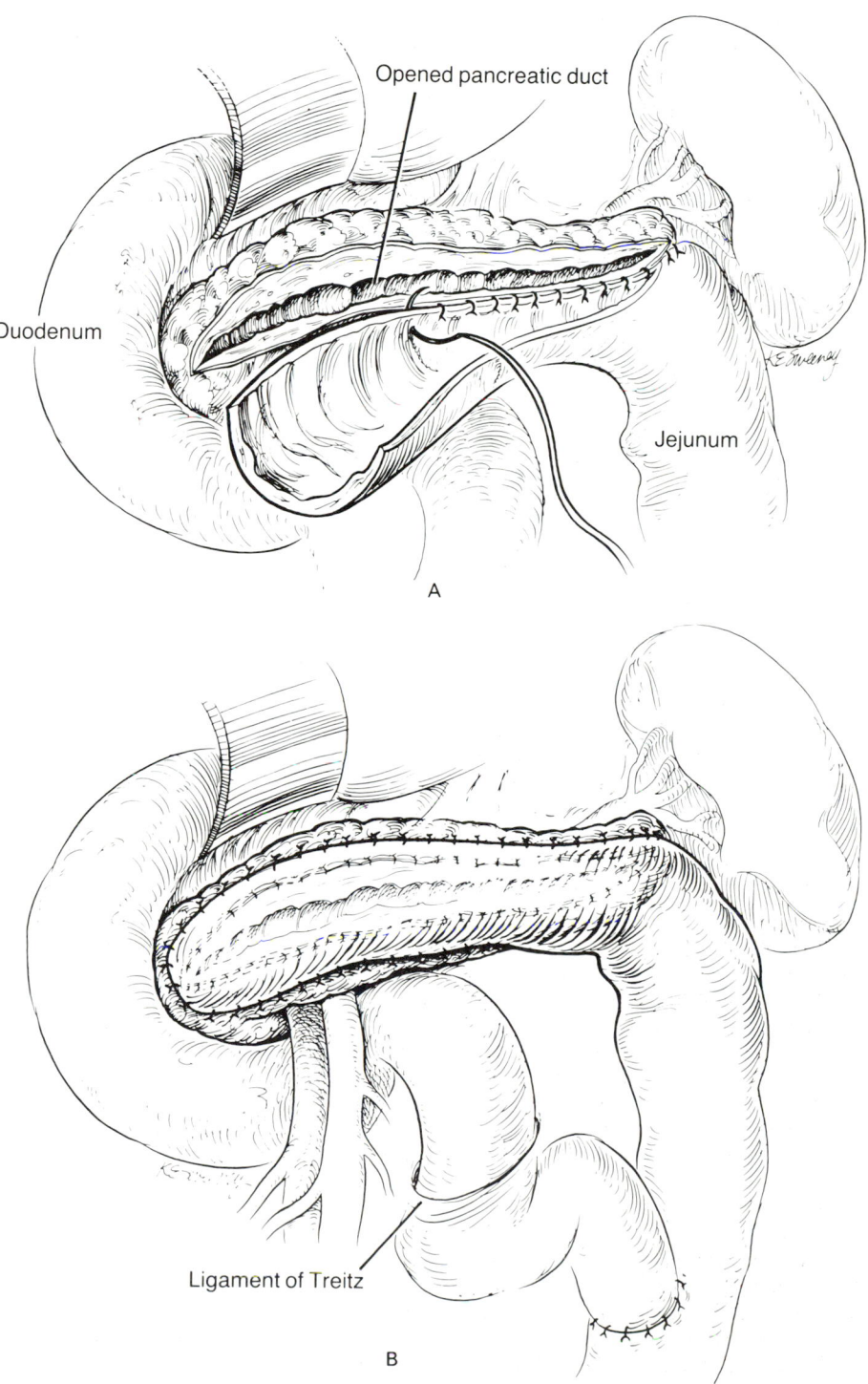

FIG. 61-6. Operative performance of pancreaticojejunostomy. **A.** The anterior surface of the pancreas has been exposed by reflecting the stomach cephalad and the transverse colon caudad. The main pancreatic duct has been opened longitudinally, exposing a grossly dilated pancreatic ductal collecting system. A Roux-en-Y limb of jejunum has been constructed. The jejunal limb has been opened longitudinally for a distance equal to that of the longitudinal opening in the pancreatic duct. A side-to-side pancreaticojejunostomy is then performed by suturing the jejunal limb to the thickened fibrotic capsule of the pancreas. **B.** Completion of pancreaticojejunostomy, showing configuration of the Roux-en-Y jejunal limb. A double-layer pancreaticojejunostomy has been constructed. Pancreatic exocrine secretion can drain through the anastomosis through the Roux-en-Y limb of the jejunum.

entire length, nearly to the ampulla of Vater. Splenectomy is unnecessary.

The operative mortality rate of pancreaticojejunostomy is low, about 4% in a compilation of several series performed by Frey (80). Late deaths following the operation are caused by diseases associated with chronic alcoholism, complications of diabetes, and various malignancies. Even though neither islet cell nor acinar tissue is destroyed in performing pancreaticojejunostomy, the incidence of diabetes and clinically symptomatic exocrine insufficiency is increased in the years following the operation (Table 61-4). This observation suggests that the chronic destruction of pancreatic tissue associated with chronic pancreatitis is not halted by decompression of the duct.

Many large series have reported the effectiveness of pancreaticojejunostomy in the treatment of pain. Complete relief or significant improvement can be expected in 70 to 80% of patients (81). Abstinence from alcohol improves the chance for pain-free survival. More than 90% of patients who do not resume alcohol intake are either pain-free or nearly so (82).

When pancreatography demonstrates normal pancreatic ducts or ducts of inadequate caliber for the performance of pancreaticojejunostomy, pancreatic resection has been performed for the treatment of pain of chronic pancreatitis. If the chronic inflammatory process is confined to the tail of the gland, distal pancreatectomy can be performed. Ideally, the extent of resection is determined by the limits of pancreatic disease. Resections of 40 to 80% of the pancreas have been most commonly employed; removal of up to 95% of the gland has also been reported (83). If the chronic inflammatory process is limited to the head of the pancreas with relatively normal tissue distally, pancreaticoduodenectomy has been performed.

The operative mortality rate of distal pancreatectomy approximates that of pancreaticojejunostomy, about 4% (80), but the operative mortality rate for pancreaticoduodenectomy is about doubled, to 9%. The higher mortality rate of proximal pancreatic resections is a result of the necessity of pancreatic-enteric reconstruction, with anastomotic leaks largely causing the difference in mortality rates. Late death rates following proximal or distal resection are similar. The incidence of postoperative diabetes varies widely from 30 to 80%, and is highly dependent on the extent of resection. Radical resection of 80 to 95% of pancreatic tissue guarantees the development of diabetes. Symptomatic fat malabsorption occurs in all patients after pancreaticoduodenectomy (84).

Reports of the success of pancreatic resection for relieving pain have varied (Table 61-4). Experienced clinicians report that approximately 50% of patients who have undergone distal pancreatectomy are symptom-free or improved after operation. A slightly lower proportion of patients is relieved of pain following resection of the head of the pancreas.

The results of operative series must be viewed from the perspective of long-term studies, which suggest that chronic pancreatitis is associated with progressive pancreatic dysfunction and eventual relief of pain in most patients, even without operation. Ammann and co-workers (76) observed that deterioration in pancreatic exocrine function was closely related in timing to the relief of chronic pain. In 85% of alcoholic patients with chronic pancreatitis, spontaneous and long-lasting relief of pain was reported in surviving patients after 5 years. Cessation of pain was noted at the point at which pancreatic function began to decline markedly. These data imply that pain in chronic pancreatitis is related to secretory capacity and, with reduction in secretory capacity below some critical level, the mechanism that initiates the pain disappears. If this supposition is correct, pancreatic resection can be effective because it decreases exocrine function, and pancreaticojejunostomy can be useful because patients with dilated ducts have already lost a critical amount of secretory capacity. Operative therapy thus does not alter the natural history of chronic pancreatitis; rather, it accelerates the symptomatic evolution of the disease.

Pancreatic Cancer (XXI-7)

Pancreatic cancer is a highly lethal disease that currently ranks as the fifth most common cause of cancer-related deaths in the United States (85). The American Cancer Society estimated that in 1986 25,500 new cases of cancer of the pancreas occurred in the United States—13,000 males and 12,500 females—while the estimates for deaths from pancreatic cancers were 24,400, 12,300, and 11,700, respectively. The number of new cases and the number of deaths have increased nearly 20% since 1980. The increasing incidence of pancreatic carcinoma takes on even more significance because the disease is highly lethal, with less than 2% of the patients surviving for 5 years.

Symptoms and Signs

Pain is the hallmark symptom in patients with cancer of the pancreas. For nearly all patients with carcinoma of the pancreas, pain becomes a management

TABLE 61-4. Operative Therapy for Chronic Pancreatitis

Procedure	Operative Mortality Rate (%)	Late Deaths (%)	Postoperative Diabetes (%)	Postoperative Steatorrhea (%)	Pain Relief (%)
Pancreatic ductal drainage pancreaticojejunostomy	4	29	20–30	20	70–80
Pancreatic resection distal pancreatectomy	4	22	30–80	20	60–75
pancreaticoduodenectomy	9	18	30–80	100	50–90

Modified from Frey, C.F.: Role of subtotal pancreatectomy and pancreaticojejunostomy in chronic pancreatitis. J. Surg. Res., 31:361, 1981.

problem at some time during their illness. Pain associated with cancer of the pancreas usually begins as a nagging discomfort in the epigastrium, but becomes rapidly and progressively more severe. The pain is gnawing, relentless, and visceral in character. Radiation to the back is noted in 25% of patients. Pain can be the only symptom associated with tumors of the body or tail of the gland; tumors in these locations can grow to a large size before causing secondary complications that prompt the correct diagnosis. Constant pain usually implies local invasion of surrounding structures and infiltration of the splanchnic nerves.

Anorexia and weight loss are frequent but nonspecific accompanying symptoms. Nausea, vomiting, and weakness are each noted in approximately 50% of patients. A palpable abdominal mass is present in 20% (86). Jaundice is present initially in 13% of patients with pancreatic cancer, although jaundice develops in 75% of these patients at some time during their illness. The presence of jaundice implies obstruction of the extrahepatic biliary system by direct neoplastic growth. Contrary to a widely held belief, the jaundice is usually not painless. In addition, a gallbladder is palpable in less than 30% of patients. At the initial examination, an enlargement of the liver is present in 33% of patients and ascites is noted in 20%.

The "hidden" retroperitoneal location of the pancreas largely accounts for the lack of specific symptoms, difficulty in physical examination, and problems in diagnosis. Most patients with cancer of the pancreas have locally or systemically disseminated disease at diagnosis. In addition, the anatomic relationship of the pancreas to other structures causes technical difficulties in the extirpation of pancreatic lesions.

Diagnosis

If pancreatic cancer is suspected, the diagnosis can be confirmed by a combination of techniques. CT scanning, endoscopic pancreatography, percutaneous biopsy, and operative exploration have important roles in the management of these patients.

The prognosis of cancer of the exocrine pancreas is grave. If the tumor has spread beyond the confines of the pancreas, surgical resection for cure is not possible, and almost every patient with unresectable cancer of the pancreas dies of the disease. Fewer than 10% of patients with pancreatic carcinoma can undergo resection. In patients who have potentially curative resections, the chance of survival for 3 years after operation is less than 15% (84).

Treatment

Currently, the only potentially curative therapy for cancer of the pancreas is surgical resection. Radiation therapy and chemotherapeutic approaches offer palliation to unresectable patients, but long-term survival is only modestly improved. Because of these considerations, symptomatic palliation is the primary goal for the great majority of patients with cancer of the pancreas.

Symptomatic palliation should be concerned with three general aspects of care: relief of anatomic complications, attention to nutritional depletion, and treatment of pain. Biliary obstruction and abnormal gastric emptying result from encroachment on the common bile duct and duodenum from tumor growth. Operative decompression of the biliary system is effective in relieving the intense pruritis associated with biliary obstruction. Gastric outlet obstruction usually requires the formation of some type of gastroenteric by-pass. The malnutrition that so commonly accompanies pancreatic malignancy should be managed, when feasible, with oral or enteral feeding regimens. Pancreatic exocrine insufficiency, usually subclinical, occasionally might require oral pancreatic enzyme supplementation.

Most patients with carcinoma of the pancreas can be maintained on oral opioids and on opioid analgesics as outpatients for most of the duration of their illness. Oral pain cocktails permit continued personal independence, with few intellectual or motor disturbances. For those patients in whom pain is not adequately controlled by oral or parenteral medication, celiac plexus block with alcohol or surgical splanchnicectomy is highly effective and should be considered if personnel skilled in these procedures are available (see page 2018). New approaches, including ambulatory epidural opioid analgesia, are discussed in Chapters 94 and 95.

REFERENCES

1. Alexander, W.F.: The innervation of the biliary system. J. Comp. Neurol., 72:357, 1946.
2. Sawchenko, P.E., and Freidman, M.I.: Sensory function of the liver—A Review. Am. J. Physiol., 236:R5, 1979.
3. Andrews, W.H., and Palmer, J.F.: Afferent nervous discharge from the canine liver. J. Exp. Physiol., 52:259, 1967.
4. Tsai, T.L.: A histological study of sensory nerves in the liver. Acta Neurosurg., 17:354, 1958.
5. Rubin, R.H., Schwartz, M.N., and Malt, R.: Hepatic abscess: Changes in clinical, bacteriological and therapeutic aspects. Am. J. Med., 57:601, 1974.
6. Butler, T.J., and McCarthy, C.F.: Pyogenic liver abscess. Gut, 10:389, 1969.
7. Friday, R.O., Barriga, T., and Crummy, A.B.: Detection and localization of intra-abdominal abscess by diagnostic ultrasound. Arch. Surg., 110:335, 1975.
8. Frick, M.P., et al.: Computer tomography, radionuclide imaging and ultrasound in hepatic mass lesions. Comput. Tomogr., 3:49, 1979.
9. Thakur, M.L., Coleman, R.E., and Welch, M.J.: Indium-111-labeled leukocytes for localization of abscess: Preparation, analysis, tissue distribution, and comparison of gallium-69 citrate in dogs. J. Lab. Clin. Med., 89:217, 1977.
10. Monif, G.R.G.: Significance of polymicrobial bacterial superinfection in the therapy of gonococcal endometritis-salpingitis-peritonitis. Obstet. Gynecol., 55S:154S, 1980.
11. Reichert, J.A., and Valle, R.F.: Fitz-Hugh Curtis syndrome. A laparoscopic approach. JAMA, 236:266, 1976.
12. Jaffe, D.M., Donegan, W.L., and Watson, F.: Factors, influencing survival in patients with untreated hepatic metastases. Surg. Gynecol. Obstet., 127:1, 1978.
13. Cade, B.: Natural history of primary and secondary tumors of the liver. Semin. Oncol., 10:127, 1983.
14. Ihde, D., et al.: Clinical manifestations of hepatoma: A review of six years at a cancer hospital. Am. J. Med., 56:83, 1974.
15. Falkson, G., et al.,: Primary liver cancer: An eastern cooperative oncology group trial. Cancer, 54:970, 1984.
16. Ramming, K.P.: The effectiveness of hepatic artery infusion in treatment of primary hepatobiliary tumors. Semin. Oncol., 10:199, 1983.
17. Patt, Y.Z., et al.: Hepatic arterial chemotherapy and occlusion for palliation of primary hepatocellular and unknown primary neoplasms in the liver. Cancer, 51:1359, 1983.

18. Lane, W.W.: Liver metastases: Analysis of autopsy data. *In* Liver Metastases. Edited by L. Weiss and H.A. Gilbert. Boston, G.K. Hall, 1981, pp. 23–30.
19. Wood, C.B.: Natural history of liver metastases. *In* Liver Metastases. Edited by C.J.H. Van de Velde and P.H. Sugarbaker. Amsterdam. Martinus Nijhoff, 1984, pp. 47–55.
20. Wagner, J.S., et al.: The natural history of hepatic metastases from colorectal cancer. A comparison with resective therapy. Ann. Surg., *199*:502, 1984.
21. Daley, J.M., et al.: Predicting tumor response in patients with colorectal hepatic metastases. Ann. Surg., *202*:284, 1985.
22. Twycross, R.G.: The use of narcotic analgesics in terminal illness. J. Med. Ethics, *1*:10, 1975.
23. Doran, F.S.A.: The sites to which pain is referred from the common bile duct in man and its implication for the theory of referred pain. Br. J. Surg., *54*:599, 1967.
24. Malagelada, J.R., et al.: Regulation of pancreatic and gallbladder functions by intraluminal fatty acids and bile acids in man. J. Clin. Invest., *58*:493, 1976.
25. Bertan, A., et al.: Effects of jejunal amino acid perfusion and exogenous cholecystokinin on the exocrine pancreatic and biliary secretions in man. Gastroenterology, *61*:686, 1971.
26. Glenn, F.: Biliary tract disease. Surg. Gynecol. Obstet., *153*:401, 1981.
27. Krook, P.M., et al.: Comparison of real-time cholecystosonography and oral cholecystography. Radiology, *135*:145, 1980.
28. Worthen, N.J., Uszler, J.M., and Funamura, J.L.: Cholecystitis: Prospective evaluation of sonography and 99m-Tc-HIDA cholescintigraphy. Am. J. Radiol., *134*:973, 1986.
29. Gunn, A., and Kaddie, N.: Some clinical observations in patients with gallstones. Lancet, *2*:239, 1972.
30. Glenn, F., and McSherry, C.K.: Secondary abdominal operations for symptoms following biliary tract surgery. Surg. Gynecol. Obstet., *121*:978, 1965.
31. Bergdahl, L., and Holmlund, D.E.W.: Retained bile duct stones. Acta Chir. Scand., *142*:145, 1976.
32. Safrany, L., and Cotton, P.B.: Endoscopic management of choledocholithiasis. Surg. Clin. North Am., *62*:825, 1982.
33. Girard, R.M., and Lagros, G.: Retained and recurrent bile duct stones. Surgical or non-surgical removal? Ann. Surg., *193*:150, 1981.
34. Way, L.W., Bernhoft, R.A., and Thomas, M.G.: Billiary stricture. Surg. Clin. North Am., *61*:963, 1981.
35. ReMine, W.H., and Ferris, D.O.: Surgery for biliary strictures. Surg. Clin. North Am., *47*:877, 1967.
36. Huibregtse, K., and Tytgat, G.N.: Palliative treatment of obstructive jaundice by transpapillary introduction of large bile duct endoprosthesis. Experience in 45 patients. Gut, *23*:371, 1982.
37. Teplick, S.K., et al.: Percutaneous transhepatic choledochoplasty and dilation of choledochoenterostomy strictures. JAMA, *244*:1240, 1980.
38. Hopkins, S.F., Bivins, V.A., and Griffen, W.O.: The problem of the cystic duct remnant. Surg. Gynecol. Obstet., *148*:531, 1979.
39. Lewicki, A.M., Kleinhaus, U., and Ozer, H.: Remnant cystic duct in T-tube cholangiography. Am. J. Roentgenol. Radium Ther. Nucl. Med., *119*:52, 1973.
40. Larmi, T.K.I., et al.: A critical analysis of the cystic duct remnant. Surg. Gynecol. Obstet., *141*:48, 1975.
41. Carr-Locke, D.L., and Gregg, J.A.: Endoscopic manometry of pancreatic and biliary sphincter zones in man. Dig. Dis. Sci., *26*:7, 1981.
42. Geenen, J.E., et al.: Intraluminal pressure recording from the human sphincter of Oddi. Gastroenterology, *78*:317, 1980.
43. Toouli, J., et al.: Action of cholecystokinin-octapeptide on the sphincter of Oddi basal pressure and phasic wave activity in humans. Surgery, *92*:497, 1982.
44. LoGiudici, J.A., Geenen, G.E., and Hogan, W.J.: Efficacy of the morphine-prostigmine test for evaluating patients with suspected papillary stenosis. Dig. Dis. Sci., *24*:455, 1979.
45. Bar-Meir, S., et al.: Biliary and pancreatic duct pressures measured by ERCP manometry in patients with suspected papillary stenosis. Dig. Dis. Sci., *24*:209, 1979.
46. Hogan, W.J., et al.: Paradoxical motor response of cholecystokinin (CCK-OP) in patients with suspected sphincter of Oddi dysfunctions. Gastroenterology, *82*:1085, 1983.
47. Shaffer, E.A., et al.: Cholescintigraphic detection of functional obstruction of the sphincter of Oddi: Effect of papillotomy. Gastroenterology, *90*:728, 1986.
48. Bar-Meir, S., Halpern, Z., and Bardan, E.: Nitrate therapy in a patient with papillary dysfunction. Am. J. Gastroenterol. *78*:94, 1983.
49. Rack, F.J., and Elkins, C.W.: Experiences with vagotomy and sympathectomy in the treatment of chronic recurrent pancreatitis. Arch. Surg., *61*:937, 1950.
50. Durr, G.H.: Acute pancreatitis. *In* The Exocrine Pancreas. Edited by H.F. Howat and H. Sarles. Philadelphia, W.B. Saunders, 1979, pp. 352–401.
51. Durbec, J.P., and Sarles, H.: Relationship between the relative risk of developing chronic pancreatitis and alcohol, protein and lipid consumption. Digestion, *18*:337, 1978.
52. Rubin, E., and Rottenberg, H.: Ethanol-induced injury and adaptation in biological membranes. Fed. Proc., 1982, *41*:2465.
53. Burke, J.P., and Rubin, E.: The effects of ethanol and acetaldehyde on the products of protein synthesis by liver mitochondria. Lab. Invest., *41*:393, 1979.
54. Majumdar, A.P. et al.: Effects of acetaldehyde administration on protein secretion from isolated pancreatic acini in rats. Physiologist, *27*:279, 1984.
55. Buch, A., et al.: Hyperlipidemia and pancreatitis. World J. Surg., *4*:307, 1980.
56. Brunzell, J.D., and Bierman, E.L.: Chylomicronemia syndrome: Interation of genetic and acquired hypertriglyceridemia. Med. Clin. North Am., *66*:455, 1982.
57. Bess, M.A., Edis, A.J., and van Heerden, J.A.: Hyperparathyroidism and pancreatitis. Chance or causal association? JAMA, *243*:246.
58. Izak, E.M., et al., Pancreatitis in association with hypercalcemia in patients receiving total parenteral nutrition. Gastroenterology, *79*:555, 1980.
59. Acosta, J.M., and Ledesma, C.L.: Gallstone migration as a cause of acute pancreatitis. N. Engl. J. Med., *290*:484, 1974.
60. Acosta, J.M., Pellegrini, C.A., and Skinner, D.B.: Etiology and pathogenesis of acute billiary pancreatitis. Surgery, *88*:118, 1980.
61. Ranson, J.H.C., Roses, D.F., and Fink, S.D.: Early respiratory insufficiencies in acute pancreatitis. Ann. Surg., *178*:75, 1973.
62. Imrie, C.W. et al.: Arterial hypoxia in acute pancreatitis. Ann. R. Coll. Surg. Engl., *58*:322, 1976.
63. Corfield, A.P., et al.: Prediction of severity in acute pancreatitis: Prospective comparison of three prognostic indices. Lancet, *2*:403, 1985.
64. Weyman, P.J., Stanley, R.J., and Levitt, R.G.: Computed tomography in evaluation of the pancreas. Semi. Roentgenol., *16*:30, 1981.
65. Stroud, W.H., Cullom, J.W., and Anderson, M.C.: Hemorrhagic complications of severe pancreatitis. Surgery, *90*:657, 1981.
66. Fuller, R.K., Levlend, J.P., and Frankel, M.H.: An evaluation of the efficacy of nasogastric suction treatment in alcoholic pancreatitis. Am. J. Gastroenterol., *75*:349, 1981.
67. Imrie, C.W., Benjamin, I.S., and Ferguson, J.C.: A single-centre-blind trial of trasylol therapy in primary acute pancreatitis. Br. J. Surg., *65*:337, 1978.
68. Regan, P.T., et al.: A prospective study of the antisecretory and therapeutic effects of cimetidine and glucagon in human acute pancreatitis. Mayo Clin. Proc., *56*:499, 1981.
69. Howes, R., Zuidema, G.D., and Cameron, J.L.: Evaluation of prophylactic antibodies in acute pancreatitis. J. Surg. Res., *18*:197, 1975.
70. Stone, H.H., Fabian, T.C., and Dunlop, W.E.: Gallstone pancreatitis: Biliary tract pathology in relation to time of operation. Ann. Surg., *194*:305, 1981.
71. Sarles, H., et al.: Observations on 205 confirmed cases of acute pancreatic, recurring pancreatitis, and chronic pancreatitis. Gut, *6*:545, 1965.
72. Sarles, H., and Sahel, J.: Pathology of chronic calcifying pancreatitis. Am. J. Gastroenterol., *66*:117, 1976.
73. Rossi, R.L., Heiss, F.W., and Braach, J.W.: Surgical management of chronic pancreatitis. Surg. Clin. North Am., *65*:79, 1985.
74. Braasch, J.W., Vito, L., and Nugen, F.W.: Total pancreatectomy for end-stage pancreatitis. Ann. Surg., *188*:317, 1978.
75. Ferucci, J.T., et al.: Computed body tomography in chronic pancreatitis. Radiology, *130*:175, 1974.
76. Ammann, R.W., et al.: Course and outcome of chronic pancreatitis: Longitudinal study of a mixed medical-surgical series of 245 patients. Gastroenterology, *86*:820, 1984.
77. White, T.T.: Pain-relieving procedures in chronic pancreatitis. Contemp. Surg., *22*:43, 1983.

78. Mallet-Guy, P.A.: Late and very late results of resections of the nervous system in the treatment of chronic relapse in chronic pancreatitis. Am. J. Surg., *145*:234, 1983.
79. Bradley, E.L., and Nasrallah, A.H.: Fat absorption after longitudinal pancreaticojejunostomy. Surgery, *95*:640, 1984.
80. Frey, C.F.: Role of sub-total pancreatectomy in pancreaticojejunostomy in chronic pancreatitis. J. Surg. Res., *31*:361, 1981.
81. Taylor, R.H., et al.: Ductal drainage or resection for chronic pancreatitis. Am. J. Surg., *141*:28, 1981.
82. Prinz, R.A., Kaufman, B.H., and Folk, F.A.: Pancreaticojejunostomy for chronic pancreatitis. Arch. Surg., *113*:520, 1978.
83. Najarian, J.S., et al.: Total or near-total pancreatectomy and autotransplantation for treatment of chronic pancreatitis. Ann. Surg., *192*:526, 1980.
84. Kalser, M.H., Leite, C.A., and Warren, W.D.: Fat assimilation after massive distal pancreatectomy. N. Engl. J. Med., *279*:570, 1968.
85. American Cancer Society: Cancer Facts and Figures, 1986. New York, American Cancer Society, 1986.
86. Macdonald, J.S., Widerlite, L., and Schein, P.S.: Biopsy, diagnosis, and chemotherapeutic management of pancreatic malignancy. Adv. Pharmacol. Chemother., *14*:107, 1977.
87. McDonald, J.S., Gunderson, L.L., and Cohn, I., Jr.: Cancer of the pancreas. *In* Cancer: Principles and Practice of Oncology. Edited by V.T. DeVita, Jr., S. Hellman, and S.A. Rosenberg. Philadelphia, J.B. Lippincott, 1982, pp. 563–589.
88. Gardner, A.M. and Solomou, G.: Relief of the pain of unresectable carcinoma of the pancreas by chemical splanchnicectomy during laparotomy. Ann. R. Coll. Surg. Engl., *66*:409, 1984.

62 · DISEASES OF THE KIDNEY AND URETER

JULIAN S. ANSELL and WILLIAM F. GEE

with contributions by

JOHN J. BONICA

No pain known to humans is more severe than the pain of acute urinary obstruction. We have collected subjective testimony on this point from patients of both sexes and varying ages, among them experts on the treatment of pain from the Pain Clinic at the University of Washington. In this chapter we emphasize those diseases of the kidney and ureter in which pain is the presenting symptom or a major problem in the management of the patient. The material is presented in two major sections: A, Basic Considerations, including the anatomy and innervation of the kidneys and ureters, the general character-istics and mechanisms of pain, and the techniques used for diagnosis of renal and ureteral diseases and B, Clinical Considerations, including a discussion of congenital, vascular, infectious, and obstructive diseases and tumors of the kidney. Bonica contributed to the section on the innervation of the kidneys and ureters, the section on characteristics and mechanisms of renal and ureteral pain, and the discussion of tumors of the kidney. The remainder of the text was written by Ansell and Gee. A more detailed discussion of the subject can be found in textbooks by Campbell (1), Wyker and Gillenwater (2), and Smith (3).

A. BASIC CONSIDERATIONS

Anatomic aspects

Figures 62-1 and 62-2 depict the gross anatomy and nerve supply of the kidneys and ureters and indicate their relationship to other structures that are important in considering the pathophysiology of renal and ureteral pain. Both structures receive sympathetic, parasympathetic, and sensory (afferent) fibers. The following description of the nerve supply of the kidneys and ureters was written by Bonica and is based on information derived from the first edition of this book (4) and from descriptions by Kunz (5) and Netter et al. (6).

Innervation of the kidneys

Sympathetic Supply

The sympathetic fibers are derived mainly from the celiac and aorticorenal ganglia and also directly from the upper portion of the lumbar sympathetic trunk. These two great collections of ganglia receive the preganglionic fibers, which convey afferent (sympathetic) impulses to the kidneys from the T10 to L1 spinal cord segments via the corresponding white rami communicantes and paravertebral ganglia and then by way of the middle (lesser) and inferior (least) thoracic splanchnic nerves and the 1st (and perhaps the 2nd) lumbar splanchnic nerves. As mentioned in Chapters 6 and 59 the middle (lesser) thoracic splanchnic nerves derive from roots given off by the 10th and 11th paravertebral ganglia and end in the ipsilateral celiac and/or aorticorenal ganglion. The inferior (least) thoracic splanchnic nerve derives from the 12th thoracic paravertebral ganglion and usually ends in the aorticorenal ganglion near the renal plexus. Within these ganglia, preganglionic neurons synapse with postgan-glionic neurons, which pass directly to form the renal plexus. Not infrequently the least splanchnic nerve and the 1st (and perhaps the 2nd) lumbar splanchnic nerve pass directly to the renal plexus to synapse in the posterior renal ganglion or in other smaller renal ganglia incorporated at nodal points in the renal plexus. The renal plexus occasionally also receives small communicating rami from the suprarenal plexus.

Parasympathetic Nerves

The parasympathetic nerve supply comes from the vagus nerves, consisting of preganglionic neurons. Most of these fibers traverse the celiac plexus, but some fibers, particularly on the right side, pass directly to the renal plexus. Within the plexus they proceed as far as the smooth muscle of the pelvis, where they synapse with short postganglionic fibers.

Afferent (Sensory) Fibers

The afferent (sensory) fibers are composed of spinal nerves whose cell bodies are located in dorsal spinal nerve root ganglia and whose central processes pass through the dorsal nerve roots of the 10th, 11th, and 12th thoracic spinal nerves to synapse with dorsal horn neurons. The distal branches of these fibers accompany sympathetic nerves and thus pass through the whole rami communicantes, the paravertebral sympathetic ganglia (without synapsing) and thence to the splanchnic nerves to reach the renal plexus.

Renal Plexus and Branches

The renal plexus consists of a fine network of sympathetic, parasympathetic, and sensory fibers surrounding the renal vessels, mostly the artery. These fibers

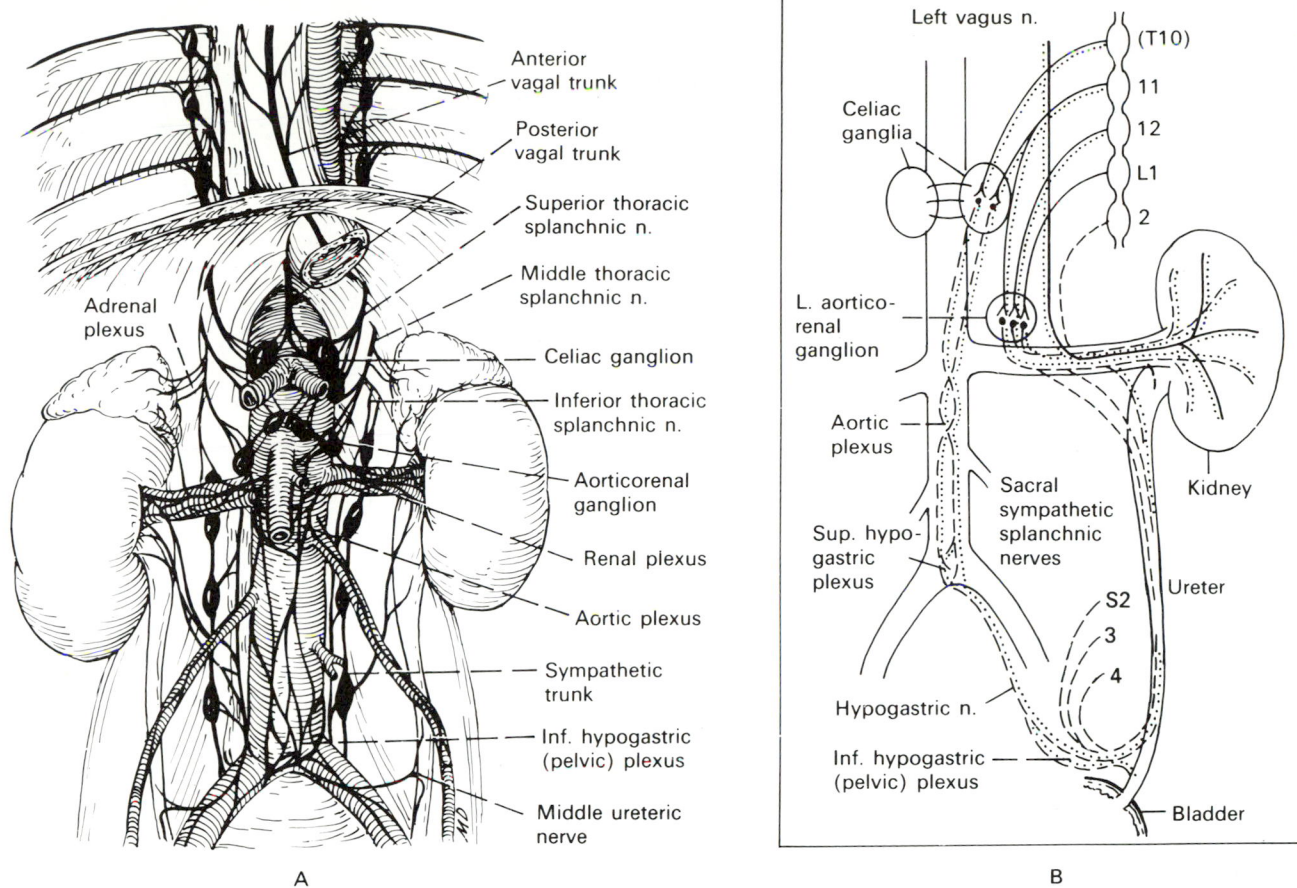

FIG. 62-1. *A.* The gross anatomy and innervation of the kidneys. *B.* Schematic illustration of the autonomic and sensory nerve pathways supplying the kidney and ureters.

thus reach the pelvis and (except for the parasympathetic fibers) the calyces and substance of the kidney by following the branches of the renal artery, some of them traveling within its muscular coat.

Intrinsic nerves

The nerves within the kidney form rich perivascular plexuses around the renal artery and its branches, continuing along even the smaller arterial branches, arterioles, and capillaries. The sympathetic postganglionic fibers are distributed to the vascular musculature and to the smooth muscles in the renal pelvis and calyces; from the slender rami associated with the interlobular arteries, strands of these fibers extend along the afferent arterioles to the juxtaglomerular apparatus. The parasympathetic postganglionic fibers supply the muscles of the pelvis and calyces and probably do not extend into the renal parenchyma. Afferent (sensory) nerve fibers terminate in the musculature of the renal pelvis, the adventitia and endothelium of the renal vessels, and the renal capsule.

The parenchyma is supplied mostly by thin unmyelinated fibers, although some small myelinated axons can be found. The renal pelvis and renal calyces also are richly supplied with unmyelinated nerve fibers, which terminate in relation to the musculature, but myelinated fibers are more abundant than in the parenchyma.

Innervation of the Ureters

The ureters receive sympathetic, parasympathetic, and sensory nerves derived from the renal, spermatic (or ovarian), and hypogastric plexuses. The upper half or two-thirds of each ureter receives the same nerve supply as the corresponding kidney. Preganglionic fibers with their cell bodies in T10–L1 (and perhaps L2) pass along the anterior roots, the white rami communicantes, the paravertebral sympathetic trunk, and thence through the splanchnic nerves that end in the aforementioned ganglia where they synapse with postganglionic fibers. The latter pass to and through the renal and spermatic (or ovarian) plexuses to reach and contribute to the upper portion of the ureteral plexus. Parasympathetic fibers to the upper portion of the ureter are derived from: vagal fibers that pass through the celiac and renal plexus and then into the wall of the ureter where they synapse with short, postganglionic fibers. The afferent (sensory) fibers to the upper portion of the ureter are derived from T11 and T12 and traverse the same structures as the sympathetic fibers without interruption to end in the muscles of the upper portion of the ureter.

The nerves to the lower portion of the ureter take a slightly different course. Preganglionic sympathetic fibers have their cell body in L1 and possibly L2 spinal segments and pass through the anterior roots, white

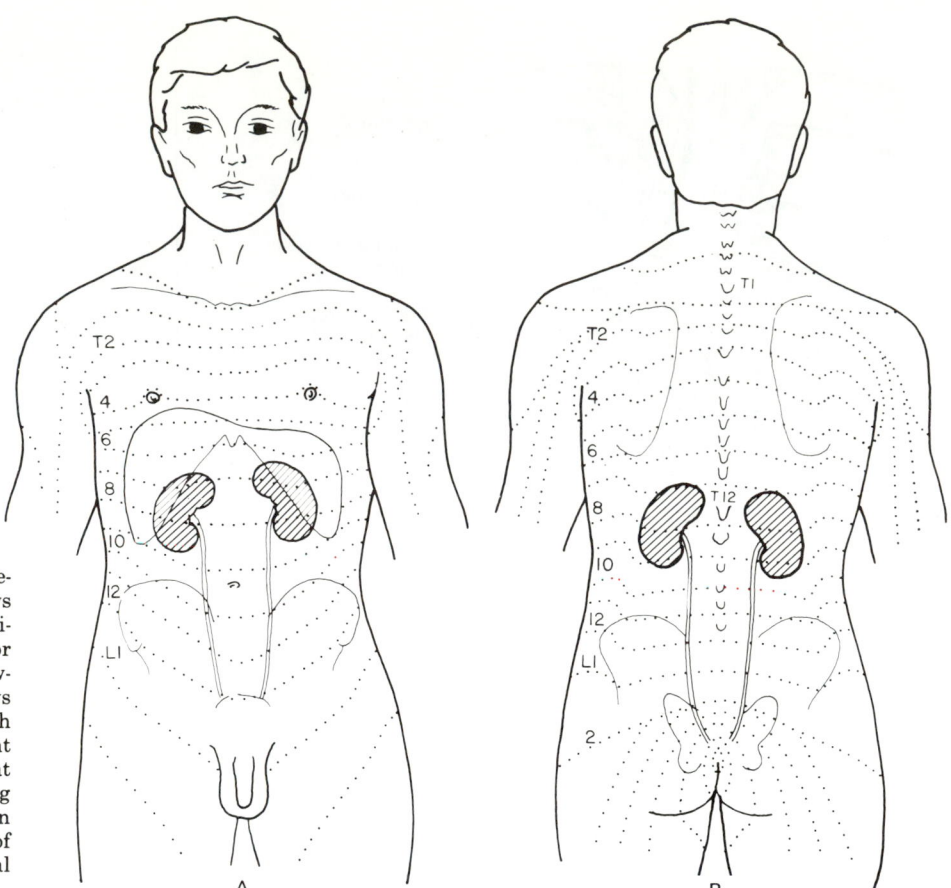

Fig. 62-2. Schematic illustrations depicting the relationship of the kidneys to the liver and the dermatomes (indicated by dotted lines and numbered for identification). **A.** anterior view showing that the skin overlying the kidneys is supplied by dermatomes T6 to T9 with the left kidney higher than the right kidney. **B.** Posterior view showing that the dermatomes in the back overlying the kidneys are one segment lower than in the front because of the migration of the posterior division of the spinal nerves (see Chapter 6 for details).

rami communicantes, and paravertebral chain within which they synapse with postganglionic fibers, some in the upper two ganglia and others in the sacral ganglia. Postganglionic fibers from the upper lumbar chain pass as lumbar splanchnic nerves to reach the aortic plexus and then pass to and through the superior hypogastric plexus and hypogastric nerves to reach the ureter. The postganglionic fibers that derive from the sacral trunk can be considered sacral splanchnic nerves and reach the inferior hypogastric plexus where they pass to the ureter. The parasympathetic nerve fibers to the lower part of the ureter arise from S2–S4 segments and pass sequentially through the pelvic splanchnic nerves (nervi erigentes) and the inferior hypogastric plexus (some go through the hypogastric nerves) to reach the lower portion of the ureter. The afferent (sensory) nerves to the lower portion of the ureter have their cell body in dorsal root ganglia of T12 and L1 (and perhaps L2); the proximal branch enters the spinal cord and distal branch passes in company of the sympathetic fibers to the lower portion of the ureter. Although these various fibers are arranged in three corresponding groups—the superior, middle, and inferior ureteral plexus—they branch freely and intercommunicate with one another.

Renal and Ureteral Pain

Location and Characteristics

Diseases of the kidneys and/or ureters, like other visceral disease, may cause localized (true) visceral

pain and referred visceral pain. Moreover, if the disease involves the parietal peritoneum, it may cause either localized or referred parietal pain. Of these, referred visceral pain is the most frequent and most important.

The distribution of referred pain caused by diseases of the ureter and kidney have been studied by several investigators. As early as 1900 (4 years after the first use of a practical cystoscope), Lennander (7) demonstrated that the distension of human kidney pelvis produced pain. Some four decades later, McLellan and Goodell (8) carried out the most definitive study to date. Figure 62-3A illustrates the ascending location of the cutaneous sites of pain caused by ascending stimulation of the ureter by dilatation with a balloon at the ureterovesical junction and then at 5, 10, 15, 20, and 25 cm above the ureteral orifice. When stimulation of the ureter was at threshold intensity, pain was discretely localized and approximately 5 cm in diameter, the location being approximately on a line drawn along the lateral edge of the rectus muscle. Stimulation of the kidney pelvis at threshold intensity caused a similar type of pain in the back at the level of the costovertebral angle (Fig. 62-3B). Increasing the intensity of the stimulus produced an even larger area of pain. Stimulation in the upper part of the ureter and pelvis often caused splinting and "spasm" of the lateral abdominal and loin muscles, which did not relax when the stimulus was removed. Several hours later some of the subjects began to have "side ache," which subsequently increased in intensity during the

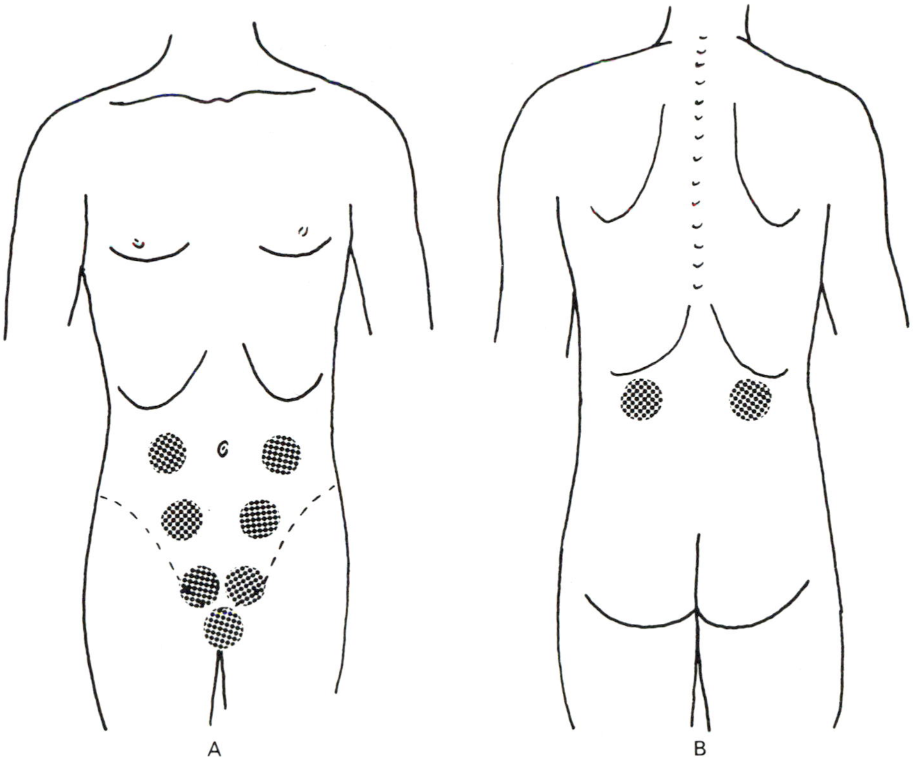

FIG. 62-3. **A.** Schematic representation of the anterior areas of pain reference to the skin from stimulation of the kidney pelves and of the ureters at the ureteral vesical junction and 5, 10, 15, 20, and 25 cm upward from there. **B.** Schematic representation of posterior area of pain reference produced by either faradic stimulation or local distension in the upper ureter or kidney pelvis, followed by contraction of skeletal muscles. About an hour after the onset of muscle contraction, subject developed aching pain, which persisted from 6 hours to 2 days. Modified from McLellan, A.N., and Goodell, H.: Pain from the bladder, the ureter and kidney pelvis. Pain (Res. Publ. Assoc. Res. Nerv. Mental Dis.). Vol. 23. Baltimore, Williams & Wilkins, 1943, pp. 252–259.

ensuing 12 hours, undoubtedly due to sustained contraction of the skeletal muscles.

Other authors also have studied the distribution of pain caused by distension of the pelvis and ureters by inflating distensible catheters in various parts of the upper urinary tract (Fig. 62-4). The following findings have been reported (1): (a) distension of the renal pelvis consistently causes pain in the region of the costovertebral angle; (b) distension of the ureteropelvic segment of the ureter produces pain adjacent to the anterior superior iliac spine; (c) distension of the mid-ureter causes pain to be felt at the middle of Poupart's ligament, whereas distension of the ureterovesical portion of the ureter produces pain in the suprapubic region. Pain of renal pelvic origin is often referred to the ipsilateral testicle or ovary. Pain due to a stone in the terminal ureter may be referred to the scrotal or labial skin, or medial thigh. When the stone is located in the terminal ureter, irritation and edema in the adjacent trigone of the bladder may produce symptoms of frequency of urination as well. In addition to pain, the patient usually experiences hyperalgesia in the dermatomes T10–L1 as well as in the testicle (Fig. 62-5).

Several colleagues who have experienced "colic" due to passage of calculi have provided a subtle subjective description of the pain that is worth repeating here. The pain starts as an expanded "bubble" located in the flank and rapidly becomes a feeling of unbearable expanding pressure that cannot be ignored. The symptom is exacerbated by concern about what might possibly be causing this growing discomfort, and the desire for relief. This sensation of something expand-

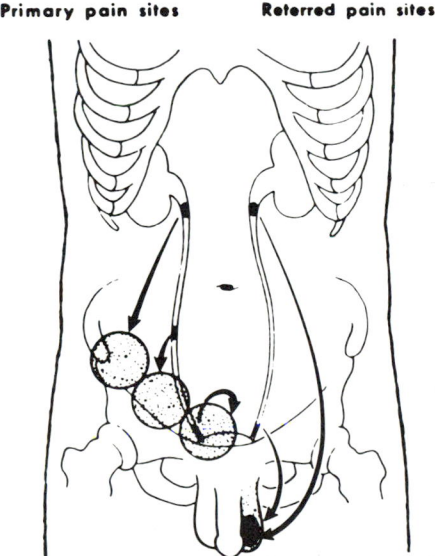

Primary pain sites   **Referred pain sites**

FIG. 62-4. Sites of referred pain noted clinically from obstruction and distension of the ureter at the pelvic junction, the mid-ureter, and the uteropelvic junction. Note that pain of renal pelvic origin may be referred to the ipsilateral testicle (or ovary) and pain due to a stone in the terminal ureter is frequently referred to the scrotal or labial skin. Modified from Wyker, A.W. and Gillenwater, J.Y.: Method of Urology, Baltimore, Williams and Wilkins, 1975, p. 3.

ing uncontrollably internally may provoke restless attempts to find a comfortable position, but no position is better than any other. The agitated activity of

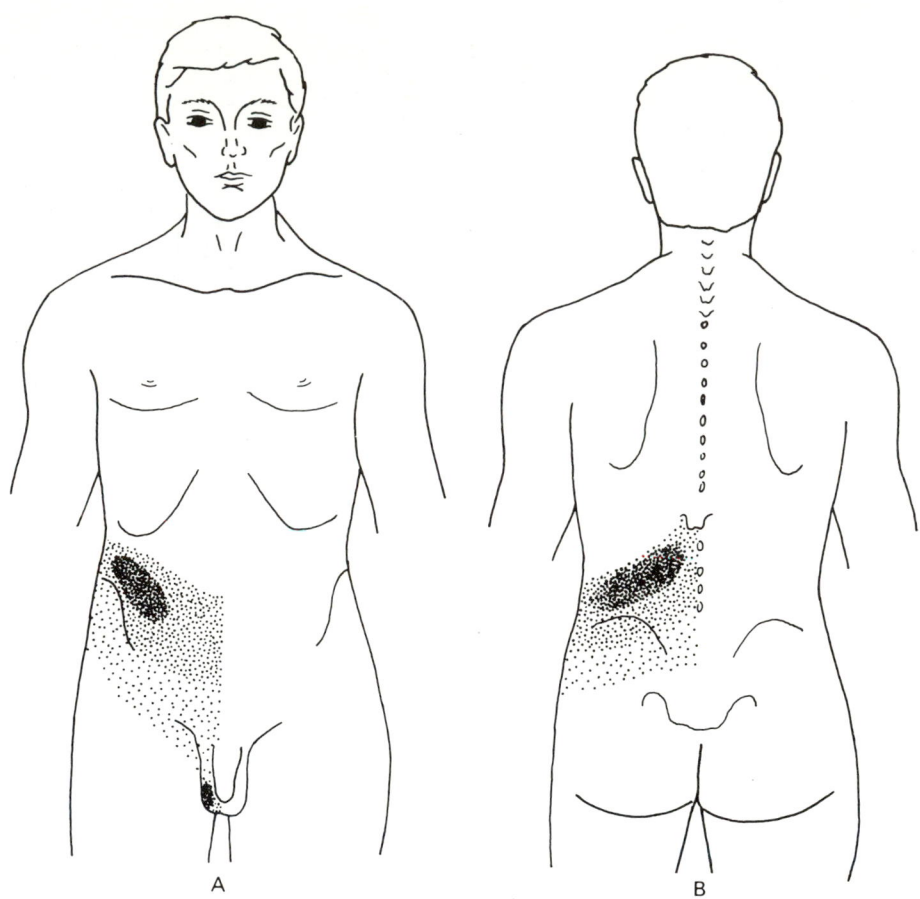

FIG. 62-5. Schematic illustration showing the anterior (*A*) and posterior (*B*) sites of pain (black areas) and hyperalgesia in the dermatomes (stippled area) caused by distension of the kidney, renal pelvis, or ureter.

A

B

the sufferer seeking relief from pain has even led to mistaken admission to the psychiatric service, from which the patient was transferred when red cells found on routine urinalysis helped in locating the source of the discomfort to the urinary tract.

Mechanisms Producing Pain

Pain related to an urinary organ may be produced by distension of the collecting system or renal capsule, extravasation of urine into the tissues, inflammation, ischemia, or traction and displacement on the pedicle of the organ itself or adjacent organs and structures. Pain related to distension is directly proportional to the rate of the distension (1). Sudden distension usually produces severe discomfort, whereas slow, progressive distension might produce little or no pain (Fig. 62-6).

The use of contrast agents, which are secreted by the kidney in highly concentrated form, has shown that the acute obstruction associated with passage of urinary calculi is often accompanied by extravasation of significant amounts of the material into the renal parenchyma, surrounding fat, lymphatics, and veins. The severest colic is accompanied by extravasation. Therefore, pain that was formerly attributed solely to distension probably also has a component due to extravasation of urine. Mild pain in the flank and costovertebral angle has long been associated with swollen kidneys affected by the inflammatory changes seen in glomerulonephritis and pyelo-

nephritis. Whether such mild pain is due to inflammation of the parenchyma itself or to the distension of the renal capsule as a result of parenchymal swelling is not clear. Nor is the source of the tenderness elicited by percussion of the costovertebral angle in such patients (Murphy's sign).

Another mechanism that produces pain related to distension of the renal capsule is subcapsular hematoma following accidental trauma. Once the bleeding has stabilized, the pain remains steady and mild until the hematoma has resolved. Renal ischemia due to arterial embolization can produce severe steady disabling pain followed by abdominal distension. This phenomenon is clearest in individuals whose renal arteries are intentionally embolized to control neoplasia or hemorrhage, but it also occurs in patients with emboli from the left ventricle (9). Frequently, patients with renal pain will place a hand, with the fingers and thumb spread in opposite directions, palm down on the affected flank as an aid in describing their pain (9).

Not only do the kidneys and ureters share autonomic and sensory nerves with adjacent viscera, but diseases that can spread to or from adjacent anatomic structures or compress or displace them will mimic pain patterns attributable to these structures and vice versa. Biliary and right renal colic are easily confused if there is no hepatic or bile duct involvement to highlight the difference. Right ureteral colic is occasionally misdiagnosed and treated as appendicitis if

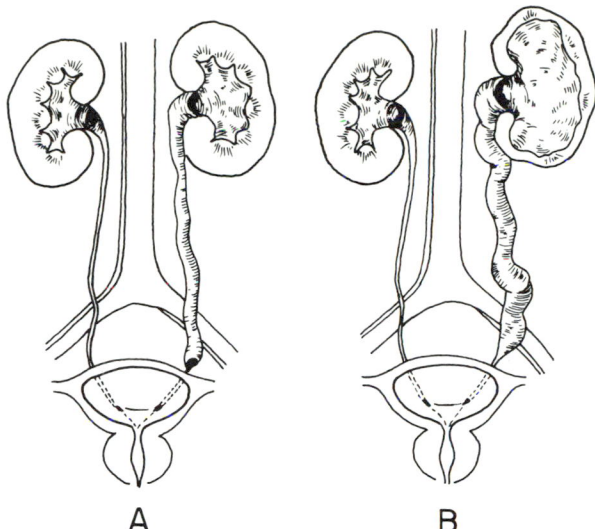

FIG. 62-6. *A.* With acute distension of the left ureter and renal pelvis above an obstructing calculus, the patient experienced severe pain requiring narcotics for relief although the ureter was only slightly dilated. *B.* When the ureter was slowly dilated over many months, the patient experienced no pain despite the fact that the ureter was greatly dilated. From Wyker, A.W., and Gillenwater, J.Y.: Method of Urology. Baltimore, Williams & Wilkins, 1975.

the urinalysis showing hematuria or pyuria is missed or ignored. Pain from pancreatitis, pancreatic calculi, or pancreatic pseudocyst can be attributed to the kidneys if these possibilities are not kept in mind and an amylase is not obtained. The duodenum, jejunum, vena cava, and hepatic or splenic colon can be partially obstructed by expanding renal masses.

A number of structures related to the kidneys can contribute to the pain. The anterior aspects of the kidneys are near the peritoneal surfaces, and infection and inflammation of kidneys and ureters can produce a mild peritoneal reaction with accompanying pain and other symptoms. Nausea and vomiting, however, usually *follow* the pain due to diseases of the urinary system, whereas nausea and vomiting usually *precede* the pain generated by disease in gastrointestinal organs.

The posterior superior aspect of each kidney is adjacent to the tendinous portions of each side of the diaphragm. Therefore, penetrating reaction to renal disease occasionally produces characteristic findings referable to the diaphragm, pleura, and lower lungs including symptoms of diaphragmatic irritation such as cough, hiccough, shoulder strap pain, pleuritis, pleural effusion, and pneumonitis. Secondary ipsilateral skeletal muscular spasms and aching have been produced by stimulating the inside of the ureter with an electrode (8, 10). The muscles on the affected side along the lateral border of the rectus muscles contracted painfully and ached for over 24 hours thereafter. Similar spasms and aching occurred in the paraspinus muscles at the level of the costovertebral angle when the renal pelvis was so stimulated. The

phenomenon is reproduced clinically by the frequent finding of spinal curvature concave to the affected side during acute obstruction.

Diagnostic Techniques

Sophisticated methods for diagnosing diseases of the upper urinary tract are available. In many cases, the pain history will direct attention to one side or the other, and physical examination may produce signs of mass or tenderness. Because the gonads and kidneys share pain pathways, the physician should carefully examine the ipsilateral testicle or ovary of an individual with occult pain thought to be of renal origin. For diagnostic purposes, it may be possible to reproduce renal or ureteral pain by retrograde catheterization and overdistension of the ureter or renal pelvis.

Response of the kidney to fluid load can be assessed by isotope renography with furosemide-induced diuresis, intravenous pyelography with fluid loading, or urodynamic measurement of pressure during constant flow through a percutaneously inserted nephrostomy catheter. If diagnostic studies made in the absence of fluid loading appear normal, the occurrence or reproduction of the characteristic pain in response to fluid load is a valuable way of establishing that the upper urinary tract is the source of the patient's pain problem. Diagnostic paravertebral somatic nerve blocks of T10–L2 spinal nerves help to establish the nociceptive pathways that are involved. These are discussed briefly later in this chapter and in detail in Chapter 94.

Computer-assisted tomography (CAT), ultrasound, and magnetic resonance imaging (MRI) produce complementary representations of the detailed anatomy and spectra of tissue densities, which are helpful in determining the cause of difficult pain problems affecting the kidneys, ureters, and adjacent structures (11–15). Positron emission imaging (PEI) will provide an additional diagnostic dimension in the future. Angiography demonstrates arterial and venous anomalies that may obstruct the collecting system directly or secondarily as a result of bleeding. Endoscopic examination of the ureter and renal pelvis and collecting system is now practical with newly designed instruments for use retrograde after introduction through the urethra and bladder or antegrade after insertion through percutaneous flank tracts.

In summary, the upper urinary tract can be displayed in intricate detail by current imaging techniques, it can be assessed hydrodynamically and functionally with the aid of pressure measurements and radioisotopes, and the urothelium can be examined almost in its entirety with instruments whose lenses magnify the surface four times. Computer-assisted imaging by means of ultrasound, radiography, radioisotopes, electromagnetic resonance, and positron emission are available to examine the upper urinary tracts in minute detail. One can make arterial and venous angiograms of the vascular supply to these organs. Functional hydrodynamics can be assessed directly and indirectly. No lesion need be missed.

B. CLINICAL CONSIDERATIONS

Congenital Renal Diseases

Polycystic Kidney Disease

Etiology

Polycystic kidney disease, a congenital disease with a familial pattern, derives from failure of the junction between the uriniferous tubules and the collecting ducts, the result being blind secretory tubules connected to glomeruli producing fluid that is unable to escape and slowly expands into huge cysts compressing the surrounding structures. The renal parenchyma is gradually destroyed, and the enlarging cysts swell the kidneys to huge masses, which may reach weights of 5 kg. Pain is produced by the weight of the organ pulling on the renal pedicle, hemorrhage into cysts, cyst rupture, or infection.

Symptoms and Signs

The commonest presentation in young people is hematuria following athletic activity. Individuals with known family history may request evaluation to rule out the disease and be discovered to have it. Patients who are first diagnosed in the fifth decade present with flank pain, which is dull, intermittent, and bilateral. Of these, 60% will be hypertensive and 30% will already be uremic. In addition to hypertension, large, palpable bilateral lobular abdominal masses may be present. Patients with infected cysts or recent hemorrhage into a cyst will be tender to palpation of the affected area.

Diagnosis and Treatment

Renal ultrasound images can differentiate polycystic kidney disease from bilateral giant hydronephrosis, the rare bilateral hypernephroma, and Wilms' tumor.

Treatment should include pain medication during passage of clots or obstruction and infection. A supporting garment or corset may help with the chronic discomfort caused by the mass of these kidneys tugging on the renal pedicles. Occasionally, nephrectomy is performed on the hypertensive patient with polycystic disease who is about to undergo dialysis or transplantation for renal failure. Infection of cysts tends to occur late in the disease and is therefore an ominous prognosticator.

Simple (Solitary) Renal Cyst

Etiology

The cause of solitary renal cyst is unknown. These cysts, in contrast to those seen in polycystic kidneys, do not destroy significant amounts of parenchyma. They do not communicate with the collecting sytem. Rarely, they cause obstruction of the collecting system by compression.

Symptoms and Signs

The typical patient is over 40 years of age and complains of intermittent dull unilateral flank pain that has been present for months or years. When such a cyst becomes infected, symptoms of sepsis will be described.

Diagnosis and Treatment

Renal ultrasound or a CAT scan provide the best means of establishing the diagnosis of simple renal cyst. In cystic renal lesions of doubtful definition, it might be necessary to puncture the cyst with a fine-gauge needle under ultrasonic or scanning image control, aspirate the contents, and perform cytological examination. The differential diagnosis includes renal neoplasm, carbuncle, hydronephrosis, and hydrocalicosis.

Percutaneous aspiration may relieve symptoms of simple renal cysts. If not, it may be necessary to explore the kidney and unroof the cyst (16).

Calyceal Diverticulum

Etiology

Calyceal diverticula are outpocketings of the kidney collecting system, which may be congenital communicating cystic lesions or be acquired by rupture of parenchymal abscess cavities into the collecting system. These then become lined with urothelium and continue to communicate with calyces, infundibula, or renal pelves.

Symptoms and Signs

Individuals with these lesions are mostly asymptomatic but may complain of chronic dull intermittent flank pain. Stones trapped in the diverticula can harbor infection with symptoms of pyelonephritis from time to time. These lesions may require retrograde pyelography for full delineation and diagnosis.

Treatment

Patients who are persistently symptomatic, or whose infections cannot be controlled with antibiotics might require surgical excision of the diverticulum (17).

Horseshoe Kidney

Pathophysiology

Because of its weight, position, and variable blood supply, congenital horseshoe kidney can produce traction on the renal vessels and other adjacent vascular structures, resulting in abdominal pain of a dull, intermittent, and vague nature. Any of the obstructive lesions found in the unfused kidney can occur in the horseshoe kidney and produce similar symptoms.

Treatment

Although successful treatment of obstructive conditions in the upper collecting systems of horseshoe kidneys depends on separation of the isthmus, this is not always feasible or desirable because of the vascular configuration (18, 19) Symptoms due to lesions that cannot be corrected may respond to medications or regional analgesia achieved with paravertebral T10–L1 blockade (18, 19).

Medullary Sponge Kidney

Etiology

Medullary sponge kidney is a congenital autosomal recessive defect in which the distal collecting tubules are dilated and visible on intravenous pyelography.

Symptoms and Signs

Most individuals with this defect are unaffected and asymptomatic (20). Pain is associated with infection and stone formation in the widened (at times cystic) collecting tubules. Since autoelimination of the stones requires erosion through a papilla into the collecting system, the pain is chronic and intermittent as well as difficult to treat.

Treatment

Nerve blocks to relieve the pain might be followed by renal denervation in selected cases. (Nerve blocks are discussed under Renal and Ureteral Calculi and Idiopathic Nephralgia.) Endourologic approaches to this disease may offer relief to the individual who suffers chronically because of pain from trapped intermittently obstructing calculi (21).

Acquired Vascular Lesions

Renal Vein Thrombosis

Etiology

Dehydration, infection, and coagulopathy are thought to be involved in renal vein thrombosis. Whatever the cause, the obstruction of venous outflow by clot causes renal swelling, capsular distension, and pain.

Symptoms and Signs

Half of the patients present with acute flank pain, hematuria, and persistent proteinuria. The other half experience a gradual onset of chronic flank pain rather than acute pain. In some patients the first symptom is that of pulmonary emboli.

Diagnosis and Treatment

Diminished function in a swollen kidney can be detected by ultrasonic or other forms of venography. If the vena cava is involved, however, venography causes emboli in many; therefore ultrasound is a safer diagnostic procedure if this problem is suspected.

Anticoagulation therapy often promotes return of full function within 4 to 6 weeks (22). Pain is relatively mild and controllable with aspirin and codeine, but the physician should be mindful of the effects of aspirin on the ongoing anticoagulation.

Renal Infarct

Etiology

Slowly progressive compromise of renal vasculature with secondary renal infarction produces no acute symptoms. Sudden infarction can occur in patients suffering from bacterial endocarditis, atrial or ventricular cardiac thrombi, severe generalized vascular disease, or acute deceleration trauma, particularly a fall onto the back.

Symptoms and Signs

The patient suffers sudden severe prostrating flank pain, similar to that seen in acute obstruction; following this the patient might go into shock. Physical examination is not specific. Urinalysis might be normal or show red cells. The affected side will not function on radioisotope urography or intravenous pyelography. Arteriography will demonstrate the lesion.

Treatment

Pain associated with renal infarct is controlled by narcotics as the shock is treated. If the situation is discovered within 2 to 4 hours, embolectomy might be considered (23).

Vesico-Ureteral Reflux into the Kidney

Renal pain occurring as a result of vesico-ureteral reflux is discussed later in this chapter.

Renal Infections

Acute Pyelonephritis

Etiology

Acute pyelonephritis is a common disease most frequently seen in females after repeated bouts of cystitis. It can also result from hematogenous spread of bacteria or through vesico-ureteral reflux.

Symptoms and Signs

Acute and constant aching over the involved flanks, accompanied by systemic symptoms of infection, agues and fever is common with this disease. Mild peritoneal signs may be present. Tenderness is present in the costovertebral angles and flanks (Murphy's sign). The urine contains pus and bacteria. The white blood count is elevated.

Diagnosis and Treatment

In the diagnosis of acute pyelonephritis, the physician should establish that there is no associated obstruction. The differential diagnosis includes obstructed pyonephrosis from urinary calculus or sloughed papilla, pancreatitis, pneumonia, and appendicitis.

Pain is relatively easily controlled by a variety of analgesics during the short period before antibiotics correct the underlying infection.

Renal Carbuncle

Etiology

Hematogenous seeding from another primary source, most commonly with Staphylococcus epidermidis from a skin carbuncle, is the usual cause of renal carbuncle.

Symptoms and Signs

Spiking fevers, often over a prolonged period, vague intermittent back pain, and weight loss generally are present. These suggest the use of a CAT scan, from which the diagnosis is made.

Treatment

Specific pain is not a prominent problem in the management of patients with renal carbuncle. They are treated with systemic antibiotics with penicillinase inhibitors for Staphylococcus, such as cephalexin (Keflex) 0.5 to 1.0 g qid for 10 days in uncomplicated cases or for 6 weeks in cases associated with structural problems (24).

Perinephric Abscess

Etiology

Perinephric abscesses, which are collections of pus between the renal capsule and Gerota's fascia, are usually secondary to chronic problems such as infected obstruction due to stones, diabetic nephropathy with abscess formation, papillary necrosis, and sickle cell disease. The expanding pockets of pus and reaction cause pain.

Diagnosis and Treatment

The possibility of perinephric abscess needs to be considered in diabetics, patients with sickle cell trait, and those with known stones who develop dull persistent flank pain and signs of low-grade sepsis. Physical findings might include a flank mass and tenderness, scoliosis to the affected side, and signs of pleural effusion. In occult cases, barium study of the colon might show displacement and compression of the colon by the extrinsic mass on the affected side. A CAT scan should demonstrate the lesion and allow differentiation from other space-occupying retroperitoneal or renal lesions.

Reflex skeletal muscle spasm associated with perinephric abscess can be relieved by analgesics and heat before drainage of the lesion, which is the definitive treatment (25).

Renal-Duodenal Syndrome

Etiology

Renal-duodenal syndrome is due to adhesions between the right kidney and duodenum that develop after repeated bouts of infection and perinephritis or as a result of surgery. The adhesions cause the normally mobile kidney to tug on the duodenum, producing nausea and at times vomiting and, in some patients, pain.

Diagnosis and Treatment

Diagnosis of this very rare condition is made in patients with appropriate signs and symptoms and a history of repeated infection or prior surgery involving the two structures.

Treatment consists of surgical lysis of the offending renal-duodenal adhesions (26).

Parasitic Infection (Echinoccocal Cyst)

In regions where Echinococcus is endemic, patients occasionally present with renal colic secondary to passage of Echinococcus down the ureter. About 3% of those with liver involvement also have renal disease (27).

Obstructions

Renal and Ureteral Calculi

Etiology

Although Pak et al. (28) demonstrated alterations of calcium absorption and excretion in chronic stone formers, the relationship of these metabolic alterations to stone formation are still under clinical investigation, as are the role of urate, oxalate, and magnesium in calcium stone formation (29, 30). In appropriately selected patients the following factors seem to reduce the number of episodes of stone passage in established stone formers: (a) alteration of calcium load in diet; (b) manipulation of tubular excretion of calcium by hydrochlorthiazide; (c) reduction of urate excretion with the aid of xanthine oxidase inhibitors such as allopurinol; and (d) liberal intake of fluids.

Symptoms and Signs

Currently, metabolic diagnosis is not a cost-effective screening method for identifying stone formers, and the physician's first contact with such individuals usually is during the acute pain caused by the passing of a calculus. As previously mentioned, pain of passage is characterized in adults as an "expanding bubble" of severe discomfort unrelieved by position changes. The site of referred pain depends on the position of the stone in the collecting system. The severity of the pain is such that maximum doses of potent narcotics (e.g., 15 mg morphine sulfate or 125 mg meperidine) might not relieve the pain. Pain from stones within the renal pelvis and its branches is referred to the costovertebral angle; stones obstructing the upper ureter refer pain to the flank and gonad; mid-ureteral stones cause referred pain in the anterior superior iliac crest and inguinal region; and with lower ureteral stones the pain is referred to the pubic area and scrotal or labial skin. Stones in the terminal ureter can also cause urinary urgency and frequency due to irritation of the trigone of the bladder.

The pain is often accompanied by hyperesthesia, allodynia, and tenderness of the kidney region and spasm of the muscles of the abdomen and flank. Not infrequently, retraction of the testicle, nausea, vomiting, urgency, and "cold sweat." and occasionally signs of shock are present. Often there is a compelling urge to urinate, and urination becomes painful.

As mentioned earlier, the mechanisms of pain are obstruction and distension of the collecting system and renal capsule, extravasation of urine into the tissues, and irritation of the mucosa. In addition to the reflex spasm of the skeletal muscles, reflex spasm of the smooth muscles of the ureteropelvic junction and ureters frequently occurs. This spasm becomes a new source of noxious stimuli that give rise to pain and other reflex mechanisms, which in turn aggravate the spasm. In this way a viscious circle is initiated, causing aggravation and persistence of the pain. In addition, reflex vasoconstriction of the renal vascular complex can occur, with further aggravation of the deranged physiology (3).

Diagnosis

Diagnosis of calculi is based on the history of the pain, which has a characteristic radiation and progression from flank to groin, along with physical findings of costovertebral angle tenderness. Gross or microscopic hematuria is typical, but in a significant percentage of individuals, the symptoms of stone passage vary from none to vague and poorly localized abdominal malaise. The patient may be cool and clammy during episodes of colic. In contrast to the patient with intestinal disease, whose problem is usually heralded by nausea and/or vomiting, the patient with renal colic usually becomes nauseated after the onset of pain (i.e., the nausea is caused by intense pain). The patient with intraperitoneal lesions that irritate the peritoneum usually tries to lie still, whereas the patient suffering from urinary colic is often restless and seeks different positions in attempts to get relief from the pain.

Plain radiographs of the abdomen and pelvis may show calcific stones of fair size but will fail to demonstrate radiolucent stones or smaller calcific densities in the presence of much gas and fecal matter in the colon. Therefore an intravenous pyelogram should be done in patients suspected to be passing a stone except for those known to be allergic to contrast agents; with these patients, radioisotope renography can safely demonstrate the obstruction. This technique is particularly useful for the occasional wily narcotics abuser who visits emergency facilities feigning renal colic in order to obtain the analgesics but claims allergy to contrast agents as a means of avoiding discovery.

Treatment

Therapy depends on the size of the stone, its location, presence or absence of sepsis, the amount of pain the individual is experiencing, and occasionally social circumstances. Ureteral stones less than 5 mm in diameter will pass spontaneously in 80% of the cases; stones that are 5 to 10 mm in diameter will pass spontaneously in about 20% of patients; stones larger than 10 mm in diameter are much less likely to pass on their own.

OPIOIDS. In most patients, relief of the severe pain is one of the primary objectives of the treatment of ureteral colic. Morphine, like all other phenanthrene derivatives of opium, tends to cause contraction of all smooth muscles with the notable exception of those of the blood vessels. Clinical studies have shown that morphine can increase intrabiliary pressure to 15 times the normal value (3). Although large doses of morphine (e.g., 15 mg intravenously, slowly) may relieve the pain through its central effects, it is likely to aggravate the smooth muscle spasm. Meperidine has a slightly less spasmogenic effect than other potent analgesics and can be used in combination with atropine given simultaneously. Dextroamphetamine given in conjunction with an opiod potentiates the latter's analgesic efficacy and thus reduces the narcotic dosage required to achieve pain relief; it also is an effective antiemetic drug (31).

REGIONAL ANALGESIA. If none of these agents provides good pain relief, serious consideration should be given to the use of one of the nerve block techniques, which interrupt the innervation of the kidney and ureter. Of the several regional analgesic techniques available, paravertebral sympathetic block and segmental epidural block are the most practical and effective. Paravertebral block, first used by Mandl (32) to successfully treat renal colic and subsequently employed by many European clinicians with very good results, has the disadvantage of requiring insertion of several needles (see 4 for references). For this reason, continuous segmental epidural analgesia, limited to T10–L1 inclusive, is the more practical procedure; it not only provides complete and persistent relief of pain as long as the analgesia is continued, but also interrupts efferent sympathetic impulses and thus eliminates the reflex spasm and any associated renal vasospasm. This in turn increases the chance of spontaneous passage of stones that are less tham 10 mm in diameter.

Bonica (4, 33, 34) has used either paravertebral sympathetic block or continuous epidural block in 53 patients, including 8 physicians, during the past four decades. In addition to providing complete pain relief, in some patients the treatment resulted in downward movement of stones that had not advanced for 18 to 36 hours prior to the block. In 23% of these patients, treatment was accompanied by passage of the stone into the bladder; in another 18% of patients with calculi that had not advanced for a number of hours, the stone moved to the ureterovesical junction, where it was extracted through a cystoscope (Fig. 62-7). An important advantage of regional analgesia is that it poses no risk of respiratory depression. In contrast, if the patient is given a narcotic and then suddenly passes the stone, the pain often promptly subsides along with the pain-induced respiratory stimulation; in this situation the patient may incur severe respiratory depression. In addition, epidural analgesia can be extended if it is necessary to treat the stone through percutaneous ultrasonic destruction or open surgery.

OTHER THERAPY. Stones accompanied by sepsis are a truly life-threatening medical emergency. A history of chills and fever and findings of preshock or shock, fever, or elevated white blood count should alert the physician to the probability of concurrent sepsis. Intravenous lines must be established immediately for infusion of antibiotics and fluids, medications, and electrolytes to combat shock. Once the patient is in stable condition, this will be a convenient route for administration of potent opioid analgesics if someone experienced in epidural analgesia is not available.

Some means of drainage of the obstructed organ must be established. It can be drained percutaneously with the aid of local anesthesia or epidural block, or endoscopically via retrograde passage of a ureteral cath-eter, again under topical or epidural analgesia. Topical anesthesia of the urethra is achieved with 2% Xylocaine jelly available from Astra. Instrumental manipulation within the bladder is made less uncomfortable by epidural block or by instillation through a small catheter of 20 ml lidocaine (Xylocaine) before cystoscopy.

Urine and blood are cultured. Pending identification of the organism and its sensitivities, broad-spectrum

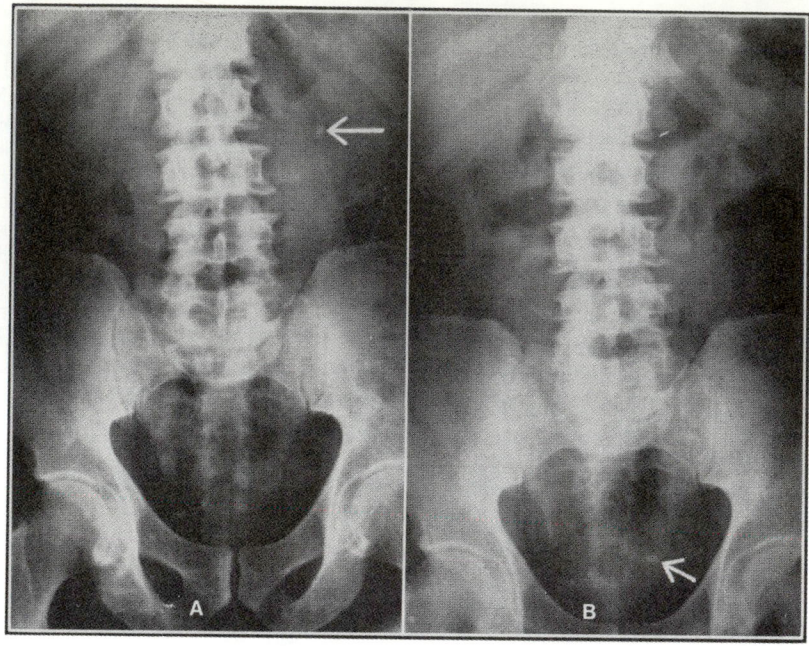

Fig. 62-7. *A.* Radiograph of a patient with a stone in the left ureter at the level of the second lumbar interspace, which produced severe colicky pain in the left flank with radiation to the left groin, testicle, and inner aspect of the thigh. The stone did not advance for 48 hours, and the pain persisted despite repeated administration of narcotics. Paravertebral sympathetic block of T10–L2 caused complete relief of pain and permitted the patient to be up and about. The nerve block was repeated in 12 hours. *B.* Radiograph taken after second nerve block showing that the calculus had descended to the ureterovesical junction. From this position, it was extracted with cystoscopic manipulation.

antibiotics are administered. Since coliforms are the most likely offenders, although cocci may also be involved, a combination of antibiotics including an aminoglycoside is a good choice (e.g., ampicillin 1 gm every 6 hours and gentamicin 1 mg per kg every 8 hours for several days). When the sepsis has been well controlled, removal of the stone by extracorporeal lithotripsy, percutaneous ultrasonic destruction, endoscopic ureteral manipulation, or open surgery can be safely carried out as indicated.

An example of a socially motivated stone removal is the airline pilot discovered to have a renal calculus as a result of a workup for microhematuria found in an annual examination urinalysis. Such individuals are barred from flying commercial aircraft if they harbor stones. Therefore, otherwise asymptomatic stones in such individuals are often manipulated into a position that will allow them to pass or be broken up by extracorporeal shock wave lithotripsy (35).

Acute Intermittent Hydronephrosis

Etiology

In acute intermittent hydronephrosis, a minimally compensated congenital or acquired constriction of the ureteropelvic segment decompensates as the result of sudden increase in local edema, angulation, or fluid load, producing acute renal colic.

Diagnosis

When prompted, the patient might remember that past episodes of colic have followed increased intake of fluids, such as bouts of beer drinking, or high intake of salty foods such as smoked ham, pickles, or saltines, which induce a sodium-load diuresis. Diagnosis is made by obtaining an emergency intravenous pyelogram during an episode of colic. Failing this, infusion pyelography with a diuretic phase induced by furosemide may reproduce the colic and show the lesion. As a diagnostic maneuver, it may be possible to reproduce the pain during cystoscopy under local anesthesia and retrograde filling and overdistension of the renal pelvis through an ureteral catheter.

Treatment

Treatment of intermittent hydronephrosis involves surgical relief of the obstruction. In the period between diagnosis and definitive treatment, the patient is instructed to avoid fluid loading of the kidney; if an episode should occur, analgesics are dispensed as needed (36).

Clot Colic

Etiology

Renal bleeding unassociated with glomerulonephritis often produces clots. During passage, the clots can obstruct the ureter, producing colic indistinguishable from that due to passage of calculi as far as symptoms are concernerd. Clot passage commonly occurs after blunt renal trauma, after renal surgery, with rupture of renal cysts, and from renal neoplasms.

Treatment

While diagnostic studies are under way, management of the pain is similar to management of pain due to acute obstruction of any kind. Analgesics are given, and if vomiting is a significant problem, intravenous fluids are administered. In the presence of severe bleeding, blood should be cross-matched in case transfusion becomes necessary, and vital signs and hematocrit should be monitored. It is wise to have venous access available as well.

Papillary Necrosis

Etiology

Those at greatest risk of developing papillary necrosis—a rare, potentially life-threatening condition—are diabetics, chronic phenacetin abusers, alcoholics, persons with the sickle cell trait, and patients with chronic pyelonephritis. The renal papilla loses its vascular integrity and sloughs. The sloughed papilla obstructs the ureter and produces colic. Because infection is a common contributing factor, the danger of an infected, closed space threatens whenever a papilla sloughs and obstructs the collecting system. If this diagnosis is suspected, prompt action to relieve the obstruction is mandatory.

Diagnosis and Treatment

If pyelography is carried out in the patient with colic who is passing a papilla, a negative filling defect in the calyx outlining the bed of the slough can be seen. The appearance of this defect has been described as the "signet ring" sign. The location of radiolucent necrotic tissue in the ureter is also seen as a filling defect.

If the ureter is obstructed, prompt relief by retrograde passage of a catheter or percutaneous nephrostomy is mandatory in the management of sepsis. The urine should be strained, and retrieved necrotic tissue should be sent to a pathologist to confirm the diagnosis (37).

Retroperitoneal Fibrosis

Etiology

Retroperitoneal fibrosis is most commonly related to leaks from aortic aneurysms or associated with retroperitoneal malignancies such as reticulum cell sarcoma. Before it was withdrawn from the market, methysergide, effective against migraine, produced a rash of cases. In over half the case of retroperitoneal fibrosis, the etiology is undetermined. A dense fibrotic process involves the retroperitoneal structures, surrounds the ureter, and compresses it. The earliest involvement usually occurs at the crossing of the iliac vessels, but later the process can extend to involve the kidneys, the great vessels, and the mediastinum.

Symptoms and Signs

The symptoms of retroperitoneal fibrosis are often nonspecific and can include moderate hypertension, vague back or abdominal pain, flank pain, scrotal swelling, and venous engorgement of the lower extremities and abdominal wall. Eventually, uremic symptoms appear after the slowly progressive bilateral renal obstruction interferes with function.

Diagnosis

The diagnosis is usually made after other organ system studies prove negative and the urinary tract has been investigated to "rule out" disease in that system. Typical findings on urography are hydronephrosis without an obvious point of obstruction and medial deviation of the lumbar course of the ureters. Retrograde passage of ureteral catheters is usually easy in spite of the antegrade obstruction.

Treatment

Treatment of retroperitoneal fibrosis involves relief of obstruction. On a temporary or semipermanent basis, ureteral stents are effective. Longer-lasting correction requires surgical lysis of the ureters and replantation to an area less likely to be affected by the disease. The ureters can be replanted laterally or intraperitoneally to remove them from the fibrotic process. The disease process is often progressive, and prognosis is guarded in spite of good initial results (38).

Hydronephrosis of Pregnancy

Etiology

At the beginning of the fourth month of pregnancy, progressive dilation of renal calyces, pelves, and ureters above the pelvic brim starts and continues until the last 2 months, when it usually regresses. At least 2 factors are involved: mechanical compression by the enlarging uterus and endocrine effects on the smooth muscle of the ureter and renal pelvis. Because the left ureter is cushioned by the sigmoid colon, it is less affected by uterine compression than the right.

Symptoms and Signs

In the absence of infection or other complicating factors, (see Ovarian Vein Syndrome), hydronephrosis of pregnancy does not cause pain or other symptoms. Complications combined with obstruction produce persistent pain.

Treatment

When persistent pain develops, care must be exercised in the use of narcotics because of the possible depressant effects on the fetus. This risk can be minimized by combining small doses of narcotics with nonsteroidal anti-inflammatory drugs and perhaps even dextroamphetamines. Because obstruction can be relieved with the aid of indwelling internal "double j" stents, which can usually be passed with the aid of topical anesthesia, the problem of long-term analgesics can be bypassed (39).

Ovarian Vein syndrome

Etiology

Initially known as the "right ovarian vein syndrome," this condition is most commonly seen in women of childbearing age following pregnancy (see previous section). Presumably, a process is set in motion during pregnancy in which an aberrant ovarian vein traps the ureter after hormonal changes, and the obstruction caused by the uterine enlargement produces ureteral dilation. The resulting constriction persists postpartum, leaving permanent hydroureteronephrosis above the level of the surrounding vein. Since hydronephrosis of pregnancy is more common (80%) and more severe on the right side, that side is more frequently involved in the ovarian vein syndrome. Symptoms are pain in the involved flank due to obstruction and those of the accompanying infection.

Diagnosis and Treatment

Postpartum pain in the right flank and/or abdomen accompanied by chills, fever, malaise, nausea, and vomiting should alert the clinician to the possibility of ovarian vein syndrome. On examination there is flank tenderness. Ultrasound or pyelography helps establish the diagnosis.

Relief of pain with analgesics is required until obstruction is bypassed by ureteral stenting and antibiotic therapy is instituted to control infection. Permanent relief is provided by surgical excision of the obstructing vein (40, 41).

Infundibular Stenosis (Fraley's Syndrome)

Etiology

In Fraley's syndrome, flank pain is caused by obstruction of the superior infundibulum and its calyces (42). The latter obstruction is produced by intrarenal vessels impinging on the infundibular channel as the secondary vessels wind around it in their course through the renal sinus.

Diagnosis and Treatment

All reported cases of Fraley's syndrome thus far have been adults. Patients complain of steady, dull pain in the costovertebral angle and flank, usually for months or years. The key to diagnosis is that the pain is relieved by lying down. Tenderness may or may not be present on examination. Upon careful review of the pyelogram, which includes oblique views, a linear filling defect caused by vascular compression is seen crossing the infundibulum to the superior calyx. A 30- or 60-min drainage film shows contrast trapped in the superior calyx.

Treatment of Fraley's syndrome requires severance and reanastomosis of the infundibulum or the occluding vessel, preferably the former (42).

Conditions Causing Pseudorenal Pain

Etiology

Ilioinguinal neuropathy and genitofemoral nerve entrapment, which cause pseudorenal pain, almost always follow inguinal surgery, most frequently herniorrhaphy. Genitofemoral entrapment is rare, but both conditions can be mistaken for renal pain by the unwary.

Symptoms and Signs

These conditions are characterized by radicular (segmental) pain in the distribution of dermatomes T10–T12 that can mimic renal pain. Unlike renal colic, however,

pseudorenal pain is usually brought on by a physical strain such as heavy lifting, sleeping in an awkward posture, or occasionally by a blow to the spine. It is relieved by a change of position, which is not the case with most renal pain (for an exception to this see Infundibular Stenosis).

Diagnosis

These conditions are rare; they are mentioned in this chapter for the sake of completeness in considering the differential diagnosis of renal pain (43, 44).

Idiopathic Nephralgia

Etiology

Idiopathic nephralgia is an extremely rare condition characterized by renal-like pain and other urologic symptoms (e.g., frequency, nocturia, and dysuria), in absence of demonstrable pathology. In former years the condition was diagnosed more frequently and was attributed to irregular and incomplete contraction of the calyces and renal pelvis resulting from uncoordinated overactivity of the sympathetic nerve supply so that impulses for peristalsis either did not reach or did not pass beyond the ureteropelvic junction (45).

As knowledge of renal pathophysiology increased and advanced diagnostic methods became available, the number of patients diagnosed with this syndrome steadily declined and now is minuscule. Nonetheless, if after comprehensive urologic, neurologic, orthopedic, psychiatric, and radiologic evaluation, no demonstrable pathology is found for persistent and disabling renal-type pain and other related symptoms, one is faced with the need for treatment. In the rare instances in which this occurs, patients should be submitted to comprehensive psychosocial evaluation, incuding psychometric testing, to eliminate pain due to psychologic problems.

Therapy

If all of the diagnostic procedures discussed so far prove negative and the patient has persistent, disabling pain, diagnostic-prognostic paravertebral nerve block of T10–L2 inclusive with a local anesthetic is carried out. At least three such procedures should be carried out using local anesthetics with different durations of action, and the patient's response carefully monitored and compared with the predicted duration of the analgesia. If the patient derives complete pain relief for the duration of the blockade, a series of such blocks might alter the behavioral response to the underlying stimulus, whatever it may be, and provide adequate relief of the pain syndrome. When such procedures provide complete but only temporary relief, renal denervation may be considered.

DENERVATION. In the early part of this century, denervation of the kidneys was achieved by periarterial stripping of the nerves. This procedure does not effect complete denervation, however, because some of the nerves run in the wall of the vessel. Moreover, because the fibers removed are postganglionic and only small sections are removed, regeneration occurs within weeks and months. These factors, together with the fact that the operation is tedious and carries an inherent risk of laceration of vessels, caused a number of clinicians to abandon this procedure and replace it with aorticorenal ganglionectomy. Fontaine et al. (46), among others, obtained good results by combining aorticorenal ganglionectomy and splanchnicectomy.

The most impressive report on the efficacy of denervation for idiopathic nephralgia is that published by Bauer (47). He noted that in a large series of cases, all but one patient was freed of persistent "idiopathic" renal pain by denervation of the kidney. More recently, White and Sweet (48) reported that four patients, in whom paravertebral block of T10–L1 (or L2) produced complete temporary relief, derived relief for 1 to 8 years after sympathetic denervation. For reasons previously mentioned, the preganglionic operation of dividing small and lesser splanchnic nerves and removing the three lower thoracic and 1st and 2nd lumbar sympathetic ganglia as well as the intervening trunks is the procedure of choice. We have performed this procedure in 1 patient with a successful outcome. As has been amply demonstrated following autotransplantation and heterotransplantation of kidneys in many patients, total denervation has little effect on renal function.

Renal and Ureteral Tumors

A variety of tumors of the kidney and ureter can cause pain in the flank and various other symptoms and signs. The most important tumors are renal cell carcinoma, carcinoma of the renal pelvis, sarcomas, oncocytoma and Wilms' tumor of the kidney and carcinoma of the ureter. For 1986, American Cancer Society estimated that there were 22,000 new cases of cancer of the kidney and "other urinary" structures (except bladder), of which 12,700 were males and 7300 were females (49). The mortality statistics were 9200, 5600, and 3600, respectively.

Renal Cell Carcinoma

Renal cell carcinoma, also called hypernephroma and Grawitz tumor, now rivals syphilis in the U.S.A. as "the great imitator" of other diseases. Because of the variety and diversity of the presenting symptoms and signs related to secondary effects of this tumor (paraneoplastic syndrome), it has been dubbed "the internist's tumor" (50). The tumor occurs in all age groups, but it is most prevalent in the sixth and seventh decades of life and has a male predominance with a ratio of 3:2 (51, 52). This tumor afflicts all races, but its highest incidence is in Scandinavia.

Etiology

Although the exact cause of renal cell carcinoma has not been defined, there is evidence for carcinogenic and genetic factors. Smoking increases the risk of renal cancer by approximately 40% and cadmium exposure has been associated with an increased risk; the presence of both factors increases the risk of renal cancer even further (52). A genetic propensity for renal carcinoma also has been demonstrated. Patients with von Hippel–Lindau disease are at significant risk of developing renal carcinoma including bilateral

multiple tumors (50). Cohen (51) described an abnormal karyotype caused by reciprocal translocation of chromosomes 3 and 8 in families in which a kidney tumor was prevalent. He reported that 8 of 10 of the family members with tumors had the chromosomal abnormality, whereas the 22 without cancer did not. These data support a multifaceted basis for renal cell carcinoma including environmental, genetic, and hormonal factors.

Although Grawitz (53) originally postulated that these tumors arose from adrenal rests because of their microscopic resemblance to adrenal tissues, which prompted him to name the tumor "hypernephroma," subsequent studies established that the tumors are of renal tubular origin (see 54 for references). Three cell types can be identified in these malignancies: (a) clear cell carcinoma, (b) granular cell carcinoma, and (c) sarcomatoid cells. Kidney tumors often are given a pathologic grade of I, II, or III, based on degree of cellular anaplasia, with grade I being least anaplastic and grade III showing the greatest degree of anaplasia. Metastatic spread occurs both by direct extension and through lymphatic and hematogenous routes. Most common sites of metastasis are lungs (55%), lymph nodes (34%), liver (33%), bone (32%), adrenal (19%), contralateral kidney (11%), brain (6%), heart (5%), spleen (5%), bowel (4%), and skin (3%) (54).

Symptoms and Signs

Renal cell carcinoma may present with a wide variety of clinical symptoms and signs including the classic triad of flank pain, hematuria, and a palpable flank mass, as well as nonspecific systemic symptoms and numerous paraneoplastic syndromes. In several series of studies, the classic triad occurred in 4 to 6% of the patients studies (52). In these studies, individual features of the triad occurred more frequently than the entire triad. Hematuria, noted in 35 to 59% of the patients reviewed, was most common. Pain directly related to the primary tumor, provoked by stretching of the renal capsule or sudden expansion due to bleeding into it, was found in about one-third of the cases (range 10 to 38%), although in one study of 309 patients, pain was present in 41% of the patients (55). Palpable mass was found in about 22% (range 2 to 35%) (54), although in the study of 309 patients, it was noted in 45% of the patients. In the series of studies cited by Bagley (52), 30% of the patients had none of the classic triad of symptoms. Thus, the disease may remain clinically silent during the early stages, and in over 50% of patients, metastatic disease is present at the time of diagnosis (54).

Hypertension and weight loss are relatively common presenting signs of renal cell carcinoma. Tumor obstructing the spermatic vein can cause a varicocele, which fails to disappear when the patient lies down. Abnormal liver function tests are found in about 15% of patients, including some without metastasis, the cause of which is unknown. A similar fraction have hypercalcemia.

The paraneoplastic syndromes associated with renal cell carcinoma constitute a large portion of the signs and symptoms associated with the initial diagnosis of the tumor. Other secondary symptoms, which may be related to systemic, toxic, or endocrine effects, include intermittent fevers, weakness, anemia, or paradoxically erythrocythemia due to overproduction of erythropoietin. Chronic spiking fever is the presenting symptom in 1/8 of the cases. Cardiac failure associated with hypertension may occur because of the arteriovenous shunting within the neovasculature of the tumor.

Diagnosis

The diagnosis of renal cell carcinoma requires thorough history and physical examination as well as radiography and other more sophisticated diagnostic procedures mentioned earlier in this chapter. The presence of a spiking fever in conjunction with regional mass makes differential diagnosis between renal tumor and renal abscess quite difficult, and radiologic findings may not distinguish between these two lesions; final diagnosis must await surgical exploration or fine needle aspiration. Currently, the tumor is as likely to be discovered incidentally by ultrasound imaging as in any other way. If the cancer is identified thus within the kidney at the time of screening for other diseases, about 65% of the patients survive 5 years. However, if one or more of the symptoms of renal cell carcinoma are present, only one-third of all patients survive 5 years (54). Once ultrasound imaging suggests diagnosis of renal carcinoma, further studies of the mass by CAT scan and angiography usually confirm the diagnosis and lead to exploration and excision. Tumors picked up incidentally in early stages by these means are much less likely to have developed a neovasculature, which lights up the angiogram in large later neoplasms.

Treatment

Surgical removal remains the only effective treatment for renal cell carcinoma. Localized stage I (tumor confined to the kidney) and stage II (tumor locally invasive but confined to Gerota's fascia) are amenable to radical nephrectomy (52, 54, 55). This procedure includes early control of the renovascular pedicles and removal of the kidney and the associated tumor, the adrenal gland and the surrounding perinephritic fat, and Gerota's fascia along with the regional lymph nodes.

METASTATIC RENAL CELL CARCINOMA. Stage III renal carcinoma, which by definition includes regional invasion of the renal vein or vena cava or both or metastasis to regional lymph nodes or a combination of these, is also treated by radical nephrectomy with excision of the regional lymph nodes around the renal vessels and the ipsilateral great vessels from the level of the superior mesenteric artery to the inferior mesenteric artery. This procedure results in 30% five-year survival (52, 54). Local extension of the tumor into the renal vein appears to have less effect on the prognosis than nodal involvement.

No uniformly satisfactory treatment exists for stage IV renal cell carcinoma, which by definition includes invasion of surrounding organs. Since as many as 50% of patients have evidence of metastatic disease at the time of diagnosis, therapy remains a major problem. In selected patients who have a proven solitary metastasis surgical excision of the primary tumor and the metastasis, may provide long-term cure, whereas in patients with widespread metastasis, the prognosis is poor even when radiation, chemotherapy, or hormonal manipulation is added to the surgery.

In patients with metastatic lesions from renal cell carcinoma, pain control is a very critical issue. Pain due to metastatic lytic lesion of the bone or periosteal elevation are best treated by irradiation of the involved area. Occasionally long-bone lesions may benefit from internal fixation. For far advanced disease with bone marrow replacement, "half-body" irradiation relieves the pain in some patients (52). Pain caused by infiltration of nerves or nerve plexuses or spread to other organs can be severe, intractable, and not relieved by oncologic therapy. In such instances symptomatic therapy as discussed in Chapter 24 should be carried out. This should include the use of nonopioid and narcotic analgesics and various adjuvant agents such as amitriptyline and other antidepressants, which have proven useful in relieving the lancinating deafferentation pain. Attempts should be made to use a multimodal approach combining pharmacologic therapy, psychologic techniques, neurostimulation techniques, nerve blocks, intraspinal opioids and neuroablative procedures as discussed in Chapter 24.

Sarcomas

Sarcomas account for only 3% of the malignancies of the kidney or renal pelvis. The majority of these lesions are leiomyosarcomas, but other histologic varieties have been reported (52). The mean age of patients who develop this type of tumor is about 50 years, with a range of 10 to 86 years.

The symptoms and signs depend on the size of the lesion. Large tumors cause pain by stretching of the renal capsule and perhaps by compression and/or irritation of intercostal nerves. No radiologic findings have been considered diagnostic. Treatment generally has consisted of excision by nephrectomy. The poor results noted, with frequent local recurrence and metastases, have prompted interest in combining surgery with radiotherapy and chemotherapy, which has been promising with sarcomas in other sites (52).

Oncocytomas

Oncocytomas are solid tumors of the renal parenchyma that have a benign course. This type of tumor accounts for 3 to 5% of all renal tumors (52). The age of patients with these tumors has ranged from the third to the ninth decade. There is a slightly higher incidence among males then females.

The signs and symptoms are somewhat similar to those of renal cell carcinoma and include flank pain, hematuria, and a palpable mass. The prognosis of patients with oncocytoma appears to be excellent.

Carcinoma of the Renal Pelvis

Carcinomas of the renal pelvis constitute 5% of all renal tumors (52, 54). These tumors first appear in the fifth and sixth decades of life with a progressive increase in incidence with advancing age. Carcinoma of the ureter is most common in older age groups being rare before 30 years of age. The incidence of carcinoma of the pelvis and ureter is greater in males than females by a ratio of 2:1.

Etiology and Pathology

Transitional epithelial cells lining the calyces and renal pelvis as well as the ureter are subject to environmental carcinogens. A strong relationship between carcinoma of the renal pelvis and a long-standing history of phenacetin ingestion has been established, as has an association betwen carcinoma of the renal pelvis and Danubian endemic familial nephropathy.

Malignant lesions of the renal pelvis can be classified into transitional cell carcinomas, squamous cell carcinomas, adenocarcinomas, and connective tissue tumors; 90% of all tumors of the renal pelvis are transitional cell tumors. In the ureter, over 70% of transitional cell carcinomas are primary transitional cell malignancies, and only 8% are squamous cell tumors (54). Transitional cell carcinoma is spread by direct extension and through blood and lymphatics. About 85% of transitional cell carcinomas of the renal pelvis are papillary, and approximately 50% of these demonstrate muscle invasion at the time of resection. The other 15% are sessile; of these, about 80% show muscle invasion at the time of resection.

Symptoms and Signs

Gross or microscopic hematuria appears in 80 to 90% of patients with renal pelvic tumors (52, 54). Pain is usually precipitated by ureteral or ureteropelvic junction obstruction secondary to the tumor mass. These patients are likely to suffer pain in the psoas, quadratus lumborum, and erector spinae muscles; if there has been extension to the vertebral column, back pain is present. Palpable flank mass in a patient with transitional cell carcinoma signifies massive extrarenal extension or hydronephrotic renal destruction secondary to obstruction.

Diagnosis

Diagnosis is helped by the appearance of a defect in the collecting system or renal pelvis on excretary pyelography. In patients with ureteral tumors, about 50% will present with urinary frequency or dysuria. Radiographically these patients will have ureteral dilatation, which develops as a result of accommodation of a slowly expanding tumor mass and reflects the absence of ureteral spasm produced by the presence of a calculus.

Treatment

Nephroureterectomy traditionally has been the treatment of choice for transitional carcinoma of the pelvis and/or ureter (52, 54). A stage I tumor of the ureter can be managed by excision of the tumor along with an uretero-ureterostomy. In patients with tumor of the renal pelvis, radical nephroureterectomy is advocated; this includes en bloc removal of the kidney, ureter with the cuff of the bladder, and the surrounding lymphatic structures. The addition of lymphadenectomy at the time of surgical resection may not provide any improved disease control but does provide information with regard to the stage of the disease, which can be used to select patients for adjunctive chemotherapy when appropriate agents have been identified. The 5-year survival rate is about 75 to 80% in grade I, about 50% in grade II, but less than 10% in grades III and IV. The prognosis in patients with transitional cell cancer of the ureter is the least favorable with patients rarely living more than 2 years after diagnosis.

Wilms' Tumor

Wilms' tumor which develops in about 500 children each year in the United States, accounts for approximately 95% of primary renal malignancies in childhood (56, 57). Moreover, it is the third most common solid tumor in childhood, following tumors of the central nervous system and neuroblastoma in incidence. During the past three decades, methods of treating this tumor have improved significantly, providing striking increases in survival rates.

Etiology and Pathology

The cause of Wilms' tumor is unknown, but the predilection of patients with certain genetic factors to develop this type of neoplasm suggests a partial genetic basis. Children with aniridia, hemihypertrophy, Von Recklinghausen's disease, or genitourinary congenital anomalies have an increased risk of developing Wilms' tumor (56).

Grossly, most Wilms' tumors are large, fleshy, soft tumors that grow in extensive fashion within an apparent "capsule." In advanced stage III of the disease, metastasis to the regional lymph nodes is present, while in stage IV of the disease, there is a hematogenous metastasis to the lung, liver, brain, or bone.

Symptoms and Signs

Most children present because of an abdominal mass first noted by a parent, (often when bathing the child). Other frequent presenting symptoms and signs include pain, anorexia, fever, or hematuria. The latter symptom is a sign of renal collecting-system involvement and is seen with much less frequency than in renal cell carcinoma. Mild hypertension is noted in many children, and plasma renin levels may be increased. Primary Wilms' tumor often undergoes extremely rapid growth in apparent size.

Diagnosis

In addition to a thorough history and physical examination, roentgenograms of the chest and intravenous urograms should be performed in all children (56, 57). The evaluation of the inferior vena cava, best performed by ultrasonography, should be done routinely to provide information about tumor size, site, and extent. Computer-assisted tomography of the lungs should also be performed. Other diagnostic procedures mentioned in the earlier part of this chapter should also be considered.

Treatment

Treatment of Wilm's tumor consists of surgical removal of the kidney and the entire tumor, a segment of the ureter, and regional lymph nodes (56, 57). This is followed by administration of a combination of actinomycin D and vincristine with or without the addition of doxorubicin (Adriamycin) and/or cyclophosphamide. Radiation is usually not used in stage I disease or in children under 2 years with stage II disease but is used postoperatively with more advanced stages of the neoplasm. Most recent studies suggest that nearly 80% of all patients with Wilms' tumor are cured with optimal current therapy. Survival is inversely proportional to the stage of the disease. The survival rate is 90 to 95% for those with stage I and 80 to 90% for those with stage II and stage III disease, whereas it is only about 30% for those who have pulmonary metastasis and even lower for the very few patients who have metastasis to the liver, bone, and brain. Metastasis to the lungs accounts for about two-thirds of the relapses, but with aggressive treatment, control of metastasis is possible in at least half of the cases.

Effective pain control before and after the surgical operation is an important part of management. Recent studies have provided impressive evidence that the prevalent misconception that children do not experience as much pain as adults, is incorrect. Pain may be managed by parenteral, oral, or intraspinal narcotics (see Chapter 24).

REFERENCES

1. Walsh, P.C., et al. (eds.): Campbell's Urology. 5th Ed. Philadelphia, W.B. Saunders, 1986.
2. Wyker, A.W., and Gillenwater, J.Y.: *In* Method of Urology, Baltimore, Williams & Wilkins, 1975, pp. 1–28.
3. Smith, D.R.: General Urology. 11th Ed. Los Altos, CA, Lange Medical, 1984.
4. Bonica, J.J.: Management of Pain. Philadephia, Lea & Febiger, 1953, pp. 1403–1409.
5. Kuntz, A.: The Automonic Nervous System. 4th Ed. Philadelphia, Lea & Febiger, 1953, pp. 269–276.
6. Netter, F.H., Shaper, R.K., and Yonkman, F.F. (eds.): Kidneys, Ureters and Urinary Bladder. Vol. 6 of The CIBA Collection of Medical Illustrations. Summit, NJ, CIBA Pharmaceutical Co. 1973, pp. 27–29.
7. Lennandier, K.G.: Ueber Lokale Anaesthesia und Ueber Sensibilitat in Organ und Geweve Weitere Beobachtunge. Mitt. Granzgeb. Med. Chir. *15*:465, 1906.
8. McLellan, A.N., and Goodell, H.: Pain from the bladder, the ureter and kidney pelvis. Pain (Res. Publ. Assoc. Res. Nerv. Mental Dis.). Vol. 23. Baltimore, Williams & Wilkins, 1943, pp. 252–259.
9. Bailey, H.: Physical Signs in Clinical Surgery. 13th Ed. Baltimore, Williams & Wilkins, 1960, pp. 430. Fig. 608.
10. Ruch, T.C.: Pathophysiology of pain. *In* Physiology and Biophysics. 19th Ed. Edited by T.C. Ruch and H.D. Patton. Philadelphia, W.B. Saunders, 1965, pp. 353–363.
11. Sandler, C.M., Raval, R., and David, C.L.: Computed tomography of the kidney. Urol. Clin. North Am., *12*(4):657, 1985.
12. Arger, P.H.: Computed tomography of the lower urinary tract. Urol. Clin. North Am. *12*(4):677, 1985.
13. Bova, J.G., Potter, J.L., and Arevalors, E.: Renal and perirenal infection: The role of computerized tomography. J. Urol., *133*:375, 1985.
14. Resnick, M.I., Willard, J.W., and Boyce, W.H.: Recent progress in ultrasonography of the bladder and prostate. J. Urol., *117*:444, 1977.
15. Williams, R.D., and Hricak, H.: Magnetic resonance imaging in urology. J. Urol., *132*:641, 1984.
16. Gernert, J.E., Stein, J., and Bischoff, A.J.: Solitary renal cysts: Experience with 100 cases. J. Urol., *100*:251, 1968.
17. Devine, C.J., Jr., Guzman, J.A., Devine, P.C., and Poutasse, E.F.: Calyceal diverticulum. J. Urol., *101*:8, 1969.
18. Gutierrez, R.: The Clinical Management of Horseshoe Kidney. New York, Paul B. Hoebar, 1934.
19. Pitts, W.R., and Muecke, E.C.: Horseshoe kidneys: A 40-year experience. J. Urol., *113*:743, 1975.
20. Kuiper, J.J.: Medullary sponge kidney. *In* Cystic Diseases of the Kidney. Edited by K.D. Gardner. New York, John Wiley and Sons, 1976.
21. Krieger, J.N., Rudd, T.G., and Mayo, M.E.: Current treatment of infection stones in high-risk patients. J. Urol. *132*:874, 1984.
22. Rosenmann, E., Pollak, V.E., and Pirani, C.L.: Renal vein thrombosis in the adult: A clinical and pathologic study based on renal biopsies. Medicine, *47*:269, 1968.
23. Halpern, M.: Acute renal artery embolus: A concept of diagnosis and treatment. J. Urol. *98*:552, 1967.
24. Cobb, O.E.: Carbuncle of the kidney. Br. J. Urol., *38*:262, 1966.
25. Cukier, J., Aubert, J., and Broc, A.: Pyonephrosis: Report of 50 cases. J. Urol. Nephrol., *77*:737, 1971.
26. Irwin, W.K.: Movable kidney. *In* Textbook of Genito-Urinary Surgery. Edited by H.P. Winsbury-White. Baltimore, Williams & Wilkins, 1948.
27. Silber, S.J., and Moyad, R.A.: Renal echinococcus. J. Urol., *108*:669, 1972.
28. Pak, C.Y.C., et al.: A simple test for the diagnosis of absorptive, resorptive, and renal hypercalciurias. N. Engl. J. Med., *292*(10):497, 1975.
29. Drach, G.W.: Urinary lithiasis. J. Urol., *123*:348, 1980.
30. Drach, G.W.: Urinary lithiasis. *In* Campbell's Urology. 4th Ed. Vol. 1. Edited by J.H. Harrison et al. Philadelphia, W.B. Saunders, 1978, pp. 779–878.
31. Forrest, W.H., et al.: Dextroamphetamine with morphine in the treatment of postoperative pain. N. Engl. J. Med., *296*:712, 1977.
32. Mandl, F.: Paravertebral Block. New York, Grune & Stratton, 1947.
33. Bonica, J.J.: Clinical Applications of Diagnostic and Therapeutic Blocks, Springfield, IL, Charles C Thomas, 1959, pp. 242–243.
34. Bonica, J.J.: Local anaesthesia and regional blocks. *In* Textbook of Pain. Edited by P.D. Wall and R. Melzack. Edinburgh, Churchill Livingstone, 1984, pp. 541–555.
35. Brannen, G.E.: Endourology update. *In* AUA Update Series. Lesson 15. Vol. V. American Urological Association, 1986, pp. 5–6.
36. Paterson, J.R., and Ansell, J.S.: Intermittent hydronephrosis. N. Engl. J. Med., *267*(8):447, 1962.
37. Jones, L.W., and Morrow, J.W.: Renal papillary necrosis: Management by ureteral catheter drainage. J. Urol., *106*:467, 1971.
38. Utz, D.C., and Henry, J.D.: Retroperitoneal fibrosis. Med. Clin. North Am., *50*:1091, 1966.
39. Gibbons, R.P.: Gibbons ureteral stents. Urol. Clin. North Am., *9*(2), 85, 1982.
40. Emmett, J.L., and Witten, D.M.: Clinical Radiography. 3rd Ed. Philadelphia, W.B. Saunders, 1971.
41. Derrick, F.C., Jr., Rosenblum, R.R., and Lynch, K.M., Jr.: Pathological association of the right ureter and right ovarian vein. J. Urol., *97*:633, 1967.
42. Fraley, E.E.: Surgical correction of intrarenal disease. I. Obstruction of the superior infundibulum. J. Urol., *98*:54, 1967.
43. Smith, D.R., and Raney, F.L., Jr.: Radiculitis distress as a mimic of renal pain. J. Urol., *116*:269, 1976.
44. Harris, B.A., DeHaas, D.R., Jr., and Starling, J.R.: Diagnosis and management of genito-femoral nerve neuralgia. Arch. Surg. *119*:339, 1984.
45. Harris, S.H., and Harris, R.G.S.: Sympatheticotonus, renal pain and renal sympathectomy. Br. J. Urol. *2*:367, 1930.
46. Fontaine, R., Forster, E., and Stefanini, C.: Resultats eloignes de 63 splanchnicectomies pour diverses affections (en dehors de l'hypertension arterielle chronique permanente). Lyon Chir. *41*:279, 1946.
47. Bauer, G.: Late results of denervation of the kidney for renal pain. Acta. Chir. Scand. *90*:460, 1944.
48. White, J.C., and Sweet, W.H.: Pain and the Neurosurgeon: A 40-year-experience. Springfield, Charles C Thomas, 1969, pp. 578–582.

49. Cancer Facts and Figures—1986. New York, American Cancer Society, 1986.
50. Bennington, J.L., and Beckwith, J.B.: Tumors of the Kidney, Renal Pelvis, and Ureter. Bethesda, MD, Armed Forces Institute of Pathology, 1975. p. 107.
51. Cohen, A.J., et al.: Hereditary renal cell carcinoma associated with a chromosomal translocation. New Engl. J. Med., *301*:592, 1979.
52. Bagley, D.H.: Renal parenchymal tumors. *In* Comprehensive Textbook of Oncology. Edited by A.R. Moossa, M.C. Robson, and S.C. Schimpff. Baltimore, Williams & Wilkins, 1986, pp. 889–900.
53. Grawitz, P. A.: Die Sogenannten Lipome der Niere. Virchows Arch. Pathol. Anat., *93*:39, 1883.
54. Paulson, D.F., Perez, C.A., and Anderson, T.: Geritourinary malignancy. *In* Cancer: Principles and Practice of Oncology. Edited by V.T. DeVita, Jr., S. Hellman, and S.A. Rosenberg, Philadelphia, J.B. Lippincott, 1982, pp. 732–785.
55. Skinner, D.G., Vermillion, C.D., and Colvin, R.B.: The surgical management of renal cell carcinoma. J. Urol., *107*:705, 1972.
56. Cassady, J.R.: Wilms' tumor. *In* Comprehensive Textbook of Oncology. Edited by A.R. Moossa, M.C. Robson, and S.C. Schimpff. Baltimore, Williams & Wilkins, 1986, pp. 1203–1210.
57. Simone, J.V., Cassady, J.R., and Filler, R.M.: Cancers of childhood: Wilms' tumor. *In* Cancer: Principles and Practice of Oncology. Edited by V.T. DeVita, Jr., S. Hellman, and S.A. Rosenberg. Philadelphia, J.B. Lippincott, 1982, pp. 1283–1291.

63 · ABDOMINAL PAIN PRIMARILY OF PSYCHOLOGIC ORIGIN

WILBERT E. FORDYCE

THIS chapter concerns abdominal pain primarily of psychologic origin and should be studied in relation to Chapters 16 through 19. The abdominal pain conditions for which psychologic factors are likely to play a major role are irritable bowel syndrome, chronic pelvic pain, chronic peptic ulcer, premenstrual syndrome, and recurrent abdominal pain (RAP) in children.

Chronic abdominal pain, like other pain problems, restricts activity and is likely to have a major adverse effect on both patient and family. Eating, sexual functioning, recreational activities, and even survival of the family unit can be at risk from the pain problem. In this chapter I first discuss A some basic considerations, including causes, epidemiology, and possible mechanisms, and B then consider the diagnosis and management of these disorders.

A. BASIC CONSIDERATIONS

Abdominal pain problems are fraught with ambiguities. Diagnostic management and therapeutic procedures must reconcile these ambiguities, a formidable task indeed. Diagnosing and treating abdominal pain are difficult for many reasons. A major reason for these difficulties might be that the gastrointestinal system is sensitive to learning, conditioning, and stress effects. The relatively high incidence of recurring abdominal pain in children and the so-called irritable bowel syndrome (IBS) in children and adults has repeatedly been shown to relate to stressful life events (1–3). Lavigne and colleagues (4, 5) performed comprehensive studies of pain problems in children, including but not restricted to abdominal pain. The relationships of stress and other psychologic factors to the other conditions mentioned above—peptic ulcer, premenstrual syndrome, and chronic pelvic pain—are more complex and not always clear.

The influence of stress on abdominal functioning, with considerable potential for producing pain, is not surprising. When stress persists, the stressful state is inevitably connected to survival activities (e.g., eating, elimination). For example, a person mobilized to flee or immobilized by fear automatically has disrupted gastrointestinal function. Repeated stress ensures repeated pairing of cues in the environment that elicit stress reactions with consequent interference in abdominal function. That pairing, and the influence of the contingent consequences to stress-related behaviors by the patient's surroundings, should be recognized and appreciated as a potent source of continued symptom behavior.

In traditional medical practice the problem can be further complicated by an initial tendency to focus on the search for an "organic" cause. This is usually a prudent course at first, but, if the "cause" is not clearly identified, the inherent ambiguities in assessment of abdominal pain present the clinician with the choice of continued pursuit of a diagnosis in medical or disease terms or of exploring the possible role of stress and, if long-persisting, of the learning effects on gastrointestinal function. This poses problems for both the physician and the patient. Levine and Rappaport (6) stated that

The recurring abdominal pain can be a taxing clinical ordeal for the primary care physician or consultant. It often is a test of stamina, of diagnostic self-confidence, of fiscal constraint, and of vigilance for rare conditions. The clinician is apt to be haunted by the lingering question: "Am I missing something?"

The choice is a difficult one. That is, patients perceived as having a psychologic or psychogenic condition often are shunted on to have their psyches examined or treated. Although this might indeed be appropriate, it can become an exercise in mind-body dualism. Either patients have abdominal pain because of some underlying pathophysiologic process or have some form of emotional or mental problem. This view risks shutting the primary physician off from a number of interventions that could be used for the benefit of patients without recourse to the more logistically formidable and often dubiously effective psychotherapeutic alternative. McGrath and associates (3) noted that "establishing a psychogenic cause is only indicated where there is positive evidence for psychological factors such as family or school stress, extreme personality characteristics, or modelling of family pain behavior."

The primary physician must keep in mind the sensitivity of abdominal processes to stress and to learning and conditioning effects. At the same time, it should be recognized that the problem could be managed by having the patient and family understand that situational factors are important and must be considered. Whether more formidable intervention is required should be determined in the individual case. With children, appropriate interventions might be relatively simple and straightforward, although this is not always the case. A more comprehensive assessment can be indicated with adults, where emotional, stress, or adverse learning problems might have been persisting for months and years.

Etiology

Because this chapter concerns the role of psychosocial causation factors in abdominal pain, discussion of such causative factors is presented below (Possible Mechanisms.)

Epidemiology

Irritable Bowel Syndrome (XXI-11)

The irritable bowel syndrome (IBS) is estimated to affect 14 to 22% of the population (7–9), though only about 30% seek medical help (10). Farrell (11) reported that recurring abdominal pain (RAP) affects 10 to 12% of school-aged children, with no organic cause identified in 90 to 95%. Sex differences have been noted. Apley and Naish (12) reported that the incidence of RAP remained at about 10 to 12% from ages 5 to 10 and declined thereafter. RAP was noted to occur in approximately 8 to 12% of girls between the ages of 5 and 8, increasing to 30% at age 9, and declining to 12 to 15% at ages 11 and 12, followed by a steady decline to near zero thereafter. Buntain (13) commented that "Chronic intermittent abdominal pain in childhood, reported to afflict 9 to 12% of all children, is an enigma of such magnitude that more than 30% of these patients reach adulthood with persistent problems and no definitive diagnosis."

Faull and Nicol (1) reported recurring abdominal pain in 24.5 to 26.9% of children "and their associations with psychiatric deviance both at home and at school." Krag (14) found that about 5% of the adult population consults a physician each year with complaints that ultimately are labeled as IBS. These occur without demonstrable organic pathology.

Chronic Pelvic Pain

The incidence and prevalence of chronic pelvic pain (CPP) are unknown. A survey of general practitioners in Denmark (15) indicated that CPP was the third most frequent reason for consultation relating to the viscera, with a rate of 12/1000 visits. The female:male ratio was 4:1. Chronic pain was more frequent than acute, reported by 72%. The Nuprin survey (16) of adult Americans reported that 40% of adult women had menstrual pain during the year preceding the study.

CPP of idiopathic origin is common. It occurred in 30% of 1194 women in a hospital sample (17). This type of CPP is frequently associated with dyspareunia and tends to persist following coitus. Exercise also often makes it worse (18), and other symptoms thought to be psychologic in nature, such as headache, are often present (19).

Chronic Peptic Ulcer

Chronic peptic ulcer (CPU) is a common disease. It is reported to have a prevalence in the general population ranging from 7.2% in Australia to 2.5% in the United States (20). Few studies have been carried out, however, to assess its intensity, quality, or relationship to psychosocial or demographic variables. According to the *Nuprin Pain Report* stomach pains tend to drop sharply with age, decreasing from a rate of 62% in 18- to 24-year-olds to 31% in those 65 or older (16).

Dysmenorrhea and Premenstrual Syndrome (XXIV-2,3)

Dysmenorrhea describes episodes of pelvic pain related to menstrual blood flow. Premenstrual syndrome describes a mood disorder related to menstruation that can be accompanied by affective, cognitive, somatic, and behavioral symptoms. Little agreement exists in regard to its diagnostic criteria, definition, or cause (19). Menstruation itself appears to be of secondary importance, because the condition persists after hysterectomy (21). This pattern further suggests that learning factors are probably implicated.

Possible Mechanisms

Psychologic factors, which are another way of denoting prior experience, can influence the emergence or persistence of abdominal pain in several ways. One such factor, aversive conditioning, is especially important in relation to abdominal pain. The ingestion of food is a crucial survival issue. It is no wonder that our nervous systems are geared to monitor and react closely to eating and digestion.

Animal research has shown that even a small amount of an aversive food can produce an enduring avoidance response (22) (Chapter 81). Seligman and Hager (23) have described a persisting aversion to certain foods because of adventitious pairing of their ingestion with highly aversive circumstances: nausea and emesis from coincident influenza. The somatic distress associated with food aversion is itself an anticipatory phenomenon. That is, the system reacts as if poison had been ingested when actual sensory input was probably restricted to visual and olfactory sensations, not even gustatory. This clearly indicates that the anticipation of possible adverse consequences on the basis of prior experience is a key factor, which in turn has powerful implications for judging whether nociception is present. The mere presence of indications of suffering clearly should not be enough to infer somewhat automatically that antecedent nociceptive stimulation is present.

Emotional intensity seems to be a critical factor. When emotional intensity is high, the ensuing conditioned response can be particularly resistant to extinction, maintained in part by the highly reinforcing effects of avoiding a highly aversive consequence. Acquisition of a conditioned response is also influenced by the extent to which a "coping" response is available that resolves the stressful problem. If requisite coping skill is lacking, conditioning becomes more likely. Davison and associates (2) compared children with recurring abdominal pain to a symptom-free age-matched control group and found the patient group "temperamentally more difficult" than controls.

Another set of factors is assumed to be significant in the persistence of abdominal pain. Abdominal pain, like any other pain problem, leads to the expression of pain behaviors or suffering behaviors. These often lead to reinforcing consequences in the environment—for example, special attention, use of analgesics, or sanctioned time out from aversive activities. Such effects can be present in relation to pain in any body part; they are not specific to abdominal pain. It is evident from the epidemiologic data cited above, however, that they are particularly likely to occur in relation to abdominal pain, and even more so in children. A more detailed discussion of the learning or conditioning process is presented in Chapter 81.

Another issue involves psychologic factors specific to abdominal pain and concerns learning or conditioning effects more likely to be associated with the abdominal region of the body. A search of the professional literature reveals few studies identifying cases of abdominal pain by gender. One study by Modan and co-workers (24) described a massive epidemic of abdominal pain of "psychogenic" cause and noted that 77% of the 949 individuals were adolescent females. Drossman (14) studied patients who were described (by nonpsychiatrists) as having psychogenic abdominal pain. Of the 24 in the study, 20 were women. The markedly skewed gender ratio noted in these two studies should be viewed in relation to several other studies. The first, done by Gross and colleagues (26), studied 100 consecutive women presenting with complaints of chronic lower quadrant abdominal pain. Of these, 98 reported sexual intercourse as being aversive before onset of the pain problem and he reported a history of sexual abuse.

Haber and Roos (27) reported a study of 53 women evaluated at a multidisciplinary pain center. They stated that "Fifty-six% of the women were found to have either severe sexual or spouse abuse before their pain problems began . . . . Women with abdominal or vaginal pain of unknown etiology had the highest percentage of previous abuse." Seidel et al. (28) reported that, of 26,000 women seen, 300 victims of sexual abuse were identified, of whom 57 presented with complaints other than sexual abuse. They went on to state that "the most common presenting complaints of these 57 patients were abdominal pain (26%) and vaginal symptoms (26%)."

The data described are limited but consistent. The studies all suggest that abdominal pain in the absence of supporting physical findings is common. It occurs with a frequency close to 10 to 12% in children, in whom it is likely to be stress-related. In adults it is somewhat more likely to occur in women and is likely to be associated with sexual or physical abuse; if sexual abuse is a factor it is likely to antedate the pain problem. This pattern strongly indicates a learning or conditioning effect.

Learning or conditioning effects should also be anticipated as a consequence of frequent major abdominal disturbance, such as repeated intestinal blockages with or without required surgeries. Intense trauma repeated a number of times almost ensures the development of anticipatory fear responses. Even minor signals from the involved part of the body could be expected to become sufficient to trigger intense distress.

Inasmuch as Chapter 16 provides a detailed discussion of the role of learning or conditioning in the onset and maintenance of pain, it is not repeated here. For the purposes of this chapter two of the more obvious sources of conditioning effects are considered briefly. First, the intense emotional trauma associated with physical or sexual abuse, or with repeated crises of abdominal malfunction, results in stimuli within the body or in the environment but associated with the trauma becoming able to elicit distress that is interpreted as pain. A second possibility is that, over the course of the patient's prior history, the highly emotionally charged area of sexual activity and close interpersonal relationships has fared poorly and residual anxieties, fears, or guilt feelings exist. Intercourse can then be aversive. Subsequently, impulses from the body interpreted as pain lead to avoidance of intercourse.

This avoidance, or "time out" from the aversive activity, is probably highly reinforcing for that person. It is a form of avoidance learning that is common in problems of abdominal pain, as noted from the data cited above. And, of course, as pertains to children, what mother has not experienced her school-aged child occasionally announcing an unwillingness to go to school because of some reported symptom? All too often that child seeks time out from anticipated aversive events in school that day.

B. CLINICAL CONSIDERATIONS

Diagnosis

An adequate medical workup is of course indicated. In view of the apparent vulnerability to conditioning effects, particularly with the extreme stress associated with sexual activity or with emotionally charged physical abuse, the absence of definitive physical findings in relation to persisting abdominal pain should be seen as an indication for full psychosocial assessment. Although the incidence of occult or nonsupported—in terms of physical findings—persisting abdominal pain is much lower in males than in females, it is reasonable to assume that similar conditioning problems might exist, and a full psychosocial assessment is indi-

cated. This in turn means that puzzling but persisting abdominal pain can probably not be evaluated adequately without also seeing the spouse or significant other.

In patients with a history of repeated abdominal crises (e.g., Crohn's disease or repeated abdominal blockage for whatever reason), it should also be anticipated that learning or conditioning effects probably have rendered the person vulnerable to tension or to emotional distress. These states can in turn aggravate abdominal disease episodes or lead to reports of pain when the problem might be more accurately labeled as emotional distress. Therefore, assessment of psychosocial factors should be considered as an integral part of the evaluation process. Procedures for carrying out psychosocial assessment are described in Chapter 33.

Treatment

Treatment contacts with patients are also teaching and learning contacts. The physician's actions, tactical and in regard to the social communication, are likely to play a significant role in the long-term outcome. This is particularly true in relation to children.

If physical findings clearly do not support the pain behaviors presented, treatment needs to address the factors that elicit pain episodes as well as any adverse side effects that have emerged with the pain problem— for example, deactivation, excessive medication consumption, excessive guarding behavior, excessive environmental reinforcement of pain behaviors, excessive illness conviction, and associated use of health care services.

Treatment of the psychologic factors that elicit pain episodes involves cognitive and behavioral methods (Chapter 82) and psychotherapy techniques (Chapter 86). These try to help the person become desensitized to cues in the environment or within the body that activate the associations leading to the sensation of pain.

The issue of treatment of adverse side effects to chronicity also needs to be addressed. These probably involve mainly illness conviction and deactivation. Illness conviction is best treated by minimizing ambiguity to the patient in regard to the natural course of the abdominal pain problem and by systematically programming a resumption of normal activities at a pace and time appropriate to expected healing time. That is, having long been overguarding or avoiding certain activities, mere insight or cognitive relabeling through desensitization or some other form of psychotherapeutic intervention is not likely to suffice. Probably the patient needs to experience the heretofore avoided activities directly without the immobilizing pain previously experienced. Procedures for bringing about deactivation and for the reduction of overguarding are described in detail in Chapter 81.

REFERENCES

1. Faull, C., and Nicol, A.: Abdominal pain in six-year-olds: An epidemiologic study in a new town. J. Child Psychiatry, 27:251, 1986.
2. Davison, I., Faull, C., and Nicol, A.: Research note: temperament and behavior in six-year-olds with recurrent abdominal pain: A follow-up. J. Child Psychiatry, 27:539, 1986.
3. McGrath, P., et al.: Recurrent abdominal pain: A psychogenic disorder? Arch. Dis. Child. 58:888, 1983.
4. Lavigne, J., Schulein, M., and Hahn, Y.: Psychological aspects of painful medical conditions in children. I. Developmental aspects and assessment. Pain, 27:133, 1986.
5. Lavigne, J., Schulein, M., and Hahn, Y.: Psychological aspects of painful medical conditions in children. II. Personality factors, family characteristics and treatment. Pain, 27:147, 1986.
6. Levine, M., and Rappaport, L.: Recurrent abdominal pain in school children: The loneliness of the long-distance physician, Pediatr. Clin. North. Am. 31:969, 1984.
7. Drossman, D., et al.: Bowel patterns among subjects not seeking health care—use of a questionnaire to identify a population with bowel dysfunction. Gastroenterology, 83:529, 1982.
8. Whitehead, W., et al.: Learned illness behaviour in patients with irritable bowel syndrome and peptic ulcer. Dig. Dis. Sci., 27:202, 1982.
9. Thomson, W., and Heaton, K.: Functional bowel disorders in apparently healthy people. Gastroenterology, 87:283, 1980.
10. Sandler, R., et al.: Symptoms, complaints and health-care seeking behavior in subjects with bowel dysfunction. Gastroenterology, 87:314, 1984.
11. Farrell, M.K.: Abdominal pain, Pediatrics, 74:955, 1984.
12. Apley, J., and Naish, N.: Recurrent abdominal pains: A field survey of 1000 school children, Arch. Dis. Child., 33:165, 1958.
13. Buntain, W.E.: Chronic relapsing pancreatitis in childhood. Am. Surg. 51:217, 1985.
14. Krag, E.: Irritable bowel syndrome: Current concepts and future trends. Scand. J. Gastroenterol. (Suppl.), 109:197, 1985.
15. Frolund, F., and Frolund, C.: Pain in general practice. Scand. J. Prim. Health Care, 4:97, 1986.
16. Harris, L., et al.: The Nuprin Pain Report. New York, Louis Harris & Associates, 1985.
17. Cunanan, R., Courey, N., and Lippers, J.: Laparoscopic findings in patients with pelvic pain. Am. J. Obstet. Gynecol., 146:589, 1983.
18. Renaer, M., et al.: Chronic pelvic pain without obvious pathology in women. Eur. J. Obstet. Gynecol. Reprod. Biol., 10:415, 1980.
19. Henker, F.O.: Diagnosis and treatment of non-organic pelvic pain. South. Med. J., 72:1132, 1979.
20. Langmar, M.J.S.: Epidemiology of peptic ulcer. In Gastroenterology, Vol. I. 3rd Ed. Edited by H.L. Bockus. Philadelphia, W.B. Saunders, 1974, pp. 611–618.
21. Scambler, A., and Scambler, G.: Menstrual symptoms, attitudes and consulting behavior. Soc. Sci. Med., 20:1065, 1985.
22. Harris, A., and Brady, J.: Animal learning: Visceral and autonomic conditioning. Ann. Rev. Psychol. 25:107, 1974.
23. Seligman, E., and Hager, J.: The biological boundaries of learning: The sauce bernaise syndrome. Psychol. Today, Aug. 1972, p. 67.
24. Modan, B., et al.: The arjenyattah epidemic. A mass phenomenon: Spread and triggering factors, Lancet, 2:1472, 1983.
25. Drossman, D.A.: Patients with psychogenic abdominal pain: Six years' observation in the medical setting. Am. J. Psychiatry, 139:1549, 1982.
26. Gross, R.: Borderline syndrome and incest in chronic pelvic pain patients. Int. J. Psychiat. Med. 10:79, 1980.
27. Haber, J., and Roos, C.: Effects of spouse abuse and/or sexual abuse in the development and maintenance of chronic pain in women. In Advances in Pain Research and Therapy, Vol. 9. Edited by H.L. Fields, et al. New York, Raven Press, 1985, pp. 889–894.
28. Seidel, J., et al.: Presentation and evaluation of sexual misuse in the emergency department. Pediatr. Emerg. Care, 2:157, 1986.

64 · ABDOMINAL PAIN CAUSED BY OTHER DISEASES

JOHN J. BONICA

with contributions by

KARL JOHANSEN *and* JOHN D. LOESER

THIS chapter discusses disorders that cause abdominal pain not considered in the preceding four chapters of this section: A, Intra-Abdominal Vascular Diseases; B, Diseases of the Peritoneum, Mesentery, and Diaphragm; C, Other Intra-Abdominal Diseases, including abscesses, neurogenic ileus, gas entrapment syndrome, and abdominal migraine; D, Systemic Disorders, including hematologic, biochemical, and biologic disorders; and E, Extra-Abdominal Diseases, including thoracic visceral disease, gynecologic disease, pain of neuropathic origin, and pain of musculoskeletal and tegumentary origin (Table 64-1). Johansen contributed part of Section A, Loeser contributed to the subsection on abdominal pain of neuropathic origin, and Bonica is responsible for the remainder of the chapter. Many disorders discussed in this chapter have been considered in more detail by Sleisenger and Fordtran (1).

A. INTRA-ABDOMINAL VASCULAR DISEASES

Abdominal pain arising from vascular causes is of special importance because it presages two different and highly lethal conditions—expansion or rupture of an arterial aneurysm and intestinal ischemia leading to infarction, perforation, and peritonitis. Recognition of the underlying cause is thus a crucial aspect of the successful management of such pain. In this section the pertinent pathophysiologic states are discussed, the symptoms associated with each are elucidated, with emphasis on pain complaints; appropriate means of diagnosis and management, both of the pain and the underlying conditions, are presented, and the natural history of these conditions, both in the untreated state and following appropriate management, are discussed. We first consider aortic aneurysm and then discuss acute and chronic intestinal ischemia and vasculitis. A more comprehensive discussion of these conditions can be found in several excellent textbooks on vascular surgery (2–4).

Intra-Abdominal Aneurysm (XVII-7)

Etiology

The vast majority of intra-abdominal aneurysms are found in the infrarenal aorta, starting 1 or 2 cm distal to the renal artery orifices and ending at or just before the aortic bifurcation (Fig. 64-1). Historically, aneurysms were once a common consequence of trauma, bacterial infection, or syphilis, but the overwhelming majority now arise as a consequence of an apparent systemic lathyrism (a collagen-elastin defect), manifested by a weakening and fragmentation of the arterial media. Causes for this collagen-elastin defect are probably multiple, including inheritance of a biochemical defect (5), inadequate nutrition because of sparse arterial vasa vasorum (6), hydraulic stresses (7), and increased lytic enzymes, either primary or secondary to such exogenous stresses as cigarette smoking (8) or operation (9). Standard teaching to the contrary, an excellent case can be made that atherosclerosis does *not* cause aneurysms (10).

Because aneurysmal dilatation is a systemic disorder, it is not surprising that other intra-abdominal vessels can occasionally (although more rarely) develop aneurysms as well (11). These are most commonly seen in the hepatic, superior mesenteric, celiac, and pancreatoduodenal arteries. Aneurysmal dilatation can also occur in a special circumstance in the splenic artery; this is a rare but serious disorder in pregnant women, unfortunately frequently presenting with hypovolemic shock following rupture (12).

Aneurysms occasionally arise as a consequence of infection, most commonly in the aorta or in one of its branches. Formerly this was usually related to embolization from subacute bacterial endocarditis, but a more recent report suggested that mycotic aneurysms arise more commonly from vascular trauma, various immunosuppressed states, and concurrent sepsis (13). An aneurysm of special importance, both because it is iatrogenic and because it heralds such potentially lethal conditions as graft infection or aortoenteric fistula, is the anastomotic aneurysm arising at the suture line of a previously placed arterial prosthetic graft (14).

Pathophysiology

Pain arising from aneurysms within the abdomen results primarily from the stretching of sensory nerves of the retroperitoneum, stimulated even more significantly with aneurysmal rupture. Because aortic aneurysmal rupture most commonly occurs to the patient's left side into the retroperitoneum beneath the sigmoid colon, stimulation of nerves of the lumbosacral plexus on the left side is common. Indeed, individuals with slowly leaking aneurysms might first be evaluated by a urologist, neurosurgeon, or orthopedist because of the initial mistaken impression of ureteral colic or lumbar

TABLE 64-1. Abdominal Pain Caused by Other Disorders

I. INTRA-ABDOMINAL VASCULAR DISEASE
A. Aneurysm
1. Aortic aneurysm and rupture
2. Aneurysm of superior mesenteric, celiac axis, hepatic, and pancreatoduodenal arteries
B. Intestinal ischemia
1. Acute mesenteric ischemia (e.g., embolism, thrombosis, nonorganic venous thrombosis)
2. Chronic mesenteric ischemia (e.g., abdominal angina, celiac band compression)
3. Vasculitis
II. DISEASES OF THE PERITONEUM, MESENTERY, AND DIAPHRAGM
A. Diseases of the peritoneum
1. Infectious peritonitis (e.g., bacterial, tuberculous, fungal, parasitic)
2. Granulomatous peritonitis
3. Familial paroxysmal polyserositis (familial Mediterranean fever)
4. Neoplasms (e.g., primary mesothelioma, secondary carcinomatosis)
5. Other disorders (e.g., vasculitis, gastoenteritis, splenosis, gynecologic problems)
B. Diseases of the mesentery and omentum
1. Mesenteric inflammatory disease
2. Mesenteric tumors
3. Torsion of the omentum
C. Diseases of the diaphragm
1. Herniation
2. Rupture
3. Tumors and cysts
III. OTHER INTRA-ABDOMINAL DISEASES
A. Intra-abdominal abscesses
1. Intraperitoneal abscess (subphrenic, subhepatic); midabdominal abscess (e.g., RLQ, LLQ, interloop)
2. Retroperitoneal abscess
3. Visceral abscesses (e.g., hepatic, splenic, pancreatic, renal)
B. Gastrointestinal disorders
1. Neurogenic intestinal obstruction (adynamic ileus)
2. Gas entrapment syndromes (e.g., gastric, hepatic flexure, splenic flexure)
3. Abdominal angina
IV. SYSTEMIC DISORDERS
A. Hematologic disorders
1. Sickle cell anemia
2. Acute hemolytic crises
3. Chronic hemolytic anemia
B. Biochemical and biologic disorders
1. Acute intermittent porphyria
2. Lead and other heavy metal poisoning
3. Spider bites
V. EXTRA-ABDOMINAL DISORDERS
A. Thoracic and pelvic visceral disease
1. Acute myocardial infarction
2. Acute pericarditis
3. Pulmonary embolism
4. Pneumonia
5. Esophageal disease
6. Gynecologic disorders
B. Pain of neuropathic origin
1. Disorders of the brain and brain stem
2. Disorders of the roots and rootlets
3. Disorders of spinal nerves
C. Pain of musculoskeletal origin
1. Slipping rib syndrome
2. Xiphoidalgia
3. Epidemic myalgia
4. Myofascial pain syndromes
5. Traumatic hematoma
D. Pain of Tegumentary Origin
1. Cutaneous cicatrices
2. Subcutaneous neuroma
3. Postoperative pain

disk disease. Erosion of an expanding aortic aneurysm into the lumbar vertebrae can cause severe back pain, probably a consequence both of irritation of lumbar nerve roots and of the overlying periosteum. On rare occasions patients with aneurysmal rupture can present with pain in the right upper quadrant so that the initial impression is that of biliary colic—as noted during the terminal illness of Albert Einstein (15).

Symptoms and Signs

Most infrarenal abdominal aortic aneurysms are symptomless until rupture. Patients occasionally complain of a dull, diffuse, poorly localized midabdominal pain, commonly not significant enough to prompt medical consultation. Rarely, aneurysms can obstruct the gastrointestinal tract or the ureter by extrinsic compression, resulting in intermittent or constant symptoms appropriate to those organs. Erosion of an aneurysm into the lumbar spine can cause symptoms either locally, presenting as chronic back pain, or as a consequence of encroachment on nerve roots, wherein projected pain might be noted in the distribution of these lumbosacral nerve roots—that is, into the pelvis, groin or scrotum, or lower extremity.

Much more commonly pain is a cardinal feature of aneurysmal rupture. The patient frequently notes sudden tearing aching pain in the midabdomen and midback, most commonly radiating into the left flank or groin for reasons noted above (Fig. 64-2). Such pain is commonly associated with the symptoms and signs of hypovolemic shock, because what might be a substantial portion of the patient's blood volume exits into the retroperitoneum. Similar tearing aching pain followed by hypovolemic shock results from the rupture of aneurysms of various intra-abdominal visceral arteries and their branches as well. The "double rupture" sign has been reported with splenic artery aneurysm rupture, seen primarily in pregnant women (see above). Severe sharp left upper quadrant pain occurs and then subsides as the initial aneurysm rupture is tamponaded in the lesser sac; further pain and shock supervene when the rupture breaks into the free peritoneal cavity (12).

Diagnosis

Aneurysms are found most commonly in elderly men; the average age for a standard population of patients with abdominal aortic aneurysm is 70, and the male:female ratio is 4:1 to 8:1 in most series. A prior history of aneurysm elsewhere strongly predicts abdominal aortic aneurysm, and hypertension and cigarette smoking are associated with greater frequency in patients with aneurysms. A recent study (16) proposed that a tendency to aneurysmal deterioration of arteries can be inherited, suggesting that the elderly relatives of aneurysm patients might be at increased risk of developing aneurysms themselves. Risk factors for the development of mycotic or anastomotic aneurysms have been mentioned.

The vast majority of intra-abdominal aneurysms are asymptomatic, and most commonly are discovered by serendipity during physical examination or on roentgenographic or other imaging evaluation performed for other purposes. For example, calcium outlining the wall of an intra-abdominal aneurysm can be

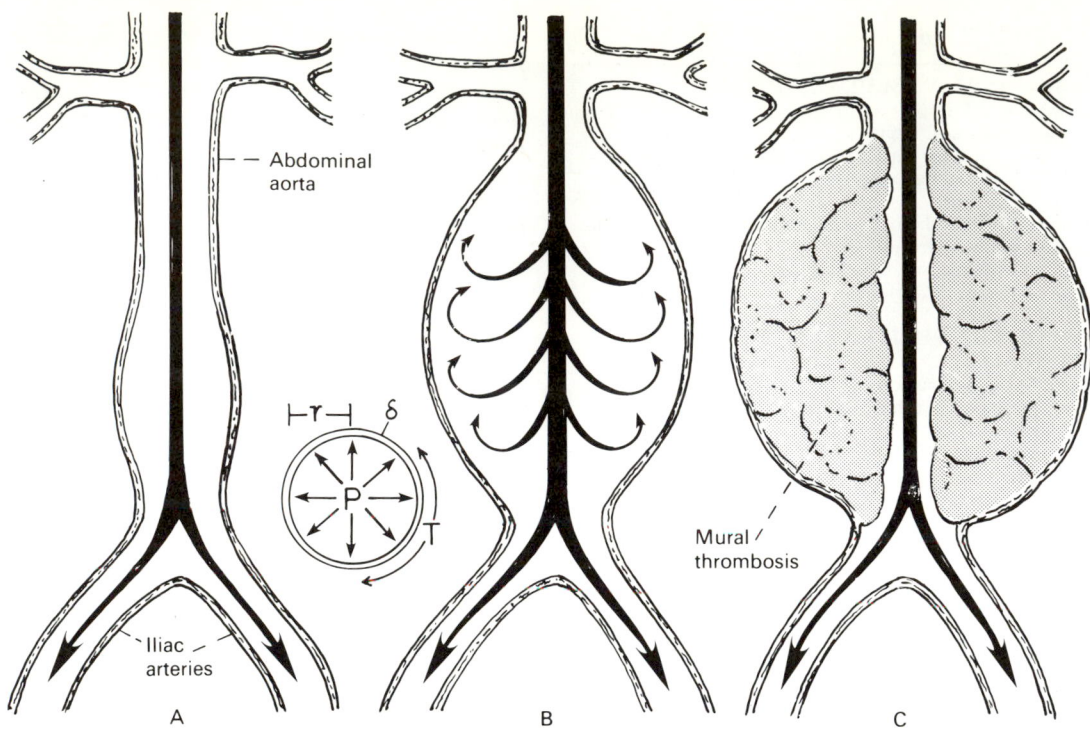

FIG. 64-1. Development and progression of an abdominal aortic aneurysm. **A.** Initial phase. The insert shows that tension (T) on the wall varies directly with the product of the intraluminal pressure (P) and the radius (r) of the lumen and inversely with the thickness (δ) of the wall. T is proportional to Pr/δ. Any slight dilatation shown in **A** increases the radius and decreases the thickness, thereby increasing the tension and progressively enlarging the aneurysm. **B.** As the artery dilates, blood near the wall flows more slowly, creating turbulence. Turbulent flow causes the wall of the vessel to vibrate, further weakening it. **C.** Both turbulence and irregularity on the lining of the damaged wall promote the formation of a mural thrombus, which significantly reduces the diameter of the lumen. Modified from Johansen, K.: Aneurysms. Sci. Am., *247*:110, 1982.

discovered on plain roentgenograms of the lumbosacral spine performed for low back pain or on excretory urograms performed for presumed ureteral colic. Abdominal ultrasonograms obtained for evaluation of possible biliary colic can demonstrate an occult abdominal aortic aneurysm.

Recalling that the aorta bifurcates at the level of the umbilicus, the physical examination should emphasize careful palpation of the epigastrium. Aneurysm is diagnosed on physical examination by evidence for a pulsatile mass substantially broader than the 2-cm upper limits for the diameter of the normal adult infrarenal aorta. Tortuosity of the abdominal aorta can sometimes mimic aneurysm formation, especially in the elderly, and overlying inflammatory or neoplastic masses can transmit the aortic pulse and cause the mistaken impression of aneurysm (17). Aneurysms of visceral arteries are rarely symptomatic until rupture. A large iliac aneurysm might occasionally be palpable on rectal examination, frequently presenting initially with urologic or gynecologic symptoms; these are sinister lesions with a dismal prognosis following rupture (18).

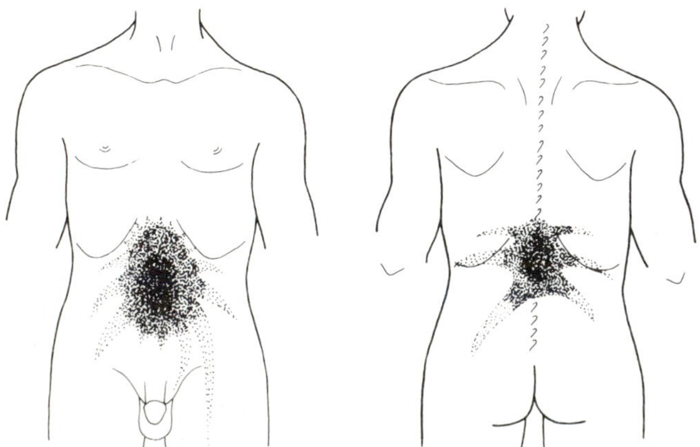

Current diagnostic procedures most important for demonstrating the presence and size of intra-abdominal aneurysms include B-mode ultrasonography (19) and computerized tomographic (CT) scanning (20). With a high sensitivity, specificity, and accuracy these can be used to define the presence of aneurysms as well as to discern their sizes, with a resolution rate of less than 1 mm. Arteriography not only has little to add in the diagnosis of aneurysms but it can be frankly misleading because aneurysms in general, and infrarenal abdominal aortic aneurysms in particular, fill circumferentially with thrombus so that the angiographic dye column can appear little different from the normal artery. Arteriography might have a particular role to play in the preoperative evaluation of

FIG. 64-2. Distribution of the pain caused by rupture of the abdominal aorta consequent to aneurysm.

certain patients with aneurysm, however, particularly those with hypertension or peripheral arterial occlusive symptoms.

Patients who rupture an aneurysm present with signs and symptoms of sudden abdominal, flank, and back pain and circulatory collapse. Thus, the astute clinician generally can differentiate this condition from several others that might resemble it superficially, including perforating peptic ulcer, visceral artery embolism, and myocardial infarction. Although the pain patterns and collapse seen with each of these conditions can be similar to those of aneurysm rupture, initially all are usually characterized by relative normovolemia (in the case of perforated ulcer or mesenteric embolism) or hypervolemia (in the case of heart attack), in contrast to the signs of profound hypovolemia that accompany ruptured aneurysm. The subacute rupture of an aneurysm can, as noted above, lead to confusion with ureteral or biliary colic or with the orthopedic or neurosurgical implications of lumbar spine disease.

Treatment

No effective nonoperative therapy for intra-abdominal aneurysms exists. Whereas hypertension and cigarette smoking can play a role in the early genesis of the arterial wall degeneration leading to aneurysm formation, once developed the arterial dilatation proceeds inexorably toward rupture in consonance with LaPlace's law (21).

In brief, the operative management of aneurysm involves proximal and distal control of the artery and, in cases of aortic or iliac aneurysms, opening of the artery and intraluminal insertion of an appropriately sized prosthetic graft. Visceral artery aneurysms can often be treated by simple ligation, although those involving the hepatic or superior mesenteric artery frequently can require bypass grafting, usually with autogenous vein. The controversial nonresectional approach to management of aortic aneurysms, promulgated by workers in Detroit (22) and at Albany Medical College (23), is designed to cause aneurysm thrombosis by iliac artery ligation and, in some cases, to cause intrasaccular thrombosis, with distal revascularization by axillobifemoral bypass graft. Not unexpectedly these patients have a substantial risk of aneurysm rupture.

When an aortic or visceral arterial aneurysm ruptures, repair must be performed under emergent circumstances in a patient who frequently is in hypovolemic shock and who requires simultaneous volume resuscitation. Initial control of the proximal aorta, usually at the aortic hiatus of the diaphragm, is crucial; the retroperitoneal hematoma accompanying aneurysm rupture can make dissection around the aneurysm neck difficult. Control of the distal thoracic aorta by left thoracotomy or by direct opening of the aneurysm and passage of a proximal balloon-tipped catheter might be necessary. In addition to their severe hypovolemia, these elderly patients are at markedly increased risk for myocardial infarction, stroke, acute renal failure, and colon ischemia (24).

OUTCOME. Surgery for intra-abdominal aneurysms is highly successful when performed on an elective

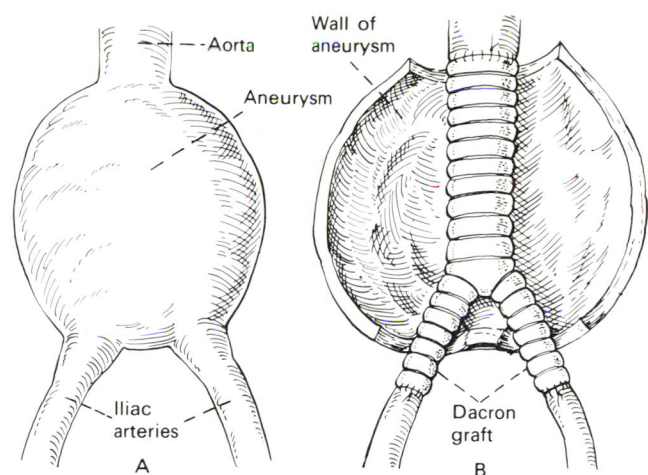

FIG. 64-3. **A.** Large aneurysm of the abdominal aorta, extending cephalad from just above the bifurcation of the aorta. The aorta above the aneurysm and the two iliac vessels are clamped, the dilated sack is opened, and a graft is sutured in place from within. **B.** Dacron prosthetic graft in place, resulting in reestablishment of blood flow. Modified from Johansen, K.: Aneurysms. Sci. Am. *247*:110, 1982.

basis (Fig. 64-3). Despite the advanced age of patients with intra-abdominal aneurysms, and the not infrequent concurrence of substantial atherosclerotic involvement of the coronary and cerebrovascular vessels, the operative mortality rate in several large series has been in the 1 to 3% range. At least three studies have demonstrated that operative mortality rates of lower than 5% can be achieved for elective aneurysmorrhaphy, even in octogenarians (25). Equivalent results have been found for the management of other intra-abdominal aneurysms approached electively.

The outcome is different for patients who suffer aneurysmal rupture prior to appropriate management. Whereas those who can undergo operation after aneurysmal rupture but before development of hypotension and shock might have an outcome little different from that of patients undergoing elective operations, these elderly patients have little cardiovascular reserve and do poorly after the development of shock, with mortality rates approaching 90% in many series (25, 26). The outcome can be equally dismal for rupture of other intra-abdominal aneurysms, frequently because they might be hidden deep in the pelvis, as in the case of iliac aneurysms, or might mimic other intra-abdominal problems and therefore delay diagnosis, as in the case of various visceral artery aneurysms. Because the mortality rate of rupture associated with splenic artery aneurysms in young women exceeds 65%, the presence of such lesions in these patients warrants an aggressive resectional approach (12).

Landmark studies by both DeBakey and colleagues (27) and by Szilagyi and associates (28) have demonstrated that successful aneurysm operation restores the patient to a life expectancy not different from that of an age-matched control population. This, and the well-documented low operative mortality rates for elective surgery, clearly support adoption of an aggressive posture toward resection of almost all intraabdominal aneurysms. On follow-up these patients must be examined serially for the development of aneurysms elsewhere, as well as for anastomotic or infectious complications of their prosthetic grafts, which occur in 1 to 2% of all patients (14).

Intestinal Ischemia (XXI-8)

Intestinal ischemia can either be acute or chronic, arising primarily from embolic phenomena to the visceral arteries (usually the superior mesenteric artery) or secondary to thrombotic occlusion of atherosclerotic stenosis of one or more of these vessels. A further poorly understood syndrome of bowel ischemia is characterized by peripheral mesenteric vasoconstriction in the absence of proximal arterial disease, the "nonorganic mesenteric ischemia" syndrome (29). Uncommon causes of pain secondary to visceral ischemia result from rare vascular disorders of the splanchnic vessels. These include the "celiac band syndrome," various forms of vasculitis, fibromuscular dysplasia, and irradiation. In this subsection we first briefly mention the anatomy and regulation of mesenteric blood flow, then consider the causes, pathophysiology, and symptoms and signs of acute ischemia and chronic ischemia, and finally discuss the diagnosis and therapy for both types of intestinal ischemia. This is followed by a brief discussion of vasculitis.

Basic Considerations

Obviously, a sound clinical approach to intestinal ischemia is necessarily based on an understanding of the anatomy and physiology of the circulation to the abdominal viscera. The gastrointestinal tract is supplied by the celiac axis and its branches, the superior and inferior mesenteric arteries (see Figs. 59-6, 59-10, and 59-11). The blood supply to the intra-abdominal portion of the gastrointestinal tract is richly endowed with several anastomotic interconnections that help to protect it against the consequences of occlusive vascular disease (30). In the presence of chronic progressive occlusive disease these anastomotic interconnections, including the pancreaticoduodenal arcades, the arch of Riolan, and the marginal artery of Drummond, usually can develop enough to permit collateral flow. On the other hand, the collateral supply might be only marginally adequate in certain areas.

The blood flow to the abdominal viscera, like blood flow in other parts of the body, is regulated by various intrinsic mechanisms, including local response to alterations in pressure or to an increase in tissue metabolites, and by the function of the extrinsic autonomic nervous system. Intrinsic or local modulation of blood flow occurs in response to changes in arteriolar transmural pressure or to alteration in tissue oxygenation to maintain adequate blood flow and oxygen delivery. This seems to involve changes in both arteriolar resistance and precapillary sphincter activity. The extrinsic neurogenic regulation of mesenteric and intestinal flow is mediated by the sympathetic postganglionic fibers supplied by the splanchnic nerves: increased activity causes vasoconstriction while decrease or inhibition of the sympathetics result in vasodilation. In addition to the intrinsic and neurogenic regulation of mesenteric blood flow, gastrointestinal hormones, as well as various endogenous or exogenous circulating vasoactive substances, can exert an important effect. Vasodilators include cholinergic stimuli, cholescystokinin, gastrin, prostaglandin E, and other gastrointestinal hormones (Chapter 59), as well as circulating beta-adrenergic stimulants. Vasoconstrictors include alpha-adrenergic stimulants, vasopressin, angiotensin II, and digitalis glycosides (31–34).

Acute Intestinal Ischemic Syndromes

Most patients with acute ischemic bowel syndromes present with an acute episode manifested by abdominal pain and other symptoms and signs. The most important syndromes are acute mesenteric arterial occlusion, mesenteric arterial embolization, nonocclusive ("nonorganic") mesenteric ischemia syndrome, and mesenteric venous thrombosis. The causes, pathophysiology, and symptoms and signs of these acute ischemic syndromes and of the chronic ischemic syndrome are discussed here before the diagnosis and treatment of both types are considered.

Etiology

Acute mesenteric arterial occlusion and the consequent ischemic necrosis are most commonly caused by advanced arteriosclerotic disease affecting at least two of the major visceral branches of the aorta, with the lesion affecting the most proximal segment of the mesenteric artery near its takeoff from the aorta.

Arterial embolization occurs most commonly in the superior mesenteric artery because of the caliber of the vessel and the obliquity of its takeoff from the abdominal aorta. Emboli to the celiac axis and the inferior mesenteric artery are less common. Most mesenteric emboli occur in patients who have valvular or atherosclerotic heart disease or mural thrombi in the heart.

Nonocclusive ("nonorganic") mesenteric ischemia syndrome is characterized by severe mesenteric malperfusion without apparent organic occlusion in the major splanchnic arterial branches (29). It is most commonly seen in elderly hemoconcentrated patients with congestive heart failure who frequently are being treated with digitalis. Other precipitating factors are shock, hypoxia, or a recent myocardial infarction. Occasionally, however, a precipitating event is not identifiable (35, 36). About 50% of patients have angiographic findings considered to be specific for the syndrome; these include a narrowed and irregular branch of the superior mesenteric artery, spasm of the arcades, and impaired filling of the intramural vessels (36, 37).

Acute mesenteric venous thrombosis occurs less frequently than arterial occlusion, affecting about 5 to 15% of patients with intestinal ischemia (38). The thrombotic process involves the superior mesenteric vein in 95% of patients with this condition. It is caused by, or is associated with, various disorders predisposing to stasis in the mesenteric venous bed, including congestive heart failure, portal hypertension, abdominal neoplasm, intra-abdominal inflammation, abdominal surgery or trauma, and hypercoagulable states such as polycythemia vera, migratory thrombophlebitis, and antithrombin III deficiency (38).

Pathophysiology

The extent, severity, and possible reversibility of ischemic processes depend on the rapidity with which the occlusion occurs and, to a lesser extent, on the anatomic characteristics of particular vessels. If occlusion of a large vessel occurs gradually adequate collateral circulation can develop, so ischemia might be minimized or prevented if the large vessel becomes completely blocked. Thus, chronic arterial occlusive diseases ordinarily do not cause symptoms or signs of ischemia unless two or more major vessels are affected because of the large number of collateral channels that interconnect the major arterial trunks. In contrast, occlusion of a vessel that occurs abruptly or over a period of time too brief to allow the development of adequate collateral circulation is likely to result in ischemic necrosis. A classic example of this is embolization to the superior mesenteric artery in a young person with mitral stenosis but normal mesenteric arteries (30).

With acute visceral ischemia ultrastructural changes are evident in the absorptive cells within 5 minutes after occlusion of the mesenteric artery, after which the epithelium becomes detached from the basement membrane, especially at the villus tips, and subepithelial blebs form (30, 39). With 30 to 60 minutes the upper portion of the villi is denuded of epithelium and the mucosa undergoes necrosis and alteration with the appearance of a variable inflammatory infiltrate, probably in response to both tissue necrosis and secondary bacterial invasion (30). Among the phenomena that characterize acute ischemic necrosis is an increase in capillary permeability followed by loss of capillary integrity, as reflected by submucosal edema and hemorrhage (40). Later, the exudation of protein-rich fluid (and ultimately bleeding) into the lumen of the bowel reflects extensive loss of vascular epithelial integrity. Eventually even the relatively resistant muscular layers become necrotic and perforation occurs, usually with consequent development of peritonitis. In those ischemic episodes that do not perforate or require immediate resection, the resolution of the acute inflammatory reaction is followed by development of granulation tissue, fibrosis, and finally a scar and stricture that frequently characterize this process.

Symptoms and Signs

Acute occlusion with consequent infarction of the small intestine produces severe, poorly localized abdominal pain that initially can be colicky in nature and periumbilical in location. Early in the clinical presentation the patient's complaint of pain often appears to be out of proportion to physical findings or laboratory studies. Generally this is soon accompanied by gastrointestinal hyperperistalsis characterized by vomiting and by the passage of loose nonbloody stools.

Development of peritonitis and specific localized pain and tenderness occur only after delay, when transmural gut infarction and perforation occur. On the other hand, patients who suffer acute mesenteric artery thrombosis on the basis of prior atherosclerotic stenosis present with steady, aching midabdominal pain with early superimposed spasm or colic, the bowel's initial response to ischemia. Again, peritonitis is a late sign, following infarction, perforation, and peritoneal soiling, at which time the patient commonly manifests symptoms and signs of sepsis, including tachycardia, hypotension, fever, and marked leukocytosis, often in excess of 30,000 mm^3 with a shift to the left. Other physical signs include severe tenderness, rebound tenderness, and abdominal muscle spasm with rigidity and other signs of peritonitis (see below, Diseases of the Peritoneum). At this point, severe and unrelenting abdominal pain persists, even if massive doses of narcotic analgesic agents are administered.

Chronic Intestinal Ischemic Syndromes (XXI-8)

In contrast to the frequently occurring acute intestinal ischemic syndromes, chronic or, more precisely, recurrent acute ischemia is uncommon and is represented by intestinal angina and celiac compression syndrome.

Etiology and Pathophysiology

Intestinal angina is caused by a gradual and progressive occlusive vascular disease, usually atherosclerotic, that affects at least two of the three major splanchnic vessels. While nutrients are undergoing digestion and absorption in the small intestine adequate vascular perfusion is required to permit increased intestinal blood flow and oxygen consumption; thus a partially or completely occluded mesenteric arterial system cannot provide ample blood flow, and a relative ischemia results. Consequently the patient experiences periods of pain that can be considered analogous to those of angina pectoris.

The celiac band compression syndrome is characterized by recurrent abdominal pain associated with a narrowing of the celiac axis alone (41). This disorder is an apparent exception to the general rule that at least two major visceral arteries must be narrowed before symptoms occur. Among patients who have been surgically explored, the celiac artery has been found to be compressed by the median arcuate ligament of the diaphragm or by neurofibrous tissue of the celiac plexus (30).

Symptoms and Signs

Intestinal angina is characterized by recurrent bouts of intermittent dull or cramping midabdominal pain that characteristically occur from 15 to 30 minutes after a meal. The relationship to meals, presumably the time when bowel blood supply cannot meet metabolic demands, leads to the descriptive term "intestinal angina." Rarely it is colicky in nature. Duration of the pain is usually less than 1 hour in the early part of the natural history of this syndrome but, as the underlying superior mesenteric artery stenosis increases, the pain becomes more severe and longer in duration until it becomes continuous. Other symptoms can include diarrhea and signs of malabsorption.

Celiac band compression syndrome, which has been found most frequently among women younger than those expected to have significant atherosclerotic disease, is characterized by epigastric pain of variable frequency and duration. The pain might or might not be related to meals and is infrequently associated with nausea and vomiting (30). The only physical finding noted with regularity is an epigastric bruit that does not radiate to the lower abdomen.

In chronic visceral ischemic syndromes the patient is often initially unaware of the relationship of pain to eating, as well as of the fact that weight loss and diminished oral intake have been subconsciously accepted to avoid recurrent abdominal pain.

Management of Intestinal Ischemic Syndromes

Diagnosis

The major predictive factors for developing mesenteric ischemia relate to a prior history of rheumatic heart disease or myocardial infarction, intracardiac thrombus, which ultimately leads to mesenteric embolus, or a picture of premature and aggressive atherosclerosis, as with acute mesenteric artery thrombosis. The clinical picture of patients with nonorganic mesenteric ischemia has been noted above. Patients with mesenteric embolization frequently can relate a history of prior embolization, and might have been on anticoagulant therapy in the past. Prior cardiac disease is noted in 90 to 95% of patients with emboli, most commonly in regard to a past history of myocardial infarction with akinetic or dyskinetic left ventricular segments (42).

The crucial diagnostic procedures in all circumstances, following a heightened sense of clinical suspicion, are the performance of contrast aortography and selective mesenteric arteriography; these can provide the bases for both diagnosis and possible treatment. The duplex scanner has been used in pilot studies to examine the origins of the mesenteric vessels successfully in a noninvasive fashion (43). Other studies, including plain roentgenography, radioisotope or malabsorption studies, and other imaging techniques, have yet to prove their value in the diagnosis of the mesenteric ischemic syndromes. It is widely believed that polymorphonuclear leukocytosis, metabolic acidosis, hyperkalemia, and hyperamylasemia can frequently be demonstrated in those with mesenteric ischemic syndromes; they are actually the consequences of bowel infarction and are thus the late manifestations of a clinical situation that, by the time they appear, can be unsalvageable.

Flush aortography with selective arteriographic injections into the orifices of the celiac axis and the origins of the superior and inferior mesenteric arteries is frequently diagnostic for the various conditions that lead to acute and chronic mesenteric ischemia. Superior mesenteric artery embolization often demonstrates a characteristic "meniscus sign" (i.e., a dye outlines the crescentic "tail" of the embolus), usually 3 to 10 cm from the origin of the superior mesenteric artery. Because this phenomenon occurs at the site of an ostial atherosclerotic stenosis, in cases of superior mesenteric artery thrombosis only a stub of artery can be seen. This is best (and sometimes only) seen on lateral aortography.

Arteriography can also demonstrate the absence of involvement of the large splanchnic arteries with peripheral arterial spasm, a sign seen most notably with nonorganic mesenteric ischemia. Contrast studies are also useful for demonstrating the celiac band syndrome, in which the crura of the diaphragm are felt to impinge on the celiac axis or superior mesenteric artery (21). Pressure studies to define gradients across the stenosis, before and after the administration of rapid-acting vasodilating agents such as papaverine, can be of further diagnostic use.

Certain features of acute mesenteric ischemia can be confused with those of perforated peptic ulcer, appendicitis, ruptured aneurysm or, occasionally, myocardial infarction. When the condition is chronic it can mimic such conditions as pancreatic or gastric cancer or chronic relapsing pancreatitis; occasionally, the profound weight loss from dietary changes that occur with chronic mesenteric ischemia can be confused with that of depression or neurosis, and unavailing treatment with pain medications, antidepressants, and tranquilizers might be continued for a substantial period of time.

Treatment

Management of acute and chronic mesenteric ischemic conditions could be initiated at the time of diagnostic arteriography. The advent of techniques for the administration of low-dose fibrinolytic agents (e.g., streptokinase, urokinase, and specific tissue plasminogen activators, TPAs) suggests that, in selected cases of intestinal ischemia *not* accompanied by impending tissue infarction, the embolic or thrombotic occlusion might be relieved nonsurgically. In the case of mesenteric thrombosis, as has been demonstrated in the peripheral arteries, lysis of an acute thrombosis can often reveal a high-grade atherosclerotic stenosis that could then be treatable by percutaneous transluminal angioplasty (PTA) (44). The angiographic catheter is probably most effective in treating the syndrome of nonorganic mesenteric ischemia; once relatively normal proximal mesenteric arteries with peripheral splanchnic vasoconstriction have been demonstrated, the administration of intra-arterial vasodilators such as papaverine has been shown (29) to be a useful therapeutic maneuver in this otherwise lethal condition.

Unfortunately, in many cases of both acute and chronic mesenteric ischemia, the onset of severe abdominal symptoms heralds tissue death, perforation, and peritonitis; therefore, the diagnosis of significant mesenteric ischemias generally requires laparotomy. The presence of superior mesenteric artery embolus frequently leads to successful treatment by a relatively straightforward embolectomy. Generally the patient has already been heparinized by the time of operation, and anticoagulation should be continued with heparin and then with warfarin indefinitely. Resection of clearly nonviable bowel is necessary; the presence of marginally viable intestine that is left in situ is thought by many to mandate a formal "second-look" operation (45). Techniques for assessing tissue viability, such as intraoperative Doppler, fluorescein clearance, and tissue oximetry, have been used, but a consensus has not been reached concerning their accuracy. Some (46) have advocated the use of postbowel resection vasodilators administered through a percutaneous catheter in an attempt to salvage such marginal tissue.

Once superior mesenteric artery stenosis or thrombosis, or both, have been identified, general management usually involves bypass grafting from the anterior surface of the aorta to the superior mesenteric artery just distal to the site of occlusion (47). Thromboendarterectomy has been used by some (48) but can require a more extensive dissection to expose the most proximal part of the superior mesenteric artery. As with mesenteric artery embolus, bowel resection might be required, and a second-look operation is prudent.

The celiac band syndrome, when identified by careful lateral aortography and pressure gradient measurements, is approached successfully by a combined complete exposure of the celiac axis, including lysis of the diaphragmatic crura at this level, as well as by bypass grafting using a saphenous vein or prosthetic graft as previously described. Some have argued that the extensive dissection in this area effectively performs a splanchnic neurectomy, thereby resulting in the pain relief noted in most patients so treated.

OUTCOME. Untreated, the natural history of mesenteric infarction leads to death in almost all circumstances. For acute mesenteric ischemia the mortality rate is still excessive, primarily because the diagnosis is often delayed and the aggressive therapy required for patient salvage frequently cannot be carried out in these desperately ill patients. Nevertheless, some patients can be treated successfully, and their follow-up requires consideration of the basic underlying pathophysiology. Patients who have suffered a mesenteric artery embolus must be indefinitely anticoagulated against the possibility of future emboli; myocardial revascularization and resection of left ventricular aneurysm might be useful to diminish the incidence of recurrent cardiogenic emboli.

In patients who have suffered mesenteric artery thrombosis superimposed on atherosclerotic stenosis, the systemic nature of this disease, and these patients' markedly elevated risk for coronary and cerebrovascular ischemic events, must be emphasized. These patients who undergo elective bypass for endarterectomy for atherosclerotic mesenteric vessel stenosis, or who have operative repair of the "celiac band" syndrome, often have a gratifying relief of their chronic pain and weight loss following resumption of normal food intake and body weight. As noted above, some believe that the inadvertent splanchnicectomy performed during dissection of the celiac axis can play a major role in postoperative pain relief.

Vasculitis

A number of diverse systemic collagen diseases associated with vasculitis can cause abdominal pain. These disorders have several common denominators that are of interest to surgeons and physicians: (a) they can involve multiple intra-abdominal organs, often producing pain; (b) they can begin suddenly, occasionally evoking a "crisis" with severe abdominal pain that can mimic that of a surgical lesion; and (c) they produce a serositis that can affect the peritoneum (49). These conditions include polyarteritis nodosa, lupus erythematosus, Henoch-Schönlein purpura, dermatomyositis, polyarteritis, and rheumatoid vasculitis.

Symptoms and Signs

POLYARTERITIS NODOSA. Abdominal pain and other gastrointestinal symptoms have been reported in up to 65% of patients with polyarteritis nodosa (50). This condition occurs most commonly in young males and is characterized by a necrotizing vasculitis of the muscular arteries that can affect not only the gastrointestinal tract but most other organs. This condition is particularly confusing because some patients experience such severe abdominal pain but no lesion can be found at surgery to explain the pain. Clinically apparent ischemic disease of bowel is more frequent and can range from massive infarction to segmental ischemia with ulceration, hemorrhage, or perforation (30). Although clinically significant liver disease is uncommon in this condition, hepatic artery thrombosis caused by polyarteritis accounts for approximately 50% of reported cases of infarction of the liver.

SYSTEMIC LUPUS ERYTHEMATOSUS. Systemic lupus erythematosus (SLE) involves the gastrointestinal tract in as many as 60% of patients (30). Nonspecific gastrointestinal symptoms such as anorexia, nausea, mild pain, and diarrhea occur in about 30% of patients. Vasculitis of the intestine is the most dangerous manifestation of SLE because it causes acute or subacute cramping pain, vomiting, and diarrhea, and leads to intestinal perforation and death in almost 50% of affected patients (51). Another gastrointestinal manifestation of SLE is a pseudo-obstruction picture in which patients present with acute cramping abdominal pain and radiographs show dilated loops of small bowel, which might be edematous. Surgery should be avoided unless true obstruction is present. Acute pancreatitis occurs with SLE and can be severe; it can result from glucocorticoid therapy or from active SLE itself (30). Abdominal pain can also be caused by serositis.

HENOCH-SCHÖNLEIN DISEASE. Henoch-Schönlein disease, also referred to as anaphylactoid purpura, is a disorder of unknown cause associated with small-vessel vasculitis. Typically it is associated with a clinical triad of palpable purpura, arthritis, and abdominal pain (30). Although the disease is usually seen in children and young adults, individuals of any age can be affected. Gastrointestinal involvement, which is seen in about 70% of pediatric patients, is characterized by colicky abdominal pain generally associated with nausea, vomiting, diarrhea, or constipation; these are frequently accompanied by passage of blood and mucus rectally. The symptoms and signs reflect localized or segmental ischemia and ulceration. Intussusception, gross infarction, and perforation rarely occur. Most patients recover completely and some do not require therapy.

DERMATOMYOSITIS. Dermatomyositis is important because of increased incidence of associated gastrointestinal malignancy with this disorder (30). The malignancy can antedate or postdate the onset of myositis by up to 2 years; this is usually classified as group III dermatomyositis. Group IV dermatomyositis is associated with vasculitis in the skin, muscles, gastrointestinal tract, and other organs and can cause ischemic infarction of the gastrointestinal tract.

LESS COMMON TYPES. A number of less common vascular disorders are associated with ischemia of the bowel. One rare syndrome of progressive occlusive vascular disease affecting the small and medium-sized arteries involves chiefly the skin and intestine, primarily affects young men, and terminates in intestinal infarction and perforation (30). The disease is recognized by its characteristic cutaneous lesions. Takayasu's disease can also affect mesenteric arteries and has been reported to occur in association with Crohn's disease, as has giant cell arteritis of the temporal arteries (30).

Diagnosis

The diagnosis is greatly helped by systemic features of each of these conditions and less so by abdominal findings, which are nonspecific. One finding that differentiates vasculitis from chronic atherosclerotic mesenteric insufficiency is that these patients can have steatorrhea in the absence of pain (30). Radiographs demonstrate a mucosal ulceration or edema ("thumbprinting") that can be indistinguishable from Crohn's disease either in appearance or location. Abdominal angiography is useful, especially in demonstrating aneurysms at the bifurcation of the medium-sized arteries, thereby suggesting the diagnosis of polyarteritis nodosa.

Treatment

The prognosis of untreated classic polyarteritis nodosa is extremely poor, with death resulting from gastrointestinal or renal complication or other causes. Aggressive therapy using corticosteroids significantly increases the 5-year survival rate (51). A combination of prednisone, 1 mg/kg day, and cyclophosphamide, 2 mg/day, during the first month of therapy, given thereafter every other day and eventually tapering it after approximately 6 months, has been reported to result in a long-term remission rate of up to 90%, even following the discontinuation of therapy (50). Similar results have been obtained with this treatment in patients with Wegener's granulomatosis and other types of vasculitis that involve the upper and lower respiratory tracts.

No cure for SLE is known; complete remissions occur but are rare, so the patient and physician should plan to control acute severe flares and to develop maintenance therapies in which symptoms are suppressed to an acceptable level (51). The patient who is disabled because of the pain and fatigue should be managed with nonsteroidal anti-inflammatory drugs (NSAIDs), including salicylates. Life-threatening and severe disabling manifestations of SLE should be treated with high doses of glucocorticoids (1 to 2 mg/kg day).

Most patients with Henoch-Schönlein purpura recover completely, and some do not require therapy. When corticosteroid therapy is required it is usually administered as 1 mg/kg/day of prednisone and tapered according to the clinical response.

If corticosteroids are not sufficiently effective in providing good pain relief for all these conditions, they should be supplemented with appropriate doses of NSAIDs alone or in combination with codeine or other mild narcotics to tide the patient over.

Many of these patients pose a dilemma to surgeons who must make the decision of whether to carry out a surgical exploration for possible infarction or perforation. If clinical signs of an acute abdomen are present, surgical exploration should be carried out. The clinical assessment is made more difficult because many patients with systemic vasculitis are already receiving corticosteroids, and these agents can mask important signs of a serious intra-abdominal process.

B. DISEASES OF THE PERITONEUM, MESENTERY, AND DIAPHRAGM

Anatomically the surface of the peritoneal membrane is $1.7 \, m^2$ and is similar to the total body surface area, although the functional work surface of this membrane is substantially less (60%) because of changes in vascularity, membrane potential, and diffusion gradient (52). Both parietal and visceral peritoneum normally secrete small quantities of serous fluid. When exposed to insult, however, their porosity increases, with a rapid outpouring of fluid from both vascular and interstitial spaces (third space) that allows the sequestration of large amounts of fluid. This impaired diffusion also allows the reverse to occur—that is, the rapid absorption of bacteria and microscopic debris that can produce a bacteremia. This exposes the perfused organs to two specific effects: (a) microscopic bacterial seeding of the offending organism and (b) the functional organ response to the shower of bacteria and endotoxins. As the process progresses, the damaged membrane leaches fluid from the vascular compartment and provides a pathway for bacteria to reach the vascular tree.

Several intraperitoneal factors mitigate against the sequence of events being constant. Gravity helps to localize all peritoneal collections in dependent locations, consisting of the pelvis and flanks. Moreover, the greater omentum acts as an initial "sealer" of perforations, and the lymphatic system is important in removing bacteria and other particulate matter. Following peritoneal insult, fibrin deposition also tends to seal visceral leaks and wall off the contaminated region. This inflammatory response, which includes the exudation of lymphocytes, neutrophils, macrophages, and opsins, occurs rapidly so that intraperitoneal bacterial phagocytosis and destruction occur immediately following the initial insult. After this protective action the fibrin can be removed from the peritoneal cavity through fibrinolysis by regeneration of mesothelial cells that demonstrate increased fibrinolytic activity, but this process is depressed in injured cells. This temporary suppression of fibrinolysis can provide time for fibroblasts to convert fibrins to fibrous adhesions. Normally, however, peritoneal injuries or defects heal without formation of fibrous adhesions unless other factors such as infection, ischemia, or foreign bodies are associated or superimposed.

Diseases of the Peritoneum

Table 64-1 lists the diseases of the peritoneum. The cardinal symptoms of peritoneal disease are abdominal pain and ascites, with fever, distension, nausea, vomiting, and altered bowel habits varying in their occurrence. Direct tenderness, rebound tenderness, and involuntary spasm of the abdominal musculature are the major signs of irritation of the parietal peritoneum. These signs and symptoms can be minimal or absent in the elderly or debilitated patients and vary depending on the location, cause, and acuteness of the underlying process. In addition to a complete history and physical examination, diagnosis of diseases of the peritoneum is helped by plain radiography, barium contrast studies, peritoneography, ultrasonography, CT scanning, and gallium-67 scanning (52). In addition, all patients with ascites and suspected peritoneal disease should undergo paracentesis to permit analysis of the ascitic fluid. Percutaneous peritoneal biopsy can also yield a tissue diagnosis of the cause of the peritoneal disease but its use is limited to patients with ascites. Peritoneoscopy is an excellent diagnostic tool for visualization and direct biopsy of observed lesions of the peritoneum.

Acute Bacterial or Chemical Peritonitis

Bacterial peritonitis most commonly results from perforation of an abdominal viscus, such as perforated ulcer or diverticulum, ruptured appendix, and during abdominal trauma (52). Chemical peritonitis is caused by perforation of an ulcer with liberation of sterile acid, enzymatically active pancreatic juice, or other chemicals.

Symptoms and Signs

Regardless of cause, abdominal pain, nausea, vomiting, tachycardia, and fever are the cardinal signs of bacterial peritonitis. The severity of these symptoms and signs is related to the extent of the peritoneal contamination. If the infection is localized, symptoms and signs can be mild, whereas with generalized peritonitis symptoms and signs are severe—as a significant third-space deficit develops, the blood pressure falls and the pulse becomes weak, rapid, and thready. Because motion is painful, patients usually lie still, preferably on their side with their hips slightly flexed, to relax their abdominal muscles.

Early in the course of the disease the abdomen is scaphoid and contracted, particularly across the epigastrium,—an appearance produced by spasm of the rectus abdominis muscle in response to motion of the diaphgram. Abdominal distension develops later. Diffuse tenderness is present, with rebound tenderness referred to the point of pressure, and abdominal muscle spasm is felt, the degree of which depends on the site of the peritonitis. In patients in whom the anterior parietal peritoneum is inflamed the abdominal musculature is usually completely unyielding, whereas rigidity is not a prominent sign if the posterior peritoneum is primarily involved, as seen with retroperitoneal or pelvic abscess. Ileus develops rapidly and is so consistent that, if normal peristalsis is heard in a patient with generalized abdominal pain, the condition is not peritonitis.

Diagnosis

Laboratory findings are not specific. Leukocytosis is present and can be marked. Hemoconcentration results from loss of fluid into the peritoneal cavity, electrolyte concentrations vary, and metabolic acidosis and respiratory alkalosis are often seen. Plain abdominal films show distension of the small and large intestines and demonstrate air-fluid levels. On upright films the air can be seen beneath the diaphragm if the viscus is perforated.

Complications of peritonitis can be local, consisting of wound infection, intraperitoneal abscess, and fistula formation, or systemic, consisting of septicemia, shock, and organ failure.

Treatment

Patients with mild forms of peritonitis, especially those in whom the process is well localized or in whom the risk of surgery is judged unacceptable, should be managed nonoperatively (52). Measures should include nasogastric suction, antibiotics, pain control with analgesics or other appropriate methods, administration of fluids, and monitoring of blood volume, acid-base, and electrolyte status, as well as of cardiopulmonary and renal function. Percutaneous drainage of the localized abscess should be given serious consideration.

In patients with generalized severe peritonitis in whom surgery is indicated, ample preoperative preparation is necessary to restore fluid balance and to stabilize circulatory and pulmonary function. In addition to nasogastric suction, which reduces distension and thus helps pulmonary function, adequate volumes of electrolyte and colloidal solutions are administered to correct the hypovolemia. Complete blood and other laboratory studies should be carried out.

Because these patients have severe abdominal pain it is best to control it with epidural opioid analgesia during the preparation. As soon as the blood volume has been restored opioids should be supplemented with low concentrations of local anesthetic to provide more effective relief and also to eliminate the intense vasoconstriction of the splanchnic region that is frequently found in such patients. Moreover, the epidural analgesia decreases the ileus and degree of muscle spasm that invariably decrease chest wall compliance and thus produce hypoxemia. In most patients the ideal anesthesia is a combined segmental epidural block with tracheal intubation carried out under topical anesthesia, followed by light inhalation or intravenous analgesics and sedatives.

Antibiotic therapy is essential and should be initiated early with a drug specific for the offending organism. In advanced peritonitis, however, a single organism is rarely found; most patients have a polymicrobial flora consisting of one or two aerobic and two or three anaerobic species (52). Approximately 30% of patients have septicemia, usually caused by Escherichia coli and Bacteroides fragilis. During surgery the patient should be monitored with urinary bladder, central venous, and pulmonary artery catheterization.

Other Types of Infectious Peritonitis

Although peritonitis is an unusual form of tuberculosis, it constitutes one of the most important diseases of the peritoneum (52). This condition is present in 1 to 1.5% of patients admitted to tuberculosis sanitaria (52). Its insidious nature and the clinical circumstances in which it occurs often cause it to be mistaken for neoplastic disease or ascites caused by cirrhosis (52).

The symptoms and signs are insidious, with the most common complaints being fever, anorexia, weakness, malaise, and weight loss. Abdominal pain is reported in only 50% of patients, and this is usually described as a vague, dull, diffuse discomfort. Abdominal tenderness is usually diffuse and present in 65% of patients (52).

With the advent of antituberculosis agents the mortality rate of tuberculous peritonitis has been reduced from 60 to almost 0%. Therapy with isoniazid and a second agent such as ethambutol or streptomycin should be continued for 18 to 24 months. Symptoms should begin to improve within 1 to 2 weeks of the onset of therapy and fever should resolve within 4 weeks. The pain is managed with nonopioid systemic analgesics.

Peritoneal inflammation caused by fungi and parasites is uncommon and pain is not a major symptom (52); therefore, it is not considered further here.

Granulomatous Peritonitis

When the peritoneum responds to a wide variety of stimuli with a granulomatous inflammatory reaction, it can be caused by such exogenous conditions as parasites or ingested organic material or it can have an endogenous cause, in which the response is a result of ruptured cystic teratomas or squamous metaplasia and, rarely, sarcoidosis. Iatrogenic causes are starch and barium peritonitis.

The symptoms and signs are consistent with those of intestinal obstruction or peritonitis and include pain, tenderness, fever, nausea, vomiting, and abdominal distension. Small bowel obstruction can occur in 25% of patients (52).

Treatment of mild cases of peritonitis should be conservative and should consist of supportive measures, pain control, fluids, and rest. Patients who have signs of intestinal obstruction or severe peritonitis require surgical therapy.

Familial Paroxysmal Polyserositis (XXII-1)

Etiology and Pathophysiology

Familial paroxysmal polyserositis (FPP), also called familial Mediterranean fever, is a disease characterized by recurring episodes of acute self-limited serositis, especially peritonitis. It is an inherited disease transmitted as an autosomal receptive trait that occurs predominantly in Mediterranean peoples, with Sephardic Jews accounting for 50% of cases, Armenians 22%, Arabs 11%, Turks 7%, and other ethnic groups the remaining 10% (53). The onset of the disease is usually within the first two decades of life but 20% of patients have their first episode after the age of 20 and 4% after the age of 30. About 60% of patients are males.

Symptoms and Signs

Disease usually appears suddenly with attacks of serositis that include peritonitis in 55% of patients, arthritis in about 25%, and pleuritis in 5%. During the course of FPP 95% of patients eventually develop peritonitis; this is the sole manifestation in 30% (52, 53). The attack consists of a sudden onset of fever, usually 101 to 103° F (38.3 to 39.4° C), with localized or diffuse abdominal pain, exquisite direct abdominal tenderness with marked rebound tenderness, and leukocytosis in almost 90% of patients. The plain film of the abdomen shows air-fluid levels. After 6 to 12 hours these signs and symptoms recede and the patient is usually well within 24 to 48 hours. The attacks occur at irregular and unpredictable intervals and the patient is entirely well between them. Except for the rapid resolution and recurrent nature of the disease, FPP presents all the characteristics of an acute surgical abdomen.

Treatment and Prognosis

The therapy that has proven to be highly effective consists of the administration of colchicine in doses of 0.6 mg bid or tid (53, 54). Studies have shown that this decreases both the severity and frequency of attacks, and long-term studies report continuous suppression of attacks with little evidence of adverse effects (54).

Prognosis of FPP is excellent and many patients have been followed for years with persistent good general health despite hundreds of attacks (53). Attacks can increase in frequency with age, perhaps with occasional remissions or periods in which the disease is quite intractable.

Neoplasm of the Peritoneum

Primary Mesothelioma

Primary mesotheliomas are tumors arising from the epithelial and mesenchymal elements of the mesothelium. About 25% of these tumors involve the peritoneum, 65% involve the pleura, and 10% are pericardial (55).

Etiology and Pathology

Asbestos is the only substance that has been shown to have an epidemiologic relationship to mesothelioma and the apparent increased incidence since the 1950s can be related to expansion of the asbestos industry (55). In addition to historical evidence of asbestos exposure, 50% of patients with mesothelioma have pathologic evidence of pulmonary asbestosis, including pulmonary fibrosis, pleural hyaline plaques, and asbestos bodies in the lungs. Because at least 30% of patients with mesothelioma have no history of asbestos exposure, however, other factors also play a role.

Mesotheliomas, especially peritoneal ones, are more common in males, possibly reflecting occupational factors. The highest incidence is in the sixth decade but the condition has been reported in young children (55).

Symptoms and Signs

Patients presenting with peritoneal primary tumors usually complain first of abdominal pain and abdominal mass or increased abdominal girth, along with anorexia, nausea, vomiting, constipation, and weight loss (55). Signs of asbestosis are evident in chest radiographs in 50% of patients and early pleural mesothelioma can be apparent, with chest pain, dyspnea, or cough.

Diagnosis and Treatment

Other than an elevated sedimentation rate, the blood count and blood chemistries are normal. Radiography is not useful. Ultrasonography and CT scanning can demonstrate sheet-like masses and ascites. Paracentesis reveals an exudate that can be hemorrhagic. Peritoneal cytologic studies and biopsy and peritoneoscopy can suggest a diagnosis, but laparoscopy is usually necessary to provide adequate biopsy samples for definitive diagnosis and to rule out a primary neoplasm. The prognosis of mesothelioma is poor, and most patients survive only 1 year after diagnosis (55). Curative surgery and radiation therapy are not helpful. Recently doxorubicin has provided encouraging results, with up to a 50% increase in the survival rate (52). Multimodal chemotherapy might prove effective (55).

Secondary Carcinomatosis

Peritoneal involvement by spread from a primary neoplasm is one of the most common causes of peritoneal disease. Pathologic studies of selected open peritoneal biopsy specimens in a large general hospital showed that about 65% were neoplastic and, of these, 75% were metastatic adenocarcinomas (56). Sarcomas, carcinoids, teratomas, and nervous tissue tumors are rare. Malignancies of lymphoid or myeloid tissue can also infiltrate the peritoneum. The most common lesions involved are malignant lymphoma, Hodgkin's lymphoma, Hodgkin's disease, and myeloid metaplasia (57).

Symptoms and Signs

Patients with peritoneal carcinomatosis present with ascites, diffuse abdominal pain, weight loss and, less frequently, nausea and vomiting (52). The pain can be produced by various interactions between the tumor and intra-abdominal organs. Barium contrast studies can show nodular indentation of the intestine or angulated fixed or displaced intestinal loops, especially if attention is paid to major areas of intraperitoneal seating. These areas include the pouch of Douglas at the rectosigmoid, the right lower quadrant at the lower end of the small bowel, the left lower quadrant along the superior border of the sigmoid mesocolon and colon, and the right paracolic gutter lateral to the cecum and ascending colon (56).

Diagnosis

In addition to barium contrast studies, other diagnostic procedures include paracentesis, ultrasonography or CT scanning, and mediastinal lymphoscintigraphy. The diagnosis is made most directly by cytology, peritoneal biopsy, or peritoneoscopy.

Treatment

Once the neoplasm has spread to the peritoneum, the prognosis is poor (52). Paracentesis is useful for removal of a large volume of fluid and is tolerated without hemodynamic problems. Cytotoxic agents, radioisotopes, and sclerosing agents have been used with varying success. The cytotoxic agents that have been used include nitrogen mustard, 5-fluorouracil, thiatepa, bleomycin, and Adriamycin; these have produced response rates ranging from 20 to 70% with a variable incidence of toxic effects, including local pain, nausea, fever, or depression (52). Installation of radioisotopes, such as ^{32}P and ^{198}Au, has also proved helpful. Peritoneovenous shunting has become more widely used as a method of palliation for malignant ascites. Surgery is not indicated except in patients with intestinal obstruction that is not responsive to conservative measures.

Diseases of the Mesentery and Omentum

Patients with mesenteric disease usually present with nonspecific symptoms such as abdominal pain, abdominal distension, or intestinal obstruction (52). The most frequent physical finding is a mass that might be mobile. Associated lymphatic obstruction can cause steatorrhea, chylous ascites, or protein-losing enteropathy, with hypoalbuminemia and edema. Of the various pathologic processes, only mesenteric inflammatory disease and mesenteric and omental tumors produce abdominal pain (52, 57).

Mesenteric inflammatory disease is characterized by recurrent episodes of cramping abdominal pain, either localized or generalized, and weight loss, nausea, vomiting, and low-grade fever. Corticosteroids have been claimed as useful therapy.

Mesenteric tumors are rare and can arise from any of the cellular elements of the mesentery. Metastatic tumors of the mesentery are more common than primary mesenteric tumors and are usually the result of an enlarged lymphomatous or carcinomatous lymph node. In contrast to mesenteric tumors, omental tumors are derived from muscle in 60% of patients and include leiomyomas, leiomyosarcomas, and hemangiopericytomas (56). These are characterized by abdominal pain, abdominal mass, and weight loss. Treatment is directed toward the type of tumor.

Torsion of the omentum is an acute condition that mimics appendicitis or cholecystitis and is characterized by abdominal pain in the right lower (80% of patients) or the right upper quadrant (10%). Tenderness, guarding, and ileus are usually present and nausea, vomiting, abdominal mass, and leukocytosis are present in 50% of patients (52). Surgical excision of the gangrenous omentum is necessary.

Diseases of the Diaphragm (XVII-8)

Diseases of the diaphragm that can cause pain are diaphragmatic hernias, rupture, and tumors.

Herniation (XIX-2)

Diaphragmatic hernias are caused by congenital abnormalities in the formation of the diaphragm (52). Most commonly the left pleural and peritoneal membrane fails to fuse with the septum transversum, causing a left posterolateral defect without a hernia sac. The fusion may be complete but a failure of muscularization posterolaterally is present. A hernia with a sac is formed, called the Bochdalek hernia. About 25%

of patients with Bochdalek hernia are asymptomatic but 50% have vague intermittent abdominal pain and 25% have chest pain, cardiovascular symptoms, and dyspnea (58). Incarceration of the intestine leads to acute sharp retrosternal pain that radiates to the left upper quadrant or back, along with the typical symptoms of intestinal obstruction.

The diagnosis can usually be made on the lateral chest film, which reveals a blunted cardiophrenic angle, a small effusion, and a gas-filled intestinal loop. Surgery is always indicated in patients with incarceration or obstruction because of the danger of strangulation (52).

Rupture

Blunt injury to the abdomen can cause diaphragmatic rupture that is said to occur in about 5% of all patients undergoing surgery for trauma (52, 59). Because the early clinical course can be dominated by signs of other injuries, signs of visceral herniation are often delayed. Patients can present many years later with postprandial fullness, chest pain, nausea, vomiting, cramps, dyspnea, or obvious bowel obstruction and strangulation, with severe epigastric and chest pain (59).

Diaphragmatic rupture should be suspected in any patient who has vague abdominal symptoms and a history of blunt abdominal trauma. Because of the high frequency of later visceral herniation, diaphragmatic laceration should be repaired surgically (52).

Tumors and Cysts

Diaphragmatic neoplasms usually cause pleuritic chest pain simulating that of intra-abdominal disease, with the pain referred primarily to the epigastrium. Chest radiographs reveal irregularity of the diaphragm or a large mass that abuts the diaphragm (52).

Diaphragmatic cysts can also cause upper abdominal pain, located primarily in the epigastrium. When located on the right side, however, they suggest possible hepatic or subphrenic abnormalities. The cysts are usually bronchogenic, mesothelial, or fibrous. They can be acquired or congenital. If pain is severe and persistent, surgical removal is necessary.

C. OTHER INTRA-ABDOMINAL DISEASES

Intra-abdominal Abscesses

The three types of intra-abdominal abscesses are intraperitoneal, retroperitoneal, and visceral, and occur with about equal frequency (60). Intraperitoneal abscesses (subdiaphragmatic, midabdominal, or pelvic) (60, 61) are localized collections of pus that can occur consequent to either generalized peritonitis or a more localized intra-abdominal disease process or injury. In the former case the normal barriers that limit the inflammatory process are inadequate and the abscess can occur at some distance from the original source of contamination. In the latter instance the spread of peritonitis is limited by contiguous viscera, omentum, and peritoneum, and the abscess develops closer to the source of contamination. Retroperitoneal abscesses can be located in the anterior or posterior part of the space. Visceral abscesses can involve the liver, pancreas, spleen, kidney, and gallbladder. Because many of these are discussed elsewhere in this section, I limit the discussion here to subdiaphragmatic, midabdominal, anterior retroperitoneal, and splenic abscesses.

Most intra-abdominal abscesses develop from infecting organisms that are a complex mixture of anaerobic and aerobic bacteria, which are part of the normal bowel flora. The most important isolates from these abscesses are aerobic gram-negative rods, such as Escherichia coli and Klebsiella spp., and anaerobes, especially Bacteroides fragilis (60, 61). Antimicrobial therapy requires agents effective against these organisms.

Subdiaphragmatic Abscess (XIX-1)

The subdiaphragmatic space, arbitrarily defined as lying below the diaphragm and above the transverse colon, consists of four subdivisions. On the right side are the suprahepatic and subhepatic spaces, while on the left side the subhepatic and suprahepatic spaces freely communicate and constitute a single combined subphrenic space. The other left-sided space behind the stomach and anterior to the pancreas is the lesser sac. A subhepatic abscess is found on either side of the falciform ligament, between the liver and the transverse colon (62). On the right side the abscess can be anterior or posterior, while on the left side posterior subhepatic abscess is synonymous with lesser sac abscess. Left anterior subhepatic abscess occurs between the left lobe of the liver and the stomach or spleen. Some clues to localization are afforded by a knowledge of the primary disease process. A right-sided abscess is more frequent after appendicitis, whereas perforated duodenal ulcer causes right anterior subhepatic abscess and pancreatic disease is more likely to result in a lesser sac abscess.

Subphrenic abscesses occur between the dome of the liver and the diaphragmatic surfaces and are referred to as right or left according to their relationship to the falciform ligament (62). Abscesses on the right side tend to localize either anteriorly or posteriorly and are designated as right anterior or right posterior subphrenic abscesses. On the left side no such distinction is made.

Symptoms and Signs

The clinical manifestations of subphrenic abscess usually begin within 2 to 6 weeks following surgery but occasionally do not appear for several months (60, 62). Fever is nearly always present and can be the only evidence of abscess. Nonspecific constitutional symptoms such as anorexia and weight loss are less common. The most frequent findings relate to the thorax and abdomen and include nonproductive cough, chest pain, dyspnea, and shoulder pain caused by the irritation of the diaphragmatic pleura. Rales, rhonchi, or a friction rub can be audible. Dullness to percussion and decreased breath sounds might be present when basilar atelectasis, pneumonia, or pleural effusion occurs. Pain, the most common abdominal complaint, is often accompanied by localized tenderness, and these are frequently associated with abdominal distension and hypoactive bowel sounds. A mass wound drainage or sinus tract of a previous abdominal incision site is sometimes present.

Subhepatic abscess usually presents with symptoms referable to the abdomen and is less likely to cause any pleural or diaphragmatic abnormality. Abdominal pain and tenderness are usually present, and a mass is occasionally found.

Diagnosis

Leukocytosis occurs in most patients with subphrenic abscess, anemia is frequent, and blood cultures are occasionally positive. Chest radiographs usually demonstrate ipsilateral pleural effusion, an elevated or immobile hemidiaphragm, pneumonitis, and atelectasis (60). Plain abdominal films can reveal extraintestinal gas in the abscess, displacement of adjacent organs, or a soft tissue density representing the abscess. Ultrasonography is especially useful in right-sided subphrenic abscess. A left-sided subphrenic area is more difficult to examine, however, because of the gas-filled stomach, splenic flexure, and aerated lung and ribs, and also because the spleen varies in size and shape and can produce a few echoes that resemble those of an abscess. CT scanning generally provides the most accurate information about the presence and extent of abscess into these areas (60).

Treatment

Treatment of these abscesses involves surgical drainage, either by open operation or by percutaneous catheter drainage (60). This relatively new approach consists of accurate localization of the abscess by ultrasonography, CT scanning, or both. The skin is punctured with a 20-gauge needle over which a flexible guide wire and then a drainage catheter are inserted into the abscess cavity. The catheter remains in place until the abscess cavity is obliterated, usually 2 to 3 weeks or longer. Antibiotics effective against both aerobic and anaerobic organisms are a good adjunct but are no substitute for drainage. Adequate nutrition is critical during the often prolonged hospital course.

Midabdominal Abscess

A midabdominal abscess can form in the peritoneal cavity anywhere between the transverse colon and pelvis (60). They are frequent in the paracolic gutters but can be located between the leaves of the small bowel and mesentery. They are referred to as right lower quadrant, left lower quadrant, or interloop abscesses according to their location.

Etiology, Symptoms, and Signs

RIGHT LOWER QUADRANT ABSCESS. Abscess in the right lower quadrant develops most commonly as a complication of acute appendicitis and less frequently from colonic diverticulitis, regional enteritis, or perforated duodenal ulcers, with drainage down the right paracolic gutter. The clinical manifestations include right lower quadrant pain and tenderness and a mass that develops following symptoms suggesting those of acute appendicitis. The mass can cause partial or complete small bowel obstruction.

LEFT LOWER QUADRANT ABSCESS. Left lower quadrant abscess usually develops from perforation of a diverticulum in the descending or sigmoid colon and less commonly from a perforated colonic carcinoma. The symptoms are those of acute diverticulitis and include left lower quadrant pain, tenderness, anorexia, and nausea followed by fever, leukocytosis, and development of a palpable mass.

INTERLOOP ABSCESS. Interloop abscess is comprised of loculations of pus between the folded surfaces of the small and large intestines and their mesenteries. It is usually a complication of bowel perforation, anastomotic disruption, or Crohn's disease. Clinical manifestations are usually subtle and consist of fever, leukocytosis, and abdominal pain and tenderness. Signs of paralytic ileus or palpable mass can develop. Plain abdominal films occasionally suggest the diagnosis by the presence of bowel wall edema, separation of bowel loops, localized ileus, and air-fluid levels on upright films.

Treatment

The therapy of midabdominal abscess includes surgical drainage and antibiotics. Reber (60) noted that, even without a firm diagnosis, a progressively enlarging painful tender abdominal mass in a febrile patient is an indication for drainage because perforation of the abscess might be imminent. Occasionally, in a gravely ill patient with no localizing findings, abdominal exploration might be necessary to find and drain the abscess. At operation the abdomen must be explored thoroughly, because these abscesses are frequently multiple. If the clinical picture does not improve promptly, re-exploration might be necessary to find missed or new abscesses.

Anterior Retroperitoneal Abscess

Etiology, Symptoms, and Signs

Abscess in the anterior retroperitoneal space is a complication of acute appendicitis, colonic perforation from diverticulitis or tumor, gastric or duodenal perforation, regional enteritis, or pancreatitis (60). The major symptoms are abdominal or flank pain, fever, nausea and vomiting, and pain in the hip, thigh, or knee from psoas muscle involvement. Physical examination usually reveals a palpable mass in addition to the abdominal or flank tenderness. Extension of the hip aggravates or causes the pain.

Diagnosis and Treatment

Diagnosis is based on the symptoms and signs, the presence of leukocytosis, and findings on plain radiographs, which show extraintestinal gas in the abscess, displacement of adjacent organs, and loss of the psoas muscle shadow. Barium studies of the intestinal tract can show displacement of adjacent viscera. CT scanning often defines retroperitoneal abscess when other studies are negative or equivocal.

Treatment usually involves surgery or percutaneous catheter drainage and antibiotics effective against enteric aerobic and anaerobic organisms. In some patients the abscess resolves with antimicrobial therapy alone.

Splenic Abscess

Etiology

Most splenic abscesses develop as a result of uncontrolled infection elsewhere. In 75% of patients they are small, multiple, and clinically silent, and are found incidentally at autopsy (63). In the remaining 25% of patients the splenic abscess is solitary and diagnosis is especially important because splenectomy is usually curative. A solitary abscess can arise from the following: systemic bacteremia that originated in another site and is now causing infection in a previously normal spleen; infection, presumably of hematogenous origin, and a spleen damaged by blunt or penetrating trauma, bland infarction such as occurs in sickle cell trait or hemoglobin sickle cell disease, or other diseases such as malaria; or extension from contiguous infection, such as subphrenic abscess. The most common infecting organisms are staphylococci, streptococci, anaerobes, and aerobic gram-negative rods, including Salmonella (61, 63).

Symptoms and Signs

The clinical manifestations include subacute onset of fever and left-sided pain that is often in the flank, upper abdomen, or lower chest and that can radiate to the left shoulder (61, 63). The left upper quadrant is commonly tender to palpation and splenomegaly is typical. Occasionally a splenic friction rub is audible. Leukocytosis is usual and blood cultures sometimes grow the infecting organisms.

Diagnosis

The signs and symptoms and radiographic findings should lead to a suspicion of diagnosis. Radiographs show a left upper quadrant mass, extraintestinal gas in the abscess from gas-forming organisms, displacement of other organs, including the kidney, colon, and stomach, elevated left hemidiaphragm, and left pleural effusion. Liver-spleen radionuclide scanning, CT scanning, and ultrasonography should demonstrate intrasplenic defects with abscesses larger than 2 to 3 cm.

Treatment

Untreated abscesses are followed by such complication as hemorrhage into the abscess cavity or rupture into the peritoneal, bowel, bronchus, or pleural space. Treatment consists of systemic antibiotics and splenectomy, which is curative (see above).

Other Gastrointestinal Disorders

Three conditions that can cause abdominal pain, distension, and other symptoms and signs of an acute abdomen are briefly discussed here. They are neurogenic intestinal obstruction (adynamic ileus), gas entrapment syndromes, and abdominal migraine. Although pain is usually not severe and the conditions are self-limited, they are considered here to emphasize simple methods of treatment usually not considered by surgeons or internists.

Neurogenic Intestinal Obstruction

In Chapter 60 Kimmey and Silverstein indicated that intestinal obstruction is a common cause of abdominal pain. In most cases the obstruction is caused by mechanical factors that require surgical intervention. A number of cases have been noted, however, in which the obstruction is caused by neurogenic factors that produce adynamic ileus, which often can be corrected by interrupting certain sympathetic pathways. Adynamic ileus is said to be the most common cause of intestinal obstruction (64). Dynamic ileus, in contrast, which is characterized by prolonged contraction or spasm of a segment of the large bowel, is uncommon.

Etiology

Adynamic ileus occurs to some degree after any intra-abdominal operation. Its severity and duration vary directly with the amount of intestinal handling and length of the operation. It usually lasts 2 to 3 days after most operative procedures but, in some cases, it can last for a longer period. The pathophysiology of this condition is discussed in detail in Chapter 25. It is the result of visceroceral, cutaneovisceral, and somatovisceral reflexes that are consequent to tissue injury, marked nociceptive input, and reflex sympathetic hyperactivity (Figs. 25-1 and 25-2).

Acute adynamic ileus also occurs after any peritoneal insult and its severity and duration are dependent to some degree on the type of peritoneal injury. Thus, hydrochloric acid, colonic contents, and pancreatic enzymes are the most irritating whereas blood and urine are less irritating. Patients with severe acute hemorrhagic pancreatitis frequently develop severe ileus that lasts for days and sometimes a week or longer.

Another common cause of severe prolonged adynamic ileus is fracture of one of the lower thoracic vertebrae. This causes severe compression of one or more nerves with consequent radiculalgia and reflex responses, including sympathetic hyperactivity in those segments adjacent to the fracture. Other retroperitoneal conditions that cause adynamic ileus include ureteral calculus, severe pyelonephritis, retroperitoneal infection, and hematoma. Thoracic disorders, including lower lobe pneumonia, fractured ribs, myocardial infarction, and pulmonary embolism, frequently produce adynamic ileus, as do electrolyte disturbances, particularly potassium depletion. Intestinal ischemia, whether it results from vascular occlusion or intestinal distension itself, can perpetuate an adynamic ileus. Dynamic ileus occurs in patients with heavy metal poisoning, porphyria, and extensive intestinal ulceration.

Pathophysiology

The pathophysiologic mechanism is predominantly an autonomic functional imbalance with an increase in sympathetic activity and perhaps a concomitant decrease in the activity of the parasympathetic nerves supplying the gastrointestinal tract. It was formerly thought that in this condition the intestinal musculature is paralyzed. This is not the case, however, because it has been repeatedly demonstrated experimentally and clinically that interruption of sympathetic supply to the gut causes a progressive decrease in the ileus and increases the ability of intestinal musculature to return to normal function. Thus, the term "paralytic ileus" should be discarded and replaced by the term "reflex inhibition ileus" (65). Obviously, adynamic ileus caused by peritonitis, with marked electrolyte imbalance (particularly hypokalemia) is exacerbated by interference with normal ionic movements during smooth muscle contractions. Certain drugs such as phenothiazines and narcotics inhibit bowel motility.

Symptoms and Signs

Clinically, acute adynamic ileus is characterized by cramping abdominal pain, distension, vomiting, absence of peristaltic sounds, and other signs and symptoms of intestinal obstruction. An important deleterious effect of severe ileus is a marked increase in intra-abdominal pressure with consequent cephalad displacement of the diaphragm, encroachment of the lower lobes of the lungs, and a constant decrease of lung capacities and pulmonary compliance. If the ileus is a result of postoperative pain or some other painful disorder, reflex responses decrease chest wall compliance; combined with the effects on the lungs atelectasis is produced, with consequent alveolar-arterial mismatch and hypoxemia that can progress to pneumonitis. As a consequence the patient develops tachypnea associated with dyspnea that results in inadequate pulmonary ventilation and produces a vicious cycle that can result in death. I personally have known of three patients who died from progressive respiratory failure resulting from postoperative ileus.

Treatment

The standard treatment for adynamic ileus is use of nasogastric suction and intravenous fluid administration to correct electrolyte imbalance, particularly hypokalemia (64). In some patients with severe or extreme distension, passage of a Cantor tube into the intestine should be tried because this method of suction provides intestinal decompression superior to that achieved with a nasogastric tube.

Although these procedures are usually effective and certainly reasonable in patients with mild ileus, the most effective therapy for severe ileus is interruption of the sympathetic supply to the bowel using a segmental epidural block with local anesthetics. The use of sympathetic blockade to increase the tone and motility of the gastrointestinal tract and enhance its function was first suggested by Wagner in 1919, who published a more extensive report containing favorable results 3 years later (65). This prompted a number of others to use spinal anesthesia and splanchnic block. In 1928 Ochsner and colleagues (66) reported that physiologic, chemical, and paralytic ileus in dogs could be relieved by injection of the splanchnic nerves, and they suggested that this method be used in the treatment of clinical ileus. Two years later they reported their extensive experience in humans. In the first edition of this book (65) a large number of reports were cited containing favorable reports of the use of

this method by many highly respected surgeons, including Ochsner and colleagues, Smithwick, Morton and Scott, J.C. White and associates, and a number of distinguished European clinicians. For the past four decades I have used continuous segmental epidural blockade as an effective method of decreasing the incidence of postoperative ileus and as an effective treatment for patients who developed it after surgery, following fractures of the thoracic vertebrae, and as a result of other conditions that provoke segmental reflex inhibition of the gastrointestinal tract. Continuous segmental block using appropriate doses of local anesthetics to block thinly myelinated and unmyelinated sympathetic and nociceptive fibers relieves the ileus and any consequent discomfort.

Sarnoff and associates (67) reported the successful use of differential spinal block to treat patients with dynamic ileus. Under the influence of sympathetic visceromotor block peristaltic action became coordinated, large amounts of flatus and feces were expelled, and the colicky pain and distension were relieved (see 65 for detail).

Gas Entrapment Syndromes

Gas entrapment syndromes occur as a result of gaseous distension of a portion of the gastrointestinal tract (68). Patients usually complain of a dull constant pain in the abdomen and frequently in the chest, bloating, distension, eructation (belching), or passage of excessively voluminous or noxious flatus that patients attribute to "too much gas in my stomach." Although this is a subject of some controversy and a number of authorities do not consider it a valid diagnosis based on experimental studies, it remains an important clinical problem. Here I briefly mention the causes, symptoms and signs, and treatment of this condition.

Etiology

Gas that is present in the gut results from swallowed air (aerophagia), production of gas in the lumen, and diffusion of gas from the blood into the lumen (69).

Aerophagia occurs normally to some degree during eating and drinking but some people unconsciously swallow repeated boluses of air at other times, especially when anxious. Most of the swallowed air is subsequently eructated and only a small amount passes into the small bowel, with the quantity apparently being influenced by posture. The esophagus empties the air into the posterior cephalad part of the stomach. Disposition of the gas then depends on the position of the patient: when the patient is upright air rises above the liquid contents of the stomach, comes in contact with the gastroesophageal junction, and is readily eructated but, when the person is supine, air is trapped below the fluid level and tends to be propelled into the duodenum.

Gas is produced in the lumen of the gastrointestinal tract by several mechanisms. Bacterial metabolism yields significant volumes of hydrogen (H_2), methane (CH_4), and carbon dioxide (CO_2). Nearly all H_2 is produced by bacterial metabolism of ingested fermentable material (i.e., carbohydrates and amino acids in the colon). Each is produced in large quantities by eating certain fruits and vegetables (e.g., baked beans, which contain indigestible carbohydrates) and by malabsorption syndromes. CH_4 is produced by bacterial metabolism of endogenous substances in the colon with the production rate only minimally influenced by food ingestion. CO_2 can also be produced by bacterial metabolism but a more important source is the reaction of bicarbonate and hydrogen ions that are derived from gastric hydrochloric acid or fatty acids released during digestion of fats from a meal.

Radiographic studies indicate that patients who complain of abdominal pain caused by gas do not have excessive amounts of gas (69). In addition, studies employing the intestinal gas washout technique in both fasting and fed individuals failed to demonstrate increased intestinal gas volumes. In 18 patients who thought they had excessive gas the mean fasting intestinal gas volume was 176 ml, which did not differ from the 199 ml found in the 10 control subjects (70). Similarly, no significant differences were observed after ingestion of a standard meal. The consumption of intestinal gas and the rate of accommodation of the five major gases (O_2, N_2O, CO_2, H_2, and CH_4) were also similar in patients with gas and in controls. The patients did differ from normal controls in that more of the inert gas that was infused into the upper small bowel refluxed back into the stomach, and they more frequently complained of severe abdominal pain during the infusion. These studies suggest that complaints of pain and bloating result from disordered intestinal motility that interferes with the orderly passage of gas through the bowel rather than from excessive bowel gas (69). Patients with such complaints also appear to have an abnormal pain response to bowel distension (71).

Pathophysiology

The location of pain and other symptoms depends on the source of the gas and on the position of the patient. Three syndromes have been recognized, depending on the location of the pain: gastric entrapment syndrome, hepatic splenic flexure entrapment syndrome, and splenic flexure entrapment syndrome (68).

Gastric distension is usually caused by aerophagia unless the patient has been drinking large quantities of carbonated beverages or beer. Aerophagia can be primary as a result of excess swallowing consequent to anxiety, tension, or poor eating practices, such as hurrying through meals, gulping of food, inadequate chewing, and talking while eating. Secondary aerophagia is usually a result of reflex esophagitis but it can also be caused by peptic ulcer disease, gastritis, or carcinoma of the stomach, pancreas, or esophagus (68).

Gas entrapment of the colon occurs in individuals with aerophagia, in those who consume large quantities of carbonated beverages or beer, and who avoid eructation (belching) or cannot do so because of the strong lower esophageal sphincter. In such people the swallowed air is carried by normal peristalsis through the small intestine to the colon, ultimately to be expelled. If peristalsis is delayed for any reason colonic distension can occur. Large bowel distension can also be caused by excessive gas production.

Symptoms and Signs

With gastric distension most of the discomfort is in the epigastrium, but this often extends into the central lower chest (Fig. 64-4A). In addition, if referred pain is in the left shoulder, it is likely caused by diaphragmatic irritation by the distended gastric fundus. The pain is dull and constant, worsening as the day progresses, and is frequently exacerbated at mealtimes because all swallowing produces some aerophagia.

In colonic distension the pain is localized mainly to the quadrant in which the distension occurs. With the hepatic flexure syndrome the pain is in the right upper quadrant (Fig. 64-4B) whereas with the splenic flexure

syndrome the pain is in the left upper quadrant (Fig. 64-4C). The pain frequently radiates to the adjacent anterior and lateral chest and, in the splenic flexure syndrome, it often radiates to the left shoulder. Occasionally the most generalized pain of small or large bowel distension can be felt across the anterior chest and above the costal margin.

Relief of any of these pains by rectal passage of gas is a diagnostic clue. Another diagnostic lead is the fact that pain frequently shifts in location. Physical examination of these patients is usually normal, although abdominal tympany is sometimes present. Plain radiographic examination of standing aerophagic patients who are seen in the emergency room can reveal excess gas in some portion of the gastrointestinal tract.

Diagnosis

Because the excessive gas or gas entrapment syndromes have such nonspecific symptoms they commonly overlap with irritable bowel syndrome as well as with organic disease, so a careful history is essential to guide the extent of medical evaluation. Long-standing symptoms in a young person who is otherwise well and has not lost weight are unlikely to be caused by serious organic disease. The older person, especially with the onset of new symptoms, merits more thorough examination before the excessive gas, real or imagined, is treated.

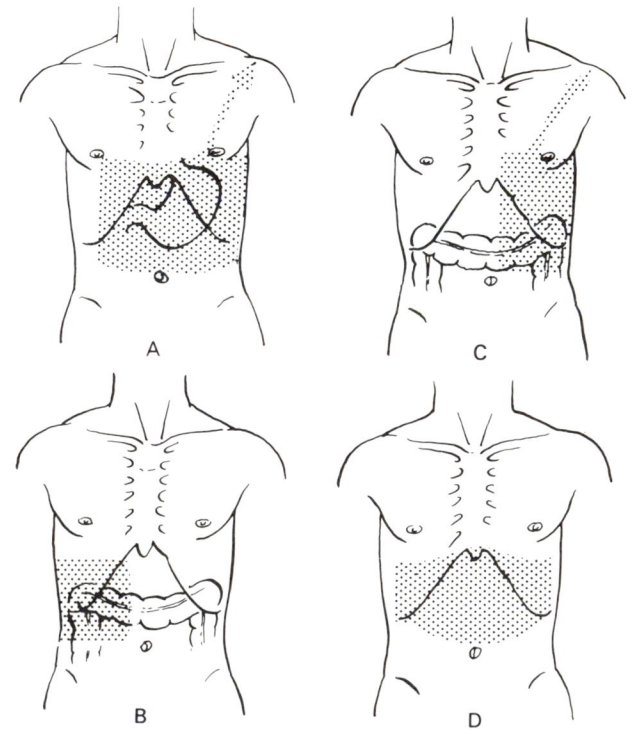

FIG. 64-4. Sites of pain caused by gas entrapment syndrome. *A.* Location of pain caused by gastric distension. *B.* Location of pain in "hepatic flexure syndrome." *C.* Location of pain in "splenic flexure syndrome." *D.* Generalized abdominal pain with gas entrapment in small bowel. Modified from Saibil, F.G., and Edmeads, J.: Chest pain arising from extrathoracic structures. *In* Chest Pain: An Integrated Diagnostic Approach. Edited by Donald L. Levene. Philadelphia, Lea & Febiger, 1977, p. 123.

Treatment

Belching, bloating and distension are difficult to relieve because most complaints are caused by unconscious aerophagia or by exaggerated sensitivity to normal amounts of gas. An attempt must be made to reduce aerophagia; the mechanisms of repeated eructation should be explained and demonstrated to minimize the amount of gas that remains in the stomach.

Foods containing nonabsorbable carbohydrates must be avoided. Milk-containing products should be excluded from the diet of patients with lactose intolerance. Several drugs have some beneficial effects. Simethicone, an agent that breaks up small gas bubbles, has been incorporated into several preparations and various anticholinergic drugs have also been used, with variable results (71). Some persons with dyspepsia and postprandial upper abdominal fullness benefit from such drugs as metoclopramide, 10 mg, or bethanechol, 5 to 25 mg, 30 minutes before meals. These drugs increase the rate of gastric emptying or increase lower esophageal sphincter tone. Roughage (e.g., bran or psyllium seed) can be added to the diet in an effort to increase colonic transit rate. Unfortunately, in some patients, the symptoms become worse. Finally, reassurance that these problems are not detrimental to health is an important step in eliminating any anxiety and emotional reactions that can aggravate the problem.

Abdominal Migraine (XXII-2)

Etiology, Symptoms, and Signs

Abdominal migraine is a migraine equivalent that occurs mostly in children. Many synonyms exist, including periodic syndrome of children, cyclic vomiting, recurrent abdominal pain and headache, and navel colic. The symptoms complex consists of recurrent and identical attacks of periumbilical pain, nausea, vomiting, headache, pallor, perspiration, slowing of the pulse, fever, occasional diarrhea, and limb pains. Attacks usually last less than 6 hours, with most occurring in children between the ages of 3 and 10, particularly in those whose parents have migraine (72). No abdominal symptoms are noted between attacks.

The close relationships between recurrent abdominal crisis and migraine was substantiated by Farquhar (73), who found that one-third of those in a series of 112 children between the ages of 3 and 15 with this syndrome suffered from associated migraine while one or more relatives of two-thirds of these children had migraine. The combination of migraine and abdominal pain was seen in 20% of 73 children aged 9 to 15 who had migraine and in 12% of 100 migraineurs aged 50 to 66 (74). It has also been noted that a significant percentage of children who have recurrent abdominal pain (crises) develop migraine during adult life.

Diagnosis and Treatment

Bruyn (72) emphasized that, if the physician takes the trouble to explore the patient's biography in detail, and a history emerges of common or classic migraine attacks, the diagnosis is made whether the abdominal attacks replace migraine attacks or are associated with them. The diagnosis is also more probable when a family member has migraine. If ergotamine is prescribed and the attacks then diminish or even cease altogether, this can be interpreted as confirmation of the diagnosis.

Because the symptoms and signs simulate those of appendicitis, biliary colic, pancreatitis, lead intoxication, and gallbladder disease, these should be excluded. Bruyn (72) cited reports of adult patients with abdominal migraine who had been mistakenly subjected to as many as five futile laparotomies and of one patient who underwent cholecystectomy and thoracic sympathectomy and subsequently became a morphine addict. Obviously, therefore, a thorough physical and laboratory examination are essential to exclude the possibility of an intra-abdominal disease.

Bruyn (72) further emphasized that the diagnosis should not be difficult if the following points are borne in mind: (a) migraine in the history of the patient or relatives; (b) repetition of identical abdominal crises; (c) attack-free intervals; (d) absence of systemic signs such as an increase in erythrocyte sedementation rate (ESR), leukocytosis, and abnormal urinalysis results during and between attacks; (e) unremarkable physical examination during and between attacks; (f) normal ECG during and between attacks; (g) positive response to ergotamine; and (h) the occasional presence of other migrainous symptoms, such as nausea, vomiting, perspiration, and body temperature changes. Prevention and treatment are similar to migraine as discussed in Chapter 39.

D. SYSTEMIC DISORDERS

A number of systemic disorders cause abdominal pain that simulates that of intra-abdominal disease but do not require surgical intervention. Laparotomy is not only unnecessary for such patients but can set the stage for postoperative problems associated with the underlying disease as well as for complications of the operation itself. Among the most important of these systemic problems are hematologic disorders and metabolic or biochemical disorders. Because they are complex they produce widespread symptoms and signs, but here only those aspects relevant to abdominal pain are considered.

Hematologic Disorders

Various hematologic conditions can produce abdominal pain as part of their symptom complex. Most have pain as a prominent feature only during a "crisis." In some, however, such as paroxysmal nocturnal hemoglobinurea, pain is a prominent constant feature.

Sickle Cell Anemia

Sickle cell anemia is a chronic hemolytic anemia occurring almost exclusively in blacks. It is characterized by the sickle-shaped red blood cells produced by homozygous inheritance of hemoglobin S (HbS). This condition is a significant cause of morbidity and mortality among blacks. About 0.15% of black children in the United States have the disease (75). The prevalence is lower among adults because patients with sickle cell anemia have a decreased life expectancy.

The protean clinical manifestions of this disorder can all be attributed to a specific molecular lesion, the substitution of valine for glutamic acid in the sixth acid of the beta chain. On exposure to low levels of oxygen a red blood cell containing HbS changes from a biconcave disk to an elongated crescent-shaped or sickle-shaped cell. In addition, sickling is precipitated by a lowering of pH and by an increase in body temperature (75, 76). As a red blood cell sickles it becomes rigid. The distorted but inflexible RBCs plug small arterioles and capillaries, leading to occlusion and infarction. Because sickled RBCs are too fragile to withstand the mechanical trauma of circulation, hemolysis occurs when they are released into the circulation. Almost all the systemic effects of this disease are related to the "sickling" phenomenon and to the increased fragility of the red cell. Severe disease is incompatible with long life and 50% of patients with severe sickle cell anemia are dead before the age of 10 (49). Those in the surviving pool of patients often develop a crisis. Recent improvement in treatment has increased survival (76).

Symptoms and Signs

With heterozygous inheritance patients have sickling trait but are normal and do not experience hemolysis, painful crises, or thrombotic complications. In contrast, the clinical manifestations in homozygotes are caused by anemia and by tissue ischemia and infarction. Anemia is usually severe but varies greatly among patients, with most patients having mild jaundice. Anemia can be exacerbated in children by acute sequestration of sickle cells in the spleen, producing splenomegaly. If the splenomegaly is severe it can cause abdominal pain because of its capsule stretching and compressing surrounding viscera or impinging on the diaphragm.

Throughout their lives the homozygotes are plagued by recurrent painful crises (76). These episodes can appear with explosive suddenness and attack various parts of the body, particularly the abdomen, chest, and joints. About one-third of the painful crises are preceded by a viral or bacterial infection. The frequency of painful crises is highly variable. A given patient might have months or even years without a crisis and then have a cluster of frequent and severe attacks. In some individuals crises occur more frequently in cold weather, perhaps precipitated by reflex vasospasm, while in others crises occur more often in warm weather when patients are likely to become dehydrated.

The episodic abdominal pain is usually severe and associated with vomiting, and is a frequent feature of the painful vaso-occlusive crisis. The organs most often involved include the liver, gallbladder, and spleen. The severity of the pain and other symptoms simulate those of acute severe intra-abdominal disorders, and thus it is often difficult to distinguish between painful sickle crisis and such acute processes as biliary colic, appendicitis, and perforated viscus. Many patients have undergone surgical exploration because they were thought to have an acute surgical problem. The clue that the patient is undergoing a sickle cell crisis rather than an acute abdomen is the presence of increased sickling on the peripheral blood smear and evidence of some degree of hemolysis. Moreover, whereas abdominal tenderness is common, the guarding is of a voluntary nature because the muscles can relax and bowel sounds are usually normal, with no rebound tenderness.

Those who are SS homozygotes frequently develop attacks of acute pleuritic chest pain with fever. Although the initial chest radiograph is usually unremarkable, an infiltrate can evolve. The important differential is between pneumonitis and pulmonary infarction. Culture and Gram's staining of the sputum help in establishing the presence of pneumonia.

Diagnosis

The diagnosis is made through the history, physical examination, and comprehensive laboratory studies of the blood. The homozygous state is determined by electrophoresis, which shows only HbS and a variable amount of HbF. The heterozygote is recognized by the presence of both HbA and HbS, with more HbA than HbS.

Treatment

Therapy is usually symptomatic. Splenectomy and hematinics have proven valueless (75). Transfusions should be given only for an anemia that is more severe than usual. The severe abdominal pain should be managed with vigorous oral intravenous hydration and with nonopioid and opioid analgesics. In those hospitals in which such services are available, patient-controlled analgesia is an excellent method of providing effective pain relief. Prophylactic antibiotics, pneumococcal vaccine, early identification and treatment of serious bacterial infection, and general prophylaxis have reduced the mortality rate, particularly during childhood (75, 76).

Acute Hemolytic Crisis

In some instances autoimmune hemolytic anemia, thrombotic thrombocytopenia, purpura, or other hemolytic disorders can begin abruptly and cause moderate to severe pain in the abdomen, back, or limbs. The abdominal pain can be severe and the accompanying muscular spasm and rigidity might simulate the signs of an acute surgical emergency (49). Profound prostration and shock can develop, followed by oliguria or anuria. Pallor, jaundice, tachycardia, and other symptoms of severe anemia can be prominent.

Such patients require careful evaluation and supportive therapy consisting of effective pain control, infusion of appropriate fluids, and other measures to prevent or treat shock.

Chronic Hemolytic Anemia

Other congenital hemolytic anemias can also cause abdominal pain as part of their complex clinical manifestations. The major features relate to anemia, jaundice, the occurrence of crises, splenomegaly, and the development of gallstones. The jaundice of hemolytic disease is acholuric, with the bilirubin being unconjugated and thus not excreted in the urine. The spleen is commonly enlarged in this group of patients but usually the degree of enlargement is mild to moderate. If the spleen assumes gigantic proportion, as in a few patients, it can produce abdominal pain described as a vague sensation of oppression or weight in the left side of the abdomen or, less commonly, is the site of an attack of acute abdominal pain (49). Crises can result from the transient failure of red cell production, so-called aplastic crises. It is the hemolytic crisis, however, that produces a manifestation of an acute abdominal catastrophe (see above, Acute Hemolytic Crisis). In these patients the abdominal pain can be severe and accompanied by muscular spasm and rigidity, possibly simulating the signs of an acute surgical emergency.

In some patients symptoms of gallbladder disease might be the initial manifestation of a hemolytic crisis because of one of these congenital hemolytic anemias and can be what brings the patient to the physician (49). The stones are of the pigmented type and are presumed to be the consequence of continuous excessive bilirubin load presented to the liver. Such patients have a progressive increase in the incidence of gallstones with age. In some disorders, particularly in hereditary spherocytosis, as many as 85% of adult patients develop stones.

The therapy of patients with congenital hemolytic anemias is usually supportive. Effective pain control with nonopioid and opioid analgesics in appropriate doses is part of the initial treatment. Fluid replacement and transfusions might be required. In cases of major thalassemia (Cooley's anemia), the obvious benefits of transfusion therapy are partially offset by the risk of iron overload hepatitis and alloimmunization. Despite these problems, children with Cooley's anemia fare better if their hemoblobin is maintained at a level greater than 9 g/dL (49). In view of the increased demand of the hyperplastic marrow, it is reasonable to maintain these patients on a daily supplement of folic acid. Because splenic sequestration contributes to shortened red blood cell survival, many patients derive some benefit from splenectomy because the need for transfusions is decreased. Splenectomy is also indicated if the size of the tumor is so great that it produces severe respiratory problems or is a source of great discomfort because of its encroachment on the diaphragm and other organs.

Biochemical and Biologic Disorders

Acute Intermittent Porphyria (XXII-3)

Acute intermittent porphyria is a dominantly transmitted inherited disorder that can exist in latent form indefinitely or be manifested as acute attacks of neurologic dysfunction precipitated by various environmental and endogenous factors (77, 78).

Etiology and Pathophysiology

The basic enzyme defect in this disease is a 50% decrease of uroporphyrinogen synthetase. Consequently, δ-aminolevulinic acid (ALA), porphobilinogen (PBG), and uroporphyrinogen are produced in excess by the liver and excreted in the urine. This metabolic abnormality is accompanied by acute attacks of mental or abdominal neurologic symptoms. It is inherited as an autosomal dominant trait with an overall prevalence of 5 to 10/100,000 population in the United States. The prevalence, however, is much higher in some countries (77); for example, in Sweden, it is 1/13,000 population (49). The frequency and severity of attacks and prevalence are greater in women (60 to 75%) than in men.

The disease exists in latent form until an attack of acute neurologic dysfunction is precipitated by one of four groups of factors—drugs, starvation, sex hormones, and infection. Drugs implicated in precipitating attacks of acute porphyria include barbiturates, sulfonamides, phenytoin, methsuximide, griseofulvin, meprobamate, amidopyrine, antipyrine, dipyrone, imipramine, ergot preparations, methyldopa, pentazocine, danazol, chloramphenicol, and chlorprotamide (77). Starvation and crash dieting precipitate attacks of porphyria. The deleterious effects of diet relate to the ability of glucose and certain other carbohydrates to block the induction of hepatic ALA synthetase. Female sex hormones are also implicated in precipitating attacks of porphyria; a small percentage (less than 5%) of women with this disorder have an attack during pregnancy. Acute attacks of porphyria can also follow bacterial and viral infections, but the mechanism is unknown.

Symptoms and Signs

Symptoms of the acute attack result from nervous system damage. Any part of the system can be involved, and the specific clinical findings depend on the areas that are affected. The outcome of the acute attack can vary through a spectrum from death to complete recovery, although some patients who recover can retain varying types of neurologic deficits. Symptoms rarely occur before puberty.

Abdominal pain is frequently the initial and most prominent symptom of the porphyric attack, occurring in about 95% of the patients. The pain can be moderate but more frequently is severe in degree and cramping or colicky in nature. It can be localized in one of the lower quadrants or in the periumbilical region, but in some cases it is felt throughout the abdomen. The pain can radiate to the back or loins and is accompanied by vomiting, constipation, and mild abdominal tenderness (77, 78). It has been suggested that the pain results from autonomic neuropathy that causes disturbed gastrointestinal motility or alternating areas of spasm and dilation. Low-grade fever and mild leukocytosis along with the pain can suggest other diagnoses. Other autonomic manifestations include labile hypertension, sinus tachycardia, postural hypotension, and sweating. Because these symptoms can be attributed to various conditions requiring emergency surgery, many patients have already been subjected to unnecessary laparotomy when seen with another acute attack.

Patients can also manifest peripheral neuropathy that is predominantly motor, but sensory components can also be present. Deep tendon reflexes are diminished or absent. Neuralgia in the extremities associated with areas of hypesthesia and paresthesia and foot or wrist drop are typical. CNS involvement can produce an organic brain syndrome, seizures, cerebellar and basal ganglia manifestations, hypothalamic dysfunction, and bulbar paralysis.

Acute attacks can last from days to months and vary in frequency and severity. The characteristic finding of this disease is increased porphyrin precursor excretion in the urine.

Diagnosis

Diagnosis is made by establishing the presence of excessive urinary porphobilinogen. These precursors can be quantitated accurately by chromatographic techniques. Clinically they can be detected by qualitative analysis using the Watson-Schwartz or Hoesch test (77). If these tests are not available, a useful technique involves collecting a sample of urine and exposing it to light and air. Because porphobilinogen is colorless the initial sample appears normal, but on exposure to light or air the urine darkens. This phenomenon is largely accounted for by the formation of porphobilin, a dark brown nonporphyrin oxidation product of porphobilinogen.

Treatment

Treatment involves prevention of attacks, treatment of symptoms, and attempts to reverse the fundamental disease process. Prevention of attacks entails instructing patients to avoid the known precipitating factors listed above. Many patients scheduled for surgery should inform both the anesthesiologist and surgeon of their condition, because they know to avoid the use of thiopental or other barbiturates for sedation or induction of anesthesia.

Pain control is the first step in symptom management. Some believe that phenothiazines can be useful for the control of abdominal pain, presumably by their effects on decreasing autonomic outflow. Usually these patients require large doses of intravenous opioids, either in incremental doses or by continuous infusion. An excellent alternative is patient-controlled analgesia. If these methods do not provide effective relief, serious consideration should be given to the induction of continuous segmental epidural analgesia with a local anesthetic (Chapter 94). This technique has the advantage of providing complete pain relief because it blocks all nociceptive input from the abdomen and interrupts sympathetic efferent impulses, thus helping to decrease the effects of the pathophysiologic process.

Other Porphyrias

Other rare types of porphyrias cause intermittent acute attacks of abdominal pain, including hereditary coproporphyria (HCP) (IASP XXII-4) and variegata porphyria (VP) (IASP XXII-5). Both can be associated with neurologic and mental disturbances. VP also causes photosensitivity and is accompanied by cutaneous lesions. Photosensitivity occurs with HCP, but not as frequently as with VP.

Other Metabolic and Biochemical Disorders

Other metabolic and biochemical disorders that cause abdominal pain include diabetes, uremia, lead and other heavy metal poisoning, food poisoning, and spider bites. In all these conditions abdominal pain is only one of many symptoms and signs. In each case the pain is controlled symptomatically with nonopioid or opioid analgesia or with a combination of these, depending on the severity of the pain.

LEAD POISONING.   Abdominal pain is an especially frequent symptom of lead poisoning in children. Obviously analgesics must be given in reduced but appropriate dosages to provide good pain relief. If the pain is expected to persist for several days or weeks, continuous epidural opioid analgesia is highly effective and has advantages over other methods of administration of these drugs (Chapter 95).

SPIDER BITE.   Spider bite first produces a momentary sharp pain at the site of bite, followed by a cramping pain that begins locally within 15 to 60 minutes and gradually spreads (79). The abdomen becomes boardlike and the waves of pain become excruciating, causing the patient to turn, toss, and cry out (79). Respirations are often labored and grunting. The pain is associated with nausea, vomiting, headache, sweating, salivation, hyperactive reflexes, twitching, tremor, paresthesia of the hands and feet and, occasionally, systolic hypertension. A mild leukocytosis is usual but many patients have high fever. After several hours the pain subsides, although a mild recurrence for 2 to 3 days is common. It can be a week before well-being is restored. Death caused by cardiac or respiratory failure has ensued mostly in children and the aged.

Treatment consists of pain relief measures and administration of antivenom. Initial treatment should begin with pain control with opioids, first administered intravenously and subsequently intramuscularly at regular intervals. If the patient is hospitalized a better alternative would be epidural opioid analgesia or segmental epidural analgesia with local anesthetics. A 10-ml vial of 10% calcium gluconate injected intravenously slowly over 10 to 20 minutes usually produces dramatic but transient cessation of cramps (79, 80). A solution of 10% methocarbamol administered intravenously can also be effective in treating the muscle spasm. When the symptoms are severe, or when the patient is a small child or is at special risk because of other associated medical problems, treatment with Latrodectus antivenom is indicated. An intravenous injection of one vial (2.5 ml) diluted in 50 ml of saline and administered over a 15-minute period is usually effective; this can be repeated within a few hours if symptoms recur (79).

E. EXTRA-ABDOMINAL DISORDERS

Abdominal pain can and often does occur as a referred phenomenon that is part of the symptoms and signs of thoracic or pelvic visceral disease, or as a projected pain phenomenon from disease of the spine or other musculoskeletal or neuropathic disorders. Because most of these are discussed in detail in Chapters

54 through 58 in Section C, Pain in the Chest) and Chapter 67 (Gynecologic Pain), only brief comments are made here in regard to the abdominal pain.

Thoracic and Pelvic Visceral Disease

Diseases arising within the thoracic cavity can produce diaphragmatic irritation or referred pain that is often indistinguishable from pain arising from the pancreas, stomach, or biliary tract. Fortunately, certain general guidelines can be used that help to differentiate a thoracic from an abdominal origin (49). Thoracic pain is almost never associated with abdominal tenderness. Bowel signs are usually present and, with careful questioning, the time sequence reveals that symptoms and signs of a cardiopulmonary or esophageal disorder preceded the development of the abdominal pain.

Acute Myocardial Infarction

Generally, acute myocardial infarction produces characteristic symptoms of retrosternal and anterior chest pain with radiation to one or both arms, neck and, occasionally, the jaw. A significant percentage of patients, however, also have radiation of pain in the epigastrium. Indeed, in some patients, the epigastric pain is the predominant symptom. It is probably caused by an inferior wall infarction that produces diaphragmatic pleuritis with pain referred to the lower chest and abdomen, associated with belching and occasionally back pain. One or more of these symptoms can mimic the initial symptoms of a penetrating ulcer, cholecystitis, or pancreatitis, and can present a difficult differential diagnosis.

In either case it is essential for the patient to be admitted to the hospital, often with a stay in the coronary care unit, while serial electrocardiograms, cardiac monitoring, and cardiac enzyme levels are obtained. The pain of myocardial infarction usually begins to decrease within 12 to 24 hours, whereas if the condition is an acute intra-abdominal problem pain continues and is associated with severe abdominal tenderness, reflex muscle spasm that produces rigid abdomen, and the absence of peristalsis.

Acute Pericarditis

Acute pericarditis of the diaphragmatic portion of the pericardium can cause irritation of the diaphragm that involves not only the central portion, supplied by the phrenic nerve, but also the peripheral part, supplied by the lower 6th and 7th thoracic spinal nerve, with consequent pain and muscle spasm in the lower chest and epigastrium. The pericardial source of the pain can be ascertained by the fact that this pain is markedly aggravated by deep breathing, is associated with dyspnea and triphasic pericardial friction rub, and radiates to the neck and trapezius ridge. On the other hand, all symptoms and signs except the pericardial friction rub can be present with a subdiaphragmatic irritation caused by subphrenic abscess, acute cholecystitis, or pancreatitis.

Pulmonary Embolism

Confusion between the pain of pulmonary embolism (PE) and that of intra-abdominal disease arises primarily with medium-sized emboli that produce a pleuritis with consequent pleuritic pain. If the pleuritis involves the diaphragmatic portion of the pleura the patient might experience pain in the epigastrium and lower part of the thorax laterally and posteriorly. Again, the pain is markedly aggravated by deep breathing and is associated with friction rub and radiographic evidence that the lesion is in the chest.

With a large central embolus the patient experiences sudden, severe, crushing central pain that can radiate to the upper epigastrium. The pre-eminence of pain in the retrosternal region, however, associated with a feeling of impending death (angor animi) that lasts from a few minutes to several hours, should suggest PE. If massive central pulmonary emboli produce certain cardiovascular collapse and death, symptoms are usually not confused with those of an acute abdomen. Other symptoms and signs that differentiate acute PE from an acute intra-abdominal disorder include dyspnea, which is found in most PE patients, hemoptysis, a history of venous disease, changes in blood viscosity, obesity, and a period of prolonged bed rest or inactivity.

Pneumonia

The clinical symptoms and signs of pneumonia include fever, cough, purulent sputum, mild dyspnea, and usually pain, which can be retrosternal or, most frequently, pleuritic, and felt in the side and back of the chest. On the other hand, if the pneumonia involves the diaphragmatic pleura, the patient experiences pain in the lower chest and upper abdomen. A differential diagnosis is aided by the fact and that the pain is exaggerated by deep breathing and coughing and by the presence of rales and other signs of pneumonic consolidation.

Upper Respiratory Infection

The symptoms and signs of upper respiratory infection (URI) in adults are located in the chest and should never cause confusion with those of abdominal disorders. On the other hand, as Kirkpatrick indicated (49), children with an upper respiratory infection can experience nonspecific abdominal pain localized in the right lower quadrant that might be mistaken for that of acute appendicitis. In such cases the lower quadrant pain is caused by a mesenteric adenitis, a relatively uncommon complication that occurs consequent to a respiratory infection and afflicts children 5 to 15 years of age, more commonly in boys than in girls. Characteristically the child has an acute pharyngitis or otitis media and develops cramping periumbilical pain during the recuperative phase. Leukocytosis ranging from 12,000 to 18,000 per mm³ and a mild fever of 99 to 100° F (37.2 to 37.8° C) suggest either appendicitis or mesenteric adenitis. Kirkpatrick (49) suggested that, if signs of URI are still present, re-evaluation as an outpatient in 12 hours should help to avoid an unnecessary operation and minimize the risk of missing appendicitis. If the URI has resolved but the pain persists, however, then hospital admission, repeat blood work, and close observation are necessary to avoid missing an attack of acute appendicitis.

Esophageal Disease

Acute and chronic esophagitis produced by chemical or infectious disorders often cause pain in the sternum that extends down into the epigastrium. The pain is usually constant with periodic increases in intensity produced by esophageal spasm, and is markedly aggravated by swallowing (odynophagia). It is rare for the pain to be located only in the epigastrium and therefore the differential diagnosis, should not be difficult especially with a history of ingestion of a chemical or other signs of esophagitis.

Esophageal motor disorders can also cause retrosternal pain with radiation to the epigastrium and back and also to the neck, jaw, teeth, or both arms, thus simulating the pain of acute myocardial infarction. The pain, which lasts seconds to many hours, is aggravated by cold liquids, solids, and emotional stress and is partially relieved by nitroglycerin. The differential diagnosis is aided by manometry, scintigraphy, and provocative tests using pharmacologic agents.

Esophageal lacerations and rupture can also cause pain in the lower sternum and epigastrium; if located in the lower part of the esophagus the epigastric pain can be the most prominent. Spontaneous rupture, called Boerhaave's syndrome, also causes excruciating, crushing, or tearing pain in the lower retrosternal region and epigastrium. Because the rupture occurs during intense vomiting following a large meal, together with other symptoms and signs, it is easily differentiated from intra-abdominal disorders.

Similarly, carcinoma of the esophagus produces moderate to severe retrosternal pain with radiation to the epigastrium when the lesions are in the lower part of the esophagus. The pain radiates to the back and interscapular region, is continuous, and is aggravated by food ingestion. The differential diagnosis is aided by the history and by radiography, CT scanning, and esophagoscopy.

Retroesophageal reflux caused by incompetent gastroesophageal sphincter also produces a symptom complex characterized by retrosternal epigastric burning pain, dysphagia, and occasional bleeding. When these signs and symptoms are present the diagnosis should be suspected from the history and confirmed by esophagoscopy, acid perfusion test, and pH monitoring.

Gynecologic Disorders

Some gynecologic conditions can mimic those of acute abdomen by producing pain in the right or left lower quadrant or in the suprapubic region, with radiation to the back. These include acute salpingitis, twisted ovarian cyst, ruptured ovarian follicle, and various other disorders (Chapter 67). To avoid a misdiagnosis it is mandatory for pelvic and rectal examinations to be carried out; if necessary, a pregnancy test is done. Pelvic examination reveals exquisite cervical tenderness (other differential diagnostic procedures are discussed in Chapter 67 and summarized in Table 65-1).

Pain of Neuropathic Origin

In Chapter 58 it was noted that most pathologic processes of the thoracic portion of the spinal cord and of the thoracic spinal nerve roots or peripheral nerves produce similar pain syndromes in the chest and the abdomen. They therefore have been discussed in detail in Chapter 58. To avoid repetition, only a few comments pertinent to abdominal pain are made here.

Brain Lesions

It is uncommon in the brain or brain stem to cause pain only in the abdomen without causing pain or other sensory disturbances in the extremities. The one exception is a rare form of epilepsy that can cause pain in the abdomen as an aura or as part of the seizure itself (81). Abdominal epilepsy is more common during childhood and can abate spontaneously in adolescence. The patient usually complains of unpleasant sensations that can vary from paresthesiae to pain. Some of these patients were described as having intussusception in association with their epileptiform disorder. Motor phenomena and a sensory deficit are usually not present (82), but autonomic phenomena are common. Most patients with this type of seizure

disorder also report environmental distortions and emotional changes.

Central pain caused by vascular lesions or by tumors of the brain and brain stem usually produce pain in the contralateral extremities and side of the trunk and other signs and symptoms of brain stem lesions. Although some of the pain can be felt in the abdominal wall on the same side, it is rarely, if ever, localized only to the abdomen.

Lesions of the Spinal Cord, Meninges, and Epidural Space

Intramedullary lesions or diseases of the lower thoracic portion of the spinal cord, including tumors, syringomyelia, trauma, multiple sclerosis, abscess, hemorrhage and other conditions, can produce pain in the trunk that includes the abdominal wall. The pain can be a spontaneous, burning, diffuse, poorly localized pain that is continuous or explosive in nature or, in some cases, the pain can have a radicular (segmental) distribution involving several segments, depending on the extent of the lesion; this is often associated with hyperalgesia, hyperpathia, and paresthesia.

Extramedullary intrathecal lesions such as primary or metastatic lesions, abscesses, and hemorrhages initially produce low back pain localized around the segments of the lesions. Subsequently, however, the pain becomes radicular and is aggravated by straining and coughing and is associated with paravertebral tenderness and paresthesia. These are followed by sensory loss, muscle weakness, and lower motor neuron signs at the level of the lesion.

Epidural spinal cord compression caused by primary or metastatic tumor, hemorrhage, posterior disk protrusion, abscess, or hemorrhage produces localized low back pain at the level of the site of lesion in 95% of patients and bilateral radicular pain involving the abdominal wall in 55% (83). The pain is aggravated by neck flexion, straight leg raising, coughing, sneezing, and the Valsalva maneuver. Deep palpation and fist pounding produce back tenderness. Early in the course of the disease no other signs are seen but muscle weakness develops later, varying from mild weakness to paraplegia. Numbness and paresthesia are noted in 50% of patients and bladder and bowel dysfunction are frequent (57%) (see Chapter 58 for details).

Arachnoiditis, characterized by inflammation and fibrosis of the arachnoid membrane, is a well-recognized cause of chronic pain. Although the cauda equina is the most common site, arachnoiditis can occur at any spinal level. It can be focal and involve only one root, thereby leading to a segmental pain syndrome with variable loss of sensory and motor function. Arachnoiditis can also affect multiple segments and lead to a more diffuse pain syndrome in the lower trunk and abdomen. The pain of arachnoiditis is constant but is worsened by physical activity. Often a dysesthetic component is present, and paresthesiae are common. Patients often report both a deep aching and a superficial sharp jabbing pain. This type of pain is not often ameliorated by narcotics.

Lesions of Roots and Trunks of the Thoracic Nerves (XX-3)

Lesion of the roots produces a radiculopathy and consequent radiculalgia or segmental pain. The pathology can be a result of an acute or chronic infectious process or of mechanical compression.

HERPES ZOSTER. Herpes zoster is an infection by the varicella-zoster virus that involves the ganglion cells, rootlets, and posterior horn. It produces a continuous aching, itching, or burning pain with superimposed bouts of severe lancinating pain. Hyperalgesia and hyperesthesia are present in the affected segments. These patients usually develop a rash in the involved segments that spreads along the entire nerve or part of the affected nerve, frequently in the upper or lower anterior abdomen. Some patients develop postherpetic neuralgia, which is a chronic condition that produces severe, intractable, continuous, unrelenting and burning pain and itching accompanied by severe spasm with stabbing lancinating pain that persists long after the acute phase. The skin of the posterior and lateral lower thoracic cavity and abdominal wall has dried white or brownish black scars that represent the healing of the vesicles. Patients experience hyperalgesia, hyperesthesia, and hyperpathia and frequently hypesthesia, depression, sleep disturbance, anorexia, lassitude, and constipation (Chapters 13 and 58).

TABES DORSALIS. Tabes dorsalis is one of the many forms of tertiary syphilis. Formerly a common affliction, the development of serologic testing and effective antibiotic therapy have made this an exceedingly rare disease in most developed nations. Pains are often the earliest signs of tabes; the vast majority of patients has typical lightning pains during the course of the disease. The electric shock-like stabbing pain might last only a brief moment or be continuous for days. Girdle-like pains about the thorax or abdomen are common, although most patients have pains in the limbs. Paresthesiae and objective sensory changes in the region of the pain occur in about 25% of patients. Most patients with tabes dorsalis have altered position sense, absent deep tendon reflexes, hypotonia, ataxia, and Argyll Robertson pupils (miotic pupils that fail to react to light but contract with accommodation).

Even worse than the intermittent lancinating pains is the pain syndrome known as *"gastric crisis."* This has been reported in about 10% of tabetics. The patient has a sudden onset of agonizing epigastric pain associated with nausea and vomiting. Such an attack can last for days, but spontaneous remission always occurs. This pain syndrome is exceedingly difficult to differentiate from renal or biliary colic or penetrating ulcer on the basis of the clinical presentation alone. A similar pain syndrome can affect the lower abdomen and pelvic areas.

COMPRESSION. Many factors can cause compression radiculopathy, including tumors, disk protrusions, vertebral fractures, osteophytes, and adhesive arachnoiditis. All of these produce a segmental sharp burning pain, hyperesthesia, hyperalgesia, hypesthesia, and dysesthesia in the segments involved.

Protrusion of the intervertebral disk deserves special note here because, contrary to former teachings, herniation of a thoracic intervertebral disk is now being recognized with increasing frequency. In most cases it involves one of the lower thoracic disks, producing radiculalgia with segmental pain in the lower abdomen. Initially the pain is vague and poorly localized and can be referred laterally or bilaterally in the abdomen. Typically the pain is aggravated by neck flexion and by an increase in intraspinal pressure resulting from coughing, sneezing, or straining. The pain is usually relieved by recumbency. Subjective numbness and paresthesia, such as coldness and a burning sensation, are early and outstanding symptoms. If the disk is posterior it produces compression of the spinal cord with weakness and heaviness of the leg. Physical signs of upper neuron damage can also be present, including hyperactive deep reflexes, spasticity, and the Babinski response. Early recognition and removal prevent irretrievable damage to the spinal cord (Chapter 58).

Other causes of the segmental abdominal pain of neuralgia are vertebral compression resulting from arthritis, metastatic or traumatic fractures, tumors of the vertebrae, osteomyelitis of normal curvature, and paravertebral compression resulting from adenopathy. All these usually produce unilateral segmental neuralgia characterized by continuous burning or sharp pain that affects part or the entire segment of the nerve and is associated with paroxysms of stabbing pain. Patients frequently have paravertebral tenderness and segmental hyperalgesia, hyperesthesia, and hypesthesia, and usually show radiographic evidence of the disease.

Intercostal Neuropathy

One or more of the lower six or seven intercostal nerves can be irritated, infected, or damaged by lesions of the ribs, which can include trauma, fractures, and primary or metastatic tumors. These conditions are characterized by superficial continuous burning pain in the lower part of the posterior and lateral chest and the abdominal wall. Pain is usually unilateral.

Abdominal Cutaneous Nerve Entrapment Syndrome (XX-5)

The cutaneous entrapment syndrome is a special type of intercostal neuropathy that deserves special mention because it causes pain in the anterior abdominal wall or can cause segmental neuralgia.

Etiology

The most common type is a result of entrapment of one or more of the anterior cutaneous branches of the thoracoabdominal intercostal nerve(s) in the rectus sheath. Applegate (84) described a small fibromuscular ring near the lateral margin of the rectus abdominis muscle through which the intercostal nerve turns sharply in an anterior direction on its terminal course through the skin in which it is firmly anchored. The nerve enters the ring accompanied by the epigastric artery and vein from which it is separated by a well-defined fatty mass. All these structures continue in a channel between the fibers of the rectus muscle and its anterior sheath, passing subcutaneously and ending at the skin (Fig. 64-5A).

In some patients the walls of the muscular channels are split or spread apart. This allows the fat and neurovascular bundle to herniate into the subcutaneous tissue, where they are intermittently compressed or become incarcerated as a tender mass that is palpable from the surface (Fig. 64-5B). The weakness of the channel is induced by sustained and increased intra-abdominal pressure or by stretching of the abdomen during pregnancy, or is consequent to severe ascites or a large intra-abdominal tumor. The weakness can also be caused by a chronic, persistent strong cough.

Contraction of the abdominal muscles causes local compression of the trapped nerve in the muscular

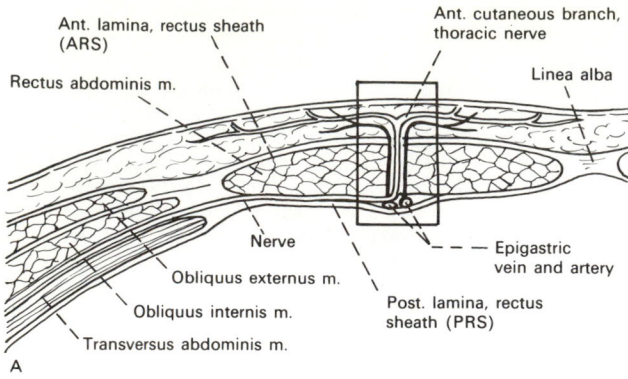

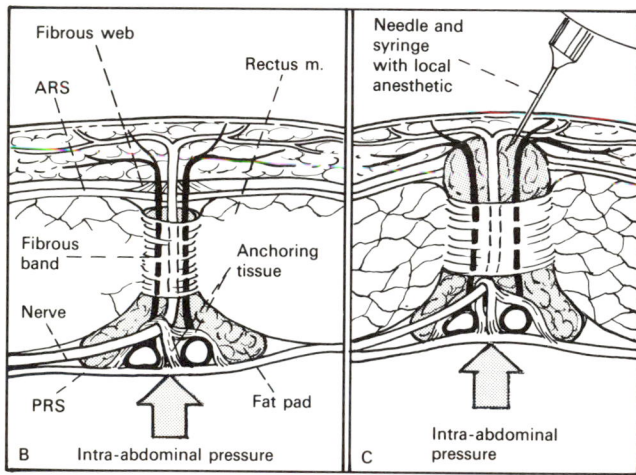

FIG. 64-5. Mechanism of abdominal cutaneous nerve entrapment syndromes. **A.** Normal anatomy of the neurovascular bundle as it passes through the fibrous muscular foramen in the rectus muscle, together with increased intra-abdominal pressure, cause the nerve, which is anchored by fibrous tissue, to be stretched. **B.** Herniation of the neurovascular bundle and the fat pad surrounding it through the fibromuscular foramen in the rectus muscle and the aponeurotic opening at the rectus margin. **C.** Technique of injecting a local anesthetic to confirm the diagnosis and as part of the treatment. Modified from Applegate, W.V.: Abdominal cutaneous nerve entrapment syndrome. Surgery, *71*:118, 1972.

channel, which provokes bouts of sharp burning pain. Pain is also produced by sudden twisting or lateral flexion of the spine away from the affected side, causing the nerve to be stretched and pressed tightly against unyielding fibrous tissue in the ring.

Entrapment of the lateral cutaneous branch of the thoracoabdominal intercostal nerves can also occur as each traverses the internal and external intercostal and serratus anterior muscles to reach the subcutaneous tissue, where it divides into anterior and posterior subdivisions (Chapter 53). Indeed, the cutaneous branch of the posterior primary division can also become trapped as it traverses the paraspinal muscle and their fascia.

Symptoms and Signs

Initially most patients experience bouts of intermittent dull aching pain that can be associated with sharp piercing pain in the distribution of the dermatome and paresthesia, hyperesthesia, and local tenderness—the characteristics of neuropathy. The distribution of the pain symptoms depends on the site of entrapment and on the number of nerves involved. In most cases one anterior cutaneous nerve is entrapped, causing pain in the medial part of the anterior abdominal wall over the rectus muscle. The pain is reproduced by localized pressure with a fingertip. Entrapment of the lateral cutaneous branch produces pain and sensory disturbance in its distribution, and is also reproduced by fingertip pressure at the midaxillary line.

Diagnosis

Pain from cutaneous nerve entrapment can be confused with acute pain caused by intra-abdominal visceral disease; the latter must be ruled out to avoid unnecessary surgery. The diagnosis is made by keeping entrapment syndromes in mind, by the characteristics (quality, location, intensity, and duration of pain), and by reproducing the pain with fingertip pressure. The anterior cutaneous syndrome is also reproduced by increasing the tension of the rectus abdominis muscles by having the patient raise the head and shoulders from the examining table. Often the symptoms are also reproduced by strong coughing efforts in the standing position. The diagnosis is confirmed by prompt and complete relief of the pain following injection of the localized tender area with 1 to 2 ml of a local anesthetic solution (Fig. 64-5C).

Treatment

Conservative measures such as heat, cold, massage, and transcutaneous electric nerve stimulation (TENS) can provide moderate but temporary relief of the pain. Repeated injection with a local anesthetic usually produces only temporary relief, although some patients experience progressively longer intervals of pain relief with a series of injections. In patients who obtained complete but only transient relief of the pain following a series of blocks, Mehta and associates (85, 86) recommended injection of a 5% aqueous phenol solution. They reported relief at 2 to 3 weeks postinjection in 60% of 103 patients treated and long-term relief in 70% of 82 patients who could be contacted several months after injection. An alternative method is surgical exploration and relief of the entrapment.

Pain Primarily of Musculoskeletal Origin

Disorders of the lower thoracic spine are likely to produce localized pain in the lower part of the back, with occasional spread to the lateral part of the thorax; rarely do they produce pain in the abdomen unless the lesion causes a radiculopathy or neuropathy. Occasionally fractures of the anterior part of the lower ribs or fracture or dislocation of the lower costal cartilages can result in upper abdominal pain. The epigastric pain can also be caused by damage, infection, or irritation of the xiphoid process. Finally, myofascial syndromes involving one or more of the abdominal muscles can cause moderate to severe continuous pain. These three conditions are discussed briefly here.

Slipping Rib Syndrome

The slipping rib syndrome, also known as a rib tip syndrome or slipped rib cartilage syndrome, is characterized by sharp stabbing pain localized to the upper quadrant or to the epigastrium. The pain is present at rest and is aggravated by movement, especially twisting, hyperextension, or raising the arm. Occasionally the pain is dull aching or burning, located below the costal margin and radiating to the back. The condition is discussed in detail in Chapter 58.

Xiphoidalgia

Xiphoidalgia, or painful tender xiphoid process, is characterized by spontaneous deep aching or sharp pain that varies in intensity from a slight to agonizing discomfort simulating that of myocardial infarction. The pain is felt in the region of the xiphoid process, with radiation to the epigastrium and occasionally to the lower chest. The pain is aggravated by movements that act on xiphoid processes such as bending, stooping, or turning or by an increase in intragastric pressure caused by a large meal. The pain can be constant or recur several times a day and last for minutes to several hours. Pressure on the xiphoid process produces spontaneous pain that is felt most severely in the region of the xiphoid process, with radiation to the epigastrium, retrosternally and occasionally to the precordium. The condition can persist for weeks or months but usually disappears spontaneously (Chapter 58).

Epidemic Myalgia

Epidemic myalgia, also known as Bornholm disease, epidemic pleurodynia, and devil's grip, has already been discussed in Chapter 55 (see Disorders of the Pleura). It is mentioned here because it affects not only the intercostal but also the abdominal muscles in many patients, and causes abdominal pain. After a nondescript course of from 1 to 10 days adult patients experience bouts of severe sharp pain in the lateral chest wall, while in children the pain involves the upper abdominal muscles. The involved muscles are usually tender. Bouts of pain are separated by symptom-free intervals. Fever, headache, and pharyngitis are present.

The illness usually lasts 3 to 7 days, but relapses can occur. Specific diagnosis is made by isolation of the virus from the throat or feces early in the course of the disease or by demonstration of a rising titer of type-specific neutralizing antibodies.

Treatment is usually conservative, consisting of pain control using systemic analgesics; these also relieve headache and reduce fever.

Myofascial Pain Syndromes

Myofascial pain syndromes are common causes of pain in various parts of the body. Their etiology, pathophysiology, characteristics of the pain, other symptoms, diagnostic procedures, and therapy are discussed in detail in Chapter 21. Here I briefly mention the characteristics of the syndromes with trigger points that can be located in the externus obliquus, transversus abdominis, and rectus abdominis muscles. Painful trigger points are frequently found in the muscle of the anterior wall and all major quadrants; in particular the rectus abdominis muscles usually contain multiple trigger points.

These syndromes are important because trigger points in these abdominal muscles can initiate somato-

visceral reflex phenomena that might induce visceral dysfunction, possibly resulting in as much distress as that induced from the referred pain (87). Symptoms referred from these myofascial trigger points commonly confuse the diagnosis by mimicking those of visceral disease. Sola (88) has successfully treated several patients with confirmed cardiospasm by injection of these trigger points (TPs) with dilute solutions of local anesthetics. In these patients the TPs were located in the left upper rectus abdominis muscles. Edegawa and Friedman (89) described a similar treatment for cardiospasm as well as for functional gastrointestinal disturbances, such as bloating, diarrhea, and constipation involving injection of all four major abdominal quadrants.

Pain patterns of TPs in the abdominal muscles, especially the obliques, are less consistent from patient to patient than are the patterns for most other muscles. Abdominal pain referred from TPs on one side frequently cause bilateral pain. In addition to the localized and referred pain, patients can complain of burning, fullness, bloating, and swelling of gas, although objective evidence is frequently missing.

Figures 64-6 and 64-7 depict the location of TPs and the areas of referred pain that they produce. The solid area of referred pain in the figures indicates the essential zone—the site of pain that is experienced by most patients. The area that is stippled indicates the spillover zone—the site of pain that is experienced by some patients. Referred pain from myofascial TPs in the abdominal musculature is likely to appear in the same quadrant and occasionally in any other quadrant of the abdomen, as well as in the back (87, 88). These TPs can initiate somatovisceral responses, including projectile vomiting, anorexia, nausea, intestinal colic, diarrhea, urinary bladder and sphincter spasm, and

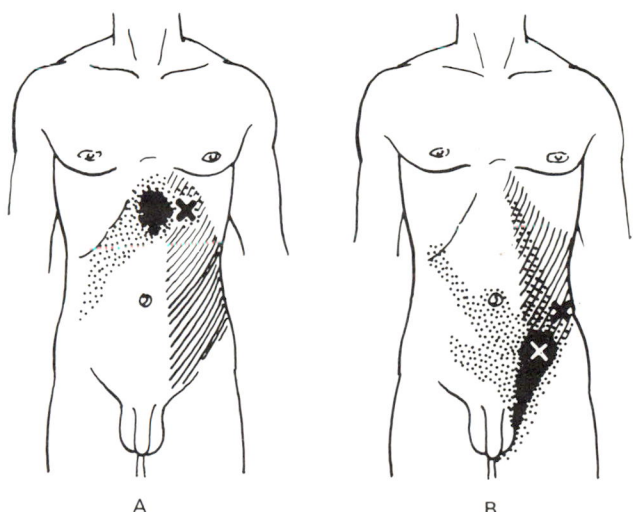

FIG. 64-6. Pain patterns produced and sustained by trigger points (X) in the abdominal muscles. *A.* Trigger point in the external oblique muscle overlying the lower part of the anterior chest wall. *B.* Pain in the groin and testicle, with radiation to the upper lateral abdominal caused by a trigger point in the lower lateral abdominal wall musculature. The solid black depicts the essential zone and the stippled pattern depicts the spillover zone. See text for details.

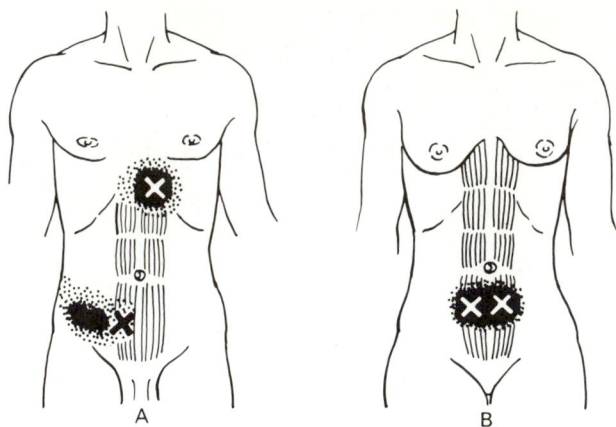

FIG. 64-7. Pain patterns produced and sustained by trigger points (X) in the rectus abdominis muscle. *A.* Right lower quadrant pain and tenderness in the region of McBurney's point caused by a trigger point in the lateral border of the ipsilateral rectus abdominis muscles and by a trigger point at the upper attachment of the rectus muscle that occasionally causes lower esophageal spasm ("cardiospasm"). *B.* Pain pattern in the hypogastric region produced by trigger points in the lower part of both rectus abdominis muscles. Through somatovisceral reflexes, the trigger point can intensify the pain of dysmenorrhea or can cause other types of visceral disfunction. The solid black depicts the essential zone and the stippled pattern depicts the spillover zone.

dysmenorrhea (87). When such visceral symptoms occur with abdominal pain and tenderness, the combination can strongly mimic the manifestations of acute visceral disease, especially appendicitis and cholecystitis.

Activation of TPs in the abdominal musculature can be a result of trauma or stress of the muscle or can represent viscerosomatic responses to visceral disease, including peptic ulcer, intestinal parasites, ulcerative colitis, diverticulosis, and cholecystitis (87). Once activated, TPs can then be perpetuated by emotional stress, occupational strain, faulty posture, and over-enthusiasm for fitness (fitness exercises).

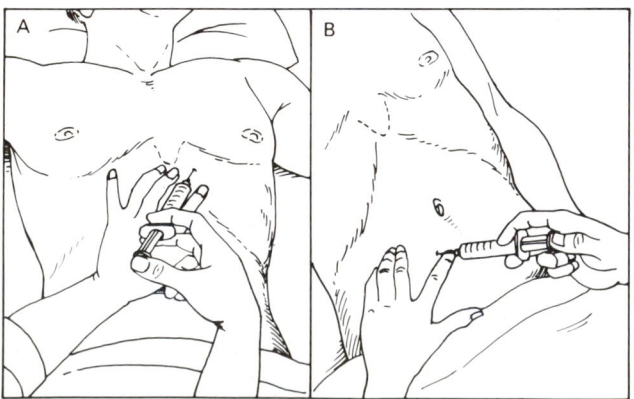

FIG. 64-8. Technique of injection in patients with myofascial syndromes caused by trigger points in the abdominal muscles. *A.* Injection of the trigger point in the upper part of the external oblique muscle responsible for the pain pattern shown in Figure 64-6A. *B.* Injection of the lower part of the right rectus muscle to eliminate the pain shown in Figure 64-7A.

TPs are located by systemic point pressure of the area in which the TPs are suspected to exist. When the pressure is applied to the TP, patients experience aggravation of pain similar to the spontaneous pain that they have had. Local muscle twitch and other signs can also be felt.

Treatment

Treatment of myofascial syndromes is discussed in detail in Chapter 21. It consists of therapy directed at decreasing the activity of the TP, supportive measures, and corrective actions. I prefer penetration of the TP and injection with a local anesthetic (Fig. 64-8), as described in detail in Chapter 21. Stretch and spray of the involved abdominal muscles involves hyperextension of the spine, protrusion of the abdomen, and a downward spray pattern. Corrective actions include self-administration of ischemic compression, learning how to breathe with the abdomen (diaphragm), and carrying out various progressive exercises (87).

Abdominal Pain of Tegumentary Origin

Painful Scars

Pain in the abdominal or flank region can be caused by post-traumatic or postoperative scars that usually contain small neuromata. These painful abdominal disorders are similar to those of post-thoracotomy and postmastectomy pain (Chapter 5). The scars can occur in any part of the abdomen but develop most frequently following a subcostal curved incision for cholecystectomy, a flank incision for operation on the kidney, and incision for appendectomy. They are especially likely to develop into painful scars if the scar drains persistently or is infected.

Patients usually complain of a continuous aching, burning pain in the region of the scar and, around it, occasional bouts of lancinating pain that can develop spontaneously with movement of the trunk, be provoked by pressure on the neuroma, or result from both. In most patients the pain is mild to moderate and can be managed with nonopioid analgesics and adjuvants. In patients with severe lancinating pain, diagnostic and prognostic blocks consisting of infiltration of small amounts of dilute solutions of a local anesthetic into the scar can be performed. If properly done these produce complete pain relief that lasts for several hours, usually beyond the duration of the pharmacologic effect of the local anesthetic. Repeated injections provide longer and longer periods of pain relief and can be curative. Injection of alcohol into a neuroma can produce prolonged relief (Chapter 94, section on local infiltration). If injection therapy does not produce prolonged pain relief, however, excision of the scar by plastic surgery should be considered.

Acute and Chronic Dermatologic Diseases

Various acute and chronic dermatologic diseases can involve the abdominal wall and flank region and cause pain (Chapter 27).

Chronic postburn pain can also involve the abdomen and cause persistent aching burning pain in the site of the postburn scar. These disorders are often difficult to treat, but if the pain is sufficiently severe, intercostal block with a long-lasting local anesthetic should be given a trial. This chronic pain syndrome might also respond to intravenous infusion of local anesthetics (Chapter 94).

Postoperative Pain

Acute postoperative pain is most severe following upper abdominal and thoracic operations and following renal surgery. The incidence and severity of pain following lower abdominal surgery are lower but moderate to severe pain occurs in a significant percentage of patients. This condition is discussed in detail in Chapter 25.

REFERENCES

1. Sleisenger, M.H., and Fordtran, J.S., (eds.): Gastrointestinal Disease: Pathophysiology, Diagnosis and Management. 3rd Ed. Philadelphia, W.B. Saunders, 1983.
2. Rutherford, R.B. (ed.): Vascular Surgery. 2nd Ed. Philadelphia, W.B. Saunders, 1984.
3. Haimovici, H. (ed.): Vascular Surgery: Principles and Techniques. New York, McGraw-Hill, 1976.
4. Moore, W.S. (ed.): Vascular Surgery: A Comprehensive Review. New York, Grune & Stratton, 1983.
5. Rowe, D.W., et al.: A sex-linked defect in the cross-linking of collagen and elastin associated with the mottled locus in mice. J. Exp. Med., 139:180, 1974.
6. Wolinsky, H., and Glagov, S.: Comparison of abdominal and thoracic aortic and medial structure in mammals—deviation of man from the usual patterns. Circ. Res., 25:677, 1969.
7. Roach, M.R.: An experimental study of the production and time course of post-stenotic dilatation in the femoral and carotid arteries of adult dogs. Circ. Res., 13:537, 1963.
8. Auerbach, O. and Garfinkel, L.: Atherosclerosis and aneurysm of aorta in relation to smoking habits and age. Chest, 78:805, 1980.
9. Swanson, R.J., et al.: Laparotomy as a precipitating factor in the rupture of abdominal aneurysms. Arch. Surg., 115:299, 1980.
10. Tilson, M.D., and Stansel, H.C.: Differences in results for aneurysms versus occlusive disease after bifurcation grafts. Arch. Surg., 115:1173, 1980.
11. Busuttil, R.W., and Brin, B.J.: The diagnosis and management of visceral artery aneurysms. Surgery, 88:619, 1980.
12. Stanley, J.C., and Fry, W.J.: Pathogenesis and clinical significance of splenic artery aneurysms. Surgery, 76:898, 1974.
13. Johansen, K., and Devin, J.: Mycotic aortic aneurysms—a reappraisal. Arch. Surg., 118:583, 1983.
14. Millili, J.J., Lanes, J.S., and Nemir, P.: A study of anastomotic aneurysms following aorto-femoral prosthetic bypass. Ann. Surg., 192:69, 1980.
15. Chandler, J.J.: Letter to the editor. The Einstein sign: The clinical picture of acute cholecystitis caused by ruptured abdominal aortic aneurysm. N. Engl. J. Med., 310:1538, 1984.
16. Johansen, K., and Koepsell, T.: Are aneurysms inherited? JAMA, 256:1934, 1986.
17. Kadir, S., et al.: Tender pulsatile abdominal mass: Abdominal aortic aneurysm or not? Arch. Surg., 115:631, 1980.
18. Lowry, W.F., and Kraft, R.O.: Isolated aneurysms of the iliac artery. Arch. Surg., 113:1289, 1978.
19. Bernstein, E.F.: Ultrasound techniques in the diagnosis and evaluation of abdominal aortic aneurysm. In Noninvasive Diagnostic Techniques in Vascular Disease. Edited by E.F. Bernstein. St. Louis, C.V. Mosby, 1978, pp. 330–338.
20. Axelbaum, S.P., et al.: Computed tomographic evaluation of aortic aneurysm. Am. J. Roentgenol., 127:75, 1976.
21. Johansen, K.: Aneurysms. Sci. Am., 247:110, 1982.
22. Berguer, R. Feldman, A.J., and Karmody, A.M.: Induced thrombosis of inoperable abdominal aortic aneurysms. Surgery, 83:425, 1978.
23. Karmody, A.M., et al. The current position of non-resective treatment for abdominal aortic aneurysm. Surgery, 94:591, 1983.
24. Bandyk, D.F., Florence, M.G., and Johansen, K.H.: Ischemia accompanying ruptured abdominal aortic aneurysms. J. Surg. Res., 30:297, 1981.
25. O'Donnell, T.F., Darling, R.D., and Linton, R.R.: Is 80 years too old for aneurysmectomy? Arch. Surg., 111:1250, 1980.
26. Hicks, G.L. et al.: Survival improvement following aortic aneurysm resection. Ann. Surg., 181:861, 1975.
27. DeBakey, M.D., et al.: Aneurysm of abdominal aorta: Analysis of graft replacement therapy 1–11 years after operation. Ann. Surg., 160:622, 1964.
28. Szilagyi, D.E., et al.: Contribution of abdominal aortic aneurysmectomy to prolongation of life. Ann. Surg., 164:678, 1966.
29. Williams, L.F.: Vascular insufficiency of the intestines. Gastroenterology, 61:757, 1971.
30. Grendell, J.H., and Ockner, R.K.: Vascular diseases of the bowel. In Gastrointestinal Disease: Pathophysiology, Diagnosis, Management. 3rd Ed. Edited by M.H. Sleisenger and J.S. Fordtran. Philadelphia, W.B. Saunders, 1983, pp. 1543.
31. Granger, D.N., et al.: Intestinal blood flow. Gastroenterology, 78:837, 1980.
32. Shepherd, A.P.: Local control of intestinal oxygenation and blood flow. Ann. Rev. Physiol., 44:13, 1982.
33. Kern, J.C., Reynolds, D.G., and Swan, K.G.: Adrenergic stimulation and blockade in mesenteric circulation of the baboon. Am. J. Physiol., 234:E457, 1978.
34. Pawlik, W., Shepherd, A.P., and Jacobson, E.D.: Effects of vasoactive agents on intestinal oxygen consumption and blood flow in dogs. J. Clin. Invest., 56:484, 1975.
35. Watt-Boolsen, S.: Non-occlusive intestinal infarction. Acta Chir. Scand., 143:365, 1977.
36. Haglund, J., and Lundgren, O.: Non-occlusive acute intestinal vascular failure. Br. J. Surg., 66:155, 1979.
37. Wittenberg, J., et al.: A radiologic approach to the patient with acute extensive bowel ischemia. Radiology, 106:13, 1973.
38. Grendell, J.H., and Ockner, R.K. Mesenteric venous thrombosis. Gastroenterology, 82:358, 1982.
39. Robinson, J.W.L., et al.: Response of the intestinal mucosa to ischemia. Gut, 22:512, 1981.
40. Granger, D.N., et al.: Effect of local arterial hypotension on cat intestinal capillary permeability. Gastroenterology, 79:474, 1980.
41. Watson, W.C., and Sadikali, F.: Celiac axis compression. Experience with 20 patients and a critical appraisal of the syndrome. Ann. Intern. Med., 86:278, 1977.
42. Silvers, L.W., Royster, T.S., and Mulcare, R.J.: Peripheral arterial emboli and factors in their recurrence rate. Ann. Surg., 192:232, 1980.
43. Nicholls, S.C., et al.: Hemodynamic parameters in the diagnosis of mesenteric insufficiency. Presented at the Symposium for Noninvasive Techniques in Vascular Disease. San Diego, February, 1979.
44. Golden, D.A., Ring, E.J., and McLean, G.K.: Percutaneous transluminal angioplasty in the treatment of abdominal angina. Am. J. Radiol., 139:247, 1982.
45. Zuidema, G.D., et al.: Superior mesenteric artery embolectomy. Ann. Surg., 159:548, 1964.
46. Athanasoulis, C.A., et al.: Vasodilatory drugs in the management of non-occlusive bowel ischemia. Gastroenterology, 68:148, 1975.
47. Reul, G.J., et al.: Surgical treatment of abdominal angina: Review of 25 patients. Surgery, 75:682, 1974.
48. Stoney, R.J., Ehrenfeld, W.K., and Wylie, E.J.: Revascularization methods in chronic visceral ischemia caused by atherosclerosis. Ann. Surg., 186:468, 1977.
49. Kirkpatrick, J.R.: The Acute Abdomen: Diagnosis and Management. Baltimore, Williams & Wilkins, 1984, p. 287.
50. Fauci, A.S., Haynes, B.F., and Katz, P.: The spectrum of vasculitis: Clinical pathologic, immunologic and therapeutic considerations. Ann. Intern. Med., 89:660, 1978.
51. Hahn, B.H.: Systemic erythematosis. In Harrison's Principles of Internal Medicine. 11th Ed. Edited by E. Braunwald, et al.: New York, McGraw-Hill, 1987, pp. 1418–1423.

52. Bender, M.D., and Ockner, R.K.: Disease of the peritoneum, mesentery and diaphragm. *In* Gastrointestinal Disease: Pathophysiology, Diagnosis, Management. 3rd Ed. Edited by M.H. Sleisenger and J.S. Fordtran. Philadelphia, W.B. Saunders, 1983, pp. 1559–1596.

53. Meyerhoff, J.: Familial Mediterranean fever: A report of a large family, review of the literature and discussion of the frequency of amyloidosis. Medicine, *59*:66, 1980.

54. Zemer, M.D., et al.: A control trial of colchicine in preventing attacks of FMF. N. Engl. J. Med., *291*:932, 1974.

55. Antman, K.H.: Clinical presentation and natural history of benign and malignant mesothelioma. Semin. Oncol., *8*:313, 1981.

56. Walsch, D., and Williams, G.: Surgical biopsy studies of omental and peritoneal nodules. Br. J. Surg., *58*:428, 1971.

57. Meyer, M.: Distribution of intra-abdominal malignant seeding. Am. J. Roentgenol., *119*:198, 1973.

58. Ahrend, T., and Thompson, B.: Hernia of the foramen of Bochdalek in the adult. Am. J. Surg., *122*:612, 1971.

59. Hood, R.: Traumatic diaphragmatic hernia. Ann. Thorac. Surg., *12*:311, 1971.

60. Reber, H.A.: Abdominal abscesses and gastrointestinal fistules. *In* Gastrointestinal Disease: Pathophysiology, Diagnosis, Management. 3rd Ed. Edited by M.H. Sleisenger and J.S. Fordtran. Philadelphia, W.B. Saunders, 1983, pp. 319–330.

61. Hirschmann, J.V.: Localized infections and abscesses. *In* Harrison's Principles of Internal Medicine. 11th Ed. Edited by E. Braunwald, et al. New York, McGraw-Hill, 1987, pp. 482–484.

62. Ariel, I.M., and Kazarian, K.K.: Classification, diagnosis and treatment of subphrenic abscesses. *In* Diagnosis and Treatment of Abdominal Abscesses. Edited by I.M. Ariel and K.K. Kazarian. Baltimore, Williams & Wilkins, 1971, p. 174.

63. Sart, M.G., and Zuidema, G.D.: Splenic abscess. Presentation, diagnosis and treatment. Surgery, *92*:480, 1982.

64. Silen, W.: Acute appendicitis. *In* Harrison's Principles of Internal Medicine. 11th Ed. Edited by E. Braunwald, et al. New York, McGraw-Hill, 1987, pp. 1304–1307.

65. Bonica, J.J.: The Management of Pain. Philadelphia, Lea & Febiger, 1953, pp. 1376–1379.

66. Ochsner, A., Gage, I.N., and Cutting, R.A.: Treatment of ileus by splanchnic anesthesia. JAMA, *90*:1847, 1928.

67. Sarnoff, S., Arrowood, J.G., and Chapman, W.P.: Differential spinal block: IV. The investigation of intestinal dyskinesia, colonicatony and visceral afferent fibers. Surg. Gynecol. Obstet., *86*:571, 1948.

68. Saibil, F.G., and Edmeads, J.: Chest pain arising from extrathoracic structures. *In* Chest Pain: An Integrated Diagnostic Approach. Edited by D.L. Levene. Philadelphia, Lea & Febiger, 1977, pp. 119–126.

69. Levitt, M.D., and Bond, J.H.: Intestinal gas. *In* Gastrointestinal Disease: Pathophysiology, Diagnosis, Management. 3rd Ed. Edited by M.H. Sleisenger and J.S. Fordtran. Philadelphia, W.B. Saunders, 1983, pp. 222–227.

70. Lasser, R.B., Bond, J.H., and Levitt, M.D.: The role of intestinal gas in functional abdominal pain. N. Engl. J. Med., *293*:524, 1975.

71. Richie, J.: Pain from distension of the pelvic colon by inflating a balloon in the irritable colon syndrome. Gut, *14*:125, 1973.

72. Bruyn, G.W.: Migraine equivalents. *In* Handbook of Clinical Neurology, Vol. 4, Headaches. Edited by F. C. Rose, et al. Amsterdam, Elsevier, 1986, pp. 158–160.

73. Farquhar, H.G.: Abdominal migraine in children. Br. Med. J., *1/2*:1082, 1956.

74. Bille, B.O.: Migraine in school children. Acta Paediatr. *51* (Suppl. 136):14, 1962.

75. Frenkel, E.P.: Sickle cell anemia. *In* The Merck Manual. 15th Ed. Edited by R. Berkow. Rahway, NJ, Merck, Sharp & Dohme Research Laboratories, 1987, pp. 1120–1122.

76. Bunn, H.F.: Disorders of hemoglobin structure, function, and synthesis. *In* Harrison's Principles of Internal Medicine. 11th Ed. Edited by E. Braunwald, et al. New York, McGraw-Hill, 1987, pp. 1518–1527.

77. Sachar, D.B.: Acute intermittent porphyria. *In* The Merck Manual. 15th Ed. Edited by R. Berkow. Rahway, NJ, Merck, Sharp & Dohme Research Laboratories, 1987, pp. 996–999.

78. Meyer, U.A.: Porphyrias. *In* Harrison's Principles of Internal Medicine. 10th Ed. Edited by R.G. Petersdorf, et al. New York, McGraw-Hill, 1983, pp. 533–539.

79. Wallace, J.F.: Disorders caused by venoms, bites and stings. *In* Harrison's Principles of Internal Medicine. 11th Ed. Edited by E. Braunwald, et al. New York, McGraw-Hill, 1987, pp. 831–838.

80. Russell, F.E.: Venomous bites and stings. *In* The Merck Manual. 15th Ed. Edited by R. Berkow. Rahway, NJ, Merck, Sharp & Dohme Research Laboratories, 1987, pp. 2565–2576.

81. Lennox, W.G., and Cobb, S.: Epilepsy. XIII. Aura in epilepsy: Statistical review of 1,359 cases. Arch. Neurol. Psychiatry, *30*:374, 1933.

82. Moore, M.T.: Paroxysmal abdominal pain: A form of focal symptomatic epilepsy. JAMA, *129*:1233–1240, 1945.

83. Posner, J.B.: Back pain and epidural spinal cord compression. Med. Clin. North Am., *71*:185, 1987.

84. Applegate, W.V.: Abdominal cutaneous nerve entrapment syndrome. Surgery, *71*:118, 1972.

85. Mehta, M.: Intractable Pain. London, W.B. Saunders, 1973, pp. 122–125.

86. Ranger, I., Mehta, M., and Pennington, M.: Abdominal wall pain due to nerve entrapment. Practitioner, *206*:791, 1971.

87. Travell, J.G., and Simons, D.G.: Myofascial Pain and Disfunction: The Trigger Point Manual. Baltimore, Williams & Wilkins, 1983, pp. 660–683.

88. Sola, A.: Trigger point therapy. *In* Clinical Procedures and Emergency Medicine. Edited by J.R. Roberts and J.I. Hedges. Philadelphia, W.B. Saunders, 1985, pp. 674–686.

89. Edegawa, N., and Friedman, L.W.: Treatment of abdominal pain. The Treatment of Disordered Function. Edited by L.W. Friedman. Smithtown, NY, Exposition Press, 1981, pp. 95–110.

65 • GENERAL CONSIDERATIONS OF PAIN IN THE PELVIS AND PERINEUM

JOHN J. BONICA

Pain arising from disorders of the viscera and of the somatic structures that comprise the pelvis and perineum is a frequent cause of discomfort and disability, especially among women. This chapter, like others that introduce considerations of pain in various body regions, provides a review of the basic essentials of pain caused by disorders of the pelvis and its contents and of pain in the perineum, and how to approach the patient with pain in these regions. The material is presented in two major sections: A, Basic

Considerations, includes a review of the anatomy and neurology of the pelvis, pelvic viscera, and perineum. B details the evaluation of the patient with pelvic or perineal pain. The table at the end of the chapter summarizes the characteristics and symptoms and signs of painful diseases of the pelvis and perineum to assist the physician in making differential diagnoses. Much of the information on anatomy and neurology is derived from the first edition of this book (1) and from several other textbooks and reviews (2–9).

A. BASIC CONSIDERATIONS

Anatomic and Neurologic Bases of Pelvic Pain

The pelvis, the lower part of the abdominal cavity, is roughly infundibular, like an inverted truncated cone, and extends posteroinferiorly from the lower end of the abdominal cavity (2). It is composed of the skeletal pelvis and its ligaments and muscles and contains the pelvic viscera. It is bounded anterolaterally by the parts of the hip bones below the pubic crests and arcuate lines and by the obturator internus muscles, posterosuperiorly by the sacrum, coccyx, and piriformis and coccygeus muscles, and inferiorly by the levatores ani muscles, which form the pelvic diaphragm with their covering fascia, and by the deep transverse perineal muscle and sphincter urethrae, which together with their fascial coverings constitute the urogenital diaphragm. The pelvis contains the urinary bladder, terminal part of the ureters, sigmoid colon, rectum and a few coils of small intestine, and internal genitalia, together with blood vessels, lymph vessels, lymph nodes, and nerves. Here I first describe the skeletal pelvis, its ligaments and muscles, and their fascia, consider the neurology of the pelvis and its viscera, and finally discuss the same aspects of the perineum.

Skeletal Pelvis

Figure 65-1 depicts the anatomy of the female and male pelvis. It is massively constructed in conformity with its primary function of withstanding the compression and other stresses caused by body weight and powerful musculature (2, 3). The pelvis is composed of two parts, the greater segment and the lesser segment, sometimes called the false and true pelvis, respectively. These are arbitrarily divided by an oblique line that passes through the sacral promontory behind and the lineae terminalis at the sides and in front. Each linea terminalis includes the arcuate line of the ilium, iliopectineal line, and crest of the pubis. These two parts are structurally continuous and the parts of the

body cavity that they enclose are continuous through the superior pelvic aperture or pelvic inlet with the abdomen proper (Chapter 59).

GREATER PELVIS. The greater (false) pelvis consists of the phalangeal parts of the iliac bones above the linea terminalis on each side and the base of the sacrum posteriorly. The bone structure along this junctional zone is particularly massive and forms the main pathway on each side from the acetabular fossae to the vertebral column around the visceral cavity. The cavity of the greater pelvis is part of the abdomen and, because of the inclination of the pelvis as a whole, the cavity has little skeletal wall anteriorly.

LESSER PELVIS. The lesser (true) pelvis encloses a true basin when the soft tissues of the pelvic floor are in place (2, 3). From the skeletal point of view it is a narrowed continuation of the greater pelvis with irregular but more complete walls bounding the pelvic cavity or canal. This cavity, which is of special obstetric importance, has an axis that is curved in the median plane. It is limited above by a superior opening, occupied in life by viscera traversing it, and limited below by the inferior opening that is largely closed by the pelvic floor and its sphincter mechanisms. Figure 65-2 depicts the boundaries and diameters of the superior pelvic aperture (Fig. 65-2A) and of the inferior pelvic aperture (Fig. 65-2B and C) and shows a sagittal section through the female pelvis depicting the planes of the inlet and outlet and their relation to each other (Fig. 65-2D). From a standing position the pelvic canal curves obliquely backward relative to the trunk and abdominal cavity. The whole pelvis is tilted forward so that the plane of the pelvic brim makes an angle of 50 to 60° with the horizontal.

Joints and Ligaments of the Pelvis

The pelvis has a complex of joints and ligaments that tie together the ilium with the sacrum and with the 5th lumbar vertebra. The two pubic bones meet in the midline plane, where they form the cartilaginous joints of the pubis symphysis.

Sacroiliac Joint

The sacroiliac articulation is synovial in between the articular surfaces of the sacrum and ilium. The

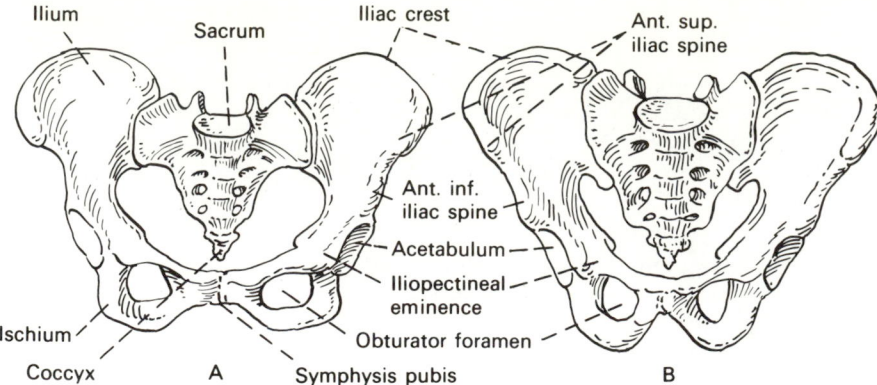

FIG. 65-1. Anterior view of the female pelvis (*A*) and male pelvis (*B*). Modified from Clemente, C.D. (ed.): Gray's Anatomy of the Human Body. 30th Ed. Philadelphia, Lea & Febiger, 1985, p. 273.

articular surfaces exhibit irregular elevations and depressions that are more pronounced in the male and fit into one another. These surfaces restrict movement but contribute to the strength of the joint that transmits weight from the vertebral column to the lower limb. The articular surface is covered by hyaline cartilage and the ilium by fibrocartilage (Fig. 65-3). The articular capsule is attached close to the margin of the articular surfaces of the sacrum and ilium (2, 3). The joint is held together by anterior, interosseous, and posterior sacroiliac ligaments (Figs. 65-3 and 65-4), which are all supplied by the posterior primary divisions of the upper three sacral nerves.

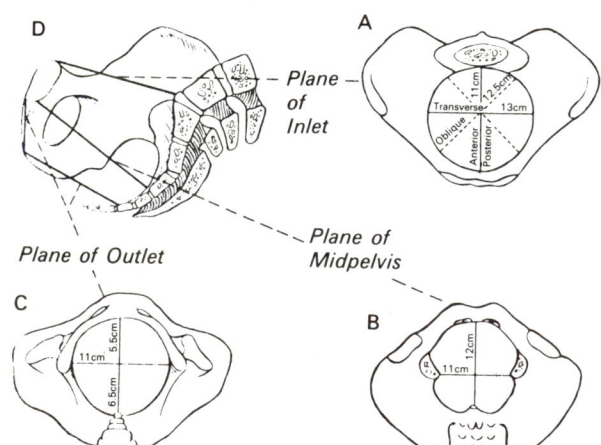

FIG. 65-2. Planes and diameters of the pelvis. **A.** Superior plane or obstetric inlet, bounded posteriorly by the promontory of the sacrum, laterally by the iliopectineal line, and anteriorly by the rami of pubic bones and the upper margin of the symphysis pubis. **B.** Midpelvic plane, bounded posteriorly by the sacrum near the junction of the S3 and S4 vertebrae, laterally by the ischial spine, and anteriorly by the inferior aspect of the symphysis. **C.** Inferior plane or obstetric outlet, composed of two triangular components. The posterior component is bounded behind by the sacrococcygeal joint, laterally by the sacrotuberous ligament, and anteriorly by the bi-ischial diameter; the anterior component is bounded by the bi-ischial diameter behind, laterally by the inner margin of the pubic arch, and anteriorly by the inferior margin of the symphysis. The floor or the pelvic outlet is composed of the soft tissues of the perineum and the structures making up the urogenital diaphragm. **D.** Sagittal view of the pelvis showing important anteroposterior diameters (*solid lines*). From Bonica, J.J.: Principles and Practice of Obstetric Analgesia, Vol. 2. Philadelphia, F.A. Davis, 1969, p. 851.

ANTERIOR SACROILIAC LIGAMENT. The anterior sacroiliac ligament is a thickening of the anterior inferior parts of the fibrous capsule. It is well developed at the level of the arcuate line and inferiorly at the level of the posterior inferior iliac spine, where it connects the base and lower part of the sacrum to the auricular surface of the ilium and preauricular sulcus.

INTEROSSEOUS SACROILIAC LIGAMENT. The interosseous sacroiliac ligament is massive and strong and forms the chief bond between the two bones. It fills the irregular space immediately above and behind the joint and is covered by the

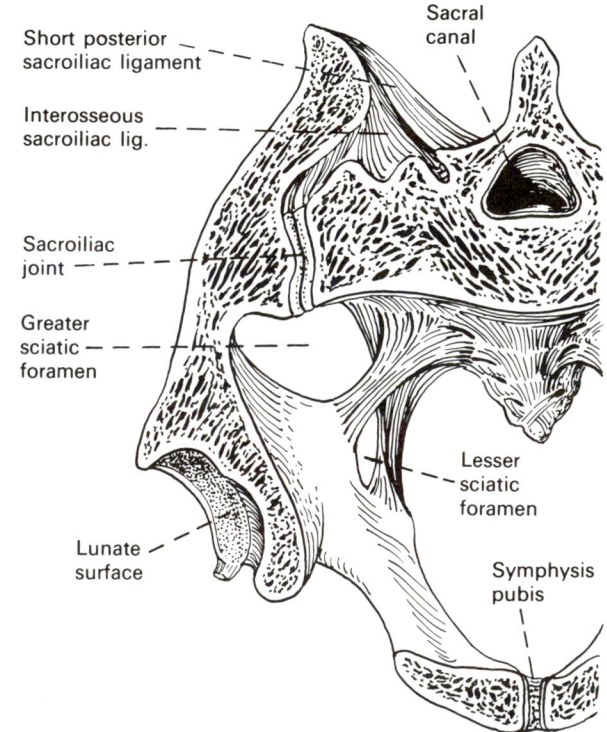

FIG. 65-3. Coronal section through the pelvis showing the sacroiliac joint through the anterior sacral segment. The anterior part of the joint is covered by hyaline cartilage on the sacral surface, and fibrocartilage overlies the surface of the ilium. The interosseous sacroiliac ligament fills the cleft above and behind the joint cavity. The joints of the surfaces are irregularly shaped and the interconnecting bones fit snugly, thus restricting movement but buttressing the weight-bearing function of the joint. Modified from Clemente, C.D. (ed.): Gray's Anatomy of the Human Body. 30th Ed. Philadelphia, Lea & Febiger, 1985, p. 360.

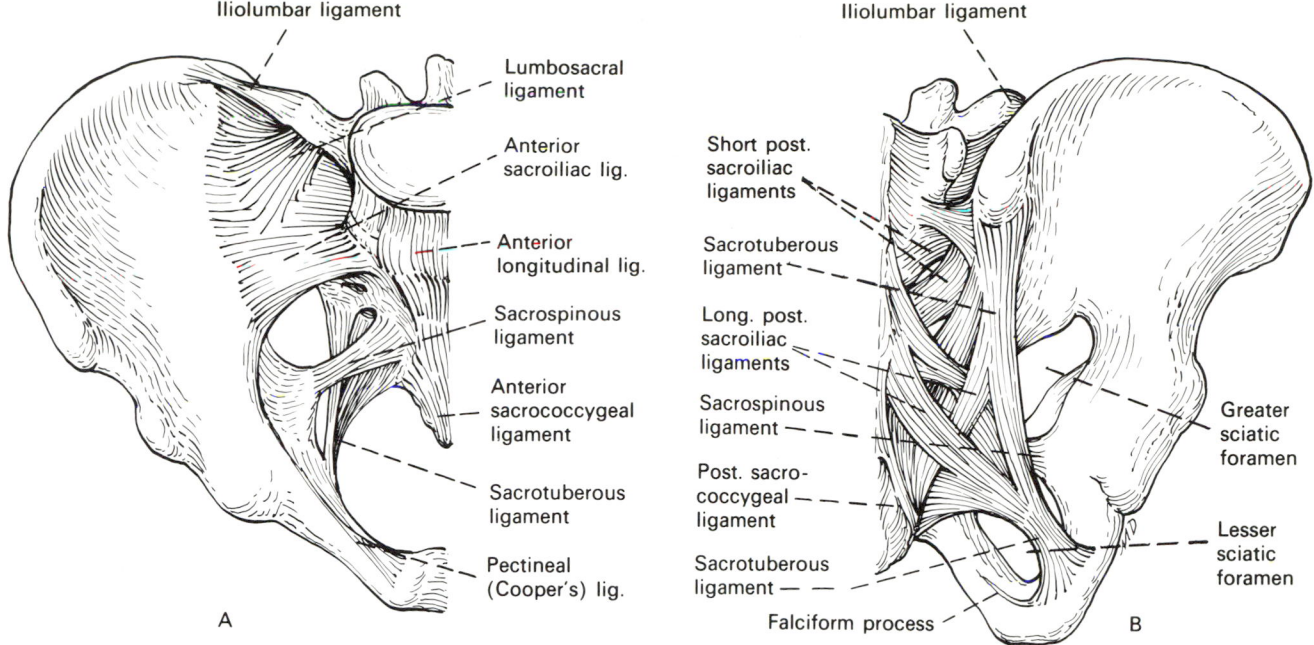

Iliolumbar ligament

Lumbosacral ligament

Anterior sacroiliac lig.

Anterior longitudinal lig.

Sacrospinous ligament

Anterior sacrococcygeal ligament

Sacrotuberous ligament

Pectineal (Cooper's) lig.

A

Iliolumbar ligament

Short post. sacroiliac ligaments

Sacrotuberous ligament

Long. post. sacroiliac ligaments

Sacrospinous ligament

Post. sacro-coccygeal ligament

Sacrotuberous ligament

Falciform process

Greater sciatic foramen

Lesser sciatic foramen

B

FIG. 65-4. Joints and ligaments of the right half of the pelvis. *A*. Anterior view. *B*. Posterior view. See text for details. Modified from Clemente, C.D. (ed.): Gray's Anatomy of the Human Body. 30th Ed. Philadelphia, Lea & Febiger, 1985, pp. 361–362.

posterior sacroiliac ligament. It consists of deeper and more superficial parts, with the deeper parts having cranial and caudal bands that pass from the depression behind the auricular surface of the sacrum to the depression in the iliac tuberosity. These bands are covered by and blend with the more superficial part, which forms a fibrous sheet connecting the cranial and posterior margins of the rough area behind the auricular surface on the sacrum with the corresponding margin of the iliac tuberosity.

POSTERIOR SACROILIAC LIGAMENT. The posterior sacroiliac ligament overlies the interosseous ligament from which it is separated by the dorsal rami of the sacral spinal nerves and vessels. It consists of several fasciculi that course in various directions. The deeper upper part is called the short posterior sacroiliac ligament and passes from the lateral sacral crest with varying degrees of obliquity to the posterior superior iliac spine and inner lip of the posterior part of the iliac crest. The lower fibers, which comprise the long posterior sacroiliac ligament, pass from the 2nd, 3rd, and 4th sacral crests to the posterior superior iliac spine. This ligament descends obliquely and becomes continuous with the sacrotuberous ligament and medially with the posterior layer of the thoracolumbar fascia.

MOVEMENT. The sacroiliac joint allows a small amount of anteroposterior rotatory movement around a transverse axis that is usually about 5 to 10 cm below the promontory of the sacrum vertically. These movements occur during flexion and extension of the trunk. The range is the same in the male and nonpregnant female but is increased considerably during pregnancy. The greatest change in position of the sacrum in relation to the iliac bones occurs when the individual arises from a recumbent to a standing position: the sacral promontory moves forward as much as 5 to 6 mm as the body weight is taken on the sacrum. The backward movement of the lower end of the sacrum is considerably less. In middle age and beyond, fibrous adhesions and a gradual obliteration of the synovial

cavity occur in both sexes, earlier in men and after menopause in women (2, 3). In old age the joints can become completely fibrosed and even ossified.

Vertebropelvic Ligaments

The ilium is connected with the L5 vertebra by the iliolumbar ligament, and the sacrum is connected to the ischium by the sacrotuberous and sacrospinous ligaments (Fig. 65-4).

ILIOLUMBAR LIGAMENT. The iliolumbar ligament is attached to the tip and to the lower and front part of the transverse process of the L5 vertebra. Sometimes it has an additional weak attachment to the transverse process of the L4 vertebra. It radiates as it passes laterally and is attached by two main bands to the pelvis. The inferior band, the lumbosacral ligament, runs from the inferior aspect of the L5 transverse process to the upper medial aspect of the ilium, blending with the anterior sacroiliac ligament. The superior band passes from the transverse process of the L5 vertebra to the posterior surface of the medial part of the iliac crest. This band gives partial origin to the quadratus lumborum muscle, which is also attached to the crest of the ilium immediately in front of the sacroiliac joint.

SACROTUBEROUS LIGAMENT. The sacrotuberous ligament is attached by a broad flat base to the posterior superior and inferior iliac spines (where it partially blends with the posterior sacroiliac ligament), to the 4th and 5th transverse tubercles of the sacrum, and to the lateral margin of the lower part of the sacrum and upper part of the coccyx (Fig. 65-4B). These fibers run obliquely downward and laterally and converge to form a thick narrow band that is fixed to the medial margin of the ischial tuberosity and then continues along the ramus of the ischium as the falciform process. The free concave edge of the falciform process blends with the fascial sheath of the internal pudendal vessels and pudendal nerve. The lowest fibers of the gluteus maximus are attached to the posterior surface of the sacrotuberous ligament. The ligament is pierced by the coccygeal branch of the gluteal artery, by the perforating cutaneous nerve, and by minute filaments of the coccygeal plexus.

SACROSPINOUS LIGAMENT. The sacrospinous ligament is a thin, triangular-shaped structure that attaches to the spine of the ischium. It attaches medially by its broad base to the lateral margin of the sacrum and coccyx in front of the sacrotuberous ligament. The pudendal nerve passes posteriorly to the point at which the ligament attaches to the spine. It is an important landmark in carrying out pudendal nerve block for vaginal delivery or during surgical procedures on the perineum.

FUNCTION. The sacrotuberous ligament and, to a lesser extent, the sacrospinous ligament, oppose upward tilting of the lower part of the sacrum under the downward thrust that is imparted to the upper end of the bone by the weight of the trunk. These two ligaments convert the sciatic notches into two foramina. The greater sciatic foramen is bounded in front and above by the greater sciatic notch, behind by the sacrotuberous ligament, and below by the sacrospinous ligament in the spine of the ischium. It is partially filled by the piriformis muscles that emerge from the pelvis through it. Above this muscle the superior gluteal vessels and nerves pass out of the pelvis while below it pass the inferior gluteal vessels and nerves, internal pudendal vessels and pudendal nerves, sciatic nerve, posterior femoral cutaneous nerve, and nerves to the obturator internus and quadratus femoris muscles. The lesser sciatic foramen is bounded in front by the body of the ischium, above by the spine of the ischium and sacrospinous ligament, and behind by the sacrotuberous ligament. It transmits the tendon of the obturator internus muscle, the nerve to this muscle, and the internal pudendal vessels and pudendal nerves.

Pubic Symphysis

The pubic symphysis is the point at which the two pubic bones meet each other in the medial plane to form a cartilaginous ligament and are connected by the superior pubic and arcuate pubic ligaments and by an interpubic disk of fibrocartilage. The superior pubic ligament connects the pubic bone superiorly and extends as far as the pubic tubercles. The arcuate ligament is a thick arch of fibers that connects the lower borders of the symphysis surface of the two pubic bones and forms the upper boundary of the pubic arch. Above, it blends with the interpubic disk and is attached laterally to the inferior rami of the pubic bone. The interpubic disk connects the adjacent surfaces of the pubic bones; each surface is covered with a thin layer of hyaline cartilage and is firmly attached to the bone, an arrangement that resists shearing forces. The opposed surfaces of the hyaline cartilage are connected by a lamina of fibrocartilage that varies in thickness. Some separation between the pubic bones occurs late in pregnancy and during childbirth.

Mechanism of the Pelvis

Although the skeletal pelvis supports and protects the contained pelvic viscera, it is primarily part of the lower limb and affords surfaces for the attachment of the muscles of the trunk and lower limbs (2, 3). Its most important mechanical function is transmission of the weight of the head, trunk, and upper limbs to the lower extremities. Movements of the sacrum are regulated by its form and ligamentous attachment. Viewed as a whole it presents the shape of a wedge, with its base upward and forward. The first component force is therefore acting against the resistance of the wedge, and its tendency to separate the iliac bones is resisted by the sacroiliac and lumbar ligaments posteriorly and by the ligaments of the symphysis pubis anteriorly. During pregnancy hormonal changes cause the pelvic ligaments and joints to become relaxed and capable of more extensive movements. This renders the locking mechanism of the sacroiliac joint less restrictive and permits greater rotation, a change that allows alteration in the diameter of the pelvis during childbirth. The less effective the locking mechanism, the more the strain of weight-bearing pulls the ligaments, frequently resulting in sacroiliac strain during and after pregnancy. After childbirth the ligaments tighten up again and the locking mechanism becomes more effective. In some cases, however, the locking occurs in the position of rotation of the hip bones that occurred during pregnancy. This so-called subluxation of the sacroiliac joint causes pain by the unusual tension that is imposed on the ligaments. Reduction by forcible manipulation after the joint is completely anesthetized can be attempted.

Pelvic Muscles and Fascia

The muscles within the pelvis are divided into two groups: (a) the piriformis and obturator internus muscles; and (b) the levator ani and coccygeus muscles that, with the corresponding muscles of the opposite side, form the pelvic diaphragm. All the fascia investing the muscles form a continuum of connective tissue that joins the fascial covering of the pelvic viscera above with the fascia of the perineum below.

PELVIC FASCIA. The pelvic fascia consists of the parietal pelvic fascia, which constitutes the fascial sheaths of the pelvic muscles, and the visceral pelvic fascia, the fascial sheaths of the pelvic viscera and of their blood vessels and nerves (see below, Anatomy and Neurology of the Perineum). The parietal pelvic fascia covering the pelvic surface of the obturator internus muscle is well differentiated as the obturator fascia. The fascia of the piriform muscle is thin and fuses with periosteum of the anterior surface of the sacrum around the margin of the anterior sacral foramina. Its sacral attachment ensheathes the nerves emerging from these foramina.

The fascia of the pelvic diaphragm extends over both surfaces of the levator ani muscles. The portion above is called the superior fascia of the pelvic diaphragm and the part below it is called the inferior fascia of the pelvic diaphragm, also known as the anal fascia. Laterally the superior fascia follows the line of attachment of the muscle and therefore varies somewhat. Anteriorly it is attached to the back of the symphysis pubis about 2 cm above its lower border. It can be traced laterally across the back of the superior ramus of the pubis for a short distance to the obturator fascia, with which it blends along a somewhat irregular line to the spine of the ischium. The inferior fascia of the pelvic diaphragm covers the medial wall of the ischiorectal fossa. Above it is continuous with the fascia of the pudendal canal and with the obturator fascia along the line of attachment of the levator ani muscle. It is continuous below with the fascia on the sphincter urethra and sphincter ani externus muscle.

Levator Ani Muscle

Figure 65-5 depicts a sagittal section of the pelvis with the viscera removed to show the pelvic aspect of the left levator ani and coccygeal muscles. The levator ani muscle is a broad thin structure attached to the inner surface of the side of the true pelvis. It unites with the opposite muscle to form the greater part of the floor of the pelvic cavity. It is attached anteriorly to the pelvic surface of the body of the pubis, lateral to the symphysis, behind to the medial surface of the spine of the ischium, and between these two points to the obturator fascia. Morphologically the levator ani can be divided into the pubococcygeus and iliococcygeus muscles.

The pubococcygeus muscle arises from the posterior surface of the pubis and from the anterior part of the obturator fascia. Its fibers are directed backward almost horizontally along the line of the anal canal and become attached to the front of the coccyx by a tendinous plate that is continuous with the anterior sacrococcygeal ligament. The medial coccygeus muscle arises from the ischial spine and from the posterior part of the tendinous arch of the levator ani muscle. Its fibers attach to the sides of the coccyx and to the opposite muscle in the median raphe on the undersurface of the tendinous plates of the pubococcygeus that contribute to the anococcygeal ligament.

The superior or pelvic surface of the levator ani is separated by its covering fascia from the bladder, prostate, rectum, and peritoneum, while its inferior or perineal surface forms the medial boundary of the ischiorectal fossa and is covered by the inferior fascia of the pelvic diaphragm. Its posterior border is free and is separated from the coccygeus muscle by areolar tissue, while the medial borders of the two muscles are separated by the visceral outlet, an interval through which the urethra, vagina, and anorectum pass from the pelvis.

The nerve supply of the levator ani muscle includes a branch from the S4 nerve, a branch that arises either from the inferior rectal nerve or from the perineal branch of the pudendal nerve. The function of the levator ani muscle is constriction of the lower end of the rectum and vagina, and probably fixation of the perineal body. The levator ani, together with the coccygei, form a muscular diaphragm that supports the pelvic viscera and opposes itself to the downward thrust produced by any increase in intra-abdominal pressure.

Coccygeus Muscle

The coccygeus muscle is posterosuperior in the same tissue plane as the levator ani muscle. It consists of a triangular sheath of muscular and tendinous fibers, arising by its apex from the pelvic surface of the spine of the ischium and sacrospinous ligament. It is attached at its base to the margin of the coccyx and side of the S5 segment. The muscle receives its nerve supply through branches from the S4 and S5 spinal nerves. The coccygeus functions in pulling forward and supporting the coccyx after it has been pressed backward during defecation or parturition. The coccygeus, together with the levator ani and piriformis muscles, closes the posterior part of the pelvic outlet.

Pelvic Viscera and Their Peritoneal Covering

The pelvic viscera consist of the urinary bladder, terminal parts of the ureters, sigmoid colon, rectum and a few coils of small intestine, blood vessels, lymph vessels, nodes, nerves, and internal genitalia. In the male the internal genitalia consists of the prostate, seminal vesicles, ejaculatory ducts, and vas deferens; in the female the internal genitalia consists of the ovaries, uterine tubes, uterus, and vagina. A description of the anatomy of each of these structures is beyond the scope of this book and is limited to the

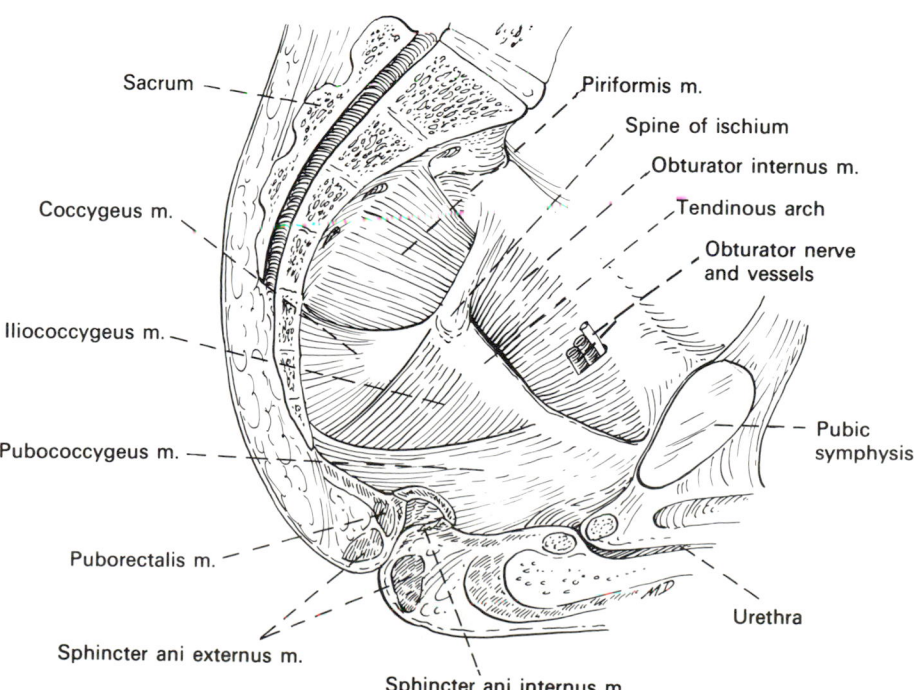

FIG. 65-5. Sagittal section of the pelvis showing the muscles of the left lateral wall of the pelvis. The obturator nerve and vessels pass through the obturator muscle, which is normally covered by fascia (not shown). Modified from Clemente, C.D. (ed.): Gray's Anatomy of the Human Body. 30th Edition. Philadelphia, Lea & Febiger, 1985, p. 499.

Labels: Sacrum, Coccygeus m., Iliococcygeus m., Pubococcygeus m., Puborectalis m., Sphincter ani externus m., Sphincter ani internus m., Piriformis m., Spine of ischium, Obturator internus m., Tendinous arch, Obturator nerve and vessels, Pubic symphysis, Urethra

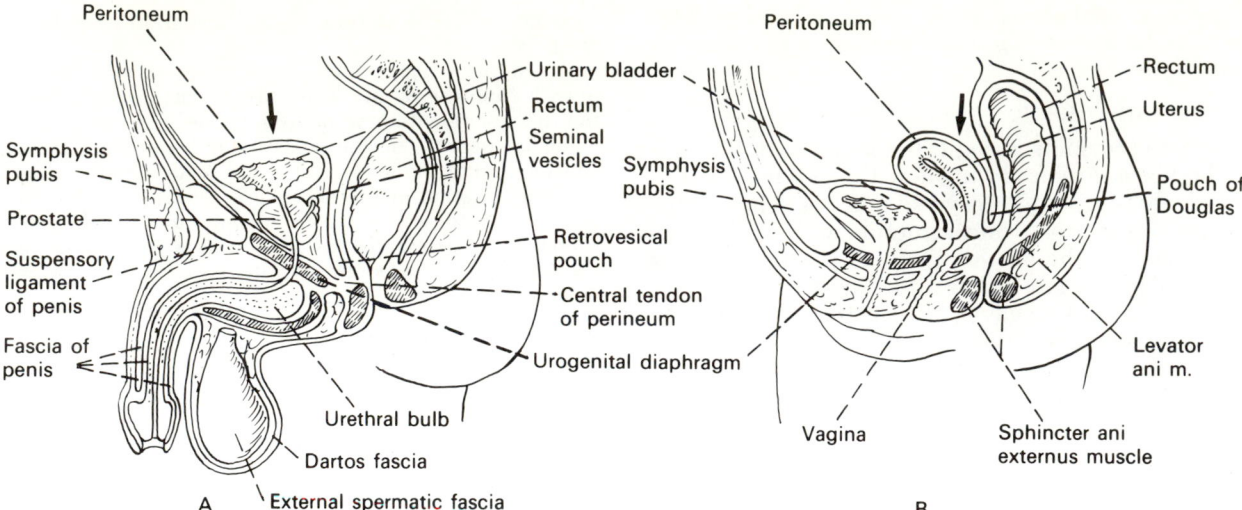

FIG. 65-6. Schematic diagram of the pelvis and perineum in the medial sagittal plane showing the fascia and some of the muscles. *A.* Male. *B.* Female. See text for details. *A* modified from Clemente, C.D. (ed.): Gray's Anatomy of the Human Body. 30th Ed. Philadelphia, Lea & Febiger, 1985, p. 502; *B* modified from Bonica, J.J.: Principles and Practices of Obstetric Analgesia and Anesthesia, Vol. 1. Philadelphia, F.A. Davis, 1967, pp. 502–503.

illustration of these organs (Figs. 65-6 and 65-11). Painful disorders of female internal genital organs are discussed in Chapter 67, while those that affect the male genital organs and the bladder are described in Chapter 68. Because pain from diseases of these organs usually involves inflammation of the pelvic peritoneum that overlies these structures, it is briefly described below. Following the suggestion by Williams and Warwick (2) to trace the peritoneum from one viscus to another and from the viscus to the parietes, it is helpful to follow its continuity in the vertical and horizontal directions. Here the discussion is limited to its vertical disposition.

Vertical Disposition of the Pelvic Peritoneum

The peritoneum descends from the abdomen proper over structures in the pelvic cavity. It is reflected from the posterior pelvic wall as the anterior layer of the sigmoid mesocolon, which invests the sigmoid colon and returns to the pelvic wall as the posterior layer of the sigmoid mesocolon. It then descends, covering the front and sides of the upper third of the rectum and the front of the middle third of the rectum.

IN THE MALE. In the male it leads to the front of the rectum (at the junction of the middle and lower thirds) and passes forward onto the upper end of the seminal vesicles and the upper surface of the urinary bladder. Between the rectum and bladder it dips slightly downward to form a recess, the rectovesical pouch, the bottom of which is a little below the level of the upper ends of the seminal vesicles and about 7.5 cm from its anal orifice (2). From the apex of the bladder it is carried along the medial umbilical ligaments to the anterior abdominal wall, up to the level of the umbilicus. When the bladder is distended the peritoneum is stripped away from the lower part of the anterior abdominal wall so that a considerable part of the anterior surface of the bladder lies directly against the abdominal wall, without the intervention of peritoneum. This permits an instrument to be passed through the abdominal wall into the distended bladder without passing through the peritoneal cavity.

IN THE FEMALE. In the female the peritoneum passes from the front of the rectum onto the posterior fornix of the

vagina and from there to the back of the cervix and body of the uterus to form the rectouterine fold. This dips downward to form the rectouterine pouch of Douglas, the bottom of which is about 5.5 cm above the anal orifice. The peritoneum continues over the fundus of the uterus and descends on its anterior (vesical) surface as far as the body of the uterus and cervix. From here it is reflected anteriorly onto the upper surface of the bladder to form a shallow recess, the vesicouterine pouch. The layers of the peritoneum on the anterior and posterior surfaces of the uterus are reflected laterally from the lateral margins of the uterus to the side walls of the pelvis to form an expanded fold on each side, the broad ligament of the uterus (see Fig. 65-7).

Uterine Ligaments

The uterus is connected to the bladder, rectum, and walls of the lesser pelvis by a number of ligaments. Some of these are merely peritoneal folds and have little supporting effect, while others consist of nonstriated muscles and fibrous tissue and function as real ties to provide some measure of dynamic control. These ligaments consist of the anterior, uterosacral (posterior), broad, round, and transverse ligaments (Fig. 65-7).

ANTERIOR AND POSTERIOR LIGAMENTS. The anterior ligament consists of the uterovesical fold of the peritoneum, which is reflected onto the surface of the bladder from the front of the uterus at the junction of the cervix and body of the uterus. The posterior ligament consists of the rectovaginal fold of peritoneum, which is reflected from the back of the posterior fornix of the vagina onto the front of the rectum. It forms the bottom of the deep rectouterine pouch that is bounded anteriorly by the posterior wall of the body of the uterus, supravaginal portion of the cervix, and posterior fornix of the vagina, posteriorly by the rectum, and laterally by two folds of the peritoneum that pass backward from the cervix, one on each side of the rectum, to the posterior wall of the lesser pelvis. These are the rectouterine folds, which contain a considerable amount of fibrous tissue and nonstriated muscular fibers, are attached to the front of

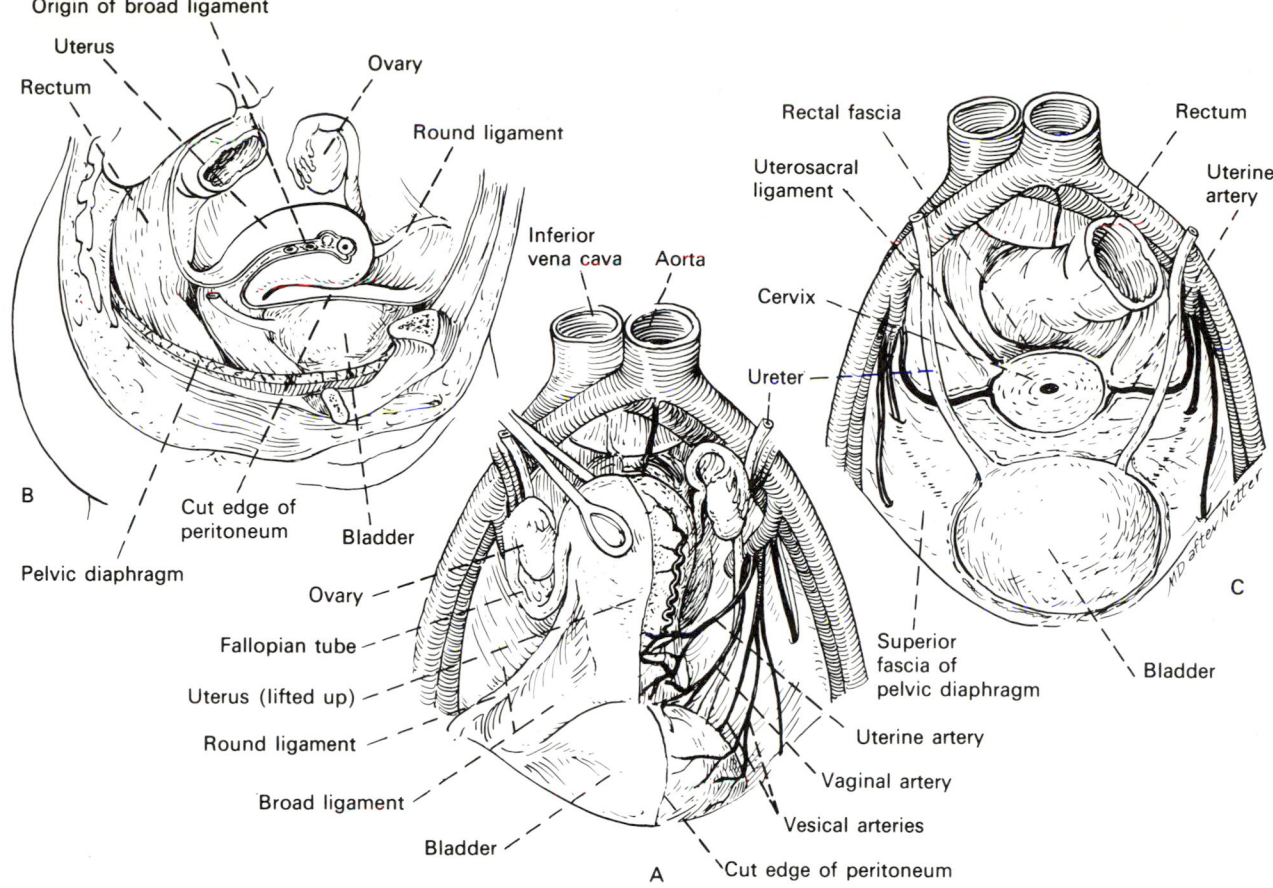

Fig. 65-7. Ligaments of the uterus. **A.** Anterior view. **B.** Parasagittal view. **C.** Superior view. Modified from Netter, F.H.: The CIBA Collection of Medical Illustrations, Vol. 2. Reproductive System. Summit, NJ, CIBA Pharmaceuticals, 1979, pp. 89, 95, and 97.

the sacrum, and constitute the uterosacral ligament. On rectal examination, the uterosacral ligaments can be palpated as they pass backward on the side of the rectum (2).

BROAD LIGAMENTS. Each of two broad ligaments passes from the side of the uterus to the lateral wall of the pelvis (Fig. 65-7). With the uterus both form a septum across the cavity of the lesser pelvis, dividing it into an anterior part containing the bladder and a posterior part containing the rectum, terminal coils of the ileum, and part of the sigmoid colon. When the bladder is empty or only slightly distended, the surface of the broad ligaments is directed superiorly and inferiorly and they have a free anterior (unattached) border. As the bladder fills, the plane of the ligaments alters and their free border become superior in position; in this condition the broad ligaments consist of anterior and posterior layers that are continuous with each other at their upper free border and diverge from each other below, where they approach the superior surface of the levator ani muscle.

The uterine tube is contained in the free border. The lateral part of the ligament between the tubes and ligament of the ovary and mesovarium is known as the mesosalpinx. The infundibulum of the uterine tube projects from the free border near its lateral extremity. The ovary is attached to the posterior layer by the mesovarium. The part of the broad ligament that extends from the infundibulum of the tube and the upper pole of the ovary to the lateral wall of the pelvis contains the ovarian vessels, nerves, and lymph vessels, and is known as the suspensory ligament of the ovary. The term "mesometrium" is applied to that part of the broad ligament extending from the pelvic floor to the ovary, ligament of the ovary, and body of the uterus. The uterine artery, vein, and

nerves pass between the layers of the broad ligaments at their inferior border about 1.5 cm lateral to the cervix and then ascend in the medial part of the broad ligament, turning laterally below the uterine tube to anastomose with the ovarian artery.

ROUND LIGAMENTS. The round ligaments of the uterus are two narrow flat bands from 10 to 12 cm long that are situated between the layers of the broad ligament in front of and below the uterine tubes. Each ligament begins at the lateral edge of the uterus and is directed anteriorly and laterally across the vesical vessels, obturator vessels and nerves, and obliterated umbilical artery, and over the externus iliac vessels. It then passes through the deep inguinal ring to hook around the beginning of the inferior epigastric artery, traversing the inguinal canal. It finally breaks up into strands that merge with the areolar tissue in the labium majus.

TRANSVERSE CERVICAL LIGAMENTS. Each transverse cervical ligament of Mackenrodt, also called the cardinal ligament, is attached to the side of the cervix uteri and to the vault and lateral fornix of the vagina. Both are continuous with the fibrous tissue that surrounds the pelvic blood vessels, and help to maintain the position of the uterus.

FUNCTION. All these ligaments act as mechanical supports for the uterus, helping to maintain it in its normal position. The levator ani and coccygei muscles, the muscles of the uterogenital diaphragm, and the perineal body appear to be of particular importance in this respect.

Neurology of the Pelvis and Its Viscera

Like other abdominal viscera, the viscera of the pelvis are supplied by sympathetic and parasympathetic nerves that contain both efferent and afferent fibers. Chapter 59 contains a description of the distribution of the celiac plexus and its subsidiary plexuses, which supply viscera in the abdomen proper. It is mentioned in Chapter 59 that the aortic plexus contributes fibers to the formation of the superior and inferior hypogastric plexuses, which totally innervate the pelvic viscera. The inferior mesenteric plexus also supplies the pelvic portion of the large bowel. These and other subsidiary plexuses supplying the pelvic viscera are briefly described here.

Superior Hypogastric Plexus

The plexus is formed above by the union of branches from the aortic plexus, with contributions by the L3 and L4 splanchnic nerves (2–7). The plexus is situated in front of the bifurcation of the abdominal aorta, left common iliac vein, median sacral vessel, body of the last lumbar vertebra, and promontory of the sacrum, and between the two common iliac arteries (Fig. 65-8). Although surgeons in the 1920s and 1930s who resected this nerve for the treatment of severe dysmenorrhea referred to it as the presacral nerve, it is rarely sufficiently condensed to resemble a sacral nerve but rather is a complex structure of intertwining fibers. Moreover, the plexus is prelumbar rather than presacral in position. It lies in the extraperitoneal connective tissue, and the parietal peritoneum can easily be stripped off its anterior surface. The plexus varies in breadth and in degree of condensation of its constituent nerves and often lies a little to one side of the median plane, more often to the left than to the right. The root of the sigmoid mesocolon containing the

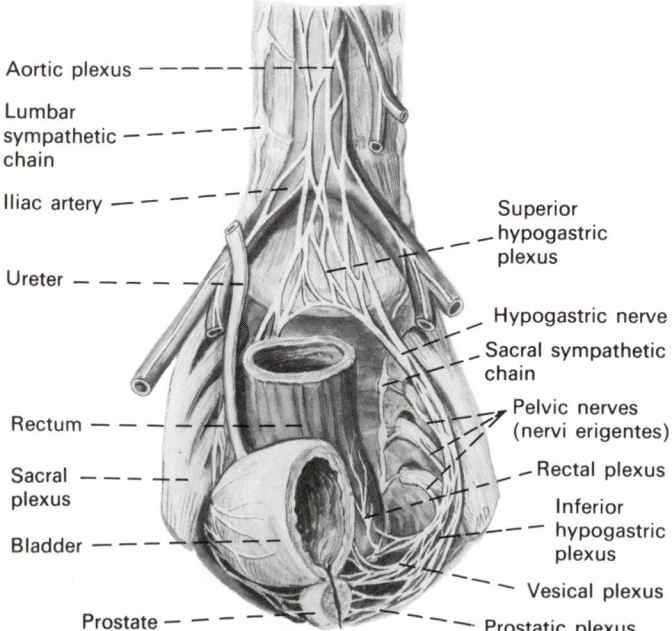

FIG. 65-8. Anatomy of the superior and inferior hypogastric plexuses and subsidiary plexuses. See text for details.

Labels: Aortic plexus — Lumbar sympathetic chain — Iliac artery — Ureter — Rectum — Sacral plexus — Bladder — Prostate — Superior hypogastric plexus — Hypogastric nerve — Sacral sympathetic chain — Pelvic nerves (nervi erigentes) — Rectal plexus — Inferior hypogastric plexus — Vesical plexus — Prostatic plexus

superior rectal vessels lies to the left side of the lower part of the plexus. Scattered nerve cells are found in the plexus.

At its lower border the plexus divides into right and left hypogastric nerves, often called the middle hypogastric plexuses, which descend to contribute to the inferior hypogastric (pelvic) plexuses. The superior hypogastric plexus gives off branches to the ureteric and testicular (or ovarian) plexuses and to those on the common iliac arteries. As emphasized in Chapter 66, the plexus contains sensory fibers that transmit nociceptive impulses from the body of the uterus and cervix that pass cephalad through the lower lumbar splanchnic nerves. In addition to the sympathetic fibers, which descend to form the superior hypogastric plexus, it contains parasympathetic fibers derived from the pelvic splanchnic nerves, which ascend from the inferior hypogastric plexus. Usually these parasympathetic fibers pass cephalad to the left of the superior hypogastric plexus, across the sigmoid vessels and branches of the left colic vessels, to become distributed partly along the branches of the inferior mesenteric artery. Parasympathetic fibers also arise directly from the pelvic splanchnic nerves and pass as independent retroperitoneal nerves to supply a short portion of the distal left part of the transverse colon, left colic (splenic) flexure, descending colon, and sigmoid colon (see Fig. 60-9). The parasympathetic supply to the distal colon is largely through these direct branches of the pelvic splanchnic nerves and not through the hypogastric and inferior mesenteric plexuses (5–8).

Hypogastric Nerves (Middle Hypogastric Plexus)

The superior hypogastric plexus divides below into right and left hypogastric "nerves," each of which runs down in the extraperitoneal connective tissue into the pelvis medial to each internal iliac artery and its branches to contribute to the formation of the inferior hypogastric (pelvic) plexus. Each nerve can be single or can form an elongated narrow plexus that consists of two or three longitudinal nerves connected by anastomosing filaments. Each nerve or plexus can be joined near its beginning by the lowest lumbar splanchnic nerve. From each hypogastric nerve branches pass to the testicular or ovarian plexus, ureteric plexus, the plexus on the internal iliac artery, and sigmoid colon.

Inferior Hypogastric (Pelvic) Plexus

Each of the two inferior hypogastric plexuses is formed by fibers contributed by the following: (a) the hypogastric nerves, which contain mostly sympathetic efferent and afferent fibers; (b) postganglionic sympathetic fibers from the sacral splanchnic nerves; and (c) para-sympathetic fibers derived from the pelvic splanchnic nerves (nervi erigentes) that have their cell bodies in the S2, S3, and S4 segments of the spinal cord (Figs. 65-8 and 65-9).

Each of the two hypogastric plexuses lies in the extraperitoneal connective tissue. In the male each plexus is situated on the rectum, seminal vesicle, prostate, and posterior part of the urinary bladder. In the female each plexus is placed on the side of the

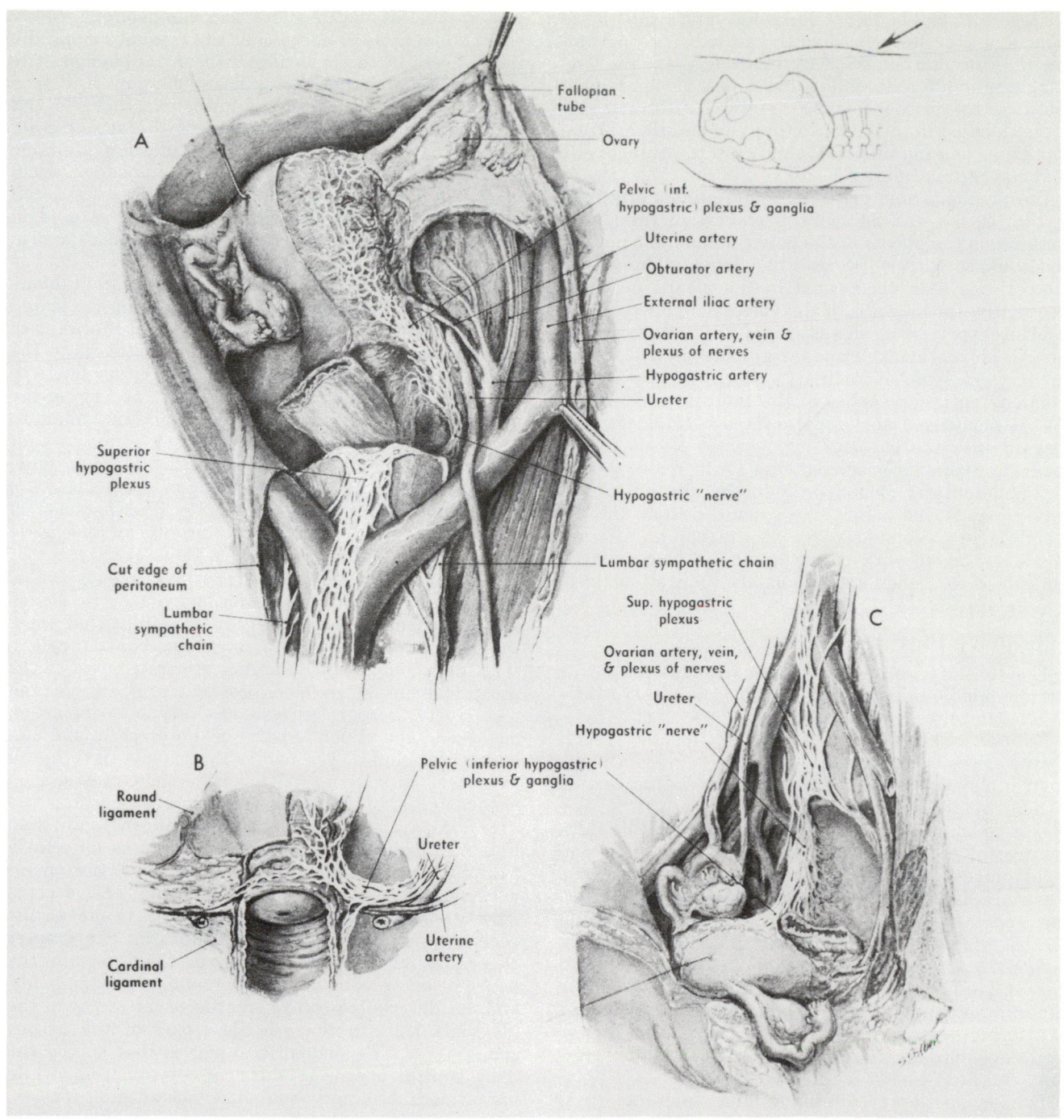

FIG. 65-9. Nerve supply of uterus. **A.** Superior view of pelvis (*inset*: *arrow*). The peritoneum has been removed to show the distribution of the lower portion of the aortic plexus, superior hypogastric plexus, and pelvic (inferior hypogastric) plexus. Note the relation of the nerve supply to the uterus. **B.** Coronal section of cervix and vagina showing distribution of the pelvic plexus in the paracervical region. Note the relation of the plexus to the uterine artery and ureter. **C.** Sagittal section of pelvis with view of its right lateral wall showing course and relation of some of the nerves to the uterus. From Bonica, J.J.: Principles and Practice of Obstetric Analgesia and Anesthesia, Vol. 1. Philadelphia, F.A. Davis, 1967, p. 513.

rectum, uterine cervix, vaginal fornix, and posterior part of the urinary bladder, and extends into the base of the broad ligaments of the uterus. Lateral to the plexus are the internal iliac vessels and their branches and tributaries and the levator ani, coccygeus, and obturator internus muscles. Behind are the sacral and coccygeal plexuses and above are the superior vesical

and obliterated umbilical arteries. The plexus contains numerous small ganglia.

The cell bodies of preganglionic efferent sympathetic fibers originate in the lower three thoracic and upper two lumbar segments of the spinal cord. Some of these lay in the ganglia in the lumbar and sacral parts of the paravertebral sympathetic trunk, while others synapse with cell bodies of postganglionic sympathetic neurons in the lower part of the aortic plexus and in the inferior and superior hypogastric plexuses. The sympathetic afferents follow the course of the sympathetic pathways in a reverse direction, with their cell bodies located in the posterior ganglia and their proximal axons passing into the spinal cord to contact cells of the superficial dorsal horn.

The preganglionic parasympathetic fibers originate in the S2, S3, and S4 sacral segments of the spinal cord, reach the plexus in the pelvic splanchnic nerves, and synapse with cell bodies of postganglionic parasympathetic neurons located in the plexus or, more frequently, in the walls of the viscera supplied by the inferior hypogastric plexus. From the inferior hypogastric plexus many branches are distributed to the pelvic (and some abdominal) viscera directly by accompanying the branches of the internal iliac artery (8). As mentioned above, parasympathetic fibers pass upward into the superior hypogastric plexus (or as separate filaments accompanying it) to reach the inferior mesenteric plexus through the medium of the aortic plexus and supply the splenic flexure and descending and sigmoid parts of the colon. Afferent fibers associated with parasympathetic fibers convey sensations for reflex action but also convey nociceptive impulses.

Subsidiary Plexuses

The subsidiaries of the inferior hypogastric plexus are the middle rectal plexus, vesical plexus, prostatic plexus, and uterovaginal plexus.

MIDDLE RECTAL PLEXUS. The middle rectal plexus arises from the upper part of the inferior hypogastric plexus, with the fibers passing to the rectum either directly or along the middle rectal artery. The plexus communicates above with branches of the superior rectal plexus (derived from the inferior mesenteric plexus) and extends inferiorly as far as the internal anal sphincter. The nerve supply of the rectum and anal canal is derived from the superior rectal plexus, middle rectal plexus, and inferior rectal (hemorrhoidal) nerves, which are branches of the pudendal nerves. Parasympathetic preganglionic fibers from the superior and middle sacral plexuses synapse with postganglionic neurons in the myenteric plexus, which is well developed in the wall of the sigmoid colon, rectum, and anal canal (see Fig. 60-9).

The sympathetic afferents and efferents pass through the plexus uninterrupted. The efferent sympathetic fibers in the rectal plexus are concerned with inhibition of expulsive musculature and contraction of the sphincter. Afferent fibers that transmit nociceptive impulses pass along both the sympathetic and parasympathetic nerves, but the parasympathetic afferent and efferent fibers are more active in controlling the defecation process. The inferior rectal nerves supply motor fibers to the external anal sphincter and sensory somatic fibers to the lower (ectodermal) part of the anal canal.

VESICAL PLEXUS. The vesical plexus arises from the anterior part of the inferior hypogastric plexus. It is composed of many nerves that accompany the vesical arteries to the bladder. Branches from the plexus

pass to the seminal vesicles and vas deferens. Many small collections of nerve cells are present among the nerve fibers in the muscular wall of the bladder. The sympathetic preganglionic efferent fibers in the plexus have their cell bodies in the lower two thoracic and the upper two lumbar segments of the spinal cord. Their axons pass through the inferior thoracic splanchnic nerve and the upper two lumbar splanchnic nerves, eventually ending to synapse with cell bodies of postganglionic fibers that are scattered in the superior and inferior hypogastric plexuses and in the wall of the bladder (see Fig. 68-1).

The parasympathetic preganglionic efferent fibers arise from the S2, S3, and S4 segments of the spinal cord and synapse with cells near to or in the walls of the bladder. These nerves convey motor fibers to the muscular coats of the bladder and inhibitory fibers to the sphincter. The efferent sympathetic nerves convey motor fibers to the sphincter and inhibitory fibers to the muscular coats. Some authorities maintain that the sympathetic fibers are mainly vasomotor in function, and that filling and emptying of the bladder are normally controlled exclusively by the parasympathetic nerves (1) (a further description of the nerve supply to the bladder is given in Chapter 68).

PROSTATIC PLEXUS. The prostatic plexus arises from the lower part of the inferior hypogastric plexus and is composed of relatively large nerves that enter the base and sides of the prostate and contain collections of nerve cells. The nerves are distributed to the prostate, seminal vesicles, prostatic urethra, ejaculatory ducts, corpora cavernosa, corpus spongiosum, membranous and penile parts of the urethra, and bulbourethral glands. The nerves that supply the corpora cavernosa form two sets, the lesser and greater cavernous nerves of the penis. These nerves arise from the anterior part of the prostatic plexus and join with branches from the pudendal nerve to pass anteriorly below the pubic arch. Filaments of the lesser cavernous nerves pierce the fibrous covering of the penis near its root and supply the erectile tissue of the corpus spongiosum and penile urethra. The greater cavernous nerves run anteriorly on the dorsum of the penis, communicate with the dorsal nerve of the penis, and are distributed to the erectile tissue. Some of the filaments pass to the erectile tissue of the corpus spongiosum. The sympathetic nerves that supply the male genital organs produce vasoconstriction, while parasympathetic nerves produce vasodilation (5).

The seminal vesicles are supplied by nerves derived from the vesical plexus, prostatic plexus, and lower part of the inferior hypogastric plexus. Nerve filaments pass from these structures to the ejaculatory ducts and vas deferens. It is generally believed that constriction of the seminal vesicles and seminal ejaculation are brought about by the sympathetic nerves (5, 6). These nerves also produce inhibition of the bladder musculature and contraction of the sphincter during ejaculation, thus preventing reflux of the seminal fluid into the bladder (a more detailed description of the nerve supply to the prostate is given in Chapter 68).

UTEROVAGINAL PLEXUS. The uterovaginal plexus arises from the inferior hypogastric plexus, predominantly from that part of the plexus lying in the base of the broad ligament (Fig. 65-9). Some nerves pass caudad from the plexus down with the vaginal arteries, others pass directly to the cervix uteri, and still others pass cephalad with or near the uterine arteries in the broad ligament. The nerves passing to the cervix form a plexus in which small paracervical ganglia are found. One ganglion is sometimes large, and is called the uterine cervical ganglion. The uterine nerves pass cephalad, with the uterine artery supplying branches to the body of the uterus. In the upper part of the broad ligament they supply branches to the uterine tube and communicate with the tubal nerves from the inferior hypogastric plexus and with the nerves of the ovarian plexus. Branches of the uterine nerves ramify in the myometrium and endometrium by accompanying blood vessels.

The efferent preganglionic sympathetic fibers supplying the uterus are derived from cell bodies located in the T10, 11, 12 (and sometimes T5-9) and L1 and (sometimes L2) segments of the cord, while the axons pass peripherally and synapse in various ganglia (6). The preganglionic parasympathetic fibers arise from the S2, S3, and S4 sacral segments of the cord and are relayed in the paracervical ganglia. The sympathetic nerves can produce uterine contractions and vasoconstriction and the parasympathetic nerves can produce uterine inhibition and vasodilation. The results of the activity of these two systems are complicated, however, by the pronounced hormonal control of uterine function (2, 6).

The vaginal plexus arises from the lower part of the pelvic and uterovaginal plexuses and follows the vaginal arteries and their branches to be distributed to the walls of the vagina, erectile tissue of the vestibular bulbs and clitoris (cavernous nerves of the clitoris), urethra, and greater vestibular glands. These nerves contain numerous parasympathetic fibers, which have a vasodilatory effect on the erectile tissue. (A more detailed description and illustrations of the nerve supply to the pelvic viscera are contained in Chapters 66 and 68.)

Anatomy and Neurology of the Perineum

Perineal Muscles and Fascia

The perineum overlies the inferior pelvic aperture, or pelvic outlet. Its deep boundaries are the pubic arch and arcuate pubic ligament anteriorly, the tip of the coccyx posteriorly, and the inferior ramus of the pubis and ramus of the ischium, ischial tuberosity, and sacrotuberous ligament laterally (2, 3). The space within these boundaries is somewhat trapezoidal in shape. The surface of the body of the perineum in the male is limited by the scrotum in front, the buttocks behind, and the medial sides of the thighs laterally, whereas in the female the external genitalia (labia majora and minora) limit the perineum anteriorly. Most anatomists divide the perineum into two parts by drawing a line transversely in front of the ischial tuberosity. The region posterior to this line contains the termination of the anal canal and is thus known as the anal region or anal triangle, while the anterior part contains the

external urogenital organs and is known as the urogenital region or urogenital triangle. The muscles and fascia of the perineum are also divided into these two groups, anal and urogenital, although these two groups meet in the perineal body and actually constitute a single morphologic unit (2, 5).

Muscles and Fascia of the Anal Region

Muscles. Figure 65-10 depicts the musculature of both the male and female perineum. Each muscle is briefly described.

The sphincter ani externus muscle surrounds the lower part of the anal canal and is intimately adherent to the skin below, whereas above it overlaps the sphincter ani internus. The muscle is composed of three parts—the subcutaneous, superficial, and deep. The subcutaneous lamina is a band of fibers that lies beneath the skin and surrounds the anal orifice. Some fibers are attached anteriorly to the perineal body and posteriorly to the anococcygeal ligament. The superficial lamina lies deep to the subcutaneous lamina and constitutes the main portion of the muscle (3). It also arises from the narrow tendinous anococcygeal ligament that stretches from the tip of the coccyx to the posterior margin of the anus. The muscle fibers then encircle the anus and meet anterior to the anus to be inserted into the perineal body. Here the muscle joins with fibers from the transversus perinei superficialis, levator ani, and bulbospongiosus muscles. The deep lamina forms a complete sphincter to the anal canal with its fibers surrounding the canal closely applied to the internal anal sphincter, while its deep fibers are interlaced with fibers of the puborectalis muscle. In front the deep part of the external anal sphincter blends with other muscles at the perineal body. This muscle is supplied by the perineal branch of the S4 spinal nerve and by twigs from the inferior rectal branch of the pudendal nerve (S2 and S3 spinal nerves).

The sphincter ani internus muscle is a muscular ring that surrounds about 2.5 cm of the anal canal. Its inferior border is in contact with, but quite separate from, the external sphincter. It is about 5 mm thick and is formed by an aggregation of the involuntary circular fibers of the large intestine. The distal border is about 6 mm from the orifice of the anus. This muscle is supplied by fibers from the middle rectal plexus (see above).

The corrugator cutis ani muscle is a thin layer of involuntary muscle and yellow elastic fibers that radiates from the orifice. It is believed that the fibers fade into the submucous tissue, while blending with the true skin laterally. By its contraction this muscle puckers the skin, raising it into ridges around the anal orifice.

FASCIA. The superficial fascia of the region is thick and areolar in texture and contains many fat cells in its meshes. On each side a pad of fatty tissue extends deeply into the lateral space between the levator ani and obturator internus muscles called the ischiorectal fossa. The deep fascia lines the ischiorectal fossa and comprises the inferior fascia of the pelvic diaphragm and the part of the obturator fascia below the attachment of the levator ani muscles (Fig. 65-10).

The ischiorectal fossa is somewhat wedge-shaped, with its space directed to the surface of the peritoneum and its thin edge at the line of meeting of the obturator internus and levator ani muscles covered by the obturator fascia and by the inferior fascia of the pelvic diaphragm. The internal pudendal vessels and their accompanying nerves are in the lateral wall of the ischiorectal fossa and are enclosed in a special sheath of fascia to form the pudendal canal. This sheath is fused with the lower part of the obturator fascia, extending upward to blend with the inferior fascia of the

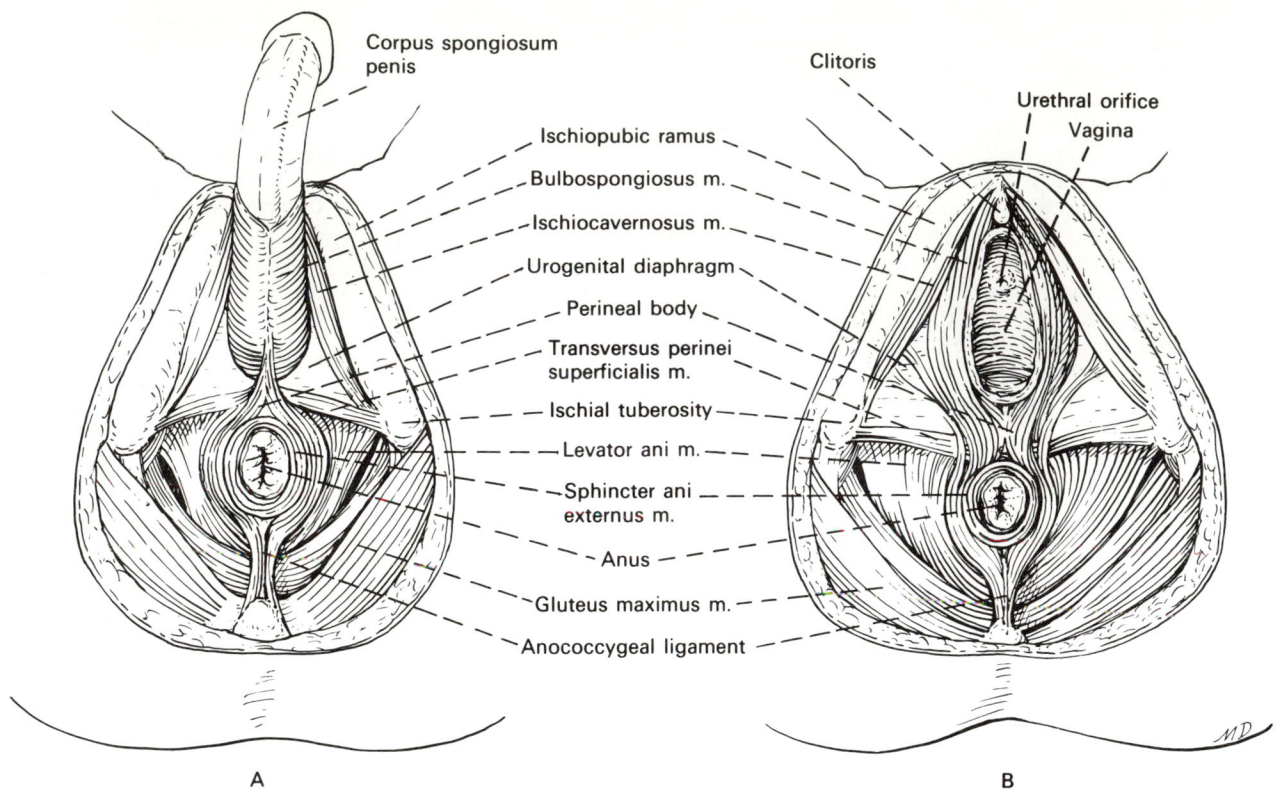

Corpus spongiosum penis

Clitoris

Urethral orifice
Vagina

Ischiopubic ramus

Bulbospongiosus m.

Ischiocavernosus m.

Urogenital diaphragm

Perineal body

Transversus perinei superficialis m.

Ischial tuberosity

Levator ani m.

Sphincter ani externus m.

Anus

Gluteus maximus m.

Anococcygeal ligament

A

B

Fig. 65-10. Muscles of the perineum. The inferior fascia of the urogenital diaphragm has been removed to depict the muscles. **A.** Muscles of the male perineum. **B.** Muscles of the female perineum.

pelvic diaphragm and downward to become continuous with the falciform process of the sacrotuberous ligament.

Muscles and Fascia of the Male Urogenital Region

MUSCLES. In both genders the muscles of the urogenital region consist of the bulbospongiosus, ischiocavernosus, transversus perinei superficialis and profundus, and sphincter urethrae. The muscles are grouped into superficial and deep layers. The superficial urogenital muscles include the midline bulbospongiosus, right and left ischiocavernosus, and right and left transversus perinei superficialis, all of which occupy the superficial perineal space. The deep perineal space is occupied by the sphincter urethra and right and left deep transversus perinei profundus, collectively known as the urogenital diaphragm (Fig. 65-11). The following review of these muscles is intended to supplement the illustration.

The transversus perinei superficialis muscles consist of a pair, each of which is composed of a narrow strip of muscle fibers that passes more or less transversely across the superficial space in front of the anus. Each arises by tendinous fibers from the medial and anterior parts of the tuberosity of the ischium. Running medially it ends in the perineal body, where it joins the muscle of the opposite side. At the perineal body it is also joined by the superficial part of the sphincter ani externus muscle posteriorly and by the bulbospongiosus muscle anteriorly.

The bulbospongiosus (bulbocavernosus) muscle is located in the medial line of the perineum in front of the anus. It consists of two symmetric parts united by a median tendinous raphe. The muscle arises from this median raphe and from the perineal body, and its fibers diverge into two halves (2, 3) (Fig. 65-10A and 65-11A). The most posterior fibers form a thin layer that is lost on the inferior fascia of the urogenital diaphram. The middle fibers encircle the bulk and adjacent part of the corpus spongiosum penis and join with fibers of the opposite side on the upper part of the corpus cavernosum penis in a strong aponeurosis. The anterior fibers spread out over the side of the corpus cavernosum penis and are inserted partly in that body, anterior to the ischiocavernosus, and partly in the tendinous expansion that covers the dorsal vessels of the penis (3). This muscle aids in emptying of the urethra after the bladder has expelled its contents. Its middle fibers assist in the erection of the corpus spongiosum penis by compressing the erectile tissue of the bulb. The anterior fibers also contribute to the erection of the penis by compressing the deep dorsal vein of the penis because their tendinous expansion is inserted into and is continuous with the deep fascia covering the deep dorsal vessels of the penis.

The ischiocavernous muscle, also called the erector penis muscle, consists of a pair, with each covering the crura of the penis (Figs. 65-10A and 65-11A). Each is an elongated muscle, broader in the middle than at either end and situated at the lateral boundary of the perineum. It is erected by tendinous and fleshy fibers from the inner surface of the ischial tuberosity behind the crus penis and from the rami of the pubis and ischium on both sides of the crus. From these points fleshy fibers course anteriorly along the crus and end in an aponeurosis that is inserted into the sides and undersurface of the crura as they become the body of the penis. This muscle compresses the crus penis and thus helps to maintain erection of the penis.

The transversus perinei profundus muscle arises from the inner surface of the ramus of the ischium and passes to the

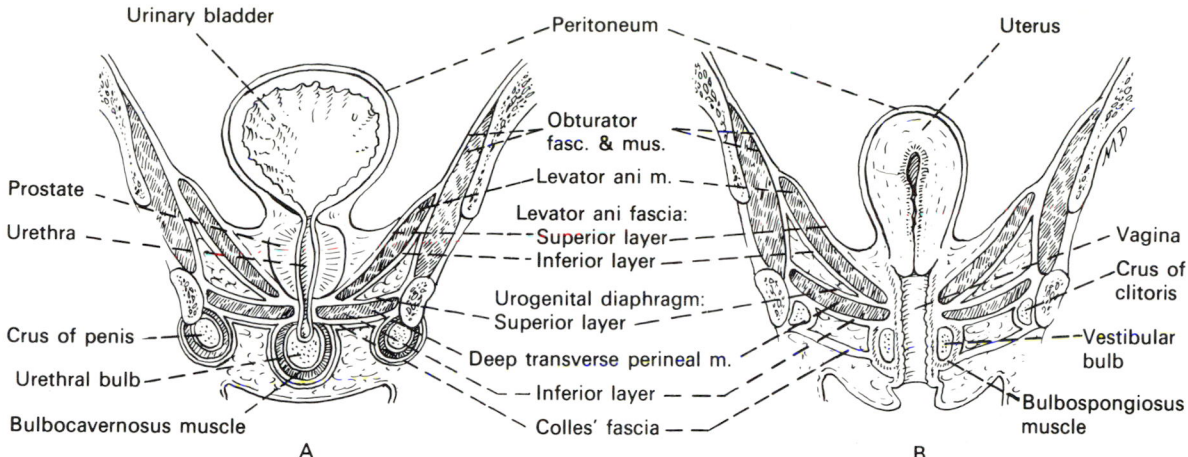

FIG. 65-11. Transverse section depicting the fascia and muscles of the male (*A*) and female (*B*) pelvic and anal regions. See text for details. Modified from Clemente, C.D. (ed.): Gray's Anatomy of the Human Body. 27th Ed. Philadelphia, Lea & Febiger, 1959, p. 476.

median line, where it interlaces in a tendinous raphe with its fellow of the opposite side. Lying in the same plane as the sphincter urethra, these two muscles are interposed between the superior and inferior fascial layers of the urogenital diaphragm and form much of the bulk of the structure (Fig. 65-11A). These two muscles were formerly described together as the constrictor urethrae. They are believed to help in steadying the perineal body and therefore are likely to contribute to the general supportive function of the region (2).

The sphincter urethrae muscles, in the male, surround the whole length of the membranous portion of the urethra and are enclosed in the fascia of the urogenital diaphragm. The superficial or external fibers arise in front of the transverse perineal ligament and from the neighboring fascia, and pass backward on each side of the urethra to converge on the perineal body. Their deep fibers arise from the inner surface of the ramus of the pubis and pass medially to form a continuous circular investment of the membranous urethra. The muscles of both sides act together as a sphincter to compress the membranous region of the urethra, particularly if the bladder contains fluid. Like the bulbospongiosus muscle during micturition, they are relaxed and only come into action at the end of the process to eject the last drops of urine. These muscles are also concerned with ejaculation. All the muscles of the urogenital region are supplied by the perineal branch of the pudendal nerve.

FASCIA. The fascia of the male urogenital diaphragm consists of a superficial (external, inferior) fascia and deep (internal, superior) fascia. The inferior fascia is a flat, triangular, membranous sheet that bridges the angular interval between the ischiopubic rami. It is attached laterally to the medial border of the rami from the arcuate pubic ligament to the ischial tuberosity. The middle portion of the fascia is pierced by the urethra. The superior fascia of the urogenital diaphragm is also a flat triangular membrane that stretches across the same interval as the superficial fascia. It lies between the transversus perinei profundus and pubococcygeus portions of the levator ani, representing the fused fascial membranes of both these muscles. It is securely attached to the symphysis pubis anteriorly and joins other perineal layers at the central tendinous point posteriorly. Laterally it is attached to the medial borders of the ischiopubic rami, where it is continuous with the obturator fascia.

Muscles and Fascia of the Female Urogenital Region

MUSCLES. This group of muscles in the female is composed of the same five paired muscles as in the male, with some difference in size and disposition because of the presence of the vagina and female external genitalia. They are similarly grouped into superficial and deep layers, with the latter constituting the urogenital diaphragm (Figs. 65-10B and 65-11B).

The transversus perinei superficialis muscle in the female is a narrow muscular slip that differs little from the corresponding muscle in the male.

The bulbospongiosus muscle surrounds the orifice of the vagina, and has been called the sphincter vaginae. Each muscle covers the lateral parts of the vestibular bulbs and is continuous posteriorly with the perineal body, where it blends with the external and sphincter muscles. Its fibers pass forward on each side of the vagina to become attached to the corpora cavernosa clitoridis. A fasciculus crosses over the body of the clitoris and compresses the deep dorsal vein. The anterior fibers contribute to the erection of the clitoris by compression of the deep dorsal vein.

The ischiocavernosus muscle in the female is smaller than in the male. It covers the unattached surface of the crus clitoridis. It is erected by tendinous and fleshy fibers from the inner surface of the tuberosity of the ischium from the surface of the crus clitoridis and from the adjacent surface of the ramus of the ischium. The muscular fibers end in an aponeurosis that is attached to the sides and undersurface of the crus clitoridis. This muscle compresses the crus clitoridis and thus retards the return of blood through the veins that help to erect the clitoris.

The transversus perinei profundus muscle in the female courses from the inferior ramus of the ischium to the side of the vagina, meeting fibers of the muscles from the opposite side. It helps to fix the perineal body.

The sphincter urethra muscle, as in the male, consists of superficial and deep fibers. The superficial fibers arise on each side from the margin of the inferior ramus of the pubis and transverse perineal ligament. These fibers are directly across the pubic arch in front of the urethra and pass around it to blend with the muscular fibers of the opposite side between the urethra and vagina. The internal fibers encircle the lower end of the urethra. The actions of these muscles are similar to those of the male.

All the muscles of the female in the genital region are supplied by the perineal branch of the pudendal nerve.

Fascia. The urogenital diaphragm in the female, as in the male, is formed by two layers of fascia between which are interposed a deep transverse perineal muscle and sphincter urethra (Fig. 65-11B). The fascial layers are not as strong in the female as in the male. The fascial layers are attached anteriorly to the pubic arch by connecting to the arcuate pubic ligament and posteriorly the two continuous deep layers of the superficial fascia surround the superficial transverse perineal muscle. In the midline the fascial layers are divided by the aperture of the vagina and blend with its external coat. The urogenital diaphragm is perforated by the urethra anterior to the midline.

Between the two fascial layers are the dorsal vein of the clitoris, a portion of the urethra, the deep transverse perineal muscle and sphincter urethrae muscle, the greater vestibular glands and their ducts, the internal pudendal vessels, the dorsal nerves of the clitoris, the arteries and nerves of the vestibular bulbs, and a plexus of veins.

Neurology of the Perineum

The perineum derives its nerve supply primarily from various branches of the pudendal nerve. It also receives some fibers from the anterior labial or scrotal branches of the ilioinguinal, genital branch of the genitofemoral, perforating cutaneous, and muscular branches of the S2, S3, and S4, and anococcygeal nerves. The perineal branches of the ilioinguinal and genitofemoral nerves are discussed in Chapter 69 in connection with the nerve supply to the lower limbs. Here I first discuss the anatomy of the pudendal plexus

and then the anatomy and distribution of the pudendal nerve.

Pudendal Plexus

The pudendal plexus is formed by the union of the anterior divisions of the S2 and S3 nerves and of the entire S4 nerve (Fig. 65-12). It lies in the lower part of the posterior wall of the pelvic cavity and the anterior surface of the piriformis muscle, where it divides into the pudendal nerve, perforating cutaneous nerve, and visceral and muscular branches. The visceral branches make up the pelvic nerve, which leaves the pudendal plexus and proceeds anteriorly to join the pelvic plexuses to contribute parasympathetic fibers.

The muscular branches of the pudendal plexus are provided mainly by the S4 nerve to supply the levator ani, coccygeus, and sphincter ani externus muscles. The nerves to the levator ani and coccygeus muscles enter these structures on their pelvic surface. The nerve to the sphincter ani externus, generally known as the perineal branch of the S4 nerve, pierces the sacrotuberous ligament and coccygeus muscle and enters the ischiorectal fossa to supply muscular branches to the sphincter and cutaneous branches to the skin between the anus and coccyx.

The perforating cutaneous branches of the S2 and S3 nerves descend in front of the coccygeus muscle and pass through it, perforate the sacrotuberous ligament, and turn around at the inferior border of the gluteus maximus to supply the skin of the buttocks. Some of the fibers, however, run anteriorly to the perineum. The anococcygeal nerve, derived from the S4 and S5

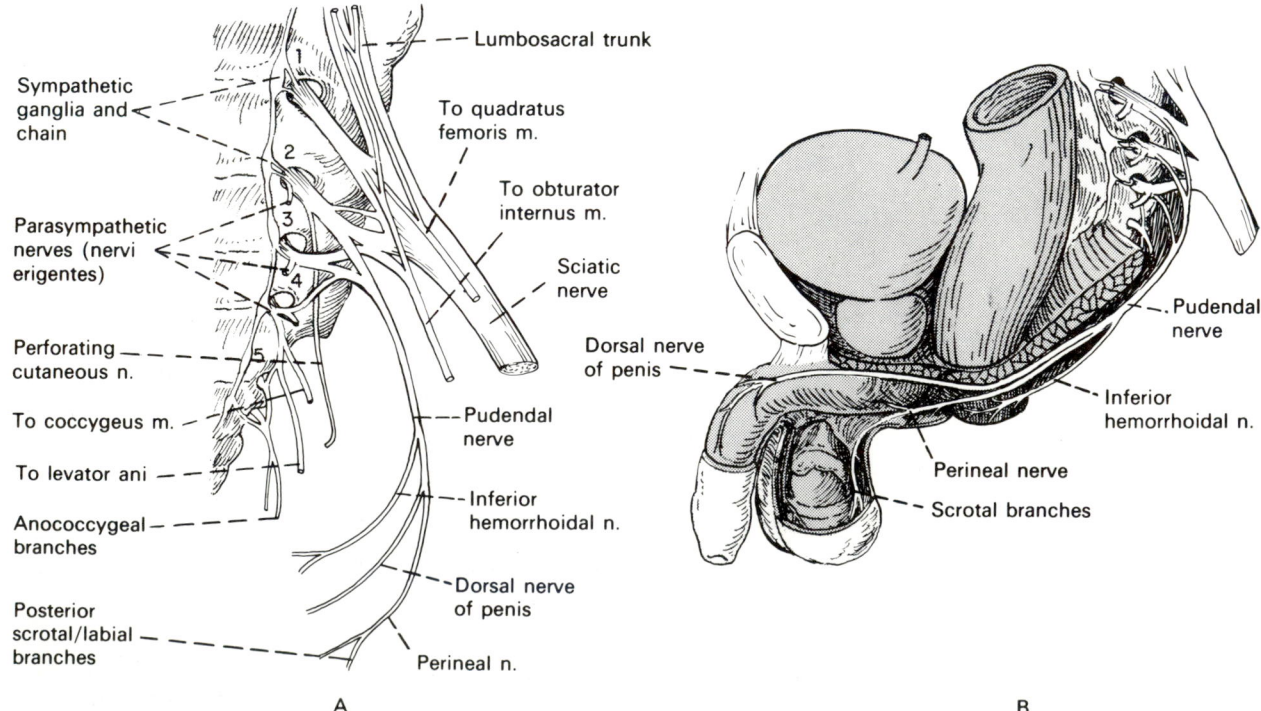

A

B

FIG. 65-12. *A.* Anatomy of the pudendal plexus and its branches. See text for details. *B.* Parasagittal view depicting the course and branches of the left pudendal nerve in the male. *A* modified from Bonica, J.J.: Principles and Practice of Obstetric Analgesia and Anesthesia, Vol. 1. Philadelphia, F.A. Davis, 1967, p. 490; and *B* modified from Netter, F.H.: The CIBA Collection of Medical Illustrations, Vol. 2. Reproductive System. Summit, NJ, CIBA Pharmaceuticals, 1979. p. 19.

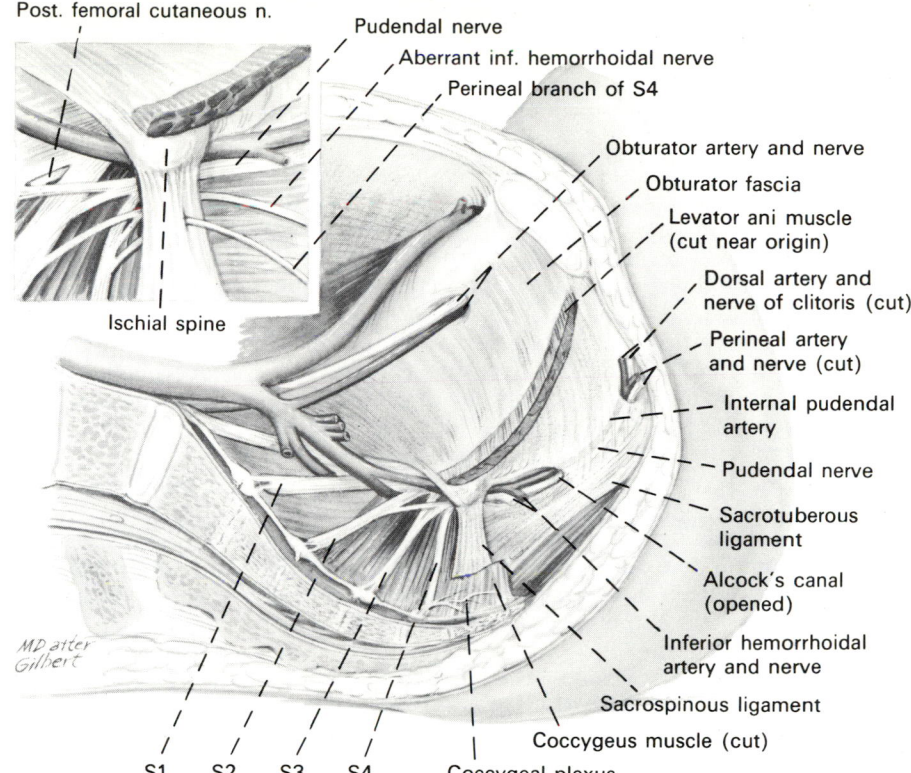

FIG. 65-13. Sagittal section of the perineum showing the origin and course of the pudendal nerve. The pudendal nerve passes posterior to the junction of the ischial spine and the sacrospinous ligament and then re-enters the pelvis to pass through Alcock's canal. *Inset*: Aberrant hemorrhoidal nerve (which occurs in 50% of individuals) and perineal branch of S4. See text for details. Modified from Bonica, J.J.: Principles and Practice of Obstetric Analgesia and Anesthesia, Vol. 1. Philadelphia, F.A. Davis, 1967, facing p. 490.

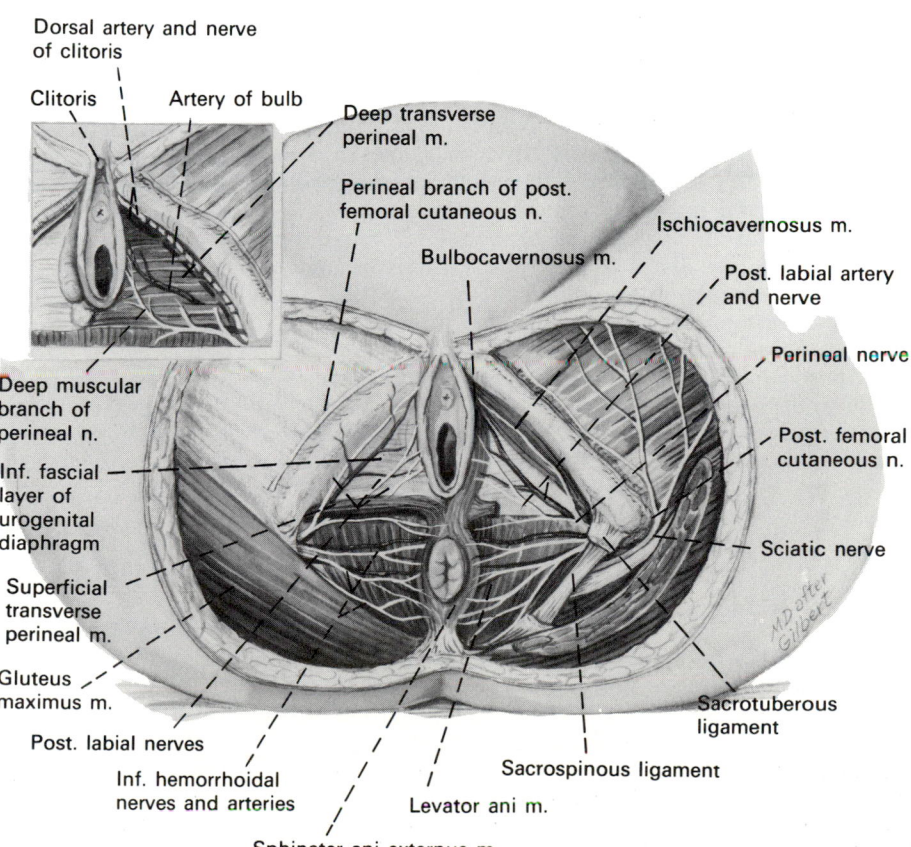

FIG. 65-14. Nerve supply of the perineum of a gravida showing the principal branches of the pudendal nerve as well as the posterior femoral cutaneous nerve and other nerves that supply sensory fibers to the skin, subcutaneous tissue, external genitalia, and muscular fibers to the various muscles. The superficial transverse perineal muscles have been cut to show the course of the perineal nerve. *Inset*: Deeper dissection after inferior (superficial) fascia of the urogenital diaphragm has been removed shows the course of the dorsal nerve of the clitoris. The posterior two-thirds of the nerve passes through the thickness of the muscle. Modified from Bonica, J.J.: Principles and Practice of Obstetric Analgesia and Anesthesia. Vol. 1. Philadelphia, F.A. Davis. 1967, facing p. 491.

and coccygeal nerves, also penetrates the sacrotuberous ligaments to supply the skin behind the anus in the anococcygeal area.

Anatomy of the Pudendal Nerve

The anatomy of the pudendal nerve is shown in Figures 65-13 and 65-14. The somatic fibers are derived from the anterior primary division of the S2, S3, and S4 nerves, while the sympathetic fibers are contributed by the sacral portion of the sympathetic chain. All these fibers combine to form a single trunk about 1 cm proximal (posterior) to the ischial spine. The formed nerve is directed anteriorly and inferiorly and leaves the pelvic cavity by passing through the greater sciatic foramen inferior to the piriformis muscle, between it and the coccygeal muscle. It then re-enters the pelvic cavity through the lesser sciatic foramen and proceeds anteriorly through Alcock's (pudendal) canal.

The nerve passes posterior to the junction between the ischial spine and sacrospinous ligament and anterior to the sacrotuberous ligament. Except when the ischial spine is long and prominent, the nerve does not pass behind the spine but rather passes diagonally across the posterior surface of the sacrospinous ligament just as it attaches to the spine (10). Here it is medial to the internal pudendal vessels that separated from the nerve to the obturator internus muscle. The posterior femoral cutaneous nerve lies lateral and posterior to the pudendal nerve, while the sciatic nerve is much more lateral and some distance away from the pudendal nerve.

The pudendal nerve trunk divides into three main branches, the inferior hemorrhoidal, perineal, and dorsal nerve to the clitoris (or to the penis). Each of these makes an important contribution to the nerve supply of the perineum.

INFERIOR HEMORRHOIDAL NERVE. In approximately 50% of individuals the inferior hemorrhoidal nerve arises directly from the S3 and S4 nerves, while in the other 50% it arises from the pudendal nerve (10, 11). In the latter instance it branches off from the parent nerve just distal to the sacrospinous ligament and then accompanies the pudendal nerve within the posterior part of Alcock's canal. The inferior hemorrhoidal nerve pierces the medial wall of Alcock's canal, crosses the ischiorectal fossa, and proceeds medially and anteriorly across the ischiorectal fossa accompanied by the inferior hemorrhoidal vessels to reach the perianal region. Midway in its course to the

anus it divides into muscular branches for the sphincter ani externus, cutaneous filaments that supply the skin around the anus, and branches that communicate with other nerves of the perineum. When the inferior hemorrhoidal nerve arises separately it does not pass through Alcock's canal but proceeds anteriorly from its origin, lying significantly more medially than the pudendal nerve.

PERINEAL NERVE. The perineal nerve is the largest of the three branches of the pudendal nerve. It arises near the base of the urogenital diaphragm, approximately 3 cm above the inferior border of the ischial tuberosity, and divides almost immediately into the superficial cutaneous and deep muscular branches. The superficial part of the perineal nerve is purely cutaneous and consists of two nerves, medial posterior and lateral posterior labial (or scrotal) nerves. These supply the skin of the perineum and the major portion of the ipsilateral labia majora and minora (or the scrotum) (see Fig. 68-2). They also communicate with the inferior hemorrhoidal nerves and with the perineal branch of the posterior femoral cutaneous nerve.

The deep branch of the perineal nerve arises at the anterior end of the ischiorectal fossa and proceeds anteriorly by passing between the superior and inferior layers of the urogenital diaphragm to reach the urethra. Its branches supply the following muscles: transversus perinei superficialis, bulbocavernosus, ischiocavernosus, transversus perinei profundus, sphincter urethrae, and anterior part of the levator ani and sphincter ani externus. It also supplies sensory fibers to the fascia of these muscles. The deep branch of the perineal nerve terminates in the urethra and supplies the erectile tissue of the bulb of the vestibule, urethra, and mucous membrane of the urethra with vasomotor nerves.

DORSAL NERVE OF THE CLITORIS (OR PENIS). The third branch of the pudendal nerve, the dorsal nerve of the clitoris in the female or of the penis in the male, emerges from the anterior end of Alcock's canal, passes through the urogenital diaphragm, and proceeds anteriorly, lying between the two layers of fascia of the diaphragm. Near the apex of the urogenital diaphragm it pierces the superficial fascial layer and proceeds anteriorly on the side of the dorsal artery of the clitoris or penis to reach the dorsum of the structure it supplies. This nerve also supplies a small branch to the corpus cavernosum muscle and carries sympathetic fibers that supply the erectile tissue (Fig. 65-12B).

B. EVALUATION OF PATIENTS WITH PELVIC AND PERINEAL PAIN

General Comments

The general approach to assessment of patients with pain in the pelvis or perineum is presented in this section because pelvic pain is a result of either urologic or gynecologic problems. Some specific comments applicable to both these areas are also presented. As emphasized in Chapter 31 and in the introductory chapters to each section of Part IV, other than in patients who require urgent operative inter-

vention, it is essential to obtain a detailed history and carry out a comprehensive physical examination, including urologic and gynecologic evaluation; in some cases it might also be necessary to include neurologic and orthopedic studies (Chapter 31 and Table 53-1). Other laboratory studies, including a complete blood count, comprehensive urinalysis, radiographic studies, and various other specialized urologic and gynecologic tests, might also be required.

History

As emphasized in Chapter 31 and elsewhere in this book, an orderly, systematic, painstakingly detailed history is the most important aspect of the assessment, and often the correct diagnosis can be made on the information obtained. In other cases the history might not be so decisive but can have so limited a diagnostic possibility that a logical program of investigation is suggested. Finally, and equally important, the history affords the physician an unequaled opportunity to establish a rapport with patients by being friendly, understanding, and courteous, by being visibly interested in the problem, by centering all attention on patients, and by appearing anxious to help.

A comprehensive history consists of the following: (a) history of the pain problem; (b) past medical history; (c) general psychologic and psychosocial history; and (d) family history. Because patients present with a painful disorder, they expect to be asked first about the pain. Initially, patients should be allowed to use their own words in describing the characteristics of the pain. Particularly important is to suggest that patients provide information about the rapidity of the onset of the pain, its location, quality, intensity, duration, and temporal characteristics, and what factors make it better and what factors relieve it. If the pain has been present for several days or longer before patients consult a physician it is important to ascertain if characteristics have changed and what time of the day the pain is better and what time it is worse. Patients should be asked specifically what effects the following activities or functions have on the pain: standing, lying, bending, eating, swallowing, coughing, straining, release of flatus, defecation, urination, lateral or forward flexion of the trunk, and other movements. Specific information should be obtained about associated symptoms and signs or phenomena such as nausea, vomiting, melena, and the presence of weakness or numbness in various parts of the body.

Next in importance is obtaining as detailed and comprehensive information as possible about past medical history, including any hospitalization and surgery, especially details of abdominal or pelvic surgery. The patient's general health should be reviewed, including the psychologic status, with particular attention to depression, anxiety, and drug abuse. Drug intake should be ascertained, with reference to allergies and especially drugs affecting the present condition. This should be followed by a family history.

Information about changes in micturition should be obtained from patients in whom pain is thought to be caused by urinary disorders (12). Because most adults void about four to six times a day, mostly in the daytime, increased frequency, unassociated with an increase in urine volume, is a symptom of lowered urinary bladder effective filling capacity. This can be a result of infection or of the presence of a foreign body, stones, or tumors that injure the bladder mucosa or underlying structures, leading to inflammatory infiltration and edema. Mild stretching of the bladder and loss of bladder elasticity results, producing a functional decrease, pain, and urgency. Information should also be obtained about urinary tenesmus, dysuria (painful urination), and nocturia, and about hesitancy, straining, decrease in force and caliber of the urinary stream, and terminal dribbling, which are common symptoms of obstruction distal to the bladder. Incontinence is usually associated with exstrophy of the bladder, vesicovaginal fistula, ectopic ureteral orifices, or congenital or acquired neuropathic bladder dysfunction, as well as with injury sustained during prostatectomy or childbirth. Incontinence with mild physical stress in women, such as coughing, laughing, running, or lifting, is commonly associated with a cystocele as a result of stretching of the pelvic floor muscles following childbirth or as a result of aging. Other important information pertains to changes in urinary output and in the appearance of urine.

The physician should also obtain information from women presenting with pelvic pain about the menstrual history, including the age of menarche of the patient (and other family members), frequency, regularity, duration, amount of flow, pain or other symptoms with or before menses, abnormal bleeding, and dates of the last two menses (13). History of pregnancy should include the number of pregnancies, dates and outcomes, and problems in becoming pregnant. Information about sexual activity and orientation is important. Questions should also be asked regarding any history of radiation therapy for benign disease, such as mastitis, menorrhagia, or skin disorders, and any prior use of diethylstilbestrol (DES) by women who were pregnant or who were born from 1947 to 1971. Information should be elicited about breast problems, including pain or growth, and general endocrine status, including abnormal hair growth, abnormal lactation, and other symptoms of endocrine dysfunction. A family history might reveal hereditary disease; ovarian, uterine, or breast cancer, diabetes, and genetic abnormalities are especially pertinent.

Physical Examination

The physical examination should begin with a simple critical inspection of the patient regarding the facies, color and degree of hydration, respiratory movements, abdominal distensions, and observation of posture during walking and sitting. The physical examination includes determination of height, weight, and blood pressure and a check of the heart, lungs, and lymph nodes. Abnormal body hair texture or distribution is noted; a thorough breast examination in both the sitting and prone positions should be done, noting maturation of the breast and any tenderness, asymmetry, retraction of the skin or nipples, and masses. It is important for the physician to have warm hands and to be gentle, and to use this occasion to instruct the patient in self-examination for early detection of malignancy.

The next step is to carry out an abdominal examination beginning at a site away from the area of pain. Using a flat hand for gentle palpation (not poking), each quadrant of the abdomen is systematically palpated to detect any tenderness, masses, or aggravation of pain. If a mass is felt it is important to note its size, location, mobility, and tenderness, the size of the liver and possible tenderness, and whether the kidneys, liver, or spleen is palpable. If tenderness is present its severity, location, and any accompanying rigidity of the abdominal wall should be noted and bowel sounds checked.

Examination of the lower part of the abdomen and pelvis is usually deferred until last. This should be preceded by having the patient empty the bladder and submit a urine specimen, which is examined by the laboratory. Rectal examination is then carried out in men to detect enlargement of the prostate or tumors in the rectum. Note should be made if the examination elicits pain and tenderness, and of their location.

Pelvic examination in women should be done in the presence of a female nurse and *after* the physician gives an unhurried explanation in a sensitive, gentle, and matter-of-fact manner to help the patient relax. These amenities not only make the patient happier but the examination can be done more thoroughly. The genital area should be inspected for hair distribution, clitoral size, vulvar lesions, discoloration, discharge, inflammation, and degree of patency of the hymenal orifice. The cervix is inspected by using a warm water-lubricated speculum inserted into the upper vagina at a 45° angle and then rotated and opened. Lubricating jelly should be avoided because it can interfere with the Papanicolaou (Pap) test, which is carried out next to detect any preinvasive as well as invasive lesions.

Bimanual palpation of the uterus is done to assess the position, size, consistency, surface contour, and mobility of the uterus (13). If the examination produces tenderness and pain the site of these symptoms should be noted and special gentleness should be used. Enlargement of the uterus can be a result of pregnancy, myoma, adenomyosis, simple hypertrophy, malignancy, or inflammation. Softening can result from pregnancy, malignancy, degenerating myoma, or sarcoma, or might be caused by a low estrogen level. Irregularities can be caused by myoma, abnormalities of the uterus, neoplasm, or adhesions of other pelvic structures, such as between the ovary and uterus. The adnexal structures are carefully palpated by approximating the fingers of the two hands and, if the patient has presented with pain in one of the lower quadrants, the nonpainful side should be examined first. Because the normal adult ovary is only $3 \times 3 \times 2$ cm, it might be difficult to feel, especially if the abdominal wall is thick or tense but, in patients who are not obese, a small enlargement is detectable. Enlargement of the ovary or an adnexal mass, including any in the uterine tubes, should be noted, and note should be made if the palpation produces pain and tenderness. The position of the cecum can be differentiated on the right side by its mobility and by the presence of gas. The cul-de-sac area behind the uterus is palpated at this point and again at the time of the rectovaginal examination. Finally, the vagina is palpated to search for vaginal cysts or nodules and the pelvic support is evaluated to determine if a cystocele, rectocele, or enterocele is present.

The rectovaginal examination is done last, with the index finger in the vagina and the second finger in the rectum, to confirm the previous findings (13). This should include palpation of the uterosacral ligament, the back of the uterus and cervix, and the contents of the posterior cul-de-sac (pouch of Douglas) and parametria to search for masses, tenderness, or induration. This part of the examination is especially important when the uterus is retroflexed. Again, any rectal lesions within the range of the examining fingers, such as hemorrhoids, fissures, polyps, masses, or the presence of blood, are noted.

Laboratory Studies

The results of the laboratory examination, including a complete blood count, urinalysis, and radiographic studies, should be integrated with the information obtained from the history and physical examination. The results of the urinalysis are critical for indicating the state of hydration and for ruling out severe renal diseases, diabetes, or urinary infection. If the history and physical examination suggest a urinary tract problem, radiographic procedures, such as plain radiography of the abdomen to demonstrate the size and location of the kidneys and perhaps urethra and bladder, are done. Intravenous urography (IVU) is used to visualize the kidneys and lower urinary tract, and retrograde pyelography might also be indicated for this purpose. Other more specialized techniques used to diagnose urinary tract problems include ultrasound (US), computed tomography (CT), and magnetic resonance imaging (MRI) (13). These are newer and expensive but are more specific diagnostic procedures for obtaining information about urinary tract disease as well as about gynecologic cancer. The indications for and efficacy of these diagnostic procedures are discussed in Chapters 67 and 68.

Key Points of Differential Diagnosis

The characteristics of pelvic pain and its associated signs and symptoms are presented in Table 65-1, intended to help in making the differential diagnosis of pain in the pelvis.

Chapter 59 presents important points about the location, distribution, rapidity of onset, duration, and other features of abdominal pain. The last sections, dealing with pain in the left iliac region, pain in the hypogastric region, and pain in the right iliac region, are relevant to pelvic pain and should be reviewed in considering the differential diagnosis.

Briefly, pain in the left iliac region is most frequently caused by acute salpingitis, chronic salpingo-oophoritis, ectopic pregnancy, twisted ovarian cyst, ruptured graafian follicle, acute oophoritis, ulcerative colitis, acute diverticulitis, left lower ureteral calculus, volvulus of the sigmoid, and intestinal obstruction. Less common causes are neurologic and musculoskeletal disorders with pain projected to the lower abdomen.

Pain in the right iliac region is most commonly caused by acute appendicitis, acute or chronic salpingitis, ruptured ectopic pregnancy, twisted ovarian cyst, ruptured graafian follicle, acute oophoritis, Meckel's diverticulitis, and colic resulting from obstruction in the lower right ureter.

Pain in the hypogastric region usually results from diseases of the urinary bladder, internal genitalia, intestinal diseases, and neurologic or musculoskeletal disorders. The most common causes include acute cystitis, urinary bladder distension, prostatitis, seminal vesiculitis, hypertrophy of the prostate, calculi in the urinary bladder, other urinary bladder diseases (e.g., carcinoma, ulcer, rupture), various diseases of the female genitalia (e.g., dysmenorrhea, acute salpingitis, ruptured ectopic pregnancy, acute or chronic endometritis, retrodisplacement or prolapse of the uterus, carcinoma of the uterus), various acute and chronic diseases of the bowel, and neuropathic or musculoskeletal disorders.

Characteristics and Causes of Pelvic Pain

Colicky pain in the pelvic region is usually caused by obstruction of the lower ureter on one side or the other. A sudden onset of pain usually occurs from ischemia, as with a twisted ovarian cyst or following sudden bowel perforation into the pelvic peritoneal cavity. A slower onset of pain (occurring over a period of minutes or hours) is caused by inflammation or obstruction such as with salpingitis, appendicitis, and intestinal obstruction (Table 59-3). *Localized pain* represents a localized inflammation or problem with one adnexa or part of the uterus, whereas pain involving the entire abdomen suggests generalized peritonitis caused by infection or chemical agents. This type of pain usually increases with movement of the abdomen, general bodily movement, bowel or bladder movement, or examination. Pain and tenderness in the adnexa of one or both sides are usually caused by ectopic pregnancy, ovarian cyst, or inflammatory mass.

Acute salpingitis is usually bilateral and causes severe lower abdominal and pelvic pain and tenderness, especially on movement of the cervix. The pain is usually accompanied by fever, leukocytosis, and purulent discharge from the cervical canal. If salpingitis persists for several days a pelvic abscess can develop, with pain most often pointing toward the vagina or rectum. A sudden easing of symptoms indicates that the abscess has ruptured intra-abdominally, and immediate laparotomy is required.

Ectopic gestation is most commonly signaled by pelvic pain, menstrual irregularity, and adnexal mass. Sudden pelvic pain in pregnant women can also be caused by associated torsion of an ovarian cyst, acute degeneration of a uterine myoma, placental abruption, or ruptured uterus or, if fever is present, by parametritis.

Ovarian cysts are usually asymptomatic, although the pressure of an abdominal mass can cause a dull aching pain or heaviness in the pelvis. Sudden sharp pain indicates rupture, hemorrhage, or torsion. Twisted ovarian cysts produce intermittent colicky pain. Malposition of the uterus rarely causes pelvic pain unless it is retrodisplaced and fixed by adhesions of scar tissue. Pain caused by an invasive neoplasm is usually caused by invasion of pelvic tissue or by infiltration of sacral nerve roots.

Endometriosis can cause pain and tenderness by direct action on nerve endings or by interfering with the function of involved or adjacent organs. The pain is characteristically worse a few days before menstruation than during the early period of flow. Midcycle pain (mittelschmerz) can cause severe hypogastric pain for a few hours that can mimic that of acute appendicitis.

Pain of urologic origin is frequently associated with urinary symptoms such as frequency, urgency, dysuria, burning, fever, chills, hematuria, and ureteral colic. Occasionally the only finding is suprapubic pain referred to the distal urethra during urination and tenderness, or tenderness in the area of the bladder trigone.

Pain of musculoskeletal origin from the spine or pelvis can cause projected pain in the pelvis. Lower back pain is a common complaint that is sometimes attributed to pelvic problems but is seldom caused by gynecologic disease except in cases of advanced carcinoma. Back and lower abdominal pain simulating that of intrapelvic disease can be caused by entrapment of the iliohypogastric or ilioinguinal nerve or by neuropathic lesions (Chapters 57 and 59).

Pain caused by disorders of the external genitalia is discussed in detail in Chapters 67 and 68.

TABLE 65-1. Pelvic and Perineal Pain: Summary of Etiology and Differential Diagnoses

Etiology (Disease)	IASP Code Ref.*	Chapter No.	Important Diagnostic Features	
			Characteristics of the Pain	Associated Symptoms and Signs
I. GYNECOLOGIC DISEASE OR DYSFUNCTION				
A. Acute pain				
1. Normal pregnancy				
a. Enlarged uterus		67	Mild to moderate lower abdominal and pelvic pain	Amenorrhea; breast enlargement and tenderness; morning nausea; urinary frequency; weight gain; fatigue; increase in human chorionic gonadotropin (hCG) level; ultrasonographic and laboratory evidence
b. Stretching of round ligament		67	Mild to moderate lower abdominal pain in second trimester	
c. Premature labor		67	Mild to moderate cramping pain at regular intervals with pain-free intervals; pain felt in second and third trimesters in low back, uterine fundus, cervix, and rectum	
2. Complication of pregnancy				
a. Ruptured ectopic pregnancy		67	Sudden severe sharp pain in lower right or left lower quadrant of the abdomen; associated with painful tender adnexa on pelvic examination	History of amenorrhea for several weeks; faintness, shock, vaginal bleeding
b. Abortion		67	Spontaneous abortion produces intermittent menstrual-like cramping pain that is initially mild but gradually increases in intensity	Vaginal bleeding accompanies cramps; in septic abortion patients have fever, chills, purulent discharge, tenderness of uterus; spread to pelvic peritoneum; nausea, constipation, reflex muscle spasm, and signs of septicemia
c. Degeneration of a fibroid		67	Mild to moderate pain; dull constant aching pain; localized at site of tumor; later becomes severe, intense, and unremitting until degeneration is complete	Tumor tender to palpation; also slight fever, moderate leukocytosis
3. Acute infections				
a. Acute endometritis	XXIV-4	67	Lower abdominal pain centrally located over pubic symphysis; cramping in nature; aggravated by palpation of uterus; adnexal area painless	Foul-smelling vaginal discharge or vaginal bleeding; frequent urination; low-grade fever
b. Acute pelvic inflammatory disease (acute PID)	XXIV-6	67	Moderate to severe lower abdominal and pelvic pain; aggravated by palpation of cervical adnexa	Rebound abdominal tenderness, nausea, diarrhea, dysuria and dyspareunia; with mixed flora infection patient seriously ill, with fever, leukocytosis
4. Adnexal disorders				
a. Recurrent painful functional ovarian cyst	XXIV-8	67	Lower abdominal pain caused by recurrent ovarian cyst; occurs in young women but rare	Laparoscopy reveals functional cyst
b. Torsion of adnexa caused by ovarian tumor		67	Regular bouts of dull unilateral aching pain; pain does not radiate or involve midline structures or organs on the contralateral side	Abdominal tenderness on palpation; pelvic examination reveals extremely tender mass on one side; leukocytosis, fever, nausea
c. Twisted ovarian cyst		67	Sudden severe pain in a lower quadrant can later spread to entire pelvis and lower abdomen	Tenderness, abdominal muscle spasm; pelvic examination reveals definite tender cystic mass; confirmed by laparoscopy
d. Bleeding of functional ovarian cysts		67	Acute moderate to severe unilateral pelvic pain; initially sharp and throbbing with no radiation, but subsides over next 12 hours and then disappears	Usually mild nausea, occasionally vomiting; with hemoperitoneum patients become pale, faint, and pain spreads to entire pelvis and lower abdomen

*See Table 2-2.

Table 65-1. (Cont.)

Etiology (Disease)	IASP Code Ref.*	Chapter No.	Important Diagnostic Features	
			Characteristics of the Pain	Associated Symptoms and Signs
e. Ruptured ovarian follicle		67	Sudden, often mild, but sometimes severe colicky pain in one of the iliac fossae; lasts a few minutes to an hour or so; then continues to spread to pelvis, lower abdomen, and sometimes shoulder	Slight tenderness and muscle rigidity; menstrual history; no fever or leukocytosis
B. Recurrent pelvic pain				
1. Mittelschmerz (midcycle pain)	XXIV-1	67	Unilateral pelvic pain varies from month to month and from one side to another; initially pain constant and lasts 2 hours to 3 or 4 days; later moves to midline	Occurs about 2 weeks before menses, around time of ovulation; pain associated with mild nausea, diarrhea, vaginal bleeding
2. Primary dysmenorrhea	XXIV-3		Cyclic pain associated with menses without demonstrable organic pathology; pain begins before menstruation and is severe as flow begins; pain cramping and localized to midportion of lower abdomen; can also involve the low back and, rarely, upper thighs	Prodromal symptoms characteristic of prostaglandin effect on other systems: diarrhea, nausea, headache, light-headedness, palpitations, diaphoresis, tremulousness, anxiety
3. Secondary dysmenorrhea	XXIV-2	67	Cyclic pain secondary to organic pelvic pathology; pain is mild to moderate but can be severe, felt deep in pelvis; usually in midline, with frequent radiation to low back and rectum; pain constant rather than cramping; aggravated by intercourse, urination, or defecation; pain usually lasts longer than menstrual period and increases in severity	Uterus can be enlarged and irregular because of fibroids; large, boggy, and tender in adenomyosis; with retroverted uterus, nodules in cul-de-sac or on uterosacral ligaments and tender masses in adnexa indicate endometriosis
C. Chronic pain				
1. Chronic endometriosis	XXIV-4	67	Persistent chronic pain felt in general area where endometrial tissue is present at abnormal sites (outside uterus) such as ovaries, tubes, ligaments, cervix, peritoneum; pain only in affected side; occasionally pain is periodic with menses (dysmenorrhea) or sexual intercourse (dyspareunia), or is continuous	Hematuria, hematochezia, bowel obstruction, or bleeding from unusual sites, such as pleural cavity or abdominal scar; history of infertility and chronic PID; confirmed by laparoscopic visualization of lesion
2. Chronic PID	XXIV-4	67	Mild to moderate pain with intercourse or heavy activity; rarely, pain is continuous; during an acute exacerbation, pain can be severe	History of prior episodes of PID; observation of pathology; fever, chills, leukocytosis, and abdominal pain during acute exacerbation
3. Developmental anomalies		67	Patients can have primary dysmenorrhea with cyclic pain or normal menses that become progressively more painful	History of cyclic or continuous pain and presence of developmental anomaly; laboratory confirmation by chromosome and other studies
4. Vascular disorders		67	Continuous pelvic pain of mild to moderate intensity; caused by congestion of vessels in broad ligament and uterus	Varicosities of pelvic veins produce throbbing burning pain that worsens on standing for long periods
5. Uterine prolapse		67	Mild pain in introitus and cervix; severe pain rare, even with extreme degrees of prolapse	Feeling of pelvic heaviness or "things are falling out"; usually relieved by lifting of uterus
6. Pelvic muscle spasm		67	Chronic persistent pain associated with intense local spasm of levator muscles; provoked by specific factors such as intercourse or pelvic examination (called "vaginismus"); pain felt deep in lower abdomen, pelvis, vagina, and sometimes in sacrum, coccyx, or rectum	History plus vaginal and rectal palpation reveal tense tender muscles; vigorous palpation reproduces or exacerbates pain

*See Table 2-2.

TABLE 65-1. (Cont.)

Etiology (Disease)	IASP Code Ref.*	Chapter No.	Important Diagnostic Features	
			Characteristics of the Pain	Associated Symptoms and Signs
D. Gynecologic cancer				
1. Cancer of the ovary		67	Asymptomatic in early stages; with advanced cancer, however, patients develop pelvic pressure, fullness associated with urinary frequency, and constipation; pain occurs with extension of disease to adnexa or tumor invasion of pelvic wall, with consequent bone involvement or infiltration of lumbosacral plexus that causes burning pain, dysesthesia, and other signs of plexopathy	In advanced disease pelvic mass palpable in 40 to 75% of patients; ascites in 20 to 30%; pleural effusion in very advanced cases; bimanual and rectovaginal examination reveals palpable mass; confirmed by laparoscopy or exploratory laparotomy
2. Cancer of the uterine cervix		67	Intraepithelial or early invasive carcinoma asymptomatic; in advanced stages, pain in pelvis or hypogastrium with tumor necrosis or associated PID; in advanced or terminal phase 75% of patients have moderate, severe, or excruciating pain	Extension to pelvic lymph nodes or lumbosacral plexus produces plexopathy with radiculalgia associated with dysesthesia, paresthesia, and other signs of plexopathy
3. Carcinoma of the endometrium		67	Little or no pain in early stages; in advanced stage, pain in bladder or rectum from extension; pain caused by distant metastasis elsewhere; initially, pain mild to moderate but eventually becomes continuous and severe	Unexpected postmenopausal vaginal bleeding or abnormal menometrorrhagia in premenopausal women; pyometria and hematometria present in patients with an enlarged uterus or blockage of cervical canal; bimanual pelvic and rectal examinations reveal presence of tumor in pelvis
E. Disorders of vulva and vagina				
1. Acute infections				
a. Furunculitis, perineal boils, bartholinitis		67	Localized moderate to severe pain confined to site of infection; with time increases in intensity; aggravated on sitting or standing	Rupture of abscess relieves pain
b. Infections of the vaginal mucosa and vulvar skin		67	Continuous moderate to severe pain and itching of the entire vaginal mucosa and vulvar skin; pain aggravated by touch of clothing or during urination	Pain associated with vaginal discharge or vulvar exudate; discharge curdy and white in moniliasis, yellow and bubbly in trichomoniasis, grayish and fishy odor in Gardnerella infections
c. Herpetic infections		67	Vaginal or cervical herpetic infection usually painless but causes pruritis or tingling; fluid-filled vesicles break leaving painful, shallow ulcer that crusts over and heals in about a week; with recurrent lesion, ulcers usually last 4 days and pain is mild	About 25% of patients become acutely ill with severe local signs and symptoms, malaise, headache, arthralgia, and fever; can cause painful swelling of inguinal lymph nodes
d. Hemophilus ducreyi infections (chancroid)		67	Painful genital ulcers with red base, ragged edges, and raised borders	Tender unilateral enlargement of inguinal nodes
e. Lymphogranuloma venereum (Chlamydia) infection		67	Painful vulvar ulcers; associated with painful inguinal adenopathy	Vulva, anal margin, and rectal mucosa can be involved; abscess can develop
f. Acute trauma (vaginal delivery, external trauma, iatrogenic, sexual activity)		67	Moderate to severe continuous sharp burning pain localized to vulva or vagina or both; if hematoma present, associated with gradual dull, aching pain that increases in severity	Visible lesions; after occult hemorrhage that dissects in vulvar tissue or rectum, large hematoma associated with symptoms and signs of hypovolemia
g. Allergic reactions (irritating agent: e.g., soap, nylon, deodorant)		67	Sudden severe pain and itching with strong allergic vulvulitis; mild and chronic with milder allergen	Redness and tenderness; severe scratching causes abrasion of vulva

*See Table 2-2.

TABLE 65-1. (Cont.)

Etiology (Disease)	IASP Code Ref.*	Chapter No.	Important Diagnostic Features	
			Characteristics of the Pain	Associated Symptoms and Signs
2. Chronic infections				
a. Ringworm, fungus, bacteria		67	Continuous vulvar and vaginal pain caused by chronic irritation secondary to infection; pain associated with severe itching provoked by irritating garments or poor perineal care	Inflammation and maceration of fragile vulvar and vaginal tissue; after discharge white and curdy with moniliasis; fishy odor with Gardnerella
b. Suppurative hydradenitis (purulent infection of apocrine glands)		67	Chronic persistent moderate or severe pain in external genitalia; localized in one area or generalized over entire vulva	Chronic infection leads to chronic abscess and sinus tract formation; generalized maceration seen on inspection of the vulva; laboratory evidence confirms presence of causative agent
3. Severe chronic itching (food, pinworms, parasites)		67	Perirectal and perineal itching that provokes scratching → abrasion → more itching → more scratching	Visible areas of abrasion; careful examination reveals pinworm or parasites
II. PELVIC AND PERINEAL PAIN OF UROLOGIC DISORDERS				
A. Diseases of the urinary bladder				
1. Acute cystitis		68	Continuous burning aching pain felt deep in pelvis, suprapubic region, and often low back; referred to distal urethra and undersurface of glans penis in men and to urethra, perimeatal skin, and clitoral region in women; responds promptly to antibiotics; with application of heat, relief of pain and other symptoms within hours	Frequent in young women; symptoms of frequency, dysuria, urgency, and often hematuria; 80% caused by E. coli
2. Chronic cystitis		68	Pain similar to that of acute cystitis but less severe; present only when bacteria are found in urine	Frequency, urgency, hematuria, nocturia
3. Interstitial cystitis		68	Continuous mild burning aching pain in suprapubic region and perineum; severe when bladder is full, partially relieved by emptying of the bladder	Frequency, urgency, nocturia, occasionally hematuria; cystoscopy reveals punctate petechiae in bladder mucosa
4. Postradiation cystitis				
a. Acute phase		68	Similar to that of acute bacterial cystitis: felt deep in pelvis; burning, aching in character; aggravated by bladder distension	Immediate inflammatory response to radiation: edema, mild infiltration, and some hemorrhage usually clears within weeks or months
b. Chronic phase		68	Similar to that of interstitial cystitis; caused by obliterative endarteritis, scar formation, ulceration of mucosa; continuous burning pain aggravated by distension of bladder	Similar to those of interstitial cystitis plus hemorrhage, which can progress to severe blood loss, with consequent hypovolemic shock.
5. Chronic tuberculous cystitis		68	Similar to that of chronic radiation cystitis: continuous burning, aching pain in pelvis; radiation to urethra	Pain of chronic radiation cystitis, plus pyuria with mixed infections
6. Schistosomal cystitis		68	Similar to that of radiation cystitis: continuous burning aching pain, plus necroturia (passage of necrotic tissue)	Initial phase accompanied by cutaneous hyperemia and itching; late phase, symptoms of urethral stricture; also scarring of glans penis and palpable fibrous masses in perineum

*See Table 2-2.

TABLE 65-1. (Cont.)

Etiology (Disease)	IASP Code Ref.*	Chapter No.	Important Diagnostic Features	
			Characteristics of the Pain	Associated Symptoms and Signs
7. Cancer of the bladder		68	Early stages painless; pain occurs in advanced disease with spread of tumor to a pelvic lymph gland or infiltration of lumbosacral plexus; one of the most common causes of bone metastasis, with consequent moderate to severe pain	Microhematuria early sign; also hematuria, pyuria, dysuria, burning, and frequency; urinary cytology positive for tumor cells; positive diagnosis by cystoscopy and transurethral resection biopsy
B. Diseases of the urethra				
1. Male urethra				
a. Acute infectious urethritis		68	Continuous mild to moderate burning pain; initially localized to urethra but later referred to perineum, urethral meatus, and glans penis; development of periurethral abscess causes severe excruciating pain that is promptly relieved by incision and evacuation of abscess	Frequency, dysuria, urgency, often hematuria; can even develop strangury and tenesmus; 80% caused by E. coli, which responds promptly to antibiotics that quickly relieve symptoms and signs
b. Trauma to urethra		68	Self-inflicted or iatrogenic (instrumentation) trauma produces acute pain that can be severe; can be referred to perineum, urethral meatus, or glans penis; chronic pain referred to perineum, urethral meatus, or glans penis	Accumulation of secretions in periurethral glands produces sensation of discomfort in perineum and rectum; acute condition associated with terminal dysuria or even strangury, at times tenesmus
2. Female urethra				
a. Acute infectious urethritis		68	Moderate to severe pain felt in urethra, urethral meatus, clitoris, sometimes referred to perineum and rectum	Acute urethritis in women independent of cystitis is most frequently caused by sexually transmitted diseases such as Chlamydia infection, herpes, trichomoniasis, and gonorrhea; frequency, dysuria, nocturia, and other symptoms (see above)
b. Female urethral syndrome (psychosomatic cystitis, chronic urethritis)		68	Continuous mild burning pain; aggravated by urination; burning pain in periurethral area or entire perineum	Pain associated with depression, dysfunctional voiding patterns, sexual frustration, vaginitis, guilt about sexual fantasies and feelings, and other "psychosomatic" symptoms and signs; also associated with various minor local problems
C. Diseases of the prostate and seminal vesicles				
1. Acute bacterial prostatitis		68	Continuous moderate to severe burning aching pain in pelvis, perineum, rectum; often referred to glans penis	Chills, high fever, urinary frequency and urgency, dysuria, decrease in stream size, occasionally nausea and vomiting; severe pain inhibits defecation; urine cloudy, containing pus and bacteria; prostate tender, enlarged, "boggy"; occasionally gross hematuria
2. Chronic prostatitis		68	Sensation of fullness of perineum; mild discomfort; burning of urethra might be related to dysuria and pain in perineum and lower pelvis; aggravated by defecation and ejaculation	Rectal examination reveals firm and fibrous or boggy prostate; secretions obtained by massage variable but usually sterile, occasionally clumps of white cells and bacteria

*See Table 2-2.

Table 65-1. (Cont.)

Etiology (Disease)	IASP Code Ref.*	Chapter No.	Important Diagnostic Features	
			Characteristics of the Pain	Associated Symptoms and Signs
3. Prostatic calculi		68	Usually asymptomatic; occasionally produces mild pain	Rectal examination reveals hardened nodules in prostate; confirmed by radiography of pelvis
4. Cancer of prostate		68	Early asymptomatic; frequent metastasis to pelvis, ribs, vertebrae, and other bones causes moderate to severe pain	Rectal examination reveals stony hard induration or nodular irregular prostate; elevated serum acid phosphatase level; confirmed by biopsy
5. Disease of seminal vesicles		68	Primary disease rare; vesiculitis secondary to prostatitis produces severe pain in groin on affected side	Tenderness in groin; possibly fever, chills, and other signs of infection
D. Acute epididymitis		68	Gradual onset of moderate dull aching burning pain in scrotum; aggravated by standing and relieved in supine position; can progress to severe pain	Scrotum is swollen, red, and tender over epididymis; chills, fever, and malaise; history of recent sexual exposure and urethral discharge
E. Diseases of the testicles				
1. Torsion of testicle and spermatic cord		68	Sudden onset of severe continuous sharp, burning, aching pain, which often occurs at night; exquisite tenderness on palpation	Testicle larger than normal size; normal urinalysis, except for leukocytosis
2. Torsion of testicular appendages		68	Sudden severe pain initially localized to upper pole of testis; later spreads to entire testis, which is extremely tender; pain relieved by infiltration of spermatic cord by local anesthetic	Early physical examination reveals blue dots seen through scrotum over twisted testis
3. Orchitis		68	Continuous sharp moderate or severe pain in testicular region; can radiate to perineum	Swollen testicle; history of viral exposure; fever; urinalysis normal except for proteinuria
4. Orchiodynia (orchidalgia, testalgia)		68	Continuous nagging aching pain in testicle; occasional bouts of severe pain	Cause unknown, but possibly history of trauma or inflammation; tenderness of testicle variable
F. Diseases of the penis				
1. Paraphimosis		68	Mild continuous aching pain in glans penis	Swollen edematous glans penis caused by redundant foreskin, which constricts corona of glans
2. Balanoposthitis (balanitis)			Initially painless; 2 to 3 days after sexual intercourse mild to moderate pain in glans penis and prepuce	Beefy red nodule, prepuce, and glans that slowly develop into rounded, elevated granulomatous mass; sites of infection: penis, scrotum, groin, and thigh; no lymphadenopathy; diagnosis confirmed by demonstration of Donovan's bodies
3. Priapism		68	Continuous mild to moderate or severe pain; associated with persistent penile erection, and not associated with sexual stimulation	Corpora cavernosa are painful, engorged but corpus spongiosum and glans are not turgid; usually idiopathic but can be secondary to medications, leukemia, lymphoma, dialysis, heparinization
4. Peyronie's disease		68	Occasionally causes painful erection	Fibrous thickening and contracture of investing fascia of corpora cavernosa of penis, characterized by induration and curving of penis; can prevent intromission

*See Table 2-2.

TABLE 65-1. (Cont.)

Etiology (Disease)	IASP Code Ref.*	Chapter No.	Important Diagnostic Features	
			Characteristics of the Pain	**Associated Symptoms and Signs**
5. Herpes progenitalis			Painful small blistering lesions on skin of shaft of penis	Common sexually transmitted disease
III. MUSCULOSKELETAL DISORDERS OF THE PELVIS				
A. Trauma				
1. Sprains		69	Mild to moderate dull aching pain; aggravated by stress of affected ligament; suprapubic pain with sprain of symphysis pubis or low back pain from sacroiliac strain; pain relieved by infiltration of ligament with local anesthetic	Tenderness in pubic region or sacroiliac joint
2. Fractures		69	Simple fractures produce moderate continuous pain localized to site of fracture and aggravated by pelvic movement or compression; severe fractures produce generalized pelvic pain with radiation to lower anterior abdomen, back, and upper thigh	Simple fracture produces tenderness and hematoma; severe fracture usually part of multiple injuries to other parts, producing severe pain in various body organs; massive hemorrhage occurs; early external or internal fixation relieves symptoms
3. Coccygodynia (sprain, fracture, infection)		69	Mild to severe pain and tenderness in coccygeal region; aggravated by movement of coccyx and by sitting; frequently radiates to perineum, gluteii, and posterior sacral region, and occasionally down posterior thigh	Moderate to severe spasms of levator ani, coccygeus, and piriformis muscles; marked tenderness to palpation
B. Infectious or inflammatory disorders of bones and joints				
1. Osteomyelitis		69	Moderate to severe pain; localized to pelvic bone involved	With acute infection, patient extremely ill: high fever, malaise, lethargy, often vomiting
2. Infectious (septic) arthritis		69	Pain localized in sacroiliac joint or symphysis pubis	Usually signs of bacterial arthritis elsewhere in body
3. Paget's disease of bone		69	Continuous dull aching pain of moderate or severe intensity in pelvis; occasionally referred to back	Radiographic evidence; increasing hydroxyproline level
C. Neoplastic bone disease				
1. Primary bone tumor (osteosarcoma, fibrosarcoma, chondrosarcoma)		69	Mild to moderate deep aching pain felt in region of primary tumor as a result of expansion of periosteum; tumor encroachment of viscera can cause pelvic pain; encroachment of sciatic or obturator nerve can produce pain along its distribution	Little evidence with small primary tumors; with large tumors, however, swelling of affected parts and tenderness on palpation; radiographic evidence.
2. Metastatic disease of pelvic bones (e.g., to breast, prostate, thyroid, kidney, rectum)		69	Progressively more severe deep aching pain; usually localized to site of tumor; more severe at night; can be relieved by shifting weight	Same as primary tumors (see above) but expansion of tumor in ischium irritates obturator or sciatic nerve, with pain and neurologic signs and symptoms in its distribution
D. Myofascial syndromes				
1. Muscle spasms: spasm of levator muscles (cause not identifiable)		67	Pain deep in lower abdomen, pelvis, vagina and sometimes in sacrum, coccyx, or rectum; can be constant or triggered by intercourse or pelvic examination (vaginismus); markedly aggravated by vigorous palpation; occurs less frequently in men	Pelvic examination in women reveals spasm of all levator muscles, which are felt to be tense and tender along pelvic side walls; spasms can be unilateral or bilateral; in men, rectal examination reveals similar findings

*See Table 2-2.

TABLE 65-1. (Cont.)

Etiology (Disease)	IASP Code Ref.*	Chapter No.	Important Diagnostic Features	
			Characteristics of the Pain	Associated Symptoms and Signs
2. Post-traumatic syndrome		23	Moderate sharp deep pain felt in perineum; radiation to coccyx, sacrum, and rectum; can be unilateral or bilateral	History of straddle injury or iatrogenic cause (e.g., instrumentation); tenderness, discoloration
3. Postepisiotomy pain		66	Mild to moderate but occasionally severe pain at site of episiotomy; with mild radiation to unilateral perineum; aggravated by standing or ambulation	Tenderness and discoloration at site of incision; can be accompanied by reflex muscle spasm
4. Postlaminectomy muscle spasm		69	Bouts of severe spasm of the gluteal and perineal muscles, as well as low back and thigh that produce severe pain; lasts only a few minutes and occurs at third or fourth postoperative day	Reflex muscle spasm brief and not associated with evidence of any other symptoms or signs; not associated with incisional pain
5. Myofascial pain syndromes				
a. Rectus abdominis syndrome		64	Trigger points in lateral border of lowermost right rectus abdominis produce pain at McBurney's point simulating that of acute appendicitis; trigger points at lowermost border of the left rectus produce pain in left lower quadrant simulating that of adnexal disease, trigger points bilaterally in lower rectus produce hypogastric pain simulating that of uterine disease	Can be accompanied by mild muscle spasm; can intensify pain of dysmenorrhea; palpation reveals trigger point(s)
b. Lower abdominal muscle syndrome		64, 69	Mild to moderate continuous aching pain in groin and testicle; radiation to lower abdominal wall and upper part of thigh	Palpation reveals tenderness and presence of trigger point
c. Trigger points in gluteii maximus, medius, and minimus and piriformis muscles		72, 77	Mild to moderate constant pain in lower back, over sacrum; spillover to perineum and thigh	Palpation reveals presence of trigger points in one or more muscles; occasionally, reflex spasms and autonomic dysfunction

IV. PAIN OF NEUROPATHIC ORIGIN

A. Central pain syndromes

1. Lesions of conus medullaris (tumor, multiple sclerosis, abscess)		69, 73	Spontaneous burning diffuse poorly localized pain in pelvis, low back, and perineum	Hyperalgesia, hyperpathia, paresthesia; other neurologic signs
2. Extramedullary intrathecal lesions (primary or metastatic neoplasm, abscess, hemorrhage)		69, 73	Initially deep aching pain in pelvis, low back; later becomes radicular; aggravated by increase in cerebrospinal fluid pressure	Paravertebral tenderness; paresthesia, sensory loss, muscle weakness, lower motor neuron signs
3. Compression of conus medullaris (tumor, hemorrhage, abscess)		69, 73	Pelvic and low back pain; frequently radiates to posterior thigh and leg	Neurologic lower motor neuron signs; sensory deficit in "saddle" area (perineum and medial thighs)
4. Arachnoiditis of lower cauda equina		69, 73	Continuous aching burning pain in lower abdomen, pelvis, sacrum, and perineal area; occasionally located only in perineum	Sensory deficit, dysesthesia, paresthesia in area of pain, often motor dysfunction

B. Lesions of roots and formed spinal nerves

1. Herpes zoster		69, 73	Usually continuous deep aching burning pain in affected segments; upper sacral segment involvement causes pain in pelvis; lower sacral segment involvement cause pain in perineum	Sensory deficit, hypesthesia, hyperesthesia; skin blebs and other signs of herpes zoster

*See Table 2-2.

TABLE 65-1. (Cont.)

Etiology (Disease)	IASP Code Ref.*	Chapter No.	Important Diagnostic Features	
			Characteristics of the Pain	Associated Symptoms and Signs
C. Peripheral neuropathy				
1. Iliohypogastric, ilioinguinal, or genitofemoral neuralgia (usually section or entrapment during operation, or compression in pervis)	XXV-1	69, 73	With iliohypogastric neuralgia, pain in inguinal and suprapubic regions, with radiation to lateral gluteal region; with ilioinguinal and genitofemoral neuralgia, pain radiates to inguinal region and anteriorly to ipsilateral vulva in female or to scrotum and root of penis in male; with genitofemoral neuralgia, internal inguinal canal painful	Hyperalgesia, hypesthesia; with iliohypogastric neuropathy, loss of lower abdominal reflex; with genitofemoral neuropathy, loss of ipsilateral cremaster reflex
2. Obstetric neuropathy (damage by presenting part or instrumentation during vaginal delivery)		69	Usually deep aching burning pain in distribution of affected nerve; with obturator or sciatic neuropathy, pain in pelvis and lower limb; with pudendal plexopathy, pain in perineum	Sensory deficit, hyperalgesia, paresthesia; frequently motor impairment ("obstetric paralysis")
3. Pudendal neuropathy caused by metastasis: tumor infiltration of lower sacrum and sacral nerves	XXV-2	69	Dull aching burning pain; initially located in midline; associated with burning or throbbing pain in soft tissue of rectum and perineal region; aggravated by sitting and lying; often progresses to bilateral involvement, usually in the fifth to seventh decade	Tenderness over sacral region of sciatic notch; sensory deficit in perianal region and genitalia; hyperpathia, hypalgesia; radiographic evidence
4. Pudendal neuralgia (injury to ischial spine by bicycle or horseback riding, straddle injury, occasionally damage from injection)		69	Mild to severe burning aching pain; associated with bouts of lancinating pain in entire perineum or limited to distribution of branch of pudendal nerve; usually unilateral but can be bilateral; complete relief by block of nerve	Hyperalgesia, hypalgesia, deep tenderness, paresthesia, tingling, subjective numbness
D. Phantom pelvic visceral pain syndromes				
1. Phantom urinary bladder pain syndrome (following cystectomy or spinal cord injury)		69	Continuous mild to moderate aching pain and feeling of "full bladder"; associated with bouts of sharp burning aching pain, usually severe; spinal cord injury and hemodialysis patients experience feelings of uncomfortable excessive bladder distension and urge to micturate	Most patients have normal social and psychologic profile except for sharp decrease in recreational and sexual activities; physical examination reveals no positive findings except for tenderness to palpation and increased pinprick pain threshold over suprapubic region
2. Phantom anus pain syndrome (following abdominoperineal resection for cancer or nonmalignant disease)		69	Moderate to severe pain in region of absent anus; radiation to the perineum; develops after days or weeks in some patients and months and years in others; described as aching, discomfort; often associated with burning, sharp, or stabbing pain; usually triggered by sitting but can be spontaneous; fatigue can contribute to pain; relieved by rest and use of cushion on sitting	Usually absence of local disease, prompting diagnosis of hysteric or psychoneurotic pain; no demonstrable cutaneous hypesthesia or hyperesthesia in perineal region
V. PAINFUL DERMATOLOGIC DISORDERS				
A. Pain in rectal and perianal regions				
1. Local lesions of rectum and anus				
a. Hemorrhoids		60	Prolapse of incarcerated and thrombosed hemorrhoids produces intense pain localized to anal region; aggravated by bowel movement, sitting, and walking	Fresh blood in stool; frequently, tenesmus

*See Table 2-2.

TABLE 65-1. (Cont.)

Etiology (Disease)	IASP Code Ref.*	Chapter No.	Important Diagnostic Features	
			Characteristics of the Pain	Associated Symptoms and Signs
b. Proctitis (infectious, traumatic, radiation therapy)		60	Continuous burning aching pain in lower rectum and anus; aggravated by defecation and wearing tight clothing; inflammation increases severity of pain	Rectal urgency, tenesmus, anal discharge with sexual infection (e.g. gonorrhea); diarrhea frequent with amebic, Campylobacter, Shigella, or Chlamydia infection
c. Anal fissures		60	Abrupt onset of acute sharp burning pain; provoked by defecation; pain localized in anal area; continuous; aggravated by sitting and further defecation	Constipation secondary to fear of provoking pain; rectal bleeding and discharge
2. Ulcers of the rectum and anus (syphilitic, tuberculous, typhoidal, dysenteric)		60	Sharp throbbing pain in rectum, anus, and perianal region; aggravated by defecation or walking	Tenesmus, diarrhea, blood, or mucus; spasm of sphincter muscle; proctoscopic evidence
3. Anorectal abscess or cellulitis (ischiorectal, perirectal, submucous proctitis, fistula in ano)		60	Continuous sharp throbbing pain in rectum or perirectal and anal regions; aggravated by defecation or walking; promptly relieved by evacuation of abscess	Acute tenderness, swelling, redness, fever; proctoscopic evidence
4. Rectal papilitis and cryptitis (infection by various bacteria)			Continuous aching burning pain; becomes sharp and lancinating during defecation	Spasm of sphincter, constipation; proctoscopic and biopsy evidence
5. Rectal carcinoma		60	Initially asymptomatic; later, sense of fullness, tenesmus, and pain during defecation; continuous localized pain unassociated with defecation can also occur	Presence of anal mass, bleeding, mucous discharge, cachexia, and other signs of cancer; proctoscopic and biospy evidence
6. Acute furunculosis and carbuncles (staphylococcal infection)		27, 69	Continuous sharp aching burning throbbing pain	Edema, tender, red area around lesion
7. Pruritus ani (pinworms and other parasites, hemorrhoids, cryptitis, papillitis)		69	Moderate to severe intractable itching of anal region; produces urge to scratch → more itch → more scratch → abrasion	Evidence of original lesion and scratch marks or abrasion
B. Dermatologic disorders of the perineum and external genitalia				
1. Superficial trauma to perineum or external genitalia		66, 67, 69	Acute sharp burning pain in area of injury	Abrasion or laceration of skin, with redness and tenderness around it
2. Ulcers, chancroid, and condylomata lata		69	Continuous burning aching pain; localized to area of bleeding	Swelling, tenderness; other signs of disease
3. Hidradenitis suppurativa (inflamation of apocrine glands)		27, 69	Continuous moderate to severe pain in genitocrural region; markedly aggravated by palpation, walking, and tight clothing	Exquisite tenderness; subcutaneous nodules; other signs of inflammation (e.g., fever, occasional chills)
VI. REFERRED PAIN				
A. Referred pelvic pain Abdominal diseases (appendicitis, pyelitis, spasm of lower bowel, passage of stone through lower ureter)		69	Pain felt in right lower quadrant simulates that of adnexal disease; bilateral pain simulates that of disease of uterus or bladder	Usually reflex muscle spasm of upper abdomen, tenderness; other signs of disease
B. Referred perineal pain				
1. Disease of rectosigmoid (ileocolitis, carcinoma, intussusception)			Pain deep in pelvis; radiation to low back, anorectal region, and posterior perineum	Tenesmus, diarrhea, or obstipation; blood, mucus, or pus; proctoscopic and radiographic evidence

*See Table 2-2.

TABLE 65-1. (Cont.)

Etiology (Disease)	IASP Code Ref.*	Chapter No.	Important Diagnostic Features	
			Characteristics of the Pain	Associated Symptoms and Signs
2. Diseases of the prostate and seminal vesicles (prostatitis, vasculitis, carcinoma)			Pain in pelvis; radiation to anorectal region; aggravated by digital rectal examination and defecation	Palpable tender mass on digital rectal examination; urethral smear diagnostic
3. Diseases of the urinary bladder			Felt deep in pelvis; radiation to distal urethra, penis, and clitoris (see above, Section II-A)	Signs and symptoms of the disease
4. Diseases of the uterus and adnexa			Pain deep in pelvis or right and left lower quadrants; radiation to perineum and external genitalia	
VII. PELVIC AND PERINEAL PAIN PRIMARILY OF PSYCHOLOGIC ORIGIN				
A. **Gynecologic pain without obvious pathology** (neurosis, hysterical personality)	XXIV-9	67	Continuous mild to moderate pain in lower abdomen, pelvis, one or both iliac fossae; exacerbation and remissions unrelated to any factor; occasionally aggravated by intercourse	Thorough physical and laboratory examinations reveal no positive findings; MMPI and other psychometric tests suggest psychopathology most frequently caused by childhood sexual and other physical abuse
B. **Pelvic, rectal, and perineal pain of psychiatric origin**	XXV-3	69	Patients can complain of continuous or intermittent pain in rectal, perineal, or genital region; can simulate that of gynecologic or urologic disease; usually patients complain of pain in other parts of body, also without pathology	Rectal and perineal or genital pain associated with severe depressive or schizophrenic illness, but can also be associated with conversion symptoms; positive evidence of psychopathology by psychiatric evaluation and psychometric testing
C. Orchiodynia		68	Continuous pain in testicle without obvious pathology; usually nagging, persistent, aching in character; mild or moderate; rarely severe and fleeting	No evidence of testicular pathology, patients might complain of mild tenderness upon palpation

*See Table 2-2.

REFERENCES

1. Bonica, J.J.: The Management of Pain. Philadelphia, Lea & Febiger, 1953, pp. 367–371, 385–386, 1403–1420.
2. Williams, P.L., and Warwick, R. (eds.): Gray's Anatomy. 36th Ed. Philadelphia, W.B. Saunders, 1980, pp. 1319.
3. Clemente, C.D. (ed): Gray's Anatomy of the Human Body. 30th Ed. Philadelphia, Lea & Febiger, 1985, pp. 270–275, 358–366, 498–512.
4. Netter, F.H.: The CIBA Collection of Medical Illustrations, Vol. 2. Reproductive System. Summit, NJ, CIBA Pharmaceuticals, 1979, pp. 89–123.
5. Kuntz, A.: The Autonomic Nervous System. 4th Ed. Philadelphia, Lea & Febiger, 1953, pp. 289–307.
6. Mitchell, G.A.G.: Anatomy of Autonomic Nervous System. Edinburgh, Livingstone, 1953.
7. Mitchell, G.A.G.: Cardiovascular Innervation. Edinburgh and London, Livingstone, 1956.
8. Mitchell, G.A.G.: Innervation of distal colon. Edin. Med. J., 42:11, 1935.
9. Woodburn, R.T.: The sacral parasympathetic innervation of the colon. Anat. Rec., 124:67, 1956.
10. Klink, E.W.: Perineal nerve block: An anatomic and clinical study in the female. Obstet. Gynecol., 1:137, 1953.
11. Hovelacque, A.: Anatomie des Nerfs Crainines et Rachidiens et du Systeme Grande Sympathique chez l'Homme. Paris, G. Doin, 1927.
12. Cutter, R.E.: Clinical evaluation of genitourinary disorders. In The Merck Manual. 15th Ed. Edited by R. Berkow, Rahway, NJ, Merck, Sharp and Dohme Research Laboratories, 1987, pp. 1552–1566.
13. Schwartz, R.W.: Gynecologic practice and approach to the patient. In The Merck Manual. 15th Ed. Edited by R. Berkow. Rahway, NJ, Merck, Sharp and Dohme Research Laboratories, 1987, pp. 1674–1678.
14. Kirkpatrick, J.R.: The Acute Abdomen: Diagnosis and Management. Baltimore, Williams & Williams, 1984, p. 287.

66 · THE PAIN OF CHILDBIRTH

JOHN J. BONICA *and* JOHN S. MCDONALD

EFFECTIVE control of the pain of childbirth, like most other acute painful problems, has long been and today remains an important health and sociologic issue worldwide. It is important for several reasons. For one thing, contrary to the claims of proponents of "natural childbirth" that labor and vaginal delivery can and should be painless, it has long been known that labor and delivery are painful events for most women. For another, misconceptions exist among the public, some physicians, nurses, midwives, and other health professionals about its nature, function, and effects, and about methods for its control. Many believe that the pain has an important biologic function and should not be relieved, and others believe that pharmacologic methods of pain relief have deleterious effects on the mother and fetus and should be avoided.

Pain has the important biologic function of indicating to the gravida that labor is beginning, but it should be effectively relieved once it has served this function because persistent severe pain has harmful effects on the mother that might also have harmful effects on the fetus and newborn. Although improperly administered analgesia and anesthesia can entail the risk of complications, it is being increasingly found that, *properly administered*, they do *not* contribute to maternal and perinatal mortality and morbidity rates but might even help to lower them. Finally, many gravidas in developed countries, having been informed of the benefits of modern analgesia by the news media and other sources, expect effective pain relief.

In this chapter we present an overview of these and other aspects of obstetric analgesia and anesthesia. The material is presented in two major sections: A, Basic Considerations, including a brief historical review, the magnitude (incidence and severity) of parturition pain, the physiologic and psychologic alterations produced by pregnancy and labor and how these are affected by pain and pain relief, and the mechanisms and pathways of parturition pain; and B, Management of the Pain of Childbirth, including a review of the basic principles of management and a review and assessment of specific current methods for controlling childbirth pain. Episiotomy pain is briefly discussed in the last section. This chapter represents an updated summary of the subject as presented in previous articles (1–3), a two-volume book (4, 5), and a monograph (6) written by Bonica. A comprehensive discussion of childbirth pain and other aspects can be found in these references and in other books on obstetric anesthesia (7–9).

A. BASIC CONSIDERATIONS

Historical Notes

Through the ages the relief of pain during childbirth has been of great interest both to physicians and to the public. Despite the misconceptions and writings of some authorities (10–12), suggesting that primitive women experienced no more pain in labor than the animals among which they fought for existence, much evidence shows that women have suffered pain in childbirth for as long as humans have existed (13–17). It is unlikely that the process of labor, and consequently the physiologic stimulus of the pain associated with it, was any different in prehistoric times from what it is now (5).

The earliest attempts to control pain in childbirth consisted of psychologic, physical, or pharmacologic methods, or of a combination of these. Physical methods in the form of brute force were used: the tribal strongman sometimes resorted to jumping on the abdomen of the pregnant woman to hasten the delivery of the child (16). Other physical measures included having the parturient tied to or suspended from a tree, with her arms tied over her head or with ropes under her armpits (16, 17). Autosuggestion was also used by our aboriginal forebears. Incantations, spells, and words of power were used by the woman in labor to enable her to put the pain demons to flight. All these methods entail the use of suggestion, distraction, and other psychologic forms of analgesia. The concentrated form of suggestion—which today we call hypnosis—was used by the Egyptians, Chinese, and other advanced cultures to relieve the pain of childbirth. Ellis (18) suggested that possibly the first recorded instance of hypnotism occurred with the proto-obstetric case found in Genesis 2:21: "And the Lord God caused a deep sleep to fall upon Adam, and he slept; and he took one of his ribs, and closed up the flesh instead thereof."

After many centuries people's idea of the cause of labor pain underwent a change; what once had been sport of evil spirits became punishment inflicted by an offended deity, perhaps explaining the prophetic curse in Genesis 3:16: "Unto the woman, I will multiply thy sorrow and thy conception; in sorrow thou shalt bring forth children." With the advent of Christianity pain became important as a means of obtaining grace or as a sacrament, and the woman in labor was expected to accept pain voluntarily. The same affirmation of physical pain was embraced by all Oriental as well as by various Western religions.

Despite these teachings, attempts to relieve childbirth pain continued. In addition to, or instead of, psychologic analgesia, numerous pharmacologic agents were used. These mainly consisted of herbal concoctions and extracts of such plants as the poppy, mandragora (mandrake), hemp, and henbane (19, 20). Alcohol in various forms was also used widely as an analgesic in childbirth. In Persian literature wine is mentioned as the agent used for the abdominal delivery of

Rustan, the semimythical hero (21). In Europe, during the Middle Ages, wine, beer, brandy, and other alcoholic beverages were kept beside the maternity bed for self-administration (22). The same methods continued to be used until the advent of modern anesthesia, initiated by the first public demonstration of the anesthetic effects of ether for a surgical operation by William T.G. Morton on October 16, 1846 (23).

The credit for the introduction of modern analgesia in obstetrics rightly belongs to Sir James Y. Simpson, a Scottish obstetrician who first used ether during childbirth on January 19, 1847, and chloroform on November 8 of the same year (24). The use of analgesia for childbirth aroused violent opposition from some physicians, the public, and particularly the clergy, who labeled Simpson a heretic, a blasphemer, and an agent of the devil. For support they cited the Biblical admonition, "In sorrow thou shalt bring forth children" (Genesis 3:16). In rebuttal, Simpson, who himself was an astute student of the Bible, cited the passage quoted above (Genesis 2:21). Simpson further added (24) "What God, Himself, did cannot be sinful" and argued "But even if . . . we were to admit that woman was, as the results of the primal curse, adjudged to the miseries of pure physical pain and agony in parturition, still, certainly under the Christian dispensation, the moral necessity of undergoing such anguish has ceased and terminated."

In 1853 the successful administration of chloroform analgesia to Queen Victoria for the birth of her eighth child, Prince Leopold, and her positive expression of pleasure with its effect, is considered to be one of the most important milestones in the history of obstetric anesthesia. The analgesia was administered by the patriarch of anesthesiology, John Snow, whose precocious concepts, painstaking research, and accurate and perspicuous writings and clinical practice did so much for the development of the field. He gave his royal patient 15-minim doses intermittently on a handkerchief and thus originated the method of "chloroforme à la reine." Although the Queen's obstetrician, Sir James Clark, wrote to Simpson about this event, it was not publicized because of the opposition of Thomas Wakley, editor of *The Lancet* (25). On April 18, 1857, however, *The Lancet* reported that Snow had safely administered chloroform to Queen Victoria for the delivery of a new princess (Beatrice). This announcement was tantamount to moral, medical, and even religious sanction of alleviation of the pain of childbirth.

Despite this auspicious beginning, obstetric analgesia and anesthesia remained a field neglected by obstetricians and subsequently by anesthesiologists for the ensuing 12 decades. During this period new techniques and more information about some aspects of childbirth pain were introduced, but pain relief was afforded only to a few patients with complicated deliveries. Usually it was administered by incompetent people, resulting in complications and occasionally death. Fortunately, during the 1940s and 1950s, a few pioneers in anesthesia became interested in the issue and made herculean efforts to promote development of this subspecialty. As a result of this and of other factors (including the increasing number of births in hospitals, the better appreciation by obstetricians of good obstetric anesthesia, the increasing interest among women in regard to obtaining effective pain relief, and the sanctioning of pain relief during childbirth by religious leaders), many anesthesiologists are now more interested and involved in research and the teaching of obstetric anesthesia. It is fair to state that, in the understanding and usage of the principles of safe obstetric analgesia and anesthesia, more has been accomplished in the past 20 than in the previous 100 years. This field has become a subspecialty of anesthesiology in the United States, Canada, and many Western European countries.

Magnitude of the Problem

Mention has been made of the misconceptions and confusion about the nature of the pain of childbirth and its treatment. This has been and continues to be a result of inadequate dissemination of information to the public about advances in knowledge and current therapeutic procedures. Many proponents of natural childbirth have compounded the problem by insisting that pain need not occur during normal labor and that when it occurs it is the product of modern cultural and environmental factors. The origin of this notion is not known, but Behan (26) was among the first to mention it, stating in 1914 that "like menstruation, childbirth naturally should be a painless process. It is only as culture advances that the labor becomes painful, for in women of primitive races pain is absent. Savages of a low degree of civilization are generally little troubled by parturiency." Nineteen years later the same argument was put forth by Dick-Read (10), who for the ensuing 25 years traveled worldwide espousing this thesis, strongly condemning pharmacologic analgesia, and encouraging the use of his method of "natural childbirth" (11). In 1950, in the USSR, Velvovski and associates (12) began to use the technique of "psychoprophylaxis," which they had developed and which was a modification of the Dick-Read method. Psychoprophylaxis was subsequently embraced by Lamaze (27) of France, who did much to popularize it in Europe and the Western hemisphere.

The claim by these clinicians and their followers that childbirth among primitive peoples is painless is disputed. Ford (13), who studied this and other problems of reproduction in 64 primitive societies, wrote that "the popular impression of childbirth in primitive society as painless and easy is definitely contradicted by our cases. As a matter of fact, it is often prolonged and painful." After studying 80 primitive groups, Freedman and Ferguson (14) reported that the pain response in these groups during childbirth was similar to that observed in American and European parturients. Similar views have been expressed by others who studied the problem of labor pain in primitive societies (15, 16). Bonica (unpublished data) observed over 24 parturients from primitive societies in Australia and Africa, most of whom manifested severe pain behavior. Finally, mention of the prevalence of pain during childbirth and its importance is found in the writings of the ancient Babylonians, Egyptians, Chinese, Hebrews, and Greeks, and in the writings of many subsequent cultures and civilizations (4).

Incidence and Intensity of Labor Pain

Although it is a common observation in obstetrics that parturients vary in the amount of suffering associated with labor and vaginal delivery, few well-designed studies on the prevalence, intensity, and quality of labor pain have been performed. Lundh (28) published a survey of several Swedish investigations, which included both primiparae and multiparae; these revealed that the incidence of intolerable severe pain ranged from 35 to 58%, with the remainder having moderate pain. Bundsen (29) found that 77% of primiparae reported that their pain during childbirth was severe or intolerable. In a study of 78 Swedish randomly selected primiparae, Nettelbladt and colleagues (30) found that 35% reported intolerable pain, 37% had severe pain, and 28% had moderate pain during labor and delivery. Records on 2700 parturients observed (and many interviewed) by Bonica while visiting or working (demonstrating obstetric anesthetic techniques) in 121 obstetric centers (with some having 100 to 150 deliveries daily) in 35 countries on six continents indicated that the frequency and intensity of labor pain was as follows: 15% had little or no pain, 35% had moderate pain, 30% had severe pain, and 20% had extremely severe pain. The data are similar to those noted among over 8000 American parturients to whom Bonica has administered or supervised anesthetic care during the past 40 years (Bonica, unpublished data).

Obviously, these surveys and observations were based on simple numeric or verbal descriptions of pain, and thus lack quantification. One of the first attempts to quantify the intensity of labor pain was made by Javert and Hardy (31), who used the Hardy-Wolff-Goodell dolorimeter to induce experimental pain and asked the parturients to compare it to the pain of their labor. The method entails the application of thermal heat, measured in millicalories (mc), to 3.5 cm², of skin for 3 seconds. The stimulus is increased in intensity stepwise until perceptible pain (pain threshold) and eventually the greatest perceivable pain (ceiling or maximum pain) are induced. They used a pain scale that ranged from 1 pain unit ("dol"), assigned to pain threshold, to $12\frac{1}{2}$ dol, denoting maximum pain, which was produced by a stimulus of sufficient intensity to produce a third-degree burn. Javert and Hardy (31) studied 26 primiparae and 6 multiparae during the course of normal labor and delivery and found that the intensity of pain in the early part (latent phase) of the first stage was 2 to 3 dol (very mild), increasing progressively to 3 to 4 dol at about 4 cm cervical dilatation, 5 to 7 dol at 6 to 8 cm, and 8 to 9 dol at full dilatation, and ranging from 9 to $10\frac{1}{2}$ dol (maximum pain) as the head of the baby dilated and stretched the perineum during the second stage of labor.

Melzack and associates (32, 33) used the McGill Pain Questionnaire (MPQ)* to measure pain during labor and delivery in 87 primiparae and 54 multiparae. They found that the mean total pain rating index (PRI) was 34 for primiparae and 30 for multiparae, thus confirming the widely held view that labor is significantly more painful for the first birth than for later births. Significant differences were also found between primiparae and multiparae for each of the four classes of words describing their pain. The sensory qualities of the pain were described as sharp, cramping, aching, throbbing, stabbing, hot, shooting, or heavy; the affective qualities were described as tiring by half and exhausting by more than a third.

*See Chapter 32 for a description of the MPQ.

Subsequently, Melzack (34) compared the mean total PRI scores for several pain syndromes obtained in an earlier study (35) with those of labor and noted that the scores for labor pain were some 8 to 10 points higher than those associated with back pain, cancer pain, phantom limb pain, or postherpetic neuralgia (Fig. 66-1A). As might be expected, although the average intensity of labor pain was extremely high, a wide range in pain scores was observed, which Melzack (34) divided into six groups within the range of the PRI scores recorded (ranging from 2 to 62) (Fig. 66-1B).

Assigning verbal descriptors of pain intensity to these data suggests that about 10% of primiparae and about 24% of multiparae experienced mild to moderate pain, about 30% of both groups rated their pain as

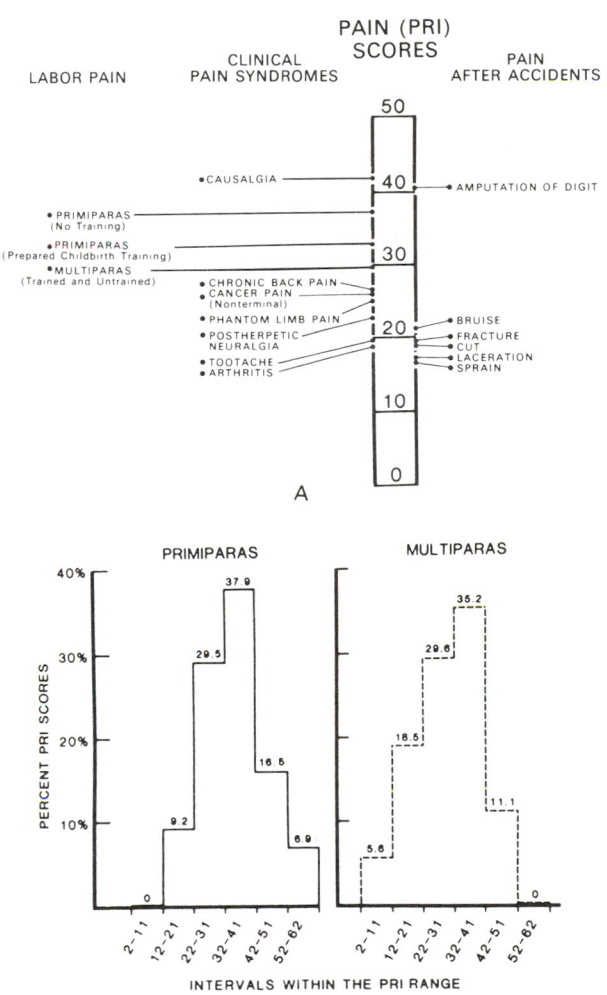

FIG. 66-1. A. Comparison of pain scores using the McGill pain questionnaire obtained from women during labor and from patients in general hospital clinics and an emergency department. The pain rating index (PRI) represents the sum of the rank values for all words chosen from 20 sets of pain descriptions. B. Distribution of PRI scores for primiparas and multiparas in six intervals of the total PRI range. A from Melzack, R.: The McGill pain questionnaire: Major properties and scoring methods. Pain, 1:277, 1975; and B from Melzack R.: The myths of painless childbirth (the John J. Bonica Lecture). Pain, 19:321, 1984.

severe, about 38% of primiparae and 35% of multi-parae felt very severe pain, and 23% of primiparae and 11% of multiparae experienced horrible or excruciating pain. The mean PRI scores of 61 primiparae who received prepared childbirth training was 33 and, for the 26 primiparae who received no training, it was 37. On the other hand, no significant difference was noted in any of the PRI measures of the 30 multiparae who had received training and 24 who received no training. Of the 28 parturients who were given successful epidural analgesia, the PRI score decreased from a mean of 28 before the block to a mean of 8 and 7.6 at 30 and 60 minutes, respectively, after induction of analgesia. These scores were based on the use of such words as numbness, pressing, and tingling.

Physiologic Alterations During Pregnancy and Labor

To provide optimal pain relief to the parturient using current techniques, it is essential for the anesthesiologist to have a thorough understanding of the remarkable maternal physiologic alterations produced by pregnancy, labor, and parturition, of the physiology and pharmacology of the fetal-placental complex, and of the forces of labor, and how these are altered by the administration of analgesics and anesthetics. From the viewpoint of anesthetic care, the changes in the mother involving circulation, respiration, acid-base and electrolyte balance, and gastrointestinal, renal, and hepatic functions are the most important. These changes, produced by placental hormones, by the mechanical effects of the growing uterus, or by both, occur because of the increasing metabolic needs of the maternal-fetal-placental complex (5). They also prepare the gravida for the stresses of parturition and for the subsequent occlusion of the placental circulation.

Circulatory Changes

Blood and Blood Volumes

Beginning at 6 to 8 weeks of pregnancy, the total blood, plasma, and red cell volumes progressively increase, reaching a maximum at 28 to 32 weeks and thereafter remaining constant until parturition (Fig. 66-2). The hypervolemia of pregnancy is accommodated by enlargement of the uterus and breasts and by increased blood flow to the kidneys, skeletal muscles, and skin, and parallels the increased cardiac output and ventilation. These changes facilitate the maternal-fetal exchange of blood gases, nutrients, and metabolites and enable the gravida to tolerate blood loss during parturition, which is 300 to 500 ml with vaginal delivery and 600 to 1000 ml with cesarean section (4, 36). The increase in plasma volume (50%) is greater than the increase in red cell mass (30%), resulting in hemodilution and a consequent decrease in red cell count, hemoglobin, and hematocrit—the so-called "physiologic anemia" of pregnancy.

Hemodynamic Changes During Pregnancy

Figure 66-3 depicts the changes in heart rate and stroke volume and consequently in caridac output. These three variables differ markedly in the lateral

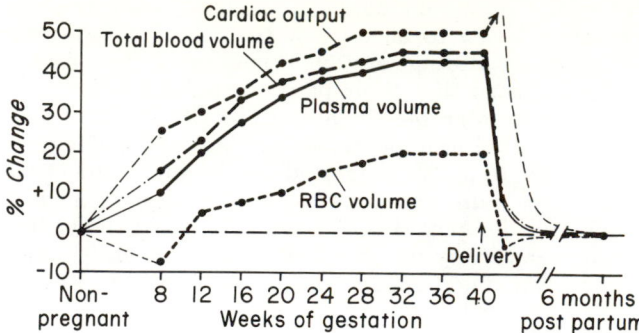

FIG. 66-2. Changes in blood volume, plasma volume, red cell volume, and cardiac output during pregnancy and in the puerperium. The curves were constructed from data in the literature and illustrate trends in terms of percentage change rather than in absolute values. From Bonica, J.J.: Obstetric Analgesia and Anesthesia. 2nd Ed. Seattle, University of Washington Press, 1980, p. 2.

and supine positions, especially during the last trimester, when the enlarged uterus compresses the inferior vena cava and other veins at the pelvic brim. This vein-compressing effect is greatest in the supine position, significantly less in the lateral position, and least in the knee-chest position. Figure 66-4 depicts the effect of the compression by the gravid uterus on the inferior vena cava and the aorta in the supine and lateral positions.

The obstruction of the inferior vena cava and pelvic vein reduces the venous return to the heart and thus reduces cardiac output. This effect is offset by two compensatory mechanisms: (a) an increase in sympathetic tone with generalized vasoconstriction, and an increase in total peripheral resistance and heart rate; and (b) diversion of some of the blood through the internal vertebral venous plexus. Consequently, in 90% of gravidas, these compensatory mechanisms are sufficiently effective to maintain arterial blood pressure at near-normal levels, but in the remaining 10% the obstruction is so great and the amount of blood

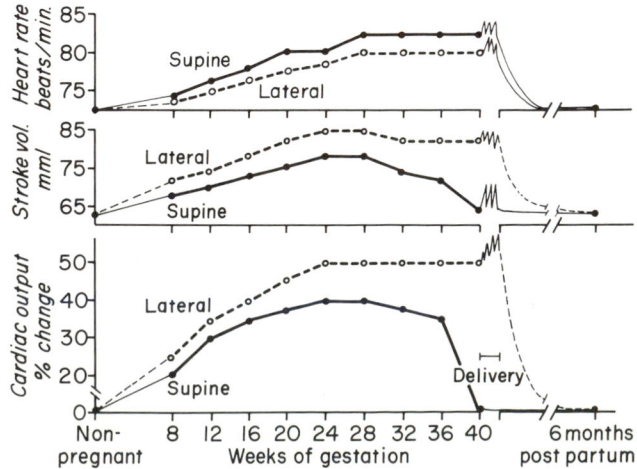

FIG. 66-3. Changes in heart rate, stroke volume, and cardiac output during pregnancy and in the puerperium. From Bonica, J.J.: Obstetric Analgesia and Anesthesia. 2nd Ed. Seattle, University of Washington Press, 1980, p. 5.

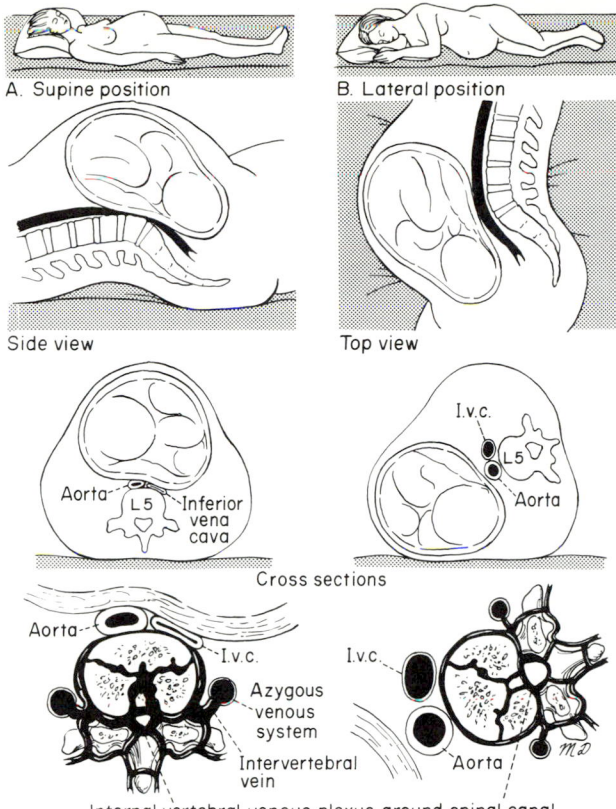

FIG. 66-4. Effects of the pregnant uterus on the inferior vena cava and the aorta in the supine position (*left*) and lateral position (*right*). The marked aortocaval compression in the supine position causes venous blood to be diverted to and through vertebral venous plexus, which becomes engorged and thus reduces the size of the epidural and subarachnoid spaces. From Bonica, J.J.: Obstetric Analgesia and Anesthesia. 2nd Ed. Seattle, University of Washington Press, 1980, p. 8.

returned to the heart and the consequent cardiac output are so low that, despite the intense vaso-constriction and tachycardia, blood pressure falls precipitously, causing the so-called supine hypotensive syndrome (37, 38).

Figure 66-5 depicts the changes in arterial blood pressure, venous pressure, and total resistance during pregnancy.

Hemodynamic Changes During Parturition

CARDIAC OUTPUT. During labor cardiac output increases above prelabor levels (Fig. 66-6). Between contractions, cardiac output during the early first stage is about 15% above that of prelabor, during the late first stage it is about 30%, during the second stage about 45%, immediately after delivery about 65%, and 1 hour after delivery it is 30 to 50% above prelabor levels (38–40). With each uterine contraction the uterus is raised by action of the uterine ligaments, and about 250 to 300 ml of blood is also squeezed out of the uterus into the central circulation. Moreover, increased venous return from the pelvis and lower limbs is made possible by a decrease in the degree of obstruction as the uterus is lifted away from the spinal column (39). Consequently, stroke volume, cardiac

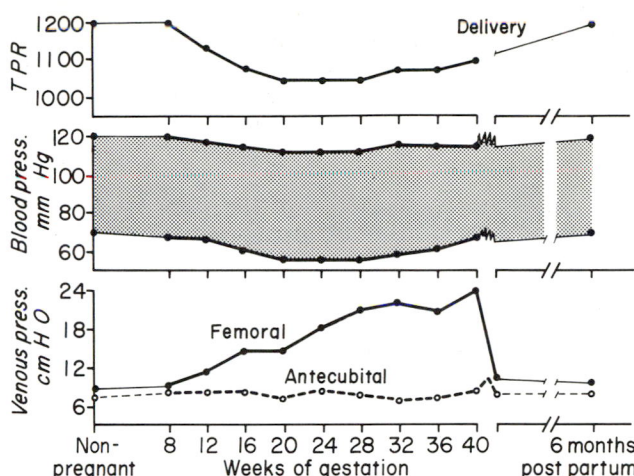

FIG. 66-5. Changes in total peripheral resistance (TPR) (*top*), systolic and diastolic blood pressures (*middle*), and venous pressure (*bottom*). Pressure in the antecubital vein remains normal but pressure in the femoral vein steadily increases because of the progressive compression of the inferior vena cava by the gravid uterus. From Bonica, J.J.: Obstetric Analgesia and Anesthesia. 2nd Ed. Seattle, University of Washington Press, 1980, p. 5.

output, and left ventricular work increase (38–41). Each contraction consistently increases cardiac output 15 to 25% above that between the contractions.

CHANGES IN PRESSURES. Figure 66-7 depicts the changes in arterial blood pressure caused by uterine contractions. The magnitude of these changes varies and depends on the intensity of the contraction and the position of the parturient, with these parameters being greater in the supine than in the lateral position. As emphasized below, pain, anxiety, and apprehension produce a significant further increase because of the release of catecholamines. During the second stage the bearing down efforts often alter blood pressure in a way similar to that produced by the Valsalva

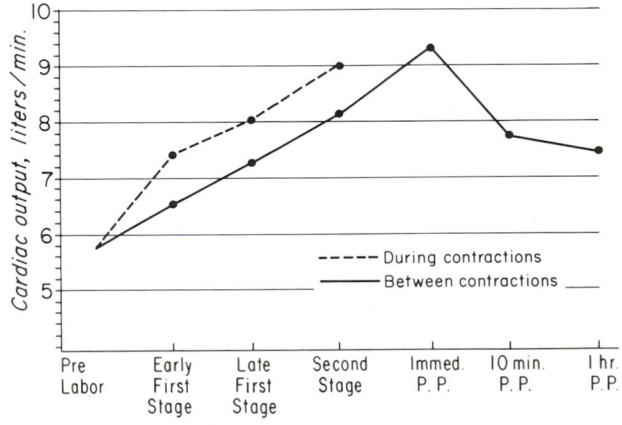

FIG. 66-6. Cardiac output during various phases of labor, between contractions and during contractions. The cardiac output progressively increases between contractions and increases 15 to 20% more during contractions. From Bonica, J.J.: Obstetric Analgesia and Anesthesia. 2nd Ed. Seattle, University of Washington Press, 1980, p. 6.

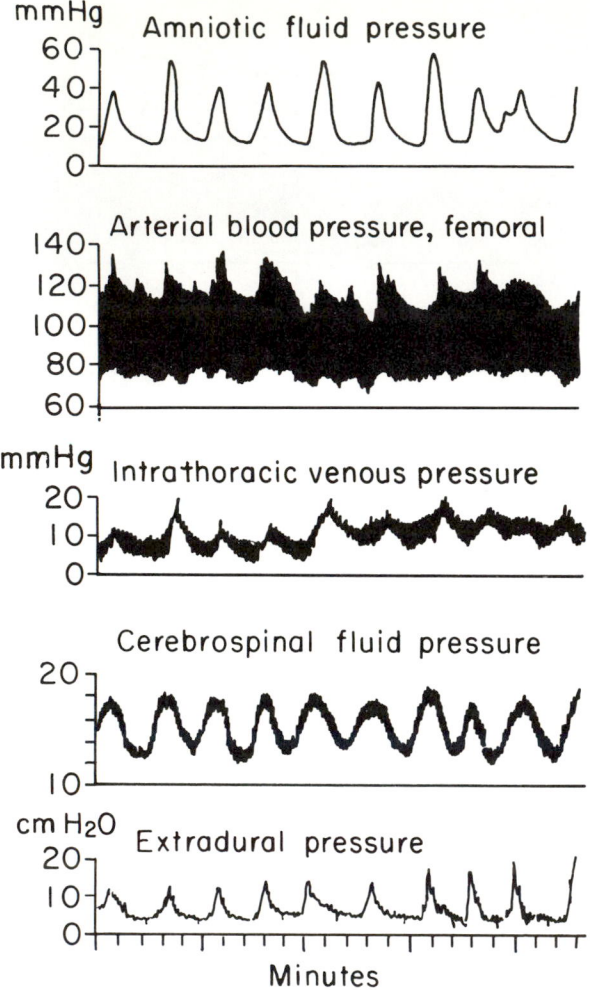

mmHg
60
40
20
0
Amniotic fluid pressure

140
120
100
80
60
Arterial blood pressure, femoral

mmHg
20
10
0
Intrathoracic venous pressure

20

10
Cerebrospinal fluid pressure

cm H₂O
20
10
0
Extradural pressure

Minutes

FIG. 66-7. Hemodynamic effects of uterine contractions. The increases in arterial blood pressure and central venous pressure are reflected in cerebrospinal fluid and extradural pressures. From Bonica, J.J.: Obstetric Analgesia and Anesthesia. 2nd Ed. Seattle, University of Washington Press, 1980, p. 7.

maneuver (39). The changes in venous pressure are rapidly transmitted to the internal vertebral venous plexus and thus cause a transient rise in the extradural and cerebrospinal fluid pressures, which have some influence on the spread of local anesthetic injection into these spaces (42).

During labor, the compression of the large veins is exaggerated by uterine contractions. As the uterus tenses and hardens and increases its pressure on the major veins and arteries across the pelvic brim, often the mother's circulation apparently improves, but with a hidden deterioration of the placental blood pressure. Each contraction tips the uterus around a fulcrum formed by the lumbosacral vertebral prominence, and aortic compression is increased, leading to a hyperdynamic circulation above the compression but a further deterioration below it. Consequently, the maternal cardiac output increases sharply, accompanied by a hypertensive rise of blood pressure above the obstruction but a marked decrease below it.

Clinical Implications

These changes in blood volume and hemodynamics produced by pregnancy, parturition, and puerperium are of significant relevance to anesthetic care. Whereas the increase in cardiac workload is tolerated by the healthy gravidas, the increase in the work of the heart in those with heart disease and consequent low myocardial reserve usually constitutes too great a strain and could precipitate pulmonary congestion. In such patients it is especially important to obviate any further increase in the work of the heart during labor caused by pain by providing effective analgesia, preferably with regional techniques. Moreover, the engorgement of the extradural space reduces its size and therefore less local anesthetic is needed to achieve epidural analgesia. Fluctuations in the cerebrospinal fluid pressure can also influence the extent of subarachnoid block. Finally, and most importantly, postural hemodynamic changes make it mandatory for gravidas to avoid the supine position during the latter phases of pregnancy and during labor. Because the induction of spinal or epidural anesthesia or other procedures that entail vasomotor blockade deprive gravidas of a compensatory vasoconstriciton, they are likely to incur much greater decreases in arterial blood pressure than nonpregnant women. Unless prophylactic measures are carried out, such severe hypotension can develop that the lives of the mother and fetus are threatened.

Changes in Respiration

Pregnancy produces impressive anatomic and physiologic changes involving the airway, lung volumes, ventilation, and dynamics of breathing. In most gravidas capillary engorgement takes place throughout the respiratory tract and the growing uterus causes the diaphragm to rise 4 cm, but this is counterbalanced by an increase of 2 cm in the anteroposterior and transverse diameters of the thoracic cage and flaring of the ribs, producing a 5 to 7 cm increase in the circumference of the thoracic cage.

Lung Volumes

Lung volumes begin to change during the fifth month of gestation, with a consequent progressive decrease in expiratory reserve volume (ERV), residual volume (RV), and functional residual capacity (FRC) (42) (Fig. 66-8). The reduction in FRC is sufficient to cause some degree of airway closure in 50% of parturients at term during normal tidal ventilation (43). Obesity, recumbency, and the lithotomy position aggravate this effect further. This can result in lowered V:Q ratios in the dependent portions of the lung and might account for the lowered arterial Pa_{O_2} seen in some parturients at term.

Ventilation

CHANGES DURING PREGNANCY. Ventilation increases significantly during pregnancy (Fig. 66-9). The changes in lung volumes and ventilation lead to a reduction of arterial and alveolar carbon dioxide pressure, which averages 32 mm Hg at term, and an increase in the oxygen tension to about 105 mm Hg.

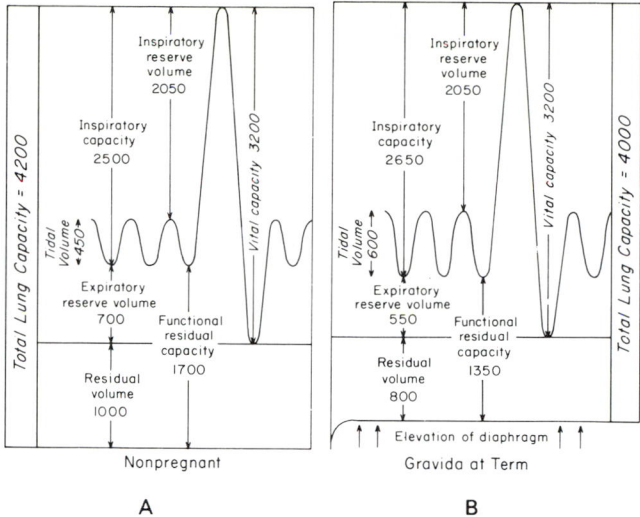

Fig. 66-8. Pulmonary volumes and capacity in the nonpregnant state (**A**) and in the gravida at term (**B**). The changes in the functional residual capacity (FRC), expiratory reserve volume (ERV), and residual volume (RV) begin after the fifth month of pregnancy and increase progressively until term. From Bonica, J.J.: Principles and Practice of Obstetric Analgesia and Anesthesia. Vol. 1. Philadelphia, F.A. Davis, 1967, p. 24.

These are accompanied by a decrease in Pa_{CO_2} and by changes in other acid-base parameters (see below).

CHANGES DURING PARTURITION. Ventilation is further increased by the pain of labor, anxiety, and apprehension, or voluntarily in patients trained in natural childbirth. The magnitude of hyperventilation varies greatly, with respiratory rates as high as 60 to 70/minute and tidal volumes of up to 2250 ml, and maximum peak inspiratory flow rates of up to 340 L/minute have been reported (44, 45). The effects of labor pain on ventilation as well as on circulation are discussed in more detail below.

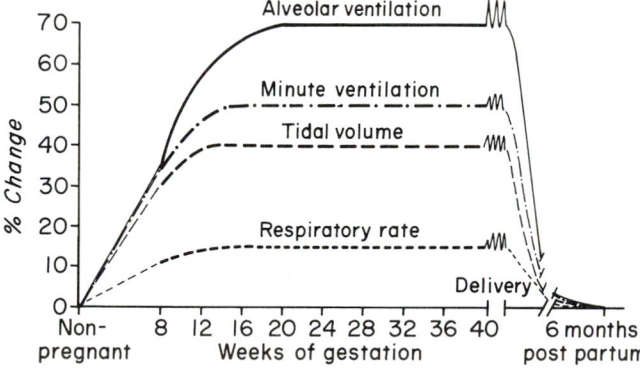

Fig. 66-9. Changes in ventilatory parameters during pregnancy. Almost maximum hyperventilation occurs as early as the second or third month of gestation. Because the respiratory rate increases to a much lesser extent than tidal volume and dead space remains normal, the percentage increase in alveolar ventilation is greater than the percentage increase in minute ventilation. From Bonica, J.J.: Obstetric Analgesia and Anesthesia. 2nd Ed. Seattle, University of Washington Press, 1980, p. 17.

Clinical Implications

These changes in ventilation have also important clinical implications. The anatomic changes are conducive to respiratory obstruction of the nasal passages, to an increased hazard of tracheal intubation, and to misinterpretation of physical findings. Changes in lung volumes and ventilation increase the efficiency of gaseous transfer between maternal blood and the alveolar air so that the carbon dioxide tension is decreased and that of oxygen is increased. Such changes, in turn, enhance the transfer of these gases between the mother and the fetus. On the other hand, these changes make gravidas more susceptible to the effects of more rapid changes in respiratory blood gas levels during respiratory complications than nonpregnant women. Hypoventilation, breath holding, or respiratory obstruction produces hypoxia, hypercapnea, and respiratory acidosis more readily in the gravidas than in nonpregnant women. Conversely, moderate to severe hyperventilation achieved spontaneously by awake gravidas or produced by the anesthesiologist with excessive positive pressure ventilation during general anesthesia can quickly lead to severe respiratory alkalosis. The respiratory alkalosis is associated with a decrease in cerebral blood flow, and possible decreased uterine blood flow, and a shift of the maternal oxygen dissociation curve to the left. Prolonged acute hypocarbia also results in diminished bicarbonate and buffer base levels that contribute to the development of metabolic acidosis during painful labor (46, 47).

Other Physiologic Changes

ACID-BASE BALANCE. The acid-base balance changes during pregnancy and labor. The total base level decreases from the normal nonpregnant level of about 155 to about 148 mEq/L, with a corresponding decrease in potassium, calcium, and magnesium concentrations. The plasma bicarbonate level decreases from an average of 25 to 21 mEq/L (Fig. 66-10). The plasma buffer base concentration, which refers to the total buffer available and includes bicarbonate, protein, and hemoglobin, decreases from a normal adult mean level of 47 to 42 mEq/L and base excess decreases to -3.0 mEq/L. In normal gravidas the pH of the blood remains at 7.4, suggesting that normal pregnant women have a compensatory alkali deficit. Some gravidas, however, have a mild metabolic acidosis, with a pH from 7.43 to 7.45.

GASTROINTESTINAL FUNCTION. During pregnancy the stomach and intestines are progressively displaced cephalad by the enlarging uterus, with consequent increases in intra-abdominal and intragastric pressures. Together with a decreased gastric emptying time and increased gastric acidity, the tendency to esophageal reflux is increased (4).

RENAL AND HEPATIC FUNCTION. During pregnancy the muscular tone and rhythmicity of the urinary tract decrease, resulting in an increase in urinary tract dead space and a progressive increase in the glomerular filtration rate (GFR) that affects the renal plasma flow (RPF), filtration fraction, and tubular reabsorption. These changes cause a decrease in the urea nitrogen concentration. Several liver

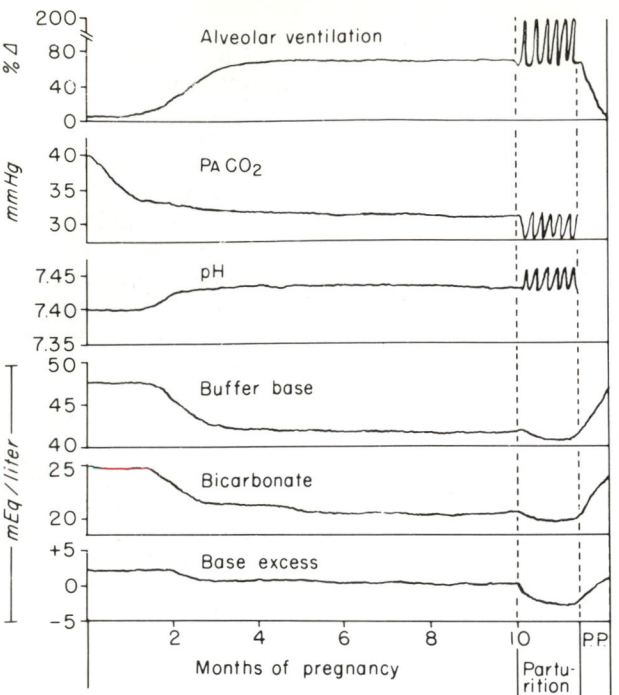

FIG. 66-10. Changes in alveolar ventilation, arterial carbon dioxide pressure, pH, and acid-base concentrations during pregnancy, parturition, and postpartum. With the nearly 80% increase in alveolar ventilation the Pa_{CO_2} decreases to levels of 32 mm Hg at term, with concomitant changes in the acid-base balance. During parturition further changes occur, especially during uterine contractions, which increase ventilation and decrease the Pa_{CO_2}. All these variables return to normal 1 to 3 weeks after delivery. From Bonica, J.J.: Maternal respiratory changes during pregnancy and parturition. *In* Parturition and Perinatology. Clinical Anesthesia Series, Vol. 10. No. 2. Edited by G.F. Marx. Philadelphia, F.A. Davis, 1973, p. 9.

function tests show abnormal values during normal pregnancy, but nonetheless the liver functions without difficulty.

METABOLIC RATE AND OXYGEN CONSUMPTION. During pregnancy the basal metabolic rate and oxygen consumption progressively increase; at term their values are 20% above normal. In addition water, protein, and minerals are retained and stored, along with retention of salts and the acquisition of fat. During parturition the metabolism and oxygen consumption increase further to satisfy the increased requirements of the uterus and, during the second stage of labor, to meet additional needs consequent to the bearing down efforts. Parturients who have inadequate pain relief have greater oxygen consumption than those who have complete pain relief, and most of the former develop a progressive metabolic acidosis and a steady rise in the free fatty acid level, as well as showing other endocrine responses to pain.

Effects of the Pain of Childbirth

Labor and vaginal delivery produce tissue damage and, like tissue injury from other causes, result in pain and local segmental, suprasegmental, and cortical responses (Chapter 7). These responses include marked stimulation of respiration, circulation, hypothalamic autonomic (predominantly sympathetic) centers of neuroendocrine function, limbic structures, and psychodynamic mechanisms of anxiety and apprehension, resulting in what has come to be known as the "stress response" to injury. As a result, the parturient incurs marked increases in respiration, circulation, and metabolism, and other body functions are altered (see Figs. 66-11, 66-12, and 66-13). These maternal changes can have a deleterious impact on the fetus and newborn. Pain and reflex responses have a predominant role in these alterations of maternal function, because blockade of the nociceptive pathways by regional analgesia with a local anesthetic greatly diminishes or eliminates them. We now summarize the impact of the pain of childbirth on the mother, uterus, and fetus and newborn, and then present data on the effects of analgesia and sedation on these changes.

Changes in Ventilation

The pain of childbirth is a powerful respiratory stimulus, causing marked increases in tidal volume and minute ventilation. In a study by Bonica in collaboration with Caldeyro-Barcia and associates in Montevideo of a group of unpremedicated primiparae who had not been prepared for childbirth, the minute ventilation increased from a normal mean of about 10 L/minute between contractions to a mean of 23 L/minute during contractions, with some parturients having a minute ventilation of 35 L/minute or more (45). Consequent to the hyperventilation, was a fall of the Pa_{CO_2} from a normal pregnant level of 32 mm Hg (4.25 kPa) to a value of 16 to 20 mm Hg (2.13 to 2.67 kPa), with some as low as 10 to 15 mm Hg (1.33 to 2 kPa), and a concomitant increase in pH to 7.55 to 7.60 (Fig. 66-11). Hyperventilation consequent to the pain of uterine contraction was also reported by Marx and associates (48), by Peabody (49), and by Huch and colleagues (50), among others. Huch and associates (50) also noted that, with the onset of the relaxation phase, pain no longer stimulated respiration, so that the hypocapnia caused a transient period of hypoventilation that decreased the maternal Pa_{O_2} by 10 to 50%, with a mean of 25%. In parturients who had received an opioid (meperidine, 100 mg IM) the depressant effects of the respiratory alkalosis was enhanced by the action of the opioid (Fig. 66-12). When the maternal Pa_{O_2} fell below 70 mm Hg (9.33 kPa) it had a significant effect on the fetus, consisting of a decrease in the fetal Pa_{O_2} and late decelerations (Fig. 66-13).

Endocrine Effects

Animal studies have shown that acute pain caused by noxious stimulation produces a significant (20 to 40%) increase in catecholamine levels, particularly norepinephrine, with a consequent 35 to 70% decrease in uterine blood flow (51, 52) (Fig. 66-14). Human studies have shown that severe pain and anxiety during active labor cause a 300 to 600% increase in the epinephrine (E) level, a 200 to 400% increase in the norepinephrine (NE) level, a 200 to 300% increase in the cortisol level, and significant increases in corticosteroid and ACTH levels during the course of labor; these reach peak values at or after delivery (53–56). Lederman and associates (54, 55) noted that, during

1320 *Pain in the Pelvis, Perineum, and Genitalia*

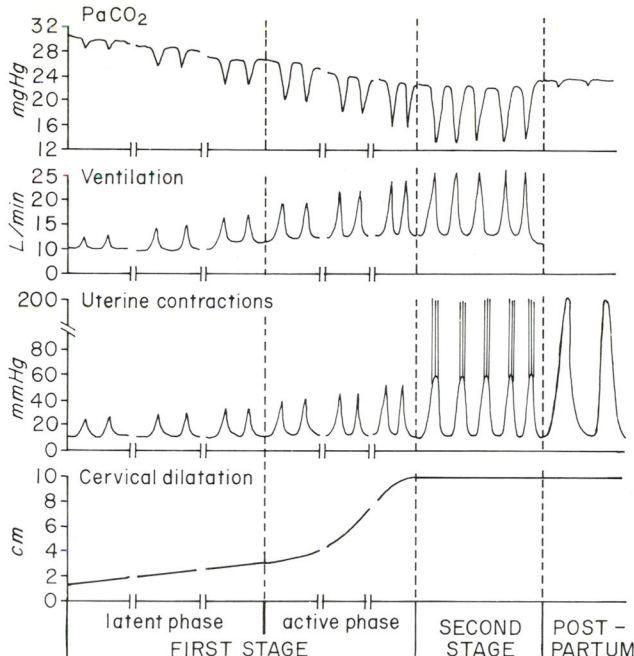

FIG. 66-11. Schematic representation of ventilatory changes during labor in an unpremedicated gravida. Note the correlation of the stages of labor as reflected by the Friedman's curve (*bottom tracing*), the frequency and intensity of uterine contractions, minute ventilation, and arterial carbon dioxide tension (*top tracing*). Early in labor uterine contractions are slight and are associated with mild pain, causing only small increases in minute ventilation and decreases in the Pa_{CO_2}. As labor progresses, however, the greater intensity of contractions causes greater changes in ventilation and Pa_{CO_2}. During the active phase, contractions with an increased intrauterine pressure of 40 to 60 mm Hg cause severe pain, which acts as an intense stimulus to ventilation with a consequent reduction of the Pa_{CO_2} to 18 to 20 mm Hg. During the second stage the reflex bearing down efforts further increase intrauterine pressure and distend the perineum, producing consequent additional pain that prompts the parturient to ventilate at a rate almost twice that of early labor and causing a commensurate reduction in the Pa_{CO_2}. Pudendal block relieves the perineal pain but the patient can still effectively bear down voluntarily. These efforts decrease the respiratory rate and consequently decrease minute volume ventilation, resulting in a smaller reduction in the Pa_{CO_2} than was present before the block. Modified from Bonica, J.J: Maternal respiratory changes during pregnancy and parturition. *In* Parturition and Perinatology. Clinical Anesthesia Series, Vol. 10, No. 2. Edited by G.F. Marx. Philadelphia, F.A. Davis, 1973.

the period of active labor, the E level increased by nearly 300%, the NE level by 150%, and the cortisol level by 200%. They noted that the higher epinephrine levels were significantly associated with uterine contractile activity at the onset of active labor (3 cm cervical dilatation) and with longer labor during the active phase (3 to 10 cm cervical dilatation). Increased epinephrine and cortisol levels were correlated significantly with anxiety and pain.

In a later study, Ohno and associates (57) carried out a comprehensive study of catecholamines and cyclic nucleotides during labor and following delivery and noted a nearly twofold increase in the dopamine level, a threefold increase in the E level, and a twofold increase in the NE as well as a small increase in the cAMP level. They noted a positive correlation be-

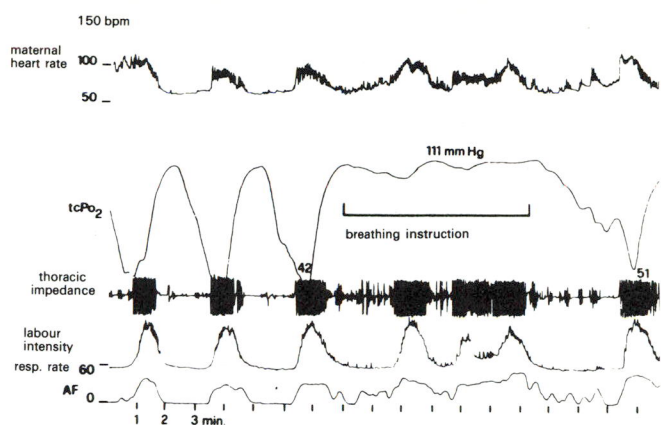

FIG. 66-12. Continuous recording of maternal heart rate, transcutaneous $(tc)P_{O_2}$ thoracic impedance, uterine pressure (labor intensity), and respiratory rate after the parturient was given 100 mg meperidine IM. With each uterine contraction marked hyperventilation caused the tcP_{O_2} to increase to 110 mm Hg but then to fall to low levels as a result of the marked respiratory alkalosis and of the respiratory depressant effect of the meperidine. The large decreases in tcP_{O_2} were avoided by giving the parturient breathing instructions during the relaxation period. From Peabody, J.L.: Transcutaneous oxygen measurement to evaluate drug effect. Clin. Perinatol., 6:109, 1979.

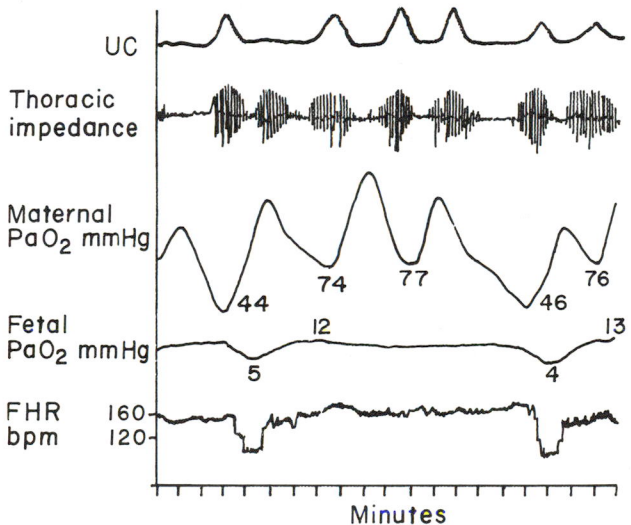

FIG. 66-13. Continuous recording of uterine contractions (UC), maternal thoracic impedance, maternal transcutaneous oxygen tension (Pa_{O_2}), fetal oxygen tension, and fetal heart rate (FHR) in a primipara 120 minutes before spontaneous delivery of an infant with an Apgar of 7. Marked hyperventilation during uterine contractions was followed by hypoventilation or apnea between contractions. With the parturient breathing air during and after the first and fourth periods of hyperventilation, the maternal Pa_{O_2} fell to 44 and 46 mm Hg, with a consequent decrease in fetal Pa_{O_2} and variable decelerations, which reflected fetal hypoxia. Modified from Huch, A., et al.: Continuous transcutaneous monitoring of foetal oxygen tension during labour. J. Obstet. Gynecol., *84*(Suppl. 1):1, 1977.

tween E on the one hand and heart rate and systolic blood pressure on the other, as well as a correlation between NE and cAMP during labor. The greater increase in E than in NE was contrasted with the findings of a previous study, which showed that NE

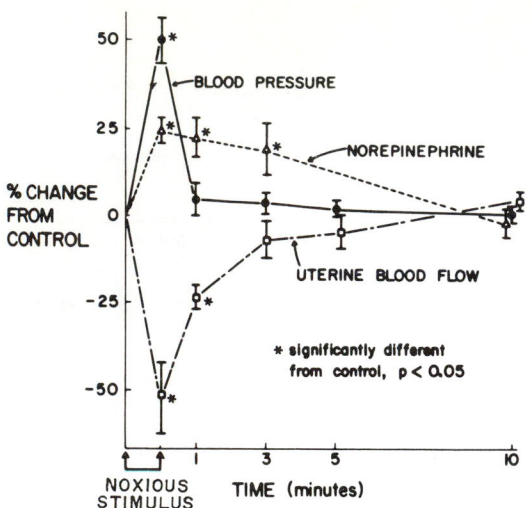

Fig. 66-14. Effects of noxious stimulus on maternal arterial blood pressure, norepinephrine blood level, and uterine blood flow. The stress was induced by application of an electric current onto the skin of an ewe at term. The increase in arterial pressure is transient but the decay in norepinephrine level is more protracted, and is reflected by a mirror image decrease in uterine blood flow. From Shnider, S.M., et al.: Uterine blood flow and plasma norepinephrine changes during maternal stress in the pregnant ewe. Anesthesiology, *50*:524, 1979.

was much greater than E during physical exercise. This led to the conclusion that elevated symphathoadrenal activity during labor is a result of pain and anxiety rather than of physical effort. Other data, however, show that although pain is a major factor in the elevation of catecholamine levels, physical effort during the second stage does contribute to the increase in catecholamine levels.

Other studies have demonstrated a progressive increase in plasma beta-endorphin, beta-lipotropin, and ACTH levels, all of which are derived from a common precursor (58–63). These values have been found to peak at delivery or in the immediate postpartum period at 4 to 10 times the prelabor and nonpregnant values. These findings have led to the speculation that plasma beta-endorphin might have an intrinsic analgesic role during parturition (64). The fact that plasma beta-endorphin levels that are considerably higher than those observed in these studies do not appear to cross the blood-brain barrier or have analgesic effects in humans (65), as well as the fact that no change in pain threshold has been demonstrated in parturients (66), detract from this hypothesis.

Cardiovascular Changes

During labor the progressive increase in cardiac output is about 40 to 50% higher than the prelabor value during the late first and second stages, and some parturients have an increase of nearly 100% with a further increase of 20 to 30% during each painful uterine contraction. Available data suggest that 40 to 50% of the increase during the contraction is caused by the extrusion of 250 to 300 ml of blood from the uterus and by increased venous return from the pelvis and lower limbs into the maternal central circulation.

The rest is caused by an increase in sympathetic activity provoked by pain, anxiety, apprehension, and the physical effort of labor, which contribute to the progressive rise in cardiac output as labor advances (39, 40). Uterine contractions in the absence of analgesia also cause increases of 20 to 30 mm Hg (2.6 to 6.4 kPa) in the systolic and diastolic blood pressures. The increases in cardiac output and systolic blood pressure lead to a significant increase in left ventricular work that is tolerated by healthy parturients but can prove deleterious if the parturients have heart disease, pregnancy-induced hypertension (pre-eclampsia), essential hypertension, pulmonary hypertension, or severe anemia.

Metabolic and Other Effects

During the first and second stages of labor free fatty acids and lactate levels increase significantly, apparently as a result of the pain-induced release of catecholamines and the consequent sympathetic-induced lipolytic metabolism (67). This assumption is based on the fact that, with complete blockade of nociceptive (afferent) and efferent pathways achieved with epidural or other forms of regional analgesia, only slight increases in maternal free fatty acid and lactate levels and acidosis are seen. During the second stage of labor maternal acidosis is a result of the pain and physical exertion inherent in the active bearing down (pushing) effort during contractions.

Increased sympathetic activity caused by labor pain and anxiety also increases metabolism and oxygen consumption and decreases gastrointestinal and urinary bladder motility. The increased oxygen consumption, plus that inherent in the work of labor, together with the loss of bicarbonate from the kidney as compensation for the pain-induced respiratory alkalosis and often reduced carbohydrate intake, produce a progressive metabolic acidosis that is transferred to the fetus. The maternal pyruvate level increases, along with an even greater increase in the lactate level and a progressive accumulation of excess lactate, which is reflected by a progressive increase in base excess (46, 47, 68).

The pain of labor also affects the function of the gastrointestinal tract. Gastrin release is stimulated during painful labor and results in an increase in gastric acid secretion (69). Moreover, the pain and associated anxiety and emotional stress produce segmental and suprasegmental reflex inhibition of gastrointestinal motility and function, and consequently a significant delay in gastric emptying. These reflex effects of nociception are aggravated by the recumbent position and by the use of opioids and other depressant drugs (4, 5, 70, 71). The combined effect of pain and depressant drugs can cause food and fluids other than water to be retained for as long as 36 hours or more, and during this period swallowed air and gastric juices accumulate progressively, with the pH of the stomach contents decreasing below the critical value of 2.5 in most parturients. Delayed gastric emptying of acidic gastric contents increases the risk of regurgitation and pulmonary aspiration, especially during the induction of general anesthesia.

Psychologic Effects

Severe labor pain can produce serious long-term emotional disturbances that might impair the parturient's mental health, negatively influence her relationship with her baby during the first few crucial days, and cause fears of future pregnancies that could affect her sexual relationship with her husband (30, 31, 72–75). Kartchner (72), Rogers (73), Melzack et al. (33), and others (74, 75) reported a significant number of women who had participated in natural childbirth developed or had aggravation of prelabor depression and other deleterious emotional reactions in the postpartum period, consequent to the pain experienced during their childbirth without analgesia. Cheetham and Rzadkowolski (74) reported that nearly two-thirds of parturients experienced some type of emotional upset characterized predominantly by a decrease in mental acuity and in social interests, and an increase in their feelings of dysphoria, depression, and anxiety. They pointed out that psychologic aspects of labor are accentuated by the well-cited triad of "fear-tension-pain," which might in turn decrease uterine activity and thus prolong labor. In addition, Melzack (34) noted that some women might experience an added burden of guilt, anger, and failure when they anticipate "natural, painless childbirth" and are then confronted with such severe pain that they require epidural analgesia. Stewart (75) reported that some women who failed to achieve "painless" childbirth and experienced such severe pain as to require epidural analgesia subsequently became miserable, depressed, and even suicidal, and lost interest in sex. In some cases, the husbands of women who anticipated "natural" childbirth had to undergo psychotherapy for serious reactions after seeing their wives experience such severe pain that they developed feelings of guilt and subsequent impotence, and phobias. Melzack (34) also mentioned other reports of similar reactions by parturients who failed to achieve painless childbirth.

Effects on Uterine Activity and Labor

Through increased secretion of catecholamines and cortisol, pain and emotional stress can either increase or decrease uterine contractility and thus influence the duration of labor. Norepinephrine increases uterine activity, whereas epinephrine and cortisol decrease it (5, 55). Morishima and colleagues (51, 76) reported that, in pregnant baboons and Rhesus monkeys, nociceptive stimulation increased uterine activity about 60 to 65%, and was associated with a decrease in fetal heart rate and oxygenation. In contrast, severe pain and anxiety in some parturients caused such an increase in epinephrine and cortisol levels that uterine activity was consequently decreased and labor was prolonged (54, 55). In a small number of parturients, pain and anxiety produce "incoordinate uterine contractions" manifested by a decrease in intensity coupled with an increase in frequency and uterine tonus (77).

Effects on the Fetus

During labor the intermittent reduction of intervillous blood flow during the peak of a contraction leads to a temporary decrease in placental gas exchange. This impairment is often further increased by pain-induced severe hyperventilation, which causes severe respiratory alkalosis (see above) and results in the following: (a) a shift (to the left) in the maternal oxygen dissociation curve, which diminishes the transfer of oxygen from mother to fetus; (b) maternal hypoxemia during uterine relaxation; (c) umbilical vasoconstriction with a consequent decrease in umbilical blood flow (78); and (d) a reduction in uterine blood flow, which is provoked by an increase in norepinephrine and cortisol release (Fig. 66-14). These deleterious effects on the fetus have been demonstrated in several species of animals and in humans (51, 55, 76, 77). Figure 66-13 depicts the deleterious effects on fetal heart rate that are caused by marked hyperventilation during a contraction and by hypoventilation between contractions. Lederman and associates (55) also noted that parturients who were anxious and had pain had a higher incidence of abnormal fetal heart rate patterns, and that their infants had lower 1- and 5-minute Apgar scores.

Under the conditions of normal labor, such series of transient and intermittent impairments of blood gas exchange are tolerated by the normal fetus because oxygen is stored in the fetal circulation and intervillous space, and is sufficient to maintain adequate fetal oxygenation during the brief period of placental hypoperfusion. Moreover, the fetus can compensate by increasing the proportion of cardiac output that is distributed to the myocardium and brain (79, 80). If the above factors are combined with an excessive increase in uterine activity, however, fetal hypoxia, hypercapnea, and acidosis develop that might still be tolerated by the normal fetus, although its ability to withstand oxygen deprivation is limited. If the fetus is already at risk because of obstetric or maternal complications (e.g., pre-eclampsia, heart disease, diabetes), the pain-induced reductions of oxygen and carbon dioxide transfer can be the critical factors that produce perinatal morbidity, and could even contribute to mortality (4, 5, 51, 76). The maternal metabolic acidosis is transferred to the fetus, making it more vulnerable to the effects of intrauterine asphyxia caused by cord compression, prolapse, or other obstetric complications (5, 76, 81).

Effects of Sedation and Analgesia

Many laboratory and clinical studies have produced impressive evidence that relief of pain and anxiety can decrease or virtually eliminate most of these maternal and fetal alterations.

Ventilation

Partial relief of pain with opioids decreases hyperventilation somewhat so that the Pa_{CO_2} is in the 22 to 25 mm Hg (3 to 3.3 kPa) range and oxygenation improves (45–48). Complete pain relief achieved with extradural analgesia prevents the transient period of hyperventilation during a contraction and prevents hypoventilation during relaxation, so that the Pa_{CO_2} remains in the range of 28 to 32 mm Hg (3.7 to 4.25 kPa) and the Pa_{O_2} increases to about 100 mm Hg (1.3 kPa) (Figs. 66-15 and 66-16).

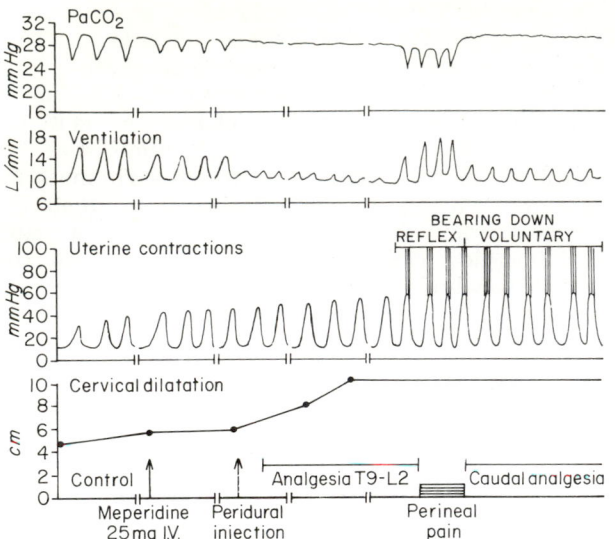

FIG. 66-15. Schematic representation of the effects of analgesia on ventilation based on measurements in a primipara. At 5-cm cervical dilatation 25 mg of meperidine IV resulted in partial relief of pain and consequently produced smaller changes in ventilation and Pa_{CO_2}. Subsequent induction of segmental epidural analgesia produced complete pain relief, which eliminated maternal hyperventilation and Pa_{CO_2} changes without affecting uterine contractions. During the second stage the onset of perineal pain and initiation of reflex bearing down efforts caused a concomitant increase in ventilation and a slight decrease in the Pa_{CO_2}, which were eliminated with the induction of low caudal (S1–S5) analgesia. From Bonica, J.J.: Obstetric Analgesia and Anesthesia. 2nd Ed. Seattle, University of Washington Press, 1980, p. 114.

Neuroendocrine Effects

Recent studies have provided impressive evidence that epidural analgesia, by blocking nociceptive input and sympathetic efferents, reduces the release of catecholamines, beta-endorphins, ACTH, and cortisol (53, 60, 61, 67, 82–85). This neuroendocrine lowering effect is primarily a result of relief of pain during labor and was demonstrated by Abboud and associates (86), who noted that spinal anesthesia at the T4

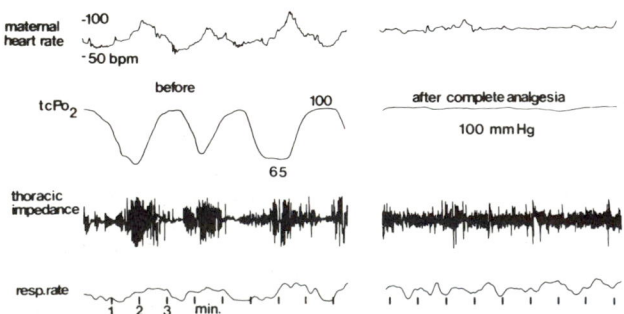

FIG. 66-16. Polygraph recording of maternal heart rate, transcutaneous oxygen tension (tcP$_{O_2}$), thoracic impedance, and respiratory rate during labor. Before the induction of epidural analgesia the pain of uterine contractions caused marked hyperventilation and a consequent increase in tcP$_{O_2}$ to 100 mm Hg kPa), which fell to 65 to 70 mm Hg (8.7–9.3 kPa) between contractions. After complete epidural analgesia all curves were more regular, and the tcP$_{O_2}$ was maintained at a stable 100 mm Hg. From Peabody, J.L.: Transcutaneous oxygen measurement to evaluate drug effect. Clin. Perinatol., 6:109, 1979.

dermatomal level decreased catecholamine levels in women in labor, but did not do so in women who were not in labor. This selectivity suggests that the mechanism by which catecholamine release is decreased is relief of maternal pain.

Epidural analgesia during labor and delivery does not decrease catecholamine and beta-endorphin release in the fetus and newborn (61, 63, 83–86), and norepinephrine predominates over epinephrine (86). This response indicates that, even during completely uncomplicated deliveries with adequate maternal analgesia, the infant is considerably distressed by the process of birth by vaginal delivery. A number of studies have suggested that catecholamines have an important role for neonatal adaptation to the extrauterine environment, including surfactant synthesis and release, lung liquid resorption, nonshivering thermogenesis, glucose homeostasis, cardiovascular changes, and water metabolism (86).

Cardiovascular Effects

By decreasing the pain-induced sympathetic hyperactivity and neuroendocrine response, epidural analgesia eliminates that portion of the increase in cardiac output and blood pressure caused by pain. Figures 66-17 and 66-18 show that epidural analgesia decreases the progressive increase in cardiac output and its further increase during uterine contractions to about 50% of that without analgesia. A similar decrease in periodic increase in blood pressure is depicted in Figure 66-19. Several studies have proven the value of epidural analgesia in dampening the increase in cardiac output, cardiac work, and blood pressure in laboring parturients with heart disease, pregnancy-induced

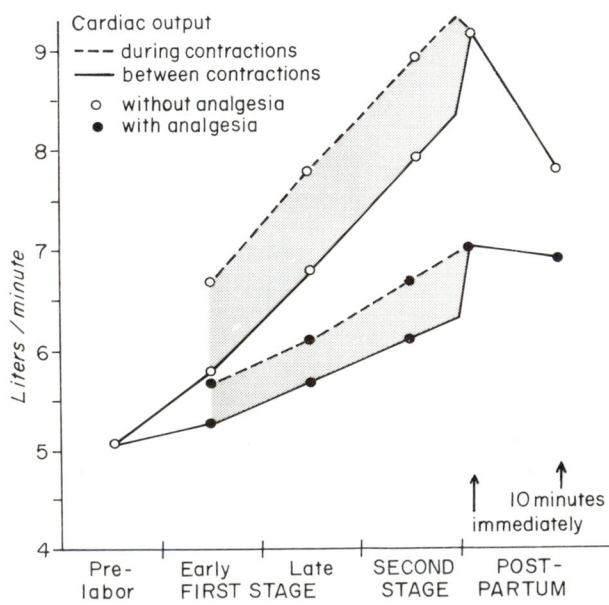

FIG. 66-17. Cardiac output during various phases of labor between contractions and during contractions. In a group of patients laboring without analgesia, the progressive increases between contractions and the further increases during each contraction were much greater than corresponding changes in a group of patients who received continuous epidural analgesia. From Bonica, J.J.: Principles and Practice of Obstetric Analgesia and Anesthesia. Philadelphia, F.A. Davis, 1967, p. 383.

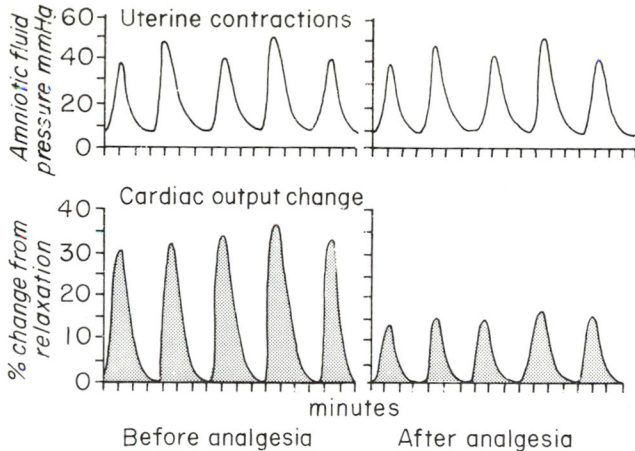

FIG. 66-18. Increases in cardiac output during each uterine contraction before and after induction of continuous epidural analgesia in a primipara. With pain relief the increases in cardiac output during contractions were about 50% of those before induction of analgesia. From Bonica, J.J.: Labour pain. *In* Textbook of Pain. Edited by P.D. Wall and R. Melzack. Edinburgh, Churchill Livingstone, 1984, pp. 327–392.

hypertension (pre-eclampsia), and pulmonary hypertension, provided of course that maternal hypotension is avoided (88, 89).

Metabolic Effects

The relief of pain and associated anxiety with continuous epidural analgesia decreases the total work of labor, maternal metabolism, and oxygen consumption. Buchan (67) showed that, during labor, epidural analgesia reduced internal stress by abolishing pain, thus eliminating the progressive increase in

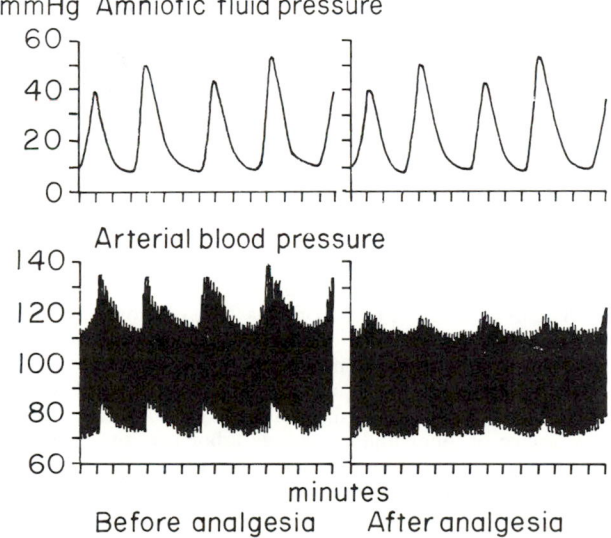

FIG. 66-19. Fluctuations in blood pressure produced by uterine contractions before and after induction of continuous epidural analgesia. Like the cardiac output changes (Fig. 66-18), complete relief of pain resulted in decreasing the contraction-induced fluctuations to nearly 50% of the values measured before analgesia. From Bonica, J.J.: Labour pain. *In* Textbook of Pain. Edited by P.D. Wall and R. Melzack. Edinburgh, Churchill Livingstone, 1984, pp. 327–392.

the 11-hydroxycorticosteroid levels normally seen throughout labor. Consequently, epidural analgesia significantly reduces maternal and fetal metabolic acidosis. The superiority of epidural analgesia over opioids and other systemic drugs in decreasing maternal work, oxygen consumption, and maternal and fetal metabolic acidosis has been impressively demonstrated by a number of investigators (46, 47, 53, 90–94) (Fig. 66-20). Because active pushing during the second stage of labor contributes to metabolic acidosis, epidural analgesia does not completely eliminate metabolic and fetal acidosis. Figure 66-20 demonstrates that epidural analgesia and elimination of the bearing down effort (pushing) during the second stage almost eliminates maternal metabolic acidosis. Moreover, under these conditions it decreases but does not eliminate the degree of fetal acidosis. Undoubtedly, this is a result of the physical stress on the fetus inherent in the process of birth.

Effects on Uterine Activity

By decreasing the sympathetic-induced hyperactivity, sedation and complete analgesia can reduce or

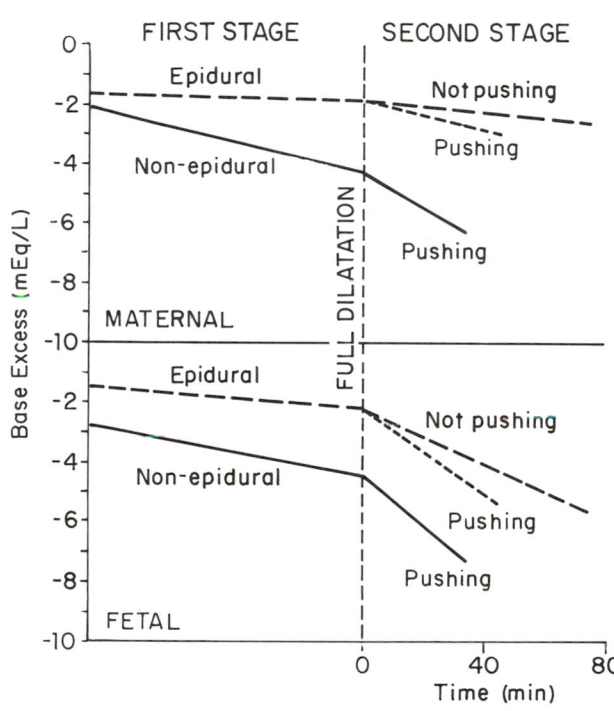

FIG. 66-20. Mean changes in extent of maternal (*above*) and fetal (*below*) metabolic acidosis during the first and second stages of labor in a group of parturients managed without lumbar epidural analgesia and in two similar groups managed with epidural analgesia, one of which retained the bearing down reflex and the other did not. The parturients were delivered by outlet forceps. Significant metabolic acidosis was experienced by those in the nonepidural group of parturients whereas those given epidural analgesia experienced little or no changes in their acid-base status. Fetuses born of mothers managed without epidural also developed metabolic acidosis during the first stage, and to an even greater degree during the second stage. In contrast, fetuses of mothers given epidural had no change in acid-base status during the first stage but showed a time-dependent increase in metabolic acidosis during the second stage. From Bonica, J.J.: Obstetric Analgesia and Anesthesia. 2nd Ed. Seattle, University of Washington Press, 1980, p. 115.

eliminate uterine hyperactivity or hypoactivity and can change incoordinate uterine contractions to a normal labor pattern (5, 77, 95) (Fig. 66-21). Equally important is the efficacy of analgesia in reducing placental hypoperfusion and any existing deterioration in uterine blood flow, thus decreasing or even eliminating any impairment of blood gas transfer that might be a result of increased catecholamines or uterine hyperactivity (5).

Effects on the Fetus

These benefits of pain relief, best achieved with regional analgesia, are likely to be of value to many infants, but they are especially important to the fetus at risk. It has been found to be the best method of analgesia for breech delivery and for multiple pregnancies (5, 7, 9). It has been shown that epidural analgesia, through its vasomotor blocking effect, increases intervillous blood flow in parturients with severe pre-eclampsia and probably also in those with hypertension, diabetes, and other conditions that decrease placental blood flow and function (5–9). Janisch and co-workers (96) found that continuous epidural analgesia administered to pre-eclamptics during their last few weeks of gestation produced a 100% increase in placental blood flow. Jouppila and colleagues (97) studied the influence of lumbar epidural analgesia that was limited to a few segments and the effect of a more extensive type of lumbar epidural block on parturients with severe pre-eclampsia. They found that the limited block increased intervillous blood flow by 34% whereas the more extensive block increased it by a mean of 77%. They attributed this effect to the relief of severe vasoconstriction by the vasomotor block. Maternal hypotension must be strictly avoided by

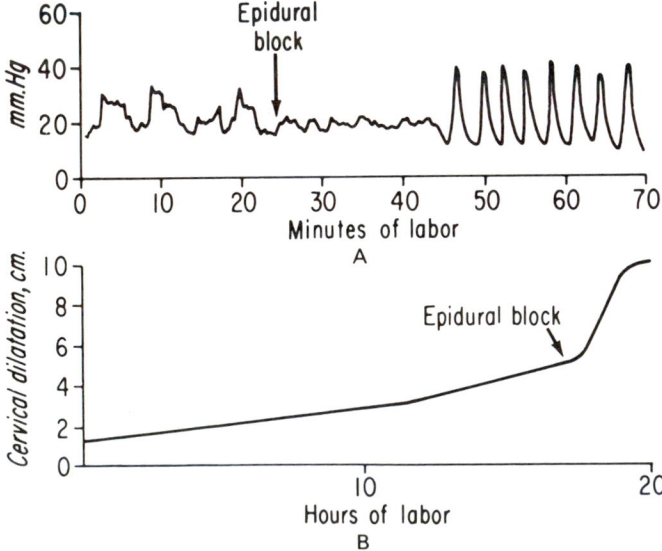

FIG. 66-21. Effect of epidural block on incoordinate uterine contractile pattern. **A.** Intrauterine pressure tracings. Note the temporary decrease in uterine contractions and the subsequent normalization of the previously irregular contractions. **B.** Cervimetric curve showing the rapid cervical dilation that followed start of the epidural block. From Bonica, J.J: Principles and Practice of Obstetric Analgesia and Anesthesia, Vol. 2. Philadelphia, F.A. Davis, 1969, p. 1200.

appropriate prophylactic measures (e.g., intravenous infusion of fluids, lateral displacement of the uterus) to achieve these benefits.

Mechanisms, Pathways, and Characteristics of the Pain of Parturition

To provide optimal pain relief with regional analgesia, it is essential for the obstetric team to understand the peripheral mechanisms and pathways of the pain of parturition and the factors that influence its intensity, duration, and quality. Most of these factors vary during the different phases and stages of labor and are therapeutically significant, so they are considered separately.

Pain of the First Stage of Labor

Intrinsic Mechanisms

During the first stage, labor pain initially is entirely in the uterus and its adnexa during contractions. Earlier, it was proposed that labor pain was caused by the following: (a) pressure on nerve endings between the muscle fibers of the body and fundus of the uterus (98); (b) contraction of the ischemic myometrium and cervix consequent to expulsion of blood from the uterus during the contraction (99) or as a result of vasoconstriction consequent to sympathetic hyperactivity (11); (c) inflammatory changes of uterine muscles (98); (d) contraction of the cervix and lower uterine segment consequent to fear-induced hyperactivity of the sympathetic nervous system (11); and (e) dilatation of the cervix and lower uterine segment (31, 99). Most data support the concept that the pain of the first stage of labor is predominantly a result of dilatation of the cervix (CX) and lower uterine segment (LUS) and of the consequent distension, stretching, and tearing of these structures during contractions. Contractions of the uterus under isometric conditions—that is, against the obstruction presented by the cervix and perineum—also probably contribute to the pain of uterine contractions.

These hypotheses are based on the following considerations:

a. Stretching of smooth muscle of a hollow viscus is an adequate stimulus for visceral pain (100).

b. The degree of CX and LUS dilatation is correlated with the rapidity with which it occurs on the one hand and with the intensity of the pain on the other (4).

c. The time of onset of uterine contractions is related to the time of onset of the pain. This lag, which is longest in the early stages of labor and lessens as labor progresses, occurs because uterine contractions need time to increase the amniotic fluid pressure to 15 mm Hg above tonus. This has been determined to be the minimum pressure required to initiate distension of the CX and LUS (101).

d. In the parturient undergoing cesarean section with abdominal field block, the exposed but unanesthetized uterus can be incised and gently palpated without discomfort to the conscious parturient (31, 99), while forceful palpation and stretching of the CX and LUS produce pain similar in quality and location to that experienced during labor (31, 99).

e. When the cervix is suddenly and widely dilated in parturients or in gynecologic patients, they feel pain similar in quality, distribution, and intensity to that experienced during uterine contractions (31, 99, 102).

The evidence that contractions of the body of the uterus contribute to the pain of labor is somewhat puzzling. Braxton-Hicks contractions of prelabor are frequently painless, even though they can attain the intensity of labor contractions, and this detracts from this hypothesis. Moreover, during the immediate postpartum period, the intensity of uterine contractions of the empty uterus might be two to three times stronger than the contractions of active labor but are associated either with much less intense pain or with no pain at all. On the other hand, strong contractions are associated with severe pain in most parturients with mechanical distortion caused by abnormal fetal positions and in those in whom the cervix dilates slowly. Because in such situations the uterine muscle is contracting under isometric conditions (i.e., its exit, the cervix and perineum, present an obstruction), the strong contractions are probably also a source of pain.

The validity of various other hypotheses is also disputed. The suggestion that pain is a result of ischemia during uterine contractions is disputed by monkey studies that showed that, although placental (intervillous) perfusion decreased to nearly 50% of control values, myometrial blood flow increased significantly during contractions (103) and increased to an even greater degree during a sustained (8-minute) contraction (104). Moreover, no evidence of an inflammatory process in the uterine muscles has been found (4). Dick-Read's (11) hypothesis that contraction of the cervix brought about by fear-induced hyperactivity of the sympathetic nervous system as the cause of pain is unwarranted in view of the fact that the cervix is composed mostly of connective tissue, with little muscle and elastic tissue (105). Moreover, during uncomplicated childbirth, the LUS and CX manifest only a small contractile force, which becomes even weaker as labor progresses (101).

Peripheral Pathways

A misconception about the peripheral nociceptive pathways of the uterus and cervix has existed for over 75 years. Based on his studies of the segments of hyperalgesia associated with various uterine disorders, as well as of hyperalgesia during the second stage of labor, Head (106) concluded that the sensory nerve supply of the uterus always involved the T11, often the T12, and not infrequently the T10 and L1 and sometimes L2 segments, and that the cervix was supplied by the S2, S3, and S4. Some 40 years later, based on animal experiments and studies of parturients, Cleland (107) concluded that in humans the sensory supply of the uterus is through the T11 and T12 spinal segments and that pain caused by stretch of the birth canal was transmitted through "undetermined sacral segments." This latter finding was interpreted to mean that the cervix and vagina are supplied by the sacral segments. As a result of these two studies it became widely taught that nociceptive impulses from the body of the uterus are transmitted through the T11 and T12 nerves, and that pain from the LUS and CX is transmitted through the pelvic nerve to the S2, S3, and S4 spinal segments.

Because Bonica's observations were at variance with this concept, he and associates carried out a study that involved 240 parturients and 35 gynecologic patients investigated over a period of 22 years (108). The study entailed the use of discrete blocks of various nociceptive pathways by paravertebral block, segmental epidural block, caudal block, and trans-sacral block of various

segments (108). Their results demonstrated conclusively that the upper part of the CX and the LUS are not supplied by sensory fibers that accompany the pelvic nerves (nervi erigentes), as stated in almost every modern anatomy and obstetric textbook (109–112). Rather, these structures are supplied by afferents that, like those that supply the body of the uterus, accompany the sympathetic nerves in the following sequence: the uterine and cervical plexus; the pelvic (inferior hypogastric) plexus; the middle hypogastric plexus or nerve; and the superior hypogastric and aortic plexuses. The nociceptive afferents then pass to the lumbar sympathetic chain and course cephalad through the lower thoracic sympathetic chain, which they leave by way of the rami communicantes associated with the T10, T11, T12, and L1 spinal nerves. Finally they pass through the posterior roots of these nerves to make synaptic contact with interneurons in the dorsal horn (Figs. 66-22 and 66-23).

Typical of the pain arising from viscera, the pain of the first stage of labor is referred to the dermatomes supplied by the same spinal cord segments that receive input from the uterus and cervix. During the latent (early) phase of the first stage the pain is felt as an ache and discomfort is limited to the T11 and T12 dermatomes (Fig. 66-24A). As labor progresses to the active phase of the first stage (usually 3 to 4 cm cervical dilatation) and the uterine contractions become more intense, the pain in the T11 and T12 dermatomes becomes more severe, is described as sharp and cramping, and spreads to the two adjacent (T10 and L1) dermatomes (Fig. 66-24B).

The distribution of the T10, T11, T12, and L1 dermatomes in the back overlies the lower three lumbar vertebrae and the upper half of the sacrum (see Fig. 6-9). This distribution of pain during the first stage

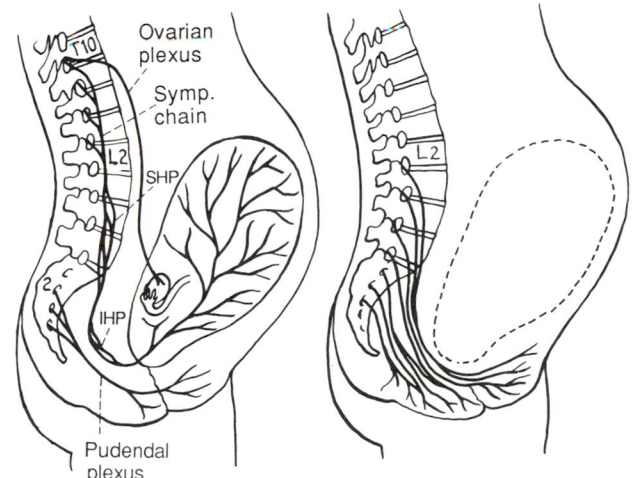

FIG. 66-22. Schematic depiction of the peripheral nociceptive pathways involved in the pain of childbirth. **A.** The uterus, including the cervix and lower uterine segments, is supplied by afferents that pass from the uterus to the spinal cord by accompanying sympathetic nerves through the inferior hypogastric plexus (IHP), the hypogastric nerve, the superior hypogastric plexus (SHP), the lumbar and lower thoracic sympathetic chain, and the nerves at T10, T11, T12, and L1. **B.** The nerves involved in transmission of nociceptive impulses are provoked by noxious stimulation of pelvic structures. See text for details.

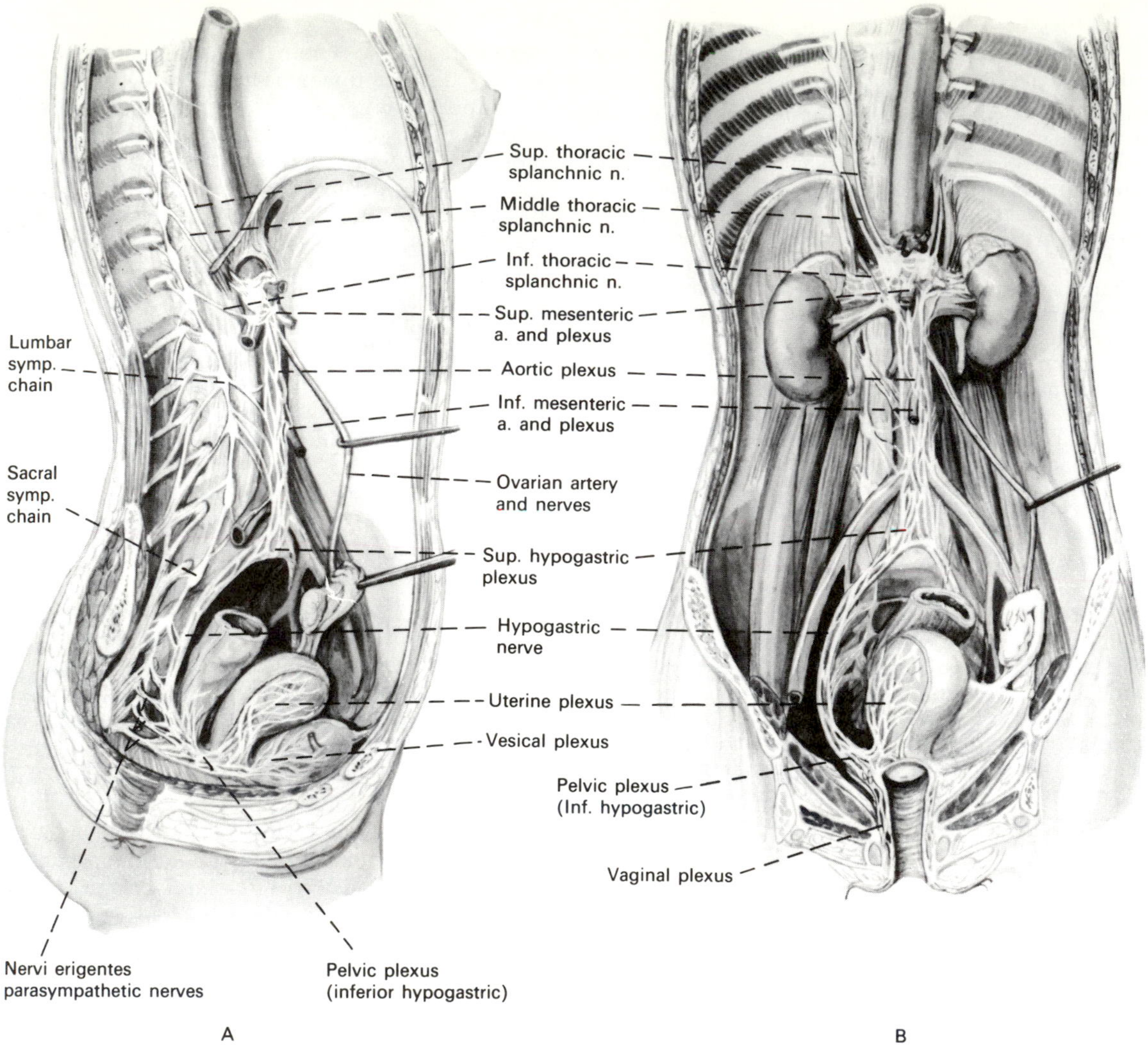

Sup. thoracic splanchnic n.
Middle thoracic splanchnic n.
Inf. thoracic splanchnic n.
Sup. mesenteric a. and plexus
Lumbar symp. chain
Aortic plexus
Inf. mesenteric a. and plexus
Sacral symp. chain
Ovarian artery and nerves
Sup. hypogastric plexus
Hypogastric nerve
Uterine plexus
Vesical plexus
Pelvic plexus (Inf. hypogastric)
Vaginal plexus
Nervi erigentes parasympathetic nerves
Pelvic plexus (inferior hypogastric)
A
B

FIG. 66-23. Gross anatomy of the nerve supply to the uterus. *A.* Lateral view. *B.* Anterior view. The uterus is shown in the nonpregnant state to permit the various nerves that supply it to be depicted. Note that the uterine and cervical plexuses are derived from the pelvic plexus, which contains parasympathetic and sympathetic efferents. The parasympathetic efferents have their cell bodies in the middle three sacral segments, and the parasympathetic afferents pass through these segments and progress cephalad through the neuraxis. The sympathetic efferents and afferents pass through the hypogastric nerve, which in turn is a continuation of the superior hypogastric and aortic plexuses. Note that fibers from the latter two plexuses pass on to the lumbar sympathetic chain, the afferents of which mediate nociceptive impulses and accompany the sympathetic fibers through these structures. From the lumbar and lower thoracic sympathetic chain the nociceptive afferents pass to the T10, T11, T12, and L1 spinal nerves and reach the spinal cord via their posterior roots and rootlets. Modified from Bonica, J.J.: Principles and Practice of Obstetric Analgesia and Anesthesia. Philadelphia, F.A. Davis, 1967. pp. 110–111.

segments. Often the pain is not referred to the entire dermatome but can be more severe in one or more patches of varying sizes within the territory of one or more dermatomes (4, 33, 34).

Second and Third Stages of Labor

Once the cervix is fully dilated, the amount of nociceptive stimulation arising in this structure decreases, but the contractions of the body of the uterus and distension of the lower uterine segment continue to cause pain in the same areas of reference as in the first stage of labor. In addition, the progressively greater pressure of the presenting part on pain-sensitive structures in the pelvis and distension of the outlet and perineum become new sources of pain. Progressively greater distension causes intense stretching and actual tearing of fascia and subcutaneous tissues and pressure on the skeletal muscles of the perineum. Like other pain caused by stimulation of superficial somatic structures, the perineal pain is sharp and well localized, predominantly to the regions supplied by the pudendal nerves, and can be eliminated by block of these nerves (5, 113) (see Fig. 66-25A and C on p. 1336).

In the late part of the first stage and during the second stage, a number of parturients develop aching, burning, or cramping discomfort in the thigh and, less frequently, in the legs (Fig. 66-24C and D). This is presumably a result of stimulation of pain-sensitive structures in the pelvic cavity, including the following: (a) traction on the pelvic parietal peritoneum and on the structures it envelops, including the uterine ligaments; (b) stretching and tension of the bladder, urethra, and rectum; (c) stretching and tension of ligaments, fascia, and muscles in the pelvic cavity; and

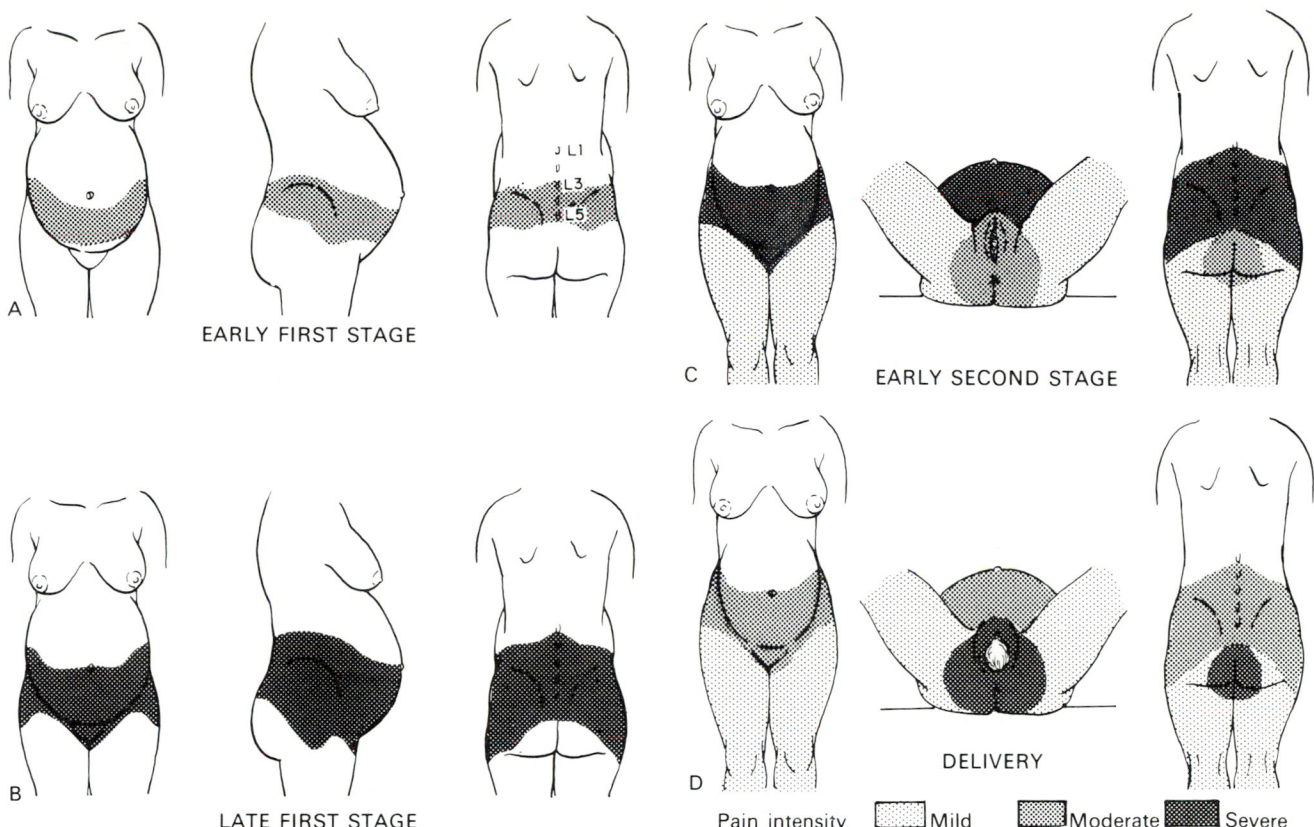

EARLY FIRST STAGE

EARLY SECOND STAGE

LATE FIRST STAGE

DELIVERY

Pain intensity ☐ Mild ▨ Moderate ■ Severe

FIG. 66-24. The intensity and distribution of parturition pain during the various phases of labor and delivery. **A.** In the early first stage the pain is referred to the T11 and T12 dermatomes. **B.** In the late first stage, however, the severe pain is also referred to the T10 to L1 dermatomes. **C.** In the early second stage uterine contractions remain intense and produce severe pain in the T10 to L1 dermatomes. At the same time the presenting part exerts pressure on pelvic structures and thus causes moderate pain in the very low back and perineum and often produces mild pain in the thighs and legs. **D.** Intensity and distribution of pain during the latter phase of the second stage and during actual delivery. The perineal component is the primary cause of pain whereas uterine contractions produce moderate pain. From Bonica, J.J.: Obstetric Analgesia and Anesthesia. 2nd Ed. Seattle, University of Washington Press, 1980, pp. 46–47.

(d) undue pressure on one or more roots of the lumbosacral plexus. These factors usually produce mild pain referred to the lower lumbar and sacral segments; (Fig. 66-22B) but, if the fetus is in an abnormal position, with undue pressure by the presenting part, the referred pain can become moderate or severe (Fig. 66-24C and D).

The transmission of the nociceptive information that arises from these various structures to the dorsal horn and then to other parts of the spinal cord and to the ascending systems to the brain is presumably similar to that of other types of acute pain. It need not be discussed further here except for one point. The pain is provoked by tissue damage in the cervix and perineum and is thought to be passed to the dorsal horn through A-delta and C nociceptive fibers. In addition to producing local tissue responses, the pain provokes segmental and suprasegmental reflex responses discussed in Chapter 7, Section F, which are responsible for the various effects discussed above.

Factors that Affect the Pain of Childbirth

In addition to the role played by such intrinsic factors as the intensity, duration, and pattern of contractions and related physiologic and biochemi-cal mechanisms, the amount or degree of pain and suffering associated with childbirth is influenced by physical, psychologic, emotional, and motivational factors (5, 6, 31, 34, 98, 111, 112).

Physical Factors

Physical factors that influence the incidence, severity, and duration of the pain of childbirth include the age, parity, and condition of the parturient, the condition of the cervix at the onset of labor, and the relationship of the size of the infant to the size of the birth canal. Many of these factors are interrelated. Generally, an older primipara experiences a longer and more painful labor than a younger primipara. The cervix of the multipara begins to soften even before the onset of labor and is less sensitive than that of the primipara. The intensity of uterine contractions in early labor tends to be higher in primiparae than in multiparae, whereas in the latter phase of labor the reverse is true. In the presence of dystocia caused by a contracted pelvis, a large baby, or abnormal presentation, the parturient experiences more pain than under normal conditions. Melzack and associates (32, 33) found that high pain levels were associated with a history of menstrual difficulties. Fatigue, loss of sleep, and general debility influence a parturient's tolerance of the painful experience and increase the pain behavior. This is particularly significant in parturients with prolonged labor.

Psychologic Factors

Psychologic factors that can and frequently do affect the incidence and intensity of parturition pain include the mentation, attitude, and mood of the parturient at the time of labor, and other emotional factors. Fear, apprehension, and anxiety probably enhance pain perception and pain behavior (4, 5, 30). One of the most frequent causes of fear and anxiety is ignorance of or misinformation about the process of pregnancy and parturition, and what the onset of labor signifies. An uninformed parturient, especially a primipara, can be disturbed by fear of the unknown, death, suffering, mutilation, possible complications, and concern for her condition or that of her fetus (4). Parturients who have had an unplanned or illegitimate pregnancy or have an ambivalent or negative reaction to gestation report more pain than those who do not (4, 30, 114). In contrast, other emotional factors such as intense motivation and cultural influences can affect modulation of sensory transmissions and certainly can influence the affective and behavioral dimensions of pain. Moreover, cognitive intervention such as giving the parturient preparatory information about labor, thus reducing uncertainty while focusing attention or producing distraction and dissociation from pain (all parts of an "educated" childbirth program) reduces pain behavior.

Cultural and Ethnic Factors

Racial, cultural, and ethnic factors have long been considered to be important in influencing pain tolerance and pain behavior. Persons of Italian and other Latin cultures or of Jewish or Mediterranean background are said to express pain in an emotive fashion and to exaggerate their verbal report, whereas those of Anglo-Saxon origin (e.g., English, third-generation Americans, Irish) as well as Scandinavians, Asians, American Indians, and Eskimos, are said to be more stoic and to manifest less pain behavior (115). Experimental data and clinical observations, however, suggest that, although racial, cultural, and ethnic differences do exist, they appear to be differences in expressiveness consequent to underlying attitudes toward the pain rather than differences in the sensory experience or pain perception.

True (116) reported that Mohave Indian women experienced a great deal of pain during childbirth but avoided expressing their suffering for fear of ridicule. In an experimental study, Meehan and colleagues (117) found no significant differences between pain tolerance of American Indians, Eskimos, and whites. In a study of Turkomenian women, Preissman and Ogoulbostan-Essenova (118) noted that they behaved calmly during childbirth and manifested no pain behavior but inquiry revealed that the process was painful. Nettelbladt and associates (30), in a study of 78 women, noted that 56% of parturients who reported intolerable pain were not rated by the midwives as having very painful deliveries. This discrepancy prob-

ably occurred because the parturients manifested less overt pain behavior than they actually felt, which is a characteristic of Scandinavian culture. Winsberg and Greenlick (119) examined pain behavior in black and white parturients who were matched on such parameters as social class or cooperation and found no differences in pain response or estimated degree of pain.

The thesis that cultural and racial differences can have some influence on pain behavior but probably not on the pain felt by parturients is supported by Bonica's studies (unpublished data) of 2700 parturients in other countries and of 8000 parturients in the United States (see above: Incidence and Intensity of Labor Pain). In Western and Eastern Europe, Latin America, Africa, Asia-Australia, the Near East, and North America parturients who were not "educated" and who were psychologically unprepared for childbirth manifested a similar incidence of pain behavior, although the patterns of behavior varied. During the contractions some women moaned, others screamed, others writhed and had facial expression of suffering with little or no verbal expression, while still others used incantations (said to be specific for labor pain in that particular country). Contrary to traditional belief, Asian women (including Japanese, Chinese, Malaysians, Indians, Cambodians, and Thais) did not remain stoic but manifested as much pain behavior as American and European parturients. Moreover, the large Oriental population of Seattle and the recent influx of refugees from Indochina afforded the opportunity to observe and interview several hundred parturients from various countries in Southeast Asia. These studies revealed that the frequency and intensity of labor pain and the request for analgesia was the same as for Occidental parturients living in Asia, and the pain behavior was similar to that observed among parturients in their native countries (Bonica, unpublished data).

The influence of education and psychologic conditioning inherent in psychoprophylaxis and natural childbirth in modifying pain behavior without significantly affecting pain sensation is now widely appreciated. During 5- to 10-day visits to obstetric centers that practiced psychoprophylaxis or natural childbirth in the Soviet Union, France, Germany, Italy, The Netherlands, Sweden, and the United States, made over a 5-month period in 1959, Bonica observed about 700 parturients (and interviewed many) who had received training in one of these methods, and over 85% of them manifested little or no pain behavior during labor and delivery. When questioned the next day, however, most of them indicated that the process had been painful but many quickly added that they were pleased to cooperate with their instructor and obstetric team (5). Especially impressive was the marked change in behavior of Italian parturients in a large obstetric center in Turin noted during two visits made 5 years apart. During the first visit, in 1954, the labor ward was a scene of cacophony caused by the screaming, pleading, and praying of the nearly 50 laboring women in the same ward. In contrast, 5 years later, one heard only an occasional moan from a similar number of parturients who had undergone an intensive course of psychoprophylaxis. Most went through the entire labor and delivery with minimal pain behavior but later stated that they had had moderate to severe pain.

Summary

It is obvious that the pain-associated responses to noxious stimulation provoked by uterine contractions and other tissue-damaging factors during labor and vaginal delivery are the net effects of highly complex interactions of various neural systems, modulating influences, and psychologic factors. Through the interaction of the afferent system and neocortical processes, the parturient receives perceptual and discriminate information that is analyzed and that usually activates motivational cognitive processes.

These, in turn, act on the motor system and initiate psychodynamic mechanisms of anxiety and apprehension that produce the complex physiologic, behavioral, and affective responses that characterize acute pain.

B. MANAGEMENT OF THE PAIN OF CHILDBIRTH

Nociception associated with labor and vaginal delivery not only produces suffering and emotional disturbances, but also induces segmental and suprasegmental reflex responses that further alter the function of the organism. The data presented also suggest that the relief of childbirth pain not only eliminates emotional reactions and suffering but decreases or eliminates some of the alterations. It is the task of the obstetric team to provide optimal relief of pain to parturients with the resources that are available.

Many drugs and techniques are currently available for providing analgesia during childbirth. The methods vary according to geographic region or country and depend on the culture, medical personnel, facilities, and other sociologic and professional factors. To be used properly, each drug and technique must be evaluated from four interrelated viewpoints: (a) analgesic potency and other therapeutic efficacy; (b) side effects on the mother; (c) effects on the fetus and newborn; and (d) effects on the forces of labor. Table 66-1 contains a critical evaluation of the various drugs and techniques in current use from these perspectives. The effects on the mother, fetus, and newborn, and the forces of labor discussed in the table are based on the use of optimal doses and routes of administration of systemic drugs and on the use of optimal concentrations and volumes of local and regional anesthetics.

General Considerations

Basic Principles

To obtain the most effective results with obstetric analgesia and anesthesia, those on the obstetric team must adhere to certain basic principles. The objective is to provide optimal relief of pain to the mother with little or no risk to her and her infant. The type of analgesia or anesthesia must be tailored to the needs of each mother and infant within the framework of the personnel and resources available. Each member of the obstetric team must be fully informed of the plans and possible problems of other members, with excellent communication, coordination, and cooperation among those on the team. The anesthetist must have a thorough understanding of the physiologic and pathophysiologic alterations caused by pregnancy and labor, and how these are affected by each type of analgesia.

Antepartal and Preanesthetic Care

The proper preparation of the gravida and her spouse during the antepartum period is one of the most important responsibilities of the obstetric team (6). She and her husband should be fully informed about the physiology and psychology of pregnancy and labor and about the psychologic and emotional effects these might produce. Understanding the changes in her circulation, respiration, endocrine function, and other systems helps the gravida to understand and accept the inconveniences, discomforts, and awkwardness of the lopsided silhouette she develops during pregnancy (4, 6). Similarly, a discussion of the physiology and clinical course of labor provides her with useful information and helps her to cooperate and participate actively during labor as well as in the many other aspects of educated childbirth. During one of the antepartum visits the obstetrician should bring up the matter of analgesia and anesthesia and, if the gravida indicates that she is interested, the advantages, disadvantages, and limitations of each technique should be clearly explained. If the gravida delivers in the hospital, it is essential that everyone who comes in contact with the patient (from the admission clerk to members of the house staff) thoroughly appreciate the importance of a friendly and reassuring attitude.

Those gravidas who indicate a desire for some form of pain relief should be seen by an anesthesiologist either prior to or soon after admission to the hospital. Proper preanesthetic care requires a thorough evaluation of the parturient, including a medical and anesthesia history, physical examination, assessment of the physiologic and emotional status of the parturient, and discussion of the various forms of analgesia and anesthesia available. Selection of the method of analgesia to be used is made in consultation with the parturient and obstetrician.

Intrapartal and Intra-Anesthetic Care

During labor the uterine contractions, cervical dilatation, and advance of the presenting part should be monitored. The cervicographic method of following the progress of labor is recommended. During a home or hospital delivery in which modern equipment is not available, the fetal heart rate (FHR) is monitored by auscultation. The limitations of this method and of palpating uterine contractions are generally recognized and emphasize the need for the clinical use of more sophisticated techniques, especially in monitoring the labor of women with high-risk pregnancies. Currently, a number of systems permit the continuous and simultaneous measurements of FHR and myometrial activity; these are simple to operate, easy to maintain, and are of reasonable cost. Combined with these are the measurements of the cervical dilatation and advance of the presenting part, recorded on a partograph that also has space for recording maternal blood pressure, respiration, and the effects of the administration of oxytocin, sedatives, systemic and regional analgesics and other drugs used during labor and delivery. During labor the parturient is made

TABLE 66-1. Pharmacology and Applications of Obstetric Analgesia and Anesthesia

Feature	Sedatives and analgesics		Regional Analgesia and Anesthesia				General Analgesia and Anesthesia	
Specific drugs or technique	Promazine; hydroxyzine	Meperidine Demerol (D) Pethidine; Morphine (M)	Spinal epidural block: standard (SEB) T10–S5; segmental (S) T10–L1; and caudal block S2–S5 double-catheter T10–L1 and caudal block S2–S5	Caudal block (CEB) (catheter tip at S1)	Subarachnoid block (SAB); standard subarachnoid block (STB) T10–S5; true saddle block (SB) S1–S5	Paracervical block (PCB); pudendal block (PB)	Inhalation analgesia	Balanced anesthesia
Optimal dose and route	50 mg IM	D, 100 mg IM M, 10 mg IM (or 50% dose IV slowly)					40–50% nitrous oxide ($N_2O + O_2$); 0.35% methoxyflurane (MF); 0.35–0.5% trichloroethylene (TC); 3–5% cyclopropane (C); 1–1.5% diethyl ether (DE); 0.25–1.25% enflurane (E)	100% O_2 for 5 minutes; 3 mg D-tubocurarine or 1 mg pancuronium → ketamine 0.4–0.5/kg and thiopental 3 mg/kg immediate cricoid pressure →; 100 mg succinylcholine (SC) IV → tracheal intubation → 40% N_2O + 0.5% H in O_2 + SC infusion until delivery → increase to 60% N_2O + 0.5% H in O_2 after delivery
Therapeutic effects	Sedation, decrease of anxiety; antiemetic	Analgesia, sedation, and decrease of anxiety as a result of pain relief	Greater degree of pain relief than with other regional techniques	Excellent pain relief	STB: analgesia for labor and delivery; SB: anesthesia for delivery only	PCB: for relief of uterine pain; PB: for relief of perineal pain	Satisfactory analgesia in 60–70% with N_2O, M, C, TC, and DE, 80% with E, and 90% with combination M and N_2O	Ensures adequate oxygenation, anesthesia, relaxation, and satisfactory maintenance
Side effects on mother	None	Respiration ↓ between contractions; delayed gastric emptying; nausea and vomiting in some	Minimal hypotension with proper management; moderate or severe hypotension in supine position	More hypotension than SEB	STB: more hypotension than SEB, CEB SB: none	None if properly done, but sedation and toxic reaction with overdose	None with analgesic concentration except occasional amnesia and confusion	Respiratory depression and paralysis; artificial ventilation required
Effects on labor	None	None	None, if initiated too early → prolonged latent phase, which can be obviated with oxytocin; bearing down reflex lost, but able to push voluntarily	Same as SEB	STB: same as SEB; SB: none except loss of bearing down reflex	PCB: transient depression of contractions, but no effect on labor progress; PB: none	None	None
Placental transfer	Rapid, within 3–5 minutes after IM or 60 seconds after IV	Same as SEB	Rapid but small amounts with analgesic concentrations (AC) of local anesthetics (LA)	Rapid but more amounts than SEB	None	PCB: rapid and more than SEB, CEB; PB: less than SEB, CEB, or PC	Rapid	IV and inhalation agents rapid; muscle relaxants little or none
Effects on fetus	Slight CNS depression (↓) Decrease or loss of beat-to-beat variability (BBV↓)	Moderate CNS ↓ and cardiovascular (CV)↓; BBV ↓	Transient BBV↓ with lidocaine (L) and mepivacaine (MP), but none with bupivacaine (B)	Same as SEB but greater effects	STB: none unless severe and sustained hypotension → fetal distress; SB: none	PCB: bradycardia BBV↓; PB: same as SEB	None	Same as SEB
Effects on newborn	Slight respiratory ↓	Moderate CNS ↓; EEG ↓; Early Neonatal Neurobehavioral Scale (ENNS)↓	ENNS ↓ with 1.5–2% L or MP, but none with AC/LA, none with B	Same as SEB but greater degree (more LA used)	None except if severe and sustained hypotension → neonatal ↓	PCB: ENNS ↓; PB: same as SEB	None or slight neonatal ↓	None with above amounts and concentrations, moderate ↓ with larger amounts or concentrations
Remarks	Used alone during latent phase and combined with narcotics during active phase	Effective analgesics for moderate pain in 70–80% of parturients	Excellent analgesia, but premature block of lower limbs and perineum with standard; sometimes inadequate perineal block with segmental; double-catheter best technique	Same as SEB plus greater perineal and limb paralysis	Simple and rapid analgesia and perineal relaxation, but premature perineal and limb paralysis and loss of reflex	PCB plus PB: good analgesia; can be done by obstetrician; no hypotension	C and DE no longer used; other agents provide satisfactory analgesia and are simple to administer	Best method of anesthesia in hypovolemic or hypotensive parturients; excellent for cesarean section and for instrumental vaginal delivery

to lie on her side and should only assume the supine position for brief periods (seconds), during which left lateral tilt or left uterine displacement is used. The induction and maintenance of regional analgesia are also carried out with the parturient on her side.

Current Methods of Obstetric Analgesia and Anesthesia

All the drugs and techniques that are currently available to provide pain relief during childbirth can be arbitrarily classified into four categories: (a) nonpharmacologic analgesia, primarily in the form of psychologic and physiologic techniques; (b) simple methods of pharmacologic analgesia; (c) inhalation analgesia and anesthesia; and (d) regional analgesia. Detailed consideration of these methods is precluded here, but the pharmacologic methods are summarized in Table 66-1.

Nonpharmacologic Techniques

The past 40 years have seen a progressive increase in the application of several methods that do not entail the use of pharmacologic agents to relieve the pain of childbirth. These include the following: (a) natural childbirth, originally proposed and practiced by the late Dick-Read (10, 11); (b) the method of psychoprophylaxis originated by Velvovski and associates in the Soviet Union (12) in the late 1940s and practiced thereafter and advocated by Lamaze (27) in Paris and worldwide since then; (c) hypnosis, which has been used sporadically in a few obstetric clinics; and (d) acupuncture and transcutaneous electrical nerve stimulation (TENS), both of which have been given clinical trials during the past 15 years.

Psychologic Analgesia

The term "psychologic analgesia" applies to both educated (natural) childbirth and psychoprophylaxis because, despite claims to the contrary by the proponents of each method, these have similar physiotherapeutic and psychophysiologic bases (4, 5). Early proponents of these techniques claimed that most patients can achieve "painless" childbirth, but most current workers in the field acknowledge the fact that pain is not completely eliminated in most parturients but can be somewhat ameliorated. The major benefits of these methods are a decrease in anxiety and apprehension, enhancement of the parturient's ability to cope with the entire process and to control her behavior, the experience of a personal sense of achievement, and enhancement of the early bonding process by immediate visual, auditory, and tactile contact between the mother and her newborn.

Analysis of published data and observations in various countries suggests that, if psychoprophylactic or natural childbirth methods are properly used by both primiparae and multiparae, the following results can be expected: (a) little or no pain is experienced by 15 to 20%, and no analgesia or anesthesia is required during the entire process; (b) the pain is decreased in an additional 15 to 20% to a moderate degree, and parturients require less pharmacologic analgesia and

anesthesia; and (c) the pain is not affected in the remainder but fear and anxiety are less, and parturients manifest less pain behavior (5, 6). Some reports (120) indicate that women who are trained in prepared childbirth methods have shorter labor, fewer operative deliveries, fewer intrapartum and postpartum complications, less blood loss, and better and happier babies than those given drug-induced analgesia or anesthesia. Other studies (including some with proper controls) indicate no significant differences regarding these variables between those in prepared and unprepared (analgesia) groups (32–34, 121, 122). Observations by Bonica (unpublished data) in hospitals in the Soviet Union, Eastern and Western Europe, and North and South America suggest that the discrepancies are a result of differences in motivation, attitude, and personality of parturients and their instructors, the practices of the obstetrician and, most importantly, the skill with which pharmacologic analgesia and anesthesia are administered. On the basis of these observations and long experience with regional analgesia, we agree with Melzack (34) in recommending that prepared childbirth training be combined with regional analgesia to achieve the best results for mothers and their infants.

Hypnosis

Most practitioners of hypnosis for pregnant women begin with early preparation at about the fifth or sixth month of pregnancy and subsequently thereafter every 2 to 4 weeks. Various techniques have been employed. The word "hypnosis" is not used; rather the term "medical relaxation" is used instead to suggest to parturients what is expected of them during preparatory sessions and at delivery. Although most women derive some benefit, only a small percentage (15 to 20%) of parturients are sufficiently susceptible to hypnotic suggestion to be able to obtain complete pain relief.

Acupuncture and Transcutaneous Electric Nerve Stimulation

Despite the great interest in China in the use of acupuncture analgesia for surgery, the use of this method in obstetrics has been limited to cesarean section (123). The Chinese have not used it for vaginal delivery because of their cultural premise that parturition is a physiologic function and does not require analgesia. This technique has been tried in Europe, North America, and other parts of Asia, with conflicting results. Several obstetric anesthesiologists have given acupuncture an adequate trial but did not obtain satisfactory results and discontinued its use.

Transcutaneous electric nerve stimulation (TENS) is another nonpharmacologic technique that has been given limited clinical trial. The first pair of electrodes is usually applied to the skin overlying the T10 to L1 vertebrae, with one electrode just lateral of the midline, while the second pair is applied bilaterally on the skin overlying the S2 to S4 vertebrae. Low-intensity high-frequency (60- to 80-Hz) stimulation is applied continuously through the upper electrodes and, as soon as more intense pain caused by the onset of uterine contractions is felt, parturients themselves increase the stimulation until tingling sensations are felt. Uncontrolled clinical trials suggest that about 40 to 60% of parturients obtain good or partial relief of pain during the first stage, but two-thirds of these require regional analgesia during the second stage and for delivery.

Simple Techniques of Pharmacologic Analgesia

In many parts of the world in which anesthetists are not available, the midwife or obstetrician must rely on the use of prepared childbirth and on simple methods of drug-induced analgesia. Mild pain during the early first stage can be relieved by using suggestion and combining it with sedatives and tranquilizers. With the onset of moderate pain during the active phase of labor, however, opioids are usually required, and these are given either intramuscularly or intravenously in small increments. Properly administered opioids produce adequate but not complete relief of moderate pain in 70 to 80% of parturients and relief of severe pain in about 35 to 60% of parturients (4–6). Opioids do not produce significant maternal respiratory depression in optimal doses but do produce neonatal depression that can be minimized. Inhalation analgesia, bilateral pudendal block, or infiltration of the perineum is used for the actual delivery.

Inhalation Analgesia and Anesthesia

Inhalation *analgesia* is a widely used method of relieving childbirth pain because it produces moderately effective pain relief without causing loss of consciousness or significant maternal or neonatal depression. The agents most commonly used are 40 to 50% nitrous oxide in oxygen or 0.35% methoxyflurane, 0.35 to 0.5% trichlorethylene, or 0.25 to 1% enflurane in either air or oxygen. Each agent can be administered intermittently during uterine contractions by the parturient or administered by the midwife or anesthetist. Premixed cylinders of 50% nitrous oxide and 50% oxygen (Entonox) are available in some areas, and these greatly facilitate the use of this agent by either the parturient or midwife. For optimal results, inhalation of the drug should begin some 10 to 15 seconds before the painful period of each contraction. Properly used, inhalation analgesia produces good pain relief in about 60% and partial relief in another 30% of parturients (4–9).

Inhalation *anesthesia* is still used for vaginal delivery because it affords maximum control of depth and duration of action and is rapidly eliminated at the end of the procedure. On the other hand, general anesthesia carries the risk of provoking regurgitation or vomiting and consequent pulmonary aspiration, the leading cause of anesthesia-related maternal mortality in Britain and the United States (7, 8). General anesthesia should therefore only be given by a properly trained anesthestist who has secured the airway by tracheal intubation. Balanced general anesthesia is used for cesarean section.

Regional Analgesia and Anesthesia

The use of regional analgesia and anesthesia during labor and for delivery has increased dramatically over the past 40 years in the United States, Great Britain and, more recently, in many European countries in which the use of pharmacologic obstetric anesthesia had been avoided. The most common techniques are continuous lumbar epidural block, subarachnoid (saddle) block, bilateral paracervical or bilateral pudendal block, or both, continuous caudal block, and double-catheter extradural block, which consists of combining segmental epidural and low caudal blocks.

Advantages, Disadvantages, and Contraindications

The popularity of regional analgesia and anesthesia is that it provides certain advantages over other methods, as follows:

In contrast to narcotics and inhalation analgesia, regional analgesia and anesthesia produces complete relief of pain in most parturients.

The hazard of pulmonary aspiration of gastric contents inherent in general anesthesia is greatly reduced or eliminated.

By blocking all nociceptive and efferent pathways, it obviates the pain-induced deleterious reflex responses noted in the previous section.

With most techniques the use of a dilute solution of local anesthetic produces block of nociceptive (A-delta and C) fibers, with minimal or no effect on the larger somatomotor and tactile fibers.

Provided it is properly administered and complications are avoided, regional analgesia and anesthesia causes no maternal or neonatal depression.

Administered properly, regional analgesia and anesthesia has no clinically significant effect on the progress of labor.

"Continuous" epidural analgesia can be extended for delivery and can even be modified for cesarean section, if necessary.

Regional analgesia permits the mother to remain awake and alert during labor and delivery so that she can experience the pleasure of actively participating in the birth process (by bearing down voluntarily) and of promptly bonding with her child.

On the other hand, the various techniques have certain disadvantages:

The use of regional analgesia and anesthesia requires greater knowledge of anatomy and greater technical skill for administration than the use of systemic drugs, inhalation agents, or general anesthesia.

Technical failures occur, although the incidence is small in experienced hands.

The vasomotor block inherent in spinal, standard epidural, and caudal block can cause significant maternal hypotension if prophylactic measures are not carried out.

Techniques that produce premature perineal muscle relaxation can interfere with the mechanism of internal rotation and might increase the incidence of occipitoposterior or occipitotransverse positions.

Techniques that produce perineal analgesia cause loss of the afferent limb of the reflex urge to bear down and, unless the parturient is instructed how to bear down effectively, it can prolong the second stage, require the use of outlet forceps, or both.

Spinal, caudal, or lumbar epidural and double-catheter techniques are relatively contraindicated in parturients with coagulopathy because of the risk of hemorrhage within the spinal canal.

Regional analgesia and anesthesia procedures can only be carried out in a hospital.

In addition to the relative contraindications of the use of regional analgesia and anesthesia in parturients with coagulation defects, other contraindications to this procedure have been noted:

The use of regional analgesia and anesthesia is contraindicated if the anesthesiologist lacks skill and experience in the technique, lacks knowledge of obstetric physiology and pathophysiology, or lacks knowledge about the prevention and treatment of complications.

Infection of the puncture site, pre-existing coagulation defects, or hemorrhagic hypovolemia or shock are contraindications, especially for subarachnoid and extradural techniques.

The parturient's refusal or intense fear of regional anesthesia is a contraindication.

A lack of experience or appreciation by the obstetrician of how regional analgesia and anesthesia influences the management of labor negates the use of these techniques.

To achieve the stated objectives of obstetric analgesia—that is, good maternal pain relief with little or no risk to the parturient or her infant—it is essential for the anesthesiologist to fulfill the following:

The anesthesiologist must have a thorough understanding of parturition pain pathways and the pharmacology of local anesthetics, must have acquired sufficient skill and experience with the various techniques, and must know how to manage the parturient during and after regional analgesia has been administered.

The anesthesiologist must know the possible complications, their prevention, and prompt treatment.

The anesthesiologist must ensure that none of the regional procedures be started without an *intravenous infusion running and without having equipment for treatment of complications and for resuscitation available for immediate use.*

The anesthesiologist should avoid using a regional technique if it is contraindicated.

Except in circumstances in which the use of regional analgesia is particularly indicated and has significant advantages over other methods, it should not be used against the wishes of the parturient.

Regional analgesia should not be started until the contractions are strong, last 35 to 40 seconds or more, and occur at intervals of 3 minutes or less (5–6). The only exceptions to this rule are the parturients who experience extreme pain during the latent phase of labor and those in whom labor has been induced and maintained with oxytocin.

The parturient should be continuously monitored during and following administration of the analgesia and her blood pressure, pulse, and respiration measured every 30 seconds during the first 15 minutes and every 5 minutes thereafter.

Frequently it is necessary to complement regional analgesia with psychologic support and, if necessary, a sedative and small doses of a narcotic.

Nursing personnel who are skilled and willing to supervise the parturient properly must be available.

Prevention of Complications

Care must be exercised to avoid three serious complications: (a) maternal hypotension; (b) systemic toxic reactions; and (c) high or total spinal anesthesia. Maternal hypotension can be avoided or minimized by infusing 1 L of fluid 10 minutes before inducing spinal, epidural, or caudal block to compensate for the increased vasodilation consequent to the vasomotor blockade. It is also essential to have the parturient labor on her side to avoid aortocaval compression inherent in the supine position. Systemic toxic reactions must be prevented by avoiding excessive doses or accidental intravenous injection of therapeutic doses. High or total spinal anesthesia might result from accidental subarachnoid injection of a local anesthetic dose intended for extradural block. The latter two complications can almost always be prevented by attempting to aspirate blood or cerebrospinal fluid and by injecting a test dose of 2 to 3 ml of a solution containing 5 to 7.5 mg of bupivacaine and 15 μg of epinephrine. If the injection is accidentally subarachnoid, the parturient develops a low (T10 to S5) spinal anesthesia, which can be used instead of the extradural block. If the injection is intravenous the epinephrine produces moderate tachycardia and hypertension within 20 to 30 seconds of the injection that lasts for 30 to 60 seconds. A large therapeutic dose should be injected only when neither occurs (see Chapter 94 for a more detailed discussion of these complications).

Paracervical and Pudendal Block

The techniques of paracervical block (PCB) combined with pudendal block (PB) are shown in Figure 66-25. These procedures, usually done by the obstetrician or physician managing the parturient, offer advantages and certain disadvantages.

Advantages of the use of PCB and PB include the following: (a) the procedures are especially useful in cases in which anesthetists are not available; (b) both procedures can be done easily, provided the physician knows the anatomy well; (c) PCB provides good relief of uterine pain during the first and second stages of labor, while PB provides good relief of perineal pain during the second stage and delivery.

Disadvantages of the use of PCB and PB include the following: (a) PCB produces transient fetal bradycardia in 5 to 20% of cases; (b) PB can impair the bearing down reflex; (c) both PCB and PB entail the risk of systemic toxicity from overdose or accidental IV injection; and (d) the degree of pain relief is less than with other regional techniques.

Subarachnoid Block

Subarachnoid block (SAB), also frequently referred to as spinal anesthesia and "modified saddle block," usually produces analgesia and anesthesia extending from the T10 to the S5 spinal segments.

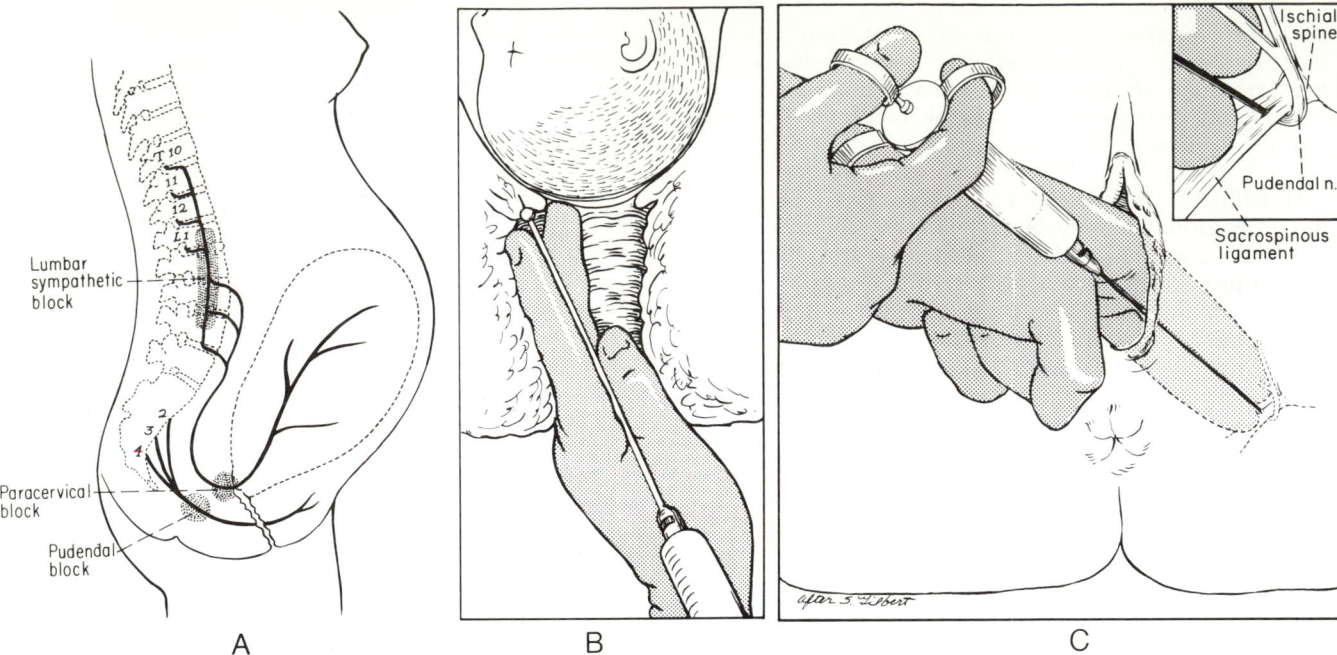

FIG. 66-25. *A.* Sites of three regional techniques for obstetric analgesia. Lumbar sympathetic block is rarely used but is highly effective in relieving pain of the first stage and can be preferable to the use of paracervical block, especially in high-risk pregnancies. *B.* Technique of paracervical block. The coronal section of the vagina and the lower part of the uterus containing the fetal head are shown. The 22-gauge needle is contained within a guide, with its point protruding only 5 to 7 mm beyond the end of the guide. This prevents the needle being inserted more than 5 to 7 mm beyond the surface of the mucosa. After negative aspiration an injection of 8 to 10 ml of 0.25% bupivacaine at 4 and 8 o'clock of the cervical fornix produces relief of uterine pain for several hours. *C.* Transvaginal technique of blocking the pudendal nerve. The two fingers of the left hand are inserted into the vagina to guide the needle point into the sacrospinous ligament. As long as the bevel of the needle is in the ligament there is some resistance to the injection of local anesthetic, but as soon as the bevel passes through the ligament there is a sudden lack of resistance, indicating that the needle point is next to the nerve. Modified from Bonica, J.J.: Principles and Practice of Obstetric Analgesia and Anesthesia, Vol. 1. Philadelphia, F.A. Davis, 1967, pp. 493, 514–515.

The advantages of the use of SAB include the following: (a) it is relatively simple to perform and is rapid and certain in its action; (b) it entails the use of small amounts of local anesthetic (e.g., 5 mg bupivacaine), thus eliminating the risk of systemic toxicity; (c) it can be initiated in the first stage of labor and carried out until delivery; and (d) it produces the most profound perineal relaxation, thus facilitating the use of forceps or other maneuvers that require perineal relaxation.

The disadvantages of the use of SAB include the following: (a) it produces a higher incidence and degree of hypotension than extradural block, although these could be reduced with the infusion of fluids prior to induction of the procedure; (b) it produces premature perineal paralysis and thus interferes with flexion and internal rotation of the presenting part; (c) it eliminates the bearing down reflex although the parturient can voluntarily bear down effectively, provided the abdominal muscles are not paralyzed; (d) it produces not only numbness but also paralysis of the lower limbs, making it impossible for the parturient to move them; and (e) it carries the risk of postpuncture headache, the incidence of which depends on the size of the needle used and on the number of punctures done. The incidence of headache should be between 1 and 5% if a 25-gauge spinal needle is used (5–8).

Continuous Caudal Analgesia and Anesthesia

Continuous caudal analgesia and anesthesia (CCB) is a form of extradural blockade that provides good pain relief during labor and produces anesthesia for vaginal delivery (Fig. 66-26).

The advantages of the use of CCB include the following: (a) it has a slower onset of vasomotor blockade than SAB and consequently produces less hypotension; (b) by using an analgesic concentration of local anesthetic (e.g., 0.25% bupivacaine) it produces less perineal and lower limb paralysis than SAB; and (c) it has no risk of postpuncture headache.

The disadvantages of the use of CCB include the following: (a) it requires larger amounts of local anesthetic than other regional techniques; (b) more anatomic anomalies occur in the sacrum than in the lumbar region and consequently it is more difficult to execute this procedure, thus entailing a greater risk of failure; and (c) if the procedure is carried out by inexperienced personnel during late labor there is a risk of puncturing the rectum and fetal head.

Continuous Spinal Epidural Block

In medical centers in the United States, Great Britain, and other countries that have specialized obstetric anesthesia services, spinal epidural blockade is the procedure of choice for most parturients because it provides effective pain relief in 85 to 95% of women in labor (4–8, 124) (Fig. 66-27). Inadequate perineal analgesia for delivery is a frequent occurence, but this can be avoided by administering a large dose of local anesthetic (LA) when delivery is imminent or by having parturients receive a top-up dose (reinjection of LA) in the sitting position about 10 to 15 minutes before delivery.

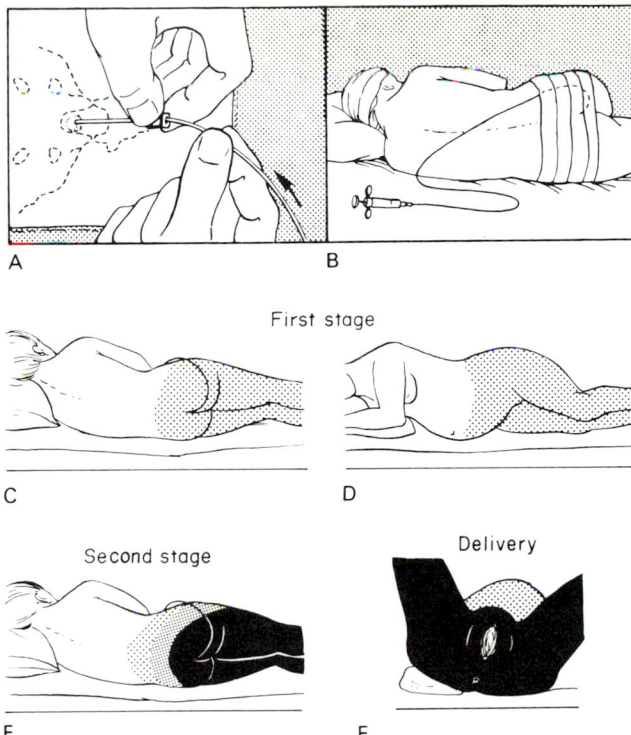

First stage

C   D

Second stage   Delivery

E   F

FIG. 66-26. Technique of continuous caudal analgesia. **A.** A special 18-gauge, thin-walled, 7-cm needle is inserted and advanced 2 cm and its shaft turned 180° so that its bevel faces the roof of the sacral canal. **B.** A plastic epidural catheter is introduced and advanced 8 to 10 cm to place its tip at the level of the S1 to L5 vertebrae. For the first stage (**C, D**) low concentrations of anesthetics are used to produce only analgesia (*light stippling*). **E, F.** After internal rotation of the presenting part, a higher concentration is injected to achieve motor block and perineal relaxation (*black*) and differential block of the T10 to T12 segments (*light stippling*) and of the lumbar segments (*heavy stippling*). From Bonica, J.J.: Obstetric Analgesia and Anesthesia. 2nd Ed. Seattle, University of Washington Press, 1980, p. 110.

It is now generally accepted that epidural analgesia does not prolong, and might even shorten, the duration of the first stage of labor (5–8, 124). Although a transitory decrease in uterine activity has been described, this is of little clinical importance. Unless the technique is carried out precisely and the parturient is coached to bear down effecively, the duration of the second stage of labor might be prolonged and instruments might be needed for delivery. Figure 66-28 and Table 66-2 summarize the technique of standard epidural analgesia and its advantages and disadvantages as compared with other forms of extradural blockade. Figure 66-29 and Table 66-3 summarize the technique of segmental epidural analgesia for the first stage of labor and the extension of this procedure to involve the perineum for the second stage of labor.

The Double-Catheter Technique

The double-catheter technique involves the insertion of one catheter into the lumbar epidural space, with its tip at the level of the T12 vertebra, and another catheter placed into the sacral canal, with its tip at the level of the S3 vertebra (Fig. 66-30 and Table

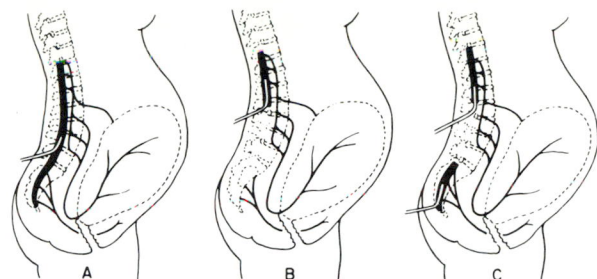

FIG. 66-27. Technique of continuous spinal epidural block. **A.** Standard technique for vaginal delivery (analgesia of T10–S5). **B.** Segmental (T10–L1) block for analgesia during first stage of labor. **C.** Double-catheter technique. (*White tube*, level of catheter; *black area in spinal canal*, diffusion of local anesthetic.) From Bonica, J.J.: Principles and Practice of Obstetric Analgesia and Anesthesia, Vol. 1. Philadelphia, F.A. Davis, 1967, p. 614.

66-4). This technique was first used and advocated by the late John Cleland (125), whose monumental studies of the pathways of uterine pain have already been mentioned. Having had extensive experience with this technique, Bonica believes it to be the ultimate in analgesia and anesthesia for labor and vaginal delivery because it provides all the advantages of regional block with few of its disadvantages. The technique permits exquisitely specific analgesia for the first and second stages of labor and produces anesthesia for the delivery.

The process is accomplished with smaller individual doses and total dose, with the following advantages: (a) hypotension and other side effects and the risk of systemic toxic reactions in the mother are minimized; (b) it causes little or no effect on uterine contractions (because of the smaller doses of local anesthetic); (c) it permits the voluntary use of the abdominal muscles because the analgesic concentrations do not produce motor blockade; (d) although the caudal analgesia interrupts the afferent limb of the reflex urge to bear down, the parturient can voluntarily exert as much increase in intra-abdominal pressure as she does reflexively and, indeed, in some instances, she can bear down more effectively because she has pain relief; and (e) the fetus receives less local anesthetic than with any other extradural technique, and therefore incurs no drug-induced cardiovascular or central nervous system depression. With this or any other extradural technique it is best to insert the catheters once it has been decided that active labor has been established, but before the parturient has experienced severe pain, so that she obtains the full benefits of the analgesia.

Intraspinal Opioids for Labor Pain

Recently both intrathecal and epidural opioids have been used during the first stage of labor to relieve the pain of uterine contractions. To date some two dozen studies on about 3000 parturients have been published. Because many of the studies have been uncontrolled, and have had conflicting results, these techniques are mentioned only briefly here. Only a few references are cited because of space limitations.

TABLE 66-2. Continuous Standard (T10–S5) Epidural Block

Technique	Comparison with Other Extradural Techniques
—Needle puncture at L4 → catheter advanced 3 cm (L3)	**Advantages:**
—Aspiration test and injection of test dose	1. Requires only one puncture and insertion of a catheter
—If negative, 10–12-ml injection of analgesic dose of local anesthetic → analgesia T10–L5	2. Puncture done in lower lumbar area:
—Continuous oxygen and frequent monitoring	a. Less risk of cord damage
—Top-up analgesic doses as soon as slight pain returns	b. Larger space → easier puncture
—Continue analgesia until after internal rotation → 10–12-ml injection of high concentration of local anesthetic (LA) to relax the perineum	3. Provides good analgesia and anesthesia as required
	Disadvantages:
—If perineal analgesia or relaxation deficient → inject with patient in Fowler's position at least 15 minutes prior to delivery	1. Premature numbness of lower limbs during first stage
	2. High concentration produces premature perineal relaxation → interferes with flexion and internal rotation
	3. Eliminates bearing down reflex (but with analgesic dose can push)
	4. Larger doses of drugs required than with segmental or double-catheter technique

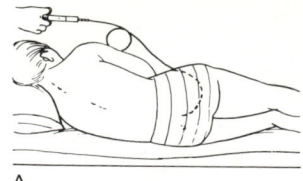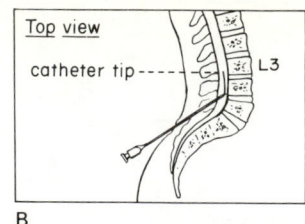

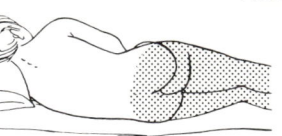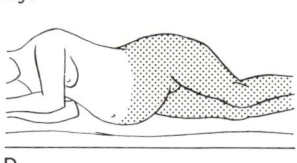

First stage

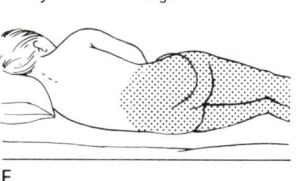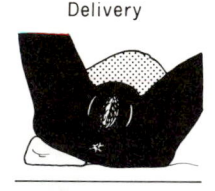

Early second stage   Delivery

FIG. 66-28. The technique of standard continuous lumbar epidural block. A preload infusion of fluid is started. *A, B.* A continuous catheter is then inserted through a needle placed in the L4 interlaminar space and advanced until its tip is at the L3 vertebra. *C.* With the onset of moderate pain a test dose is injected and, if negative, 10 to 12 ml of analgesic concentrations of local anesthetic (ACLA) (e.g., 0.25 bupivacaine) are injected to produce analgesia extending from T10 to S5. *C–E.* The patient is then made to lie on her side and given oxygen and frequent monitoring, top-up analgesia doses are injected as soon as pain returns to produce continuous pain relief. *F.* After flexion and internal rotation of the presenting part has occurred, a higher concentration of LA (0.5% bupivacaine) is injected with the patient in the semirecumbent position to produce perineal relaxation and anesthesia (*black*). A wedge is placed under the right buttock for delivery to displace the uterus toward the left, away from the inferior vena cava. (Table 66-4 summarizes the techniques, advantages, and disadvantages of the procedure.) From Bonica, J.J.: Obstetric Analgesia and Anesthesia. 2nd Ed. Seattle, University of Washington Press, 1980, p. 105.

Intrathecal Opioids

Morphine in doses ranging from 0.5 to 2 mg injected intrathecally has apparently provided fairly good relief from uterine contraction pain, lasting for several hours (126). The onset of analgesia was slow, however, and analgesia during the delivery was poor, requiring supplementary pain relief. The serious disadvantages of the use of intrathecal morphine in labor is the high incidence of adverse side effects, including pruritus, nausea, urinary retention, and respiratory depression (see Chapter 95).

Epidural Opioids

Epidural morphine has been used in doses ranging from 2 to 10 mg (127, 128). Most reports suggest that analgesia was poor, even in the high-dose range, and, in many cases, was ineffective in relieving the pain of uterine contractions (129). Like intrathecal morphine, the onset of analgesia was slow and supplementary analgesia was needed during delivery. Moreover, side effects similar to those seen with intrathecal morphine have been encountered.

Epidural meperidine has been found to produce analgesia within 10 minutes and has been more consistent and reliable than morphine. Both the efficacy and duration of analgesia are dose-dependent: with an injection of 25 mg, analgesia was less reliable than that produced by 0.125% bupivacaine (130) and lasted less than 1 hour (131). Increasing the dose to 50 or 100 mg provided analgesia that was almost equivalent to that obtained with 0.25% bupivacaine for about 2 hours, but these higher doses were associated with a higher incidence of side effects (132).

Epidural fentanyl in doses ranging from 0.15 to 0.20 mg also provided effective analgesia for the pain caused by uterine contractions within 10 minutes, and lasted for 90 to 130 minutes during labor (133). Perineal analgesia was poor and side effects also occurred. The addition of 0.8 mg of fentanyl to a test dose of bupivacaine provided a more rapid and complete onset of analgesia and significantly prolonged the duration of the effect of the local anesthetic (133).

TABLE 66-3. Single-Catheter Continuous Segmental Block

Technique	Comparison with Other Extradural Techniques
—Needle puncture at L3 → catheter advanced 3 cm (L2)	Advantages:
—Aspiration test and injection of test dose	1. Requires less drug than standard technique
—If negative at 5 minutes, inject 5–6 ml of dilute (analgesic) solution of local anesthetic → analgesia T10–L1	2. No effect on uterine contractions
	3. No premature numbness of the limbs
—Continuous oxygen and frequent monitoring	4. No premature perineal relaxation → no interference with flexion or rotation
—Top-up analgesic dose as soon as slight pain returns	5. Less effect of local anesthetic on mother and fetus
—When pain in limbs and perineum inject 10–12 ml of analgesic concentration with patient in Fowler's position	Disadvantages:
	1. Can produce incomplete analgesia or relaxation of perineum
—After internal rotation inject higher concentration to relax perineum	2. Requires Fowler's or sitting-up position

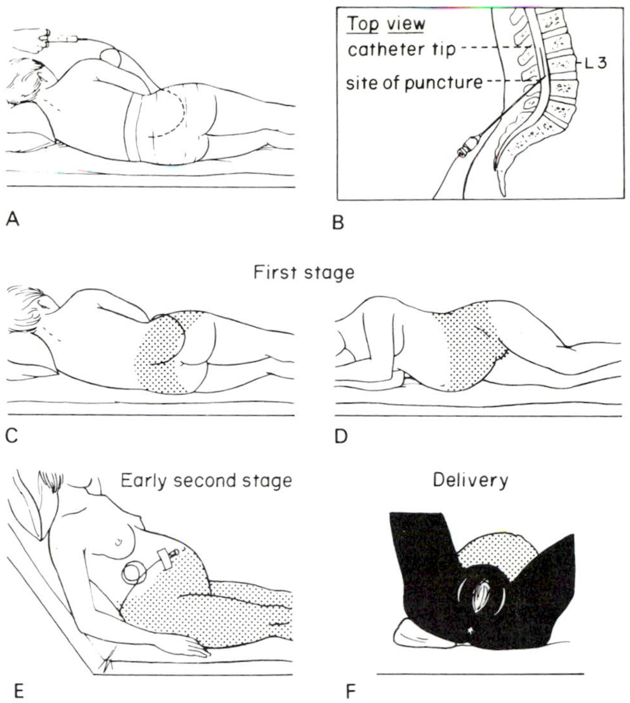

FIG. 66-29. Technique of continuous segmental epidural analgesia and anesthesia. After a preload infusion of fluid is started, a continuous catheter is inserted through a needle placed in the L3 interspace and advanced so that its tip is at L2. *A*, *B*. With the onset of moderate pain a test dose is injected and, if negative, 4 to 6 ml of local analgesic solution is injected to produce segmental analgesia (*C*, *D*). *E*. For the second stage the analgesia is extended to the sacral segments by injecting a larger volume of the same concentration of local anesthetic, with the patient in the semirecumbent position. *F*. After internal rotation an injection is made of a higher concentration of local anesthetic to produce motor block of the sacral segments and thus achieve perineal relaxation and anesthesia (*black*). The wedge under the right buttock causes the uterus to displace to the left. From Bonica, J.J.: Obstetric Analgesia and Anesthesia. 2nd Ed. Seattle, University of Washington Press, 1980, p. 107.

Epidural Opioids and Local Anesthetics

Very recently a number of obstetric anesthesiologists have used a combination of opioids and dilute solutions of local anesthetics (e.g., 0.125% bupivacaine) with significant success. It is likely that this technique will become widely used (see Chapter 95).

Episiotomy Pain

Many obstetricians and midwives carry out an episiotomy incision to facilitate delivery, especially in primiparae, although it is also frequently done in multiparae. Prophylactic episiotomy is done to decrease the duration of the second stage of labor, to protect against tears, and to facilitate the introduction of forceps if their use becomes necessary. The pain caused by this procedure is also transmitted by branches of the pudendal nerve and can be obviated with local infiltration or pudendal block or with other types of regional anesthesia.

In a comprehensive review, Thacker and Banta (134) discussed the benefits and risks of episiotomy in labor and delivery as recorded in the English-language literature (350 books and articles published between 1860 and 1980). They cited the fact that, in 1979, an episiotomy was performed in nearly 63% of vaginal deliveries in the United States. It was determined, however, that episiotomy did not offer a clear benefit to women in terms of decreased number of lacerations. Moreover, in reviewing the extensive literature, it was noted that the role of episiotomy in preventing serious pelvic relaxation has not been adequately studied. In fact, women who did not have an episiotomy had little risk of pelvic relaxation. In regard to the issue of doing an episiotomy to protect the brain of infants, it was noted that it is beneficial in extreme cases, such as when the fetus is large and labor is prolonged (134). The probable benefit, however, does not necessarily mean that most routine episiotomies can be justified. The risks of episiotomy include extension of the episiotomy by tear of tissues, unsatisfactory anatomic results, blood loss, pain, edema, and infection (134). It was concluded that risks of episiotomy are more severe than many obstetricians appreciate. Although rarely associated with a life-threatening problem, complications of this procedure can be a source of serious morbidity to young mothers, who already have major personal and social adjustments to undergo.

One study in Great Britain by Kitzinger and Walters (135) revealed that, among 717 women who had had an episiotomy, 45% stated that the perineum

TABLE 66-4. Double-Catheter Epidural Block

Technique	Comparison with Other Extradural Techniques
—Needle puncture at L2–L1 → catheter advanced 3 cm (T12)	Advantages:
—Needle puncture in sacrum at S4 → advance catheter to S3	1. Requires less drug than standard or single-catheter techniques
—Aspiration test and injection of test dose	2. Most specific technique for labor and delivery
—If negative at 5 minutes, inject 4 to 5 ml analgesic solution of local anesthetic in upper catheter → analgesia T10–L1	3. Least effect on mother and fetus 4. No effects on newborn
—Continuous oxygen and frequent monitoring	5. No premature numbness or weakness of limbs
—Top-up analgesic dose in the upper catheter as soon as uterine pain returns	6. No premature perineal relaxation → no interference with flexion and internal rotation
—With onset of pain in limbs and perineum inject 5 to 7 ml of analgesic solution through caudal catheter → analgesia in limbs and perineum	7. "Rolls Royce" of obstetric analgesia Disadvantages:
—Continue analgesia until after internal rotation → 5 to 7 ml 0.75% bupivacaine or 1.5% etidocaine through lower catheter → profound perineal muscle relaxation	1. Two catheters are required → greater risk of complication and failure 2. (Obviated by skilled anesthetist)

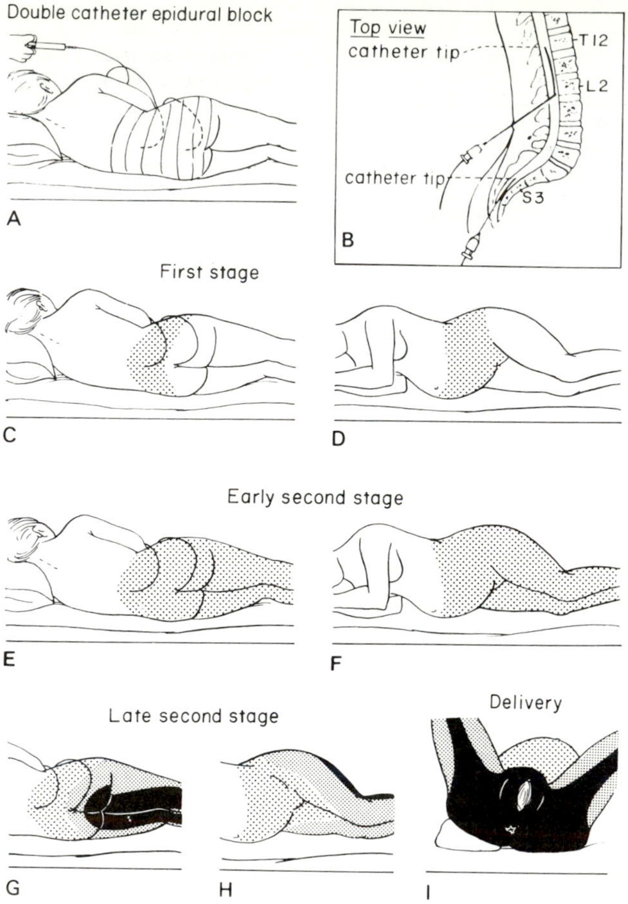

FIG. 66-30. Double-catheter technique for extradural analgesia and anesthesia. *A, B.* The two catheters are inserted: the upper catheter is inserted through the L2 interspace and advanced so that its tip is at T12; the second catheter is inserted into the sacral canal and advanced so that its tip is at S3. C, D. As soon as contractions produce moderate pain, small volumes (4 to 5 ml) of analgesic concentrations of local anesthetic (ACLA) are injected through the upper catheter to relieve the pain. Similar injections are repeated throughout labor. *E, F.* When the presenting part exerts pressure on the pelvic structures and perineum, causing pain in the lower lumbar and sacral segments, 5- to 7-ml volumes of ACLA are injected through the lower catheter. *G–I.* After flexion and internal rotation are completed a high concentration of the local anesthetic is injected through the lower catheter to produce perineal muscle relaxation and anesthesia of the sacral segments (*black*). From Bonica, J.J.: Obstetric Analgesia and Anesthesia. 2nd Ed. Seattle, University of Washington Press, 1980, p. 113.

was moderately uncomfortable at the end of the first week, 19% thought it was painful, and 9% thought it was very painful. The figures among 341 women who had had perineal tears (no episiotomy) were 39, 11, and 4% respectively. Moreover, in 17% of those who had had an episiotomy the pain often distracted them when breast feeding and 22% could not sit comfortably when holding the baby. Many of the women who had had an episiotomy experienced pain during sexual intercourse that persisted for more than 3 months in some. It was also concluded (135) that, although episiotomy might be necessary in special cases (e.g., when it is necessary to hasten delivery), it is not necessary in most women and, when done, causes unnecessary pain for varying periods following delivery.

In one report it was suggested that local infiltration with saline solution before the episiotomy repair decreases the severity of postepisiotomy pain (136). It was postulated that the pain is a result of tight enclosure caused by the edema of inflammation which can be accommodated under less pressure if "slack" is created by prior distension of the tissues. The pain is treated with cold or hot sitz baths. In women who have moderate to severe pain, nonopioid analgesics, given alone or combined with weak opioids, can be used, but care must be exercised in prescribing these or any other drugs in women who are breast feeding. Some studies have shown that an episiotomy is unnecessary, especially when perineal massage etc. is done during labor and delivery (137).

REFERENCES

1. Bonica, J.J.: The nature of pain of parturition. Clin. Obstet. Gynecol., *2*:499, 1975.
2. Bonica, J.J.: Pain of parturition. Clin. Anesthesiol., *4*:1, 1986.
3. Bonica, J.J.: Labour pain. *In* Textbook of Pain. Edited by P.D. Wall and R. Melzack. Edinburgh, Churchill, Livingstone, 1984, pp. 377–392.
4. Bonica, J.J.: Principles and Practice of Obstetric Analgesia and Anesthesia, Vol. 1. Philadelphia, F.A. Davis, 1967.

5. Bonica, J.J.: Principles and Practice of Obstetric Analgesia and Anesthesia, Vol. 2. Philadelphia, F.A. Davis, 1967.
6. Bonica, J.J.: Obstetric Analgesia and Anaesthesia. 2nd Ed. Amsterdam, World Federation of Societies of Anaesthesiologists, 1980.
7. Crawford, J.S.: Principles and Practice of Obstetric Anesthesia. 5th Ed. Oxford, Blackwell Scientic, 1984.
8. Albright, G.A.: Anesthesia and Obstetrics: Maternal, Fetal and Neonatal Aspects. 2nd Ed. Boston, Butterworths, 1986.
9. Shnider, S.M., and Levinson, G.: Anesthesia for Obstetrics. Baltimore, Williams & Wilkins, 1984.
10. Dick-Read, G.: Natural Childbirth. London, William Heinemann, 1933.
11. Dick-Read, G.: Childbirth without Fear. New York, Harper, 1953.
12. Velvovski, I.Z., Chougom, E.A., and Plotitcher, V.A.: The psychoprophylactic and psychotherapeutic method in painless childbirth. Pediatriia, Akusherstvo i Ginekologiia, 1:32, 1950.
13. Ford, C.S.: A Comparative Study of Human Reproduction. Yale University Publications in Anthropology. New Haven, CT, Yale University Press, 1945.
14. Freedman, L.Z., and Ferguson, V.S.: The question of "painless childbirth" in primitive cultures. Am. J. Orthopsychiatry, 20:363, 1950.
15. Jochelson, W.: The Yukaghir and the Youkaghirized Tungus: Vol. XIII of the Memoirs of American Museum of Natural History which constitutes at the same time Vol. IX, Part I, of the Jesup North Pacific expedition. New York and Leiden, Am. Museum of Natural History, 1910.
16. Levy-Strauss, C.: Sorciers et psychanalyse. Geneva, LeCourier de l'Unesco, 1956, pp. 808–810.
17. Englemann, G.J.: Labor among Primitive Peoples. 2nd Ed. St. Louis, J.H. Chambers, 1883.
18. Ellis, E.H.: Ancient Anodynes. Primitive Anesthesia and Allied Conditions. London, William Heinemann, 1946, p. 16.
19. Macht, D.I.: The history of opium and some of its preparations and alkaloids. JAMA, 64:477, 1915.
20. Tainter, M.L.: Pain. Ann. N.Y. Acad. Sci., 51:3, 1948.
21. Claye, A.M.: The Evolution of Obstetric Analgesia. London, Oxford University Press, 1939.
22. Heaton, C.E.: The history of anesthesia and analgesia in obstetrics. J. Hist. Med., 1:567, 1946.
23. Warren, J.C.: Inhalation of aethereal vapor for the prevention of pain in surgical operation. Boston Med. Soc. J., 35:375, 1846.
24. Priestley, W.O., and Storer, H.R.: The Obstetric Memoirs and Contributions of James Y. Simpson, Vol. 2. Edinburgh, A. & C. Black, 1856.
25. Sykes, W.S.: Essays of the First One Hundred Years of Anesthesia, Vol. 1. Edinburgh, E. & S. Livingston, 1960, pp. 77–83.
26. Behan, R.J.: Pain. New York, Appleton, 1914, pp. 738–739.
27. Lamaze, F.: Qu'est-ce que l'Accouchement sans Douleur par la Méthode Psychoprophylactique? Ses Principes, sa Réalisation, ses Résultats. Paris, Savoir et Connaitre, 1956.
28. Lundh, W.: Modraundervisning, Forlossningstraning eller foraldrakunskap? Ph.D. Dissertation, Pedagogiska Institutionen, Stockholms Universitet, 1974.
29. Bundsen, P.: Subjectiva resultat av smartlindring under forlossning-En enkatundersokning. Lakartidningen, 3:129, 1975.
30. Nettelbladt, P., Fagerstrom, C.F., and Uddenberg, N.: The significance of reported childbirth pain. J. Psychol. Res., 20:215, 1976.
31. Javert, C.T., and Hardy, J.D.: Measurement of pain intensity in labour and its physiologic, neurologic and pharmacologic implications. Am. J. Obstet. Gynecol., 60:552, 1950.
32. Melzack, R., et al.: Labour is still painful after prepared childbirth training. Can. Med. Assoc. J., 125:357, 1981.
33. Melzack, R., et al.: Severity of labour pain: Influence of physical as well as psychological variables. Can. Med. Assoc. J., 130:579, 1984.
34. Melzack, R.: The myth of painless childbirth (the John J. Bonica Lecture). Pain, 19:321, 1984.
35. Melzack, R.: The McGill pain questionnaire: Major properties and scoring methods. Pain, 1:277, 1975.
36. Ueland, K., and Hansen, J.M.: Maternal cardiovascular dynamics, II. Posture and uterine contractions. Am. J. Obstet. Gynecol., 103:1, 1969.
37. Holmes, F.: Incidence of the supine hypotensive syndrome in late pregnancy. J. Obstet. Gynaecol. [Br.], 67:254, 1960.
38. Adams, J.Q., and Alexander, A.M.: Alterations in cardiovascular physiology during labor. Obstet. Gynecol., 12:542, 1958.
39. Hansen, J.M., and Ueland, K.: The influence of caudal analgesia on cardiovascular dynamics during normal labor and delivery. Acta Anaesthesiol. Scand. 23(Suppl. 10):449, 1966.
40. Lees, M.M., Scott, D.B., and Kerr, M.G.: Haemodynamic changes associated with labour. J. Obstet. Gynaecol. [Br.], 77:29, 1970.
41. Hendricks, C.H., and Quilligan, E.J.: Cardiac output during labour. Am. J. Obstet. Gynecol. 71:953, 1956.
42. Cugell, D.W.: Pulmonary function in pregnancy: Serial observations in normal women. Am. Rev. Tuberc., 67:568, 1953.
43. Russell, I.F., and Chambers, W.A.: Closing volume in normal pregnancy. Br. J. Anaesth., 53:1043, 1981.
44. Cole, P.V., and Nainby-Luxmoore, R.C.: Respiratory volumes in labour. Br. Med. J., 1:1118, 1962.
45. Bonica, J.J.: Maternal respiratory changes during pregnancy and parturition. In Parturition and Perinatology. Clinical Anesthesia Series, Vol. 10, No. 2. Edited by G.F. Marx. Philadelphia, F.A. Davis, 1973, pp. 9–21.
46. Pearson, J.F., and Davies, P.: The effect of continuous lumbar epidural analgesia on the acid-base status of maternal arterial blood during the first stage of labour. J. Obstet. Gynaecol. [Br.], 80:218, 1973.
47. Pearson, J.F., and Davies, P.: The effect of continuous lumbar epidural analgesia on maternal acid-base balance and arterial lactate concentration during the second stage of labour. J. Obstet. Gynaecol. [Br.], 80:225, 1973.
48. Marx, G.F., et al.: Effect of pain relief on arterial blood gas values during labor. N.Y. J. Med., 69:819, 1969.
49. Peabody, J.L.: Transcutaneous oxygen measurement to evaluate drug effect. Clin. Perinatol., 6:109, 1979.
50. Huch, A., et al.: Continuous transcutaneous monitoring of foetal oxygen tension during labour. Br. J. Obstet. Gynecol., 84(Suppl. 1):1, 1977.
51. Morishima, H.O., Pedersen, H., and Finster, M.: The influence of maternal psychological stress on the fetus. Am. J. Obstet. Gynecol., 134:286, 1978.
52. Shnider, S.M., et al.: Uterine blood flow and plasma norepinephrine changes during maternal stress in the pregnant ewe. Anesthesiology, 50:524, 1979.
53. Joupplila, R., and Hollmen, A.: The effect of segmental epidural analgesia on maternal and foetal acid-base balance, lactate, serum potassium and creatine phosphokinase during labour. Acta Anaesthesiol. Scand., 20:259, 1976.
54. Lederman, R.P., et al.: Endogenous plasma epinephrine and norepinephrine in last-trimester pregnancy and labour. Am. J. Obstet. Gynecol., 129:5, 1977.
55. Lederman, R.P., et al.: The relationship of maternal anxiety, plasma catecholamines, and plasma cortisol to progress in labour. Am. J. Obstet. Gynecol., 132:495, 1978.
56. Falconer, A.D., and Powles, A.B.: Plasma noradrenaline levels during labour. Anesthesiology, 37:416, 1982.
57. Ohno, H., et al.: Maternal plasma concentrations of catecholamines and cyclic nucleotides during labor and following delivery. Res. Commun. Chem. Pathol. Pharmacol., 51:183, 1986.
58. Csontos, K., Rust, M., and Hollt, V.: The role of endorphins during parturition. Rockville, MD, National Institute of Drug Abuse Research, Monograph Series, 1980, pp. 264–271.
59. Goland, R.S., et al.: Human plasma beta-endorphin during pregnancy, labour and delivery. J. Clin. Endocrinol. Metabol., 52:74, 1981.
60. Abbound, T.K., et al.: Effects of epidural anesthesia during labor on maternal plasma beta-endorphin levels. Anesthesiology, 59:1, 1983.
61. Browning, A.J., et al.: Maternal and cord plasma concentrations of beta-lipotrophin, beta-endorphin and γ-lipotrophin at delivery: Effect of analgesia. Br. J. Obstet. Gynaecol., 90:1152, 1983.
62. Fettes, I., et al.: Plasma levels of immunoreactive beta-endorphin and adrenocorticotropic hormone during labor and delivery. Obstet. Gynecol., 64:359, 1984.
63. Goebelsmann, U., et al.: Beta-endorphin in pregnancy. Eur. J. Obstet. Gynecol. Reprod. Biol., 17:77, 1984.
64. Gintzler, A.R.: Endorphin-mediated increases in pain threshold during pregnancy. Science, 210:913, 1980.
65. Foley, K.M., et al.: β-endorphin: Analgesic and hormonal effects in humans. Proc. Natl. Acad. Sci. USA, 76:5377, 1979.

66. Sepgupta, P., and Nielsen, M.: The effect of labour and epidural analgesia on pain threshold. Anaesthesia, 39:982, 1984.
67. Buchan, P.C.: Emotional stress in childbirth and its modification by variations in obstetric management—epidural analgesia and stress in labor. Acta. Obstet. Gynecol. Scand., 59:319, 1980.
68. Marx, G.F., and Greene, N.M.: Maternal lactate, pyruvate and excess lactate production during labour and delivery. Am. J. Obstet. Gynecol., 90:786, 1964.
69. Hayes, J.R., et al.: Stimulation of gastrin release by catecholamines. Lancet, 1:1, 1972.
70. Holdsworth, J.D.: Relationships between stomach contents and analgesia in labour. Br. J. Anaesth., 50:1145, 1978.
71. Nimmo, W.S., Wilson, J., and Prescott, L.F.: Narcotic analgesics and delayed gastric emptying during labour. Lancet, 1:890, 1975.
72. Kartchner, F.D.: A study of the emotional reactions during labour. Am. J. Obstet. Gynecol., 60:19, 1950.
73. Rogers, F.S.: Dangers of the Read method in patients with major personality problems. Am. J. Obstet. Gynecol., 71:1236, 1956.
74. Cheetham, R.W., and Rzadkowolski, A.: Psychiatric aspects of labour and the puerperium. S. Afr. Med. J., 58:814, 1980.
75. Stewart, D.E., Psychiatric symptoms following attempted natural childbirth. Can. Med. Assoc. J., 127:713, 1982.
76. Morishima, H.O., Pedersen, H., and Finster, M.: Effects of pain on mother, labour and fetus, In Obstetric Analgesia and Anaesthesia. Edited by G.F. Marx and G.M. Bassell. Amsterdam, Elsevier North Holland, 1980, pp. 197–210.
77. Bonica, J.J., and Hunter, C.A., Jr.: Management in dysfunction of the forces of labor. In Principles of Obstetric Analgesia and Anesthesia, Vol. 2. Philadelphia, F.A. Davis, 1969, pp. 1188–1208.
78. Motoyama, E.K., et al.: The effects of changes in maternal pH and P_{CO_2} on the P_{O_2} of fetal lambs. Anesthesiology, 28:891, 1967.
79. Assali, N.S., Holm, I.W., and Sehgal, N.: Hemodynamic changes in foetal lamb in utero in response to asphyxia, hypoxia and hypercapnia. Circ. Res., 11:423, 1962.
80. Cohn, H.E., et al.: Cardiovascular responses to hypoxemia and acidemia in foetal lambs. Am. J. Obstet. Gynecol., 120:817, 1974.
81. Beard, R.W., Morris, E.D., and Clayton, S.G.: pH of foetal capillary blood as an indication of the conditions of foetus. J. Obstet. Gynaecol. [Br.], 74:812, 1967.
82. Shnider, S.M., et al.: Maternal catecholamines decrease during labor after lumbar epidural anesthesia. Am. J. Obstet. Gynecol., 147:13, 1983.
83. Raisanen, I., et al.: Beta-endorphin in maternal and umbilical cord plasma at elective cesarean section and in spontaneous labor. Obstet. Gynecol., 67:384, 1986.
84. Westgren, M., Lindahl, S.G.E., and Norden, N.E.: Maternal and fetal endocrine stress response at vaginal delivery with and without an epidural block. J. Perinat. Med., 14:235, 1986.
85. Neumark, J., Hammerle, A.F., and Biegelmayer, C.: Effects of epidural analgesia on plasma catecholamines and cortisol in parturition. Acta Anaesthesiol. Scand., 29:555, 1985.
86. Abboud, T.K., et al.: Effects of spinal anesthesia on maternal circulating catecholamines. Am. J. Obstet. Gynecol., 142:252, 1982.
87. Abboud, T.K., et al.: Effect of epidural analgesia during labor on fetal plasma catecholamine release. Reg. Anaesth., 10:170, 1985.
88. Bonica, J.J., and Ueland, K.: Heart disease. In Principles and Practice of Obstetric Analgesia and Anaesthesia, Vol. 2. Edited by J.J. Bonica. Philadelphia, F.A. Davis, 1969, pp. 941–977.
89. Sorenson, M.B., et al.: The use of epidural analgesia for delivery in a patient with pulmonary hypertension. Acta Anaesthesiol. Scand., 26:180, 1982.
90. Pearson, J.F., and Davies, P.: The effect of continuous lumbar epidural analgesia upon fetal acid-base status during the first stage of labour. J. Obstet. Gynaecol. [Br.], 81:971, 1974.
91. Pearson, J.F., and Davies, P.: The effect of continuous lumbar epidural analgesia upon fetal acid-base status of maternal arterial blood during the first stage of labour. J. Obstet. Gynaecol. [Br.], 81:975, 1974.
92. Thalme, B., Belfrage, P., and Raabe, N.: Lumbar epidural analgesia in labour. Acta Obstet. Gynaecol. Scand., 53:27, 1974.
93. Thalme, B., Raabe, N., and Belfrage, P.: Lumbar epidural analgesia in labour. Acta Obstet. Gynaecol. Scand., 53:113, 1974.
94. Zador, G., et al.: Low dose intermittent epidural anaesthesia with lidocaine for vaginal delivery. Acta Obstet. Gynaecol. Scand. 34(Suppl.):17, 1974.
95. Moir, D.D., and Willocks, J.: Management of incoordinate uterine action under continuous epidural analgesia. Br. Med. J., 3:396, 1967.
96. Janisch, H., et al.: Der Einfluss der kontinuierlichen Epiduralanaesthesia auf die uteroplazentare Durchblutung. Z. Gerburtshilfe Perinatol., 182:343, 1978.
97. Jouppila, P., et al.: Lumbar epidural analgesia to improve intervillous blood flow during labour in severe pre-eclampsia. Obstet. Gynecol., 59:158, 1982.
98. Reynolds, S.R.M.: Physiology of the Uterus. 2nd Ed. New York, Paul B. Hoeber, 1949.
99. Moir, C.: The nature of the pain of labour. J. Obstet. Gynaecol. [Br.], 46:409, 1939.
100. Hurst, A.F.: The Sensibility of the Alimentary Canal. Oxford, Oxford University Press, 1911.
101. Caldeyro-Barcia, R., and Poseiro, J.J.: Physiology of the uterine contraction. Clin. Obstet. Gynaecol., 3:386, 1960.
102. Paul, W.M., et al.: Clinical tone and pain threshold. Am. J. Obstet. Gynecol., 7:510, 1956.
103. Lees, M.H., et al.: Maternal placental and myometrial blood flow of the rhesus monkey during uterine contractions. Am. J. Obstet. Gynecol., 110:68, 1971.
104. Novey, M.J.: The effect of sustained uterine contractions on myometrial and placental blood flow in the rhesus monkey. In Respiratory Gas Exchange and Blood Flow in the Placenta. Edited by L.D. Longo and H. Bartels. Bethesda, MD, Department of Health, Education and Welfare, 1972, Publ. No. (NIH)7–361, pp. 143–152.
105. Danforth, D.N.: Distribution and functional significance of the cervical musculature. Am. J. Obstet. Gynecol., 68:1261, 1954.
106. Head, H.: On disturbances of sensation with special reference to the pain of visceral disease. Brain, 16:1, 1893.
107. Cleland, J.G.P.: Paravertebral anaesthesia in obstetrics. Surg. Gynaecol. Obstet., 57:51, 1933.
108. Bonica, J.J.: The nature of pain in parturition. Clin. Obstet. Gynaecol., 2:499, 1975.
109. Williams, P.L., and Warwick, R. (eds.): Gray's Anatomy. 36th Ed. Philadelphia, W.B. Saunders, 1980, pp. 1319–1324.
110. Clemente, C.D. (ed.): Gray's Anatomy of the Human Body. 30th Ed. Philadelphia, Lea & Febiger, 1985.
111. Pritchard, J.A., MacDonald, P.C., and Gant, N.F. (eds.): Williams Obstetrics. 17th Ed. Norwalk, CT, Appleton-Century-Crofts, 1985.
112. Greenhill, J.P.: Obstetrics. 13th Ed. Philadelphia, W.B. Saunders, 1965, pp. 379–427.
113. Klink, E.W.: Perineal nerve block, an anatomic and clinical study in the female. Obstet. Gynecol., 1:137, 1953.
114. Deutsch, H.: Psychology of pregnancy, labour and puerperium. In Obstetrics. 11th Ed. Edited by J.P. Greenhill. Philadelphia, W.B. Saunders, 1955, pp. 349–360.
115. Wolff, B.B., and Langley, S.: Cultural factors and the response to pain: A review. In Pain: Clinical and Experimental Perspectives. Edited by M. Weisenberg. St. Louis, C.V. Mosby, 1975, pp. 144–151.
116. True, R.M.: Obstetrical hypnoanalgesia. Am. J. Obstet. Gynecol., 67:373, 1953.
117. Meehan, J.P., Stoll, A.M., and Hardy, J.D.: Cutaneous pain threshold in Native Alaskan Indians and Eskimos. J. Appl. Physiol., 6:397, 1954.
118. Preissman, A.B., and Ogoulbostan-Essenova: Some details of psychoprophylactic preparation for childbirth in the Turkomenian. S.S.R. Kieve Congress, 90:66, 1956.
119. Winsberg, B., and Greenlick, M.: Pain response in Negro and white obstetrical patients. J. Health Soc. Behav., 8:222, 1967.
120. Hughey, M.J., McElin, T.W., and Young, T.: Maternal and fetal outcome of Lamaze-prepared patients. Obstet. Gynecol., 51:643, 1978.
121. Davenport-Slack, B., and Boylan, C.H.: Psychological correlates of childbirth pain. Psychosom. Med., 36:215, 1974.
122. Scott, J.R., and Rose, N.B.: Effect of psychoprophylaxis (Lamaze preparation) on labor and delivery in primiparas. N. Engl. J. Med., 294:1205, 1976.

123. Bonica, J.J.: Acupuncture anesthesia in the Peoples' Republic of China: Implications for American medicine. JAMA, *229*:1317, 1974.
124. Crawford, J.S.: The second thousand epidural blocks in an obstetric hospital practice. Br. J. Anaesth., *44*:1277, 1972.
125. Cleland, J.G.P.: Continuous peridural and caudal analgesia and obstetrics. Curr. Res. Anesth. Analg., *28*:61, 1949.
126. Abboud, T.K., et al.: Intrathecal administration of hyperbaric morphine for the relief of pain in labour. Br. J. Anaesth., *56*:1351, 1984.
127. Crawford, J.S.: Experiences with epidural morphine in obstetrics. Anesthesiology, *36*:207, 1981.
128. Husemeyer, R.P., O'Connor, M.C., and Davenport, H.T.: Failure of epidural morphine to relieve pain in labour. Anesthesiology, *35*:161, 1980.
129. Nybell-Lindahl, G., et al.: Maternal and fetal concentrations of morphine after epidural administration during labor. Am. J. Obstet. Gynecol., *139*:20, 1981.
130. Hammonds, W., et al.: A comparison of epidural meperidine and bupivacaine for relief of labor pain. Anesth. Analg., *61*:187, 1982.
131. Perris, B.W.: Epidural pethidine in labour: A study of dose requirements. Anesthesiology, *35*:380, 1980.
132. Baraka, A., Maktabi, M., and Noueihid, R.: Epidural meperidine-bupivacaine for obstetric analgesia. Anesth. Analg., *61*:652, 1982.
133. Youngstrom, P., et al.: Epidural fentanyl and bupivacaine in labor: Double-blind study (Abstr.). Anesthesiology, *61*:414, 1984.
134. Thacker, S.B., and Banta, H.D.: Benefits and risks of episiotomy: An interpretative review of the English language literature, 1860–1980. Obstet. Gynecol. Survey *38*:322, 1983.
135. Kitzinger, S., and Walters, R.: Some women's experiences of episiotomy. London, National Childbirth Trust, 1981.
136. Khan, G.Q., and Lilford, R.J.: Wound pain may be reduced by prior infiltration of the episiotomy site after delivery under epidural analgesia. *94*:341, 1987.
137. Kitzinger, S., and Simkin, P. (eds.): Episiotomy and the Second Stage of Labor. Seattle, Pennypress, 1984.

67 · GYNECOLOGIC PAIN

GAY M. GUZINSKI

with contributions by

JOHN J. BONICA *and* JOHN S. MCDONALD

PAIN is one of the most frequent complaints brought by patients to the gynecologist for evaluation. Patients with acute pain might be slightly dysfunctional or, at the other end of the spectrum, severely handicapped physically and emotionally, with survival depending on proper diagnosis and prompt therapy. Episodic pain can make it impossible for patients to perform their normal activities at work, at home, or at school; chronic pain can force some to focus their entire lives on this problem. Extrapolation of data from the National Center for Health Statistics (NCHS) (1, 2) suggests that in the United States painful disorders of gynecologic origin afflicted 11 million women in 1986 and caused 700 million days of bed disability and over 60 million days of work lost. Moreover, in 1986, 3.0 million gynecologic operations and 4.7 million obstetric procedures were performed, most of which had pain as a prominent symptom. The total cost to the American people has been estimated to be over $15 billion. Data on the most frequent causes of painful gynecologic disorders are presented in the discussion of each condition.

This chapter discusses the causes, pathophysiology, mechanisms, symptoms and signs, diagnosis, and treatment of gynecologic pain, which can be acute, recurrent, or chronic. The material is presented in three sections: A, Acute Pain; B, Recurrent Pain; and C, Chronic Pain. More detailed information on each subject can be found in specialized gynecologic textbooks (3–7).

A. ACUTE PAIN

A number of conditions of obstetric and gynecologic origin can cause acute pain, including the following:

a. Normal pregnancy: early pregnancy—growth of uterus and corpus luteum; late pregnancy—stretch of round ligament, premature labor
b. Complications of pregnancy: abortion; ectopic pregnancy; degenerating fibroid
c. Infection: endometritis; pelvic inflammatory disease (PID)
d. Adnexal disorders: torsion of the adnexa; bleeding from adnexal pathology; neoplasia
e. Coexisting nongynecologic visceral disease: appendicitis; pyelitis and pyelonephritis; diverticulitis; ureteral stone; cystitis
f. Disease or trauma to vulva and vagina: infection; trauma; allergic reactions

In general, these problems relate to normal or abnormal pregnancy, infection, mechanical disorders, or neoplasia. Coexisting nongynecologic pathologic conditions can also cause acute pain that simulates that of gynecologic origin. Acute pain usually has a rapid or sudden onset and rapid remission once the underlying condition has been treated.

Normal Pregnancy

Etiology and Pathophysiology

Several conditions can cause pain early in normal pregnancy. Abdominal and pelvic pain can occur early in normal intrauterine pregnancy as the uterus gradually enlarges and growth of the corpus luteum of pregnancy distends the ovary.

Mild to moderate lower abdominal pain in the second trimester of normal pregnancy can result from *stretch-ing of the round ligament* as the uterine fundus grows out of the pelvis into the abdominal cavity.

Pain that is crampy and regular in the second or third trimester can signal the onset of labor. Such pain is caused by contraction of the uterine muscles and by the gradual dilatation and effacement of the cervix (Chapter 66).

Symptoms and Signs

The patient experiencing painful uterine enlargement from a normal pregnancy can complain of a dull suprapubic ache that is usually present during waking hours. Pain from an enlarging corpus luteum is also dull and constant but is localized to one side in the lower abdomen.

Pain of the uterine round ligament is generally dull and bilateral, occurring along the course of this structure from the cornu to its insertion in the labium majus. Movement from side to side can relieve pain on one side but increase it on the other side as one ligament and then the other is stretched by movement of the uterus.

The pain of premature labor is usually similar to that of menstrual cramps and begins in the uterine fundus. Pain descends towards the cervix, producing discomfort deep in the pelvis or even in the rectum. Low back pain, vaginal bleeding, or even rupture of the fetal membranes can also occur.

Physical examination reveals the presence of an enlarged, soft, tender uterus. The uterine round ligament that is causing the pain can also be palpated.

Diagnosis

The clinician must know if the patient is pregnant to diagnose any of the above mentioned pregnancy-related conditions. The classic symptoms of amenorrhea, breast enlargement and tenderness, morning nausea, urinary frequency, weight gain, and fatigue can be present totally or in part. If the diagnosis of pregnancy is in question, a test specific for human chorionic gonadotropin (hCG) is indicated. The hCG test is usually performed on a daily basis (and sometimes on an emergency basis) in most laboratories. In one study early uterine pregnancies were usually associated with an increase in the hCG level of 66% over 48 hours; also, in a normal pregnancy, a level above 6500 mIU/ml was most always associated with a normal intrauterine gestational sac (8). Decreased or increased hCG levels suggest an abnormal gestation, such as a blighted ovum or ectopic pregnancy.

Ultrasonography of the pelvic organs can also be used to determine the presence or absence of an intrauterine gestational sac as early as 5 or 6 weeks. Ultrasound can also be used to elucidate the corpus luteum of pregnancy and to detect uterine myomata and fluid in the cul-de-sac. This information, however, should always be evaluated in light of the clinical picture.

Laboratory studies such as determination of hematocrit and hemoglobin level can be useful in assessing whether bleeding has occurred, provided the results are correlated with the clinical picture and past history. Because the white blood cell count varies considerably during pregnancy, other signs (cultures and direct examination of body fluids) should be sought to corroborate infection.

In a late normally progressing pregnancy, the differential diagnosis of acute pain necessarily focuses on causes of pain other than pregnancy itself.

Treatment

The treatment of pain caused by a normal pregnancy with uterine enlargement or a corpus luteum of pregnancy is simply reassurance and careful follow-up as long as the corpus luteum is intact. Rupture of the corpus luteum can necessitate laparoscopy, exploratory surgery, or both to stop the bleeding.

The pregnant patient with uterine round ligament pain, which is usually mild and episodic, can sometimes gain relief from changes in position, administration of appropriate analgesics, and reassurance.

Premature labor pain should be recognized and managed by those on the high-risk obstetric team. If circumstances warrant, tocolytic agents such as ritodrine hydrochloride should be used to suppress uterine activity. The patient might need initial parenteral treatment, followed by maintenance on oral medication. The pain of preterm labor is usually managed effectively by this class of agents; narcotic medication is neither necessary nor desirable.

Complications of Pregnancy

Ectopic Pregnancy

Etiology and Pathophysiology

Another cause of pain in early pregnancy is abnormal or ectopic pregnancy, in which the conceptus implants itself outside the uterine cavity—for example, in the uterine cornu, along the uterine tube, in the

ovary, or on the abdominal and pelvic peritoneum. In 98% of cases the ectopic pregnancy is a tubal pregnancy and occurs whenever the migration of the fertilized ovum toward the uterine cavity is unduly delayed, either by extrinsic or intrinsic tubal factors. It has an incidence of about 1 in 200 pregnancies; its frequency seems to have increased recently, probably as a result of the increasing incidence of acute salpingitis (9).

Ectopic pregnancy in the cornu, uterine tube, or ovary is painful because these structures and their visceral peritoneum are stretched and distended. Later, when rupture occurs, pain is largely caused by blood in the peritoneal cavity. Similarly, severe pain in the first trimester often indicates an acute abdomen and anemia, which necessitate surgery. Surgery confirms the diagnosis of ectopic pregnancy with implantation at some point outside the uterine cavity.

Symptoms and Signs

Pelvic pain is the most common presenting symptom of ectopic pregnancy (10). At first, pain is limited to the site of implantation and probably represents stretching of the visceral peritoneum over the organ involved. If hemorrhage occurs, however, and is contained within the ectopic site, pain increases and becomes less limited. Once the trophoblast grows through the supporting organ, hemorrhage occurs into the peritoneal cavity. The accompanying pain is initially localized deep in the pelvis as blood collects in the cul-de-sac (pouch of Douglas). If the patient is supine and blood runs upward along the lateral border of the peritoneal cavity, irritation of the diaphragm can cause intense bilateral shoulder pain.

In addition to the pain, the patient can feel faint; physical examination will reveal that the patient is pale and manifests other signs of hypovolemic shock. Evidence of abdominal distension and tenderness on palpation is also found, especially over the iliac fossa where the pain starts. Pelvic examination is difficult because of the tenderness of the abdomen, the disease adnexum, and the pouch of Douglas. Usually a bulging posterior cul-de-sac can be palpated.

Diagnosis

Early recognition of ectopic pregnancy is imperative because it is a significant cause of maternal mortality (11). Usually the diagnosis is not difficult and is made through the history, physical examination, and laboratory studies. Aspiration of the bulging posterior cul-de-sac through a large needle yields nonclotting blood—that is, blood that has already clotted and lysed. As previously mentioned, decreased and increased hCG levels suggest an abnormal gestation, such as ectopic pregnancy. Although ultrasonography is less accurate in identifying extrauterine gestation than intrauterine pregnancy, an experienced sonographer can provide helpful information regarding this condition.

Because pain in early pregnancy can be caused by either a normal or abnormal gestation, the clinician should attempt to make this distinction based on history, physical findings, and appropriate laboratory studies (see above). Signs of shock indicate intraperitoneal or vaginal blood loss.

Treatment

Treatment of ectopic pregnancy pain involves a correct diagnosis and a surgical procedure appropriate to the individual patient and the operative findings. Current conservative surgical therapy includes opening the tube and removing the conceptus or simply excising the conceptus and rejoining the tube to retain the reproductive abilities of the patient (9). The surgeon must be fully aware of the patient's desires regarding this matter before operating because, even in a patient with a ruptured uterine tube, some portion of the organ might be salvageable. Removal of the conceptus, regardless of its location, usually eliminates the pain. Postoperative pain can be controlled with administration of narcotics (e.g., intermittent injection, patient-controlled anesthesia, or lumbar epidural opioid analgesia).

Abortion

Spontaneous abortion is associated with pain caused by uterine muscle contractions and by attempts to expel the conceptus from the endometrial cavity.

Symptoms and Signs

Spontaneous abortion usually produces intermittent menstrual-like cramping pain that is mild initially but gradually increases in intensity. Later, vaginal bleeding, which can be profuse, and passage of placental tissue from the vagina accompany the cramps.

In *septic abortion* signs of infection are also present, such as fever, occasional chills, a purulent discharge, and tenderness of the uterus. When the infection spreads to the adnexa and pelvic peritoneum, signs of peritoneal inflammation appear, including nausea, constipation, reflex muscle spasm, and even signs of septicemia.

Diagnosis

Diagnosis is made by the history and physical findings. A patient with septic abortion reveals laboratory signs of infection. Ultrasonography can be used to reveal a fragmental gestational sac, a low implantation of the sac, and absence of fetal heart movements. Radioimmunoassay for luteinizing hormone (LH)-hCG is positive, denoting the presence of functional placental tissue.

Treatment

A patient with a threatened abortion, a closed os, no passage of tissue, and vaginal bleeding needs close observation but no immediate intervention. Pain usually stops once the threat of abortion passes, the abortus is passed, or pregnancy is terminated surgically (usually by dilatation and curettage). In the instance of a threatened abortion the patient's pain and bleeding increase until she completely passes all tissue, which terminates the gestation, or until dilatation and curettage. The pain subsides once this process is complete, although uterine cramps can persist if an oxytocic agent is administered after the procedure to keep the uterus well contracted.

Degeneration of a Fibroid

During pregnancy, estrogen secretion by the placenta causes uterine myomata "fibroids" to enlarge, often without a concomitant increase in blood supply. Consequently an aseptic degeneration within the tumor can occur.

Symptoms and Signs

Aseptic degeneration of a myoma causes pain that is localized at the site of the tumor. Initially the discomfort is a dull constant ache, but it usually progresses to an intense unremitting pain that prevents the patient from all activity, including sleep. The location of the pain depends on the location of the fibroid. The tumor is usually tender on palpation, possibly accompanied by slight fever and a moderate leukocytosis.

Diagnosis and Treatment

The diagnosis is usually made through careful evaluation of the pain and its location and by physical examination. Because the pain is usually unremitting until degeneration is complete, administration of narcotics such as morphine might be necessary to relieve the pain. Analgesia and bed rest are continued until the pain ceases.

Coexisting Nongynecologic Visceral Disease

A number of coexisting visceral diseases can occur during pregnancy and cause pain. Although these conditions are discussed in detail elsewhere in this book, they are mentioned here for the sake of completeness.

Etiology and Pathophysiology

Inflammation of the appendix and surrounding structures produces the pain of appendicitis. Spasms of the bowel from acute infection or a chronic bowel disorder produce generalized crampy abdominal discomfort. The pain of acute pyelitis stems from accumulation of the products of infection in and around the kidney. Passage of a kidney stone is extremely painful because the stone obstructs the ureter while passing from kidney to bladder. In acute cystitis pain results from infection and irritation of the bladder and of the urethral mucosa and musculature.

Symptoms and Signs

Although the pain of appendicitis can present as it usually does—at McBurney's point—early in pregnancy, the growing uterus can lift the appendix out of the pelvis and thus cause pain that is much higher and more lateral in the abdomen.

Pyelonephritis presents initially as mild and continuous unilateral or bilateral flank pain. In pregnancy this flank pain can progress rapidly to severe back and abdominopelvic pain. High fevers and abnormally high white blood cell counts occur early in the course of pyelonephritis. Casts and bacteria are seen in the urine. Patients complain of a feeling of general malaise and lassitude.

The pain of a ureteral stone is intense and colicky from the onset and can be localized unilaterally anywhere along the course of the affected ureter. Low-grade fever can be present.

Cystitis produces mild to intense suprapubic discomfort that is accompanied by intense pain in the urethra and lower pelvis after voiding. The frequency of urination increases, little urine is passed, and nocturia can occur.

Diagnosis

Diagnosis of these various visceral conditions has been discussed in detail (Part IV, Section D). To differentiate these from other acute painful conditions it is necessary to elicit a good history, perform a comprehensive physical examination, and carry out appropriate laboratory studies, as already mentioned.

Treatment

Treatment of appendicitis in pregnancy can be conservative or surgical. It is best managed jointly by the obstetrician and general surgeon. In acute appendicitis surgery is the most reliable way to relieve pain. Chronic appendicitis can require the use of narcotics for relief of the pain.

The pain of pyelonephritis in pregnancy can be severe. Once appropriate antibiotic therapy has been instituted, pain usually subsides within 24 to 48 hours. The pain of a ureteral stone usually requires narcotic analgesics while the stone is being passed, after which time pain usually subsides promptly. Severe pain caused by a ureteral stone is best managed with segmental epidural analgesia achieved with a dilute solution of a local anesthetic (Chapter 94) or with an opioid (epidural opiate analgesia is discussed in Chapter 95).

Cystitis can be treated by sulfisoxazole in doses of 8 g initially, followed by 4 g daily by mouth for 10 days in the nonpregnant patient, or by ampicillin in doses of 2 g by mouth daily for 10 days in the pregnant patient. The pain itself might require phenazopyridine in doses of 100 mg by mouth tid for 2 or 3 days until irritation of the bladder lining subsides.

Any treatment given during pregnancy should be instituted under supervision of the patient's obstetrician to ensure that both mother and fetus are in optimal condition.

Infections

Acute Endometritis

Etiology and Pathophysiology

Acute endometritis is distinguished from pelvic inflammatory disease (PID) because the former involves only the uterus. Endometritis (infection of the uterus) results when bacteria invade the uterus and multiply. The pain of acute endometritis is caused by multiplication of infecting organisms and accumulation of the products of infection.

Ordinarily, the cervix presents an impenetrable barrier to invasive organisms. When the cervix has been breached by surgical instrumentation (e.g., as in dilatation and curettage) or the passage of a pregnancy (spontaneous abortion or a term pregnancy), however, the uterus is open to colonization by organisms. The offending organism can be one of the normal vaginal flora or can be a more virulent organism introduced by sexual activity, such as Neisseria gonorrhoeae, Chlamydia trachomatis, or Bacteroides. A pregnant uterus most often becomes infected after attempted evacuation of a failed pregnancy.

Symptoms and Signs

The initial symptoms are lower abdominal pain centrally located over the pubic symphysis. The pain can become crampy in nature, accompanied by foul-smelling vaginal discharge or vaginal bleeding. Urinary frequency can occur as the bladder becomes irritated, and a low-grade fever might be present.

In endometritis pain occurs on manipulation of the uterus during the vaginal examination and is confined to the uterus; the adnexal areas are relatively free of pain.

Diagnosis

A recent pregnancy or uterine instrumentation combined with the appropriate symptoms and signs are the bases for the diagnosis of endometritis. Visualization of the cervix with culture of the exudate, particularly for organisms causing sexually transmitted diseases, should be performed.

Endometritis must be differentiated from uterine cramping without infection, and from cystitis. The patient experiencing uterine pain without infection usually is afebrile, and the white blood cell count is elevated only slightly. Such elevation can be confusing, however, because pregnancy itself causes a leukocytosis. In endometritis, however, the purulent and foul-smelling cervical discharge can show growth when culture and sensitivity tests are performed, or can reveal organisms with Gram's stain.

Cystitis is distinguished by the presence of red and white blood cells and bacteria in the urine. These organisms can usually be cultured.

Treatment

Mild endometritis is usually treated on an outpatient basis with oral medication to eliminate the organisms typically found in gynecologic infections. Such medication generally includes an immediate dose of penicillin or cephalosporin followed by doxycycline or tetracycline for 10 days (see below, Acute Pelvic Inflammatory Disease: Treatment). Septic abortion requires hospitalization and parenteral antibiotics along with appropriate support if gram-negative sepsis develops.

Treatment of chronic endometriosis is discussed below (see Chronic Endometriosis).

Acute Pelvic Inflammatory Disease

Acute pelvic inflammatory disease (PID) is an ascending infection involving the intra-abdominal pelvic organs and contiguous structures. PID poses a serious threat to the health and welfare of women because an estimated 1 million cases occur annually in the United States and are a major cause of ectopic pregnancies and infertility (12).

Etiology and Pathophysiology

The responsible organisms can be aerobic or anaerobic bacteria that are normally found in the cervical or vaginal flora, sexually transmitted agents (e.g., Neisseria gonorrhoeae, Chlamydia trachomatis, and Mycoplasma hominis), or a combination of these organisms, either sequentially or concurrently. These organisms gain access to the upper genital tract through the cervix, perhaps by cervical instrumentation or through loss of the cervical mucous plug during menstruation.

Sexual activity is the common denominator for women who acquire this infection (13); women who have multiple sex partners are more likely to have PID than those who have one partner. A previous episode of PID also predisposes a person to a subsequent episode (12). The use of an intrauterine device (IUD), particularly the Dalkon shield, has been associated with a significantly higher risk of PID. Use of other intrauterine devices has produced a slight increase in the risk of subsequent PID, to a greater degree in nulliparous women than in multiparous ones (14). One published survey showed only a slight risk of infection in the first 4 months after insertion of the device (15). Although IUDs are not presently manufactured for use in the US, some women continue to use them. Use of oral contraceptive tablets, however, seems to decrease the incidence of PID because this changes the cervical mucus (16).

Sexual contact with a partner who has gonorrhea is also a factor in acquiring PID (17). Instrumentation of the uterus for diagnostic purposes or termination of pregnancy can spread an infection of the lower genital tract upward to involve the entire abdominopelvic cavity.

The pain of PID is caused by multiplication of the infecting agent within the pelvic organs. Tissue is destroyed, and accumulation of cells and products of infection irritates both the organs and peritoneal surfaces. The edema occurring in response to infection causes further tissue damage and distortion. Some patients have pain from adhesions that develop secondarily between damaged intra-abdominal organs or between these organs and the abdominal wall. Although such adhesions usually occur in the lower abdominopelvic cavity, perihepatic lesions have been reported, such as in the Fitz-Hugh-Curtis syndrome (perihepatitis occurring as a complication of gonorrhea in women). When movement occurs between tissues fixed by these adhesions, pain results. These adhesions are more friable in acute infection and increase with the severity and number of infections.

Symptoms and Signs

Patients with acute PID usually have abdominal and pelvic pain, tenderness of the adnexa, rebound tenderness, and discomfort on motion of the cervix. Some patients have severe abdominal pain, nausea, and diarrhea.

Acute gonorrhea usually produces severe pain soon after menses. In contrast, chlamydial infection usually produces no symptoms at all; sometimes mild pain lasts several weeks. Patients with mixed flora, particularly an anaerobic infection, are often febrile and appear seriously ill as well as in pain. Dysuria and dyspareunia are common in patients with PID.

Among the possible complications of acute PID are abscess in the pouch of Douglas or tubo-ovarian abscess, recurrent episodes of PID, infertility, ectopic pregnancy, and chronic lower abdominal pain, which develops later.

Diagnosis

The clinical diagnosis of PID depends on the presence of abdominal pain, rebound tenderness, discomfort on motion of the cervix, tenderness of the adnexa, and the presence of at least one of the following: gram-negative intracellular diplococci found on culture of cervical discharge; bacteria and white blood cells found in the fluid obtained by culdocentesis; a pelvic or adnexal mass; or leukocytosis (white blood cell count 10,500 mm^3), fever of 38° C (100.4° F), and an erythrocyte sedimentation rate (ESR) higher than 15 mm/hour.

The use of these clinical criteria, however, even by experienced clinicians, is not uniformly accurate in diagnosing PID. Laparoscopy performed by Weström (18) and Jacobson and Weström (19) in Sweden revealed that, of 3000 patients presumed to have acute salpingitis (on the basis of lower abdominal pain, increased pain on pelvic examination, and lower genital tract infection diagnosed by increased white blood cell count on wet mount of vaginal contents), only 65% actually had acute salpingitis; 12% had some other pathologic condition of the pelvis, and 23% had no abnormal condition of the pelvis. Although these data suggest that it would be desirable to perform laparoscopy whenever PID is suspected, the cost of doing this procedure (in the hospital) in the United States is high and it entails certain risks, so it is not done routinely.

Pelvic inflammatory disease must be differentiated from other conditions causing pelvic pain or masses, including early pregnancy (intrauterine and ectopic), endometriosis, ovarian neoplasia, appendicitis, diverticulitis, bowel disease, cystitis, and pyelonephritis.

Use of ultrasound and measurement of the beta-subunit of hCG by radioimmunoassay aid in distinguishing pain caused by pregnancy from pain caused by infection. Assessment of the presence of peritoneal fluid and performance of a pregnancy test can help to eliminate pregnancy as a cause of symptoms. Of course, if culdocentesis produces blood instead of purulent material, an accident of pregnancy or a ruptured ovarian cyst should be suspected rather than PID, and further steps should be undertaken to determine the source of bleeding. A history of prior severe dysmenorrhea, tenesmus, and dyspareunia suggests endometriosis. Ovarian neoplasia sometimes (but not always) produces calcification that can be seen in radiographs.

Although appendicitis can present with signs and symptoms that closely resemble those of PID, the pain of appendicitis is usually unilateral, and periumbilical and gastrointestinal symptoms such as nausea and vomiting usually occur early in the course of the disease. If the appendix is retrocecal, a mass can be felt more clearly on rectal than on vaginal examination.

Because regional ileitis (Crohn's disease) is a chronic disease, patients with pain from this bowel problem often have a history of this condition that facilitates diagnosis. Also, such patients do not customarily have the organisms of a sexually transmitted disease present with Gram's stain or culture.

Urinary tract infections, particularly acute cystitis and severe pyelonephritis, can be confused with PID. The discovery of significant amounts of bacteria, white and red blood cells, or cast, or a combination of these, in an aseptically collected urine specimen strongly suggests the presence of a urinary tract infection. The pain of cystitis is usually low and central, whereas the pain of severe pyelonephritis can be bilateral and low in the groin and costovertebral angles. The back should always be examined and a centrifuged urine sample analyzed to rule out urinary tract disorders when confirming the cause of acute lower abdominal pain.

Treatment

Treatment of PID centers around eradicating infection. Pain gradually subsides once the process of tissue damage stops. Such damage results from multiplication of the infectious agent, accumulation of the products of infection, and the body's defenses against this invasion. Treatment takes approximately 48 to 72 hours, even with parenteral antibiotic therapy. During this time pain should be managed with a nonsteroidal anti-inflammatory drug (NSAID) and codeine or a potent opioid, depending on the severity of the pain. Although many clinicians believe that analgesia should not be used because pain is used to monitor the efficacy of treatment, this is not a valid reason to have a patient suffer severe pain. NSAIDs and opioids in usual therapeutic doses rarely, if ever, relieve severe pain completely. Consequently, they can be given and titrated to provide the patient with ample (but not complete) relief without eliminating the prognostic value of the pain. Because fever is another parameter for monitoring the efficacy of treatment, it is not treated unless it constitutes a danger to the health of the patient. One author maintained that immediate diagnosis and treatment are crucial to the future reproductive health of the affected woman and that the polymicrobic nature of PID must be recognized and treated with appropriate parenteral therapy (20).

Some patients with PID can be treated on an outpatient basis, such as those with a first episode of PID who have a temperature lower than 38° C. These patients must be able to walk and eat, and must have no pelvic mass suggestive of abscess. The following conditions require admission of the outpatient with PID to a hospital for parenteral antibiotic therapy: failure to respond to oral medication, inability to take oral medication or walk because of severe infection, a greatly elevated temperature, upper abdominal signs, a suspected or diagnosed abscess, pregnancy, or ongoing use of an IUD. When the diagnosis of PID is uncertain further diagnostic study, such as laparoscopy, is necessary.

Many antibiotic treatment regimens have been recommended for PID. The Centers for Disease Control have presented guidelines for the treatment of acute PID (21).

On an inpatient basis the following treatment regimen is suggested (21):

a. Doxycycline 100 mg IV q12h and cefoxitin 2 g IV q6h for 4 days minimum (48 hours after defervescence), followed by doxycycline 100 mg PO bid for 10 to 14 days
b. Clindamycin 600 mg IV q6h and tobramycin or gentamycin 2 mg/kg (loading dose), then 1.5 mg/kg IV q8h for 4 days minimum (48 hours after defervescence) followed by clindamycin 450 mg PO qid for 10 to 14 days
c. Doxycycline 100 mg IV q12h and metronidazole 1 g IV q12h for 4 days minimum (48 hours after defervescence), followed by doxycycline 100 mg PO bid and metronidazole 1 g PO bid for 10 to 14 days

On an outpatient basis initial medication should include one of the following (21):

a. Cefoxitin 2.0 g IM
b. Aqueous procaine penicillin G 4.8 mU IM with 1 g probenecid PO
c. Ampicillin 3.5 g PO
d. Amoxicillin 3.0 g PO
e. Spectinomycin 2.0 g for known penicillinase-producing GC

This should be followed by one of the following (21):

a. Doxycycline 100 mg PO bid for 10 to 14 days
b. Tetracycline 500 mg PO qid for 10 to 14 days
c. Erythromycin 500 mg PO qid for 7 days (patient unable to tolerate doxycycline or tetracycline or pregnant)

Most patients improve within 48 hours with parenteral antibiotic therapy. Some patients, however, require surgical intervention because they are seriously ill and have failed to respond to antibiotics, or because they have become even more ill in spite of 48 hours of antibiotic therapy. Surgery is almost always indicated for patients who are admitted with a pelvic mass that has disappeared, or who are moribund on admission; both conditions suggest a ruptured pelvic abscess. Other patients might require exploratory surgery to establish a diagnosis of PID if the pelvic examination shows no abnormalities and if pain fails to resolve after antibiotic therapy.

Surgery for PID should be tailored to the patient's condition and desires for conservation of reproductive ability. The use of new and more potent antibiotics has decreased the incidence of life-threatening ruptured abscesses. The advent of more advanced techniques for treating infertility (e.g., tubal microsurgery and in vitro fertilization) has decreased the number of surgical procedures that remove all pelvic organs if a conservative approach is requested by the patient, and these procedures can be carried out without undue hazard to health (22, 23).

Treatment of chronic PID is discussed below (see Chronic Pelvic Inflammatory Disease).

Adnexal Disorders

Torsion of Adnexa Produced by Ovarian Tumor

Etiology and Pathophysiology

The uterine adnexa consist of the uterine tubes, the ovaries, the peritoneum, and the blood vessels supplying these organs. These fragile tubes are anchored firmly only at their proximal ends, whereas the distal ends of the tubes (with the ovaries attached) hang freely in the pelvic cavity. Therefore, enlargement of the ovary (as occurs in ovarian tumors) can twist the tube on movement and cause ischemia in the distal structures. Necrosis and pain result.

Torsion can produce intermittent pain if the tube twists and untwists, or acute progressive pain if necrosis occurs. Normal adnexal organs rarely undergo torsion.

Symptoms and Signs

Torsion of the adnexa causes a dull unilateral ache that can come and go. The pain does not radiate or involve the midline structures or organs on the other side. The pain can be accompanied by nausea and fever that are mild to severe.

Diagnosis

The presence of an extremely tender mass in one adnexal area on pelvic examination suggests the diagnosis of torsion of the adnexa. If tenderness makes delineation of the mass by pelvic examination difficult, ultrasonic imaging of the pelvis can be useful. The diagnosis of torsion of the adnexa is also supported by mild elevation of the white blood cell count and by the presence of fever and nausea. Also, the patient might have a history of recurrent episodes of similar pain.

Torsion of the adnexa must be differentiated from other causes of adnexal masses and pain, such as ectopic pregnancy, functional ovarian cysts, endometriomas, ovarian neoplasia and, less frequently, pelvic infection.

Treatment

Once torsion has been diagnosed, surgical confirmation or treatment must be considered. If the diagnosis is questionable and the mass is quite small (4 cm) or indistinct, laparoscopy can be undertaken to visualize pelvic organs. If a discrete painful adnexal mass is present, however, or if the mass is sufficiently large to warrant operation, laparotomy should be performed.

When the abdomen has been entered and the pelvic organs visualized, care must be taken to determine the nature and extent of the problem in accordance with the patient's wishes to have children. If the adnexa have indeed twisted and the structures involved are gangrenous, the mass should be excised completely without untwisting it. This practice prevents clots from being squeezed from the venous complex involved into the general circulation.

If the patient wishes to preserve the adnexa, the surgeon must carefully evaluate the viability of the organs. Narcotic medication might be needed to relieve pain if the diagnosis is in question or if surgery must be delayed.

Bleeding of Functional Ovarian Cysts (XXIV-8)

Etiology and Pathophysiology

The functioning ovary produces two cysts each month, a follicle cyst and a corpus luteum cyst. The follicle ruptures at the stigma and produces an egg. The remaining cells coalesce and undergo changes to become a corpus luteum. If a pregnancy ensues, the corpus luteum persists and enlarges; without pregnancy, the corpus luteum degenerates, usually within 14 days.

Symptoms and Signs

At the time of ovulation the patient can have acute unilateral pelvic pain. The pain is initially sharp and throbbing, with no radiation. The pain can subside gradually over the next 12 hours and then disappear completely, or it can decrease in intensity but become generalized to the lower abdomen and pelvic area. In some patients pain occurs in the shoulder.

The acute unilateral pain is initially caused by rupture of the ovarian follicle through the capsule. Subsequent pain comes from blood escaping from this site and collecting in the pelvis and eventually in the abdomen. The shoulder pain has its origin in the diaphragm, which becomes irritated by blood collecting under it.

In addition to unilateral pelvic pain, the patient can have mild nausea that usually subsides in a day or so. If a hemoperitoneum develops the patient can experience faintness in addition to generalized pain.

Diagnosis

The diagnosis of a leaking ovarian cyst should be considered when symptoms occur in the last half of the menstrual cycle and an adnexal mass is palpated. A ruptured ovarian cyst should be suspected when an adnexal mass reported to be present "disappears" on subsequent pelvic examination. The presence of intraperitoneal fluid can be detected by ultrasonic imaging. If signs of hypovolemia (e.g., unstable vital signs with orthostatic hypotension) are present, a hemoperitoneum should be suspected and diagnosed by culdocentesis. With this technique fluid is aspirated from the cul-de-sac through a needle placed through the posterior vaginal fornix. If blood is obtained on aspiration, however, the source of the bleeding must be located by direct visualization. Although laparoscopy can be used, the presence of a significant amount of blood can make visualization of pelvic organs difficult. Under these circumstances laparotomy should be undertaken, both for diagnosis and for treatment.

Bleeding ovarian cysts must be distinguished from other causes of intraperitoneal bleeding, adnexal masses, and pain. These causes are usually pregnancy and endometriosis. Pregnancy should be suspected if the patient is sexually active but does not use effective contraception. The usual signs and symptoms of pregnancy should be elicited and an accurate menstrual history taken. Measurement of the beta-subunit of serum hCG can be ordered on an emergency basis if the signs and symptoms suggest pregnancy as a cause of pain.

Although endometriosis is a possible cause, pain from this condition usually occurs closer to the onset of menses.

Treatment

A ruptured cyst accompanied by pain that subsides without evidence of a progressive hemoperitoneum needs no treatment, although the pain might require narcotic medication during the acute phase. If recurring monthly pain of this nature is severe enough to warrant suppression of ovulation, the risks and benefits should be weighed in light of the patient's need for contraception.

Hemoperitoneum requires evacuation, drainage, and surgical removal or repair of the site of bleeding. The patient's wishes regarding reproductive ability should be known before proceeding in case further pathologic conditions requiring surgery are found at the time of operation.

Painful Disorders of the Vulva and Vagina

Acute pain in the vulva and vagina can be produced by infectious diseases, injury, or allergic reaction. Each of these is discussed separately.

Infection

Etiology and Pathophysiology

A wide variety of agents (e.g., viruses, arthropods, fungi, and bacteria) can produce painful infections of the vulva and vagina. Most of these agents are sexually transmitted. In viral or bacterial infections pain is caused by tissue destruction and nerve involvement. In folliculitis or bartholinitis pain is caused by accumulation of the products of infection within a closed space. In trichomoniasis and Gardnerella infections pain is caused by irritation of vulvovaginal tissue by the infectious agent.

Symptoms and Signs

In furunculitis, perineal boils, and bartholinitis, the pain of infection is generally confined to the site of infection. Pain begins as a dull ache that builds in intensity but does not radiate. Sometimes the abscess ruptures and drains spontaneously, greatly lessening pain. At other times the abscess remains intact and causes intense local discomfort when the patient attempts to sit or stand.

Infections of the vaginal mucosa and vulvar skin can produce pain and itching of the entire organ. This can be accompanied by a vaginal discharge or vulvar exudate that is curdy and white in moniliasis, yellow and bubbly in trichomoniasis, and grayish and fishy in odor in Gardnerella infections. The vagina and vulva can feel "raw " and sting or burn when touched by clothing or urine.

The pain of herpetic infection is most intense in the ulcers that occur on the vulva or introitus. Vaginal or cervical involvement is usually painless. The usual sequence is nonlocalized pruritus or tingling and then development of a fluid-filled vesicle that breaks, leaving a painful shallow ulcer. The ulcer then crusts over and heals, the whole process taking about a week. With recurrent lesions the ulcers usually last about 4 days and pain is mild (24). Lesions of the upper vaginal canal are generally painless. Some herpes infections cause a painful swelling of the inguinal lymph nodes that might be mistaken for a hernia. In approximately 25% of primary infections the patient becomes acutely ill, with severe local signs and symptoms, malaise, headache, arthralgias, and fevers (25). This severe clinical situation can last 2 to 3 weeks, with gradual resolution taking approximately 6 weeks.

Infection by Hemophilus ducreyi produces chancroid, a condition characterized by painful genital ulcers that have a red base, ragged edges, and a raised border. These are usually accompanied by tender unilateral enlargement of the inguinal nodes.

In lymphogranuloma venereum, vulvar ulcers are caused by a Chlamydia trachomatis infection, which also produces painful inguinal adenopathy. The vulva, anal margin, and rectal mucosa can be involved, with irregular swelling of these tissues. The lymphatic infection can become an abscess that drains and leads to fistula formation in the vulvar, inguinal, or perirectal areas.

Diagnosis

Vulvovaginal pain caused by infections is usually suspected from history and visualization of the tissue involved. Diagnoses of folliculitis and abscess of Bartholin's gland are also made by visualization of the infected structures. It is not really helpful to culture abscesses of the Bartholin's gland because common skin flora are generally involved; drainage is the treatment of choice.

In all generalized vulvovaginitis with discharge, however, a wet preparation of the exudate with saline solution should be examined under the microscope for identification of the responsible organisms. The discharge in moniliasis is curdy and white, and spores and hyphae strands can be seen under high magnification. These features are revealed more clearly if a few drops of 10% potassium hydroxide solution are used to hydrolyze other material on the slide. The wet preparation also shows motile trichomonads and "clue cells" of a Gardnerella infection—that is, epithelial cells with indistinct borders covered with the organisms. The discharge caused by Gardnerella infection has a fishy odor when potassium hydroxide solution is added to the slide (24, 25).

Acute painful ulcerative lesions of the vulva and vagina should be cultured for herpes and chlamydia. If granuloma inguinale is suspected, a biopsy can be taken and silver stain used to demonstrate the presence of Donovan bodies.

To rule out tumors and establish the differential diagnosis of ulcerative lesions of this area, cultures should be made for suspected agents and biopsy performed if the lesion is chronic or persistent. Although other conditions, such as Behçet's syndrome, granuloma inguinale, and syphilis also cause genital ulcers, these conditions are usually painless. In Behçet's syndrome lesions occur on not only the genitalia but also on the eye and mouth. If syphilis is suspected a dark-field microscopic examination of secretions from the lesion and serologic tests can be performed to determine if the infection is present.

Treatment

Furunculitis can be treated by applying heat locally to encourage spontaneous drainage and by using an antibacterial skin cleanser. Preparations with chlorhexidine are particularly effective for severe infections. In the patient with diabetes or a severe or persistent infection, the addition of antistaphylococcic antibiotics might be necessary. Although abscess of the Bartholin's gland can open and drain spontaneously, it might need to be drained and kept open by marsupialization (6), packing, or insertion of a Ward catheter (26). Antibiotics are usually not necessary, because the infection subsides promptly. Sitz baths, followed by air drying twice a day, decrease the pain considerably.

Each of the common vulvovaginal infectious agents has a specific recommended treatment (see above, Acute PID: Treatment). The newer antifungal agents have a high cure rate (90%) and should be used instead of older medications. Because of potential teratogenic effects, metronidazole should be avoided during the first 20 weeks of pregnancy. Persistent infections are more likely to be caused by not treating the patient's partner than by failure of metronidazole therapy. This fact, coupled with the mild disulfiram-like effect of metronidazole, makes longer treatment regimens with this drug less desirable today than previously (27). The treatment of Gardnerella infection is not uniformly successful, with cure rates ranging from 65 to 85% (28).

The initial episode of the ulcers of herpes can be treated with oral acyclovir, an agent that reduces the duration of the acute infection and promotes lesion healing (29). In severe episodes it is important to start therapy as early as possible. In one study, patients with frequent recurrences who were given acyclovir had a decrease in the rate of recurrences of up to 6 months (30). Because of potential teratogenicity, this drug should not be used during pregnancy and should be avoided in the nursing mother. Acutely ill patients with an initial episode might require hospital admission and intravenous medication. The patient with acute herpes might require oral administration of narcotic analgesics such as meperidine (75 to 100 mg every 3 to 4 hours) during the initial phase; if hospitalized, intravenous administration of analgesics such as meperidine (25 to 40 g) or hydroxyzine pamoate (25 mg every 5 to 6 hours) might be necessary to control pain.

The pain of an infectious process usually subsides once appropriate therapy has been instituted. General measures that relieve vulvar discomfort are applicable for various vulvar conditions. One measure is keeping the area clean by soaking it in tepid water, in water with baking soda, or in Burow's solution (aluminum acetate solution). The wearing of all-cotton underwear or at least cotton-crotch underwear increases water absorption and promotes dryness. Nylon underwear should particularly be avoided because it produces a skin irritant, formaldehyde, on contact with perspiration. The wearing of loose clothing promotes circulation of air and drying of tissue. Intermittent exposure of the perineum to light can significantly decrease bacterial or fungal infection and increase comfort (a goose-necked desk lamp can easily be adapted for this purpose). Powder can be used to keep the area dry, but products containing a scent or deodorant should be avoided. Baby powder and cornstarch are the most acceptable alternatives.

Trauma

Etiology and Pathophysiology

Vulvovaginal pain can occur secondary to acute tissue damage. The initiating event might have been a vaginal delivery, trauma from straddle injuries, or sexual activity. The acute pain is caused by tissue destruction and distortion of normal anatomy by hematoma formation within a closed space. Figure 67-1 depicts a typical straddle injury with hematoma formation, anatomic distortion that caused considerable pain, and urinary retention caused by blockade of the urethra. Surgical removal of the hematoma and hemostasis were necessary for successful treatment of the patient (Fig. 67-1).

Symptoms and Signs

Acute trauma can cause visible painful lacerations of the vulva and vagina. Such injury can produce an

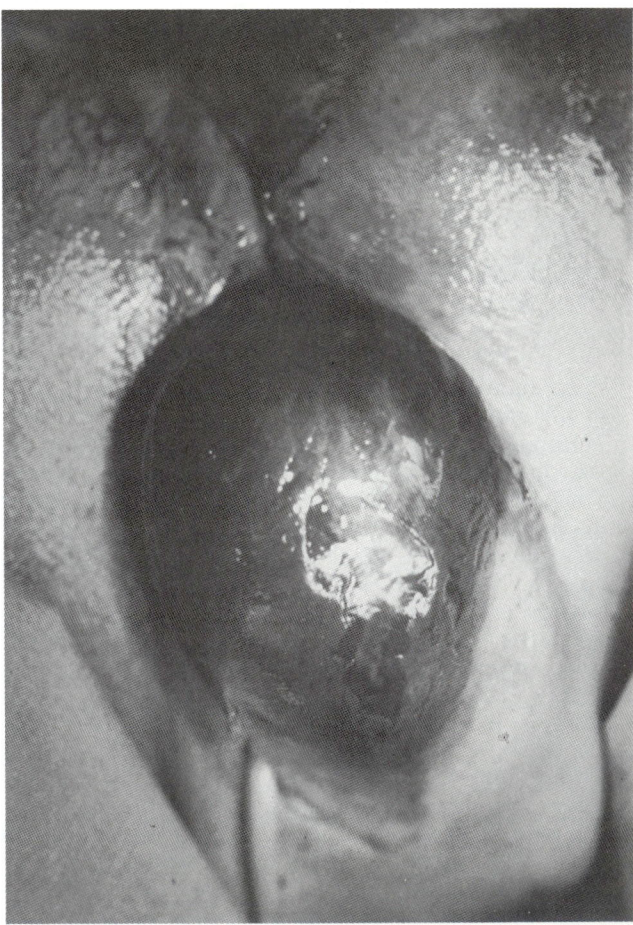

FIG. 67-1. Acute traumatic vulvovaginal hematoma. The patient was seen for intense pain and inability to urinate. Treatment consisted of immediate evacuation of the hematoma and ligation of the bleeding sites by figure-eight sutures. The patient's recovery was rapid and uneventful.

occult hematoma that dissects into the vulvar tissue or, less commonly, along the rectum or retroperitoneally into the abdomen. The pain of a hematoma usually develops gradually as a dull ache that becomes more intense as more tissue is involved. The skin over the hematoma becomes discolored, taut, and painful to touch, and eventually can become necrotic and slough off. If the injury has been extensive or severe a large amount of blood can collect in this area, and symptoms and signs of hypovolemia develop.

Diagnosis

Hematomas and lacerations are usually obvious. Occasionally, however, injury from intercourse is presented as a confusing or unclear story of vague pain because the patient wishes to conceal the real nature of the event. Careful examination of the tissue can be difficult because of pain or lack of cooperation. Caudal or general anesthesia might be necessary to perform an adequate examination, assess the extent of the damage, and effect repair.

Visible lacerations and hematomas are rarely mistaken for something else. Concealed hematomas can sometimes be misdiagnosed as infection of the internal organs. A careful history, examination, and laboratory studies help to differentiate these conditions.

Treatment

The treatment of vaginal laceration is surgical closure if the laceration is large, bleeding, or both. Vulvovaginal hematomas might need incision and drainage if they are painful and enlarging. The bleeding sites in the base of the lesion must be identified by careful removal of the clot and irrigation of tissue. Often a single vessel cannot be identified, and figure-of-eight sutures with chromic catgut must be used to occlude several areas of oozing. If the hematoma is stable and acute bleeding into the lesion has obviously stopped, consideration can be given to waiting for drainage until liquification of the clot has occurred and active bleeding has subsided. A patient with a large hematoma might need narcotic medication for pain if drainage is delayed.

Allergic Reactions

Etiology and Pathophysiology

Allergic reactions can also occur after these damaged tissues come in contact with irritating agents such as soap, clothing (particularly nylon), perfumes, and deodorants. Also, foods such as strawberries, tomatoes, and chocolate sometimes cause vulvar pruritus. In such cases, pain results from local release of histamines and other products of cell breakdown in response to allergens.

Symptoms and Signs

The pain of allergic vulvitis can be intense and sudden if the entire vulva is involved. Pain can be milder and chronic if the allergen is less potent or is applied continuously. Two examples of such allergens are the formaldehyde that develops when nylon underwear comes in contact with skin and the dye in colored toilet paper. In allergic vulvitis itching can be more prominent than pain.

Diagnosis

If an allergic response is suspected, a careful history of possible exposure must be taken to determine the agent. Intravaginal agents, deodorants, powders, perfumes, toilet tissue, clothing, soaps, laundry compounds, and foods are all possible allergens.

Allergic reactions usually produce itching and pain of the entire vulva. Itching of just the hair-bearing areas indicates the possiblity of pubic lice and scabies.

Treatment

Allergic reactions are best treated by determining and removing the allergen. This process can require several changes of clothing or changes in personal habits and diet. Bland local cleansing agents such as mineral oil and tub soaks with colloidal oatmeal or baking soda can be helpful. The use of a topical steroid might decrease discomfort and promote healing if no infection is present. The more potent topical steroids such as betamethasone or triamcinolone give results more promptly, and the clinician should become familiar with the use of at least one of these agents. Pain generally responds to local measures, and narcotic pain medication is usually not necessary.

B. RECURRENT PAIN

If pelvic pain recurs acutely, it is usually in relation to the menstrual cycle. Mittelschmerz and dysmenorrhea are the significant types of recurrent pelvic pain, and are frequent causes of discomfort and suffering among women. The Nuprin Pain Report (31), which contains data from a 1985 national survey of various painful disorders among Americans, indicated that 40% of adult women suffered premenstrual or menstrual pain during the previous 12 months. The incidence of pain was 81% among those 18 to 24 years old, 69% among those 25 to 34, 45% among those 35 to 49, and 7% among those 50 to 64. Moreover, among those who had pain, 15% said they could not work, sleep, or engage in routine activities for from 1 to 5 days, 5% could not do so for 6 to 10 days, 7.5% for 11 to 30 days, and 2.5% for 31 to 100 days. Among the entire population, nearly 75 million workdays were lost, lost including 25 million by adult women employed full time.

Mittelschmerz (XXIV-1)

Etiology and Pathophysiology

Midcycle pain, or mittelschmerz, occurs about 2 weeks before the menses, usually around the time of ovulation, and is believed to be caused by the rupture of the ovarian follicle with disruption of the capsule. Some blood can leak out and cause peritoneal irritation, particularly if blood collects in the cul-de-sac. The patient can also experience the pain of uterine contractions because the follicular fluid, which is rich in prostaglandins E and F, is released into the peritoneal cavity.

Symptoms and Signs

Mittelschmerz is usually unilateral and can vary monthly from side to side or can remain on the same side. Initially it is a constant pain on one side, low in the abdomen, that lasts several hours or up to 3 or 4 days. The pain can subsequently change to a more mid-line distribution with menstrual-like cramps that last for a day or so. Sometimes mild nausea, diarrhea, and vaginal bleeding occur.

Diagnosis

The hallmark of mittelschmerz is its timing relative to the menstrual cycle. The pain must occur in the middle of a cycle and recur at the same relative time each month. If the patient notes basal body temperature on a daily basis, it is possible to relate pain to the ovulatory rise and to confirm the diagnosis of mittelschmerz.

Other gynecologic conditions such as endometriosis, ovarian cysts, and pelvic infection should be considered. In general, only the pain of enlarging or leaking ovarian cysts recurs in relation to the menstrual cycle, but that type of pain usually does not occur with every cycle. The other conditions (endometriosis and pelvic infection) produce a more generalized pain that is unrelated to the cycle. In addition, pelvic infection usually is accompanied by fever and by an elevated white blood count and erythrocyte sedimentation rate. If pain is on the right side, consideration should be given to the possibility of appendicitis. The absence of guarding and rigidity and the occurrence of progressive nausea and fever should eliminate appendicitis as a cause.

Treatment

Treatment of mittelschmerz must be based on the degree of disability from pain and on the patient's desire to conceive. If the pain is severe and the patient wants to remain ovulating, administration of narcotic pain medication such as acetaminophen with codeine or meperidine (100 mg PO every 4 to 5 hours for 1 or 2 days) might suffice. Use of antiprostaglandin agents on the day before and the day of anticipated pain can decrease symptoms. The patient who does not currently want to become pregnant can obtain complete pain relief by suppressing ovulation with oral contraceptives.

Dysmenorrhea

Dysmenorrhea (cyclic pain associated with menses) is usually said to be primary if no pelvic or structural abnormalities are found as causes, and secondary if organic pathology exists; these definitions are used in this section. Some authorities designate dysmenorrhea as being primary if it has existed since shortly after menarche, and secondary if it began suddenly after a long interval of pain-free menses (32). Dysmenorrhea is a frequent disorder, with as many as 50% of young women experiencing the symptom, and up to 10% being unable to function normally for some time each month (32). The pain associated with menses can begin a few

hours or days before bleeding and usually lasts through the initial flow; pain can even last throughout the entire period.

Primary Dysmenorrhea (XXIV-3)

Etiology and Pathophysiology

The pain of dysmenorrhea not associated with pelvic structural abnormalities can be caused by relative uterine ischemia from hypercontractility of the myometrium (33, 34), which can be a result of excess prostaglandins or possibly vasopressin. Prostaglandins can act by increasing uterine contractility and also by sensitizing nerve endings to the pain-producing effects of other compounds, such as bradykinins. Although the vasopressin theory has not been documented clinically, the excess prostaglandin theory has received support both in the laboratory and because administration of prostaglandin synthetase inhibitors has resulted in significant pain relief in women with dysmenorrhea (35).

Pain in primary dysmenorrhea can also be a result of ovulatory cycles. Pain is not caused by ovulation itself but probably by the amount of prostaglandin E_2 stored in the thickened endometrium. When the patient is ovulating, pain can also be intensified in ovulatory cycles because the uterine muscle is sensitized to prostaglandins.

Symptoms and Signs

Dysmenorrhea usually begins immediately before menstruation and is severe as flow begins. It is cramping in nature and localized in the midportion of the lower abdomen. It can then involve the lower back and, on rare occasion, the upper thighs. Patients with primary dysmenorrhea often have prodromal symptoms characteristic of the prostaglandin effect on other systems: diarrhea, nausea, headache, lightheadedness, palpitations, diaphoresis, tremulousness, and anxiety. Some patients have mittelschmerz (midcycle pain) as well.

Diagnosis

Patients who report menstrual pain originating shortly after menarche and those who report subsequent dysmenorrhea with the symptoms described above should be evaluated for primary dysmenorrhea. A pelvic examination that produces completely normal and age-appropriate results would support this diagnosis. Some conditions that cause secondary dysmenorrhea (e.g., uterine polyps and endometriosis), however, can be present despite a normal pelvic examination, and only examination of the uterine and pelvic cavities rules out these conditions.

Treatment

The most recent theory of the cause of the pain of dysmenorrhea incriminates uterine ischemia and sensitization of uterine pain fibers resulting from excessive myometrial contractility after prostaglandin stimulation. Prostaglandin synthetase inhibitors, such as NSAIDs, block cyclo-oxygenase, which is an enzyme of the arachidonic acid pathway, and are thus effective therapy for primary dysmenorrhea (36). As noted, the mainstay in the treatment of primary dysmenorrhea is

TABLE 67-1. Nonopioid Analgesics

Drug (Proprietary Name)	Dosage
Ibuprofen (Motrin)	300 or 600 mg tid PO, tailored to individual symptoms and response
Naproxen sodium (Anaprox)	Initial dose 2 tablets 250 mg PO, then 1 tab q6–8h
Naproxen (Naprosyn)	250 mg PO bid
Mefenamic acid (Ponstel)	Initial dose of 2 250-mg tablets PO, followed by 250 mg q6h (for not more than 1 week)

the administration of antiprostaglandin drugs (Table 67-1). The action of these agents is somewhat similar except for mefenamic acid, which in addition to inhibiting prostaglandin synthetase aids in the breakdown of prostaglandins. All these drugs cause gastrointestinal irritation as a side effect. Although aspirin inhibits prostaglandin synthetase it acts primarily as a prostaglandin synthesizer in platelets and is not particularly effective in the uterus (37).

Oral contraceptives sometimes relieve dysmenorrhea through a decrease in the amount of prostaglandin F_2 stored in the endometrium and released into the menstrual blood (38). Oral contraceptives also make the myometrium less sensitive to prostaglandins, as shown by one study that demonstrated decreased motility in response to exogenously administered prostaglandins (39). Although suppression of ovulation can be beneficial in relieving dysmenorrhea, the patient must be willing to accept the risks, however minimal, of oral contraceptives. Young nonsmokers are at low risk whereas smokers, particularly those over 35, must accept a significantly higher risk of death from circulatory disease; these risks should be discussed with the patient before instituting therapy.

Inhalation of terbutaline has also been used for alleviation of the pain of dysmenorrhea. In one double-blind crossover study significant pain relief was experienced in the 14 women tested (40). One recent study, which used meclofenamate therapy and found it to be effective, differentiated patient response to placebo versus drug by using a discriminatory test for pain relief as opposed to objective uterine activity (41).

Secondary Dysmenorrhea (XXIV-2)

Etiology and Pathophysiology

Secondary dysmenorrhea originates in organic pelvic pathology. Pain can be intrauterine in origin, such as that occurring with submucosal fibroids, polyps of the endometrium, or use of an intrauterine device. In these cases pain is thought to be caused by contractions generated by the uterus trying to expel its contents. Although narrowing of the cervical canal was once thought to be a significant factor, studies of canal width in dysmenorrheic and normal women showed no difference (42). Relative stenosis can occur, however, if the endometrial lining sloughs off in large chunks, a

condition called "membranous dysmenorrhea." Other intrauterine possibilities for acute abdominal pain include deterioration of a myoma, which is either subserosal or intramuscular. Such an infarction can cause significant distress and even simulate an acute abdomen as a result of the intensity of pain. Other differential diagnoses must be entertained, however, because infarction of other intra-abdominal organs can also simulate uterine fibroid infarction (43).

Secondary dysmenorrhea can also be related to adenomyosis, the presence of endometrial glands deep within the myometrial tissue. When menstruation occurs menstrual blood is released directly into myometrial tissue, thereby increasing cramping and irritation of the fibers themselves.

Endometriosis, the presence of endometrial tissue in abnormal locations in the pelvis, is a common cause of secondary dysmenorrhea. The mechanism of pain in this condition is not well understood but probably includes a combination of excess prostaglandin production, increased peritoneal sensitivity, chemical irritation of the peritoneum, and bleeding in sites of endometriosis, such as the rectovaginal septum or ovary.

Symptoms and Signs

In some cases secondary dysmenorrhea resembles primary dysmenorrhea and is accompanied by symptoms and signs suggestive of prostaglandin excess. In other cases, the pain of endometriosis can be considered, because the pain begins several days before menstrual flow. The pain can be located in the low back and rectum and tends to be more dull and constant rather than cramping in nature. Pain can also occur with intercourse or on urination or defecation. This pain can last longer than the menstrual period, and the pain level can progressively increase over time.

Diagnosis

Pelvic examination often reveals abnormalities that indicate the cause of secondary dysmenorrhea. An enlarged and irregular uterus suggests the presence of fibroids, whereas a visible string from the cervical os corroborates the presence of an intrauterine device. A large, boggy, tender uterus suggests adenomyosis, whereas a fixed retroverted uterus, nodules in the cul-de-sac or on the uterosacral ligaments, and tender masses in the adnexa indicate endometriosis. A recent study of endometriosis, which used the cell surface antigen CA-125 as measured by serum radioimmunoassay, revealed a most remarkable correlation to women with mild, moderate, severe and very severe endometriosis with levels of 13.6, 22.8, 27, and 50 U/ml, respectively (44). In comparison, women with normal laparoscopic examinations had CA-125 levels of only 7.8 U/ml. It appears that this might be a valuable assay for the diagnosis and management of endometriosis.

Special studies examining the uterine cavity (e.g., hysterosalpingography, direct visualization with the hysteroscope, or cervical dilatation and uterine curettage) delineate pathologic conditions such as submucosal fibroids or endometrial polyps. Laparoscopy or laparotomy is needed to visualize the pelvis and to determine if endometriosis is present.

Treatment

Treatment of secondary dysmenorrhea centers on ameliorating or eliminating pathologic pelvic conditions. Intrauterine devices, fibroids, and polyps can all be removed. Endometriosis requires special treatment (see next section). Although adenomyosis can be managed by making the endometrial tissue quiescent in the same ways as those described for endometriosis, definitive management is by hysterectomy. Antiprostaglandin agents might be beneficial in some cases of secondary dysmenorrhea, as described for primary dysmenorrhea.

C. CHRONIC PAIN

Chronic pelvic pain can have a number of gynecologic causes, including the following: endometriosis; chronic pelvic inflammatory disease; developmental anomalies; vascular problems; uterine prolapse; pelvic muscle spasm; gynecologic cancer; vulvovaginal disorders; and chronic pain without obvious pathology. Many of these have been discussed. Some patients have pain without apparent sufficient underlying cause (see below, Chronic Pelvic Pain Without Obvious Pathology).

Chronic Endometriosis

The earlier section on acute pain from infection also describes endometriosis (see Acute Endometriosis).

Etiology and Pathophysiology

Endometriosis is the presence of functioning endometrial tissue at abnormal sites, such as outside the uterus. The most common of these sites are the ovaries, the cul-de-sac, the uterine tubes, the supporting ligaments of the uterus, the pelvic peritoneum, the rectovaginal septum, the cervix, and the surface of the bowel (45). Although the pathogenesis of endometriosis is unknown, several theories have been proposed. The most likely theory is that of retrograde menstruation, with implantation of endometrial tissue onto peritoneal surfaces (46). Endometrial metaplasia in the serosa has been discussed (47) but not proven. Spread of endometrial implants by the lymphatic system has been postulated and reported (48). Hematogenous spread of viable endometrial tissue has also been hypothesized (49).

The pain of endometriosis can occur with menses or sexual intercourse, or can always be present. The mechanisms causing pain are not well established but probably involve not only release of prostaglandins into the peritoneal fluid from the ectopic endometrium but also chemical irritation of the peritoneal surfaces by the products of menstruation. Pain can also be caused by swelling and stretching of the tissue to accommodate an endometrioma, or by nerve damage secondary to the scarring that occurs around implants.

Symptoms and Signs

The patient with endometriosis can have dysmenorrhea, dyspareunia, chronic pelvic pain, or all three. In addition, she can be infertile. Other symptoms include hematuria, hematochezia, bowel obstruction, or bleeding from unusual sites such as the pleural cavity or an abdominal scar; all are related to the location of the lesions.

Diagnosis

Occurrence of the pain symptoms described, coupled with infertility, should suggest the possibility of endometriosis. Definitive diagnosis of endometriosis is made by visualization of the lesions. Histologic confirmation is not necessary and is often difficult to obtain because the endometriotic implants might not contain active glandular tissue. Although implants can be present on the cervix and visible on vaginal examination, they more commonly occur on the ovary and peritoneal surface and thus require an operative procedure for diagnosis.

To confirm diagnosis, endometriotic implants—and not just adhesions, which can be caused by pelvic inflammatory disease or previous surgery—must be seen. The classification system described by the American Fertility Society should be used to determine the stage of the disease (Fig. 67-2, pp. 1358, 1359).

Treatment

Therapy for painful endometriosis depends on the extent of the disease and on the patient's desire to have children. If avoiding infertility is the prime consideration, measures should be undertaken to preserve and enhance the ability to conceive. If childbearing is to be delayed and relief of pain is the main concern, medical measures are appropriate for mild and moderate stages of the disease.

The object of medical treatment is to render the endometrial tissue quiescent. The mainstay of current therapy is danazol, a mildly androgenic compound that stops menstruation by inhibiting ovulation. Danazol is given orally in doses of 200 mg qid for 6 to 12 months. The major side effects are some increase in acne and weight, nausea, and irregular vaginal bleeding. A less common side effect is an increase in androgenic effects such as hirsutism, increase in libido, and decrease in breast size. Menstruation usually returns spontaneously within 1 or 2 months of cessation of therapy. Pregnancy rates after danazol therapy are reported to be higher than after other medical regimens for management of endometriosis. One disadvantage is that the drug is expensive.

Another acceptable method of treating endometriosis is keeping the patient on a continuous regimen of oral contraceptives of the combination type—that is, a synthetic estrogen and a synthetic progestogen. This treatment suppresses ovulation and endogenous estrogen production and decidualizes the endometrium. The patient on oral contraceptives might experience nausea, fluid retention, and an initial increase in pelvic pain; these conditions subside after the first 2 months of treatment. Although the use of progestogens alone had been recommended, this practice was found to be associated with a higher rate of irregular vaginal bleeding, sometimes necessitating treatment with estrogen. Administration of androgens alone, once a recommended treatment, is no longer popular because of the significant incidence of adverse side effects and the effectiveness of newer regimens. The treatment regimen selected usually continues for 9 to 10 months. Pregnancy rates are somewhat lower after therapy with oral contraceptives than after therapy with danazol.

Surgical removal of implants is usually indicated for moderate endometriosis. This process is generally accomplished using laparoscopy or laparotomy, and the patient can be placed on danazol postoperatively if she does not wish to conceive. Presacral neurectomy produces variable results and should only be considered in the young woman with disabling dysmenorrhea who has not responded to other measures (50).

More severe degrees of endometriosis need more aggressive surgical treatment. In some patients pain relief can be achieved only by total abdominal hysterectomy and bilateral salpingo-oophorectomy to eliminate the cyclic production of ovarian hormones. For the young woman, preservation of the ovaries is sometimes considered, but this might allow endometriosis to continue under the influence of cyclic ovarian hormones. The patient might then need oophorectomy and further surgery at a later date. Removal of the ovaries avoids this but does produce menopausal symptoms. Consideration should be given to treating these patients with low-dose noncyclic estrogen or progesterone replacement (50).

Chronic Pelvic Inflammatory Disease

The earlier section on acute pain from infection also describes PID (see Acute Pelvic Inflammatory Disease).

Etiology and Pathophysiology

The scarring, tissue damage, and adhesions resulting from chronic PID can cause chronic pelvic pain. The nerves to the intra-abdominal pelvic organs and contiguous structures can be damaged, or the structures can adhere in such a way that painful stretching is produced by activities such as exercise, sexual intercourse, or passage of digested food along the bowel.

Symptoms and Signs

Patients with adhesions and damage from chronic (or repeated) pelvic infections can have pain with intercourse or heavy activity, pain related to food consumption or, more rarely, continuous pain. During an acute exacerbation they have classic signs and symptoms of an acute infection, such as fever, chills, elevated white cell count, and abdominal pain.

Diagnosis

The diagnosis of chronic PID is based on a documented history of prior episodes of the disease and on visualization of current damage sufficient to account for the pain. The presence of pain on pelvic examination with no other findings and a history of being treated for a pelvic infection without documentation of disease are insufficient bases for a diagnosis of chronic PID.

Treatment

Major structural damage secondary to infection, such as hydrosalpinx, dense adhesions of the adnexa to the cul-de-sac and posterior aspect of the uterus, or adhesions of bowel and bladder to grossly abnormal adnexal structures, requires surgical treatment. Although the damage is surgically removable or at least partially correctable, all healing involves some scar tissue and any intra-abdominal manipulation can lead to further adhesions. Moreover, no direct correlation between visible pathology and pain has been found. Therefore great care should be exercised not to promise complete pain relief from any surgical procedure. Anatomy can be restored to normal while function is still impaired. Less severe abnormalities such as filmy adhesions in the pelvis also require surgery for treatment. Again, pain relief is not guaranteed. If the pelvic organs are visibly normal, surgery is not indicated for pain relief.

Presumptive treatment of "chronic pelvic infection" with long-term antibiotic therapy without documentation of an active infection is not indicated and is unlikely to relieve pain.

Developmental Anomalies

Etiology and Pathophysiology

On rare occasions chronic pelvic pain arises from various failures in normal development of the paramesonephric (müllerian) ducts. If one of these ducts becomes blocked during menses the organs above the blockage fill with blood, because menstrual blood has no direct egress from the body. Distension and pain result. The blockage can occur at the hymen or above, at a transverse septum. Such accumulation of blood in the vagina is called hematocolpos and, in both the vagina and uterus, is known as hematocolpometra.

Another developmental anomaly that often causes chronic pain is failure of the two uterine horns to fuse normally. That is, a "blind horn" can be present that gradually distends with menstrual blood.

Symptoms and Signs

Patients with these problems can have primary amenorrhea with cyclic pain or can have normal menses that gradually become more and more painful. Patients with primary amenorrhea can have normal secondary sex characteristics but no menarche. If a blind uterine horn is involved, the patient can have an adnexal mass that causes unilateral pain while menstruating from the other horn.

Diagnosis

The patient with an intact hymen and normal upper genital organs must be differentiated from one with Rokitansky-Küster-Hauser (RKH) syndrome or testicular feminization. Chromosome studies, determination of testosterone levels, ultrasonography, and pelvic examination help to diagnose these conditions. A patient with an XX karyotype has an intact hymen with internal pelvic organs and a vagina distended with blood. The patient with testicular feminization has an XY karyotype, an apparently intact hymen but no internal female genitalia, and testes located (usually) in the groin. The patient with RKH syndrome is chromosomally female but has no vagina and only a rudimentary uterus. Ultrasonography aids in identifying internal

Patient's Name _____ Date _____

Stage I   (Minimal) - 1–5

Stage II (Mild)   - 6–15

Stage III (Moderate) - 16–40

Stage IV (Severe)   - >40

Laparoscopy _____ Laparotomy _____ Photography _____

Recommended Treatment _____

Prognosis _____

Total _____

PERITONEUM	ENDOMETRIOSIS		<1 cm	1–3 cm	>3 cm
		Superficial	1	2	4
		Deep	2	4	6
OVARY	R	Superficial	1	2	4
		Deep	4	16	20
	L	Superficial	1	2	4
		Deep	4	16	20

	POSTERIOR CUL-DE-SAC OBLITERATION		Partial		Complete
			4		40

	ADHESIONS		<1/3 Enclosure	1/3–2/3 Enclosure	>2/3 Enclosure
OVARY	R	Filmy	1	2	4
		Dense	4	8	16
	L	Filmy	1	2	4
		Dense	4	8	16
TUBE	R	Filmy	1	2	4
		Dense	1˙	8˙	16
	L	Filmy	1	2	4
		Dense	4˙	8˙	16

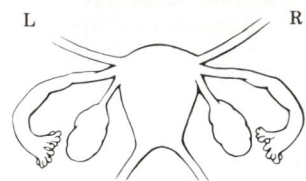

To Be Used with Normal Tubes and Ovaries

L   R

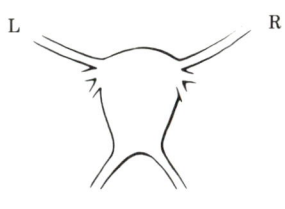

To Be Used with Abnormal Tubes and/or Ovaries

L   R

˙ If the fimbriated end of the fallopian tube is completely enclosed, change the point assignment to 16.

Additional Endometriosis: _____ Associated Pathology: _____

_____

_____

A

STAGE I (MINIMAL)

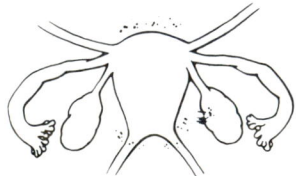

PERITONEUM
Superficial Endo   1–3 cm   2
R. OVARY
Superficial Endo   <1 cm   1
Filmy Adhesions   <1/3   1
TOTAL POINTS   4

STAGE II (MILD)

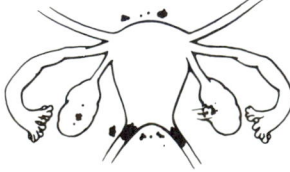

PERITONEUM
Deep Endo   <1 cm   6
R. OVARY
Superficial Endo   <1 cm   1
Filmy Adhesions   <1/3   1
L. OVARY
Superficial Endo   <1 cm   1
TOTAL POINTS   9

STAGE III (MODERATE)

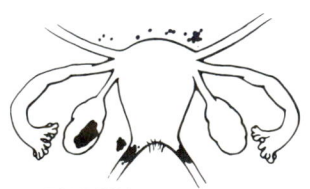

PERITONEUM
Deep Endo   >3 cm   6
CUL-DE-SAC
Partial Obliteration   4
L. OVARY
Deep Endo   1–3 cm   16
TOTAL POINTS   26

STAGE III (MODERATE)

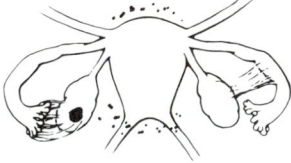

PERITONEUM
Superficial Endo   >3 cm   3
R. TUBE
Filmy Adhesions   <1/3   1
R. OVARY
Filmy Adhesions   <1/3   1
L. TUBE
Dense Adhesions   <1/3   16˙
L. OVARY
Deep Endo   <1/3   4
Dense Adhesions   <1/3   4
TOTAL POINTS   29

STAGE IV (SEVERE)

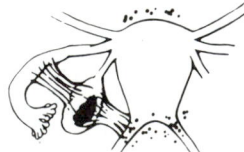

PERITONEUM
Superficial Endo   >3 cm   3
L. OVARY
Deep Endo   1–3 cm   32˙˙
Dense Adhesions   <1–3   8˙˙
L. TUBE
Dense Adhesions   <1/3   8˙˙
TOTAL POINTS   51

˙Point assignment changed to 16
˙˙Point assignment doubled

STAGE IV (SEVERE)

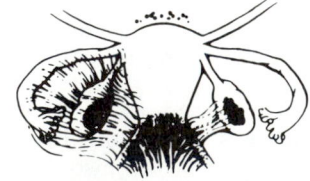

PERITONEUM
Deep Endo   >3 cm   6
CUL-DE-SAC
Complete Obliteration   40
R. OVARY
Deep Endo   1–3 cm   16
Dense Adhesions   <1/3   4
L. TUBE
Dense Adhesions   >2/3   16
L. OVARY
Deep Endo   1–3 cm   16
Dense Adhesions   >2/3   16
TOTAL POINTS   114

B

pelvic organs and a vaginal canal. Laparoscopy should also be considered to visualize internal pelvic organs and to identify anomalies such as a blind uterine horn.

Treatment

Hymenotomy is the procedure of choice for the patient with a vagina and internal genitalia. Making a cruciate incision and tacking back the edges is the preferred treatment for repairing an imperforate hymen. Surgical removal is appropriate for patients with a blind uterine horn. Patients with testicular feminization or RKH syndrome rarely have pain but might require other surgical, medical, and psychologic treatment and support. Some patients might be candidates for a nonsurgical approach (e.g., gradual dilatation to create a neovagina).

Vascular Problems

Etiology and Pathophysiology

Congestion of the vessels in the broad ligament and uterus has been discussed by several authors as a possible cause of pelvic pain (51, 52). Distension of the veins themselves and the lack of free drainage of blood from the pelvic organs can cause pain. Some doubts have been raised, however, about this causal relationship. In one study, more control patients than pain patients had large pelvic veins (53).

Symptoms and Signs

The pain of varicosities in other areas of the body is throbbing and burning in nature and worsens when patients stand for long periods of time. Patients can report this type of pain in the pelvis or lower abdomen.

Diagnosis

Direct visualization of the veins by laparoscopy or laparotomy is the most accurate way of documenting the presence of varicosities. Radiographic visualization by introducing dye into the pelvic venous system is another, but this study must be performed by an experienced radiologist.

Treatment

Injection sclerotherapy and ligation have been used to treat varicosities in other areas of the body but not in the pelvis. Hysterectomy is still the only procedure

suggested. The technique of using biofeedback to alter blood flow in patients with Raynaud's disease might prove useful for pelvic varicosities if pelvic blood flow could be made visible or audible to the patient.

Uterine Prolapse

Etiology and Pathophysiology

Tearing or stretching of the ligaments supporting the uterus can allow this organ to become displaced from its normal location inside the peritoneal cavity. Tension on nerves and blood vessels in these stretched or torn ligaments is thought to produce pain, but minor disruptions of the uterine supports probably do not contribute significantly to pelvic pain.

Symptoms and Signs

Although uterine prolapse often occurs without symptoms, some patients report feeling that "things are falling out." Severe pain is rare, even when the uterus is outside the introitus and the cervix is ulcerated. A dull ache and feeling of pelvic heaviness can occur.

Diagnosis

Lifting of the uterus by a pessary can relieve symptoms. If the symptoms are significantly changed by this maneuver, permanent relief by surgery should be considered.

Treatment

Uterine prolapse is usually treated by hysterectomy if patients have finished bearing children. Suspension from above might be considered if the patients have many symptoms and signs and wish to retain their childbearing potential. Elevation of the uterus and obliteration of the vagina below has been used by LaForte (54) in elderly patients who do not need a functional vagina and who have total uterine prolapse.

Pelvic Muscle Spasm

Etiology and Pathology

Tension myalgia of the levator can cause pelvic, back, and rectal pain (55–57). The actual spasm of the muscle and the accumulation of the products of metabolism, with tension on the attached ligaments and joints, are thought to be responsible for the pain.

FIG. 67-2. Classification of endometriosis. *A.* Suggested questionnaire and sketches of pelvic organs to aid in determination of stage of endometriosis. *B.* Examples and guidelines for use of point system. Determination of the stage or degree of endometrial involvement is based on a weighted point system. Distribution of points has been arbitrarily determined and may require further revision or refinement as knowledge of the disease increases.

To ensure complete evaluation, inspection of the pelvis in a clockwise or counterclockwise fashion is encouraged. Number, size, and location of endometrial implants, plaques, endometriomas, and/or adhesions are noted. For example, five separate 0.5-cm superficial implants on the peritoneum (2.5 cm total) would be assigned 2 points. (The surface of the uterus should be considered peritoneum.) The severity of the endometriosis or adhesions should be assigned only the highest score for peritoneum, ovary, tube, or cul-de-sac. For example, a 4-cm superficial and a 2-cm deep implant of the peritoneum should be given a score of 6 (not 7). A 4-cm deep endometrioma of the ovary associated with more than 3 cm of superficial disease should be scored 20 (not 24).

In patients with only one adnexum, points applied to disease of the remaining tube and ovary should be multiplied by 2 (**). Points assigned may be circled and totaled. Aggregation of points indicates stage of disease (minimal, mild, moderate, or severe).

The presence of endometriosis of the bowel, urinary tract, fallopian tube, vagina, cervix, skin, etc. should be documented under "additional endometriosis." Other pathology such as tubal occlusion, leiomyomata, uterine anomaly, etc. should be documented under "associated pathology." All pathology should be depicted as specifically as possible on the sketch of pelvic organs, and means of observation should be noted. Modified from The American Fertility Society: Revised American Fertility Society classification of endometriosis. Fertil. Steril., *43*:351, 1985.

Although the exact cause of the spasm is unknown, poor posture, trauma, infection, and emotional tension are possible factors.

Symptoms and Signs

The condition, characterized by intense local spasms of levator muscles in response to specific situations such as sexual intercourse or pelvic examination, is called vaginismus. Generalized spasm of these muscles can be chronic but without an identifiable situational trigger. The spasm produces chronic pain more like that of a tension headache or "charley horse." The pain is described as being deep in the lower abdomen, the pelvis, the vagina, and sometimes in the sacrum, coccyx, or rectum. In some cases pain is always present at a low level, with exacerbations. It can be worse after intercourse, and local heat in the form of baths or a heaing pad can decrease the pain.

Diagnosis

The diagnosis is based on vaginal or rectal palpation of tense, tender muscles along the pelvic side walls. The spasms can be unilateral or bilateral. Vigorous palpation reproduces or exacerbates the patient's pain and causes the patient to move away or cry out.

Treatment

In spite of the description of various therapies, no permanent cures have been reported. Traditional therapy for muscle spasm consists of injection of local anesthetics, application of deep heat, and massage. Some experts have tried high-voltage electrogalvanic stimulation (58) and hypnosis (59). Muscle relaxants can be helpful; agents such as carisoprodol (Soma) and methocarbamol (Robaxin) are probably preferable to diazepam because they do not produce as much depression. Behavioral approaches such as stress management and muscle relaxation techniques should be part of the general management plan. Little information from controlled treatment trials is available to date, however, and the clinician probably should arrive at the best combination in an individual patient by trying several treatments, singly or in combination.

Gynecologic Cancer

Gynecologic malignant tumors constitute nearly 16% of all new cancers among the American female population and are the fourth leading cause of death. Table 67-2 lists the 1986 American Cancer Society estimates for gynecologic cancers. Many of the tumors do not cause pain in the early phase of the disease but, in the advanced terminal stages, gynecologic cancer causes moderate to severe pain in some 75% of patients (Table 24-3). Cancer of the ovary, cervix, endometrium, and external genitalia is discussed briefly in this section.

Cancer of the Ovary

Ovarian cancer is the leading cause of death from gynecologic malignancy and the fifth leading cause of death among American females (60). The age-adjusted death rates have steadily increased over the past 25 years, not only in the United States but also in other

TABLE 67-2. 1986 Estimates of New Cases and Deaths from Cancer of the Female Genital Tract

Site of Cancer	Number of New Cases	Number of Deaths
Cervix uteri*	14,000	6,800
Corpus uteri (endometrium)	36,000	2,900
Ovary	19,000	11,600
Other types	4,400	1,100
All:	73,400	22,400

*Invasive cancer only.
American Cancer Society: 1986 Cancer Facts and Figures. New York, American Cancer Society, 1986.

industrialized nations (61). Unfortunately, ovarian cancer is often detected only when it has spread throughout the peritoneal cavity and, despite aggressive surgical resection and adjunctive therapy, most patients succumb in a period of months from malnutrition and small bowel obstruction caused by intraperitoneal tumor.

Pathology

Epithelial ovarian carcinoma, arising from the germinal epithelium of the ovary, comprises more than 80% of the ovarian cancers. This type of cancer can be subclassified by cell type to include scirrhous, mucinous, endometroid, mesonephroid, and undifferentiated carcinoma. Although in the past a better prognosis was affixed to the mucinous and endometroid varieties, it is now apparent that these different histologic types behave similarly stage for stage and grade for grade (60).

Other malignancies of the ovary include the following: primary stromal tumor (e.g., cystadenofibroma, fibrocystadenoma, and Brenner type); granulosatheca cell tumor; Sertoli-Leydig cell tumor; stromal tumors of mesenchymal origin (e.g., thecoma, fibrothecoma, fibroma, sarcoma), most of which occur in later life; metastatic tumors to the ovary, in particular from the gastrointestinal tract (Krukenberg tumor) and breast.

The most common mechanism of spread is by continuity and intraperitoneal dissemination. A number of studies indicate that tumor cells in the peritoneal cavity are drained by diaphragmatic lymphatics, which occurs well in advance of clinical ascites (60, 62). Ascites appears to be related to impaired diaphragmatic drainage. In addition, spread occurs through the ovarian lymphatics, which pass cephalad and terminate in periaortic nodes. This results in spread of metastatic ovarian cancer to the peritoneum, omentum, and bowel, as well as to other parts of the genitourinary tract, particularly the uterus and the fallopian tube, the latter by direct extension rather than by lymphatic permeation. Involvement of the opposite ovary occurs in 50% of cases of epithelial ovarian cancer, in two-thirds of cases of scirrhous carcinoma, and in 25% of those with mucinous adenocarcinoma (62). Among the distant organs that can be involved with ovarian carcinoma, in order of decreasing frequency, are the liver, lung, pleura, kidney, bone, adrenal, bladder, and spleen (62).

Carcinoma of the ovary has been classified into four stages and several substages. Stage 1 is growth limited to the ovaries; stage 2 is growth limited to one or both ovaries, with pelvic extension; stage 3 is growth involving one or both ovaries, with intraperitoneal metastasis outside the pelvis, or positive retroperitoneal nodes, or both; and stage 4 is growth involving one or both ovaries, with distant metastasis (60).

Symptoms and Signs

As mentioned above, ovarian cancer is generally asymptomatic in the early stages of the disease. With advanced ovarian cancer patients develop pelvic pressure and fullness associated with urinary frequency and constipation. Increasing abdominal girth occurs because of ascites or a mass rising out of the pelvis. Pain is an unusual symptom in the early stages of the disease; when it occurs it is caused by a portion of the adnexa or actual tumor invasion of the pelvic side wall, with consequent bone involvement, or by pressure on the lumbosacral plexus, which is likely to cause burning sensation and dysesthesia along a course of nerves derived from the plexus. Mixed germ cell tumors of the ovary, which occur in those in the younger age group, have abdominal pain as the most common denominator in regard to symptoms. In one study the mean age of patients was 16 years and pain was present in 90% of patients (63).

Physical findings in patients with ovarian carcinoma usually include a pelvic mass with a palpable abdominal mass in about 40 to 75% of the cases. Ascites can be detected clinically in from 20 to 30% of patients and, in more advanced cases, pleural effusion can be noted (62). Only approximately 1 to 2% of patients with ovarian cancer have an entirely negative physical examination, except in the early stages of the disease.

Diagnosis

A careful bimanual and rectal-vaginal examination is the most productive diagnostic test for the detection of ovarian carcinoma. Because the ovary might not be palpable in postmenopausal women, the finding of even a just palpable mass indicates further investigation. The diagnosis is confirmed either by laparoscopy or exploratory laparotomy. Identification of the tumor is made by tissue biopsy and confirmation of specific type is made by microscopic examination, most often in the form of a frozen section analysis. In addition, the functional ovarian neoplasms with feminizing or masculinizing potential are carefully evaluated preoperatively by attention to history and hormone analysis.

Treatment

Treatment regimens for these neoplasms consist of a combination of surgical exploration with careful attention to involvement of surrounding tissues, extirpation of the tumor, often by complete total abdominal hysterectomy, and bilateral oophorectomy (60). Identification of tumor borders is often made by surgical clips, which can later be visualized radiographically. Radiation can then be directed subsequently toward the high-risk areas. In addition to surgical extirpation and radiation, chemotherapy plays a major role in the aggressive management of such tumors (62).

Cancer of the Uterine Cervix

Except for ovarian carcinoma, more deaths occur annually among women from carcinoma of the cervix than from any other gynecologic malignancy. In its early stages cervical cancer is relatively curable but, as it becomes more advanced locally to involve the parametrium, pelvic side walls, and vagina, the probability of local control with radiation therapy decreases and the risk of periaortic lymph node involvement increases (64). Consequently, the potential for cure decreases when extensive localized disease is present.

Etiology and Pathology

No causative agent has been identified for cervical carcinoma but predisposing associated factors have been well identified (64). These include a history of sexual promiscuity, large number of pregnancies, low socioeconomic status, and a history of diethylstilbesterol ingestion by women during the first trimester of pregnancy. All have been shown to cause an increased incidence of carcinoma of the cervix.

The lesion is frequently associated with a history of chronic cervicitis, severe dysplasia, and carcinoma in situ. This progression from chronic cervicitis to severe dysplasia to carcinoma in situ to invasive carcinoma can take from 10 to 20 years (64). Of untreated patients with carcinoma in situ, 30 to 70% develop invasive lesions 10 years after diagnosis of the in situ carcinoma. When the carcinoma has broken through the basement membrane of the epithelium and invaded the underlying stroma, it is classified as stage 1. With more advanced disease, the cancer can spread into the vaginal fornices of the paracervical or parametrial tissue or, occasionally, into the lower uterine segment of the endometrial cavity (stage 2). Once tumor has extended to the pelvic side wall or lower third of the vagina, fixation of the uterus and paracervical tissue can occur (stage 3). Finally, tumor can invade the bladder or rectum directly or cause hydronephrosis by ureteral compression; the periaortic lymph nodes are probably involved, as well as distant metastases (stage 4). Spread of the cancer is through the paracervical and parametrial lymphatics and also by the ascending periaortic lymphatic system to involve the periaortic nodes. In advanced cases hematogenous dissemination to the venous plexus and paracervical veins occurs less frequently, with the most common metastatic sites being the lungs, the mediastinal and supraclavicular lymph nodes, the bones, and the liver (64).

Symptoms and Signs

Intraepithelial or early invasive carcinoma of the cervix is asymptomatic, and a small central superficial ulceration might be the only finding on examination. The first manifestation of abnormality in cervical carcinoma is postcoital spotting, which later can increase to limited metrorrhagia and still later to menorrhagia. In the patient with invasive carcinoma, a vaginal serosanguineous or yellowish foul-smelling discharge intermixed with profuse bleeding, can occur, and the patient might develop anemia with consequent complaint of fatigue.

Pain, usually in the pelvis or the hypogastrium, is experienced when tumor necrosis or associated pelvic inflammatory disease is present. Some patients complain of pain in the lumbosacral area, probably caused by periaortic lymph node involvement with extension into the lumbosacral plexus. Occasionally, epigastric pain can be a result of high periaortic metastases to the lymph nodes. In an epidemiologic study carried out by Greenwald, Bonica, and Bergner (65) on 536 patients with four cancers (lung, prostate, cervix, pancreas) it was found that among patients with carcinoma of the cervix in stages 1, 2, and 3, 56% had pain and, of these, 68% stated that their pain had been moderate to severe or excruciating during the week prior to the interview. During the preceding 2 months 47% had mild pain, 11% had moderate pain, and 47% had severe to excruciating pain. Among patients with advanced or terminal cancer of the cervix, 75% had moderate to severe pain (Table 24-3). Urinary and rectal symptoms can appear in advanced stages as a consequence of invasion of the bladder or rectum by the cancer. In such instances hematorrhea or rectal bleeding can occur.

Diagnosis

Early invasive carcinoma of the cervix can only be detected through periodic cytologic (Papanicolaou) smears. The early detection of cervical carcinoma through screening cytology has resulted in a lower number of advanced cases and consequently a lower overall mortality rate. Other procedures that help to detect carcinoma of the cervix include colposcopy, conization, biopsy, and dilatation and curettage.

Every patient with carcinoma of the cervix should be jointly evaluated and staged by a radiation oncologist and gynecologist, and should have a complete physical and detailed pelvic and rectal examinations. If a biopsy reveals cervical carcinoma, additional workup should be done, including an intravenous pyelogram and chest roentgenogram, complete blood count, blood urea, nitrogen, creatinine, and uric acid tests, and liver function studies at the time of the physical examination, which is best done with regional or general anesthesia. In addition to the pelvic examination, most patients have cystoscopy and sigmoidoscopy (64).

Treatment

Early lesions are highly curable either with radiation therapy or surgery, but more advanced lesions need higher doses of radiation to control the disease. Even when lesions are advanced, they can still remain localized and are potentially curable (64). With careful attention to patient anatomy, high doses of radiation both by external beam and intracavitary application can produce local control, even for advanced tumors. In some centers preoperative radiation combined with a radical hysterectomy has been used. Chemotherapy is being tried for this type of lesion. A more comprehensive discussion of therapy can be found elsewhere (64, 66). The management of pain of cancer of the cervix, as well as other gynecologic cancers, is discussed in detail in Chapter 24.

Carcinoma of the Endometrium

Endometrial cancer is the most common invasive malignancy of the female reproductive tract. Despite its high incidence the prognosis is very good, with the annual mortality rate being about 8% of the incidence rate. Most cases occur in postmenopausal women, in whom the presenting complaint is almost always abnormal vaginal bleeding.

Etiology and Pathophysiology

A number of risk factors have been identified in association with carcinoma of the endometrium, including diabetes mellitus, obesity, and exogenous estrogen intake (67), and it occurs more frequently in Jewish women than in women of other ethnic groups. It occurs more commonly in unmarried women and women of low parity (67).

At least 90% of malignant tumors of the uterine corpus are adenocarcinomas, usually arising within the uterine fundus, and are polypoid or infiltrative. Tumors can infiltrate the uterus from the mucosal surface all the way through the serosa (67). In stage 1 the carcinoma is confined to the corpus, while in stage 2 the tumor involves the corpus and the cervix. Metastatic spread to pelvic and periaortic lymph nodes causes the lesion to extend outside of the uterus but, as long as it remains within the true pelvis, it is considered to be in stage 3. When the lesion extends outside the true pelvis or involves the mucosa of the bladder or rectum it is considered to be in stage 4. Metastasis to peritoneal surfaces and omentum, as well as ascites, are uncommon at the time of presentation but are frequent manifestations of recurrent disease. It can spread to the bloodstream and cause metastasis to the lungs, liver, bones, brain, and other structures.

Symptoms and Signs

The most common presenting complaint is unexpected postmenopausal vaginal bleeding or abnormal menometrorrhagia in those of premenopausal age. The patient can also complain of a yellowish or serosanguineous vaginal discharge, and pyometra and hematometra can be present in patients with an enlarged uterus or blockage of the cervical canal.

As in the case of other gynecologic cancers, carcinoma of the endometrium in its early stages is associated with a low incidence of pain. Hypogastric or pelvic pain is occasionally reported, which is probably caused by concomitant presence of myomata in the uterus. Periaortic lymph node metastasis not infrequently causes lumbosacral pain. In advanced stages of the disease the patient has bladder or rectal pain or pain resulting from distant metastatic lesions, which eventually becomes severe and requires effective therapy.

Diagnosis

The diagnosis is made through history and a complete physical examination, including a detailed bimanual pelvic and rectal examination, preferably done under regional or general anesthesia. Routine laboratory workup should include a hemogram, blood chemistry profile (SMA-12), and urinalysis. Fractional dilatation and curettage should always be performed if endometrial pathology is suspected. Other diagnostic procedures include chest roentgenography and IV pyelography. Cystoscopy and proctosigmoidoscopy are done in patients with clinical stage 2 or advanced disease. In patients with advanced disease, additional studies such as liver function tests, bone scan, whole lung tomography, CT scanning, barium enema, and hysterography should be carried out.

Treatment

Total abdominal hysterectomy with bilateral salpingo-oophorectomy is the mainstay of treatment of early carcinoma of the endometrium (67). Adjuvant intracavitary or external beam radiation (or both) is used to prevent vaginal recurrence and destroy potential microbial causes of disease in pelvic lymph nodes and other pelvic structures. Patients with well-differentiated tumors and little or no myometrial invasion have an excellent prognosis, with an 85 to 95% 5-year survival rate. In stage 2 of the disease the combined therapy produces a 60 to 65% survival rate, while in stage 3 the survival rate ranges from 20 to 80%, depending on whether the lesion is confined to the ovary and fallopian tubes or extends beyond these organs to other pelvic structures. The most common systemic therapy in stage 4 and in recurrent adenocarcinoma of the endometrium is the use of progestational agents, which produces an average response rate of 30 to 35% (67).

Other Gynecologic Cancers

Other much less frequently occurring gynecologic cancers include carcinoma of the fallopian tube, which is the least frequent of all malignant tumors of the female genital tract and comprises from 0.5 to 1% of all gynecologic malignancies, carcinoma of the vagina, which accounts for less than 2% of all these lesions, and carcinoma of the vulva, which accounts for 3 to 4% of all female primary genital malignancies (66).

Pathology

Adenocarcinoma is the most common histologic type of primary carcinoma of the fallopian tube, although such rare tumors as sarcoma, mixed mesodermal tumors, lymphomas, and carcinosarcoma have been reported (66). Over 90% of all vaginal tumors are epidermoid carcinomas, while 90% of cancers of the vulva are squamous cell carcinomas.

Symptoms and Signs

Abnormal vaginal bleeding associated with pelvic and abdominal pain are the most common symptoms of carcinoma of the fallopian tube (66). Most invasive squamous cell carcinomas of the vagina present with vaginal bleeding, and only in more advanced stages, in which tumor has spread to adjacent organs, are symptoms present that are associated with dysuria and pelvic pain. The most common presenting complaint of vulvar carcinoma is the presence of a mass or growth in the vulvar area associated with pruritus vulva, bleeding, and pain (66).

Diagnosis and Treatment

The diagnostic procedures are similar to those discussed for other gynecologic cancers.

The primary treatment of carcinoma of the fallopian tube is surgical, consisting of total abdominal hysterectomy and bilateral salpingo-oophorectomy (66). If the tumor invades adjacent pelvic organs or extends directly into the lower abdomen with separate metastasis en bloc, excision of all the tumor is carried out, in addition to the aforementioned operations.

Primary therapy for carcinoma of the vagina is radiation therapy. Although some authorities advocate a surgical approach, this should be discouraged because of the excellent tumor control and good functional results obtained with adequate radiation therapy.

Treatment of cancer of the vulva should be tailored to the stage of the disease. Nevertheless, operative intervention is the primary therapy and extends from wide local incision for carcinoma in situ to total vulvectomy for more advanced lesions. Detailed discussion of these and other therapeutic procedures can be found elsewhere (66).

Other Painful Disorders

Chronic Pain of External Genital Organs

Etiology and Pathophysiology

Vulvovaginal pain can be caused by chronic irritation secondary to infection from ringworm or other fungus or, less commonly, from bacteria. Maceration of these fragile tissues by improper garments and poor perineal care also causes pain. Loss of the epithelium can expose nerve endings to chronic stimulation by clothing or furniture; this stimulation can be compounded by scratching, which releases irritating algogenic agents such as bradykinin and histamine into the skin.

Certain foods (e.g., coffee, tea, cola, chocolate, citrus fruit, tomatoes, alcohol, milk) produce perirectal and perineal itching in susceptible individuals. Pinworm infestation causes perianal itching, particularly at night. Spasms of the levator muscle can cause perirectal and vulvar pain. Hidradenitis suppurativa (purulent infection of the apocrine glands) can lead to chronic abscess, sinus tract formation, and chronic pain.

Symptoms and Signs

The patient with chronic vulvar pain might complain that clothing irritates her or that the vulva is always moist and sensitive. The pain can be localized to one area or generalized to the entire vulva. Draining sinuses or painful abscesses can be present.

Diagnosis

The essential diagnostic element is visualization of the external genitalia and determination of whether a discrete lesion is present. Infectious agents such as ringworm produce a classic red lesion with a serpiginous border of flaking skin. These flakes of skin can be examined for fungus by suspending them in a drop of potassium hydroxide or by examining the skin directly under a Wood's light—fluorescence indicates infection. The most common vulvovaginal fungus,

Candida albicans, can also be seen on a potassium hydroxide preparation.

Generalized maceration can be seen on visual inspection of the vulva. Bacterial cultures should be taken if a purulent exudate is present or if abscesses are seen.

A history of pruritus ani suggests that a stool sample be examined for ova and parasites to detect pinworm.

Treatment

Specific infections should be treated with appropriate antibiotics or antifungal agents. General vulvar maceration requires mild cleansing with oil and less frequent immersion of tissues in water. Use of loose absorbent clothing is encouraged, as is dusting the area with cornstarch to absorb moisture. Products containing scents or deodorants should be avoided.

A thorough history of dietary habits should be obtained and offending items omitted in an attempt to reduce pruritus. It might be necessary to eliminate all questionable items and then add them gradually one by one to determine which, if any, are causing the problem.

Chronic abscess of the apocrine glands requires surgical drainage and administration of systemic antibiotics. This disease is kept active by estrogen, however, and probably does not subside permanently until menopause.

Chronic Pelvic Pain Without Obvious Pathology (CPPWOP) (XXIV-9)

In a significant number of patients who present with pelvic pain with characteristics of pain of gynecologic origin, no obvious organic pathology can be found, even with comprehensive clinical laboratory examination. This condition, recognized for over a century and called by various names, has prompted various speculations and hypotheses regarding its causes, which are considered here briefly.

Etiology

In the late 1940s and early 1950s several authorities proposed hypotheses to explain pelvic pain without obvious pathology. Taylor (68), one of the most prominent, suggested dysfunction of the autonomic and sensory nervous systems. He studied a series of ten patients who presented with the syndrome; blood flow probes were placed in the vagina, and an increased blood flow was noted during emotionally stressful situations. Although significant psychopathology was seen the pain was attributed to two types of pelvic autonomic disorders—one that Taylor called "vascular dysfunction of pelvic congestion" and the other "sensory change," otherwise known as hypogastric plexalgia (69). In the former, the mechanism of pain was thought to be a combination of venous distension with interstitial edema, followed possibly by fibrosis of the uterus. In the latter type, the patient could have ultrasensitivity of the pelvic organs and tissues on a hereditary basis.

Theobald (70) called this syndrome "the pelvic sympathetic syndrome," suggesting that abnormal sympathetic dysfunction might produce ischemia, dilatation of the hollow viscus, chemical irritation in the pelvis, or a combination of these, which in themselves cause pain. Others have suggested that nerve endings from previously damaged structures that were removed can still produce nociceptive impulses, and "phantom organ sensation" and "phantom pain" might ensue (71).

Allen and Masters (72) suggested that the syndrome is caused by small traumatic lacerations of the sacral uterine ligament or of a posterior leaf of the broad ligament. Subsequently, DeBrux and associates (73) examined 25 patients with chronic pelvic pain without obvious pathology in whom large biopsies were taken from the broad ligament, the uterosacral ligaments, and the peritoneum of the pouch of Douglas. They found microscopic lesions indicative of recurrent pelvic peritonitis in several patients. Microscopic findings of endometriosis were found in half of these patients, a hemangioma in two, and a neuroma in one. Renaer (74–77) disputed this hypothesis because real tears in the supporting structure of the uterus are rare; when they do occur their role in chronic pain without pelvic pathology syndrome is negligible.

Ample evidence now exists that the pain of most patients presenting with pelvic pain and associated symptoms without obvious pathology is most likely caused by the presence of psychopathology. In a follow-up report, Duncan and Taylor (78) studied 35 patients with pelvic pain without obvious pathology, and found that all but a few had significant psychopathology. They reported that these patients had in common large families and a disturbed childhood in the form of lack of maternal warmth. Moreover, in 34 of the 35 patients, the onset of pain was associated with depression and major life stresses, including major marital and family problems. In another study, Taylor and colleagues (79) found that 34 of 40 patients with pelvic pain without obvious pathology were diagnosed either as having schizophrenia, borderline syndrome, or severe neurosis, while only 12 in the control group had these diagnoses. In relating early childhood experience to the later development of pelvic pain, it was found that those in the group with pelvic pain experienced significantly more physical pain and psychic trauma than those in the control group. It was concluded that patients with pelvic pain functioned poorly in many ways and demonstrated constricted affect, depressive trends, somatization, and conflicts involving femininity. It was postulated that patients with this syndrome could not establish and preserve that unconscious sense of "femininity, identity with which permits the unhampered execution of so-called feminine function," and inferred that early severe anxiety about female functioning had been subjected to massive repression, denial, and projection, and that both phobic avoidance and magical thinking were employed in relation to men (78). Epidemiologic data from other recent studies and detailed discussion of the psychologic mechanisms of chronic pelvic pain without pathology are presented in Chapter 63 by Fordyce.

Benson and associates (80) studied 35 patients with pelvic pain, also without definite organic cause. Of these, 29 were diagnosed as neurotic, with most having hysterical personality disorders, and 6 were found to be psychotic. A significant relationship was noted between the pelvic pain and life stress events preceding the occurrence of the pain. In a study by Renaer (74) of 108 patients with pelvic pain, 28 patients were found with no obvious pelvic pathology. A psychiatric evaluation was done by a psychiatrist in 24 of the 28 patients, and definite psychopathologic problems were found in 20 of these patients.

Finally, the senior author, in collaboration with a psychiatrist, social worker, and psychologist, studied 25 gynecologic patients with pelvic pain of at least 6 months' duration (81). Gynecologic examination revealed that 15 (60%) had normal pelvic examinations, while 10 (40%) were found to have minor degrees of abnormality. Psychiatric evaluation showed 9 patients with borderline syndrome, 9 with severe or moderate hysterical character disorder, 4 with adolescent adjustment syndrome, 2 with passive-aggressive character disorder, and 1 with narcissistic character disorder. The social worker's interview revealed significant early childhood family dysfunction as well as adult family dysfunction. An unexpected finding of the study revealed that 9 of the 25 patients had a history of childhood incest and that 6 of 9 had a diagnosis of borderline syndrome. Psychologic testing using the Minnesota Multiphasic Personality Inventory (MMPI) showed four significant clusters, objectively corroborating the occurrence of severe psychopathology.

Symptoms and Signs

The most important symptom of this syndrome is lower abdominal pain and, less frequently, low back pain. Low abdominal pain can be felt either in the whole lower abdomen, in both iliac fossae, or unilaterally (Fig. 67-3). The pain is usually described as a vague discomfort that is continuously present at low levels, but exacerbation and remissions occur unrelated to anything the patient can identify. The pain can be brought on with intercourse or made worse by it (dyspareunia), but this does not prevent the patient from being sexually active. Various other gynecologic problems might be present such as dysmenorrhea, ovarian cysts, past infections, or infertility.

Patients can exhibit classic signs and symptoms of depression, such as loss of appetite, fatigue, insomnia, and loss of libido, or might only have a lack of ability to enjoy anything. Some patients can have a high energy level and poor impulse control, acting out anger in sociopathic ways sometimes directed against the physician. Others can somatize all emotions, dealing with stress by denial and repression and presenting a bland contented face to the world. As previously mentioned, a significant portion of these patients have experienced sexual abuse as children and as adults (81).

Some patients manifest abnormal illness behavior (82–84). They have a bodily preoccupation and conviction that they suffer from illness or disease, and they do not respond to reassurance by the physician. They maintain their symptoms—in this case, pain—to meet their psychologic needs to be dependent yet in control of the situation. Although they seek cure they continue to have their presenting complaint of pain in spite of all efforts to diagnose and treat it.

Some patients with chronic pelvic pain without obvious pathology have persistent pain as a result of positive or negative environmental factors (Chapter 16). In

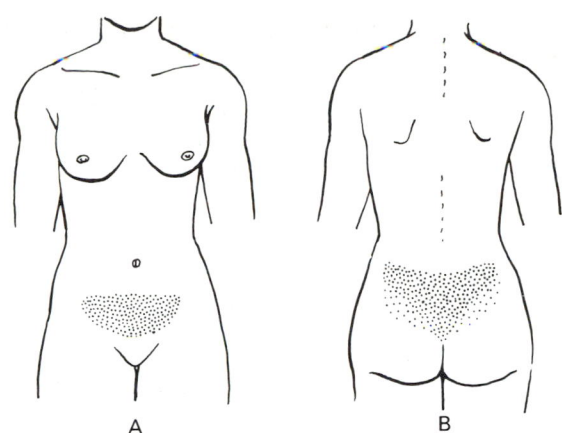

FIG. 67-3. Usual localization of chronic pain of gynecologic origin. **A.** Ventral zone. This generally does not extend above the level of the anterior superior iliac spines. **B.** Dorsal zone. This is localized in the skin overlying the cephalad half of the sacrum; it also extends laterally over the gluteal region.

our social system, physical illness elicits noncritical sympathy and support in which patients are cared for and absolved of all responsibility for their condition. In gynecologic patients (as in patients with other disease states), strong positive or negative reinforcing influences in the environment can cause the patient to develop "chronic pain behavior" or "learned pain," which persists beyond the time of cure of the gynecologic disorder.

Diagnosis

Patients who present with chronic pelvic pain without obvious pathology are a diagnostic challenge. Because all chronic illness and pain patients have significant behavioral components to their illness, these aspects of pain should be routinely evaluated. Serious psychopathology was found equally in patients both with and without organic pathology, so a psychologic and behavioral evaluation should be done on all chronic pelvic pain patients by a clinical psychologist with experience and expertise in managing patients with chronic pain (Chapter 33). Diagnostic measures to rule out all previously described organic problems should be employed appropriately in selective fashion and concurrently with the psychologic and psychosocial evaluation. Because many patients consider the suggestion that psychologic factors might be present as demeaning, criticizing, and threatening, it is important at the outset of the evaluation to make clear to patients that psychosocial evaluations are standard and routine in the evaluation of all patients. This often overlooked procedure, in addition to the psychologic focusing during the evaluation process, helps to prepare the patient for biologic, psychologic, and social impressions of the pelvic pain.

The findings of physical and psychologic evaluation should be presented by the gynecologist and a psychologist to the patient, and should include the patient's husband or partner to make the problem of pelvic pain overtly a family problem or joint concern.

If the pelvic examination is normal, these findings should be presented to the patient, and the benefits and risks of visualizing the pelvic organs by laparoscopy should be discussed. Some authors have advocated not doing so (77), but others have shown that pathology can be present even when a comprehensive pelvic examination reveals no abnormality. Moreover, most patients are unwilling to accept the diagnosis that nothing serious is wrong with their pelvic organs unless a gynecologist has verified this by carefully visualizing the pelvis. This information is also useful to the multiple health care providers usually involved with these patients, because it allows effective treatment programs to be proposed on a more rational basis.

Treatment

Both biologic and behavioral therapies can be employed for these patients. Organic problems should receive a conservative approach, and no treatment should be done without sufficient biologic justification merely in the hope that it will make the pain go away. The physician should avoid promises that any treatment will cure the pain because patients might need the pain to meet compelling psychologic needs. Successful treatment of chronic pain, however, involves identification and management of all factors contributing to the pain, including psychologic and behavioral disturbances. Appropriate therapeutic procedures should be suggested; these might include the use of antidepressants, antipsychotics, stress management, biofeedback, marital counseling, or a combination of these (85). Indeed, it is best to manage these patients with a multidisciplinary approach. In the study by Gross, Guzinski, and associates (81), at the time of follow-up (6 to 12 months after the evaluation), 53% of patients reported that pain was gone, 21% reported pain as less than before, and 26% reported that the pain was unchanged.

Great care should be taken not to perform surgical procedures or prescribe courses of medicine that are not directly and specifically indicated by the organic pathology present. These measures are likely to do more harm than good if insufficient organic pathology exists to justify them. The physician who treats those with chronic pelvic pain frequently finds it helpful to combine both the "disease model" and "the learning model" to understand and manage these difficult problems. Frequent follow-up, consistency of opinion, and behavioral support comprise the most workable plan for these difficult patients. More details of the psychologic management of these patients are found in Chapter 63 and Chapters 81 through 83.

REFERENCES

1. National Center for Health Statistics: Health. United States 1985. Department of Health and Human Services, Hyattsville, MD, 1985, Publ. No. (PHS) 86-1232.
2. National Center for Health Statistics: Advance Data. 1986 Summary: National Hospital Discharge Survey. Hyattsville, MD, Department of Health and Human Services, 1987, p. 112.
3. Sciarra, J.J., Droegemueller, W., and McElin, J.W. (eds.): Gynecology and Obstetrics. Philadelphia, Harper & Row, 1982.
4. Jeffcoate, N.: Principles of Gynaecology. 4th Ed. London, Butterworths, 1975.
5. Monif, G.R.G. (ed.): Infectious Diseases in Obstetrics and Gynecology. 2nd Ed. Philadelphia, Harper & Row, 1982.
6. Friedrich, E.G., Jr.: Vulvar Disease. Philadelphia, W.B. Saunders, 1976.
7. Pritchard, J.A., and MacDonald, P.C.: Williams Obstetrics. 16th Ed. New York, Appleton-Century-Crofts, 1980.
8. Kadar, N., Devore, G., and Romero, R.: Discriminating hCG zone: Its use in the sonographic evaluation for ectopic pregnancy. Obstet. Gynecol., 58:156, 1981.
9. Taylor, P.J., Leader, A., and Pattinson, H.A.: Conservative management of the unruptured tubal pregnancy. Int. J. Fertil., 29:149, 1984.
10. Weinstein, L., et al.: Ectopic pregnancy—a new surgical epidemic. Obstet. Gynecol., 61:698, 1983.
11. Dorfman, S.F.: Deaths from ectopic pregnancy, United States, 1979 to 1980. Obstet. Gynecol., 62:334, 1983.
12. Weström, L.: Effect of acute pelvic inflammatory disease on fertility. Am. J. Obstet. Gynecol., 121:707, 1975.
13. Eschenbach, D.A.: Epidemiology and diagnosis of acute pelvic inflammatory disease. Obstet. Gynecol., 55:132S, 1980.
14. Eschenbach, D.A., Harnisch, J.P., and Holmes, K.K.: Pathogenesis of acute pelvic inflammatory disease: Role of contraception and other risk factors. Am. J. Obstet. Gynecol., 128:838, 1977.
15. Lee, N.C., et al.: Type of intrauterine device and the risk of pelvic inflammatory disease. Obstet. Gynecol., 62:1, 1983.
16. Mishell, D.R., Jr.: Noncontraceptive health benefits of oral steroidal contraceptives. Am. J. Obstet. Gynecol., 142:809, 1982.
17. Eschenbach, D.A., et al.: Polymicrobial etiology of acute pelvic inflammatory disease. N. Engl. J. Med., 293:166, 1975.
18. Weström, L.: Clinical manifestations and diagnosis of pelvic inflammatory disease. J. Reprod. Med., 28:703, 1983.
19. Jacobson, L., and Weström, L.: Objectionalized diagnosis of acute pelvic inflammatory disease. Am. J. Obstet. Gynecol., 142:809, 1982.
20. Sweet, R.L.: Pelvic inflammatory disease. Sex. Transm. Dis., 13:192, 1986.
21. Centers for Disease Control: Sexually transmitted disease treatment guidelines. C.D.C. Morbid. Mortal. Weekly Rep. 31(Suppl.):335, 1982.
22. Ledger, W.: Surgical treatment of salpingo-oophoritis patients. J. Reprod. Med., 28:716, 1983.
23. Roberts, W., and Dockery, J.L.: Operative and conservative treatment of tubo-ovarian abscess due to pelvic inflammatory disease. South Med. J., 77:860, 1984.
24. Guinan, M.E., et al.: The course of untreated recurrent genital herpes simplex infection in 27 women. N. Engl. J. Med., 304:759, 1981.
25. Fiumara, J.J.: Herpes Simplex, Varicella, and Herpes Zoster. Current Concepts. Kalamazoo, Upjohn Co., 1983.
26. Ward, B.: New instrument for office treatment of cyst and abscess of Bartholin's gland. JAMA, 190:777, 1964.
27. Hager, W., et al.: Metronidazole for vaginal trichomoniasis: Seven-day vs. single-dose regimens. JAMA, 244:1219, 1980.
28. Eschenbach, D.: Vulvovaginal discharge. In Signs and Symptoms in Gynecology. Edited by B.M. Peckham and S.S. Shapiro. Philadelphia, J.B. Lippincott, 1983, pp. 254–261.
29. Nilsen, A., et al.: Efficacy of oral acyclovir in the treatment of initial and recurrent genital herpes. Lancet, 2:57, 1982.
30. Straus, S., et al.: Suppression of frequently recurring genital herpes: A placebo-controlled double-blind trial of oral acyclovir. N. Engl. J. Med., 310:1545, 1984.
31. Taylor, H.: The Nuprin Pain Report. New York, Lou Harris & Associates, 1985.
32. Lamb, E.: Clinical features of primary dysmenorrhea. In Dysmenorrhea. Edited by M.Y. Dawood. Baltimore, Williams & Wilkins, 1981, pp. 107–129.
33. Akerlund, M., Andersson, K., and Ingemarsson, J.: Effects of terbutaline on myometrial activity, endometrial flow, and lower abdominal pain in women with primary dysmenorrhea. Br. J. Obstet. Gynaecol., 83:673, 1976.
34. Filler, W., and Hall, J.: Dysmenorrhea and its therapy; a uterine contractility study. Am. J. Obstet. Gynecol., 106:104, 1970.
35. Chan, W.Y., Dawood, M.Y., and Fuchs, F.: Ibuprofin: Effect on prostaglandin levels in menstrual fluid. Am. J. Obstet. Gynecol., 135:102, 1979.
36. Dawood, M.Y.: Current concepts in the etiology and treatment of primary dysmenorrhea. Acta Obstet. Gynaecol. Scand. (Suppl.), 138:7, 1986.
37. Tolman, E.L.: Data presented at International Symposium on Premenstrual Tension and Dysmenorrhea, Kiawah Island, SC, 1983.

38. Pickels, V.R.: Prostaglandins in the human endometrium. Int. J. Fertil., *12*:335, 1967.
39. Moawad, A., and Bengtsson, L.: *In vitro* studies of the motility patterns of the nonpregnant human uterus. III. The effect of anovulatory pills. Am. J. Obstet. Gynecol., *106*:104, 1970.
40. Kullander, S., and Svanberg, L.: Terbutaline inhalation for alleviation of severe pain in essential dysmenorrhea. Acta Obstet. Gynaecol. Scand., *50*:425, 1981.
41. Smith, R.P.: Objective changes in intrauterine pressure during placebo treatment of dysmenorrhea. Pain, *29*:59, 1987.
42. Asplund, J.: The uterine cervix and isthmus under normal and pathological conditions. Acta Radiol., *91*(Suppl.):1, 1952.
43. Boerlum, K.G.: Infarction of an accessory spleen presenting as a uterine fibroid with necrosis. Am. J. Obstet. Gynecol., *143*:974, 1982.
44. Pittaway, D.E., and Fayez, J.A.: The use of CA-125 in the diagnosis and management of endometriosis. Fertil. Steril., *46*:790, 1986.
45. Fayez, J.A., and Taylor, R.B.: Endometriosis: Staging and management. Hosp. Physician, Nov. 26, 1984.
46. Sampson, J.A.: Peritoneal endometriosis due to the menstrual dissemination of endometrial tissue into the peritoneal cavity. Am. J. Obstet. Gynecol., *14*:422, 1927.
47. Gruenwald, P.: Origin of endometriosis from the mesenchyme of the coelomic walls. Am. J. Obstet. Gynecol., *44*:470, 1942.
48. Javert, C.T.: Observations on the pathology and spread of endometriosis based on the theory of benign metastasis. Am. J. Obstet. Gynecol., *62*:477, 1951.
49. Hobbs, J.E., and Bortnick, A.R.: Endometriosis of the lungs. Am. J. Obstet. Gynecol., *40*:832, 1940.
50. Darowski, W.P., and Scommegna, A.: The appropriate uses of medical and surgical therapy in endometriosis. *In* Reid's Controversy in Obstetrics and Gynecology, Vol. 3. Edited by F.P. Zuspan and C.D. Christian. Philadelphia, W.B. Saunders, 1983, pp. 543–553.
51. Taylor, H.C., Jr.: Vascular congestion and hyperemia. Am. J. Obstet. Gynecol., *57*:211, 1949.
52. Beard, R.W., et al.: Diagnosis of pelvic varicosities in women with chronic pelvic pain. Lancet, *2*:946, 1984.
53. Kresch, A.J., et al.: Laparoscopy in 100 women with chronic pelvic pain. Obstet. Gynecol., *64*:672, 1984.
54. Mattingly, R.F., and Thompson, J.D.: TeLinde's Operative Gynecology, 6th Ed. Philadelphia, J.B. Lippincott, 1985. pp. 561.
55. Thiels, G.H.: Coccygodynia and pain in the superior gluteal region. JAMA, *109*:1274, 1937.
56. McGivney, J.Q., and Cleveland, B.R.: The levator syndrome and its treatment. South. Med. J., *58*:505, 1965.
57. Sinaki, M., Merritt, J.L., and Stillwell, G.K.: Tension myalgia of the pelvic floor. Mayo Clin. Proc., *52*:717, 1977.
58. Sohn, N., Weinstein, M.A., and Robbins, R.D.: The levator syndrome and its treatment with high voltage electrogalvanic stimulation. Am. J. Surg., *144*:580, 1982.
59. Holst, J.: Hypnotic treatment in the levator ani(?) spasm syndrome. J. Psychosom. Obstet. Gynecol., *2*:111, 1983.
60. Clarke-Pearson, D.L., and Creasman, W.T.: Ovarian cancer. *In* Comprehensive Textbook of Oncology. Edited by A.R. Moossa, M.C. Robson, and S.C. Schimpff. Baltimore, Williams & Wilkins, 1986, pp. 845–854.
61. Doll, R., Muir, C., and Waterhouse, J. (eds.): International Union Against Cancer: Cancer Incidence in Five Continents, Vol. 2. Berlin, Springer-Verlag, 1970.
62. Young, R.C., Knapp, R.C., and Perez, C.A.: Cancer of the ovary. *In* Cancer: Principles and Practice of Oncology. Edited by V.T. DeVita, Jr., S. Hellman, and S.A. Rosenberg. Philadelphia, J.P. Lippincott, 1982, pp. 884–913.
63. Gershenson, D.M., et al.: Mixed germ cell tumors of the ovary. Obstet. Gynecol., *64*:200, 1984.
64. Mauch, P.M., and Bloomer, W.D.: Cancer of the uterine cervix. *In* Comprehensive Textbook of Oncology. Edited by A.R. Moossa, M.C. Robson, and S.C. Schimpff. Baltimore, Williams & Wilkins, 1986, pp. 855–863.
65. Greenwald, H.P., Bonica, J.J., and Bergner, M.: The prevalence of pain in four cancers. Cancer, *60*:2563, 1987.
66. Perez, C.A., Knapp, R.C., and Young, R.C.: Gynecologic tumors. *In* Principles and Practice of Oncology. Edited by V.T. DeVita, Jr., S. Hellman, and S.A. Rosenberg. Philadelphia, J.P. Lippincott, 1982, pp. 823–883.
67. Bloomer, W.D., and Mauch, P.M.: Carcinoma of the Endometrioma. *In* Comprehensive Textbook of Oncology. Edited by A.R. Moossa, M.C. Robson, and S.C. Schimpff. Baltimore, Williams & Wilkins, 1986, pp. 864–870.
68. Taylor, H.C., Jr.: Vascular congestion and hyperemia. Am. J. Obstet. Gynecol., *57*:637, 1949.
69. Taylor, H.C., Jr.: Pelvic pain based on vascular and autonomic nervous system disorder. Am. J. Obstet. Gynecol., *67*:1177, 1954.
70. Theobald, G.W.: Pelvic sympathetic syndrome. J. Obstet. Gynaecol., Br. Empire, *58*:733, 1951.
71. Dorpat, T.L.: Phantom sensations of internal organs. Compr. Psychiatry, *12*:27, 1971.
72. Allen, W.M., and Masters, W.H.: Traumatic laceration of uterine support. Am. J. Obstet. Gynecol., *70*:500, 1955.
73. DeBrux, J.A., et al.: Recurrent pelvic peritonitis. Am. J. Obstet. Gynecol., *102*:501, 1968.
74. Renaer, M., et al.: Psychic aspects of chronic pelvic pain in women. Am. J. Obstet. Gynecol., *134*:75, 1979.
75. Renaer, M.: Chronische pelvische et pijn zonder duidelijke pathologit. T. Geneesk., *32*:53, 1976.
76. Renaer, M.: Chronic Pelvic Pain in Women. Berlin, Springer-Verlag, 1981.
77. Renaer, M., and Guzinski, G.M.: Pain in gynecologic practice. Pain, *5*:305, 1978.
78. Duncan, C.H., and Taylor, H.C., Jr.: Psychosomatic study of pelvic congestion. Am. J. Obstet. Gynecol., *64*:1, 1952.
79. Gidro-Frank, L., Gordon, T., and Taylor, H.C., Jr.: Pelvic pain and female identity: A study of emotional factors in 40 patients. Am. J. Obstet. Gynecol., *79*:1184, 1960.
80. Benson, R.C., Hanson, K.H., and Matarazzo, J.D.: Atypical pelvic pain in women: Gynecologic-psychiatric considerations. Am. J. Obstet. Gynecol., *77*:806, 1959.
81. Gross, R.J., et al.: Borderline syndrome and incest in chronic pelvic pain patients. Int. J. Psychiatry Med., *10*:79, 1980–1981.
82. Pilowsky, I., and Spence, N.D.: Patterns of illness behavior in patients with intractable pain. J. Psychosom. Res., *19*:279, 1975.
83. Rosenthal, R.H., et al.: Chronic pelvic pain: Psychological features and laparoscopic findings. Psychosomatics, *25*:833, 1984.
84. DeVries, L., Levitan, Z., and Elbschitz, I.: Psychological evaluation in chronic pelvic pain (letter to the editor). J. Psychosom. Obstet. Gynecol., *2*:115, 1983.
85. Fordyce, W.E., Roberts, A.H., and Sternbach, R.D.: The behavioral management of chronic pain: A response to critics. Pain, *22*:113, 1985.

68 · PELVIC AND PERINEAL PAIN OF UROLOGIC ORIGIN

WILLIAM F. GEE *and* JULIAN S. ANSELL

with contributions by

JOHN J. BONICA

IN this chapter we discuss pain arising in the male urogenital organs and female urinary tract and related structures located in the bony pelvis. We cover afflictions directly attributable to diseases of the bony pelvis, ovarian tubes, uterus, or rectosigmoid colon only if they affect the urinary system or male genitalia. About 75% of patients seeking treatment for urinary symptoms suffer primarily or secondarily from infection (1). Approximately 3% of all women have positive urine cultures in clean voided specimens taken in surveys, but less than half are symptomatic, and only a small percentage have significant associated anatomic lesions (2). Less than 0.3% of males so surveyed are infected, but about half of those discovered to have infection have underlying uropathology (3).

Most painful conditions in the pelvis and perineum occur as a result of infection or distension of the bladder and/or perineum, but expanding neoplasms or extravasation of urine and seminal products outside the normal ducts and channels into the tissues can cause severe pain. Extravasation of seminal fluid may occur after vasectomy and produces disabling lancinating local pain. Extravasation of fluid into the perivesical structures during transurethral surgery produces pain even in patients anesthetized below the 9th thoracic nerve dermatome by subarachnoid block. This serves as a useful warning to the anesthesiologist and surgeon of the presence of extravasation and the need to consider early termination of the procedure to prevent the occurrence of the TUR syndrome of fluid overload and hyponatremia. Such pain is presumably mediated through the somatic nerves supplying the parietal peritoneum over the dome of the bladder and perhaps through the afferent sympathetic nerves that enter the spinal cord above the 10th thoracic segment. Unfortunately, some of the gravest chronic urinary tract diseases (e.g., massive dilation due to prolonged obstruction or advanced tuberculosis) may be accompanied by very little pain, possibly because the nerves mediating painful sensations have been altered or destroyed by the disease process.

The first part of this chapter includes discussion of the innervation of the pelvic urologic organs and male genitalia and some general comments about the pathology and symptoms of pain related to disorders of these structures. We then discuss the pathophysiology, symptoms and signs, diagnosis, and treatment of specific painful states of the bladder and urethra in males and females and of the prostate, seminal vesicles, epididymis and funiculus, testicle and appendages, and the penis. Although we make no attempt to provide a complete catalogue of diseases of the male and female urinary system and male generative tract, we try to mention those pathologic states and problems most likely to concern the physician trying to cope with patients with severe or unusually prolonged or difficult pain symptoms referrable to these organs. For a more complete understanding of urologic problems, the reader is referred to texts by Walsh et al. (3) and Smith (4). Ilioinguinal and genitofemoral nerve neuralgias are covered in other chapters of this book.

BASIC CONSIDERATIONS

Anatomic and Physiologic Aspects

Innervation of the Bladder and Urethra

Figure 68-1 depicts the nerve supply to the bladder, prostate, seminal vesicles, testicles, and penis, which constitutes a complex network involving many nerve pathways. The following discussion, which was written by Bonica, is derived from the first edition of this book (5). It is based on descriptions by Kuntz (6), Mitchell (7), Netter (8), and Ruch (9) and should be reviewed after study of the nerve supply to the entire pelvis as described in Chapter 65.

The Bladder

SYMPATHETIC NERVES. The peripheral sympathetic fibers to the bladder originate in the anterolat-eral cell column of the spinal cord at T12, L1, and L2 (and sometimes at T11) segments (Fig. 68-1B). They then pass sequentially through the anterior roots, the formed nerves, the white rami communicante, the lowest thoracic and upper two lumbar paravertebral sympathetic ganglia, and thence either through the lower (lesser) thoracic and upper two lumbar splanchnic nerves to the aortic plexus or caudad to the sacral sympathetic trunk. Those fibers that pass to the aortic plexus proceed caudally to the superior hypogastric plexus, the left and right hypogastric nerves, and the inferior hypogastric (pelvic) plexus to end in the vesical plexus. Some pre- and postganglionic fibers synapse in the inferior mesenteric ganglion and some in the superior hypogastric plexus, but the majority synapse in the extrinsic or intrinsic vesical plexuses. Those that pass to the sacral sympathetic trunk synapse therein with

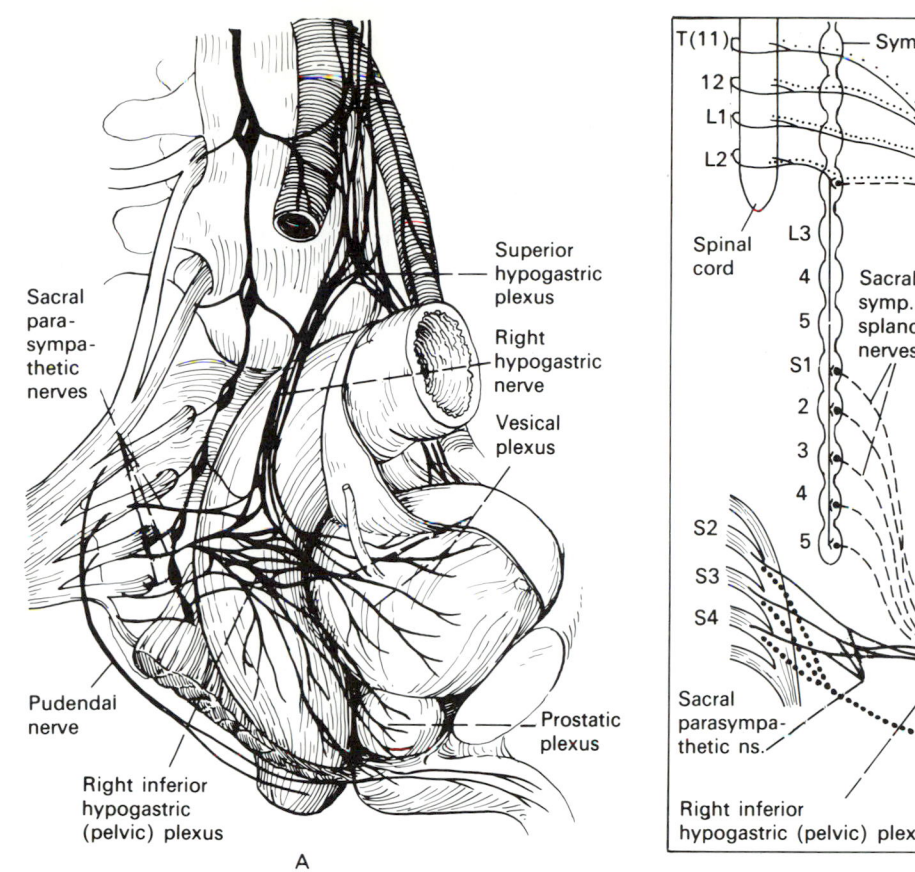

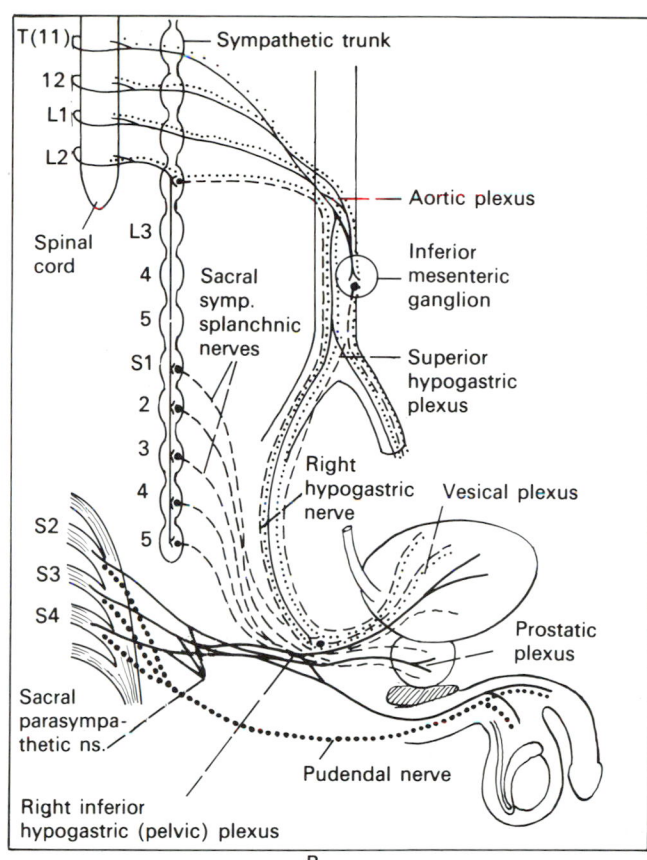

FIG. 68-1. *A.* Nerve supply of the urinary bladder and prostate showing the relationship of the various nerve structures to the large intestine and their distribution in the bladder and prostate. *B.* Schematic illustration showing the segmental nerve supply to the bladder, penis, and scrotum. Solid lines = preganglionic fibers; dashed lines = postganglionic fibers; and dotted lines = sensory fibers.

postganglionic fibers that proceed through the sacral sympathetic splanchnic nerves to also join the inferior hypogastric plexus.

PARASYMPATHETIC NERVES. The preganglionic parasympathetic neurons have their cell bodies in the 2nd, 3rd, and 4th sacral spinal cord segments. Their axons pass through the right and left pelvic splanchnic nerves (nervi erigentis) to end in the extrinsic and intrinsic vesical plexus where they synapse with the short postganglionic fibers.

AFFERENT NERVES. Afferent (sensory) nerves accompany both the sympathetic and parasympathetic efferent pathways. Many parasympathetic afferent fibers pass to the spinal cord via the ventral roots (see Chapter 3), and the rest pass through the usual course via the dorsal roots. In addition, the pudendal nerve supplies afferent fibers to the external and internal vesical sphincters and adjacent parts of the bladder. The peritoneum of the dome of the bladder is supplied by afferent fibers of T11 to L1 spinal nerves. The function of these nerves is discussed later.

INTRINSIC NERVES. The external vesical plexus containing sympathetic, parasympathetic, and afferent fibers penetrates the wall of the bladder to join the intrinsic plexus, which includes numerous ganglia. The intramural ganglia are most abundant in the trigone; they become less frequent as the distance from the trigone increases and are probably absent in the fundic area. The larger intramural ganglia and some of the

smaller ones are situated just below the serosa; other small ganglia are located between muscle bundles. These ganglia constitute relay stations between pre- and postganglionic fibers for both parasympathetic and sympathetic pathways. Most of the nerve fibers in the bladder wall are small and unmyelinated, although some are myelinated. Nerve endings with receptors are widely distributed in the mucosa and the submucosa; most of those in the trigone and adjacent areas are connected with afferent fibers that pass to the spinal cord with sympathetic nerves, whereas most of those farther removed from the base of the bladder are connected with afferent components of the pelvic nerves. Experiments further suggest that the parasympathetic fibers supply the detrusor muscle and that the sympathetic fibers supply blood vessels, Bell's muscle (pyloric muscle of the ureters), and the crista of the urethra.

NERVE FUNCTION. Animal and human studies (7) have revealed that stimulation of the entire sympathetic supply to the bladder results in powerful contraction of the orifices of the ureters, increased tonus in the trigone and contraction of the internal sphincter, and inhibition of the detrusor muscle. Temporary interruption of the sympathetic supply produces relaxation of the orifices, entire trigone, and internal sphincter and some increase in detrusor muscle activity. In contrast, parasympathetic stimulation elicits contraction of the detrusor muscle and relaxation of the trigone and sphincters.

The nociceptive (pain) pathways to the bladder and urethra are composed predominantly of the afferent fibers contained in the pelvic nerves with their cell body in the dorsal root ganglion of S2, S3, and S4. Numerous human studies detailed in the first edition of this book (5) demonstrated that following resection of the superior hypogastric plexus, there is no diminution of pain caused by distension of the bladder or application of tactile, thermal, or nociceptive stimuli to the bladder mucosa. In contrast, section of the posterior roots of S2, S3, and S4 or injuries of the conus medullaris or the pelvic nerves produce loss of all painful sensation. Langworthy et al. (10) reported vague sensation due to filling of the bladder in cases of paralysis or resection of the sacral nerves, but they regarded conduction of nociceptive impulses from the bladder through the superior hypogastric plexus as highly improbable. Although early clinical evidence seemed to indicate that resection of the superior hypogastric plexus produces relief of severe pain of vesical origin (11), the procedure eliminated spasm of the internal vesical sphincter and produced vasodilation.

The Male Urethra

The male urethra is innervated through the prostatic and cavernous plexuses, both of which are part of the pelvic plexus and include parasympathetic, sympathetic, and afferent fibers (Fig. 68-1). All of these have a similar course as the nerve supply to the bladder. The prostatic plexus is contiguous with the vesical plexus, lies in intimate contact with the prostate gland, and supplies fibers to the neck of the bladder, the prostate, and the prostatic urethra. The cavernous plexus, which may be regarded as an extension of the prostatic plexus along the urethra, gives off branches that communicate with branches of the pudendal nerves to supply the membranous and cavernous portion of the urethra.

The Female Urethra

The female urethra is innervated through the vaginal plexus, which is derived from the pelvic plexus, and contains sympathetic, parasympathetic, and afferent fibers. It is described in detail in Chapters 65 and 66.

Innervation of the Male Genitalia

Figure 68-2 shows the nerve supply to the male genitalia. The innervation of specific organs is described in the following sections.

The Testis and Spermatic Cord

The testis and the contents of the spermatic cord, which include the ductus deferens, are supplied by branches of the spermatic plexus, which is derived primarily from the aortic plexus but also from the renal and superior hypogastric plexuses. The spermatic plexus invests the spermatic artery throughout its course and includes chiefly sympathetic postganglionic and afferent fibers. Three groups of nerves contribute to the spermatic plexus: the rostral, intermediate, and caudal groups. Fibers in the rostral group are derived from the aortic and renal plexuses, extend along the spermatic artery, and terminate in the testis. Fibers of the intermediate group arise from the proximal portion of the superior hypogastric plexus, reach and enter the internal inguinal ring to course along the spermatic cord, and finally terminate by supplying the epididymis and the proximal portion of the vas deferens. Fibers in the caudal group are derived in part from a neural complex around the distal portion of the ureter and in part from fibers of the vesical plexus; they supply the distal portion of the vas deferens and epididymis and the seminal vesicles.

The nerves derived from the spermatic plexus are predominantly sympathetic and afferent fibers and transmit nociceptive impulses, whereas those that are

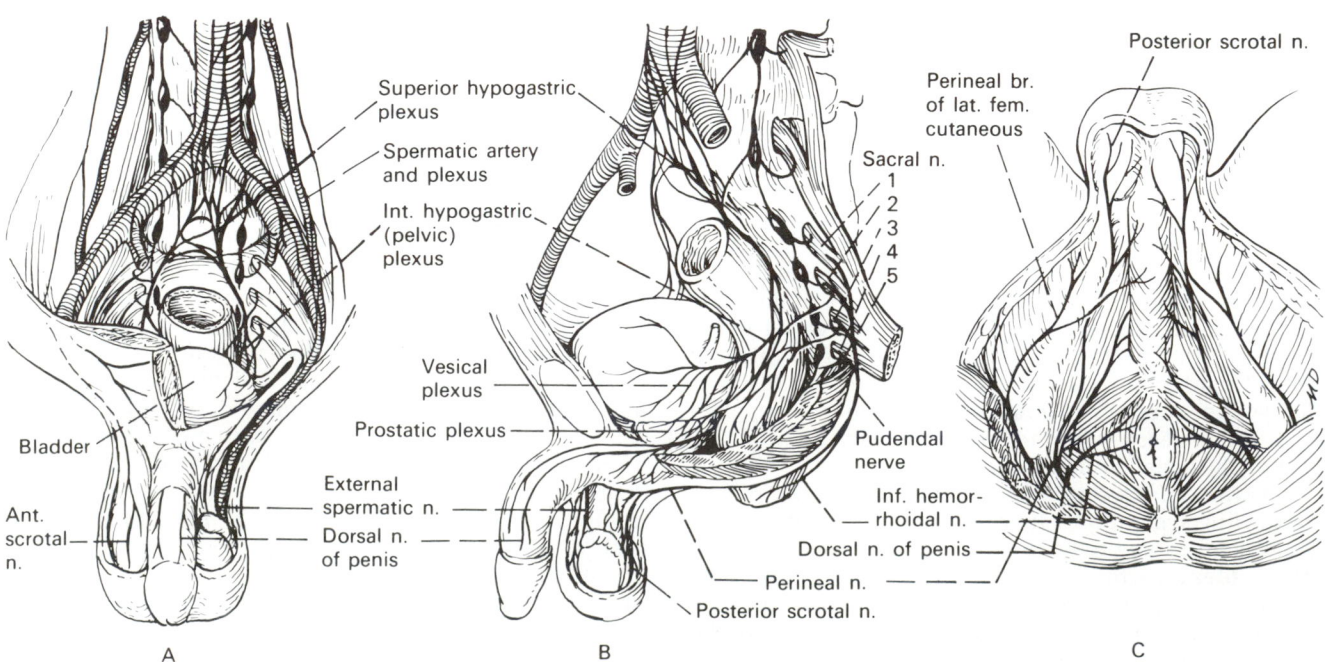

FIG. 68-2. Nerve supply of the male genitalia. *A.* Anterior view. *B.* Sagittal view. *C.* Perineal view.

derived from the vesical plexus contain parasympathetic fibers and contribute importantly to the supply of the vas deferens and also of the seminal vesicles. Preganglionic sympathetic neurons, which convey efferent impulses to these structures, have their cell bodies in the T10–L1 (and perhaps L2) segments. Most of the afferent fibers of the testes are components of the 10th thoracic spinal nerve; those that supply the epididymis reach the spinal cord at the T11 and T12 segments, while those that supply the vas deferens enter the spinal cord at T10–L1.

The Prostate

The prostate is supplied by the prostatic plexus, which is derived from the pelvic plexus and contains sympathetic, parasympathetic, and afferent (sensory) fibers. The course of these nerves to and from the spinal cord is similar to that described for the urinary bladder. Some of the fibers also supply the seminal vesicles and constitute an important supply to the penis.

The Scrotum

The skin and subcutaneous tissue and fascia of the scrotum are supplied by (a) small branches of the ilio-inguinal nerve; (b) the genital branch of the genito-femoral nerve; (c) the lateral posterior and medial posterior scrotal branches of the perineal nerve, which is a major branch of the pudendal nerve; and (d) the inferior pudendal branch of the posterior femoral cutaneous nerve.

The Penis

The sensory nerves of the glans and the skin covering the penis are contributed primarily by branches of the left and right dorsal nerves of the penis, which in turn are branches of the pudendal nerves and consist of fibers derived from the 3rd and 4th sacral nerves. The root of the penis also is supplied by filaments from the ilioinguinal nerves. The compressor urethrae, the ischio-cavernous, and the bulbocavernous muscles, which are the voluntary muscles employed in the act of ejaculation, are also innervated through branches of the pudendal nerve. The corpora are supplied by two sets of nerves, the greater and lesser cavernous nerves, which constitute the cavernous plexus and arise from the anterior part of the prostatic plexus; these are the nerves involved in penile erection. The greater cavernous nerve passes forward along the dorsum of the penis, joins the dorsal nerves of the penis, and is distributed to the corpus cavernosum of the penis; the lesser cavernous nerves perforate the fibrous covering of the penis and its root and are distributed to the corpora cavernosa and the corpus spongiosum of the urethra and the penile urethra. Vasoconstrictive fibers derived from the hypogastric plexuses join the pudendal nerves to be distributed through its branches to the blood vessels of the penis.

Physiologic Aspects

Micturition

Normal micturition is in part reflex and in part a voluntary act. The micturition reflex involves afferent and efferent fibers that send impulses to and from the middle three sacral segments where the reflex center is located in the conus medullaris of the spinal cord, which is found at the level of the 1st lumbar vertebral body (12). These centers in turn are under cortical control, which can either facilitate or inhibit the voiding reflex. Habib (13) studied the effects of stimulating the individual sacral nerves involved in the voiding reflex and found that the 2nd sacral nerve played no function, whereas stimulation of the 3rd and 4th sacral nerves caused detrussor contraction and concomitant decreased sphincter resistance. Stimulation of the 4th sacral nerve, however, caused better voiding because of the decreased resistance by the sphincters. Apparently the sympathetic nerves play no role in voiding, whereas the pudendal nerves, via their control of the external urinary sphincter, allow a person to voluntarily shut off his or her urinary stream.

Ejaculation

In males, stimulation of the sympathetic nerves causes the expulsion of semen from the ejaculary tract by contraction of the musculature of the seminal vesicles and expulsion of secretions from the prostatic duct by contraction of the smooth muscles of the prostate gland.

Erection

Penile erection, as is well known, can occur as a purely reflex action in response to psychic stimulation. It is mediated primarily through parasympathetic nerves, which reach the cavernous tissue through the prostatic plexus. Although the cavernous tissue also is supplied by sympathetic fibers, these are not essential for erection. Moreover, their stimulation generally tends to inhibit erection by producing arteriolar constriction and a consequent decrease in blood flow into the cavernous tissue. Erection is characterized by dilatation of the arterioles, which coincides with inhibition of the smooth muscles in the walls of the venous sinuses and partial closure of their outlets through the small smooth channels. Afferent fibers in the pudendal nerves are also important for erection, and severance of these nerves causes loss of erection as well as ejaculation due to paralysis of the compressor urethra, ischiaocavernosus, and bulbocavernosus muscles.

Failure of semen to be discharged through the urethra following lumbar sympathectomy in males led to the initial conclusion that ejaculation is abolished by denervation of the upper lumbar sympathetic chain. However, in a study of male patients who had had bilateral extirpation of the sympathetic trunk from the T9 to the L3 segment, Retief (14) found that ejaculation took place, but that semen was discharged into the urinary bladder instead of distally into the urethra. The reason for this was that the internal vesical sphincter was not closed at the time of ejaculation due to the absence of impulses conducted through the sympathetic nerves. Kedia et al. (50) showed that denervation of the deferential ducts prevents peristalsis and aspermia results.

Pathophysiology and Symptoms

Disorders of the bladder neck and trigone produce pain referred to the urethra, perineum, and glans of the penis or clitoris, whereas pain of prostatic origin is most often referred to the perineum behind the scrotum or to the rectum. The close association of all the pelvic viscera and their nerve supply, however, often results in direct spread of inflammatory changes to adjacent structures or mediation of severe pain by adjacent pathways in such a manner as to make the localization of the disease process on the basis of subjective symptoms a most difficult task.

Discomfort in the organs of the pelvis is generally relieved by warmth and exacerbated by cold temperatures. Patients with urinary symptoms are best off staying in warm surroundings, taking hot sitz baths, and applying heat locally. Medications that increase the frequency of urination (e.g., diuretics) or increase central awareness exacerbate symptoms referable to the urinary system. Thus, caffeine-containing foods and drinks (coffee, tea, colas, chocolate) should be avoided because they are both central stimulants and diuretics.

Pain Related to the Bladder and Urethra

Pain related to urination (dysuria) is most often described as burning or scalding in character and can occur at the beginning of urination (initial), throughout urination (total), or in a terminal crescendo, which may persist for a time after voiding is completed. Initial dysuria is most likely to be related to lesions causing breaks in the mucosa of the urethra or denudation of perineal skin such as gonococcal mucositis, herpetic ulcerations, and excorations incurred as a result of scratching during a pinworm infestation. When hypertonic solutions such as urine wet mucosal or epidermal surfaces that have been stripped of their protective covering, a painful stimulus occurs. Total dysuria probably localizes the offending process to the urethra and bladder. Terminal discomfort may be caused by lesions of the bladder, urethra or prostate. Strangury—the excruciatingly painful, difficult, and slow passage of urine accompanied by spasm of the urethra and bladder—is usually the result of severe inflammation.

Bladder Disorders

In males, pain caused by bladder disorders may be referred to the distal urethra, or under the surface and glans of the penis. The latter occurs particularly when the bladder neck and prostatic urethra are the affected parts. In females, bladder lesions commonly produce referred pain in the urethra, perimeatal skin, and clitoral region.

Urinary frequency commonly accompanies other urinary symptoms and may be a symptom of infection or bladder obstruction when it occurs both at night and in the daytime. Nocturnal frequency, unaccompanied by daytime symptoms, is more likely associated with cardiac problems and nocturnal mobilization of fluid than disease of pelvic organs. Enuresis is not painful per se, but a good deal of social unease accompanies such accidents. Urinary urgency, almost uncontrollable desire to urinate immediately, is another irritative symptom due to inflammation, and about 10% of all individuals have a degree of bladder instability manifested as urgency (16). Adults who manifest daytime urinary frequency and urgency but do not have nocturia may be reacting to emotional or other stress.

Pain due to distension of the bladder has two compo-

nents. The first is the intrinsic response to stretch and is felt suprapubically as an uncomfortable need to void. The second is due to lifting and stretching of the peritoneum overlying the bladder dome and is a more visceral and vague discomfort. This visceral sensation, mediated by the splanchnic nerves, is useful to paraplegics and others whose pudendal afferents and sacral nerve connections have been severed because they can readily learn to interpret this sensation as a need to empty the bladder. It may also contribute to the autonomic dysreflexia occasionally seen in such individuals.

Positional discomfort or pain related to activity can occur in patients with bladder calculi. The portion of the bladder with the greatest concentration of nerve endings in relation to area is the trigone. Therefore, patients with bladder stones may experience relief of irritation in the supine position when the stone rolls off the trigone onto another surface, or exacerbation of symptoms with jogging due to the stone bouncing on the trigone. Submucosal extravasation of urine through tears or cracks may be a part of the discomfort felt in interstitial cystitis and other entities. In these conditions, fixation of the normally mobile and elastic mucosal lining may occur as a result of scarring with secondary tearing as the bladder distends and pulls the mucosa away from a point of abnormal fixation.

Urethral Disorders

The urethra has a mucosal lining and contains compound glands and ducts in the walls. Pain can occur as a result of acute inflammation secondary to infection, the presence of irritating chemicals (bubble bath, cyclophosphamide) or foreign bodies, and trauma, which may be self-inflicted or produced by iatrogenic instrumentation. Accumulation of secretions in one of the glands lining the urethra can also produce a sensation of fullness or discomfort in the perineum, vagina, or rectum, which, although rarely excruciating, can be severely annoying if it persists. Acute conditions are usually associated with terminal dysuria or even strangury and at times tenesmus. Chronic pain is referred to the perineum, urethral meatus, clitoris, or glans penis.

Pain Related to the Prostate and Seminal Vesicles

An inflamed or distended prostate may evoke complaints of rectal fullness or discomfort, tenesmus, perineal pain and fullness, difficulty in voiding, decrease in stream size, frequency due to trigonal stretch, and ultimately retention of urine, which is severely painful. Marked enlargement of the prostate can intrude upon and compress the rectal lumen to the point of obstructing the passage of stool. On the other hand, severe perineal discomfort and spasm of the levator or perineal diaphragmatic muscles can precipitate urinary retention. This is most likely to occur in males following hemorrhoidectomy or in females after gynecologic surgery.

Disorders of the seminal vesicles can be associated with ipsilateral lower abdominal or groin pain as well as referred pain to the gonad, perineum, and phallus. Significant lesions of the seminal vesicles unassociated with disease of the contiguous prostate are extremely rare.

Pain Related to the Scrotal Contents and Penis

Infection is the most common cause of distension of the epididymis, which results in pain and tenderness. Chemical inflammation can occur as a result of retrograde flow of urine down the ejaculatory ducts, which occasionally takes place traumatically during contact sports or when congenital or acquired obstructing urethral lesions create high proximal voiding pressures. Recently, some experimental drugs have been reported to cause painful distension of the epididymis (17).

Pain caused by distension of the epididymis may radiate up the affected spermatic cord into the groin. Since the embryonic origin and nerve supply are almost the same as those of the kidney and renal pelvis, it should not be surprising that the pain may mimic renal colic. The physician should examine the genitalia of any patient with flank pain and, conversely, suspect organs in the flank of patients with labial or scrotal pain when there is no local pathology.

Testicular pain can occur as a result of infection, typically viral, or by extension from epididymides infected with sexually transmitted diseases; in association with traumatic rupture or hematoma; and infarction from torsion. Such pain is severe and may be accompanied by nausea and vomiting. Acute congestion of the male gonadal structures as a result of sexual stimulation can also be painful. Smooth muscle, which contracts the tough tunica albiginea of the testicle, can produce such pain by increasing intratesticular pressure.

As indicated already, pain is frequently referred to the penis from the bladder (particularly bladder neck and trigone), urethra, prostate, and occasionally the seminal vesicles. Thus referred pain is the commonest pain experienced. Primary pain of the penis is associated with specific lesions to be discussed in later sections.

PELVIC UROLOGIC DISORDERS

Diseases of the Bladder

Acute Bacterial Cystitis

Acute uncomplicated cystitis is a common problem, particularly in young women, with characteristic symptoms of urinary frequency and urgency, dysuria, and often hematuria. About 80% of cases are due to sensitive E. coli and respond promptly to antibiotics (18). If response to treatment is not prompt or symptoms recur rapidly following completion of a 5- to 10-day course of appropriate therapy, or if the symptoms return three or more times within a year, further evaluation is indicated to rule out the possibility that underlying structural problems are involved. At a minimum, some test of renal function and imaging of the urinary tract are indicated in such individuals. Women who have flank pain and fever accompanying their cystitis and all males with cystitis also should have an imaging evaluation. The pain of acute cystitis leaves within hours in response to antibiotic control of the infection. Hot sitz baths or warm heating pads to the perineum relieve some of the associated muscular spasm. Pain of urination can also be diminished if the patient urinates while in a warm tub.

Chronic Cystitis

Etiology

Chronic cystitis occurs at any age in either sex but is most common among women who are middle aged and older. The differential diagnosis must include interstitial cystitis, female urethral syndrome, and urinary symptoms of psychosocial origin. The major diagnostic criterion of chronic cystitis is persistence of organisms in the urine on culture, but this is not as straightforward as it sounds. In patients with the chronic disease, the commonly accepted colony count of 100,000 organisms per ml of urine does not serve to separate infected from uninfected individuals. In chronic cases, persistent cultures of the same organisms in counts as low as 1000 colonies per ml may be significant (17). Also under these conditions, organisms usually regarded as nonpathogens (e.g., Staphylococcus epidermidis, alpha-hemolytic streptococci, and yeast) can be offending pathogens if cultured repeatedly in relatively pure growth. An important cocriterion is the presence of white blood cells in the urine.

Patients with chronic cystitis need complete evaluation of their urinary tracts to rule out associated anatomic lesions such as vesicoureteral reflux, ureterocele, bladder diverticula, urethral diverticula, and vesicovaginal fistula as well as chronic upper tract problems such as infected stones, which might be seeding the bladder with bacteria.

Diagnosis and Treatment

The symptoms of chronic cystitis are similar to those of acute cystitis, only less severe, and occur when bacteria are cultured from the urine. When the patient is bacteria-free, the symptoms usually are absent. In contrast to patients with psychosocial problems who rarely have nocturia, patients with chronic infection almost always have nocturia while infected. Depression can play a role in both conditions. The urine is usually clear of significant sediment and bacteria in interstitial cystitis. Pus can often be expressed from urethral diverticula by gently stripping the urethra on physical examination.

Causes of depression, if present, should be sought and treated. At the same time, treatment is started with a loading dosage of an appropriate antibiotic, which is maintained in chronic low dosage for 6 months to years in some patients. A typical regimen would be nitrofurantoin (Macrodantin) 50 mg bid or trimethoprim and sulfamethoxazole 1 regular strength tablet twice a day. Pain almost always subsides with appropriate antibiotic therapy.

Interstitial Cystitis

Etiology

The cause of interstitial cystitis is unknown, but the disease is characterized by fibrosis of all the layers of the bladder. Late in the disease in severe cases the entire bladder may be markedly scarred and contracted. Walsh (19) stated, "Interstitial cystitis is a disease of extremes: extremely severe symptoms; extremes of overdiagnosis and underdiagnosis; etiologic theories varying from the abstruse to the fashionable; treatment ranging from the alpha of vitamin prescription to the omega of radical bladder substitution surgery; and sadly often, extreme confusion in medical thinking." The disease is 10 times more common in women than in men and more common in the middle-aged individual, but it does occur in children. Oravisto (20) found in a complete survey of the disease in Finland that only 1 in 10 cases was considered severe. In Oravisto's series, the disease initially progressed rapidly then stabilized at a given individual plateau from which it subsequently varied little in most patients. The disease seemed milder in men. The presence of antinuclear antibodies in many patients (19–22) suggests that an autoimmune disorder is an important etiologic factor.

Diagnosis

The symptomatic hallmark for interstitial cystitis is pain, which is usually most severe when the bladder is full and is most often suprapubic in location, although it can have perineal components, particularly in males. The pain is relieved by emptying the bladder. No significant organisms grow in culture, and the urinalysis is unremarkable unless there is coincidental bacterial infection. Diagnosis requires endoscopy and overdistension of the bladder under regional or general anesthesia. Ordinarily these patients experience such pain with bladder filling that they cannot tolerate cystoscopy under local anesthesia. To make the diagnosis, the bladder must be examined while only partly filled following overdistension. The typical punctate petecchiae seen in many places in the bladder mucosa establish the diagnosis. Bladder biopsies must always be taken in these patients to rule out the occasional individual with in situ bladder cancer, which can present with the same symptoms and have a similar appearance endoscopically.

Treatment

DILATION. Treatment of this painful entity is at times frustrating for both patient and physician. The standard treatment over the years has been periodic overdistension of the bladder under anesthesia when urinary frequency or suprapubic pain becomes unbearable. Most clinicians allow the patient's symptoms to direct the frequency of dilation because stretching on a regularly timed or prophylactic basis does not seem to improve results. Dilation may be done hydraulically with simple gravity flow or with the aid of a distensible balloon in the bladder whose pressure is carefully monitored. Bladder rupture has been reported under these circumstances (23). Although intentional rupture has not been advocated as therapy, Higson et al. (24) noted that patients whose bladders have been accidentally ruptured in this way do much better for a long period afterwards than those whose bladders remain intact during stretching.

DRUG THERAPY. As might be expected, a great variety of medications have been used to treat interstitial cystitis. The established inflammatory response and the finding of antinuclear antibodies in these patients would seem to favor anti-inflammatory therapy, yet treatment with steroidal and nonsteroidal anti-inflammatory agents has not given lasting benefit in the vast majority of cases in which these have been applied locally or given systemically.

Topical application of dimethyl sulfoxide (DMSO) in a 50% solution was reported to provide relief in 60 to 70% of cases, being statistically significantly better than placebo (25). The DMSO solution has been applied to the skin of the lower abdomen by the patient in some studies, but most suggest instilling DMSO solution into the bladder through a catheter and having the patient hold it in the bladder for 30 to 60 min.

DENERVATION. In the first edition of this book, Bonica (5) noted that in the 1930s a number of respected clinicians, including Leriche and Mandl, reported relief of pain associated with severe chronic cystitis following a lumbar sympathetic blockade. Bonica also described his own experience with this procedure, which provided only some improvement in a small series of patients. These procedures had been prompted in part by the reports of Learmonth and Braasch (26), Nesbit and McLellan (11), and others that resection of the superior hypogastric plexus gave uniformly good results in patients with chronic intractable pain due to cystitis and associated vesical spasm. In view of the fact that sensory supply to the bladder is primarily through the sacral segments, these authors suggested that relief of vesical pain following the operation was caused not by interruption of nociceptive pathways but by alteration in the blood supply and reduction of spasm in the region of the trigone and bladder neck. A decade later, however, Jacobsen et al. (27) concluded that "although partial or temporary relief of vesical pain often is observed, permanent relief followed only occasionally, and in this respect, the operation has been found wanting." Similar opinions have been expressed by White and Sweet (28).

Bonica (5) reported that patients with severe vesical spasm accompanied by intractable pain, in whom lumbar sympathetic block had failed to produce relief, experienced complete temporary relief after transacral block of the 2nd, 3rd, and 4th sacral nerves with 0.15% tetracaine, which produces prolonged analgesia. He also used continuous caudal block to provide highly effective but only temporary relief of severe intractable bladder pain. Although others suggested prolonged blockade with neurolytic agents, this procedure as well as posterior rhizotomy of the segments causes loss of bladder and rectal sensation and penile erection and orgasm; therefore, these procedures are impractical for definitive therapy.

SURGERY. Relief for those with severely contracted bladders has been achieved by resecting all the bladder except the trigone and anastomosing the cecum or small bowel to the remaining trigone to serve as a substitute reservoir (29). In other patients, urine has been diverted to the colon or through an intestinal conduit to the skin, where the urine is collected in a plastic receptacle (30). Attempts at supratrigonal denervation by resecting the bladder from its trigone and reanastomosing it afterwards have resulted in contracted useless bladders in some patients.

Radiation Cystitis and Postirradiation Contracted Bladder

Etiology

The effects of radiation on the bladder can be separated into two phases. The acute phase is an immediate inflammatory response to radiation consisting of edema, mild infiltration, and some hemorrhage, which usually clears in weeks to months. The chronic phase is a delayed obliterative endarteritis accompanied by scar formation, varying degrees of contraction of the bladder, and ulceration of the mucosa, which can occur from 1 to several years following radiation therapy but usually within 3 years. The increasing use of radiation in the treatment of pelvic malignancy has resulted in more disorders of this nature, although better control of radiation fields has kept the increased incidence of chronic radiation cystitis well below that expected by the increased usage of radiation for pelvic neoplasms.

Symptoms and Treatment

ACUTE PHASE. The acute phase of radiation cystitis presents with symptoms that are similar to those of acute bacterial cystitis; frequency, dysuria, and urgency the common triad. The urine is usually sterile. Treatment with anticholinergic drugs such as propantheline 15 mg qid or oxybutenone 1 tablet qid sometimes is helpful. Some patients require added sedatives systemically such as barbiturates and codeine. Aspirin is not advised because it is largely excreted in the urine and can be locally irritating, and because of its effects on platelet function, which may worsen the bleeding propensity of irradiated mucosa.

Belladonna and opiate (B&O) suppositories taken per rectum every 4 hours give relief in some stubborn cases. If at all possible, bladder catheterization is avoided while radiation therapy is ongoing because the risk of infection is increased by the presence of a foreign body, as is the local irritation and trauma. Also to be avoided if possible are known irritants and diuretics. If superimposed infection is proven by culture, appropriate antibiotics should be prescribed. The acute phase can progress to the chronic phase and ultimately to a contracted bladder.

CHRONIC PHASE. Treatment of contracted bladder, which can occur in the chronic phase of postirradiation cystitis, is difficult. Symptoms are similar to those of interstitial cystitis with the added problem of hemorrhage, which at times causes clot retention and life-threatening loss of blood. If blood loss is massive, endoscopic fulguration of bleeding sites is required. When diffuse oozing is present, other methods have been tried including balloon inflation within the bladder under regional anesthesia or instillation of protein-precipitating agents, such as 5% silver nitrate or even 10% formalin, in desperate circumstances. Augmentation cystoplasty with small or large bowel has also been used with some success in selected patients. Palliative diversion of urine is not helpful unless the bladder is also removed because hemorrhage and discomfort often persist in spite of urinary diversion.

At least partial pain relief can be obtained by regional nerve blocks followed by section of the 3rd sacral nerve roots or cordotomy in severe cases with limited projected life span (31).

Chronic Tuberculous Cystitis

Tuberculous cystitis, if severe, can present with symptoms and problems very similar to those of chronic radiation cystitis. These patients are most commonly found to have pyuria with mixed infections, but the pyuria fails to clear with control of the usual pathogens. The patient's history should be reviewed for significant tuberculosis contacts. If positive, tuberculosis should be sought by culture and biopsy; the latter often yields the diagnosis first.

Patients with chronic tuberculous cystitis often respond to antituberculosis drugs with symptomatic relief. Periodic evaluation of the upper urinary tracts during therapy is necessary because ureteral scarring and stenosis can occur in the presence of antituberculosis drugs and result in upper-tract damage if not suspected and treated by ureteral stenting or other measures. Should the disease progress to the contracted bladder stage in spite of therapy, augmentation cystoplasty or diversion sometimes is necessary. Treatment of this condition with nerve blocks has been tried only occasionally but may be worth trial.

Schistosomal Bladder Infection

Symptoms and Signs

Schistosomal infection of the bladder, caused by Schistosoma haematobium, produces symptoms similar to those seen in tuberculous and postirradiation cystitis with the additional symptoms of necroturia (passage of necrotic tissue) and urethral stricture in advanced cases. The initial episodes of infection are usually accompanied by cutaneous hyperemia and itching; the late stages, depending on the degree of involvement, may duplicate the spectrum of symptoms seen in other chronic inflammatory processes involving the bladder with additional symptoms of urethral stricture, since the urethra is often affected also. Pitting and scarring of the glans penis and palpable fibrous masses in the perineum sometimes are present.

Diagnosis and Treatment

The differential diagnosis is aided by a history of exposure to S. haematobium in endemic regions of North Africa and the Middle East. Radiographs of the urinary tract may show submucosal and/or intramural calcification of the affected bladder, ureters, seminal vesicles, and prostate. The disease has as a late complication the development of squamous carcinoma of the bladder, which is treated in the same way as other types of bladder cancer.

Treatment of schistosomiasis (bilharziasis) now is simplified by the development of specific antischistosomal agents such as trichlorfon (Bilarcil) and praziquantel (Biltricide) for use orally. Chronic and advanced cases may require any or all of the measures described for tuberculous and radiation cystitis along with removal of calculi and treatment of urethral strictures. Ideally, endoscopy should be performed periodically on a prophylactic basis to remove stones and observe for the development of secondary cancer.

Pain control is complicated by the protean involvement of the urinary tract and male accessory genitalia. The chronic and slow progress of the disease may destroy some of the nociceptive fibers. Measures such as nerve blocks, rhizotomy, and cordotomy can help some victims of this terrible disease. The prognosis in this disease is as grave as that in cancer of the bladder.

Cancer of the Bladder

In its early stages transitional cell cancer of the bladder is typically painless. Pain occurs late in the disease due to spread of tumor, scarring, or postirradiation changes similar to those discussed previously. Pain due to metastatic bone disease, which can occur in any part of the skeleton, is treated in a fashion similar to bony metastases from other visceral mucosal tumors. Radiation of locally painful metastases and chemotherapeutic agents, with their low yields of tumor control, are all we can offer.

Pain due to ureteral obstruction by intrinsic or extrinsic tumor growth may be relieved, when possible, by local transurethral resection of the blocking tumor or by passing a stent endoscopically through the obstructed channel to the kidney. Such Silastic stents can be left in place for months and changed as needed. When it is impossible to achieve relief of obstruction by retrograde catheterization, drainage can be achieved through percutaneous nephrostomy and antegrade passage of guide wires followed by stenting Silastic catheters. The percutaneous procedure can be performed with the aid of local infiltration anesthesia and the retrograde catheterization with the use of topical lidocaine (Xylocaine) jelly in high-risk individuals.

Erectile dysfunction is one of the less often discussed side effects of cystoprostatectomy, cordotomy, presacral neurectomy, and pelvic irradiation. The loss of ability to perform sexually because of erectile dysfunction can be relieved by implantation of simple rodlike prostheses in the corpora cavernosa, which allow the patient to overcome iatrogenic erectile inadequacy. The simplest of these devices can be placed with regional anesthesia including local infiltration.

Diseases of the Urethra

Acute Urethritis in Males

Sexually transmitted disease is by far the commonest cause of acute urethritis in males, and its symptoms respond dramatically to specific antibiotic therapy. Chlamydia infections can become chronic, but the symptoms are usually so mild that reassurance about the natural history of the disease is enough to satisfy all but the most guilt-ridden sufferers.

Only rarely does sufficient pain develop to require more than the usual management of acute pain. If the pain becomes severe and is unrelieved with the use of analgesic medication, several blocks of the pudendal nerve with a local anesthetic or continuous caudal analgesia limited to the sacral segments can be used for several days to provide relief. In the extremely rare patient who has severe persistent and disabling pain that is not relieved with temporary pudendal blocks, alcohol block or neurectomy can be considered. It is important to note, however, that destructive procedures provide relief for only 6 to 12 months, after which the pain returns. Moreover, the neurolytic block is often followed by postchemical neuropathy and indirectly can cause a neuroma, which is likely to involve additional and even more severe pain (see Chapter 73).

Acute Urethritis in Females

Acute urethritis in females independent of cystitis is most frequently associated with sexually transmitted diseases such as Chlamydia infection, herpes, trichomoniasis, and gonorrhea. As in males, the usual response to specific antimicrobial treatment is prompt and gratifying pain relief. Genital herpes may recur with chronically painful lesions, which often require systemic relaxants; if absolutely necessary, potent narcotics such as methadone can be given by mouth. Because of the problem of physical dependence and possible addiction, patients on this therapeutic regimen must be closely monitored. The principles of this therapy are described in Chapter 67A. Urethral inflammation can also be produced chemically by "bubble bath" soaps (32).

Female Urethral Syndrome

Etiology

The symptom complex termed urethral syndrome, which is also called psychosomatic cystitis and chronic urethritis, is the female equivalent of chronic prostatitis in males and probably acutely affects as many as half of the women aged 15 to 50 years who are said to have cystitis (17). Because the causes of chronic urethral syndrome are multiple, treatment directed only at a single specific cause often fails. Depression and stress appear to contribute to this entity, as do local trauma, dysfunctional voiding patterns, sexual frustration, vaginitis, concerns about sexually transmitted diseases, and guilt about sexual fantasies and feelings. It is also probable that a variety of minor local problems are operative including blocked and distended urethral glands, prolapsing urethral mucosa, postmenopausal epithelial changes, inflammatory polyps in the urethral mucosa, urinary frequency related to menstrual fluid retention and its diuresis, previous experience with cystitis or sexually transmitted disease, and fear of recurrence or cancerophobia triggered by minimal urethral symptoms.

Symptoms and Diagnosis

Characteristic symptoms are dysuria, burning on urination, or a burning or irritated sensation in the periurethral area or perineum not necessarily associated with urination but perhaps exacerbated by it. The symptoms are most prominent during waking hours with little or no nocturnal disturbance. Typically, the urinary sediment is unremarkable, and urine cultures grow limited quantities of mixed flora or nothing. The following conditions must be considered in the differential diagnosis: interstitial cystitis, urethral diverticulum, urethral caruncle, stricture, vesicovaginal or urethrovaginal fistulae, vaginitis, vulvar and perineal cutaneous problems, chronic yeast infestation, pinworm infestation, postmenopausal mucosal and skin alterations, diabetic neuropathy, and tuberculosis.

If the primary involvement is vaginal, a vaginal discharge usually precedes the urinary symptoms. Vaginal discharge occurring after treatment with antibiotics for urinary symptoms usually is secondary to yeast infestation. Examination of the perineum may reveal excoriation, herpetic lesions, urethral caruncle, or mucosal prolapse. In the case of a urethral diverticulum, gentle stripping of the urethra by stroking through the anterior vaginal wall may express pus through the urethral meatus.

In patients with persistent symptoms of this type, an intravenous pyelogram should be obtained to make certain that there are no lesions of the upper urinary tracts producing referred symptoms. Allowing contrast medium to accumulate in the bladder and looking at a voiding film of the urethra is the least traumatic way of imaging the organ. Cystourethroscopy also is required in many of these patients to provide absolute assurance that no serious disease process is present to account for the symptoms (33–35).

Treatment

The most important aspect of treatment for female urethral syndrome is the process of ruling out serious illness or any potential for serious illness in the organs of the region. Carefully listening to the patient, who needs to feel that she is really being heard, followed by a gentle and thorough physical examination enhances the patient's confidence in the physician. Then appropriate diagnostic studies to confirm or deny the presence of local pathology must be obtained and reviewed. Lesions found must be discussed and addressed. These diagnostic and therapeutic maneuvers may take several sessions with the patient.

If the problem is dysfunctional voiding or sexual behavior, retraining should be considered. Communication problems between partners should be discussed, and strategies for dealing with them laid out. The patient can learn to relax the perineal musculature during urination by voiding while in a hot tub. Encouraging the patient to raise her concerns about premature ejaculation or inadequate foreplay directly with her partner may be all the help necessary. Reassurance that no sexually transmitted disease is present is effective. A frank and practical discussion of the ways of dealing with a persistent problem such as herpes and referral to an appropriate support group may allow the patient to cope.

Oral nystatin (Mycostatin) to clear the intestinal source of a perineal yeast infestation along with Lactinex powder to reseed the lactobacilli that may have been driven out by previous antibiotic therapy can considerably reduce the local "noise." If postmenopausal changes in the perineal skin and mucous membranes are seen and there is no contraindication, a combination of estrogens and periodic progestational treatment may be useful. Such treatment should be carried out under the supervision or support of a gynecologist. Conjugated estrogens (Premarin) 0.625 mg/day and medroxyprogesterone acetate (Provera) 10 mg taken from the tenth to the twentieth of the month provide satisfactory replacement. Before prescribing these, the physician must be aware of potential thrombotic complications and carcinogenicity. The female internal and external genitalia are equaled by their counterparts in the male in hormonal response.

Diseases of the Prostate and Seminal Vesicles

Acute Prostatitis

Etiology

In middle-aged males acute prostatitis is mostly of bacterial origin. Coliforms are the leading offender, though Staphyloccocus epidermidis runs a close second and is probably the most common agent in diabetics and those with immunodeficiency disorders. Posterior urethritis and therefore (at least technically) prostatitis accompany 80% of the urethritis associated with sexually transmitted diseases. In younger males, the most common cause is sexually transmitted disease, with chlamydial infection and gonorrhea being the leading offenders.

Diagnosis

The patient has chills, fever, pain in the perineum and rectum sometimes severe enough to inhibit defecation, along with urinary frequency, dysuria, and decrease in stream size and possibly nausea and vomiting. If secondary seminal vesiculitis occurs, there may be pain in the groin. The urine is cloudy, and its sediment is loaded with pus and bacteria. The patient is sweaty, febrile, and obviously ill. The prostate is very tender and enlarged and has a "boggy" consistency, which is similar to the sensation encountered on palpating pitting edema of an extremity. If acute or subacute prostatitis is part of the differential diagnosis, rectal palpation of the prostate must be done with extreme care and gentleness as the potential is high for precipitating a bacterial shower into the blood stream with sudden septicemia and shock.

Treatment

Treatment for acute prostatitis includes bedrest, extra fluids, appropriate antibiotics, and pain medication. Usually oral nonsteroidal anti-inflammatory agents alone or in combination with codeine are sufficient, but occasionally parenteral narcotics are required. Hot sitz baths are helpful, and belladonna and opiate suppositories relieve bladder irritability and tenesmus. If retention occurs that necessitates catheterization, it is best to avoid the urethra and place a catheter into the bladder percutaneously above the symphysis with the aid of local infiltration anesthesia. If a urethral catheter must be used, the smallest one possible should be selected. Acute prostatitis rarely causes significant problems with pain relief; chronic prostatitis is another matter.

Chronic Prostatitis

Etiology and Symptoms

Chronic prostatitis, like urethral syndrome in the female, probably involves several different underlying processes with similar symptoms, which are merged under one diagnostic label. Patients complain of fullness in the perineum, urethral burning which may or may not be related to urination, rectal discomfort, and discomfort on ejaculation. In some patients, blocked ducts and trapped secretions in distended prostate glands probably are responsible for the symptoms. Loci of microscopic inflammation may create symptoms in others. These same lesions, however, may be found incidentally in asymptomatic individuals whose prostates are histologically examined for unrelated reasons such as death due to trauma or coronary disease. Low back pain is such a common complaint among the general population that it probably is coincidental to chronic prostatitis, or it reflects a musculoskeletal response to the primary problem. Driving trucks, tractors, and construction equipment seems to exacerbate such symptoms.

Diagnosis

On examination, the prostate tends to be firm and fibrous or boggy. Secretions obtained at massage are variable, but in some patients white cells are found in large clumps. Prostate secretions should be cultured. They are normally absolutely sterile, so the presence of even a few organisms is significant, particularly if they are pathogens. Before the prostate is massaged to obtain secretions for culture, the urethra must be cleansed by partially emptying the bladder. The specimen so obtained is divided into two parts. The first 5 to 10 ml of urine is collected in a tube labeled VB1 (voided bladder urine 1). Without interrupting the voiding process, the next 150 ml or so is collected in a container, and the last 5 to 10 ml of this portion is collected in a culture tube and labeled VB2. Voiding is interrupted, the prostate is then massaged, and secretions are collected in a sterile receptacle held under the meatus. This is labeled EP1 (expressed prostatic secretion 1).

If no secretions are obtained, the patient is instructed to void additional urine, which is collected in two parts, the first part being labeled VB3 and the last part VB4. If, when cultured, there is a higher colony count in EP1 or in VB3 than in VB1 or VB4, the bacteria almost surely originate in the prostate.

Therapy

When the 4-glass test is positive (36), sensitivities on the culture should be obtained and appropriate antibiotic therapy used (trimethoprim and sulfamethoxazole, reg strength tab qid for 5 days to load and bid for the next 45 days). Young individuals should be cultured for Chlamydia also. A 6-week course of tetracycline may be reasonable if one suspects chlamydial etiology. Patients who do not respond to such measures may be helped if accumulated secretions are expressed by periodic prostatic massage. Occasionally, such individuals have a urethral stricture that responds to dilation. Pain due to chronic prostatitis is usually persistent and annoying but not of an intensity to require potent narcotic analgesics. Most individuals are more concerned about cancer or some other long-term danger. If they can be reassured that these are not present, they are generally willing to live with the problem (37).

Prostatic Calculi

Patients with prostatic calculi are rarely symptomatic, and often are picked up when hard nodules are palpated on routine rectal examination. If the stones are multiple, in contact with each other, and crepitate when palpated, the diagnosis is made on physical examination. A radiograph of the pelvis usually reveals the offending calcification in the region of the prostate, thus differentiating it from cancer. Patients with prostatic cancer occasionally are misdiagnosed as having calculi. This is most likely to occur if the physician overlooks changes in the size or character of palpable nodules on re-examination. If prostatic calculi become infected or symptomatic, they can be removed by resecting the tissue between the stone and the urethra, which frees the stone into the urethra or bladder, and then crushing the stone and evacuating the fragments (38).

Benign Prostatic Hypertrophy

Benign prostatic hypertrophy is included only for completeness. Other than the pain of urinary retention, for which treatment is straightforward, pain is not a characteristic problem of this disease. Common symptoms are perineal or rectal fullness and, of course, urinary frequency and dysuria. All of these disappear with removal of the underlying obstruction.

Cancer of the Prostate

Epidemiology

The cause of cancer of the prostate is unknown, but this cancer affects all races and ethnic groups. Findings of occult cancer of the prostate in autopsy series increases dramatically after 50 years of age to over 80% of those above 80 years of age (39). Only 1 in 400 individuals over the age of 80 dies because of cancer of the prostate, whereas 10% of those discovered with the disease under age 60 succumb from it. According to Breslow et al. (40), the incidence of large latent cancer of the prostate is the same as the death rate from the disease in several different racial groups, whereas the incidence of small latent cancer is the same as the general mortality for these groups. The implication of this study is that large latent cancer behaves in a malignant fashion whereas small latent cancer does not.

Diagnosis

Many patients with cancer of the prostate are asymptomatic, their disease being discovered on screening rectal examination. Others present with characteristic obstructive symptoms, which tend to be more unrelentingly progressive than those of benign prostatic hypertrophy. Approximately 15 to 20% present with lumbar spine or pelvic pain due to metastatic bone disease as their first symptom. The prostate characteristically is hard or contains hard nodules on rectal examination, and biopsy of these areas of the prostate yields tissue that is positive for adenocarcinoma.

Serum acid phosphatase may be elevated. Osteoblastic lesions may be seen on radiographs of the lumbar spine and bony pelvis and/or a positive bone scan will be obtained.

Treatment

Pain associated with cancer of the prostate is usually related to obstruction or metastases. Advanced or acute obstruction can be relieved by catheter drainage and resection of obstructing tissue. Less acute obstruction in patients unsuitable for excision can be relieved by hormonal control therapy. Hormonal control therapy for pain from metastatic disease provides objective as well as subjective improvement in about 70% of the cases. Synthetic estrogen (stilbestrol) given daily is effective but may take 30 to 60 days to achieve complete palliation, whereas the dramatic relief resulting from orchiectomy occurs within a week after the procedure.

Subsequent recurrence of pain may respond to alteration in estrogen dosage or in the type of estrogen. Recent dramatic claims for luteinizing hormone releasing hormone (LHRH) may prove to be exaggerated, but this drug, like orchiectomy, does not produce salt retention or thrombotic problems, which are common side effects of estrogens.

Pain in localized areas of bone involvement, particularly periosteal elevation, responds well to irradiation. Patients with bone marrow replacement respond to transfusion and irradiation for varying periods. Thus far, the use of antimetabolites in advanced prostatic cancer has yielded disappointing results. The management of patients with pain due to advanced or terminal cancer is discussed in Chapter 24.

Seminal Vesicle Diseases

Primary disease of the seminal vesicles is extremely rare. Secondary disease related to congenital anomalies of the urinary collecting system is also rare. More common is involvement secondary to prostate infection or cancer. Symptoms are pain in the groin on the affected side. The differential diagnosis should include ilioinguinal and genitofemoral neuralgias in patients who have had recent flank or groin surgery (41).

Treatment is directed at the primary disease such as prostatitis and cancer of the prostate.

DISORDERS OF THE EXTERNAL MALE GENITALIA

Diseases of the Epididymis

Acute Epididymitis

Etiology

Acute epididymitis is characteristically due to chlamydial organisms in men under 40 and coliform bacteria in older men; thus it is a sexually transmitted disease in sexually active young males, whereas in older patients it is usually secondary to obstruction or other changes. In prepubertal males it is also associated with urethral obstruction (42, 43).

Symptoms and Signs

Typically, the history is one of gradual onset of dull pain in the scrotum followed in hours or days by tenderness in the affected epididymis, swelling, redness in the scrotum, and then chills, fever, and malaise. The pain is partially relieved in the supine position. The pain, inflammation, tenderness, and swelling may radiate up the spermatic cord. There is usually a history of recent sexual exposure and urethral discharge. On examination, the scrotum is often swollen, red, and tender, particularly over the epididymis, which should lie posterolaterally even though it is three or four times normal size.

Differential Diagnosis

Acute epididymitis must be distinguished from torsion of the testicle or one of its appendages (44), mumps orchitis, incarcerated hernia or sudden hemorrhage into the testicle, and possibly neoplasm. Pain associated with torsion is sudden in onset and often occurs at night; there is no discharge and the urinary sediment is normal with torsion. The twisted testicle is higher than the nonaffected organ, and the pain is not particularly relieved by elevation. One might hear bowel tones on auscultation over the scrotum of a patient with an incarcerated hernia. If the scrotal mass is herniated bowel, the testicle and epididymis should be normal.

Patients with mumps orchitis should have a history of exposure, parotitis, and perhaps elevated serum amylase. The testicle should be principally involved, not the epididymis. Patients suffering an acute hemorrhage into the testicle often have a history of trauma, and the epididymis is normal. If the ipsilateral spermatic cord is not involved, dramatic relief of pain may be achieved by infiltration of the cord structures with 0.5 to 1% lidocaine or 0.25% bupivacaine. This may also permit the patient to undergo a more thorough examination to determine the location of the epididymis in order to establish the presence or absence of torsion.

Radioisotope studies of the testicle may be helpful in differentiating torsion from other disorders. At the University of Washington Medical Center, ultrasound has been less satisfactory. If there is legitimate concern that the diagnosis may be torsion, the safest course is exploration. We have not seen any scrotal morbidity in individuals with epididymitis who were explored in order to rule out torsion, but we have saved some testicles in patients who would have lost them if their torsion had been treated as epididymitis.

Treatment

Since most young males with acute epididymitis are infected with Chlamydia, the logical treatment is tetracycline therapy. Males over 40 years of age should be treated with an antibiotic effective against coliform organisms pending identification and sensitivities. Acute epididymitis is not a trivial disease for those who engage in heavy physical activity at work or in sports. In addition to 50 days of antibiotics, treatment requires scrotal support and bedrest with some privileges for 10 to 14 days and restricted activity for 4 to 6 weeks. If activities are resumed too early or antibiotics are given for shorter periods, the end result may be development of chronic epididymitis, which may take months of limited activity or an epididymectomy to resolve.

Chronic Epididymitis

Chronic epididymitis, the end stage of unresolved acute epididymitis, is a disabling condition. The epididymis is chronically swollen, painful, and extremely tender to palpation. This disorder also is likely to develop in patients with bacterial prostatitis or congenital defects of the urethra.

Treatment of chronic epididymitis involves prolonged use of a scrotal support, several months of limited physical activity, and antibiotic therapy. A few patients will develop chronic orchidodynia (see later section). Some will require epididymectomy, and some removal of both testicle and epididymis. Before removal, several local anesthetic infiltration blocks of the spermatic cord should be tried to see if the pain cycle can be interrupted and relieved permanently (see Orchiodynia). Infection of the spermatic cord (funiculitis) occasionally accompanies epididymitis. It is almost never seen independently and is usually treated by the same regimen employed for epididymitis.

Diseases of the Testicle

Torsion of the Testicle and Spermatic Cord

Etiology

Torsion is primarily a disease of adolescence and young adulthood, although it occasionally occurs in the newborn and has been reported in a 78-year-old man (44). The incidence in a busy general hospital is three or four cases a year. The left side is involved twice as often as the right. The cause of torsion is a congenitally high insertion of the tunica vaginalis onto the spermatic cord, which allows the testicle to turn within the tunic. Depending on the degree of twist (90 to 720°), vascular compromise with ischemia and necrosis of the testicle and epididymis results. Put more correctly, the torsion is of the spermatic cord, and the testicle is infarcted.

Diagnosis and Treatment

Pain in the testicle is the cardinal presenting symptom of the twisted testicle. It is sudden in onset, often at night, severe in degree, and followed by exquisite tenderness. Many patients have had a previous similar episode or episodes of less severity, which have resolved spontaneously. On physical examination the affected testicle is often higher than the normal one, whereas in epididymitis, it hangs lower. In the twisted testicle, the epididymis is in some position other than the normal dorsolateral location, and the degree of swelling and tenderness varies. Urinalysis is usually normal in patients with torsion, whereas the urine of patients with epididymitis usually contains white blood cells. Local infiltration of local anesthetic around the spermatic cord relieves symptoms and tenderness, allowing a more careful examination of the scrotal contents and possibly manual detorsion.

The treatment is immediate detorsion. This must be accompanied by surgical fixation to prevent subsequent episodes. The contralateral side must also be suture fixated prophylactically, since the congenital defect underlying the condition is usually present bilaterally.

Torsion of the Testicular Appendages

Although there are four testicular appendages, the appendix testis, a vestigial structure on the upper pole of the testis, is involved in 95% of the cases of torsion. This small (0.1 to 0.5 cm in diameter) pedunculated structure twists on its pedicle, and ischemia with necrosis follows. The highest incidence is in prepubertal patients 10 to 13 years of age (44).

The patient presents with pain of sudden onset, initially localized to the upper pole of the testis. After several hours, however, the pain may be difficult to distinguish from that of torsion of the testicle and cord. Early, on physical examination, a blue dot may be seen through the scrotum over the twisted appendix testis. Local infiltration blockade of the spermatic cord permits careful examination, which is necessary to make the diagnosis and temporarily relieves the pain. The urinalysis is normal.

Surgical excision results in prompt relief of pain and can resolve any diagnostic doubts about the possibility of torsion of the spermatic cord.

Orchitis

As an independent entity, orchitis is most commonly caused by a virus and occurs only after puberty. Mumps is the most common cause, but Coxsackie and other viruses have been implicated. Pain results from swelling of the testicular parenchyma within an unyielding tunic. History of viral exposure and involvement of other organs usually precedes the testicular pain. There are no urinary symptoms, and except for proteinuria the urinalysis is normal. Fever to 39°C is common.

Infiltration of 1% lidocaine into and around the spermatic cord at the external inguinal ring may resolve pain and swelling due to orchitis. Local measures such as heat and support also help some patients.

Orchiodynia

Orchiodynia—also known as orchidalgia, orchialgia, and testalgia—is a rare disease of unknown etiology characterized by chronic pain in the testicle. Some patients have a history of trauma to the testicle, and occasionally this disorder occurs following vasectomy. The pain is usually nagging, persistent, and achy but only rarely and fleetingly severe. The pain may be perceived in the testicle but tenderness is variable. If the patient has a history of trauma or inflammation, scarring or atrophy may be evident on examination of the testicle.

Often simple reassurance that no malignancy or other serious or transmittable disease is present will encourage the patient to live with the minor discomfort of orchiodynia. Two of the three patients seen by us with this disorder were relieved with infiltration of local anesthetics around the spermatic cord at the external inguinal ring. The injections were repeated two to three times at weekly intervals. Removal of the testicle in these cases is not recommended because the pain usually persists after the testicle is gone. For example, one 91-year-old whom we have seen for years continues to complain periodically of pain in the testicle forty years after that organ's removal and thirty years after an ipsilateral seminal vesiculectomy.

Diseases of the Penis

Paraphimosis

In paraphimosis, the redundant foreskin retracts behind the corona of the glans penis and constricts it. The result is similar to that of a tourniquet. Further swelling and edema of the glans make diagnosis and treatment difficult for those unaware of the mechanism of this disorder.

Reduction of the foreskin often is possible after pressure over the glans has reduced the edema and swelling. This is aided by judicious use of local anesthesia infiltrated under the skin and subcutaneous tissue circumferentially at the base of the penile shaft and around the dorsal nerves of the penis and the deep corporeal nerves. Since the nerves to the coronal skin and glans reach them via the corpus spongiosum, it is necessary to infiltrate the corona circumferentially as well. (These same maneuvers apply when anesthetising locally for purposes of circumcision.) If the edema is great, the foreskin may be reduced following local block with the aid of Babcock clamps placed on the contraction ring, or it may be necessary to perform a dorsal slit at the bedside. When the patient has recovered and the swelling is considerably reduced, elective circumcision is indicated (45).

Priapism

Priapism, a prolonged painful erection not associated with sexual stimulation, can occur idiopathically or secondary to medications or other disease processes. Patients with leukemia and lymphoma, those undergoing dialysis, and those being treated by heparinization are at increased risk. An initial prolonged episode usually is preceded by a number of short bouts of this disorder. On physical examination the corpora cavernosa are painfully engorged, but the corpus spongiosum and glans are not turgid.

All successful therapy of persistent priapism establishes some form of shunting mechanism between the corpora cavernosa, whose venous outflow is obstructed, and the corpus spongiosum of the glans or urethra, whose venous drainage is normal. In its simplest form, this is accomplished by needle excision of cores of tissue between glans and corpora cavernosa (46). If that fails, a formal shunt will have to be created between the corpus spongiosum and the cavernous bodies, or perhaps a corporosaphenous shunt. Unfortunately, impotence often follows such procedures (47), but this is correctable by insertion of one of the penile prostheses now available (48). Control of pain due to priapism may require administration of opioids or continuous caudal block. Various anesthetics and local measures formerly used in an attempt to treat the problem are not warranted by the meager clinical results obtained.

Peyronie's Disease

Peyronie's disease is characterized by induration and sometimes curving of the corpora cavernosa of the penis. An autosomal dominant inheritable form of the disease has been identified by Nyberg et al. (49). An HLA linkage and association with Dupuytren's contractures also have been established for this inherited form, which occurs as early as the third decade; the more common, less obviously inherited form presents in the fifth and sixth decades. Patients often have no symptoms, but the discovery of a hard plaque in the dorsal shaft raises fears of a malignant process. Some patients notice incomplete erection distal to the lesion and then discover the plaque. Others have severe angulation on erection, making intromission painful or impossible. Characteristically the symptoms wax and wane over time, making assessment of treatment results difficult.

The patients most likely to be satisfied with surgical correction are those unable to intromit because of severe angulation due to the plaque and those whose distal erectile dysfunction also creates problems with intromission. Both will probably require penile prostheses in the course of treatment. Those with minor degrees of deformity or curvature usually do well when informed of the natural history of the disease and realize the prognosis for them is good.

Herpes Progenitalis

Herpes progenitalis, one of the most common of the sexually transmitted diseases, causes pain due to the chronic recurrence of small blistering lesions on the skin of the shaft. The painful character of the skin lesion is short-lived, but the pain of the social impact of the disease on the individual's life is not.

Treatment with 5% acyclovir (Zovirax) ointment applied locally may increase the interval between recurrence of lesions. Most large communities have support groups that are helpful for patients with herpes.

REFERENCES

1. Kunin, C.M., Polyak, F., and Postel, E.: Periurethral bacterial flora in women: Prolonged intermittent colonization with Escherichia coli. JAMA, 243:134, 1980.
2. Kunin, C.M.: The natural history of recurrent bacteriuria in schoolgirls. N. Engl. J. Med., 282:1443, 1978.
3. Walsh, P.C., et al. (eds.): Campbell's Textbook of Urology. 5th Ed. Vol. 1. Philadelphia, W.B. Saunders, 1986.
4. Smith, D.R.: General Urology. 11th Ed. Los Altos, CA, Lange Medical, 1984.
5. Bonica, J.J.: Management of Pain. 1st Ed. Philadelphia, Lea & Febiger, 1953.
6. Kuntz, A.: The Autonomic Nervous System. 4th Ed. Philadelphia, Lea & Febiger, 1953, pp. 289–307.
7. Mitchell, G.A.G.: Anatomy of the Autonomic Nervous System. Edinburgh, E. & S. Livingstone, 1956.
8. Netter, F.H.: CIBA Collection of Medical Illustrations. Vol. 6: Kidneys, Ureters and Urinary Bladder. Summit, NJ, CIBA-Geigy Corp., 1973.
9. Ruch, T.C.: Pathophysiology of pain. In Physiology and Biophysics. 19th Ed. Edited by T.C. Ruch and H.D. Patton. Philadelphia, W.B. Saunders, 1965, pp. 353–363.
10. Langworthy, O.R., Kolb, L.C., and Lewis, L.G.: Physiology and Micturition. Baltimore, Williams & Wilkins, 1940.

11. Nesbit, R.M., and McLellan, F.C.: Sympathectomy for the relief of vesical spasm and pain resulting from intractable bladder infection. Surg. Gynecol. Obstet., 68:540, 1939.
12. Wyker, A.W.: Neurogenic bladder. *In* Method of Urology. Edited by A.W. Wyker and J.Y. Gillenwater. Baltimore, Williams & Wilkins, 1975, pp. 1–28.
13. Habib, H.N.: Experience and recent contributions in sacral nerve stimulation for voiding both human and animal. Br. J. Urol., 39:73, 1967.
14. Retief, P.J.M.: Physiology of micturition and ejaculation. So. Afr. Med. J., 24:509, 1950.
15. Kedia, K.R., Markland, C., and Fraley, E.E.: Sexual function following high retroperitoneal lymphadenectomy. J. Urol., 114:237, 1975.
16. Mayo, M.E., and Ansell, J.S.: Urodynamic assessment of incontinence after prostatectomy. J. Urol., 122:60, 1979.
17. Gasparich, J.P., et al.: Noninfectious epididymitis associated with amiodarone therapy. J. Urol., 133:971, 1985.
18. Hooten, T.M., Running, K., and Stamm, W.E.: Single dose therapy for cystitis in women. JAMA, 253:387, 1985.
19. Walsh, A.: Interstitial cystitis. *In* Campbell's Urology. 4th Ed. Vol. 1. Edited by J.H. Harrison et al. Philadelphia, W.B. Saunders, 1978, pp. 693–707.
20. Oravisto, K.J.: Epidemiology of interstitial cystitis. Ann. Chir. Gynaecol. 64:75, 1975.
21. Oravisto, K.J., Alfthan, O.S., and Jokinen, E.J.: Interstitial cystitis: Clinical and immunological findings. Scand. J. Urol. Nephrol., 4:37, 1970.
22. Gordon, H.L., Rossen, R.D., Hersh, E.M., and Yium, J.J.: Immunologic aspects of interstitial cystitis. J. Urol., 109:228, 1973.
23. Dunn, M., et al.: Interstitial cystitis treated by prolonged bladder distension. Br. J. Urol., 49:641, 1977.
24. Higson, R.H., Smith, J.C., and Wilson, P.: Bladder rupture: An acceptable complication of distension therapy. Br. J. Urol., 50:529, 1978.
25. Shirley, S.W., Stewart, B.H., and Mirelman, S.: Dimethyl sulfoxide in treatment of inflammatory genitourinary disorders. Urology, 11:215, 1978.
26. Learmonth, J.R., and Braasch, W.F.: Clinical and surgical aspects of nerve lesions involving the lower part of the urinary tract. Z. Urol. Chir., 36:195, 1933.
27. Jacobsen, C.E., Braasch, W.F., and Love, J.C.: Presacral neurectomy for intractable vesical pain and neurogenic vesical dysfunction. Surg. Gynecol. Obstet., 79:21, 1944.
28. White, J.C., and Sweet, W.H.: Pain and the Neurosurgeon: A 40-Year Experience. Springfield, IL, Charles C Thomas, 1969.
29. Goldwasser, R., and Webster, G.D.: Augmentation and substitution enterocystoplasty. J. Urol., 135:215, 1986.
30. Badenoch, A.W.: Chronic interstitial cystitis. Br. J. Urol., 43:718, 1971.
31. Mallik, M.K.B.: Study of radiation necrosis of the urinary bladder following treatment of carcinoma of the cervix. Am. J. Obstet. Gynecol., 83:393, 1962.
32. Csonka, G.W.: Non-gonococcal urethritis. Br. J. Vener. Dis., 41:1, 1965.
33. O'Grady, F.W., et al.: Introital enterobacteria, urinary infection and the urethral syndrome. Lancet, 2:1208–1210, 1970.
34. Pfau, A.: The rape of the female urethra. Urol. Dig., 11:11, 1972.
35. Evans, A.T.: Etiology of the urethral syndrome: Preliminary report. J. Urol., 105:245, 1971.
36. Meares, E.M., and Stamey, T.A.: Bacteriologic localization patterns in bacterial prostatitis and urethritis. Invest. Urol., 5:492, 1968.
37. Jewett, H.J., and Colston, J.A.C.: Urethritis, cystitis and prostatitis: Diagnosis and treatment. Med. Clin. North Am., 45:1547, 1961.
38. Fox, M.: The natural history and significance of stone formation in the prostate gland. J. Urol., 89:716, 1963.
39. Klein, L.A.: Medical progress: Prostatic carcinoma. N. Engl. J. Med., 15:824, 1979.
40. Breslow, C.W., et al.: Latent carcinoma of prostate at autopsy in seven areas. Int. J. Cancer, 20:680, 1977.
41. Harms, B.A., DeHaas, D.R., Jr., and Starling, J.R.: Diagnosis and management of genitofemoral neuralgia. Arch. Surg., 119:339, 1985.
42. Berger, R.E., et al.: Chlamydia trachomatis as a cause of acute "idiopathic epididymitis." N. Engl. J. Med., 298:301, 1978.
43. Kiviat, M.D., Shurtleff, D.B., and Ansell, J.S.: Urinary reflux via the vas deferens: Unusual cause of epididymitis in infancy. J. Pediatr., 80:476, 1972.
44. Skoglund, R.W., McRoberts, J.W., and Ragde, H.: Torsion of the spermatic cord: A review of the literature and analysis of 70 new cases. J. Urol., 104:604, 1970.
45. Skoglund, R.W., and Chapman, W.H.: Reduction of paraphimosis. J. Urol., 104:137, 1970.
46. Winter, C.C.: Priapism cured by creation of fistulas between glans penis and corpora cavernosa. J. Urol., 119:227, 1978.
47. Falk, D., and Loos, D.C.: Spongiocavernosum shunt in the surgical treatment of idiopathic persistent priapism. J. Urol., 108:101, 1972.
48. Gee, W.F., McRoberts, J.W., Raney, J.O., and Ansell, J.S.: The impotent patient: Surgical treatment with penile prosthesis and psychiatric evaluation. J. Urol., 111:41, 1974.
49. Nyberg, L.M., Bias, W.B., Hochberg, M.C., and Walsh, P.C.: Identification of an inherited form of Peyronie's disease with autosomal dominant inheritance and association with Dupuytren's contracture and histocompatibility B7 cross-reacting antigens. J. Urol., 128:48, 1982.
50. Kedia, K.R., Markland, C., and Fraley, E.E.: Sexual function following high retroperitoneal lymphadenectomy. J. Urol., 114:237, 1975.

69 • PELVIC AND PERINEAL PAIN CAUSED BY OTHER DISORDERS

JOHN J. BONICA

The preceding three chapters discuss various acute and chronic painful conditions caused by diseases of the pelvic viscera and by other gynecologic and urologic disorders. This chapter discusses a pain caused by disorders of bone, joints, muscles of the pelvis, nerves, and skin, and pain referred to the pelvis from other regions. Because many of these conditions occur in various parts of the body, they are discussed elsewhere in this book (see Part II and also Part III, Chapters 40, 52, 58, and 77). Therefore, only comments relevant to the pelvis and perineum are presented in this chapter. The material is presented in five sections: A, Musculoskeletal Disorders; B, Pain of Neuropathic Origin; C, Painful Visceral and Dermatologic Disorders; D, Referred Pain; and E, Pain Primarily of Psychologic Origin.

A. MUSCULOSKELETAL DISORDERS

Pain in the pelvis is frequently associated with trauma, infection, metabolic disease, or neoplasm involving the bones and joints of the pelvis. Muscular spasm and myofascial syndromes involving some of the muscles in the pelvis, particularly the pelvic diaphragm, are also a frequent cause of pain.

Trauma

Sprains

Etiology and Symptoms and Signs

Sprains of one or more of the numerous ligaments of the pelvis as a result of accidental trauma or some other unusual exertion can be a source of pain. One of the most frequent types is sprain of the ligaments of the symphysis pubis (Fig. 65-4). During pregnancy the ligamentous tissues of the pelvis relax and stretch and, with an unusually large fetus or multiple fetuses, sufficient stress might be placed on the symphysis to be a source of pain. The pain is usually dull and aching in character, of mild to moderate intensity, and associated with localized tenderness in the pubic region. Occasionally direct impact can cause bleeding, with consequent subcutaneous hematoma.

Sacroiliac joint sprain can occur as a result of excessive stress on the joint or because of injury. This condition usually produces pain in the low back and thigh (Chapter 72).

Treatment

If the patient is seen soon after injury, application of ice to the region is useful to decrease bleeding. The pain can usually be controlled by nonsteroidal antiinflammatory drugs (NSAIDs), given alone or combined with codeine or a more potent opioid. In patients who experience moderate to severe pain, it is useful to infiltrate the joint with a local anesthetic (e.g., 0.25% bupivacaine) combined with a steroid. The local anesthetic produces relief of pain for 6 to 8 hours, and the steroid decreases the degree of post-traumatic inflammation.

Fractures

Direct force applied to the pelvis can fracture this structure anywhere. Fractures that involve the pelvic ring are typically produced by compression and can either be single or multiple (1, 2). Because a fracture tends to occur across a weaker part of the ring, it is especially likely to be at the obturator foramen or across the wing of the ilium, from the crest to the margin of the greater sciatic foramen. A single fracture in either location allows parts to lift and separate, and treatment is conservative. The pain is usually moderate and can be controlled by NSAIDs alone or in combination with a weak or strong opioid.

In contrast, severe trauma invariably produces an unstable pelvic ring fracture as part of multiple trauma. Fu and Mears (3) have noted that formerly patients with multiple trauma were managed in a community hospital setting, in which expert trauma surgeons were not available, with a consequent high incidence of morbidity and mortality. The advent of rapid transport to specialized trauma centers and the development of effective techniques of external fixation have markedly decreased these morbidity and mortality rates and have proven effective in reducing the pain, resulting in early mobilization with a consequent decrease in post-traumatic complications, earlier ambulation, and shorter hospitalization.

Pathophysiology

Watson-Jones (2) and, much more recently, Pennal and Massiah (4), have classified unstable pelvic ring fractures according to the mechanism of injury. The most frequently encountered mechanism is a lateral compressive force that can produce one of several patterns of anterior or posterior injury. The anterior disruption can be a fracture of one or more pelvic rami, a dislocation of the symphysis pubis, or both (3, 4). The posterior injury disrupts the ipsilateral or contralateral ilium, sacroiliac joint, or sacrum. Occasionally multiple posterior disruptions occur. The second mechanism involves an anteroposterior compressive force, which usually disrupts the symphysis pubis, with a wide diastasis. A third type of injury, the vertical shear disruption, is generally produced by the most violent indirect forces. Usually the disruptive force is transmitted through a lower extremity by way of the hip joint to the pelvic ring (3). Radiologic evidence of a vertical shear fracture includes an avulsion fracture of the ischial spine, with superior migration of the entire hemipelvis. Injury of one or more branches of the lumbosacral plexus, particularly the L5 root segment, is a frequent accompaniment to this type of injury.

Symptoms and Signs

Invariably patients who present with an unstable pelvic ring fracture show evidence of other serious injuries to the intra-abdominal organs, intrathoracic viscera, central nervous system, or limbs. Depending on the degree and severity of CNS injury, patients experience severe pain in various body organs. Massive hemorrhage might have occurred, manifested by the signs and symptoms of hypovolemic shock.

Diagnosis

Unless multiple radiographic views are taken, a pelvic instability might not be evident in the conventional anteroposterior pelvic view (3). Radiography should include pelvic inlet and outlet projections; if available, CT scanning is most useful because it reveals the pattern and degree of disruption of a severe pelvic ring fracture (3, 4). Indeed, bone scans have revealed a number of so-called stable pelvic ring fractures accompanied by undisplaced fracture adjacent to the sacroiliac joint, and this appears to accompany every injury in which multiple pelvic rami are fractured.

Treatment

Fu and Mears (3) have presented impressive evidence that nonsurgical methods do not control osseous bleeding from the fracture site and do not permit early mobilization of patients. Consequently patients have a high incidence of serious mental, urinary, and pulmonary complications, the latter causing delayed death in 10 to 30% of patients. Moreover, nonoperative procedures have been associated with a high incidence of serious chronic disabilities.

On the basis of these results and personal experience, Fu and Mears (3) have suggested that these patients undergo immediate reduction and stabilization of the fracture to minimize pain and hemorrhage, late pulmonary complications, and various chronic musculoskeletal disorders, which are frequently associated with these massive traumatic insults. Reduction and stabilization are best achieved by external skeletal fixation using an anterior fixation frame, which is simple to apply. In patients who are receiving emergency room care and who are in unstable hypovolemic condition, rigid external pelvic fixation should be done as soon as blood and fluids have been replaced by IV administration. In patients who are stable, primary internal or external fixation of the posterior or anterior site of pelvic disruption should be carried out. In reporting their experiences with 20 patients, Fu and Mears (3) noted that 14 obtained marked relief of pain

within a day after application of the frame, and an equal number were out of bed within a week after surgery.

Coccygodynia

Coccygodynia is a common problem and is characterized by pain in the "tail bone," with radiation to the lower sacral and perineal areas. The condition afflicts women more frequently than men.

Etiology

Coccygodynia usually follows a fall in the sitting position in which one lands on the coccyx, such as astride a log, or it can follow a direct blow or kick to this region. One of the most frequent causes of coccygodynia is damage to the sacrococcygeal ligament during a difficult vaginal delivery (5, 6). Any of these factors can cause a fracture or ligamentous sprain. Because the coccyx is quite movable and is supported by the sacrococcygeal ligaments, fracture is not as common as a sprain. A chronic sprain can follow repeated microtraumata caused by poor sitting habits, in which pressure is centered on the coccyx. Arthritis, osteitis, osteomyelitis, and other skeletal disorders involving the coccyx and lower sacrum, although rare, have been reported as causative factors. In my experience with patients referred to me with coccygodynia, trauma from a fall or a difficult delivery had been the most common cause. Traut (7) reported that at least 50% of patients gave no history of trauma. Holmes (8) believed that the condition had primarily a psychologic basis, particularly in women.

Symptoms and Signs

Pain and tenderness at the tip of the spine or in the coccyx is the most frequent complaint. The pain can be severe, as in fractures, or it can be a dull ache accompanied by bouts of lancinating pain. The pain frequently radiates to the perineal, gluteal, and posterior sacral regions and occasionally down the posterior thigh along the course of the sciatic nerve. The pain and tenderness are aggravated by sitting on a hard chair, particularly in thin individuals with poorly developed gluteal muscles, and by movement of the coccyx by the examining index finger inserted into the rectum. The levator ani, coccygeus, and piriformis muscles are frequently in moderate to severe spasm. The tenderness and spasm are generalized and involve all the myofascial and ligamentous structures of the posterior wall of the pelvis.

Diagnosis

Diagnosis is based on the symptoms and signs and on the results of rectal examination. Occasionally radiography reveals fracture, malalignment of the coccyx, or arthritic changes involving the sacrococcygeal joint. Infectious process can be present.

Treatment

Treatment consists of massage, local heat, injection of the joint with a local anesthetic and steroid, and, whenever indicated, psychotherapy. Thiele (9) and Traut (7) reported permanent relief in most patients following a series of treatments consisting of massage performed through the rectum and hot sitz baths or diathermy. Usually six treatments given at 3- to 5-day intervals were sufficient. Local injection of hydrocortisone has been reported as effective. If the pain is severe, local infiltration, coccygeal nerve block, or a low caudal block, involving only the S5 and coccygeal nerves, is effective. This can be repeated several times using a local anesthetic. If the block provides complete but only transient relief of pain, the procedure is done with alcohol or with a cryoprobe (10) (Chapter 96). Because many of these patients are tense, apprehensive, and nervous, reassurance, encouragement, and other psychotherapeutic measures constitute an important phase of treatment.

Infectious and Inflammatory Disorders

Osteomyelitis

Osteomyelitis in one or more of the bones of the pelvis, although rare, can cause pain localized to the pelvis. With acute infection patients are usually extremely ill, with high fever, malaise, lethargy, and often vomiting (11). Most patients have tenderness over the affected bone, which can be palpated. This condition is infrequently a cause of pain in the pelvis and is discussed in detail in Chapter 23, so no further comments are made here.

Arthritides

Infectious or septic arthritis and osteoarthritis frequently involve a sacroiliac joint, causing pain in the hips and buttocks with reference to the groin. Degeneration of the interpubic disk can also cause pubic pain. Sutro (12) noted that pregnancy accentuated a degenerative process in the interpubic disk, and these patients can develop localized pain later in life. These conditions are all discussed in detail in Chapter 20.

Paget's Disease of Bone

Paget's disease of bone, also known as osteitis deformans, is a localized disorder characterized by initial excessive resorption and subsequent active deposition of bone. The cause of Paget's disease is unknown. Because no disturbance of mineral or protein metabolism has been demonstrated it is not considered as a metabolic bone disease. The condition is rare in those below the age of 40; among those over 40 the prevalence is said to be approximately 3%, men being affected slightly more frequently than women (13). The pelvic bones are the most commonly involved, followed by the femur, skull, tibia, lumbosacral spine, dorsal spine, clavicle, and ribs (13, 14).

Symptoms and Signs

The most common presenting symptom is pain, which can be bone pain from the active disease process or pain arising from secondary complications such as nerve compression, fracture, or osteoarthritis. The bone pain is usually continuous and often interferes with sleep. When the pelvis is involved patients usually experience pelvic or back pain, or both.

Diagnosis

Diagnosis of Paget's disease is usually not difficult because of the bone deformity (13, 14). Radiographic studies demonstrate lytic, sclerotic, or mixed changes. Laboratory studies might reveal an increase in the urinary hydroxyproline level, reflecting increased degradation of bone collagen consequent to elevated bone resorption.

Treatment

Treatment is directed at inhibition of osteoclastic activity, which produces symptomatic improvement and restoration of normal bone architecture. Three classes of drugs are now used to achieve this therapeutic objective: hormones, diphosphonates, and antibiotics. Calcitonin, a polypeptide hormone produced in the perifollicular cells of the thyroid, blocks bone absorption, decreasing skeletal turnover and leading to a mild hypocalcemia (13–15). The drug is given parenterally; symptomatic improvement is noted in a few weeks, reflected by a decrease in the serum alkaline phosphatase and hydroxyproline levels to 50% of pretreatment levels (15). Treatment of this condition is discussed in detail in Chapter 23.

Neoplastic Diseases

Primary Bone Tumors

The most common types of primary bone tumors of the pelvis are chondrosarcoma, followed by osteosarcoma, fibrosarcoma, giant cell tumor, and chondroblastoma (16, 17). These neoplasms can produce pain that is usually continuous, dull and aching in character, of moderate to severe degree, and generally localized to the region of the primary tumor. If the tumor encroaches on the sciatic nerve, obturator nerve, or both, however, the pain is accompanied by neurologic symptoms and signs.

Diagnosis

Because patients with primary bone tumors of the pelvis might be candidates for local resection of the pelvis or for hemipelvectomy, it is essential for the surgeon to determine the local extent of the tumor as precisely as possible (17). Only then can the surgeon accurately predict whether patients require a local resection of part of the pelvis or hemipelvectomy. For a primary bone tumor it is necessary to ascertain the intraosseous and extraosseous extent of the tumor, which cannot be done by physical examination alone. Consequently it is essential to carry out extensive diagnostic imaging. The use of conventional radiography to determine the extent of the tumor is complicated by the depth of the pelvis and by its obstruction by soft tissue. Therefore, radiographs taken at 45° of an anterior and posterior rotation provide more information than conventional anteroposterior views (17). Moreover, conventional tomography is more useful than conventional radiography for visualizing the intraosseous extent of the tumor. Skeletal scintigraphy is moderately useful for demonstrating the local intraosseous extent of the tumor in the pelvis. Angiography is helpful for defining the relationship of the tumor to the major intrapelvic vessels. CT scanning is the single most reliable diagnostic procedure for viewing the soft tissue extent of a primary pelvic bone tumor (17).

Treatment

Local pelvic resection can be used for removal of a primary bone tumor. Marginal excision—a section at the periphery (margin) of the pseudocapsular tumor—is usually chosen for a benign tumor and also for a locally aggressive tumor such as a giant cell tumor or chondroblastoma (17). A wide excision is usually indicated for a low-grade malignancy such as a low-grade chondrosarcoma or a recurrent aggressive Paget's tumor, such as a giant cell tumor. Radical resection (in which the plane of dissection leaves a cuff of normal tissue and continuity with the tumor outside a normal anatomic compartment) is indicated for a high-grade malignant tumor. If the operative procedure is going to be used as an adjunct to other forms of treatment, as in the case of Ewing's sarcoma, the surgeon might elect to decrease the extent of the surgical incision from a radical to a wide excision. Local pelvic resection should not be performed for palliation or in the presence of metastasis because recovery is slow (17). A decision regarding the best therapeutic strategy for particular patients with specific primary bone tumors in the pelvis should always depend on the personnel and resources available and on a collaborative multidisciplinary and interdisciplinary effort.

Metastatic Disease of the Pelvis

Numerous studies have shown that the pelvis is one of the most important and frequent sites of metastasis from such primary tumors as breast, prostate and, less frequently, thyroid, kidney, bronchial, and rectal tumors (18). Thus, Lenz and Freid (19) carried out radiologic and postmortem studies of 81 patients with skeletal metastasis from breast cancer and found that the pelvis was affected in 51 patients (63%). Kaufmann (20) found that 62% of patients with prostatic carcinoma had metastasis to the pelvis. Among 50 patients with advanced breast cancer, metastasis to the pelvis occurred in 66% of patients (21, 22).

Symptoms and Signs

The most frequent symptom associated with bone metastasis is pain, which characteristically develops gradually over weeks or months and becomes progressively more severe. The pain is usually localized and is typically more severe at night. Percussion tenderness at the site of involvement is a highly reliable clinical sign (23). Stretching of the periosteum of the involved bone, either by direct tumor expansion or by weakening of the bone by mechanical stress at the tumor site, precipitates pain in many patients. In most patients bone metastasis is likely to involve other sites, and the initial site of pain might be elsewhere. In such cases radiographs must be obtained to rule out a pathologic fracture.

Pain is often positional in nature and can be temporarily relieved by shifting weight from the involved area. Expansion of a tumor located in the ischium can cause encroachment on the obturator or the sciatic nerve, or both, causing pain and neurologic deficits in the distribution of these nerves.

Diagnosis and Evaluation

The physical examination is one of the most important elements in the evaluation of patients with osseous metastasis. Patients with severe pain are often heavily medicated, and precise location of the pain requires interviewing and examining patients just before the next dose of medication is administered (23). Multiple areas of pain are often noted in patients with extensive bone metastasis. Routine radiographs do not reveal bone metastasis until the bone density has changed by 30 to 50%, so it is necessary to use more sophisticated radiographic imaging techniques such as computerized bone scanning tomography, and, in centers where it is available, magnetic resonance imaging (MRI). Occasionally patients develop pain without bone scan or radiographic evidence. It might be necessary to carry out a biopsy, if this is feasible.

Treatment

In general, bone metastasis requires treatment directed toward relieving the pain and preventing fracture of weight-bearing bones. Mauch (23) has firmly stated that, with few exceptions, a radical curative approach to the treatment of bone metastasis is unrealistic and its attempt only risks treatment complications in patients with incurable disease. Before relying solely on opioid medication, anticancer therapy should be attempted (Chapter 24). Localized radiation therapy is a highly effective measure in treatment of bone pain, offering partial or complete relief in 75% of patients (Chapter 89). The chance of producing good pain relief appears to be slightly better with metastatic breast cancer than with metastasis from carcinoma of the kidney or prostate. Mauch (23) presented data that low-dose short-fraction irradiation (500 to 2000 rad in one to five fractions) appears to be as effective and long-lasting in relieving pain as more protracted irradiation (3000 to 4500 rad over $2\frac{1}{2}$ to $4\frac{1}{2}$ weeks). Because radiation from metastasis of the pelvis is likely to involve a portion of the small and large bowels, any fractionation greater than 300 to 400 rad should not be employed. Hemibody radiation might be necessary for patients who have pelvic bone metastasis as part of an extensive metastasis.

During radiation therapy for cancer, pain should be controlled with appropriate doses of systemic analgesics consisting of NSAIDs, which are specifically effective in the relief of bone pain and, if necessary, supplementation by weak or strong opioids (Chapters 24 and 89). In patients whose pain is severe or excruciating, and in whom radiation therapy is being done on an inpatient basis, the use of continuous epidural opioid therapy achieved by the insertion of a catheter into the epidural space and by injection of an opioid should be considered. Because various bones of the pelvis are supplied by nerve fibers derived from L2 to S1, the catheter should ideally be placed through the L5–S1 interspace; with the catheter tip at the L3 level, 4 ml of opioid solution is injected. If difficulty is encountered the catheter can be inserted into the sacral canal and advanced 8 cm to place its tip at the S1 vertebral level. By adhering strictly to aseptic technique the catheter can be maintained for the several weeks required for the radiation therapy. (Chapter 95).

Myofascial Disorders

Muscle Spasms

Pelvic muscle spasm in females was discussed in Chapter 67. A similar condition occurs in males, who experience pain in the perineum, rectum, and back that is associated with intense local spasm of the levator muscles. Acute transient muscle spasm can develop following injury to the perineum. In such cases the pain might be moderate but occasionally is severe enough to disable patients completely. The pain is usually sharp and felt deeply in the perineum, with radiation to the coccyx, sacrum, and rectum. Patients respond to application of deep heat and massage. If the pain is severe enough, injection of local anesthetic into the spastic muscles might be required (Chapter 94).

An alternate procedure involves administration of a low caudal analgesia limited to the lower three sacral segments. This is done by injecting 4 to 5 ml of a long-acting local anesthetic (e.g., 0.25% bupivacaine with epinephrine 1:200,000), which provides complete pain relief for 8 to 10 hours. In some patients it might be necessary to insert an epidural catheter through the sacrococcygeal hiatus and advance it to the S3 level. This permits repeated injection of the local anesthetic or continuous infusion using an infusion pump.

Generalized perineal muscle spasm unrelated to trauma can persist and produce chronic dull aching pain felt deep in the lower abdomen, pelvis, perineum, rectum, and lower part of the sacrum (Chapter 67). In many patients the pain is of mild to moderate intensity, and can be exacerbated by intercourse and emotional tension. Drinkwater and associates (24) studied 14 patients with chronic perineal pain who had gained no lasting relief from various therapies and were considered to be on a "nothing further can be done" status. They examined the profile of pain personality, nonpain problems, and attitudes to treatment parameters. In addition to the clinical interview schedule they administered the McGill Pain Questionnaire, Cattell's 16 PF Questionnaire, and the Claybury Battery. They found that the means of all variables in the McGill Pain Questionnaire exceeded (indicated more pain) than those quoted by Melzack for menstrual, arthritic, cancer, dental, back, phantom limb, and postherpetic pain (see Fig. 66-1). On the average, the affective subclasses were more frequently used than the sensory subclasses. The mean other-problem total was low compared to that in psychiatric groups, and the mean 16 PF profile showed significant desurgency and conscientiousness. They found that all 14 patients were more responsive to behavioral psychologic intervention than to psychotherapy. Apparently, most of the patients studied had perineal pain primarily as a result of psychologic factors, and behavioral approaches such as stress management and muscle relaxation techniques were part of the general management plan. In some selected patients the use of continuous

or intermittent caudal analgesia as a "psychologic crutch" might prove beneficial.

Postoperative Muscle Spasm

Surgery on perineal structures or pelvic viscera, like operations on other parts of the body, invariably produces reflex spasm of skeletal muscles that results in moderate to severe pain. Usually the muscle spasm and pain occur during the first and the second postoperative days. The treatment of such pain is discussed in detail in Chapter 25.

Some patients who undergo laminectomy for removal of a herniated disk or for spinal stenosis have repeated bouts of severe muscle spasm in the low back, perineum, and upper thighs. Rather perplexingly, the reflex muscle spasm does not occur during the first 2 days after the procedure, but begins as soon as patients ambulate, perhaps on the third or fourth postoperative day. The spasm and associated severe pain last only a few minutes. These bouts are triggered by movement of the trunk, especially the pelvis, although sometimes they occur while patients lie in bed. On the basis of personal experience with this type of pain, which followed a laminectomy for spinal stenosis and removal of a herniated disk 2 years later, I can attest to the severity and excruciating nature of this condition.

The mechanism of such abnormal reflex responses is unknown, but they might result from sensitization of the spinal cord neurons involved in reflex mechanisms, which is initiated by the surgery and sustained by a postoperative nociceptive barrage. Surprisingly, this problem is not discussed in textbooks of orthopedic surgery.

Therapy is directed toward decreasing the hyperreflexia with pharmacologic agents. Diazepam, given in doses of 10 mg every 4 hours, has proven to be highly effective in terminating the spasm and associated pain. Because this problem follows low back surgery it is discussed in more detail in Chapter 73.

Myofascial Pain Syndromes

Pain in the pelvis and perineum can be provoked by myofascial pain syndromes with trigger points. Because the causes, pathophysiology, diagnosis, and treatment of myofascial pain syndromes with trigger points are discussed in detail in Chapter 21 only brief mention is made here of several syndromes that produce pain in the pelvis and gluteal region with reference to the perineum. These include trigger points in the lowermost portion of the external abdominal oblique, the lower part of the rectus abdominis, gluteus maximus, gluteus medius, and gluteus minimus (25–27). The pattern of pain produced by trigger points in the lowermost portion of the abdominal wall is depicted in Figure 64-6B. Pain is produced in the groin and testicle, with some radiation to the lower abdominal wall and upper part of the interior thigh.

Trigger points in the lateral border of the rectus abdominis muscle produce pain in the right or left lower quadrant, depending on which side the trigger point is located. Trigger points in the right lower rectus abdominis produce pain and tenderness in the region of McBurney's point, which simulates the pain of acute appendicitis (Fig. 64-7A). Trigger points in the lowermost part of the rectus abdominis bilaterally produce pain in the hypogastric region. Through somatovisceral reflexes, trigger points can intensify the pain of dysmenorrhea or can cause other types of dysfunction of the pelvic viscera (26).

Trigger points in one or more of the gluteal muscles and in the piriformis muscle frequently produce pain in the lower back over the sacrum and in the glutei with spillover pain to the perineum and thigh. Because these syndromes produce pain primarily in the low back, lower limbs, or both, they are discussed in Chapters 73 and 77.

B. PAIN OF NEUROPATHIC ORIGIN

Pain in the pelvis and perineum can be caused by various neuropathic disorders, including lesions of the lowermost portion of the spinal cord or conus medullaris, by pathology of surrounding meninges, or by lesions in the lumbar epidural space and sacral canal, with consequent compression and irritation of the nerves that supply the pelvis, perineum, and the lower limb. Nerves to these regions can also be involved in peripheral neuropathic conditions that produce pain as well as sensory and motor deficits. The pathophysiology, diagnosis, and treatment of most of these conditions are discussed in Chapter 73, so a brief description of several conditions is presented here for the sake of completeness. Several peripheral neuropathies not considered in Chapter 73 are discussed in detail.

Central Pain Syndromes

Lesions of the Spinal Cord, Meninges, and Epidural Space (XXVI-7)

Intramedullary lesions, or disease of the lowest portion of the conus medullaris, such as tumor, multiple sclerosis, syringomyelia, abscess, trauma, or a combination of these, can produce pain in the pelvis and perineum. The pain is usually spontaneous, burning, diffuse, and poorly localized, is continuous or explosive in nature, and is frequently associated with hyperalgesia, hyperpathia, and paresthesia.

Extramedullary intrathecal lesions, such as primary or metastatic neoplasms, abscesses, and hemorrhages, initially produce pain localized to the low back and pelvis. The pain subsequently becomes radicular, however, is aggravated by straining and coughing, and is associated with paravertebral tenderness, paresthesia, sensory loss, muscle weakness, and lower motor neuron signs involving those lumbosacral spinal cord segments in which the lesion is located.

Epidural spinal cord compression caused by primary or metastatic tumor, hemorrhage, or abscess that produces pressure of the conus medullaris invariably produces low back and pelvic pain, but often it also involves the lower limbs. I have learned of cases of patients who had been heparinized and in whom puncture for subarachnoid or epidural block was followed by hemorrhage in the lower lumbar and sacral canals, with consequent neurologic, sensory, and motor dysfunction in the pelvis, lower limbs, and perineum.

Arachnoiditis of the cauda equina is a condition characterized by inflammation and fibrosis of the arachnoid membrane. In most patients the condition involves many segments of the cauda equina, but occasionally it is limited to the rootlets and roots of the lower three sacral and coccygeal nerves. It is manifested by pain, sensory deficits, and motor dysfunction in the "saddle region," and is often associated with dysesthesia and paresthesia.

Lesions of the Roots or Spinal Nerves of the Lumbosacral Segments

Lesions of the roots or rootlets produce a radiculopathy, consequent radiculalgia, or segmental pain. They are caused by acute and infectious processes such as herpes zoster, chronic infection, or metabolic or toxic neuropathy, or by compression of nerve roots or formed nerves by tumors, disk protrusions, vertebral fractures, osteophytes, and arthropathies (Chapters 10 and 73).

Peripheral Neuropathy
Iliohypogastric, Ilioinguinal, or Genitofemoral Neuralgia (XXV-1)
Etiology and Pathophysiology

Neuralgia of the iliohypogastric, ilioinguinal, or genitofemoral nerve, or a combination of these, can be provoked by a large pelvic tumor that compresses these nerves in a course along the lateral edge of the pelvis, becoming subcutaneous near the anterior superior iliac spine. More frequently, neuralgia is consequent to unintentional section of one or more nerves, with consequent development of neuroma. The nerve can also be ligated or entrapped by a tear, resulting in endoneural fibrosis (28).

Symptoms and Signs

Neuralgia of one or more of these nerves is characterized by a burning, aching pain in the distribution of the affected nerve. If the hypogastric nerve is involved, pain is produced in the inguinal and suprapubic regions, with occasional reference to the hip region. If the injury involves the ilioinguinal and genitofemoral nerves, the pain radiates to the inguinal region and to the anterior part of the labia majora in the female or to the scrotum and root of the penis in the male, as well as to the inner and anterior surfaces of the thigh. The pain is usually continuous but can be aggravated by forcible stretching of the hip joint, coughing, sneezing, or general tension in the abdominal muscles, or sexual intercourse. The patient frequently adopts a posture that eases discomfort, with a slight flexure of the hip and a slight forward inclination of the trunk.

On examination, pain can be triggered by pressure in a narrowly circumscribed area of the operative scar (28). Usually tenderness extends along the course of the nerve from the anterior superior iliac spine to the external genitalia. When the genitofemoral nerve is involved, the internal ring of the inguinal canal can be painful. Associated with pain is cutaneous hyperalgesia and occasionally hypesthesia, especially to cold stimuli. In some patients scratching the skin produces less or no reddening on the affected side as compared to the normal side, indicating the degeneration of afferent C fibers. A lesion of the hypogastric nerve is associated with decrease or loss of the lower abdominal reflex, whereas the cremaster reflex is absent on the affected side with involvement of the genital branch of the genitofemoral nerve.

Diagnosis

Diagnosis is made by history, characteristics of the pain, and physical findings. Infiltration of the affected nerve with a local anesthetic eliminates the pain and thus helps to confirm the diagnosis.

Treatment

Without treatment the pain can persist for several years without any tendency to improve (28). A series of blocks of the affected nerve with a long-acting local anesthetic, such as 0.25% bupivacaine with epinephrine, done on a biweekly basis for 3 to 4 weeks, should be tried; occasionally this produces prolonged or permanent relief. If a sensitive neuroma is found, and its palpation produces aggravation of the pain, injection of a local anesthetic into the neuroma can relieve the pain and associated symptoms. If repeated injections of the neuroma produce only transient relief, the neuroma can be injected with 0.5 ml of alcohol or phenol; this has been reported to be effective in providing prolonged relief but carries the risk of producing postinjection neuropathy with neuralgia. Before neurolytic agents are used, local anesthetic block and transcutaneous electrical nerve stimulation (TENS) should be tried. If none of these conservative therapies is helpful, surgical repair of the nerve is said to be the most effective therapy.

Obstetric Neuropathy

Many cases of maternal obstetric neuropathy consequent to vaginal delivery have been reported. The frequency is reported to be 1 in 2500 deliveries (29).

Etiology

Neuropathy of the obturator or sciatic nerve, or of the pudendal plexus, can be caused by continuous pressure by the presenting part during a prolonged labor and vaginal delivery; or it can be caused by direct damage by the edges of the obstetric forceps during forceps delivery (30). Usually one or more nerves on one side are involved, but occasionally bilateral involvement occurs. Although obstetricians generally tend to attribute the neuropathy to local anesthesia, most reported incidents have occurred with general anesthesia or no anesthesia at all (30). In some cases the condition developed in parturients who were managed with subarachnoid or epidural anesthesia, but careful evaluation of the symptoms and signs eliminated this cause (see below).

Symptoms and Signs

Usually, soon after delivery, or 1 or 2 days later, the patient has a burning, aching pain in the distribution of the affected nerve and frequently motor impairment or loss—hence the term "obstetric paralysis."

Diagnosis

Differential diagnosis is simple if one considers that the symptoms and signs in obstetric neuropathy have a peripheral nerve distribution. Involvement of the rootlets and roots of a single peripheral nerve and sparing of other nerves supplied by the same lumbosacral spinal segments is impossible as a complication of subarachnoid or epidural block because, with these procedures, the neurotoxic effect of the local anesthetic is bilateral and involves the rootlets of all anesthetized nerves.

Treatment

Treatment of obstetric neuropathy consists of rest, together with a splint or cast to prevent footdrop. Recovery is usually slow but is complete in most patients. Pain is controlled with NSAIDs given over several weeks. If these are not sufficient they can be supplemented with opioids for 2 to 3 weeks.

Tumor Infiltration of the Lower Sacrum and Sacral Nerves (XXV-2)

Etiology

Metastasis of neoplasm to the lower half of the sacrum can result in compression of the nerves that contribute to the pudendal plexus and nerves. In other cases the lumbosacral plexus can be compressed by the tumor, or marked lymphadenopathy is present.

Symptoms and Signs

Pain in the distribution of the sacral nerves occurring in patients in their fifth, sixth, or seventh decade is frequently the result of the spread of bladder, gynecologic, or colonic cancer. The pain is dull, aching, and burning in character, is frequently located in the midline, and is associated with a burning or throbbing pain in the soft tissues of the rectal and perineal regions. The pain is aggravated by sitting and lying.

Examination reveals tenderness over the sacrum and region of the sciatic notch associated with sensory loss in the perianal region and in the genitalia, and can be accompanied by hyperpathia. The pain and sensory deficit can initially be unilateral but later can progress to bilateral sacral nerve involvement, with consequent sphincter incontinence and impotence.

Diagnosis

Diagnosis is made through the history, physical examination, and radiography, including CT scanning of the pelvis, which shows sacral erosion with a presacral mass.

Treatment

Treatment should begin with anticancer therapies (Chapters 24 and 89). Pharmacologic agents, regional anesthesia, neurostimulation techniques, or a combination of these can be used to control the pain, depending on the severity of the pain and on the resources available. In patients who have severe unilateral pain it is best to give trial to subarachnoid local anesthetic block followed by subarachnoid neurolysis (Chapter 96). With precise technique and skill the analgesia can be produced predominantly on one side. In patients in good physical condition a percutaneous cervical cordotomy is indicated. If the pain is bilateral, percutaneous cordotomy is done on one side and a subarachnoid neurolysis on the other. In patients with bladder or anal sphincter dysfunction, alternative procedures (Chapter 96) include administration of a low caudal block, preferably with a local anesthetic; if relief is complete it is followed by injection of 5% aqueous phenol, phenol in glycerin, or 25% alcohol. Cryoanalgesia is another alternative.

Pudendal Neuralgia

Etiology

Unilateral pudendal neuropathy with neuralgia can result from trauma that causes fracture of the ischial spine, which lies just anterior to the origin of the pudendal nerve. It can also result from entrapment of the nerve or of some of its branches, which pass through the sacrospinous ligament, or the nerve can be compressed during its course in Alcock's canal. Finally, damage to the nerve during pudendal nerve block can occur if the nerve is penetrated with a large dull needle with a hook on its bevel, a condition in which axons are sectioned in a jagged fashion and cause intraneural hemorrhage.

Bilateral pudendal neuralgia is extremely rare and can be caused by trauma during injection or, more frequently, by trauma to the perineum, such as during bicycle or horseback riding, or following injury of the type that occurs when the patient falls and straddles a sharp object. In addition, one or more branches of the pudendal nerve can become involved when surgical or traumatic scars in the perineal area are produced.

Symptoms and Signs

Pudendal neuralgia is characterized by a mild to severe burning pain with occasional bouts of lancinating pain, cutaneous hyperalgesia, hypalgesia, deep tenderness (particularly in the course of the nerve), paresthesia, tingling, and subjective numbness. The cutaneous tenderness can be so severe as to prevent the patient from sitting or from engaging in sexual intercourse. Paresthesia can cause the patient to scratch, resulting in irritation of the skin and soon creating a vicious circle (see below, Pruritus Ani).

Diagnosis

Diagnosis is made on the basis of the history and physical examination and, in the case of trauma or fracture, by radiographic evidence, or palpation can reveal a scar involving the nerve or one of its branches. Diagnostic pudendal nerve block with a local anesthetic confirms the diagnosis.

Treatment

Post-traumatic neuropathy consequent to needle penetration usually resolves over a period of weeks. Severe nerve damage by fracture can cause the neuropathy to persist for months. If the neuralgic pain is mild to moderate it can be controlled with NSAIDs and tricyclic antidepressants such as amitriptyline,

which has been found to be helpful in managing the pain of various neuropathies. Periods of severe pain can be controlled by pudendal block achieved with 0.25% bupivacaine with epinephrine, using extreme care not to damage the nerve further with the needle.

Chronic Postepisiotomy Pain

Earlier in this chapter acute postepisiotomy pain was mentioned, and this is discussed in detail in Chapter 66. Because this type of pain usually lasts several days it can be adequately managed with NSAIDs. In a small number of patients, however, the pain persists and becomes chronic. It is usually continuous and burning in character, with occasional bouts of lancinating pain, and is aggravated by intercourse or vaginal douching. Although the pain is usually mild, in some instances it is sufficiently intense to disable the puerpera partially or completely. In such patients, the episiotomy scar is usually extremely tender, large, and firm, and is associated with a burning, aching pain that either is localized to the region of the scar or more frequently is spread over the ipsilateral perineum. The pain is associated with hyperalgesia and deep tenderness of the perineum.

Diagnosis

The diagnosis is made through the history and examination of the perineum. Infiltration of the scar with a local anesthetic should provide complete relief of pain, whether localized or spread over the perineum.

Treatment

If the pain is mild to moderate, conservative management consists of NSAIDs combined with antidepressants and sitz baths three times daily for several weeks. If these measures are ineffective or if the pain is severe, a series of injections of the scar with a long-lasting local anesthetic twice weekly for several weeks can help to provide relief or at least decrease the intensity of the pain and eliminate hyperalgesia and tenderness. If these procedures provide complete but transient pain relief, the problem can be resolved either by plastic revision of the scar or by infiltration of the scar with a small amount of neurolytic agent provided the patient has been thoroughly informed of possible complications (Chapter 96).

Phantom Pelvic Visceral Pain Syndromes

Phantom Urinary Bladder Pain Syndrome (I-3)

Review of the literature reveals that phantom urinary phenomena occur rarely following cystectomy, spinal cord injury, and hemodialysis, in which previous disease of the kidney, urethra, and urinary bladder was present.

Symptoms and Signs

Brena and Sammons (31) reported a case of a 38-year-old woman who complained of midline suprapubic pain that had started 1 year previously following removal of the bladder for chronic severe cystitis. The patient described the pain as being continuous and feeling like "having a very full bladder," with recurrent episodes of sharp, burning acute pain. She rated the degree of pain as 90 on a scale of 0 to 100 (0, no pain; 100, intensity of pain comparable to that of labor pain), and further stated that the discomfort was "tearing her nervous system apart." Treatment with oxycodone, diazepam, and other mild analgesics was ineffective.

The patient's past medical history and social profile appeared normal except for a sharp decrease in social, recreational, and sexual activities because of the continuing pain (31). Physical examination revealed no abnormalities other than tenderness to palpation and a decreased pinprick pain threshold over the suprapubic region in both lower quadrants. She also had tenderness to palpation in the right flank, with a number of trigger points over the paravertebral area in the lumbar back region. Neurologic examination revealed no abnormalities. Brena and Sammons (31) made the important point that their patient had had continuous pain caused by the urinary tract infection prior to surgery.

Brena and Sammons (31) cited three other reports pertaining to this phenomenon. One involved phantom urinary bladder following cystectomy for recurrent bladder tumors. Another report described 7 patients with spinal cord injury who had experienced sensations of unpleasant urinary bladder distension after drinking water. The third report concerned 24 of 35 patients undergoing hemodialysis because of severe renal damage, with average urinary outputs of no more than 500 ml. These 24 patients experienced feelings of discomfort, bladder distension, and an urge to micturate. Brena and Sammons (31) then briefly mentioned the possible mechanisms, which are similar to those discussed in Chapter 12.

Treatment

Brena and Sammons (31) managed their patient with a series of six lumbar sympathetic blocks with 0.25% bupivacaine combined with a course of six applications of TENS, and relaxation-assertiveness training, given over a 10-day period. At the end of the treatment and at 3- and 6-months follow-up, the patient reported that the phantom bladder sensation had been reduced to 25% of previous levels and that the suprapubic burning pain and tenderness were no longer present. It has also been reported that regional analgesia carried out for several days prior to amputation in patients who had pain in the limb before the surgery and continued for several days postoperatively markedly decreases the incidence of painful phantom sensations (Chapter 94). This would suggest that patients who have severe urinary bladder pain (or severe pain as a result of other pelvic visceral disease) should receive continuous epidural analgesia extending from T9 to S5 for 48 hours prior to removal of the viscus and for 2 to 3 days postoperatively. Although the literature review suggests that these cases are rare, it is likely that the condition has been under-reported. Notwithstanding its low frequency, aggressive management with regional analgesia should be considered to relieve the discomfort of patients who experience these phenomena.

Phantom Anus Pain Syndrome

Boas (32) reported that, among 177 patients who had undergone abdominoperineal surgical resection, 40 patients (23%) developed characteristics of phantom anus perineal pain. Analysis of the characteristics of the pain, and especially of the time of onset, revealed that these patients fell into two subgroups, early onset and late onset.

Symptoms and Signs

Patients in the early group experienced phantom anus perineal pain within days or weeks of the surgery, and the pain was rated as having an intensity of 2.1 ± 0.8 on a scale of 0 to 4 (32). Of those in this group, 18 patients (75%) experienced aching pain, 8 (33%) had burning pain, and 4 (17%) had sharp or stabbing pain. In a considerable number of those in this early group (7 patients) the pain was mild, but, among those with burning pain about the nonexistent anus, the pain was of high intensity, having a score of 2.6 ± 0.5.

In the 16 patients who experienced pain months or years after the surgery, the pain had greater intensity (2.4 ± 0.9). In 14 of these 16 patients (88%) the pain was aching, 2 (13%) experienced burning pain, and 6 (38%) had a sharp or stabbing component to the pain; those in this last group (with the sharp stabbing pain) recorded high scores (2.8 ± 0.9).

The most common factor that initiated or aggravated the pain in the entire group was sitting on hard surfaces, with tiredness being a significant contributing factor in 25% of all patients. Spontaneous pain was experienced by 9 patients (38%) in the early group and by 4 (25%) in the late group. None of the patients experienced cutaneous numbness or hyperesthesia around the perineal scar. None of the patients in the first group had recurrence of pain, while 4 (25%) in the late group had recurrence of the cancer.

Treatment

Fifty-eight percent of those in the early group and 69% of those in the late group noted that rest and use of cushions relieved the pain. Systemic analgesic drugs proved to be almost totally ineffective for the relief of early onset-type pain, but helped some in the late onset group. Boas (32) reported that IV lidocaine administered in doses of 1.5 to 2 ml/kg totally abolished the phantom anal pain for several hours. Subarachnoid block, with small doses of a hyperbaric solution of lidocaine, reduced the pain intensity but did not abolish the phantom sensation until the block extended to the T10 to T12 spinal cord levels. Boas (32) also noted that the phantom pain could be relieved by a combination of tricyclic antidepressants and antiepileptic drugs.

C. PAINFUL VISCERAL AND DERMATOLOGIC DISORDERS

Various painful disorders of the skin and subcutaneous tissue can cause pain in the rectum, perianal region, perineum, and external genitalia. Most of these have been discussed in Chapters 60, 67, and 68, so here I briefly mention those that, although unusual, deserve to be considered in the differential diagnosis.

Rectal and Anal Pain

Etiology and Symptoms and Signs

In addition to fissure in ano and hemorrhoids, superficial ulcers of the rectum and anus can be caused by syphilis, tuberculosis, typhoid, dysentery and, of course, malignant lesions. These conditions cause pain in the rectum, anus, and perianal region that is sharp and burning in character and is aggravated by defecation. These patients have tenesmus, diarrhea, blood or mucus, and spasm of the sphincter muscle, and proctoscopic examination reveals characteristics of the lesion.

SUBMUCOUS PROCTITIS AND PERIPROCTITIS. Submucous proctitis and periproctitis, fistula in ano, and rectal papillitis and cryptitis produce a sharp throbbing pain in the perirectal and perianal regions aggravated by defecation or walking. The pain is associated with acute tenderness, swelling, and redness and, if the infection is severe, with fever, malaise, and other systemic symptoms.

PRURITUS ANI. Pruritus ani from pinworms and other parasites, hemorrhoids, cryptitis, papillitis, and other superficial lesions causes moderate to severe intractable itching of the anal region. This produces the urge to scratch and initiates the vicious circle of scratch → more itch → more scratch → abrasion of the region.

FURUNCLES AND CARBUNCLES. The perianal region can also be the site of acute furuncles and carbuncles, which are painful staphylococcal abscesses of one or more hair follicles in the hair-bearing area around the anus. The furuncle can commence as a superficial pustular infection of the osteum of a hair follicle and then can extend down to produce a painful, red, swollen lesion surrounding a deeper abscess and surmounted by a central pustule. A carbuncle results from the dissection of a furuncle in the subcutaneous space to adjacent follicles and the ultimate development of abscesses in a number of adjacent follicles. This leads to a more edematous, larger, and much more painful red lesion surmounted by numerous follicular pustules.

Treatment

Treatment of most of these dermatologic disorders is considered in Chapter 27. Obviously, if the condition is caused by bacteria, antibacterial drugs constitute the first phase of treatment. Patients with an infectious process, such as periproctitis, furuncles, or carbuncles, should have cultures made of the superficial pustules to determine the antibiotic sensitivity of the causative agent. During the primary therapy it is essential to control the pain, which can range in intensity from a minor annoyance to disabling discomfort, with appropriate systemic analgesics, including opioids if the pain is severe enough.

In case of severe excruciating pain it might be useful to administer a continuous low caudal block *provided* that the sacrococcygeal area is not infected. This procedure is especially useful for those with pruritus ani because it provides complete relief of itching for several days and thus breaks the vicious circle mentioned above. Usually a low caudal block with 0.25% bupivacaine given in volumes of 3 to 4 ml produces analgesia of the last two or three sacral and coccygeal nerves, and thus eliminates the abnormal sensory input from this region. Patients who have severe tenesmus should be given a trial on lumbar sympathetic block; if this is effective in relieving the condition, chemical sympathectomy should be carried out because it can provide long-term relief. Bristow and Foster (33) reported that 10 of 12 patients with severe spasmodic painful tenesmus were relieved with chemical sympathectomy and the relief lasted as long as 7 months at follow-up.

Dermatologic Disorders of the Perineum and External Genitalia

Etiology and Symptoms and Signs

Injury to the skin caused by superficial trauma and dermatologic conditions can also involve the rest of the perineal area including the female external genitalia, or the scrotum and penis. Conditions include condyloma lata, which produces pain and tenderness if the warts are ulcerated and is associated with muscle spasms. Pain caused by trauma to the female perineum and genitalia is discussed in Chapter 67. In addition to injury, ulcers, chancroid, and condylomata lata cause localized pain and swelling in the scrotum.

Another condition that can cause pain and discomfort in the pelvic perineal area is hydrenadenitis suppurativa, a chronic painful suppurative inflammatory disease of the apocrine glands in the genitocrural area. This condition is thought to be caused by occlusion of the apocrine duct, which leads to an inflammatory foreign body reaction and eventually results in a mixed secondary bacterial infection. The pain is usually moderate to severe and is associated with exquisite tenderness and subcutaneous nodules. Unless treated promptly the condition progresses to development of deep abscesses that dissect with scarring and suppuration to adjacent follicles and apocrine glands, ultimately forming sinus tracts that cause symptoms and signs to wax and wane for years (Chapter 27).

Treatment

Treatment of infectious processes and trauma in the external female genitalia and vagina is discussed in detail in Chapter 67. Obviously, treatment of trauma to male genitalia requires debridement and surgical closure of lacerations. If a hematoma is present it needs to be incised and drained. Treatment of infectious dermatologic disorders in the perineum and scrotum requires appropriate antimicrobial therapy.

Hydrenadenitis suppurativa requires incision and draining of abscesses and palliative intralesional corticosteroid irrigation. Because this condition is often caused by multiple types of organisms a broad-spectrum antibiotic should be used. The therapy of choice in recent years has been prompt diagnosis and surgical extirpation of the affected skin and subcutaneous tissue (Chapter 27).

During the primary therapy for the condition, pain and suffering should be controlled with NSAIDs and, if necessary, by opioids for short periods. Again, if the pain is severe, or very severe, continuous low caudal analgesia achieved with 0.25% bupivacaine with epinephrine is highly effective. A steady level of analgesia can be achieved either with repeated boluses or continuous infusion.

D. REFERRED PAIN

Pain Referred to the Pelvis

Pain in the pelvis can be referred from diseases of the abdomen, especially acute appendicitis, acute renal pyelitis, spasm of the lower bowel from acute infection or chronic bowel disorders, which produce generalized cramping and abdominal discomfort, ulcerative colitis, disease of the kidney and pelvis, pelvic peritonitis, chronic colitis, Meckel's diverticulum, regional enteritis, and lower rectoperineal tumor. Because all these conditions are discussed in detail in Chapters 60, 62, and 64, no further comments are made here except that they must be considered in the differential diagnosis in patients complaining of pain in the pelvis.

Less common pain referred to the pelvis includes diseases of the hip and sacroiliac joint, left psoas abscess, aneurysm of the left iliac artery, strangulated retroperitoneal hernia, lower abdominal abscess, and chemical or infectious peritonitis (Chapters 64, 72, and 73).

Pain Referred to the Perineum

Pain referred to the perineum is frequently present with various pelvic gynecologic and urologic disorders, such as cystitis, prostatitis, and diseases of the uterus, and with other conditions (Chapters 67 and 68). Similarly, diseases of the hip joint or upper thigh can cause pain radiating to the perineum (Chapters 73 and 74).

E. PAIN PRIMARILY OF PSYCHOLOGIC ORIGIN

Chronic Pelvic Pain Without Obvious Pathology (XXIV-9)

In a significant number of patients who present with pelvic pain having characteristics of pain of gynecologic origin no obvious organic pathology can be found, even with comprehensive clinical and laboratory examination (Chapter 67). During the 1940s and 1950s various causative factors and hypotheses were presented, including pelvic vascular congestion, functional disturbance of sensory nerves, disturbance of the pelvic sympathetic system, and microscopic lacerations of the uterine ligaments, among others.

During the past decade, however, ample evidence has accumulated to suggest strongly that pelvic pain and associated symptoms without obvious pathology are caused primarily by psychopathology of one form or another. Psychiatric evaluation has shown that most of these women have borderline syndrome, neurosis, severe anxiety, depressive trends, somatization, and conflicts involving femininity. One study showed the unexpected findings of a history of childhood incest (34). Psychologic testing using the Minnesota Multiphasic Personality Inventory (MMPI) showed four significant clusters, objectively corroborating the occurrence of severe psychopathology. Other studies have shown that many of these patients experienced sexual and physical abuse as children and some as adults, while others had serious marital problems. (For a more detailed discussion of this problem refer to the last subsection of Chapter 67.)

Orchiodynia (XXV-1)

Orchiodynia, also known as orchidalgia and orchialgia, is characterized by chronic pain in one or both testicles without any obvious pathology found, even when the most modern methods of evaluation and laboratory testing are carried out. Although some patients give a vague history of an incidence of injury or vasectomy many years before, no abnormality can be found at the time of complaint. The pain is usually nagging, persistent, and achy, but only rarely and fleetingly severe. Unfortunately, no serious effort has been made to subject these patients to psychologic and psychiatric evaluation, which probably would reveal an underlying psychopathologic basis for the chronic complaints.

Rectal and Perineal Pain of Psychiatric Origin (XXV-3)

About 10% of psychiatric patients who complain of pain have rectal or perineal pain, although this is usually mentioned as a secondary site of pain (28). Only about 2% of patients report pain in these parts as the primary site and, in such cases, the rectal pain is usually associated with severe depressive or schizophrenic illness, although it can be associated with conversion symptoms. Conversion pain in these patients is usually accompanied by pain experienced elsewhere in the body.

Usually two types of pain are of psychiatric origin (Chapter 19), delusional or hallucinatory and hysteric or hypochondriac. Hallucinatory pain is attributed by the patient to a specific delusional cause, such as pain or a painful object in the rectum or perineum or in the vagina or penis. This type of pain varies from mild to severe and lasts in accordance with the causal psychologic illness. The pain can be aggravated by psychologic stress. A comprehensive physical and laboratory examination reveals no "organic pathology."

Hysteric or hypochondriac pain is specifically attributable to the thought processes, emotional state, or personality of patients in the absence of an organic or delusional cause, or to a tension mechanism (24, 28). This type of pain can be felt anywhere in the perineum or rectum, but, like other types of chronic pain of psychologic origin, is extremely rare. In general, females experience this type of pain more frequently than males. Pain is described in simple sensory terms but complex or affective descriptions are given by some patients. The pain is usually continuous throughout most of the waking hours but fluctuates somewhat in intensity, does not awaken patients from sleep, and usually lasts for more than 6 months. Pain is often present in other areas and can be associated with loss of function without a physical basis (e.g., anesthesia, paralyses).

REFERENCES

1. Hollinshead, W.H.: Anatomy for Surgeons, Vol. 3. The Back and Limbs. 3rd Ed. Philadelphia, Harper & Row, 1982, pp. 623–628.
2. Watson-Jones, R.: Dislocations and fracture dislocations of the pelvis. Br. J. Surg., 25:773, 1938.
3. Fu, F.H., and Mears, D.C.: Nonacetabular fractures of the pelvis. In Surgery of the Musculoskeletal System, Vol. 2. Edited by C. Evarts. New York, Churchill Livingstone, 1983, pp. 5:35–5:51.
4. Pennal, G.F., and Massiah, K.A.: Nonunion and delayed union of fractures of the pelvis. Clin. Orthop., 151:124, 1980.
5. Bonica, J.J.: Principles and Practice of Obstetric Analgesia and Anesthesia. Philadelphia, F.A. Davis, 1967, p. 95.
6. Greenhill, J.P.: Obstetrics. 13th Ed. Philadelphia, W.B. Saunders, 1965, p. 944.
7. Traut, E.F.: Rheumatic Diseases. St. Louis, C.V. Mosby, 1952.
8. Holmes, T.H.: Back muscle spasm, professional cramp and backache. In Textbook of Medicine. Edited by R.L. Cecil and R.F. Loeb. Philadelphia, W.B. Saunders, 1951.
9. Thiele, G.H.: Coccygodynia and pain in the gluteal region and down the back of the thighs. JAMA, 109:1271, 1937.
10. Lloyd, J.W., Barnard, J.D.W., and Glynn, C.J.: Cryoanalgesia: A new approach to pain relief. Lancet, 2:932, 1976.
11. Clawson, D.K.: Bacterial infection of bones and joints. In The Musculoskeletal System in Health and Disease. Edited by C. Rosse and D.K. Clawson. Hagerstown, MD, Harper & Row, 1980, pp. 363–374.
12. Sutro, C.J.: The pubic bones and the symphysis. Arch. Surg., 32:823. 1936.
13. Krane, S.M.: Paget's disease of the bone. In Harrison's Principles of Internal Medicine. Edited by R.G. Petersdorf et al. New York, McGraw-Hill, 1983, pp. 1960–1963.
14. Singer, F.R., et al.: Paget's disease of the bone. In Metabolic Bone Disease, Vol 2. Edited by L.V. Avioli and S.M. Krane. New York, Academic Press, 1978, p. 489.
15. DeRose, J., et al.: Response of Paget's disease to porcine and salmon calcitonins: Effect of long-term treatment. Am. J. Med., 56:858, 1974.
16. Rosse, C., and Clawson, D.K.: Neoplasia. In The Musculoskeletal System in Health and Disease. Edited by C. Rosse and D.K. Clawson. Hagerstown, MD, Harper & Row, 1980, pp. 421–430.
17. Neff, J.: Primary tumors of bone: An overview in adults. In Comprehensive Textbook of Oncology. Edited by A.R. Moossa, M.G. Robson, and S.C. Schimpff. Baltimore, Williams & Wilkins, 1986, pp. 641–656.
18. Weiss, L., and Gilbert, H.A. (eds.): Bone Metastasis. Boston, J.K. Hall, 1981, pp. 1–61.
19. Lenz, J., and Freid, J.R.: Metastases to skeleton, brain and spinal cord from cancer of the breast and effect of radiotherapy. Ann. Surg., 93:278, 1931.
20. Kaufmann, E.: Pathologische Anatomie der Malignen Neoplasmen der Prostata. Dtsch. Chir., 53:381, 1902.
21. Galasko, C.S.B.: Skeletal metastases and mammary cancer. Ann. R. Coll. Surg. Engl., 50:3, 1972.
22. Galasko, C.S.B., and Doyle, F.H.: The detection of skeletal metastases from mammary cancer. A regional comparison between radiology and scintigraphy. Clin. Radiol, 23:295, 1972.
23. Mauch, P.M.: Treatment of metastatic cancer to bone. In Cancer: Principles and Practices of Oncology. Edited by V.T. DeVita, S. Helman, and S.A. Rosenburg. Philadelphia, J.B. Lippincott, 1982, pp. 1564–1568.
24. Drinkwater, J.E., et al.: Psychologic characteristics of chronic perineal pain patients. Pain (Suppl.), 4:(S61):117, 1987.
25. Bonica, J.J.: Management of myofascial pain syndromes in general practice. JAMA, 164:732, 1957.
26. Travell, J.G., and Simons, D.J.: Myofascial Pain and Dysfunction: The Trigger Point Manual. Baltimore, Williams & Wilkins, 1983, pp. 660–683.
27. Sola, A.E.: Treatment of myofascial pain syndromes. In Recent Advances in Pain Research and Therapy, Vol. 7. Edited by C. Benedetti et al. New York, Raven Press, 1984, pp. 467–485.
28. Merskey, H. (ed.): Classification of chronic pain: Description of chronic pain syndromes and definition of pain terms. Pain (Suppl.), 3:PS45–46, S203, 1986.
29. Hill, E.C.: Maternal obstetric paralysis. Am. J. Obstet. Gynecol., 83:1452, 1962.
30. Bonica, J.J.: Principles and Practice of Obstetric Analgesia and Anesthesia, Vol. 1. Philadelphia, F.A. Davis, 1967, p. 733.
31. Brena, S.F., and Sammons, E.E.: Phantom urinary bladder pain—case report. Pain, 7:197, 1979.
32. Boas, R.A.: Phantom anus pain syndrome. In Advances in Pain Research and Therapy, Vol. 5. Edited by J.J. Bonica, U. Lindblom, and A. Iggo. New York, Raven Press, 1983, pp. 947–951.
33. Bristow, A., and Foster, J.M.G.: Lumbar sympathectomy in the management of rectal tenesmoid pain. Ann. Royal College Surg. Engl., 70:38, 1988.
34. Gross, R.G., et al.: Borderline syndrome and incest in chronic pelvic pain patients. Int. J. Psychiatr. Med., 10:79, 1980–1981.

70 • GENERAL CONSIDERATIONS OF PAIN IN THE LOW BACK, HIPS, AND LOWER EXTREMITIES

JOHN J. BONICA

DISORDERS of the lumbosacral portion of the spine or hip and of the lower limbs cause pain, suffering, and disability more frequently than disorders in any other part of the body. The most frequent cause of pain and disability in this region is musculoskeletal disease or dysfunction of the low back and lower limbs, followed by neuropathic disorders and peripheral vascular disease. It is essential to know the causes, pathophysiology, and symptoms and signs to make a correct diagnosis and to develop an effective therapeutic strategy. The clinician should have a thorough knowledge of the functional anatomy and biomechanics of the lumbar spine, sacrum, and various parts of the lower limbs, of the anatomy and function of the lumbar and lumbosacral plexuses and the major nerves derived therefrom, and of the vasculature to these structures.

This first chapter of Section F, like other chapters that introduce the managment of pain in various regions of the body, discusses these issues in five sections: A, The Lumbosacral Spine, including its functional anatomy and biomechanics; B, The Vertebral (Spinal) Canal and Its Contents, specifically a description of the spinal cord and its relation to the various parts of the vertebral canal; C, Nerves to the Lumbar Spine, Pelvis, and Lower Limbs; D, Sympathetic and Somatic Segmental and Peripheral Nerve Supply to the Hips and Lower Limbs; and E, Evaluation of the Patient, with an outline summarizing the most important aspects and a table summarizing the pain characteristics and other symptoms and signs to help make a differential diagnosis. The functional anatomy and biomechanics of the hip joints and adjacent structures are presented in Chapter 74, of the thigh and knee in Chapter 75, and of the leg, ankle, and foot in Chapter 76. The material in this chapter updates information from the first edition of this book (1) and summarizes more detailed discussions on these various subjects, presented elsewhere (2–6).

A. THE LUMBOSACRAL SPINE

Anatomy

This section presents the clinically relevant aspects of the anatomy of the lumbar spine and sacrum, including a brief description of the vertebrae, joints, ligaments, muscles, mobility, and biomechanics of the lumbar spine. Some of this is also presented in Chapters 46 and 53, which are concerned with the cervical and thoracic spines. Although the embryologic development of the three parts of the vertebral column is similar, the anatomy of the lumbar spine has characteristics different from those of the thoracic and cervical spines (Chapter 46). For example, the lumbar vertebrae are the largest of the true immovable vertebrae and are also large in comparison with their own vertebral canal. Additionally, the lumbar vertebrae have no articular facets on the sides of their centra as do the thoracic vertebrae, and have no foramina in their transverse processes, as do the cervical vertebrae. Figure 70-1 depicts the anatomy of a lumbar vertebra.

The body of the vertebra is large and is wider transversely than anteroposteriorly and a little thicker anteriorly than posteriorly (3). The cranial (superior) and caudal (inferior) surfaces are flat or slightly concave, while the sides of the centrum are definitely concave. Strong but short pedicles unite on the cranial part of the body and leave deep inferior vertebral notches. The laminae are broad, short, and strong and the vertebral (spinal) canal is triangular, and is larger than in the thoracic spine but smaller than in the cervical region. The spinous processes are thick, broad, and somewhat quadrilateral, ending in a rough uneven border that is thickest caudally, where it is occasionally notched (3). The transverse processes of the upper three vertebrae arise from junctions of the pedicles and laminae and are horizontal, while the transverse processes in the caudal two vertebrae arise from the pedicles and posterior parts of the body and are inclined posteriorly. Situated anterior to the articular processes, instead of posterior, as in the thoracic vertebrae, the transverse processes can be considered to be homologous with the ribs.

The articular processes are well defined and project from the junctions of the pedicles and laminae. The facets on the superior processes are concave and face medially and somewhat posteriorly, while those on the inferior processes are convex and are directed laterally and somewhat anteriorly. The superior facets are wider apart than the inferior and, in the articulated column, the inferior articular processes are embraced by the superior processes of the subjacent vertebrae. On the posterior borders of the large superior articular processes are rounded enlargements called the mammillary processes. Arising from the posterior portions of the bases of the transverse processes are small, rough elevations called accessory processes (Fig. 70-1A and B).

The L5 vertebra is massive in its structure and its body is much thicker anteriorly, which accords with the prominent sacrovertebral angle formed at the lumbosacral articulation (3). The spinous processes are smaller than those of other lumbar vertebrae, but the transverse processes are bulky, short, and thick and arise from the body as well as from the pedicle.

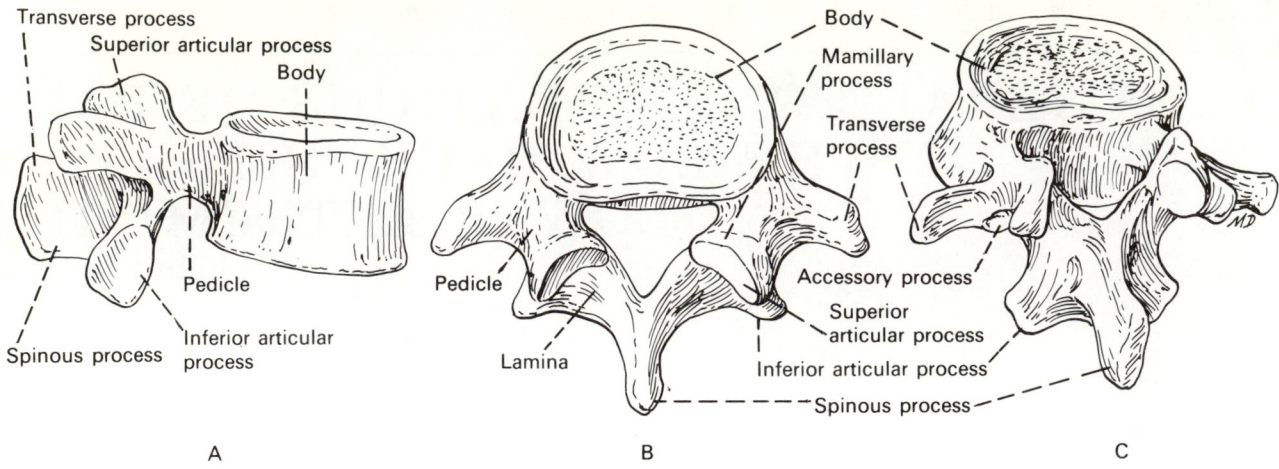

FIG. 70-1. Anatomy of a lumbar vertebra. **A.** Laterial view. **B.** Superior inferior view. **C.** Superior (cranial) aspect. The body is wider transversely than anteroposteriorly, and the spinal canal is triangle-shaped. Note the directions of the articular facets. See text for more details.

Sacrum

The sacrum is a large triangular bone situated in the lowermost part of the vertebral column that forms the posterior bony wall of the true pelvis. The broad superior end of the bone, considered as its base, articulates with the last lumbar vertebra while its more narrow apex articulates inferiorly with the coccyx. Inserted like a wedge between the two hip bones, its base projects anteriorly and forms the prominent sacrovertebral angle when articulated with the last lumbar vertebra. Figure 70-2 depicts the anatomy of the sacrum and coccyx, and Figure 70-3 illustrates the shape of the sacral canal.

Ligaments

Interconnecting each succeeding vertebra from the axis to the sacrum is a series of cartilaginous joints, which unite each adjacent pair of vertebral bodies by longitudinal ligaments and an intervertebral disk, and a series of synovial joints reinforced by ligaments, which unite the vertebral arches of the vertebrae at their interfacing articular processes. Figure 70-5 depicts the ligaments of the lumbar spine, and Figure 70-6 shows the sacral ligaments of the pelvis.

Functional Anatomy

The vertebral column is an aggregate of articulated superimposed segments, each of which is a functional unit (Chapter 46). The vertebral column functions to support two-legged humans in an upright position; it is mechanically balanced to conform to the stress of gravity, at the same time permitting locomotion and assisting in purposeful movement (2). The functional unit is composed of two segments (Chapter 46): the anterior segment, which contains two adjacent vertebral bodies, one superincumbent on the other and separated by the intervertebral disk, and a posterior neural segment (2). The anterior segment is essentially a weight-bearing, shock-absorbing, flexible structure while the posterior segment is a nonweight-bearing triangular structure that contains and protects the spinal cord, its coverings, and the rootlets and roots of

the spinal nerves, and contains a pair of joints that direct the movements of the unit (Fig. 70-4).

Anterior Portion of the Functional Unit

The anterior portion of the functional unit of the lumbar spine is well constructed for its weight-bearing and shock-absorbing function (2). The unit is comprised of two large vertebral bodies that are capable of

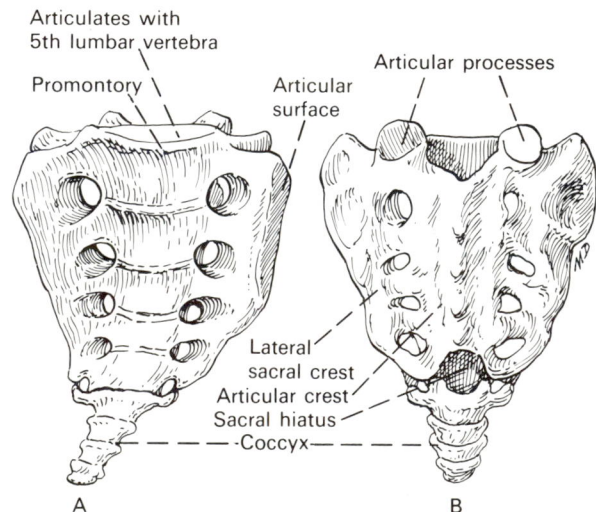

FIG. 70-2. Anatomy of the sacrum and coccyx. **A.** Anterior view. The anterior (pelvic) surface is concave, which provides increased capacity to the pelvic cavity, and is crossed by four transverse ridges that separate the five segments of vertebral bodies. The four pairs of rounded anterior (pelvic) sacral foramina communicate with the sacral canal by the intervertebral foramina, through which course the anterior primary divisions of the first four sacral nerves and the lateral sacral arteries and veins. The coccyx is a triangular structure composed of four rudimentary vertebrae. **B.** Posterior view. The posterior surface is convex and is narrower than the anterior surface. In the midline is the median sacral crest, on which are mounted three or four tubercles of the rudimentary spinous processes of the upper three or four sacral segments. The posterior sacral foramina are located between the intermediate and lateral sacral crests, through which pass the posterior primary divisions of the upper four sacral nerves. Between the sacrum and coccyx is the sacrococcygeal hiatus.

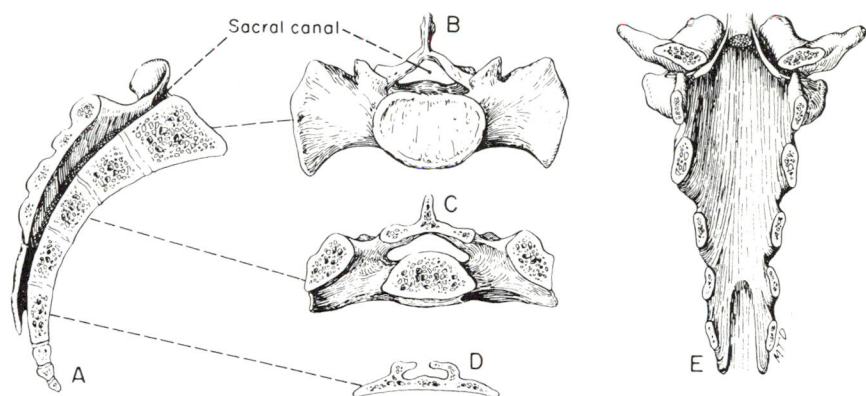

FIG. 70-3. Sacral canal. *A.* Sagittal view. *B.* Superior view showing the triangular canal. *C.* Horizontal cross section at the level of the 2nd pair of foramina. The anteroposterior diameter is short. The groove present on its posterior wall in the midline permits the catheter inserted into the canal to be advanced rostrally without deviation. Normally the anterior primary divisions of the lower three sacral nerves lie on the anterior surface of the canal. *D.* Cross-sectional view at the level of the S5 vertebra, where the canal is the upper part of the sacrococcygeal hiatus. This is covered by the posterior sacrococcygeal ligament, and a needle can be inserted through it for injection of local anesthetic solution into the canal. *E.* Roof of the sacral canal, as seen from within. From Bonica, J.J.: Principles and Practice of Obstetric Analgesia and Anesthesia. Vol. 1. Philadelphia, F.A. Davis, 1967.

sustaining extreme compressive stresses. These are separated by a "hydraulic system"—the intervertebral disk. The anterior portion of the lumbar spine has several structural differences from the anterior portion of the cervical unit (Chapter 46). Whereas the vertebral cartilaginous plates in the cervical spine are definitely concave and convex, and the nucleus pulposus is located in the anterior portion of the disk, the end plates in the lumbar spine are flat or slightly concave and the nucleus is centrally located in the disk. The relationship of the end plates and their shapes, plus the location of the nucleus, permits a rocker movement between the vertebrae in the lumbar region, whereas in the cervical region they permit a forward and backward gliding motion of the adjacent vertebrae. The

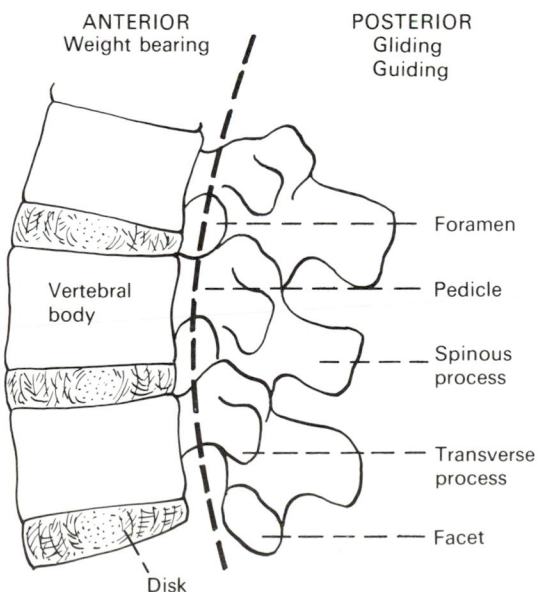

FIG. 70-4. Lumbar spine. Shown are parts of the anterior and posterior functional units.

anterior functional units of the lumbar spine, as in the cervical region, are bound together by the anterior and posterior longitudinal ligaments.

ANTERIOR LONGITUDINAL LIGAMENT. The anterior longitudinal ligament (ALL) is a broad strong band of fibers that extends along the anterior surfaces of the bodies of the vertebrae from the axis to the sacrum. The ligament is narrower in the cervical region but it broadens as it descends and is widest and strongest in the lumbar region, where it has the important function of helping to maintain an erect posture (see below) (3). The ligament is slightly narrowed but thicker as it passes over the vertebral bodies than over the intervertebral disk. It consists of dense longitudinal fibers that are intimately adherent to the intervertebral disks and the margins of the vertebrae but are not attached firmly to the middle parts of the bodies. The ligament is composed of several layers of fibers that vary in length but that are closely interrelated with each other, with the most superficial fibers being the longest, extending across four or five vertebrae. A second subjacent set of fibers extends between two or three vertebrae while a third set, the shortest and deepest, reaches from one vertebra to the other.

POSTERIOR LONGITUDINAL LIGAMENT. The posterior longitudinal ligament (PLL) extends along the posterior surface of the body of the vertebra from the axis to the sacrum and contributes to the anterior wall of the vertebral (spinal) canal (3). Of functional and potential pathologic significance is the fact that the PLL is intact and broad throughout the length of the vertebral column until it reaches the lumbar vertebrae (2). At the L1 vertebral level it begins to narrow progressively so that, on reaching the last lumbar and first sacral (L5–S1) interspace, it is only half of its original width (Fig. 70-5D; also see Fig. 70-7). This ultimate narrow posterior ligamentous reinforcement contributes to an inherent structural weakness at the level of greatest static stress and most spinal movement, producing the greatest kinetic strain (L5–S1) (2). The PLL is composed of longitudinal fibers that are denser and more compact than those of the ALL.

INTERVERTEBRAL DISKS. Although the anatomy of the intervertebral disk is described in detail in Chapter 46 its importance, particularly in the lumbar

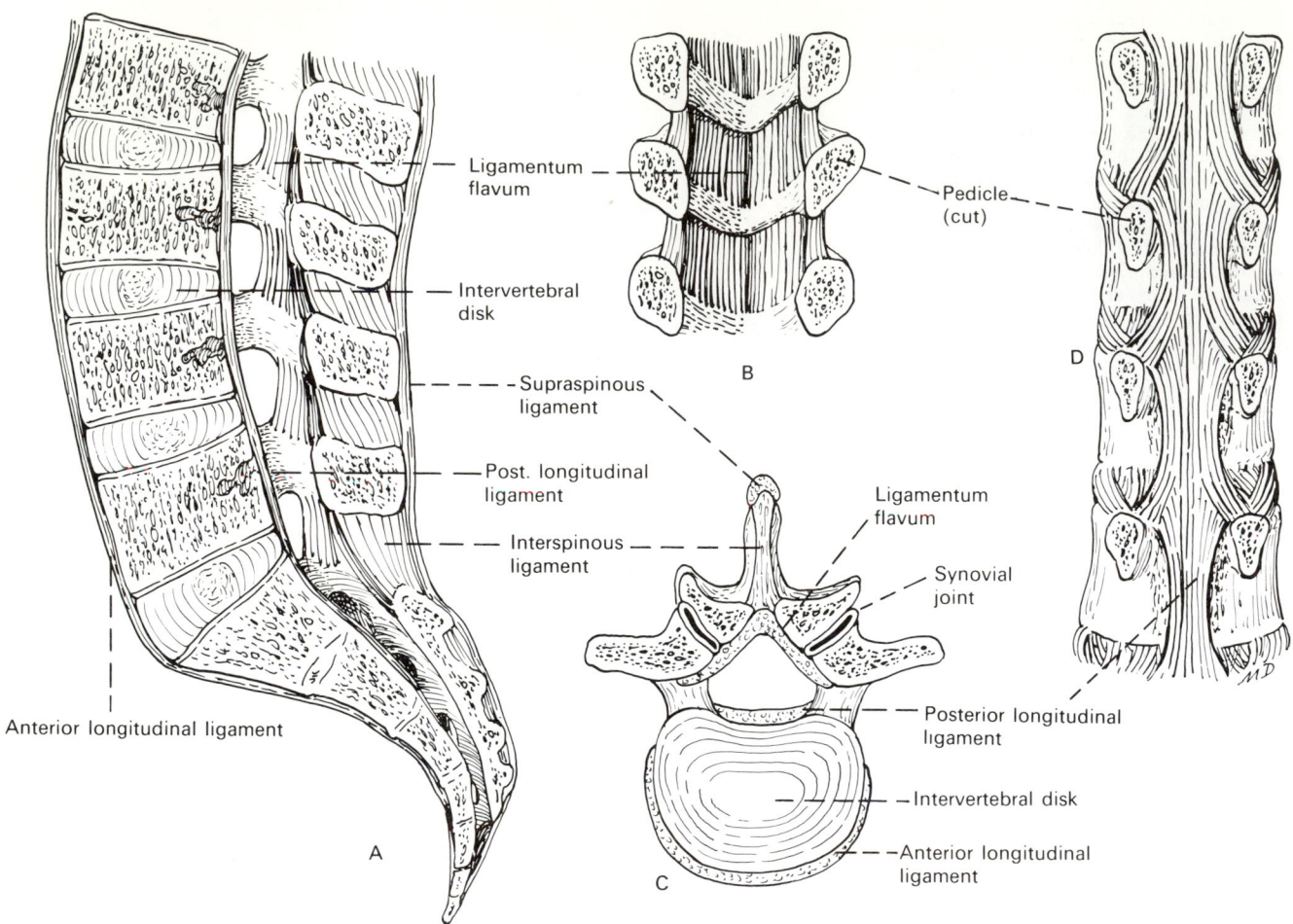

FIG. 70-5. Ligaments of the lumbar vertebrae. **A.** Medial sagittal section of three lumbar vertebrae and their ligaments. The vertebral bodies are slightly higher anteriorly than posteriorly and the intervertebral disk is also higher anteriorly than posteriorly. The interspinous ligaments are thin and membranous and interconnect with adjoining spinous processes, with their attachments extending from the root to the apex of each spinous process. Here they meet the ligamentum flavum anteriorly and the supraspinous ligament posteriorly. Whereas they are narrow and elongated in the thoracic region, they are broad, thick, and quadrilateral-shaped in the lumbar region to conform to the shape of the spinous process. The supraspinous ligament is a strong fibrous cord that connects the apices of the spinous processes the vertebrae. Fibrocartilage is developed in the ligament at its point of attachment to the tips of the spinous processes. The supraspinous ligament is thicker and broader in the lumbar than in the thoracic region. The most superficial fibers of the supraspinous ligament extend over three or four vertebrae, those coursing more deeply pass between two or three, and the deepest ones connect the spinous processes of neighboring vertebrae and become continuous with the interspinous ligament. **B.** Anteroposterior view of the laminae and intervening ligamenta flava in the lumbar region. The ligamenta flava connect the laminae of adjacent vertebrae and are thickest and strongest in the lumbar region. Each ligament consists of two lateral portions that begin on each side of the root of the articular process surrounded by the capsule and extend posteriorly to the point where the two laminae meet to form the spinous process. Each ligamentum flavum consists of yellow elastic tissue, the fibers of which are almost perpendicular to and are attached to the anterior and inferior surfaces of the lamina above and to the superior and posterior surfaces of the lamina below. **C.** Superior view of a lumbar vertebra showing the positions of the various ligaments in the lumbar region. The anterior longitudinal ligament almost covers the anterior surface of the body of the vertebra, whereas the posterior longitudinal ligament covers only a portion of the posterior surface of the vertebra. Note also the cut supraspinous and interspinous ligaments, ligamenta flava, and articular joints. **D.** Posterior aspect of the vertebral body. The laminae and spinous process have been removed to show the posterior longitudinal ligament in the lumbar region. The ligament broadens and becomes intimately adherent as it passes over each of the intervertebral disks and over contiguous margins of the vertebrae. It is narrow and thick over the center of the body, however, from which it is separated by the basivertebral veins. This ligament is broad in the cervical region but at the L1 vertebral level it begins to narrow progressively, so that on reaching the last lumbar and first sacral interspace it is only half of its original width. See text for a discussion of the implications.

region, requires that certain points be re-emphasized. Each disk, composed of a tough peripheral fibrocartilaginous ring, the annulus fibrosus, and of a more pliable intergelatinous mass, the nucleus pulposus, is a self-contained fluid system that absorbs shock, permits transient compression, and allows movement (2–5).

The superior and inferior plates of the disk are the end plates of the vertebral bodies which are composed of articular hyaline cartilage in direct contact and adherent to the underlying resilient bone of the vertebral body (2). In their normal state these end plates are firm, flat, circular, inflexible surfaces that form the cephalad and caudad portions of the disk, to which the encircling annulus fibrosus is attached.

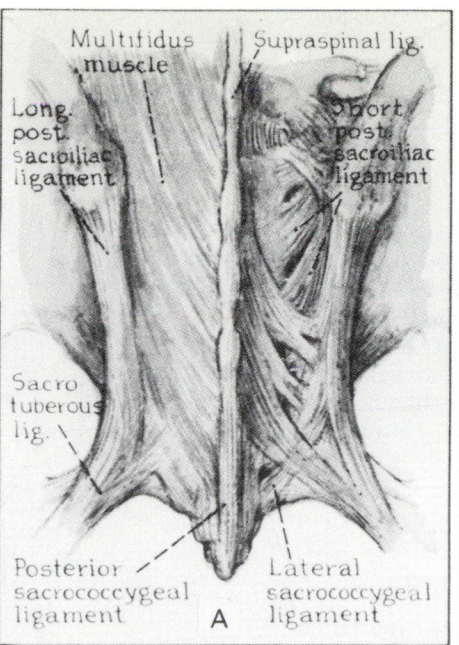
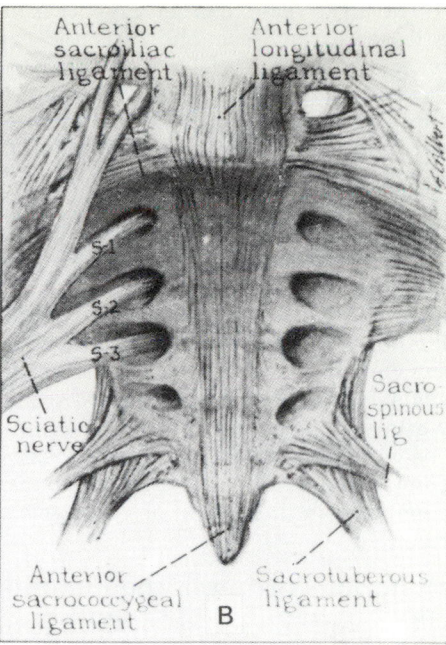

FIG. 70-6. *A.* Posterior view of the sacrum showing the ligaments and some of the muscles covering the posterior surface. *B.* Anterior view of the sacrum showing the ligaments and also the exit of the upper three sacral nerves. Note the direction and large size of the anterior sacral foramina. Blood vessels and loose areolar tissue that surround the nerves as they exit the foramina have been removed. (Compare with Fig. 65-4) From Bonica, J.J.: Principles and Practice of Obstetric Analgesia and Anesthesia. Vol. 1. Philadelphia, F.A. Davis, 1967.

The annulus is an intertwined fibroelastic mesh that encapsulates the gelatinous matrix of the disk, the nucleus pulposus (Fig. 70-7). The annulus fibers are attached around the entire circumference of both upper and lower end plates and intertwine in crisscross oblique directions, thus permitting movement of one vertebra on the other in a rocker motion, in a rotatory direction, and in a horizontal translational motion.

Because the nucleus pulposus is about 88% fluid, which is contained within the fibrous resilient wall of the annulus and between the floor and ceiling formed by the end plates of the vertebrae, it cannot be compressed. Thus, it conforms with Pascal's law, which states that "any external force exerted on a unit area of a confined liquid is transmitted undiminished to every unit area of the interior of the containing vessel." Consequently, any external force exerted on one unit area is transmitted undiminished to every unit area of the interior of the annulus (2).

The young or undamaged intervertebral disk has predominantly fibroelastic tissue, but the effect of aging or injury to the disk (or both) causes more and more fibrous tissue to replace the young, highly elastic collagen fibers. Consequently, the "older" disk container is less elastic and its hydraulic recoil mechanism weakens.

The colloidal gel of the nucleus pulposus is a mucopolysaccharide with a physicochemical action: it can imbibe external fluid and maintain its intrinsic water balance. At birth the disk contains 88% water but it dehydrates with age and trauma, so that in senescence it is 80% water. This causes a decrease in the protein polysaccharide level and thus a loss in the imbibitory property of the gel. Loss of the intradiskal fluid and the decrease of annular elasticity results in a decrease in pressure.

In the lumbar region the intervertebral disks comprise about 30% of the length of the column (4), as compared to 20 to 25% in the thoracic and cervical regions. The disks dehydrate (shrink) consequent to weight-bearing during the day and rehydrate during rest at night. The intervertebral disk is higher at its anterior portion than its posterior part, the greatest difference occurring in the L5 (L5–S1) disk. Through

its decidedly wedge shape the L5 disk contributes markedly to the lumbrosacral angle (4). Thus, in the upper part of the lumbar column, the normal curve is almost entirely a result of the wedge shape of the disks, whereas in the lower part the shape of the vertebral bodies is also a contributing factor, the last lumbar vertebra being the most wedge-shaped (4).

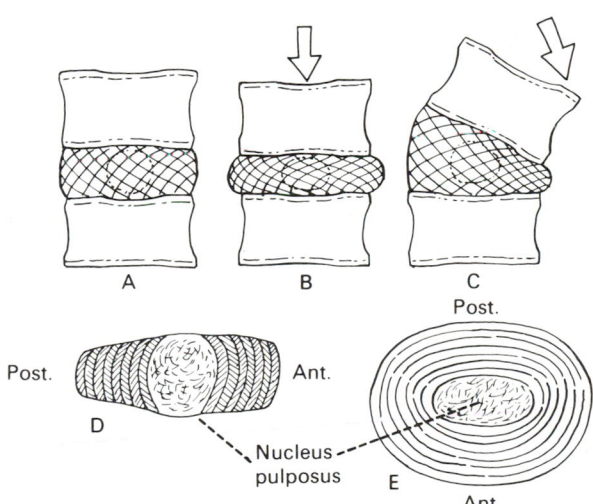

FIG. 70-7. Structure of the intervertebral disk. *A.* A crisscross arrangement of collagen fiber bundles in the annulus fibrosus permits rotation between the vertebrae and also allows for bulging when the nucleus pulposus is compressed (*B* and *C*). *D.* Side view of a lumbar intervertebral disk. The anterior part of the disk is higher than the posterior part and the outer part is composed of layers of intertwining fibroelastic tissue. *E.* Superior view showing the circumferential annular fibers around the centrally located nucleus pulposus. Modified from Rosse, C.: The vertebral column. *In* The Musculoskeletal System in Health and Disease. Edited by C. Rosse and D.K. Clawson. Hagerstown, MD, Harper & Row, 1980.

The disks receive great support from the ALL and to a lesser extent from the PLL and the muscles of the back.

The blood supply to the disk is important. In the fetus the blood supply to the disk reaches it both from its periphery and from vessels in the bodies of adjacent vertebrae, which grow through the cartilaginous plates and run toward but do not reach the nucleus pulposus (2, 3). Soon after birth, however, the vascular supply begins to diminish; after the second decade and by the third decade the disk is almost avascular. Thereafter it receives its nutrition by diffusion of solutes, lymph, and other fluids through the central portion of the vertebral end plate and through the annulus fibrosus. Glucose and oxygen enter through the end plates while sulfate enters through the annulus to form glucosaminoglycans. This is made possible by alternating compression and relaxation of the elastic container in a manner similar to that of a sponge being squeezed and released.

Posterior Portion of the Functional Unit

The posterior portion of the functional unit in the lumbar region is composed of two vertebral arches, two transverse processes, a central posterior spinous process, and a paired articulation. The transverse processes and posterior spinous processes are bony sites of attachment of back muscles and are also sites of attachment for supporting ligaments.

The ligaments of the posterior portion of the functional unit are also extremely important in stabilizing the vertebral column. The ligamenta flava connect the laminae of adjacent vertebrae and are thickest and strongest in the lumbar region. Their marked elasticity permits separation of laminae during flexion of the vertebral column and also serves to preserve the upright posture.

The supraspinous ligament is also a strong fibrous cord that connects the apices of the spinous processes of each vertebra. The interspinous ligaments are thin and membranous and interconnect adjoining spinous processes (3). The intertransverse ligaments are interposed between transverse processes. Whereas in the thoracic region they are rounded cords intimately connected with the deep muscles of the back, they are thin and membranous in the lumbar region.

THE POSTERIOR ARTICULATION. The posterior articulations, or facets, are comprised of two arthrodial joints that are lined with synovium and lubricated by synovial fluid within the joint capsule. The orientation of the facets of these intervertebral joints determines the direction of motion of the motion segment (4–6). Throughout the spine this orientation changes in relation to the transverse and frontal planes (Fig. 70-8). In the thoracic spine the facets are convex-concave and lie essentially in the horizontal plane, thus permitting lateral flexing, such as side bending and rotation, about a vertical line. In the upper part of the lumbar spine the facet planes lie in a vertical sagittal plane and permit flexion and extension but prevent lateral flexion or bending in the lordotic curve. As the facet joints are followed from the thoracolumbar to the lumbrosacral regions, however, the superior articular processes gradually undergo a transition to face more posteriorly

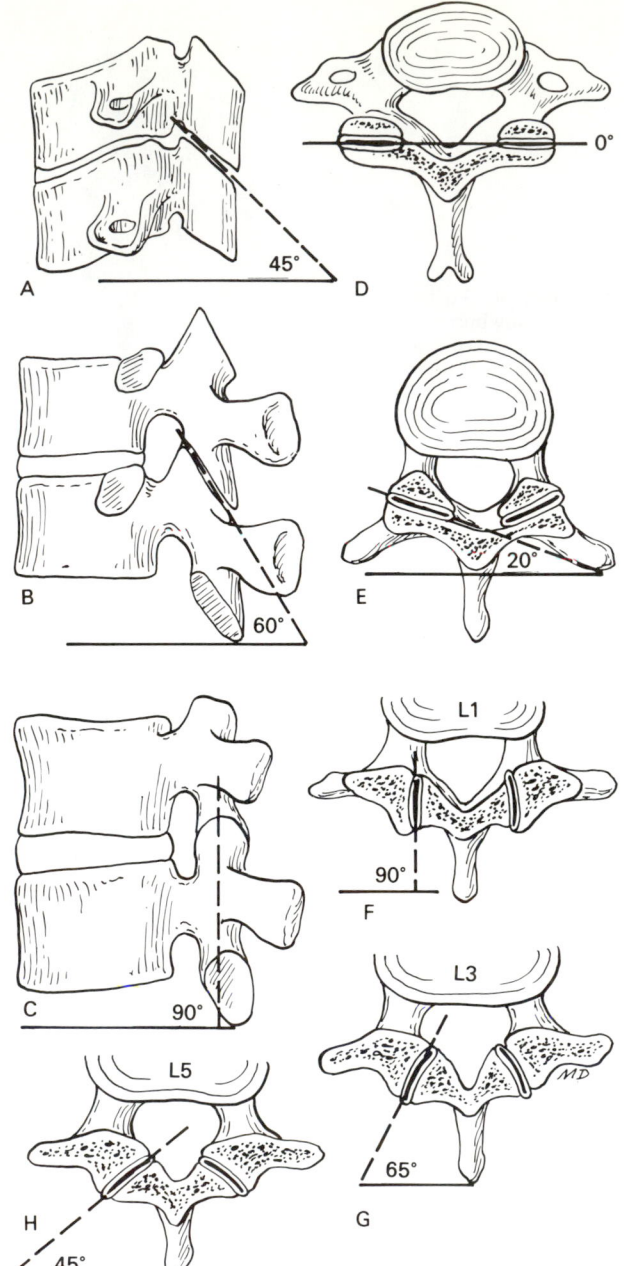

FIG. 70-8. Planes of the articular facet surfaces of the vertebral arch joints. Lateral views show the angulation that determines the direction of movement permitted by the vertebral facet in the cervical (*A*), thoracic (*B*), and lumbar (*C*) regions. *D–H.* Depiction of the superior surfaces to show the facet planes horizontally. In the cervical region (*D*) they allow anterior flexion and extension, in the thoracic region (*E*) their angle permits an appreciable amount of rotation between consecutive vertebrae, and the upper lumbar vertebrae (*F*) the facet planes are vertical. As they proceed caudad (*G, H*), however, there tends to be a gradual transition in the angle of the superior articular process, which gradually faces more posteriorly and less medially, while the inferior articular process gradually faces more anteriorly and less laterally. The lumbosacral joint, the part farthest from the sagittal plane, allows some rotation of the lower part of the lumbar spine. Modified from Hollinshead, W.H.: Anatomy for Surgeons. 3rd Ed. Vol. 3, The Back and Limbs. Philadelphia, Harper & Row, 1982; and from Lindh, M.: Biomechanics of the lumbar spine. *In* Basic Biomechanics of the Skeletal System. Edited by V.H. Frankel and M. Nordin. Philadelphia, Lea & Febiger, 1980.

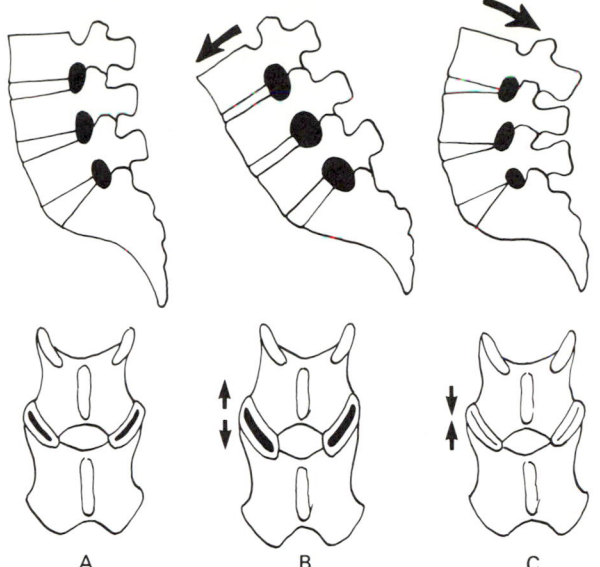

FIG. 70-9. Flexion and hyperextension in the lumbar region. **A.** Normal posture showing the relation of the facets as well as the size of the intervertebral foramina and the configuration of the intervertebral disks. **B.** Flexion causes the facets to separate, thus allowing movement in the lumbar area in both lateral and rotatory directions. The intervertebral foramina enlarge and the anterior portions of the disks are compressed. **C.** Hyperextension. Facets approximate each other, thus completely eliminating any lateral rotatory movement and causing a significant decrease in the size of the intervertebral foramen. Modified from Cailliet, R.: Low Back Pain Syndromes. 3rd Ed. Philadelphia, F.A. Davis, 1981.

and less medially, while the inferior articular processes gradually face more anteriorly and less laterally (4) (Fig. 70-9). The lumbosacral joint typically departs farthest from the sagittal plane, although it varies in different individuals (4). This allows some rotation of the lower part of the lumbar spine. Moreover, in a slightly forward flexed position, the facets of the other lumbar vertebrae separate and thus permit a modest degree of lateral and rotatory movements.

Nerve and Blood Supply of the Lumbar Spine

Nerve Supply

The lumbar spine and the contents of the spinal canal are supplied by the meningeal (recurrent) nerves, which are derived from the spinal nerves, and by articular and ligamentous branches, which are derived from the posterior primary division (Fig. 70-10). The distribution of these nerves has been studied by a number of investigators (7–9). Pedersen and associates (7) studied the distribution of the posterior primary division and of the meningeal branches of the lumbosacral spinal nerves to various structures of the lumbosacral spine.

ARTICULAR NERVES. It was found that, in addition to the cutaneous and muscular distribution, the posterior primary division provides sensory fibers to fascia, ligaments, periosteum, and intervertebral (facet) joints of the posterior functional unit (7). Adjacent divisions overlap their area of supply, and the interspinous ligaments are supplied mainly by branches from the next cranial level. This important branch of the posterior primary division runs in the groove formed by the junction between the transverse process and superior articular process, being located first on the lateral aspect of the superior articular process and then on the medial aspect of the inferior articular process. During its course it gives off branches to these various parts of the posterior functional unit and to the erector spinae muscles (Fig. 70-10A).

MENINGEAL NERVES. The meningeal nerves (Fig. 70-10), also called the sinovertebral or recurrent nerves of Luschka, supply many structures within the spinal canal and also the longitudinal ligaments. These nerves arise from the spinal nerves close to, or in common with, the rami communicantes, and consist of both somatic afferent and sympathetic fibers (4). After the meningeal nerve enters the vertebral canal

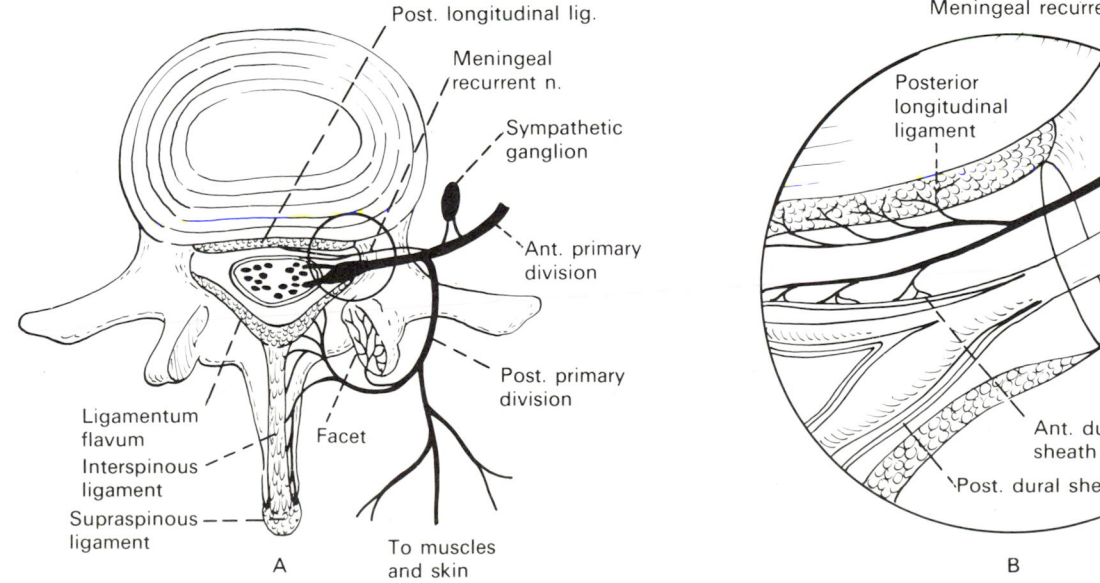

FIG. 70-10. A. Nerve supply to the lumbar vertebrae, consisting of the meningeal branch of the spinal nerve and the articular branch of the posterior primary division. **B.** Enlargement of the part circled in **A** showing details of the distribution of the meningeal recurrent nerve. See text for details.

through the intervertebral foramen its branches proceed toward the PLL and both ascend and descend. Thus, the nerve endings at any level are derived from at least two segmental levels (7). Both Stilwell (8) and Hirsch and colleagues (9) reported finding free nerve endings that probably transmit nociceptive information in both anterior and posterior longitudinal ligaments, in the periosteum of the vertebral bodies, in the anterior and posterior parts of the dura mater, along blood vessels that supply these structures, and in the spinal cord. Many nerve endings have been found both in and on the surface of the PLL and on the outermost layers of the annulus fibrosus directly adjacent the undersurface of the PLL. These fibers and their endings probably belong to the same system of nerves that supplies the PLL. No fibers have been found within this structure of the nucleus pulposus, other than on the most superficial layer of the annulus fibrosus.

Hirsch and co-workers (9) studied human lumbar spine sections by the intravital staining method using methylene blue. They found free nerve endings of small (usually less than 3 μm in diameter) myelinated fibers and complex unencapsulated endings, which are nerve terminations derived from medium-sized myelinated fibers (5 to 12 μm in diameter), with various types of organ endings. They also noted unmyelinated fibers associated with blood vessels that they believed to be postganglionic sympathetic fibers. Fine free fiber endings and complex unencapsulated endings were found in the lumbar dorsal fascia, supraspinous ligaments, interspinous ligaments, and anterior and posterior longitudinal ligaments. They also found fine free nerve endings on the posterior surface of the ligamentum flavum but not in the deeper substance of the structure. Both fine free fiber endings and complex unencapsulated endings were found in the vertebral periosteum. Small myelinated and unmyelinated fibers (not associated with blood vessels) were also found in the subchondral bony trabeculae. Stilwell (8) found nerve bundles that enter the many vascular foramina in the lumbar vertebrae of monkeys. The intervertebral joint capsules are innervated by the full triad of nerve endings: fine free nerve endings, complex unencapsulated endings, and small encapsulated endings. In this respect these joint capsules have similar innervation as other joint capsules.

Blood Supply

Each lumbar vertebra is supplied by a pair of segmental lumbar arteries that arise from the aorta and are accompanied by the venous system (Fig. 70-11). The arteries are close to and surround the middle of each vertebra and anastomose freely with the large vessels that enter the vertebra posteriorly (Fig. 70-11). The posterior branch of the segmental artery, close to the intervertebral foramen, gives rise to spinal branches that enter the foramen and divide into three terminal branches—posterior, intermediate, and anterior (4) (Fig. 70-11A).

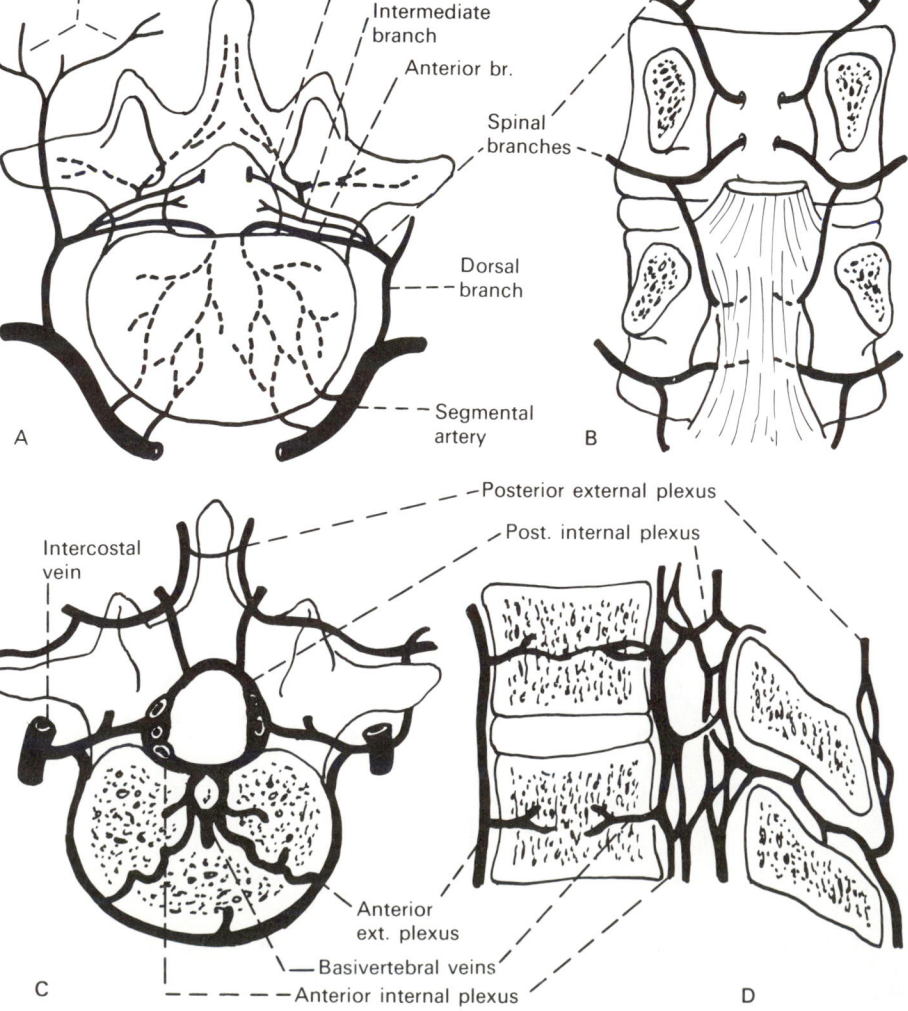

FIG. 70-11. Blood supply to a lumbar vertebra. A. Inferior view of a lumbar vertebra surrounded by the two segmental arteries derived from the aorta. These contribute branches that pass through the anterior surface of the body and, importantly, provide the spinal branch, which breaks up into three branches that supply the body of the vertebra, the contents of the spinal canal, and the ipsilateral lamina and spinous process. The posterior branch also gives off branches that supply the paravertebral muscles and cutaneous tissue. B. Posteroanterior view of the body of the vertebra showing arterial branches to the vertebral bodies. The cut surfaces of the pedicles are recognizable and part of the posterior longitudinal ligament has been removed. C, D. Venous drainage of the vertebrae by the external and internal vertebral venous plexuses. Note the complex drainage within the spinal canal. A and B modified from Hollinshead, W.H.: Anatomy for Surgeons. 3rd Ed. Vol. 3, The Back and Limbs Philadelphia, Harper & Row, 1982; C and D modified from Clemente, C.D. (ed.): Gray's Anatomy of the Human Body. 30th Am. Ed. Philadelphia, Lea & Febiger, 1985.

The posterior branches of the spinal arteries help supply the spinal dura and the tissue of the epidural space. They anastomose with similar branches above and below them to form small channels that accompany the posterior internal vertebral venous plexuses and, in general, lie posterolateral to the dura. The largest part of each posterior branch enters the vertebral arch and supplies the pedicles, transverse process, lamina, and spinous process—all part of the posterior functional unit.

The intermediate (middle) branch of the spinal artery supplies the dura of the associated nerve roots. Its radicular branch can pierce the dura, continue along nerve roots and rootlets intradurally, and help to supply the spinal cord.

The anterior branches of the spinal artery supply the vertebral bodies. They give off twigs to the anterolateral part of the spinal dura mater and to the tissue of the epidural space but, most importantly, they supply the body of the vertebra. Typically, an anterior branch is divided into two major terminals, ascending and descending. These run obliquely cephalad or caudad toward the center of the two adjacent vertebral bodies (Fig. 70-11B), pass deep to the posterior longitudinal ligament between this structure and the posterior aspect of the vertebral bodies, and pierce each body toward its middle under cover of the ligament. Thus, on its posterior aspect, each vertebral body receives blood from four arteries, two from each side, one ascending and one descending.

The posterior branches of the segmental arteries also supply the muscles of the back.

The vertebral column is intimately associated with interconnecting venous plexuses and the venous drainage of the bones into the plexuses.

Internal and external vertebral venous plexuses are shown in Figure 70-11C and D.

Musculature of the Lumbosacral Spine

The range and type of movement possible in each region of the spine is determined by the facet joints, but the control and strength of the movement depend on muscles that are also essential for the stability of the spine (6). Generally, the muscles are of two types, extensors and flexors, and both can also rotate and bend the spinal column laterally (Fig. 70-12).

Extensors

The extensors of the spine are placed posterior to the laminae and transverse processes and span the entire back between the sacrum and occiput. The numerous individual muscles, which are collectively known as the erector spinae or sacrospinalis muscles, have the primary function of restoring the spine to an erect position and, by producing extension, control flexion of the spine. Deep to the sacrospinalis is the transversospinalis muscle group. These various muscles cross each other in different layers to establish a system of guy ropes or trusses in an arrangement that is ideal for providing lateral stability to the vertebral column. If this mechanism is effective only on one side, a pathologic lateral curvature or scoliosis results.

The subdivision of this muscle mass by numerous connective tissue planes and the multiple attachment of tendons over small areas of periosteum on vertebral processes suggest why pain and spasm are so common in the extensive musculature of the spine and why it is difficult to offer a specific anatomic explanation for it (10). The strong fascia that envelops the entire erector spinae in the lumbar region is known as the thoracolumbar fascia, and many muscle fibers of the erector spinae originate from it. The anterior layer of this fascia is anchored to the transverse processes, and the anterior and posterior layers meet along the lateral edge of the muscle mass, where muscles of the anterior abdominal wall arise.

NERVE AND BLOOD SUPPLY. All the muscles that comprise the erector spinae are supplied by the posterior primary division of the spinal nerves. Stimulation of a single formed spinal nerve or its posterior primary division can lead to segmental spasm and pain. Conversely, segments of the muscle can go into spasm to guard against movement when a painful lesion is present, whether it is in the intraspinal or paravertebral part of the nerve. The muscles receive their blood supply by way of the posterior (dorsal) branches of the lumbar segmental arteries.

Flexors

The flexor muscles are virtually confined to the cervical and lumbar regions of the spine, reflecting the fact that these are the most mobile regions of the vertebral column. Because gravity plays a major part in flexion, the flexor muscles of the spine are best demonstrated when they are made to function against gravity, as when raising the head or trunk from a supine position.

As emphasized by Rosse (10), the prevertebral musculature is anatomically the flexor counterpart of the erector spinae, but, because of their poor mechanical advantage, the muscles that are in close opposition to the vertebral column anteriorly are ineffectual as flexor units. These prevertebral flexors retain their original function only in the cevical region, where they are chiefly represented by the longus colli and scalene muscles. No prevertebral muscles are found in the thoracic region, while in the lumbar spine the prevertebral musculature is represented by the psoas major, which no longer functions as a flexor of the spine, but helps to flex the entire trunk on the lower limbs at the hips.

The flexors of the lumbar spine are the anterior abdominal muscles, consisting of the two rectus abdominal muscles assisted by the external and internal oblique muscles, which approximate the rib cage to the pelvis. The muscles are put to work during sit-ups when the hips and knees are kept flexed. With extended hips, sit-ups mainly exercise the psoas muscle.

All the prevertebral and anterior abdominal wall muscles are innervated by the anterior primary division of the spinal nerves (Chapters 53 and 59). These muscles receive arterial blood supply from the lumbar segmental and posterior intercostal arteries.

Lateral Flexors (Bending)

Unilateral contraction of spinal flexors, extensors, or both, produces lateral flexion or bending.

Biomechanics

Total Spine

The entire vertebral column constitutes supraincumbent functional units in an erect jointed column balanced against gravity and capable of movement. The column has four anatomic curves. A forward convexity in the lumbar and cervical regions of the spinal column is known as lordosis, and an opposing curvature with posterior convexity in the thoracic and sacrococcygeal regions is known as kyphosis. Because the sacrococcygeal component has no effect on a person's attempt

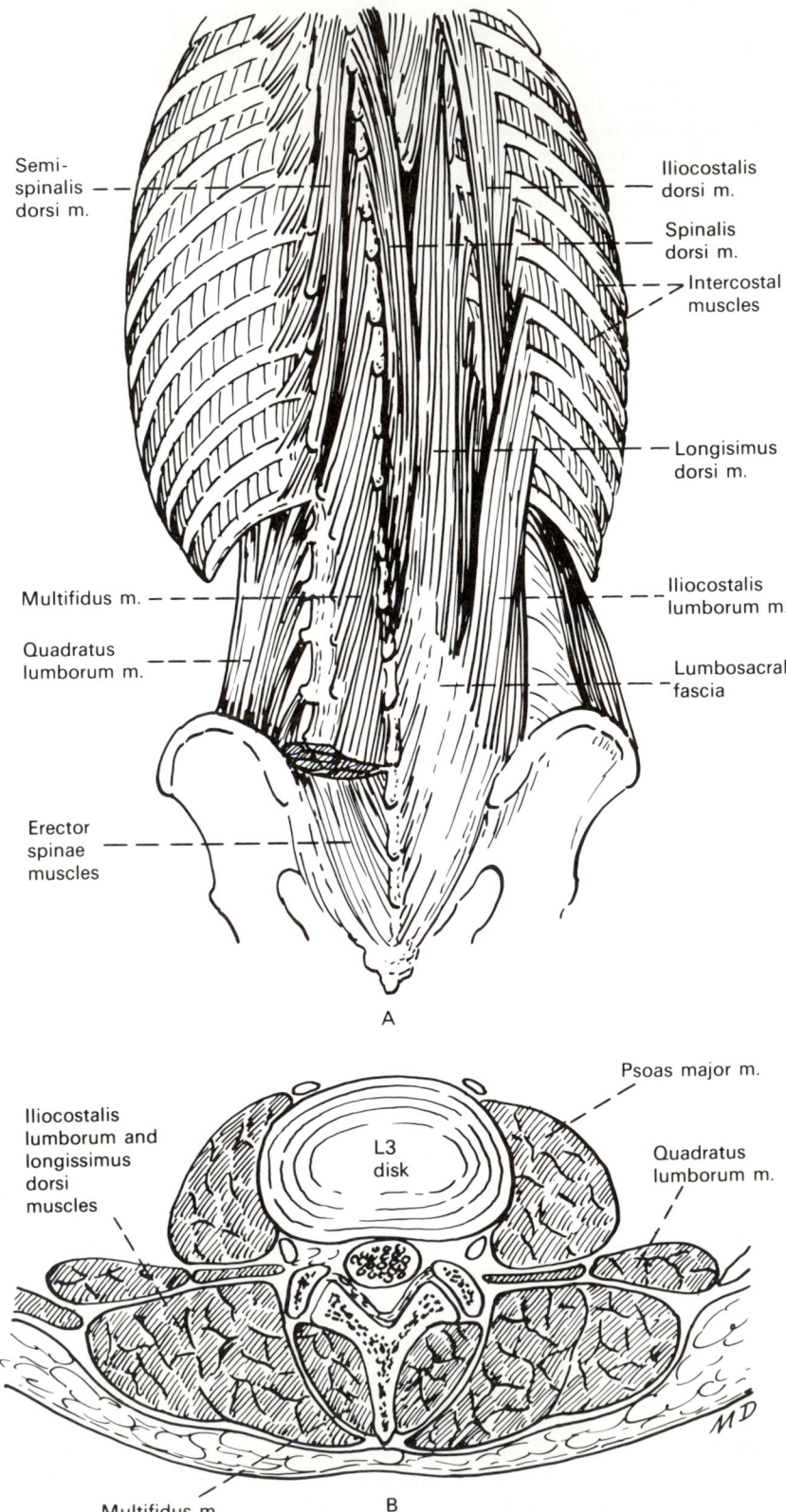

FIG. 70-12. Erector spinae (sacro-spinalis) and transversospinalis muscles of the back. **A.** The erector spinae muscles, which have been cut on the left to show the deeper muscles, originate from the last two thoracic vertebrae, all the lumbar vertebrae, the sacral spine, the sacrum, the sacroiliac ligament, and the entire medial aspect of the iliac crest. At the level of the 12th rib the erector spinae (sacrospinalis) muscles split into three columns. The iliocostalis, or lateral band, is inserted into the angles of the lower six or seven ribs. The longissimus, or intermediate band, has a double insertion on each of the lower nine or ten ribs and on the tips of the transverse processes of the corresponding vertebrae. The spinalis, or medial band, is essentially a flat aponeurosis; its medial border is attached to the posterior spines of the thoracic vertebrae while the lateral margin is free. On the left side are shown two layers of the transversospinalis muscle. A semispinalis (superficial) layer arises from the tips of the transverse processes and inserts into the tips of the spinous processes spanning three to five segments in the thoracic and cervical regions. A multifidus or deeper layer of muscle arises with a thick fleshy mass on the dorsum of the sacrum and from the overlying erector spinae aponeurosis and all the transverse processes, and then spans three segments to attach to the inferior borders of the spinous processes. **B.** Transverse section to show the muscles of the back.

Labels in figure A: Semi-spinalis dorsi m.; Iliocostalis dorsi m.; Spinalis dorsi m.; Intercostal muscles; Longisimus dorsi m.; Multifidus m.; Iliocostalis lumborum m.; Quadratus lumborum m.; Lumbosacral fascia; Erector spinae muscles; A

Labels in figure B: Psoas major m.; Iliocostalis lumborum and longissimus dorsi muscles; L3 disk; Quadratus lumborum m.; Multifidus m.; B

to maintain balance in the erect position, it is not considered in the study of physiologic curves. The side view of the three physiologic curves comprises what is referred to as posture (2).

In the erect posture the entire vertebral column is supported on an oblique sacral base that oscillates between the two hip joints. Because the sacrum is firmly attached to both ilia these bones move together as one unit and constitute the pelvis, which is centrally balanced on a transverse axis between the two ball-bearing joints. These joints are formed by the rounded heads of the femurs fitting into the acetabular sockets, which permits a rotary motion in the anteroposterior plane (2). By pivoting in a rotating manner between these two lateral points the pelvis can rotate back and forth, simultaneously rocking and changing the sacral angle (determined as a line drawn parallel to the superior border of the sacrum and measured in relation to a horizontal line). The entire vertebral column, with all its physiologic curves, is balanced on this sacral base. Consequently, all curves depend on the lumbosacral angle to retain their balance with respect to the center of gravity. The degree of the lumbosacral angle varies, depending on cultural, genetic, and racial differences. It can also be affected by faulty habits, ligamentous laxity, and poor muscular tone.

Erect Posture

An erect posture requires biomechanical balance (2). In individuals who have a normal spinal column and whose body segments are in good alignment, erect posture is maintained mainly by ligamentous support with minimal but adequate muscular activity (Fig. 70-13). The lumbar curve extends into greater lordosis, placing its support on the strong, broad ALL and posteriorly on the facet joints and ligaments of the posterior functional unit (2). The pelvis is held in ligamentous balance by the anterior hip joint and iliofemoral ligament (or Y ligament of Bigelow), which is a fibrous reinforcement of the anterior portion of the hip joint that prevents hyperextension of the hip. Thus, the hip can remain extended with little muscular activity. The pelvis is further supported by the tensor fascia latae, consisting of fascial bands that mechanically assist the Y ligament and limit lateral shift of the pelvis. Their course from the iliac crest downward and backward to insert at the iliotibial band at the knee lends itself well to the reinforcement of the Y ligament and helps to lock the knee.

The knee joint can similarly be "locked" in extension by the posterior popliteal tissues, which prevent overextension of the knee (2). This position eliminates the need for muscular effort on the part of the quadratus femoris. Only the ankle cannot be immobilized and supported by ligaments. To remain in the erect weight-bearing position, the ankle requires alternating isometric contraction of the anterior dorsi flexors muscles and of the posterior gastrocnemius-soleus muscle groups (2).

Although their activity is kept at a minimum, postural muscles are always active in the standing position (11). The center of gravity of the upper part of the body is anterior to the spine, with the line of gravity for the trunk passing anterior to the center of the L4

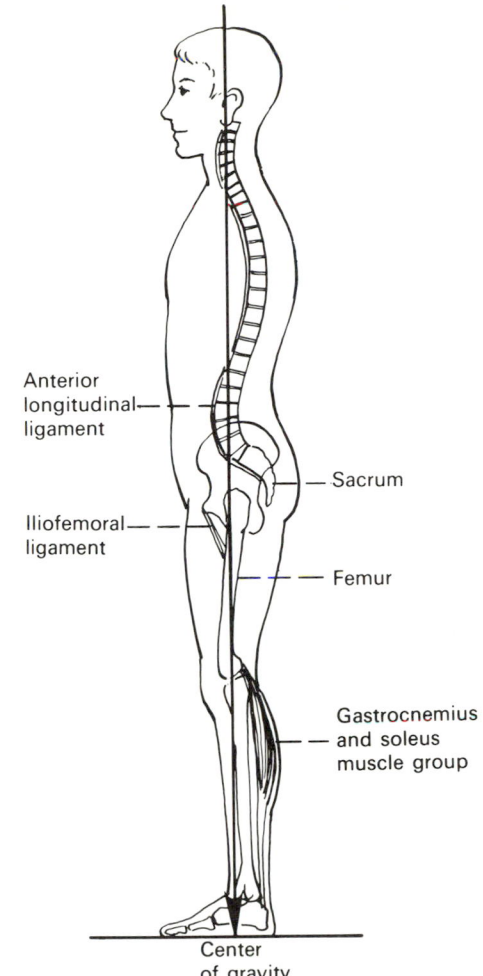

FIG. 70-13. Subject in erect posture depicting the most important structures that support the static spine, including the anterior longitudinal ligament, which supports the lumbar lordosis, and the iliofemoral (Y) ligament, which reinforces the anterior portion of the hip joint to prevent hyperextension of the hip. The knee joint can be locked in place by the posterior popliteal tissues, while the gastrocnemius soleus muscle lends support to the ankle. The line of gravity is usually ventral to the transverse axis of motion and passes ventral to the center of the force from the vertebral bodies. Modified from Cailliet, R.: Low Back Pain Syndrome. 3rd Ed. Philadelphia, F.A. Davis, 1981.

vertebral body (12). This means that the line of gravity falls anterior to the transverse axis of motion at all spinal levels, subjecting the motion segment to a forward bending movement that must be counterbalanced by ligament forces and back muscle forces (11) (Fig. 70-13). Standing is not a completely static position even when the body is well balanced, and any displacement of the line of gravity creates a moment that must be counterbalanced by muscle activity for the body to remain in equilibrium. Consequently, postural sway occurs intermittently and involves not only the erector spinae muscles but also the abdominal muscles and the vertebral portion of the psoas muscles (11, 13).

During relaxed standing the base of the sacrum is inclined forward and downward about 30° to the trans-

General Considerations of Pain in the Low Back, Hips, and Lower Extremities   **1405**

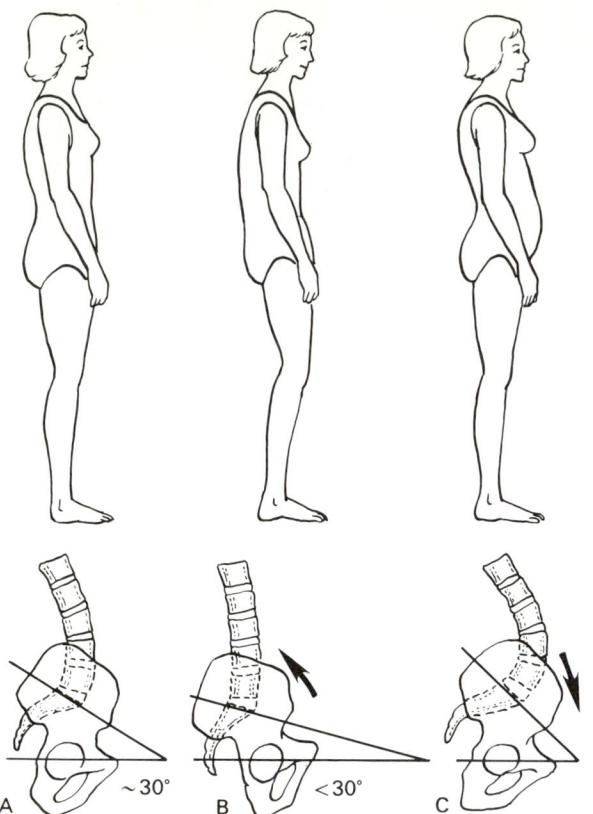

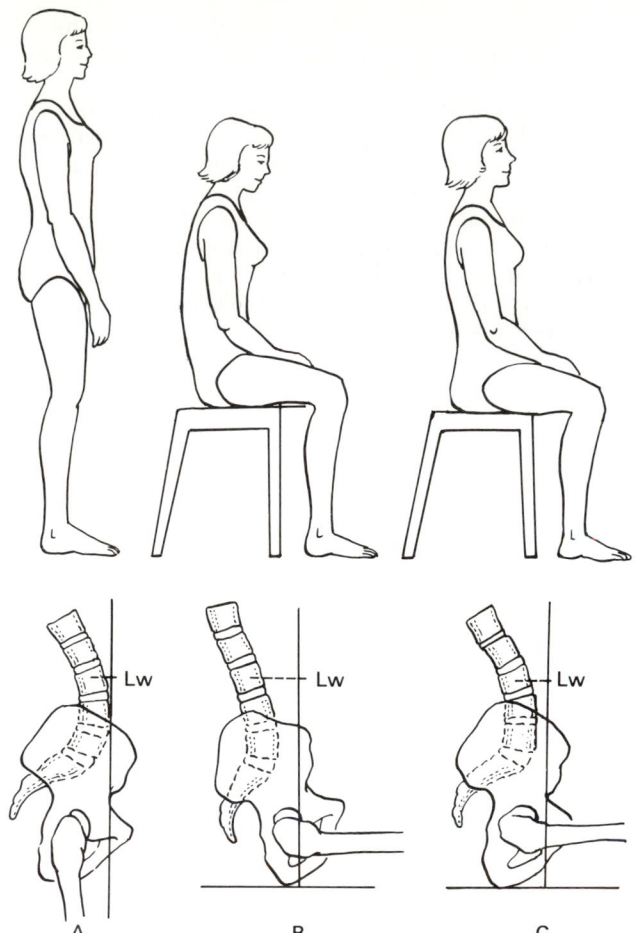

FIG. 70-14. Effect of pelvic tilting on the sacral angle during upright standing. **A.** During relaxed standing the sacral angle is about 30°. **B.** Backward tilting of the pelvis decreases the sacral angle and flattens the lumbar spine. **C.** Forward tilting of the pelvis increases the sacral angle and increases the lumbar lordosis. Modified from Lindh, M.: Biomechanics of the lumbar spine. *In* Basic Biomechanics of the Skeletal System. Edited by V.H. Frankel and M. Nordin. Philadelphia, Lea & Febiger, 1980.

FIG. 70-15. Comparison of various sitting positions and relaxed upright standing. **A.** The subject is in the relaxed standing posture. The line of gravity for the upper body is near the lumbar spine. **B.** The subject is in a relaxed but unsupported sitting position. The line of gravity shifts further ventrally as the pelvis tilts backward and the lumbar lordosis flattens. This shift creates a longer lever arm (Lw) for the force exerted by the weight of the upper body. **C.** During erect sitting the backward pelvic tilt is reduced and the lever arm (Lw) is shortened but is still slightly longer than that during the relaxed upright standing. Modified from Lindh, M.: Biomechanics of the lumbar spine. *In* Basic Biomechanics of the Skeletal System. Edited by V.H. Frankel and M. Nordin. Philadelphia, Lea & Febiger, 1980.

verse plane (Fig. 70-14). This inclination is partly compensated for by the wedge-shaped lumbosacral disk, which is much higher on the anterior and lateral aspects than posteriorly and thus gives the lowest lumbar vertebra a less inclined position (11). Tilting of the pelvis about the transverse axis between the hip joints changes the sacral angle. When the pelvis is tilted backward the angle decreases, lumbar lordosis decreases, and a slight extension of the thoracic spine occurs to adjust the center of gravity. When the pelvis is tilted forward the lumbosacral angle increases, causing an increase in lumbar lordosis and thoracic kyphosis (Fig. 70-14).

Effects of Body Positions on the Load of the Lumbar Spine

Because the lumbar spine is the main load-bearing part of the vertebral column, spinal loads have been estimated for this region. The in vivo disk pressure during relaxed upright standing is a function of the intrinsic pressure on the disk, the body weight above the measured level, and the muscles acting over the motion segment. Nachemson and associates (13–15) have measured the intradisk pressure and found that, in a man weighing 70 kg, the load on the L3 disk

calculated from the disk pressure is 70 kilograms. This is almost twice the weight of the body above the measured level, which is about 60% of total body weight or 40 kg. Flexion of the trunk increases the load by increasing the forward bending movement, making the disk bulge and protrude anteriorly and then contract and become depressed posteriorly. Nachemson and colleagues (12–15) have also studied loads on the lumbar spine in the relaxed upright standing, unsupported sitting, supported sitting, and supine positions and they have been summarized by Lindh (11) (Figs. 70-15, 70-16, and 70-17). As noted for the standing relaxed position, the intradisk pressure is lower than in the sitting or forward bending position. Moreover, the addition of a back support, as well as a backward inclination of the back rest, alone or with a support, decreases disk pressure (Fig. 70-17). In the

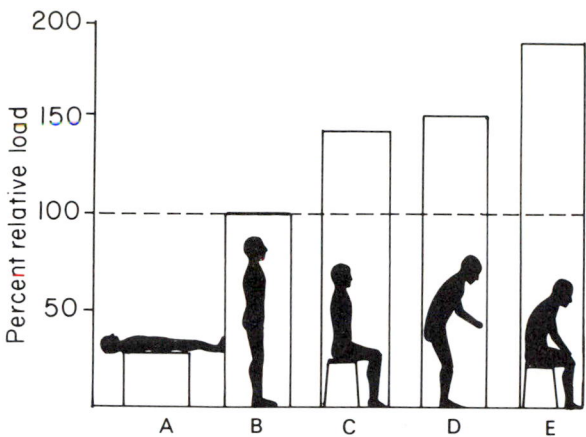

FIG. 70-16. Relative loads on the L3 disk for various body positions compared with the load during upright standing. *A.* With the subject lying the load decreases significantly. *B.* Upright standing (100% of relative load). *C.* In the sitting position, and with the back straight, the load shows about 40% increase above relaxed standing. *D.* With the subject bending the load shows about a 50% increase. *E.* With the patient sitting, back unsupported and bending over, the load shows an even greater increase. Modified from Lindh, M.: Biomechanics of the lumbar spine. *In* Basic Biomechanics of the Skeletal System. Edited by V.H. Frankel and M. Nordin. Philadelphia, Lea & Febiger, 1980.

supine position loads on the spine produced by the body are less than in the standing or sitting position. When the knees are extended, however, the pull of the vertebral portion of the psoas muscle produces some load on the lumbar spine (Fig. 70-18A) but, when the hips and knees are bent, the psoas muscle relaxes, thus decreasing the load on the lumbar spine (Fig. 70-18B). Table 70-1 lists the load on the L3 disk in kilograms in 70-kg males during different positions, movements, and exercises.

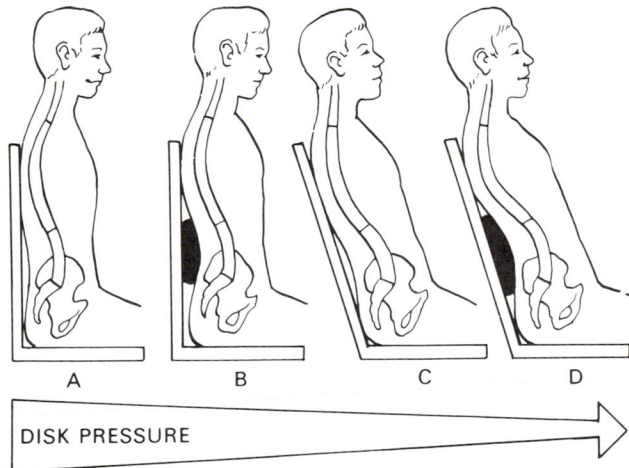

FIG. 70-17. Influence of back rest inclination and back support on loads on the lumbar spine in terms of pressure in the L3 disk during supported sitting. *A.* The back rest inclination is 90° and the disk pressure is at a maximum. *B.* Addition of a lumbar support decreases the disk pressure. *C.* Backward inclination of the back rest to 110°, but with no lumbar support, produces less disk pressure. *D.* Addition of a lumbar support, with the back rest to 100° inclination, produces the lowest load on the disk. Modified from Lindh, M.: Biomechanics of the lumbar spine. *In* Basic Biomechanics of the Skeletal System. Edited by V.H. Frankel and M. Nordin. Philadelphia, Lea & Febiger, 1980.

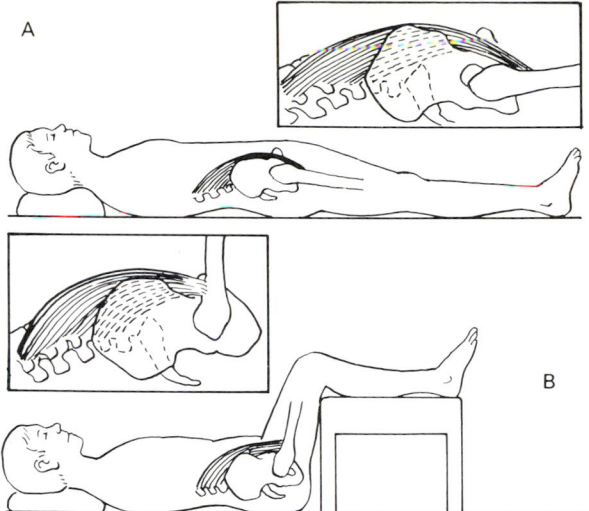

FIG. 70-18. Load on the lumbar spine in the supine position. *A.* Legs straight. *B.* Hips and knees bent. In *A* some load on the lumbar spine is produced by the pull of the vertebral portion of the psoas muscle whereas in *B* the psoas muscle is relaxed, thus decreasing the load on the lumbar spine. Modified from Lindh, M.: Biomechanics of the lumbar spine. *In* Basic Biomechanics of the Skeletal System. Edited by V.H. Frankel and M. Nordin. Philadelphia, Lea & Febiger, 1980.

Movement

Whereas the erect stance is a posture that primarily depends on ligamentous support, anterior or posterior movement from the center of gravity requires muscular activity. In forward flexion the erector spinae muscles elongate to decelerate forward flexion (Fig. 70-19). Once the body reaches full forward flexion, further movement is restricted by ligamentous connective tissue. To return to the full erect posture the extensor muscles must shorten until the full erect posture of the ligamentous support is achieved, thus reversing the process.

TABLE 70-1. Approximate Load on L3 Disk in 70-kg Individual in Different Positions, Movements, and Maneuvers

Activity	Load (kg)
Supine	30
Standing	70
Upright sitting, no support	100
Walking	85
Twisting	90
Bending sideways	95
Coughing	110
Jumping	110
Straining	120
Laughing	120
Bending forward 20°	120
Lifting of 20 kg, back straight, knees bent	210
Lifting of 20 kg, back bent, knees straight	340
Bilateral straight leg raising, supine	120
Sit-up exercise with knees bent	180
Sit-up exercise with knees extended	175
Isometric abdominal muscle exercise	110
Active back hyperextension prone	150

From Nachemson, A.L.: Pathophysiology and treatment of back pain: A critical look at the different types of treatment. *In* Approaches to the Validation of Manipulation Therapy. Edited by A.A. Buerger and J.S. Tobis. Springfield, Charles C Thomas, 1977, pp. 49-50.

Motion in the lumbar spine is produced by a coordinated action of nerves and muscles. Agonistic muscles (prime movers) initiate and carry out motion, whereas antagonistic muscles often control and modify it (11). The range of motion differs at various levels of the spine, depending on the orientation of the intervertebral joint facets at each level. Spinal movements are always a combined action of several segments. Skeletal structures that influence spinal motion include the rib cage, which limits thoracic motion, and the pelvis, whose tilting increases trunk movements (11).

Flexion and Extension

Flexion and extension involve the simultaneous movement of the lumbar spine and pelvis in one plane, which Cailliet (2) has called the "lumbar-pelvic rhythm." The lumbar portion of the rhythm initially involves a flattening of the lumbar spine and a gradual reversal of an arc that is not a perfect sphere (2). This reversal thus does not occur to the same degree at all points along the spine but occurs mainly in the lowermost motion segment of the L5–S1 joint and to a lesser extent in the L4–5 joint.

The first 45 to 50° of spinal flexion occur primarily in the lumbar spine, mostly in the lowermost motion segment (75%), the lumbosacral joint, and at the L4–L5 segment (20%). Forward tilting of the pelvis allows further flexion (Fig. 70-20). The thoracic spine contributes little to the flexion of the total spine because of the orientation of the facets, the almost vertical orientation of the spinous processes, and the restriction to motion imposed by the rib cage (11). Flexion is initiated by the abdominal muscles and by the vertebral portion of the psoas muscle (12). The weight of the body then produces further flexion, which is controlled by the gradually increasing activity of the erector spinae muscles as the moment of the force

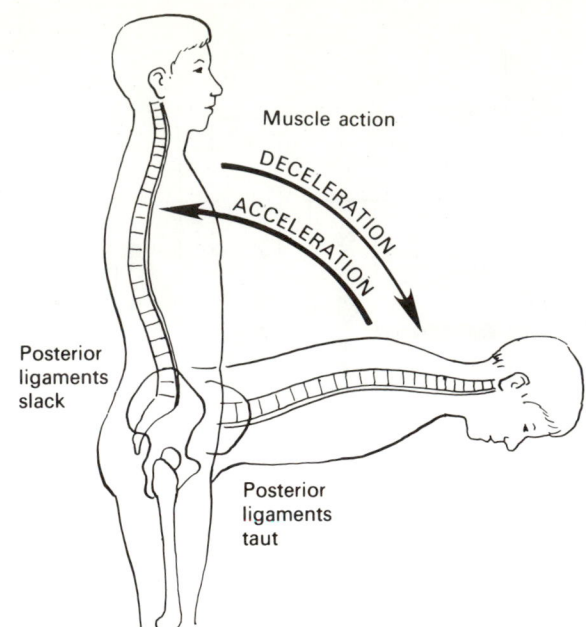

FIG. 70-19. Forward flexion in the erect position is made possible by deceleration of the erector spinae muscle, whereas the muscle must shorten by acceleration in returning to the erect position.

increases. The posterior hip muscles are active in controlling the forward tilting of the pelvis (16) but, in full flexion, the erector spinae muscles become inactive. This forward bending is passively balanced by the posterior ligaments which are initially slack but then become taut at this point as a result of spinal elongation. Almost all flexion in the lumbar spine occurs by the time the trunk is inclined 45° forward (Fig. 70-20C) with the remainder of forward flexion caused by rotation of the pelvis (Fig. 70-20).

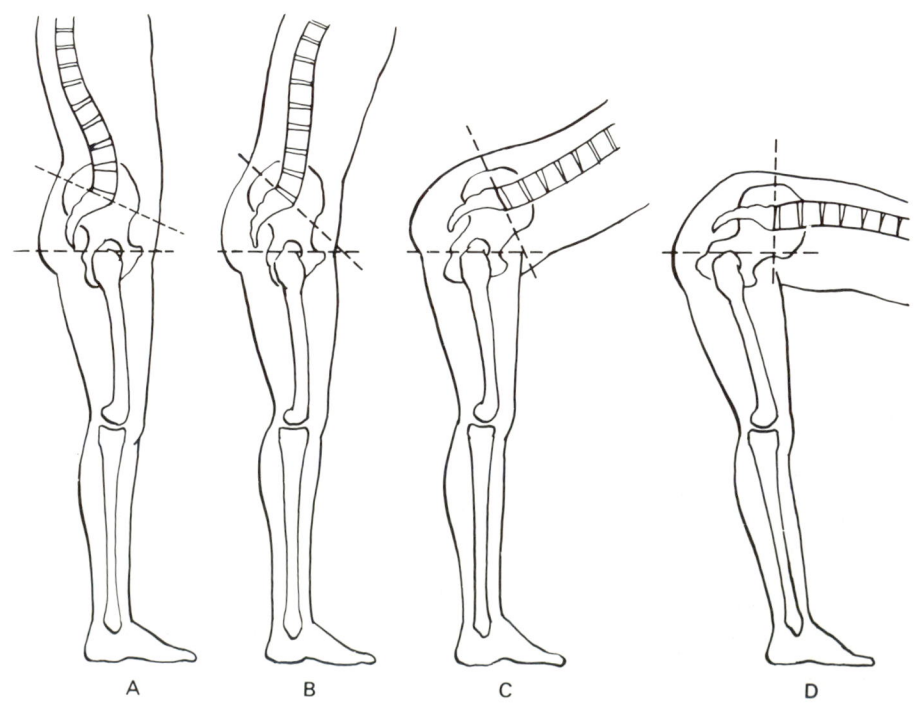

FIG. 70-20. The lumbar-pelvic rhythm. A. Normal position showing normal lumbar lordosis in a 30° lumbosacral angle. B. Initially the first 45° to 50° of flexion occurs in the lumbar spine, particularly at the L5–S1 and L4–L5 segments. C. With more than 45° of flexion the pelvis begins to tilt, with a consequent significant increase in the lumbosacral angle. D. In extreme flexion at 90° the pelvis rotates almost completely to a 90° lumbosacral angle. Modified from Lindh, M.: Biomechanics of the lumbar spine. In Basic Biomechanics of the Skeletal System. Edited by V.H. Frankel and M. Nordin. Philadelphia, Lea & Febiger, 1980; and from Cailliet, R.: Low Back Pain Syndromes. 3rd Ed. Philadelphia, F. A. Davis, 1981.

A   B   C   D

Extension from full flexion to the upright position of the trunk is brought about by a reverse sequence: the pelvis first tilts backward and the spine then extends. When the trunk is extended from the upright position the back muscles are active during the initial phase of the motion but, with further extension, the activity decreases and the abdominal muscles become active to control and modify the motion (11). In extreme or forced extension, activity of the extensor muscles is again required. The degree of maximum flexion is less than that of maximum extension, primarily because the intervertebral disks in the lower part of the lumbar spine are thicker anteriorly than posteriorly.

Effects of Lifting

The movements of flexion and extension while lifting or lowering a heavy object place additional stress on muscles and ligaments. In lifting a heavy object the pelvis at first rotates, with the ligaments of the lumbar spine bearing the brunt of the stress until 45° of flexion is reached, at which point the muscles of the back become active (2). During these movements flexing the hips and knees places the hip extensors at a mechanical advantage and allows the quadriceps femoris muscles to assist in the lifting and simultaneously tensing the iliotibial band, which is the site of attachment of the glutei muscles. By flexing the hips and knees the distance between the weight being lifted and the center of gravity decreases (17) (Fig. 70-21). As the spine flexes the shoulder girdle and pelvis (hip joint) come closer together and consequently decrease the length of arm for lifting. The shorter the lever arm is for the force produced by the weight of a given object, the lower the magnitude of the forward-bending moment and thus the lower the load on the lumbar spine (18, 19).

When an object is held with the body in a forward bending position, not only the force produced by the weight of the object but also that produced by the weight of the upper body create a bending movement on the disk, resulting in an increased load on the spine (11). Lifting while bending the knees reduces the load on the spine if the object is close to the trunk and consequently closer to the center of motion in the spine (Fig. 70-21B). If the object is held out in front of the knees, however, rather than between the knees (i.e., farther away from the center of motion), lifting a load increases rather than decreases the load on the spine despite the bent knees (11) (Fig. 70-21C).

Lateral Flexion and Rotation

During lateral flexion of the trunk, motion can predominate in the thoracic or lumbar spine (11). Although the orientation of the facet joints in the thoracic spine allows lateral flexion, motion is restricted by the rib cage to a varying degree in different individuals (11). In the lumbar spine the wedge-shaped spaces of the intervertebral joints show variation during motion.

Rotation is consistently combined with thoracic lateral flexion; this combined motion is most marked in the upper thoracic spine, where each vertebral body usually rotates toward the concavity of the lateral curve of the spine. A combined pattern of rotation with lateral flexion also exists in the lumbar spine, but the vertebral body rotates toward the convexity of the curve. Rotation occurs both in the thoracic spine and at the lumbosacral level, where it is moderate because of the orientation of the facets. During rotation the back and abdominal muscles are active on both sides of the spine, because both ipsilateral and contralateral muscles have coordinated motion. Pelvic motion is essential for increasing the range of functional rotation of the trunk.

Functional trunk movements are not only a combination of motion of different parts of the spine but also depend on coordination by the pelvis.

Fig. 70-21. Effect of different positions used in lifting loads on the lumbar spine. **A.** The upper body is flexed forward so that the lever arm of the force produced by the weight of the object (Lp) is 40 cm, creating a forward bending moment of 80 newton-meters (Nm) (200 N × 0.4 m). To this is added the weight of the upper part of the body (lever arm Lw), resulting in a total forward-bending moment of 192.5 Nm. **B.** Flexing the hips and knees and holding the weight closer to the trunk causes a decrease in the length of the lever arm of the force produced by the weight of the object (Lp) (as well as Lw), resulting in a significant decrease in the forward-bending moment applied to the lumbar spine (151 Nm). **C.** The knees and hips are bent, but the subject is attempting to lift the load in front of the knees, thus increasing the lever arm of the weight (Lp) and increasing the forward-bending moment to 212.5 Nm. Modified from Lindh, M.: Biomechanics of the lumbar spine. *In* Basic Biomechanics of the Skeletal System. Edited by V.H. Frankel and M. Nordin. Philadelphia, Lea & Febiger, 1980.

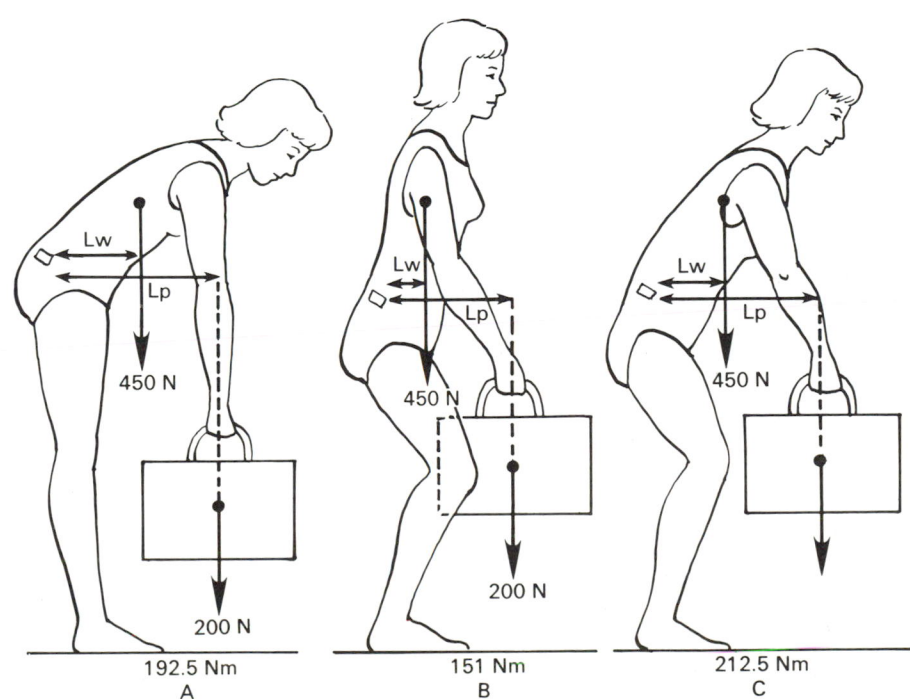

B. THE VERTEBRAL (SPINAL) CANAL AND ITS CONTENTS

The vertebral or spinal canal extends from the foramen magnum to the sacrococcygeal hiatus. It is bounded anteriorly by the posterior surface of the vertebral body, intervertebral disk and overlying posterior longitudinal ligament, laterally by the pedicles, laminae, ligamenta flava, and the lateral vertebral ligaments, and posteriorly by the anterior surfaces of the vertebral arches, laminae, and the ligamenta flava. Its shape and size vary in different parts of the vertebral column to conform to the shape of the spinal cord. It is triangularly prismatic and large in the cervical and lumbar regions to conform to the cervical and lumbar enlargements of the spinal cord, while in the thoracic region it is cylindrical and somewhat smaller. The length of the canal varies and depends, of course, on the height of the individual. The diameters of the cervical portion of the spinal canal are given in Chapter 46. The diameters of the thoracic portions of the canal are 17 mm transversely and 17 mm antero-posteriorly, while in the lumbar region they are 23 and 18 mm, respectively. The size of the canal is about twice the size of the spinal cord (see below). Figure 70-22 illustrates the posterior aspects of the lower thoracic and lumbosacral spines.

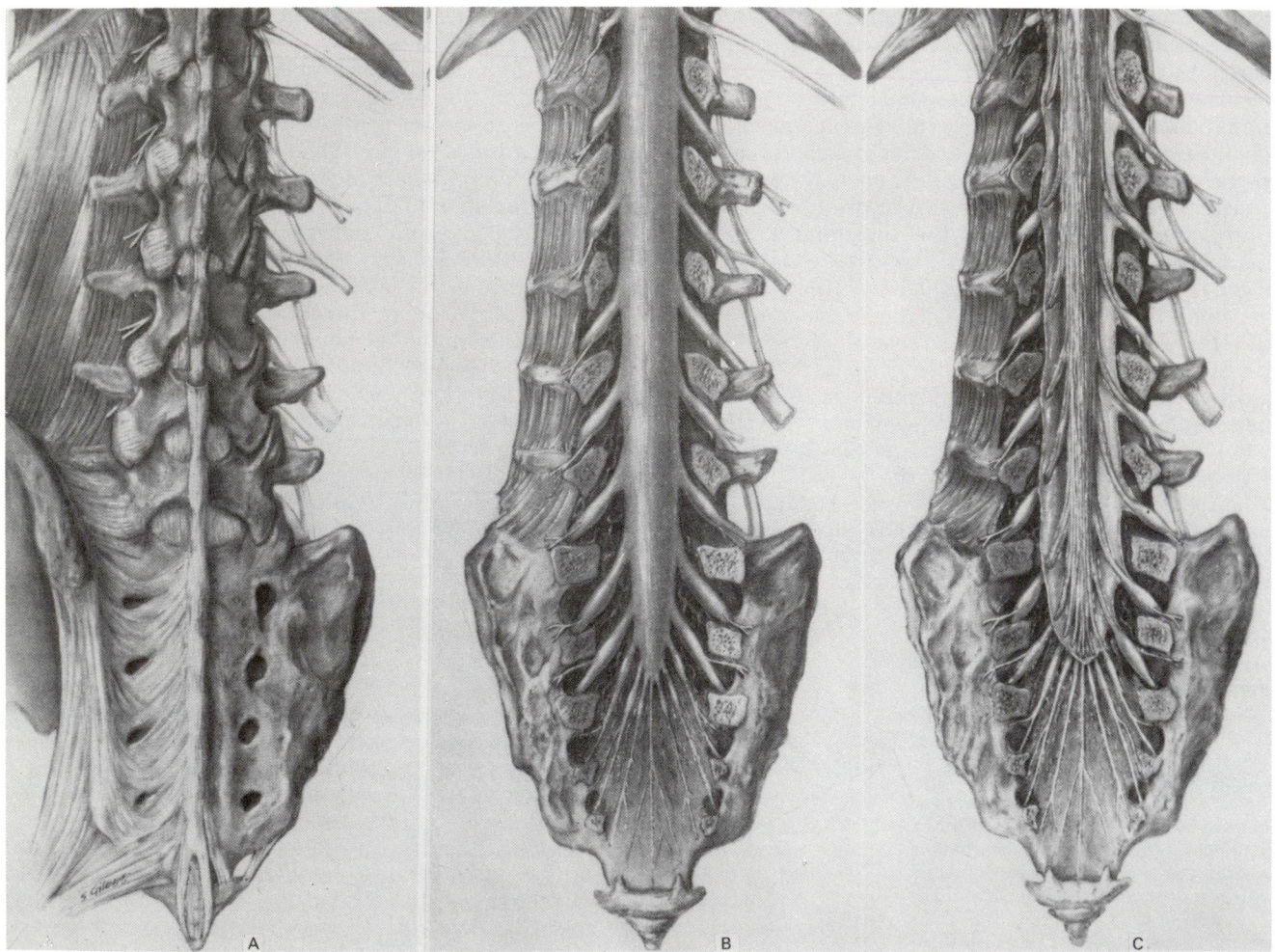

FIG. 70-22. Posterior view of the lower thoracic and lumbosacral spines and their contents. **A.** The vertebral column showing the ligamentous structure of the lumbar spine, including the supraspinous ligament and the deeper ligamentum flavum and the relationship of the transverse processes of the lumbar spine to the lumbar plexus and lumbosacral trunk. Note also the posterior sacral foramina through which the posterior division of the sacral nerves emerges to supply the bones, ligaments, and muscles of the lower back. **B.** Deeper dissection. The contents of the epidural space have been removed to show the position of the dural sac, which ends at the S2 vertebral level. The lumbar nerves formed by the merging of the anterior and posterior roots at the outer edge of the intervertebral foramina are covered by the dura, which fuses at that point with the epineurium of the nerve. The S1 and S2 nerves are located within the sacral canal and the trans-sacral foramina, while the lower three sacral nerves and the coccygeal nerve are contained in the sacral canal. **C.** The dura arachnoid has been opened and the cerebrospinal fluid removed to show the conus medullaris and cauda equina. In this subject the spinal cord ended at the level of the L1 vertebra. On the right the dural cuff has been opened to show the fusion with the epineurium of the formed nerves. From Bonica, J.J.: Principles and Practice of Obstetric Analgesia and Anesthesia, Vol. 1. Philadelphia, F.A. Davis, 1967.

Epidural Space

The epidural space is the interval between the periosteum that lines the vertebral canal and the dura mater that surrounds the spinal cord in its extension from the foramen magnum to the lower end of the dural sac at the level of the S2 vertebra. Caudad to this is the sacral canal. Through its length the space is bound anteriorly by the PLL and vertebral bodies; it is bound anteriorly by the PLL of the vertebral bodies and laterally by the pedicles and the 48 intervertebral foramina, which permit it to communicate with the paravertebral spaces, posteriorly by the laminae and ligamenta flava, and inferiorly by its continuation with the sacral canal.

The size of the epidural space varies greatly. The anterior portion is narrow (1 mm) because the dura is near the PLL throughout the length of the spinal canal. The posterolateral portion, between the dura, ligamenta flava, and laminae, is wider—1.5 to 2 mm in the cervical region, 3 to 5 mm in the thoracic region, and 4 to 6 mm in the lumbar region. In the lumbar region it is triangular, with the apex of the triangle corresponding to the posterior midline of the vertebral canal, where the right and left ligamenta flava come close together (Fig. 94-54). In contrast, at the lumbosacral junction, the epidural space is narrow (about 2 mm).

The contents of the epidural space include fat and loose areolar tissue, through which run the internal vertebral venous plexus, the spinal branches of the segmental arteries, the lymphatics, and the dura-arachnoid projections that surround the spinal nerve roots. Fat is abundant in the posterolateral space, where it forms small pads that intervene between the dura, laminae, and yellow ligament.

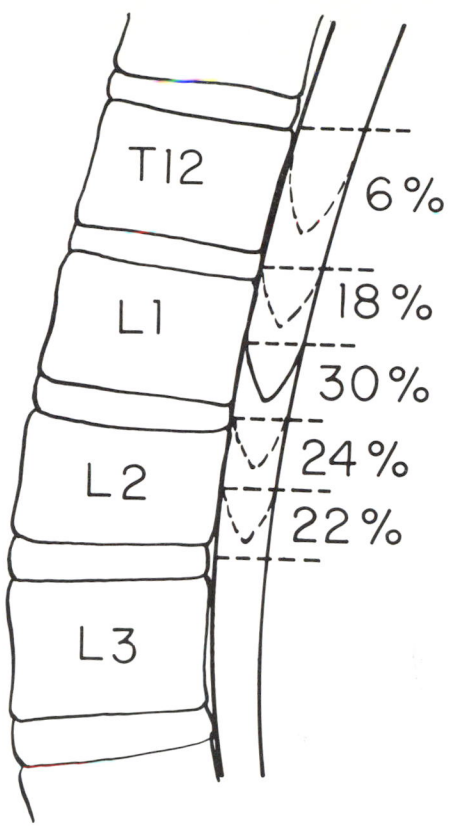

FIG. 70-23. Various levels of the lowermost termination of the spinal cord shown in percentages as found in several autopsy studies.

Spinal Cord

The spinal cord in the adult occupies the upper two-thirds of the vertebral canal, being continuous above with the brain stem and ending below in a conical extremity, the conus medullaris, usually at the level of the lower border of the L1 vertebra. Figure 70-23 shows the variation in the lower caudal termination of the spinal cord. Because the cord is a great deal shorter than the vertebral column in adult life, the spinal cord segments do not lie exactly opposite the correspondingly named vertebrae. Figure 6-2 shows these relationships, and it can be seen that the eight cervical spinal cord segments are opposite the upper six cervical vertebrae, the upper six thoracic segments are opposite the C7 and upper four thoracic vertebrae, the lower six thoracic segments are opposite the T5 to T9 vertebrae, the five lumbar segments are opposite the T10, T11, and upper half of the T12 vertebra, and the 5 sacral and one coccygyeal segments are opposite the lower half of the T12 and the entire L1 vertebrae. In those in whom the spinal cord ends lower, these relationships between cord segments and vertebrae are lower. As a result of this unequal growth between the spinal cord and spinal column, the spinal nerve rootlets and roots course more and more obliquely in a caudal direction from their points of origin in the cord to the same intervertebral foramina through which they made their exits in the fetus before the vertebral column lengthened. Thus, the lumbar, sacral, and coc-

cygeal nerves descend vertically, occupying the subarachnoid space below the conus medullaris in a voluminous group of fibers, the cauda equina.

The spinal cord presents two fusiform enlargements: an upper, or cervical, enlargement, which extends from the C3 to the T2 vertebrae and corresponds to the attachments of the nerves that supply the upper extremities and a lower, or lumbar enlargement, which extends from the T9 to the upper border of the L1 vertebrae and corresponds to the attachments of the nerves that make up the lumbar and lumbosacral plexuses, the branches of which supply the lower extremities (Fig. 70-22). Below the lower enlargement the spinal cord tapers rapidly into the conus medullaris, from whose apex a fibrous cord, the filum terminale, arises. The latter descends first inside the dura and then extradurally in the sacral canal to become attached to the posterior surface of the 1st coccygeal vertebra.

The spinal cord only partially fills the spinal canal, with its diameter being about half that of the canal. It is surrounded by three membranes, the meninges, with a fluid compartment between the arachnoid and pia mater and the epidural space around the dura mater. The spinal cord is fixed in place by several mechanisms, which more or less ensure its relationship within the spinal canal: above, it is suspended at the foramen magnum, which prevents the larger medulla oblongata with which the cord is continuous from moving caudad;

below, it is fixed by a series of nerve roots, the dentate ligaments, and the filum terminale.

Although no trace of transverse segmentation of the spinal cord can be noted macroscopically, it is convenient to regard it as being composed of a series of segments, to each of which are connected a pair of spinal nerves. Because the extent of attachment of these nerves varies in different parts, it follows that the segments are of varying lengths. In the cervical region the length of each of the eight segments is about 12 to 13 mm so that the entire cervical portion of the cord is about 10 cm long; in the thoracic region the length of each segment averages about 20 mm so that the entire thoracic portion is about 24 cm long; in the lumbar region the length of each segment averages about 12 mm so that the lumbar portion of the cord is about 6 cm long; and in the sacrococcygeal region the length of each segment is about 5 mm so that this portion of the cord is about 3 cm long. The cross-sectional diameters of the thoracic spinal cord are 5 mm transversely and 7 mm anteroposteriorly and in the lumbosacral enlargement the diameters are 9.6 and 8.0 mm, respectively—about half the size of the spinal canal. The total length of the spinal cord averages 45 cm in men and 42 cm in women.

Spinal Nerve Roots and Rootlets

Each of the 31 pairs of symmetrically arranged spinal nerves is attached to the spinal cord by two roots, an anterior and a posterior. The smaller anterior root emerges from the anterolateral surface of the cord as two to three rows of rootlets, which form irregular rows over an area 3 to 5 mm wide. These soon converge into a single compact root that extends laterally toward the intervertebral foramen, where it meets the posterior root. The larger posterior root is composed of 7 to 10 rootlets called the fila radicularia, which are attached to the spinal cord in a linear series along the posterolateral sulcus. These rootlets converge peripherally into two bundles, the fasciculi radiculi, which in turn unite near the dorsal root ganglion to form the posterior root.

The spinal root ganglia, which are composed of nerve cells, are oval reddish structures that are situated in their respective intervertebral foramina, immediately outside the point at which the nerve roots preforate the dura mater (Fig. 70-24). The ganglia of the C1, C2, and all the sacral nerves are exceptions to this, with the former usually being situated on the vertebral arches of the C1 and C2 vertebrae and the latter being situated within the sacral canal.

Each nerve root is covered by a sleeve-like investment composed of a closely adherent layer of pia mater, a loose layer of arachnoid, and a layer of dura mater, with cerebrospinal fluid being present between the pia-arachnoid membrane and the arachnoid-dural sheaths. These cover the roots as far as the intervertebral foramen, where the coverings fuse and become continuous with the epineurium of the formed spinal nerve.

The roots of the lumbar and sacral nerves are the largest and longest, and their filaments the most numerous, of all the spinal nerves. The roots of the lumbar and sacral nerves extend the height of 5 to 10 vertebral bodies. The roots of the coccygeal nerve are the smallest, but the longest, having their origin at the end of the conus medullaris at the lower end of the L1 vertebra and making their exit at the level of the 1st coccygeal vertebra.

Meninges of the Spinal Cord

PIA MATER. The pia mater is a thin, delicate vascular membrane composed mostly of minute blood vessels held together by fine areolar tissue and mesothelial cells. It is a continuation of the pia mater of the brain, and, like the latter, closely invests the structure it surrounds. Thus, it is intimately adherent to the spinal cord, dipping into all the depressions, carrying with it the numerous blood vessels that nourish the cord, and forming their adventitial tissue. The pia ensheaths the spinal nerve roots to form a sleeve-like investment that is closely adherent to the nerve tissue and extends as far as the intervertebral foramen. In addition it sends out prolongations laterally, anteriorly, posteriorly, and inferiorly, all of which reach and become attached to the dura.

A condensation of the lateral prolongation occurs at the midcoronal line and is known as the denticulate (or dentate) ligaments, or the lateral suspensory ligaments of the cord. These are triangular processes with their base fixed to the pia and cord and their apex fixed at intervals to the dura mater. The dentate ligaments, 21 on either side, separate the anterior from the posterior roots. A condensation of the prolongation known as the linea splendens occurs at the anterior midline and stretches across the anterior median fissure, and another at the posterior midline, the septum posticum or dorsal suspensory ligament of the cord, extends to the dura. The condensation of the pia mater, which occurs below the conus medullaris, is called the filum terminale. This slender filament descends through the center of the cauda equina as far as the end of the dural sac at the level of the S2 vertebra, where it blends with the dura and proceeds downward as far as the base of the coccyx, to which it is attached by fusion with the periosteum. The filum terminale is often referred to as the central ligament of the cord because it assists in maintaining the latter in position during movements of the trunk. When the patient's spine is acutely flexed this ligament tends to pull the cord anteriorly.

ARACHNOID MATER. The arachnoid mater is a thin, delicate membrane that loosely invests the spinal cord, each of the spinal nerve roots, and the accompanying blood vessels as far as the intervertebral foramen. It also invests the denticulate ligaments and the septum posticum. The spinal arachnoid is continuous with the arachnoid membrane of the brain, and below it widens out and invests the cauda equina. It is composed of two layers of white fibrous and elastic connective tissue, the internal visceral and the outer parietal layers. The internal visceral layer is thin and transparent and forms a film on the pia (hence, it is often called the pia-arachnoid membrane). The outer parietal layer lines the dura and is adherent to it. The space between the two layers is known as the subarachnoid (arachnoid) space; it is filled with cerebrospinal fluid. Crossing this space and connecting the two layers of arachnoid are many trabeculae, which form a sponge-like mass in the subarachnoid space that results in the formation of innumerable channels that are lined by mesothelial cells and contain the cerebrospinal fluid. These trabeculae aid in the mixing of any fluid injected into the subarachnoid space. The subarachnoid space and its fluid contents encircle the spinal cord along its length, being continuous below the conus medullaris as the so-called cisterna terminale and continuous above with the cranial subarachnoid space.

DURA MATER. The dura mater covering the spinal cord is a tough fibroelastic tube that forms a loose sheath around the spinal cord. It is composed principally of longitudinal

Fig. 70-24. Detailed anatomy of the nerve rootlets and roots of the lumbar, sacral, and coccygeal nerves. **A.** Posterior view. **B.** Lateral view at midthoracic vertebral level. **C.** Lateral view of the lumbar spine. The rootlets and roots of the lumbar, sacral, and coccygeal nerves course some distance before they leave the spinal canal. Gathered from their respective rootlets, they proceed caudad toward their respective intervertebral foramina and traverse the subarachnoid space within the dura-arachnoid sac in their own separate dura-arachnoid sleeves. As the nerve roots of the lumbar nerves descend in the spinal canal they cross the disk immediately above the foramina through which they exit and then enter the foramina beneath the pedicles. After entry into the foramina on their extravertebral course each root invaginates the dura-arachnoid and carries the sheath of each into the foramen, so that each of the two roots has its own separate investment of dura-arachnoid as far as lateral to the spinal root ganglion where the roots unite. At this point the two separate sheaths likewise merge so that the formed spinal nerve is invested by a single sheath, which continues for a short distance before it fuses with the epineurium of the spinal nerves. Within the foramen part of the dura fuses with connective tissue and thus anchors the dural sleeve to protect the nerve root from being stretched during movements of the spine. **C.** Within the foramen the smaller anterior (motor) root is located anteriorly and inferiorly near the intervertebral disk. After leaving the foramina the lumbar nerves incline caudad, laterally and slightly anteriorly. The roots and dorsal ganglia of the S1, S2, and S3 nerves lie in sheaths immediately external to the arachnoid-dura cisterna or cul de sac, while the roots and ganglia of the S4, S5, and coccygeal nerves lie within their sheaths in the bony sacral canal at a considerable distance from the dural cul de sac.

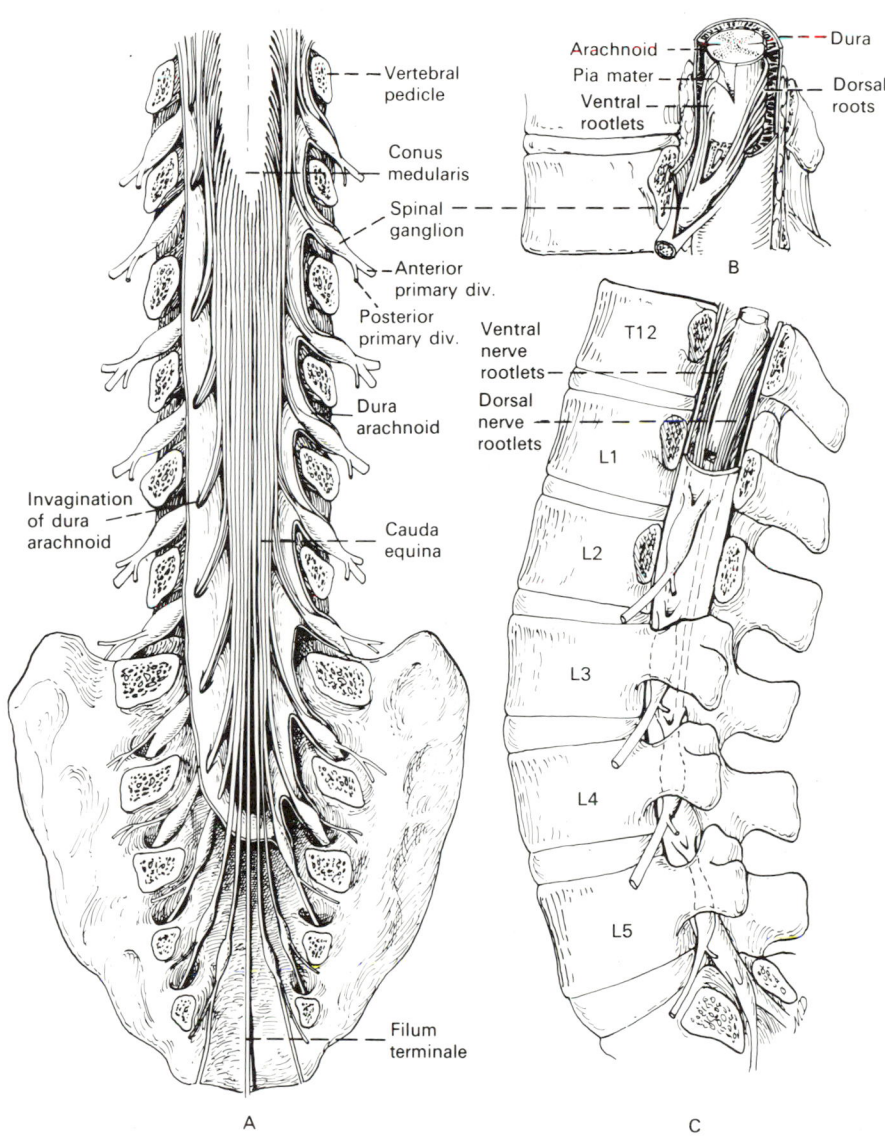

connective tissue fibers, with a proportionately small amount of circular yellow elastic tissue fibers. The spinal dura mater extends from the foramen magnum, to which it is closely adherent by its outer surface, to the S2 vertebra, where it ends in a cul-de-sac. Below this level the dura mater closely invests the filum terminale and descends to the back of the base of the coccyx, where it fuses with the periosteum.

The dura mater, like the arachnoid and pia mater, sends out sleeve-like prolongations that surround the spinal nerve roots. Each spinal nerve root receives a special separate investment of dura-arachnoid. Thus, the anterior and posterior roots, as they approach each other, are encased in separate sheaths as far as the lateral extremity of the spinal root ganglion, where the roots unite. At this point the two separate sheaths likewise merge, so that the formed spinal nerve is invested by a single sheath that continues for a short distance before it fuses with the epineurium of the nerve. These prolongations occasionally extend beyond the intervertebral foramina. They are usually short in the upper part of the vertebral column but gradually become longer below, enclosing the roots of the lower spinal nerves. The roots and dorsal ganglia of the S1, S2, and S3 nerves lie in sheaths immediately external to the cul-de-sac, while part of the roots and ganglia of the S4, S5, and coccygeal nerves lie within their sheaths in the bony sacral canal at a considerable distance caudad to the lower end of the cisterna terminalis.

CEREBROSPINAL FLUID. The cerebrospinal fluid is a colorless transparent watery fluid, a form of lymph, which is found in the arachnoid space, surrounding the entire central nervous system, and in the ventricles of the brain. It has a specific gravity of about 1.0065 and is mildly alkaline in reaction (pH 7.6). Two or three lymphocytes/mm³ can be found in it, and each 100 ml of fluid contains about 25 mg of albumin, 50 mg of sugar, 750 mg of sodium chloride, and 20 to 30 mg of urea. Usually a total volume of 120 to 150 ml of fluid is in the average adult, of which 60 to 75 ml are in the ventricles, 35 to 40 ml in the large reservoirs at the base of the brain, and 20 to 35 ml in the spinal portion of the subarachnoid space. With the patient in the lateral position the cerebrospinal fluid pressure is 10 to 15 cm H_2O.

C. NERVES TO THE LUMBAR SPINE, PELVIS, AND LOWER LIMBS

Somatic Lumbar Nerves

The lumbar nerves are five pairs of typical spinal nerves derived from that part of the spinal cord located between the T10 and T12 vertebrae. Each nerve, on emerging from its respective intervertebral foramen, gives off a recurrent branch that returns to supply the homologous vertebra, its ligaments, and the meninges of the cord (see above: A. The Lumbosacral Spine). Each nerve then divides into posterior and anterior primary divisions.

The posterior primary divisions proceed posteriorly and divide into major medial and lateral branches and also give off an articular branch. The medial branch runs close to the articular process of the vertebra to end in the multifidus muscle and the skin over the upper sacral region, while the lateral branch goes through the sacrospinalis muscle, to which it gives off muscular filaments. The lateral branches of the posterior divisions of the upper three lumbar nerves terminate as the superior clunial nerves to supply the skin over the upper part of the buttock. The articular branch of the posterior primary division provides the nerve supply to the posterior part of the functional unit of the lumbar spine (see above).

The anterior primary divisions leave their posterior fellows and run laterally, inferiorly, and slightly anteriorly in front of the transverse processes of the lumbar vertebrae to enter the substance of the psoas muscles. Within the muscles the first four inosculate to form the lumbar plexus and the 4th and 5th unite to form the lumbosacral trunk. Before uniting each primary division gives off muscular filaments to the intertransversarii and quadratus lumborum muscles, the primary divisions of the 2nd and 3rd give off filaments to the psoas muscles, the primary divisions of the 1st and 2nd give off white rami communicantes to the lumbar sympathetic ganglia and all the primary divisions receive gray rami communicantes from the sympathetic ganglia. These gray rami communicantes supply sympathetic fibers to the lower abdominal wall and lower limbs.

Lumbar Plexus

The lumbar plexus (and its constituent nerves) is formed by the union of the anterior primary divisions of the upper four lumbar nerves and often a filament contributed by the T12 nerve (Fig. 70-25). Thus, by means of these constituent nerves, the lumbar plexus supplies the lower abdominal wall, inguinal region, part of the external genitalia, gluteal region, anterior part of the thigh, and anteromedial part of the leg and foot.

Iliohypogastric Nerve

The iliohypogastric nerve arises together with the ilioinguinal nerve from the upper branch of the anterior primary division of the L1 nerve. Its course is similar to and parallel with the T12 nerve above and the ilioinguinal nerve below. It proceeds laterally and inferiorly through the psoas muscles and then between the quadratus lumborum muscle and parietal peritoneum to reach the region above the iliac crest,

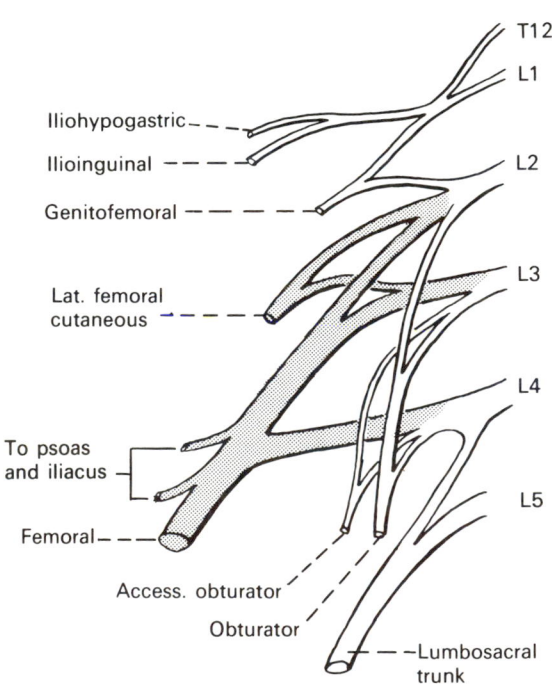

FIG. 70-25. The lumbar plexus. The anterior primary division of the L1 nerve splits into upper and lower branches, with the upper branch joined by a filament from the T12 nerve to form the common trunk of the iliohypogastric and ilioinguinal nerves. The lower branch joins a branch of the L2 nerve to form the genitofemoral nerve. The anterior primary division of the L2 nerve also splits into upper and lower branches. The smaller upper branch takes part in the formation of the genitofemoral nerve while the lower branch takes part in the formation of the femoral, lateral femoral cutaneous, and obturator nerves. The lower branch of the L2 nerve, the upper branch of the L4 nerve, and the undivided L3 anterior primary division split into ventral and dorsal subdivisions. The smaller branch of the anterior primary division of the L4 nerve joins the undivided anterior primary division of the L5 nerve to form the lumbo-sacral trunk or nervus furcalis, which takes part in the formation of the sacral plexus.

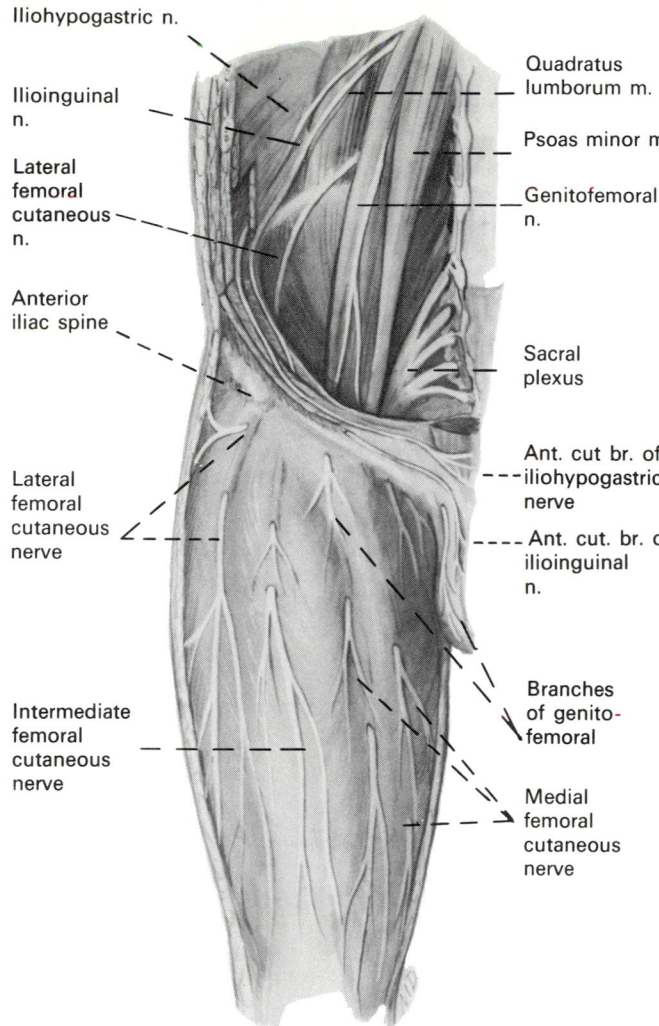

Iliohypogastric n.

Ilioinguinal n.

Lateral femoral cutaneous n.

Anterior iliac spine

Lateral femoral cutaneous nerve

Intermediate femoral cutaneous nerve

Quadratus lumborum m.

Psoas minor m.

Genitofemoral n.

Sacral plexus

Ant. cut. br. of iliohypogastric nerve

Ant. cut. br. of ilioinguinal n.

Branches of genito-femoral

Medial femoral cutaneous nerve

FIG. 70-26. Anatomy of the iliohypogastric, ilioinguinal, genitofemoral, and lateral, intermediate, and medial femoral cutaneous nerves. See text for details.

where it pierces the transversus abdominis to become situated between this muscle and the internal oblique (Fig. 70-26). At this point it gives off the iliac branch, which corresponds to the lateral cutaneous branch of the thoracic nerves and supplies the anterior gluteal region. The hypogastric nerve then continues within the interval between the two muscles to a point above the anterior superior spine of the ilium, where it pierces the internal oblique muscle. It proceeds further along the aponeurosis of the external oblique to terminate as an anterior cutaneous branch, which supplies the suprapubic region. Along its course it gives off filaments to the abdominal muscles.

Ilioinguinal Nerve

The origin of the ilioinguinal nerve is the same as that of the iliohypogastric. After arising from the upper branch of the anterior primary division of the L1 nerve it circles the trunk by coursing parallel and inferior to the iliohypogastric nerve (Fig. 70-26). It remains subperitoneal as far as the anterior part of the iliac crest, where it pierces the transversus abdominis to join the iliohypogastric, with which it inosculates. It then pierces the obliquus internus, enters and traverses the inguinal canal on the anterior aspect of the

spermatic cord, and makes its exit through the external inguinal ring to terminate as cutaneous branches, which supply the skin overlying the symphysis of the pubis, root and dorsum of the penis, upper part of the scrotum (mons pubis and labium majus in the female), and upper medial part of the thigh. It gives off muscular branches to the transversus abdominis and obliquus internus and often a lateral recurrent branch after the nerve leaves the inguinal canal and returns to innervate a strip of skin over the inguinal ligaments.

Genitofemoral Nerve

The genitofemoral nerve arises from the anterior primary divisions of the L1 and L2 nerves, passes obliquely downward through the substance of the psoas, and emerges on the anteromedial surface of this muscle, on which it descends behind the peritoneum to reach the internal inguinal ring. Here it divides into genital and femoral branches (Fig. 70-26). The genital or extenal spermatic branch (derived from the L1 segment) enters and proceeds within the inguinal canal on the posterior aspect of the spermatic cord, emerging through the external inguinal ring to become distributed to the skin of the scrotum and adjacent part of the thigh and to the cremaster muscle. The femoral, or lumboinguinal, branch (derived from the L2 segment) descends on the external iliac artery beneath Poupart's ligament and into the thigh, where it penetrates the fascia lata to supply the skin over the femoral triangle.

Lateral Femoral Cutaneous Nerve

The laterial femoral cutaneous nerve arises from the anterior primary division of the L2 and L3 lumbar nerves and enters and traverses the psoas muscle obliquely downward and laterally to emerge on the anterolateral surface of this muscle. It then runs across the iliacus muscle and the false pelvis beneath the iliac fascia to enter the thigh by passing beneath the lateral end of the inguinal ligament 1 cm medial to the anterior superior iliac spine. In the thigh it proceeds downward by first crossing over or passing through the tendinous origin of the sartorius muscle and then runs beneath the fascia lata to a point 10 cm below the inguinal ligament, where it pierces the fascia to become subcutaneous. At this level the nerve divides into a larger anterior branch, which supplies the skin of the anterolateral part of the thigh as far as the knee, and a posterior branch, which supplies the skin of the lateral aspect of the buttock below the greater trochanter and the upper two-thirds of the lateral side of the thigh (Fig. 70-26).

Femoral Nerve

The femoral nerve, the largest constituent of the lumbar plexus, is formed in front of the transverse process of the L4 vertebra by the union of the anterior primary divisions of the L2, L3, and L4 lumbar nerves (Fig. 70-27). The formed nerve descends in a groove formed by the psoas and iliacus muscles behind the iliac fascia and then enters the thigh by passing behind the inguinal ligament lateral to the femoral artery, from which it is usually separated by slip of the psoas muscle or fascia. While within the abdomen the femoral nerve gives a branch to the iliacus muscle and a branch that supplies the upper part of the femoral artery. Just behind or a little below the inguinal ligament, while within the femoral triangle, the femoral nerve divides into its anterior and posterior groups of branches.

The anterior or superficial group consists of the intermediate and medial femoral cutaneous nerves and several

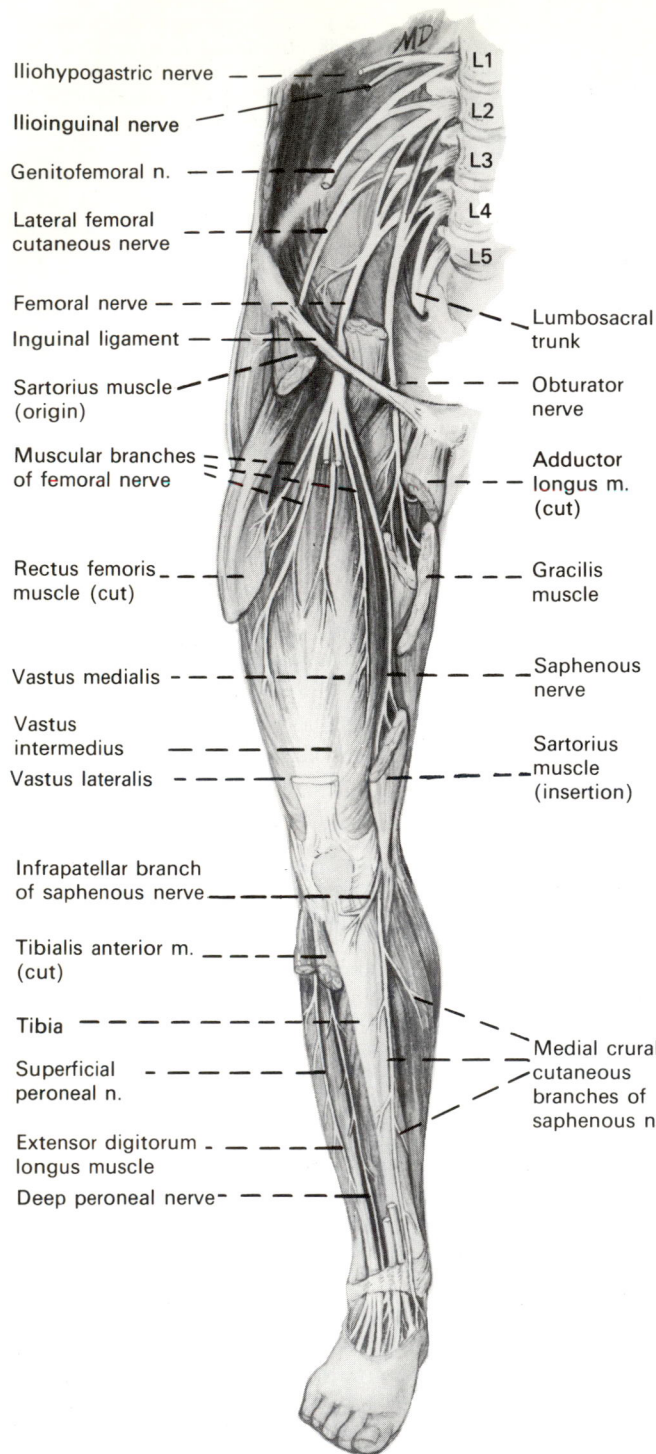

Iliohypogastric nerve

Ilioinguinal nerve

Genitofemoral n.

Lateral femoral
cutaneous nerve

Femoral nerve

Inguinal ligament

Sartorius muscle
(origin)

Muscular branches
of femoral nerve

Rectus femoris
muscle (cut)

Vastus medialis

Vastus
intermedius

Vastus lateralis

Infrapatellar branch
of saphenous nerve

Tibialis anterior m.
(cut)

Tibia

Superficial
peroneal n.

Extensor digitorum
longus muscle

Deep peroneal nerve

L1
L2
L3
L4
L5

Lumbosacral
trunk

Obturator
nerve

Adductor
longus m.
(cut)

Gracilis
muscle

Saphenous
nerve

Sartorius
muscle
(insertion)

Medial crural
cutaneous
branches of
saphenous n.

FIG. 70-27. Anatomy of the femoral nerves. See text for details.

branches that supply the pectineus and sartorius muscles (Fig. 70-26). The intermediate femoral cutaneous nerve pierces the fascia lata about 7 to 10 cm below the inguinal ligament, gives off a filament that inosculates with the lumboinguinal branch of the genitofemoral, and then divides into medial and lateral branches, both of which descend to supply the skin of the anterior aspect of the thigh as far as the knee.

The medial femoral cutaneous nerve passes obliquely across the upper part of the sheath of the femoral artery

below the apex of the femoral triangle, where it divides into anterior and posterior branches. The anterior branch runs downward on the sartorius muscle, pierces the fascia lata at the junction of the middle and lower thirds of the thigh, and divides into two branches. One branch supplies the skin on the medial aspect of the lower third of the thigh as low as the knee and another crosses to the lateral side of the patella to take part in the formation of the patellar plexus. The posterior branch of the medial femoral cutaneous nerve descends along the posteromedial border of the sartorius as far as the knee, where it pierces the fascia lata, communicates with the saphenous and obturator nerves to form the subsartorial plexus, and gives off several cutaneous branches that supply the medial side of the lower thigh, knee, and upper part of the leg. Before the medial cutaneous nerve divides into its anterior and posterior branches it gives off several filaments that pierce the fascia lata to supply the skin of the medial side of the thigh.

The posterior or deep group of branches consists of muscular fibers to the quadriceps femoris, articular branches to the hip and knee joints, and the saphenous nerve. The muscular branches consist of individual nerves, one or more of which supply the rectus femoris, vastus lateralis, vastus intermedius, and vastus medialis. The articular branches are usually derived from the muscular branches, with the one to the hip joint being derived from the nerve to the rectus femoris and the knee joint receiving filaments from each of the nerves to the vastus lateralis, vastus intermedius, and vastus medialis. The latter joint also receives filaments from the articulatio genu and the saphenous nerve (see Figs. 74-6 and 75-11).

Saphenous Nerve

Because of its size the saphenous nerve is often regarded as the terminal branch of the femoral nerve. After it arises within the femoral triangle it descends on the lateral side of the femoral artery outside the femoral sheath, in which relation it enters the adductor canal. Within the canal it crosses obliquely in front of the artery to become situated medial to the femoral vessels, which it accompanies as far as the lower end of the canal and there quits the artery and pierces the aponeurotic covering of the canal. It then descends vertically to cross in front of the tendon of the adductor magnus to the medial side of the knee behind the sartorius, pierces the fascia lata, and becomes superficial by passing between the sartorius and gracilis muscles. The nerve then descends along the tibial side of the leg accompanied by the great saphenous vein to the lower third of the leg, where it divides into two branches. One branch continues along the medial border of the tibia to end at the ankle and the other passes in front of the medial malleolus to become distributed to the skin over the medial side of the foot as far as the metatarsophalangeal joint. Here the saphenous nerve communicates with the medial branch of the superficial peroneal nerve. Along its course the saphenous nerve gives off several branches, some of which inosculate with other nerves. The first of these filaments is given off within the adductor canal and takes part in the formation of the subsartorial plexus. The second branch, the large infrapatellar nerve, is also given off within the canal and supplies the skin over the anteromedial part of the patella and the upper part of the leg. The third group of filaments is given off at the medial side of the knee and communicates with the medial, intermediate, and lateral femoral cutaneous nerves to form the patellar plexus. The fourth group of filaments communicates with branches of the obturator or femoral cutaneous nerve to supply the skin of the medial side of the upper leg. The saphenous nerve also gives off an articular filament at the knee and ankle joints and medial aspects of intertarsal, metatarsal, and interphalangeal joints.

From this detailed description, it is evident that the femoral nerve supplies all the muscles of the anterior part of the thigh that extend the leg and aid in flexion, adduction, and external rotation of the thigh, and also the skin over the anteromedial aspect of the thigh, leg, and foot (Fig. 70-27).

Obturator Nerve

The obturator nerve is formed within the substance of the psoas major muscle by the union of the ventral branches of the anterior primary divisions of the L2, L3, and L4 nerves. The formed nerve emerges from the medial border of the muscle near the brim of the false pelvis and descends downward, first behind the common iliac vessels and then on the lateral side of the hypogastric vessels (Fig. 70-28). It runs on the medial surface of the obturator muscle across the lateral wall of the true pelvis within the obturator groove, accompanied by the obturator vessels, to reach the upper part of the obturator foramen, through which it leaves the pelvis to enter the thigh (Fig. 70-28). While within the foramen it lies below the horizontal ramus of the pubis, where it is usually most easily accessible to the block needle. Here it divides into anterior and posterior branches which are separated from each other by the obturator externus muscle and later by the adductor brevis.

The anterior branch of the obturator descends anterior to the obturator externus and adductor brevis and posterior to the pectineus and adductor longus. At the lower border of the adductor longus it divides into two terminal branches; one supplies the femoral artery and the other supplies the skin of the medial aspect of the lower thigh. It gives off branches to the adductor longus, gracilis, usually the adductor brevis, and rarely the pectineus muscles. Just below the obturator foramen it gives off one or more articular branches to the hip joint (Fig. 74-6).

The posterior branch of the obturator nerve pierces the anterior part of the obturator externus and passes posterior to the adductor brevis, anterior to the adductor magnus, and then through the fibers of the latter muscle to reach the upper part of the popliteal fossa, where it lies on the popliteal artery for a short distance before it splits up into terminal filaments that supply the artery and the knee joint. It also supplies the obturator externus, adductor magnus, and adductor brevis when the latter does not receive filaments from the anterior branch of the obturator nerve. About one-third of people have an accessory obturator nerve, which sends a significant branch to the hip joint and one to the pectineus. In those who have no accessory obturator, the obturator nerve sends two branches to the hip joint.

Sacral and Coccygeal Nerves

The five pairs of sacral and the one pair of coccygeal nerves are derived from the homologous segments located within the lower half of the T12 and L1 vertebrae (or at L2 in 46% of persons). These nerves course downward within the spinal canal as the cauda equina, first within the dura and then within the sacral canal, to reach their respective intervertebral foramina. They leave the canal through these foramina and immediately divide into anterior and posterior primary divisions.

The posterior primary divisions of the upper four sacral nerves pass posteriorly through the posterior sacral foramina, while those of the S5 and coccygeal nerves emerge

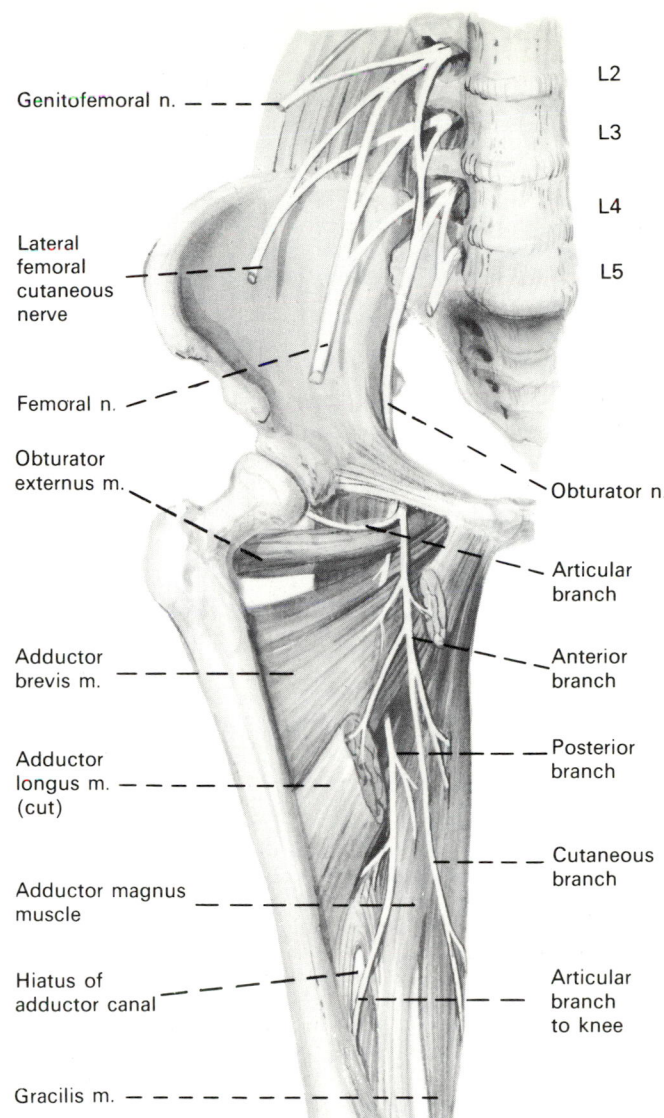

FIG. 70-28. Anatomy of the obturator nerve. See text for details.

through the sacral hiatus (Fig. 70-24). The posterior divisions of the upper three sacral nerves divide into medial branches, which are distributed to the muiltifidus muscle, and lateral branches, which become the posterior sacral plexus and supply the skin over the medial part of the gluteus maximus. The posterior primary divisions of the lower two sacral nerves and that of the coccygeal nerve unite to form the posterior anococcygeal nerve, which supplies the skin over the coccyx.

The anterior primary divisions (APD) of the upper four sacral nerves pass anteriorly into the pelvis through the anterior sacral foramina, that of the S5 nerve emerges from the sacral canal through the sacral hiatus just below the sacral cornu and passes anteriorly by curving around between the lower borders of what can be considered as the transverse process of the S5 vertebra and the coccyx, and that of the coccygeal nerve curves anteriorly below the rudimentary transverse process of the 1st coccygeal vertebra (Fig. 70-22). Except for S3, the APD divide into anterior (ventral) and posterior (dorsal) subdivisions (or branches). The anterior subdivisions of the upper three sacrals unite with the lumbosacral trunk (derived from the anterior primary divisions of the L4 and L5 nerves) to form the sacral plexus, the anterior subdivisions of S2, S3, and S4 form the pudendal plexus, and the dorsal subdivisions of S4 and S5 unite with the coccygeal nerve to form the coccygeal plexus. Parasympathetic white rami communicantes pass from the S2, S3, and S4 nerves and unite to form the nervus erigens, which supplies the lower abdominal and pelvic viscera. All the sacral nerves receive a sympathetic gray ramus communicans that follows the nerves to supply the homologous somatic segments. The sacral nerves, together with the lumbar nerves, supply the lower extremities.

Sacral Plexus

The sacral plexus is formed by an intricate interlacement of the anterior primary divisions of the L4 and L5 nerves (lumbosacral trunk) and those of the S1, S2, and S3 nerves. These unite to form two terminal and six collateral branches, all of which constitute the sacral plexus (Fig. 70-29).

Collateral Branches

The nerve to the quadratus femoris and gemellus inferior, which arises from the anterior subdivisions of the L4, L5, and S1 nerves, leaves the pelvis through the greater sciatic foramen below the piriformis, runs inferiorly in front of the sciatic nerve, gives off an articular filament to the hip joint, and then enters and terminates within the two muscles that it supplies.

The nerve to the obturator internus and gemellus inferior, which arises from the anterior subdivision of the L5, S1, and S2 nerves, leaves the pelvis through the greater sciatic foramen, gives off a branch that enters the posterior surface of the gemellus superior, crosses posterior to the ischial spine, and then re-enters the pelvis through the lesser sciatic foramen to reach and pierce the pelvic surface of the obturator internus.

The nerve to the piriformis arises from the posterior subdivision of the S1 (not shown in Fig. 70-29) and S2 nerves and supplies the piriformis muscle.

The superior and inferior gluteal nerves arise from the posterior subdivision of the L4, L5, S1, and S2 nerves and leave the pelvis through the greater sciatic foramen (the superior above and the inferior below the piriformis muscle) to reach the gluteal muscles. The superior gluteal nerve supplies the gluteus minimus and medius and the tensor fascia lata, while the inferior gluteal nerve supplies the gluteus maximus.

The posterior femoral cutaneous nerve, often called the small sciatic nerve, arises from the posterior subdivisions of the S1 and S2 nerves and from the anterior subdivision of the S2 and S3 nerves and leaves the pelvis through the greater sciatic foramen below the piriformis, accompanied by the great sciatic nerve, to descend beneath the gluteus maximus to the back of the thigh. It runs down beneath the fascia lata and over the long head of the biceps femoris to the back of the knee, where it pierces the deep fascia to become subcutaneous; it then travels subcutaneously to about the middle of the posterior part of the calf. The posterior femoral cutaneous nerve gives off several gluteal branches, which supply the skin covering the lower and lateral parts of the gluteus maximus, two or three *perineal branches*, which supply the skin of the upper and medial parts of the thigh and part of the skin of the scrotum (male) or labium majus (female), and *posterior femoral cutaneous branches*, which supply the skin of the posterior aspect of the thigh, popliteal fossa, and upper part of the back of the leg.

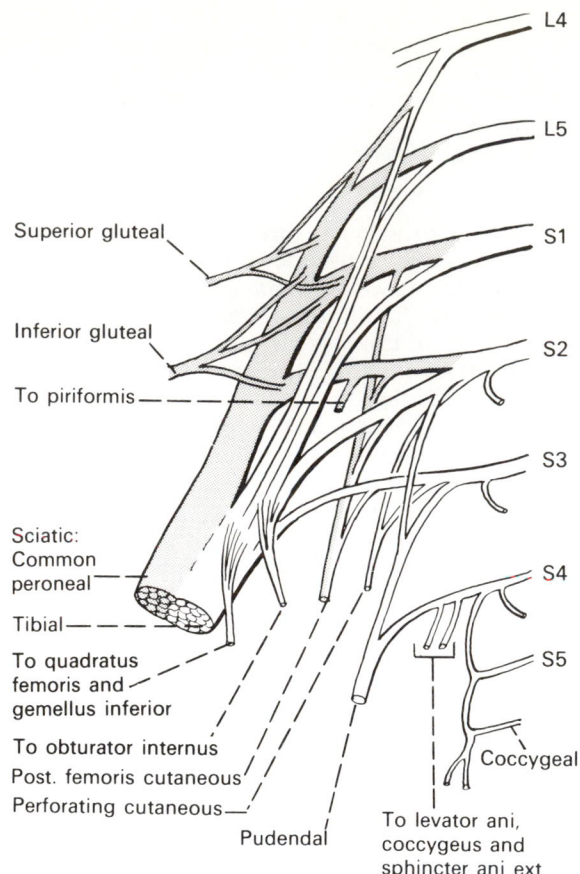

FIG. 70-29. The sacral plexus. The large tibial nerve, the nerve to the quadratus femoris and gemellus inferior, the nerve to the obturator internus and gemellus superior, and part of the posterior femoral cutaneous nerve are derived from the anterior subdivisions. The common peroneal nerve, the nerve to the piriformis, the superior gluteal, the inferior gluteal, and part of the posterior femoral cutaneous nerves are derived from the posterior subdivision. The tibial and common peroneal nerves are the two terminal branches and are usually fused together as far as the posterior part of the thigh into what is commonly known as the great sciatic nerve (see Fig. 70-30). Modified from Clemente, C.D. (ed.): Gray's Anatomy of the Human Body. 30th Am. Ed. Philadelphia, Lea & Febiger, 1985, p. 471.

Sciatic Nerve

The sciatic is the largest nerve in the body, measuring about 2 cm in width at its point of origin (Fig. 70-30). It is the continuation of the flattened head of the sacral plexus and actually consists of two separate nerves, the common peroneal and the tibial nerves, which are enclosed within a common sheath. The common nerve trunk leaves the pelvis through the greater sciatic foramen below the piriformis muscle and descends toward the posterior aspect of the thigh, coming to lie in the hollow between the ischial tuberosity and the greater trochanter of the femur in a position corresponding to the junction of the medial and middle thirds of the line connecting these two points. The sciatic nerve is often blocked here (see Fig. 94-37). In this region it is situated posterior to the ischium, obturator internus, gemelli, and quadratus femoris muscles, and anterior to the gluteus maximus.

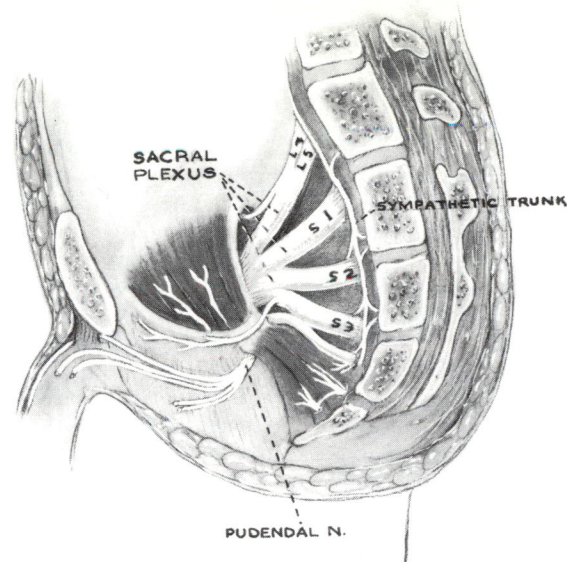

the larger of the two, thereafter begins its own course in the upper part of the popliteal space and passes along the vertical diagonal of this space to the lower part of the popliteal muscle. It then passes beneath the arch of the soleus and continues to run along the posterior aspect of the leg accompanied by the

FIG. 70-30. Sagittal view of the right pelvis showing the position of the sacral plexus, which is a large, broad, triangular structure lying in the posterior part of the true pelvis in front of the sacrum, from which it is separated by the piriformis muscle. Its broad base is formed by the anterior primary divisions and therefore coincides with the row of anterior sacral foramina and with the L5 and L4 paravertebral spaces, while its apex is composed of the great sciatic nerve as it lies in the great sciatic notch. The plexus is covered by the pelvic fascia and is in close relation with the pelvic viscera. Anterior to the plexus are the hypogastric vessels and some of their branches, the ureter, and the sigmoid colon. Some branches of the hypogastric vessels run between the anterior primary divisions before they unite to form the plexus.

It proceeds downward to reach the upper part of the posterior thigh where, at the inferior aspect of the buttock, it occupies a more superficial position. It continues its descent down the posterior aspect of the thigh between the adductor magnus and the hamstring muscles to the upper part of the popliteal fossa; here, at a variable point, the two nerves comprising the sciatic diverge from each other to follow separate courses. The common peroneal nerve courses around the side of the leg below the knee, where it finally becomes distributed to the posterior part of the leg and the plantar aspect of the foot.

Along its course the sciatic nerve gives off several articular and muscular branches. The articular branches arise from the upper part of the nerve and supply the hip joint. The muscular branches, which are given off at various points along its course, supply the biceps femoris, semitendinosus, semimembranosus, and adductor magnus. The nerve to the short head of the biceps arises from the common peroneal nerve, while the other muscular branches are given off by the tibial portion of the sciatic nerve.

Tibial Nerve

The tibial nerve (also called the posterior tibial and formerly called the internal popliteal) arises from all five ventral subdivisions of the sacral plexus and proceeds distally together with and in the same sheath as the common peroneal nerve as far as the popliteal space, where these two components of the sciatic nerve take separate courses. The tibial nerve, which is

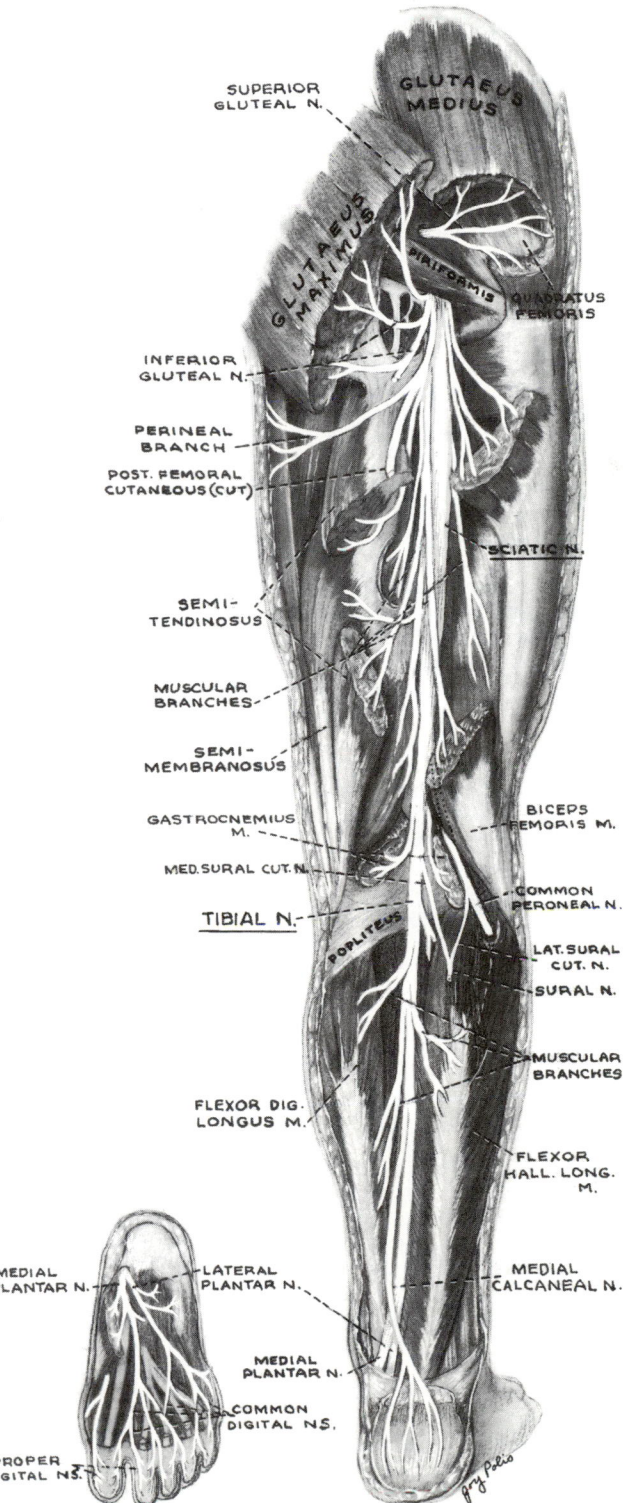

FIG. 70-31. A. Anatomy and distribution of the sciatic nerve and its branches, including the tibial and common peroneal nerves. B. The plantar surface of the foot, depicting distribution of the two plantar nerves and their branches.

posterior popliteal vessels to reach the interval between the medial malleolus and the heel on the posteromedial aspect of the ankle, where it divides beneath the laciniate ligament into the medial and lateral plantar nerves (Fig. 70-30).

In the thigh the tibial nerve lies lateral to and some distance from the popliteal vessels and beneath the hamstring muscles. As it approaches the posterior aspect of the knee it crosses superficial to the vessels from their lateral to their medial side; lower down in back of the calf, it again crosses obliquely to the lateral side of the vessels, in which relation it reaches the posteromedial aspect of the ankle. In the popliteal fossa it is rather superficial, being covered by the skin, and superficial and deep fascia. In the upper part of the leg it lies on the deep muscles and is covered by the superficial muscles of the calf, while lower down it again becomes superficial and is covered by the skin and superficial and deep fascia. In the lower part of the leg it runs parallel and medial to the medial border of the Achilles tendon.

The upper portion of the tibial nerve gives off articular branches to the knee joint and muscular branches to the gastrocnemius, plantaris, soleus, and popliteal muscles. It also gives off the medial sural cutaneous nerve, which descends between the two heads of the gastrocnemius to the middle of the back of the leg, where it pierces the deep fascia and inosculates with the anastomotic branch of the common peroneal nerve to form the sural nerve. The latter passes down the posterolateral aspect of the leg to the interval between the lateral malleolus and the calcaneus and then turns forward to the dorsolateral aspect of the foot as the lateral dorsal cutaneous nerve. The sural nerve is the cutaneous nerve to the posterolateral aspect of the leg and to the dorsolateral aspect of the foot and little toe.

The lower portion of the tibial nerve gives off muscular branches to the soleus, tibialis posterior, flexor digitorum longus, and flexor hallucis longus muscles; the medial calcaneal branches, which supply the ball and posterior portion of the sole of the foot; and two terminal branches, the medial and lateral plantar nerves.

The medial plantar nerve is homologous (or has a similar distribution) to the median nerve of the hand. It gives off cutaneous branches to the medial portion of the sole, articular branches to the tarsal and metatarsal articulations, muscular branches to the adductor hallucis, flexor digitorum brevis, flexor hallucis brevis, and 1st lumbricales: It also gives off the proper digital nerve to the great toe and the three common digital nerves, each of which splits into two proper digital nerves to supply the adjacent sides of the 1st, 2nd, 3rd, and 4th toes. Each proper digital nerve gives off a cutaneous and articular branch to the plantar surface of the toes and, opposite the last phalanx, gives off a dorsal branch, which supplies the structures around the nail.

The lateral plantar nerve is homologous to the ulnar branches in the hand. It supplies the skin of the 5th toe and of the lateral half of the 4th toe, as well as most of the deep muscles. It runs obliquely across from the medial to the lateral side of the sole, where it splits into superficial and deep branches. The superficial branch splits into a proper digital and a common digital nerve; the former supplies the lateral side of the little toe, the flexor digiti quinti, and the two interossei of the 4th intermetatarsal space, while the latter communicates with the 3rd common digital nerve of the medial plantar and then splits into two proper digital nerves, which supply the adjacent sides of the 4th and 5th toes. The deep branch of the lateral plantar nerve proceeds to the deep part of the sole to supply all the interossei except those of the 4th intermetatarsal space, the adductor hallucis, and the 2nd, 3rd, and 4th lumbricales.

Common Peroneal Nerve

The common peroneal nerve is formed by the union of the upper four posterior subdivisions of the sacral plexus and therefore derives its fibers from the L4, L5, S1, and S2 segments. In the thigh, it is a component of the sciatic nerve as far as the upper part of the popliteal space, where it parts from the tibial nerve and begins its independent course. It descends diagonally across the posterior aspect of the knee and along the lateral border of the popliteal fossa close to the posteromedial margin of the biceps femoris muscle as far as the upper external portion of the leg, where it winds around the neck of the fibula between the peroneus longus muscle and the bone (Fig. 70-30). Here the common peroneal nerve divides into three terminal branches—the recurrent articular, the deep peroneal, and the superficial peroneal nerves. While in the popliteal space the nerve gives off superior and inferior articular branches to the knee joint and the lateral sural cutaneous nerve, which supplies the skin of the posterolateral surface of the leg. The lateral sural cutaneous nerve gives off the peroneal anastomotic branch, which joins the medial sural cutaneous branch of the tibial nerve to form the sural nerve.

The recurrent articular nerve accompanies the anterior tibial recurrent artery to supply the knee and tibiofibular joints.

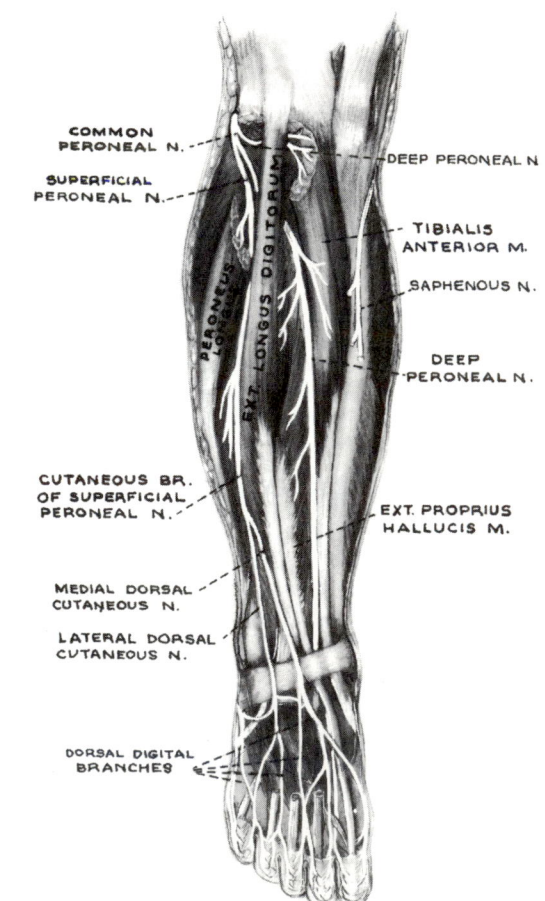

FIG. 70-32. Anterior view of the leg showing the course and distribution of the common peroneal nerve into the superficial and deep peroneal nerves and their branches.

The deep peroneal (anterior tibial) nerve (Fig. 70-30) parts from the superficial peroneal nerve at the neck of the fibula beneath the upper part of the peroneus longus and passes obliquely in an anterior direction beneath the extensor digitorum longus to the front part of the leg, where it pursues its course in front of the upper part of the interosseous membrane and then in front of the lower third of the tibia as far as the ankle joint. At the ankle it passes beneath the superior extensor retinaculum just lateral to the tendon of the extensor hallucis proprius and medial to the anterior tibial artery, in which relation it gains the dorsal aspect of the foot where it divides into medial and lateral terminal branches. The medial branch proceeds distally, medial to and accompanied by, the dorsalis pedis artery to the 1st interosseous space, where it communicates with the medial dorsal cutaneous nerve of the superficial peroneal nerve. It then divides into two dorsal digital nerves that supply the adjacent sides of the great and 2nd toes, the meta-tarsophalangeal joint of the great toe, and the 1st interosseous muscle.

The lateral branch of the deep peroneal nerve passes across the tarsus beneath the extensor digitorum brevis to supply this muscle and the metatarsophalangeal joints of the 2nd, 3rd, and 4th toes. While in the leg the deep peroneal nerve gives off muscular branches to the tibialis anterior, extensor digitorum longus, peroneus tertius, and extensor hallucis proprius and articular branches to the ankle joint.

The superficial peroneal (musculocutaneous) nerve leaves the deep nerve and descends between the peronei and extensor digitorum longus along the intermuscular septum to the lower third of the leg, where it pierces the deep fascia to enter the subcutaneous plane, wherein it descends for a short distance before it divides into two terminal branches, the medial and intermediate dorsal cutaneous nerves. The medial cutaneous nerve passes obliquely across the ankle joint superficial to the superior and inferior extensor retinacula and divides into two dorsal digital branches, one of which supplies the medial and lateral sides of the great toe, while the other supplies the adjacent sides of the 2nd and 3rd toes. It also communicates with the saphenous and deep peroneal nerves to supply indirectly the skin of the medial side of the foot. The intermediate dorsal cutaneous nerve passes along and supplies the skin of the dorsolateral aspect of the ankle and foot, and then divides into dorsal digital branches, which supply the adjacent sides of the 3rd, 4th, and 5th toes. The superficial cutaneous nerves therefore supply the skin of the anterolateral aspect of the lower half of the leg and ankle, the dorsal surface of the foot, and all of the toes, except the lateral side of the little toe and the contiguous sides of the great toe and 2nd toe, the former being supplied by the lateral dorsal cutaneous branch of the sural nerve and the latter by the medial branch of the deep peroneal nerve.

D. SYMPATHETIC AND SOMATIC SEGMENTAL AND PERIPHERAL NERVE SUPPLY TO THE HIPS AND LOWER LIMBS

This section summarizes the sympathetic and the segmental and peripheral somatic nerve supply to various structures of the lumbosacral spine, hips, and lower limbs. First a detailed description of the sympathetic nerve supply to the vessels of the lower limbs is presented. This is followed by illustrations depicting the segmental somatic nerve supply (Fig. 70-35) and the peripheral somatic nerve supply (Fig. 70-36) to these structures. The peripheral and segmental innervation of various muscle groups of the lower limb is presented in tables in Chapters 74, 75, and 76.

Sympathetic Nerve Supply to Vessels in the Lower Limbs

The vessels of the lower limbs receive sympathetic and sensory fibers in a pattern somewhat similar to that of the upper extremities. The preganglionic sympathetic neurons have their cell bodies in the anterolateral horn of the spinal cord at the T10, T11, T12, L1, L2, and sometimes the L3 spinal cord segments (1, 20, 21) (Fig. 70-33). Their axons pass by way of the anterior root of the corresponding spinal nerves and the white rami communicantes to reach the sympathetic trunk. They then descend to the lower three lumbar and upper three sacral sympathetic ganglia, where they synapse with postganglionic neurons. A small percentage of postganglionic fibers pass directly to the aortic and hypogastric plexuses. Most of the postganglionic fibers, however, leave the sympathetic trunk as gray rami communicantes (GRCs) and join the L1 nerve, which contributes to the iliohypogastric and genitofemoral nerves, and the L2 to the L5 and upper three sacral nerves, which form the lumbosacral plexus. These GRCs then pass peripherally through their constituent nerves, which supply the lower limbs. Some

sympathetic fibers do not pass through the sympathetic trunk but pass directly to the lumbosacral plexus and its branches (20, 21). Intermediary ganglia are also

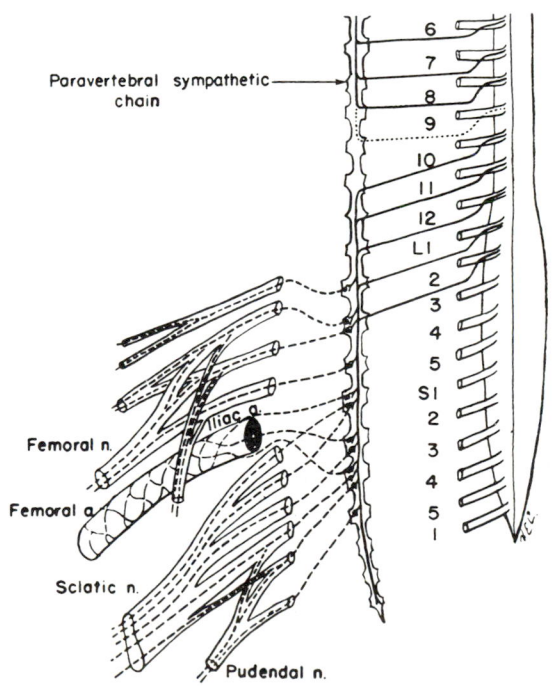

FIG 70-33. Origin and course of preganglionic (solid lines) and postganglionic (dashed lines) sympathetic fibers that supply the lower limbs. Preganglionic fibers at the T6–T9 spinal cord levels pass cephalad to join those from T2–T5 to supply the upper limb. From Bonica, J.J.: Clinical Applications of Diagnostic and Therapeutic Nerve Blocks. Springfield, IL, Charles C Thomas, 1959.

present (22). The S1 and S2 nerves contain the largest number of gray rami communicantes (23).

The last thoracic and upper two lumbar spinal nerves receive two sets of rami: one group ascends from the sympathetic trunk to the spinal nerves, consists histologically of myelinated fibers, and represents white rami communicantes, while the other group of rami travels from the sympathetic trunk to the spinal nerves in a descending or transverse course. These rami, which are present in all levels of the lumbosacral region, represent gray rami communicantes consisting of vasomotor, pilomotor, and sudomotor postganglionic fibers. Each root of the lumbosacral plexus receives one group of gray rami communicantes but the S1, S2, and S3 nerves receive several groups of GRCs, because these eventually reach the vessels in the lower part of the leg and foot and consequently provide the largest number of GRCs and accompanying sensory fibers.

INNERVATION OF THE COMMON ILIAC ARTERY. The common iliac artery (Fig. 70-34) is innervated in a variable manner by branches of the aortic plexus and by filaments given off by the lumbar sympathetic ganglia. Some authorities (21, 24) have claimed that all nerves to the common iliac artery originate mainly from the L3 and to a lesser extent from the L2 and L4 sympathetic ganglia. Some of these branches pass directly to the anterior and posterior surfaces of the artery, while others join the aortic plexus first and are later given off as a distinct nerve to the common iliac artery and its branches (24).

INNERVATION OF THE EXTERNAL ILIAC ARTERY. The external iliac artery represents the limit between the areas, of vascular innervation from visceral and parietal sources, because the proximal part is supplied by an extension of the common iliac plexus while the distal part is supplied by branches from the genitofemoral nerve (23, 25) (Fig. 70-34). Lazorthes (24) found that proximal branches of the genitofemoral nerve interlace with the extension of the common iliac nerve plexuses, whereas the distal nerve filaments of the genitofemoral nerve supply the external iliac artery near the inguinal ligament.

Others (26) have found additional nerve filaments from the pelvic portion of the femoral nerve to the external iliac artery.

Nerve Supply of the Femoral Artery of the Thigh

The femoral artery (Fig. 70-34) is innervated chiefly by the femoral nerve but, at the beginning and end of the femoral blood vessel, the innervation is reinforced by accession of nerve filaments from other sources (21). The upper portion of the femoral artery—that is, the part between the inguinal ligament and the offshoot of the profunda femoris—is richly supplied by a variable number of branches from the femoral nerve (21, 24, 25) and also by filaments supplied by the lumboinguinal branch of the genitofemoral nerve and by an extension of the external iliac plexus, and occasionally from the lumbar plexus and the lateral femoral cutaneous nerve (25). The medial femoral circumflex artery and the profunda femoris artery are supplied by filaments derived from the medial cutaneous and intermediate cutaneous nerves and the nerve to the pectineus muscle, all of which are branches of the femoral nerve (24–26).

The middle portion of the femoral artery has a meager nerve supply, receiving fine twigs from the medial femoral cutaneous and saphenous nerves (25, 26), while the inferior portion of the artery has a more conspicuous nerve supply from a nerve plexus derived from the saphenous nerve, anterior division of the obturator nerve, and some filaments from the popliteal nerve.

Nerve Supply of the Leg and Foot

Below the knee the vessels are supplied by filaments given off at irregular intervals by the saphenous nerve (cutaneous vessels only) and especially the tibial and peroneal nerves and all their terminal branches (Fig. 70-34). As in the upper extremity, these fibers run mostly parallel to one another from the nerves to the vessels. The distal portions of the arterial tree and venous system, especially the feet and toes, receive more sympathetic and sensory fibers than the proximal parts of the limbs, and these are given off at more frequent intervals. As in the upper extremity, the sympathetic and sensory supply is somewhat demarcated into zones supplied by various cutaneous nerves.

INNERVATION OF THE POPLITEAL ARTERY. The popliteal artery receives sympathetic and sensory branches from the posterior division of the obturator nerve and from the saphenous and sciatic nerves. According to Lazorthes (24), the posterior branch of the obturator nerve provides the filament of the origin of the popliteal artery by passing through the nerve to the adductor magnus muscle. After a course of several centimeters this filament divides into two terminal branches—an external branch, which passes along the middle genicular artery to the posterior fibrous capsule of the knee joint, and an internal branch, which accompanies the superior internal genicular blood vessel. This internal ramus of the obturator nerve anastomoses with branches of the saphenous nerve, which supply the distal part of the artery, and of the sciatic nerve, which supply the proximal part of the artery. The superior external genicular artery is innervated by the trunk of the sciatic nerve, the inferior internal genicular artery is innervated by the tibial nerve, and the inferior external genicular artery is innervated by the peroneal nerve. Most muscular branches of the popliteal artery are innervated by filaments from the tibial nerve (26, 27).

TIBIOPERONEAL ARTERIAL TRUNK. This arterial trunk has a rich nerve supply (24), which includes the following: (a) a vascular filament from the nerve to the popliteal muscle; (b) an occasional filament from the main nerve trunk to the popliteal and posterior tibial muscles; and (c) a single or double "nerve of the division of the tibioperoneal trunk" (2) that, in a variable manner, arises independently from the tibial nerve, from the nerve to the flexor digitorum communis, or from the nerve to the posterior tibial muscle.

POSTERIOR TIBIAL ARTERY. The proximal portion of the posterior tibial artery is abundantly innervated by the nerve of the division of the tibioperoneal trunk (21). The middle portion has a scanty innervation from two or three small twigs of the nerve to the flexor digitorum communis, while the inferior portion of this artery has a conspicuous nerve supply from the retromalleolar plexus. This in turn is formed by contributions from the tibial nerve, the articular branch to the ankle joint, and the medial and lateral plantar nerves.

PERONEAL ARTERY. The proximal segment of the peroneal artery is supplied by branches derived from the division of the tibioperoneal trunk, the middle portion is supplied by a twig from the nerve of the soleus muscle, and the inferior part is supplied by filaments from the nerve to the flexor hallucis longus muscle.

PLANTAR ARTERIES. The lateral plantar artery receives two to four branches from the lateral plantar nerve and the medial plantar artery receives one or two twigs from the medial plantar nerve. Lazorthes (24) emphasized the meager nerve supply to the plantar vessels, which is in contrast to the abundant nerve supply of the palmar vessels in the hand (27).

ANTERIOR TIBIAL ARTERY. The upper portion of the anterior tibial artery, still placed in the posterior muscular compartment, receives a twig from the nerve to the popliteal muscle and another from the articular branch to the tibiofibular joint (21, 24). The middle and distal portions of the deep peroneal artery are innervated by direct branches from

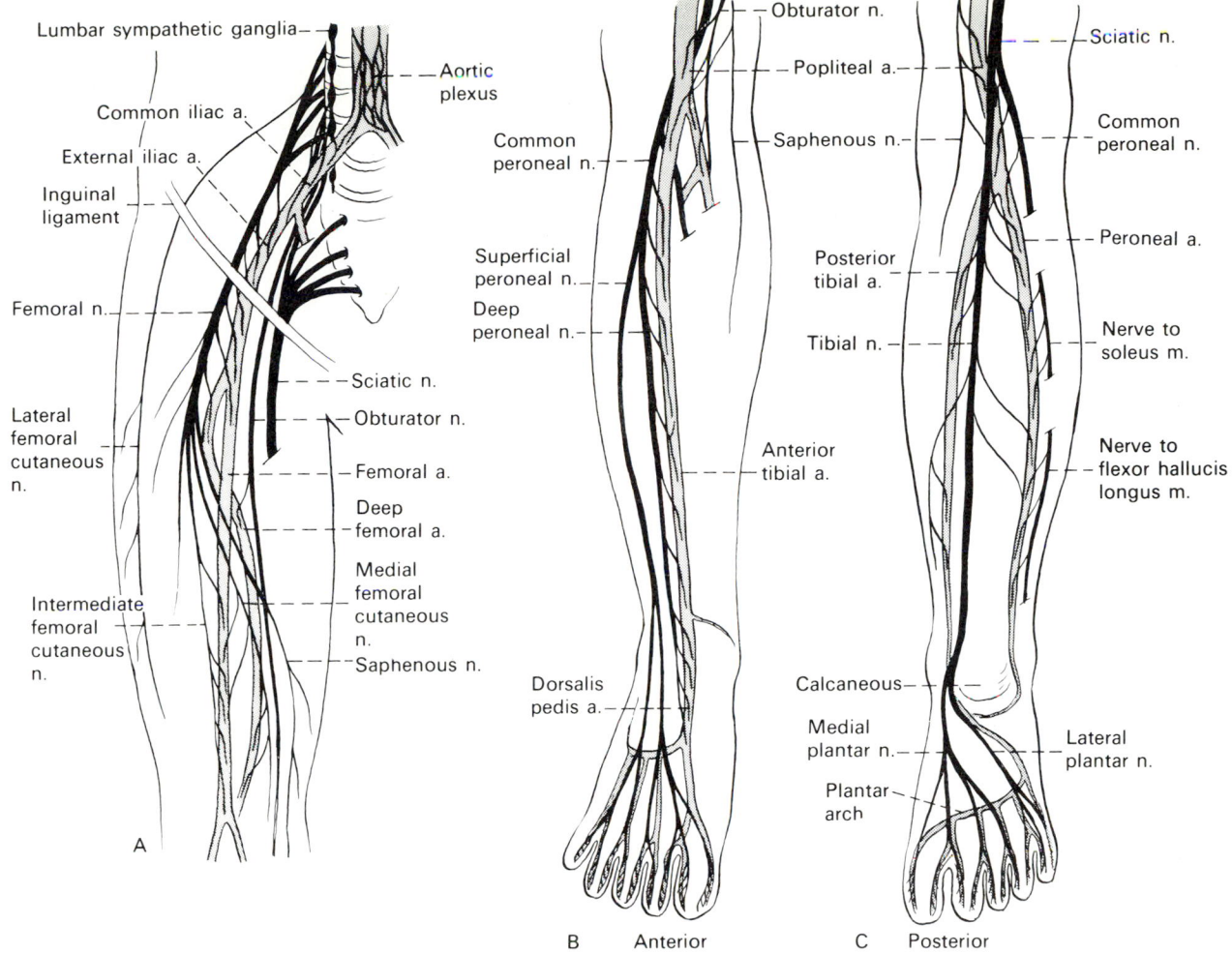

FIG. 70-34. Nerve supply to the blood vessels of the lower limbs. **A.** Anterior view of the pelvis and thigh showing the nervelets from the aortic plexus that supply the common iliac artery and the external iliac artery, which is also supplied by the femoral nerve, which gives many branches to the femoral artery and all of its subdivisions. **B.** Anterior view of the leg to show the nerve supply to the anterior tibial artery derived from the common and deep peroneal nerves. **C.** Posterior view of the leg showing the nervelets derived from the tibial nerve with some also being supplied by the common peroneal nerve in some of its branches. See text for details.

the anterior tibial nerve and by numerous offshoots from the nerves to the muscles of the front of the leg.

ARTERIES IN THE DORSUM OF THE FOOT. The dorsalis pedis artery is supplied by the deep peroneal nerve, and the other branches of the anterior tibial artery are innervated by the continuation of the anterior tibial artery. The endings of the dorsal metatarsal and interdigital arteries and veins over the medial two-thirds of the dorsum of the foot are supplied by extremely thin nervelets, which originate chiefly from the medial branch of the superficial peroneal nerve (29). The sural nerve issues strong branches to

the lateral interdigital, metatarsal, and lateral calcaneal arteries.

DISTRIBUTION AND PHYSIOLOGY. Distribution of the sympathetic nerves to the walls of the vessels of the lower limbs and physiology of these nerves are similar to those of the upper limb (Chapter 46).

Somatic Nerve Supply

Figure 70-35 depicts the segmental nerve supply to the lower limb, and Figure 70-36 shows the peripheral nerve supply.

E. EVALUATION OF THE PATIENT

To diagnose the cause of pain in the low back, parts of the lower extremity, or both areas, it is necessary to obtain a detailed history and to carry out a comprehensive physical examination, including orthopedic and neurologic studies (Chapter 31). In contrast to the format used with other introductory chapters in this book, which contain a detailed dis-

cussion of the evaluation process, here I present only an outline. I do this because each region would require a complicated workup and result in a long section, and because it is better to consider each region separately. Therefore, in addition to the following, a detailed evaluation of patients with pain in the low back is presented in Chapter 71, evaluation of patients

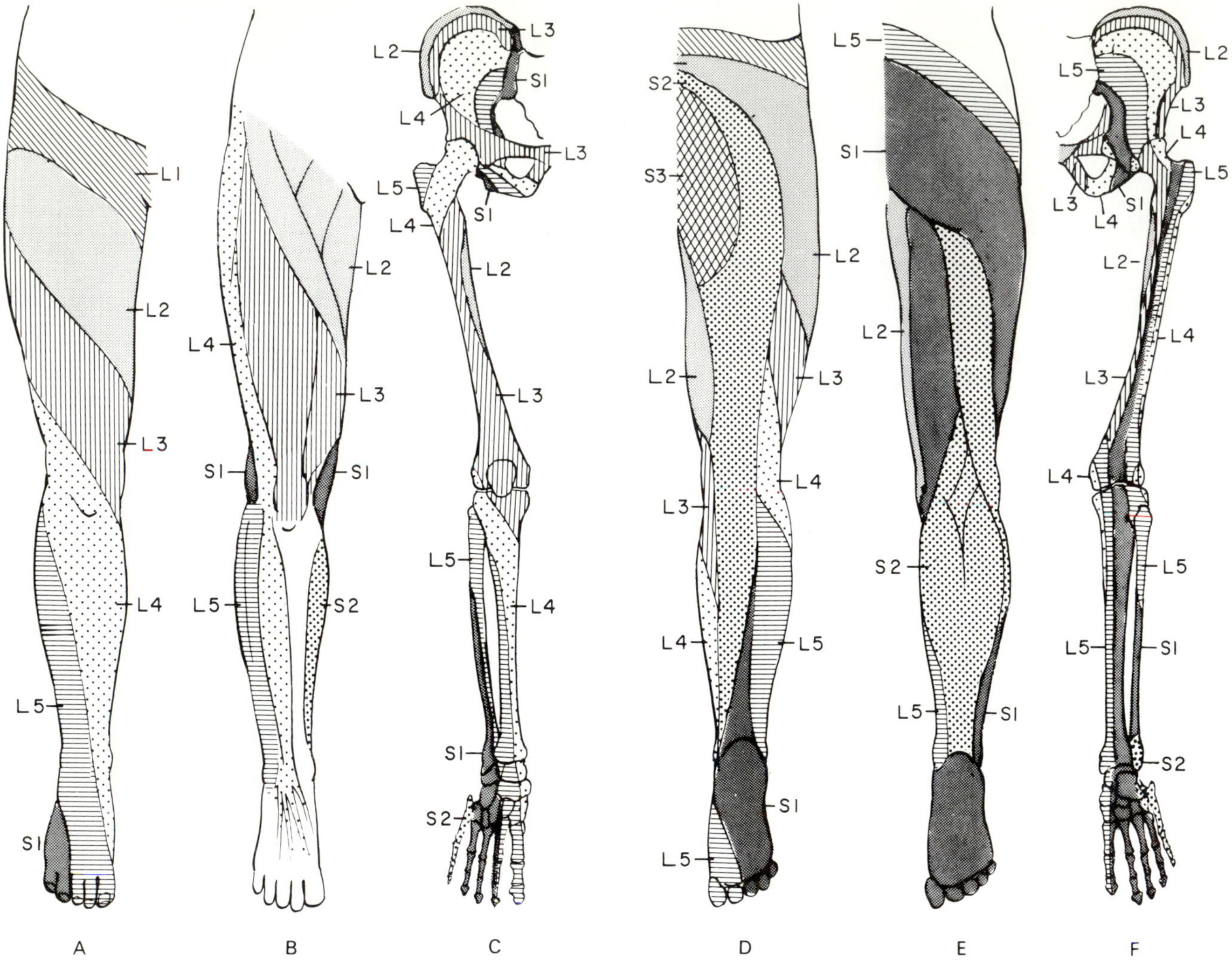

FIG. 70-35. Segmental nerve supply to the lower limbs. **A.** Anterior view showing dematomes, **B.** Anterior view showing myotomes. **C.** Anterior view showing sclerotomes. **D.** Posterior view showing dermatomes. **E.** Posterior view showing myotomes. **F.** Posterior view showing sclerotomes. See Chapter 6.

with pain in the hip is presented in Chapter 74, evaluation of those with pain in the thigh and knee is given in Chapter 75, and evaluation of those with pain in the leg, ankle, and foot is discussed in Chapter 76.

Summary of History and Examination

A detailed history of the pain and of associated phenomena usually provides sufficient information to make the diagnosis. Because pain is usually caused by musculoskeletal, neurologic, or peripheral vascular disorders, emphasis should be placed on diagnostic points that generally indicate whether the cause is in one of these categories. Pain that is sudden and lancinating in character, begins in the low back, and "shoots" down the entire extremity to the foot is probably of neuropathic origin. The patient is then questioned further in an attempt to locate the site of the lesion. If the pain is aggravated by coughing,

straining, and sneezing it is probably intraspinal, whereas if it is aggravated by movement of the lumbosacral spine it is probably a compression neuritis secondary to a vertebral lesion. Pain that is circumscribed, does not radiate along segmental or peripheral nerve distribution, and is aggravated by motion of the extremity is probably musculoskeletal. Pain of peripheral vascular disease has a peculiar history of onset, has definite characteristics, is associated with changes in the color and temperature of skin, alteration of peripheral pulses, trophic changes, and swelling, and is modified by walking or dependency or elevation of the leg.

The examination is similar to that described for the upper extremities. Because lesions that produce pain in the lower limbs also cause low back pain, it is often necessary to perform a detailed examination of both regions. Therefore, the same outline can be used for both regions. Of course, for pain in the upper back, it might not be necessary to perform some of the parts

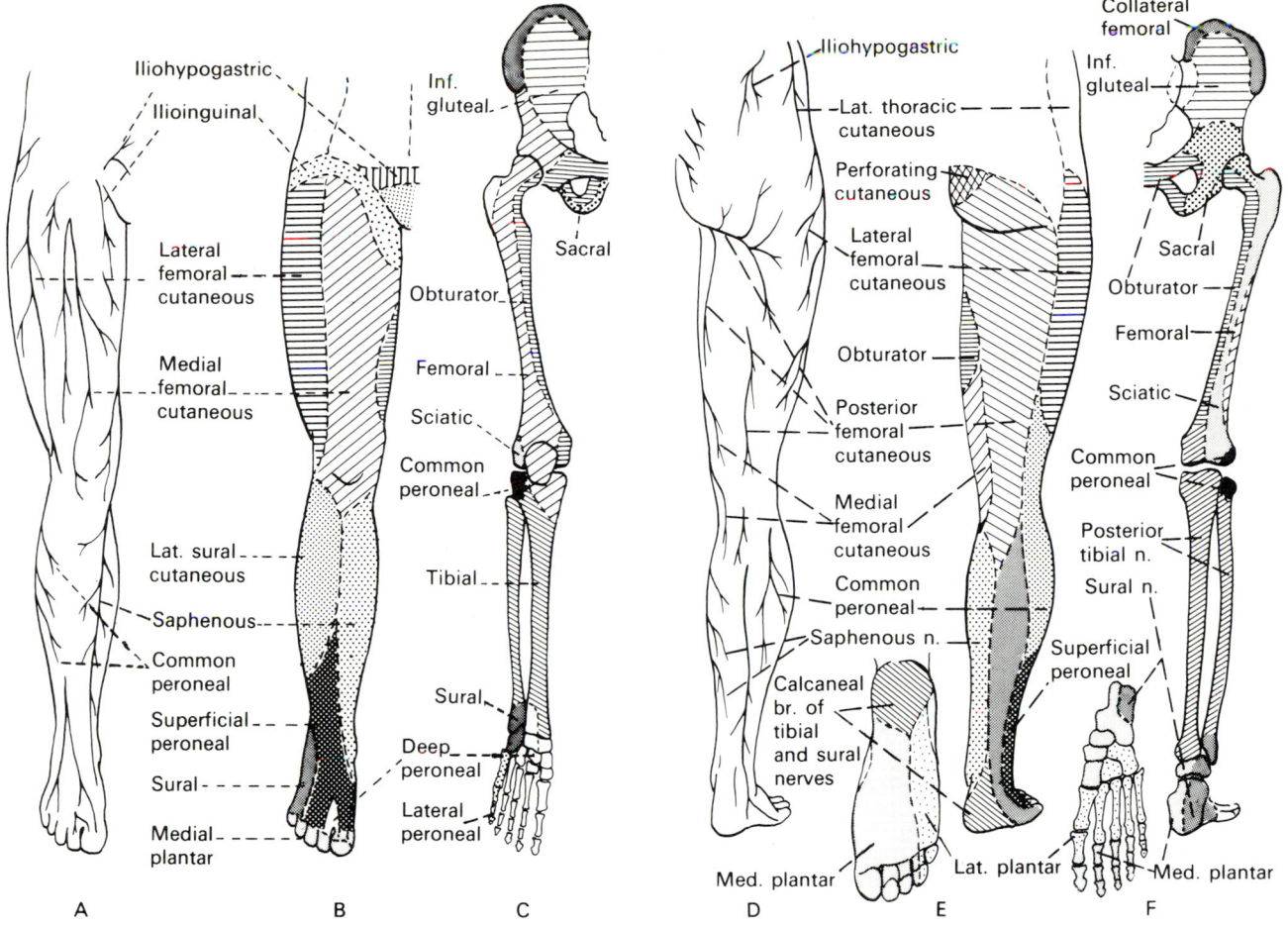

FIG. 70-36. Peripheral nerve supply to the lower extremities. *A–C.* Anterior views. *A.* Cutaneous branches. *B.* Territories of cutaneous branches. *C.* Distribution of peripheral nerves to bones. *D–F.* Posterior views.

of the examination for the lower extremities and, conversely, in certain cases of pain in the lower limbs, it is not necessary to perform a detailed examination of the cervical and thoracic spine.

The lower extremities must be examined with the patient in the standing and supine positions. With the patient standing, the length of both limbs is measured from the internal malleolus to the anterior superior iliac spine and also to the umbilicus. The weight-bearing line must be noted and recorded. The levels of both iliac crests, gluteal creases, and patellae must also be noted and recorded. Each part of both limbs is inspected and note is made of any abnormality. The patient is asked to perform certain movements to test muscle and joint function. Particular note is made of

limited motion. The color, texture, and moisture of the skin, character and distribution of the hairs, presence or absence of dilated or tortuous veins, presence of trophic lesions and ulcers, and pigmentation should be noted and recorded.

The extremities are examined again when the patient is in the supine position. In addition to close inspection, the skin, muscles, peripheral pulses, bones, and joints are carefully palpated to detect abnormalities and the circumference of the various parts of each extremity is measured. These and other important points in examining the lower extremities are presented in Table 70-2.

Table 70-3 is a summary of the differential diagnosis of painful disorders of the low back, hip, and lower extremities.

TABLE 70-2. Outline of History and Examination

I. HISTORY
  A. History of the pain
  1. Characteristics and precipitating factors of pain at onset
  2. Characteristics of pain since onset
  3. Pain at the present time:
     a. Location and distribution—local, segmental, or peripheral
     b. Quality and intensity—sharp, dull, aching, shooting, severe, moderate, mild
     c. Temporal characteristics—continuous or intermittent, pain worse in morning, evening, or night
  4. Effect on pain of coughing, sneezing, straining, activity, standing, sitting

General Considerations of Pain in the Low Back, Hips, and Lower Extremities **1425**

TABLE 70-2. (Cont.)

B. **Associated phenomena**
  1. Sensory: numbness, paresthesia, anesthesia, other
  2. Motor: weakness, paralysis (in what muscles?)
  3. Autonomic: vasoconstriction, cyanosis, vasodilatation, hyperhidrosis, trophic disturbances
  4. Sphincter control: vesical (normal or abnormal), anorectal (normal or abnormal)
C. **Past medical history:** history of previous painful and nonpainful diseases

II. EXAMINATION OF THE BACK

A. **Standing**
  1. Body type, gait, coordination, Romberg's sign
  2. Posture: comparison of levels of both shoulders, angle of scapulae, costovertebral angles, iliac crests, gluteal creases, knees
B. **Spine:** physiologic curves—lordosis, scoliosis, kyphosis, gibbous or other prominences
C. **Entire back:** muscle spasm, round shoulders, atrophy, hypertrophy, tumors, other
D. **Upper extremities:** normal, abnormal
E. **Chest:** normal, abnormal
F. **Abdomen:** normal, pendulous
G. **Active motion:** note degree of limitation of painful region
H. **Neck:** flexion, extension, rotation, pain
I. **Shoulders:** right and left—abduction, rotation, swing, pain
J. **Trunk**
  1. Forward flexion: stooping, extension, pain
  2. Lateral flexion: right, left torsion
  3. Squatting, other movements
K. **Sitting**
  1. Forward bending, lateral flexion to right and left
  2. Right and left torsion, extension
L. **Lying supine**
  1. Raising the head from the table: normal, limited, pain
  2. Compression on chest and abdomen; pain, dyspnea, other
  3. Sit ups: active, raising head, shoulders, and touching toes with fingers
  4. Hip flexion with knee flexed
M. **Special tests of both lower limbs:** straight leg raising; Goldthwait's, Gaenslen's, Kernig's, Lasègue's signs; other nerve stretching tests; Patrick's, Freiberg's, other tests (specify)
N. **Lying prone**
  1. Palpation and percussion (specify location of pain and tenderness): spinous processes, paravertebral region, neck, back of chest, lumbar region, sacral region, coccyx
  2. Pain: localized, radiating (where), trigger points (indicate on diagram)
  3. Active extension of spine: normal, limited, pain
O. **Lying on right side**
  1. Compression of iliac crests: normal, pain (site)
  2. Torsion of spine: hip forward, shoulder fixed, normal or pain; hip backward, shoulder fixed, normal or pain
P. **Lying on left side**
  1. Compression of iliac crests: normal or pain
  2. Torsion of spine: hip forward, shoulder fixed, normal or pain; hip backward, shoulder fixed, normal or pain

III. EXAMINATION OF LOWER EXTREMITIES

A. **Standing**
  1. Weight bearing
  2. Shape
  3. Length: malleolus to superior iliac spine, malleolus to umbilicus
  4. Skin color and texture
  5. Veins or deformities (specify)
  6. Motion: straight leg raising, squatting
B. **Recumbent position**
  1. Length: malleolus to spine, malleolus to umbilicus
  2. Circumference and site: foot—at the arch; ankle—1 cm above malleolus; leg—10 cm above malleolus; knee—superior border of patella; thigh—lower, 8 cm above patella; upper, 15 cm above patella
  3. Sensory examination: pain—pinprick, pin scratch, pinch; temperature, touch, vibration
  4. Hip motion: abduction, adduction, flexion; internal rotation, external rotation; abnormal motion; pain or tenderness
  5. Thighs: femoral pulse; cremasteric reflex; atrophy, swelling; pain, tenderness; trigger points
  6. Knees: popliteal pulse; swelling; tender points; flexion and extension; abnormal motion; patellar reflex
  7. Legs: calf tenderness; atrophy or swelling; skin temperature, skin moisture
  8. Ankles: pain, joint tenderness, swelling; trigger points; motion; anterior tibial pulse, posterior tibial pulse; Achilles reflex
  9. Feet: skin color—horizontal, elevated, dependent; temperature (palpation), moisture; trophic changes; ulcers, gangrene; color and shape of nails; swelling, tenderness: general, trigger points; arches, heels; abnormalities (deformity, corns, other)

IV. ANORECTAL, VAGINAL, AND CYSTOSCOPIC EXAMINATION: findings (specify)

V. SPECIAL TESTS

A. **Lumbar puncture:** date, findings
B. **Biopsy:** date, findings
C. **Examination of stool:** date, findings
D. **Roentgenography (including myelography):** date, findings, summary

TABLE 70-3. Pain in the Low Back, Hip, and Lower Extremities: Summary of Etiology and Differential Diagnosis

Etiology (Disease)	IASP Code Ref.*	Chapter No.	Important Diagnostic Features	
			Characteristics of the Pain	Associated Symptoms and Signs
I. LOCALIZED LOW BACK PAIN WITHOUT RADIATION TO LOWER LIMBS				
A. Static (postural) disorders (poor postural habits; occupational postural stress; obesity; muscular deficiency; congenital anomalies—scoliosis, lordosis, short leg)	XXVII-6	72	Constant diffuse pain in low back; aggravated by activity, prolonged standing, sitting, or recumbency; worse on motion after prolonged rest; occasional bouts of acute pain lasting hours or days provoked by trauma or by excessive activity	Stiffness; muscle spasm or increased muscle tension; postural deformity or muscle imbalance present—abnormal curves (e.g., lordosis, scoliosis); occupational history; physical and radiographic evidence of deformity
B. Myofascial pain with trigger points (TPs)				
1. Quadratus lumborum, iliocostalis, multifidus, rotatores, rectus abdominus	XXVII-13	72	Moderate to severe pain in low back; elicited by systematic forefinger pressure on the entire low back; aggravated by motion of muscle and pressure on TP; relieved completely by injection of TP	Maximum tenderness at trigger area; tenderness and muscle spasm in area of reference; decreased range of motion; autonomic disturbances frequently present
2. Gluteus maximus and medius	XXVII-14	72		
C. Increased muscle tension or spasm (major trauma; microtrauma; reflex response of neurolgic, deep somatic, or visceral disease; emotional stress)	XXVII-6	72	Localized or diffuse pain, frequently severe; aggravated by movement and palpation; pain and other symptoms relieved by surface or infiltration analgesia or paravertebral somatic nerve block	Tenderness on palpation; palpation reveals spastic muscle and limitation of movement; no radiographic evidence of skeletal pathology or dysfunction
D. Postoperative reflex spasm		72	Unexpected bouts of severe excruciating pain in lumbar paraspinal and gluteal muscles lasting 2 to 15 minutes; usual onset second or third postoperative day	Usually occurs after laminectomy by noxious stimulation of periosteum, deep muscles and damage to nerves and tendons
E. Traumatic lesions (Violent blow or excessive effort—lifting, twisting)	XXVII-8	72		
1. Muscle strain		72	Diffuse dull aching pain, sometimes occurring after injury; aggravated by motion	Stiffness, or diffuse localized tenderness (TPs), and muscle spasm; history of trauma; fracture ruled out by radiography
2. Lumbosacral sprain or strain (common)	XXVII-6	72	Moderate to severe pain and tenderness in lumbosacral junction; aggravated by motion; onset can be sudden, severe, disabling with severe trauma; relieved by local injection of lumbosacral joint	Tenderness over joint; obliteration of lumbar curve; negative Patrick's tests, Goldthwait's and Gaenslen's signs
3. Dislocation or fracture without nerve compression	XXVI-5	71	Sudden severe pain and tenderness; localized to site of injury; aggravated by movement	Muscle spasm; localized tenderness over spinous process or paravertebral region; history of trauma; radiographic evidence

*See Table 2-2.

TABLE 70-3. (Cont.)

Etiology (Disease)	IASP Code Ref.*	Chapter No.	Important Diagnostic Features	
			Characteristics of the Pain	Associated Symptoms and Signs
4. Post-traumatic spondylosis	XXVII-2	71	Sudden onset of acute deep aching pain; poorly localized in lumbosacral region; recedes over time	Limited motion of lumbosacral spine but no specific findings; radiographic evidence late
F. Developmental disorders				
1. Vertebral epiphysitis (Scheuermann's disease)		72	Chronic, aching pain; localized over involved area (usually dorsal and upper lumbar); aggravated by exertion, fatigue, percussion	Mainly affects adolescents; exaggerated dorsal kyphosis; radiographic evidence
2. Secondary or idiopathic scoliosis		71	Chronic dull aching pain	Early, fatigue; progressive curvature, with loss of height; later, signs of degenerative arthritis
G. Arthritides				
1. Rheumatoid arthritis of lumbar spine	I-10	20, 71	Diffuse deep aching, burning pain in low back; moderately severe; usually intermittent, with exacerbations and remissions; aggravated by spine motion	Morning stiffness; tenderness to palpation; typical radiographic changes; positive test for rheumatoid factor
2. Osteoarthritis (degenerative)	I-11	20, 71	Deep aching pain in low back; markedly aggravated by anterior or lateral flexion or extension	Other joints involved with radiographic evidence
3. Rheumatoid arthritis of sacroiliac joint		72	Pain on one side of back (joint usually affected first)	Radiographic and laboratory evidence
4. Infectious arthritis (staphylococcal, gonococcal, tuberculous, others)		20, 71	Acute moderate to severe deep aching pain localized in low back; aggravated by deep palpation or fist pound over spinous processes and paraspinal region	Muscle spasm, severe tenderness, fever, leukocytosis, malaise, and other signs of infection; laboratory and radiographic evidence
H. Destructive lesion of bone				
1. Metabolic (osteoporosis—senile, menopausal; osteopenia; osteomalacia)		22, 71	Chronic persistent dull aching pain in thoracic and lumbar spine; can radiate anteriorly; aggravated by exertion; trivial injury can cause sudden severe localized pain	Generalized tenderness to spine; later exaggeration of dorsal kyphosis; radiographic evidence
2. Infections of vertebrae (osteomyelitis, tuberculosis, brucellosis, actinomycosis, blastomycocis, syphilis)		22, 71	Constant localized pain and tenderness that gradually worsens; aggravated by percussion over spinous process, forceful compression of spine, any motion of spine; worse at night (night crises)	Severe muscle spasm, chills, fever, leukocytosis; history of exposure and other signs and symptoms of disease; radiographic evidence
3. Neoplasm of spine a. Primary tumor: osteoid osteoma (hemangioma, giant cell tumor); osteogenic sarcoma; chondrosarcoma b. Metastatic carcinoma		22, 71	Constant pain (initially at night), fever, palpable mass; later, constant persistent severe back pain, expansive or boring in character; aggravated by motion of spine and weight bearing; progressively more severe and intractable	The first category usually affects those in the younger age group, and is considered to be benign, occurring in the posterior element; secondary lesions also affect spine; metastatic carcinoma usually occurs after age 50, with weight loss

*See Table 2-2.

TABLE 70-3. (Cont.)

Etiology (Disease)	IASP Code Ref.*	Chapter No.	Important Diagnostic Features	
			Characteristics of the Pain	Associated Symptoms and Signs
I. Low back pain caused by operant mechanisms		71	Deep, aching, and mild pain, or sharp and severe; located over entire low back or in one part of back; usually persists beyond healing time; sustained by reinforcing influences in environment, with psychosocial factors playing major role in pain and disability; one of the most frequent causes of chronic low back pain	Unusual degree of fatigue, disability; frequently associated with depression; presence of three or more of Waddell's five signs (Chapter 71)
J. Pain of psychologic origin				
1. Psychophysiologic low back pain	XXIX	15, 72	Moderate to severe pain; usually localized to lumbosacral region	Stiffness and muscle spasm; anxiety, emotional stress, abnormal EMG; signs of autonomic hyperactivity (e.g., palpitations, tachycardia)
2. Low back pain and psychiatric illness	XXIX	15, 72	Low back pain manifested with delusion or hallucination, higher incidence with hysteric or hypochondriac disorders (now called somatoform condition); occurs more frequently than formerly, but still rare	
K. Referred pain				
1. Diseases of the abdomen				
a. Retrocecal appendicitis		61	Sudden acute low back pain	Signs of "acute abdomen"; see Table 59-6
b. Diseases of the kidney (renal tumors, pyelonephritis, pyelitis, carbuncle or furuncle, renal tuberculosis, aneurysm of renal artery)		63	Continuous dull aching pain in lower thoracic and lumbar paravertebral regions and costovertebral angle of affected side; radiation anteriorly and to thigh; aggravated by deep palpation and percussion	Nausea, vomiting, fever, leukocytosis, hematuria, pyuria, albuminuria, palpable tumor; other signs and symptoms of disease
c. Calculi and other obstructive lesions of renal artery (embolism, acute glomerulonephritis, arteriosclerosis)		63	Sudden sharp severe, agonizing pain in lumbar region of affected side; radiation to groin, inner side of thigh, and testis or labium	Same as above
d. Retroperitoneal masses (lymphosarcoma, Hodgkin's disease, carcinomatous lymphadenopathy, aneurysm of abdominal aorta)		65	Continuous moderate to severe boring pain in thoracolumbar region of back	Other signs and symptoms of disease; radiographic evidence
2. Diseases of the pelvic viscera	XXIV	67		
a. Diseases of the uterus and adnexae (tumors; ovarian cysts; infections; dysmenorrhea; retrodisplacement of uterus)		67	Chronic continuous ache or pain in lumbosacral region of back	Palpable tumor or evidence of infection on vaginal examination

*See Table 2-2.

TABLE 70-3. (Cont.)

Etiology (Disease)	IASP Code Ref.*	Chapter No.	Important Diagnostic Features	
			Characteristics of the Pain	Associated Symptoms and Signs
b. Diseases of the rectosigmoid (cancer and other tumors; distension; fecal impaction; ulcer; hemorrhoids)		67	Continuous dull aching pain in low back; somewhat relieved by defecation	Evidence on digital or proctoscopic examination
c. Prostate (prostatitis; urethritis; cancer; other disorders)		68	Persistent chronic low backache or pain	Evidence on rectal or cystoscopic examination
3. Referred somatic pain (diseases of the hip— osteoarthritis, infectious arthritis, fractures)		74	Pain in hip and thigh; radiation to low back	See Chapter 74
II. LOW BACK PAIN WITH RADIATION TO THE THIGH AND LEG WITH LITTLE OR NO NEUROLOGIC DEFICIT				
A. Spinal stenosis	XXVII-3	71	Moderate to severe deep aching cramping pain in low back, buttocks, thigh, and leg; brought on by walking a varying distance; not relieved by standing still; relieved with flexing of the lumbar spine by bending over or sitting; increases in severity as pathologic process progresses, becomes more cramping and is then associated with paresthesia and numbness; with severe stenosis pain can be constant and is markedly increased by walking as little as 50 yards, at which point pain becomes intolerable	Incidence usually increases with age with loss of disk height, leading to end folding of the ligamenta flava that encroach on the spinal canal and cause ischemia of the cauda equina; nerve root dysfunction with advanced stenosis demonstrated by somatosensory evoked potential (SEP); radiographic examination reveals extensive changes in disks and facet joints, spondylosis, and characteristic myelographic changes
B. Spondylolisthesis		71	Usually dull aching low back pain; radiation to thigh and leg with severe degrees of disorder; aggravated by activity; relieved by rest	Stiffness in lumbosacral junction; markedly increased lordosis; antalgic gait, tight hamstring muscles; in advanced cases nerve roots at or below level of slip can be irritated and produce radiculopathy
C. Ankylosing spondylitis				
1. Primary	XXVII-12	20, 71	Gradually progressive severe localizing aching pain and stiffness in back; worse on awakening; improved with activity; later, pain radiates to buttocks, back of thigh, knee; onset in second or third decade	Increased erythrocyte sedimentation rate (ESR); positive HLA-B27 in 90%; normocytic anemia; elevated alkaline phosphatase level; radiographic evidence of sacroiliitis
2. Secondary— psoriatic spondylitis, colitic spondylitis		20	Joints of limbs usually involved, but some patients develop sacroiliitis with pain in low back; radiation to lower limbs	Other joints involved; increased ESR; positive HLA-B27 in small percentage

*See Table 2-2.

TABLE 70-3. (Cont.)

Etiology (Disease)	IASP Code Ref.*	Chapter No.	Important Diagnostic Features	
			Characteristics of the Pain	Associated Symptoms and Signs
D. Sacroiliac joint disorders (sprain, infection, arthritis)		72	Pain located in region of sacroiliac joint; radiation to posterior gluteal region, posterior pain of thigh as far as knee, occasional involvement of posterior part of leg; aggravated by flexion and extension, compression test, and maneuver of spreading the iliac crests apart (Fig. 72-24)	Varying degrees of tenderness depending on the disorder; possible swelling; exquisite tenderness to pressure over joint with inflammatory condition; hamstring and low back muscles are usually in spasm, producing stiffness and limitation of motion; patient usually lists to affected side; positive Gaenslen's sign
E. Myofascial pain syndrome with TPs (longissimus thoracis, iliopsoas, obturator internus, gluteus medius, piriformis, gluteus minimus)	XXI-9	72	Moderate to severe pain; located in low back; radiation to posterior, lateral, or anterior aspect of thigh depending on site of TP; deep fingertip palpation on TP brings on pain and aggravates spontaneous pain; also aggravated by stress of muscle; completely relieved by injection of TP	Tenderness and muscle spasm in area of pain reference, with maximum tenderness on TP; autonomic disturbances frequently present
F. Fibromyalgia	I-9	72	Generalized musculoskeletal pain with multiple localized pain (tender spots) in the paraspinal muscles	Local tenderness in various parts of body, including low back, thigh, knee, and leg; disturbed sleep, morning fatigue, stiffness; Raynaud's phenomenon often present
G. Chronic muscle contracture		72	Chronic muscular contracture caused by trauma or prolonged spasm, or by mild radiculopathy consequent to spondylosis (Chapted 90); involvement of lower segments produces pain in low back; radiation to thigh	Increased muscle tone; tenderness over motor points, tender palpable contractures; frequently signs of autonomic disturbance manifested by vasomotor, sudomotor, and somatomotor changes
H. Injury or inflammation of the joints and ligaments of the lumbosacral spine				
1. Acute conditions or chronic degenerative conditions	XXVII	72	Dull aching pain of varying severity; located in low back with reference to thigh, leg, or foot, depending on level of injury; injury of joints and interspinous or ligamentum flava or inflammation of periosteum of upper lumbar level produces back pain and referred pain in anterior thigh; injury at L4–L5 produces pain in lateral aspect of thigh and leg; injury of ligaments in 1st and 2nd sacral segments produces pain in posterior thigh and leg	History of injury to low back or signs of inflammation; palpation produces tenderness and can reveal muscle spasm; no radiographic evidence of bony pathology
2. Facet syndrome		72	Pain in low back; frequent reference to thigh or leg; if one joint involved, pain localized to ipsilateral side of back and gluteal region, with reference to thigh and occasionally leg; with multiple joint involvement pain can be bilateral; usually aggravated by hyperextension of spine; completely relieved by injection of nerve supply to joint or injection into joint with local anesthetic	Palpation of back produces tenderness over affected facet joint; possible swelling, muscle spasm; occasionally deep tendon reflexes are depressed and straight leg raising is limited simulating radiculalgia

*See Table 2-2.

TABLE 70-3. (Cont.)

Etiology (Disease)	IASP Code Ref.*	Chapter No.	Important Diagnostic Features	
			Characteristics of the Pain	Associated Symptoms and Signs
3. Contracture of fascia lata and iliotibial band			Pain in low back and thigh, occasionally extending as far as leg simulating sciatic pain (caused by trauma or inflammation). Radiation to back of thigh and leg, with sciatic radiation; contracted fascia and band cause compression and tension on gluteal and piriformis muscles and occasionally on sciatic nerve	Palpation reveals contracted fascia and compression and tension of gluteal and piriformis muscles; positive Ober's test
4. Aortoiliac obstruction (thrombosis or severe arteriosclerosis)			Increasing pain in gluteal region, thigh, leg during walking; pain is sharp and can become disabling with prolonged exercise of muscles; ceases within a minute or two of cessation of activity	Absent femoral pulses; other signs of arterial insufficiency in lower limbs
5. Epidural abscess			Presence of abscess in the lumbar region produces low back pain; radiation to thigh and even leg	Often history of bacteremia following surgical procedure or infection of the pelvic area; no neurologic deficits initially, but eventually compression of rootlets causes neurologic symptoms and signs and other signs of epidural spinal cord compression
III. BACK PAIN WITH RADIATION TO THE THIGHS, LEGS, AND FEET ASSOCIATED WITH NEUROLOGIC DEFICITS (NEUROPATHIC PAIN)				
A. Diseases of the spinal cord				
1. Intrinsic tumors of lower spinal cord or cauda equina (most common lesion of spinal cord causing back pain)	XXVI-4	73	Constant moderate to severe pain in low back, not affected by position or movement; later, radiculopathy results from stretching and compression of intradural dorsal roots, leading to bilateral segmental pain radiating to gluteal region and lower limbs; aggravated by coughing, sneezing, straining	Sensory deficit, muscular weakness, reflex changes, sphincter and sexual dysfunction; spinal fluid evidence; positive Queckenstedt's sign; myelographic, CT scan, MRI evidence
2. Other less common intrinsic lesions (syringomyelia, myelitis, abscess, cyst, hemorrhage, vascular malformation)				
3. Extramedullary intradural lesions (ependymoma of conus, meningioma, meningeal carcinomatosis, epidural abscess)	XXVI-7	73	Pain in lumbosacral region with abscess pain, usually in midline, with or without radicular pain; carcinomatosis produces severe back and radicular pain, with radiation to gluteal region and lower limbs	Other neurologic signs and symptoms; signs of infection with abscess; muscle weakness; CT scan, MRI, laboratory evidence

*See Table 2-2.

TABLE 70-3. (Cont.)

Etiology (Disease)	IASP Code Ref.*	Chapter No.	Important Diagnostic Features	
			Characteristics of the Pain	Associated Symptoms and Signs
B. Lesions of the spinal nerve roots (radiculopathy)				
1. Protruded or herniated intervertebral disk (most common neurologic disorder causing pain in low back and lower limbs)	XXVI-7	73	Several episodes of low back pain occur before radiculalgia develops; severe sharp, lancinating, intermittent burning pain along distribution of involved segment; S1 most frequently involved, so pain radiates from low back to buttocks, posterior thigh, lateral leg, lateral ankle and foot, and 5th toe with L5 (2nd toe most frequently involved); radiation to low back, posterolateral thigh, dorsal foot, and medial toes (Fig. 70-3 shows distribution)	History of previous episodes of "lame duck" low back pain and tenderness along distribution of sciatic nerve; patient stands with list to normal side; segmental paresthesia, hypalgesia, or anesthesia; positive Lasègue and other straight leg raising signs; decreased or absent deep tendon reflex; muscle weakness
2. Vertebral fracture or dislocation (osteoporosis, neoplasm, trauma) with compression of nerve roots	XXVI-5	73		
3. Other causes of radiculopathy				
a. Osteophyte	XXVII-1	73	Sharp, burning pain in low back with bouts of lancinating pain, especially with tabes dorsalis and postherpetic neuralgia; aggravated by flexion to affected side with osteophytic or arthritic changes	Radiculalgia in distribution of affected segment; frequently, segmental paresthesia, hyperalgesia, anesthesia; reflex changes, muscle weakness, or atrophy, depending on segment involved; herpes associated with eruption; postherpetic neuralgia with scarring of skin
b. Osteoarthritis of spine				
c. Arachnoiditis				
d. Herpes zoster	XXVI-2	73		
e. Postherpetic neuralgia	XXVI-3	73		
f. Tabes dorsalis				
C. Lesions of the lumbar and lumbosacral nerves and plexuses— neuralgia (vertebral fracture or dislocation; pelvic neoplasm— neurofibroma, schwannoma; other pelvic tumors—fibroid cysts, abscess; lumbosacral plexitis—viral inflammation; traumatic stretching or complete avulsion; postradiation plexopathy)			Continuous burning aching pain in gluteal region, with bouts of lancinating pain and radiation to anterior and anterolateral thigh (lumbar plexus), or in low back with radiation to back of thigh, calf, and outer side of sole of foot (lumbosacral plexus); with radiation plexopathy, pain constant and progressive	Skin changes with radiation plexopathy; sensory, motor, reflex changes; limitation of motion of lower extremities; atrophy of affected muscles; CT scan, MRI, EMG evidence

IV. PAIN IN THE HIP

A. Traumatic lesions

1. Fracture in older patients			Sudden severe sharp, aching, burning pain in greater trochanter, groin, buttocks; frequently referred to knee and part of thigh	Inability to bear weight; extreme tenderness to palpation, pressure laterally or posteriorly; can be swelling caused by hemorrhage; radiographic evidence; muscle spasm

*See Table 2-2.

Table 70-3. (Cont.)

Etiology (Disease)	IASP Code Ref.*	Chapter No.	Important Diagnostic Features	
			Characteristics of the Pain	**Associated Symptoms and Signs**
2. Fractures in younger patients (major trauma, stress fracture)			Severe fracture with dislocation produces sudden sharp, severe pain in greater trochanter, groin, buttocks, with some radiation to knee and thigh; with stress fracture pain is mild, aching; aggravated by movement	History of major trauma or unusual stress, such as running; localized tenderness, antalgic gait; radiographic evidence
3. Dislocation of the hip (fall, motor vehicle accident)			Transient mild to moderate or even severe sharp pain at time of injury in groin, posterior gluteal region, or medial upper thigh	History and evidence of trauma; swelling, ecchymosis, muscle spasm; limitation of motion and other physical signs; radiographic evidence
B. Acute arthritides				
1. Acute arthritis (rheumatic fever; infection—staphylococcus, streptococcus, gonococcus and, rarely, mycosis, brucellosis, dysentery)		20, 74	Acute moderate to severe pain in hip joint; aggravated by motion of joint; often referred to knee; symmetric joint involvement, with pain in both joints	Swelling and redness of hip joint; fever, malaise, leukocytosis; other signs and symptoms of acute febrile disease; laboratory evidence (agglutination tests, sedimentation rate, hyperuricemia)
2. Tuberculosis (formerly common, but currently rare)			Moderate to severe continuous pain in hip; aggravated by motion; often worse at night; night cries; usually occurs in children	Tenderness, limitation of motion; history and evidence of disease
3. Infections of hip in infants (hematogenous dissemination to metaphyseal bone within hip capsule)		74	Occurs in young infants; pain usually aggravated by palpation, which can provoke pain reaction	Decreased use of involved extremity; leukocytosis, fever; increased ESR; laboratory evidence of organism
4. Hemarthrosis (hemophilia, other blood dyscrasias)		74	Pain and swelling in joint resulting from hemorrhage following trivial injury	Aspiration of blood
5. Transient synovitis		74	Pain of mild to moderate severity in region of joint; aggravated by motion; affects boys under 10 years of age	Limitation of motion and limp; radiographs are normal; no organisms retrieved
C. Chronic inflammatory arthritides				
1. Rheumatoid arthritis	I-10	20, 74	Mild to moderate continuous aching pain in hip, groin, and buttock; reference to thigh and knee; aggravated by motion; relieved by rest	Limitation of motion; mild to moderate muscle spasm; evidence of other joint involvement; radiographic and laboratory evidence
2. Gouty arthrosis	I-13	20, 74		
3. Psoriatic arthrosis				
4. Degenerative osteoarthritis (primary arthritis)	I-11	20, 74	Usually occurs in those over 60; dull pain, aching in character; gradual onset; poorly localized to groin, buttock, thigh, but almost always to knee; early pain provoked by increased activity, and decreases or disappears with rest; in more advanced cases rest pain, increasing limb pain, and deformity become apparent	Early, narrow joint space; later, total loss of joint space; frequently, cyst formation on femoral head and acetabulum; radiographic evidence
5. Pigmented villonodular synovitis		74	Typical patient 20 to 40 years of age; pain aggravated by movement	Limitation of motion of hip joint; early, radiographs negative; later, cyst formation, synovial tumefactions of lobular outline; aspiration of joint reveals hemosiderin-stained aspirate

*See Table 2-2.

TABLE 70-3. (Cont.)

Etiology (Disease)	IASP Code Ref.*	Chapter No.	Important Diagnostic Features	
			Characteristics of the Pain	Associated Symptoms and Signs
D. Apophyseal disorders				
1. Legg-Calvé-Perthes disease (coxa plana)		74	Affects children from 3 to 11; four phases: early, only limp associated with vague aching pain in groin, medial aspect of thigh, side of knee; aggravated by movement of hip, increased by walking and running; relieved by rest	Motion limited in all directions, especially abduction and internal rotation. Muscle spasm apparent in early phase; radiographic evidence
2. Slipped capital femoral epiphysis		74	Occurs during period of rapid growth, usually in boys; usual complaint is of mild discomfort or weakness of lower limb; referred to knee and, in long-standing cases, in buttock and groin	Limp; decreased range of motion, especially internal rotation, and decreased flexion and abduction; radiographic evidence
E. Extra-articular disorders				
1. Trochanteric bursitis	XXXI-2	74	Mild to moderate discomfort localized over greater trochanter and lateral thigh; aggravated by active abduction of hip	Swelling, erythema, and exquisite tenderness on palpation of bursa
2. Iliopectineal bursitis		74	Pain of mild to moderate severe degree in lateral part of Scarpa's triangle; inflammation can irritate adjacent femoral nerve, producing pain referred to anterior thigh as far as medial aspect of leg; aggravated by tensing iliopsoas muscle and by active flexion of hip	Tenderness on palpation; swelling sufficient to obliterate inguinal groove
3. Ischiogluteal bursitis	XXXI-1	74	Pain in area of ischial tuberosity; aggravated by sitting; relieved by standing	Local tenderness, swelling, heat; irritation of adjacent sciatic nerve can produce symptoms and signs simulating those of sciatica
4. Neoplasm (primary or metastatic)		74	Continuous deep dull aching pain in hip joint; radiation to groin, thigh, and knee; worse in evening or at night	Some large neoplasms can be palpated but radiographic evidence usually necessary, such as CT scan, bone scan
F. Metabolic/endocrine disorders				
1. Paget's disease (not metabolic disorder)		23, 74	Significant pain in hip joint, when affected; pain and discomfort in other areas of body affected by the disease	Radiographic (bone scan) evidence; elevated serum alkaline phosphatase and urinary hydroxyproline levels
2. Osteonecrosis (avascular necrosis of the femoral head)		74	Aching pain in groin or buttock on weight bearing; often referred to knee and occasionally to thigh; some patients have pain at rest	Subtle loss of extremes of motion; internal rotation aggravates pain; MRI helpful (more sensitive imaging)
V. PAIN IN THE THIGH				
A. Musculoskeletal disorders				
1. Traumatic lesions of the femur (fracture of femur, dislocation or fracture of hip or knee joints, posttraumatic subperiosteal hemorrhage)		75	Moderate to severe continuous dull aching pain in thigh; often, radiation to hip and knee; worse at night; with fracture, pain is sudden, severe, usually localized	History and evidence of trauma; ecchymosis, swelling, tenderness, muscle spasm

*See Table 2-2.

TABLE 70-3. (Cont.)

Etiology (Disease)	IASP Code Ref.*	Chapter No.	Important Diagnostic Features	
			Characteristics of the Pain	Associated Symptoms and Signs
2. Infections of the femur (osteomyelitis, tuberculosis, syphilis, mycotic disease, typhoid, others)			Moderate to severe throbbing pain in thigh; often radiation to other parts of extremity; much worse at night	History and other physical signs and symptoms of infection: fever, leukocytosis, other laboratory evidence; radiographic evidence of pathology
3. Neoplastic diseases of the femur (sarcoma, osteoid osteoma, metastatic carcinoma, eosinophilic granuloma, leukemia, myeloma)			Mild to deep dull aching and boring pain in thigh, usually circumscribed; worse at night	Swelling often present; radiographic and laboratory evidence
4. Other diseases of the femur (hemorrhagic diathesis with subperiosteal hemorrhage, osteitis fibrocystica and deformans, Gaucher's disease, scurvy, rickets)			Localized sharp or diffuse dull aching pain in thigh; severe with scurvy or rickets	Other signs and symptoms of disease; laboratory and radiographic evidence
5. Myofascial disorders a. Myofascial syndrome with TPs				
(1) Gluteus medius, gluteus minimus, piriformis, vastus lateralis, biceps femoris		74	Mild aching pain of various severity in posterior thigh; aggravated by palpation of TP	Tenderness, muscle spasm; presence of TPs; history of major trauma or microtrauma and perpetuating factors; increased muscle load; injection of TP with local anesthetic produces complete relief
(2) Gluteus minimus, vastus lateralis, tensor fascia lata		74	Pain in distribution of lateral aspect of thigh	
(3) Adductor longus, rectus femoris, vastus intermedius, vastus medius			Pain primarily in anterior thigh	
b. Postoperative spasm of the quadriceps			Following major hip surgery patient develops unexpected bouts of severe spasm of quadriceps, which produce excruciating pain lasting 2 to 10 minutes or longer; bouts provoked by movement of pelvis or are spontaneous	History of surgery in hip joint, usually arthroplasty
c. Contusion of quadriceps or other muscles		74	Localized dull aching burning pain in site of injury; aggravated by flexion of knee greater than 90°	Tenderness and swelling with palpation; limp; restricted daily activities
d. Rupture of the quadriceps		74	Major impact injury can result in complete rupture producing sudden severe pain that subsides in a few minutes; later, continuous burning aching pain; disabling pain on contraction of muscles	Marked tenderness, muscle spasm; swelling in midline of middle third of thigh consisting of retractable muscle fibers with large ruptures; gap in muscle can be palpated; minor injuries of rectus femoris
6. Other muscle disorders (myositis, tenosynovitis, abscess of thigh, contracted fascia, obturator hernia; fibromyalgia)		74	Mild dull diffuse aching pain in thigh, often spreading to knee; aggravated by motion and pressure; relieved by rest; localized to site of lesion with strain, obturator hernia; pain and multiple tender points with fibromyalgia	Tenderness, muscle spasm, fever (abscess myositis); disturbed sleep; fatigue and stiffness with fibromyalgia

*See Table 2-2.

TABLE 70-3. (Cont.)

Etiology (Disease)	IASP Code Ref.*	Chapter No.	Important Diagnostic Features	
			Characteristics of the Pain	Associated Symptoms and Signs
B. Pain of neuropathic origin (entrapment syndromes)				
1. Meralgia paresthetica—lateral femoral cutaneous neuralgia (entrapment, trauma)	XXX-1	73	Burning tingling pain in anterolateral surface of thigh; aggravated by standing, walking; relieved by recumbency and flexion of hip	Paresthesia; hyperesthesia, hyperalgesia, or hypalgesia and tenderness of nerve at anterior superior iliac spine or along its course
2. Femoral neuralgia (pelvic tumors, inflammation; tumors at inguinal region—hernia, lymphadenopathy, aneurysm, neoplasms, hematoma)	XXX-3	73	Continuous burning or transient sharp lancinating pain in anteromedial part of thigh; aggravated by hyperextension of thigh	Tenderness of nerve trunk; hyperalgesia or hypalgesia and other sensory disturbances; weakness of quadriceps, deficit of patellar reflex
3. Sciatic neuralgia—entrapment by spasm of piriformis; intrapelvic pathology, (tumors along its course—osteoma, neoplasm, aneurysm, abscess)	XXX-4	73	Continuous burning or transient sharp lancinating pain in back of thigh, calf, and outer and plantar side of foot; aggravated by flexion of thigh with knee extended	Tenderness of nerve trunk; sensory, motor, and reflex disturbances; often, positive Lasègue's sign and its modifications; frequently spasm of piriformis muscle
4. Obturator neuralgia—entrapment at obturator membrane; trauma	XXX-2	73	Pain continuous burning or transient sharp lancinating pain in medial aspect of thigh	Weakness of adductor muscles results in wide-based gait with leg in abduction
C. Referred pain from the hips, knees, low back, low abdomen		75	Pain in thigh associated with pain in affected region	Signs and symptoms of specific disease or disorder
VI. PAIN IN THE KNEE				
A. Traumatic lesions				
1. Dislocation or fracture of patella, upper tibia, or lower femur		75	Sudden onset of sharp pain at time of injury localized to knee joint; later, continuous aching pain with frequent spread to hip, thigh, and leg; aggravated by motion	Extreme limitation of motion; tenderness, swelling, ecchymosis of knee; spasm of adjacent muscles; history of trauma; radiographic evidence
2. Ligamentous or capsular injuries (medial, lateral, anterior; mild, moderate, severe)			Mild sprain: mild to moderate pain, aggravated by palpation or stressing of injured ligaments; moderate strain: more severe pain, some instability; severe sprain: moderate to severe sharp pain, markedly aggravated by pressure and movement of ankle	Localized tenderness and swelling but no effusion or locking with mild sprain; with moderate or severe sprain, "locking" of the joint, instability, joint effusion, or hemarthrosis
3. Meniscal injuries		75	Sudden sharp pain in medial or lateral aspect of knee; later, continuous dull aching pain, but compression of menisci reproduces sharp pain	Exquisite tenderness, effusion, "locking" of knee; impaired range of motion

*See Table 2-2.

TABLE 70-3. (Cont.)

Etiology (Disease)	IASP Code Ref.*	Chapter No.	Important Diagnostic Features	
			Characteristics of the Pain	Associated Symptoms and Signs
4. Rupture of the quadriceps muscle (violent muscular action or gross injury)		85	Rectus femoris most frequently involved; sudden severe disabling pain on contraction of muscles, which is sharp, burning, aching; markedly aggravated by extension and flexion of the knee	Deep tenderness; palpable gap at site of rupture; discoloration of skin; swelling from hemorrhage
B. Arthritides				
1. Infection or inflammation (rheumatoid, tuberculosis, rheumatic fever, gonococcal or staphylococcal, gout, others)	I-10	75	Continuous, sharp, throbbing pain in knee; often radiation to thigh, hip, and leg; aggravated by motion; relieved by rest; usually severe in all conditions except tuberculosis and syphilis	Exquisite tenderness, swelling, and redness with acute arthritis; limitation of motion with all; often other joints involved; history and other physical signs of disease; laboratory and radiographic evidence
2. Degenerative osteoarthritis	XXXII-2	75	Early, asymptomatic until synovitis develops, associated with mild pain; later, inflammatory changes; moderate dull aching poorly localized pain around knee	Morning stiffness improves with activity; atrophy and weakness of quadriceps with limitation of motion; crepitus on flexion of knee; later, loss of ligament and muscle support leads to unstable knee and difficulty in walking; radiographic evidence
3. Arthrosis— hemarthrosis (hemophilia, Henoch's purpura, sickle cell anemia), intermittent hydrarthrosis, neuropathic arthropathy			Continuous dull aching or sharp throbbing pain in knee of moderate to severe degree; can radiate to lower thigh or upper leg; aggravated by flexion and extension	Some tenderness; marked swelling with hemarthrosis and hydrarthrosis; fever, leukocytosis or radiographic evidence; aspiration reveals blood or fluid
4. Arthralgia (allergy—serum sickness, general disease, measles)			Acute pain and some swelling of knee and other joints, with little or no tenderness	Other signs and symptoms of allergy or generalized disease; no radiographic evidence
C. Bursitis (prepatellar, infrapatellar, posterior bursa, gastrocnemius, Baker's cyst)			With acute bursitis, moderate to severe aching burning pain in region of affected bursa; with chronic bursitis, pain mild, dull, aching; aggravated by flexion or direct pressure on bursa	Local tenderness, swelling, inflammation
D. Synovitis acute or chronic synovitis, pigmented villonodular synovitis			Continuous aching pain of mild to moderate severity; aggravated by flexion and extension movements of knee joints	Moderate tenderness, effusion; limitation of motion can cause atrophy of quadriceps muscle; with villonodular type, widespread synovial thickening and voluminous swelling
E. Other articular disorders				
1. Osteochondritis dissecans		75	Knee joint most affected; usually occurs in adolescents; moderate to severe pain in knee after exercise; aggravated by movement	Separation of loose bodies leads to recurrent sudden "locking" of joints; intermittent swelling of joint; insecurity; atrophy of quadriceps and impairment of movement
2. Loose bodies		75	Sudden unexpected severe sharp aching pain; relieved by disengagement of loose body	Effusion of joint with frequent recurrence; some atrophy of quadriceps muscle

*See Table 2-2.

TABLE 70-3. (Cont.)

Etiology (Disease)	IASP Code Ref.*	Chapter No.	Important Diagnostic Features	
			Characteristics of the Pain	Associated Symptoms and Signs
3. Spontaneous osteonecrosis (osteochondritis dissecans of the elderly)		75	Sudden onset of intense pain at medial condyle of femur; pain subsequently decreased to moderate degree, but aggravated at limit of forced flexion	Tenderness to deep pressure; synovial effusion
4. Chondromalacia patellae		75	Moderate to severe aching pain in or under patella; aggravated by movement that opposes patella and femur; localized aching after periods of immobility	Stiffness of joint; crepitation and grinding felt on palpation
F. **Tumors of the knee** (benign tumors—osteo-chondromatosis, osteoid osteoma; malignant tumors—osteosarcoma, chondrosarcoma, fibrosarcoma)		75	Continuous or intermittent pain that progresses in severity; with osteoid osteoma, pain intense and worse at night; malignant tumors have pain as most frequent presenting symptom	Swelling, stiffness, and possibly locking of joint with benign tumors; swelling and limitation of movement in knee joint with malignant tumors; radiographic evidence
G. **Myofascial pain syndromes (MPS)**				
1. Trigger point (TP) syndromes of thigh muscles produce referred pain to knee		77	Moderate to severe pain in back of knee produced by MPS of gluteus minimus or biceps femoris; pain in front of knee by MPS of vastus medialis, rectus femoris, or adductor longus	Tenderness and spasm of affected muscles; pressure on TPs aggravates pain, autonomic disturbances. Complete relief with injection of TP with local anesthetic
2. Rupture of tendon of quadriceps		75	Sudden severe sharp pain in knee (see above, rupture of muscle)	Tenderness, limitation of muscle; palpable gap at site of rupture
H. **Other painful disorders of the knee joint**				
1. Painful subpatellar fat pad		75	Pain in knee associated with tender fullness on each side of patellar ligament	Possible history of chronic microtraumata
2. Chronic painful knees			Pain in knee in obese, older patients	Degenerative changes
3. Cysts or swelling of the posterior capsule, aneurysm of the popliteal artery			Pain in popliteal fossa and around the knee	Cystic swelling or pulsating tumor
VII. **PAIN IN THE LEG**				
A. **Traumatic disorders**				
1. Fracture or dislocation of tibia or fibula			Sudden severe sharp pain localized to site of lesion; aggravated by weight bearing or palpation	History of trauma; tenderness, swelling, deformity; radiographic evidence
2. Rupture of gastrocnemius muscle			Sudden severe pain and snapping sensation in calf caused by abnormal or excessive effort with consequent abnormal muscle loading; aggravated by plantar flexion of foot and flexion of knee	Local tenderness in calf; inability to walk without limp or crutches; palpable gap at site of lesion; large hematoma beneath fascia

*See Table 2-2.

TABLE 70-3. (Cont.)

Etiology (Disease)	IASP Code Ref.*	Chapter No.	Important Diagnostic Features	
			Characteristics of the Pain	Associated Symptoms and Signs
3. Rupture of muscle tendons—calcaneal (CR), tibialis anterior (TA), tibialis posterior (TP)			Sudden severe agonizing pain in ankle located in back with CR, anteriorly with TA, and medially with TP; caused by excessive effort (running, jumping); aggravated by plantar flexion (CR), dorsiflexion (TA), or inversion of foot (TP)	Tenderness at site of rupture; effusion, edema; difficulty in walking without limp or crutches; inability to plantar flex with CR; no dorsiflexion with TA; instability with painful flat feet with TP
4. Compartmental syndrome		22, 76	Severe pain in anterior, posterior, or anterolateral aspect of leg; caused by swelling with ischemia of muscle and nerve, usually resulting from excessive running	Some swelling; numbness in distribution of affected nerve; usually no tenderness; dorsalis pedis pulse normal; history of onset of pain after running a certain distance
B. Bone disorders				
1. Infections (osteomyelitis, tuberculosis, typhoid fever, trench fever, mycosis, others)		23, 76	Mild to severe throbbing or boring pain in tibia or fibula; worse at night; aggravated by palpation	Local tenderness, fever, other signs of infection; laboratory and radiographic evidence
2. Neoplasms (benign—osteoma, giant cell; malignant—osteosarcoma, Ewing's sarcoma; metastatic)		23, 76	Dull deep-seated aching boring pain; often worse at night; fracture of bone can produce sudden severe sharp pain; decreases to aching pain over time	Palpation can reveal enlarged mass; possible weight loss and other signs of malignant disease; radiographic evidence
3. Other disorders (epiphysitis; subperiosteal hemorrhage; periostitis— syphilis; metaplasia—bone cysts, osteitis deformans, hypertrophic pulmonary osteoarthropathy, sickle cell anemia)		76	Localized aching or boring pain; often worse at night; aggravated by local pressure; severe with subperiosteal hemorrhage	Slight swelling can be palpable; some tenderness; laboratory and radiographic evidence of disease
C. Other muscle disorders				
1. Myofascial pain syndromes with TPs—gastrocnemius (G), soleus (S), peroneus longus (PL), tibialis anterior (TA)		20, 77	Pain in posterior part of the leg with TPs in G and S, lateral part of leg with PL, anteriorly with TA, varies from slight ache to severe unrelenting disabling pain; aggravated by pressure on TPs; completely relieved by injection of TPs	Tenderness, muscle spasm, autonomic disturbances; impairment of muscle function
2. Intermittent claudication (arteriosclerosis, Buerger's disease)	XV-1	28, 77	Intermittent calf pain on walking or exercise; relieved by rest	See below, section IX, for details
3. Tenosynovitis		22	Moderate to severe pain along tendon; aggravated by muscle function	Exquisite tenderness and swelling, redness along tendon
4. Generalized myalgia (phlebitis, generalized infection, myositis)		23	Continuous generalized pain in leg; aggravated by function of leg muscles; with fibromyalgia, multiple localized pain aggravated by pressure	Tenderness and some swelling in leg; Homans' sign (phlebitis); with fibromyalgia, disturbed sleep, morning fatigue and stiffness, and Raynaud's phenomenon
5. Fibromyalgia		23, 77		

*See Table 2-2.

TABLE 70-3. (Cont.)

Etiology (Disease)	IASP Code Ref.*	Chapter No.	Important Diagnostic Features	
			Characteristics of the Pain	Associated Symptoms and Signs
6. Abscess		23	Severe throbbing localized pain and tenderness in leg	Localized tenderness, swelling, redness, fever
7. Muscle spasm		22, 77	Sudden onset of severe calf pain; caused by trauma or abnormal effort on plantar flexion	Tenderness and palpable spasm of calf muscle
D. Pain of neuropathic origin (entrapment syndromes)				
1. Saphenous neuralgia		73	Burning aching pain in anteromedial part of leg and entire distribution of saphenous nerve	Paresthesia, hyperalgesia, or hypalgesia
2. Peroneal neuralgia (entrapment in neck of fibula)		73	Deep aching burning pain in lateral distal part of knee, anterolateral aspect of leg, and dorsum of foot	Slowly progressive sensory changes in lateral leg and dorsum of foot; weakness of dorsiflexors; EMG evidence
3. Tibial neuralgia (entrapment in calf)		73	Burning aching pain in posterolateral aspect of leg and lateral aspect of foot	Paresthesia, hyperesthesia in distribution of sural nerve; weakness of plantar flexors; twisting or aching in legs with involuntary movements of foot, especially of the toes
4. Other disorders (painful legs and moving toes; causalgia; postamputation pain)			See below, section IXB	
E. Peripheral vascular disease			See below, section IXA	
VIII. PAIN IN THE ANKLE AND FOOT				
A. Pain in the ankle and heel				
1. Traumatic				
a. Fracture, dislocation; ankle sprain		76	Sudden sharp pain localized to ankle—lateral, medial, anteroposterior, depending on site of lesion; aggravated by movement	Exquisite tenderness to palpation, swelling, ecchymosis; inability to bear full weight and ambulate
b. Ankle laxity		76	Follows recurrent ankle sprain with continuous mild aching pain; aggravated by movement	Chronic swelling, and slight tenderness to palpation; weakness of muscles
2. Arthritides	I-10	20, 76		
a. Inflammation (rheumatoid, gout, pyogenic, gonococcal, tuberculous)		76	Moderate to severe localized pain in or about involved joint; possibly aggravated by movement	Tenderness, swelling, and redness; involvement of other joints (rheumatoid); hyperuricemia (gout); fever and laboratory evidence with infection; radiographic evidence
b. Degenerative osteoarthritis	I-11	76	Localized pain; slowly increases over months or years	Limp; joint thickened from bony hypertrophy; limited movements; radiographic evidence
c. Other arthritides (hemophilic, neuropathic)		76	Localized ankle pain; aggravated by movement	Tenderness, swelling; aspiration of blood (hemophilic arthritis)
3. Bursitis: posterior calcaneal or subcalcaneal		76	Acute moderate to severe pain localized in posterior aspect of the heel; aggravated by direct palpation and pressure	Exquisite tenderness, swelling

*See Table 2-2.

TABLE 70-3. (Cont.)

Etiology (Disease)	IASP Code Ref.*	Chapter No.	Important Diagnostic Features	
			Characteristics of the Pain	Associated Symptoms and Signs
4. Dislocation of peroneal tendon		76	Moderate to severe sharp pain in lateral aspect of ankle	Palpation over lateral malleolus reveals tenderness at subluxing tendon; difficulty in walking
5. Osteochondritis dissecans		76	Initial state has mild to moderate ankle pain with "catching" with motion; when bone lesion becomes loose, chronic continuous pain and intermittent "locking"	Early, none; middle stage, small osteochondral defect; late, radiographic evidence of loose body
6. Calcaneal paratendinitis		76	Pain in Achilles tendon; aggravated by running, dancing	Palpation produces tenderness; local thickening; can be swollen, distended; crepitation
B. Pain in the hindfoot				
1. Plantar fasciitis	XXXII-4	76	Pain and tenderness beneath posterior and anterior portion of the heel; radiation into sole of foot	Deep tenderness at anterior medial area of calcaneus
2. Tarsal coalition		76	Moderate to severe pain in hindfoot caused by effusion between bones of hindfoot and midfoot; aggravated by subtalar joint motion and weight bearing; relieved by rest	Deep pressure causes tenderness and crepitation
3. Painful heel pad (heel pad deficiency)		76	Moderate to severe pain over entire calcaneal pad	Palpation produces tenderness and reveals loss of fat and fibrous pad
4. Tarsal tunnel syndrome (plantar nerve entrapment)		76	Paresthetic burning pain in area of medial or lateral plantar nerve or both, depending on site of entrapment; can be relieved on reclining, but aggravated by standing	Tenderness on deep palpation; positive Tinel's sign elicited by palpating nerve posterior to medial malleolus
5. Subtalar arthritis		76	Mild to moderate pain in heel referred from arthritic subtalar joint; aggravated by motion of joint	Pressure over sinus tarsi produces tenderness; crepitation during joint motion; radiographic evidence
C. Pain in the midfoot				
1. Medial arch strain		76	Mild to moderate aching pain felt in foot; caused by prolonged standing on hard surface or unaccustomed prolonged walking	Palpation reveals calcaneus in eversion and pronation; plantar ligament and fascia can be tender
2. Lisfranc's joint instability (injury to metatarsal cuneiform joint)		76	Severe inversion plantar flexion injury causes pain in area of the midfoot; aggravated by palpation	Swelling and tenderness over affected joint
3. Posterior tendon insufficiency		76	Tendon insufficiency produces progressive breakdown in the structure of midfoot, causing dull aching pain; aggravated by pressure, standing, walking	Frequently, tenderness and swelling
4. Ganglion		76	Mucus-filled cyst arising from joint or tendon sheath causes pain because of pressure from shoe; aggravated by palpation, pressure, ambulation	Tenderness on palpation
5. Osteochondritis of navicular bone (Köhler's disease)		76	Condition affects only children 3 to 5 years old; complaint of pain in midtarsal part of the foot	Limp; slight swelling in midtarsal region; tenderness to firm palpation over navicular bone; radiographic evidence

*See Table 2-2.

TABLE 70-3. (Cont.)

Etiology (Disease)	IASP Code Ref.*	Chapter No.	Important Diagnostic Features	
			Characteristics of the Pain	Associated Symptoms and Signs
D. Pain in the forefoot				
1. Stress fracture (march fracture)		76	Unaccustomed prolonged walking, running, or aerobic dancing causes fracture of neck of one or more metatarsal bones, most frequently of the 2nd; initially, dull aching pain in foot during running or dancing, but later pain when walking; aggravated by pressure, weight bearing	Exquisite tenderness on palpation at site of fracture; early radiographs negative but stress fracture appears in 3 to 4 weeks
2. Metatarsalgia		76	Moderate to severe pain in forefoot; most intense in region of heads of 1st and 2nd metatarsals because they bear disproportionate amount of body weight; aggravated by pressure of affected bone, weight bearing, walking	Callus over 2nd and 3rd metatarsals; palpation causes tenderness, which is aggravated when examiner squeezes metatarsal head between thumb and index finger
3. Osteochondritis of a metatarsal head (Freiberg's disease)		76	Usually found in patients 14 to 18 years of age, who experience pain in the affected metatarsophalangeal (MP) joint; aggravated by standing or walking	Thickening of head of metatarsal, which is tender on pressure; restricted and painful movements of MP joint; early radiographs negative, but later reveal increased density
E. Disorders of the great toe				
1. Hallux valgus		76	Pain only when walking with shoes	Obvious deformity; joint is hard, red, and tender; later, limited and painful motion, and osteoarthritis of MP joint produces anterior flatfoot, with further discomfort
2. Hallux rigidus (osteoarthritis of MP joint)		76	Gradual onset of mild to moderate pain that increases with walking, even without shoes; aggravated by dorsiflexion of great toe or by toe push-off	Palpation causes tenderness; restricted dorsiflexion but usually no restriction of plantar flexion
3. Gout	I-13	76	Acute gouty arthritis of 1st MP joint causes severe pain, markedly aggravated by palpation and movement of toe	Swollen, red MP joint; restricted motion; hyperuricemia
4. Sesamoiditis		76	Inflammation of sesamoid metatarsal head complex causes pain; aggravated by dorsiflexion of MP joint	Palpation produces tenderness, swelling; other signs of inflammation
F. Disorders of the small toes				
1. Interdigital neuroma (Morton's metatarsalgia)	XXX-5	76	Neuroma of digital nerve, most frequently between 3rd and 4th metatarsals, causes pain in forefoot; aggravated by standing and walking; sharp, burning, piercing in character, associated with bouts of lancinating pain; frequently radiates to contiguous side of 3rd and 4th toes; pressure aggravates pain and causes bouts of lancinating pain	Forefoot often splayed (anterior flatfoot); palpation reveals thickening of digital nerve
2. Hammer toe, claw toe		76	Hammer toes and claw toes are deformities that cause painful corns and callosities and interfere with their shared weight-bearing function on the metatarsal heads	Deformity obvious; later, intractable keratoses develop
3. Ingrown toenail		76	Exquisite sharp burning pain; aggravated by pressure from shoe	Inspection shows obvious pathology

*See Table 2-2.

Table 70-3. (Cont.)

Etiology (Disease)	IASP Code Ref.*	Chapter No.	Important Diagnostic Features	
			Characteristics of the Pain	Associated Symptoms and Signs
G. Disorders that influence the entire foot				
1. Rheumatoid arthritis	I-10	20, 76	As described above, for one or more joints of foot	Other characteristics of various types of arthritis
2. Osteoarthritis	I-11			
3. Deformities				
a. Pes cavus (hollow foot)		76	Painful callosities beneath metatarsal heads often produced; pain in tarsal region from osteoarthritis of tarsal joint	High arch, clawed toes, prominence of metatarsal heads in sole; tenderness over deformed toes from pressure against shoe
b. Pes planus (flat foot)		76	Condition asymptomatic in children and even in adults; in adults, however, foot strain results, with consequent pain; later, pain can arise from osteoarthritis of tarsal joints	Pathophysiology obvious on inspection
IX. OTHER DISORDERS OF THE LOWER LIMBS				
A. Peripheral vascular disease				
1. Sudden arterial occlusion (embolism, thrombosis, ligation, trauma)		28, 77	Sudden sharp excruciating pain in toes, foot, and leg or thigh, depending on site of occlusion	Numbness, marked coldness, pallor; paresthesia, anesthesia of foot and lower part of leg; pulse distal to occlusion absent; vasomotor and temperature changes
2. Chronic arterial occlusive disease				
a. Arteriosclerosis obliterans	XV-1, 2	28, 77	Intermittent claudication of calf characterized by extreme fatigue, cramping, tightness of muscle that progresses to sharp excruciating pain and occasionally numbness; brought on by walking; relieved within a few minutes by rest; with advanced disease, rest pain in toes and distal foot; burning pain, constant and severe; worse at night, but later pain throughout day; relieved by dependency of limb; aggravated by elevation of limb	Skin cold and white on elevation; red with dependency; trophic changes in toes and foot with ulceration or gangrene; diminished or absent pulse distal to lesion
b. Thromboangiitis obliterans (Buerger's disease)	XIV-2	28, 77	Intermittent claudication varying in intensity from an ache or sense of fatigue to persistent cramp or severe aching squeezing pain; increased during walking, relieved by rest; in advanced cases ischemic rest pain in toes and feet; often severe, burning, unrelenting; aggravated by elevation of limb; relieved by dependency of limb	Usually bilateral involvement, manifested by cold sensitivity (Raynaud's phenomenon); in advanced cases ischemic neuropathy, with pain involving most of limb
3. Diseases of the small arteries and microcirculation				
a. Vasospastic disease				
(1) Cold injuries				
(a) Pernio (chilblain)	XII-4	28, 77	Pain and itching, burning sensation after exposure to cold; aggravated by burning	Skin reddish, cyanotic, edematous; small pigmented or purpuric spot

*See Table 2-2.

TABLE 70-3. (Cont.)

Etiology (Disease)	IASP Code Ref.*	Chapter No.	Important Diagnostic Features	
			Characteristics of the Pain	Associated Symptoms and Signs
(b) Frostbite	XII-3	28, 77	Severe burning pain in digits; the more severe the degree, the more severe the pain	Pallor and numbness followed by cyanosis and redness; hyperhidrosis; sensitivity to cold; chronic stage, hyperesthesia, paresthesia, dysesthesia
(c) Trench foot (immersion foot)		28, 77	In initial vasospastic ischemic phase pain moderate to severe and aching; in intermediate hyperemic phase, intense burning lancinating pain; in late vasospastic ischemic phase, severe deep aching pain	Initial phase: feet and toes pale or cyanotic and cold, decreased arterial pulses, edema; intermediate phase: toes and feet red and hot, bounding pulses, increasing edema, paresthesia; late phase: limb pale, cold, hyperhidrosis, stiffness, sensitivity to cold (Raynaud's phenomenon)
(2) Raynaud's disease, Raynaud's phenomenon	XII-1	28, 77	Attacks of aching, burning pain in digits; occasionally in toes; aggravated by emotional stress, exposure to cold	Triphasic color changes— white to blue to red; numbness and hyperesthesia frequent; in severe advanced cases, ulcers of tips of toes; initially unilateral, later bilateral
(3) Acrocyanosis	XII-5	28, 77	Continuous deep aching pain in toes and foot; markedly aggravated by exposure to cold; worse in winter	Persistent coldness; bluish-purple discoloration of toes and feet; pulses normal; no trophic changes
(4) Livedo reticularis	XII-6	28, 77	Dull deep aching pain; with severe cases, painful ulcers on dorsum of foot	Paresthesia; persistent bluish to bluish-red mottling; reticular (fishnet) skin of both feet and legs, can extend to thigh; when present, ulcers slow to heal; dorsalis pedis, posterior tibial, and popliteal pulses normal
(5) Collagen disease, scleroderma	XIII-1	28	Intermittent ischemic aching pain ranging from mild to severe, then changing to burning dysesthesia with reactive hyperemia	Intermittent vasospasm associated with soreness, stiffness, or swelling of peripheral joints of toes caused by collagen disease of skin; skin cold, pale with reactive hyperemia, increase in temperature, redness
b. Vasodilating disease (erythromelalgia: primary— idiopathic; secondary— complication of polycythemia, arteriosclerosis)	XIV-1	28	Severe burning pain in toes, foot, leg, and as high as thigh; usually bilateral; affects middle-aged men; markedly aggravated by increased temperature to "critical point" (usually 32 to 36°C); relieved by decreasing temperature below critical point; pain greater during summer months	Skin red, its temperature often raised above normal; flushed with venous engorgement; often hyperalgesia and hyperesthesia; trophic changes, alteration of ganglia uncommon in primary disease, but can occur in secondary disease, with arterial occlusion
4. Diseases of veins a. Acute thrombophlebitis		28	Acute moderate to severe pain; calf pain severe; Homan's sign present (calf pain on dorsiflexion of foot); usually unilateral	Exquisite tenderness along region of inflamed vein; perivenous erythema along involved vein; edema involving lower part of limb; dilated superficial vein; decreased ankle pulses; systemic symptoms of fever, tachycardia, general malaise

*See Table 2-2.

TABLE 70-3. (Cont.)

Etiology (Disease)	IASP Code Ref.*	Chapter No.	Important Diagnostic Features	
			Characteristics of the Pain	Associated Symptoms and Signs
b. Acute deep venous thrombosis		28, 77	Moderate to severe pain and tenderness in calf; aggravated by dorsiflexion of foot (Homan's sign) and palpation of calf	Edema, increased tissue turgor; increased skin temperature affecting limb because of diversion of blood to superficial veins, which are dilated; skin cyanotic; fever, tachycardia; condition "clinically silent" in 30 to 50% of patients
c. Postphlebitic syndrome	XIV-3	28, 77	Mild to moderate deep aching pain; always relieved by elevation of limbs	Feeling of heaviness and early fatigability of legs; edema, swelling, hyperpigmentation; secondary varicose veins; cutaneous ulcers
B. Pain of neuropathic origin				
1. Causalgia	I-4	11, 77	Incomplete severance of sciatic or peroneal or tibial nerve, usually caused by high-velocity missile injury; severe, continuous, burning, aching pain; allodynia, hyperpathia; initially in region of hand supplied by injured nerve; later, spread to entire hand and forearm; aggravated by light touch, stress, temperature change, movement of limb, visual and auditory stimuli; relieved by sympathetic interruption	History of nerve injury, vasomotor, sudomotor changes; sensory and motor deficits in affected part of limb; later, trophic changes of skin, nail, hair, and bone; radiographic evidence of bony atrophy
2. Reflex sympathetic dystrophy	I-4	11, 77	Continuous aching burning pain in foot caused by accidental or iatrogenic injury or disease; possible radiation to leg; severity of pain depends on grade and stage of disease	Vasomotor and sudomotor changes; edema; hyperhidrosis; later, trophic changes of skin, soft tissue, and bone
3. Postamputation pain				
a. Phantom limb pain	I-3	12, 77	Pain in foot and usually in leg; can develop promptly after amputation or several days or weeks later; burning, throbbing pain not unlike that of causalgia, described as foot held too close to a fire, or as extremely abnormal position of phantom limb that is very uncomfortable—foot feels painfully twisted, cramped, rigid, or fixed in a posture that patient cannot release; pain and other symptoms aggravated by exposure of stump to cold, changes in weather	Patient can feel pins or needles, warmth or coldness, paresthesia
b. Stump pain	I-4	12, 77	Constant diffuse burning or throbbing pain similar to that of causalgia or paroxysm, lancinating shooting discomfort with a segmental peripheral nerve distribution, or a combination of these; aggravated by palpation of neuroma	Vasomotor and sudomotor disturbances; frequently manifested by coldness, cyanosis, edema, signs of vasoconstriction and hyperhidrosis. Edema may be diffuse or localized
4. Painful legs and moving toes	XXX-7	77	Deep often gnawing, piercing, or aching pain in leg; most intense in lower leg and foot, occasionally in great toe; usually severe, deep, poorly localized; in some patients is more severe in leg than in periphery; can be relieved by activity but aggravated by exercise	Involuntary movements of limb, especially of the toes; movement of the toes can be marked or almost imperceptible; irregular, involuntary, and sometimes writhing movements of the toes, which cannot be imitated voluntarily but can be suppressed for a minute or two by voluntary effort; can be unilateral or bilateral

*See Table 2-2.

TABLE 70-3. (Cont.)

Etiology (Disease)	IASP Code Ref.*	Chapter No.	Important Diagnostic Features	
			Characteristics of the Pain	Associated Symptoms and Signs
C. Pain of cutaneous origin				
1. Traumatic (burns, contusions, lacerations)			Continuous sharp burning pain	History and evidence of trauma
2. Ulcers			Continuous mild pain and itching	Presence of scar or ulcer
3. Scars			Continuous mild to moderate pain; if neuroma present, pain lancinating and sharp	Presence of scar or ulcer

*See Table 2-2.

REFERENCES

1. Bonica, J.J.: The Management of Pain. 1st Ed. Philadelphia, Lea & Febiger, 1953.
2. Cailliet, R.: Low Back Pain Syndromes. 3rd Ed. Philadelphia, F.A. Davis, 1981, pp. 1–53.
3. Gray, H.: Anatomy of the Human Body. 30th Am. Ed. Edited by C.D. Clemente. Philadelphia, Lea & Febiger, 1985, pp. 137–144, 346–350, 464–473.
4. Hollinshead, W.H.: Anatomy for Surgeons. Vol. 3. The Back and Limbs. 3rd Ed. Philadelphia, Harper & Row, 1982, pp. 77–193.
5. Rosse, C., and Clawson, D.K.: The Musculoskeletal System in Health and Disease. Hagerstown, MD, Harper & Row, 1980, pp. 119–160.
6. Ruge, D., and Wiltse, L.L. (eds): Spinal Disorders, Diagnosis and Treatment. Philadelphia, Lea & Febiger, 1977.
7. Pedersen, H.E., Blunck, C.F.J., and Gardner, E.: The anatomy of the lumbosacral posterior rami and meningeal branches of the spinal nerves (sinuvertebral nerves): With an experimental study of their functions. J. Bone Joint Surg. [Am.] 38:377, 1956.
8. Stilwell, D.L., Jr.: The nerve supply of the vertebral column and its associated structures in the monkey. Anat. Rec., 125:139, 1956.
9. Hirsch, C., Inglemark, B.E., and Miller, M.: The anatomical basis for low back pain: Studies on the presence of sensory nerve endings in ligaments, capsular and intervertebral disk structures in the human lumbar spine. Acta Orthop. Scand., 1:33, 1963–1964.
10. Rosse, C.: The vertebral column. In The Musculoskeletal System in Health and Disease. Edited by C. Rosse and D.K. Clawson. Hagerstown, MD, Harper & Row, 1980, pp. 119–145.
11. Lindh, M.: Biomechanics of the lumbar spine. In Basic Biomechanics of the Skeletal System. Edited by V.H. Frankel and M. Nordin. Philadelphia, Lea & Febiger, 1980, pp. 255–290.
12. Nachemson, A.: Electromyographic studies on the vertebral portion of the psoas muscle, with special reference to its stabilizing function of the lumbar spine. Acta. Orthop. Scand., 37:177, 1966.
13. Nachemson, A., and Morris, J.M.: In vivo measurement of intraviscal pressure: Discometry, a method for determina-

tion of pressure in the lower lumbar disks. J. Bone Joint Surg. [Am.] 46:1077, 1964.
14. Nachemson, A., and Elfström, G.: Intravital Dynamic Pressure Measurement in Lumbar Disks: A Study of Common Movements, Maneuvers and Exercises. Stockholm, Almquist & Wikstell, 1970.
15. Nachemson, A.: Towards a better understanding of back pain: A review of the mechanics of the lumbar disk. Rheumatol. Rehabil., 14:129, 1975.
16. Carlsöö, S.: The static muscle load in different work positions: An electromyographic study. Ergonomics, 4:193, 1961.
17. Farfan, H.F.: Muscular mechanism of the lumbar spine in the position of power and efficiency. Orthop. Clin. North Am., 6:135, 1975.
18. Floyd, W.F., and Silver, P.H.F.: The function of the erector spinae muscle in certain movements and postures in man. J. Physiol., 129 184, 1955.
19. Farfan, H.F.: The biomechanical advantage of lordosis and hip extension for upright activity. Spine, 3:336, 1978.
20. White, J.C., Smithwick, R.H., and Simeone, F.A.: The Autonomic Nervous System. 3rd. Ed. New York, Macmillan, 1952.
21. Pick, J.: The Autonomic Nervous System: Morphological, Comparative, Clinical and Surgical Aspects. Philadelphia, J.B. Lippincott, 1970, pp. 351–358.
22. Monroe, P.A.G.: Sympathectomy. London, Oxford University Press, 1959, 290.
23. Kuntz, A.: Autonomic Nervous System. 4th Ed. Philadelphia, Lea & Febiger, 1953, pp. 152–157.
24. Lazorthes, G.: Le système neurovasculaire. Étude Anatomique, Physiologique, Pathologique et Chirurgicale. Paris, Masson, 1949, p. 300.
25. Hovelacque, A.: Anatomie des Nerfs Crainiens et Rachidiens et du Système Grand Sympathique chez l'Homme. Paris, G. Doin & Cie, 1927, p. 873.
26. Wilde, F.R.: The perivascular neural pattern of the femoral region. Br. J. Surg., 39:96, 1951.
27. Mitchell, G.A.G.: Anatomy of the Autonomic Nervous System. London, E. & S. Livingstone, 1953.
28. Ray, B.S.: Sympathectomy of the upper extremity. Evaluation of surgical methods. J. Neurosurg., 10:624, 1953.
29. Mustalish, A.C., and Pick, J.: On the innervation of the blood vessels in the human foot. Anat. Rec., 149:587, 1964.

71 · LOW BACK PAIN

JOHN D. LOESER, STANLEY J. BIGOS, WILBERT E. FORDYCE, *and* ERNEST P. VOLINN

PEOPLE in the industrialized nations are seeking help for low back pains in epidemic proportions and an even larger number say that they suffer from low back pain but do not use health care services or lose time from their jobs. Low back pain is a major expense to society and is the most common disabling problem of those of working age (1–3). Knowledge about the causes of low back pain and effective treatment is rudimentary, but some strategies are available to minimize the risk of disability. Many common treatments advocated for this condition lack evidence of efficacy; in fact, they might even prolong the period of symptoms and disability (4). The importance of the back in human endeavor is not often appreciated, so it is worthwhile to remember Melville:

For I believe that much of a man's character will be found betoken in the backbone. I would rather feel your spine than your skull, whoever you are. A thin joist of a spine never yet upheld a full and noble soul. I rejoice in my spine, as in the firm audacious staff of that flag which I fling half out to the world.

Moby Dick

In this chapter we discuss the epidemiology, etiology, pathophysiology, symptoms and signs, diagnosis, and treatment of low back pain. The material in this chapter is presented in five major sections: A, basic considerations, including classification, patient evaluation, psychosocial factors that influence low back pain, B, mechanisms of low back pain, C, general comments on management of low back pain, D, specific chronic low back pain syndromes, and E, summary of approaches to treatment of low back pain. Other aspects of the low back pain problem are found elsewhere in this book, and many other books and articles address this topic (5–8).

A. BASIC CONSIDERATIONS

Epidemiology

The incidence, prevalence, and costs of low back pain have been the subject of numerous reports, but so has the absence of meaningful data on these topics. Precise figures are certainly not available and the differences among countries and regions of a country are almost certainly significant. Epidemiologic studies of low back pain have several other inherent problems:

a. "Pain" is not a discrete, objective entity that can be measured exactly.

b. The physician only knows that someone has pain if they report it verbally or act in ways that an observer can assess as manifesting pain (see Chapter 16).

c. Almost no studies have been done that validate the accuracy of reports on the presence or absence of pain in survey responses. Eyewitnesses are notoriously unreliable and patients are eyewitnesses; reporting on their own health status, they do not necessarily convey an accurate picture of past events.

d. The phenomena that contribute to pain include a heterogeneous set of events, such as tissue damage, central processing of sensory information, cognitive interpretations of the sensory data, and the responses to these events (either reflexive, verbal, or motor, or a combination of these). Estimates of the presence and degree of pain are indirect and reflect the experiencing of a complex phenomenon by the subject.

e. The methodologies of epidemiologic studies create fragmented pictures of the population; it is difficult to compare studies that use different types of survey strategies.

For example, surveys of the population at large, by telephone or personal interview, produce one set of data. Other studies are undertaken by assessing health care consumption, either by using survey data or by reviewing health care providers' records. Another common methodology involves reviewing the effects of low back pain on the work place, again by survey, by review of employers' records, or by review of insurance or administrative records. Each type of study provides a piece of the overall picture, but it is difficult to integrate the pieces into a meaningful whole. Cost data are notoriously difficult to compare because of inflation, fluctuating currency conversion rates, and changes in the relative costs of health care as new technologies are introduced. Each data collection method is subject to bias or selectivity according to what questions are asked and in what form. Measurement errors, of course, are always present.

In this section we divide epidemiologic data into three generic types: (a) population-based surveys; (b) health care consumption surveys; and (c) industrial low back pain surveys.

Population Surveys

Population-based surveys are often conducted by governmental agencies and have large sample sizes. They usually include few questions related specifically to low back pain and generally fail to differentiate the mere presence of this complaint from health care consumption and disability, issues that are costly both to the respondent and to society. Other population-based surveys are concerned with the residents of a particular region or use some other selection process. Surveys

TABLE 71-1. Self-Reported Low Back Pain*

No. of Those with Pain for 1 or More Days (% of total)	No. of Days in Previous 12 Months with Pain as Reported by Those Who Had any Low Back Pain (%)						
	1–5	6–10	11–30	31–100	101+	None	Not Sure
56	22	7	12	6	9	43	1

Data from Taylor, H., and Curran, N.M.: The Nuprin Pain Report. New York, Louis Harris & Associates, 1985.
*As reported for the 12 months preceding the survey by a total of 1254 respondents. Of all those in the sample, 3% claimed to have had low back pain for more than 31 days in the past year.

can be conducted by mail or telephone, but how the data obtained from such studies relate to formal population-based interview surveys is not known.

Incidence and Prevalence

The Nuprin Pain Report (9), which was conducted by telephone interview, suggested that 56% of American adults had some back pain in the year preceding the survey. The number of days of pain reported is listed in Table 71-1. The vast majority of those with low back pain had used health care services and reported impairment in their daily activities. The incidence of low back pain decreases with advancing age, but the percentage of those with more than 100 days of backache is higher in those over 50 years old.

Holbrook and colleagues (10), in a report summarizing data from the National Center for Health Statistics, indicated that in 1977 8,681,000 Americans had an impairment (defined as a chronic deficit leading to loss of functional abilities) of the back or spine. Of these, 81% had no bed disability days and 7.7% had more than 8 days in bed (Table 71-2). The data do not differentiate cervical and thoracic pain from low back pain and are based on interviews and self-reports; how the data relate to other surveys of the National Center for Health Statistics is unclear.

Another survey in the United States conducted from 1970 to 1977 indicated that 17% of the adult population complained of back pain at any one time. These people claimed to have spent 77,534,000 days in bed annually because of back pain; the average stay in bed was 12 days. Using this rate of 17% and estimating the number of people in the United States over the age of 18 as approximately 178,000,000, it can be extrapolated that 30,000,000 Americans claim some back pain (10).

TABLE 71-2. Impairments Reported in 1977 Health Interview Survey Caused by Back or Spine Conditions

No. Impaired	Bed Disability Days in Past Year (% of number impaired)			
	None	1–7	8–30	More Than 30
8,681,000	81.3	11.0	5.5	2.2

Data from Holbrook, T.L., et al.: The Frequency of Occurrence, Impact and Cost of Selected Musculoskeletal Conditions in the United States. Chicago, American Academy of Orthopedic Surgeons, 1984.

A study of members of a large health maintenance organization estimated that 85% will experience back pain at some time in their lives (11). Another study of men aged 18 to 55 who were patients in a family medicine clinic indicated that 70% had experienced back pain at some time (12). Deyo and Tsui-Wu (13) reviewed data from the National Health and Nutrition Examination Survey (NHANES II) and found that 14% of the respondents over the age of 25 (21 million, extrapolating to the 1986 United States population) had had an episode of back pain that lasted 2 weeks or more. Ten percent (15 million) said they had had back pain for 2 weeks or more some time in the prior year. At any specific time, 6.8% of the respondents claimed to have low back pain. Approximately one-third of the respondents reported that their pain lasted less than 1 month, one-third said 1 to 6 months, and one-third said longer than 6 months (13). Another report indicated that 18% of those in the sample (approximately 32 million adults, extrapolating to the 1986 United States population) reported that they were "often bothered" by back pain (14).

Several reports from Sweden contain data on the incidence and prevalence of low back pain. In the 1950s Hult (15) found that over 80% of Swedish industrial and forest workers had a history of low back pain and that over 50% of these workers had incapacitating low back or leg pain at some time. Another study by the same author found that men aged 25 to 69 reported a 60% cumulative incidence of low back pain and that 16% had been incapacitated for 3 weeks to 6 months (16). A more recent report indicated that Swedish men aged 40 to 47 had a cumulative incidence of back pain of 61% (3). About 4% of respondents claimed to be unable to work at the time of the survey.

Wood and Badley (17) have reviewed epidemiologic data from Great Britain and have also noted the difficulties with epidemiologic studies of back pain. Of those surveyed 21% claimed to have low back pain in the 2 weeks prior to interview, and 4.3% had consulted a general practitioner for low back pain in the preceding year. It was found that both the incidence of low back pain and the number of days lost from work had increased significantly between 1961 and 1972 (17).

Data are available from a few other countries. The incidence of back pain in Denmark appeared to be similar to that of Sweden in one study, but the incidence in men in Copenhagen seemed to be 50% of that reported in the United States and Sweden in another (18, 19). The lowest reported rate appeared to be in Israel, where Magora (20) reported a lifetime incidence of 13%. Different questions and survey techniques might be responsible for these discrepancies.

Conflicting data have been obtained from population surveys in third-world countries. One study claimed that low back pain was rare in rural India, whereas another found that it was common in Jamaica (21, 22). The disability caused by low back pain in Jamaica was less than that found in the United Kingdom.

Disability

The amount of disability caused by reported back pain is difficult to determine because most epidemiologic studies have not discriminated between short-term and long-term disability and have relied almost exclusively on self-report. The United States Census Bureau estimated that in 1984 to 1985 1.8 million Americans could not work at any one time because of back pain (23).

The Nuprin Pain Report (9) suggested that 14% (25 million) of American adults could not work 1 or more days annually because of back pain. In 1985, 1,308 million workdays were lost because of back pain in the adult United States population of 174 million. Adults employed full time lost 89 million workdays.

Long-term disability caused by back pain appears to be increasing sharply in the United States. The National Center for Health Statistics estimated a 163% increase between 1970 and 1981 (24) (Table 71-3). Back pain is the leading cause of disability for both men and women under the age of 45. Similar increases in disability caused by low back pain have been reported in the United Kingdom and Sweden; in Sweden it now accounts for 25% of all disability pensions (17, 25, 26).

Health Care Consumption Surveys

Even though most treatments for low back pain have little or no demonstrated efficacy, back pain is the second most common symptomatic reason for visiting a physician in the United States and accounted for 32 million visits in 1979, 3% of all physician visits (27). Annual hospital discharges for back pain from 1972 to 1978 were about 6.7 million (10). The advent of the DRG (diagnosis-related groups) system in the

TABLE 71-4. Incidence and Health Care Consumption of Low Back Pain*

Parameter	Percentage (of total)	No. (approx.)
Population of United States	100	225,000,000
Had any episode of low back pain lasting more than 2 weeks	13.8	31,050,000
Sought health care	84.6	26,268,300
Admitted to hospital	30.9	9,594,450
Underwent back surgery	11.6	3,601,800

From Deyo, R.A., and Tsui-Wu, Y.-J.: Descriptive epidemiology of low back pain and its related medical care in the United States. Spine, 12:264, 1987.
*NHANES II, 1976–1980.

United States led to the realization that "medical back problem" is the leading symptomatic cause of hospital admission and accounts for 2.8% of all hospital discharges (28).

Deyo and Hsui-Wu reported that 85% of Americans who had had back pain for 2 weeks had consulted a health care provider (13). Of those in this group, 31% had been hospitalized and 11.6% had undergone a surgical procedure (Table 71-4). These data are now over 10 years old and both the incidence of back pain and the number of operations performed have increased significantly, so these percentages and the absolute numbers are considerably below present levels.

Some estimates of the costs of health care for back pain in the United States are available. The three types of cost generally considered are wage replacement, wages lost, and health care costs. It is difficult to compare studies on these topics, but estimates by Bonica (29) for 1979 suggested that back pain cost a total of 17 billion dollars in the United States, including costs for health care, loss of work, compensation, litigation, and quack therapies. Holbrook and associates (10) estimated the cost for 1984 to be 16 billion dollars, of which 13 billion dollars were for direct health care costs and 3 billion were for loss of earnings. They did not consider the costs of compensation and litigation. In Chapter 8 Bonica estimated the cost of back pain in 1986 to be 20 billion dollars, of which 7 billion dollars were for litigation, compensation, and loss of earnings (Table 8-1). The effects of time lost on manufacturing productivity and of lost wages on tax

TABLE 71-3. Self-Reported Chronic Back Pain for 1969–1970 and 1981*

Year	Population Age 18 and Over (in millions)	All Ages No. with Total Disability	All Ages No. with Partial Disability
1969–1970	133.6	237,102	1,375,937
1981	162.8	618,562	2,536,346

From National Center for Health Statistics: National Health Interview Study. Unpublished data, 1983.
*Because disability is not reported as a function of age, we have assumed that a negligible number are disabled under the age of 18.

contributions could also be considered but data are not available.

The rate of surgery for low back pain is clearly higher in the United States than in any other country (W.J. Kane, unpublished data, 1985). This appears to be increasing in spite of widespread concern that too much back surgery is being performed (E. Volinn et al., unpublished data, 1988). A survey of American men indicated that 3.4% had undergone surgery for low back pain, compared to only 0.8% of Swedish men (3, 12).

Industrial Low Back Pain Surveys

Many studies of low back pain and its effects on workers have been carried out. The feature that distinguishes low back pain from other pain complaints and from most other health issues is the number of days of disability it causes in those of working age. Data from Sweden indicate that between 50 and 80% of the working population have suffered from low back pain (30). Other studies indicate that 10 to 20% of all sickness absence days can be ascribed to low back pain (26), representing 1% of all workdays lost yearly. Similar findings have been reported in the United States (1). During a 10-year study at an industrial plant in New York, Rowe (31) found that low back pain was second only to upper respiratory tract illness as a cause of time lost from the job, with 4 hours lost per worker annually because of low back symptoms. Over one-third of employees had used company health care facilities because of back pain during this 10-year period.

In Great Britain in the mid-1970s 750,000 episodes of disability were reported annually and 19,200,000 workdays were lost because of low back pain in a population of approximately 40,000,000 (17). Almost 1.8% of all workers lost time from work each year because of low back pain. Furthermore, 10,000 were off work for 6 months or more and 4,500 were disabled for over 2 years at any given time because of low back problems.

A well-done study in Quebec indicated that 14% of disability claims in 1981 were for spinal disorders and 70% of these claims were for low back pain (Table 71-5) (4). Low back disorders represented 10% of total claims. Although 74% of workers were absent for less than 1 month, 4.3% were absent for 1 year or more. Claims for disability related to spinal disorders were filed by 1.69% of all workers. The cost of claims for spinal disorders was 150 million dollars (Canadian) in 1981. The incidence of claims peaked at ages 20 to 24 for both men and women and declined steadily with age to 25% of the peak incidence by ages 55 to 64 (4). The presentation of data in the Quebec study, however, did not indicate allocation of costs and incidence of claims to that portion of the claimants who had low back pain. Somewhat different incidence data have been reported in other studies.

From the time of the pioneering studies of Hult in 1954, it has been recognized that both back pain symptoms and claims for disability have some relation to the proportion of workers involved in heavy physical labor (15, 16). Static work postures, frequent bending and twisting, lifting, forceful movements, repetitive work, and vibrations are some documented contributing factors to low back pain but not necessarily to claims for disability (26). The literature on individual risk factors is contradictory. Age certainly influences the incidence of claims for low back pain; young and elderly workers have fewer claims for disability. Symptoms of low back pain among workers are equally common in men and women. The incidence of low back pain symptoms (not claims) for Denmark, England, and Sweden appears to be about 25% annually (32).

In England, Benn and Wood reported that 3.6% of all sickness absence days in 1969 to 1970 were ascribed to low back pain (33), which represented more days lost than those caused by strikes. Another study contrasted mine workers with office workers: the incidence and prevalence of low back pain were found to be slightly higher for miners (34). No history of low back pain was reported by 31% of miners and 42% of office workers. Interestingly, 43% of the miners but only 27% of the office workers with back pain consulted a physician for relief of their symptoms, indicating that pain and what individuals choose to do about their symptoms are not directly related.

A study from Israel found that 12.9% of workers in eight occupations from clerks to heavy industry workers had low back pain in a 1-year period (35). Low back pain was much more common in workers who were not satisfied with their present occupation or social status, who were tense and fatigued after work, or who were stressed by too much responsibility or mental concentration. A Finnish study indicated that back pain occurred in 37% of heavy laborers and 27% of house painters in the year preceding the study; their

TABLE 71-5. Frequency of Compensated Claims in Quebec (1981)

Parameter	No. Not Absent from Work (medical care only)	No. Absent From Work*	Total
Employed population			2,719,575
Number of compensated claims			320,157
Spinal disorder claims	8,670 (18.9%)	37,188 (81.1%)	45,858
Incidence (%)	0.32	1.37	1.69
Low back claims			32,101

Data from Spitzer, W.O.: Scientific approach to the assessment and management of activity-related spinal disorders. Spine, 12(Suppl. 1):1, 1987.
*Absent from work at least 1 day.

lifetime incidences of back pain were 51% and 39%, respectively (36). Physical, emotional, and environmental factors seem to contribute to the incidence and prevalence of low back pain.

Many studies have been undertaken in the United States concerning the problem of industrial low back pain (30). The overall incidence of claims for low back pain disability has been estimated to be between 1 and 2% of those in the work force covered by industrial health insurance (37). Risk factors similar to those mentioned above have been elucidated for many of these claims, but others have demonstrated the profound effects of social factors not often considered contributory to the incidence of low back pain or to claims for disability. For example, the study by Volinn and co-workers (38) noted that in the state of Washington approximately one-third of the county-by-county variance in claims for disability resulting from low back pain could be ascribed to socioeconomic factors such as the unemployment rate, the percentage receiving food stamps, and per capita income. This study was controlled for the size of the labor force and for the proportion of workers in occupations at high risk for low back pain.

Spengler and colleagues reviewed claims for work-related injuries at the Boeing Airplane Company in Seattle over a 15-month period (39). Approximately 31,000 employees filed 4,645 claims, of which 900 were for low back injuries (Table 71-6). The mean cost per claim for a back injury was $2,054, whereas the cost for other injuries was $712 per claim. The low back claims, which were 19% of the total claims, were responsible for 41% of the total costs. Claims of more than $10,000 were four times as common for low back injuries. A small number of high-cost claims were responsible for 84% of the total costs of all claims. This study confirmed several prior observations that low back injuries and claims for disability were common in industry and that they were disproportionately expensive in regard to both health care and wage replacement. Leavitt and associates had long before demonstrated that 25% of the claims for low back pain were responsible for 75% of the total costs (40); the Quebec study demonstrated a similar trend (4).

Another survey (41), reported by a major insurance company, found that back injuries were responsible for 20% of occupational injuries; this type of injury, however, was responsible for 33% of the costs. Extrapolating from the insurance company data, $8.7 million was spent each working day in 1980 for low back pain—an annual total of $2.17 billion. Bauer (30) reported that 1 to 2% of workers have a job-related low back injury each year, accounting for 40% of all workdays lost. He also estimated that the incidence and costs of claims were increasing rapidly and by 1983 had reached $56 billion. This figure is now almost certainly too low, because the costs of health care have escalated rapidly.

A review of several other studies indicates that the costs of a claim are directly related to the duration of disability (4, 30). This should not be surprising, because the likelihood of ever returning to work decreases in proportion to the duration of disability. D. Johnson (unpublished data, 1978) reported that the 16% of workers in Washington who had time loss of more than 181 days per year for low back pain received 85% of the compensation dollars.

The costs of low back pain in the United States have been the subject of several review articles (37, 42), with the following estimates made: in 1976, $14 billion (37); in 1983, $25 billion (37); in 1984, $16 billion (30); and in 1985, $25 to 56 billion (42). All these estimates are suspiciously low; health care and wage replacement rates continue to escalate yearly, and none of them included the costs of federal disability payments made through SSDI. Approximately 2% of those in the work force have suffered a compensable low back injury (400,000 claims) (37); the total cost of compensation payments was at least $5 billion (42). Those working in heavy industry are responsible for more claims than office workers. Methodologic differences make comparisons between studies hazardous.

In conclusion, low back pain and claims for disability caused by low back pain are common in the working population. A small fraction of injured workers with low back pain receive an inordinate amount of the health care and wage replacement dollars (Table 71-7) (Volinn and Loeser, unpublished data, 1988). An excellent survey of available epidemiologic data has been published by the Institute of Medicine (43). Only a few of the relevant variables have been quantified, but clearly factors other than those related to the physical environment and work effort play a major role. Low back pain occurs in most adults; whether it becomes a health care and social policy issue is a function of the actions they take in response to their symptoms.

Classification

Until recently the terminology of the various conditions that can lead to low back pain has exhibited a notable lack of uniformity. In 1953 Bonica (44) presented a classification of low back pain based on standard orthopedic taxonomy. Unfortunately, practitioners and researchers continued to use different terms to describe the same condition and, even worse, the same terms to describe different conditions. In 1982 Nachemson and Anderson (45) proposed a classification of low back pain based mainly on clinical

TABLE 71-6. Disability Claims at Boeing Aircraft, Seattle

Parameter	Back	Nonback	Total
Number of claims	900	3,745	4,645
Percentage of claims	19	81	100
Total costs ($)	1,848,670	2,665,332	
Mean cost/claim ($)	2,054	712	972
Percentage of costs for all claims	41	59	100
Number of claims with costs > $2,054	124		
Percentage of claims with costs > $2,054	14		
Percentage of costs for claims > $2,054	84		

From Spengler, D.M., et al.: Back injuries in industry: A retrospective study. Spine, 11:241, 1986.

TABLE 71-7. Claims for Industrial Back Injury: Disproportionate Costs of a Minority of Claimants

Source	Year of Report	Claimants (% of total)	Costs (% of total)
Leavitt et al. (40)	1972	25.0	87
Johnson*	1978	4.5	36.5
Snook (42)	1982	25.0	90.0
Spengler et al. (39)	1986	10.0	79.0
Spitzer et al. (4)	1987	7.4	86.0
Volinn and Loeser†	1988	13	88

*Unpublished data, 1978.
†Unpublished data, 1988.

findings, which has proven useful for epidemiologic studies. More recently the International Association for the Study of Pain (IASP) developed a taxonomy to describe various painful disorders (Chapter 2), but the section on low back pain of this taxonomy requires extensive revision to be clinically useful. The following classifications, developed by Bonica (personal communication), are based on these important works. Table 71-8 lists several general classifications for low back pain, and Table 71-9 presents a more detailed classification based on the system involved and on the disorder that is believed to be the cause of the low back pain.

A wide array of health care providers treat back symptoms. The pain is usually ascribed to structures that fall into the domain of the musculoskeletal specialist to treat, yet primary care practitioners must initiate effective therapy during the acute phase of the illness. The natural history of back pain is such that patients who do not get over their symptoms in 4 to 6 weeks need referral to a specialist to rule out uncommon but treatable medical conditions and to ascertain whether environmental or psychologic factors are delaying recovery. A dramatic change in the health care offered to low back pain patients is required because

TABLE 71-8. General Classification of Low Back Pain (LBP)

I. ACCORDING TO SYSTEM INVOLVED AND ETIOLOGY

A. Musculoskeletal
B. Neurologic
C. Visceral or vascular
D. Psychologic
E. Idiopathic

Degenerative
Inflammatory
Metabolic
Neoplastic
Traumatic
Congenital
Infectious

II. ACCORDING TO DURATION AND INTENSITY

A. Acute: 0–3 months
B. Chronic: more than 3 months
  1. Early phase—3 to 6 months
  2. Intermediate phase—6 to 24 months
  3. Late phase—more than 2 years

Mild
Moderate
Severe
Excruciating

III. ACCORDING TO SYMPTOMS AND SIGNS AND CLINICAL AND RADIOLOGIC FINDINGS

A. Low back pain
B. Radiculopathy
C. Sciatica
D. Low back pain and radiculopathy or sciatica

most standard treatments that are currently available have no proven efficacy, are expensive, and can even delay recovery (4, 46). The task is made even more difficult by the fact that an accurate diagnosis can only be established in a small fraction of patients with acute low back pain. Patients with chronic low back pain often have the additional problem of ineffective treatment superimposed on their initiating symptoms, and accurate diagnosis is then often impossible.

Patient Evaluation

History

Obtaining the patient's history is the most important element of the evaluation of low back pain. It not only offers guidance for the subsequent physical examination and provides diagnostic suggestions but it also begins the communication process between the patient and physician. Important insights into the patient's expectations can also be obtained from the history, and these can be major determinants of treatment outcome. Decisions about diagnostic testing and management also can be made on the basis of the history and physical examination.

Interview technique is important. Patients must be allowed to present their own chronology and present status. Prior diagnostic studies and treatments must be carefully elucidated. Questions should be specific but not directive, or the examiner might actually be testing patients' willingness to please the physician rather than determining an accurate description of symptoms.

Written questionnaires filled out prior to the physician interview can be timesaving and lead to increased accuracy. Topics covered should include past medical history, family history, review of organ systems, and socioeconomic and employment data. If a questionnaire is used it should be reviewed with the patient at the time of the initial interview. A diary of pain levels, physical activities, and medication consumption for the 2 weeks prior to the interview is helpful, particularly with chronic pain patients.

History of the Pain

It is important to ascertain the history of the onset of the patient's pain, its course since that time, and factors that aggravate and relieve the pain. The precise location of the pain and its patterns of radiation are important diagnostic clues. Because low back pain

TABLE 71-9. Classification of Low Back Pain According to System Involved, Etiology, and IASP Code

I. MUSCULOSKELETAL ORIGIN

A. Spondylogenic (vertebral column)
1. Degenerative
   a. Osteoarthritis
   b. Spinal stenosis (XXVII-3)
   c. Spondylolisthesis
   d. Lumbar spondylosis (XXVII-2)
   e. Degenerative disk disease
   f. Degenerative joint disease
   g. Facet joint disease (facet tropism) (XXVII-3)
2. Inflammatory
   a. Rheumatoid arthritis
   b. Juvenile rheumatoid arthritis
   c. Ankylosing spondylitis (XXVII-2)
   d. Reiter's syndrome
   e. Psoriatic arthritis (sacroiliitis)
   f. Seronegative spondyloarthropathy
3. Metabolic
   a. Osteoporosis
   b. Osteopenia
   c. Osteomalacia
   d. Osteitis fibrocystica
   e. Ochronotic spondylosis
   f. Juvenile osteochondrosis
4. Neoplastic
   a. Benign
   b. Malignant
   c. Metastatic
5. Infectious
   a. Bacterial
   b. Tuberculosis (Pott's disease)
   c. Septic arthritis
   d. Other infections
6. Traumatic (XXVII-8)
   a. Fractures
   b. Dislocation or subluxation
   c. Lumbosacral joint sprain
   d. Sacroiliac joint sprain
   e. Apophyseal (facet) joint disorder
   f. Intervertebral disk
   g. Coccygodynia
7. Congenital
   a. Scoliosis
   b. Spondylolisthesis
   c. Vertebral epiphysitis
   d. Interspinous pseudarthrosis
8. Muscular disorders
   a. Acute strain (XXVII-6)
   b. Chronic strain (XXVII-7)
   c. Acute reflex muscle spasm
   d. Acute muscle fatigue
   e. Myofascial pain syndrome with trigger points (XXVII-13, XXVII-14)
   f. Disuse muscle atrophy

II. PRIMARY NEUROLOGIC ORIGIN

A. Radiculopathy or neuropathy
1. Herniated intervertebral disk (XXVI-1)
2. Osteophyte (XXVII-1)
3. Tumor (benign or metastatic) (XXVI-8)
4. Epidural abscess (XXVI-7)
5. Fracture or dislocation of lumbar vertebra (XXVI-5)

B. Inflammation of the nerve roots or formed nerves
1. Herpes zoster (XXVI-2)
2. Other radiculitis
3. Neuritis

C. Fibrosis of the nerve roots or formed nerves
1. Arachnoiditis
2. Epineural fibrosis (root sleeve fibrosis)
3. Intraneural fibrosis

D. Diseases or disorders of the neuraxis
1. Intradural and epidural tumors (XXVI-4)
2. Meningeal carcinomatosis (XXVI-II)
3. Tumor infiltration of lumbar plexus (XXVI-12)
4. Diseases or disorders of the neuraxis

III. REFERRED LBP CAUSED BY INTRA-ABDOMINAL DISEASES OR DISORDERS

A. Visceral diseases or disorders
1. Kidney or ureter
2. Uterus and adnexa
3. Urinary bladder and prostate
4. Descending and rectosigmoid colon (XXVIII-1)

B. Vascular diseases
1. Aneurysm of lower abdominal aorta
2. Obstruction of abdominal aorta or common iliac arteries
3. Embolism of renal artery

C. Retroperitoneal masses
1. Lymphosarcoma
2. Hodgkin's disease
3. Carcinomatous lymphadenopathy

IV. PAIN PRIMARILY CAUSED BY PSYCHOLOGIC OR ENVIRONMENTAL FACTORS (XXIX)

V. IDIOPATHIC BACK PAIN

---

can be a symptom of disease of other organ systems, a complete medical history is essential. Psychosocial and environmental factors must be considered, and it is also helpful to know whether others in the patient's family have had significant pain complaints and use of health care services.

Herniated Lumbar Disk

Characteristic findings in the history of the patient with a herniated lumbar disk have long been recognized. Pain is increased by sitting and relieved by lying, walking, or standing. Intermittent low back pain usually precedes the initial episode of pain that radiates into the lower extremity. The pain is increased by sneezing, coughing, or straining during defecation. Using the back for lifting or twisting usually increases the pain. Numbness and tingling into the leg are commonly reported if there is significant nerve root compression. Paresthesias are the best localizers of the level of nerve root involvement, and the patient should always be questioned carefully about their existence (Chapter 73).

Spinal Stenosis

A patient with significant spinal stenosis usually reports the gradual onset of low back pain, with lower extremity radiation. The pain is relieved by flexion and increased by extension of the spine. The pain is brought on by walking, but riding a bicycle in the flexed position is not painful. Unlike the typically younger patient with a herniated disk, the older patient with stenosis is relieved by the sitting position.

Spinal Instability

No typical history of pain is associated with spinal instability. A history of significant trauma, infection, neoplasm, congenital malformation, or surgery can be a clue to this diagnosis. The pain can increase with physical activity or specific positions.

Other Anatomic Factors

The medical history helps to determine additional questions that must be asked in regard to diseases that can include low back pain and their symptoms. Constant back pain that is unrelated to position, activity, or time of day is often a clue to the systemic illness affecting the spine; screening questionnaires are helpful in this regard. The general medical and family history must also be reviewed (see Chapter 31, which discusses the general aspects of historic information).

Psychosocial History

The psychosocial history in the evaluation of the patient with low back pain is of utmost importance. Initial observations include the patient's responses to the general medical questions, the way interactions with former health care providers are related, how prior diagnoses and treatments are described, and the consistency of the story. It is important to ascertain the patient's goals and expectations and whether the patient feels any responsibility for present problems.

The extent to which the problem intrudes on the patient's daily living activities must be ascertained. How have interactions with family and employment been affected? Does the patient believe that someone else is responsible for the condition? A good way to begin the interview is to ask "What can I do for you today?" The prudent physician is put on guard by such responses as "Cure me," "Do something for me," "My attorney sent me," "I'm fed up with my prior doctors," and "I've heard that you are the best doctor in town." The patient who manifests indications of responsibility for the condition is much more likely to have a favorable outcome, regardless of the eventual diagnosis of the cause of the low back pain.

Physical Examination

A thorough examination of the back is essential and should be done in a standardized fashion to ensure that it is complete. General health problems that can lead to low back pain must be assessed in both the history and the physical examination. Even though a poor correlation between physical findings, symptoms, and outcome of treatment might be found, it is essential that as much information as possible be collected so that the best management decisions can be made.

Inspection

The prudent examiner pays attention to patients from the moment they enter the office, noting how they walk, sit down, undress, and dress. Examination of the back must be undertaken with patients clad only in their undergarments. Herpes zoster often presents with pain that precedes the vesicular eruptions; if a segmental low back pain presents suddenly, patients should be carefully inspected over several days to see if the pathognomonic rash occurs.

The patient should be observed both from the side and back, noting any deviation of the spinous processes, scoliosis, height of the iliac crests, and motion when the patient is asked to flex and extend the spine. Schober's method of measuring the flexibility of the lumbar spine involves marking the S1 spinous process and marking a point 5 cm higher with the patient erect, and then measuring the distance with the spine flexed. This can document the motion of the lumbar spine (47). The range of flexibility in normal individuals is great.

Palpation

The spine and its surrounding muscles should be palpated to ascertain any focal tenderness or abnormal mass. Because low back pain can also result from sacroiliac joint disease, palpation to determine local tenderness over the joint can be helpful. In addition, the three maneuvers described by Newton can be used (48). The first is performed with the patient lying on the side and pressure is applied to the upper iliac wing. The second is performed with the patient supine, and pressure is applied to both anterior superior iliac spines in an attempt to spread them apart. The third is performed with the patient prone, and pressure is applied to the sacrum. The movements provoked by these tests can also stress the lumbar spine, so the findings must be integrated with all the other diagnostic information; none of these tests is pathognomonic for sacroiliac disease.

Some patients present with a pain complaint that sounds like sciatica but the disease is in the hip and not in the back. The greater trochanteric bursa should be palpated and the range of motion of this joint ascertained. The examination and diagnosis of hip pain are discussed in Chapters 70 and 74.

Testing Muscle Function

It is usually easiest to begin by evaluating the gait and then asking the patient to stand on each leg. Quadriceps function is observed by asking the patient to squat and then stand. Heel and toe walking tests leg muscle strength, sit-ups test abdominal muscle strength, and arching the back in the prone position tests back muscles. Range of motion at each joint should be assessed at this time.

Instability of a spinal motion segment can be detected by the presence of spinous process tenderness during flexion or by observation of cogwheel movements of the back. Local spinous process tenderness can also be a clue to the site of pathology.

Manual testing of individual muscle strength is undertaken with the patient either sitting or supine. The bulk of thigh and leg muscles is measured by marking a point 20 cm above the knee and 15 cm below the knee and determining the circumferences at these levels. A difference of more than 1 cm between the two sides is probably significant. Limb length can also be measured.

Tests of muscle strength rely on the patient's cooperation and motivation; they are all subjective to some degree even if expensive mechanical devices are used. Giveaway weakness usually indicates lack of effort by the patient. Any discrepancies between the results of manual muscle testing and spontaneous gait should be noted.

Neurologic Examination

Detailed information about the neurologic examination is found in Chapters 31 and 70. Essential points for the assessment of low back pain include determining the responses to light touch and pinprick from the umbilicus distally, including the genital and perianal areas, and observing the superficial abdominal reflexes, tendon reflexes at the knee and ankle, and presence of pathologic reflexes (Babinski's sign, or equivalents).

Mechanical back sign tests help to detect irritation of the roots that form the lumbosacral plexus. All are based on the fact that the normal lumbar and sciatic roots move several centimeters when the extended leg is moved from the neutral position to full flexion. Any mechanical obstruction to this movement produces pain. A herniated disk is the most likely cause, but tumors and infection can also lead to positive findings. The most common method of evaluating normal movements of the nerve roots is the straight leg raising test.

Straight leg raising is performed initially with the patient supine; the body is flat on the bed and both legs are fully extended. The patient is instructed to relax, and the examiner lifts the leg from the bed with the knee fully extended and the ankle in the neutral position (Fig. 71-1). When the patient complains of pain, the degree of angulation of the leg is noted, preferably with a hydrogoniometer. It is essential to record the site of the pain. Test results are confirmed by plantar flexion and then dorsiflexion of the ankle; only dorsiflexion should increase the pain. These findings are also confirmed by repeating the test at a later time with the patient seated on the edge of the bed or examining table. The correlation between the degree of straight leg raising in the supine and seated positions is a feature of Waddell's signs (see below, Nonorganic Signs).

The results of straight leg raising tests can be interpreted as follows: (a) pain at less than 30° suggests anticipation of pain or major psychosocial issues, although on rare occasions a large herniated disk is present; (b) pain between 30 and 70° usually indicates root compression; and (c) pain at greater than 90° can be caused by lumbar motion. Pain in the leg opposite to the one being elevated is even more reliable than ipsilateral straight leg raising as a sign of nerve root compression. False-positive test results are well documented; management decisions should not be made on the basis of the results of straight leg raising alone without considering all other information available about the patient.

Visceral and Vascular Examination

Palpation of the abdomen and a rectal examination should be part of every initial evaluation for low back pain. The assessment of rectal sphincter tone is an important part of neurologic testing. If any neurologic abnormalities involving the sacral segments are suggested, the bulbocavernosus reflex should be tested. Pelvic examination of women should be reserved for those cases in which gynecologic disease is suspected as a cause of low back pain.

A vascular examination is particularly important in older patients in whom the differential diagnosis of vascular claudication and spinal claudication must be established. Examining hair distribution, skin texture and temperature, capillary refilling, and arterial pulsations in the extremities can provide clues to help in carrying out a more thorough evaluation of the vascular supply to the lower extremities. Venous engorgement might suggest abdominal venous compression secondary to tumor or infection. Bruits heard

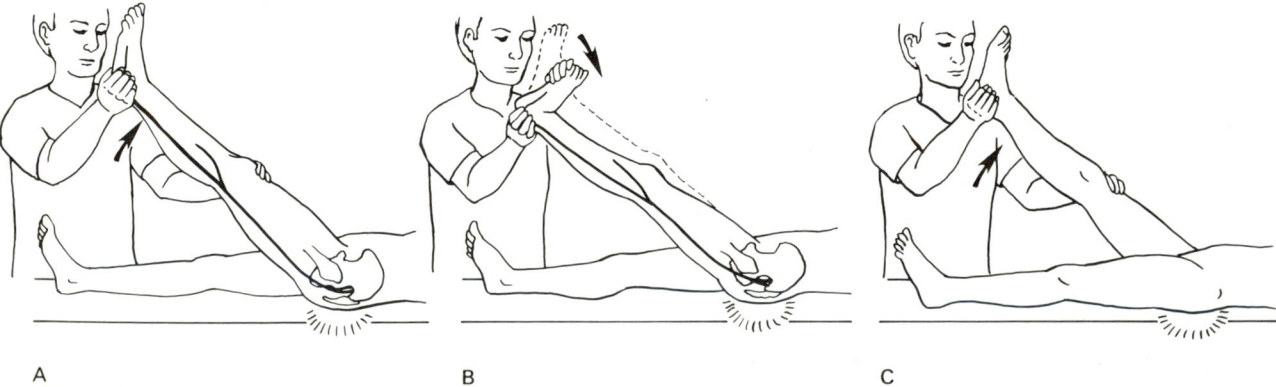

A   B   C

FIG. 71-1. *A.* Straight leg raising test on a patient suspected of left-sided pathology. With the left knee in full extension and the ankle in neutral position, the affected left leg is gradually raised. This stretches the roots of the lumbosacral plexus; the degree of hip flexion at the time the patient complains of back and leg pain is noted. *B.* Laséque's sign. Dorsiflexion of the left ankle increases stretch on the lumbosacral plexus roots and augments back and leg pain. This confirms findings of the straight leg raising test. *C.* Crossed straight leg raising test. When patient reports back and leg pain with straight leg raising of opposite leg (unaffected right), likelihood of a herniated disk on the painful side is high.

over the abdomen or groin can indicate disease of major arteries.

Nonorganic Signs

The prudent examiner should be aware of clues elaborated by the patient suggesting that something in addition to the events occurring in the back is generating the pain behavior. This is often relegated to clinical intuition, but recent work by Waddell has led to the validation of five types of findings that greatly increase the likelihood that psychosocial factors are playing a major role in the patient's complaints (49).

The first sign is superficial nonanatomic tenderness. Lightly pinching and rolling the skin over the back should not alter deep structures; the complaint of increased low back pain is a positive finding (Fig. 71-2).

The second sign is the positive simulation response. Axial loading of the head by lightly placing one's hand on the top of the patient's head should not significantly increase the pressure on the low back (Fig. 71-3). Rotation of both hips and shoulders without twisting the torso does not stress the low back. Increased low back pain with either of these maneuvers is a positive finding.

The third test is distraction. A significant discrepancy between straight leg raising in the seated and supine positions is a positive response. Determination of straight leg raising in the seated position is made when ostensibly evaluating foot or leg function (Fig. 71-4).

The fourth test looks for nonphysiologic regional disturbances of sensation, distribution of pain, or weakness. The pain drawing can be a helpful adjunct to the patient's history and physical examination (Fig. 71-5).

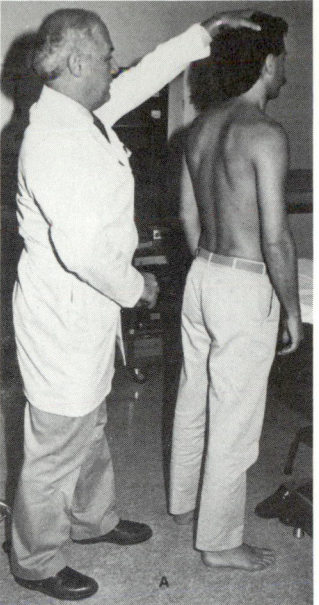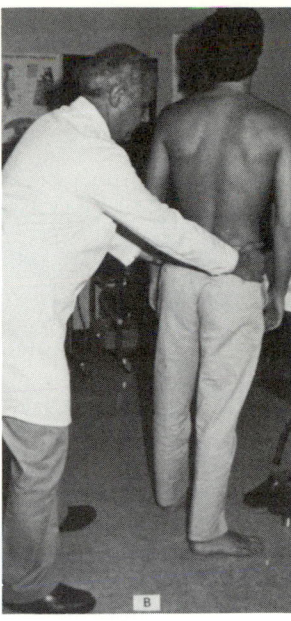

FIG. 71-3. Waddell's sign: positive simulation test. **A.** Axial loading. **B.** Hip rotation. Increased back pain reported by the patient is not likely to be caused by structural abnormalities in the spine.

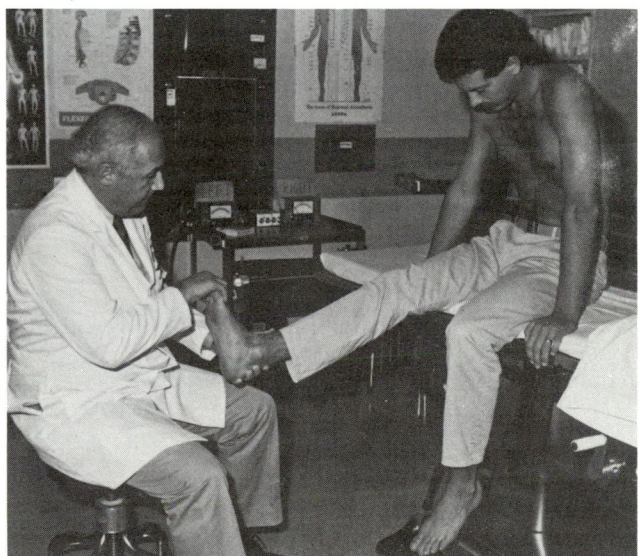

FIG. 71-4. Waddell's signs: distraction test for discrepancy between straight leg raising test when the patient is lying down and sitting up. The examiner is ostensibly testing foot strength but actually is evaluating the patient's response to straight leg raising in the seated position.

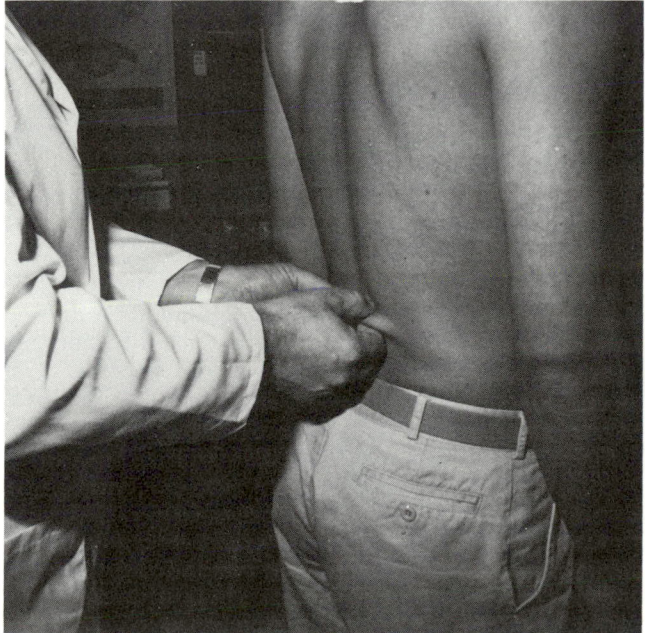

FIG. 71-2. Waddell's signs: skin roll test. Increased back pain reported by the patient is not likely to be caused by structural abnormalities in the spine.

The fifth test is for over-reaction, such as excessive verbalization, facial grimacing, and other pain behaviors out of proportion to the test stimulus and the findings on history and physical examination. Allowances must be made for the patient's age, sex, and cultural background before evaluating such pain behaviors.

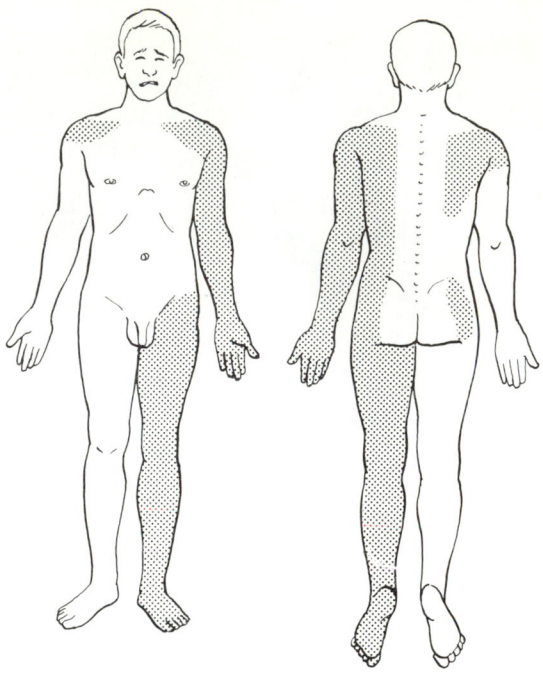

FIG. 71-5. Waddell's signs: pain drawing. This reveals a nonphysiologic pattern of pain. A structural lesion is not likely to cause pain in this distribution.

Patients with three or more positive test results did not respond favorably to any form of physical treatment, and surgery was not often beneficial (49). These are not tests of malingering; they only indicate that the patient's pain behaviors cannot be ascribed solely to structural lesions within the spine.

Special Studies

Patients with low back pain should be considered for additional diagnostic studies such as radiography, CT scanning, MRI, myelography, electromyography, or bone scanning when the history and physical findings suggest that a specific diagnosis can be established, leading to an effective management program, or when the course of the patient's illness deviates from the natural history so that recovery has not occurred as expected. No diagnostic test can replace the history and physical examination, however; management is based on the patient's symptoms and *not* on test results.

Radiography

Although radiographs of the lumbosacral region continue to be commonly ordered for patients with low back pain, they are rarely helpful in establishing a diagnosis and expose patients to significant radiation (15, 50–55). Indications for plain radiography include the suggestion of major trauma, infection, or tumor (Fig. 71-6). Patients with typical acute low back pain should not have radiographs taken unless their symptoms fail to abate during the 6 to 8 weeks after the initial examination. The physician should resist demands by patients or insurance companies that repeated radiographs of the spine be obtained. In the absence of a history of severe trauma or pre-existing

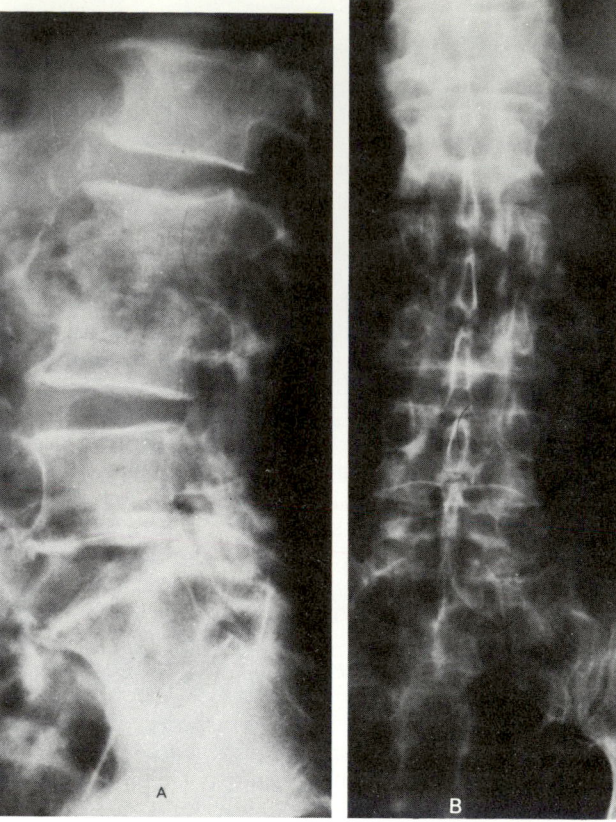

FIG. 71-6. Radiograph showing tuberculous osteomyelitis at the L3–L4 level in a patient with chronic low back pain radiating into both hips and thighs. **A.** Lateral view. **B.** Anteroposterior view. Note the loss of the cartilaginous end plates and destruction of the L3–L4 interspace. The bone in L3 and L4 is also being destroyed.

malignancy, radiography of the back is rarely helpful in establishing a cause for the pain or in planning therapy.

MYELOGRAPHY. The introduction of a radiopaque substance into the cerebrospinal fluid to delineate the anatomy of the dural sac and its contents is known as myelography. Modern techniques use water-soluble media that provide better definition and do not entail the risk of causing arachnoiditis, as do oil-based media. Myelography involves significant radiation exposure, and its use should be restricted to patients who are being considered for surgery. The conus must always be visualized, because tumors of the distal spinal cord and the cauda equina can present with signs and symptoms suggestive of lumbar disk disease. Current myelographic procedures are 95% accurate for disk herniation, but it must be remembered that the defect seen might not always be responsible for the symptoms (Figs. 71-7 and 71-8) (55–57). Disk herniations without any symptoms can be found on myelography (58). Additional information can be obtained if CT scanning is performed immediately after myelography; lesions seen on the myelogram can be more carefully delineated by CT scan.

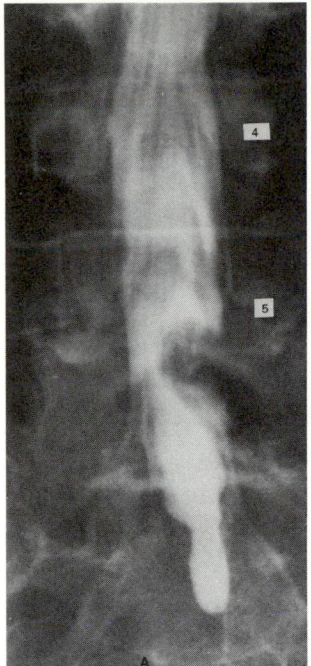
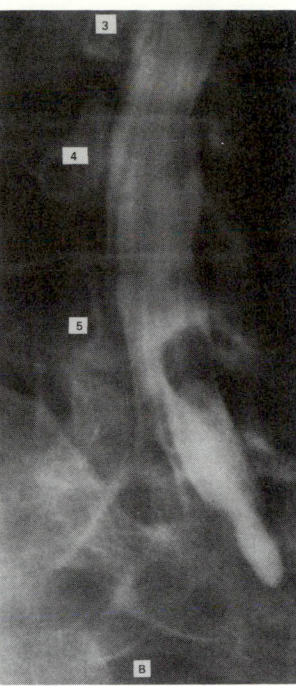

FIG. 71-7. Myelograms showing L5 neurofibroma. **A.** Anteroposterior view. **B.** Oblique view. Until the myelograms were obtained, the patient was thought to have a herniated disk. Symptoms included pain radiating to the large toe, weakness, and numbness in the L5 dermatome. The filling defect does not overlie an interspace and its margins suggest an intradural lesion.

DISKOGRAPHY. A contrast medium can be injected into the intervertebral disk to evaluate its integrity and to determine if the patient's symptoms can be reproduced, thereby verifying the source of the pain (59, 60). Varying results concerning the accuracy of this test, known as diskography, have been reported (4, 61, 62). CT scanning in conjunction with diskography can increase the diagnostic power of this procedure. It is certainly useful in documenting the placement of the needle for chymopapain injection, but it is difficult to say whether its use improves patient management. Abnormal diskograms are probably responsible for much unnecessary low back surgery.

VENOGRAPHY. Epidural venography is performed by catheterizing the femoral vein and injecting a radiopaque substance into the lumbar epidural veins. These are anatomically constant and are sensitive to compression by an intraspinal but extradural mass lesion, such as disk herniation (63, 64). Venography is particularly valuable in the assessment of the L5–S1 interspace, which is often difficult to delineate by myelography. Prior surgery renders this test of little value, because scar and disk cannot be distinguished. As with any other anatomic study, the findings must be correlated with the patient's history and physical examination.

CT SCANNING. CT scanning has become the most common method of assessing the lumbosacral spine (65–67). CT findings are not well correlated with the gross anatomy, diagnosis, aging process, or treatment

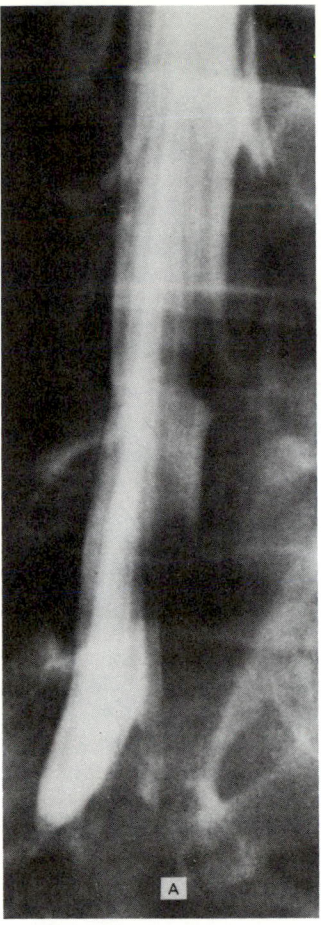
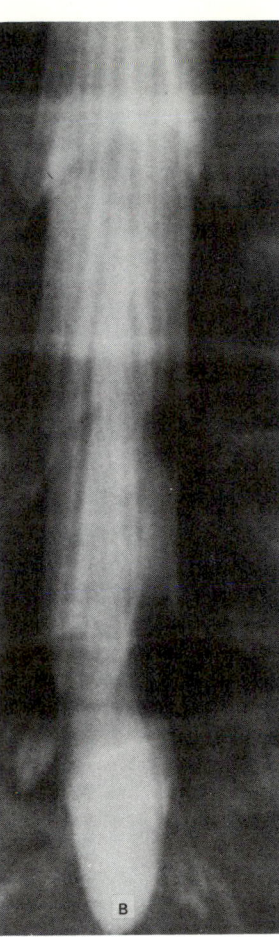

FIG. 71-8. Myelograms showing herniated disk at L4–L5 and L5–S1 in a patient with low back pain radiating to the right foot, with associated sensory and reflex changes. **A.** Oblique view. **B.** Anteroposterior view. The defects are ventrolaterally placed and overlie the interspaces. The margins suggest an extradural defect.

outcome, but are helpful in establishing the diagnosis of tumor, infection, and trauma (Figs. 71-9, 71-10 and 71-11). CT findings are also a major determinant in the diagnosis of spinal stenosis.

Late model CT scanners can image soft tissues efficiently and can help to establish the diagnosis of a herniated disk without intravenous or intrathecal contrast enhancement. When a CT scan is obtained, appropriate scout films must be made and the gantry should be tilted so that the central beam passes parallel to the disk spaces at each level under investigation. Software packages allow reconstruction of images in several planes, which is of great help in determining the anatomy of the structures adjacent to the nerve roots and dura.

MAGNETIC RESONANCE IMAGING. Magnetic resonance imaging (MRI) involves no exposure to ionizing radiation. The development of stronger magnetic fields and surface coils has made this the most powerful examination tool for the spine. Because primary images can be made in the sagittal and coronal planes, MRI is more practical than CT scanning for surveying the spine over multiple levels. Its resolution exceeds

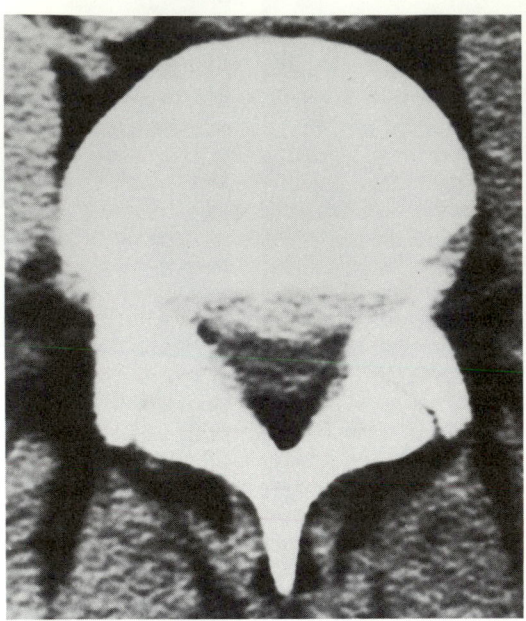

FIG. 71-9. CT scan at the L4–L5 level demonstrating a large midline disk protrusion. The patient had low back and bilateral leg pain. The dural sac is displaced posteriorly; root sleeves and the adjacent fat cannot be seen.

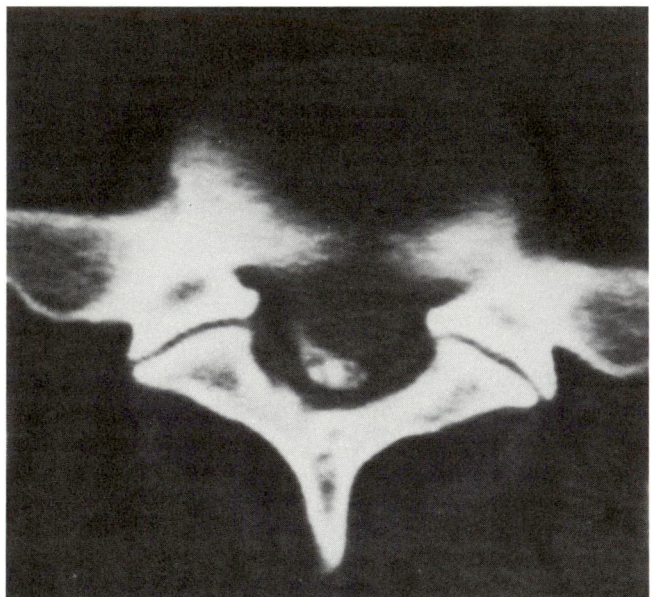

FIG. 71-10. CT scan showing free fragment disk herniation at the L5–S1 level. The patient had severe back and leg pain and inability to void. The contrast medium has been injected into the lumbar theca; the dural sac is compressed and displaced posteriorly by a large mass extending into the bony canal.

that of CT scanning or myelography, and we believe that it is highly likely to replace both of these and radiography to become the sole morphologic test used for the evaluation of low back pain. So many anatomic abnormalities have been seen that we do not yet know how to interpret the significance of many of these

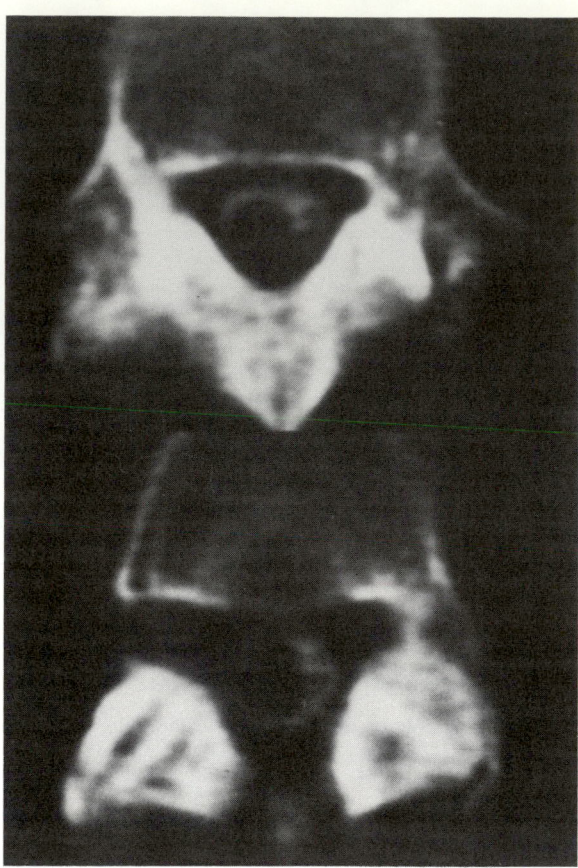

FIG. 71-11. CT scan with intrathecal contrast demonstrating an L5 neurofibroma (same patient as in Fig. 71-7). Two adjacent images are shown. The globular tumor mass is intradural; other nerve roots are displaced, but the thecal sac is in its normal position.

changes. To date, the correlation between described MRI changes and the patient's symptoms has been sporadic.

ULTRASONOGRAPHY. Ultrasonic imaging of the spinal canal was introduced by Porter and colleagues in 1978 (68). The B-scanning mode provides pictures of echoes reflected from the spinal canal that can be used to determine the intralaminar space, and some correlation with symptoms has been seen. The reliability of the technique has not been fully determined, but it has the distinct advantage of being inexpensive and without health hazard. Developments in both hardware and software might make this a valuable diagnostic procedure, especially for older patients suspected of having spinal stenosis.

BONE SCAN. A bone scan is a relatively benign procedure that can be used as a screening technique for occult abnormalities of the spine. It can also be used to determine the extent of known pathology. The most commonly used isotope for lumbar spine imaging is ^{99m}Tc-diphosphate, which reflects blood flow as well as osteoblastic activity (69). Technetium-99m scanning reveals infection, tumor, or inflammation earlier than plain radiography (Fig. 71-12). The procedure can also be used to localize an occult fracture and to discriminate between a congenital or remotely acquired pars

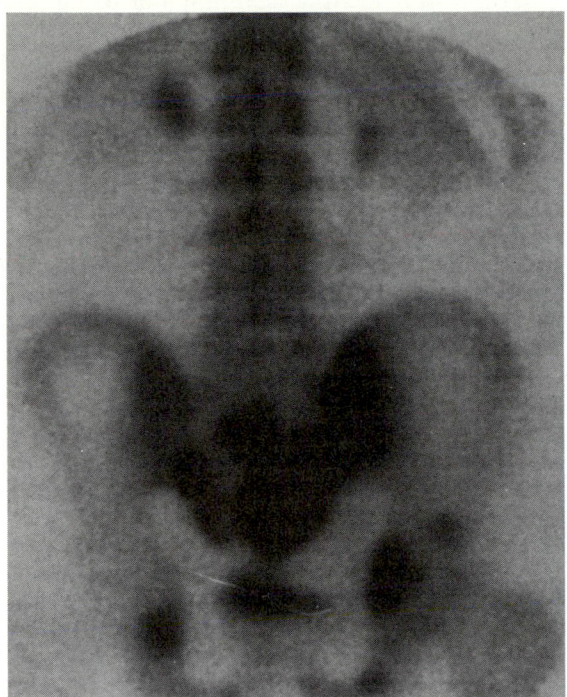

FIG. 71-12. Bone scan with ^{99m}Tc revealing multiple metastases to the spine and pelvis from prostatic carcinoma. The patient presented with insidiously progressive low back pain.

interarticularis defect and a recent fracture (70). Technetium-99m bone scanning is not 100% reliable because both false-positive and false-negative results can be obtained, but it is a very helpful diagnostic adjunct.

Electrodiagnostic Studies

Electromyography (EMG) provides physiologic information about the functional motor unit and can help to evaluate neurologic function in patients with low back pain. Somatosensory evoked potentials (SEP) are also useful in localizing the site of neural dysfunction to peripheral nerves, the cauda equina, or the spinal cord. The techniques and interpretation of the results of EMG and SEP are discussed in Chapter 35. Electrodiagnostic studies are particularly valuable in patients who have had prior surgery and whose morphologic studies are likely to be ambiguous.

Thermography

Thermography is a noninvasive technique used to determine the temperature of the body surface, and some have claimed it to be a method for measuring pain. It does not measure pain, but it might have some usefulness in assessing patients with low back pain. The thermogram is abnormal if the body part has abnormal circulation to it or if the innervation of the skin is damaged. Thermography can therefore be useful in the evaluation of vascular disease or injuries to the nervous system. Great care must be taken to ensure that the procedure is carried out properly to rule out spurious findings (Chapter 34).

Diagnostic Local Anesthetic Injections

Diagnostic injections of local anesthetic into different structures can help to delineate the cause of pain and focus treatment efforts. The use of nerve blocks is discussed in Chapter 94. The response to a diagnostic injection does not necessarily reflect only the pharmacology of events at the tip of the needle. Blocks must be interpreted with caution and must be repeated several times before management decisions can be made.

GRADUATED SPINAL ANESTHESIA. Serial injections of increasing concentrations of local anesthetic are made into the lumbar subarachnoid space to determine the neurologic component of the patient's reported pain relief. Some anesthesiologists believe that the source of the pain can be localized by this technique, but others are dubious. A placebo response prevents one from obtaining any meaningful information with this test. Failure to abolish the pain with a complete high-level spinal block suggests that no surgical or pharmacologic procedure can alleviate the pain because the generator lies higher in the nervous system. It has been argued that if the pain is abolished when only the sympathetic fibers are blocked, one can focus on the treatment of sympathetically mediated pain, but this concept is not universally accepted. Just how this procedure alters the provision of care for low back pain patients is not clear; its use should be restricted to selected patients.

PARAVERTEBRAL SPINAL NERVE BLOCK. Local anesthetic can be placed around the formed spinal nerves as they exit from the intervertebral foramen to determine the effect of blocking a single segmental nerve on the pain. The procedure must be performed under fluoroscopic or radiographic control to ensure that the needle is suitably placed. It is helpful in assessing lateral recess stenosis and in dealing with the patient with a multiply operated back who is being considered for another surgical procedure. Decisions should not be based on the results of paravertebral blocks unless repeated blocks yield consistent findings.

JOINT AND LIGAMENT INJECTIONS. Instilling a local anesthetic solution into or adjacent to the *facet joint* can help to determine the source of low back pain and whether denervation of that joint might provide long-term relief (71). The efficacy of procedures directed at the facet joints remains controversial; criteria for patient selection have not been well established. Local anesthetic can be injected into and around the *sacroiliac joint* to determine if it is the source of the pain. Some patients with low back pain can be helped by injection of local anesthetic into the *interspinous ligaments* and surrounding small muscles. This clarifies the pathogenesis of the pain syndrome and can help to establish a management program.

TRIGGER POINT INJECTION. Palpable tender areas in the back and legs can be the source of pain. Infiltration with local anesthetic or dry needling can establish a diagnosis and help to direct therapy (Chapters 21 and 77A). More diffuse infiltration of a muscle can also help to pinpoint a cause of pain.

Epidural Block. Epidural local anesthetic can be used to localize the source of noxious input and thereby focus further diagnostic and therapeutic efforts. Epidural or intrathecal opioids can be used to determine if the patient's pain syndrome depends on the nociceptive afferent system or if it is generated by activity elsewhere in the nervous system. It must be ascertained whether the patient has consistent responses to repeated blocks prior to interpreting the results.

Psychologic Testing

The known role of environmental and psychologic factors in both acute and chronic low back pain mandates their assessment as part of a comprehensive evaluation. Any patient who does not promptly get over acute low back pain and every patient with chronic low back pain needs this type of evaluation. Various formal tests can be carried out but a structured interview by a trained professional is also valuable. The Minnesota Multiphasic Personality Inventory (MMPI) is probably the most widely used diagnostic test; it has the advantage of being readily scored and interpreted. Pain drawings are also helpful. Almost every psychometric test has been used to study those with low back pain. Here we focus on the most common instruments (also see Chapter 33).

Minnesota Multiphasic Personality Inventory. MMPI results have been used to select patients for surgical treatment (72–75). Indeed, if one wishes to assess the likelihood of return to work after a diskectomy, the MMPI is a better predictor than any other diagnostic test or the findings at surgery (54). If a single psychometric test is to be the only method of assessing this aspect of the situation, the MMPI is probably the best choice.

Pain Drawings. The pain drawing is a useful method of identifying patients who must have a more thorough psychologic evaluation before undergoing medical or surgical treatment, and it can be highly correlated with the MMPI results (76). Drawings that suggest nonanatomic pain patterns should alert the physician to the possibility that psychologic or environmental factors are playing a large role in the patient's complaints.

B. MECHANISMS OF LOW BACK PAIN

In this section we discuss general issues and then proceed to characterize the management of specific diagnostic entities.

Psychosocial Factors

Accurate diagnosis is possible for only a small fraction of patients with low back pain. It has become increasingly apparent that psychosocial factors play a major role in low back pain. The observations by Mixter and Barr (77) in 1934 that a ruptured disk could cause lumbago and sciatica led to 30 years' pursuit of the surgical cure of low back pain. In the past 20 years, the growing crisis of disability resulting from low back pain has led to the recognition that the problem cannot be solved by better or more frequent surgery. This section addresses the role of psychosocial factors in the mechanisms, diagnosis, and treatment of acute and chronic low back pain.

Pathogenesis

The role of psychosocial factors in the persistence of back pain into chronicity is better understood by examining early management issues in acute back pain and their possible contribution to the evolution of chronicity. Only one reported study has directly addressed the role of psychosocial factors in the treatment of acute back pain (78). It is considered here in some detail to provide an underpinning for the hypotheses presented subsequently about psychosocial mechanisms underlying chronic back pain. (A more detailed discussion is presented in Chapter 16.)

A study of the effects of behavioral concepts on the early management of acute back pain was carried out by Fordyce and colleagues (78). The methods used were derived from behavioral methods used to treat chronic back pain (Chapter 81). Patients coming to any of four clinics with complaints of recent onset back pain and who agreed to participate were included in the study. Onset was never more remote than 7 to 10 days and was usually within 12 to 36 hours of first being seen. Using a control group design, patients were randomly assigned to traditional regimens (group A) or to regimens based on behavioral concepts (group B). The same physicians treated those in both groups; the differences were in details of the regimens. In group A, analgesics or other pain-related medications, if prescribed, were delivered on a demand or as-needed schedule, with renewal of the prescription subject to negotiation between patients and physicians. Medications for those in group B, however, if prescribed, were to be taken on a fixed time schedule (e.g., q6h) and for a fixed number of days, with no renewal of prescription.

If activity limitations were prescribed for those in group A they were pain-contingent—i.e., "let pain be your guide" as to when to terminate those limitations. That is, when patients resumed activity, if pain were experienced and deemed sufficient *by the patients* to warrant protective action, they were encouraged to stop. Activity limitations for those in group B were to be followed for a fixed number of days, based on physician estimates of probable healing time. Therefore, resumption of activity for those in group B was on a time-contingent and not a pain-contingent basis.

Exercise was handled in a manner similar to that used for prescribed activity limitations. If exercises were prescribed for group A patients, the amount done was again dictated by patients' assessment of acceptable pain levels. Thus, the basis for deciding whether to continue to exercise or to stop and resume guarding or protective behaviors was left to the patients. If prescribed, exercises for those in group B were specified as to the day on which to begin, the number of repetitions of each exercise to perform, and the daily increment rate in those repetitions. In short, the B regimen, unlike the A, included a component directed toward reactivation that was programmed on a time-contingent and not a pain-contingent basis.

The unifying theme of the differences between the two regimens was that group A patients themselves acted as judges of whether healing had occurred and resumption of activity was appropriate. In contrast, the physicians of the group B patients estimated probable healing time and decided when healing could be expected to have been adequately completed and when resumption of activity was appropriate. Thus, the B regimen entailed *physicians'* labeling the problem as ended, thereby attaching a different meaning to whatever pain might be experienced on resumption of activity. For those in group B, pain was not to be interpreted as a warning that healing was not sufficiently completed or that guarding behavior was the appropriate action.

Those in the A and B groups were also compared in regard to their use of health care measures at 6 weeks and on patient-reported measures at approximately 1 year, which included activity diary, frequency checklists of common activities as measures of activity level, vocational status, use of health care, claimed impairment, and pain drawings (76). The drawings served as a measure of patients' claims of the extent of involvement of their body in pain. All but the activity measures were combined into a single "sick-well" score.

No differences were found between group A and group B patients in measures of activity level. Linton (79) has reported data indicating the lack of a relationship between patient-reported activity and report of

pain in chronic pain. Fordyce and associates (80) also found no relationship between activity measures and patients reports of pain intensity. The lack of differences in activity measures (78) might reflect a lack of true differences or of reliability of the actual activity measures, so that what people say about their pain does not necessarily correspond with what they do (as assessed by activity measures). This has important implications for the diagnosis of back pain (see below).

Other findings reveal an interesting pattern. As shown in Figure 71-13, group B patients described themselves as less "sick," as having better vocational status, a lesser degree of claimed impairment, and less of their bodies implicated in pain than the group A patients. All differences were statistically significant except for the vocational status measure.

A second finding, the "claimed impairment" variable is particularly germane. This measure refers to what patients report as limitations in their activities. It compares claimed impairment in the month preceding the 1-year follow-up point with that in the week preceding entry into the study. As shown in Figure 71-14, the results indicated that group A patients described themselves at 1-year follow-up as more impaired than group B patients and also as more impaired than they were prior to participating in the study. In contrast, group B patients described themselves (in terms of claimed impairment) as having returned at 1-year follow-up to precisely where they were prior to onset of pain. This suggests that, in terms of what patients say about themselves, the A regimen resulted in a worsened condition whereas the B regimen restored patients to preinjury levels.

Two inferences can be drawn from the results of this study. The first is that physician prescription of termination of medications, activity limitations, and reactivation, all of which serve implicitly to label the problem as ended, results in a more favorable outcome. The second is that, although perhaps not differing in actual activity level, group A patients (on average)

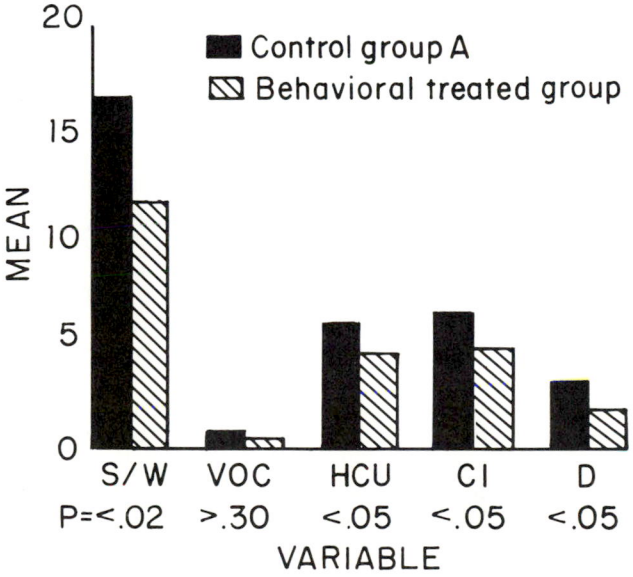

FIG. 71-13. Study of effects of behavior and acute back pain management. Shown are the outcome scores for groups A and B. S/W (Sick/Well status), overall score based on sum of VOC, HCU, CI, and D; VOC, vocational status; HCU, health care utilization; CI, claimed impairment (amount of interference in function claimed by patient); and D, pain drawings (amount of body implicated by patient). (See text for details.) From Fordyce, W., et al.: Acute back pain: A control group comparison of behavioral vs. traditional management modes. J. Behav. Med., *9*:127, 1986.

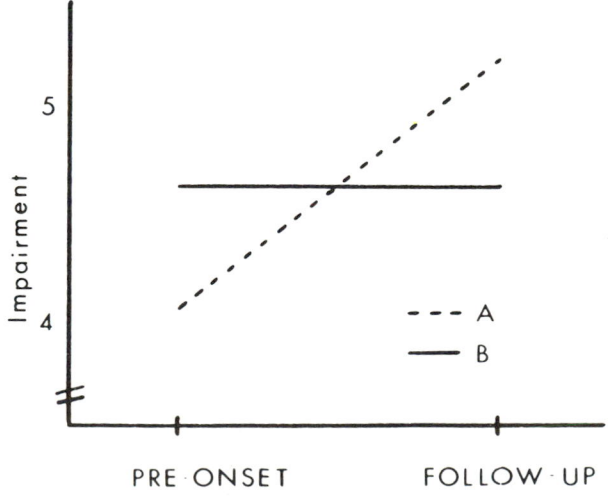

FIG. 71-14. Claimed impairment of activities for subjects in groups A and B. (See text for details.) From Fordyce, W., et al.: Acute back pain: A control group comparison of behavioral vs. traditional management modes. J. Behav. Med., *9*:127, 1986.

saw themselves as more impaired and reported more use of health care under a regimen that failed to define a treatment goal clearly.

The findings of this study have gained confirmation from a report by Deyo and co-workers (46). Their findings indicated that a group of recent-onset back pain patients who were prescribed 2 days of bed rest had a more favorable outcome than patients who were prescribed 7 days of bed rest.

As noted above, the dictum of "let pain be your guide" and the prescription of medications and activity limitations on a pain behavior-contingent basis in part leaves the task of determining when the problem has ended to the patient. This can be regarded as a labeling problem. Patients often fail to distinguish hurt from harm (Chapters 16 and 81). When patients move and experience pain they might conclude that healing has not occurred, thus perceiving themselves as having an unhealed pain problem. They might also conclude that further damage is produced by continued movement but in so doing they fail to recognize that healing is promoted by movement and that the "pain" they experience might reflect the effects of disuse.

This takes us back to the issue of labeling (Chapter 16). The essential points about the labeling issue in this context are the following:

a. No inherent relationship between what people say and what they do about the pain they claim to have has been found.

b. No inherent relationship between what people say or do about "pain" and nociception or physical findings has been found.

c. How the problem is labeled can influence significantly the course of the problem (e.g., how much patients suffer, how much guarding or activity limitation is displayed, as inferred from what they say or do, or both, and subsequent health care use).

d. How the problem (i.e., the body sensations) is labeled can be influenced by cues from the immediate environment (e.g., the prescription of analgesics, rest, or avoidance of activity on a pain-contingent basis, the patient's expectations from prior experience with pain, and actions and expectations of family members or significant others).

e. The labeling problem mainly seems to concern the failure to distinguish hurt from harm, whether by the patient, physician, or family members. Thus, healing and restoration of activity levels are unduly impaired and disuse is promoted.

In summary, early management strategies can inadvertently promote the persistence of a pain problem into chronicity because the physician might prescribe in ways that increase the chances of the patient labeling posthealing pain sensations as indicating an unhealed problem and because the regimen might fail to provide a specific reactivation component.

Acute Low Back Pain

The diagnosis of acute low back pain is not likely to necessitate close attention to psychosocial factors unless it is known that the patient has a history of chronic pain, particularly back pain. If the patient does have a history of pain, diagnostic procedures for acute back pain should be used, and then diagnostic procedures for chronic back pain should be done if normal activity is not resumed soon after the estimated healing time interval. This plan requires that, at the initial workup, a follow-up appointment be made to assess whether normal activities are being resumed. If the patient persists in guarding behavior and undue limitation of activity, and physical findings indicate that healing should have been completed sufficiently to conclude that resumption of activity does not provide significant risk of further injury, prompt action is indicated. The problem can prudently be seen as one of potential chronicity for which the diagnostic procedures specific to chronicity should be carried out.

A distinction is being made here in regard to avoidance of activity because of diminished risk of creating further tissue damage and avoidance of activity because it might produce pain. This brings us back to the distinction between hurt and harm. It takes only a few days (80) for activity limitation to result in the shortening of muscle fibers and to increase the risk that activity will produce pain. The patient must recognize that pain experienced with movement of the involved body parts after the healing time essential for restoration of tissue integrity does not indicate failed healing. Moreover, at that point in time when tissue integrity is not threatened by prudent amounts of activity, healing is promoted by activation, not threatened. Estimated healing time provides the framework for structuring early management and defines when reactivation should begin and normal activities should be resumed. This strategy also minimizes disuse effects and helps the patient and family to distinguish hurt from harm.

Chronic Low Back Pain

In regard to psychosocial issues, diagnostic procedures for chronic low back pain differ in several respects from those for acute back pain. The central issue is why pain behaviors continue to occur past the expected healing time. The diagnostic process serves to differentiate pain behaviors occurring mainly as a consequence of nociception from those occurring for other reasons likely to reflect psychosocial factors. Procedures to follow in the determination of these factors are described in detail in Chapter 16, and additional points pertaining specifically to back pain are discussed here.

The distinction between operants and respondents is essential. Pain behaviors are operants and can be subject to voluntary control. They can be said to be "effort-dependent" in the sense that the behavior in which the patient is expected to engage as part of the back examination, from which the examining physician can draw inferences about pain or nociception, depends potentially on the amount of effort put into the maneuver or on the extent of distress communicated when the patient is attempting to perform. Flexing a limb is an example. Most components of the clinical back examination involve operants.

Pain behaviors that are also respondents are those that occur essentially in a reflex fashion, with little or no potential influence from voluntary control. They can be said to be "effort-independent." Examples are the results of radiographic, CT, and other diagnostic procedures, because the patient is required to do no more than be a passive participant in the procedure. Assessment for determining the distribution of sensory loss, however, is not entirely one in which the patient is only a passive participant. A verbal report or some form of nonverbal action makes up part of the data—that is, operants are involved—so the procedure is partly effort-dependent. This is another way of stating that prior conditioning, anticipated consequences, or both, can exert a significant influence on a patient's responses.

The distinction between effort-dependent and effort-independent components of the diagnostic process is crucial to the proper evaluation of chronic back pain. It can be illustrated further by noting the differences when observing a patient engaging in lateral bending or in flexing forward in an effort to touch the floor with the fingers, and in palpating a muscle spasm as distinguished from a tight muscle. Lateral bending or flexing forward both involve operants or movements subject to

voluntary control—they are effort-dependent. This in turn means that the observed performance bears no inherent relationship to nociception. Such behaviors as limitation, grimacing, moaning, and gasping might reflect underlying pathophysiology, but they also might reflect pain behaviors that have come under the control of social contingencies.

Pain behaviors, guarding, or nonperformance of a body maneuver during a back examination, however compelling they might seem, are *not* an index of nociception or of lack of healing.

The problem of the potentially obfuscating influence of conditioning effects on performance of operants during a back examination has been studied by Waddell and colleagues (49). Waddell's signs (see above, Nonorganic Signs) are an attempt to separate pain behaviors occurring during a back examination because of nociception from those occurring for other reasons. Waddell's signs should become an integral part of all clinical examinations of chronic back pain patients.

C. MANAGEMENT OF LOW BACK PAIN

Effective Treatments

The Quebec Task Force on Spinal Disorders, as reported by Spitzer (4), has reviewed all the published literature on the diagnosis and treatment of cervical and lumbar pain syndromes. This magnum opus should lead to a reconsideration of all our diagnostic and management programs because it clearly shows that traditional health care provider strategies lack demonstrable efficacy.

Treatments for acute back pain that do seem to be effective include the following: back school, brief (under 3 days) bed rest, endurance training, and, in carefully selected patients, diskectomy (81–85). Few proven therapies exist for chronic low back pain. Therefore, management strategies should not impair the natural healing process; they rarely seem to improve on the outcome unless a highly specific diagnosis can be made. Criteria for such diagnoses have been published, but many health care providers appear to ignore them.

A recent study from Gothenberg, Sweden has confirmed the value of a comprehensive and aggressive management program for patients with low back pain (86). Patients who had been off work for 4 to 6 weeks because of low back pain participated in a program consisting of back school, fitness training, early return to work, and judicious surgery. Long-term disability was 50% less than that seen in back pain patients elsewhere in the same city who did not participate in such a structured program.

The role of physical fitness in preventing low back pain and its associated disability has been demonstrated by Cady and associates in their program for firefighters (85, 87). Back injuries were one-ninth as common in the fit, and compensation costs were reduced by 25% for those in this group.

The efficacy of surgical removal of a ruptured disk has been demonstrated by Weber (82–84). A controlled prospective study of patients who met the diagnostic criteria for a disk herniation showed that the surgical

results were superior for the first 4 years; thereafter, operated and nonoperated patients had an 85% success rate and a 95% success rate, respectively, at 10-year follow-up. Diskectomy is valuable for patients with sciatica, but patients with low back pain alone have not been shown to benefit from surgery (3, 16, 88). Spangfort showed that, if a disk herniation was not found at surgery, the course was much worse than the natural history of low back pain patients (57). Long showed that most chronic low back pain patients who failed to improve after surgery did not meet reasonable criteria for their initial operation (89).

Three components of a management program seem to reduce chronic low back pain and its accompanying disability: education related to return-to-work activities, cardiovascular endurance training, and judicious use of surgery.

Unproven Treatment Methods

The vast majority of treatments commonly used for patients with low back pain have no demonstrable effect, either on hastening recovery or on prevention of subsequent episodes. Most patients recover quickly without medical intervention. Prospective controlled trials have failed to demonstrate the value of any specific exercise program, diathermy, ultrasonography, muscle relaxants, anti-inflammatory drugs, injection of steriods, or local anesthetics (4). Manipulation, which is the mainstay of the treatments offered by chiropractors, has never been shown to be more effective than placebo.

Bed rest is frequently prescribed for patients with low back pain, but the only studies available show that the shorter the period of bed rest, the more rapid the return to work (46). In addition, the deleterious effects of bed rest on bone, muscle, and joint are well known. Bed rest is not indicated for the management of low back pain patients; moderation of mechanical stresses on the back usually controls symptoms.

No good evidence has been found to indicate that any of the physical modalities commonly used to treat low back pain improve the natural history of the course of the problem (4). This can also be said for injections, trigger point injections, acupuncture, electrical stimulation, and diets.

Causes for Delay of Recovery from Acute Low Back Pain

When the patient with acute back pain does not recover quickly, the problem usually can be traced to one of three causes: (a) a structural problem in the back; (b) a general medical problem that is affecting the back; or (c) psychosocial factors.

Structural Problems in the Back

NERVE ROOT COMPRESSION. Compression of a nerve root by a herniated disk or spinal stenosis can lead to persistent low back and leg pain (Chapter 73). Only a small percentage of patients with low back pain have a herniated disk or lumbar stenosis, and the initial management of either of these conditions is conservative. Nerve root compression is generally indicated by low back pain that radiates to the buttock and from there down the leg into the foot. Signs of sensory and motor dysfunction can be present. Maneuvers to increase the stretch of the roots of the lumbosacral plexus increase the pain. Flexion often alleviates the radicular signs, particularly in patients with stenosis.

SPINAL INSTABILITY. Even though many lumbosacral fusions are performed for low back pain, there is very little evidence that instability itself is a cause of low back pain in the absence of major trauma, infection, or tumor of the spine. Prior surgical intervention is, of course, one type of major trauma to the spine. It is generally agreed that at least 4 mm of translation on lateral radiographs or 11° of rotary motion are required to establish the diagnosis of instability. When abnormal motility is suspected as the cause of continued low back pain, a trial of external immobilization should be undertaken before any consideration is given to surgical fusion. A small percentage of patients with spondylolisthesis develop symptomatic instability and fail to respond to conservative measures for low back pain.

Medical Factors

Neoplasm, infection, inflammatory disease, metabolic bone disease, and referred pain from the pelvic, abdominal, or thoracic region are best detected by a thorough history and physical examination (see below). Such disorders are not often discovered on the initial visit, so a repeat history and physical examination is prudent when dealing with patients who have not responded to conservative therapy within a few weeks. The incidence of such disorders is small when contrasted with the vast number of patients with low back pain, so expensive diagnostic tests are not warranted on the initial visit.

Psychosocial Factors

Psychosocial factors can also play a major role in the perpetuation of low back pain. The loss of one's youthful back can be a cause of grief and frustration. The patient's psychologic makeup and environmental interactions can be determinants of failure to respond to therapy or to the natural healing process.

Treatment of Acute Back Pain

Problems in healing acute back pain include the management of any structural damage that accompanies the injury and the nociception and suffering presumably associated with it. Additional problems can occur but these are probably not present yet, except perhaps as byproducts of the patient's earlier and protracted experiences with back pain. They reside in the situation like ashes smoldering in a fireplace, and can readily be fanned into flame—they are disuse and the mislabeling of posthealing pain as indicative of lack of healing (see above).

The points made in this section are aimed specifically at those cases of recent-onset back pain in which the results of the diagnostic workup indicate no severe or potentially permanent structural defect or one that requires surgical intervention. How much they apply to back injuries in which a residual structural defect appears depends mainly on the extent to which reactivation is essential to management. It becomes a matter of the physician's judgment in each case as to how much to modify or amend the points made below.

Figure 71-15 illustrates a method for organizing the management of back pain from a psychosocial perspective. It serves to distinguish treatment strategies for acute back pain from those appropriate for chronic back pain. As shown in Figure 71-15, the various treatment measures or strategies applied early in treatment should be understood clearly by the patient as being relevant during the healing period and not thereafter, except in regard to any residual structural defect relating to the original injury. The patient should also realize that early management strategies for acute back pain can be harmful if used for chronic back pain.

Care must be exercised by the treating physician in describing or labeling the elements and meaning of each component of the management regimen. A few illustrations of how these issues might be addressed

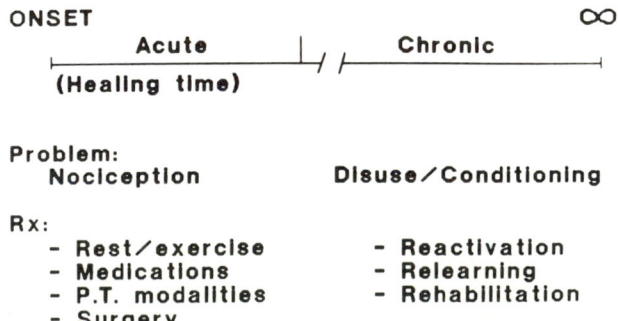

FIG. 71-15. Scheme for discriminating acute and chronic low back pain and their pathogenesis and management. (See text for details.)

early in treatment can be useful. To help the patient understand the importance of reactivation, note the difference between these two statements: "I want you to go home and take it easy until the pain is gone," and "This is a problem that can be expected to last only a certain number (e.g., 3 to 5 or 6 to 8) of days. During that time, take it easy. Thereafter it is important to resume activity to promote further healing and restore your strength."

The patient can also be made to understand that pain in the involved body parts experienced past healing time does not mean failed healing:

I will give you a few days (try to specify a number of days corresponding to your estimate of essential healing time) to protect the healing tissues until they have begun to knit. But, after that, to be sure they heal fully and can then regain full strength, it is important to begin to use them. Therefore, on day X, I want you to begin to do the following (specify activities or exercises, including amounts, daily frequency, and increment rates). You will probably experience some pain when you begin. That is to be expected, and it tells you that healing is occurring and that your activity is helping to restore muscle strength.

The process of helping patient and family to relabel the problem can be helped further by commenting on the issue of the adverse effects of disuse. For example, one might say

It is important to recognize that muscle and ligament fibers will shorten very rapidly unless they are stretched and used. That will happen to you as you take it easy for these next X days. Then, when you begin again to use and stretch those muscles, that will almost certainly produce pain. That tells you that you are getting those muscles and ligaments back into shape. Remember the phrase "use it or lose it."

Use of pain medications in early management also presents a problem in regard to patients' misunderstanding their function. Narcotics, sedative-hypnotics, and muscle relaxants do not treat pain; they provide an element of respite from suffering while healing is underway. Thereafter they have no useful purpose and can make many harmful contributions to the pain problem. Many patients and their families do not understand this but labor under the misconception that pain medications treat pain in a way analogous to an antibiotic treating an infectious process. This common misunderstanding should be made clear to patients. For example, if choosing to prescribe narcotics, sedative-hypnotics, or muscle relaxants, one might say

I will prescribe these (medications) to make things easier for you during healing time. You need to recognize that these won't treat the cause of your pain or in any way make that better. They will simply help you not to feel so much discomfort as healing occurs. Using these medications for more than a few days will not promote healing, and continued use is likely to make it more difficult for you to regain your normal activities. If taken long enough, they are capable of impairing brain function and, in some instances, lead to long-term difficulties. Therefore, I want you to take them for only X days, although you may stop using them sooner than that if you wish.

Thus, the following points should be considered in early management:

a. Estimate a probable healing time. If in doubt, err on the conservative side—that is, allow the least amount of time for healing in which you judge confidently that tissue integrity can be restored.

b. Communicate clearly to your patient the date when pronounced guarding or activity limitation is no longer necessary and in fact risks promoting further disability through the adverse effects of disuse.

c. If analgesics, sedative-hypnotics, or muscle relaxants are to be used, prescribe them on a fixed time schedule and with a termination date specified for their discontinuation.

d. Include specific exercises or activities in the management regimen: when to start, how many times per day to do them, how many repetitions or amounts, and how rapidly to increase them.

Treatment of Chronic Low Back Pain

Treatment procedures described in this section address issues common to chronic back pain that augment information provided in Chapter 81. These procedures, and the issues they address, pertain to those chronic back pain problems that began with tissue injury but in which pain behaviors and activity limitations occur in the absence of residual physical findings beyond healing time, or in which the magnitude of pain behavior and activity limitation is beyond that warranted by the physical findings. (i.e., pain problems reflecting operant pain, as discussed in Chapters 8 and 16).

Chapter 81 provides a detailed description of procedures to be used in medication management, in restoration of activity levels through reactivation procedures, and in the modification of the social feedback or reinforcement by others of pain behaviors or their failure to reinforce activity and well behavior adequately. Chapter 81 also discusses the importance of vocational planning and re-engagement in treating chronic pain.

What remains to be addressed? The major additional problem that the chronic back pain patient is likely to present concerns illness conviction. The probable long history of diagnostic procedures and failed treatment programs virtually ensure that patients and their family are skeptical about the diagnostic acumen and treatment efficacy of those in the health care system. Therefore any proposed treatment regimen, particularly in regard to reactivation, is likely to be approached reluctantly, if accepted at all. Moreover, some patients are somewhat committed to maintaining their sick role. The sanctioned "time out" from aversive activities that the pain problem might represent can make it an attractive role. If wage replacement funding is adequate, the response cost of being identified as disabled is also reduced. Finally, if the pain problem and resulting disability status have continued for many months or years, patients might understandably be doubtful about their ability to cope adequately with the role of being well on the basis of sheer protracted disuse alone.

It is prudent to expect that the illness conviction issue is important in the treatment of chronic back pain. Procedures for striving to prevent undue chronicity in the early management of back injury are described above. These procedures were developed over the course of years of research and clinical experience in the treatment of chronic pain, including mainly chronic back pain. Because procedures for avoiding chronicity and its inevitable corollary, illness conviction, have already been considered, only a brief discussion is given here.

It should be assumed at the outset of undertaking treatment of a chronic back pain patient who displays significant amounts of operant pain that illness conviction problems are present in both patient and spouse. The exceptions are too few to be concerned about.

The most expeditious way of dealing with illness conviction is through an integrated didactic approach of teaching and reactivation. A direct statement such as "Your back is now healed and the only treatment indicated is reactivation" rarely suffices, even if said to patient and spouse together. Clinical experience indicates that a more powerful approach involves providing a lecture-discussion format in which several specific topics are addressed, including the following:

a. The nature of healing and how long it takes
b. The adverse effects of disuse
c. The explanation that pain experienced on movement, past healing time, does not indicate failed healing but rather the effects of fiber shortening from disuse
d. The limited role of pain medications in relation to healing and their adverse effects on restoration of full function

e. The adverse effects of protracted communication to others about pain and limitation

Use of the schematic diagram shown in Figure 71-15, or some variation of it, can probably be a helpful heuristic device. The teaching component can be done with considerable advantage in a group setting, either of the patient alone or the patient and spouse, but teaching can become an abstract set of concepts in the mind of the patient if it is not integrated with reactivation. As teaching progresses, so should reactivation. Among other things, reactivation represents an in vivo demonstration that it *is* safe to move and therefore serves to validate the concepts presented in teaching. This is true both for patient and spouse.

In conclusion, the importance of facilitating reactivation in the treatment of back pain, acute or chronic, can hardly be overstated. Guarding, deactivation, and the fear of free movement are an inherent part of having back pain. Unless those working with the patient stress reactivation in an appropriately designed and paced way, undue pain and disability are almost inevitable. Equally important is the recognition that few nonprofessionals are sufficiently aware of the distinction between hurt and harm and of the implications of this distinction when back pain arises. It is almost impossible to discover an adult who does not sometimes have a sore back. This does not mean that the pain associated with the sore back should inevitably be interpreted as a warning signal that guarding and protective action is indicated. Such action *might* be indicated, but only for a brief interval to permit healing.

D. SPECIFIC CHRONIC LOW BACK PAIN SYNDROMES

Spinal Stenosis

Spinal stenosis is an uncommon condition whose incidence increases with age. The likelihood of establishing this diagnosis is a function of the aggressiveness of the search for surgical patients.

Etiology and Pathophysiology

Usually a gradual diminution of space for the neural elements occurs because of aging changes. The loss of disk height leads to infolding of the ligamentum flavum and capsular ligaments, and causes a gradual choking of the nerve roots. Symptoms are brought on by exercise; ischemia of the cauda equina, possibly as a result of mechanical compression, is thought to be a pathophysiologic mechanism. Nerve root dysfunction seems to be better demonstrated with the use of SEP than with EMG; denervation might not be noted. Because nerves swell slightly when they are active, this might be a factor. The most significant factor is, however, restricted space for the cauda equina or the nerve roots secondary to spondylosis.

Symptoms and Signs

The most commonly reported manifestations are low back, buttock, thigh, and leg pain and paresthesiae after walking less than 300 m. These are not relieved by standing still but are relieved by flexing the lumbar

spine when the patient is sitting or bending over. Sitting is usually well tolerated. The pain increases with exercise and becomes so severe as to force the patient to sit or flex the body. It is usually described as deep, aching, or cramping and radiates from the back into both thighs and legs. Radiating radicular shock-like pains can also occur. Flexion usually relieves the pain in a few minutes, but in severe stenosis the pain can be constant.

Diagnosis

The history should conform to the pattern for stenosis, and the physical examination should include a complete neurologic examination using EMG and SEP. The intention is to exclude occlusive arterial disease and disk hernia, and to confirm the radiologic diagnosis of spinal stenosis. The cerebrospinal fluid should be analyzed if multifocal neurologic disease is suspected. Venous occlusion, plethysmography, oscillometry, and temperature measurements might be needed to exclude vascular disease. The patient's ability to walk, preferably on a treadmill, should be assessed, noting the distance at which the leg pain begins and when the patient is unable to proceed. A neurologic examination performed immediately after walking has been reported to be of value (90).

RADIOGRAPHIC EXAMINATION. Radiology of the spine usually demonstrates rather extensive aging changes: multiple-level disk degeneration, spondylosis, hypertrophic facet joints, pseudospondylolisthesis or spondylolisthesis, and retrolisthesis (91). Radiographic measurements of canal dimensions on ordinary film are difficult to perform and yield uncertain results, although many attempts have been made (92).

A proper diagnosis can usually be made by the history, neurologic verification, and ordinary myelographic films of the spine (93–95). A diminishing anteroposterior diameter of the dural sac is almost always seen in patients with definite spinal stenosis. Sortland and associates (95) have defined the measurements obtained in a large group of patients with neurogenic claudication that helps explain the positional symptoms. In flexion the anteroposterior diameter at the level of the disks was 13 to 14 mm, compared with 19 to 20 mm in a control group, while in extension patients with symptoms of spinal stenosis had diameters of less than 8 mm, compared with the normal value of 18 mm.

Metrizamide-augmented CT scanning allows better visualization and measurement of the dimensions of the dural sac and the impressions made on it by the soft tissue and bone of the spinal canal and nerve root foramen. The use of MRI is rapidly becoming the procedure of choice for evaluating spinal stenosis. It probably will replace CT scanning and myelography once surface coils, stronger magnets, and better software are more widely available.

Ultrasonography has also been tried but is still in its infancy; a spinal canal diameter by this method exceeding 14 mm seems to exclude a myelographic measurement of ⩽9 mm with 95% accuracy (96).

EMG AND SEP. EMG changes are sporadically associated with symptoms of spinal stenosis, with or without claudication. Larson (97) has recommended that, when the EMG is negative, further information can be gained through the use of SEP. Larson indicated that posture-sensitive SEP changes were helpful in determining neurologic compromise in spinal stensois.

Treatment

The conservative treatment of spinal stenosis advocated by some includes the use of a semirigid or rigid corset in a flexed position (the Raney jacket or the Boston modified back pain brace) and ordinary pain-reducing measures. These patients, however, usually do not respond to ordinary physical therapy. By contrast, patients with true vascular claudication can considerably increase their walking distance through exercises. In moderately severe cases bicycling is the exercise advised because it can be done with the spine flexed to stimulate activity and increase the pain threshold. Often the use of SEP can help the surgeon to decide whether partial or total laminectomy is required.

EPIDURAL BLOCKS. Epidural administration of saline solution with or without steriods has been found to have limited value in the treatment of nerve root compression in young adults. In older patients with degenerative changes and symptoms of spinal stenosis, however, the results of the use of epidural steroid injections have been encouraging (98). Although this technique seems helpful in delaying the need for more radical treatment, it is imperative that a proper workup aimed at detecting tumor and infection be performed before epidural steroids are administered. In well-controlled trials, Dilke and co-workers (98) found epidural steroid injections to be helpful in patients with sciatic syndromes, whereas Snoek and associates (99) found no difference between injections of saline alone or with steroid added in patients with myelographically demonstrated disk hernias. It has been our experience that epidural blocks and steroids seem to work best in older patients who do not have severe signs of spinal stenosis.

SURGICAL THERAPY. If symptoms are severe and the patient's activity level is hampered to an unacceptable level surgical treatment is indicated, assuming that diagnostic studies clearly demonstrate spinal stenosis. Extensive surgical decompression of all involved levels is the treatment of choice (100–102). The result is usually good with regard to pseudoclaudication—that is, the walking distance is significantly increased after surgery and leg pain is diminished, although some back pain usually remains. The patient should be told of the probable outcome before surgery. A fusion procedure is generally not performed on the older patients in this age group (usually about 60 to 70 years old), because decompression is already an extensive operation. The motion segments in question are usually rather immobile with significantly diminished disk heights and osteophytes limiting the danger of future instability.

Summary

Spinal stenosis is not as common as previously thought but is a rather unusual diagnosis with a typical clinical appearance and a definite radiographically demonstrable pathology. Because it can be effectively treated the physician must be aware of this diagnosis, especially in older patients with severe back and leg pain. Root canal or foraminal stenosis has not as yet been properly defined, either clinically or radiologically. These stenoses undoubtedly exist, however, and disk hernia surgery should never be done without excluding stenosis farther laterally along the course of the nerve root.

Diseases of the Intervertebral Disk

Intervertebral disk disease is what most physicians and patients think of when they are concerned about low back pain. About 1% of low back pain sufferers have surgical lumbar disk disease. We know that asymptomatic disk disease can occur, and seems to be a function of age (21).

Pathophysiology

The intervertebral disk joint is devoid of direct blood supply from the time of cesation of growth and is the largest avascular structure in adults (103). Aging changes begin fairly early in this joint (104, 105). The difference between normal and pathologic aging, which is commonly termed "degenerative joint disease," has never been demonstrated. A wide variation exists in regard to the amount of degeneration, its onset, and its relationship to symptoms. Some patients retain normal-looking disk spaces throughout old age, with no apparent correlation between aging changes (if present) and symptoms (106). Biomechanical testing has shown that the mechanical behavior of the motion segment changes significantly with aging and degenerative changes of the disk (107). The small muscles of the motion segment, the nerves, and the different aspects of the subchondral bones and facet joints can experience variable degrees of stress and strain as these aging changes occur, but studies have been unable to pinpoint the precise manner by which the disk causes pain. It has been shown indirectly, however, that back pain can result from changes that occur within the disk (5):

a. Disk hernia is usually preceded by one or more attacks of low back pain.

b. Intradiskal injections of either hypertonic saline solution or contrast medium often give formerly symptom-free patients complaints similar to those that occur naturally (106, 108).

c. Radiating ruptures are known to occur in the posterior part of the annulus toward the area in which naked nerve endings are located (104, 105, 109, 110). Such single ruptures in the lumbar disk are first seen around the age of 25, when low back pain becomes clinically important. Various theories exist as to how these ruptures elicit pain (105, 110).

d. Only the disk shows the early changes that could account anatomically for the clinical syndromes that are seen at such a relatively young age. Similar changes in other structures in the region generally show up much later in life, and then generally only secondary to severe degeneration (111, 112).

This only indicates that the disk is pathoanatomically the weakest part of the motion segment, which would be expected considering that it has no blood supply. Changes that occur because of aging within the intervertebral disk can irritate structures outside the disk proper—for example, the vertebral bone, facet joints, sinuvertebral nerve, and even the neural contents of the spinal canal and the nerve root foramina.

Symptoms and Signs

The patient with nerve root compression caused by a herniated disk complains of low back pain that radiates to the buttock and from there down the leg, often into the foot. Paresthesiae can be present and represent the best clue to the level of nerve root involvement. Sensory and motor losses are noted to a varying degree. Signs of nerve root irritation on examination of the back and straight leg raising are usually present. The pain is augmented by coughing, sneezing, or straining (see Chapter 73 for a more detailed description of these symptoms and signs).

Diagnosis

The diagnosis of a herniated lumbar intervertebral disk is made on the basis of the history and physical examination. When the patient fails to respond to conservative therapy a surgical procedure might be indicated. Both anatomic and physiologic studies are helpful in planning the surgery and confirming the clinical diagnosis.

Electromyography is valuable in the assessment of disk disease. Fibrillation potentials and positive waves can localize the involved nerve root. Not all patients with a herniated disk have positive changes on EMG (Chapter 35). After laminectomy has been performed the paravertebral muscles are usually permanently denervated. The interpretation of a postoperative EMG is subtle.

Myelography has been the standard test for diagnosis of a herniated lumbar disk. Appropriate lateral, anteroposterior, and oblique views are required, and the conus must always be visualized. Far lateral herniations or midline herniations at the lumbosacral junction might not be detected. CT scanning adds to the diagnostic power of myelography and increases the amount of anatomic information that can be obtained; MRI, however, will soon render these two studies obsolete because it is risk-free and provides greater spatial and density resolution.

The interpretation of myelograms, CT scans, and MRI scans is more difficult in the previously operated patient. Comparison with prior studies is helpful but often does not resolve the issue of scar or recurrent disk herniation (113).

Treatment

CONSERVATIVE THERAPY. Little scientific evidence has been found to show that treatment for a herniated lumbar intervertebral disk alters the natural history of the disease. Surgery, in properly selected patients, shortens the period of disability but does not alter the long-term outcome (84). Because the vast majority of patients do not require an operation and get over their symptoms spontaneously, what should patients be told when this diagnosis has been established? The honest answer is that no program of rest or exercise has any demonstrated usefulness. Symptomatic relief should be provided with the least potent medication that is effective. The short-term use of narcotics is acceptable. Epidural blockade with local anesthetic or opioid provides dramatic symptomatic relief, but obviously this is not an appropriate long-term management strategy. Braces and corsets have not been found to be helpful. Traction only serves to keep the patient in bed, and prolonged bed rest is certainly deleterious. Our recommended management involves education of patients about the nature of their disease and the high likelihood of a favorable outcome. We recommend the avoidance of heavy lifting or strenuous exercise during the acute phase but encourage some activity and rapid return to full activity. Symptomatic relief with analgesic medications is appropriate. Muscle relaxants and sedative-hypnotics are usually not helpful.

SURGERY. The results of disk surgery to decompress lumbar nerve roots can be most dramatic and rewarding. Given proper indications, removal of a herniated disk to decompress the nerve root has been proven effective in speeding recovery from radicular nerve compression (114). In a controlled study Weber (82–84) found that 85% of patients were asymptomatic at 4 years following surgery and about 95% were asymptomatic by 10 years; those who received no surgical treatment, however, had similar success and recovery rates. The major accomplishment of back surgery was to speed recovery of function and reduce recurrences during the first 4 years.

Using the best surgical indications, early relief of symptoms can be obtained for 85 to 95% of patients, a success rate that seems to level out to about 85% after 4 years (55). But what if the workup shows that indications for surgery are not so definitive? Spangfort reported that the long-term success rate plunged to 38% if disk hernia was not found at surgery (57). Surgery thus carries a high cost:benefit ratio. Weber's long-term follow-up study (84) also indicated that patients with poor results, either surgically or nonsurgically, had mostly recovered physically after 10 years but continued to be socially devastated (84). Thus, when considering disk surgery to decompress nerve roots, surgical and nonsurgical combined results would probably be better if too few patients were operated on rather than too many. Correct technical performance of disk surgery is as critical as the decision making. The importance of proper decision making and surgical precision cannot be overemphasized when the poor success rates from second, third, and fourth surgeries are considered—reported to be as low as 30, 15, and 5% respectively (115–117).

Failed Back Surgery Syndrome

A substantial number of patients have failed to return to normal activities and to lose their pain complaints after lumbar spine surgery (115). The magnitude of this problem is unclear but it is far greater than standard neurosurgery and orthopedics textbooks would lead the neophyte to believe. It is worthwhile to remember Finneson's (118) marvelous statement: "No matter how severe or intractable the pain, it can always be made worse by surgery." Although few seem to disagree on the indications for surgery, considerable evidence has shown that those indications are not always respected by the neurosurgeon or orthopedist (117, 119–121).

Epidemiology

The determination of the success rate of surgery for low back pain is complex, because no common outcome measure has been determined. In addition, long-term follow-up has not been the characteristic of most surgical reports. Finally, most studies do not provide population-based statistics and are subject to large selection biases. It has been estimated that the failure rate is in excess of 15% in the United States (115), but if return to the same occupation is used as the outcome measure the failure rate can be as high as 30% (122). The rate of reoperation for lumbar disk disease seems to be about 5%; whether this is an optimal rate is unclear (123). A significant percentage of patients who undergo lumbar diskectomy do not achieve what they and their surgeons agree to be a satisfactory result. It is probably more prudent to speak of "failed back surgery syndrome" than "failed back syndrome" when considering this issue.

Etiology

The three main causes of failed back surgery syndrome are incorrect diagnosis, improper or inadequate surgery, and complications of surgery or of diagnostic procedures. The first is probably the most important because neurosurgeons and orthopedists often overlook the role of environmental and affective factors in the genesis of pain behavior (Chapters 8 and 33). Most reports by these specialists have emphasized inaccurate diagnosis and inadequate surgery as the major causes of recurrent pain and disability. The following differential diagnoses should be considered in the analysis of recurrent low back pain (115, 124, 125): flabby back; pseudomeningocele; diskitis; transaponeurotic fat herniation; trauma; arthritis; fusion pseudoarthrosis, fusion osteomyelitis, or fusion stenosis; spinal instability; ruptured disk at another level; psychologic or environmental factors; epidural scar; degenerative disk disease; facet syndrome; muscle spasm; trigger point pain; spinal stenosis; neoplasm; osteoporosis; radiculitis; and retained disk fragment.

INCORRECT DIAGNOSIS. Most failed back surgery syndrome patients are ascribed to another surgeon's poor patient selection criteria. Long and colleagues found that only one-third of patients seen for chronic low back pain following surgery met reasonable criteria for their initial operation (89, 121). Because the prior operation(s) cannot be undone, treating physicians can only curse their predecessors, but this does not resolve the current problem. Finneson (118) has stated that "the single most striking factor influencing the outcome of surgery is poor patient selection prior to the initial operative procedure." Various studies have identified some factors that make a patient a poor candidate for surgery; these are relevant whether one is considering a first or subsequent operation (118, 120, 121, 126). Indeed, psychologic evaluation seems more predictive of the outcome of surgery than the diagnostic studies or surgical findings.

IMPROPER OR INADEQUATE SURGERY. When the patient fails to respond to an operation and seeks help elsewhere, both the patient and the new physician suspect that the problem has been caused by the former surgeon's errors in the operating room. Although this is possible it is rarely the case. When the patient's examination fails to reveal significant neurologic or mechanical signs it is even less probable that operative misadventure was the cause of the patient's present complaints. The assessment of this diagnostic possibility requires that the treating physician obtain complete medical records to determine the patient's preoperative and postoperative status, review the relevant diagnostic studies, and be absolutely certain that the pain complaints and neurologic findings are ascribable to a pathologic process that was not adequately addressed by the prior surgeon. A good initial response to surgery that has lasted months or years followed by a recurrence of symptoms might indicate the development of a new pathologic process. This temporal course has a greater likelihood of the patient having a favorable response to further surgery than the patient who showed no improvement after the initial operation.

The use of CT scanning and MRI has led to a clearer understanding of the relationships between disk rupture, nerve root compression, and spinal stenosis (127). Some treatment failures occur because the involved nerve root was not adequately decompressed as a result of the lateral disk protrusion or stenosis going unrecognized.

COMPLICATIONS OF SURGERY OR DIAGNOSTIC STUDIES. All surgical procedures and invasive diagnostic studies can result in complications that perpetuate the patient's pain complaints and often add to the neurologic abnormalities. Careful studies are required to identify preventable complications. One of the most disabling complications is arachnoiditis, which seems to be less common since the use of oil-based myelography has been replaced by the use of water-soluble media, CT scanning, and MRI (128). Surgical trauma, infection, inflammation, and bleeding can also lead to arachnoiditis (Chapter 73). Not every patient with the pathologic changes typical of arachnoiditis has low back pain, so much has yet to be learned about who hurts and who does not.

Spinal surgery can result in damage to the nerves, dura, joints, and muscles, all of which can cause continued pain. A detailed history and appropriate diagnostic studies are required to identify such damage; CT scanning, MRI, and electrodiagnostic studies are often helpful (Chapter 35).

Treatment

The patient who has not been relieved of symptoms after low back surgery requires meticulous assessment. Clinical observations must discriminate the symptoms and signs of physical disease from those of psychologic distress and illness behavior (25). The physician must not allow the decision-making process to be swayed by the duration or intensity of the patient's complaints or by the failure of prior conservative management. The outcome of subsequent surgery depends on the accuracy of diagnosis of a lesion that can be successfully treated by surgery.

The workup commences with a detailed history and physical examination (Chapter 31). All relevant reports of previous surgery and diagnostic studies must also be scrutinized. When diagnostic tests have not been done since the last operation, or if new signs and symptoms are present, additional diagnostic studies are indicated. All diagnostic studies have risks and costs, however, and reinforce the belief held by many patients that the pain and disability are caused by some internal broken part. In addition, the relentless repetition of diagnostic studies can increase illness behavior.

Frequently anatomic and physiologic abnormalities are revealed by the physical examination and diagnostic studies. The question is not their existence, however, but how they relate to the patient's current symptoms and whether they are amenable to surgical treatment. If surgery is performed, careful attention to excellence should eliminate the possibility of future surgery being necessary to correct overlooked pathology or postoperative complications.

Several studies have shown that fusion is not an effective procedure for the treatment of failed back surgery syndrome unless major instability can be demonstrated (117, 123, 125, 129, 130). Repairing a pseudoarthrosis also yields disappointing results. Some have advocated a wide decompression and fusion as the operation of choice for the failed back surgery syndrome, but evidence of support for this viewpoint is tenuous.

The patient with a failed back surgery syndrome is usually a prototypic chronic pain patient who deserves the most thorough evaluation before further surgery. A comprehensive multidisciplinary evaluation in a pain center is a good starting point; careful orthopedic and neurosurgical consultation should be included in this assessment. A trial of behavioral and physical management should precede any surgical therapy unless the most dramatic and clear-cut indications for surgery are present. Only the presence of a cauda equina syndrome creates a mandatory need for surgical exploration. The role of other measures, such as injection of local anesthetics and steroids, manipulation, and electrical stimulation, is not clear. The administration of long-term analgesic or sedative-hypnotic medications rarely resolves the patient's complaints.

The failed back surgery syndrome is an iatrogenic disease; the goal should be prevention, not salvage. The patient who fails to respond to a surgical procedure has a far worse course than the natural history of low back pain.

Spondylolisthesis

Spondylolisthesis is the anterior slippage of one vertebral body forward onto the adjacent vertebra. Spondylolisthesis has many forms, but the most common is the isthmic lytic type secondary to spondylolysis.

Epidemiology

The reported incidence of spondylolysthesis is 6 to 10% except for the coastal Eskimos of Greenland, who have a reported incidence of 40% (53, 131–133). Approximately 3% of those with spondylolysis eventually develop spondylolisthesis, most slips measuring less than 25%. Slips tend to occur by the age of 18, and only in the few slips of more than 25% does progression occur during adulthood. Adult progression is rare.

Etiology

The common precursor of spondylolisthesis is spondylolysis, a break in the pars interarticularis and the posterior elements of the vertebral segment between the superior and inferior articular facets. Its cause is unknown but is probably traumatic. Laboratory studies have shown that spondylolysis can be caused by both flexion and extension (134, 135). Another indirect proof of a traumatic or biomechanical element is that spondylolysis is common in top gymnasts, with an incidence of up to 50 to 60% in gymnasts from the United States, Japan, and Bulgaria (136, 137). It also occurs commonly in athletes who participate in other strenuous sports (138). A 40% chance exists of an offspring having the disorder if the parent does, but the specific genetic expression has not yet been elucidated. Spondylolysis has not been found in newborns, and its incidence seems to increase with age. Five percent of the population have spondylosis at age 7, 6% at age 15, and approximately 6% at age 60, indicating that it is probably a problem of susceptibility to trauma during growth.

Symptoms and Signs

Typical symptoms of spondylolisthesis seem to depend on the age of onset and severity. In question is whether those with grade I slips have a higher incidence of back discomfort than the 80 to 85% of adults in the general population who do not have spondylolisthesis. Symptoms can include both low back and leg pain, especially in those with severe spondylolisthesis. These patients usually have increased lordosis, commonly walk with an antalgic gait, and have tightness of the hamstrings, which can produce radiculopathy. The nerve roots at or below the level of the slip can be irritated by spondylolisthesis or by the hypertrophic scarring at the break in the pars interarticularis (139). The L5 level is involved in 95% of cases of spondylolisthesis, with 2 to 3% of cases at L4; patients with involvement above the L3 level are rarely seen.

Diagnosis

Patients who have many findings on physical examination might not have any symptoms or might have some other explanation for their back pain. Careful diagnostic assessment is required, because most people with spondylolisthesis are asymptomatic.

Treatment

The conservative treatment of spondylolisthesis is the same as for all back problems. First, symptoms are controlled by decreasing mechanical stress on the spine and then measures are taken to restore function. A lumbosacral corset or brace is commonly used, followed by an aggressive physical therapy program. If a patient does not respond, has a severe slip of more than 50%, or meets radiographic criteria of possible instability, spinal fusion and its 4 to 12 months of convalescence can be considered.

Postulated Causes of Symptoms from the Lumbar Spine

The common dilemma of patients with back symptoms but no objective abnormalities has prompted many theories as to which areas of the spine cause symptoms. To date these hypotheses have not been measurably associated with a pattern of discomfort, have not been vertified with special tests, and have not been documented by a measurable response to specific treatment. For example, it is not uncommon for patients to obtain some relief after injection of different anatomic areas. Because 30% of those in the general population are placebo responders and have a diminution of symptoms for a short period of time, even with the injection of saline solution, it can be difficult to evaluate treatment efficacy and presumed pathophysiology.

Lumbar Instability

Etiology and Pathophysiology

The diagnosis of instability has markedly increased in popularity, especially among orthopedic surgeons (140, 141). A major factor promoting the use of this term is the controversy about the clinical effectiveness of lumbar fusion. Texts on back pain list a wide variety of symptoms and signs under the heading of "lumbar motion and stability" (6, 142, 143), but the diagnosis has yet to be definitively defined (5). Many attempts have been made to develop radiographic criteria and to provide reliable measures for evaluating instability.

Major textbooks describe how instability caused by fracture and traumatic dislocation jeopardizes the neural elements of the spine. Gross instability, however, does not produce a significant diagnostic dilemma. This section is concerned with other causes of instability, including degenerative conditions, postoperative problems, and spondylolisthesis.

DEGENERATIVE CONDITIONS. Degenerative spondylolisthesis rarely occurs before 40 years of age unless a major traumatic event has occurred. It is a variation of the normal aging process. Increased mobility seems to occur during the degenerative process, as verified by laboratory studies (144–147). Traction spurs are seen in early degenerative joint disease and are usually asymptomatic. Some have suggested that traction spurs increase the susceptibility to external forces and the likelihood of the back becoming symptomatic (148, 149).

Using laboratory data, Kirkaldy-Willis and Farfan (150) hypothetically divided the degenerative process of the spine into three stages—a temporary dysfunction phase, an unstable phase, and a stabilization phase, which leads to the stiffer spine that is part of a normal progression during adulthood. This type of developmental degenerative instability is commonly seen at the first motion segment above an area of surgical or congenital fusion at which motion forces are concentrated. The most common type of developmental instability occurs after a previous operation, such as laminectomy, and is related to facetectomy, vigorous diskectomy, or surgery at multiple levels involving removal of the laminae and posterior disruption with excessive muscle stripping.

SPONDYLOLISTHESIS. The greatest confusion centers around spondylolisthesis (from *Spondylo*, vertebra and *olisthanein*, to slip), which might result in instability. One vertebral body is positioned forward in its relationship to the vertebra below, which does not necessarily mean that it is unstable at the time of evaluation but that some motion had to occur to allow it to slip to that level. Spondylolisthesis and "abnormal motion" are not synonymous.

Comparing the flexion to the extension view also allows an evaluation of the rotatory angulation of one vertebra in relation to the adjacent vertebra through its particular motion segment. Instability can be ruled out with less than 4 mm of translation of one vertebra in relationship to the other, or with 11° or less angulation of one motion segment compared to other motion segments. Not all patients with this much motion, however, are symptomatic.

Scoliosis

Epidemiology and Etiology

Opinion varies on how to treat adult patients with back pain caused by scoliosis (151–153). Long-term studies of cases of untreated scoliosis, in which more than 90% of the original patients were followed for more than 30 years, did not reveal severe low back pain to be a major complaint (154, 155).

Kostuik's review of a series of radiographs from patients with kidney problems showed that the incidence of back pain in patients with 15 to 20° of lumbar scoliosis did not exceed that expected in the general population of those without scoliosis (156). Kostuick did find, however, that pain was more severe and lasted longer in patients with lumbar scoliosis, but found no correlation between thoracic and lumbar curvature. Furthermore, no correlation was found between scoliosis and pain in the few patients with lumbar scoliosis who had been awarded disability benefits, or in older patients 60 to 70 years of age in whom scoliosis could develop de novo (153, 157). One correlation with low back pain was found in patients with thoracolumbar scoliosis who had been fused at the L4 and L5 levels. Retrolisthesis was commonly found at the area of the lowest vertebra fused (158). It has been reported, though, that more severe pain syndromes occur in patients with lumbar scoliosis with severe rotatory subluxation of the spine with degenerative changes (157). Patients with painful scoliosis tend to be middle-aged patients with lumbar scoliosis or adults who have had previous surgery. In such patients the pain tends to be local and nonradiating and in older patients the symptoms are similar to those of instability and spinal stenosis, which can develop from scoliosis (159–161). Back pain seems to be no more common in patients with scoliosis than in those without.

Symptoms and Signs

The symptoms and signs are similar to those in people who have straight spines without increased curvature. The pain is usually localized to the back and does not radiate. Progressive curvature is characterized by loss of height, which can be more apparent to the patient than the actual increased curvature of the spine.

Treatment

Pain associated with scoliosis requires almost the same conservative treatment as any other back problem—that is, symptom control through the decrease of mechanical stress on the back augmented with analgesics and physical restoration. The emphasis should be on activities that do not overstress the back but that help to build endurance and stamina. According to controlled studies, stamina is a key to reducing the frequency and severity of any future back problems. Fusion is occasionally indicated for symptom control.

Isolated Disk Resorption and Canal Stenosis

Crock has described a new clinical entity: rapidly increasing disk degeneration, occurring particularly in middle-aged women who have complained of severe back pain over several years' time, and with increasing leg involvement (162). This degeneration usually occurs at the L5–S1 level. Treatment is controversial in this rare entity. No fusion is necessary because the disk has almost disappeared, and surgical therapy should be based on documented neural compression rather than on findings in the disk space.

Lordosis

Another area of controversy regarding pain and spinal posture focuses on the extent of lordosis (hyperlordosis or hypolordosis). *Hyperlordosis* is commonly thought to be related to increased lower back symptoms and is even the basis for elaborate physical treatment programs, but a correlation between lordotic posture and low back pain has never been documented. Exercises are no more effective in reducing lordosis than an attempt to change the shape and size of the nose by pressing on it three times a day. Epidemiologic studies have indicated that up to 80° of lumbar lordosis does not seem to be associated with an increased susceptibility to back pain (5).

On the other hand, a sharp kyphotic deformity in the lumbar spine exceeding 30° (*hypolordosis*) usually results from trauma and causes increased low back symptoms. Furthermore, Scheuermann's disease, which causes a developmental decrease in lumbar lordosis, increases the incidence of incapacitating back pain (163–164). Both these findings have heightened awareness of a relationship between decreased lumbar lordosis and back pain. Hypolordosis can be defined as less than 20° of angulation measured from the top of the sacrum to the top of the L1 vertebra. Patients seem to be more susceptible to back discomfort during activities that are stressful to the spine. Why patients who lack normal lordosis tend to have back pain is unknown, and no effective treatment has been described. Patients with Scheuermann's disease (changes involving two or more lumbar vertebrae or involving the thoracolumbar junction with wedging of two or more vertebrae and the presence of Schmorl's nodules), should probably be advised to avoid occupations involving heavy manual labor.

General Disorders or Nonregional Causes of Low Back Pain

Arthritides

Approximately 1% of patients with low back pain have been found to have inflammatory arthritides (165–166). These are described in Chapter 20, so only the highlights as they relate to low back pain are discussed here. The term "seronegative spondyloarthropathies," which refers to the lack of serum rheumatoid agglutinin, discriminates these conditions from rheumatoid arthritis. Four conditions, all associated with the presence of HLA-B27 antigen, can lead to low back pain: ankylosing spondylitis, Reiter's syndrome, psoriatic spondylitis, and colitic spondylitis. These disorders all have familial tendencies, so, because symptoms can precede radiologically observable changes, it is important to obtain a thorough family history.

Ankylosing spondylitis is most common in young men. Symptoms are relentlessly progressive, are worse on awakening, and improve with activity. Pain and joint stiffness are present. Diagnosis is aided by radiographs of the sacroiliac joints, and CT scanning can be more helpful. Characteristic changes in the spine are also usually present. An elevated erythrocyte sedimentation rate, positive HLA-B27, normocytic anemia, and an elevated alkaline phosphatase level are usually noted. The typical patient is a man under 40 years of age who reports progressive low back pain and stiffness without a specific antecedent, and whose symptoms are worse on awakening than later in the day. The other seronegative spondylopathies do not produce unique low back symptoms but are associated with various systemic diseases.

Treatment should emphasize programs to maintain posture and flexibility; NSAIDs can alleviate symptoms. Only a small percentage of these patients need spinal surgery. Occult fractures must be considered when sudden new pain develops.

Tumor

Neoplastic bone lesions of the spine in the adult can be separated into two major groups according to the age of the patient. Lesions in those in the younger group (about 21 to 50 years old) seem to be carryovers from the preadolescent period and are commonly benign, whereas lesions in those in the older age group (over 50 years old) tend to be malignant. Bone tumors cause some unique technical problems in the spine, but their behavior and microscopic appearance are similar to those of osseous lesions in other parts of the body.

Symptoms and Signs

Night pain, fever, a palpable mass, or a combination of these, are the usual presenting symptoms in patients with spinal neoplasms. The involved segment is often tender to palpation. The symptoms can be related to bony involvement, pressure on neurologic or vascular elements, or an inherent property of lesions such as aneurysmal bone cyst or hemangioma or of Paget's disease (167). Tumor or infection should be suspected if low back pain is nonmechanical and persistent and responds poorly to rest.

Sometimes patients report a need to walk the floor at night to relieve the intensity of their pain (166). Tumor and infection must be considered in any patient in whom weight loss, fever, chills, significant neurologic involvement, or atypical blood or urine test are present.

Diagnosis

The clinical approach to tumors of the spine is similar to that for other bone tumors. Generally, the differential diagnosis can be made by radiography, consideration of the patient's age, the area in which the lesion is located (anterior or posterior elements of the spine), the density of the lesion (increased density indicates ivory vertebra, whereas lytic appearance implies multiple myeloma), the type of deformity (expansion if found in aneurysmal bone cyst, osteoblastoma, or Paget's disease), and the host reaction

(disappearing bones with diffuse margins signal giant cell tumor, whereas well-demarcated lesions suggest osteoid osteoma (Fig. 71-16).

In young adults bone tumors have been found to have a statistically greater affinity for the posterior elements (168). Most bone tumors are aneurysmal bone cysts, osteoid osteomas, or osteoblastomas. Osteoid osteomas are commonly associated with painful scoliosis but aneurysmal bone cysts and osteoblastomas are more likely to be expansile and destructive in nature (168–170). Osteoid osteoma and osteoblastoma are most unusual in the anterior elements but aneurysmal bone cyst is reported in the vertebral body in 40% of all patients (169). Hemangioma, with its usual loculated striated appearance, is the most frequently encountered tumor in the vertebral bodies of young adults (171). Giant cell tumor involving the vertebral body can also occur during young adulthood; it is usually lytic in nature and benign, unless recurrence follows previous treatment (168). Most spinal tumors in young adults are classified as benign but approximately 1% of osteogenic sarcomas involve the spine, and even Ewing's sarcoma can have a spinal origin (168, 172).

In those in the older age group, the area of the vertebra in which the tumor occurs is a less helpful clue. After the age of 50 metastatic lesions comprise most of the tumorous processes in the spine, as in

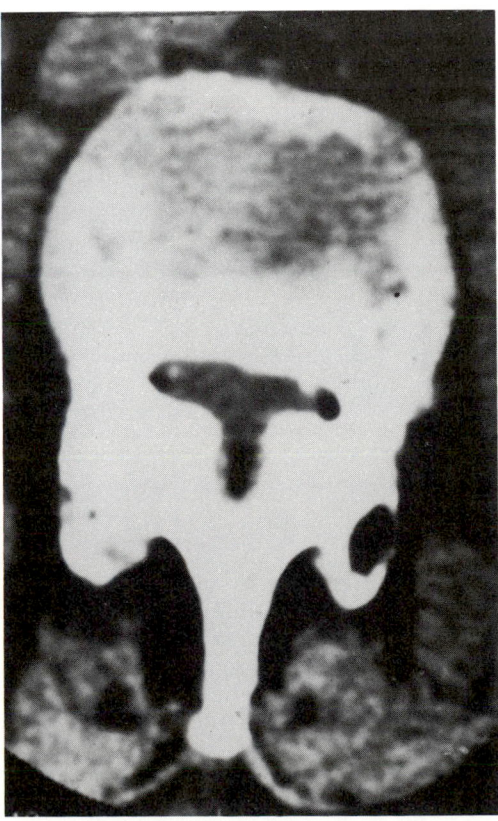

Fig. 71-16. CT scan showing severe spinal stenosis secondary to Paget's disease in a patient with chronic low back pain that increased dramatically with exercise. The trefoil spinal canal compromises both roots exiting at this level and those traveling caudally.

other parts of the body. Although the primary source of the spinal tumor is not always found it usually is the lung, breast, prostate, thyroid, gastrointestinal tract, kidney, or female reproductive tract. Whenever a metastatic tumor is suspected multiple myeloma must also be considered. Primary hematologic tumors, such as reticulum cell sarcoma, lymphoma, and leukemia, frequently cause bone destruction. Although these lesions are usually most noticeable in the vertebral body, the posterior element is commonly involved.

One particular entity, ivory vertebra, should heighten suspicion of one of four entities: Paget's disease, cancer of the prostate, carcinomatosis, or Hodgkin's disease. Although most cases of prostate cancer involve osteoblastic lesions, other metastatic tumors can also express themselves in an osteoblastic pattern. Prostatic cancer and other metastatic carcinomatoses must be considered in the differential diagnosis of ivory vertebra. If the ivory vertebra is enlarged Paget's disease should be suspected (173). Of unknown etiology, Paget's disease is characterized by excessive bone resorption followed by excessive bone formation. It is seen as a lytic lesion early in the course of the disease and as a blastic lesion later (174). Paget's disease can degenerate into sarcoma, commonly heralded by increased pain.

Chondrosarcoma occurs in a small percentage of patients and also has a poor prognosis in the spine (175). A chordoma can appear anywhere in the spinal column but is most commonly reported at the ends of the spine, at the occipitocervical and sacrococcygeal junctions. This slow-growing malignant tumor, believed to originate in the cell remnants of the notochord, constitutes about 15% of all tumors of the sacrococcygeal area. Although it can appear at any time it is usually first diagnosed in middle age (171). Metastasis usually occurs late through the bloodstream, if at all. Extirpation is usually not possible by the general orthopedic surgeon because of the location of this tumor. Recently, however, Stener and Gunterberg (176) demonstrated that extended radical approaches of these tumors in the spine and sacrum are feasible in highly skilled hands, and can prevent recurrences.

Treatment

The treatment of neoplasms of the spine must be based on a knowledge of the histology of the lesion. Some tumors are treatable by radiation therapy, some by chemotherapy, and some by surgical excision. Combinations of these measures are frequently useful. The speed at which diagnosis and treatment are undertaken is related to the presence or absence of signs of spinal cord and nerve root dysfunction. Unless the neoplasm is sensitive to radiation or chemotherapy, compression of neural elements usually indicates urgent surgical decompression. If the tumor has created an unstable vertebral column consideration should be given to fusion at the time of surgical decompression. Back pain is often most efficiently alleviated by surgical decompression of nerve roots.

Infection

Bone lesions can also result from infectious processes, most commonly bacterial or fungal. Vertebral bacterial infection usually involves the end-plates of the adjacent disk spaces and occurs early in the disease process. By contrast mycobacterial infections (tuberculosis) usually involve the end-plate and disk space late in the course of the disease.

Diagnosis

Early loss of disk space height is a good indicator of bacterial infection, whereas significant bone involvement without adjacent space destruction tends to implicate tuberculous infection. Tuberculous infection usually involves two or three vertebral bodies without diminishing the disk space (177) and is more commonly associated with gibbus formation and paraplegia (178). The diagnosis of infection of the bones of the spine is based on the presence of fever, pain, and local tenderness associated with systemic and local signs of infection. Bone scanning, radiography, CT scanning, and MRI are helpful in localizing the pathology. Symptoms can precede discernible changes in the bone.

Treatment

Treatment involves accurate diagnosis, either by determination of the organism from blood culture or by needle biopsy of the involved area. Antibiotics and immobilization usually suffice, but drainage of large abscesses might be required. Spread of infection to the epidural space can constitute a surgical emergency.

The pain associated with spinal infection can be severe. Immobilization is an important step in pain management. Narcotics and muscle relaxants are useful initially until the infection has been controlled by antibiotics and movement reduced by immobilization. The pain usually does not require long-term narcotics, because it generally abates with appropriate treatment. A sudden increase of pain can indicate a pathologic fracture or spread of infection to epidural tissues, and mandates careful observation.

Metabolic Bone Disease

Metabolic bone disease is relatively common. Its incidence increases with age and is associated with various metabolic diseases originating in other organs. The only common metabolic disease of bone related to low back pain is osteoporosis. Osteoporosis and related disorders can be classified as follows:

a. Common forms without known cause: idiopathic (juvenile and adult); severe postmenopausal (type I); age-related (type II)

b. Disorders in which osteoporosis is a common feature and pathogenesis is only partially understood: hypogonadism; hyperadrenocorticism; thyrotoxicosis; malabsorption; scurvy; calcium deficiency; immobilization; heparin administration (chronic); systemic mastocytosis; hypophosphatasia (adult); other bone diseases

c. As a feature of an inherited disorder of connective tissue

d. Disorders in which osteoporosis is sometimes an associated feature but pathogenesis is not understood: rheumatoid arthritis; malnutrition; alcoholism; epilepsy; diabetes; chronic obstructive pulmonary disease; Menkes' syndrome.

Symptoms and Signs

The major clinical manifestation of osteoporosis is fracture of a vertebra or of the wrist, hip, humerus, or tibia. Pain in the back and deformity of the spine are common; pain is secondary to fracture and is usually acute in onset. It can be localized to the back or radiate around the flank. Pain is usually relieved by bed rest and usually abates in a month or two.

Neurologic signs are rare. Tenderness over the fractured vertebra is common. Most patients are pain-free between acute fractures. The course and frequency of fractures vary.

Diagnosis

The bones of the skeleton and of the spine in particular show a reduced mineral density on plain radiographs. Biconcave deformity of the vertebral bodies is typical, and collapse of the upper lumbar vertebral bodies is common. Because plain radiographs might not be diagnostic until more than 30% of the bone mass has been lost, single or dual photon absorptionometry or other sophisticated studies are more powerful. Most blood tests are normal with uncomplicated osteoporosis. Decreased bone mass is typical in postmenopausal women so it can be difficult to establish the diagnosis of osteoporosis as a disease state. It is important to rule out neoplasia as a cause of the osteoporosis.

Treatment

Osteoporosis is a group of disease states with presumably different causes and prognoses. No therapy has been found to be ideal and claims for the efficacy of various regimens are often dubious. In general, bed rest and analgesic medications are helpful for an acute vertebral fracture secondary to osteoporosis. Epidural or paravertebral nerve blocks can be useful if the pain is debilitating and not controllable by oral medications (Chapter 94). Progressive activities should be initiated as soon as the pain has been sufficiently relieved. Estrogens have a mildly beneficial effect in postmenopausal women and androgens are useful in hypogonadal men, but no data support the use of a combination of these hormones. Oral calcium supplements and vitamin D appear to be beneficial.

Other Metabolic Bone Disorders

Rickets and osteomalacia rarely lead to low back pain, although most patients have diffuse complaints of pain in the major weight-bearing joints. Vitamin D is the usual treatment. Secondary degenerative joint disease can follow childhood rickets or long-standing osteomalacia.

Nerve Disorders

The neurologic aspects of low back pain are discussed in Chapter 73. Any disease process involving the spine can secondarily involve the lumbar nerve

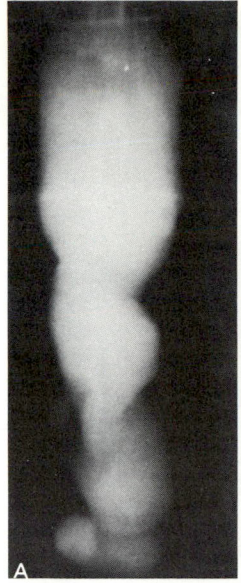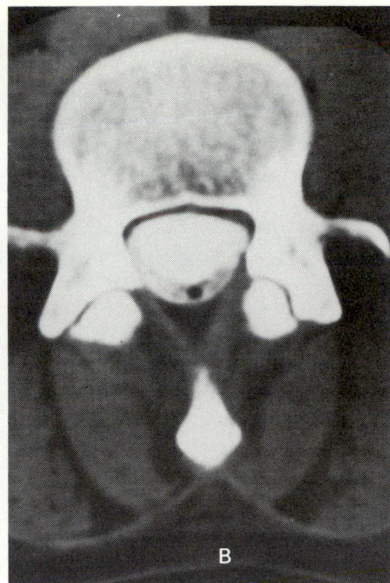

FIG. 71-17. Arachnoiditis in a patient who had chronic low back pain after several operations and myelograms. **A.** Myelogram, anteroposterior view. The irregular contour of the thecal sac and loss of root sleeve filling are typical of arachnoiditis. **B.** CT scan. Note the matting of roots posteriorly.

roots or the conus medullaris if it is at the upper lumbar level. Primary lesions of the spinal cord and nerves can cause low back pain. The patient who has had multiple myelograms and surgeries for low back pain is highly likely to develop a new source of back pain that is iatrogenic—arachnoiditis, perineural fibrosis, or both (Fig. 71-17). Neoplasms of the conus and cauda equina also present as low back pain and must be considered in the differential diagnosis.

Muscle Disorders

The muscles in the back are subjected to significant biomechanical forces while protecting themselves, the neurologic elements, and the bones and joints that they span. It should not be thought that the muscles of the back are less susceptible to injury than other muscles in the body. Injuries can occur to different parts of a muscular unit, such as the origin or insertion, the tendon, the musculotendinous complex, the belly of the muscle, and the adjacent bursa. Unfortunately, current technologic limitations hinder our ability to evaluate muscles in the spine, and such injuries cannot be verified or demonstrated directly. Furthermore, recovery from back pain does not seem to parallel what is known about muscle injury recovery in other parts of the body. For example, a major hamstring injury usually requires rest for 3 to 10 days, followed by active treatment. Low-load high-repetition therapeutic exercises generally produce good results in 6 to 12 weeks. By contrast, most back injuries become asymptomatic much sooner.

Muscle Spasm

Muscular guarding, such as that seen with chronic back problems, is commonly termed a spasm and has not been well documented. Protective guarding occurs

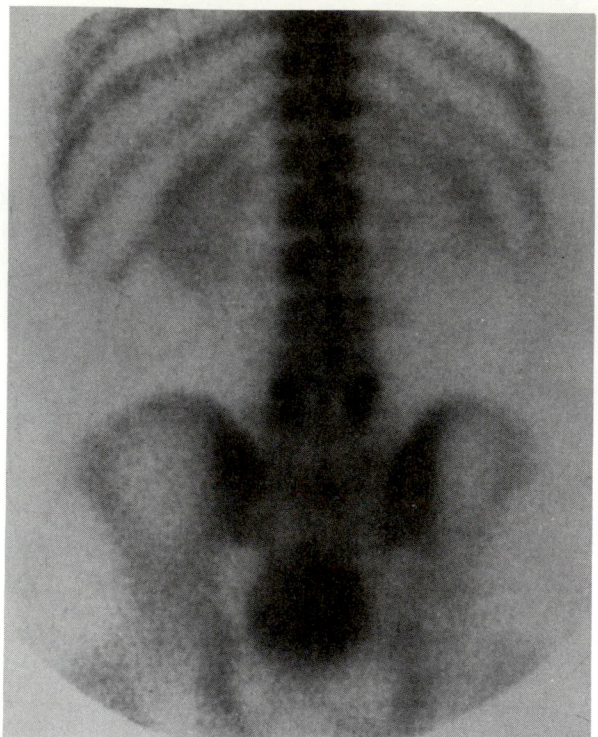

FIG. 71-18. ^{99m}Tc bone scan demonstrating increased uptake in the region of facet joints bilaterally at L4–L5. The patient had chronic low back pain; an attempted fusion resulted in pseudoarthrosis.

when a muscle is protecting itself or any part of the motion segment or adjacent neural elements that it spans (180).

Fatigue

Discomfort is well accepted as a common aspect of muscular fatigue. Exercising a muscle until it fatigues causes symptoms not only in the area of the muscle but also in areas near its origin, and produces nonspecific symptoms. For instance, doing rapid toe raises on one foot until the gastrocnemius-soleus fatigues causes calf discomfort. If the exercise is continued the discomfort eventually ascends the hamstring to the gluteal area. The phenomenon of muscle fatigue has been described as the cause of tension headaches and can also be associated with back pain.

Other changes also occur with muscle fatigue. The ability of the muscle to generate tension is reduced and the response to stimulus or command is slowed. Thus, muscular fatigue might not only be a source of potential aching but can also increase the risk of structural damage in the muscle itself or in the segment that it is attempting to protect, and whose motion it reinforces and guides.

Myofascial Pain Syndromes

Localized regions of tenderness (trigger points) with radiation of pain can be found in the superficial and deep muscles of the low back. Patients often report pain relief when these areas are infiltrated with local anesthetic solutions or stimulated by "dry needling." Pain can radiate from such regions into the buttocks and legs, and myofascial pain must be considered in the differential diagnosis of patients with low back pain who do not have any specific neurologic abnormalities (Chapters 21 and 72).

Disorders of the Facet Joints

Although the facet joints are commonly invoked as a cause of low back pain, the evidence to support this concept is not convincing. It is known that the joints are innervated and are subjected to degenerative changes in association with almost any type of pathology that can occur in the lumbar spine (181, 182) (Fig. 71-18). Changes in the morphology of these joints increase with age.

Facet joint syndromes are discussed in Chapter 72 and are only briefly considered here.

Referred Low Back Pain Syndromes

Pain can be referred to the low back from diseases of the abdominal and pelvic viscera and major blood vessels (Chapters 28, 60, and 61). A detailed history usually indicates that the pain is gradually progressive and is not related to position, activity, or time of day, nor is the pain altered during the examination of the back. Neurologic findings are absent. Appropriate examination of the abdomen and pelvis generally reveals signs of local pathology; CT scanning is particularly helpful in identifying mass lesions in the abdomen and pelvis.

E. SUMMARY OF APPROACHES TO TREATMENT OF LOW BACK PAIN

Because low back pain usually has a probable and not a definite cause, treatment cannot be based on a simple cookbook approach. We must be practical and reasonable about pursuing a diagnosis before beginning treatment. For example, in those in the 20 to 50 age group, our pathoanatomic diagnostic rate is only 12 to 15% and more than 50% of our patients are symptom-free after 1 month. Thus, without a history of significant trauma, tumor, or infection, we can usually begin treatment to control symptoms and attain physi-

cal restoration for 1 month before carrying out radiography or specific studies. Diagnoses can be made in more that 60% of cases involving children, and tumor and infection become more common after the age of 50, so we should be more aggressive in our diagnostic approaches to both children and the elderly.

Every patient we see with acute or chronic complaints deserves practical, effective treatment measures that are not debilitating or time-wasting. These have three goals: symptom control; restoration of function; and resolution of bone, joint, nerve, or general health problems that can block recovery or hinder restorative activities needed to maintain their general health and back health in the future.

Symptom Control

The mainstay of symptom control is a decrease in the mechanical stress on the spine. No magic bullet is available that allows the patient to perform strenuous activities. Medications are only an adjunct to taking the edge off of symptoms while decreasing the mechanical back stress of performing activities for physical restoration. After 3 days symptoms are commonly controlled by a combination of acetaminophen, NSAIDs, and aspirin.

Considerable information is available about the biomechanics of different body positions and activities and their relationship to symptoms (5). Most of this information comes from the work of Nachemson and colleagues (145, 153, 154), whose 30 years of research have provided a scientific basis for controlling symptoms in patients with back problems (Chapter 70). By inserting pressure-sensitive needles into the lumbar disks they quantified stress on the lumbar spine and obtained results that still represent the most scientific objective comparison between different positions and activities. If the intradiskal pressure measurement (ipm) of standing is rated at 100%, then the ipm of bed rest while lying on the side is 75% and the biomechanical stress of the sitting position is given as an ipm of 140 to 180% of standing. Walking or even jogging and jumping up and down does not mechanically stress the back as much as sitting. Thus, we can make the following recommendations to our patients for control of symptoms:

a. If incapacitated by back symptoms, avoid sitting (ipm—140 to 180% of standing).
b. Begin walking as soon as possible to limit debilitating effects of inactivity (ipm = 100% of standing).
c. Eat in the standing position and avoid weight gain.

Patients who do not have a specific diagnosis must understand that controlling the mechanical stress on the back seems to be the key to limiting back symptoms. Mild analgesics are an adjunct that cannot take the place of controlled activity for keeping symptoms under control. No study has yet found any pain medication to be significantly better than plain Tylenol, including Tylenol with 60 mg of codeine, for treatment of back symptoms preoperatively or postoperatively (4,183). Tylenol, NSAIDs, and aspirin are usually successful in providing some relief of the discomfort. Even for patients with the most severe symptoms, we can usually recommend nonopioid analgesics after the first several days.

If patients want to use other measures such as heat, cold, or massage, which they feel to have been helpful before, they can administer these at home. The advantages include cost savings and greater convenience, and reinforcing illness behavior through the institutional use of these unproven treatments is also avoided.

Restoration of Function

At least four controlled studies have indicated that building stamina is the major component of future protection from back problems or of speeding recovery (18, 85–87). No controlled studies have been reported for other treatment strategies. In addition, endurance training has been proven to provide many advantages for general health and can be performed with activities that exert much less stress on the spine than unproven strengthening or stretching techniques. Endurance training requires little in regard to special equipment, thus improving its availability to the patient without the extra expense of travel or special facilities.

Restoration of function should begin as soon as possible. Because sitting is so much more stressful on the back than many activities that can be recommended for maintaining or building endurance, the patient can usually begin endurance exercises rather soon.

Even patients with the most severe symptoms can be started on standing and walking activities by the third day after onset of symptoms. We have found that a 20- to 30-minute walk for every 3 hours of lying down during the day is well tolerated by almost all patients. As soon as patients succumb to the social pressures of sitting (e.g., as when eating), we recommend activities that place minimal load on the spine that are less stressful, including speed walking, upright arm-supported stationary cycling, swimming, and even jogging. Speed walking and stationary biking are most commonly recommended, whereas jogging is usually reserved for younger patients or those with less pain. Jogging should usually be done for 20 minutes; other activities should be done for 30 to 40 minutes at an intensity that maintains the heart rate above 130 beats/minute for those under the age of 40 and 120 beats/minute for those 40 years of age or older. Patients should be encouraged to exercise a minimum of 5 times/week until asymptomatic or for a maximum of 6 weeks before starting activities that are more stressful.

The basis for symptom control and physical restoration is the provision of guidelines for safely increasing the overall activity level. The most important aspect of a treatment program is education; as physicians we offer information and patients make the decisions. Such information can significantly influence patients' views about their health, their expectations for recovery, and their fears about how the environment can influence their symptoms. An educational program should stress the good news, the expectation of recovery, and also convey the facts about back pain: that 85% of adults have back problems by the age of 50 that interfere with work or recreation, and that as many as 30% of those between 30 and 50 have back discomfort at the time they are surveyed. Most patients understand that by 50 their backs won't tolerate stressful activities without some discomfort, and can also be reminded that only about 20% of patients associate the onset of their back problem with an accident, injury, or unusual activity that occurred within the previous 12 hours.

Patients also need a better understanding of what the health care system can offer. They must be made aware of the difference between proven effective and unproven treatment methods and warned about medicine's contributions to continuing back pain disability: excessive bed rest, medications, and surgery. Patients should be informed that standing is a reasonable resting position for the back and that bed rest can weaken muscle effectiveness twice as fast as maximal muscle power can be restored; in addition they could rapidly and perhaps permanently lose bone density in their spine.

Patients must realize that medications can be habit-forming and dangerous and that inappropriate surgery not only might not relieve their symptoms but also make them worse. Physicians should emphasize that operations on the back for the most part are attempts to speed up recovery rather than to ensure a better long-term outlook. Patients have to understand that the major factor in symptom control is control of the mechanical stress on the spine. For example, while lifting a heavy object, patients should be taught to keep it close to the abdomen.

Special studies are often necessary to determine reasons for delayed recovery. Guidelines for chronic care can be directed toward patients who continue to have symptoms despite no obvious bone, joint, nerve, or general health explanation. When complaints are chronic psychosocial problems must be suspected. These patients still seek care for their back, however, not just advice about how to live with it. They do not need unproven treatment methods

dispensed to keep them busy or given with the misguided notion of keeping their mind off their pain. Chronic back pain patients still deserve the best that can be provided in the form of proven effective treatment methods. Clinical guidelines include time-contingent treatment and visits, but office visits or medications should not become the reward for increasing complaints. Such patients need clearly stated expectations regarding the natural history of back pain, its expected course, and the response to treatment.

Any complications that occur because of performing endurance activities which are less stressful than sitting are unusual, as is a continued lack of response to treatment. Let these patients know that they deserve the best treatment available and discourage reliance on the latest fad that they might have heard or read about. Remind them about the poor results of surgery for chronic back problems. Most importantly, patients need to understand that no passive treatments for chronic back problems are available; only patients themselves can carry out treatment. Physicians must always be aware of the problems of overresting and overmedicating, which are commonly associated with depression. Patients should constantly be reminded about the realities of back pain and that the goal is to tolerate activities of daily living; regaining the back's youthful condition is usually unreasonable and impossible. It is pointless to blame someone else for the problem, because almost everyone is limited by back problems before the age of 50.

REFERENCES

1. Kelsey, J.L., et al.: The impact of musculoskeletal disorders on the population of the United States. J. Bone Joint Surg. [Am.], 61:959, 1979.
2. Gibson, E.S., Martin, R.H., and Terry, C.W.: Incidence of low back pain and pre-placement x-ray screening. J. Occup. Med., 22:515, 1980.
3. Svensson, H.O., and Andersson, G.B.J.: Low back pain in 40- 47-year-old men: Frequency of occurrence and impact on medical services. Scan. J. Rehabil. Med., 14:47, 1982.
4. Spitzer, W.O.: Scientific approach to the assessment and management of activity-related spinal disorders. Spine, 12(Suppl. 1):1, 1987.
5. Nachemson, A.L., and Bigos, S.: The low back. In Adult Orthopedics, Vol. 2. Edited by J. Cruess and W.R.J. Rennie. New York, Churchill Livingstone, 1984, pp. 843–937.
6. Rothman, R.H., and Simeone, J.A.: The Spine. Philadelphia, W.B. Saunders, 1975.
7. MacNab, I.: Back Ache. Baltimore, Williams & Wilkins, 1977.
8. Jayson, M.I.V.: The Lumbar Spine and Back Pain. 2nd Ed., Kent, England, Medical Ltd., 1980.
9. Taylor, H., and Curran, N.M.: The Nuprin Pain Report. New York, Louis Harris & Associates, 1985.
10. Holbrook, T.L., et al.: The Frequency of Occurrence, Impact and Cost of Selected Musculoskeletal Conditions in the United States. Chicago, American Academy of Orthopedic Surgeons, 1984.
11. Von Korff, M., et al.: An epidemiologic comparison of pain complaints. Pain, 32:173, 1988.
12. Frymoyer, J.W., et al.: Risk factors in low back pain. J. Bone Joint Surg. [Am.], 65:213, 1983.
13. Deyo, R.A., and Tsui-Wu, Y.-J.: Descriptive epidemiology of low back pain and its related medical care in the United States. Spine, 12:264, 1987.
14. Nagi, S.Z., Riley, L.E., and Newby, L.G.: A social epidemiology of back pain in a general population. J. Chron. Dis., 26:769, 1973.

15. Hult, L.: The Munkfors investigation. Acta Orthop. Scand. [Suppl.], 16:1–76, 1954.
16. Hult, L.: Cervical dorsal and lumbar spine syndromes: A field investigation of a non-selected material of 1200 workers in different occupations with special reference to disc degeneration and so-called muscular rheumatism. Acta. Orthop. Scand. [Suppl.], 173:1–102, 1954.
17. Wood, P.H.N., and Badley, E.M.: Epidemiology of back pain. In The Lumbar Spine and Back Pain. Edited by M.J.V. Jayson. London, Pitman Medical, 1980, pp. 29–55.
18. Biering-Sorensen, F.: Low back trouble in a general population of 30-, 40-, 50-, and 60-year-old men and women: Study design, representativeness and basic results. Dan. Med. Bull., 29:289, 1982.
19. Gyntelberg, F.: One-year incidence of low back pain among male residents of Copenhagen aged 40–50. Dan. Med. Bull., 21:30, 1974.
20. Magora, A.: Investigation of the relation between low back pain and occupation. Ind. Med., 39:31, 1970.
21. Fahrni, W.H.: Conservative treatment of lumbar disc degeneration: Our primary responsibility. Orthop. Clin. North Am., 6:93, 1975.
22. Bremner, J.M., Lawrence, J.S., and Miall, W.E.: Degenerative joint disease in a Jamaican rural population. Ann. Rheum. Dis., 27:326, 1968.
23. Disability, Functional Limitation, and Health Insurance Coverage: 1984/1985. Current Population Reports, Household Economic Studies Series P-70, No. 8. Washington, DC, U.S. Department of Commerce, 1986.
24. Statistical Abstracts of the United States: Table 189:124, 1984.
25. Waddell, G.: A new clinical model for the treatment of low back pain. Spine, 12:632, 1987.
26. Andersson, G.B.J.: Epidemiologic aspects on low-back pain in industry. Spine, 6:53, 1981.
27. Cypress, B.K.: Characteristics of physician visits for back symptoms: A national perspective. Am. J. Pub. Health, 73:389, 1983.

28. Porkos, R.: Diagnosis-related groups using data from the National Hospital Discharge Survery: United States, 1981. Advance Data from Vital and Health Statistics, No. 98. Washington, DC, DHHS Publ. No. (PHS) 84-1250, July 20, 1984.
29. Bonica, J.J.: Pain research and therapy: Past status and future needs. In Pain, Discomfort and Humanitarian Care. Edited by L.K.Y. Ng, and J.J. Bonica. Amsterdam, Elsevier-North Holland, 1980, pp. 1–48.
30. Bauer, W.I.: Scope of industrial low back pain. In Industrial Low Back Pain. Edited by S.W. Wiesel, H.W. Feffer, and R.H. Rothman. Charlottesville, NC, Michie, 1985, pp. 1–35.
31. Rowe, M.L.: Low back pain in industry. A position paper. J. Occup. Med., 11:161, 1979.
32. Anderson, J.A.D.: Rheumatism in industry: A review. Br. J. Ind. Med., 28:103, 1971.
33. Benn, R.T., and Wood, P.H.N.: Pain in the back. Rheumatol. Rehabil., 14:121, 1975.
34. Lloyd, M.H., Gauld, S., and Soutar, C.A.: Epidemiologic study of back pain in miners and office workers. Spine, 11:136, 1986.
35. Magora, A.: Investigation of the relation between low back pain and occupation. Scand. J. Rehab. Med., 5:191, 1973.
36. Riihumaki, H.: Back pain and heavy physical work: A comparative study of concrete reinforcement workers and maintenance house painters. Br. J. Ind. Med., 42:226, 1985.
37. Klein, B.P., Jensen, R.C., and Sanderson, L.M.: Assessment of workers' compensation claims for back strains/sprains. J. Occup. Med., 26:443, 1984.
38. Volinn, E., et al.: When back pain becomes disabling: A regional analysis. Pain, 33:33, 1988.
39. Spengler, D.M., et al.: Back injuries in industry: A retrospective study. Spine, 11:241, 1986.
40. Leavitt, S.S., Johnston, T.L., and Beyer, R.D.: The process of recovery: Patterns in industrial back injury: 1. Costs and other quantitative measures of effort. Ind. Med. Surg., 40:7, 1971.
41. Antonakes, J.A.: Claims costs of back pain. Best's Review, 82:36, 1985.
42. Snook, S.H.: The costs of back pain in industry. State of the art review. Spine, 2:1, 1987.
43. Osterweis, M., Klerman, A., and Mechanic, D.: Pain and Disability. National Academy Press, DC Washington, 1987.
44. Bonica, J.J.: The Management of Pain. Philadelphia, Lea & Febiger, 1953, pp. 1176–1204.
45. Nachemson, A.L., and Anderson, G.B.J.: Classification of low-back pain. Scand. J. Work Environ. Health, 8:134, 1982.
46. Deyo, R.A., Diehl, A.K., and Rosenthal, M.: How many days of bed rest for acute low back pain? N. Engl. J. Med., 315:1064, 1986.
47. Schober, P.: Lendenwirbelsaule und Kreuzschmerzen. Munch. Med. Wochenschr., 84:336, 1937.
48. Newton, D.R.L.: Discussion of the clinical and radiological aspects of sacro-iliac disease. Proc. R. Soc. Med., 50:850, 1957.
49. Waddell, G., et al.: Non-organic physical signs in low back pain. Spine, 5:117, 1980.
50. Magora, A., and Schwartz, A.: Relation between the low back pain syndrome and x-ray findings. 1. Degenerative osteoarthritis. Scand. J. Rehabil. Med., 8:115, 1976.
51. Fullenlove, T.M., and Williams, A.J.: Comparative roentgen findings in symptomatic and asymptomatic backs. Radiology, 63:572, 1957.
52. Magora, A., and Schwartz, A.: Relation between the low back pain and x-ray findings. 2. Transitional vertebra (mainly sacralization). Scand. J. Rehabil. Med., 10:135, 1978.
53. Magora, A., and Schwartz, A.: Relation between low back pain and x-ray changes. 4. Lysis and olisthesis. Scand. J. Rehabil. Med., 12:47, 1980.
54. Spengler, D.M., and Freeman, C.W.: Patient seclection for lumbar discectomy. Spine, 4:129, 1979.
55. Nachemson, A.: The lumbar spine—an orthopaedic challenge. Spine, 1:59, 1976.
56. Irstam, L.: Lumbar myelography with Amipaque. Spine, 3:70, 1978.
57. Spangfort, E.V.: The lumbar disc herniation: A computer-aided analysis of 2054 operations. Acta Orthop. Scand. [Suppl.], 142:1, 1972.
58. Hitselberger, W.E., and Witten, R.M.: Abnormalities in myelograms in asyptomatic patients. J. Neurosurg., 28:204, 1968.
59. Hirsch, C.: An attempt to diagnose the level of disc lesion clinically by disc puncture. Acta Orthop. Scand., 18:132, 1948.
60. Simmons, E.H., and Segil, C.M.: An evaluation of discography in the localization of symptomatic levels in discogenic disease of the spine. Clin. Orthop., 108:57, 1975.
61. Gresham, J.L., and Miller, R.: Evaluation of the lumbar spine by discography. Clin. Orthop., 67:29, 1969.
62. Holt, E.P.: The question of lumbar discography. J. Bone Joint Surg. [Am.], 50:720, 1968.
63. Gargano, F.P., Meyer, J.D., and Sheldon, J.J.: Transfemoral ascending lumbar catheterization of the epidural veins in lumbar disc disease. Radiology, 111:329, 1974.
64. Theron, J., et al.: Lumbar phlebography by catheterization of the lateral sacral and ascending lumbar veins with abdominal compression. Neuroradiology, 11:175, 1976.
65. Burton, C.V.: Computed tomographic scanning and the lumbar spine. Part I: Economic and historic review. Spine, 4:353, 1979.
66. Burton, C.V., et al.: Computed tomographic scanning and the lumbar spine. Part II: Clinical considerations. Spine, 4:356, 1979.
67. Gargano, F.P.: Transverse axial tomography of the spine. Crit. Rev. Clin. Radiol. Nucl. Med., 8:279, 1976.
68. Porter, R.W., Wicks, M., and Ottewell, D.: Measurement of the spinal canal by diagnostic ultrasound. J. Bone Joint Surg. [Br.], 60:481, 1978.
69. Galasko, C.S.B.: The pathological basis for skeletal scintigraphy. J. Bone Joint Surg. [Br.], 57:353, 1975.
70. Patton, D.D., and Woolfenden, J.M.: Radionuclide bone scanning in diseases of the spine. Radiol. Clin. North Am., 15:177, 1977.
71. Mooney, V., and Robertson, J.: The facet syndrome. Clin. Orthop., 115:149, 1976.
72. Dennis, M.D., et al.: The Minnesota Multiphasic Personality Inventory: General guidelines to its use and interpretation in orthopaedics. Clin. Orthop., 150:125, 1980.
73. Fordyce, W.E.: Behavioral Methods for Chronic Back Pain and Illness. St. Louis, C.V. Mosby, 1976.
74. Wiltse, L.L., and Rocchio, P.D.: Preoperative psychological test as predictors of success of chemonucleolysis in the treatment of low-back syndrome. J. Bone Joint Surg. [Am.], 57:478, 1975.
75. Pheasant, H.D., et al.: The MMPI as a predictor of outcome in low-back surgery. Spine, 4:78, 1979.
76. Ransford, A.O., Cairns, D., and Mooney, V.: The pain drawing as an aid to psychological evaluation of the patient with low back pain. Spine, 1:127, 1976.
77. Mixter, W.J., and Barr, J.S.: Rupture of the intervertebral disc with involvement of the spinal canal. N. Engl. J. Med., 211:210, 1934.
78. Fordyce, W., et al.: Acute back pain: A control group comparison of behavioral vs. traditional management modes. J. Behav. Med., 9:127, 1986.
79. Linton, S.: The relationship between activity and chronic back pain. Pain, 21:289, 1985.
80. Fordyce, W., et al.: Pain complaint—exercise performance relationship in chronic pain. Pain, 10:311, 1981.
81. Berquist-Ullman, M., and Larsson, U.: Acute low back pain in industry (thesis). Acta Orthop. Scand. [Suppl.], 170:1–150, 1977.
82. Weber, H.: Lumbar disc herniation. Part I. J. Oslo City Hosp., 28:33, 1978.
83. Weber, H.: Lumbar disc herniation. Part II. J. Oslo City Hosp., 28:89, 1978.
84. Weber, H.: Lumbar disc herniation. A controlled, prospective study with ten years of observation. Spine, 8:131, 1983.
85. Cady, L.D., et al.: Strength and fitness and subsequent back injuries in firefighters. J. Occup. Med., 21:269, 1979.
86. Choler, U., et al.: Ony y ryggen: Forsok med vardprogram for patienter med lumbala smarttillstand. Stockholm, SPRI, Rapport 188, 1985.
87. Cady, L.D.: Program for screening health and physical fitness of firefighters. J. Occup. Med., 27:110, 1985.
88. Dzioba, R.B., Neville, C., and Doxey, C.: A prospective investigation into the orthopaedic and psychologic predictors of outcome of first lumbar surgery following industrial injury. Spine, 9:614, 1984.
89. Long, D.M., et al.: Clinical features of the failed-back syndrome. J. Neurosurgery, 69:61, 1988.
90. Wilson, C.B.: Significance of the small lumbar canal: Cauda equina compression syndromes due to spondylosis. J. Neurosurg., 3:499, 1969.

91. Newman, P.H.: Stenosis of the lumbar spine in spondylolisthesis. Clin. Orthop., *115*:116, 1976.
92. Ramani, P.S.: Variation of the size of the bony lumbar canal in patients with prolapse of the lumbar intervertebral discs. Clin. Radiol., *27*:301, 1976.
93. McIvor, G.W.D., and Kirkaldy-Willis, W.H.: Pathological and myelographic changes in the major types of lumbar spinal stenosis. Clin. Orthop., *115*:72, 1976.
94. Morris, L.: Water-soluble contrast myelography in spinal canal stenosis and nerve entrapment. Clin. Orthop., *115*:49, 1976.
95. Sortland, O., Mangaes, B., and Hauge, I.: Functional myelography with metrizamide in the diagnosis of lumbar spinal stenosis. Acta Radiol. [Diagn.] (Stockh.), *355*:42, 1977.
96. Porter, W.: Measurement of the spinal canal by diagnostic ultrasound. *In* The Lumbar Spine and Back Pain. 2nd Ed. Edited by M.I.V. Jayson. Kent, England, Medical Ltd., 1980, pp. 231–245.
97. Larson, S.J.: Somatosensory evoked potentials in lumbar stenosis (abstr.). Presented to The International Society for the Study of the Lumbar Spine. Toronto, 1982.
98. Dilke, T.F.W., Burry, H.C., and Grahame, R.: Extradural corticosteroid injection in the management of lumbar nerve root compression. Br. Med. J., *2*:635, 1973.
99. Snoek, W., Weber, H., and Jorgensen, B.: Double-blind evaluation of extra-dural methyl prednisolone for herniated lumbar disc. Acta Orthop. Scand., *48*:635, 1977.
100. Cauchoix, J., Benoist, M., and Chassaing, V.: Degenerative spondylolisthesis. Clin. Orthop., *115*:122, 1976.
101. Tile, M., et al.: Spinal stenosis. Results of treatment. Clin. Orthop., *115*:104, 1976.
102. Wiltse, L.L., Kirkaldy-Willis, W.H., and McIvor, G.W.D.: The treatment of spinal stenosis. Clin. Orthop., *115*:83, 1976.
103. Urban, J.P.G., et al.: Nutrition of the intervertebral disc. An in vivo study of solute transport. Clin. Orthop., *129*:101, 1977.
104. Hirsch, C., and Schajowicz, F.: Studies on structural changes in the lumbar annulus fibrosus. Acta Orthop. Scand., *22*:184, 1953.
105. Hirsch, C., Ingelmark, B.E., and Miller, M.: The anatomical basis for low back pain. Acta Orthop. Scand., *33*:1, 1963.
106. Valkenburg, H.A., and Haanen, H.C.N.: The epidemiology of low back pain. *In* Symposium on Idiopathic Low Back Pain. Edited by A.A. White and S.L. Gordon. St. Louis, C.V. Mosby, 1982, pp. 9–22.
107. White, A.A., and Panjabi, M.M.: Clinical Biomechanics of the Spine. Philadelphia, J.B. Lippincott, 1978.
108. Holt, E.P.: The question of lumbar discography. J. Bone Joint Surg. [Am.], *50*:720, 1968.
109. Jayson, M.I.V., and Barks, J.S.: Structural changes in the intervertebral disc. Ann. Rheum. Dis., *32*:10, 1973.
110. Rothman, R.H.: The pathophysiology of disc degeneration. Clin. Neurosurg., *20*:174, 1973.
111. Ramani, P.S., Perry, R.H., and Tomlinson, B.E.: Role of ligamentum flavum in the symptomatology of prolapsed lumbar intervertebral discs. J. Neurol. Neurosurg. Psychiatry, *38*:550, 1975.
112. Rissanen, P.M.: The surgical anatomy and pathology of the supraspinous and interspinous ligaments of the lumbar spine with special reference to ligament ruptures. Acta Orthop. Scand. [Suppl.], *46*:1–100, 1960.
113. Blaser, S.I., et al.: Disks, degeneration, and MRI. MRI Decisions, *2*:18, 1988.
114. Hakelius, A.: Prognosis in sciatica. A clinical follow-up of surgical and non-surgical treatment. Acta Orthop. Scand. [Suppl.], *129*:1, 1970.
115. Pheasant, H.C., and Dyck, P.: Failed lumbar disc surgery. Clin. Orthop., *184*:93, 1982.
116. Rothman, R.H., and Booth, R.: Failures of spinal fusion. Orthop. Clin. North Am., *6*:299, 1975.
117. Waddell, G., et al.: Failed lumbar disc surgery and repeat surgery following industrial injuries. J. Bone Joint Surg. [Am.], *61*:120, 1979.
118. Finneson, B.E.: A lumbar disc surgery predictive score card. Spine, *3*:186, 1978.
119. Loeser, J.D.: Low back pain. *In* Pain. Edited by J.J. Bonica. New York, Raven Press, 1980, pp. 363–372.
120. Spengler, D.M., et al.: Low back pain following multiple lumbar spine procedures. Spine, *4*:356, 1980.
121. Fager, C.A., and Freidberg, S.R.: Analysis of failures and poor results of lumbar spine surgery. Spine, *5*:87, 1980.
122. Salenius, P., and Laurent, L.E.: Results of operative treatment of lumbar disk herniation. Acta Orthop. Scand., *48*:630, 1977.
123. Cauchoix, J., Ficat, C., and Girard, B.: Repeat surgery after disc excision. Spine, *3*:256, 1978.
124. Wilkinson, H.A.: The Failed Back Syndrome. Philadelphia, Harper & Row, 1983.
125. Lehmann, T.R., and LaRocca, H.S.: Repeat lumbar surgery. Spine, *6*:615, 1981.
126. Blumetti, A.E., and Modesti, L.M.: Psychological predictors of success or failure of surgical intervention for intractable back pain. *In* Advances in Pain Research and Therapy. Vol. 1. Edited by J.J. Bonica and D. Albe-Fessard. New York, Raven Press, 1976, pp. 323–326.
127. Burton, C.V., et al.: Causes of failure of surgery on the lumbar spine. Clin. Orthop., *157*:191, 1981.
128. Burton, C.V.: Lumbosacral arachnoiditis. Spine, *3*:24, 1978.
129. Frymoyer, J.W., et al.: Disc excision and spine fusion in the management of lumbar disc disease. Spine, *3*:1, 1978.
130. Frymoyer, J.W., et al.: Failed lumbar disc surgery requiring second operation. Spine, *3*:7, 1978.
131. Bleck, E.E.: Spondylolisthesis: Acquired, congenital or developmental. Dev. Med. Child Neurol., *16*:680, 1974.
132. Kalbak, K., Andersen, S., and Winckler, F.: Incidence of spondylolisthesis among natives of Greenland over the age of 40 years. Ugeskr Laeger, *134*:2532, 1972.
133. Kono, S., et al.: A study on the etiology of spondylolysis with reference to athletic activities. J. Jpn. Orthop. Assoc., *49*:125, 1975.
134. Farfan, H.F., Osteria, V., and Lamy, C.: The mechanical etiology of spondylolysis and spondylolisthesis. Clin. Orthop., *117*:40, 1976.
135. Troup, J.D.G.: Mechanical factors in spondylolisthesis and spondylolysis. Clin. Orthop., *117*:59, 1976.
136. Jackson, D.W., Wiltse, L.L., and Cirincione, R.J.: Spondylolysis in the female gymnast. Clin. Orthop., *117*:68, 1976.
137. Kotani, P.T., et al.: Studies of spondylolysis found among weight lifters. Med. Sport (Roma), *25*:154, 1972.
138. Russin, L.A., and Sheldon, J.: Spinal stenosis. Report of series and long term follow-up. Clin. Orthop., *115*:101, 1976.
139. Davis, I.S., and Bailey, R.W.: Spondylolisthesis. Indications for lumbar nerve root decompression and operative technique. Clin. Orthop., *117*:129, 1976.
140. Knutsson, F.: The instability associated with disc degeneration in the lumbar spine. Acta Radiol., *25*:593, 1944.
141. Symposium: The role of spine fusion for low-back pain. Presented at The International Society for the Study of the Lumbar Spine. New Orleans, May 27, 1980. Spine, *6*:277, 1981.
142. Finneson, B.E.: Low Back Pain. Philadelphia, J.B. Lippincott, 1973.
143. Helfet, A.J., and Grubel, L.D.M.: Disorders of the Lumbar Spine. Philadelphia, J.B. Lippincott, 1978.
144. Berkson, M.H., Nachemson, A.L., and Schultz, A.B.: Mechanical properties of human lumbar spine segments. Part II: Responses in compression and shear; influence of gross morphology. J. Biomech. Eng., *101*:53, 1979.
145. Nachemson, A.L., Schultz, A.B., and Berkson, M.H.: Mechanical properties of human lumbar spine motion segments. Influences of age, sex, disc level, and degeneration. Spine, *4*:1, 1979.
146. Posner, I., et al.: A biomechanical analysis of the clinical stability of the lumbar and lumbosacral spine. Spine, *7*:374, 1982.
147. Schultz, A., et al.: Mechanical properties of human lumbar spine motion segments. Part I: Responses in flexion, extension, lateral bending, and torsion. J. Biomech. Eng., *101*:46, 1979.
148. Kirkaldy-Willis, W.H., et al.: Pathology and pathogenesis of lumbar spondylosis and stenosis. Spine, *3*:319, 1978.
149. Ruge, D., and Wiltse, L.L.: Spinal Disorders. Philadelphia, Lea & Febiger, 1977.
150. Kirkaldy-Willis, W.H., and Farfan, H.F.: Instability of the lumbar spine. Clin. Orthop., *165*:110, 1982.
151. Kostuik, J.P., Israel, J., and Hall, J.E.: Scoliosis surgery in adults. Clin. Orthop., *93*:225, 1973.
152. Leatherman, K.D., and Dickson, R.A.: Spinal deformity in adults. Changing concepts. J. Bone Surg. [Am.], *58*:729, 1976.
153. Nachemson, A.: Adult scoliosis and back pain. Spine, *4*:513, 1979.
154. Nachemson, A.: A long-term follow-up study of non-treated scoliosis. Acta Orthop. Scand., *39*:446, 1968.

155. Nilsonne, U., and Lundgren, K.D.: Long-term prognosis in idiopathic scoliosis. Acta Orthop. Scand., *39*:456, 1968.
156. Kostuik, J.P., and Bentivoglo, J.: The incidence of low-back pain in adult scoliosis. Spine, *6*:268, 1981.
157. Robin, G., et al.: Scoliosis in the elderly: A follow-up study. Spine, *7*:355, 1982.
158. Nachemson, A., and Cochran, T.P.: Anatomic changes and function of the lumbar spine in patients five or more years after conventional treatment for idiopathic scoliosis. Orthop. Trans., *6*:53, 1982.
159. Benner, B., and Ehni, G.: Degenerative lumbar scoliosis. Spine, *4*:548, 1979.
160. Bjure, J., and Nachemson, A.: Non-treated scoliosis. Clin. Orthop., *93*:44, 1973.
161. Edgar, M.A., and Mehta, M.: Back pain assessment from a long-term follow-up of operated and unoperated patients with adolescent idiopathic scoliosis (abstr.). Spine, *4*:519, 1979.
162. Crock, H.V.: Isolated lumbar disk resorption as a cause of nerve root canal stenosis. Clin. Orthop., *115*:109, 1976.
163. Sorensen, K.H.: Scheuermann's Juvenile Kyphosis. Clinical Appearances, Radiography, Aetiology, and Prognosis. Copenhagen, Munksgaard, 1964, p. 7.
164. Stoddard, A., and Osborne, J.F.: Scheuermann's disease or spinal osteochondrosis: Its frequency and relationship with spondylosis. J. Bone Joint Surg. [Br.], *61*:56, 1979.
165. Kellgren, J.H.: The epidemiology of rheumatic diseases. Ann. Rheum. Dis., *23*:109, 1964.
166. Quinet, R.J., and Hadler, N.M.: Diagnosis and treatment of backache. Semin. Arthritis Rheum., *8*:261, 1979.
167. Jaffe, H.L.: Tumors and Tumorous Conditions of the Bones and Joints. Philadelphia, Lea & Febiger, 1958.
168. Horal, J.: The clinical appearance of low back disorders in the city of Gothenburg, Sweden. Acta Orthop. Scand. [Suppl.], *118*:1, 1969.
169. Hay, M.C., Patterson, D.O., and Taylor, T.K.F.: Aneurysmal bone cysts of the spine. J. Bone Joint Surg. [Br.], *60*:406, 1978.
170. Keim, H.A.: Osteoid osteoma as a cause of scoliosis. J. Bone Joint Surg. [Am.], *57*:159, 1975.
171. Luck, J.V., and Monsen, C.G.: Bone tumors and tumor-like lesions of vertebrae. *In* Spinal Disorders: Diagnosis and Treatment. Edited by D. Ruge and L.L. Wiltse. Philadelphia, Lea & Febiger, 1977.
172. Dahlin, D.C.: Bone Tumors, General Aspects and Data on 3987 Cases. 3rd Ed. Springfield, IL, Charles C Thomas, 1978.
173. Harris, D.J., and Fornasier, V.L.: An ivory vertebra. Clin. Orthop., *136*:173, 1978.
174. Jaffe, H.L.: Metabolic, Degenerative, and Inflammatory Diseases of Bones and Joints. Philadelphia, Lea & Febiger, 1972.
175. Camins, M.B., et al.: Chondrosarcoma of the spine. Spine, *3*:202, 1978.
176. Stener, B., and Gunterberg, B.: High amputation of the sacrum for extirpation of tumors. Principles and technique. Spine, *3*:351, 1978.
177. Hodgson, A.R., Wong, W., and Yau, A.: X-ray Appearances of Tuberculosis of the Spine. Springfield, IL, Charles C Thomas, 1969.
178. Hodgson, A.R., Skinsnes, O.K., and Leong, C.Y.: The pathogenesis of Pott's paraplegia. J. Bone Joint Surg. [Am.], *49*:1147, 1967.
179. Krane, S.M., and Holick, M.F.: Metabolic bone disease. *In* Principles of Internal Medicine. 11th Ed. Edited by E. Braunwald et al. New York, McGraw-Hill, 1987, pp. 1889–1899.
180. Frymoyer, J.W., et al.: Disc excision and spine fusion in the management of lumbar disc disease. A minimum ten-year follow-up. Spine, *3*:1, 1978.
181. Fairbank, J.C.T., et al.: Apophyseal joint injection of local anesthetic as a diagnostic aid in primary low-back pain syndromes. Spine, *6*:598, 1981.
182. Wyke, B.: The neurology of low back pain. *In* The Lumbar Spine and Back Pain. 2nd Ed. Edited by M.I.V. Jayson. London, Pitman Medical, 1980, pp. 265–339.
183. Weber, H., and Aasand, G.: The effect of phenylbutazone on patients with acute lumbago-sciatica: A double-blind trial. J. Oslo City Hosp., *30*:69, 1980.

72 · OTHER PAINFUL DISORDERS OF THE LOW BACK

JOHN J. BONICA

with contributions by ANDERS E. SOLA

THIS chapter discusses a number of painful disorders of the low back not discussed in the preceding chapter and also provides further discussion of some conditions mentioned only briefly there. It consists of five major sections: A, Low Back Pain Caused by Muscle Dysfunction; B, Painful Disorders of Joints and Ligaments; C, Low Back Pain Primarily of Psychologic Origin; D, Other Disorders That Cause Low Back Pain; and E, Multidisciplinary Approach to Diagnosis and Treatment of Low Back Pain. Because the evaluation of patients with low back pain is summarized in Chapter 70 and discussed in detail in Chapter 71, it is not considered here except to emphasize the critical importance of a thorough assessment to arrive at a correct diagnosis and to plan the most effective therapeutic strategy. This is important because 80 to 85% of patients with acute or chronic low back pain do not have objective evidence of neuropathic or skeletal pathology of the lumbosacral spine that can be proven to be the cause of the pain (1–3).

Chapter 71 emphasizes psychosocial and environmental factors as causes of chronic low back pain, but many patients can also develop chronic low back pain from improper therapy of conditions discussed in this chapter (4–7). Joints, ligaments, and arteries of muscles are richly endowed with unmyelinated and myelinated nociceptive afferents that can be activated by ischemia combined with stress or by inflammation or injury, so it would be surprising if pain did not arise from these structures when they are subjected to these processes. Rosomoff (8) noted that all disease processes that affect the low back must have associated soft tissue abnormalities because the protective covering offered by the muscles represents the bulk of the anatomy affected, and the continuity of bony structures and the forces of movement and maintenance depend heavily on the muscles and their attachments. When forces are applied to the bony spine or when anatomic changes occur that result in altered strength and characteristics, spinal stenosis, or injury, these forces must pass through the overlying soft tissue that binds the spine together as a functional unit. Abnormal stress or strain produces tissue injury, with consequent pain and hyperalgesia.

This chapter also presents evidence for the high prevalence of myofascial syndromes with TPs, muscle deficiency, and other types of muscle dysfunction, and of the favorable response to appropriate therapy. Unfortunately, some orthopedic authorities (9, 10) have referred to this large group of disorders as "idiopathic low back pain"—that is, "pain of spontaneous origin," the cause of which cannot be demonstrated.* Some have summarily denied that these conditions exist by stating that "such terms are the result of armchair speculation" (1, 10, 11). With few exceptions orthopedic surgeons, family physicians, and internists—the three groups that first see low back pain patients—have not obtained information from the available literature and have no experience in managing these conditions. Correctly diagnosed and treated early, patients with these conditions are not only promptly relieved of their pain, but enjoy restoration of normal function and can return to work sooner.

The format of this chapter is similar to other chapters in that each painful condition is discussed in regard to etiology, pathophysiology, symptoms and signs, diagnosis, and primary treatment. Chronic low back pain is a complex clinical problem, however, because of its various interrelated causes (e.g., physical, psychologic, behavioral, and psychosocial factors), so the last section of this chapter presents a brief discussion of the multidisciplinary approach to patients with chronic low back pain. Table 72-1 lists the causes of low back pain presented in this chapter. Sola provided information for the subsection on myofascial pain syndromes.

A. LOW BACK PAIN CAUSED BY MUSCLE DYSFUNCTION

Pain in the low back can be caused by acute or persistent muscle strain, muscle spasm provoked by direct injury to the muscle, reflex spasm consequent to visceral disease or vertebral fracture, or iatrogenic (postoperative) muscle spasm (4, 7). Other disorders of muscles that can cause acute or chronic pain include increased muscle tension resulting from emotional or psychologic disorders, muscle deficiency caused by disuse or nonuse of muscles, myofascial pain syndromes with trigger points (TPs), fibromyalgia, and muscle contractures (4–7, 12–15). These are discussed in Chapters 21 and 23 and elsewhere in this book, but they are considered here because of their importance in causing acute and chronic low back pain.

Muscle Spasm, Tension, and Deficiency

Painful Muscle Spasm (XXVII-6)

Muscle spasm is defined as sustained involuntary and usually painful contraction of a muscle that

---

*This term, long discarded and not currently used in the literature, really means that the health professional cannot make a correct diagnosis.

TABLE 72-1. Other Causes of Low Back Pain

A. Pain Caused by Dysfunction of Muscles
  1. Painful muscle spasm
  2. Postoperative muscle spasm
  3. Increased muscle tension
  4. Muscle deficiency (fatigue)
  5. Myofascial pain syndromes with TPs
  6. Fibromyalgia
  7. Chronic muscle contractures

B. Disorders of Joints, Ligaments, and Muscles
  1. Lumbosacral sprain or strain
  2. Sacroiliac sprain
  3. Zygapophyseal joint disorder (facet syndrome)

C. Pain Caused Primarily by Psychologic or Psychiatric Disease
  1. Psychologic stress-induced low back pain
  2. Premenstrual syndrome and low back pain
  3. Pain caused by environmental and learning factors
  4. Pain and psychiatric illness

D. Other Causes of Low Back Pain
  1. Aortoiliac stenosis (Leriche syndrome)
  2. Referred pain
     a. From pelvic visceral disease
     b. From disease of the colon
     c. From retroperitoneal disease
     d. From disease of the hip

cannot be alleviated by voluntary effort and that is usually caused by injury or disease (12). Spasm of paraspinal skeletal muscles of the low back is a major cause of low back pain; depending on the cause and rapidity of onset, pain can be sharp, severe, and well localized, or it can be dull and aching in quality, of mild to moderate severity, and somewhat diffuse (4, 7, 12). The pain is always aggravated by increased activity of affected muscles and is associated with deep and cutaneous tenderness and frequently with alteration of autonomic function.

Etiology and Pathophysiology

Spasm of striated (skeletal) muscles can be caused by acute macrotrauma or chronic microtrauma or it can be a reflex manifestation of neurologic, deep somatic, visceral, or psychologic disorders, or a combination of these. Severe reflex spasm of the back and abdominal muscles caused by vertebral fracture and consequent marked compression of the formed spinal nerves is an example of a neurologic disorder. Diseases of the viscera often cause reflex spasm of the skeletal muscle supplied by the spinal segments that also supply the diseased viscus. The role of psychologic stress in causing muscle spasm is discussed below.

Spasm of the paraspinal muscles has long been accepted as a cause of low back pain, but one study reported equivocal findings about the relationship between absolute lumbar paravertebral electromyographic (EMG) patterns and low back pain, especially during static postures such as standing (16). On the basis of these findings, some orthopedic surgeons and other physicians have disputed the hypothesis that spasm of the lumbar paravertebral muscles causes low back pain (1, 16). The Committee on Pain, Disability and Illness Behavior of the Institute of Medicine (17) and the Quebec Task Force on Spinal Disorders (18), however, in their comprehensive studies and reports, acknowledged spasm as a cause of low back pain and listed therapeutic modalities that are used to decrease or eliminate muscle spasm.

Fischer and Chang (19) carried out EMG monitoring of normal and spasmodic lumbar paravertebral muscles during a day-night cycle using continuous 24-hour recording. Nine patients with low back pain and unilateral or mostly one-sided palpable paraspinal muscle spasm and a control group of 12 participants without pain or palpable spasm were studied. The 9 patients had pain for 1 month to 25 years and had a diagnosis of low back sprain or myofascial syndrome following laminectomy. It was found that normal subjects without low back pain had no EMG activity in the lumbar paraspinal muscle during sleep. In patients with low back pain and palpable spasm, however, EMG activity on the predominant spastic side was 11.67 units (SD, 5.32) compared to 0.22 values (SD, 0.75) in control subjects. This study of a 24-hour continuous recording was the first to document muscle spasm under normal conditions in positions that were assumed by patients without any special instructions. In addition to confirming that normal muscles at rest produce no electrical activity, the main advantage of the 24-hour recording in patients with low back pain lies in documentation of high electrical activity during sleep, which completely eliminates any voluntary action or interference. Fischer and Chang (19) also noted that overactivity of spasmodic muscles occurred during the day and led to a relatively higher EMG output on the spasmodic side during movement as compared to the nonspasmodic side. This has important implications for management of patients with muscle spasm and pain, because it indicated that spasm can be aggravated by use of the involved muscle. Fischer and Chang concluded that failure to demonstrate EMG activity at rest in painful conditions that were called muscle spasm probably can be explained best by the absence of spasm and that the pain was a result of other disorders.

Ahern and associates (20) compared 40 chronic low back pain patients and 40 matched nonpatient controls using lumbar paravertebral EMG during mechanically stabilized static and dynamic postures. The two groups did not differ on absolute levels of EMG during quiet standing, but there was a significant difference for EMG patterns during dynamic postures. In addition, most patients did show the flexion-relaxation response or the expected pattern of EMG responses during trunk rotation, probably because of restricted range of motion, compensatory posture, or both. These findings provide further support for the biomechanical model of chronic pain.

Symptoms and Signs

In addition to the pain, which is frequently severe, untreated skeletal muscle spasm locks the patient into a vicious cycle of pain-induced increased muscle contraction, which in turn further increases the pain and severely limits movement. Consequently, the patient tends to assume and maintain whatever position feels most comfortable and exerts the least strain on the affected muscle (4). Although it is generally believed that such spasm has a protective function, there is impressive evidence that this vicious cycle can lead to nonuse of the limb and cause muscle deficiency, which is a frequent cause of chronic pain.

Diagnosis

Diagnosis is made through the history and physical examination, which should include careful palpation of the muscles and comparison to the contralateral

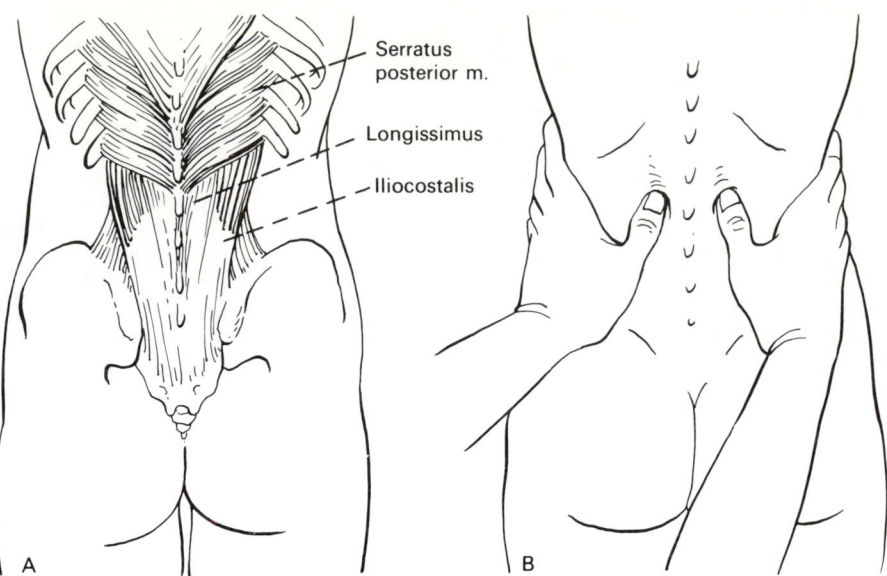

Serratus
posterior m.

Longissimus

Iliocostalis

A   B

Fig. 72-1. Method of palpating the lumbar paraspinal muscles to detect segments of muscle spasm or contracture.

side (Fig. 72-1). Unless the palpation is done carefully the muscle spasm can be missed. Fischer (21) has developed a tissue compliance meter (TCM) to permit clinicians to obtain objective, quantitative documentation of muscle spasm. The TCM is a hand-held mechanical instrument that measures the consistency (softness or firmness) of soft tissue. A 1-cm² rubber tip is pressed into the tissue to be assessed, and the force employed is monitored on an attached gauge while the depth of penetration of the rubber tip is recorded by a disk that slides up on the shaft of the force gauge. The depth of penetration per kilogram of force is known as the compliance of the tissue. Contraction of muscle increases the resistance (decreases compliance); this can be used not only for diagnosis, but also for determining the efficacy of treatment.

Treatment

In view of the above, it is essential to relieve the pain promptly and initiate "immediate controlled mobilization" after the pain is relieved, by one of the methods discussed on page 388 or by the use of ethyl chloride spray over the area of pain (4). The exercises are intended to restore elasticity and to increase the length and relaxation of the muscle. Kraus (4) and Fischer (12) also used electrical stimulation employing tetanizing and sinusoidal currents to relieve the muscle spasm. Kraus (4) suggested placing the electrode over the painful area and turning up the tetanizing current gradually until the affected muscle contracts adequately, but without discomfort, for 10 minutes, after which it is turned off. With the electrodes remaining in the same position, the sinusoidal current is gradually applied until muscle contraction is produced, and it is continued for 10 minutes. As mentioned in Chapter 21, Travell and Simons (5) use fluoromethane as a coolant spray whereas others use ice applied to the spastic muscle.

I believe that regional anesthesia is the most effective and fastest way of relieving excruciating pain caused by skeletal muscle spasm not relieved by more conservative measures. This can be achieved by infiltration of the spastic muscle with a dilute solution of a long-lasting local anesthetic (e.g., 0.125% bupivacaine) or by paravertebral block of the primary nerve(s) supplying the affected muscle. Continuous epidural analgesia with a combination of 0.125% bupivacaine and an opioid eliminates the spasm and pain within 5 to 10 minutes of the initial injection and can be sustained by continuous infusion. Most patients retain enough muscle power to carry out "prompt mobilization." Although some (4) have expressed the belief that local anesthetics produce general aftereffects, this does not occur if a proper volume of dilute solutions is injected into the muscle or around the nerve(s).

Postoperative Muscle Spasm

Severe excruciating pain follows major operations on the back and major joints (Chapters 7, 25, and 69). In this section I discuss the skeletal muscle spasm that follows surgery on the low back for herniated disk, and laminectomy for spinal stenosis or other pathologic processes. Because this is not discussed in orthopedic textbooks and no surveys have been published, I can only cite my own experiences with four back operations and interviews with about 450 others who have had such operations. These have led me to the firm conviction that the majority of patients who have had this type of surgery experience unexpected bouts of severe spasm, not only of the lumbar paraspinal muscles (particularly the segments of the erector spinae muscles), but also the gluteus maximus, medius, and minimus, piriformis, and upper thigh muscles. Rather perplexingly the reflex muscle spasm does not occur on the first or second day after surgery, but begins as soon as patients are ambulatory, perhaps on the second, third, or fourth postoperative day, because patients are usually receiving intramuscular or epidural opioids 1 or 2 days after surgery. The pain, which is sharp and searing in quality, occasionally with a burning component, can last from 2 to 3 minutes to as long as 10 minutes. The bouts of muscle spasm are triggered by movement of the trunk, especially the pelvis, although sometimes they occur while patients lie in bed.

Based on personal experience with this type of pain, which followed two laminectomies for spinal stenosis done 2 years apart, and also occurred after removal of herniated disks, the first between the two laminectomies and the second in 1988, I can attest to the severity and excruciating nature of this condition. Because I received continuous epidural opioids during the first 3 days, the bouts of muscle spasm began soon after the catheter was removed late on the third postoperative day and lasted until the sixth day of hospitalization, during which time I was ambulating and attempting to regain balance and strength. By the sixth postoperative day the intensity of the bouts of pain decreased and the intervals between them increased sufficiently for me to be discharged from the hospital. Soon after arrival home I began to resume desk work. After 15 minutes of sitting, however, severe bouts of pain and spasm returned, and despite 4 hours of bed rest, they increased to such a degree that it was necessary for an ambulance to return me to the hospital. The pain and spasm were controlled with large doses of diazepam. In Chapter 74 I describe severe spasm of the quadriceps muscles that produced excruciating pain following my last three hip procedures, which were done under general anesthesia. This phenomenon did not occur during my first eight hip surgeries, which were carried out with regional anesthesia that was continued for 48 to 72 hours postoperatively.

Mechanisms

The mechanisms of such abnormal reflex responses and of the associated pain are not known. Data from animal experiments and clinical observations, however, suggest that during back operations carried out with general anesthesia, a massive nociceptive input into the spinal cord occurs from noxious stimulation of afferents, particularly of the C fibers that supply periosteum, richly innervated joints, muscles, and structures around them. This massive afferent barrage produces sensitization (decrease in threshold), not only of peripheral nociceptors but also of dorsal horn neurons, interneurons, and anterior motoneurons (22, 23). Moreover, these operations entail severance or injury of small peripheral nerves, which generate a brief, maximal injury discharge that triggers prolonged spinal cord hyperexcitability (22, 24). This massive nociceptive input also produces a large expansion of the cutaneous receptive fields of the motoneurons (25) and a decrease in the mechanical threshold of these cutaneous fields. The input can convert spinal cord nociceptive-specific cells to cells that respond to light as well as to intense stimulation (wide dynamic range, WDR, neurons) (22, 26). This facilitation is triggered by the arrival of impulses in C fibers from the deeper tissue, but is sustained by an intrinsic spinal cord process (23). Consequently, tactile and proprioceptive afferent activity by non-noxious stimuli, such as touch or movement, causes intense activity of the anterior horn cells that produce the muscle

spasm. This, together with activation of dorsal horn WDR neurons, causes the excruciating pain. Once established, the prolonged changes of cord excitability can only be suppressed by large doses of narcotics (27). Carrying out the operation with regional anesthesia, however, interrupts almost all afferents to the spinal cord. This blocks the massive nociceptive input so that no afferent signals are set off during the operation, thus preventing the onset and maintenance of the spinal cord hyperexcitability and the consequent painful skeletal muscle spasm.

Prophylaxis and Treatment

It has now been shown that the use of regional anesthesia alone or combined with general anesthesia greatly delays and decreases the incidence of postoperative pain, tenderness, and hyperalgesia (28–30), and eliminates or at least markedly reduces the incidence of bouts of intense skeletal muscle spasm and associated pain. These findings strongly suggest that operations requiring general anesthesia should be supplemented with local infiltration or regional anesthesia of the operative field to prevent these pathophysiologic effects.

If severe reflex spasm and associated pain develop, they can be treated by continuous epidural analgesia achieved with a dilute solution of a local anesthetic alone or combined with epidural opioids. This usually decreases the intensity or completely eliminates the reflex muscle spasm and promptly relieves the pain. If these methods are not available, therapy is directed toward decreasing the excitability and hyper-reflexia with a pharmacologic agent, such as diazepam, given in a 10-mg dose every 4 hours. The initial dose should be given intravenously and subsequent doses intramuscularly. The reflex spasm usually decreases in intensity within the first 4 hours and is eliminated completely several hours thereafter.

Prolonged Increased Muscle Tension

Etiology and Pathophysiology

Prolonged contraction of the muscles or muscle groups beyond functional and postural needs results in increased tension, and tension-induced pain is a frequent cause of pain in the back. The most common cause of increased muscle tension is emotional conflict or increased emotional stress related to work or family (Chapter 23). Through psychophysiologic mechanisms these emotional disorders cause increased tension, which can be demonstrated by EMG (19, 21, 31, 32). Increased tension caused by postural defects occurs when a certain posture of the body, such as leaning over a desk for hours or squeezing the telephone between the shoulder and ear, is repeated frequently and for prolonged periods of time (4). Maintaining a fixed position for long periods or holding muscles rigidly while under stress produces muscle tension, stiffness and pain. Many occupations, such as occupational driver, typist, and telephone operator, require repeated movements (e.g., repeatedly turning to one side to reach for a telephone, raising the shoulders when typing, or using a computer), and can cause local tension. Injured muscles remain susceptible to tension and pain, especially after prolonged immobilization.

Biopsy studies of tense muscles done by Mielke and colleagues (33) showed no change in structure, but some increase in fibrous tissue and trigger points (TPs) could be detected after long-lasting increased tension.

Symptoms and Signs

Increased tension is not only painful, but is often a precursor of muscle spasm and a contributing cause of injury. Relaxation and stretching of tight muscles are therefore essential before a person engages in sports or in any other physical activity (4, 13). Injured muscles remain susceptible to tension and pain, especially after prolonged immobilization, and particular attention must be paid to these aftereffects. The critical role of emotional stress as a cause of low back pain in patients with premenstrual syndrome is discussed below.

Diagnosis

The diagnosis of increased muscle tension requires a thorough history, with special emphasis on psychosocial factors that could contribute to the patient's emotional stress, which in turn produces pain. Specific questions about interactions at work and at home should be asked to elicit information about emotional tension, anxiety, anger, and other factors that might be involved in the psychophysiologic mechanisms that cause low back pain. The examiner should inquire about the type of work the patient does, especially in regard to position and movements required, and whether it entails prolonged periods of immobility. The physical examination is carried out as described in Chapter 70, but it should also include palpation of the muscles of the low back and the use of the TCM (see above).

Treatment

Information and counseling are essential for patients with increased muscle tension caused by emotional factors. Psychologic therapy, such as relaxation, biofeedback, and other methods (Chapters 82 to 85), is effective in producing long-term relief. Relief can usually be obtained through pharmacologic means for patients with moderate to severe pain. Some authorities have advocated the use of tranquilizers such as diazepam (Valium), 2 to 5 mg bid to qid, chlordiazepoxide hydrochloride (Librium), 5 to 10 mg bid daily, or meprobamate (Equanil), 200 to 400 mg qid (4, 13, 19). These drugs should be used only for a limited period of time. In patients with severe pain and increased tension that is progressing to muscle spasm, it is most effective to break the vicious circle by infiltrating the muscle with a dilute solute of a local anesthetic (e.g., 0.125% bupivacaine; see above).

Muscle Deficiency (Fatigue)

Etiology

The use of muscles beyond their accustomed limit of exertion causes muscle fatigue and pain. The person who is not accustomed to taking long hikes can de-

velop pain in the low back and lower limbs and buttocks immediately after a long walk or several hours later. Similarly, sitting for a long time without moving about, such as during a long automobile or airplane trip, overtaxes and fatigues muscles of the low back, and causes stiffness and decreased flexibility of the hamstrings. In addition to stressing the muscles of the low back and other parts of the body, sitting increases the intradiskal pressure in the L3 disk to nearly 50% above that of standing upright (2). If the sitting is in a slouched position, the pressure can be almost double that of standing upright. Moreover, lifting a fairly heavy object with the arms well in front of the body not only can increase the intradiskal pressure threefold, but can cause severe loading and sprain of the paraspinal muscles (see Fig. 70-21). Low back pain occurs in patients who are not physically fit; even minor injuries to the low back in such patients can produce back pain. This could be caused by rupture of muscle fibers or of the musculotendinous junction. Although data from double-blind controlled clinical trials are not available to support the hypothesis of muscle injury as a source of low back pain (1, 2), indirect evidence has shown this to be the case.

Kraus (4) summarized the results of two studies involving 5000 patients, all of whom complained of low back pain. The studies were carried out in the rehabilitation departments of two major New York hospitals. Comprehensive physical and radiologic examinations revealed no pathologic findings in 83% of patients, whereas the remaining 17% had specific lesions for which a well-defined diagnosis could be made (Fig. 72-2). The investigators then subjected those without pathology to do the Kraus-Weber tests (34) (Fig. 72-3) and noted that they failed one or more of these six basic tests for minimum muscular fitness. The patients were managed first by surface or infiltration analgesia to relieve their pain and were then prescribed a gradually increasing exercise program under supervision of members of the management team, which included physiatrists, other physicians, and physical therapists.

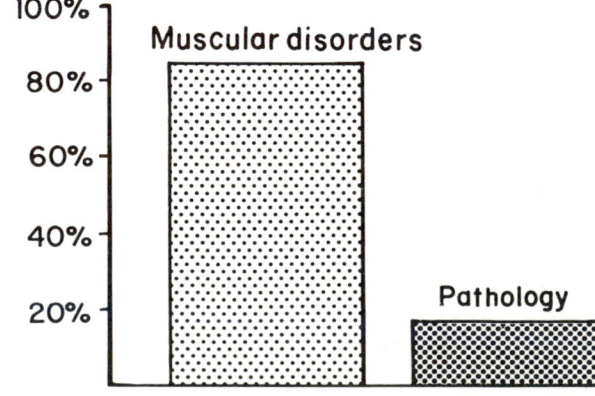

FIG. 72-2. Findings of a comprehensive examination of 3000 patients referred to a back clinic. Only 13% had obvious pathology of the lumbar spine, whereas 83% had muscular disorders. Modified from Kraus, H.: Diagnosis and Treatment of Muscle Pain. Chicago, Quintessence Publishing, 1988.

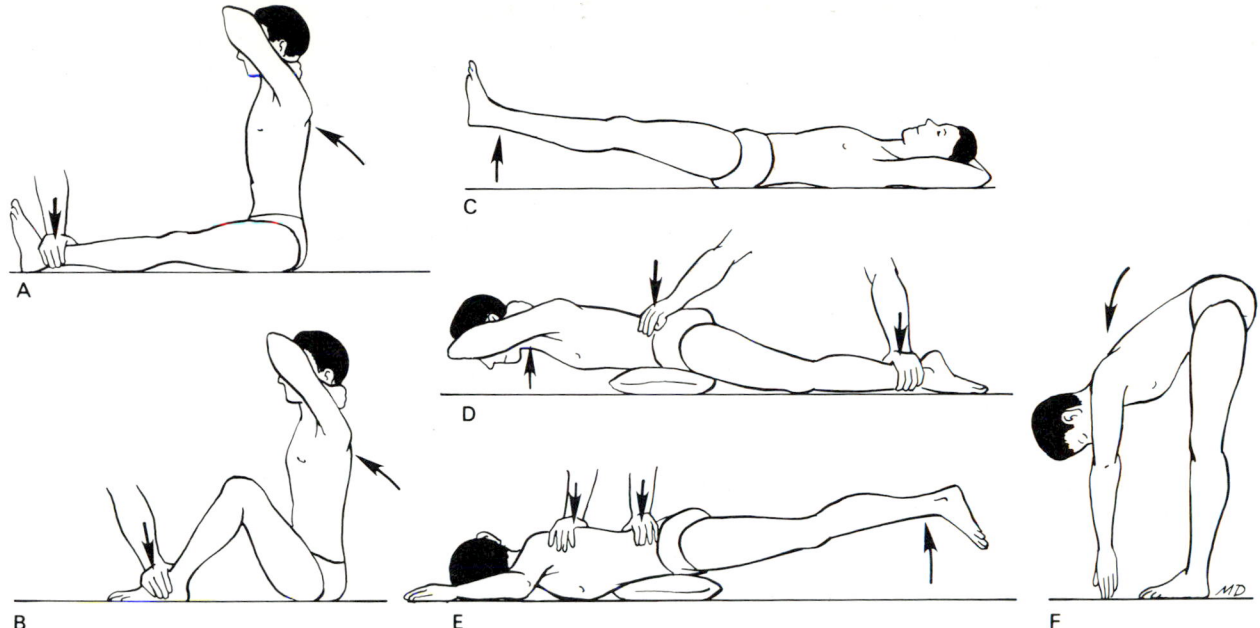

FIG. 72-3. Kraus-Weber test for evaluation of minimum muscular fitness. *A.* The subject sits up from the prone position with the hands behind the back, legs straight, and ankles held down. *B.* Same position as in *A*, but with knees flexed. *C.* Both legs are raised straight to a 30° angle and held for 10 seconds. *D.* The subject lies prone with a pillow under the hips, the trunk raised, and the hands behind the neck, and the position is held for 10 seconds. *E.* Same position as in *D*, but with both legs raised; this is held for 10 seconds. *F.* From a standing position, and with the knees straight, the subject slowly reaches toward the floor. Points at which the individual's body should be stabilized by another person are shown by arrows. Modified from Kraus, H.: Diagnosis and Treatment of Muscle Pain. Chicago, Quintessence Publishing, 1988.

The results of the exercise therapy program were assessed at the end of treatment and at intervals during a 2- to 8-year follow-up period, during which patients were encouraged to continue their therapeutic exercises and physical therapy. Figure 72-4 shows the results at the end of treatment and at 2- to 8-year follow-up for 233 of the patients. After termination of treatment, 65% of patients no longer had low back pain and had increased muscle strength and flexibility, 26% had fair results (partial pain relief and improvement), and 9% had poor results. At 8-year follow-up 82% had reported good results, 15% had fair results, and the remaining 3% had poor results. Generally, a strong correlation between muscle strength on the one

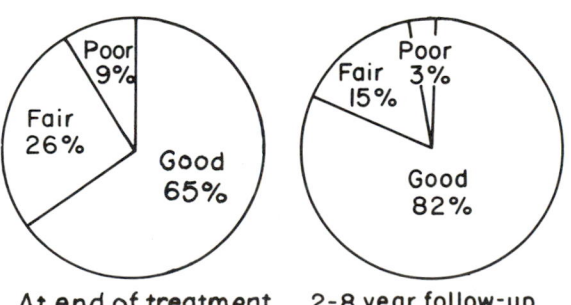

At end of treatment   2-8 year follow-up

FIG. 72-4. Results of a comprehensive therapy program, which included relief of pain by various means and an exercise program to improve strength or flexibility of muscle groups found wanting in the Kraus-Weber test in 233 patients suffering from low back pain. Modified from Kraus, H.: Diagnosis and treatment of low back pain. Gen. Pract., *5*:55, 1952.

hand and pain relief and return of functional ability on the other was found. This finding supports the more recent work by Cady and colleagues (35), who found a strong relationship between physical fitness and the incidence, recurrence, and severity of low back injuries. Data published by Frymoyer (36) suggest that vibrational influences increase the rate of fatigue, which might explain why the rate of low back injuries increases three- to five-fold in commuter driving (more than 2 hours per day), occupational driving, and working with vibrating tools, such as power saws (1).

Treatment

Muscle deficiency or fatigue requires fitness training for relief of symptoms. Nachemson and Bigos (1) emphasized that, even if the musculature is not severely injured at the time of onset of low back pain symptoms, a subsequent decrease in activity would undoubtedly have a negative effect on endurance, stamina, and fitness. Therefore, from this standpoint, aerobic exercise can be justified as part of the rehabilitation process in patients who complain of low back pain with varying degrees of muscle fatigue or weakness. They (1) cited reports showing that aerobic exercise can help decrease depression, a common finding in some patients with chronic low back pain, and also noted some studies that claimed that aerobic exercises increase endorphin levels in the cerebrospinal fluid and bloodstream. This not only can decrease the severity of the pain but can have a positive effect on stamina, sleep, mental alertness, and self-image, and can reverse activity levels compatible with chronic pain.

Myofascial Pain Syndromes

Historical Perspective

Myofascial pain syndrome with trigger points (TPs) as a common cause of low back pain was recognized more that 50 years ago by Arthur Steindler, one of the foremost American orthopedic authorities of the twentieth century. As early as 1937 Steindler and Luck (37) suggested that many patients with low back pain suffered from what they labeled the "posterior division syndrome," designated as such because the soft tissue and ligaments in this region are supplied by the posterior division of the lumbar and sacral nerves. They noted that TPs can be found in most patients with this myofascial disorder, and believed that these focal areas of tenderness represent a deep ligamentous injury or a myofascitis. On the basis of this and other studies Steindler (38) set forth the possible location of these TPs and designated each general location as a syndrome (Fig. 72-5). In a relatively high percentage of cases these TPs initiated a reflex mechanism that produced referred pain, tenderness, and muscle spasm in the lower extremity (37, 38) (see below).

Four years later William Livingston (39), another giant in the study of pain in the twentieth century, reported a series of cases in which TPs were found within the lowest portion of the multifidus muscle. He labeled this the "multifidus syndrome" and suggested that it was caused by injuries to the muscle. In the subsequent 20 years myofascial syndrome studies were reported by Travell and Rinzler (40), Bonica (41), Sola (42), Michele (another orthopedic surgeon) (43), and others. In 1952 Travell and Rinzler (44) published a comprehensive review of the most common myofascial syndromes, all of which were included in the first edition of this book (41). On the basis of many studies and reports, especially by Simons (45, 46), Simons and Travell (47), and Travell and Simons (5), these syndromes increasingly became recognized as causes of acute and chronic pain in various parts of the body.

Recently the ubiquitous nature of myofascial pain syndromes has been recognized by many rheumatologists, physiatrists, anesthesiologists, family physicians, dentists with an interest in the temporomandibular joint and in myofascial syndromes of the face, and others. Rosomoff (8), a neurosurgeon who directs the University of Miami Comprehensive Pain and Rehabilitation Center, stated that myofascial pain syndromes are the most frequent cause of chronic low back pain that he has treated. Fishbain and associates (48) reported that 85% of 283 consecutive admissions to the Miami Comprehensive Pain Center were assigned a primary organic diagnosis of myofascial syndromes, with the diagnosis being made independently by a neurosurgeon and a physiatrist based on physical examination of soft tissue findings (see below).

Rosomoff and associates (49) studied a subgroup of 283 patients and demonstrated objective physical findings in patients with "chronic intractable benign pain (CIBP, which is defined as a non-neoplastic pain of greater than 6 months' duration without known nociceptive peripheral input)" (see page 20 for an explanation of why such a term is unfortunate). To fit the CIPB definition, patients with a proven diagnosis of deafferentation pain, degenerative disease, spinal stenosis, radiculopathy, malignancy, or a finding of root compression syndrome were removed from the study group. This left 111 patients who were examined independently by a neurosurgeon and physiatrist, and only congruent physical findings were quoted. Each of these 111 patients was found to have abnormal physical findings in seven categories: decreased ranges of motion (including hip motion), TPs, rigid musculature,

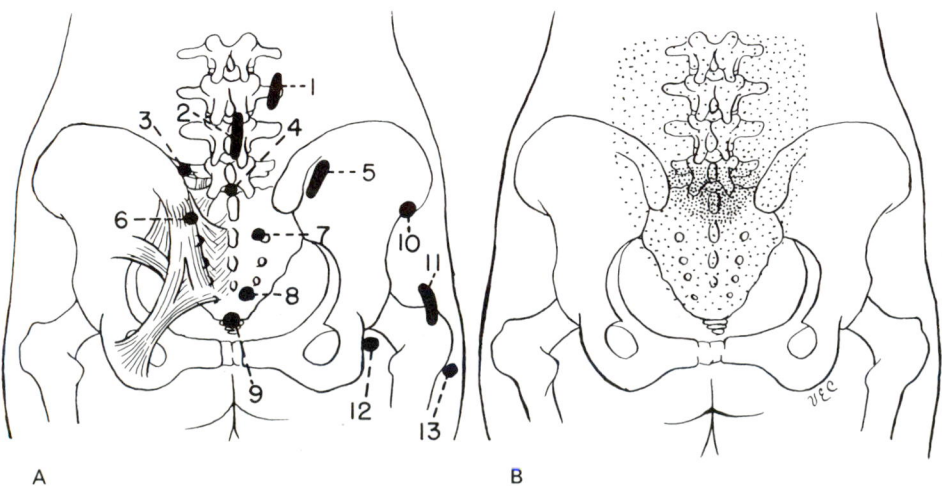

FIG. 72-5. **A.** Location of tender areas in the low back region involved in various types of musculoskeletal pain: iliocostalis syndrome (1), myofascial syndrome (2), transversosacral syndrome (Steindler) (3), lumbosacral syndrome (4), gluteal syndrome (5), sacroiliac syndrome (6), sacrospinalis syndrome (7), multifidus syndrome (8), coccygodynia (9), gluteus minimus syndrome (10), tensor fascia lata syndrome (11), piriformis syndrome (12), and trochanteric bursitis (after Steindler) (13). **B.** Location of pain and tenderness in acute low back pain (*stippled area*).

nonanatomic sensory loss, gait disturbances, and miscellaneous non-neurologic signs. Review of their past medical workup revealed that these patients had been referred to the center for treatment of behavioral or psychologic disturbances caused by operant mechanisms or that they had been labeled as "idiopathic low back pain" patients.

Further support for the existence of myofascial syndrome comes from other sources. A primary diagnosis of myofascial pain syndrome was made in over 55% of 296 patients referred to a dental clinic for chronic orofacial pain of at least 6 months' duration (50). Skootsky (51) reported that myofascial syndromes were prevalent in general practice: in 61 consecutive consultations of follow-up patients seen by those in an internal medicine group, 10% of all patients and 31% of those presenting with pain complaints had myofascial TPs that were primarily responsible for their symptoms. Reynolds (52) noted that patients with early rheumatoid arthritis had TPs that produced myofascial syndromes, the pain of which was added to the pain of the arthritis. Moreover, well-recognized criteria now exist for the diagnosis and treatment of these conditions, which are enumerated below (5–7, 41–46).

Recent evidence has shown that the therapeutic efficacy of TP injection (TPI) with a local anesthetic occurs through stimulation of an endogenous opioid mechanism. Fine and associates (53) carried out a double-blind crossover study on 10 patients with myofascial TPs who were experiencing acute or long-standing muscle pain that could be aggravated or elicited by palpation of the TPs. The 10 patients were randomly assigned to a naloxone or a placebo group during alternate (crossover) phases of assessment and TPI therapy trials, with a 1- to 2-week interval between the first and second phases. TPI with 0.25% bupivacaine decreased pain in all subjects and increased the range of motion in subjects who at initial assessment demonstrated limitation of movement of the affected part(s). Allodynia and palpable bands preceding TPI, when present, also decreased after TPI. All improvements afforded by TPI were significantly reversed with 10 mg of naloxone given intravenously as compared to no reversal with intravenous placebo. The results demonstrated a naloxone reversal mechanism in TPI therapy and suggested an endogenous opioid system as the mediator for the decreased pain and improved physical findings.

In view of all these findings, it is surprising that some orthopedic authorities and others dispute the existence of myofascial pain syndromes (1). Stoeckle and Boyd (54), members of the Committee on Pain, Disability, and Chronic Illness Behavior of the Institute of Medicine, reported that, during the committee's discussion of myofascial pain syndromes, opposing views were expressed and discussion was "heated." Although all the clinicians acknowledged the existence of muscular involvement in back pain, some expressed strong doubts about the existence of myofascial TPs and were apparently unaware of recently developed tools that provide objective evidence. Similarly, the Quebec Task Force on Spinal Disorders (18) listed local medications and included infiltration of TPs as "common practice but no scientific evidence," on the basis that no randomized or nonrandomized control trials have demonstrated its efficacy. Indeed, review of their matrix reveals that only 8 of 32 therapeutic modalities used for treatment of spinal disorders had fulfilled these criteria. The report (18) properly stated, however, that "the matrices should not be considered the final word because they were prepared on the basis of current knowledge and subjective scientific validation. The efficacy of some treatment has not been verified through scientific studies, but this does not mean that the treatments prescribed because of a known biologic effect are useless." In reviewing the list of 763 articles studied by the Quebec group, only 2 pertain to myofascial pain syndromes.

I believe that this lack of recognition of myofascial pain syndromes occurs mainly because primary care physicians, who treat about 60% of back pain patients, orthopedists, who treat another 25% (55), and internists, who care for the rest, are completely unaware of their existence. Consequently, their patients are treated improperly for other conditions, with the result that they progress to a chronic pain state. Correctly diagnosed and treated, however, it has been found that patients are not only quickly relieved of pain, but their function is restored and they return to work sooner. An example is that of a well-known national leader who was injured during World War II and consequently developed a chronic back disorder from which he suffered for nearly a decade, despite consultation and treatment by some of the most respected orthopedic surgeons in the United States. It was only when several authorities with expertise in myofascial syndromes were consulted that the correct diagnosis was made. With TPI and other treatments, his pain and suffering decreased and he was able to lead a very active and productive life.

When we wrote Chapter 21 we were not aware of the controversy over the existence of myofascial pain syndromes and therefore failed to include this historical review and the criteria for the diagnosis of myofascial pain syndromes. TPs can develop in any of the approximately 5000 skeletal muscles, although only about 15% of these are commonly involved. Myofascial syndromes have the following cardinal features that distinguish them from other musculoskeletal disorders (5–7, 41, 44–47):

a. The pain is muscle-oriented so that it consistently relates to the use of a specific muscle(s).

b. TPs are characterized by hypersensitivity so that when pressure is applied they produce or aggravate the pain and tenderness. These phenomena are reproducible and the TPs are consistently found in the same part of the muscle. The same amount of pressure on the contralateral muscle, if not involved in the syndrome, does not produce pain or tenderness.

c. Stimulation of the TP produces pain that is felt locally, is referred in a pattern distant from the TP, or both. The referred pain and tenderness are projected in a pattern characteristic of that particular muscle and reproduces part of the patient's complaint. The patterns of referred pain are frequently different from those expected on the basis of nerve root compression alone.

d. Hardening of a taut band of muscle fibers passing through the tender spot in a shortened muscle can be palpated.

e. When the TP is stimulated by snapping palpation or needle penetration a local twitch response of the taut band of muscle is produced.

f. Injection of a local anesthetic into the TP promptly eliminates the pain, tenderness, and other symptoms and signs.

Before discussing specific syndromes that produce low back pain, their causes, pathophysiology, symptoms and signs, diagnosis, and treatment are presented. A more detailed discussion of these aspects of myofascial syndromes is found in Chapter 21.

Clinical Aspects

Etiology and Pathophysiology

TPs are small, tender nodules of degenerated muscle tissue produced by major trauma or by persistent mechanical stress with consequent microtrauma resulting from repetitive or continuous use of one or more muscles during work or certain athletic activities. They can also result from poor posture, degenerative joint disease, emotional stress, and endocrine imbalance (5, 45–47). Usually one factor initiates TP activity, and mechanical or systemic factors, or both, perpetuate it. Myofascial syndromes in the low back and lower limbs can be perpetuated by four structural inadequacies: a short leg, a small hemipelvis, a short arm, or relatively long 2nd and short 1st metatarsal bones (41, 45–47).

Neither the exact pathogenesis of TP pain, dysfunction, and associated physical findings nor the mechanisms of action for the therapeutic efficacy of TPI have been fully elucidated. Sola and William (6, 42) have postulated that an injury to the muscles initiates nociceptive impulses that are transmitted to the central nervous system (CNS). This nociceptive barrage to the CNS in turn produces increased muscle tension and vasoconstriction with consequent local ischemia, increased vascular permeability, release of algesic agents, and osmotic and pH changes, all of which increase the sensitivity or activity of nociceptors in the area. This increases sympathetic activity and a vicious cycle is established, with increased vasoconstriction producing further histologic and histochemical changes in muscle fibers that lead to even more vasoconstriction. Their hypothesis has been supported by Bengtsson and Bengtsson (56), who demonstrated in a controlled study that regional sympathetic block (which produces vasodilation) eliminates a number of tender or trigger points.

Symptoms and Signs

The pain of myofascial syndromes in the low back varies from a slight, mild ache to a severe, unrelenting, and disabling pain. The pain can be sharp or dull; it can be located around the trigger area, referred to distant parts, or a combination of these. TP hypersensitivity in the paraspinal muscles, gluteii muscles, and other muscles of the low back, pelvis, and thigh also

causes limited range of motion and decreased strength of these muscles.

In the absence of specific clinical findings in patients who complain of back pain, the paraspinal muscles and the muscles of the gluteal region, the thigh, and the lower thorax and abdomen should be examined carefully for hyperactive tender points. Physicians who are not aware of these disorders usually concentrate on gross examination of the muscles, range of motion, and the lumbosacral spine. TPs are likely to be activated as a secondary cause of pain in association with any injury or strain; failure to diagnose and treat hyperactive TPs intensifies the pain, delays healing, and makes rehabilitation more difficult, with possible progression to chronic low back pain.

Diagnosis

Screening of myofascial pain syndromes should include a complete history and thorough physical examination (Chapters 21 and 31). Disorders that must be ruled out include various other specific musculoskeletal conditions (Chapter 71). A thorough assessment of neuromuscular function, including passive and active range of motion of the muscles of the trunk, thigh, and leg, should be undertaken.

To identify TPs of specific muscles, the examiner systematically palpates the suspected muscle(s) with a finger or blunt object and compares the particular muscle with the contralateral muscle (Fig. 72-6). It is important to note signs of local and ipsilateral hand coolness, sweating, edema, and piloerection. To determine the location of the TP, the patient should be positioned so that the muscles of the back, buttocks, and thighs are relaxed. The muscles that harbor TPs

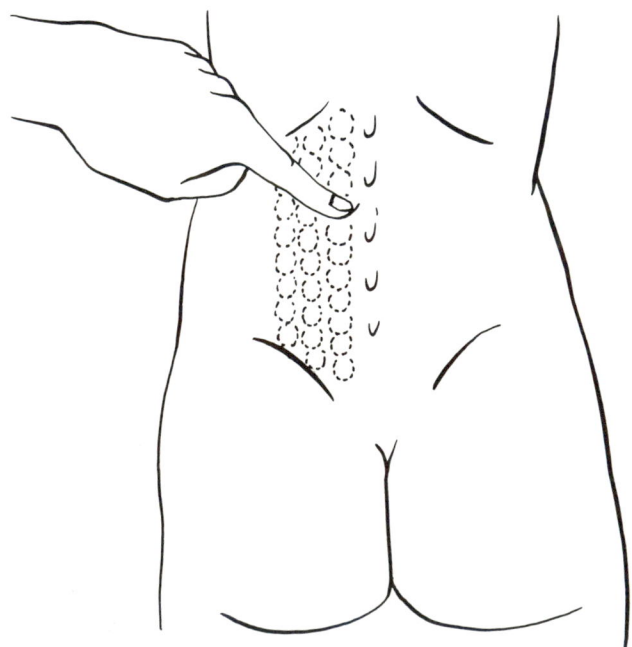

FIG. 72-6. Method of palpating one side of the back in a patient in whom a myofascial syndrome is suspected. The 2nd finger is pressed forcefully and deeply to detect TPs in the deeper muscles. The entire area of pain should be systematically palpated as indicated by the confluent circles above, below, and to the side of the palpating finger.

contain taut fibers that form a palpable band (or bands) which tighten and shorten the muscle. A sudden change in pressure on the TP by brisk rolling of the band under the finger causes a brief contraction of the fibers within the taut band, the so-called "local twitch response." When pressure is exerted on the most tender point that is a TP, the patient manifests a "jump sign" consisting of movement and vocalization.

Once a TP is localized it is helpful to use Fisher's pressure gauge (Chapter 21). The gauge is pressed gently and steadily after instructing the patient to inform the examiner when the pressure becomes painful. The pain threshold value of one side should be compared with that of the contralateral side. Because of the especially important role myofascial pain syndromes play in low back pain, they are described in more detail than those that affect most other regions. Description of the syndromes is based on personal observations and publications of Simons and Travell (47) and of Sola and associates (42, 57). Sola also provided advice on some of the illustrations that follow.

Specific Myofascial Pain Syndromes (XXVII-13, XXVII-14)

Quadratus Lumborum Syndrome

The quadratus lumborum muscle is one of the most common of the back muscles to develop active and latent TPs that produce low back pain. Sola and Kuitert (57) found this to be the most common myofascial syndrome that produces low back pain, and it was invariably involved in patients with low back pain in whom other pathologic skeletal disorders had been ruled out. They attributed its high frequency of involvement to the fact that, of all the lumbar muscles, the quadratus lumborum is the only one under active tension during walking, sitting, and lying. The "slump" position, as often assumed in driving an automobile for long distance, accentuates stress on the attachments of the muscle.

The fibers of the quadratus lumborum are attached above to the 12th rib (Fig. 72-7A), below to the posterior third of the iliac crest and to the iliolumbar ligament, and medially to the transverse processes of the upper four lumbar vertebrae. Because of its position it is one of the key muscles of the trunk, and is involved in all bending and rotating movements. Acting unilaterally, its longitudinal fibers flex the spine laterally toward the same side and, if the spine is held straight, elevate the homolateral pelvis. The pair of quadratus muscles depresses the 12th rib during forced expiration and coughing and, acting bilaterally and in concert, all quadratus lumborum fibers extend the spine.

ETIOLOGY. Factors that can precipitate development of active and latent TPs include active strain of the quadratus lumborum muscle from a quick stooping

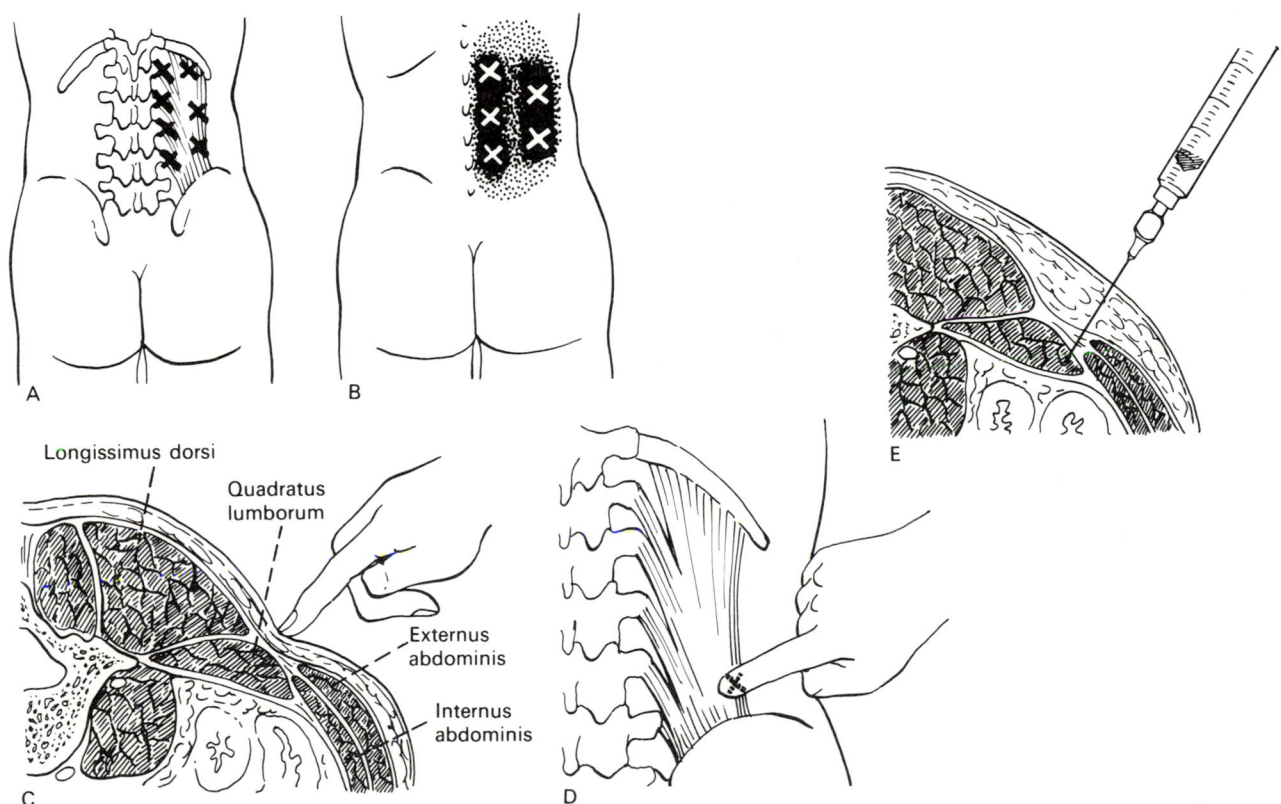

FIG. 72-7. Quadratus lumborum myofascial pain syndrome. **A.** Anatomy of the quadratus lumborum and its attachment. Trigger points (TPs) are shown by X. **B.** Pattern of pain caused by TPs in the lateral part of the muscle and in its attachment to the tranverse processes of the lumbar vertebrae. In the black areas (the essential zones) the pain is most intense and is felt by all patients; in the stippled areas (the spillover zones) not all patients experience pain and, if they do, it is of lesser intensity. **C, D.** Palpation of the area to locate the TP. **E.** Technique of injecting the TP with local anesthetic. This pattern of the quadratus lumborum syndrome was first described by Sola (Chapter 12).

movement when the torso is twisted somewhat to one side, or strain from a fall or other accident. Active TPs in this muscle can also develop after sustained and repetitive overload as in gardening, scrubbing, or prolonged automobile driving. The TPs are most frequently found in the lateral margins and on the attachment of the muscle to the vertebrae, iliac crest, and 12th rib.

SYMPTOMS AND SIGNS. The most frequent pattern of pain is shown in Figure 72-7B. This pattern involves a large lumbar paravertebral region that extends laterally to the posterolateral aspect of the trunk. In some patients pain is also referred over the iliac crest and greater trochanter and anteriorly to the lower abdomen and groin. Travell and Simons (45–47) described a pattern of pain in the low gluteal and sacroiliac regions caused by TPs in the deeper diagonal fibers that attach to the transverse processes of the lumbar vertebrae.

Patients frequently complain of pain when walking, twisting, stooping, turning over in bed, rising from a chair, coughing, sneezing, or climbing the stairs while facing forward. The quality and intensity of pain vary from a low-grade burning, aching feeling to a sharp, knife-like, excruciating pain. Rest pain, especially at night, can be severe, whereas in the morning patients might have to crawl on their hands and knees to reach the bathroom.

DIAGNOSIS. Diagnosis is made through history and physical examination, which should include careful inspection and palpation. The patient manifests guarded movements when walking, lying down on the bed, or getting up from a chair, and the pelvis lists to one side when the patient is standing. Because the muscle lies deep to the erector spinae, the quadratus lumborum myofascial syndrome is easily overlooked on examination. For proper palpation the patient should lie on the examining table on the uninvolved side in a manner that separates the 12th rib from the iliac crest. To stimulate TPs it is necessary to use firm pressure with the 2nd finger (Fig. 72-7C and D) and, if necessary, to reinforce it by also using the thumb or fingers of the other hand, thus combining the pressure of both hands.

TREATMENT. Treatment includes penetration of the TP and injection of a dilute solution (0.125%) of bupivacaine under pressure to disrupt (rupture) the TP (Fig. 72-7E). In thin individuals, a 3-cm 25-gauge needle is sufficient, but in most patients it is necessary to use a 5-cm 25-gauge needle. For obese or more muscular patients an 8-cm 22-gauge spinal needle can be used. If the stretch-and-spray technique is used the patient's muscle must be relaxed. After several sweeps of the vapocoolant have been passed slowly in parallel lines downward over the quadratus lumborum muscle, the thigh is extended and adducted at the hip as far as can be tolerated by the patient. If the patient has spillover pain over the iliac crest and abdomen, sweeps of spray are extended to cover all pain reference zones. Maximal stretch of the quadratus lumborum requires that the thigh be fully adducted to produce full tilt of the pelvis while the rib cage is elevated.

Following injection a hot pack is applied to the treated region. After the muscles have relaxed, active and passive ranges of motion are carried out without loading or sustained effort. The perpetuating factors must then be treated. Any structural inadequacies that are sources of muscular overload (see above) are corrected with appropriate supports. If the syndrome is caused by postural stress and muscular deficiency, a series of appropriate exercises must be carried out.

Superficial Lumbar Paraspinal Muscle Syndromes

The superficial paraspinal muscles include the more lateral iliocostalis lumborum and iliocostalis thoracis and the more medial longissimus thoracis muscles. These muscles primarily function to extend the spine and are therefore stretched by flexion. TPs in these muscles can be caused by macrotrauma to the muscles, prolonged stress resulting from structural inadequacies, or maintaining a prolonged position that overloads the muscles.

Referred pain patterns can be caused by TPs in the lower part of the *iliocostalis thoracis* (Fig. 72-8B). The most intense pain occurs in the upper part of the low back at the level of the 11th and 12th ribs with spillover to the lumbar paraspinal region, frequently to the upper part of the chest, and anteriorly to the suprainguinal region. The essential zone is in the flank, simulating pain caused by renal disease. Because of this similarity it can confound the examiner. The myofascial syndrome can be differentiated, however, by localizing the TP and then injecting it with a local anesthetic, causing prompt disappearance of the pain.

Pain patterns can be produced by TPs in the upper part of the *iliocostalis lumborum* at the level of the L1

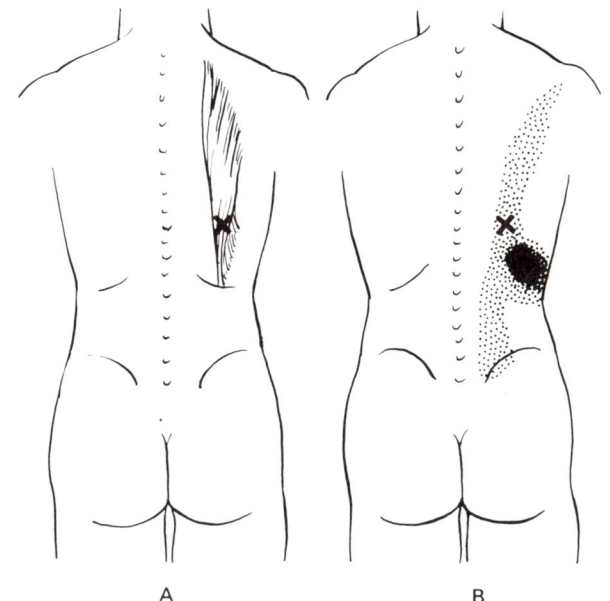

A   B

FIG. 72-8. Iliocostalis thoracis myofascial pain syndrome. *A.* Anatomy of the iliocostalis thoracis and the location of the TP (X). *B.* Pattern of pain produced by the TP. For explanation of the black and stippled areas see legend for Fig. 72-7. Modified from Simons, D.G., and Travell, J.G.: Myofascial origins of low back pain. Postgrad. Med., *73*:82, 1983.

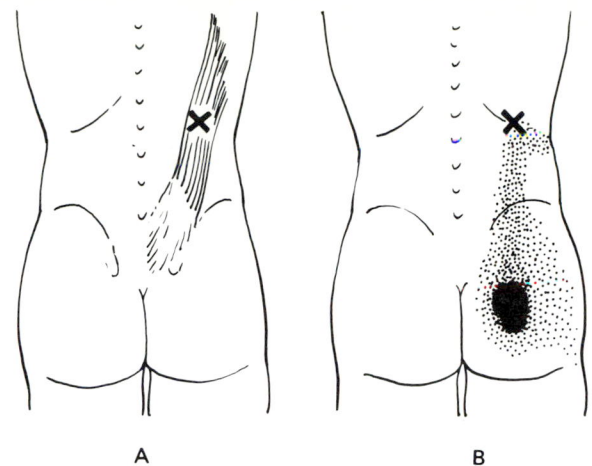

FIG. 72-9. Iliocostalis lumborum myofascial pain syndrome. **A.** Anatomy of the iliocostalis lumborum and the location of the TP (X). **B.** Pattern of pain produced by the TP. For explanation of the black and stippled areas see legend for Fig. 72-7. Modified from Simons, D.G., and Travell, J.G.: Myofascial origins of low back pain. Postgrad. Med., *73*:82, 1983.

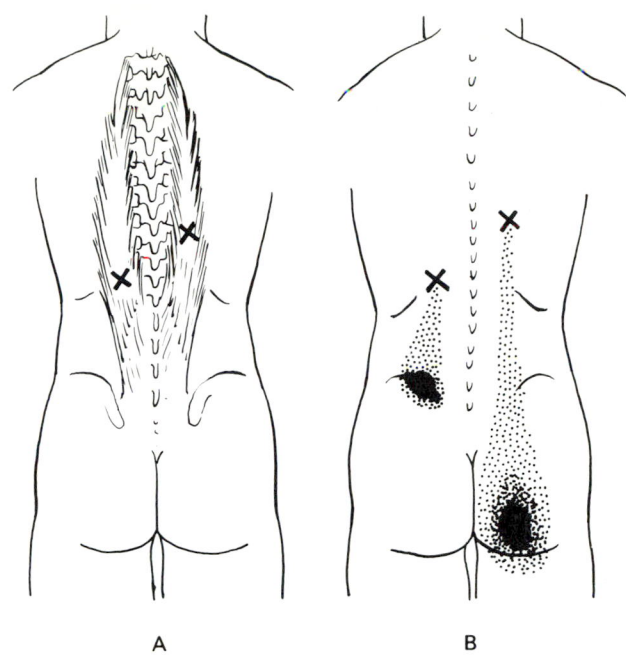

FIG. 72-10. Longissimus thoracis myofascial pain syndrome. **A.** Anatomy of the longissimus thoracis and the location of the TPs (X). **B.** Patterns of pain produced by the TPs at the level of T10 vertebra on the right and the L1 on the left. For explanation of the black and the stippled areas see legend for Fig. 72-7. Modified from Simons, D.G., and Travell, J.G.: Myofascial origins of low back pain. Postgrad Med., *73*:82, 1983.

or L2 vertebra (Fig. 72-9B). Pain occurs in the essential zone, in the posterior midgluteal region, with spillover involving the entire posterior and lateral gluteal regions and the lateral paralumbar region. In some patients the TP is located lower down, but the pattern of pain is similar.

The *longissimus thoracis* muscle, the longest part of the erector spinae, located between the iliocostalis thoracis and iliocostalis lumborum, frequently develops TPs at the level of one or more of the lumbar vertebrae and also along the lower thoracic paravertebral level. Two different patterns can be provoked by TPs at different levels of the muscle (Fig. 72-10). The pattern on the left in Figure 71-10B is caused by a TP at the level of the L1 vertebra, while the pattern on the right is caused by a TP at the level of the T10 or T11 segment.

DIAGNOSIS. Diagnosis of these three syndromes is made through history and physical examination, which should include observation and palpation. TPs develop from major trauma or, more commonly, from muscle overload when one lifts a heavy object while facing forward. Patients with one of these syndromes move with their spine stiffened protectively. Palpation reveals tense, exquisitely tender bands and provokes a strong local twitch response.

TREATMENT. Treatment is with needle penetration of the TPs and injection of 2 to 3 ml of 0.125% bupivacaine. The injection must be carried out forcibly to rupture the trigger area. This invariably provokes transient, severe pain locally and in the area of reference for about 2 to 3 minutes until the local anesthetic exerts its analgesic effect. During TPI of the lower iliocostalis thoracis or longissimus thoracis, located in the posterior chest, care must be exercised to avoid penetration of the parietal pleura and possible pneumothorax. This complication can prevented by using a short, thin needle, such as a 3-cm 25-gauge needle. (In patients who are obese or muscular it is necessary to use a 5-cm 25-gauge needle.) Use of a thin needle

markedly minimizes the risk of pneumothorax even if the needle penetrates the parietal pleura because of the small size of the puncture. On the other hand, if a thin needle has a hook that can rupture or tear the pleura, the risk of pneumothorax increases. This can and should be avoided by placing the 2nd and 3rd fingers of one hand over the intercostal spaces adjacent to the TP and carrying out TPI with the other hand.

Stretch and spray is carried out with the patient sitting on the table with the feet on the floor and leaning far forward, flexing the head maximally and letting the arms hang loosely between the legs. The spray is started in the midthoracic area and continued in a downward sweep over the affected muscles and their pain reference zones. After treatment heat is applied and, a few minutes later, the muscle is stretched. Adjunctive therapies are described in Chapter 21. It is essential to inform ("educate") these patients about the mechanics of the back and to prescribe a program of active exercise at home.

Multifidi and Rotatores Syndromes

The multifidus consists of a number of fleshy, tendinous fasciculi that fill the groove on both sides of the spinous process of the vertebra from the sacrum to the thoracic and cervical regions. In the sacral region the fasciculi arise from the back of the sacrum as low as the S4 foramen. Acting alone the multifidus muscle bends and laterally flexes the vertebral column and rotates it to the opposite side. When the multifidi on both sides act together, the vertebral column is

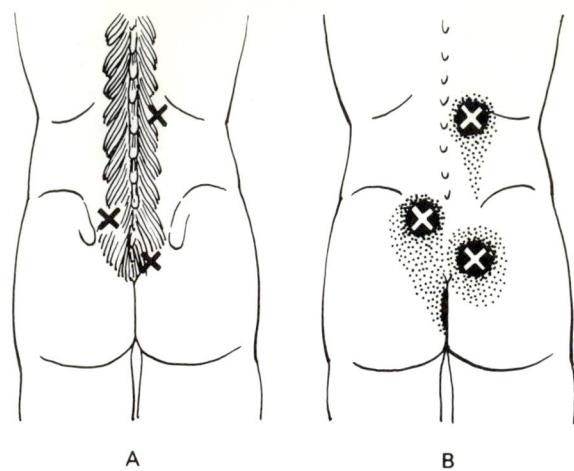

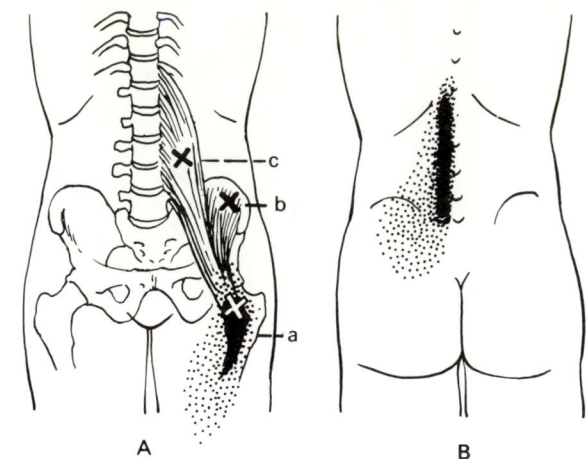

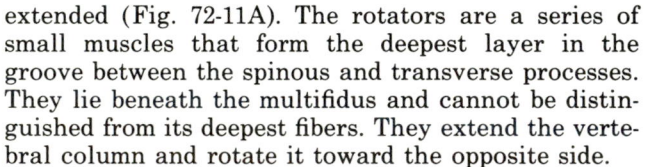

A   B

FIG. 72-11. Multifidi rotatores myofascial pain syndromes. These muscles constitute the deepest layer of the back muscles. **A.** Anatomy of the multifidi rotatores and the location of three TPs (X). **B.** Patterns of pain produced by the TPs. Modified from Simons, D.G., and Travell, J.G.: Myofascial origins of low back pain. Postgrad. Med., *73*:82, 1983.

A   B

FIG. 72-12. Iliopsoas myofascial pain syndrome. **A.** Anatomy of the iliopsoas and the location of TPs (X) at three levels: (a) just above the femoral attachment of the iliopsoas tendon, producing pain in the anterior upper thigh; (b) in the iliacus; and (c) in the psoas. **B.** Pattern of pain produced by the TPs in b and a. This distinctive vertical pattern is homolateral along the lumbosacral spine and extends down to the sacroiliac region. Modified from Simons, D.G., and Travell, J.G.: Myofascial origins of low back pain. Postgrad Med., *73*:82, 1983.

extended (Fig. 72-11A). The rotators are a series of small muscles that form the deepest layer in the groove between the spinous and transverse processes. They lie beneath the multifidus and cannot be distinguished from its deepest fibers. They extend the vertebral column and rotate it toward the opposite side.

TPs can be produced by major trauma from the impact of external objects, by lifting heavy objects, or by flexing and rotating the trunk rapidly. Figure 72-11A and B depict TPs at the level of the sacral segment and at the level of the L2 vertebra. The essential zone of the pain overlies the TP, whereas the spillover zone can involve the lower medial gluteal region, the posterior part of the thigh, and occasionally the anterior part of the abdomen.

It is difficult to stretch and spray these muscles because of the strong passive rotation and flexion that are required to stretch them fully. Injection of these TPs is usually effective if the needle penetrates to the depth of the vertebral column to reach all involved TPs. Injection to such a depth requires a 5-cm 23-gauge needle in thin individuals and an 8-cm 23-gauge needle for muscular or obese persons.

Iliopsoas Muscle Syndrome

When the iliopsoas muscle develops TPs and a myofascial pain syndrome evolves, the quadratus lumborum is usually also affected (47). Therefore, for lasting relief, TPs in both muscles must be inactivated. Acting unilaterally the iliopsoas flexes the thigh and assists in external rotation at the hip joint, whereas when acting bilaterally the psoas muscles flex the lower lumbar spine (Fig. 72-12A). Macrotrauma or prolonged unusual stress of these muscles can provoke TPs in these regions. Figure 72-12B depicts the pain pattern provoked by TPs in different parts of the iliopsoas muscle. The pain referred from these TPs forms a distinctive vertical pattern that is homolateral along the lumbosacral spine and extends downward to

the sacroiliac, ipsilateral inguinal, and upper anterior thigh regions (9).

DIAGNOSIS. Diagnosis is made through the history and physical examination, which usually reveals that the muscles are shortened. This causes patients to walk with the thigh in external rotation, and is associated with a slight flexion at the hip and consequent flattening of the normal lordotic lumbar curve (47). These patients maintain a stooped posture and psoatic gait because of the limited extension and internal rotation of the thigh and the restricted extension of the lumbar spine (47). This posture is distinguished from that caused by bony kyphosis by radiographic examination of the spine.

On physical examination exquisite tenderness or TPs are found in three sites: (Fig. 72-12A) (a) immediately above the femoral attachment of the iliopsoas tendon, which requires deep pressure along the medial wall of the femoral triangle toward the lesser trochanter; (b) in the iliacus muscle, which can be identified when pressure is applied against the iliac fossa just medial to the brim of the pelvis halfway between the anterior and posterior superior iliac spines; and (c) in the psoas muscle. To identify this last TP a medial thrust is added to deep abdominal pressure exerted laterally to the lateral edge of the rectus abdominus muscle, just below the level of the umbilicus (47).

TREATMENT. Treatment with penetration and injection of the TP can easily be done in the lower two areas. For injection of the lowest TP, the thigh of the supine patient is abducted and externally rotated and the pulsating femoral artery is located medial to the tender spot in the muscles (47). Penetration of the middle TP requires inserting the needle through the skin just above the anterior third of the iliac crest and directing the needle posteriorly and slightly medially. If these two injections do not relieve the pain it is

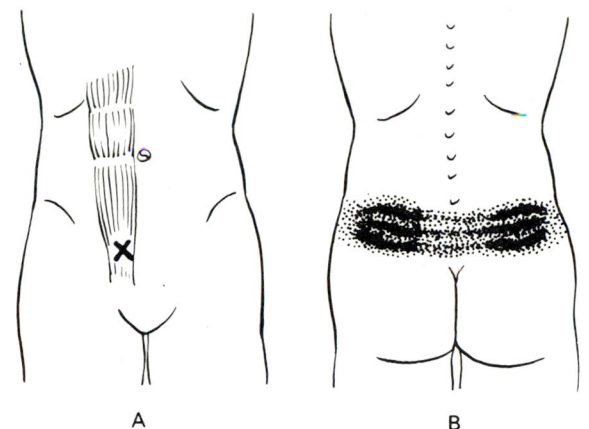

FIG. 72-13. Rectus abdominis myofascial pain syndrome. **A.** Anatomy of the rectus abdominis and the location of the TP (X) in its lowermost segment. **B.** Pattern of pain produced by the TP. Modified from Simons, D.G., and Travell, J.G.: Myofascial origins of low back pain. Postgrad. Med., *73*:82, 1983.

DIAGNOSIS. Diagnosis is made through the characteristics of the pain pattern, by mapping them, and by palpating the muscle for TPs, reproducing the pain with sustained pressure on the TP.

TREATMENT. For complete relief TPs must be penetrated and local anesthetic injected under pressure to rupture them. Stretch and spray is initiated at the upper part of the muscles and continued with a downward sweep that covers the entire area of the pain pattern.

Gluteus Medius Syndrome

A myofascial pain syndrome can be provoked by TPs in the gluteus medius (Fig. 72-15). The most intense pain is along the posterior part of the iliac crest and sacrum, with spillover to the posterior and lateral gluteal regions and the posterior thigh. The pattern of pain in the essential zone can easily be mistaken for pain caused by dysfunction or disease of the sacroiliac

necessary to penetrate the uppermost TP by a posterior paravertebral approach.

For stretch and spray of the iliopsoas muscle, the patient lies supine with the hands under the small of the back and with the thigh of the involved side moderately abducted and extended over the side of the table. After several initial sweeps of spray the physician gradually extends and rotates the thigh internally while continuing to spray the vapocoolant caudally in a long parallel sweep to cover the pain pattern.

Lower Rectus Abdominis Syndrome

TPs in the lower rectus abdominis (Chapter 64) cause low back pain (Fig. 72-13; also Figs. 64-7 and 64-8).

Gluteus Maximus Syndrome

Pain patterns can be provoked by TPs in two different locations of the lower gluteus maximus (Fig. 72-14). The most important essential zones are in the lower medial and lateral aspects of the buttock. A TP in the lowest fibers of the muscle can cause pain deep in the coccyx. In addition to pain these patients have restricted straight leg raising caused by tightness of the hamstring and gluteus maximus muscle.

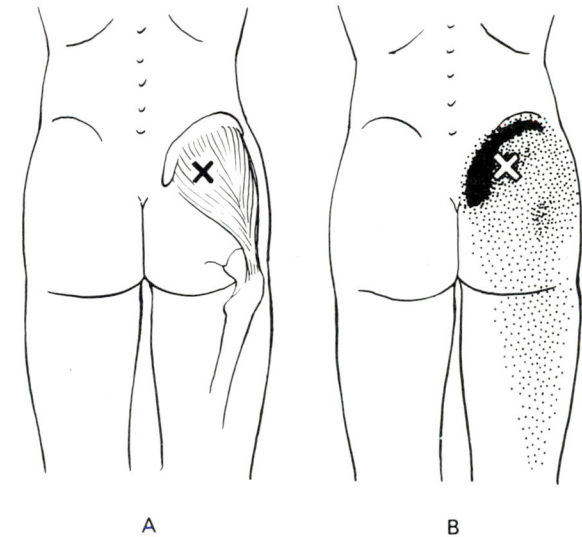

FIG. 72-15. Gluteus medius myofascial pain syndrome. **A.** Anatomy of the gluteus medius and the location of the TP (X). **B.** Pattern of pain produced by the TP. Modified from Simons, D.G., and Travell, J.G.: Myofascial origins of low back pain. Postgrad. Med., *73*:82, 1983.

FIG. 72-14. Gluteus maximus myofascial pain syndromes. **A.** Anatomy of the muscle and location of three TPs (X) in different areas. **B, C.** Patterns of pain produced by TPs in the lowermost fibers of the muscle. Modified from Simons, D.G., and Travell, J.G.: Myofascial origins of low back pain. Postgrad. Med., *73*:82, 1983.

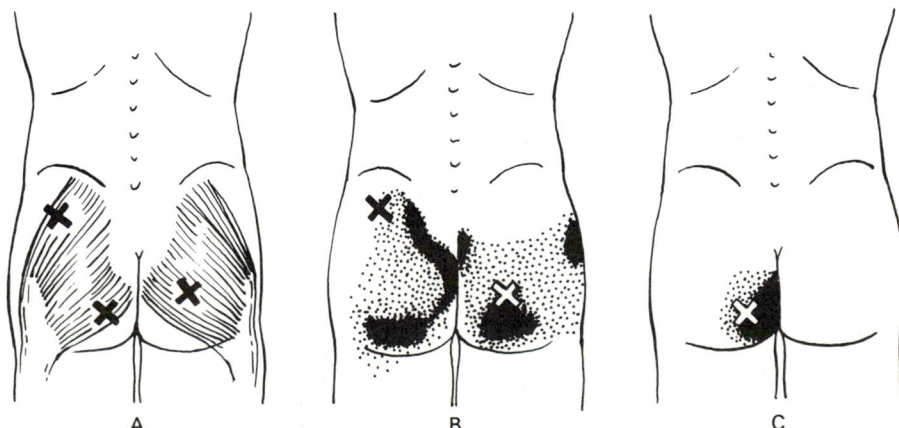

joint. A differential diagnosis can readily be made by relieving the pain by injection of TPs in the muscle.

Gluteus Minimus and Piriformis Syndromes

TPs in the gluteus minimus produce the most severe pain in the lower part of the gluteal region and in the posterior part of the thigh and leg. A TP in the piriformis muscle also produces pain in the lateral and posterior gluteal regions, with spillover to the posterior thigh and calf (see Fig. 77-1 and Chapter 77). These syndromes are mentioned here because the pattern of pain simulates that of a sciatic distribution and those who are not acquainted with myofascial syndromes might attribute the pain to a radiculopathy caused by vertebral pathology. Myofascial syndromes usually do not have the reflex changes and sensory deficits characteristic of a radiculopathy. In addition, TPI of both muscles relieves the pain and eliminates associated symptoms and signs, thus facilitating the differential diagnosis.

Levator Ani and Obturator Internus Syndromes

Pain patterns can be provoked by TPs in the levator ani and obturator internus (Fig. 72-16), resulting in myofascial pain syndromes.

Conclusion

Myofascial pain syndromes with TPs are among the most frequent causes of acute low back pain. If properly treated with several injections the pain and associated pathophysiology are relieved. If the syndromes are not recognized, however, and the pain is treated as if it had another cause, the patient can develop fibrotic changes (scar tissue) within the TP that can progress to persistent pain and a further decrease in muscle function. At this stage therapy should include elimination of pathology through breaking up the fibrotic tissue by repetitive needling combined with infiltration of local anesthetics (12). Fischer (12) also suggested multiple needling of the entire pain area at this stage, as well as of the hypersensitive band extending from both ends of the maximally sensitive spot. Repeated insertion and withdrawal of the needle, combined with deposits of small amount of local anesthetic, breaks up the scar tissue and can result in complete healing. Moreover, disruption of the pathologic tissue combined with local anesthesia prevents muscle spasm and discomfort after injection.

Promptly after injection of TPs it is essential to apply heat to the affected muscle and to carry out passive and active motions of the part; these are considered to be essential to therapy. Patients should be made to recognize the importance of their active participation in treatment and be encouraged to undertake the specific, appropriate forms of exercise. The involved muscle must not be activated too rapidly or moved to a painful degree. Fischer (12), an experienced clinician in this field, recommended that, promptly after injection, patients should receive 2 days of physiotherapy consisting of hot packs and electrical stimulation with sinusoidal surging currents for 15 minutes, thus inducing strong contraction of the muscle. Periodic contraction and relaxation squeezes out the local swelling, promotes the circulation, and relaxes the muscle, thus preventing it from going to spasm (12). The therapy session is concluded by limbering exercises, sometimes combined with an ethyl chloride spray over the areas that are painful on movement. Exercises for limbering and maintaining and improving flexibility of the body should be performed by patients at least three times daily.

In patients with acute myofascial syndromes (i.e., the symptoms are of recent onset and caused by major trauma), two or three treatments are often sufficient to provide permanent relief. Patients with long-standing myofascial syndromes associated with severe pain caused by activation of latent TPs might require 3 to 6 weeks of intensive therapy consisting of TPIs and physical therapy. In such patients TPIs can be given three times each week, with each being followed by three sessions of physiotherapy (see above). When patients improve TPIs are reduced to once weekly or biweekly. Physiotherapy is recommended at least three times weekly until being tapered to the individual response. Consult Chapter 21 for a detailed discussion of all aspects of myofascial pain syndromes.

Other Painful Musculofascial Disorders

Primary Fibromyalgia Syndrome

Primary fibromyalgia syndrome (PFS), known as "fibrositis" and other terms for many years (Chapter 23), is said to be a frequent cause of diffuse, generalized musculoskeletal pain associated with multiple, discrete, predictable tender points and stiffness (41, 14, 58–60). After reviewing the chronology of this condition, Travell and Simons (5) stated that it is an ambiguous diagnosis because of its multiple, incompatible meanings and is best avoided. Others have continued to insist, however, and have provided evidence that PFS can be differentiated from myofascial pain syndromes (MPS) (14, 58–64). Like myofascial pain syndromes, the precise pathogenesis of PFS is unknown. Hypoxia caused by vasoconstriction and other biochemical changes have been found (58) but their role is not clear.

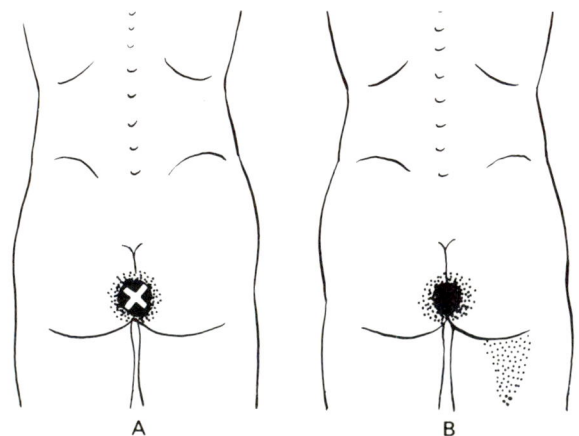

FIG. 72-16. Levator ani and obturator internus myofascial pain syndromes. *A.* Location of the TP (X) in the levator ani muscle and pattern of pain produced. *B.* The pattern of pain produced by TP in the obturator internus, which is not shown because the TP is located internally. Modified from Simons, D.G., and Travell, J.G.: Myofascial origins of low back pain. Postgrad. Med., *73*:82, 1983.

Symptoms and Signs

In addition to diffuse, generalized musculoskeletal pain, PFS is characterized by local tenderness in 12 or 14 specified sites with widespread pain and aching of more than 3 months' duration, whereas MPS is characterized by the presence of specific TPs in one or several muscles. Other criteria differentiate PFS from MPS with TPs (Chapter 23), including disturbed sleep, morning fatigue and stiffness, and absence of laboratory evidence of inflammation or muscle damage (normal ESR, SGOT, rheumatoid factor—RF, and muscle enzyme levels) (60). Formerly the only demonstrable laboratory markers for fibromyalgia were IgG deposition at the dermoepidermal junction (61) and a high prevalence (28%) of HLA-B27 tissue antigen, associated with ankylosing spondylitis. The latter suggests that it might be a prodrome of classic inflammatory rheumatic disease, but PFS is a seronegative condition (60).

A recent study by Vaerøy and collaborators (62) revealed that patients with fibromyalgia (FM) had elevated levels of substance P (sP) and a high incidence of Raynaud's phenomenon (RP). Among the 30 patients studied, sP levels were 36.1 ± 2.7 fmol/ml (range, 16.5 to 79.1) compared with values of 10 to 12 fmol/ml for healthy volunteers, and nearly 53% of patients had RP. Among those with FM and RP, sP levels were 34 ± 2.9 fmol/ml and, in those without RP, sP levels were 38.0 ± 4.7 fmol/ml. Because sP is considered to be a neurotransmitter of nociceptive information, the results provide evidence for the basis of generalized pain. The high incidence of RP suggests sympathetically-induced vasoconstriction, a hypothesis that is supported by the findings of Bengtsson and Bengtsson (56).

An important criterion for FM is demonstration of bilateral tender points in at least six areas, including the interspinous ligament of L5–S1 and the upper outer buttock over the gluteus medius. These tender points are likely to cause low back pain. Indeed, two studies showed that the low back was the first or second most common site of aches, pain, and stiffness (63, 64). Figure 72-17 depicts the sites of common tender points in PFS patients (64). After the knee, the low back area contains the most sites of tender points.

Treatment

Recent studies have indicated that relief of pain and stiffness, as well as improvement in sleep, can be achieved by reassuring patients and explaining the nature of the illness and the possible mechanisms of pain, by symptomatic treatment with heat or massage, and by encouraging moderate aerobic exercise (60). Modest relief of pain, a decrease in the number of tender spots, and overall improvement have been reported with the use of tricyclic antidepressants. One study showed that sympathetic block also markedly reduces the number of TPs and decreases rest pain (56).

In their review article, McCain and Scudds (14) cited two well-controlled studies of the beneficial effects of amitriptyline. In one study the effects of amitriptyline, given in doses of 50 mg, were compared with those of placebo in a 9-week double-blind trial (65). Amitriptyline produced overall improvement in 75% of patients at 5 weeks and in 70% at 9 weeks, whereas placebo produced improvement in 43% and 50% respectively. The second study also showed that amitriptyline alone or combined with naproxen given in doses of 500 mg bid produced significant improvement in global assessment, pain scores, and fibrotic tender point scores. A collaborative clinical trial in 120 patients with primary and secondary PFS compared cyclobenzaprine with placebo in a double-blind crossover study (66). The drug produced significant improvement, both in the total number of active fibrotic tender points and in the objective measurement of pain threshold over the fibrotic tender points. The musculoskeletal pain scores improved, sleep disturbances were relieved, and duration of fatigue decreased during the study. It has also been found that strenuous physical exercise produces not only improvement in cardiovascular fitness, but also a significant improvement in fibrotic tender point scores (14).

Bengtsson and Bengtsson (56) studied 21 patients with PFS who were divided into four groups. Eight patients received a regional (stellate ganglion) blockade with bupivacaine and 14 days later received an intravenous regional sympathetic blockade with guanethidine. Ten patients received a sham block with saline solution and another 10 received bupivacaine intramuscularly. The efficacy of the block in interrupting sympathetic function was measured by various well-known techniques. Tender points and rest pain in the arm, shoulders, and neck were evaluated 4 hours after injection, whereas the results of the guanethidine block were evaluated 24 hours after injection by counting TPs and tender points and by assessing rest pain in the hand and forearm. Complete sympathetic blockade produced by stellate ganglion block significantly reduced a number of TPs and resulted in a decrease in rest pain. Guanethidine blockade reduced the number of tender points but had no effect on rest pain. The beneficial effects of sympathetic block were attributed to improvement in microcirculation, and it was concluded that sympathetic hyperactivity in some patients contributes to the pathogenesis of primary fibromyalgia.

In view of these findings, patients with severe low back pain (or severe upper arm and neck pain) caused by proven primary fibromyalgia can be managed with lumbar sympathetic blocks achieved either paravertebrally or through a continuous epidural catheter. If this proves effective chemical sympathectomy might be considered but only in patients with severe pain that can be completely relieved by three or four prognostic blocks for at least 3 days.

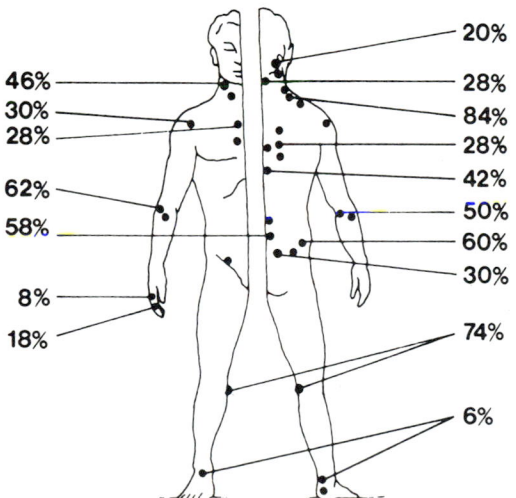

FIG. 72-17. Common tender points in patients with primary fibromyalgia syndrome on the right anterior and posterior parts of the body. From Yunus, M., et al.: Primary fibromyalgia (fibrositis): Clinical study of 50 patients with matched normal controls. Semin. Arthritis Rheum., 11:151, 1981.

Muscle Contractures

Pathophysiology and Symptoms and Signs

Chapters 23 and 90 discuss the Gunn hypothesis of musculoskeletal pain caused by spondylitic radiculopathy, which results in supersensitivity phenomena in membranes of nerves and muscles that generate ectopic impulses that produce pain. Muscle contractures develop and cause pain by squeezing intramuscular vessels containing nociceptors that can be activated by the ischemia. When paraspinal contractures compress nerve roots they can create a vicious cycle of pain. Moreover, sustained contracture leads to degeneration and secondary pain. If physical activity stresses various parts of the body the pain is markedly aggravated. This is particularly true of the low back, where contractures involve the long paraspinal muscles. Low back pain is most common at the L5–S1 level, but higher segmental levels are often involved and the pain frequently reaches the lower thoracic levels.

Most injuries to nerves are minor and the neuropathy is minimal and transient, so that the pain resolves spontaneously with time. The use of analgesics or the application of simple physical therapy measures, such as heat or massage, is generally all that is necessary. When such measures fail, however, it is necessary to release the contractures by insertion of acupuncture needles (these are thin and solid—see Fig. 90-2) into motor points in the musculotendinous junctions, which generally correspond to traditional acupuncture points (67). A motor point is the skin region at which an innervated muscle is most accessible to percutaneous electrical excitation at the lowest intensity (68). This point generally overlies the muscle motor band of innervation, and points belonging to the affected myotome(s) are chosen for treatment. For example, in treating an injury between the L3 and L4 vertebrae that affects the L3 nerve root, points in muscles belonging to the L3 myotome would be treated. When pain is of purely musculoskeletal origin, response to this treatment can be rewarding.

Diagnosis

Gunn (Chapter 90) emphasizes that examination of the lumbar region must go beyond the standard determination of signs of denervation, such as straight leg raising, Lasègue's sign, attenuated reflexes, sensory deficit, and muscle atrophy. In most back patients with early neuropathy these are generally negative and the examiner must search for more subtle signs of trophedema, tenderness on motor points, increased muscle tone, and autonomic effects (see pages 569 to 572 for more details). The key to successful treatment of persistent low back pain of musculoskeletal origin is that the entire lumbar back, including the upper lumbar and lower thoracic levels, must be examined as well as the lower limbs.

Treatment

Treatment aims to release contractures, promote healing, and remove the source of irritation and pain. This is best achieved through insertion of solid acupuncture needles into motor points. The advantage of dry or acupuncture needling is that it produces prolonged stimulation through generation of a current of injury that can last for days (68). Needle therapy might also have a unique beneficial feature—Gunn speculated that it can promote healing by local release of the platelet-derived growth hormone (69).

Treatment points in the lower back include motor points in the quadratus lumborum and erector spinae, including the iliocostalis lumborum, iliocostalis thoracis, iliocostalis longissimus, and multifidus muscles, which are supplied by all of the lumbar nerves. Insertion of the needle provides a useful and unique diagnostic tool for revealing the presence of any deep muscle spasm.

Treatment points in the buttocks include the gluteus maximus (L5, S1, S2), medius, and minimus (L4–S1), the superior and inferior gemellus, the piriformis, and the quadratus femoris muscles. Various motor points must be penetrated to relieve low back pain caused by muscle contractures (Fig. 72-18).

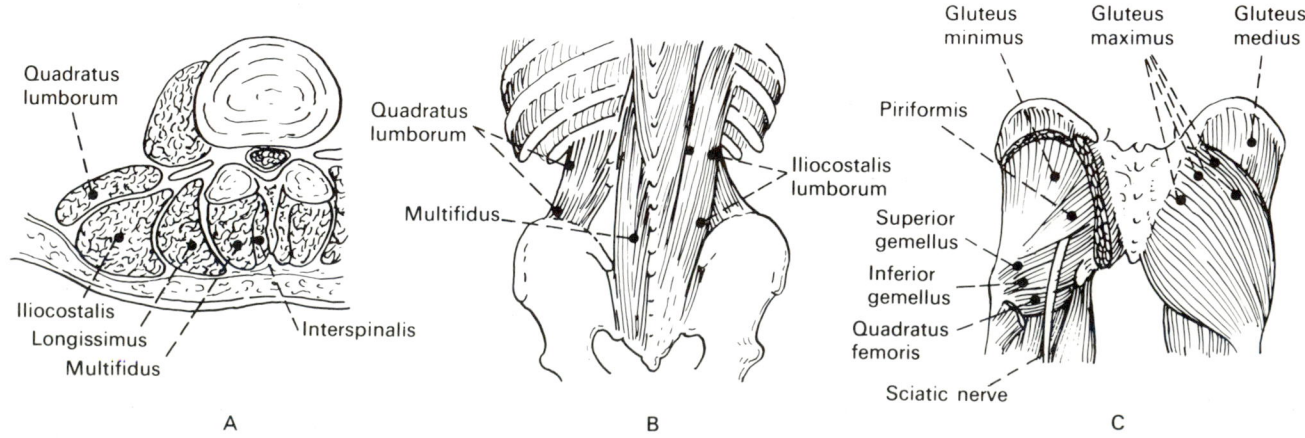

FIG. 72-18. Motor points commonly used for insertion of acupuncture needles. These motor points are often found near TPs in various parts of the body.

B. PAINFUL DISORDERS OF JOINTS AND LIGAMENTS

Disorders of joints and ligaments and of surrounding muscles of the lumbosacral spine can also cause low back pain. Other than those discussed in Chapter 71, the lumbosacral, sacroiliac, and apophyseal joints can be susceptible to injury or inflammatory changes and thus produce low back pain. In addition to arthritides and other pathologic processes (Chapter 71), sprain of the ligaments and strain of the surrounding muscles of one or more of these joints can cause low back pain. Although some authorities have disputed that sprain of these joints causes back pain, based primarily on controversial pathoanatomic findings (1), consideration of the anatomic and pathophysiologic substrates and clinical evidence support the notion that they can cause low back pain. These joints have a rich nerve supply, including nociceptive afferents that can be activated by injury or disease. They can be subjected to inflammatory changes, infections, and traumatically induced dysfunction, like other joints. When correctly diagnosed and treated, patients are relieved of pain. On the other hand, when patients are improperly diagnosed and treated, particularly with surgery, prolonged pain and disability can result. In this section I first discuss lumbosacral and sacroiliac sprain and strain and then discuss painful disorders caused by facet joint pathology.

Acute Lumbosacral Sprain or Strain (XXVII-6)

Acute lumbosacral sprain or strain is characterized by pain that varies in quality and severity, depending on the causative factors. Minor injuries produce a few dull, aching, cramping pains, whereas severe injuries cause severe, sharp, knife-like back pain.

Etiology and Pathophysiology

Recently the lumbosacral joint has assumed a more important role in the causation of low back pain, and the sacroiliac joint has become less important. This has probably occurred because of its position—the lumbosacral joint is subjected to more strain and stress than any other part of the spine (70). Marked alteration in normal lumbar lordosis and in the mechanical relationship between the lumbar spine and the sacrum, which can be produced by severe postural disturbances, places stress on the joint and causes static lumbosacral sprain or strain. Lumbosacral sprain and strain can also be caused by abnormal kinetic factors (70).

STATIC SPINE. Cailliet (70) noted that an excessive increase in lumbar lordosis produces static or postural low back pain. A normal lumbosacral angle of 30° is associated with a shearing stress of 50% of the superincumbent weight, whereas an increase to 40 or 50° increases the shearing stress to 65% or 75%, respectively, of the superincumbent weight.

Because the anterior longitudinal ligament limits the degree of extension of the lumbar spine and thus limits excessive opening of the interspace, any further extension of the spine results in a decrease or closure of the posterior disk space and in the approximation of the posterior articulations. This in turn causes a gliding of the facets into each other, which produces an increase in the axial load that is borne by the facet joint (normally 20% of the total load) (71).

When this occurs the joint surfaces are compressed and the resulting synovial irritation and inflammation produce pain. Moreover, the increase in inclination causes greater shearing stress on the facets, which further compromises the articular synovial lining. Certain pathologic processes, such as spondylolisthesis and disk degeneration, can cause approximation and stress and compression of the articular facets. Severe hyperextension of the lumbosacral segment can also cause nerve root compression and posterior disk protrusion (Fig. 72-19).

Some authorities (1), on the basis of radiologic studies, which suggested that an increase in lordosis of up to 80% of the lumbosacral angle is questionably related to low back pain, have disputed that hyperlordosis can cause back pain. A significant percentage of gravidas, however, suffer low back pain during the latter part of pregnancy (71). The pain usually radiates to the buttocks and in some women it is referred to the legs (71), but this disappears soon after delivery. The pain is presumably caused by the increase in lordosis and some have suggested that it can predispose these patients to herniated disk later in life (72).

KINETIC LOW BACK PAIN. Kinetic low back pain is caused by abnormal strain on a normal back, normal stress on an abnormal back, or normal stress on an unprepared normal back (70). *Abnormal strain on a normal back* can be caused by holding a heavy weight away from the body for an unusually long period of time, by standing in a forward flexed posture of 10 to 15° for a prolonged period, or by prolonged driving in such a posture, all of which cause excessive loading on the lumbar ligaments and intervertebral disks (Fig. 70-20). When the muscular contracture needed to sustain such a posture becomes exhausted the brunt of the stress falls on the ligaments, which have a limited resiliency, and pain can result. When the resiliency of the ligaments becomes exhausted, the brunt of the stress falls on the joints, which can subluxate. Sustained muscular contraction can produce ischemia in the muscle tissue, which in turn causes pain. Any overwhelming stress that stretches the ligaments of the functional unit and exceeds the movement within the unit ultimately stretches the long ligaments throughout the entire spine.

Normal strain on an abnormal back implies improper use of a structurally defective back. The defect can be in the bony structure, the articular portion of the spine, the ligaments, the muscular tissue, or any combination of these. It can occur with structural scoliosis with facet impingement or with tight hamstring muscles (70).

The third concept of body mechanics dysfunction that can result in low back pain proposed by Cailliet (70) is that of *normal stress imposed on a normal back*, but imposed when the back is unprepared for such a stress. Either isometric or isotonic muscle contraction is needed to initiate movement; under normal conditions an impending movement evokes appropriate action. The anticipated movement must be graded to the required intensity of contraction, to the rapidity of the contemplated action, and to the extent of contraction necessary for time and distance. A contraction can "overshoot the mark" and cause excessive movement that exceeds the physiologic limit imposed by ligaments and capsular and articular tissue. Consequently damage occurs that can be minor or major but nevertheless results in disability.

A degenerative lesion or an anatomic defect, such as spondylolisthesis, abnormal facet, or other pathologic process, can also make the joints especially susceptible to injuries. A fatigued or weak muscle is susceptible to injury, even without the presence of pathologic process. If the trunk muscles preposition the spine before it is loaded, a slowness in muscle action caused by fatigue can find the spine unprepared for the task, leading to injury (1). When an injury is

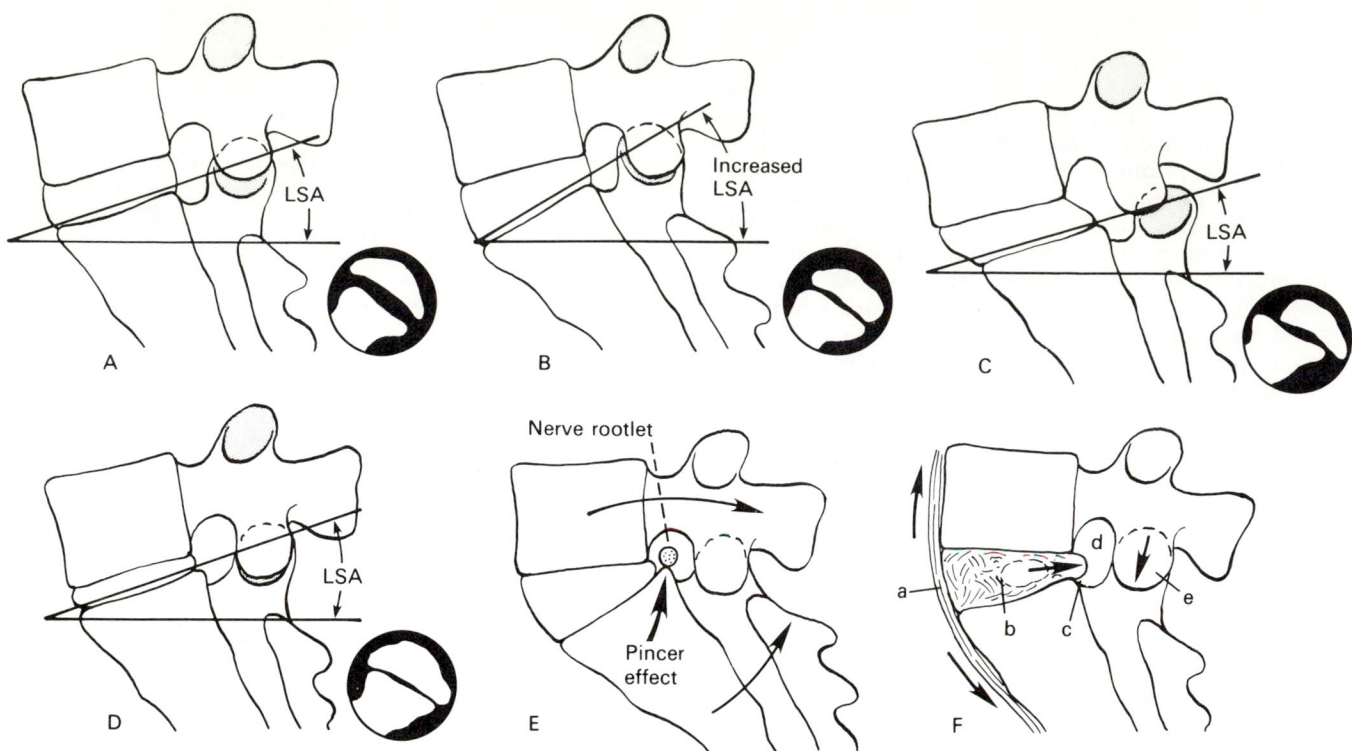

FIG. 72-19. Variations in posterior articular relationship. Side views of L5 and upper sacrum showing lumbosacral angle and effect of its changes on the zygapophyseal (facet) joint. The insets in black and white provide craniocaudal views of the facet joints. *A.* Normal lumbosacral angle with intact disk and normal relationship between articular facets. *B.* Increased lumbosacral angle (LSA) with posterior closure of the facets. *C.* Spondylolisthesis with a normal LSA. Traction is exerted on the posterior longitudinal ligament, and facet alignment is disrupted. *D.* Disk degeneration with narrowing of the intervertebral space and approximation of the facets. *E.* Nerve root impingement due to hyperextension of the lumbar spine with an increase in the sacral angle (arrow). With a degenerated disk a greater degree of impingement can be expected. *F.* Disk protrusion posteriorly during lumbosacral hyperextension. The anterior longitudinal ligament (a) restricts further extension. The nucleus (b) has deformed to the maximum and cannot migrate further anteriorly, so it moves posteriorly. This causes a bulge (c) with encroachment into the intervertebral foramen (d). The facets overlap (e) which also narrows the foramen and causes pain on weight bearing. Modified from Cailliet, R.: Low Back Pain Syndrome. 3rd Ed. Philadelphia, F.A. Davis, 1981.

added to existing weak muscles or to a pathologic process it produces acute lumbosacral sprain or strain that can involve the supraspinous and interspinous ligaments, capsular ligaments, ligamenta flava, and perhaps the iliolumbar ligaments, short and long sacroiliac ligaments, and the overlying mass of muscles.

Severe injuries can be caused by direct impact by a large object, by falling on the low back, or by excessively strenuous effort during forward bending while the body is in an unbalanced position. Lifting, twisting, or falling can result from brief, unexpectedly high-magnitude forces or by loads applied suddenly. A high proportion of injuries occur at work and lifting and twisting are said to be the leading causes, whereas gardening is first on the list of leisure time activities that produce acute low back pain, probably consequent to lumbosacral sprain or strain (1, 73–76).

Symptoms and Signs

Symptoms and signs vary according to the degree of injury. With partial tear of the ligaments and strain of the overlying muscle immediate, severe, disabling pain, tenderness, and muscle spasm are experienced. The pain is most intense in the region of the lumbosacral joints but also radiates to the gluteal region and to the lateral and posterior parts of the thigh. Pressure on the tips of the spinous process of the L5 and L4 vertebrae or on the lumbosacral or iliolumbar

joints markedly aggravates the pain and causes exquisite tenderness. The rigidity of the spine is usually marked and the lumbar lordotic curve is decreased or obliterated. All movements involved in the spine are restricted. Flexing the hip with the legs extended beyond the point of stretching the gluteal muscles or moving the pelvis or lumbar spine produces severe pain in the lumbosacral area. Extension of the straight leg causes as much pain as flexion. Forcing the patient's heel to touch the buttocks causes the pelvis to rise from the table. This is a positive Ely's sign and indicates a lumbosacral lesion. Neurologic examination produces no positive findings.

Diagnosis

Diagnosis is made through the history and physical findings. Radiography can demonstrate extreme lumbar lordosis. Because CT scans and myelograms are usually negative they should not be considered unless evidence of a neurologic problem is found. Injection of a dilute solution of local anesthetic (e.g., 0.25% bupivacaine) into the most tender areas in the muscle or ligament relieves the pain without involvement of major nerves.

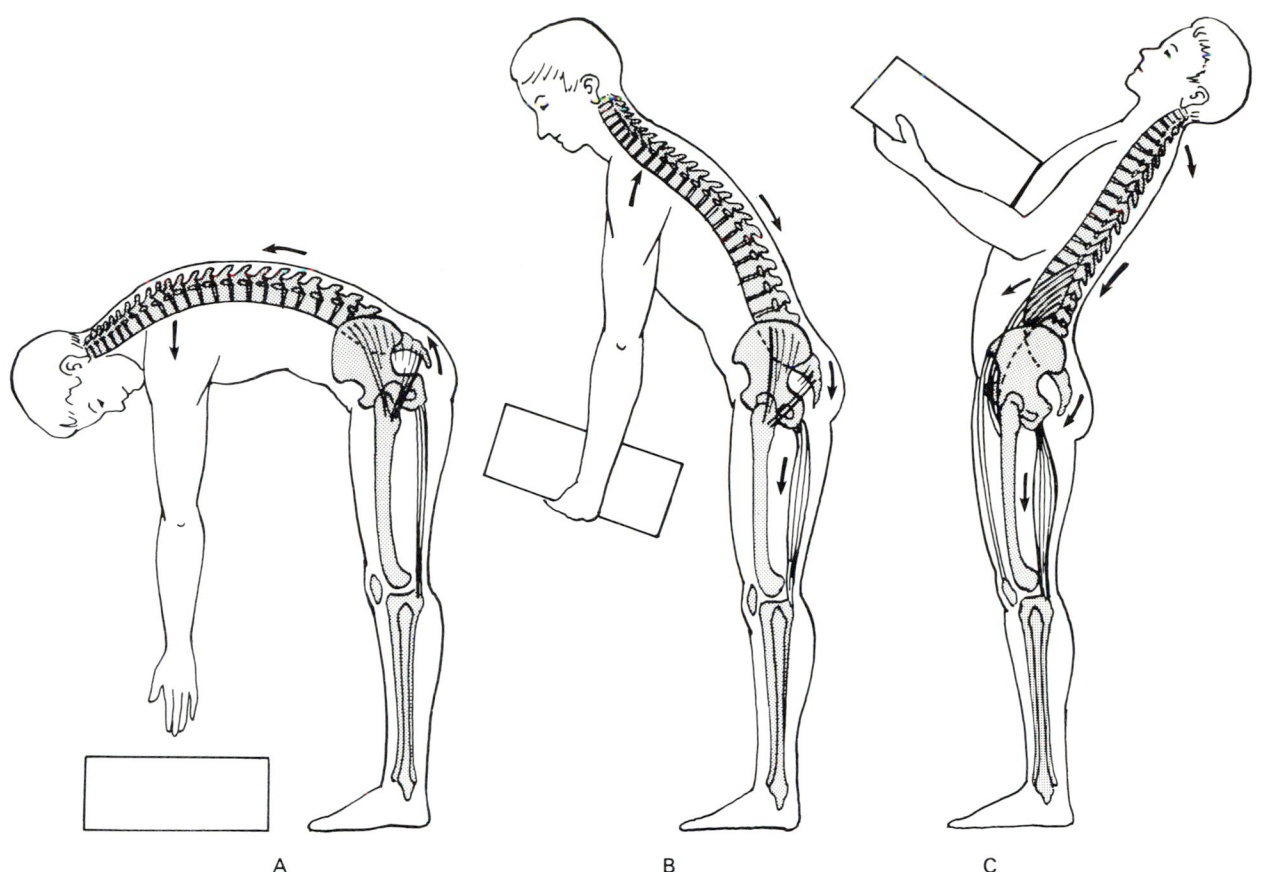

Fig. 72-20. Analysis of injuries caused by lifting and hyperextension movements of the spine. **A.** In bending forward to lift an object the spine flexes, the intervertebral disks compress anteriorly, and the spinous processes separate. This stretches the supraspinous, interspinous, and capsular ligaments and causes the hamstring muscles to tighten as the pelvis tilts forward. Onset of pain during this phase of movement indicates sprain of these ligaments. **B.** As the load is lifted the erector spinae muscles contract and the spine deflexes, causing the spinous processes to become approximated and the posterior ligaments to become relaxed. Onset of pain, indicative of injury during this act of lifting, cannot be accounted for by ligamentous sprain because the posterior ligaments are being relaxed. Any pain is the result of strain of the erector spinae muscles. **C.** Hyperextension brings about an approximation of the spinous processes and articular facets. Extreme injurious hyperextension can produce compression injury of the posterior ligaments or fracture of the spinous processes, laminae, or articular facets.

Treatment

Patients with minor trauma have symptoms and signs that resolve within a few days, provided they avoid physical activity initially and use physical therapy measures such as heat, massage, and NSAIDs for pain relief. Patients with major trauma who have moderate to severe pain should be put to bed, preferably a bed with a thin sponge rubber or air mattress reinforced by an underlying board. Shifting the mattress to the floor is often a good substitute if such a board is not available. A pillow behind the knees can assist in relaxation.

In patients who have severe pain, regional infiltration with a long-acting local anesthetic or continuous lumbosacral epidural analgesia for a few days provides complete pain relief and relaxation of the spastic muscles and facilitates the application of physical therapy measures. The use of traction is questionable because it induces immobilization and results in loss of muscle strength. The period of bed rest should be limited to 2 to 4 days; patients should be allowed up with instructions to avoid any movements that can place further stress on the muscles of the low back. Periods of sitting should be short and patients should be made to walk around. This is followed by a period of progressive exercises to reinforce the musculature that might have become weakened as a result of the injury and the immobility. Overtreatment with systemic medication and premature surgical intervention because of mistaken diagnosis should be avoided at all costs because these measures usually lead to chronic low back pain. Current evidence suggests that pain subsides in most patients rather quickly, so that 90% of patients are well within 4 to 6 weeks (median, 4 weeks) (1). It has also been shown that the risk of recurrence of acute low back pain as a result of injury is approximately 60%, with the next one or two attacks having a shorter and more benign course.

Recurrent Back Pain Caused by Sprain or Strain (XXVII-7)

Recurrent lumbosacral sprain or strain associated with low back pain occurs rather frequently, but usually is not as severe as the first attack. The pain is usually mild to moderate and is dull, aching, or burning in quality. The recurrence can be provoked by prolonged sitting or standing or by repetitive awkward movements or postures, or can be caused by lifting or twisting at work. Data published by Troup (75) suggest that pain caused by work-related accidents takes longer to subside, both during the first attack and with recurrences. In contrast, attacks not associated with work-related accidents are less common during the third year than the first 2 years. Nachemson and Bigos (1) pointed out that this demonstrates a tendency for low back pain to last for a couple of years and then subside.

Symptoms and Signs

The mild to moderate dull, aching pain, which is fluctuating or continuous in nature, is felt in the lumbosacral region, buttocks, and posterior thighs. Pain is usually greatest at the end of the day or at the end of the working shift. No significant structural abnormalities are usually present. Some cases can be associated with mild degrees of muscle spasm, decrease of normal lordosis, and limitation of movements.

Treatment

The primary goal of treatment of low back sprain or strain is to instruct the patient to avoid those movements that can aggravate the pain. Pain is generally well controlled with NSAIDs. It is essential to have the patient avoid activities that provoke recurrence and at the same time participate in a progressive exercise program to strengthen the back muscles.

Chronic Lumbosacral Sprain or Strain (XXVII-9)

Chronic lumbosacral sprain is probably the most common cause of low back pain. The condition usually develops as a result of improper treatment of acute or recurrent lumbosacral pain. Duration beyond 6 months is likely to be provoked by environmental reinforcing factors and is associated with significant impairment of daily living and work activities.

Symptoms and Signs

Symptoms can vary from a mild backache to moderately severe, gnawing, constant low back pain aggravated by bending, lifting, and other similar activities. The pain is relieved by rest. In mild cases no limitation of motion is found, but extreme motions are painful and trigger areas are present. As the severity of this condition increases additional signs are present, such as restriction of straight leg raising, loss of motion, muscle spasm, and abnormal posture. A markedly reduced tolerance for sitting, standing, or walking is also present, and most patients experience depression and sleep disturbances. Physical examination reveals weak abdominal musculature, loss of normal lordosis, and impairment of movement of the low back. Some patients can develop a mild neurologic deficit that can be confirmed by EMG.

Treatment

Treatment of patients with long-standing low back pain caused by lumbosacral sprain or strain or other disorders requires a multidisciplinary team approach (see below, Section E).

Sacroiliac Sprain

Etiology and Pathophysiology

Formerly the diagnosis of sacroiliac sprain was made frequently, but recent experience suggests that it occurs infrequently. Involvement of the sacroiliac synchondrosis is unusual and occurs with specific disorders or degenerative lesions of the joint, such as rheumatoid arthritis, osteoarthritis, and infections (77). Although the sacroiliac joint is an extremely stable structure in the vertical plane it is vulnerable to rotation or torsion, so torsion sprains of this joint can occur. Acute sacroiliac sprain is caused by vigorous muscular effort of the low back when the individual is in an awkward position, such as raising a window that is stuck, lifting a heavy object, or suddenly and forcibly applying the brakes of an automobile.

The congruity of the two irregular articulations between the sacrum and ilium tends to increase their stability, making up somewhat for the relatively inefficient active (muscular) and passive (ligamentous) supporting structures. The sacroiliac ligaments are weakest anteriorly, where they consist of a slight thickening of the periosteum. Lifting or any other movement that involves contraction or tension of the hamstring muscles causes them to tighten, thus preventing the pelvis from tilting further anteriorly. Their full traction on the pelvis tends to cause the ischium to rotate downward and

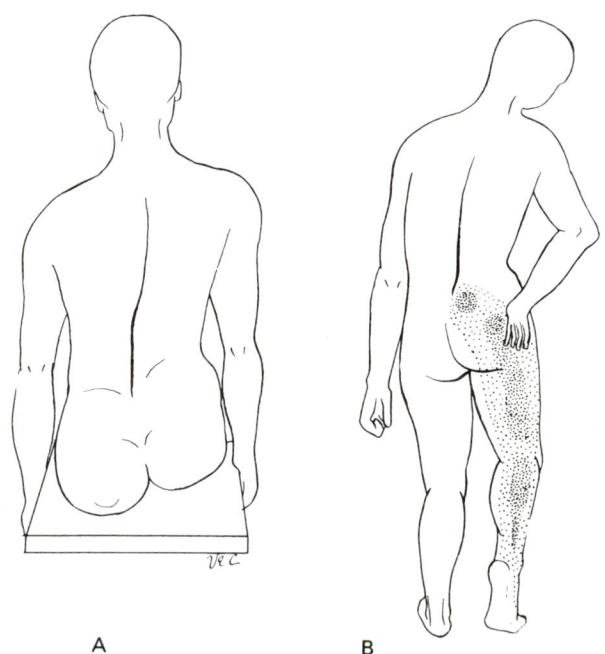

A   B

FIG. 72-21. Position of patient with acute sacroiliac sprain. **A.** Sitting position. **B.** Standing. The stippling indicates the radiation of pain.

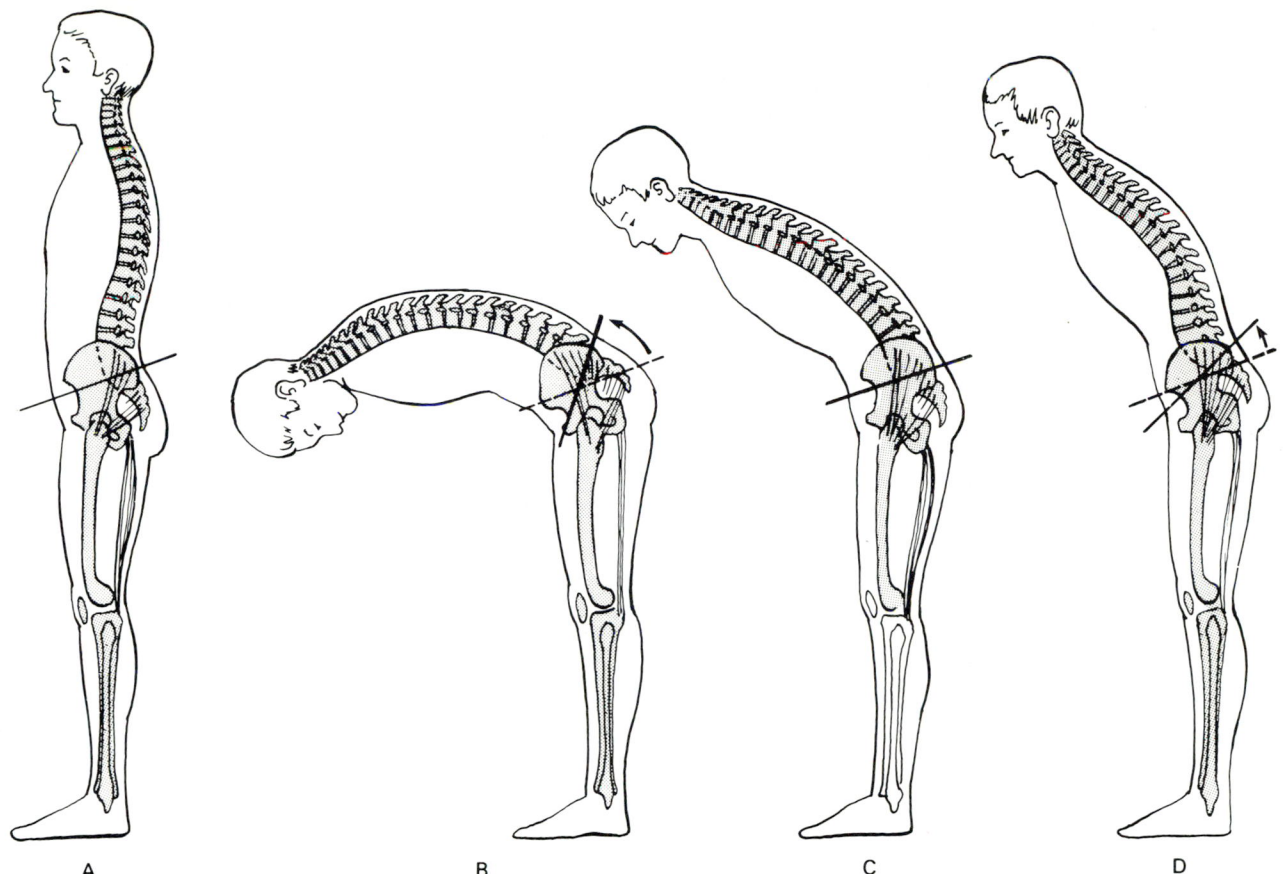

FIG. 72-22. Characteristic forward bending in sacroiliac and lumbosacral disorders. **A.** Normal standing position. **B.** When the spine is normal, bending results in flattening of the lumbar curve and exaggeration of the thoracic curve. **C.** A patient with sacroiliac disorders bends forward so as to avoid hamstring leverage transmitted through the pelvis and consequently flexes the lumbar spine to the limit of its elasticity, but stops as soon as the pelvis begins to tilt forward and the hamstrings begin to tighten. **D.** In a patient with lumbosacral sprain motion takes place in the T12-L1 segment of the spine and hip joint. The pelvis pivots forward to avoid further tension on the posterior ligaments, articular joints, or erector spinae muscles.

forward and the ilium to rotate backward away from the sacrum. Because this is the type of leverage to which the sacroiliac joints are most susceptible, a slip or subluxation results.

Symptoms and Signs

Sacroiliac sprain caused by a slip or subluxation causes pain localized along the posterior border of the ilium directly over the sacroiliac joint that radiates to the back of the hips and thighs, usually as far as the knees. The patient stands favoring the affected extremity, exhibits a list to the unaffected side (Fig. 72-21), and experiences exquisite tenderness to pressure over the inferior part of the joint and the hamstring muscles. The low back muscles are usually in spasm, which produces stiffness and limitation of motion. Extremes of hip joint motion on the affected side produce or aggravate the pain. Lying on the affected side of the low back produces discomfort.

Diagnosis

Diagnosis is made through a comprehensive history and physical examination (Chapters 70 and 71). The physical examination should include careful palpation of the back, especially the sacroiliac joints, and the

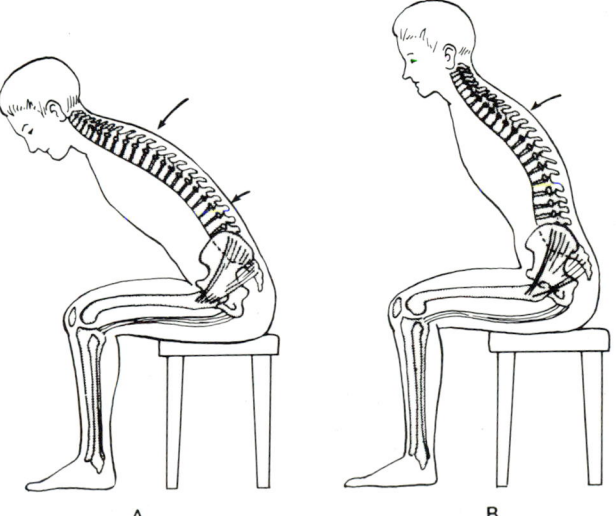

FIG. 72-23. Characteristic forward bending in the sitting position in sacroiliac and lumbosacral disorders. **A.** Because the hamstrings are relaxed in the sitting position as a result of flexion of the knees, patients with sacroiliac disorders can bend freely and painlessly. **B.** Lumbosacral lesions prevent bending, as in the standing position (see Fig. 72-22D).

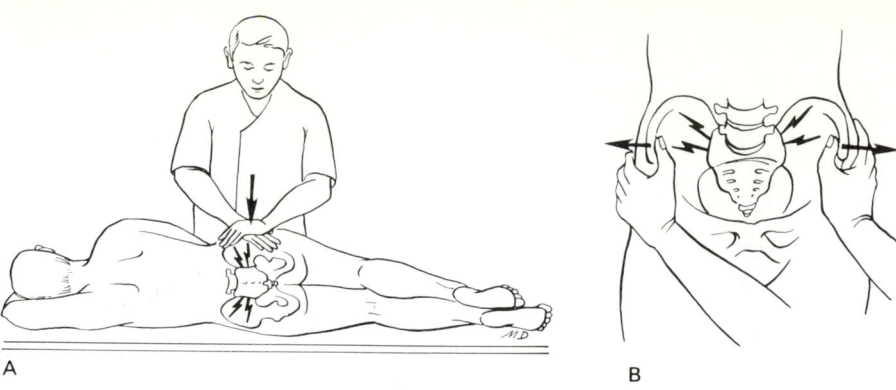

FIG. 72-24. Diagnosis of sacroiliac disorders. **A.** Iliac compression test. With the patient comfortably on the lateral side, downward pressure is exerted on the iliac crest. **B.** The Newton test for eliciting sacroiliac stress. With the patient supine on the examining table the examiner places his hand on the iliac crest, with the thumbs over the anterior superior iliac spines. Pressure is applied downward in an attempt to spread them apart.

use of special tests to determine sacroiliac joint dysfunction and other tests to differentiate sacroiliac disorders from lumbosacral disorders (Figs. 72-22 and 72-23). Other tests include the Lasègue maneuver (Fig. 71-1), compression tests (Fig. 72-24), and the Gaenslen maneuver (78) (Fig. 72-25). Chronic sacroiliac sprain usually involves both joints and causes mild, aching pain that originates in the back and both hips and radiates down both thighs. The results of all these maneuvers, although suggestive of disorders of the sacroiliac joints, must be integrated into a comprehensive examination (Chapters 70 and 71).

Treatment

Treatment of acute sprain consists of bed rest for a few days, the application of ice soon after injury, and relief of pain with NSAIDs. If the pain is severe it is promptly and most effectively relieved by infiltrating the joint with a dilute solution of a long-acting local anesthetic (e.g., 0.125% bupivacaine) and one dose of a long-acting steroid compound (see Fig. 94-5). Chronic

pain requires pain control measures and postural exercises. Acute and chronic low back pain patients should participate in a back school program, which provides information about the biomechanics of the back and ergonomic advice.

Disorders of the Zygapophyseal Joint

Historical Overview

Although the lumbar zygapophyseal joints were suggested as a cause of low back pain in the early part of the twentieth century, it was not until 1933 that Ghormley (79) considered these joints, especially at the lumbosacral level, to be a source of low back pain, and introduced the term "facet syndrome." During the early period other authorities disputed that sprain or changes in the apophyseal joints could occur, because these joints are deeply seated and strongly supported by the primary capsular ligament and accessory ligaments around the vertebral column. Others believed that they could be injured by unusual twisting movements, especially when degenerative intervertebral disks permitted an abnormal range of motion.

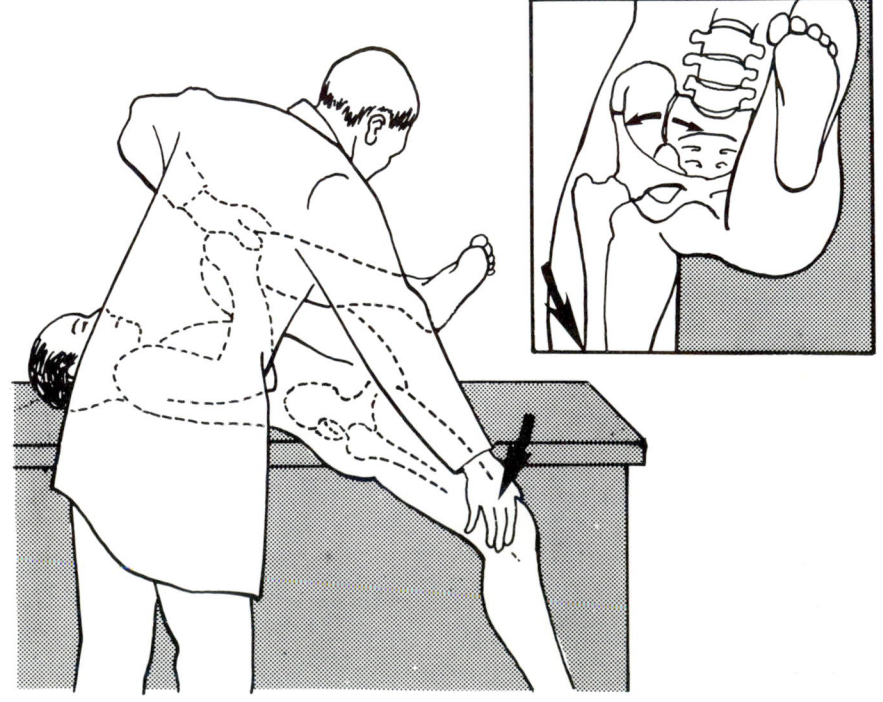

FIG. 72-25. Gaenslen's test. This diagnostic maneuver is helpful in differentiating between sacroiliac and lumbosacral lesions. With the patient lying supine the left hip and knee are flexed acutely to fix the pelvis and lumbar spine of the opposite side and the right hip is forcibly hyperextended downward on the edge of the table or bed. This exerts a rotating force on the ipsilateral half of the pelvis in the sagittal plane through the transverse axis of the sacroiliac joint, which produces or exaggerates pain in sacroiliac lesions but not in lumbosacral lesions.

It was assumed that, following injury or violent muscular effort, subluxation or "slipping" occurred and resulted in tear of the capsule and ligaments. This was said to produce pain and severe protective muscle spasm that "locked" or bound the articular facets together (80). Later, traumatic arthritis or synovitis of the facet joint was thought to develop, which produced persistent pain. More recent epidemiologic studies, however, showed that the degenerative joint diseases that had been considered to be the diagnostic criterion for the facet syndrome did not correlate with symptoms, because an almost equal incidence of such changes was found in symptomatic and asymptomatic persons (81). This lack of correlation led to doubts that the zygapophyseal joint was a significant source of pain (82).

The "facet syndrome" remained a disregarded diagnosis until the mid 1970s, when interest in this syndrome was resurrected and clinicians began to treat some patients' low back pain sucessfully by denervating the lumbar zygapophyseal joints. Prompted by these favorable results, Mooney and Robertson (83) provided the first scientific evidence that the zygapophyseal joints could cause back pain and referred pain in the lower limbs by stimulating lower lumbar zygapophyseal joints in normal volunteers. An important aspect of these experimental studies, which were subsequently corroborated by others (84), was that pain produced in normal volunteers was remarkably similar in quality and distribution to pain suffered clinically by many patients with low back syndrome. This prompted several clinicians to develop techniques of blocking the nerve supply to the zygapophyseal joints, either by injecting the medial branches of the posterior primary division of the lumbar nerves or by injecting local anesthetics into the joint itself. In the 1980s many clinicians reported the successful relief of low back pain syndromes by use of these diagnostic blocks (see ref. 85 for review and references). Techniques were subsequently developed for blocking these nerves and for administering facet intra-articular injections in the cervical region, with similarly favorable results. The techniques for these blocks in the lumbar and cervical regions are depicted in Figure 94-5.

Symptoms and Signs

Patients with proven facet syndrome complain of pain in the back, buttocks, and thighs. The area overlying the affected facet can be tender, and muscle spasm is frequently present. The pain is usually aggravated by hyperextension of the spine, simulating that of spinal stenosis. Occasionally the deep tendon reflexes are depressed and straight leg raising is limited, causing confusion with intervertebral disk syndrome. The neurologic deficits are not of the same degree as intervertebral disk syndrome, however, and the pain of facet syndrome is eliminated by facet injection with a local anesthetic.

The results obtained with diagnostic blocks and those obtained with percutaneous thermocoagulation, as well as open surgery, indicate that in some patients disorders of the zygapophyseal joints cause pain in the lumbar, cervical, or thoracic region. Injection into a joint can be a valuable diagnostic tool in determining whether pathophysiologic changes in the joint are the source of the pain. Unfortunately, no reliable clinical criteria have been developed to diagnose the facet syndrome precisely. Although the pain experienced in the volunteers was similar to that in patients (see above), the area of pain reference varied (83, 84). Pain most commonly occurs in the gluteal region or thigh, but it can also be felt anywhere in the leg. Moreover,

considerable variation and overlap in the distribution of the referred pain after stimulation of joint at different segmental levels are seen, and this distribution is in no way characteristic of the segment stimulated. Features such as aggravation of pain on extension or lateral flexion of the spine occur more frequently in patients with facet syndrome, but can also occur in patients with other causes and sites of pain; thus, they cannot be used to distinguish patients with facet syndrome from patients with other disorders (86). Certain features have been seen on CT scans of patients with facet syndrome, such as joint asymmetry, joint space narrowing, subchondral sclerosis, erosion, and facet hypertrophy (87), but no studies have demonstrated that these changes are pathognomonic of pain-producing joints.

Diagnostic and Prognostic Blocks

In the absence of precise diagnostic clinical features or criteria, the diagnosis of facet syndromes relies exclusively on the results of diagnostic blocks (85). The following points should be considered (Chapter 94):

a. The block procedure must produce *complete* pain relief to support the presumptive diagnosis.

b. At least two and preferably three blocks must be done on different days using local anesthetics that have different durations of action.

c. Each joint is supplied by articular filaments from the medial nerves above and below the joint and occasionally by those from three levels (83). Therefore, if medial block is used, it is necessary to inject both the upper and lower parts of the facet joint and perhaps adjacent segments also.

d. A permanent record of the segments injected must be obtained by radiography to show the segment blocked. Some clinicians inject a small volume (0.2 ml) of metrizamide, especially for intra-articular administration.

e. If complete pain relief is obtained, the patient should be instructed to note and record the duration of the relief with each of the various blocks.

Used in this fashion, diagnostic blocks can be invaluable in determining whether the zygapophyseal joint is the source of pain. If the patient's response is appropriate to the expected action of the drug used, the reliability of the response can be accepted (85). Conversely, an inappropriate response can prevent a reliable positive diagnosis from being made, and can indicate that the patient needs to be examined for possible unrecognized psychologic components of the pain.

Treatment

In patients in whom diagnostic blocks prove that the joints are the source of pain, one of three forms of therapy can be considered: (a) intra-articular injection of steroids; (b) percutaneous thermocoagulation of the nerves; or (c) open surgical facet denervation. The value of steroid injection into the facet joint as a therapeutic measure remains controversial. Some clinicians have reported persistent relief of pain for at least 6 months in 25 to 63% of patients (87–89) following steroid injection, with the reported duration of relief ranging from 2 weeks to 6 months in one study (90) and from 3 days to 13 months in another (91).

The procedure of percutaneous radiofrequency denervation of the joint was devised on the premise that, if diagnostic blocks produced complete pain relief, prolonged relief could be achieved by coagulation of the nerves to the joint. Despite the valid rationale and an extensive literature, cited in detail by Bogduk (85), percutaneous radiofrequency denervation of the facet joints remains controversial for two reasons. First, in the early phase of use of the procedure, anatomically inaccurate target points were employed, resulting in failure. Even though more accurate target points were later adopted, a recent study has shown that the direction in which electrodes are applied to the target nerves greatly affects the reliability with which the nerves can be coagulated (92). Second, coagulation does not produce a permanent "cure" of

the pain because the nerve eventually regenerates, usually within 12 to 18 months. Although denervation can be repeated when pain recurs, many clinicians believe that repeating the procedure every 12 months is unacceptable.

Nachemson and Bigos (1) reported that open facet denervation done through a midline approach provides a more accurate way to denervate the joint by electrocoagulation. They cited the findings of others, and their own, that nerves regenerate (and presumably the pain returns) about 2 years after open denervation. They proposed that, in view of the discovery that some of the joints have a triple nerve supply (83), an open approach is warranted and is preferable to the blind or semiblind radiofrequency destruction.

C. LOW BACK PAIN PRIMARILY OF PSYCHOLOGIC ORIGIN (XXIX)

Tension-Induced Back Pain

The important role that emotional stress plays in causing increased tension of low back muscles has been noted (see above, Prolonged and Increased Muscle Tension). Sarno (93) stated that increased tension caused by psychophysiologic mechanisms (what he referred to as "psychosomatic backache," which is now known to represent a general somatization process; Chapter 15) is the cause of low back pain in 80% of those in the low back pain population. He insisted that what other authorities have called myofascial pain syndromes with TPs, fibromyalgia, fibrositis, or muscle strain really represent "tension myositis," which is primarily the result of emotional stress. This is erroneous and unfortunate, because the approach to the diagnosis and treatment of increased tension caused by emotional stress is different from the diagnosis and treatment of these other musculoskeletal conditions.

Premenstrual Low Back Pain

Etiology

Emotional stress prior to and during menstruation can cause low back pain and pain in other parts of the body. Scambler and Scambler (94) reported that 30% of the women sampled had experienced pain prior to or during menstruation, the premenstrual syndrome (PMS).

Kessler (95) proposed that back pain results when the paraspinal muscles tense as a protective mechanism, and with the increased low back muscle tension there is exacerbation of pain. It has been hypothesized that muscles that have been contracted for long periods can contribute to sensations of tenderness and pain long after the actual contraction has subsided (see page 170 and Fig. 7-14).

Through psychophysiologic mechanisms, emotional stress can cause spasm in different parts of the body. Recently, Dickson-Parnell and Zeichner (96) reported on the psychophysiologic concomitants of perceived emotional stress and low back pain in patients with PMS during three phases of the menstrual cycle: premenstrual, menstrual, and intermenstrual. They studied 39 women who reported the following: either PMS or severe premenstrual low back pain (group I); PMS with moderate premenstrual low back pain (group II); or neither condition (group III). During each of the three menstrual phase-specific assessment sessions participants were exposed to a neutral stimulus, an experimentally induced stressor, and two personally relevant stressors in a randomized order. Concomitant monitoring of low back EMG activity and heart interbeat interval was carried out. Results indicated that participants in group I evidenced greater EMG changes in response to personal stressors compared to the neutral stimulus and experimentally induced stress during the premenstrual phase. EMG activity in response to personal stress was also significantly higher during the premenstrual phase than during the menstrual or intermenstrual phase for group I, and higher than EMG changes evidenced by those in groups II and III during the same phase. Participants in group II, although not reporting severe premenstrual back pain, as did those in group I, reported moderate levels of back pain and evidenced greater physiologic activity (EMG changes) after exposure to a personal stressor than did those in group III. These findings emphasize the relationship between personally relevant stressors and concomitant physiologic responsivity as measured by EMG, and show the role that this arousal can play in maintaining and exacerbating premenstrual low back pain.

Treatment

Treatment of premenstrual low back pain includes NSAIDs for pain relief, education, and counseling. Oral contraceptives can be used to decrease the amount of prostaglandin F_2 produced by the myometrium and can also be used for other reasons (see Chapter 67, which discusses premenstrual and menstrual syndromes in detail).

Chronic Pain Caused by Environmental Factors

The critical role of environmental reinforcing factors and learning (operant mechanisms) in causing a progression from acute low back pain to chronic low back pain is discussed elsewhere (Chapter 71). Environmental factors play an important role in the development and sustenance of chronic low back pain in a significant segment of the population.

Low Back Pain Primarily Caused by Psychologic or Psychiatric Illness

The incidence of low back pain caused solely by psychiatric illness is unknown but, according to Merskey (97) (Chapter 19) it is low compared to the overall incidence of low back pain problems. Although psychologic factors are important in persistent or protracted low back pain in a significant number of patients they are rarely the sole cause of the pain, nor will the diagnosis emphasize them in the first instance (89).

D. OTHER DISORDERS THAT CAUSE LOW BACK PAIN

Vascular Disease (XV-1/624-X8c)

Stenosis of the lower aorta, aortic bifurcation, and of the iliac arteries caused by arteriosclerosis or a thrombus causes severe, intermittent claudication in the gluteal region, low back, groin, hips, thighs, and calves that is brought on by walking but promptly relieved by rest (Fig. 28-4A and B). If patients insist on continuing walking the pain becomes excruciating and disabling, but vanishes after a few minutes of rest. The quality and distribution of the pain are somewhat similar to those produced by spinal stenosis on walking. The differential diagnosis is facilitated by palpation of the femoral arteries, which reveals the absence of pulses in aortoiliac arteries. In patients who might have decreased pulses and spinal stenosis, the differential diagnosis can be made by having them ride a bicycle with the back flexed. This relieves the pain of spinal stenosis, but not the pain of aortoiliac arterial disease. Because both conditions occur in elderly people, palpation of the arterial trunk should be included as part of the routine back examination. This condition is discussed in Chapter 28.

Referred Pain from Visceral Structures (XXVIII-1)

Pain referred to the back can be caused by disease of a pelvic viscus or by disorders of the lower bowel or of retroperitoneal structures. In women the most usual condition is a retroverted uterus, although disease of the ovaries or fallopian tube can also cause back pain. The low back pain associated with premenstrual syndrome has already been mentioned. Other diseases of the uterus that produce referred back pain include tumors, ovarian cysts, and infections. In men prostatic disorders such as prostatitis, urethritis, and cancer and other disorders can cause referred low back pain. Diseases of the rectosigmoid that can cause pain referred to the low back include cancers and other tumors, distension, fecal impaction, ulcers, and hemorrhoids.

Diseases of the hip, including osteoarthritis, infection, rheumatoid arthritis, and fracture, can cause pain in the hip and thigh that can radiate to the low back. Retroperitoneal neoplasm can cause low back pain associated with anorexia and weight loss. In most of these patients the back findings are insufficient to explain the symptoms, but in elderly patients pain associated with degenerative disorders can complicate the picture and test the diagnostic acumen of the attending physician.

Differential diagnosis to distinguish between disorders of the back and referred pain is made through a careful history and physical examination of the abdomen and pelvis, which usually reveals signs of local pathology. CT scanning is particularly helpful in identifying mass lesions in the abdomen and pelvis (Chapter 71).

E. MULTIDISCIPLINARY APPROACH TO DIAGNOSIS AND TREATMENT OF LOW BACK PAIN

In Chapter 71 Loeser and colleagues provide excellent guidelines for the correct management of patients with acute low back pain, of those with chronic low back pain caused by a specific pathologic process, and of those with chronic low back pain resulting from operant or environmental mechanisms. Although it is noted that this is best done in a multidisciplinary/interdisciplinary rehabilitation program, they do not elaborate on the concept in that chapter. In Chapter 100, however, Loeser and associates discuss two teams of this type that carry out activities for the diagnosis and treatment of all chronic pain syndrome patients and of those with chronic pain caused by operant mechanisms. In their recent monograph, Loeser and Egan (98), together with other members of the University of Washington (UW) Multidisciplinary Pain Center, described in great detail the theory, organization, and function of the UW center. Because low back pain is a most complex diagnostic and therapeutic problem with a multifactorial basis, I believe it is appropriate to re-emphasize here the importance of the multidisciplinary approach in managing not only patients whose pain is caused by operant mechanisms but also patients with failed back surgery pain, spinal stenosis, and other pathologic factors.

Obviously, most patients with acute low back pain are usually managed by a family physician, internist, or orthopedic surgeon. As noted in many studies, about 75% of patients with acute low back pain get well and return to work or to other activities in which they were involved before the injury, usually within 4 weeks (99–101). This high rate of return to work occurs because of the natural course of the disease or injury, proper treatment, or both. Two studies (99, 100) showed that, at 2 months after injury, 30% of patients injured at work still had pain, whereas the report of the Quebec Task Force (18), using data from many studies, suggested that, at 7 weeks, 16% of patients still had pain and by 3 months this decreased to 12%. One study showed that 10% of patients who still had pain at 2 months accounted for 80% of the total cost of health care and compensation (102). This extraordinary impact on the cost of health care in many industrialized nations is of great concern to society and to certain segments of the health care professions.

The magnitude of the low back pain problem prompted two groups to develop guidelines for the proper treatment of low back pain. In the United States the prestigious Institute of Medicine appointed a Committee on Pain, Disability and Chronic Illness Behavior to consider the various aspects of chronic pain and disability (17). In Canada the Quebec Task Force on Spinal Disorders focused on pain in all parts of the spine, with emphasis on the incidence of such disorders among workers in Quebec (18). The Quebec group proposed a classification of activity-related* disorders, which included 11 categories (Table 72-2). Unfortunately, and to my great distress, they included the "chronic pain syndrome," which is pain that persists over 6 months, in category 10. The term "chronic pain syndrome" (see page 19 of this book), which was coined in 1975 by my former colleague R.G. Black (103) (and which was wrongly attributed to others by the Task Force), was intended for "patients who suffer

*"Activity-related" refers to those injured at work.

persistent intractable pain complaints, many of which are inappropriate to existing physical problems or illness" and suggested operant or learned pain. My concern is provoked by the fact that this term has been used inappropriately and has caused much confusion, because there are many chronic pain syndromes and most of these are listed in the taxonomy of the International Association for the Study of Pain (89). LaRocca (editor-in-chief of the journal *Spine*) apparently shares my concern, as expressed in an editoral that preceded the Task Force report (104):

A sense of disquiet is generated by too broad a use of the term "chronic pain syndrome" if only because the connotation implies hopelessness. Many patients with symptoms of six months' duration or more can still have intractable organic disease without significant psychologic components. Every effort must be made to identify them so that they are not automatically included under this rubric. Further, modern algology has identified distinct differences between acute and chronic pain in which the latter is not merely a continuation of the former over time. Instead, a host of organic changes occur in the neuraxis in response to nociception that perpetuate pain independent of psychosocial consideration. This information has hardly been introduced into the clinical setting.

Other than this unwarranted term, the Task Force has published what Loeser (Chapter 71) calls a "magnum opus," which includes matrices for diagnosis and evaluation of therapeutic modalities based on data contained in 763 published reports. Perhaps the most important part of the report is contained in Chapter 5, which includes management guidelines; Table 72-3 summarizes the goal-oriented management of back

TABLE 72-2. Classification of Activity-Related Spinal Disorders

Classification	Symptoms	Duration of Symptoms From Onset	Working Status at Time of Evaluation
1	Pain without radiation	a (<7 days)	W (working)
2	Pain + radiation to extremity, proximally	b (7 days–7 weeks)	I (idle)
3	Pain + radiation to extremity, distally*	c (>7 weeks)	
4	Pain + radiation to upper/lower limb neurologic signs		
5	Presumptive compression of a spinal nerve root on a simple roentgenogram (i.e. spinal instability or fracture)		
6	Compression of a spinal nerve root confirmed by Specific imaging techniques (i.e., computerized axial tomography, myelography, or magnetic resonance imaging) Other diagnostic techniques (e.g., electromyography, venography)		
7	Spinal stenosis		
8	Postsurgical status, 1–6 months after intervention		
9	Postsurgical status, >6 months after intervention 9.1 Asymptomatic 9.2 Symptomatic		
10	Chronic pain syndrome		W (working)
11	Other diagnoses		I (idle)

From LaRocca, H. (ed.): Scientific approach to the assessment and management of activity-related spinal disorders: A monograph for clinicians. Spine, 12 (Suppl. 1):S32, 1987.
*Not applicable to the thoracic segment.

TABLE 72-3. Goal-Oriented Management of Spinal Disorders

Time From Onset	Involved Professional	Goals
0–4 weeks	Treating physician	Rule out specific disease process; conservative treatment oriented toward return to work
4 weeks	Treating physician	Complete re-evaluation; rule out specific disease process; pursue conservative measures oriented toward return to work
7 weeks	Treating physician	Seek consultation; act on recommendations
	Consultant	Promote functional recovery; rule out specific disease process
3–6 months	Treating physician	Seek multidisciplinary evaluation; act on recommendations
	Multidisciplinary team	Assess psychosocial aspects of pain; assess ergonomic aspects; promote functional recovery and return to work before 6 months

From LaRocca, H. (ed.): Scientific approach to the assessment and management of activity-related spinal disorders: A monograph for clinicians. Spine, *12*(Suppl. 1):S32, 1987.

pain as suggested by the Task Force. In reviewing this fine document I feel compelled to express a difference of opinion about several issues. One concerns the difference between the recommendations of the Task Force and those given in Chapter 71 regarding when a psychosocial evaluation should be done. The Task Force suggested that assessment of psychologic and psychosocial factors be the main responsibility of the multidisciplinary team, which is not consulted until more than 3 months after the onset of pain, whereas I believe that this assessment should be included in the initial workup. Stoeckle and Boyd (54) emphasized the importance of eliciting information about the patient's work and personal and family life during the initial interview.

Another difference involves what the Task Force labeled "nonspecific diagnosis" as a cause of most low back pain. I believe that most patients in this category have soft tissue pathology in the form of one or more conditions discussed in this chapter. They can be specifically diagnosed if the initial treating physician bears them in mind and includes maneuvers for their diagnosis in the physical examination. Admittedly, diagnosis cannot be made in a small percentage of patients, and the label "idiopathic back pain" is for such cases.

If systematic medication needs to be given it should *not* be administered prn but at a fixed time, with the interval dependent on the pharmacokinetic and pharmacodynamic characteristics of the drug, a point repeatedly emphasized by Fordyce (Chapters 16 and 81). Similarly, activity limitations are prescribed for a fixed number of days based on the physician's estimates of probable healing time. Fordyce stressed that exercises should be prescribed *not* on the basis of "let pain be your guide" but must be specified as to the day when they should be begun, the number of repetitions, and the daily increments. This type of regimen is likely to enhance restoration of function and an earlier return to normal activities, and helps to prevent the development of chronic pain resulting from operant mechanisms.

The Task Force report (18) recommended that, if management by the treating physician and a consultant specialist is not successful and patients still have pain after 3 months, they should be referred to a multidisciplinary team. According to the report, the team should focus primarily on the psychologic and psychosocial factors in the hope of making a diagnosis and treating the patients effectively to prevent the "chronic pain syndrome." Virtually all of the discussion of this part of the pathway was on psychologic and psychosocial factors associated with spinal disorders, particularly among workers, and on the therapies to be used to prevent the "chronic pain syndrome." Nothing was mentioned, however, about reassessment for pathophysiologic factors. While it is well known that persistent pain caused by "organic" lesions can cause serious psychologic and psychosocial disorders, I believe that the multidisciplinary team has an equal responsibility to re-evaluate patients for physical and pathophysiologic processes that might have been missed and that might be responsible for the persistent pain and consequent psychologic and psychosocial dysfunction. LaRocca (104) has stated that at 3 months and even at 6 months there may be pathologic processes that are contributing to the pain and disability, and that these can be reversed by a comprehensive rehabilitation program. In addition to pathology involving the musculoskeletal system, it has now been shown that massive nociceptive barrage to the CNS caused by injury or surgery, especially if peripheral nerves have been injured or cut, causes prolonged excitability of the spinal cord and even postsynaptic morphologic changes, which can result in persistent pain (22–27).

The importance of unrecognized or improperly treated pathophysiologic processes in patients with low back pain that persists for months and years, and that cause psychologic and psychosocial problems, has been recognized by the staff of a number of multidisciplinary pain programs. Among 111 patients referred to Fishbain and associates (48) and Rosomoff and colleagues (49) with a diagnosis of idiopathic back pain or back pain caused by operant mechanisms, all of them were found to have one or more physical disorders that had been missed by previous examiners. Stoeckle and Boyd (54) also mentioned patients with chronic low back pain in whom the diagnosis of an underlying physical illness was missed because of inadequate diagnostic assessment or because the assessment was carried out too early, before identification of the disease process was possible. They cited three studies that reported morbidity and the rate of undiagnosed physical illness presenting as psychiatric disease.

Rosomoff and co-workers (9, 105–108) have noted that most patients referred to their center had muscle spasm; reduced range of motion of joints; reduced muscle strength; shortening and contracture of muscles, ligaments, tendons, and joint capsules; and poor postural or abnormal posture that produced pain in structures not originally involved. They emphasized that the multidisciplinary team must include therapies to reverse these pathophysiologic changes. Rosomoff (107) and Rosomoff and Rosomoff (108) reported that patients with lumbar spinal stenosis and patients with herniated disks were successfully treated by nonsurgical aggressive therapy. They reported patients with pain of years duration who had pathologic findings revealed by modern imaging techniques, findings that had been missed until then because such tests were not yet available. The Miami center (106) consists of a large group of health professionals, including a number of individuals who carry out ergonomic evaluation of patients and make recommendations for future occupational activities and research. The staff uses a comprehensive multifaceted and multimodal program, as described by Loeser et al. (Chapter 100) and as carried out in the UW Pain Center.

Recently many follow-up reports have been published by the staff of multidisciplinary pain programs, indicating a global improvement in a significant portion of patients with chronic low back pain of 2 to 5 years' duration, or longer. The improvement was shown by a significant reduction of pain scores, elimination of drug intake, and return to normal function and productive life. For example, Mayer and colleagues (109) reported the results of a prospective study in which 87% of patients were working 2 years following discharge, whereas only 41% of those in the untreated group were employed. Similar results have been obtained by Addison, and by Seres and associates and others (see Chapter 100 for data and additional references).

To summarize, if the treating physicians and specialists are unsuccessful with one or at most two attempts at surgery or other medical therapy, they should seriously consider referring the patient to a multidisciplinary/interdisciplinary pain center that can carry out well-coordinated efforts in making the diagnosis and in developing the most appropriate and most effective therapeutic strategy. Such comprehensive centers were formerly regarded as a "court of last appeal" for the treatment of chronic pain. They have been found to be successful, though, and health professionals should refer patients with complex pain problems early to prevent the development of "chronic pain syndrome" and, most important, to reduce the suffering of the millions of patients with chronic pain. The success rate reported by a number of such programs suggests that the increasing use of such facilities can prevent multiple, often useless, and at times mutilating surgeries and attendant complications.

Recently, Loeser and colleagues (personal communication 1989) were referred a patient who had had 46 operations for low back pain or for complications of previous surgery. At the time of the interview, she was taking over 60 medications daily, given by 15 different doctors. Review of her records revealed that the initial operation for the back pain that had led to this almost incredible series of misadventures was not indicated. I would think that the physicians who had seen the patient after the third or fourth operation should have reached the conclusion that further surgery might not be the answer to the problem and would have referred this unfortunate woman to a multidisciplinary pain rehabilitation program for more beneficial treatment.

REFERENCES

1. Kraus, H.: Diagnosis and Treatment of Muscle Pain. Chicago, Quintessence, 1988, pp. 11–50.
2. Nachemson, A.: The lumbar spine—an orthopaedic challenge. Spine, 1:59, 1976.
3. Nachemson, A.: A critical look at the treatment for low back pain. Scand. J. Rehabil. Med., 11:143, 1979.
4. Kraus, H.: Diagnosis and Treatment of Muscle Pain. Chicago, Quintessence Publishing, 1988, pp. 11–50.
5. Travell, J., and Simons, D.: Myofascial Pain and Dysfunction: The Trigger Point Manual. Baltimore, Williams & Wilkins, 1983.
6. Sola, A.E.: Treatment of myofascial pain syndromes. In Recent Advances in Pain Research and Therapy, Vol. 7. Edited by C. Benedetti, et al. New York, Raven Press, 1984, pp. 467–485.
7. Bonica, J.J.: Management of myofascial pain syndromes in general practice. JAMA, 164:732, 1957.
8. Rosomoff, H.L.: Nonoperative treatment of the failed back syndrome presenting with chronic pain. Curr. Ther. Neurol. Surg., 209, 1985.
9. White, A.A., III, and Gordon, S.L. (eds.): Symposium on Idiopathic Low Back Pain. St. Louis, C.V. Mosby, 1982.
10. Nachemson, A.: The natural course of low back pain. In Symposium on Idiopathic Low Back Pain. Edited by A.A.

White, III, and S.L. Gordon. St. Louis, C.V. Mosby, 1982, pp. 46–51.
11. White, A.A., and Gordon, S.L.: Synopsis. Workshop on idiopathic low-back pain. Spine, 7:141, 1982.
12. Fischer, A.A.: Documentation of muscle pain in soft tissue pathology. In Diagnosis and Treatment of Muscle Pain. Edited by H. Kraus. Chicago, Quintessence Publishing, 1988, pp. 55–65.
13. Kraus, H.: Clinical Treatment of Back and Neck Pain. New York, McGraw-Hill, 1970.
14. McCain, G.A., and Scudds, R.A.: The concept of primary fibromyalgia (fibrositis): Clinical value, relation and significance to other chronic musculoskeletal pain syndromes. Pain, 33:273, 1988.
15. Gunn, C.C.: Neuropathic pain—a new theory for chronic pain of intrinsic origin. Ann. R. Coll. Phys. Surg. Canada, 22:327, 1989.
16. Nouwen, A., and Bush, C.: The relationship between paraspinal EMG and chronic low back pain. Pain, 20:109, 1984.
17. Osterweis, M., Kleinman, A., and Mechanic, D.: Pain and Disability. Washington, National Academy Press, 1987.
18. Spitzer, W.O., et al.: Scientific approach to the assessment and management of activity-related spinal disorders. Spine, 12 (Suppl. 1), 1987.
19. Fischer, A.A., and Chang, C.H.: Electromyographic evidence

of paraspinal muscle spasm during sleep in patients with low back pain. Clin. J. Pain, *1*:147, 1985.

20. Ahern, D.K., et al.: Comparison of lumbar paravertebral EMG patterns and chronic low back pain patients and non-patient controls. Pain, *34*:153, 1988.

21. Fischer, A.A.: Clinical use of tissue compliance meter for documentation of soft tissue pathology. Clin. J. Pain, *3*:23, 1987.

22. Woolf, C.J.: Long-term alterations in the excitability of the flexion reflex produced by peripheral tissue injury in the chronic decerebrate rat. Pain, *18*:325, 1984.

23. Woolf, C.J.: Evidence for a central component of post-injury pain hypersensitivity. Nature, *306*:686, 1983.

24. Wall, P.D., and Woolf, C.J.: Muscle but not cutaneous C-afferent input produces prolonged increases in the excitability of the flexion reflex in the rat. J. Physiol. (Lond.), *356*:443, 1984.

25. Cook, A.J., et al.: Expansion of cutaneous receptive fields of dorsal horn neurones following C-primary afferent fibre inputs. Nature, *325*:151, 1987.

26. Woolf, C.J., and Wall, P.D.: The brief and the prolonged facilitatory effects of unmyelinated afferent input on the rat spinal cord are independently influenced by peripheral nerve injury. Neuroscience, *17*:1199, 1986.

27. Woolf, C.J., and Wall, P.D.: A dissociation between the analgesic and antinociceptive effects of morphine. Neurosci. Lett., *64*:238, 1986.

28. McQuay, H.J., Carroll, D., and Moore, R.A.: Postoperative orthopaedic pain—the effect of opiate premedication and local anesthetic blocks. Pain, *33*:291, 1988.

29. Smith, B.E., et al.: Rectus sheath block for diagnostic laparoscopy. Anaesthesia, *43*:947, 1988.

30. Chung, F., et al.: Postoperative recovery after general anaesthesia with and without retrobulbar block in retinal detachment surgery. Anaesthesia, *43*:943, 1988.

31. Sainsbury, P., and Gibson, J.G.: Symptoms of anxiety and tension and accompanying physiological changes in the muscular system. J. Neurol. Neurosurg. Psychiatry, *17*:216, 1954.

32. Dickson-Parnell, B., and Zeichner, A.: The premenstrual syndrome: Psychophysiologic concomitants of perceived stress and low back pain. Pain, *34*:153, 1988.

33. Miehlke, K., Schulze, G., and Eger, W.: Clinical and experimental studies on the fibrositis syndrome. Z. Rheumaforsch, *19*:310, 1960.

34. Kraus, H.: Therapeutic Exercise. Springfield, IL, Charles C Thomas, 1949, pp. 58–60.

35. Cady, L.D., et al.: Strength and fitness and subsequent back injuries in firefighters. J. Occup. Med., *21*:269, 1979.

36. Frymoyer, J.W., et al.: Epidemiologic studies of low back pain. Spine, *5*:419, 1980.

37. Steindler, A., and Luck, J.V.: Differential diagnosis of pain low in the back. JAMA, *110*:106, 1938.

38. Steindler, A.: Lectures on the Interpretation of Pain in Orthopaedic Practice. Springfield, IL, Charles C Thomas, 1959.

39. Livingston, W.K.: Back disabilities due to strain of the multifidus muscle. West. J. Surg., *49*:259, 1941.

40. Travell, J., and Rinzler, S.H.: Pain syndromes of the chest muscles: Resemblance to effort angina and myocardial infarction and relief by local block. Can. Med. Assoc. J., *59*:333, 1948.

41. Bonica, J.J.: The Management of Pain. Philadelphia, Lea & Febiger, 1953, pp. 1106–1112, 1137–1141, 1162, 1191, 1211–1214.

42. Sola, A.E., and William, R.L.: Myofascial pain syndromes. Neurology, *6*:91, 1956.

43. Michele, A.A., et al.: Scapulocostal syndrome. NY State J. Med., *50*:1353, 1950.

44. Travell, J., and Rinzler, S.H.: The myofascial genesis of pain. Postgrad. Med., *11*:425, 1952.

45. Simons, D.G.: Muscle pain syndromes—Part I. Am. J. Phys. Med., *54*:289, 1975.

46. Simons, D.G.: Muscle pain syndromes—Part II. Am. J. Phys. Med., *55*:15, 1976.

47. Simons, D.G., and Travell, J.G.: Myofascial origins of low back pain. Parts 1, 2, and 3. Postgrad. Med., *73*:66, 1983.

48. Fishbain, A.A., et al.: Male and female chronic pain patients categorized by DSM-III psychiatric diagnostic criteria. Pain, *26*:181, 1986.

49. Rosomoff, H.L., et al.: Physical findings in patients with chronic intractable benign pain (Abstr.). Pain, *4*(Suppl. 4):S120, 1987.

50. Fricton, J.R., et al.: Myofascial pain syndrome of the head and neck: A review of clinical characteristics of 164 patients. Oral Surg., *60*:615, 1985.

51. Skootsky, S.: Incidence of myofascial pain in an internal medical group practice. Presented to the American Pain Society, Washington, DC, November 6–9, 1986.

52. Reynolds, M.D.: Myofascial trigger point syndromes in the practice of rheumatology. Arch. Phys. Med. Rehabil., *62*:111, 1981.

53. Fine, P.G., Milano, R., and Hare, B.D.: The effects of myofascial trigger point injections are naloxone reversible. Pain, *32*:15, 1988.

54. Stoeckle, J.D., and Boyd, R.: Chronic pain in medical practice. In Pain and Disability. Edited by M. Osterweis, A. Kleinman, and D. Mechanic. Washington, DC, National Academy Press, 1987, pp. 189–210.

55. Cypress, B.K.: The characteristics of physician visits for back symptoms: A national perspective. Am. J. Publ. Health, *73*:389, 1983.

56. Bengtsson, A., and Bengtsson, M.: Regional sympathetic blockade in primary fibromyalgia. Pain, *33*:161, 1988.

57. Sola, A.E., and Kuitert, J.H.: Quadratus lumborum myofascitis. Northwest Med., *53*:1003, 1954.

58. Bengtsson, A.: Fibromyalgia. A clinical laboratory study. Linköping, Sweden, Linköping University Medical School, Dissertation No. 224, 1986, pp. 1–59.

59. Smythe, H.A., and Moldofsky, H.: Two contributions to the understanding of the 'fibrositis' syndrome. Bull. Rheum. Dis., *28*:928, 1977–1978.

60. Symthe, H.A.: Nonarticular rheumatism and psychogenic musculoskeletal syndromes. In Arthritis and Allied Conditions. 11th Ed. Edited by D.J. McCarty. Phildelphia, Lea & Febiger, 1989, pp. 1241–1254.

61. Caro, X.J., et al.: A controlled and blinded study of immunoreactant deposition at the dermal-epidermal junction of patients with primary fibrositis syndrome. J. Rheumatol., *13*:1086, 1986.

62. Vaerøy, H., et al.: Elevated CSF levels of substance P and high incidence of Raynaud phenomenon in patients with fibromyalgia: New features for diagnosis. Pain, *32*:21, 1988.

63. McCain, G.A.: Fibromyositis. Mod. Med., *38*:197, 1983.

64. Yunus, M., et al.: Primary fibromyalgia (fibrositis): Clinical study of 50 patients with matched normal control. Semin. Arthritis Rheum., *11*:151, 1981.

65. Carette, S., et al.: A double-blind study of amitriptyline versus placebo in patients with primary fibrositis. Arthritis Rheum., *29*:655, 1986.

66. Campbell, S.M., et al.: A double-blind study of cyclobenzaprine versus placebo in patients with fibrositis (Abstr.). Arthritis Rheum., *27*:S76, 1984.

67. Melzack, R., Stillwell, D.M., and Fox, E.J.: Trigger points and acupuncture points for pain: Correlations and implications. Pain, *3*:3, 1977.

68. Gunn, C.C.: Transcutaneous neural stimulation, acupuncture and the current of injury. Am. J. Acupunct., *6*:191, 1978.

69. Ross, R., and Vogel, A.: The platelet-derived growth factor. Cell, *14*:203, 1978.

70. Cailliet, R.: Low Back Pain Syndrome. 3rd Ed. Philadelphia, F.A. Davis, 1981, pp. 53–68.

71. Fast, A., et al.: Low back pain in pregnancy. Spine, *12*:368, 1987.

72. Kelsey, J.L., et al.: Pregnancy and the syndrome of herniated lumbar intervertebral disk: An epidemiological study. Yale J. Biol. Med., *48*:361, 1975.

73. Magora, A.: Investigation of the relation between low back pain and occupation. 4. Physical requirements: Bending, rotation, reaching and sudden maximal efforts. Scand. J. Rehabil. Med., *5*:186, 1973.

74. Magora, A.: Investigation of the relation between low back pain and occupation. 6. Medical history and symptoms. Scand. J. Rehabil. Med., *6*:81, 1974.

75. Troup, J.D.G.: Relation of lumbar spine disorders to heavy manual work and lifting. Lancet, *1*:857, 1965.

76. Valkenburg, H.A., and Haanen, H.C.N.: The epidemiology of low back pain. In Symposium on Idiopathic Low Back Pain. Edited by A.A. White and S.L. Gordon. St. Louis, C.V. Mosby, 1982, pp. 9–22.

77. Newton, D.R.L.: Discussion of the clinical and radiological aspects of sacro-iliac disease. Proc. R. Soc. Med., *50*:850, 1957.

78. Hoppenfeld, S.: Physical Examination of the Spine and Extremities. New York, Appleton-Century-Crofts, 1976, pp. 261–262.

79. Ghormley, R.K.: Low back pain with special reference to the articular facets with presentation of an operative procedure. JAMA, 101:1773, 1933.
80. Mennell, J.: The Signs and Art of Joint Manipulation. New York, Blakiston, 1952.
81. Magora, A., and Schwartz, A.: Relation between the low back pain syndrome and X-ray findings. I. Degenerative osteoarthritis. Scand. J. Rehabil. Med., 8:115, 1976.
82. Lawrence, J.S., Bremner, J.M., and Bier, F.: Osteoarthrosis: Prevalence in the population and relationship between symptoms and X-ray changes. Ann. Rheum. Dis., 25:1, 1966.
83. Mooney, V., and Robertson, J.: The facet syndrome. Clin. Orthop., 115:149, 1976.
84. McCall, I.W., Park, W.M., and O'Brien, J.P.: Induced pain referral from posterior lumbar elements in normal subjects. Spine, 4:441, 1979.
85. Bogduk, N.: Back pain: Zygapophyseal blocks and epidural steriods. In Neural Blockade in Clinical Anesthesia and Management of Pain. 2nd Ed. Edited by M.J. Cousins and P.O. Bridenbaugh. Philadelphia, J.D. Lippincott, 1988, pp. 935–954.
86. Fairbank, J.C.T., et al.: Apophyseal injection of local anesthetic as a diagnostic aid in primary low-back pain syndromes. Spine, 6:598, 1981.
87. Carrera, G.F., and Williams, A.L.: Current concepts in evaluation of the lumbar facet joints. CRC Crit. Rev. Diagn. Imaging, 21:85, 1984.
88. Lynch, M.C., and Taylor, J.F.: Facet injection for low back pain. J. Bone Joint Surg. [Br.], 68:138, 1986.
89. Destouet, J.M., et al.: Lumbar facet joint injection: Indication, technique, clinical correlation and preliminary results. Radiology, 145:321, 1982.
90. Wedel, D.J., and Wilson, P.R.: Cervical facet arthrography. Reg. Anaesth, 10:7, 1985.
91. Dory, M.A.: Arthrography of the cervical facet joints. Radiology, 148:379, 1983.
92. Bogduk, N., Macintosh, J.E., and Marsland, A.: A technical limitation to the efficacy of radiofrequency neurotomy for spinal pain. Neurosurgery, 20:529, 1987.
93. Sarno, J.: Psychosomatic back ache. J. Fam. Pract., 53:353, 1977.
94. Scambler, A., and Scambler, G.: Menstrual symptoms, attitudes and consulting behaviour. Soc. Sci. Med., 20:1065, 1985.
95. Kessler, H.: Low Back Pain in Industry: A Study Prepared for the Special Committee on Workman's Compensation. New York, New York Commerce and Industry Association, 1955.
96. Dickson-Parnell, B., and Zeichner, A.: The premenstrual syndrome: Psychophysiologic concomitants of perceived stress and low back pain. Pain, 34:161, 1988.
97. Merskey, H.: Classification of chronic pain: Description of chronic pain syndromes and definition of terms. Pain (Suppl. 3), S45:203, 1986.
98. Loeser, J.D., and Egan, K.J.: Managing the Chronic Pain Patient: Theory and Practice at the University of Washington Multidisciplinary Pain Center. New York, Raven Press, 1989.
99. Dixon, A.S.J.: Progress and problems in back pain research. Rheumatol. Rehabil., 12:165, 1973.
100. Wood, P.H.N., and Badley, M.: Epidemiology of back pain. In The Lumbar Spine and Back Pain. Edited by M. Jayson. London, Pitman Medical, 1980, pp. 29–55.
101. Andersson, J.A.D.: Back pain and occupation. In The Lumbar Spine and Back Pain. Edited by M. Jayson. London, Pitman Medical, 1980, pp. 57–82.
102. Bigos, S.J., et al.: Back injuries in industry (Abstr.). Toronto, The International Society for the Study of the Lumbar Spine, 1982.
103. Black, R.G.: The chronic pain syndrome. Surg. Clin. North Am., 55:999, 1975.
104. LaRocca, H.: Editorial. Scientific approach to the assessment and management of activity-related spinal disorders. Spine, 12(Suppl. 1):S8, 1987.
105. Rosomoff, H.L., Green, C.J., and Silbret, M.: The multidisciplinary team approach to the diagnosis and treatment of chronic low back pain. In Radiographic Evaluation of the Spine. Edited by M.J.D. Post, New York, Masson, 1980, pp. 672–679.
106. Rosomoff, H.L., et al.: Pain and low back rehabilitation program at the University of Miami School of Medicine. In New Approaches to Treatment of Chronic Pain: A Review of Multidisciplinary Pain Clinics and Pain Centers. 36 Monogr. Ser. Edited by L.K.Y. Ng. National Institute on Drug Abuse Research, 1981, p. 92.
107. Rosomoff, H.L.: Do herniated disks produce pain? In Advances in Pain Research and Therapy, Vol. 9. Edited by H.L. Fields, R. Dubner, and F. Cervero. New York, Raven Press, 1985, pp. 457–461.
108. Rosomoff, H.L., and Rosomoff, R.S.: Nonsurgical aggressive treatment of lumbar spinal stenosis. Spine, 1:383, 1987.
109. Mayer, T.G., et al.: A prospective two-year study of functional restoration in industrial low back injury. JAMA, 258:1763, 1987.

73 • PAIN OF NEUROLOGIC ORIGIN IN THE HIPS AND LOWER EXTREMITIES

JOHN D. LOESER

PAIN of neurologic origin in the hips and lower extremities, often referred to as lumbar and lumbosacral neuralgia, is a broad category of painful conditions localized to the lumbar and first two sacral nerve distributions. Neuralgia restricted to the lumbar area is relatively uncommon; most of these pains also involve sacral segments. These pain syndromes are thought to be caused by pathologic processes that involve the lumbar and sacral segments of the spinal cord, the nerve roots, the lumbosacral plexus, or the peripheral nerves (see Fig. 70-20). The information in this chapter is presented in two major sections: A, General Considerations, including an overview of etiology, symptoms and signs, diagnosis, and treatment; and B, Specific Causes of Lumbosacral Neuralgia. More detailed information can be found elsewhere (1, 2).

A. GENERAL CONSIDERATIONS

Etiology

Pain of neurologic origin in the hips and lower extremities is a symptom secondary to diseases that most commonly involve the nerve roots or the lumbosacral plexus. Pathology in the spinal cord or peripheral nerves is identified less often. Although sciatica is written about as if it were common, most low back and leg pain originating in the back is not caused by radicular disease at the L5 and S1 levels, and most of what is called "sciatica" is a misnomer. The vast majority of hip and leg pains are of musculoskeletal origin, and their pathophysiology is not well understood. Further discussion of this topic can be found in Chapter 71.

Pain of neurologic origin in the hips and legs can be best considered on the basis of the site of pathology: (a) lesions of the spinal cord and dura; (b) lesions of the spinal nerve roots; (c) lesions of the formed spinal nerves; (d) lesions of the lumbosacral plexus; and (e) lesions of one or more peripheral nerves.

Symptoms and Signs

The characteristics of the pain in these conditions are a function of the location of the offending lesion. Intrinsic lesions of the spinal cord rarely present with pain, but are more likely to be characterized by motor and sensory loss. Bowel and bladder dysfunction is usually an early sign; in the male, sexual dysfunction is common. Lesions of the dorsal roots usually produce a pain syndrome that has a dermatomal pattern and is exacerbated by mechanical factors. Lesions of the formed spinal nerves are uncommon; in addition to dermatomal pain, the motor and sensory changes are a function of the nerve involved. Lumbosacral plexus lesions are relatively rare and cause both local and referred pain, as well as sensory and motor changes. Peripheral nerve lesions are characterized by focal pain at the site of nerve damage and pain referred into the distribution of the nerve. Sensory and motor deficits are determined by the innervation pattern of the involved nerve.

Sensory alterations generally accompany the pain of any lesion involving the nervous system. Variations in the type of sensory loss are not terribly helpful in locating the lesion. Anesthesia, hypesthesia, paresthesia, hyperesthesia, hyperalgesia, and dysesthesia can all be associated with almost any type of lesion.

Motor deficits are frequently observed. Weakness of the muscles, loss of tone, atrophy, and reflex changes can all be seen. If the ventral root axons are significantly compromised, fasciculations can be observed. Abnormalities of sympathetic nerve function are common when the nerves to the legs are involved, including loss of sweating and piloerection and a cool extremity. A diffuse, deep, aching pain in the hip can also indicate sympathetic involvement.

Local tenderness can help to indicate the site of the lesion. Movements of the lumbar spine and hip that lead to increased mechanical pressure can exacerbate the pain. If a nerve in the leg is mechanically traumatized, movements and local pressure can aggravate the symptoms.

If the lesion has been present for a month or more and the nerve damage has been sufficient to disrupt axons, a *neuroma* sign can be present at the lesion site. Percussion over the nerve in this area produces paresthesias that are perceived in the cutaneous distribution of the nerve. If the lesion has been present long enough for some regeneration to occur distal to the site of the injury, *Tinel's sign* can be elicited: percussion over the nerve distal to the injury site results in paresthesias in the cutaneous territory of the nerve. Tinel's sign can be used as an indication of the continuity of the nerve and the presence of some regenerating axons.

If the offending lesion is near the body surface it can be palpated, or the overlying skin contours can be altered. Deeper lesions might not be accessible to physical examination. The lesion itself can cause local pain because of tissue damage.

Diagnosis

The diagnosis of the cause of pain of neurologic origin in the hips and legs is based primarily on the history and physical examination. The strategies for obtaining a thorough history and carrying out a detailed physical examination are discussed in Chapters 31 to 33. Neurodiagnostic studies such as electromyography, nerve conduction velocity and reflex tests, somatosensory evoked potentials, and thermography are often valuable adjuncts that can help to locate the lesion precisely (Chapters 34 and 35).

When the history has been obtained and the general physical examination has been done, the examiner should focus on the region of pain. The back, abdomen, groin, buttocks, and entire lower extremities should be inspected, searching for a loss of normal contours, muscular atrophy, or other deformities. Rectal or vaginal examination is important when sacral segments are involved in a chronic pain syndrome. Atrophy should be documented by measurement of the thigh and calf circumferences a fixed distance above and below the patella. Painful areas should then be palpated to locate regions of tenderness or of pain reproduction. The effects of movement at the major joints must be ascertained. Limitation of movement usually suggests disease of the joint or of the surrounding muscles, tendons, or ligaments. Most pains in this area are found to be in the low back, buttock, hip, and proximal leg. They are most often of musculoskeletal origin, in spite of the pattern of radiation which suggests sciatic nerve involvement.

Examination of the lumbar and sacral neural segments is obviously critical in patients with pain symptoms in the lower body and legs. A knowledge of the dermatomes and patterns of muscular innervation is required (Chapter 6).

Radiographic and imaging studies can be helpful in delineating mass lesions and sites of trauma. CT scanning and magnetic resonance scanning have helped greatly in locating internal pathologic processes. Myelography is useful when a lesion of the spinal cord or nerve roots is suspected.

Paravertebral somatic nerve blocks with a local anesthetic can be helpful in locating a lesion when other studies are not conclusive (Chapter 94). If myofascial pains are suspected, trigger point injections can be both diagnostic and therapeutic. Indeed, presumptive treatment with physical measures can allow the cause of the pain to abate; vague pain states without specific findings do not need to be studied in great detail the first time that the patient is seen.

B. SPECIFIC CAUSES OF LUMBOSACRAL NEURALGIA

Lesions of the Spinal Cord

Intrinsic Spinal Cord Lesions (XXVI-4)

Neoplasms or cysts of the thoracolumbar spinal cord can lead to pain in the abdomen, low back, perineum, and lower extremities. Lesions intrinsic to the spinal cord rarely present with pain; neurologic deficits are usually the initial complaint, and profound sensory and motor loss can be found without any pain complaints. Segmental pains can be present, and are probably caused by stretching of the dorsal roots by the enlarging intrinsic mass. In the male, sexual dysfunction is a frequent early sign. Because the pain can involve the lower lumbar segments, the patient might be thought to have disk disease; for this reason myelograms should always include the conus.

The common cause of an intrinsic spinal cord lesion is a tumor. Other causes include syringomyelia, congenital or post-traumatic cysts, and vascular malformations. Patients who have been operated on for meningomyelocele or for some other congenital abnormality of the spinal cord can develop pain and neurologic deficit in later life caused by tethering of the spinal cord in scar. Surgical repair usually alleviates the symptoms and prevents further neurologic loss. Unrecognized congenital abnormalities of the spinal cord can also produce low back pain and neurologic deficit; CT or MRI scanning and other studies can help to establish the diagnosis. A significant percentage of patients with repaired meningomyelocele or lumbosacral lipomeningomyelocele develop tethered spinal cord; pain and progressive neurologic deficit are the common presentation of such a condition (3). Midline cutaneous and subcutaneous abnormalities should alert the physician to the possibility of an underlying congenital abnormality of the spinal cord.

Extramedullary Intradural Lesions

Lesions extrinsic to the spinal cord but within the dura are not common; most occur in the thoracic region and not in the lumbar and sacral segments. Neurofibroma and meningioma are the most common neoplasms, but almost any tumor of neural or glial origin, as well as congenital cysts, can be present (4). Neurofibromas usually start on a root and present relatively early, with radicular pain and neurologic loss. Meningiomas usually start ventral or dorsal to the spinal cord, and radicular signs are often late to develop. Ependymoma of the conus region can begin within the spinal cord but can expand into the subarachnoid space and compress nerve roots, leading to pain and neurologic deficits. Radicular lumbosacral pain is too often assumed to be caused by herniated nucleus pulposus at L5 or S1; a tumor at the level of the conus medullaris can also produce radicular pain and neurologic loss. For this reason, every myelogram performed for suspected lumbar disk disease should also include views of the conus.

Diagnosis of extramedullary intradural lesions is established by myelography, CT, or MRI. Electrodiagnostic studies can also be helpful. Treatment is exclusively by surgical removal, because these lesions are almost all benign and they are not sensitive to radiation or chemotherapy (Fig. 73-1).

Meningeal Carcinomatosis (XXVI-11)

Leptomeningeal metastases from solid tumors elsewhere in the body can produce severe radicular pain

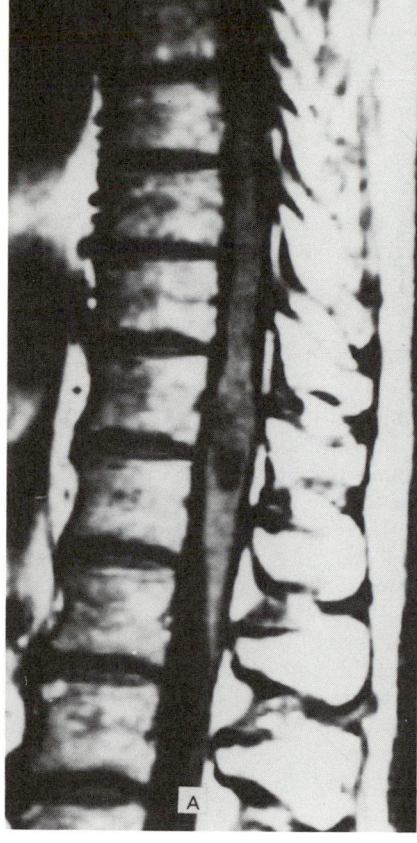
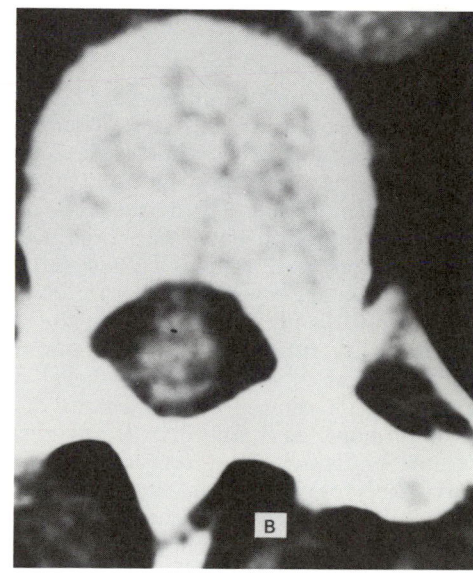

FIG. 73-1. *A.* Intramedullary tumor (hemangioblastoma) at T10–T11 as seen on midsagittal projection of MRI scan. The tumor is the low-signal ovoid region within the higher-signal spinal cord. In this scan, cerebrospinal fluid is dark; fat and bones are white. *B.* Axial CT scan with intravenous enhancement at T10–T11. Swollen spinal cord with enhancing mass is obvious.

and loss of function. The pathology is direct invasion of the nerve roots by tumor cells; a discrete mass might not be present. The most common primary tumors are carcinoma of the lung or breast, malignant melanoma, lymphoma, and leukemia. Both children and adults can suffer from this type of tumor spread. Diffuse spinal pain and headache are common. The diagnosis is confirmed by finding malignant cells in the spinal fluid. Treatment is by radiation or chemotherapy, depending on the primary lesion. Pain relief is sometimes obtained with narcotics; anticonvulsants can also be helpful (5).

Extradural Spinal Lesions (XXVI-4)

Herniated lumbar disk (see below) is probably the most common type of extradural lesion; tumors and abscesses also occur in this space. Extradural neoplasms are probably metastases from a primary lesion elsewhere in the body. Lung, breast, prostate, and thyroid neoplasms are the most common solid tumors. The patient usually has back pain before the development of signs of nerve root or spinal cord compression. The epidural deposit might be the first sign of the malignancy, or it might occur late in the course of the patient's disease. Diagnosis is established by myelography, CT, or MRI scan. Chemotherapy, radiation therapy, and decompressive laminectomy can all be used; the histology of the lesion determines the most effective therapy.

Epidural abscess is less common in the present antibiotic era than it was 50 years ago. There is often a history of bacteremia following a surgical procedure or of infection in the pelvic area, although epidural abscess can occur without any recognized antecedent infection. The patient almost always has severe back pain; neurologic deficits follow the pain if the lesion is not treated aggressively. The use of surgical decompression and appropriate antibiotics usually yields good results if the decompression is done before devastating neurologic loss has occurred (6).

Lesions of the Nerve Roots
Herniated Nucleus Pulposus (XXVI-1)

Certainly the most popular cause of lumbosacral radiculopathy, herniated nucleus pulposus ("ruptured disk"), is now recognized as a relatively uncommon cause of lumbago and sciatica. The pioneering work of Mixter and Barr (7) led to the realization that these common symptoms could be a result of extrusion of a fragment of disk into the spinal canal; formerly, surgeons had observed disk material in the spinal canal but thought it to be a form of neoplasm. Mixter and Barr (7) also described the value of myelography in establishing the diagnosis of ruptured disk.

In the past 20 years it has been recognized that many other structures in the back can produce both low back pain and pain referred to the sciatic nerve distribution. It is also well established that the pathologic changes that have been described in older texts as the basis for chronic pain are, in fact, found in many people who have never had any symptoms. Hence, there is only a loose association between the structural lesions and the patient's symptoms. Nonetheless, compression of the dorsal roots or of the dorsal root ganglion can lead to pain; herniated nucleus pulposus is a common cause of this syndrome (8). The role of herniated nucleus pulposus in low back pain is discussed in Chapter 71.

Etiology

Herniated nucleus pulposus is caused by trauma, the aging process, or both. If workers are compensated for on-the-job injuries, almost all disk disease will be ascribed to some type of minor traumatic event that happened at work. The actual role of trauma is not well understood, because ruptured disks can occur in sedentary as well as heavy labor settings. Degrees of disk disease are seen: degeneration of the disk, bulging of the annulus fibrosis, rupture of the disk through the annulus, and free fragment rupture of the disk into the spinal canal (Fig. 73-2). In general, the severity of symptoms is related to the extent of the pathology. Furthermore, as Spangfort (9) has clearly shown, the results of diskectomy are much better in patients who have free fragment disk ruptures. Disk degeneration and bulging of the annulus are a part of the aging process and occur in everyone to some degree.

Symptoms and Signs

The outstanding symptom of herniated nucleus pulposus is pain. Most patients have had several episodes of low back pain before they develop pain that radiates to the buttock and leg in a segmental pattern. A specific episode of lifting, straining, or twisting is identified as the cause by most patients. The exact distribution of the pain depends on the root involved (Fig. 73-3). The S1 root is most frequently compressed and leads to pain that radiates from the low back to the buttock, posterior thigh, lateral leg, lateral ankle, lateral foot, and 5th toe. The L5 root is the next most frequently compressed and leads to pain in the low back, posterolateral thigh, dorsal foot, and medial toes. The L4 root is the third most commonly involved and leads to pain in the low back, anterolateral thigh, and medial leg and foot to the 1st toe. Only rarely are more rostral nerve roots compressed by a herniated nucleus pulposus, because ruptures of disks above the L3–L4 interspace are uncommon. The pain is aggravated by sitting, twisting, or lifting and is usually relieved by walking or lying down. Coughing, sneezing, and straining on the toilet typically exaggerate the pain.

Paresthesias are often perceived in the distribution of the compressed nerve root. These are of greater localizing value than the pain or sensory or motor deficits. Decreased light touch and pinprick sensations are sometimes noted. Motor changes are usually subtle but can be more pronounced. Weakness, atrophy, fasciculations, and reflex changes can occur (Table 73-1).

Mechanical signs of nerve root irritation are also present. These include reproduction of the pain on straight leg raising, tenderness to percussion over the adjacent spinous processes to the herniated nucleus pulposus, paravertebral muscle spasm, lumbar scoliosis, and loss of lordosis.

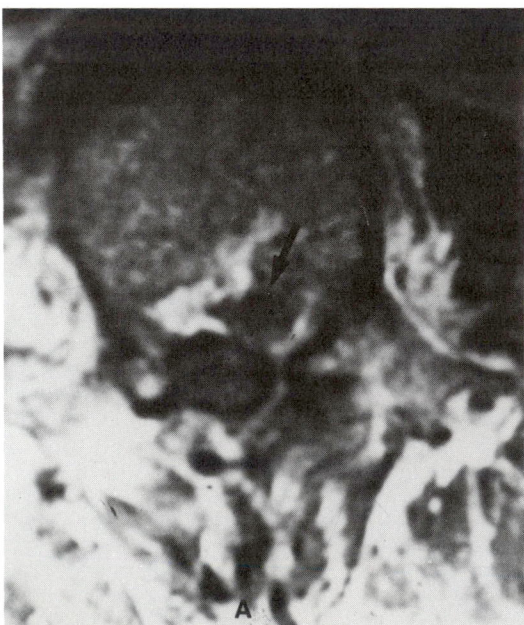
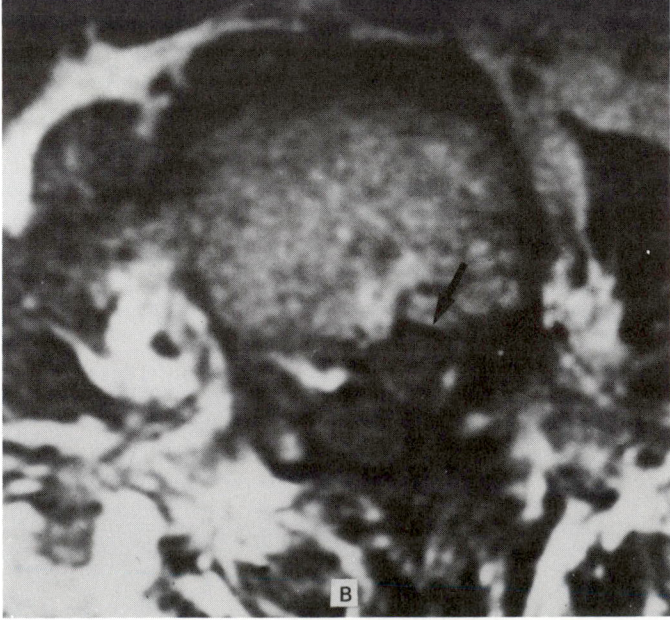

FIG. 73-2. Free fragment disk L2–L3 rupture as seen on axial MRI scan. Scar tissue from prior surgery enhances; disk fragment does not. *A.* Unenhanced scan. *B.* Gadolinium-enhanced scan. Arrow points to free fragment of disk. The patient had severe left L2 radicular pain and paresthesia.

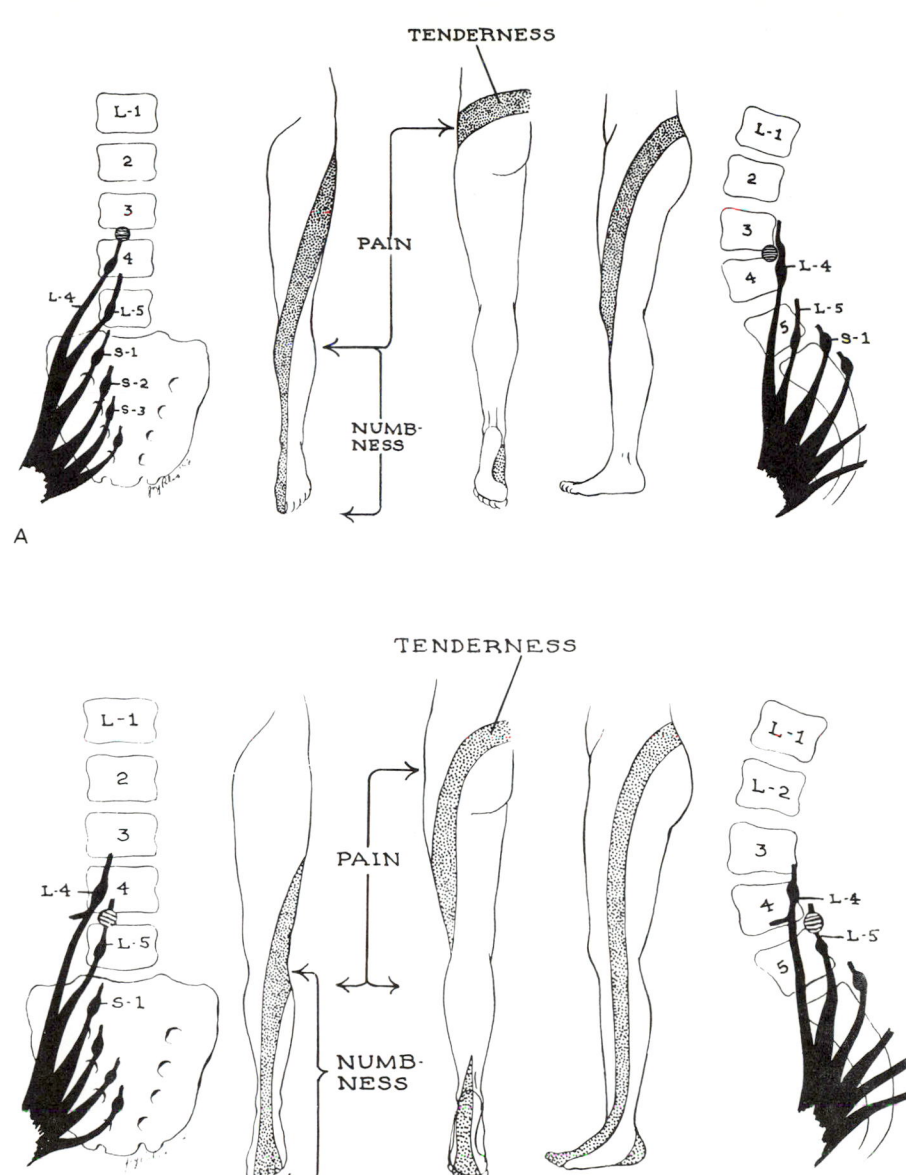

FIG. 73-3. Dermatome hypalgesia, pain, and tenderness in the distribution of the lower limb from herniation of intervertebral disks. *A.* Pattern of distribution of the L4 segment from herniation of the L3 intervertebral disk. *B.* Dermatome hypalgesia, pain and tenderness in the distribution of the L5 segment resulting from herniation of the L4 intervertebral disk. *C.* Dermatome hyperalgesia, pain, and tenderness in the distribution of the S1 segment resulting from herniation of the L5 intervertebral disk. Modified from Keegan, J.J.: Dermatome hyperalgesia associated with herniation of the lumbar intervertebral disc. J. Bone Joint Surg., *26*: 238, 1944.

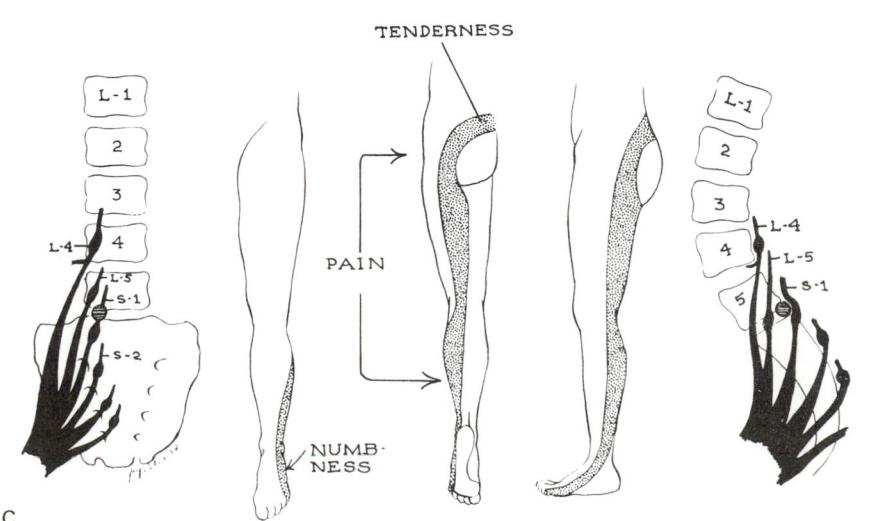

TABLE 73-1. Single Nerve Root Syndromes of the Lower Lumbar and Upper Sacral Segments

Symptoms and Signs	Location		
	L4	L5	S1
Pain	In gluteal ("hip") region below iliac crest	In gluteal ("hip") region between ischial tuberosity and femoral trochanter	In medial gluteal ("hip") region over ischial tuberosity
Pain radiation	Anterior thigh and leg	Lateral thigh and leg	Posterior thigh and leg
Tenderness	Over spinous and transverse processes of vertebrae	Over spinous and transverse processes of vertebrae	Over spinous and transverse processes of vertebrae
Subjective numbness	Anterior leg, great toe	Lateral leg, three middle toes	Posterior leg, little toe
Hypalgesia	Over entire segment	Over entire segment	Over entire segment
Reflex changes	Patellar tendon reduced or absent	Usually no alteration	Achilles tendon reduced or absent
Motor weakness	Dorsiflexors of great toe	Dorsiflexors of ankle and toes	Plantar flexors

A small percentage of patients sustain a massive free fragment rupture of a disk and suffer from a cauda equina syndrome, with multiple nerve root involvement and severe pain. This is the only case in which a herniated nucleus pulposus is a surgical emergency.

Diagnosis

Classic presentations of lumbar disk disease can be diagnosed from the history and physical examination. Atypical cases can be more difficult to discriminate from other pathologic processes that involve the back. Careful neurologic examination will usually locate the lesion. Radiculopathy caused by disk disease rarely involves more than one nerve root, and the signs and symptoms are usually unilateral. Low back pain usually precedes the development of leg pain.

Bowel and bladder symptoms are uncommon except in cases of large free fragment rupture, although subtle cystometrographic abnormalities have been well described in many patients with typical single-level disk disease. Intradural and epidural neoplasms, spinal infections and neoplasms, and retroperitoneal neoplasms and infection must be considered in the differential diagnosis. All these are much rarer than herniated nucleus pulposus. In addition, pain syndromes originating from the joints of the spine, ligaments, or muscles must also be kept in mind. Pain that radiates into the lower extremity is not pathognomonic of herniated nucleus pulposus and nerve root compression.

Treatment

CONSERVATIVE THERAPY. The treatment of herniated nucleus pulposus should always be conservative, except in the case of a massive free fragment rupture with cauda equina compression. There is little evidence to show that any form of therapy improves on the natural history (Chapter 71). The role of steroids is equivocal (10, 11). Although some studies have indicated that the use of oral or epidural steroids hastens recovery from radicular pain caused by disk prolapse, others have not been confirmatory. Furthermore, the influence on later symptoms and signs (i.e., is the natural history of the disease altered?) remains to be determined. As is so often the case, what is lacking is not the results of treatment but, instead, the natural history of the disease being treated. Prolonged bed rest and inactivity are deleterious. Narcotics and sedative-hypnotics can be of value for a few days, but their long-term use adds to the patient's disability. The patient should be told to avoid strenuous activities that stir up the pain but to resume normal activities as soon as possible.

SURGICAL THERAPY. The major problem with lumbar disk disease is pain. The severity of the neurologic deficit rarely mandates surgical therapy. Only when the pain complaints are severe and unremitting should a surgical procedure be considered. If the diagnosis is straightforward, a diagnostic study such as myelography, CT or MRI scan or electromyography is only warranted when the decision has been made to operate. Such studies only locate the lesion, and it should be remembered that they play no role in determining who needs surgery. All the myelographic, CT, and MRI changes that characterize lumbar disk disease are often found in people who do not have and might never have had significant low back and leg pain. These diagnostic studies never determine the need for surgery; they only locate the pathology in a patient who has already met the criteria for diskectomy (Fig. 73-4).

The traditional open surgical method of removing a herniated lumbar disk has seen several modifications

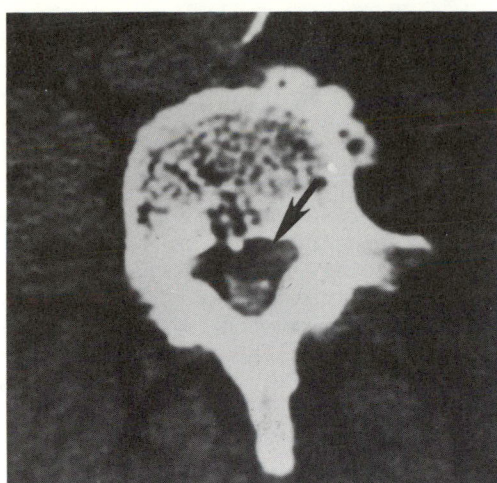

FIG. 73-4. Axial CT scan using intrathecal contrast agent showing that the dural sac is displaced posteriorly by a larger, herniated disk fragment (arrow). The patient had low back pain radiating to both legs, which was made worse by standing or walking.

in the past 20 years. Microdiskectomy has its proponents; recently, a percutaneous technique for mechanically removing the disk has been described (12, 13). Enzymatic degradation of the nucleus pulposus by injection of chymopapain has also been popular. All of these procedures remove the disk, but none has been shown to offer major advantages. Each method carries some risk of complications (9). No matter how one removes a disk, the key to success is patient selection. Spangfort (9) showed that the relief of both leg and back pain was correlated with the findings at surgery: free fragment disk ruptures had a 90% likelihood of relief of sciatica; bulging disks had a 60% likelihood of pain relief; and leg pain was more likely to be relieved than low back pain. The lack of randomized prospective allocation trials prohibits comparisons of results of different surgical strategies.

Relief of leg or back pain is not synonymous with return to work. Little evidence has shown that fusion of an otherwise normal lumbar spine improves the outcome for patients who have had a herniated nucleus pulposus and a diskectomy.

Spinal Stenosis (XXVII-3)

Spinal stenosis, also known as neurogenic claudication, is a painful syndrome that was first clearly described by Verbiest in 1954 (14). Bilateral lower extremity numbness, weakness, and pain, in association with low back pain, are present in varying degrees after walking or when standing erect. The symptoms are exercise-induced and rapidly clear with rest. Vascular claudication occurs after exercise regardless of posture; neurogenic claudication occurs only in the erect position (15). The severity of the pain complaint usually exceeds the magnitude of the neurologic deficits.

The diagnosis can be confirmed by provocative physical testing and corroborated by myelography, CT, or MRI scanning (Fig. 73-5). Decompressive surgery is the only effective treatment; stenosis of the spinal

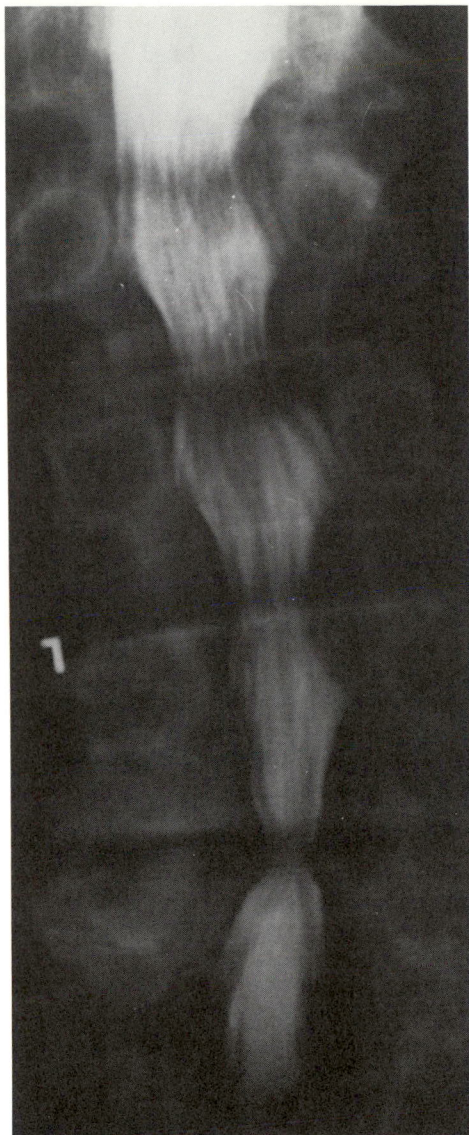

FIG. 73-5. Myelogram showing pattern of spinal stenosis. The segmental narrowing is caused by encroachment of the enlarged ligamenta flava.

canal and of the neural foramina can be present to a varying degree, and surgical therapy must resolve the anatomic problems in each patient. A well-performed operation almost always significantly relieves the symptoms (16, 17). Spinal stenosis is discussed in Chapter 71.

Arachnoiditis (XXVII-10)

One of the most disastrous complications of disk disease, myelography, trauma, subarachnoid hemorrhage, infection, or spinal surgery is the development of arachnoiditis involving the cauda equina (18). It is not understood why only a small percentage of patients who have one of these inciting causes develop inflammatory changes in the nerve roots and the surrounding arachnoid. Furthermore, not everyone with the histologic findings of arachnoiditis has a pain syndrome.

Etiology

Although any of the causes listed above can precede the development of arachnoiditis, none of them do so with any regularity. In addition to these factors, the following causative influences are thought to be involved: syphilis; bacterial, fungal, or disk space infection; intrathecal drug therapy; herniated nucleus pulposus; spinal stenosis; radiation therapy; intradural tumor; and spinal anesthesia. It is not known whether patients who develop inflammation in the arachnoid that progresses to fibrosis have an alteration in their immunologic responses. The initial inflammatory process can proceed to severe scarring, both within the arachnoid and within the nerve roots themselves. The process can be restricted to one nerve root or can involve various parts of the cauda equina.

Symptoms and Signs

The major problem with arachnoiditis is severe, unremitting pain in the low back and legs. Varying degrees of motor and sensory loss can be present, and in some patients the scarring process in the arachnoid is associated with progressive, profound neurologic loss, although this is relatively uncommon. The pain is aggravated by movements or positions that stretch the lumbar nerve roots. Most patients say that exercise aggravates their pain and rest relieves it.

Diagnosis

The development of chronic low back and leg pain in a patient who has been exposed to any of the causative factors should lead to the suspicion of arachnoiditis. Patchy neurologic deficits that involve multiple nerve roots are common. Diagnostic studies should reveal the absence of other structural lesions and the presence of nerve root matting or clumping and filling defects in the arachnoid. This is often a diagnosis of exclusion and is sometimes made without any real evidence.

Treatment

No controlled studies have demonstrated effective treatments for arachnoiditis. Some patients have responded to epidural and intrathecal steroids, usually administered with a local anesthetic. Because steroids do not affect collagen that has already been laid down to form a scar, it is hard to explain their purported efficacy in arachnoiditis (19). Surgical lysing of the scarred nerve roots has also been undertaken, with variable results at best (20, 21). Some patients lose neurologic function after this operation. Because arachnoiditis is probably a form of deafferentation pain, ablative surgical procedures are not indicated in most patients. Spinal cord stimulation has led to symptomatic improvement in many but not all patients (22, 23).

Fractured Lumbar Spine (XXVI-5)

Fractures of the lumbar spine represent major trauma. They are associated with acute pain that can be expected to abate as the injury heals, but some patients develop a chronic pain syndrome. Persistent pain should raise the suspicion of instability at the site of injury. Trauma to the lumbar and sacral spine can also result in damage to the cauda equina and lead to deafferentation pain. Arachnoiditis and nerve root scarring can also follow trauma, and severe pain can ensue.

Lumbosacral Plexus Avulsion

Avulsion of the lumbosacral plexus or contusion of the roots that form the plexus is less common than major injuries to the branchial plexus. The lumbosacral plexus is more protected than the brachial plexus, and avulsion only occurs with massive trauma. These roots originate in the conus medullaris; avulsion can lead to myelopathy because of compromise of the blood vessels that feed the spinal cord and enter the dura in association with the nerve roots. A history of major trauma is almost always present, and the neurologic deficits occur immediately. Pain is present initially, and in some patients a denervation pain develops in the anesthetic areas of the body.

The management of this chronic pain is difficult. It does not respond well to narcotics, but anticonvulsants are sometimes valuable. Ablative surgical procedures are usually not helpful; a new form of surgery, dorsal root entry zone lesions, might be the most effective (Chapter 98C).

Postherpetic Neuralgia (XXVI-3)

Herpes zoster can involve the lumbar and sacral dermatomes and can lead to severe pain in the acute phase and chronic pain if postherpetic neuralgia develops. This common pain syndrome is discussed in Chapter 13; nothing is unique about its occurrence in the lower extremities. Inflammatory and degenerative changes are found in the peripheral nerves, dorsal roots, and dorsal horn of the spinal cord. Medical and surgical management can be difficult.

Tabes Dorsalis (XXVI-9)

Tabes dorsalis (tabetic neurosyphilis) is the cause of lancinating pains in a radicular pattern that can involve the lumbar and sacral dermatomes (24). It is much less common in the present antibiotic era, occurring predominantly in those of middle age, because it takes several decades for the infection to progress to this stage. Patients describe severe, shock-like pains that are of brief duration but can recur frequently. Both hypesthesia and hyperesthesia can be found in the areas of pain. Signs of spinal cord dysfunction are usually present. This pain syndrome is almost pathognomonic; tests for syphilis are positive.

The lightning pains can be ameliorated by anticonvulsants; diphenylhydantoin or carbamazepine are most commonly used (Chapter 14). Cordotomy has been reported to have a high success rate for cases in which medications are not effective.

Diabetic Pseudotabes (XXVI-9)

Diabetics can develop various neuropathies and myelopathies, including what is called "diabetic pseudotabes." The exact cause of the neurologic signs and symptoms is not understood. The patient has signs of posterior column dysfunction (proprioceptive loss), radicular sensory loss, and radicular lancinating pains. Pseudotabes is distinguished from tabes dorsalis by the presence of abnormalities of sugar metabolism and the absence of positive tests for syphilis. Optimal management of diabetes seems to lessen the likelihood of occurrence of this form of neuropathy. Symptomatic relief can sometimes be obtained with anticonvulsants (Chapter 14).

Lesions of the Lumbosacral Plexus

Lesions of the lumbosacral plexus are rare, because its location protects it from most trauma. Any lesion of the plexus can produce pain that is increased by deep palpation or by exercise that stretches the plexus or involves the psoas muscle. A sudden onset of severe pain and unilateral lumbosacral plexopathy can be a result of rupture of an abdominal aortic aneurysm or of the development of a retroperitoneal hemorrhage in a patient who is taking anticoagulants. Most other causes of plexopathy are of gradual onset.

Neoplasms (XXVI-8/503X4b)

INTRINSIC TUMORS. Tumors of the lumbosacral plexus present with neurologic deficits and pain that is usually referred to the distribution of the involved nerves. Most of these intrinsic lesions are benign schwannomas or neurofibromas, which can be solitary or part of a more generalized phakomatosis. Malignant degeneration rarely occurs. CT and MRI scanning are of great diagnostic assistance; electromyography localizes the lesion functionally. Treatment involves surgical excision and repair of the plexus with cable grafts, when appropriate. Pain from a tumor of the plexus is sometimes relieved by narcotics; anticonvulsants can also be helpful because often a component of deafferentation pain is also present.

EXTRINSIC TUMORS. Retroperitoneal neoplasms can invade the lumbosacral plexus and produce severe pain and progressive neurologic deficits. Lymphoma, sarcoma, and uterine carcinoma (in women) are the most common types of tumors that invade the plexus and produce pain. Typically, the pain is perceived both deep in the abdomen and pelvis and in the distribution of the plexus to the groin and lower extremities. Aggressive medical (and sometimes surgical) treatment is needed to alleviate this type of cancer pain (Chapter 24).

Lumbosacral Plexitis

Pain and neurologic deficits can develop rapidly in the lumbosacral plexus without any apparent injury or anatomic lesion, and are assumed to be caused by a viral inflammation of the lumbosacral plexus. The disease is self-limiting and usually has a favorable prognosis. Symptomatic therapy is indicated; some have advocated the use of steroids (25).

Postradiation Plexopathy

Radiation therapy of the lower abdomen and pelvis can lead to lumbosacral plexopathy secondary to fibrosis. It is sometimes difficult to discriminate between tumor recurrence, surgical scarring, and radiation-induced fibrosis. MRI or CT scanning helps to rule out tumor recurrence and make the diagnosis of plexopathy more likely. Radiation-induced pain rarely develops in less than a year after therapy; the latency period can be several years (1).

Symptoms and Signs

Sensory changes are usually found earliest in those with radiation-induced plexopathy; the amount of sensory and motor loss vary and can be slowly progressive. Radiation-induced skin changes are almost always observed.

Treatment

The treatment of radiation-induced plexopathy is not successful in most patients. The condition is rare, and proven therapies do not exist. Some patients respond favorably to analgesics, and others are helped by anticonvulsants and antidepressants. Ablative surgical procedures are sometimes helpful; neurostimulation of either spinal cord or brain has been reported to be successful.

Contusion or Stretching

The lumbosacral plexus is not often contused or stretched by external trauma because it is well protected. The most common cause of such an injury is childbirth—hence the female preponderance. Either the fetal head or the forceps used to deliver the head can contuse or stretch the plexus; the lower segments are more likely to be involved. The pain and neurologic deficits are usually of several months duration and abate spontaneously. The upper portion of the plexus can be damaged during delivery if the hips are maintained in flexion and abduction for a prolonged period.

Penetrating Trauma

Either gunshot wounds or low-velocity penetrating injuries can directly damage the lumbosacral plexus, but this is a rare traumatic injury. Neuromas and scarring around the plexus can follow the acute injury and lead to chronic pain. Proper management requires adequate visualization of the plexus at the time of debridement so that the nature of the injury can be identified and plans for restorative surgery can be developed. Repair of the damaged plexus is the best method of preventing chronic pain. Secondary procedures to lyse the scar from within and around the nerve are sometimes helpful. Some patients respond to pharmacologic management with narcotics, anticonvulsants, or antidepressants. Ablative surgical procedures are rarely indicated. Electrical stimulation of the spinal cord or brain is sometimes helpful.

Lesions of the Peripheral Nerves

Acute Trauma

Any of the nerves of the leg can be injured by blunt or penetrating trauma. The injury itself is painful because of the surrounding tissue damage, and neurapraxia develops immediately. The likelihood of neurologic deficit and of the development of chronic pain is a function of the severity of the nerve injury. Chronic pain can develop if a neuroma is formed at the site of axonal disruption or if the nerve becomes chronically entrapped in a scar.

Prevention of chronic pain is associated with prompt repair of the nerve (26). If surgical exploration does not result in pain relief, local injections of steroids can be helpful for some patients.

Chronic Trauma

The most common cause of chronic nerve trauma is mechanical compression by surrounding structures; these are known as entrapment syndromes (27). Although it is possible for any nerve at any point in its course to be entrapped, in fact most entrapments occur at specific sites on specific nerves. The more common lower extremity entrapment syndromes are described in Table 73-2.

Etiology

The pathophysiology of nerve entrapment is almost certainly ischemia of the nerve. A mild degree of pressure for a short period produces a rapidly reversible dysfunction. Variations in the amount of pressure might be responsible for the intermittent symptoms that are so characteristic of these lesions. The lesion is electrophysiologically characterized by slowing of conduction velocities; histologic findings include segmental demyelination and remyelination (28).

Symptoms and Signs

Entrapment neuropathies are responsible for focal neurologic deficits, local and radiating pain, and paresthesias. Any of these three components can predominate, or they can be absent. The lost axons probably cause the motor and sensory loss; the paresthesias and pain of course require functional axons. Thus, the electrophysiologic changes do not correlate well with the pain or paresthesias (29).

Usually the symptoms of an entrapment neuropathy develop after unusual exercise of the appropriate body part. Once present, the symptoms frequently wax and wane without obvious cause. The neurologic deficits are usually slowly progressive; the pain and paresthesias vary. The pain might not only be local, but can radiate proximally and distally from the site of entrapment.

Diagnosis

Entrapment neuropathies can be diagnosed on the basis of history and physical findings and are corroborated by electrodiagnostic studies (30). Both early and late responses of nerve conduction and electromyography might be required for accurate location (Chapter 35).

Treatment

Both nonsurgical and surgical therapies have been effective for entrapment neuropathies. Mild lesions related to repetitive movements can be managed by appropriate changes in occupation or recreation. Splinting or bracing can be effective for some lesions. Local injection of steroids can be beneficial. When these measures fail, surgical decompression is often curative. If major damage to the nerve has already occurred, decompression might not alleviate the loss of function or the pain.

TABLE 73-2. Lower Extremity Entrapment Syndromes

Nerve	Location of Pain	Sensory Changes	Weakness	Usual Cause
Lateral femoral cutaneous (meralgia paresthetica)	Anterolateral thigh	Anterolateral thigh	None	Entrapment under inguinal ligament
Saphenous	Medial leg, knee	Medial calf	None	Entrapment at subsartorial tunnel
Obturator	Proximal medial	Proximal medial	Adductors	Entrapment at obturator canal
Sciatic (piriformis syndrome)	Buttock, lateral and posterior leg, foot	Lateral and posterior leg and foot	Hamstrings, all distal muscles	Entrapment by piriformis muscle
Peroneal	Lateral knee, into leg and foot	Lateral leg, dorsum of foot	Foot dorsiflexors	Entrapment at fibular head
Deep peroneal (anterior tarsal tunnel)	Dorsum of foot	1st dorsal web	None	Entrapment by flexor retinaculum
Posterior tibial (posterior tarsal tunnel)	Plantar foot and toes	Plantar foot and toes	Intrinsic flexors	Entrapment at tarsal tunnel
Interdigital (Morton's neuroma)	Toes (usually 3rd and 4th)	Apposing toe surfaces	None	Entrapment at metatarsal (?)

Specific Nerve Entrapment Syndromes

Lateral Femoral Nerve Entrapment (XXX-1)

Entrapment of the lateral femoral cutaneous nerve is known as meralgia paresthetica. It was one of the earliest entrapment syndromes to be described. The nerve is derived from the L2 and L3 roots and travels across the pelvic side wall to enter the thigh at the lateral end of the inguinal ligament, which is the common site of entrapment. This nerve has no motor fibers; the symptoms are purely sensory.

Etiology

Entrapment usually occurs where the nerve passes underneath or through the inguinal ligament at the origin of the ligament and attaches to the anterior superior iliac spine. Human studies have revealed that in a significant percentage of individuals the nerve passes from the pelvis to the thigh through the fibers of the inguinal ligament rather than below it (30) (Fig. 73-6). Other causes are chronic trauma in those in certain occupations, intrapelvic pathology with compression along the long course of the nerve, and occupations that require standing with the side of the

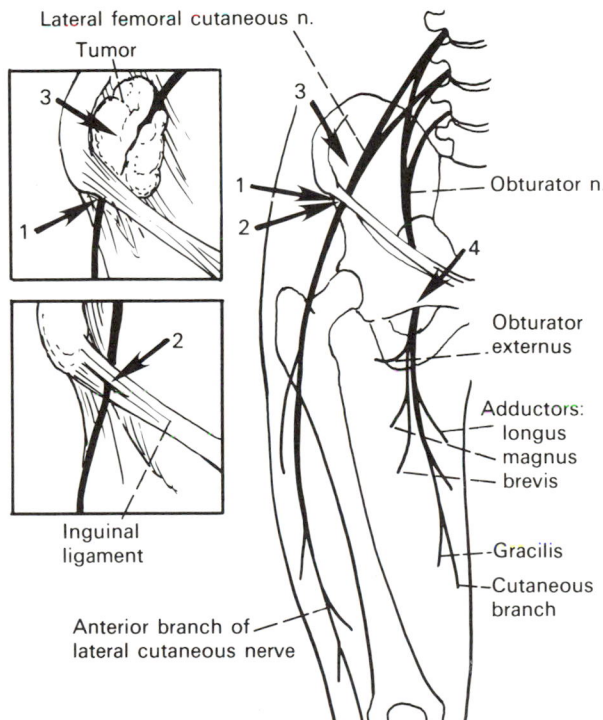

FIG. 73-6. Sites of entrapment of the lateral femoral cutaneous and obturator nerves: the most common site of entrapment of the lateral femoral cutaneous nerve as it passes below the inguinal ligament (1); site of entrapment of the lateral femoral cutaneous nerve as it passes within the ligament (2); site of entrapment of the lateral femoral cutaneous nerve in the pelvis by a tumor (3); site of entrapment of the obturator nerve (4). Developed by J.J. Bonica and M. Domenowske from data in Kopell, H.P., and Thompson, W.A.L.: Peripheral Entrapment Neuropathies. Baltimore, Williams & Wilkins, 1963.

anterior superior spine held against a hard object (e.g., barbers) (31).

Signs and Symptoms

The patient usually complains of both pain and paresthesias in the upper lateral thigh. The pain is described as burning or tingling and is localized to the skin and not to deep structures. Light stimulation of the skin is often described as very unpleasant (allesthesia). The pain and paresthesias are aggravated by standing and walking or by extending the hip; sitting or lying with the hip flexed can alleviate the symptoms. Many patients complain of the paresthesias without describing pain in the thigh; others have neither pain nor paresthesias but only sensory loss. The area of sensory loss is usually only in the center of the large territory of this nerve; the region of altered response to stimulation is often greater.

Diagnosis

Sensory action potentials can demonstrate conduction delay, temporal dispersion, or absence of responses (Chapter 35). Electromyography should not reveal abnormalities of the quadriceps muscle or femoral nerve. No motor or sensory abnormalities should be present elsewhere in the leg. Retroperitoneal mass lesions should be excluded by physical examination or appropriate imaging studies. In fact, the presentation of burning and tingling in the lateral thigh is rarely caused by anything other than entrapment of the lateral femoral cutaneous nerve.

Treatment

Symptoms are usually mild, and reassurance and accurate diagnosis often suffice. Patients should be advised not to wear constricting garments such as corsets or belts. Obese patients should be advised to lose weight. If the onset of symptoms is associated with a new exercise activity, patients should be advised to find another, less stressful exercise.

The role of nerve blocks with or without steroids at the level of the inguinal ligament is unclear, because no controlled studies have been carried out. Whether temporary relief of symptoms alters the long-term prognosis is unknown. Some patients have remission of their complaints without any treatment. Although surgical decompression and nerve resection were once common, they are often not successful. Indeed, the pain complaints usually increase after transection of this or any other peripheral nerve.

Femoral Nerve Entrapment (XXX-3)

The femoral nerve can be compressed by various neoplasms and vascular diseases, but it is not involved in an idiopathic entrapment syndrome. Most of these lesions are intrapelvic and not occult. The nerve can also be damaged by extreme flexion or hyperextension at the hip. The femoral nerve is derived from the L2, L3, and L4 roots and travels across the retroperitoneal space to exit the pelvis at the femoral triangle in close proximity to the femoral artery and vein.

Signs and Symptoms

Pain is not usually a symptom of femoral nerve entrapment. The major findings are quadriceps weakness with severe gait impairment and decreased sensation over the anterior thigh and medial calf. Pain can be at the site of the causative lesion rather than in the distribution of the nerve itself.

Diagnosis

The presence of hip flexor weakness indicates a lesion of the lumbosacral plexus or spinal roots and discriminates femoral nerve entrapment from femoral neuropathy. Electromyography, sensory action potentials, and nerve conduction velocity studies can help to locate the lesion. Imaging studies (CT scanning or MRI) can be helpful in identifying intrapelvic or retroperitoneal pathology.

Treatment

Because entrapment is almost always caused by a pathologic lesion impinging on the nerve, treatment is aimed at that lesion. Explorative surgery to relieve pain is usually fruitless.

Saphenous Nerve Entrapment

The saphenous nerve is a sensory branch of the femoral nerve that travels through the adductor canal of the thigh and penetrates the fascia just above the knee to supply the skin of the medial calf and ankle and often the medial portion of the foot dorsum. Idiopathic entrapment occurs where the nerve exits from the adductor canal in the distal thigh (subsartorial tunnel).

Symptoms and Signs

Saphenous nerve entrapment is characterized by burning or aching pain in the medial calf, which can radiate into the entire distribution of this nerve. The patient does not have any weakness. Use of the knee can exacerbate the pain or the sensory changes.

Diagnosis

The diagnosis of saphenous nerve entrapment is based on the complaint of pain and sensory changes in the territory of this nerve without involvement of any other branches of the femoral nerve. Sensory action potentials can be helpful; mass lesions in the adductor canal can be seen on CT scan or with MRI. Prior surgery in the area of the knee can lead to entrapment in the postoperative scar.

Treatment

Severe symptoms have been treated successfully by exploration and decompression of the exit zone of the saphenous nerve from the adductor canal. This is a rare entrapment neuropathy, and few data are available concerning its natural history and treatment outcomes.

Obturator Nerve Entrapment (XXX-3)

Entrapment of the obturator nerve usually occurs at the obturator membrane as this nerve leaves the pelvis and enters the thigh (Fig. 73-6). Most obturator nerve lesions are traumatic; idiopathic entrapment is rare. Sacroiliac and sacrum pathology can encroach on the obturator nerve as it traverses the pelvis.

Symptoms and Signs

The patient complains of pain in the upper medial thigh, with possible associated sensory loss in the medial thigh and weakness of the adductor muscles. The latter can lead to a wide-based gait with the leg held in an abducted position. Rarely, the pain radiates to the knee or even below it.

Diagnosis

Sensory and motor findings can be confirmed by electromyography and nerve conduction studies. Space-occupying lesions in the retroperitoneal or pelvic regions can be seen with MRI or on CT scan.

Treatment

Most obturator nerve entrapment is caused by a lesion, and extirpation of the lesion is the goal of therapy. Entrapment at the obturator membrane can be approached surgically.

Sciatic Nerve Entrapment (XXX-4)

The sciatic nerve can be compressed at many sites along its course from the sciatic notch to the point at which it divides into the peroneal and posterior tibial nerves, just above the popliteal fossa. This nerve is derived from the L4 and L5 roots and the S1, S2, and S3 sacral roots. The nerve leaves the pelvis through the sciatic notch, where it immediately underlies the piriformis muscle and is above the obturator internus muscle. This is the most frequent site of sciatic nerve entrapment, where it has been called the piriformis syndrome (Fig. 73-7).

Symptoms and Signs

Sciatic nerve entrapment by the piriformis syndrome can lead to buttock pain and pain that radiates in the distribution of the sciatic nerve to the foot. Motor loss can lead to instability of the foot and a severe gait dysfunction. The pain is usually described as aching and cramping. Paresthesias can be present in the sciatic nerve sensory territory.

Diagnosis

Piriformis syndrome can be diagnosed by determining the site of sciatic nerve compression on clinical and electrodiagnostic grounds. The nerves and muscles innervated by the nerve roots prior to the lumbosacral plexus are spared; electromyography can be helpful in showing no involvement of the paraspinal muscles. Electromyography and nerve conduction velocity studies in the extremity, however, cannot locate the site of the lesion between the plexus and midthigh. The physical findings and history so typical of herniated nucleus pulposus are not found in patients with sciatic nerve entrapment (Chapter 71). Unilateral symptoms and signs are rare in patients with spinal stenosis. Unfortunately, many patients with sciatic nerve entrapment are initially treated as if they had a herniated nucleus pulposus.

FIG. 73-7. Sites of entrapment of the sciatic nerve. **A.** Posterior view of lower limb showing the position of the sciatic nerve and its branches. Arrows indicate sites of sciatic nerve entrapment. **B.** Insets with details. Inset 1. Arrow shows the most frequent site of entrapment. This occurs because of compression by the piriformis muscle, which lies just above the sciatic nerve as it passes from the pelvis through the greater sciatic foramen; beneath the nerve itself is the obturator internus muscle. It has been shown that inward rotation of the thigh causes compression of the sciatic nerve against the tendinous origin of the piriformis muscle. Spasm of the piriformis muscle (inset 1) can also cause compression. In 12% of individuals the nerve passes between parts of the piriformis muscle (insets 2 and 3), the peroneal nerve portion of the sciatic nerve being most frequently involved. Compression can also be caused by a myofascial band in the distal portion of the thigh between the biceps femoris and the adductor magnus muscles trapping the nerve (arrow, inset 4). Other causes include muscle fibrosis induced by repeated injections of pentazocine, compression of the nerve in the pelvis during anticoagulant therapy, and compression of the nerve from leakage of acrylic plastic into the region posterior to the hip joint during total hip replacement. Developed by J.J. Bonica and M. Domenowske from data in Kopell, H.P., and Thompson, W.A.L.: Peripheral Entrapment Neuropathies. Baltimore, Williams & Wilkins, 1963.

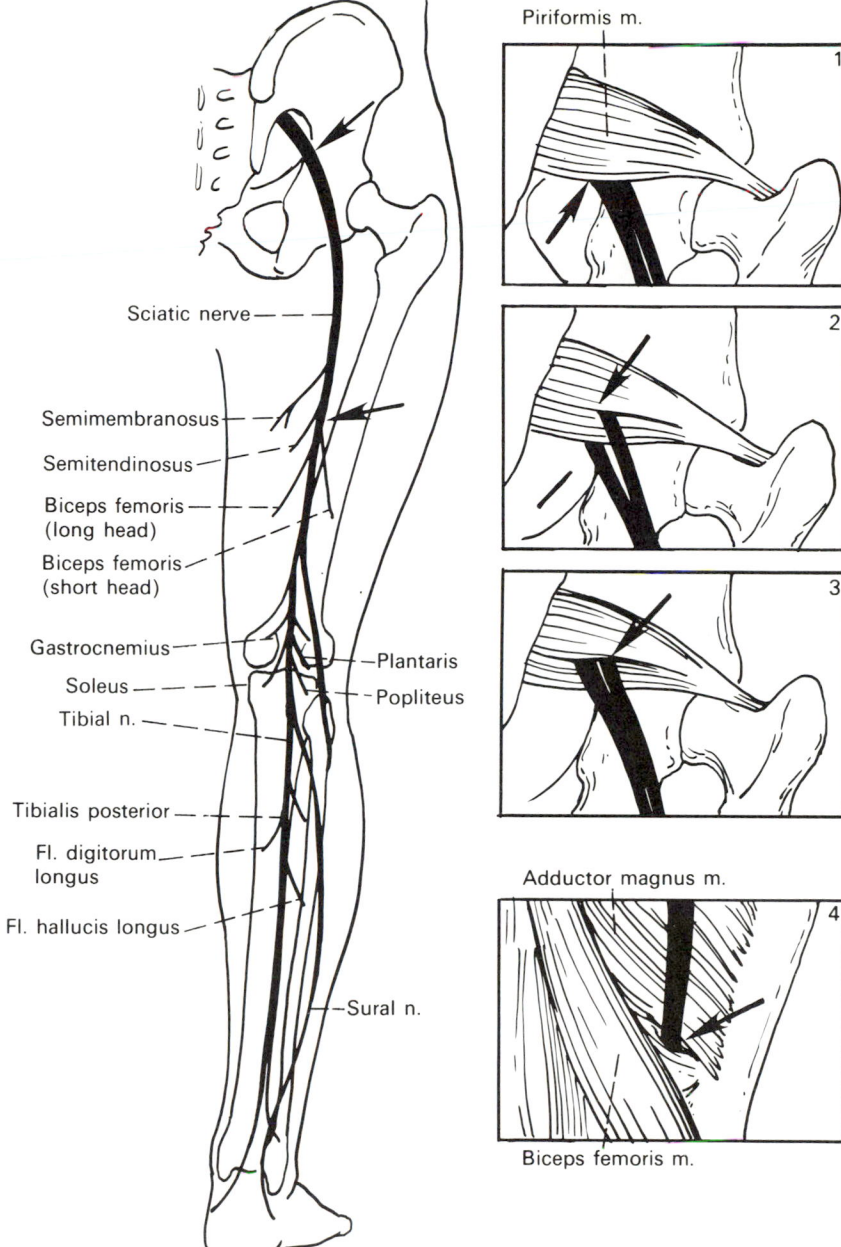

Treatment

If the diagnosis of piriformis syndrome is confirmed by diagnostic studies and the patient has significant neuropathic signs, the piriformis muscle should be detached from its origin and any fascial bands constricting the nerve should be transected.

Peroneal Nerve Entrapment

The peroneal nerve is a component of the sciatic nerve; it separates from the posterior tibial nerve about 8 cm proximal to the popliteal fossa. The peroneal nerve can be compressed as it courses around the fibular head in the upper calf and passes through a fibrous tunnel between the edge of the peroneus longus muscle and the fibula (Fig. 73-8). Trauma is a more common cause of peroneal neuropathy. Other causes include compression from improperly applied plaster casts, tight stockings, bandages, or garters. Peroneal damage can result from certain practices that produce compression and ischemia of the nerve, such as sitting, squatting, or kneeling when picking strawberries or weeding a garden for long periods, which result in compression by the tendon of the posterior part of the peroneus longus at the level of the head of the fibula. The peroneal nerve can also be compressed by various masses, including tumors of the nerve itself or tumors of the bone or ganglia arising from the superior tibiofibular joint.

Symptoms and Signs

Entrapment of the peroneal nerve usually presents with a deep, aching pain in the lateral distal knee.

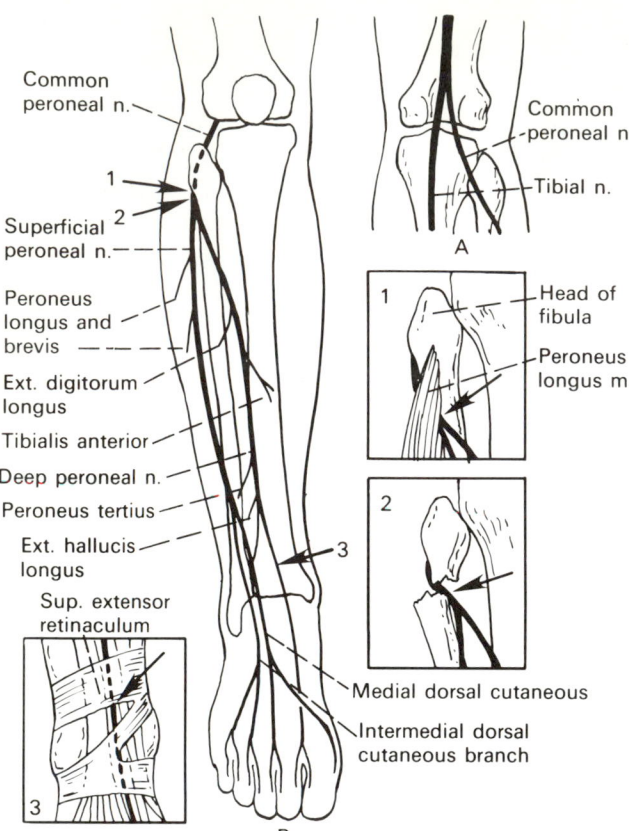

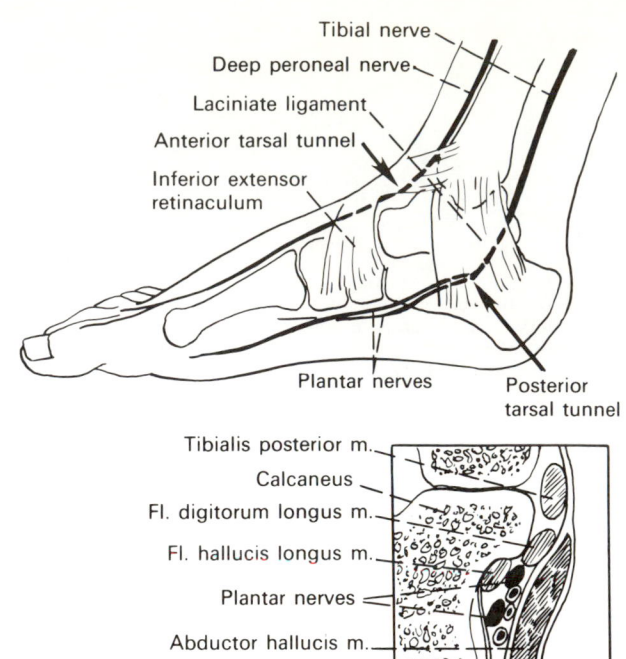

FIG. 73-8 Entrapment of the peroneal nerve. **A.** Posterior view of the knee depicting the beginning of the common peroneal nerve as it separates from the tibial nerve and winds around the head of the fibula. **B.** Anterior view of the lower leg showing the common peroneal nerve winding around the head of the fibula and then dividing into superficial and deep branches. Arrows indicate sites of nerve entrapment. Inset 1 shows entrapment as the nerve passes through a fibrous tunnel between the edge of the peroneus longus muscle and the fibula. Inset 2 shows entrapment caused by fracture of the fibula. Inset 3 shows entrapment of the deep peroneal nerve by the superior extensor retinaculum. Developed by J.J. Bonica and M. Domenowske from data in Kopell, H.P., and Thompson, W.A.L.: Peripheral Entrapment Neuropathies. Baltimore, Williams & Wilkins, 1963.

Pain can radiate into the foot, especially with pain at the fibular head, and slowly progressive sensory and motor loss is common. The sensory loss can vary from no loss to anesthesia over the lateral calf and dorsolateral surface of the foot. The skin distribution of the peroneal nerve is variable, but hypesthesia is commonly noted in the lateral calf and foot dorsum, including the medial three toes. Weakness of the foot dorsiflexors and everters can be present. Peroneal palsies caused by trauma are usually painless. Electrodiagnostic studies show both motor and sensory changes restricted to the peroneal nerve distribution. If the posterior tibial nerve is spared and both the superficial and deep branches of the peroneal nerve are involved, the lesion is at the fibular head.

Treatment

If entrapment of the peroneal nerve is confirmed, surgical decompression is warranted. Pain can be relieved effectively and return of peroneal nerve func-

FIG. 73-9. Entrapment of the tibial nerve in the posterior tarsal tunnel, which contains the tibial nerve, its posterior tibial artery, and tendons of the tibialis posterior, flexor digitorum longus, and flexor hallucis longus. The syndrome usually has a traumatic basis such as fracture and dislocation of the ankle, but symptoms might not develop until some time after the injury. Nonspecific tenosynovitis or thrombophlebitis can affect other contents of the tarsal tunnel and produce compression of the nerve. The anterior tarsal syndrome is an entrapment of the terminal portion of the deep peroneal nerve as it runs below the dense superficial fascia of the ankle. *Inset.* Cross section of the ankle showing the contents of the posterior tarsal tunnel. Developed by J.J. Bonica and M. Domenowske from data in Kopell, H.P., and Thompson, W.A.L.: Peripheral Entrapment Neuropathies. Baltimore, Williams & Wilkins, 1963.

tion is commonly seen. Significant peroneal nerve dysfunction mandates a foot brace so that the patient can ambulate effectively.

Entrapment Neuropathies of the Foot (XXX-5)

Three entrapment neuropathies of the nerves of the foot have been well described: the deep peroneal nerve can be compromised in the anterior tarsal tunnel, the posterior tibial nerve can be damaged in the posterior tarsal tunnel (Fig. 73-9), and the interdigital nerves can be damaged by adjacent metatarsal heads (Morton's neuroma). Local anesthetic injections can help to establish the diagnosis; electrodiagnostic studies have not been reported in significant number. Surgical decompression of tarsal tunnel syndrome has been reported to yield good results (27). Morton's neuroma is treated by excision of the common interdigital nerve when conservative measures have failed to relieve the metatarsal pain.

Neoplasms

Tumors of the peripheral nerves can present with both local and referred pain and with sensory and motor changes in the distribution of the nerve (32). The typical history is of gradually progressive sensory and motor loss and pain in the region of the tumor.

These tumors are usually slow-growing benign lesions, although they can become sarcomatous. Treatment is by surgical excision.

REFERENCES

1. Dyck, P.J., et al.: Peripheral Neuropathy. Philadelphia, W.B. Saunders, 1984, pp. 1498–1501.
2. Spence, A.M.: Pain and sensory disturbances in the extremities: Radiculopathies, plexopathies and mononeuropathies. *In* Signs and Symptoms in Neurology. Edited by P.D. Swanson. Philadelphia, J.B. Lippincott, 1984, pp. 245–280.
3. Loeser, J.D., and Lewin, R.A.: Lumbosacral lipoma in the adult. J. Neurosurg., *29*:405, 1968.
4. Connolly, E.S.: Spinal cord tumors in adults. *In* Neurological Surgery. Edited by J.R. Youmans. Philadelphia, W.B. Saunders, 1982, pp. 3196–3214.
5. Swerdlow, M.: Anticonvulsant drugs and chronic pain. Clin. Neuropharmacol., *7*:51, 1984.
6. Baker, A.S., et al.: Spinal epidural abscess. N. Engl. J. Med., *293*:463, 1975.
7. Mixter, W.J., and Barr, J.S.: Rupture of the intervertebral disk with involvement of the spinal canal. N. Engl. J. Med., *211*:210, 1934.
8. Howe, J.F., Loeser, J.D., and Calvin, W.H.: Mechanosensitivity of dorsal root ganglia and chronically injured axons: A physiological basis for radicular pain of nerve root compression. Pain, *3*:25, 1977.
9. Spangfort, E.: Disc surgery. *In* Textbook of Pain. Edited by P.D. Wall and R. Melzack. Edinburgh, Churchill Livingstone, 1984, pp. 601–607.
10. Green, L.N.: Dexamethasone in the management of symptoms due to herniated lumbar disc. J. Neurol. Neurosurg. Psychiatry, *38*:1211, 1975.
11. Johnson, E.W., and Fletcher, E.R.: Lumbosacral radiculopathy: Review of 100 consecutive cases. Arch. Phys. Med. Rehabil., *62*:321, 1981.
12. Onik, G., et al.: Percutaneous lumbar discectomy using a new aspiration probe. Am. J. Neuroradiol., *6*:290, 1985.
13. Maroon, J.D., and Onik, G.: Percutaneous automated discectomy: A new method for lumbar disc removal. J. Neurosurg., *66*:143, 1987.
14. Verbiest, H.: A radicular syndrome from developmental narrowing of the lumbar vertebral canal. J. Bone Joint Surg. [Br.], *36*:230, 1954.
15. Hawkes, C.H., and Roberts, G.M.: Neurogenic and vascular claudication. J. Neurol. Sci., *38*:337, 1978.
16. Hall, S., et al.: Lumbar spinal stenosis. Ann. Intern. Med., *103*:271, 1985.
17. Lombardi, J.S., et al.: Treatment of degenerative spondylolisthesis. Spine, *10*:821, 1985.
18. Ransford, A.O., and Harries, B.J.: Localised arachnoiditis complicating lumbar disc lesions. J. Bone Joint Surg. [Br.], *54*:656, 1972.
19. Howland, W.J., and Curry, J.L.: Pantopaque arachnoiditis. Experimental study of blood as a potentiating agent and corticosteroids as an ameliorating agent. Acta Radiol., *5*:1032, 1966.
20. Johnston, J.D.H., and Matheny, J.B.: Microscopic lysis of lumbar adhesive arachnoiditis. Spine, *3*:35, 1978.
21. Wilkenson, H.A., and Schuman, N.: Results of surgical lysis of lumbar adhesive arachnoiditis. Neurosurgery, *4*:401, 1979.
22. Meglio, M., and Cioni, B.: Personal experience with spinal cord stimulation in chronic pain management. Appl. Neurophysiol., *45*:195, 1982.
23. Siegfried, J., and Lazorthes, Y.: Long-term follow-up of dorsal cord stimulation for chronic pain syndrome after multiple lumbar operations. Appl. Neurophysiol., *45*:201, 1982.
24. Storm-Mathison, A.: Syphilis. *In* Handbook of Clinical Neurology. Edited by P.J. Vinken and G.W. Bruyn. Amsterdam, North-Holland, 1978, pp. 335–394.
25. Evans, B.A., Stevens, J.C., and Dyck, P.J.: Lumbosacral plexus neuropathy. Neurology, *31*:1327, 1981.
26. Sunderland, S.: Nerve and Nerve Injuries. London, Churchill Livingstone, 1972, pp. 558–563.
27. Dawson, D.M., Hallett, M., and Millender, L.H.: Entrapment Neuropathies. Boston, Little, Brown, & Company, 1983, pp. 5–194.
28. Gilliatt, R.W.: Peripheral nerve compression and entrapment. *In* Eleventh Symposium on Advanced Medicine. Edited by A.F. Lant. Tunbridge Wells, Kent, Pitman Medical Publishing, 1975.
29. Ochoa, J., et al.: Abnormal spontaneous activity in single sensory fibers in humans. Muscle Nerve, *5*:S74, 1982.
30. Kopell, H.P., and Thompson, W.A.L.: Peripheral Entrapment Neuropathies. Baltimore, Williams & Wilkins, 1963.
31. Bonica, J.J.: The Management of Pain. Philadelphia, Lea & Febiger, 1953, pp. 876–880.
32. Marmor, L.: Solitary peripheral nerve tumors. Clin. Orthop., *43*:183, 1965.

74 • PAINFUL DISORDERS OF THE HIP REGION

JOHN J. BONICA *and* DAN M. SPENGLER

DISORDERS of the hip region, including the buttocks, are among the most important and frequent causes of prolonged pain, suffering, and serious disability. The exact incidence of pain in the hip region cannot be accurately documented because these complaints often overlap with those of pain and other symptoms and signs caused by disorders of the lumbosacral spine and lumbosacral plexus. These pain complaints do, however, result in a substantial number of days of restricted activity and in time lost from productivity. A 1977 survey by the National Center for Health Statistics revealed that impairment related to the hips and lower extremities account for nearly one-third of the total number of impairments affecting the entire musculoskeletal system (1). About 10% of those who reported chronic conditions in this region and in the lower limbs reported activity limitations, and nearly 4% reported bed disability for 1 to 7 days, 3% for 8 to 30 days, and 2% for more than 1 month. Moreover, in 32%, the condition produced a great deal of discomfort, while in another 48% the condition was bothersome to some degree. In addition to the significant impact caused by chronic conditions, acute fractures, dislocations, and other acute painful conditions of the hip also resulted in significant activity restriction and impairment.

Disorders of the hip region affect persons of all age groups—infants, children, young and middle-aged adults, and especially the elderly—more than most other parts of the body. Because these pain complaints can represent a constellation of underlying causes, the physician must consider an exhaustive differential diagnosis to identify the precise cause properly. This in turn requires a thorough knowledge of the anatomy and biomechanics of the hip region. In this chapter we discuss these issues as well as specific disorders. The material is presented in two major sections: A, Basic Considerations, which includes a classification of painful hip diseases, a discussion of the anatomy, biomechanics, and function of the hip joint and region; B, Evaluation of the Patient, which complements the information in Chapter 70; and C, Clinical Considerations, which describes painful hip disorders of various causes. More detailed information can be found elsewhere (2–7).

A. BASIC CONSIDERATIONS

Classification

Table 74-1 classifies various painful disorders of the hip according to whether the condition is articular or extra-articular in the hip region. Moreover, some categories are classified as acute conditions or chronic disorders. Each condition is discussed separately below in Part B, including the causes, pathophysiology, symptoms and signs, diagnosis, and treatment.

Anatomy, Biomechanics, and Function of the Hip Region

In contrast to the prehensile and sensory functions of the upper limbs, the lower limbs of humans bear the entire body weight and serve the purpose of locomotion. As pointed out by Rosse (7), although the anatomy of the upper and lower limbs conforms to the same major plan, differential functional requirements of the lower limbs are reflected in the structural adaptation of the pelvic girdle, hips, and knee and ankle joints, and in the architecture of the foot (Fig. 74-1). The anatomy of the pelvis (Fig. 74-2) is considered in detail in Chapter 65. The anatomy and biomechanics of the knee joint are considered in Chapter 75, and those of the ankle joint and foot are presented in Chapter 76. Here we review the anatomy of the proximal end of the femur and of the hip joint, including its nerve and blood supply and the muscles important in its function.

Anatomy of the Proximal End of the Femur

The upper end of the femur consists of the head, neck, and two trochanters, of which only the greater trochanter is palpable (7). It is directly inferior to the tubercle of the iliac crest and is level with the tubercle. The femoral head, neck, and lesser trochanter are deeply buried in muscles of the head and can be palpated through the overlying muscles halfway between the pubic symphysis and the anterior superior iliac spine (Fig. 74-3).

The head of the femur, which is somewhat globular in shape, is covered with hyaline cartilage except over an ovoid depression or pit near its center, the fovea of the head of the femur, where the ligamentum teres is attached (8). The neck of the femur is considerably smaller in diameter than the head and is rather flattened anteroposteriorly, usually being thinner in its middle than at either end. It flares out considerably as it attaches to the shaft of the femur in the region of the trochanter.

TABLE 74-1. Classification of Painful Disorders of the Hip

Trauma
Fractures in older patients
Fractures in younger patients
Dislocation of the hip
Infection/inflammation
Infectious arthritis
Rheumatoid arthritis
Transient synovitis
Pigmented villonodular synovitis
Infection of the hip in infants and children
Infection of the hip in older children and adults
Developmental disorders
Congenital dislocation of the hip
Epiphyseal disorders
Legg-Calvé-Perthes disease
Slipped capital femoral epiphysitis
Extra-articular Disorders
Trochanteric bursitis
Iliopectineal bursitis
Ischiogluteal bursitis
Neoplasms
Primary
Metastatic
Metabolic/Endocrine Disorders
Paget's disease
Osteonecrosis
Referred Pain

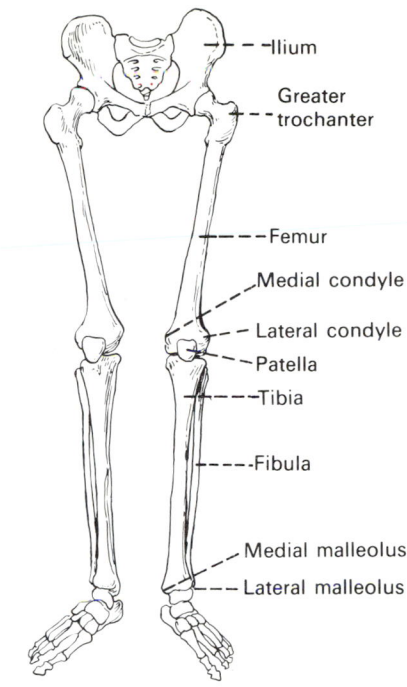

FIG. 74-1. Skeletal structure of the pelvis and lower limbs showing the relationship of the bones of the leg, ankle, and foot.

Fig. 74-2. The bony pelvis. **A.** Anterior view. **B.** Posterior view. The two hip or coxal bones are separated posteriorly by the sacrum, thus making the pelvic girdle. Each hip bone consists of the ilium, ischium, and pubis, which are shaded differently. The three bones diverge from the acetabulum in different directions, with the wing-like ilium projecting upward from the acetabulum. Its iliac crest, palpable along its length, terminates anteriorly in the anterior superior iliac spine and posteriorly in the posterior superior iliac spine. The posterior superior iliac spines are at the level of the S2 spinous process and indicate the position of the sacroiliac joint, which cannot be palpated. The summit of the iliac crest is at the level of the L4 spinous process. The ischium projects posteriorly and has two important landmarks, the ischial tuberosity and the ischial spine. Note the sacrospinous and sacrotuberous and other ligaments and the greater and lesser sciatic foramina. The body of the pubic articulates anteriorly with its fellow of the opposite side across the public symphysis, which is in the medial plane while posteriorly the superior ramus fuses with the ischium and ilium in the acetabulum and the inferior ramus fuses with the ramus of the ischium. The two pubic rami embrace the obturator foramen, which is almost completely filled by the obturator membrane. From Hollinshead, W.H.: Anatomy for Surgeons, Vol. 3. 3rd Ed. Philadelphia, Harper & Row, 1982.

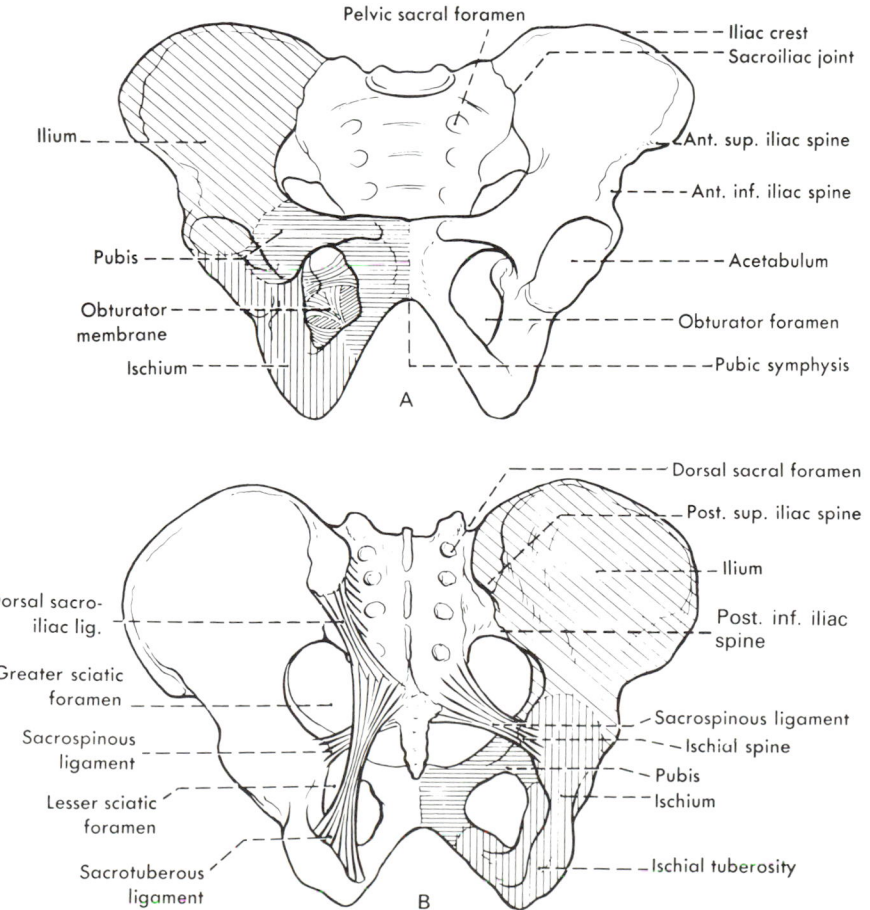

The femoral neck is about 5 cm long and projects from the shaft medially, cephalad, and slightly anteriorly. These angulations between the neck and shaft are important because they influence where the gravitational line of force falls in relation to the hip and the knee (7). The angle of the medial and cephalad projection, measured as the angle between the long axis of the neck and shaft of the femur, is known as the angle of inclination. The angle of inclination decreases from about 150° at birth to 125° in male adults and to 120° in old age (Fig. 74-4). Because of the increased width of the pelvis in the female, the angle of inclination is somewhat less (115 to 120°). Considerable variation exists, however, depending on the height of the individual as well as on the body build. A deformity caused by a decrease in the angle of inclination, known as coxa vara, shortens the leg and also limits hip abduction (7). Because of the medial displacement of the line of force acting on the hip joint in relation to the knee, the knee tends to be forced into valgus (bow legs). An increase in the angle of inclination, known as coxa valga, lengthens the limb, mimics hip abduction contracture, and results in lateral displacement of the weight-bearing force line, causing the knee to become predisposed to a varus deformity.

The angle of the anterior projection measured by the angle made by the longitudinal axis of the neck with a line drawn through the centers of the two femoral condyles is known as the angle of declination, or torsion. The angle of torsion is normally about 12°. If this angle increases (anteversion) it tends to produce a gait with "toeing in," whereas a decrease in the angle (retroversion) causes "toeing out" (7). Moreover, anteversion displaces the body center of mass anteriorly in relation to the knee, predisposing it to hyperextension, whereas retroversion produces knee flexion and recruits knee extensors to stabilize the joint.

Hip Joint

The hip is a polyaxial synovial joint in which the closely fitting ball-and-socket-shaped articular facet is formed by the reception of the head of the femur into the cup-shaped cavity of the acetabulum (2, 3). Unlike the shoulder joints, which depend on the strength and stabilization of the surrounding muscles, the hip joints are inherently strong and their structures well adapted to support the weight of the trunk, with minimal or no expenditure of muscular energy, and permit movement in all directions. Deeply molded articular surfaces and strong ligaments are key factors in the stability of the hip joints (6).

The head of the femur forms more than half of a sphere and its articular cartilage, thicker at the center than at the circumference, covers its entire surface, except for the shallow fovea of the femoral head. The inner surface of the acetabulum is characterized by a horseshoe-shaped region, the lunate (articular) surface, which is also covered by articular cartilage. Within the lunate surface is a circular depression devoid of cartilage that is occupied by fatty tissue covered by synovial membrane (2). The acetabular labrum is a fibrocartilaginous lip that significantly deepens the socket, and the joint is encased in an articular capsule reinforced by ligaments. The labrum is completed inferiorly by the transverse ligament of the acetabulum, which bridges the notch that exists in the lower rim of the socket (Figs. 74-5 and 74-6).

Capsule and Ligaments

The ligamentous structures of the hip joint include the capsule, with the synovial membrane lining its inner surface, and the iliofemoral, ischiofemoral, and bulbofemoral ligaments, which surround and reinforce the capsule.

ARTICULAR CAPSULE. The articular capsule is a thick fibrous structure that encloses a voluminous joint cavity, which contains the acetabular labrum, the head and neck of the femur, and the ligament of the head (ligamentum teres), with a fat pad that surrounds it. The fibers of the capsule run mostly longitudinally between the pelvis and the femur, although some deeper fibers, called the zona orbicularis, run

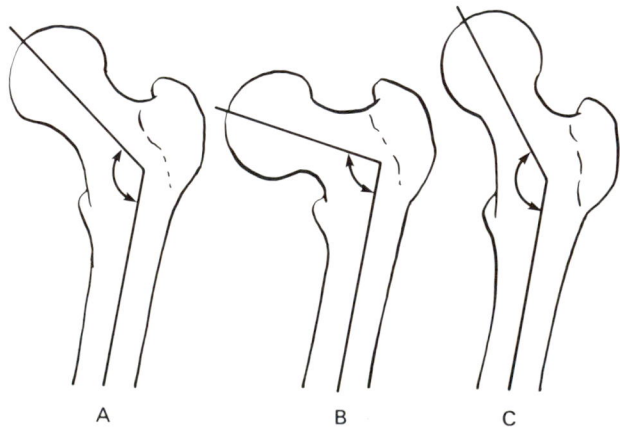

Fig. 74-4. **A.** Normal angle of inclination of the femoral neck to the shaft in the frontal plane. This is called the "neck-shaft angle," and is approximately 125°. **B.** Neck-shaft angle in coxa vara. The angle is less than 125°. **C.** Neck-shaft angle in coxa valga. The angle is greater than 125°. Modified from Nordin, M., and Frankel, V.H.: Biomechanics of the hip. *In* Basic Biomechanics of the Skeletal System. Edited by V.H. Frankel and M. Nordin. Philadelphia, Lea & Febiger, 1980.

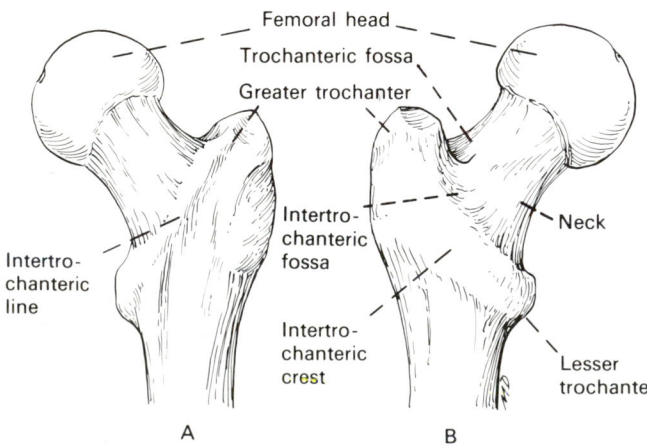

Fig. 74-3. Head, neck, and proximal portion of femur. **A.** Anterior view. **B.** Posterior view. The head fits into the acetabulum (shown in figure 74-2).

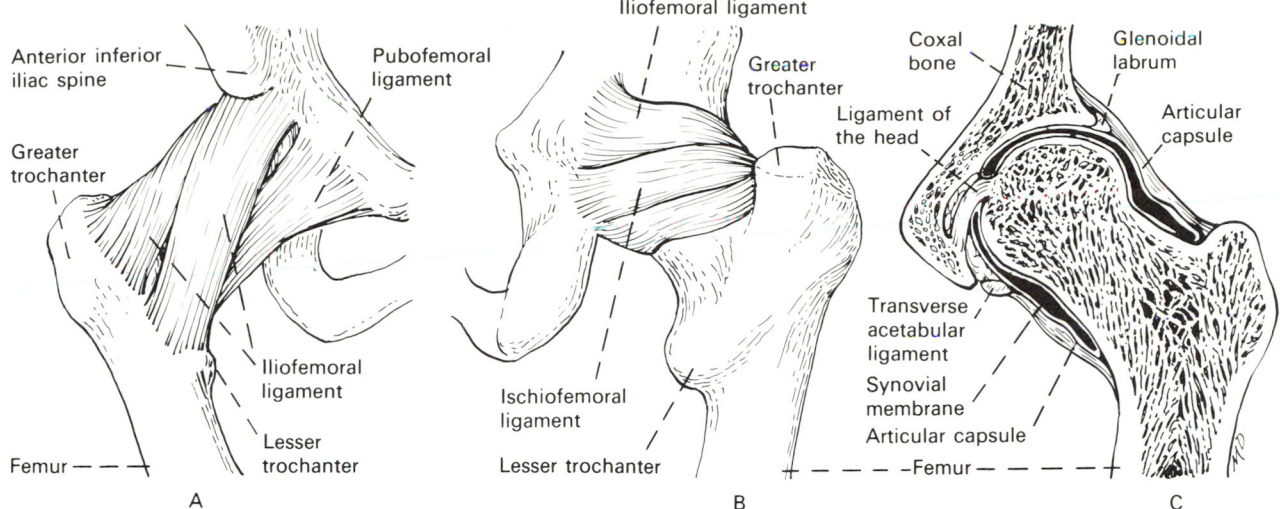

Fig. 74-5. Chief ligaments of the capsule of the hip joint. **A.** Anterior view. **B.** Posterior view. **C.** Schematic coronal section through the hip joint showing the synovial membrane, which lines the capsule and covers the femoral head, ligament of the head, and intra-articular fat. **A** and **B** modified from Clemente, C.D. (ed.): Gray's Anatomy of the Human Body. 30th Am. Ed. Philadelphia, Lea & Febiger, 1985; **C** modified from Hollinshead, W.H.: Anatomy for Surgeons. Vol. 3, The Back and Limbs. Philadelphia, Harper & Row, 1982.

circularly (3). These circular fibers are more abundant at the distal and posterior parts of the capsule and form a sling or collar around the neck of the femur (Figs. 74-5C and 74-6A).

The attachments of the articular capsule to the femur extend far beyond the articular margin (Fig. 74-5). Anteriorly the capsule is attached between the bases of the two trochanters along the intertrochanteric line and posteriorly to the base of the neck, excluding the trochanteric fossa from the joint cavity. An important clinical fact pointed out by Rosse (7) is that, up to the age of 18 or 19 years, the epiphyseal cartilage of the greater trochanter is partially intracapsular and that of the femoral head completely intracapsular.

SYNOVIAL MEMBRANE. The synovial membrane lines the capsule and reflects at the femoral capsular attachment, which invests the femoral neck in a synovial sleeve (7) (Fig. 74-6A). The synovium is attached to the edges of the articular margins on both the femur and acetabulum, thus excluding the intra-articular fat, the ligament of the head, and the femoral neck from direct contact with synovial fluid. The joint cavity sometimes communicates with the subtendinous iliac bursa, which lies deep to the tendon of the psoas major. If present, the communication is found anteriorly between the pubofemoral ligament and the more medially oriented band of the iliofemoral ligament (2).

LIGAMENTS. The iliofemoral ligament is a thick structure that is considered to be the strongest ligament in the body (7). It is triangular, similar to an inverted Y, with its stem attached to the anterior inferior iliac spine and its two arms fanning out in continuity along the intertrochanteric line. This ligament is the primary counterbalance to gravitational force during relaxed standing—because it falls behind the transverse axis of the hip joints, it would tend to tilt the pelvis backward on the femoral head. The ligament is longest when it is taut in extension and medial rotation; this is important in limiting these movements.

The ischiofemoral ligament consists of a triangular band of fibers that springs from the body of the ischium below and behind the acetabulum to blend with the circular fibers of the capsule (2). Its upper fibers are oriented horizontally across the joint while its lower fibers spiral upward and laterally, attaching to the femoral neck just medial to the greater trochanter. Cephalad its fibers blend with the iliofemoral ligament.

The pubofemoral ligament arises above from the body of the pubis near the acetabulum and from the adjacent superior pubic ramus. Below it passes anteriorly to the head of the femur to reach the femoral neck, where it blends with the capsule and with the deep surface of the more medial band of the iliofemoral ligament. A pubofemoral ligament, similar to the iliofemoral ligament, assists in preventing hyperextension as well as in checking excessive abduction of the thigh.

The ligament of the head of the femur is a triangular, somewhat flattened band, implanted by its apex into the fovea of the femur; its base is attached by two bands, one on each end of the acetabular notch (Fig. 74-6B). This ligament is ensheathed by the synovial membrane and varies greatly in strength. It is of doubtful importance and is occasionally absent (7).

Nerve and Blood Supply

NERVES. Sensory fibers, including those that convey proprioception and nociception, and vasomotor fibers reach the hip joint in the articular branches of the nerves that supply the prime muscle movers of the joint (2, 3, 7). These include branches from the femoral nerve of one or more of its muscular branches and branches from the obturator, accessory obturator (when present), and superior gluteal nerves, and one or two branches from the nerve to the quadratus femoris derived from the lumbosacral plexus (Fig. 74-7). The branches from the femoral nerves are distributed largely to the region of the lower part of the iliofemoral ligament, with some also distributed to the posterosuperior part of the capsule near the pubofemoral ligament. The obturator and accessory obturator nerves are also distributed to the region of the pubofemoral ligament (2, 8, 9). The branch of the superior gluteal nerve supplies the superior and lateral parts of the capsule, while the branch from the nerve to the quadratus femoris supplies the posterior part of the capsule (3, 10, 11). Minor variations of the origin of the nerves to the joint exist, with the branch (or branches) from the obturator nerve being particularly likely to differ (3).

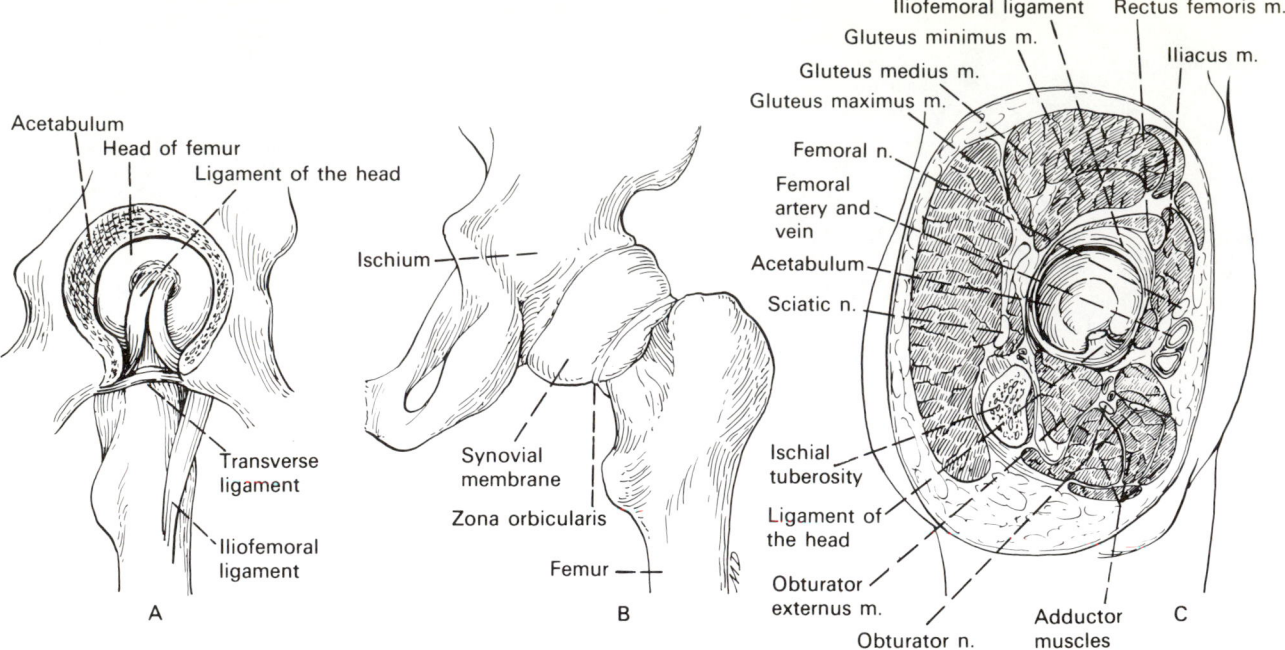

Fig. 74-6. Anatomy of the hip joint. *A.* The joint has been opened from within the pelvis by removal of the floor of the acetabulum to show the articular surface of the head of the femur, the ligament of the head, and the transverse acetabular ligament. *B.* Posterior view of the joint showing the synovial membrane of the capsule of the hip joint (distended). *C.* Sagittal section through the hip joint and the surrounding muscles and nerves. Note the position of the sciatic, femoral, and obturator nerves and of the femoral vessels Modified from Clemente, C.D. (ed.): Gray's Anatomy of the Human Body. 30th Am. Ed. Philadelphia, Lea & Febiger, 1985.

BLOOD SUPPLY. The hip, like all other joints, receives its blood supply primarily from a periarticular arterial anastomosis, which includes the following: medial and lateral femoral circumflex arteries, which are branches of the deep femoral artery; branches from the obturator artery; and articular branches of the superior and inferior gluteal arteries, which are contributed by the internal iliac artery (2, 3, 7). Usually the first perforating branch of the deep femoral artery also sends a branch upward to the hip joint. Most vessels to the capsule of the joint are twigs from the branches that supply the upper end of the femur (Fig. 74-8).

The vessels to the upper end of the femur are derived primarily from the two femoral circumflex arteries and give off small twigs to the lower part of the capsule of the joint. The acetabular branch of the obturator or medial femoral circumflex artery, or both, supply one or more branches to the head of the femur and also to tissues of the acetabular fossa. Branches of the superior gluteal artery supply an upper portion of the acetabulum, an upper portion of the fibrous capsule of the hip joint, and a small portion of the greater trochanter (3). Branches of the inferior gluteal artery supply the inferior and posterior portions of the acetabular rim and the adjacent fibrous capsule, but apparently do not enter the femur. Twigs from branches of the first perforating artery to the hip joint supply the posterior surfaces of the two trochanters and the adjacent capsule (3). All the intra-articular structures depend on this arterial anastomosis for their blood supply; an adequate blood supply is most critical to bone, especially to the proximal femoral epiphysis during its growth (7).

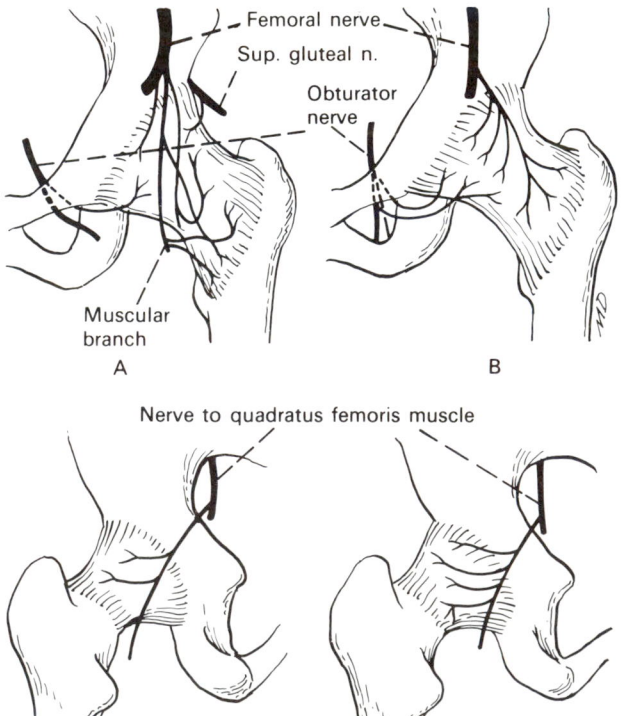

Fig. 74-7. Nerve supply to the hip joint *A, B.* Anterior views. Note the major contribution made by muscular branches of the femoral and obturator nerves. *C, D.* Posterior views. The major nerve supply to the posterior part of the capsule and joint is derived from the nerve to the quadratus femoris and the nerve to the superior gluteal muscles (not shown). Modified from Gardner, E.: The innervation of the hip joint. Anat. Rec., *101*:353, 1948.

Fig. 74-8. Arterial blood supply to the hip. This is derived from the periarticular anastomosis, which is composed of branches of the lateral and medial femoral circumflex arteries that are branches of the deep femoral artery, branches of the obturator artery, and superior gluteal branches of the internal iliac artery. Branches of the anastomosis pierce the capsule at its femoral attachment and surround the femoral neck as they proceed cephalad toward the head of the femur and beneath the synovial membrane to supply the underlying bone. These are the retinacular or capital vessels. Branches from the obturator artery supply the acetabulum and a small artery to the ligament of the head. Before closure of the epiphyseal plate the retinacular vessels reach the femoral head only through the periosteum, which bridges the avascular epiphyseal cartilage between the neck and the head of the femur. After closure the anastomosis is established between the epiphyseal and metaphyseal vessels within the cancellous bone, but further distally little or no anastomosis exists between the nutrient artery of the shaft and the vascular bed of the neck. If the retinacular vessels in the periosteum are damaged, ischemic necrosis of the femoral head occurs. Modified from Clemente, C.D. (ed.): Gray's Anatomy of the Human Body. 30th Am. Ed. Philadelphia, Lea & Febiger, 1985; and from Hollinshead, W.H.: Anatomy for Surgeons. Vol. 3, The Back and Limbs. Philadelphia, Harper & Row, 1982.

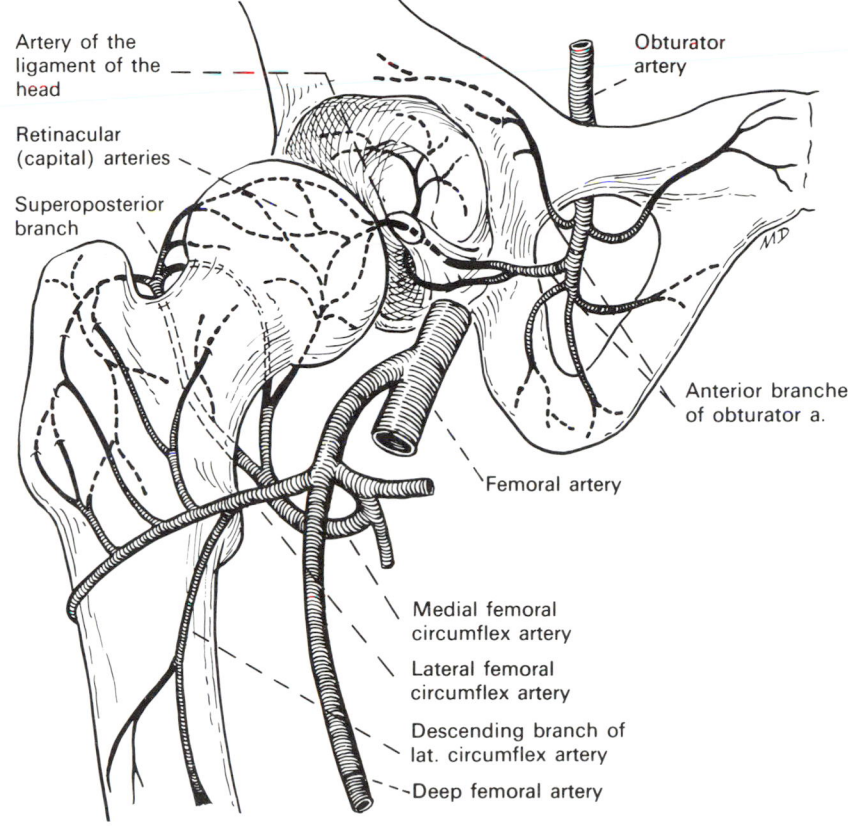

Artery of the ligament of the head

Retinacular (capital) arteries

Superoposterior branch

Obturator artery

Anterior branches of obturator a.

Femoral artery

Medial femoral circumflex artery

Lateral femoral circumflex artery

Descending branch of lat. circumflex artery

Deep femoral artery

Stability and Movement at the Hip Joint

The entire weight of the trunk is supported by the rounded femoral heads. In slight flexion of the hip joints, when the line through the center of gravity lies in front of them, the pelvis is prevented from rolling downward onto the femoral heads by the action of the posterior hamstrings (3). The more powerful gluteus maximus muscles apparently do not function at all as postural muscles (12). A stable position of the hip joint is reached only when the thighs extend it and when the line of gravity of the body is passing behind the hip joint and anterior to the knee and ankle joints. When the hip joint is stable the posterior muscles can relax and the strain is placed primarily on structures at the front of the joint, especially the iliofemoral ligament and the covering iliopsoas muscle. During standing the iliacus part of the iliopsoas does function as a postural muscle, which shows continuous slight to moderate electrical activity, but the psoas major does not (7). Stability of the hip joint in extension is increased by tightening of the ligaments, which occurs as the limb is extended (3) (see Fig. 70-14).

The hip, like all ball-and-socket joints, allows all movements, including flexion and extension, abduction and adduction, circumduction, and external and internal rotation. Because of the structure of the hip joint and its covering muscles, however, some of these movements are more limited than others. Flexion and extension occur in the sagittal plane and are produced by the spin of the femoral head within the acetabulum, with the mechanical axis of the movements being the femoral neck (7). The femoral shaft to which the muscles attach serves as a lever for these movements. Flexion and extension provide the largest range of motion in the hip, with a range of flexion from 0 to about 120° and to as much as 140° (12) and a range of extension from 0 to 15° (7, 12). In the frontal plane abduction ranges from 0 to 30 or 40° and adduction ranges from 0 to 25 or 30° (7, 13). In the transverse plane external rotation ranges from 0 to 90° and internal rotation ranges from 0 to 70° when the hip joint is flexed (12). Less rotation occurs when the hip joint is extended because of the restricting action of the soft tissue (see Fig. 74-9). All of these movements come into play during the normal gait cycle, and any limitation caused by deformity, contracture, or paralysis results in an abnormal gait pattern that is characterized by compensatory adaptations (6). It is therefore particularly important to test motion ranges at the hip.

Range of motion of the hip joint can be evaluated with the patient supine and walking. The passive range of hip flexion with the patient in the supine

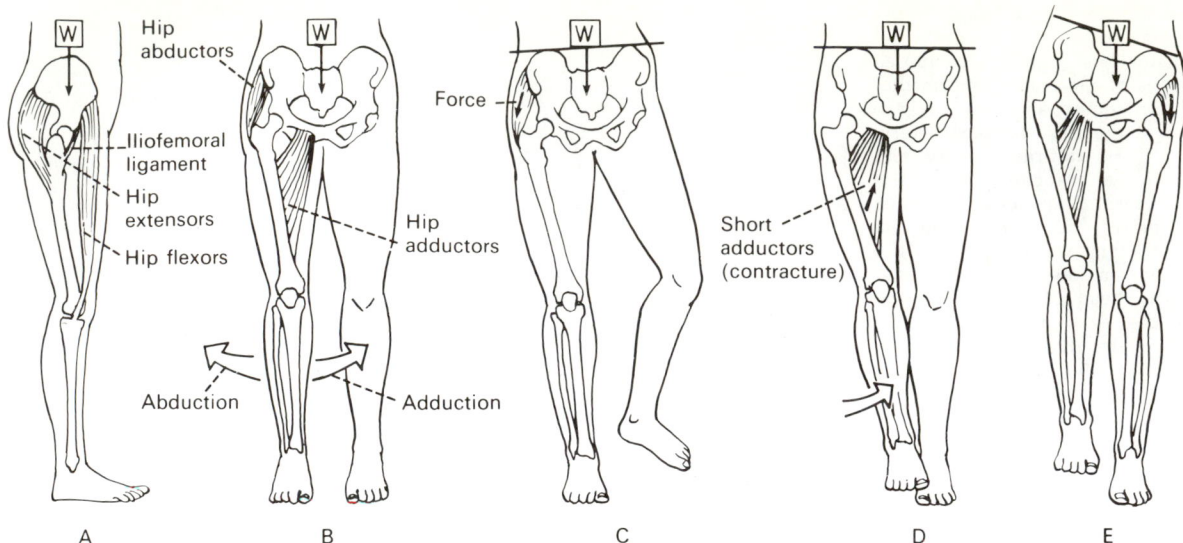

Fig. 74-9. Simplified schematic of the pelvis and lower limbs and their relation to the major muscle groups at the hip. *A.* Lateral view showing the flexors and extensors. *B.* Anterior view showing the abductors and adductors. *C.* Abductors of the hip on one side balance the pelvis when the opposite leg is lifted. (The force exerted by these muscles; this operates at the hip in addition to the weight of the body, W.) *D.* Contracture of hip adductors prevents the leg from achieving the neutral (vertical) position in the abduction-adduction plane. *E.* Because walking requires the walking limb to be vertical, an adductor contracture causes the pelvis to be elevated, thus producing a fixed tilt that results in an apparent shortening of the leg. Modified from Rosse, C.: The hip region and the lumbosacral plexus. *In* The Musculoskeletal System in Health and Disease. Edited by C. Rosse and D.K. Clawson. Hagerstown, MD, Harper & Row, 1980.

position is achieved by applying force to the flexed knee, and is greater than that of active flexion. Its limitation can be a result of bony deformity or of contractures of the hip extensors (7) (Fig. 74-9A). Indeed, hip flexion is limited when the knee is extended, which puts the hamstrings under tension.

Extension is limited by the lengths of the iliofemoral ligament and of the hip flexors. Pathologic shortening of these muscles or of the ligament (hip flexion contracture) reduces the range of extension, causing forward lifting of the pelvis and displacing the gravitational force line forward (7). This is usually compensated for by an increased lumbar lordosis, which produces abnormal gait.

The range of movement in abduction and adduction is limited by the ultimate length of the muscles, because ligamentous restraints of the joint in these planes is minimal (7) (Fig. 74-9B). Abductors of the hip on one side balance the pelvis when the opposite leg is lifted off the ground (Fig. 74-9C). If the adductor muscle group is pathologically shortened, as in adductor contracture, the range of abduction is limited and a deformity results (Fig. 74-9D and E).

Medial and lateral rotations of the femoral shaft result from anteroposterior swings and slides of the femoral head in the acetabulum, which can occur in any position of flexion and extension. The range of rotation, which should be tested in the flexed and extended positions of the hip, increases as flexion is increased because of relaxation of the ligaments (7).

Muscles

The muscles responsible for the various motions of the hip joint and thighs are listed in Table 74-2 and illustrated in Figures 74-10 to 74-12. The most impor-

tant functional muscle groups around the hip are the flexors, which accelerate the thigh as it is swung into motion during the gait cycle, and the abductors, which stabilize the pelvis when the body is supported on only one leg (Fig. 74-9C) (7). Other prime movers include extensors, abductors, and external (lateral) and internal (medial) rotators. Frequently a number of these muscles are called into action as antagonists to the force of gravity to control and prevent movements that are the opposite of those of their own prime mover action. Table 74-2 lists the nerve supply to these various muscle groups.

FLEXORS. As noted in Table 74-2, the most important flexors are the iliacus and psoas major, which form a common tendon (the iliopsoas) that crosses the hip anteriorly and inserts on the lesser trochanter (7). The two muscles produce hip flexion when the trunk or legs are stabilized. A low level of electrical activity is present in these muscles during relaxed standing because they assist the iliofemoral ligament in counterbalancing the force of gravity (Fig. 74-10A).

The rectus femoris is primarily an extensor of the knee. Because it is the only head of the quadriceps that crosses the hip it is an effective hip flexor, especially when the knee is also flexed. The sartorius, adductor brevis, adductor longus, and tensor fascia latae contribute to hip flexion.

EXTENSORS. The most powerful extensor of the hip is the gluteus maximus (Fig. 74-10B), but this is only called into action during rapid and powerful extension or when resistance has to be overcome (7). In a normal gait cycle hip extension is achieved primarily by the hamstring muscles, which include the semitendinosus, semimembranosus, and both the long and short heads of the biceps femoris. Paralysis of the gluteus maximus, the largest muscle in the body, does not seriously compromise ambulation on ground level, but its function is required for hip extension in climbing and going

Fig. 74-10. Muscles of the hip. **A.** Anterior view showing the flexors and adductors of the hip and extensors of the knee. The iliacus, together with the psoas major, forms a chief flexor. The iliacus originates from the pelvic surface of the ilium and then joins the psoas major, which originates from the last thoracic and all lumbar vertebrae. The common tendon inserts on the lesser trochanter. The rectus femoris, although primarily an extensor of the knee, is an effective hip flexor. The pectineus arises from the pectineal line of the pubis and inserts along the line leading from the lesser trochanter to the linea aspera. The sartorius arises from the anterior superior iliac spine and inserts on the proximal part of the medial surface of the tibia. The abductors also contribute to hip flexion. **B.** Posterior view showing extensors of the hip. The gluteus maximus originates over a wide area of the back of the bony pelvis and inserts into the gluteal tuberosity of the femur. The hamstring muscles, the semimembranosus, the semitendinosus, and the biceps femoris originate in the ischial tuberosity and insert below the knee. Consequently they also act as flexors of the knee joint. From Hollinshead, W.H.: Anatomy for Surgeons. Vol. 3, The Back and Limbs. Philadelphia, Harper & Row, 1982.

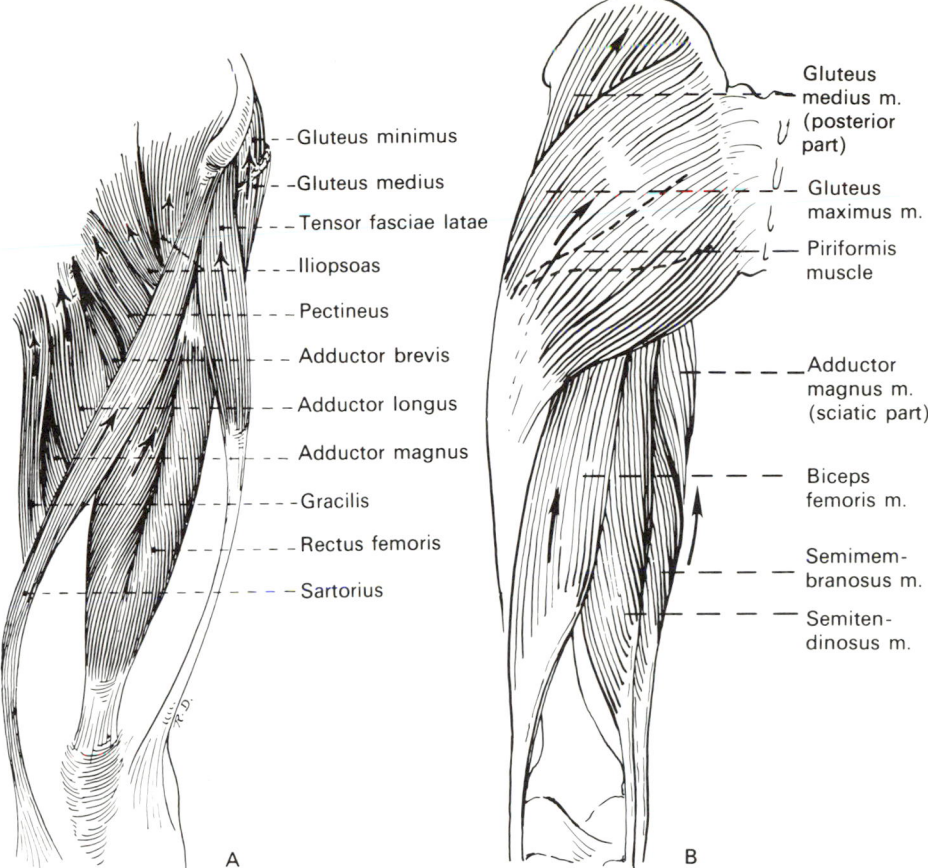

TABLE 74-2. Nerve Supply of Muscles Responsible for Movement of the Hip Joint and Thigh

Region/ Muscle Group/ Function	Peripheral Nerve Supply	Segmental Nerve Supply	Region/ Muscle Group/ Function	Peripheral Nerve Supply	Segmental Nerve Supply
Extension			**Adduction**		
Gluteus maximus	Inferior gluteal	L5, *S1*, S2	Adductor longus	Obturator	L2, 3, *4*
Semitendinosus	Sciatic (tibial)	*L5*, S1	Adductor brevis	Obturator	L2, 3, *4*
Semimembranosus	Sciatic (tibial)	*L5*, S1	Adductor magnus	Obturator/tibial	L3, 4, 5
Biceps femoris (long head)	Sciatic (tibial)	L5, *S1*	Gluteus maximus (lower fibers)	Inferior gluteal	L5, *S1*, 2
Biceps femoris (short head)	Sciatic (peroneal)	L5, *S1*	Pectineus	Femoral	L2, *3*, 4
Flexion			**Medial rotation (of free leg)**		
Iliopsoas	Branches fr. lumbar plexus and femoral	L2, *3*, 4	Tensor fascia latae	Superior gluteal	L4, *5*, S1
Rectus femoris	Femoral	L2, *3*, 4	Gluteus minimus	Superior gluteal	L4, *5*, S1
Adductor brevis	Obturator	L2, 3, *4*	Gluteus medius (ant. fibers)	Superior gluteal	L4, *5*, S1
Sartorius	Femoral	L2, 3, *4*	Semitendinosus	Sciatic (tibial)	*L5*, S1
Adductor longus	Obturator	L2, 3, *4*	Semimembranosus	Sciatic (tibial)	*L5*, S1
Tensor fascia latae	Superior gluteal	L4, *5*, S1	**Lateral rotation**	Inferior gluteal	L5, *S1*, 2
Abduction			Gluteus maximus	Inferior gluteal	L4–S3 *L5*, S*1*
Gluteus medius	Superior gluteal	L4, *5*, S1	Piriformis	To piriformis	L4–S2, *S1*, 2
Gluteus minimus	Superior gluteal	L4, *5*, S1	Obturator externus	Obturator	L2–L5 *L3*, 4
Tensor fascia latae	Superior gluteal	L4, *5*, S1	Obturator internus ⎫ Superior gemellus ⎬	Nerve to obturator internus and superior gemellus	L4–S3 *L5*, S1, 2
Gluteus maximus	Superior gluteal	L5, *S1*	Inferior gemellus ⎫ Quadratus femoris ⎬	Nerve to inferior gemellus and quadratus femoris	L4–S1 *L5*, S1

*Italics indicate main roots.

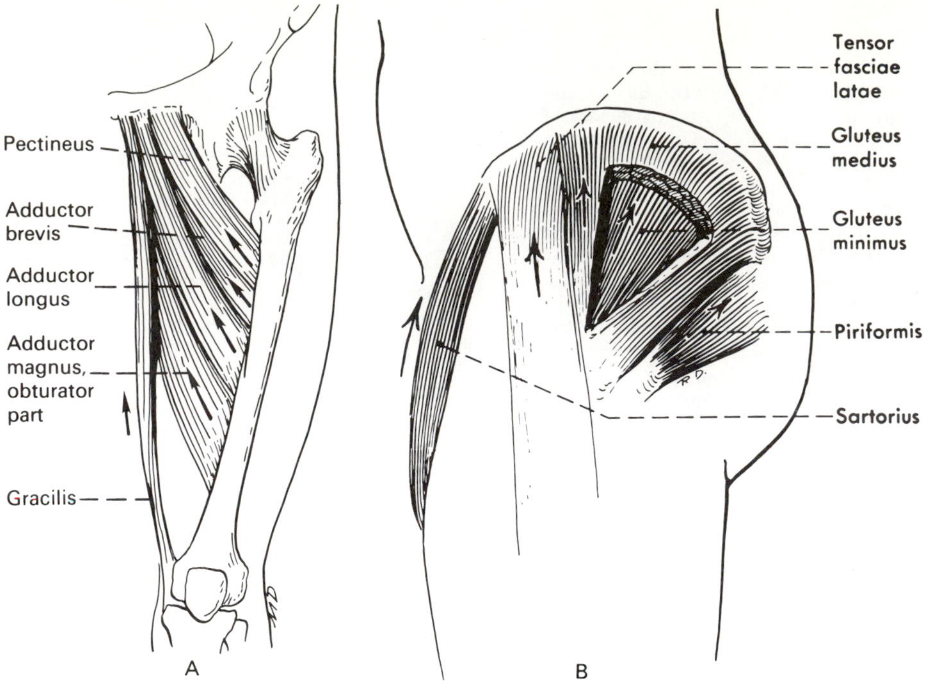

Fig. 74-11. Muscles of the hip joint. **A.** Adductors arise from the body of the pubis as a conjoint tendon and insert into the linea aspera of the femur. **B.** Abductors include the gluteus medius and gluteus minimus. These are two fan-shaped muscles that arise from the lateral surface of the ilium and insert by separate tendons into the greater trochanter. Between these tendons is the trochanteric bursa. **A** modified from and **B** from Hollinshead, W.H.: Anatomy for Surgeons. Vol. 3, The Back and Limbs. Philadelphia, Harper & Row, 1982.

up stairs and also in getting up from a squatting position. Both the hamstrings and glutei contract when the trunk is swayed anteriorly, and they continue to be active as long as the gravitational force from the body center mass falls anterior to the hip. As soon as the trunk is restored to a vertical position above the hip the hamstrings and glutei cease contracting. Acting through the iliotibial tract the gluteus maximus, together with the tensor fasciae latae, controls anteroposterior tilting of the pelvis when the body weight is supported on one leg. These two muscles are recruited if the leg is slightly flexed at the hip and knee, foregoing the stabilizing effect of the ligaments at these joints.

ABDUCTORS. The main abductors of the hip are the gluteus medius and gluteus mimimus muscles (Fig. 74-11A). These muscles are relaxed when the body weight is supported on both legs but otherwise they are in constant use, despite the fact that abduction of the femur as such seems an unusual movement during regular daily activities (7). During walking the alternating contractions of the abductors on the right and left sides can be confirmed by placing the hands over the muscles just below the iliac crest. The contraction occurs on the side of the stance leg and it acts to prevent the pelvis from sagging on the opposite side. When standing on one leg voluntary relaxation of the abductors results in tilting of the pelvis downward on the unsupported side, mimicking abductor weakness or paralysis, while a voluntary increase in contraction tips the pelvis upward, mimicking contracture. During clinical evaluation, efficacy of the abductors can be tested by observing the level of the two anterior and posterior superior iliac spines while the patient is standing on one leg. If the abductors are weak the anterior and posterior superior iliac spines sag on the opposite side (positive Trendelenburg test). The power of the abductors of one side can be assessed more accurately when the patient lies on the contralateral side and abducts the thigh against gravity and against the resistance of the examiner's hand.

ADDUCTORS. The adductors of the thigh are listed in Table 74-2. These include the adductors longus, brevis, and magnus and the lower fibers of the gluteus maximus and pectineus (Fig. 74-11B). The use of these muscles as prime movers is limited and they appear to be activated by postural reflexes during ambulation (7). They stabilize the pelvis on the femora during the phase of the gait cycle when both feet are on the ground (double support) and also stabilize the femur when the knee is forcefully flexed or extended. During these efforts the contraction of these muscles is palpable. The power of the adductors can be assessed clinically by trying to force the extended leg up while the patient attempts to keep the thighs together (Fig. 74-23).

ROTATORS. Many muscles have a rotatory action on the femoral shaft, but only a few function primarily as rotators (7). The external (lateral) rotators are situated in the gluteal region deep to the gluteus maximus; these include the gluteus maximus, piriformis, obturator internus, superior and inferior gemelli, quadratus femoris, and obturator externus (Fig. 74-12A). Internal (medial) rotators include the anterior fibers of the gluteus medius, gluteus minimus, tensor fascia latae and, to a lesser extent, the semitendinosus, semimembranosus, and adductors (Fig. 74-12B).

Biomechanics

Gait Cycle

The function of the hip joint (and of the knee and ankle joints) has been studied during the gait cycle. The following information is derived from Stolov (14). The gait cycle consists of the stance phase (the limb is in contact with the ground) and the swing phase (the limb is in the air). The duration of the gait cycle for any one limb extends from the time the heel contacts the ground (heel strike, HS) until the same heel contacts the ground again. The stance phase begins with the HS and ends with the toe leaving the ground (toe-off, TO), and the swing phase begins with TO and ends with HS. The stance phase occupies 60% and the swing phase 40% of a single gait cycle. Figure 74-13 shows a full gait cycle for the left and right legs along the same axis. A period of double support (DS) exists

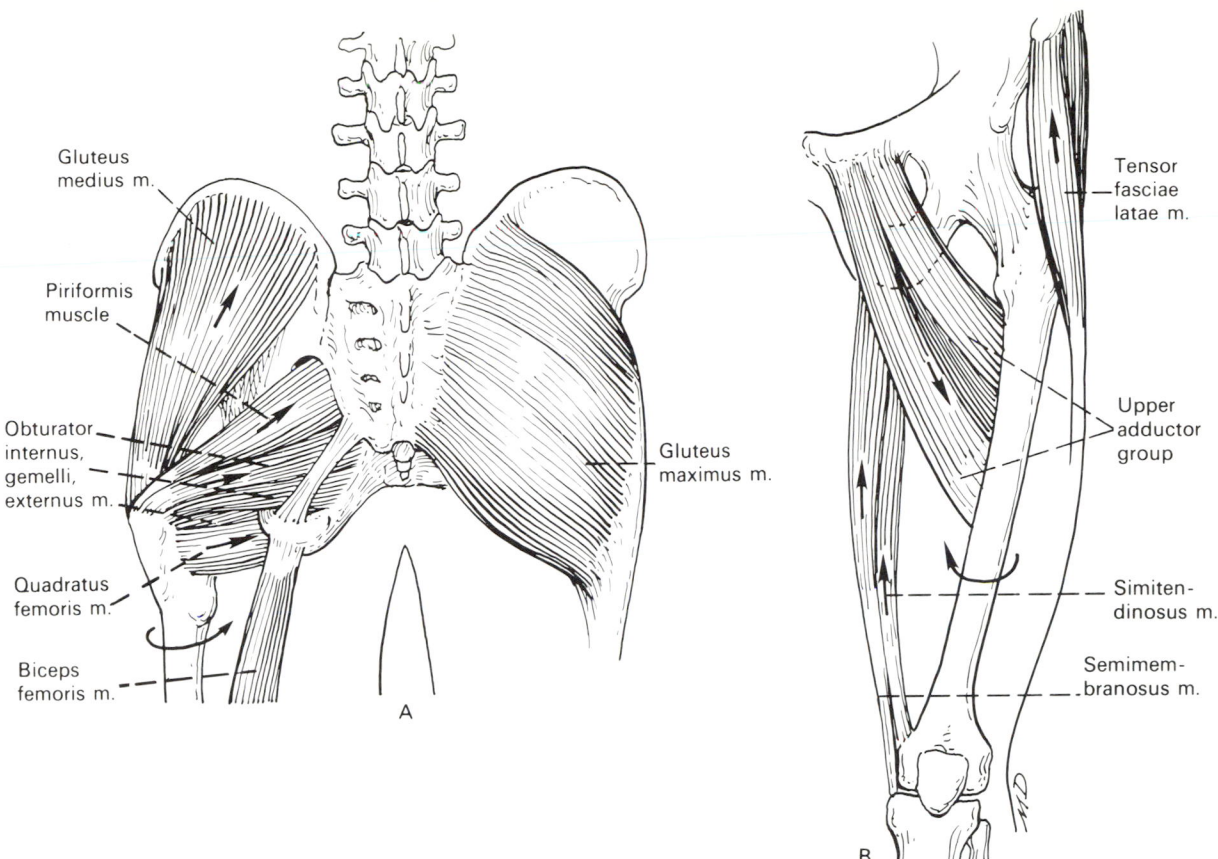

Fig. 74-12. Muscles of the hip joint. **A.** External rotators. The piriformis, obturator internus and externus, superior and inferior gemelli and quadratus femoris arise from the anterior aspect of the pelvis and insert on the medial surface of the greater trochanter proximal to the trochanteric fossa. **B.** Internal rotators. From Hollinshead, W.H.: Anatomy for Surgeons. Vol. 3, The Back and Limbs. Philadelphia, Harper & Row, 1982.

when both limbs are in the stance phase. This period accounts for about 15% of the cycle in normal comfortable walking and extends from the onset of HS of one limb to TO of the other. As the speed of walking increases the ratio of the duration of the DS period to the duration of the entire gait cycle decreases.

The first portion of the stance phase extends from HS to foot-flat (FF). Midstance (MST) lasts from FF to heel-off (HO), with the entire foot being in contact with the ground. The last period of stance phase is from HO to TO. The swing phase consists of an initial period of acceleration, beginning with TO, while the second half of the swing is a period of deceleration, ending with HS. Midswing (MSW) is the transition between acceleration and deceleration.

Range of Motion

The range of motion of the hip joint has been studied electrogoniometrically. In the sagittal plane the hip joint is maximally flexed during gait in the late swing phase as the limb moves forward for HS (12, 15). As the body moves forward at the beginning of the standing phase the hip joint extends, with maximum extension being reached at heel off. During the swing phase the joint reverses into flexion and reaches maximal flexion of 35 to 40° prior to HS (Fig. 74-14A).

In the frontal plane abduction of the hip joint occurs

during the swing phase and is at a maximum just after TO (15, 16). At HS the hip joint reverses into adduction, which continues until the late stance phase. In the transverse plane the hip joint is externally rotated throughout the swing phase; it rotates internally just before HS and remains internally rotated until the late stance phase, when external rotation again occurs (12, 16). The average ranges of motion recorded for 33 normal men in a study by Johnston and Smidt (16) were 12° for the frontal plane and 13° for the transverse plane.

With aging the gait pattern changes and less of the range of motion is used in the hip joint and in other joints of the lower limbs. Older men have shorter leg lengths, a decreased range of hip flexion and extension, decreased plantar flexion of the ankle, and decreased heel-floor angle of the tracking limb.

Surface Joint Motion

Surface motion in the hip joint can be considered to be a sliding of the femoral head on the acetabulum (12). The pivoting of the ball and socket in three planes around the center of the rotation of the femoral head produces the sliding of the joint surfaces. If incongruity is present in the femoral head, sliding might not occur parallel or tangential to the surface and the joint cartilage might be abnormally compressed or distracted.

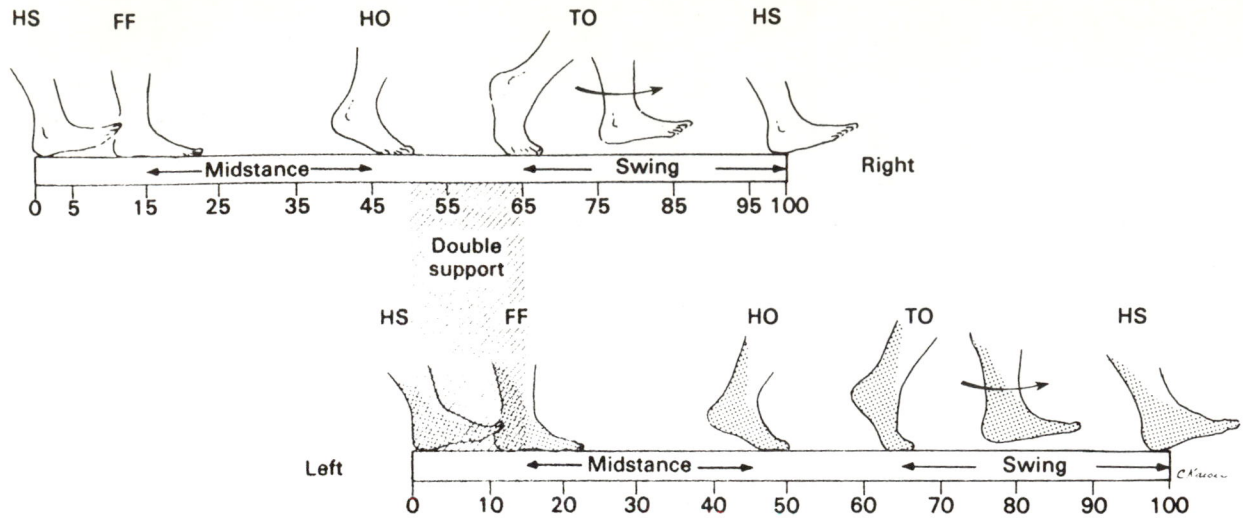

Fig. 74-13. Phases of the gait cycle shown on the same time axis for the left and right legs. HS, heel strike; FF, foot flat; HO, heel off; TO, toe off (leaving the ground). From Stolov, W.C.: Normal and pathologic ambulation. *In* The Musculoskeletal System in Health and Disease. Edited by C. Rosse and D.K. Clawson, Hagerstown, MD, Harper & Row, 1980.

Kinetics

Knowledge of the load acting on the hip joint is important in the management of patients with hip disorders because large forces act on the joint during simple activities. Nordin and Frankel (12) have summarized the kinetics of the hip joint as follows:

a. A joint reaction of approximately three times the body weight acts on the hip joint during a single-leg stance with the pelvis in a neutral position; its magnitude varies with a change in position of the upper body.

b. The magnitude of the hip joint reaction force is influenced by the ratio of the abductor muscle force to the gravitational force lever arms. A small ratio indicates a higher joint reaction force than a large ratio.

c. The hip joint reaction force during gait reaches levels of six times body weight or more in the stance phase, and is approximately equal to body weight during the swing phase.

d. An increase in gait velocity increases the magnitude of the hip joint reaction force in both the swing and stance phases.

e. The forces acting on an internal fixation device during the activities of daily living vary greatly, depending on the nursing and therapeutic activities undergone by the patient.

f. The use of a leg brace can alter the magnitude of the hip joint reaction force.

B. EVALUATION OF THE PATIENT

According to Rosse (6) the hip is the joint most frequently affected by disease throughout life, and most of its abnormalities characteristically afflict those in distinct age groups. Failure to establish an early diagnosis, particularly in the young, causes prolonged suffering and serious disability. The conditions that affect those in these age groups are discussed in the next section. Because Chapter 70 contains an extensive outline and discussion of the evaluation of the patient with pain in the lower limbs, only points relevant to the hips are discussed here.

History

A thorough history of the pain should be elicited, including the distribution, intensity, quality, and temporal characteristics at the time of onset, during the interval between onset and the time the patient is first seen, and at the time of evaluation (Chapter 31). The patient should be asked about the circumstances that brought the pain on and about what factors relieve and aggravate the pain. The physician must also elicit a past medical history and family history. Because pain felt in the region of the hip can be caused by disorders of the lumbosacral spine or inguinal region, or by vascular diseases in the thigh, it is essential to determine the history and carry out a physical examination of these regions. Moreover, because a number of the important disorders of the hip occur in childhood, often at a particular period, it is important to determine the age of the patient at the onset of symptoms. Adams (5) has suggested the use of Table 74-3 to help in this determination.

Painful limb is generally the initial clinical presentation in most acute disorders of the hip (7). Refusal by a child to use a limb can be the first sign that the disease is causing severe pain. Pain caused by pathology in the hip joint is usually referred to the medial side of the thigh and more frequently to the knee, with radiation to the inguinal region. These areas of referral are explained by the overlapping innervation of the knee and hip joint and by the innervation of the inguinal region by the upper lumbar segments, which contribute to the innervation of the hip. Intensity of the pain depends on the degree of pathology and on the presence or absence of inflammation, and can be mild, moderate, or severe. Invariably the pain is aggravated by weight bearing. It is usually deep and aching, typical of referred pain from deep somatic structures.

The patient can complain of the painful hip when no pathology is present in the joint; this might be a result of pathology in the groin, such as femoral inguinal hernia, inflamed inguinal lymph nodes, or a psoas abscess (7). Pain can be referred to the hip region from the lumbar spine, sacroiliac joints, or pelvis. The referred pain is usually felt in

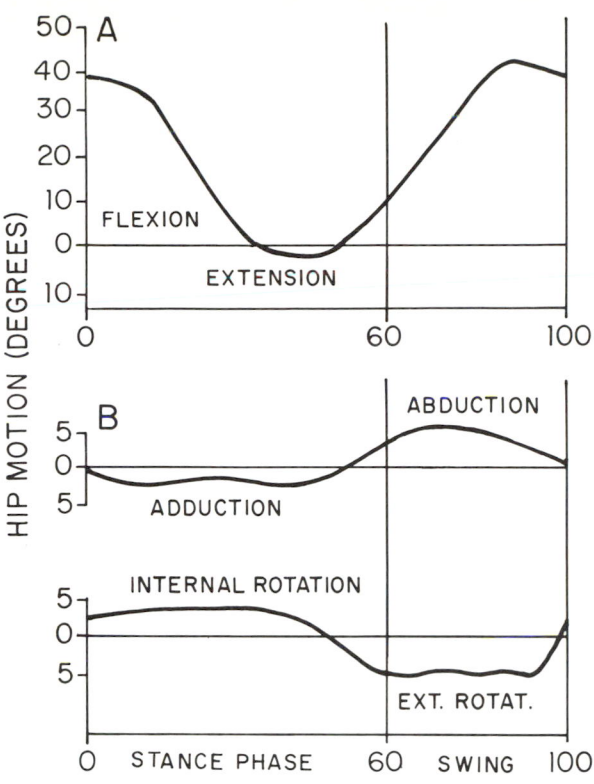

Fig. 74-14. Range of hip motion in various planes in one gait cycle, obtained from a study of 30 normal men during level walking. **A.** Typical pattern in sagittal plane. **B.** Typical pattern in frontal plane (*top*) and transverse plane (*bottom*). **A** modified from Murray, M.P.: Gait as a total pattern of movement. Am. J. Phys. Med., *46*:290, 1967; **B** modified from Johnston, R.C., and Smidt, G.L.: Measurement of the hip joint motion during walking: An evaluation of an electrogoniometric method. J. Bone Joint Surg. [Am.], *51*:1083, 1969.

the gluteal region and radiates down the back or outer side of the thigh. This type of pain is aggravated by activities such as stooping and lifting and is often eased by walking. In contrast, pain caused by ischemia of the gluteal muscles consequent to vascular disease (internal iliac artery) produces severe pain in the buttocks during walking and obviously is a form of intermittent claudication, frequently referred to as Leriche's syndrome (Chapter 28).

Physical Examination

For proper examination of the hip patients should remove their clothes, except for a pelvic split or underpants and, in

TABLE 74-3. Usual Age Incidence of Common Hip Disorders at Time of Diagnosis

Age at Time of Diagnosis (years)	Disease
0 to 2	Congenital dislocation
2 to 5	Tuberculous arthritis; transient synovitis
5 to 10	Perthes' disease; transient synovitis
10 to 20	Slipped upper femoral epiphysis
20 to 50	Osteoarthritis (secondary to previous injury or disease)
50 to 100	Osteoarthritis (primary)

From Adams, J.C.: The hip region. *In* Outline of Orthopaedics. 10th Ed. By J.C. Adams. New York, Churchill Livingstone, 1986.

TABLE 74-4. Evaluation for Painful Hip Disorders

I. HISTORY

A. Present history
1. Characteristics of the pain: distribution; intensity; quality; temporal characteristics
2. Factors that aggravate, relieve, and have no effect on the pain

B. Past medical and family history

II. PHYSICAL EXAMINATION

A. Patient standing
1. Inspection: lumbar curve; pelvis; thighs; legs; feet
2. Palpation (bilateral): swelling; tenderness; skin temperature; position of iliac crests; anterior and posterior superior iliac spines; pubic crests; greater trochanter; ischial tuberosity; muscles of buttocks and thighs

B. Patient recumbent
1. Inspection: level of the pelvis; contour of soft tissue and bones; color and texture of skin; presence of scars or sinuses (bilateral)
2. Palpation: hip joint and upper thighs; skin temperature; soft tissue and bone contours; local tenderness
3. Inguinal region: presence of glands; femoral pulses; iliopsoas muscle; hip joint; sciatic nerve
4. Measurement of limb length
   a. Real or true length: measure from anterior superior iliac spine to medial malleolus (angle between pelvis and limbs should be equal on each side)
   b. If discrepancy is found, determine site of shortening:
      (1) Above trochanter (Bryant's triangle; Nelaton's line; Shoemaker's line)
      (2) Below trochanter (measure each bone)
   c. "Apparent" or false discrepancy: measure from xiphisterum to medial malleolus (limbs should be parallel and in line with trunk)

women, a brassiere. Examination of the hip should begin with observation of the gait. Table 74-4 lists the sequence for the clinical examination in patients suspected of disorders of the hip. Inspection and palpation are first done with patients standing and then recumbent on the examining table.

Patient Standing

INSPECTION. In addition to observation of the hip during walking, the following should be observed from the front, back, and side (7). First, posture of the spine is observed, noting especially any degree of scoliosis, lordosis, or kyphosis, as well as deviation of the entire trunk to one or the other side. These abnormal spinal postures can be secondary to fixed pelvic deformity or to hip pain.

Next, the physician should observe the orientation of the pelvis, judging lateral tilt by comparing the alignment of the two anterior or two posterior iliac spines (Fig. 74-15A). Anteroposterior tilt is assessed by the vertical alignment of the anterior superior iliac spines and the pubic tubercles as well as by flattening or exaggeration of the normal lumbar curve.

Following evaluation of the pelvis the posture of the leg should be observed, noting the position adopted in relaxed standing by the hip, knee, and foot. It is important to note if any joints are flexed or hyperextended, the entire soles of both feet are in contact with the ground, and the legs are wide apart. In normal individuals both feet and both patella face symmetrically anteriorly.

Next, any asymmetry in the soft tissues of the thighs and buttocks should be assessed, particularly in regard to signs

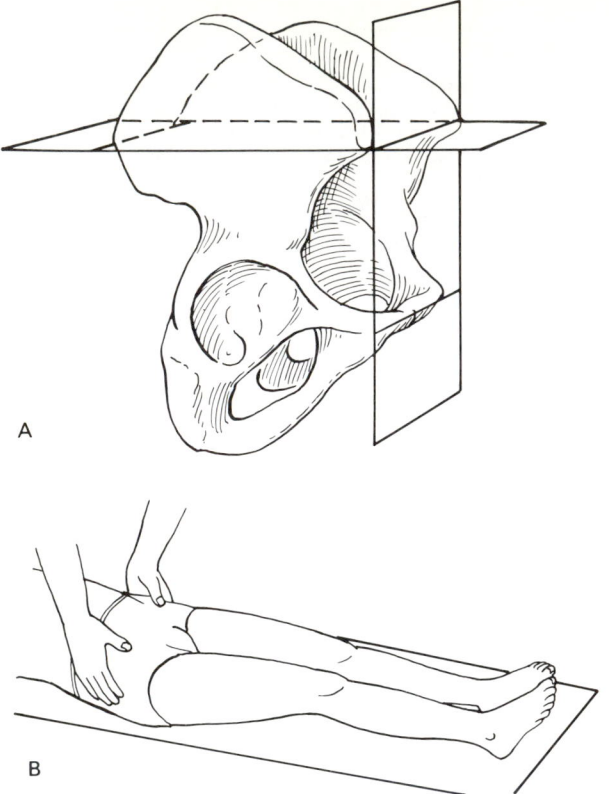

Fig. 74-15. *A.* Schematic depiction of orientation of the pelvis with the patient standing. The four superior iliac spines lie in the same horizontal plane while the anterior superior iliac spines and the pubic tubercles are in the same vertical plane. *B.* Determination of the lie of the pelvis with the patient supine. The anterior superior iliac spine is palpated to determine whether the pelvis is lying square with the limbs; if it is not, an attempt is made to set it square. If this is not possible, the adduction or abduction at one hip or the other is incorrectable. *A* modified from Rosse, C.: The hip region and the lumbosacral plexus. *In* The Musculoskeletal System in Health and Disease. Edited by C. Rosse and D.K. Clawson. Hagerstown, MD, Harper & Row, 1980: *B* modified from Adams, J.C.: Outline of Orthopaedics. 10th Ed. Edinburgh, Churchill Livingstone, 1986.

of atrophy or asymmetry in the two gluteal folds and to skin creases that delineate the buttocks from the thigh posteriorly. Any swelling, redness, scars, or sinuses in the hip region should be noted.

PALPATION. Palpation should proceed bilaterally by comparing the two sides and by noting any swelling, tenderness, or increase in skin temperature. All bony points available for palpation should be felt, including the two iliac crests with their anterior and posterior spines, the pubic crests and tubercles, the greater trochanters, and the ischial tuberosities. Moreover, the muscles of the buttocks and thighs should be compared by palpation on the two sides.

Patient Recumbent

PALPATION. With the patient recumbent the inguinal region and femoral triangle should be palpated and the pulse of the femoral arteries (each is halfway between the symphysis pubis and anterior superior iliac spine) should be assessed. Deep to the artery are the iliopsoas and the hip joint, and a swelling in this region inferior to the inguinal ligament is likely to be a psoas abscess or perhaps a neoplasm (7). With the patient's hip flexed the sciatic nerve should be

palpated through the gluteus maximus (the nerve lies halfway between the ischial tuberosity and greater trochanter). Palpation of the trochanter can elicit tenderness, which might be caused by trochanteric bursitis.

MEASUREMENT OF LIMB LENGTH. The supine position is best for measuring any discrepancy between the lengths of the two limbs. Limb length can be measured clinically with an error of 1 cm but, if greater accuracy is needed, radiographic measurement is recommended (5). The true length of each limb must be measured to determine any "apparent" or false discrepancy in the length of the limbs from fixed pelvic tilt.

True limb length is measured in centimeters, with a tape extending from the anterior superior iliac spine to the medial malleolus (Fig. 74-16). To prevent errors, the following should be considered: (a) accurate fixing of the tape measure on the points shown in Figure 74-15; (b) ensuring that the angle between the limb and pelvis is the same. If the pelvis is tilted, with consequent adduction of one limb, the length is greater, whereas abduction decreases the length (Fig. 74-17). To obtain an accurate comparison of the true lengths by surface measurement, the two limbs must be placed in comparable positions relative to the pelvis (Fig. 74-17C).

Shortening of limb length can be a result of a short tibia or femur, dislocation of the hip, or coxa vara. The lengths of the femora can be compared by measuring between the tips of the greater trochanters and the femoral condyles, while the lengths of both tibias are compared by measuring between the tibial condyles and the medial malleoli, using them as reference points (7). Tests for shortening above the trochanteric level include the construction of Nelaton's and Shoemaker's lines (Fig. 74-18). Dislocation of the hip and coxa vara displaces the greater trochanter above Nelaton's line, indicating that the femur has been displaced cephalad. A similar conclusion can be made about cephalad displacement of the femur if Shoemaker's line passes below the umbilicus. Shortening distal to the trochanter can be detected by measuring the length of the femur and tibia.

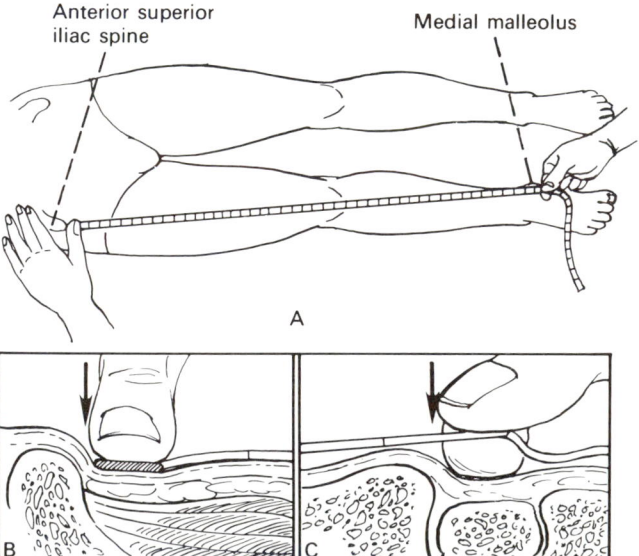

Fig. 74-16. *A.* Technique of measuring the length of the limb with the patient supine. *B.* The tape measure is fixed at the anterior superior iliac spine, with the end of the tape being placed immediately distal to the spine and pushed up against it. *C.* The tape is fixed at the level of the medial malleolus. The arrows indicate the exact point of measurement. Modified from Adams, J.C.: Outline of Orthopaedics. 10th Ed. Edinburgh, Churchill Livingstone, 1986.

Fig. 74-17. Positions of the pelvis in relation to the limbs. *A.* The pelvis is square with the limbs. This is indicated by the fact that a line above both iliac crests makes an angle of 90° with the vertical. *B.* Apparent or false discrepancy in limb length, caused entirely by tilting of the pelvis. Tilt of the pelvis results in a discrepancy in the distance between the anterior superior iliac spine and the medial malleolus. Here the left leg appears to be shorter because of the pelvic tilt. Adduction of the left limb makes the length appear to be shorter while abduction of the right limb carries the foot away from the spine and increases the length. Therefore, measurement of the true length taken from the anterior superior spine is inaccurate if the angle of abduction or adduction is not equal on both sides. *C.* Correct method of measuring the true length if a fixed adduction deformity of the left hip is present. This is done by adducting the right hip to an equal angle. The position of the tape measurement is shown by the dashed lines. Modified from Adams; J.C.: Outline of Orthopaedics. 10th Ed. Edinburgh, Churchill Livingstone, 1986. Figure 74-17 shows another method of making a correct measurement.

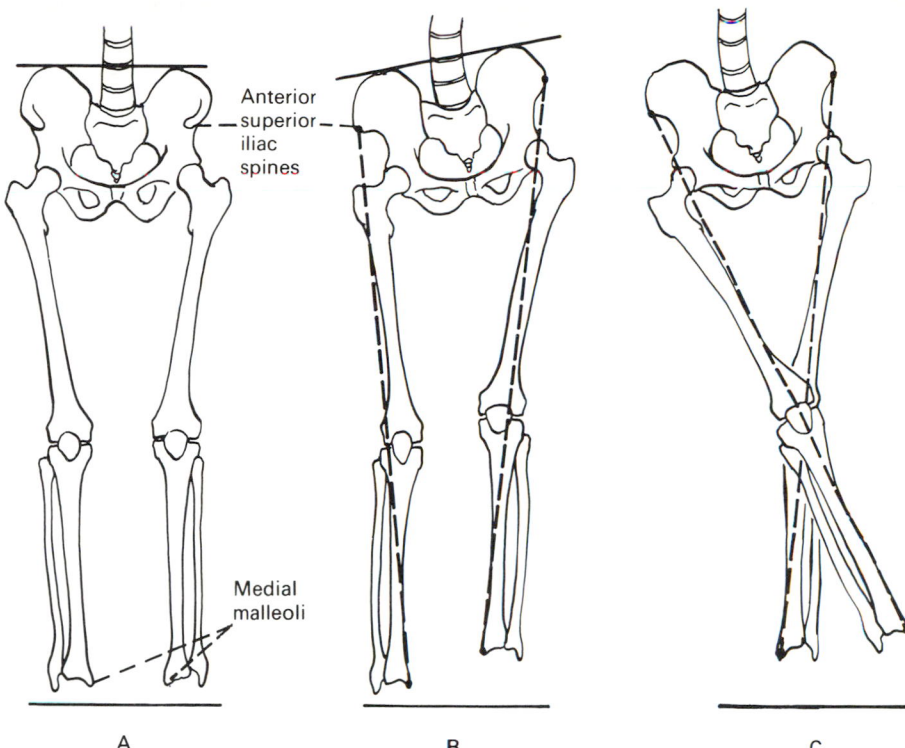

Anterior superior iliac spines

Medial malleoli

A   B   C

Apparent limb length inequality is caused entirely by fixed lateral pelvic tilting caused either by a fixed adduction deformity at one hip, which gives the appearance of shortening on that side, or by a fixed abduction deformity, which gives an appearance of lengthening (4). To measure apparent limb length discrepancy, the limbs of the supine patient are placed parallel to one another and in a line with the trunk. Measurement is made from each medial malleolus and from any fixed point in the midline of the trunk, such as the xiphisternal junction or the umbilicus (4, 6) (Fig. 74-18).

EXAMINATION FOR FIXED DEFORMITY. Contracture of the joint capsule or of muscles can cause fixed deformity at the hip, preventing it from being placed in a neutral position. Arthritis of the joint is a common cause of fixed flexion, fixed adduction, and fixed lateral rotation. A fixed adduction deformity is assessed by judging the relationship between the pelvis and limbs. The transverse axis of the pelvis (as indicated by a line joining the two anterior superior spines) cannot be set at right angles to the affected limb, but lies at an acute angle with it (5)—that is, the angle is less than 90°.

Fig. 74-18. *A.* Nelaton's line. With the patient lying supine a tape measure or string is stretched on the affected side from the ischial tuberosity to the anterior superior iliac spine of the ilium. Normally the tip of the greater trochanter is on or posterior to (below) the line. When the trochanter lies above the line as shown here, the femur has been displaced upward. *B.* Shoemaker's line. A line is projected on each side of the body from the greater trochanter through and beyond the anterior superior iliac spines. Normally the two lines meet in the midline above the umbilicus. If one femur is displaced upward because of shortening above the greater trochanter, however, the lines meet away from the midline on the opposite side. If both femurs are displaced upward the lines meet at or near the midline but below the umbilicus. Modified from Adams, J.C.: Outline of Orthopaedics. 10th Ed. Edinburgh, Churchill Livingstone, 1986.

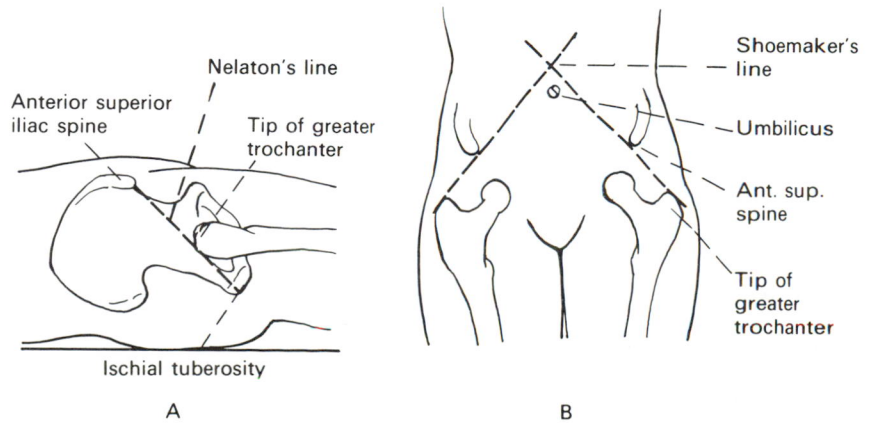

Anterior superior iliac spine   Nelaton's line   Tip of greater trochanter

Ischial tuberosity

A

Shoemaker's line   Umbilicus   Ant. sup. spine   Tip of greater trochanter

B

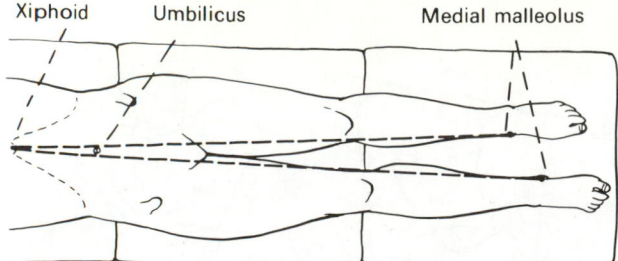

Xiphoid   Umbilicus   Medial malleolus

Fig. 74-19. Correct measurement of "apparent" discrepancy in limb length. Measurement is between the medial malleolus and the xiphoid process or the umbilicus. Modified from Adams, J.C.: Outline of Orthopaedics. 10th Ed. Edinburgh, Churchill Livingstone, 1986.

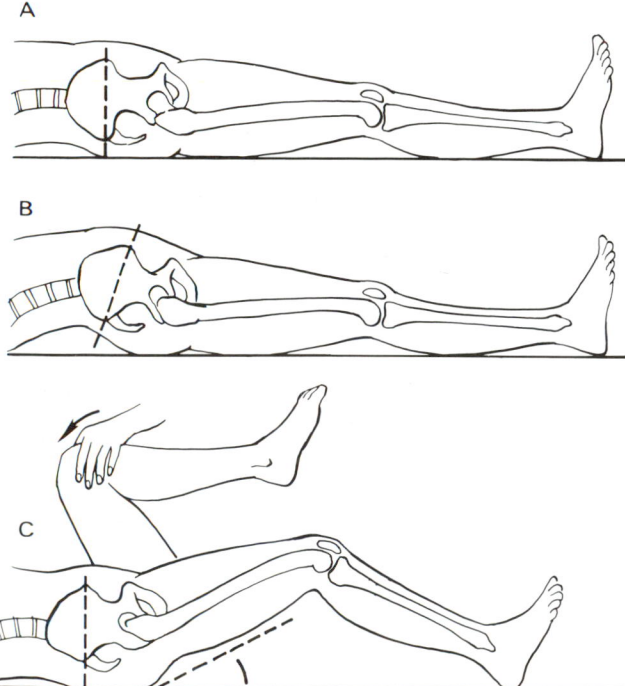

Fig. 74-20. Diagnosis of hip flexion contracture using the Thomas test. *A.* The patient lies supine on a hard surface with the hips and knees extended. If no contracture is present the pelvis remains neutral, with the anterior superior iliac spine lying vertically above the posterior superior iliac spine (dashed line). *B.* The patient has a flexion contracture, so the patient must arch the back to keep the legs on the table, thus compensating for the forward tilt of the pelvis. *C.* The Thomas test. To test the right hip, the left thigh is flexed passively until the anterior superior iliac spine lies directly over the posterior superior iliac spine. This places the pelvis in the neutral position and brings the lumbar spine down flat on the table. If a flexion contracture is present the right thigh cannot remain on the table and makes an angle with it that equals the angle of the deformity. Modified from Rosse, C.: The hip region and the lumbosacral plexus. *In* The Musculoskeletal System in Health and Disease. Edited by C. Rosse and D.K. Clawson. Hagerstown, MD, Harper & Row, 1980.

A fixed abduction deformity is present if the angle between the transverse axis of the pelvis and limb is greater than 90°.

A fixed flexion deformity is determined by the Thomas test (Fig. 74-20). A fixed lateral or medial rotation of the limbs should be considered if the limb cannot be rotated to the neutral position. Normally the patella points anteriorly

when the hip is in the neutral position. The angle by which the limb falls short of the neutral position when rotated as far as possible is the angle of the fixed rotation deformity (5).

Range of Movement and Muscle Strength

FLEXION. Passive range of hip flexion is best assessed by the examiner grasping the leg with one hand and the crest of the ilium with the other, gently flexing the thigh on the body (Fig. 74-21A). The normal range of flexion is about 120°. The strength of the chief hip flexors is tested by opposing the flexion movement with resistance applied to the distal end of the femur as the patient exerts maximum effort to flex one hip and then the other (Fig. 74-21B). This maneuver can be done with the patient supine or seated, with the legs hanging over the edge of the table.

ABDUCTION. To test passive abduction, the limb is supported by one hand while the other bridges the pelvis from one anterior superior spine to the other anterior superior spine (Fig. 74-22A). This permits the differentiation of true abduction of the hip from false abduction, which is imparted by tilting of the pelvis. The normal range of true abduction at the hip is about 30° and is even greater in children. The strength of the abductors is assessed by having the patient abduct the limb against the resistance applied by the examiner, who places the hands laterally and exerts pressure toward the midline (Fig. 74-22B). It is important to ask the patient to exert maximum effort during the maneuver.

Arthritis of the hips often restricts abduction in flexion. This is assessed by having the patient flex the hips and knees, drawing the heels toward the buttocks, and allowing the knees to fall away from one another laterally toward the top of the table. The normal range is about 70° in adults and 90° in young children.

ADDUCTION. Passive range of adduction is assessed by the examiner grasping the ankle and gently moving toward the midline and then beyond, over the lower limb (Fig. 74-23A). The strength of the adductors is assessed clinically by trying to force the extended limbs apart while the patient exerts maximum effort to keep the thighs together (Fig. 74-23B).

ROTATION. Medial and lateral rotation of the femur are assessed with the patient sitting with the hips flexed, and legs over the side of the table (Fig. 74-24). Both ranges of movement should also be tested with the patient lying prone,

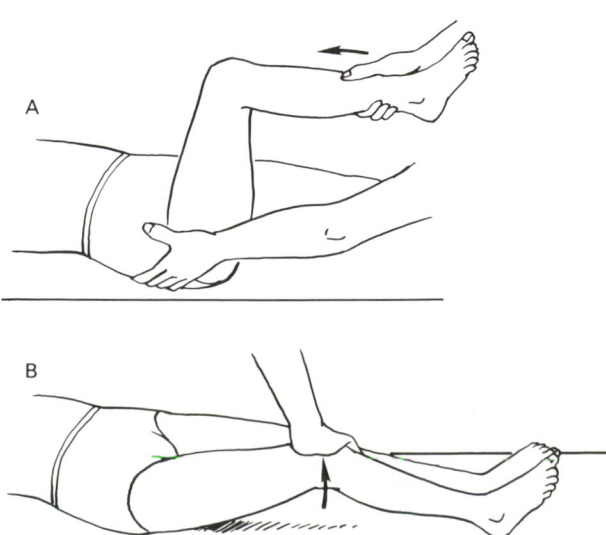

Fig. 74-21. *A.* Testing the passive range of hip flexion. *B.* Testing the strength of the chief hip flexors. See text for details.

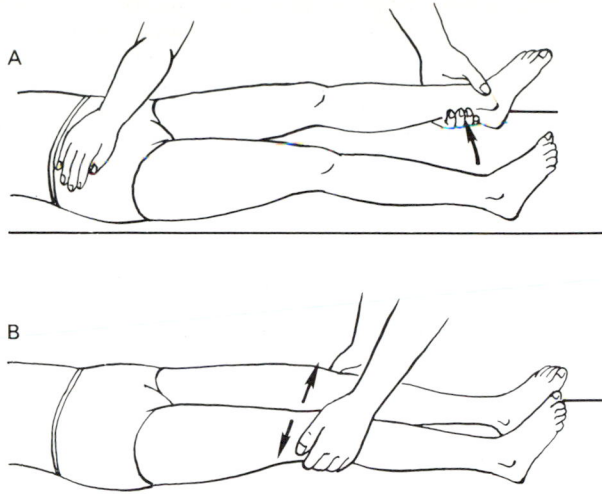

Fig. 74-22. *A.* Testing the passive range of motion of the abductors. *B.* Testing the strength of the abductors. See text for details.

the hips extended, and the knees flexed to 90°. The normal range of each movement is about 40° (4).

EXTENSION. Adams (5) has noted that, contrary to what is often written, extension of the hip joints beyond the neutral position is prevented by the strong anterior capsule and the reinforcing Y-shaped ligament, and consequently the range of extension at the hip is almost 0°. What appears to be posterior movement of the thigh is in fact contributed entirely by rotation of the pelvis and extension of the spine, and not by extension at the hip joint proper (5).

Determination of Postural Stability

To test postural stability the Trendelenburg maneuver is used (Fig. 74-25). There are three fundamental reasons for a positive Trendelenburg test result: (a) paralysis of the abductors—for example, as caused by poliomyelitis; (b) marked approximation of the insertion of the muscles to their origin by upward displacement of the greater trochanter so that the muscles are flat, as with severe coxa vara or congenital dislocation of the hip; and (c) absence of

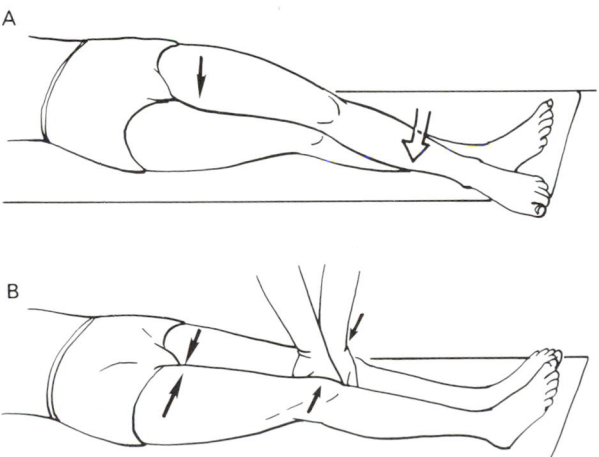

Fig. 74-23. *A.* Testing the passive range of motion of the adductors. *B.* Testing the strength of the adductors. See text for details.

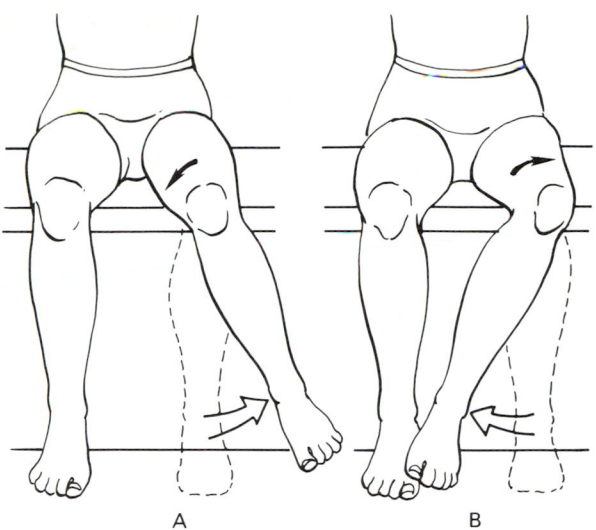

Fig. 74-24. Testing the rotators of the hip and femur. The patient is sitting so that the hip is flexed and the legs are hanging over the edge of the table. *A.* Medial rotation. *B.* Lateral rotation. Modified from Rosse, C.: The hip region and the lumbosacral plexus. *In* The Musculoskeletal System in Health and Disease. Edited by C. Rosse and D.K. Clawson. Hagerstown, MD, Harper & Row, 1980.

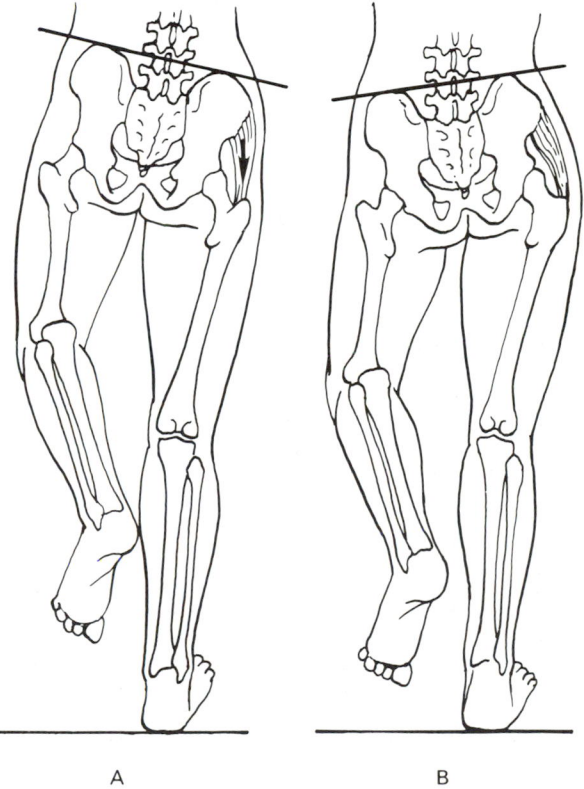

Fig. 74-25. Testing postural stability using the Trendelenburg test. *A.* If one leg is raised from the ground and the pelvis tilts upward on that side through the action of the hip abductors of the standing limb, the test result is negative. *B.* A positive test result is obtained when the abductors are inefficient and cannot sustain the pelvis against the body weight, causing it to tilt downward instead of raising it on the side of the lifted leg. Modified from Adams, J.C.: Outline of Orthopaedics. 10th Ed. Edinburgh, Churchill Livingstone, 1986.

a stable fulcrum—for example, as caused by ununited fracture of the femoral head (4). Sometimes two of these factors are operative concurrently.

Other Parts of the Physical Examination

After completion of the foregoing examination of the hip region it is also essential to evaluate the anatomy and function of the lumbar spine and sacroiliac joints, carry out a neurologic assessment, especially of the lower limbs, examine the pelvis, and do a rectal and bimanual vaginal examination. It is also important to carry out a brief examination of the abdomen and to assess the vascular system by palpating the pulses and noting the color, texture, and temperature of the skin of the lower limbs. This phase of the examination is necessary to rule out disorders outside of the hip joint that might be causing referred pain to this region.

Imaging

RADIOGRAPHIC EXAMINATION. Plain radiographs should include an anteroposterior projection, showing the whole pelvis with both hips, and lateral films of each hip separately (4, 6). The lateral films should be obtained by having the patient abduct the affected hip slightly and directing the x-ray beam horizontally beneath the opposite flexed thigh. In special cases tomography and arthrography might be indicated. If the physical examination suggests that the pain and other symptoms are referred from disorders of the back, radiographs of the spine and sacroiliac joint should be obtained.

RADIOISOTOPE BONE SCANNING. Radioisotope bone scanning is of special value in the early diagnosis of metastatic neoplastic lesions of the pelvis or upper end of the femur. This procedure is also helpful in the diagnosis of inflammatory lesions in or about the hip.

COMPUTERIZED TOMOGRAPHY. CT scanning provides clear cross-sectional images of the pelvis and thigh and is useful in special circumstances. It is used to outline bony or soft tissue tumors in or about the pelvis or hips, and can show the orientation (degree of anteversion) of the acetabulum or neck of the femur accurately (3–5). Magnetic resonance imaging (MRI) is also useful in diagnosis of a number of painful conditions of the hip.

C. CLINICAL CONSIDERATIONS

Trauma

The hip and upper part of the thigh are frequently injured as a result of high-speed vehicular accidents, falls from ladders, or athletic injuries. Fractures about the hip and femur are easily recognized in the acute, painful presentation of a patient with a history of a high-energy event. Confusion can arise, however, when both disruption of the femoral shaft and a dislocation (or fracture) of the hip occur in the same extremity. Careful examination, including appropriate radiographs of both femurs and hips, usually establishes the diagnosis.

Fractures in Older Patients

On the basis of data published by Holbrook and associates (17) obtained from the Health Interview Survey of 1970–1977 and extrapolation of the rates to the 1986 population (18), fracture of the hip including the neck and upper shaft of the femur was sustained by over 861,000 patients in 1986. The data also show that 72% of these fractures occurred in persons 65 years of age and older. Fractures in all the patients caused over 9.4 million days of restricted activity, about 3 million days of bed disability, and 1.56 million days lost from work, primarily in patients 18 to 64 years of age (18). Moreover, fractures of the hip including neck and upper shaft of the femur required 1.52 million visits to physicians, of which 54% were made by patients 65 years of age or older. Fracture of the hip including neck and upper shaft of the femur caused 1.3 million patients to be hospitalized in 1986, for a total of 14.3 million days. These included 185,000 patients over the age of 65 whose hospitalizations totaled 4.1 million hospital days. About 70% of fractures in those in the older age group were sustained by women, undoubtedly because they have diminished bone mass as compared to that of men in the same age group.

Pathophysiology

Fractures of the hip joint are produced by forces applied to the distal femur or greater trochanter and are transmitted by the femoral head to the hip capsule or to the innominate bone (19). Both intracapsular and extracapsular fractures of the hip are common in elderly persons who suffer from diminished bone mass. This is especially true of fracture of the neck that might result not only from accidents but falls and even fatigue fractures as well. Griffiths and associates (20) produced fatigue fractures in bones from elderly persons by applying loads within the range of normal activity, and found that at least sometimes a fracture leads to a fall, rather than the reverse. Intracapsular fractures can be close to the head (subcapital) or through the neck proper (transcervical or midcervical) (3, 19). Such fractures nearly always endanger the blood supply of the upper fragment of the neck and head. Extracapsular fractures include fractures of the greater or lesser trochanter and fractures at the base of the femoral neck.

Symptoms and Signs

After a fall or near fall, a patient might consult a physician complaining of inability to bear weight on the extremity and significant pain in the greater trochanter, groin, buttocks, or in more than one of these areas. Examination might reveal a shortened deformed extremity, with increased pain even on gentle internal and external rotation of the hip. Patients with minimally displaced fractures, however, do not demonstrate the classic signs of "shortening and external rotation." Often such patients exhibit only mild signs of hip irritability (e.g., pain with rotation). Thus, nondisplaced and minimally displaced fractures are occasionally difficult to recognize.

Diagnosis

Physical examination usually indicates the cause of the symptoms and signs, and this can be confirmed by radiography. Differential diagnosis of fractures of the hip in the older person includes fractures of the pelvic ring and fractures about the acetabulum. In addition, pre-existing metastatic disease might result in a pathologic fracture, which must be differentiated from fracture that is not associated with an underlying lesion.

Treatment

PAIN CONTROL. The initial phase of management of elderly patients with fracture of the hip involves prompt relief of the pain, which is often associated with reflex spasm of the musculature around the hip joint and invariably produces segmental and suprasegmental sympathetic hyperactivity and marked neuroendocrine responses (Chapter 7). Because the pain is usually severe it is necessary to administer strong opioids, preferably in small IV increments so that patients can be titrated. This minimizes the magnitude of side effects, especially respiratory depression, nausea, vomiting, and further inhibition of gastrointestinal tone. Proper administration of opioids provides adequate pain relief but unfortunately does not impair, nor eliminate the segmental and suprasegmental reflex responses and marked neuroendocrine and metabolic alterations consequent to their use (Chapter 7).

The optimal method of providing pain relief before, during, and after surgery is continuous epidural block with a local anesthetic that extends from the T10 to S1 spinal segments (Fig. 94-61). This provides complete pain relief and interruption of the afferent and efferent limbs of the reflex responses, thus obviating the aforementioned alterations. Moreover, a number of studies have shown that this form of anesthesia for surgical procedures markedly reduces blood loss and the risk of thromboembolism and shortens hospitalization (21, 22). Unless the level of analgesia extends much higher than the T10 spinal segment the degree of vasomotor paralysis and consequent hypotension are minimal, and indeed are favorable in regard to blood loss.

ORTHOPEDIC MANAGEMENT. Definitive treatment of these fractures involves orthopedic management. Intratrochanteric fractures are usually best treated by reduction and stabilization, generally using a sliding device with a side plate. The aim of surgery is attainment of sufficient apposition of the fragments to minimize long-term complications such as device cutout or failure of the implant-bone interface. Technically, the results of treatment of intertrochanteric hip fractures are good. Because many patients are elderly, however, nearly 30% do not survive the first 12 months (21).

Surgical stabilization of intracapsular fractures usually includes combinations of pins and screws to secure the displaced fragment(s) to the shaft and neck. When extreme comminution or extreme displacement is encountered, or some other pre-existing factor such as osteonecrosis is recognized, replacement arthroplasty is often preferable. Either an endoprosthesis or a total hip replacement arthroplasty can be considered. Again, because a large number of these patients are elderly, many do not survive the first 12 months following injury (23).

Fractures in Younger Patients

Fracture of the hip and the upper thigh occurs less frequently in younger persons.

On the basis of data published by Holbrook et al. (17) based on the Health Interview Survey of 1970–1977 (18) and extrapolated to 1986, it is estimated that of 780,000 fractures of the head, neck, and upper part of the femur, only 25,400 occurred in children 15 years old or younger, 7,620 occurred in persons 15 to 44, and about 15,000 occurred in persons 45 to 64.

Pathophysiology

Younger patients who present with complaints in the hip and upper thigh as a result of trauma need to be evaluated carefully for stress or fatigue fractures. Such overuse syndromes of the skeleton can be difficult to recognize without the use of enhanced imaging techniques such as bone scanning. Typical patients are runners who have recently increased the number of miles they run each week at too rapid a rate. Mild, aching, localized pain then develops over the bony stress fracture. Stress fracture of bone indicates a biologic response characterized by an increase in microdamage of bone in excess of the usual rate of physiologic repair. Other common sites for stress fractures include the metatarsals, tibia, os calcis, and femur.

Symptoms and Signs

Patients who sustain stress fractures about the hip typically complain of a dull aching pain, rather than the sharp burning pain associated with acute trauma. The most important factors in the recognition of stress fractures include localized tenderness, an antalgic gait, and a high index of suspicion.

Diagnosis

Stress fracture of the femoral neck must be recognized early to prevent catastrophic failure, displacement, and subsequent osteonecrosis of the femoral head caused by the loss of vascularity. Differential diagnosis includes bony disruptions of the pelvis and overuse conditions affecting muscles, such as adductor strain.

Treatment

PAIN CONTROL. Pain control is usually achieved with parenteral narcotics consisting of one or more IV boluses initially, followed by IM injections. Provided they are properly administered they do provide good pain relief, but as previously mentioned they do not affect the associated reflex responses. As with elderly patients, continuous epidural analgesia provides better pain relief and eliminates the usual responses. Bonica and Benedetti (24) have been able to control pain in children with continuous epidural blockade achieved by introducing the catheter into the sacral canal and advancing it to the S1 segments. Anxiolytic or sedative drugs (or both) should also be given to young children, who usually are more anxious and apprehensive than older patients. The procedures can also be used for surgical intervention if this is contemplated. In young and middle-aged adults a continuous segmental epidural block can be achieved by introducing the catheter through a needle placed in the lower lumbar interspace and advancing it to the L3 vertebra.

ORTHOPEDIC MANAGEMENT. Orthopedic treatment remains somewhat controversial. If any questions exist regarding stability of the fracture, stabilization is recommended. For a nondisplaced stress fracture, cutaneous pins can be placed from the greater trochanter through the femoral neck into the femoral head, with minimal morbidity. If the stress failure is on the inferior femoral neck, some authors have suggested that nonoperative treatment with crutches is adequate.

Dislocation of the Hip

Traumatic dislocation of the hip generally occurs in a younger population, usually in those 15 to 40 years old (19). Dislocation can occur medially, anteriorly, or posteriorly, with posterior dislocation being the most common. This usually occurs with a direct blow to the flexed knee while the hip is flexed and abducted. The position assumed by the limb after dislocation (flexion adduction and internal rotation) is also the position in which the reduced hip is likely to redislocate. If the dislocation occurs without fracture, the major threat to the hip joint is avascular necrosis of the femoral head, presumably because of strangulation of the neck by the tight joint capsule through which the femoral head has buttonholed. Anterior hip dislocations are less common than posterior dislocations and occur as a result of forced abduction of the hip. The femoral head is usually lifted out of the acetabulum anteriorly as the greater trochanter and femoral neck impinge on the acetabular rim posteriorly. Femoral head necrosis, in common with posterior dislocation, is the major problem developing from this injury.

Symptoms and Signs

Patients with dislocation of the hip usually have a history of a significant fall or motor vehicle accident followed by deformity and rather severe acute pain. Patients who sustain obturator dislocation generally have a widely abducted position of the lower limb, which makes transportation to the hospital difficult.

Diagnosis

Diagnosis is made by the history and physical findings. Few conditions can masquerade as a hip dislocation, although the dislocation can often be complicated by other fractures, including those of the knee, patella, femur, acetabulum, and pubic and ischial rami.

Treatment

Dislocation of the hip is a true emergency situation. A direct relationship exists between the time the hip is dislocated and the likelihood for developing osteonecrosis of the femoral head secondary to impaired vascular flow. Thus, individuals who have sustained a dislocation of the hip should be transferred as soon as possible to a health care facility in which prompt reduction can be carried out.

Radiography is necessary prior to the reduction to exclude associated fractures. Occasionally a patient is encountered who has both a dislocation of the hip and a fracture of the femoral neck; this requires prompt reduction and fixation. If any question remains as to the stability of the hip after reduction, stabilization of the offending acetabular fragment is usually required to gain a stable, pain-free hip. Follow-up CT scans are useful to ensure that no free fragments of bone remain within the hip joint. Any such fragments must be removed to prevent the consequences of post-traumatic arthritis. A careful neurologic examination is also indicated, because many hip dislocations affect sciatic nerve function adversely.

Because most patients who require urgent operative intervention usually have undigested food in their stomach, it is best to avoid general anesthesia and to carry out surgery with subarachnoid or continuous epidural block, extending from T9 to S5, which is supplemented with an anxiolytic or sedative drug. If possible, the regional anesthetic should be started even before the operation to prevent aggravation of pain during radiographic and physical examination. In addition to producing a marked decrease in the risk of aspiration of gastric contents and of pulmonary complications associated with general anesthesia, it provides complete muscular relaxation in the region and facilitates the reduction. Postoperative pain relief can be achieved with a continuous epidural block using a local anesthetic or intraspinal opioids (Chapter 95).

Infection and Inflammation

Arthritis

The hip joint is a major synovial-diarthrodial joint and can be adversely affected by a host of local and systemic processes. Pyogenic infections of the hip joint are more common in infants, younger children, and adults whose immunologic system has been compromised (25, 26). Chronic infections of the hip joint can also be recognized in healthy individuals who develop acute symptoms referable to a hip infection secondary to seeding from other involved areas of the body, such as from a furuncle or abscessed tooth. Pyogenic infections of the hip can also develop from osteomyelitis of the femoral head or neck. The hip joint anatomy is unique in that metaphyseal areas are included within the articular capsule. Because metaphyseal bone has an excellent blood supply, a systemic infection can disseminate hematogenously. Because the hip joint capsule encloses metaphyseal bone, perforation of the intracapsular cortical shell creates a pyarthrosis of the hip immediately.

The type of organism involved varies with age. Infants often develop gram-negative infections, while younger children and adults generally develop infections caused by staphylococci, streptococci, or both. Tuberculous arthritis can also involve the hip joint, although this condition is now less common in the United States. Tuberculous arthritis usually affects a child or young adult who presents with pain and a limp. Radiographic evaluation generally reveals a diffuse rarefaction in the area of the hip. Because of the declining incidence of this condition, a high index of suspicion must be entertained to obtain a correct diagnosis promptly and to obtain tissues for culture and sensitivity testing. The treatment of infections of the hip joint is discussed below.

Rheumatoid Arthritis

The hip joint can often be affected in a systemic inflammatory process such as rheumatoid arthritis. Diagnosis is seldom difficult in the rheumatoid patient because the hip joint is not generally involved primarily but rather secondarily, after diagnosis has been confirmed. Patients present with pain, synovitis, a limp, and restricted hip motion. Radiography often reveals osteopenia and joint space narrowing. Symmetric joint involvement usually occurs. The treatment of rheumatoid arthritis is discussed in Chapter 20.

Transient Synovitis

The diagnosis of transient synovitis of the hip must also be considered when evaluating young children with hip pain (27, 28) and is based primarily on exclusion. The cause is unknown but is possibly related to minor trauma. Transient synovitis of the hip appears to affect primarily children under the age of 10, with a male predominance. Children generally present with pain, limitation of motion, and a limp. Radiographs are normal. No organisms are retrieved with hip aspiration. The prognosis for patients with transient synovitis of the hip is excellent; full recovery and normal hip motion usually occur within 1 or 2 months.

Pigmented Villonodular Synovitis

Pigmented villonodular synovitis (PVN) also occurs in the hip joint although the prevalence is less than 2/1,000,000 population (29). The typical PVN patient is an adult, 20 to 40 years old, who presents with pain and limitation of motion of the hip. Radiographs range from no findings to extensive early cyst formation, synovial tumefactions of the lobular outline, and varying bone density. Aspiration of the hip joint reveals a hemosiderin-stained aspirate (deep xanthochromic) that is characteristic for this condition. Once diagnosis has been confirmed local surgical debridement is recommended for the localized disease, with total synovectomy being more appropriate for patients with diffuse disease.

Infections of the Hip in Infants and Children

Etiology

Infections involving the hip joint in infants and young children are generally caused by hematogenous dissemination to metaphyseal bone within the hip joint capsule. Subsequent suppuration into the synovial cavity results in pyarthrosis in which both bony structure of the hip and the synovial joint are involved. Such infections are more common in premature infants and in infants and children whose immunologic responses have been compromised. Infections can also occur in a healthy child, with seeding from pharyngitis or an infection involving the soft tissues and skin.

Symptoms and Signs

The premature infant or newborn who suffers from a septic process in the hip or femur can present with few observable findings except for decreased use of the involved extremity, which can be misinterpreted as a nerve palsy. Even the typical manifestations of infection in older children and adults, including elevation of the leukocyte count and of body temperature, can be absent.

Diagnosis

The infant or child suspected of having a septic process involving the proximal femur, hip, or both, must undergo aspiration of the hip joint under fluoroscopic guidance. Cultures must be obtained for fungi and acid-fast and pyogenic bacteria, both aerobic and anaerobic, because many different organisms can be responsible for the infectious process.

Treatment

Once diagnosis has been confirmed, the most appropriate management for infections involving the hip joint is surgical drainage. Frequent aspirations can be effective in managing selected patients with knee infections, but they are not effective in treating infections involving the deeper hip joint. If diagnosis or treatment is delayed significant destruction of the hip joint can occur, with permanent irreversible damage. The rate of destruction of the joint appears to be a function of the organism involved, staphylococci being the most rapidly destructive. Antibiotic coverage is mandatory in conjunction with surgical drainage of the hip. Immobilization is also recommended to facilitate the healing process. Pain is usually well controlled with the use of NSAIDs administered alone or in combination with a weak opioid such as codeine.

Infections of the Hip in the Older Child and Adult

Pathophysiology

Infections of the hip joint in the older child and adult generally involve hematogenous dissemination from other sites. Bony infections can also occur simultaneously with the pyarthrosis, although either can occur independently.

Symptoms and Signs

Adults with infections of the hip often present with acute groin pain, a limp, and marked restriction of hip mobility. In addition, physical examination often reveals extreme irritability of the hip when the hip is passively rotated internally or externally. Infections of the hip joint are also more commonly encountered in adults who have a compromised immunologic response. In these patients the classic signs are less recognizable and a higher index of suspicion is necessary.

Diagnosis

Diagnosis of hip joint infections is generally suspected after a thorough history and physical examination. Plain radiography might reveal some asymmetry of the tissue planes but often no evidence of bony destruction is seen, so other diagnostic approaches must be implemented. The most direct way to confirm diagnosis is to perform a hip aspiration under fluoroscopic control. This procedure is not difficult as long as the bony landmarks are recognized and the anatomy of the hip is understood. The examiner must ensure that the needle is placed within the confines of the hip joint, necessitating radiographic control. If fluid is recovered, cultures are obtained for pyogenic and acid-fast bacteria and for fungi. Differential diagnosis includes retroperitoneal infections in the iliopsoas muscle. These infections are usually apparent with magnetic resonance imaging and with CT scanning of the pelvis. Surgical drainage of the abscess is recommended.

Treatment

Treatment of infections involving the deep hip joint includes antibiotic coverage and surgical drainage. These infections represent an emergency situation. Prompt treatment is required to minimize the tissue damage and destruction caused by the process. Pain is usually controlled with NSAIDs alone or in combination with codeine.

Degenerative Osteoarthritis (XXXI-3)

Degenerative osteoarthritis involving the hip joint is a common pathologic process (30). Osteoarthritis can arise in a joint that has been previously injured. Conditions such as Perthes' disease, slipped capital femoral epiphysis, and dislocations of the hip can all lead to degenerative changes, generally observed in those in the fifth to sixth decades of life. Primary osteoarthritis involves elderly patients, usually those over 60. In those patients who do not respond to ambulatory aids and mild analgesics, and who incur a significant decrease in their quality of life, total joint replacement arthroplasty, because of its widespread success, has become the treatment of choice. Approximately 100,000 total hip replacement arthroplasties are performed in the United States annually (30).

Etiology and Pathophysiology

Osteoarthritis of the hip joint can develop in individuals with a previous injury. Slipped capital femoral epiphysis, Perthes' disease, congenital dislocation of the hip, and prior trauma are all predisposing factors for the development of arthritis of the hip. These changes are generally recognized in those in the fifth to seventh decades of life. Primary osteoarthritis of the hip in those with no previous injury generally develops de novo in persons over the age of 60 (30).

Arthritis of the hip can also be associated with previous anatomic defects, congenital or developmental anomalies, and possibly metabolic abnormalities. When no prior cause can be readily identified, primary osteoarthritis (OA) is diagnosed. Treatment of primary OA continues to be directed toward improvement of the quality of life rather than prevention and cure, because a precise causative factor has not been identified. Three types of theories with respect to the cause of osteoarthritis have been delineated (30): the role of physical forces and biomaterial failure of articular cartilage; failing articular chondrocytic responses involving both degradation and repair; and bony remodeling, synovial responses, microfractures, vascular changes, and other extracartilaginous factors. Many of these factors probably interact and lead to the development of osteoarthritis of the hip.

Symptoms and Signs

The pain associated with osteoarthritis is often dull and of gradual onset, and can be poorly localized to the thigh, groin, and buttock. Knee pain frequently occurs, probably as a result of referred pain through the anterior branch of the obturator nerve. On initial presentation the pain is typically associated with increased activity and decreases gradually with rest. As the disease becomes more advanced, rest pain can be reported and an increasing limp and even deformity might become apparent.

Diagnosis

Osteoarthritis is usually diagnosed radiographically. Patients who have clinical symptoms and a characteristic history can present with any number of radiographic changes. Early in the course of the disease the joint space is usually narrowed slightly with evidence of spur formation and mild deformity of the femoral head. Later in the disease total loss of joint space can be observed, as well as marked ossification and bony changes. In addition, advanced changes of osteoarthritis often include significant deformity of the femoral head and acetabulum. Cyst formation within both the femoral head and the acetabulum is not uncommon. Differential diagnosis includes other causes of inflammatory arthritis, osteonecrosis, and pigmented villonodular synovitis. Infectious processes and neuropathic arthropathy should also be considered in the differential diagnosis.

Treatment

CONSERVATIVE TREATMENT. Patients who initially present with mild symptoms and a minimal limp are best treated with decreased load-bearing and mild anti-inflammatory agents. Medication selection should be thoughtful and include a careful assessment of the risk factors for particular patients. Mechanical stresses can be relieved across the symptomatic joint by the use of a cane, crutches, or walker. In addition, patients should be well informed about all aspects of the disease. Such an approach improves the patients' insight into the pathologic process and encourages compliance. The activity level can be determined by the symptoms. Complete bed rest is seldom indicated, but intermittent rest might be appropriate. Avoidance of activities that constantly exacerbate symptoms is helpful.

SURGICAL TREATMENT. Surgical management for osteoarthritis of the hip must be based not only on patient factors, which include weight, activity level, and compliance, but also on the experience and technical ability of the surgeon. Currently, arthrodesis of the hip for osteoarthritis is seldom indicated in the United States. Arthrodesis might be appropriate, however, for a few well-selected younger individuals with significant disease who are engaged in labor-intensive occupations. Nevertheless, this approach is controversial, and many surgeons do not recommend it at present.

Intertrochanteric osteotomy and other osteotomies about the hip are often recommended for individuals in the younger age group (under 50) or perhaps even in patients 50 to 60 years old (31). Results of studies done in Switzerland have suggested that osteotomy might postpone the need for other interventions for 5 years (31). An osteotomy is generally viewed as a delaying tactic, although in selected cases outstanding long-term results have been reported.

Conventional total hip replacement arthroplasty remains the treatment of choice for most elderly individuals with symptomatic hip disease. Recently the prosthetic design of implants and the materials used have been changing rapidly (32). Original reports by Charnley suggested a revision rate of only 1.5% at 11-year follow-up (33). Other authors have suggested a higher incidence of earlier revision, primarily because of a patient population that is younger on average. Although complications can occur with any procedure, the results of a well-performed hip total replacement arthroplasty are excellent in more than 90% of patients (32–34). In patients over 65 years of age the results of this standard procedure are predictable and most effective. Interested health care personnel must maintain close familiarity with the medical literature because the technology and the implants are changing appreciably every year.

Developmental Disorders

Congenital Dislocation of the Hip

Congenital dislocation or subluxation of the hip (CDH) is common, with an incidence of 1.5/1,000 live births (35). More than 50% of affected children develop bilateral problems.

Etiology

Most authorities agree that congenital dislocation of the hip is a result of a combination of genetic and environmental factors (5). Other possibly significant factors, which remain controversial, include capsular laxity, that either is genetically determined or is consequent to the increased secretion of relaxin, the relaxing hormone secreted by the fetus in utero in response to esterone and progesterone reaching the fetal circulation (5). Other factors include a tendency toward subluxation or dislocation of the hip in utero or during birth and a genetically determined dysplasia of the hip.

Pathophysiology

If persistent dislocation of the bony nucleus appears late and its development is retarded, the femoral head is dislocated upward and laterally from the acetabulum (5). In most cases the neck is anteverted beyond the normal angle for infants, which is 25°. Late development of the ossification center for the roof of the acetabulum, like that for the femoral head, is another feature. Consequently the bone slopes upward at a steep angle instead of forming a nearly horizontal roof for the acetabulum. A fibrocartilaginous labrum is often folded into the cavity of the acetabulum, impeding complete reduction of the dislocation, and the capsule is gradually elongated as the femoral head is displaced upwards (5).

Clinical Features

Girls are affected six to eight times as often as boys and, in one-third of patients, both hips are affected (5). Unless it is especially looked for the abnormality might not be noticed until the child begins to walk. Walking is often delayed and a limp or waddling gait is present. Physical examination of unilateral dislocation reveals asymmetry, notably of the buttock folds, shortening of the affected leg, and restricted abduction and flexion. Striking features of bilateral dislocation are widening of the perineum and marked lumbar lordosis. The range of joint movement is full except for abduction in flexion, which is characteristically slightly restricted (5).

Diagnosis

Early diagnosis is essential to prevent the consequences of delayed treatment. The most important period for recognizing the dislocation is the first 3 months following delivery. Careful examination of every newborn infant must be performed to recognize the hip abnormality. None of these dislocations is obvious. Indeed, infants who have bilateral hip dislocations are often more difficult to diagnose on physical examination than infants who have a single dislocation because the examiner does not have a normal hip to compare with the abnormal hip. Plain radiography reveals the pathologic changes. If the diagnosis is suspected, ultrasound of the newborn is useful in determining the position of the femoral head (36).

Treatment

Treatment is based on the time of recognition. If recognized early, most infants can be treated in a hip flexion–abduction device that prevents active and passive extension of the hips. The most common device in current use is the Pavlik harness. Infants and children in whom the diagnosis of CDH has not been rendered early often require surgical procedures to centralize the femoral head to ensure acetabular coverage and to facilitate the development of a well-contained hip (37).

Epiphyseal Disorders

Legg-Calvé-Perthes Disease

Legg-Calvé-Perthes disease (coxa plana) is osteochondritis of the epiphysis of the femoral head. It occurs most commonly in those between the ages of 3 and 11 with peak at 6 years (38). Boys are approximately four times more likely to develop this disease than girls. The disease is bilateral in approximately 15% of affected children.

Pathophysiology

Several phases have been recognized in the evolution of Legg-Calvé-Perthes disease (39). The initial phase of avascularity is characterized by obliteration of blood vessels to the epiphysis. This phase is followed by a phase of revascularization, with bone deposition and resorption. Phase three is characterized primarily by a bony healing response, with decreasing resorption and increasing deposition. The final phase is described as the phase of residual deformity, which can be associated with joint incongruity and limitation of motion; in fact, it can lead to the gradual development of degenerative disease later in life.

Symptoms and Signs

Patients with early Legg-Calvé-Perthes disease present with a limp that is initially slight but gradually becomes pronounced. Patients can complain of a vague pain described as an ache in the groin, medial aspect of the thigh, and inner side of the knee (5). The pain is aggravated by movement of the hip, increased walking and running, and is relieved by rest. Patients can limp without any complaint of discomfort, although in most instances this becomes obvious. Stiffness is also a complaint.

Motion is limited in all directions, especially abduction and internal rotation; pain is aggravated at the extremes of these movements. Muscle spasm is apparent in the early stage.

Diagnosis

The diagnosis can be suspected clinically in those in the appropriate age group but can only be confirmed by radiographic evaluation. Radiography early in the course of the disease generally reveals the diminished size of the epiphysis and an apparent widening of the joint space. As the disease progresses fragmentation of the head can become apparent, as well as progressive deformity.

Treatment

The primary goal of treatment in Legg-Calvé-Perthes disease is prevention of deformity of the femoral head (40). Methods of treatment generally focus on containing the femoral head within the acetabulum. Abduction braces are commonly used, as are the more classic Toronto brace and the Petrie abduction cast (41). The prognosis varies but seems to improve when the condition is initially recognized in younger children. Children in whom diagnosis is made beyond the age of 7 years have a more guarded prognosis.

Slipped Capital Femoral Epiphysis

Slipped capital femoral epiphysis (SCFE) occurs as either a sudden or a gradual process, with the superior epiphyseal plate of the femur slipping downward and backward in relation to the neck of the femur. The condition appears to occur as a result of a combination of biomechanical shear forces and an inherent weakness in the epiphyseal plate of indeterminate cause (42, 43).

Etiology and Pathophysiology

The prevalence of SCFE in the general population is approximately 2/100,000 (44). The prevalence of SCFE appears to be higher in blacks and higher in the eastern United States. When the slip is recognized in one hip there is a 30% chance of the same condition occurring in the opposite hip. Although the slip appears to occur predominantly in the hypertrophic zone of the epiphyseal plate, its precise cause remains unknown.

Symptoms and Signs

SCFE occurs more frequently during the period of rapid growth (5, 44), with a male:female predominance of 2.5:1. Children who develop slips usually complain of mild discomfort, weakness of the lower extremity, or both. A limp might also be observed after exertion. Pain can be referred to the knee, so children can present with knee pain. In the clinical evaluation SCFE is usually classified into four categories: preslip, acute, acute or chronic, and chronic.

In the early phases the most consistent physical finding is the lack of medial rotation. When a child is placed in the supine position on the table hip flexion generally results in a fairly significant external rotation of the involved hip.

Patients who present with chronic SCFE generally have a history of long-standing buttock and groin discomfort. Physical examination again demonstrates decreased range of motion, especially decreased internal rotation, but also decreased flexion and abduction. Lateral rotation and abduction are often increased (5). Calf and thigh atrophy can also be observed.

Diagnosis

The diagnosis should be suspected after a thorough history and physical examination. It is confirmed by radiography, which demonstrates a widening and irregularity, or at least a fuzziness, of the epiphyseal plate. Furthermore, as displacement occurs, the hip slips inferiorly and posteriorly and slipping is more readily seen in the lateral view than in the anterior view.

Treatment

The main objective of treatment of individuals suffering from SCFE is the prevention of additional slips. With minimal slips, stabilization in situ using pin fixation is recommended (45). Patients who present with acute slips can be gently manipulated in an attempt to improve position. Stabilization can then be completed using pin fixation. The treatment of chronic slips remains somewhat controversial, with some authors reporting good results with cuneiform osteotomies (46) and others recommending extracapsular osteotomies (47). The major risk of any osteotomy within the femoral neck is additional disruption of the blood supply, with resultant osteonecrosis.

Extra-Articular Disorders

Trochanteric Bursitis (XXXI-2)

Trochanteric bursitis is a common musculoskeletal condition in which the pathogenesis and cause are ill defined. The diagnosis is best made by exclusion. Treatment is usually successful when the diagnosis is correct.

Etiology

The cause of trochanteric bursitis remains unknown. Like most inflammatory processes, minor bouts of trauma and a higher propensity with increasing age are typical.

Pathophysiology

Trochanteric bursitis appears to be more common in sedentary individuals who have transient bursts of slightly increased activity. Once the disorder becomes symptomatic, treatment is usually required for successful abatement of symptoms.

Symptoms and Signs

Patients who experience the symptoms of trochanteric bursitis often complain of discomfort well localized over the greater trochanteric area and lateral thigh. Occasionally the symptoms are similar to those seen in patients who present with early degenerative osteoarthritis of the hip. Active abduction of the hip usually exacerbates the symptoms of trochanteric bursitis. Slight swelling and erythema can sometimes be perceived over an inflamed bursa lateral and slightly inferior to the greater trochanter.

Diagnosis

Diagnosis should be one of exclusion. A thorough assessment is necessary to exclude osteoarthritis of the hip as well as referred pain from lumbar spine disorders and neoplastic processes. The diagnosis can usually be reaffirmed when a symptomatic patient is dramatically relieved by anti-inflammatory medications, local injections, or both.

Treatment

Once the diagnosis has been made, initial treatment can be attempted with anti-inflammatory agents such as salicylates, NSAIDs, or both. The use of intramuscular or oral steroid therapy is contraindicated. Patients who do not respond to oral anti-inflammatory agents or who are extremely symptomatic can be treated by injection into the symptomatic bursa using a combination of a local anesthetic and a steroid (Chapter 94).

Iliopectineal Bursitis (XXXI-1)

The iliopectineal bursa is the largest and most common bursa about the hip, lying between the iliopsoas muscle anteriorly and the iliopectineal eminence posteriorly (42). Inflammation of this bursa causes pain and tenderness in the lateral part of Scarpa's triangle. Occasionally the swelling is sufficient to obliterate the inguinal groove. The inflammation can irritate the adjacent femoral nerve and produce pain referred along the anterior thigh as far as the upper inner aspect of the leg. The pain is aggravated by tensing the iliopsoas by contraction, as when actively flexing the hip, or by stretching the muscle, as when extending the hip. Conservative treatment is similar to that discussed for trochanteric bursitis. If conservative treatment fails it is necessary to either excise or drain the bursa of infection; proper exposure of the bursa is essential (5).

Ischiogluteal Bursitis

The ischiogluteal bursa overlies the ischial tuberosity and becomes inflamed in occupations demanding long sitting (e.g., tailor's or weaver's bottom). Irritation in the adjacent sciatic nerve produces symptoms of sciatica (42).

Treatment should be conservative and includes avoidance of pressure, which generally relieves the symptoms. The pain usually responds also to NSAIDs. Patients who do not respond to this form of therapy can be treated by local injection into the bursa using a combination of a local anesthetic and a steroid. If conservative treatment does not provide relief it might be necessary to incise or remove the bursa.

Neoplasms

Types and Pathology

Primary or metastatic malignancies account for a small but consistent percentage of patients who present with complaints of hip and thigh pain. Common soft tissue tumors that can be encountered about the hip and thigh include rhabdomyosarcoma, malignant fibrous histiocytoma, and liposarcoma. Primary bone lesions about the hip and thigh most commonly include osteosarcoma and chondrosarcoma. Primary tumors that metastasize to the hip joint and upper femur generally originate from the breast and prostate, although bladder and gynecologic cancer can spread to this region (48).

Symptoms and Signs

Patients with primary metastatic tumors of the hip joint or upper femur experience continuous deep, dull aching pain in the hip joint, and perhaps in the groin, thigh, and knee. The pain is often worse in the evening or at night. Other symptoms and signs of malignancy are frequently present.

Diagnosis

Careful examination for soft tissue masses is essential in the routine evaluation of patients with hip, thigh, and back complaints. Early metastatic disease and early primary neoplasm can be difficult to recognize on plain radiographs. Bone scans and laboratory tests, including serum calcium, phosphorus, and alkaline phosphatase determinations, are helpful as ancillary diagnostic aids. CT scanning of areas of questionable involvement is helpful for delineating the extent of bony changes and confirming clinical suspicion. Magnetic resonance imaging is a helpful diagnostic adjunct for delineating the extent of soft tissue involvement.

Treatment

Once recognized, these lesions should be managed by an orthopedist who has special expertise in musculoskeletal oncology. The patient should preferably be referred prior to biopsy because an inappropriate biopsy can contaminate tissue planes, which could circumvent local resection and mandate amputation. In addition, protocols that use newer chemotherapeutic agents, as well as enhanced radiation therapy protocols, should be used if appropriate.

Because many lesions might be found, careful assessment and biopsy are indicated prior to recommending therapy for a primary bony tumor. Limb salvage procedures are often possible in selected patients with primary bone neoplasms. Because of the complexity of the treatment protocols and the emphasis on knowing the specific extent of the lesion, referral to a musculo-skeletal oncologist represents the best quality of care. (See Chapter 24 for a discussion of treatment of the pain associated with these neoplastic conditions.)

Metabolic and Endocrine Disorders

Many endocrinopathies and metabolic processes can produce pain about the hip and thigh. These conditions include Paget's disease (which is not considered a metabolic bone disease—see Chapter 23) and hyperthyroidism complicated by brown tumors.

Paget's Disease

Etiology and Pathophysiology

Paget's disease, or osteitis deformans, is characterized by slowly progressive involvement of multiple bones. The precise cause of Paget's disease is unknown. A "slow virus" that affects osteoclasts has been theorized as a causative factor. The condition is best characterized by an increase in bone turnover, with both osteoclastic resorption of bone and excessive osteoblastic deposition. Bones that are more commonly involved in Paget's disease include the pelvis, tibia, femur, vertebral bodies, and skull. Pathognomonic histologic features include the replacement of the normal lamellar pattern of bone with a mosaic pattern of alternating mature and immature bone. In rare instances malignant changes occur in areas affected by Paget's disease. When malignant transformation occurs the prognosis is guarded because of the anaplastic nature of the neoplasm.

Symptoms and Signs

Patients with Paget's disease usually report significant pain that is not always related to physical activity. Areas of pain parallel areas of bony involvement. Patients usually also have pain and discomfort in other areas of the body affected by the disease.

Diagnosis

Radiography often suggests the diagnosis of Paget's disease. Bone scans also reveal an increase in radionuclide uptake in the areas involved. Serum alkaline phosphatase and urinary hydroxyproline levels are usually higher in patients who have multiple areas of involvement. These studies might be normal, however, in patients with early localized conditions.

Treatment

Treatment generally consists of the use of medications in an attempt to decrease bone resorption and bone deposition. Such therapy is generic and is not specific for Paget's disease. Effective agents include calcitonin, diphosphonates, and mithramycin. Combinations of these agents have also been investigated and might represent even more effective approaches to the management of patients with multiple skeletal involvement. (See Chapter 23 for a more detailed description of this condition.)

Osteonecrosis

Osteonecrosis, or avascular necrosis of the femoral head, can occasionally be identified in individuals with no history of prior trauma. This condition is widely recognized and is classified as idiopathic osteonecrosis (49). Although no apparent cause can be identified in most patients, associated hematologic processes, exogenous administration of steroids, alcoholism, and other conditions have been identified as being associated with osteonecrosis of the femoral head.

Etiology and Pathophysiology

Individuals who develop osteonecrosis do so over a relatively long period of time, encompassing years. Meyers (49) has recognized five stages (I–V) in the evolution of osteonecrosis. In stage I radiography can reveal mottled densities in the anterior-superior portion of the femoral head. Stage I can also be used when no radiographic changes are discernible. Because magnetic resonance imaging is more sensitive than radiography, an MRI scan can detect early osteonecrosis even if radiographs are normal. Stage II reflects a well-demarcated area of infarction. In stage III flattening of the articular surface can be observed. A radiolucent "crescent" sign is also observed in this stage. In stage IV the avascular segment has collapsed and a step-off is observed at the level of the infarct. In stage V degenerative changes are apparent on the acetabular side, as is the segmental collapse of the femoral head. Classification of osteonecrosis is important because treatment options and decision analysis are different for the different stages.

Symptoms and Signs

Patients complain of aching pain in the groin or buttock on weight-bearing and can also report similar complaints at rest. Pain also always is referred to the knee area, so that patients with early osteonecrosis of the hip can actually present with symptoms along the thigh or knee region. Physical examination generally reveals some moderate hip irritability and pain with rotation, especially internal rotation. In addition, subtle loss of the extremes of motion can be observed.

Diagnosis

Osteonecrosis of the femoral head can be diagnosed earlier when the examiner possesses a high index of suspicion for the recognition of high-risk patients. Magnetic resonance imaging is probably the most sensitive imaging study for detecting early osteonecrosis. Bone scans can also provide supportive diagnostic information. Patients with more advanced stages of osteonecrosis can easily be classified from the radiographic appearance alone.

Treatment

Treatment generally depends on the stage of the disease recognized. For stage I Meyers (49) has recommended a core biopsy and drilling of the head and neck of the femur. For stage II core biopsy and drilling of the head and neck of the femur are again recommended, with the addition of an autograft (49). Several treatment options exist for stages III and IV, ranging from osteochondral allografts to total hip replacement arthroplasty. Osteotomy and endoprosthetic replacement can also be considered. Most authors agree that total hip replacement arthroplasty represents the procedure of choice for stage V. Not all authors readily endorse the concept of core decompression for treatment of this condition. In fact, Camp and Colwell (50) have reported that core decompression should be considered to be a relatively ineffective procedure with significant morbidity. Additional long-term follow-up studies are needed to accurately identify the risks and effectiveness of various treatment options.

Referred Pain

The concept of referred pain is discussed elsewhere (Chapter 7). Because this is an important category of differential diagnosis in patients who present with hip and thigh discomfort, several common categories of referred pain are mentioned here.

Patients with significant vascular disease of the abdominal aorta and iliac vessels can present with hip and thigh discomfort. Careful physical examination with attention to pulses and bruits usually facilitates the diagnosis. Doppler studies of the peripheral vessels can also be useful. The definitive diagnosis is generally made on the basis of arteriographic evaluation.

Patients who experience lumbar disk herniations, lateral root entrapment secondary to degenerative disorders of the lumbar spine, or both, or spinal stenosis, can also present with complaints of cramping pain in the hip and thigh. Patients with these conditions can be recognized by a thorough radiographic evaluation of the lower back and lumbar spine. Electromyography, CT scanning, magnetic resonance imaging, and lumbar myelography might all be necessary to delineate the diagnosis in appropriately symptomatic patients.

REFERENCES

1. Health Interview Survey: Prevalence of Selected Impairments United States 1977. Series 10, No. 134. Hyattsville, MD, National Center for Health Statistics, 1981.
2. Clemente, C.D. (Ed.): Gray's Anatomy of the Human Body, 30th American Ed. Philadelphia, Lea & Febiger, 1985, pp. 275–277, 390–396.
3. Hollinshead, W.H.: Anatomy for Surgeons. Vol. 3. The Back and Limbs. Philadelphia, Harper & Row, 1982, pp. 619–668.
4. Rosse, C., and Clawson, D.K.: The Musculoskeletal System in Health and Disease. Hagerstown, MD, Harper & Row, 1980.
5. Adams, J.C.: Outline of Orthopaedics, 10th Ed. Edinburgh, Churchill Livingstone, 1986, pp. 326–375.
6. Hoppenfeld, S.: Physical examination of the spine and extremities. New York, Appleton-Century Crofts, 1976.
7. Rosse, C.: The hip region and the lumbosacral plexus. In The Musculoskeletal System in Health and Disease. Edited by C. Rosse and D.K. Clawson. Hagerstown, MD, Harper & Row, 1980, pp. 253–268.
8. Pick, J.W., Stack, J.K., and Anson, B.J.: Measurements in the human femur. Q. Bull. Northwestern Univ. Med. School, 15:281, 1941.
9. Pick, J.W., Stack, J.K., and Anson, B.J.: Measurements in the human femur. Q. Bull. Northwestern Univ. Med. School, 17:121, 1943.
10. Gardner, E.: The innervation of the hip joint. Anat. Rec., 101:353, 1948.
11. Werthelimer, L.G.: The sensory nerves of the hip joint. J. Bone Joint Surg. [Am.], 34:477, 1952.
12. Nordin, M., and Frankel, V.H.: Biomechanics of the hip. In Basic Biomechanics of the Skeletal System. Edited by V.H. Frankel and M. Nordin. Philadelphia, Lea & Febiger, 1980, pp. 149–176.
13. Joseph, J., and Williams, P.L.: Electromyography of certain hip muscles. J. Anat., 91:286, 1957.
14. Stolov, W.C.: Normal and pathologic ambulation. In The Musculoskeletal System in Health and Disease. Edited by C. Rosse and D.K. Clawson. Hagerstown, MD, Harper & Row, 1980, pp. 315–334.
15. Murray, M.P.: Gait as a total pattern of movement. Am. J. Phys. Med., 46:290, 1967.
16. Johnston, R.C., and Smidt, G.L.: Measurement of hip-joint motion during walking: An evaluation of an electrogoniometric method. J. Bone Joint Surg. [Am.], 51:1083, 1969.
17. Holbrook, T.L., et al.: The frequency of occurrence, impact and cost of selected musculoskeletal conditions in the United States. Chicago, American Academy of Orthopedic Surgeons, 1984, pp. 73–119.
18. National Center for Health Statistics: Current Estimates from the National Health Interview Survey. United States, 1986. DHHS Publ. # PHS 87-1592. Hyattsville, MD, 1987.
19. Laros, G.S.: Dislocation of the hip and fracture of the acetabulum. In Surgery of the Musculoskeletal System. Vol. 2. Edited by C.M. Evarts. New York, Churchill Livingstone, 1983, pp. 5:53; 5:74.
20. Griffiths, W.E., Swanson, S.A.V., and Freeman, M.A.R.: Experimental fatigue fracture of the human femoral neck. J. Bone Joint Surg. [Br.], 53:136, 1971.
21. Modig, J.: Thromboembolism and blood loss: Continuous epidural block vs. general anesthesia with controlled ventilation. Reg. Anesth., 7:S84, 1982.
22. Pflug, A.E., et al.: The effects of postoperative peridural analgesia on pulmonary therapy and pulmonary complications. Anesthesiology, 41:8, 1974.
23. Miller, C.W.: Survival and ambulation following hip fracture. J. Bone Joint Surg. [Am.], 60:930, 1978.
24. Bonica, J.J., and Benedetti, C.: Postoperative pain. In Surgical Care: A Physiologic Approach to Clinical Management. Edited by R.E. Condon and J.J. DeCosse. Philadelphia, Lea & Febiger, 1980, pp. 394–414.
25. Eyre-Brook, A.: Septic arthritis of the hip and osteomyelitis of the upper end of the femur in infants. J. Bone Joint Surg. [Br.], 42:11, 1960.
26. Lloyd-Roberts, G.C.: Suppurative arthritis of infancy. J. Bone Joint Surg. [Br.], 42:706, 1960.
27. Edwards, E.G.: Transient synovitis of the hip joint in children: Report of 13 cases. JAMA, 148:30, 1952.
28. Hardinger, K.: Etiology of transient synovitis of the hip in childhood. J. Bone Joint Surg. [Br.], 52:100, 1970.
29. Flandry, F., and Hughston, J.: Pigmented villonodular synovitis. J. Bone Joint Surg. [Am.], 69:942, 1987.
30. Moskowitz, R., et al.: Osteoarthritis. Philadelphia, W.B. Saunders, 1987.
31. Morscher, E.W.: Intertrochanteric osteotomy in OA of the hip. In The Hip Society: The Hip: Proceedings of the Eighth Open Scientific Meeting of the Hip Society. St. Louis, C.V. Mosby, 1980.
32. Stinchfield, F.E.: Total hip replacement: An overview. In Surgery of the Musculoskeletal System. Vol. 3. Edited by C.M. Evarts. New York, Churchill Livingstone, 1983, pp. 6:157–172.
33. Cupic, Z.: Long term followup of Charnley arthroplasty of the hip. Clin. Orthop., 141:28, 1979.
34. Stillwell, W.: The Art of Total Hip Arthroplasty. Orlando, Grune and Stratton, 1987.
35. Blockey, N.J.: Congenital dislocation of the hip. J. Bone Jt. Surg. [Br.], 64:152, 1942.
36. Bertol, P., McNichol, M.F., and Mitchell, G.P.: Radiographic features of neonatal congenital dislocation of the hip. J. Bone Joint Surg. [Br.], 64:176, 1982.
37. Berkeley, M.E., et al.: Surgical therapy for congenital dislocation of the hip in patients who are 12 to 36 months old. J. Bone Joint Surg. [Am.], 66:412, 1984.
38. Fisher, R.L.: Epidemiologic study of Legg-Perthes disease. J. Bone Joint Surg. [Am.], 54:69, 1972.
39. Jonsäter, S.: Coxa plana. A histologic, pathologic, and arthrographic study. Acta Orthop. Scand. [Suppl.], 12, 1953.
40. Katz, J.F.: Conservative treatment of Legg-Calvé-Perthes disease. J. Bone Joint Surg. [Am.], 49:1043, 1967.
41. Salter, R.B.: Textbook of Disorders and Injuries of the Musculoskeletal System. Baltimore, Williams & Wilkins, 1983.

42. Turek, S.L.: Orthopaedics: Principles and Their Applications. 3rd Ed. Philadelphia, J.B. Lippincott, 1977, p. 1081.
43. Weinstein, S.: Slipped capital femoral epiphysis. *In* Inst. Course Lectures, Vol. 33. Edited by J.A. Murray. St. Louis, C.V. Mosby, 1984, pp. 310–318.
44. Klein, A.: Slipped Capital Femoral Epiphysis. Springfield, IL, Charles C Thomas, 1953.
45. Morrissy, R.: In situ fixation of chronic slipped capital femoral epiphysis. *In* Inst. Course Lectures, Vol. 33. Edited by J.A. Murray. St. Louis, C.V. Mosby, 1984, pp. 319–327.
46. Fish, J.B.: Cuneiform osteotomy in treatment of SLFE. NY State J. Med., *72*:2633, 1972.
47. Southwick, W.O.: Compressive fixation after biplane intertrochanteric osteotomy for SCFE. J. Bone Joint Surg. [Am.], *55*:1218, 1973.
48. Weiss, L., and Gilberts, H.A. (eds.): Bone Metastasis. Boston, G.K. Hall, 1981, pp. 54–63.
49. Meyers, M.: Surgical treatment of osteonecrosis of the femoral head. *In* Inst. Course Lectures, Vol. 32. Edited by C.M. Evarts. St. Louis, C.V. Mosby, 1983, pp. 260–271.
50. Camp, J., and Colwell, C.: Core decompression of the femoral head for osteonecrosis. J. Bone Joint Surg. [Am.], *68*:1313, 1986.

75 · PAINFUL DISORDERS OF THE THIGH AND KNEE

JOHN J. BONICA
with contributions by
WILLIAM L. LANZER

THE thigh and knee joint and their investing soft tissue structures allow us to resist gravity and provide for both stability and mobility in locomotion. The bony geometry of the knee joint is unique in that it allows stability in three planes while maintaining a stable weight-bearing platform. In addition, the muscles of the thigh, which control its function, allow us to climb stairs, accelerate and run, decelerate, and change direction laterally whenever we wish. Essential to the changing motions and forces about the knee are the muscles of the thigh and soft tissues such as the capsule, ligaments, and menisci. These provide the shock-absorbing and restraining qualities that keep the bony architecture in proper alignment.

Any disease process or injury that affects the femur or bones of the knee joint, muscles of the thighs, or soft tissues about the knee results in decreased function of these structures. The thigh and knee joints are most commonly involved in musculoskeletal disorders because they must function under adverse circumstances such as the stress of athletic competition and are frequently involved in injuries caused by vehicular accidents and falls from heights. Moreover, the knee is a frequent site of degenerative changes, infections and inflammation, and primary neoplastic disease. Most of these conditions produce pain, suffering, and disability that can persist for prolonged periods.

The proper diagnosis and treatment of disorders of the knee joint and thigh are essential for a successful return to optimal function. Proper diagnosis requires a thorough knowledge of the anatomy and biomechanics of these structures and of the pathophysiology and mechanisms of injury and disease.

This chapter is comprised of three major sections: A, Basic Considerations, including a classification of painful disorders of the knee and thigh, a discussion of the anatomy, biomechanics, and function of these structures; B, Clinical Evaluation of the Patient; C, Painful Disorders of the Thigh; and D, Painful Disorders of the Knee, including some general comments by Lanzer. More detailed information can be found elsewhere (1–9).

A. BASIC CONSIDERATIONS

Classification of Disorders

Tables 75-1 and 75-2 classify various painful conditions of the thigh and knee primarily according to their causes and pathophysiology. Almost all conditions causing pain about the thigh and knee result from traumatic, degenerative, vascular, metabolic, and infectious processes. Pain caused by peripheral vascular diseases, neurologic disorders, reflex sympathetic dystrophy, and myofascial syndromes is discussed in Chapter 77. The remainder of the conditions listed in Tables 75-1 and 75-2 are discussed in the last two sections of this chapter.

Epidemiology

The epidemiology of the conditions listed in Tables 75-1 and 75-2 is not known precisely because, with few exceptions, data specifically related to the thigh, knee, or both are not available from the National Center for Health Statistics or other sources. Usually the data in the Current Estimates from the National Health Interview Survey have one figure for fractures, one figure for sprains, one figure for arthritis, etc. However, I was able to make the following estimates on the basis of data published by Holbrook and associates (10) extrapolated to 1986 using data published by the National Center for Health Statistics (11). Extrapolation of these data suggests that in 1986 there were about 176,000 fractures of the femur. Patients who visited a physician incurred about 2.9 million restricted activity days, 1.6 million bed disability days, and about 610,000 days lost from work or school in individuals between 4 and 64 years of age. This group made 188,000 visits to physicians, and there were 86,000 hospitalizations, for a total of 2 million hospital days. In 1986 it is estimated that 1.6 million patients incurred sprains of the knee, and these caused 16 million days of restricted activity, 3.4 million days of bed disability, and some 4.7 million days lost from work or school in individuals 6 to 64 years of age. Among this group nearly 1 million visited physicians and some 33,000 were hospitalized, for a total of 215,000 hospital days.

Extrapolation of 1981–1982 data from the National Ambulatory Medical Care Survey (12) to the 1986 population suggests that 2.3 million patients visited a doctor because of chronic knee pain, and there were 1.64 million visits for new or acute pain (13). In 1986 there were over 100,000 arthroplasties

TABLE 75-1. Classification of Painful Disorders of the Thigh

Type of Disorder	Examples
Traumatic	Fracture; rupture of the quadratus femoris; muscle contusion; reflex muscle spasm; myofascial pain syndromes
Infectious	Acute osteomyelitis; chronic osteomyelitis; other bone infections
Metabolic or endocrine	Paget's disease; osteomalacia; osteoporosis
Neoplastic	Benign tumors: osteoma, chondroma; malignant primary tumors: giant cell tumor, osteosarcoma, Ewing's tumor, multiple myeloma; metastatic cancer

TABLE 75-2. Classification of Painful Intra-Articular Disorders of the Knee Joint

Type of Disorder	Examples
Traumatic	Fracture; dislocation; meniscal tear; capsular or ligamentous tear; rupture of the quadriceps tendon
Inflammatory or degenerative	Arthritis: pyogenic arthritis, rheumatoid arthritis, osteoarthritis, tuberculous arthritis, hemophilic arthritis, neuropathic arthritis; synovitis: acute traumatic synovitis, pigmented villonodular synovitis, osteochondromatosis, chronic synovitis, recurrent synovitis; bursitis: prepatellar bursitis, deep patellar bursitis, posterior bursitis, Baker's cyst
Avascular or necrotic	Osteonecrosis; embolism; circulatory insufficiency
Congenital	"Laxity" syndromes: Ehlers-Danlos; Blount's disease; varus-valgus deformities
Developmental	Patellar alignment; Osgood-Schlatter disease
Neoplastic	Primary benign tumors: osteoid osteoma, primary malignant tumors; osteosarcoma, chondrosarcoma, fibrosarcoma, giant cell tumor, Ewing's tumor, multiple myeloma
Miscellaneous	Osteochondritis dissecans; loose bodies in the knee; Pellegrini-Stieda disease
Referred pain	Diseases of the hip; spinal stenosis; other lumbosacral spinal disorders

and replacements of the knee and about 180,000 arthroscopies (14). Obviously these data indicate that painful conditions of the thigh and knee constitute an important health problem that has a major sociologic and economic impact on the American population.

Anatomy, Biomechanics, and Function of the Thigh and Knee

Rosse (3) has emphasized that the human thigh is distinguished from the arm and thigh of other primates by its massive musculature, which reflects the bipedal mode of existence. This muscle mass functions primarily to extend the knee, raising the body into the upright posture and allowing it to balance on the tibial condyles, femur, and pelvis, which support the rest of the body. Because the knee is a weight-bearing joint that allows movement, it converts the lower limb into a solid pillar in the fully extended position and allows for stability on its ligaments and to a lesser extent on the gastrocnemius muscle. In all other positions, however, muscle power is required to maintain balance at the knee during both standing and locomotion.

Anatomy of the Thigh

Femur

Figure 75-1 illustrates the anatomy of the femur, the largest of the long bones, and the muscles that arise as insertions on it. Because the upper end of the femur has been described in Chapter 74, here I mention important features of the body and the lower end of the femur only briefly. The body or shaft of the femur is slightly bowed anteriorly and below the trochanters departs only a little from a tubular shape (2). In the normal standing position the body of the femur inclines medially and produces an angle of obliquity, partially overcoming the angle of inclination of the neck by shifting the weight-bearing articular surface of the knee closer to the center of gravity. The angle of obliquity is measured between the longitudinal axis of the femur and a line drawn perpendicularly to the horizontal line across the lower surfaces of the femoral condyles. It varies from 3 to 15° with a mean of about 10° (2).

The lower end of the femur consists of two rounded condyles that project only a little in front of the body of the femur, but markedly behind. Their long axes are not parallel and are more widely separated posteriorly than anteriorly. The medial condyle projects about 0.5 cm below the lateral condyle when the femur is held vertically, a compensation for the obliquity of the bone. The articular surfaces of both condyles are described below in connection with the knee joint.

BLOOD AND NERVE SUPPLY. The blood supply to the upper part of the femur is described in Chapter 74. As is true of other long bones, the body of the femur can derive its blood supply from small periosteal vessels but usually obtains it from one or more nutrient arteries. These arteries enter the upper half of the femur and give off long descending branches, which supply the lower part of the shaft.

The nerves that supply the periosteum of the body of the femur consist of nerve filaments derived from the nerves that supply the muscles surrounding the bone. The nerves to the lower end of the body are derived from nerves that supply the knee joint (see below).

MUSCLES. The muscles of the thigh that move the knee consist of the quadriceps, composed of the rectus femoris, the three vasti, and the sartorius muscles, and flexion of the leg is controlled by the hamstring muscles. These are discussed below.

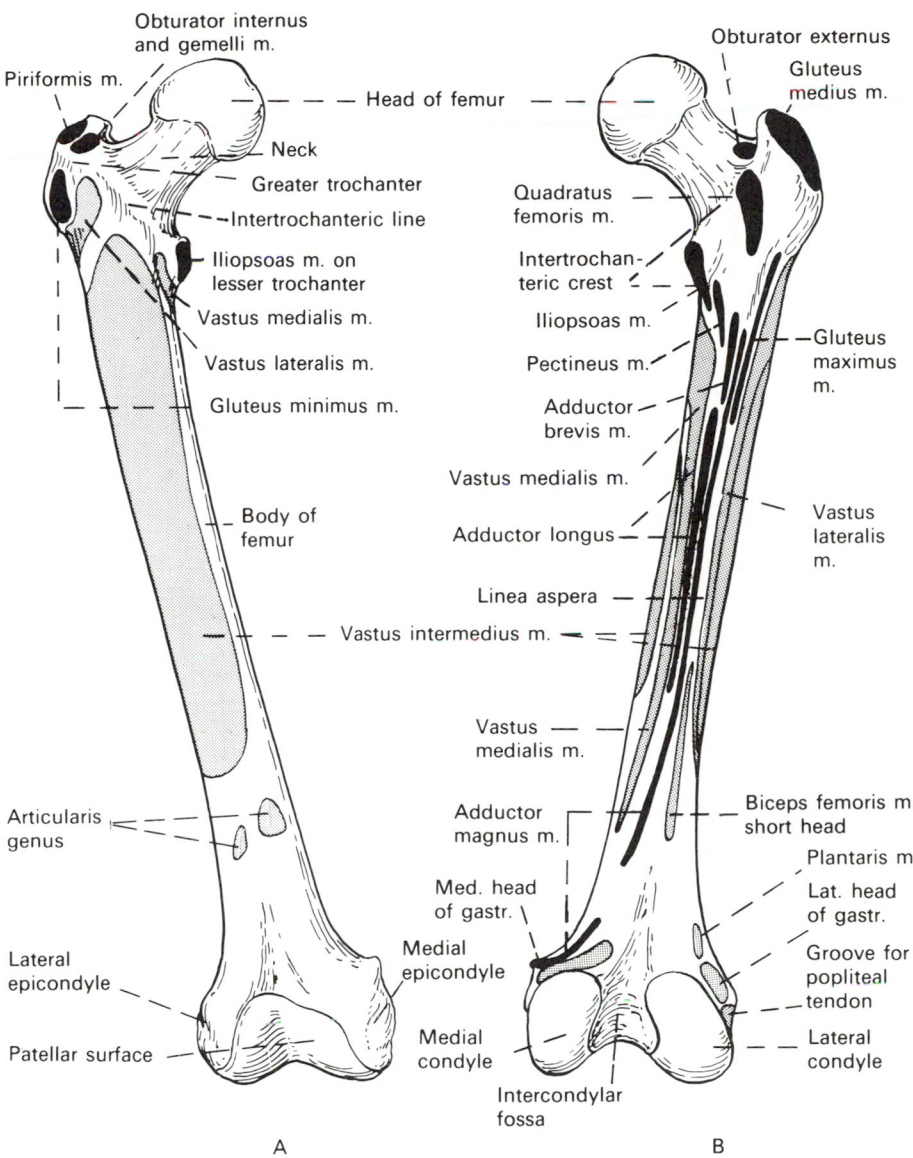

FIG. 75-1. Anatomy of the femur and its muscular attachments. **A.** Anterior view. **B.** Posterior view. The body or shaft of the femur is almost cylindric, but is a little broader proximally than in the center and is broadest and flattest distally. It is slightly arched, convex anteriorly, and concave posteriorly, where it is strengthened by a prominent longitudinal ridge, the linea aspera. This forms the prominent posterior border of the shaft and projects as an elevated longitudinal ridge or crest along the posterior aspect of the middle third of the bone. This crest consists of medial and lateral lips and a narrow rough intervening band. The distal extremity of the bone is greatly expanded in all directions to form the medial and lateral condyles, which are joined together anteriorly but separated posteriorly by the intercondylar fossa. The black areas are muscle insertions and the stippled areas are sites of origin of muscles. The upper three-quarters of the anterior surface gives rise to the vastus intermedius while the lower quarter of the bone surface is separated from the muscle by the intervention of the synovial membrane from the knee joint and by the suprapatellar bursa. The articularis genus muscle arises above the bursa. **B.** On the posterior surface the medial lip of the linea aspera gives rise to the vastus medialis while the lateral lip and its prolongation give rise to the vastus lateralis. The adductor magnus is inserted into the linea aspera. Two muscles are attached between the vastus lateralis and adductor magnus, the gluteus maximus above and the short head of the biceps femoris below. Four muscles are inserted between the adductor magnus and vastus medialis, the iliacus and pectineus proximally and the adductor brevis and adductor longus distally. From Hollinshead, W.H.: Anatomy for Surgeons. 3rd Ed. Vol. 3, The Back and Limbs. Philadelphia, Harper & Row, 1982, pp. 631, 633.

Compartments

Figure 75-2 shows the division of the musculature of the thigh into compartments and indicates the positions of various muscle groups, major nerves, and blood vessels. In contrast to the upper extremity, in which the humerus and intermuscular septa to the arm separate it clearly into flexor and extensor compartments, the extensor muscles in the thigh almost completely surround the femur as they arise from it, leaving only the linea aspera for the attachment of other muscles. With the exception of the relatively short head of the biceps femoris, the flexor muscles do not attach to the femur but extend from the ischial tuberosity to the knee. The adductors occupy a large medial compartment that inserts to the femur as far

distally as the adductor tubercle. Other relationships are shown in Figure 75-5.

The fascia lata—the deep fascia of the thigh—forms a strong fibrous sheath around the thigh. It is attached superiorly along the iliac crest, inguinal ligament, conjoint ramus, ischial tuberosity, sacrotuberous ligament, and sacrum and inferiorly to the body points around the knee (3). Just below the inguinal ligament the fascia lata covers the femoral triangle, where branches of the femoral artery, tributaries of the femoral vein, and lymph vessels pass through the saphenous opening—an aperture in the fascia lata. At the back of the knee the fascia lata covers the popliteal fascia, which covers the popliteal fossa.

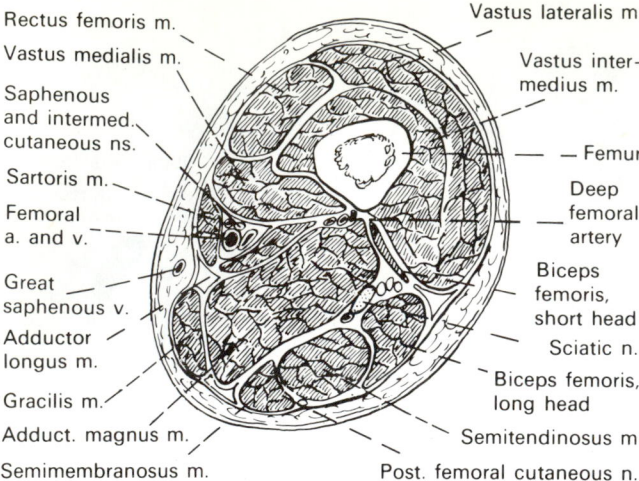

FIG. 75-2. Transverse section through the middle third of the right thigh showing the division of the musculature into compartments and the position of the arteries and vessels. The vastus intermedius covers almost the entire circumference of the femur, except for the linea aspera posteriorly. The sciatic nerve is located deep in the posterior compartment that underlies the biceps femoris and semitendinosus muscles. At this level the branches of the femoral nerves include the saphenous and intermedius cutaneous nerves, which are on the medial aspect of the thigh. From Clemente, C.D. (ed.): Gray's Anatomy of the Human Body. 30th Am. Ed. Philadelphia, Lea & Febiger, 1985, p. 561.

Muscles

The prime movers of the knee joint are the bulk of the thigh muscles, which in addition to producing knee flexion and extension are important in stabilizing the joint when it is in loose pack (Figs. 75-3 and 75-4) (3). A number of these thigh muscles, which can exert force across the knee, also move the hip, thus playing an important role in coordinating movements between the two joints. Through postural reflexes they can recruit appropriate muscles for stabilizing the joints and balancing the trunk at the hip and knee (Chapter 74). In addition to flexion and extension these muscles permit a range of accessory movements and active rotation of the tibia. Table 75-3 lists the most important muscles that control motion of the knee and leg and their nerve supply.

EXTENSORS. The major muscle of the extensor group is the quadriceps femoris. This is composed of four heads, the rectus femoris and the three vasti—the medialis, lateralis, and intermedius. The sartorius muscles also help to extend the knee (Fig. 75-3). Acting in unison, these muscles extend and stabilize the knee. When full extension of the knee is maintained with the foot off the ground the muscle is tonically contracted but, if the fully extended knee supports the body weight, the quadriceps is completely relaxed (3).

FLEXORS. The chief flexors of the knee are the semimembranosus, semitendinosus, and biceps femoris, collectively known as the hamstring muscles (Fig. 75-4). In addition, the gracilis not only adducts the thigh but also flexes the leg at the knee; after it is flexed it assists in its medial rotation (2). Similarly, the gastrocnemius also helps to flex the leg, produce the plantar reflex, and supinate the foot.

ROTATORS. In the loose-packed position of the knee the tibia can be rotated medially and laterally (3). Medial rotation of the tibia or the femur is produced by the semimembranosus, semitendinosus, sartorius, and gracilis muscles, whereas lateral rotation is produced by the biceps femoris and popliteus muscles.

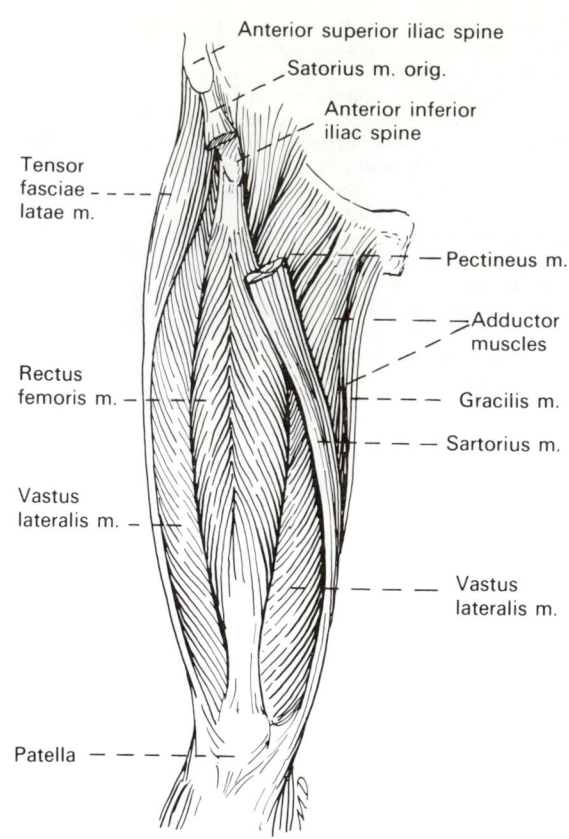

FIG. 75-3. Extensor muscles of the knee. The rectus femoris originates from the anterior inferior iliac spine while the vasti arise from the shaft of the femur. All four muscles converge onto a common tendon that crosses the knee joint and attaches to the tibial tuberosity by way of the patella. The common tendon of the quadriceps femoris is comprised of three lamina—the superficial layer from the rectus, the middle layer from the tendons of the vastus lateralis and medialis, and the deep layer from the vastus intermedius. The sartorius, a ribbon-like muscle, passes across the length of the thigh superficial to the quadriceps. It arises at the anterior superior iliac spine and inserts into the anterosuperior medial portion of the tibia. See Figure 75-1 for sites of origin and Figure 76-1 for sites of insertion of these muscles. Modified from Hollinshead, W.H.: Anatomy for Surgeons. 3rd Ed. Vol. 3, The Back and Limbs. Philadelphia, Harper & Row, 1982.

Nerves and Blood Vessels of the Thigh

The blood vessels of the thigh are shown in Figure 75-5. The segmental and peripheral nerve supplies to the skin, muscles, and bones of the thigh are described in detail elsewhere (Chapter 70 and Figs. 70-26 to 70-35). Major blood vessels supply all the structures of the thigh, especially the deep femoral artery and deep femoral and saphenous veins (Fig. 75-5). The sympathetic nerve supply to these vessels is also described in Chapter 70 and shown in Figure 70-34.

Anatomy of the Knee

The knee joint is the largest joint in the body (2). Although structurally it resembles a single hinge joint its movements are more complex, because rotation and gliding movements also occur at the knee. The knee joint is vulnerable to injury because of the incongruence of the opposing articular surfaces, but its great

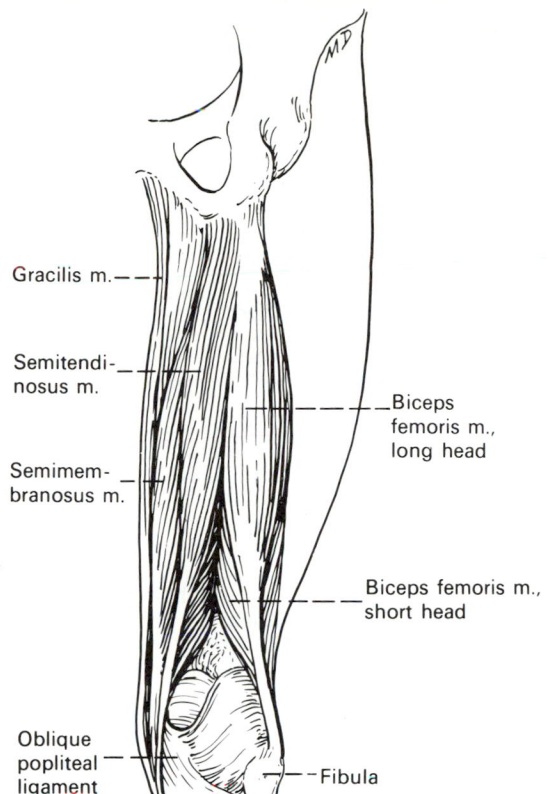

FIG. 75-4. Flexor muscles of the knee. All three of the hamstring muscles arise from the ischial tuberosity and insert into the following structures. The semitendinosus muscle inserts into the medial aspect of the body of the tibia just posterior to the insertion of the gracilis and sartorius. These three muscles form a tendon complex sometimes called the *pesanserinus*, to which the anserina bursa is associated. The semimembranosus muscle inserts into the back of the medial tibial condyle, with the straight part of the tendon attaching to the medial meniscus as it crosses it. As it goes through its insertion it gives off an expansion that runs obliquely, superiorly, and laterally across the posterior aspect of the knee joint to form the oblique popliteal ligament. The long head of the biceps femoris wraps around the lateral posterior medial side of the attachment of the fibular collateral ligament to the fibula while the short head is attached to the tibia and to the fibular collateral ligament. The gracilis muscle is a long strap-like structure located on the medial side of the thigh that arises from the lower part of the body of the pubis close to the symphysis and inserts into the medial surface at the upper end of the tibia below the medial condyle. See Figure 75-1 for sites of origin and Figure 76-1 for sites of insertion of these muscles. Modified from Hollinshead, W.H.: Anatomy for Surgeons. 3rd Ed. Vol. 3, The Back and Limbs. Philadelphia, Harper & Row, 1982.

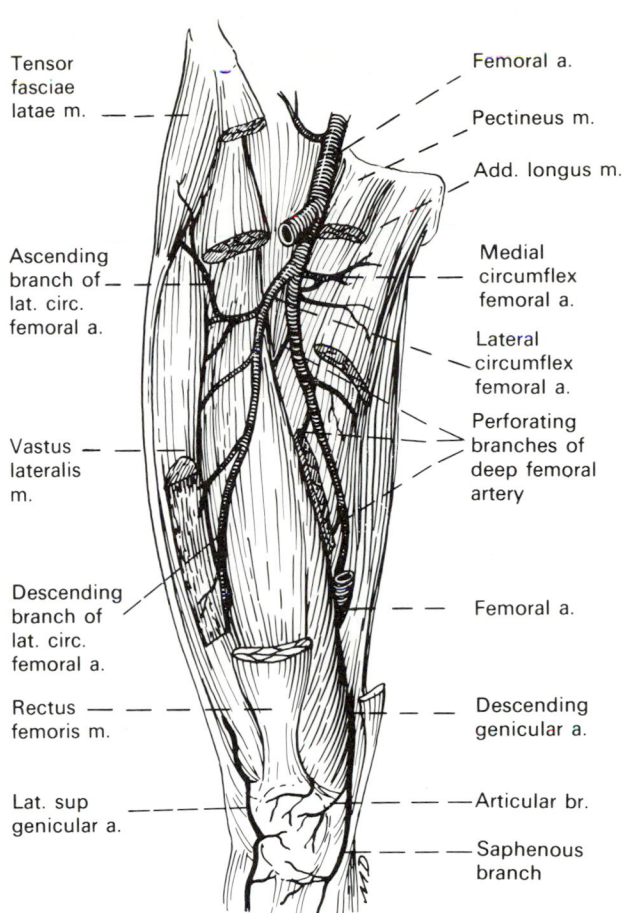

FIG. 75-5. Anatomy of the femoral artery and its branches. The femoral artery, a continuation of the external iliac artery, enters the femoral triangle midway between the symphysis pubis and anterior superior iliac spine as its emerges from underneath the inguinal ligament, which forms the base of the triangle. In the femoral triangle the artery is medial to the femoral nerve before it breaks up into its many branches. At the lower end of the femoral triangle the femoral artery is cut to show the takeoff of the deep femoral artery, which is the chief source of blood for the thigh and its musculature. The lateral and medial circumflex arteries are branches of the deep femoral artery and encircle the proximal end of the femur to supply the hip joint. The deep femoral artery then descends posteriorly to the floor of the adductor canal; as it descends it gives off muscular branches and perforating arteries, which arise throughout its course. These perforate the adductor magnus and distribute blood to muscles in the posterior compartment.

stability is maintained by the arrangement and strength of the ligaments, muscles, and tendons that pass across the joint.

The knee joint is a compound joint and could be regarded as consisting of three articulations with a common joint cavity (2). Three condyloid joints are in the knee joint, one between each condyle of the femur and the corresponding condyle of the tibia, and a third between the patella and femur, which is a saddle or sellar type of joint. Each condyloid joint is partially divided by a fibrocartilaginous meniscus interposed between the corresponding articular condyles.

Articular Surfaces

Figure 75-6 illustrates the articular surfaces of the knee joint. Of particular relevance is the fact that the two rounded femoral condyles are eccentrically curved, being more curved posteriorly than anteriorly. Moreover, the curve of the lateral condyle is slightly greater, especially anteriorly, than that of the medial condyle, but it is also slightly shorter. This difference in curvature produces a difference in the movement of the two condyles and accounts for the medial rotation of the femur on the tibia that occurs on full extension of the knee. The two femoral articular surfaces are confluent anteriorly through the articular surface of

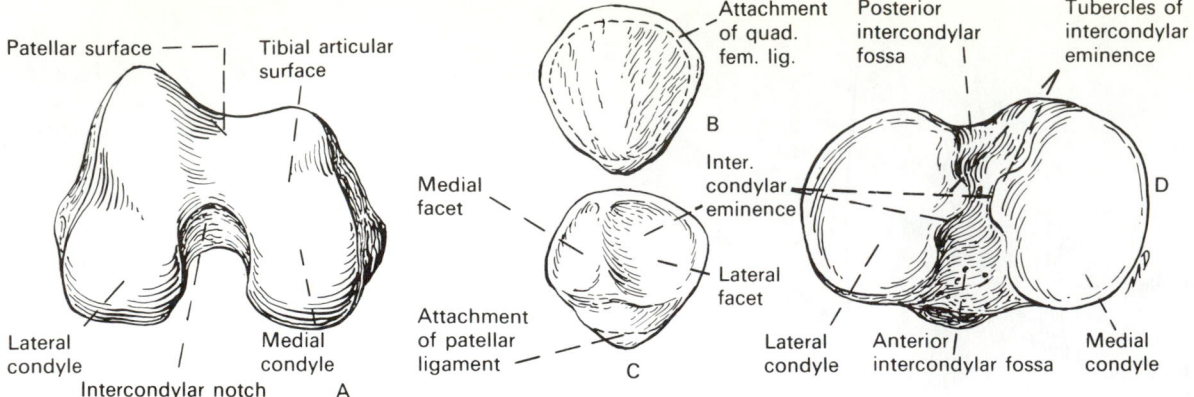

FIG. 75-6. Articular surfaces of the knee joint. **A.** The articular surfaces of both condyles of the femur participate in the formation of the articular surface of the patella, which is larger on the lateral than on the medial condyle. Posteriorly they are separated from each other below the intercondylar line by a deep intercondylar fossa. The articular surface of the lateral condyle is wide while that of the medial condyle is longer and more highly curved posteriorly. **B.** Anterior surface of the patella: To its periphery is attached the quadratus femoral ligament. **C.** Posterior surface of the patella. This presents a smooth articular area covered with cartilage and divided into two facets by a vertical ridge, which lies adjacent to the groove on the anterior surface of the femur. The lateral patellar facet is broader and deeper than the medial facet. **D.** The upper surface of each tibial condyle is an articular surface that is almost ovoid and slightly concave. The two condyles and their articular surfaces are separated anteriorly by a slight depression of the anterior intercondylar fossa (or notch), which runs from the anterior to the superior surface of the bone, and posteriorly by a more marked depression, the posterior intercondylar fossa (or notch). Between the anterior and posterior intercondylar fossae the condyles and their articular surfaces are separated by a raised area, the intercondylar eminence, which has medial and lateral tubercles. Posteriorly the articular cartilage extends over the smooth lip of the lateral condyle, but otherwise the articular surfaces are confined to the tibial plateau.

the patella but are widely separated posteroinferiorly and posteriorly by the intercondylar fossa (notch). The two epicondyles are two roughened convex prominences that surround the condyles proximally. The medial epicondyle receives the attachment of the tibial collateral ligament of the knee joint. In the upper part of the medial epicondyle and posteriorly are the insertion of the adductor magnus and the origin of the medial head of the gastrocnemius. The lateral epicondyle provides attachment for the fibular collateral ligament.

The tibial condyles also consist of medial and lateral parts, which form the top of the upper expanded end of the tibia. Posterolaterally the lateral condyle presents an articular surface for the head of the fibula. The upper surface of each condyle is an articular surface that is almost ovoid and almost flat, but slightly concave. Between the femoral and tibial condyles (attached primarily to the latter) are the fibrocartilaginous menisci, which prevent direct contact between much of the tibial and femoral articular facets.

The patella, commonly called the knee cap, is a flat, smooth, triangular bone situated on the front of the knee joint and embedded onto the deep aspects of the tendon on the quadriceps femoris (Fig. 75-6). On the periphery of its convex anterior surface is the attachment of the quadriceps femoris, while most of its surface is covered by a bursa. Its posterior surface is a smooth, oval, articular area covered with cartilage and divided into facets by a vertical ridge.

Articular Capsule and Its Ligaments

ARTICULAR CAPSULE. The articular capsule of the knee is a complex structure that does not form a complete fibrous sac or sleeve around the joint, as in most other synovial joints. Instead, throughout most

of its extent, the fibrous capsule consists of muscle tendons or tendinous expansions between which a few capsule fibers are found that interconnect the articulating bones (2). Its inner surface is lined by synovial membrane, but this synovial lining is often separated from the fibrous-ligamentous layer by other structures within the joint such as fat pads and menisci.

The articular capsule is shown in Figure 75-7. In the anterior view (Fig. 75-7A) the fibrous layers of the capsule are seen to be completely lacking above the patella and deep to the tendon of the quadriceps femoris muscle. The fibrous capsule blends with the tendons of the vasti medialis and lateralis, the fascia lata, and its iliotibial band, which constitutes the medial and lateral patellar retinacula (Fig. 75-7B). Anteriorly the capsule is reinforced by the patellar ligament, which is the central portion of the common tendon of the quadriceps femoris that is continued from the patella to the tuberosity of the tibia.

Posteriorly the capsule consists of vertical fibers that arise above from the margins of the femoral condyles and from the borders of the intercondylar fossa of the femur and descend to attach to the posterior margin of the tibial condyles. Laterally capsule fibers stretch from the border of the lateral femoral condyle above to the aspect of the tibial condyle and head of the fibula below. Medially the articular capsule attaches above to the margin of the medial femoral condyle and below to the corresponding margin of the tibial condyle.

The posterior surface of the patellar ligament is separated from the synovial membrane of the joint by a large infrapatellar pad of fat and from the tibia by a bursa (see below Figs. 75-11C and 75-12D). The capsule is also reinforced posteriorly, as well as on each side. The posterior reinforcement is derived largely from a tendinous expansion of the semimembranosus and is known as the oblique popliteal ligament. The lateral and medial reinforcements are intrinsic to the capsule and represent the deep or capsular component of the tibial and fibular collateral ligaments.

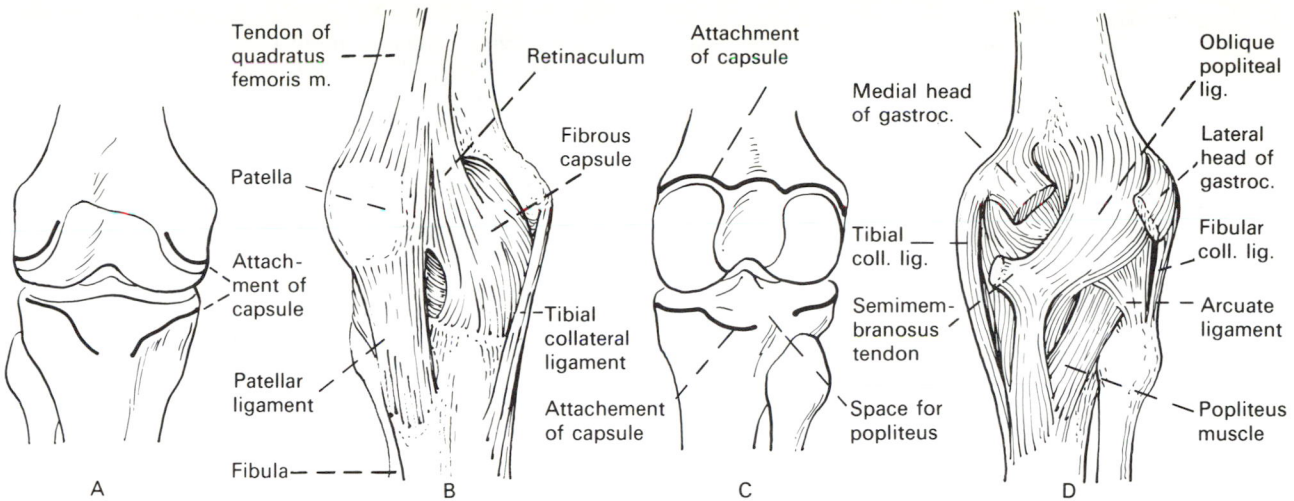

FIG. 75-7. Articular capsule and some external ligaments of the knee joint. *A.* Anterior view. As shown by the thicker lines the fibrous layers of the capsule are completely lacking above the patella. The synovial membrane is found deep to the tendon of the quadriceps. *B.* Anterior view. At the level of and inferior to the patella the anteromedial and anterolateral aspects of the fibrous capsule blend with the expansion of the tendons of the vastus medialis and vastus lateralis muscles, as well as with the fascia lata and its iliotibial band. These structures constitute the medial and lateral patellar retinacula, which fill the intervals between the patellar and collateral ligaments and descend to attach to the anterior rim of the tibial condyle. The patellar ligament is the central portion of the common tendon of the quadriceps femoris that is continued from the patella to the tuberosity of the tibia. The ligament is a strong flat band about 8 cm long that is attached above to the apex and ajoining margins of the patella and the rough depression, on its anterior surface and below to the tuberosity of the tibia. Superficial fibers are continuous over the front of the patella with those of the tendon of the quadriceps, whereas the medial and lateral portions of the tendon pass from each side to the patella to be inserted into the proximal extremity of the tibia along the side of its tuberosity. These portions merge into the capsule to form the medial and lateral patellar retinacula. *C.* Lines of attachment of the capsule on the side and posterior to the cruciate ligaments. The gap in the tibial attachment of the capsule provides a hiatus for the exit of the popliteus muscle from the joint. *D.* Posterior view. The capsule consists of vertical fibers that arise above from the margins of the femoral condyles and from the border of the intercondylar fossa of the femur and descend to attach to the posterior margin of the tibial condyles. Blending with the capsule fibers posteriorly and above are the tendons of origin of the two heads of the gastrocnemius muscle. The popliteus muscle arises by a strong tendon about 2.5 cm long from a depression at the anterior part of the groove on the lateral condyle of the femur. The edge of the capsule, which arches over the muscle, is known as the arcuate ligament.

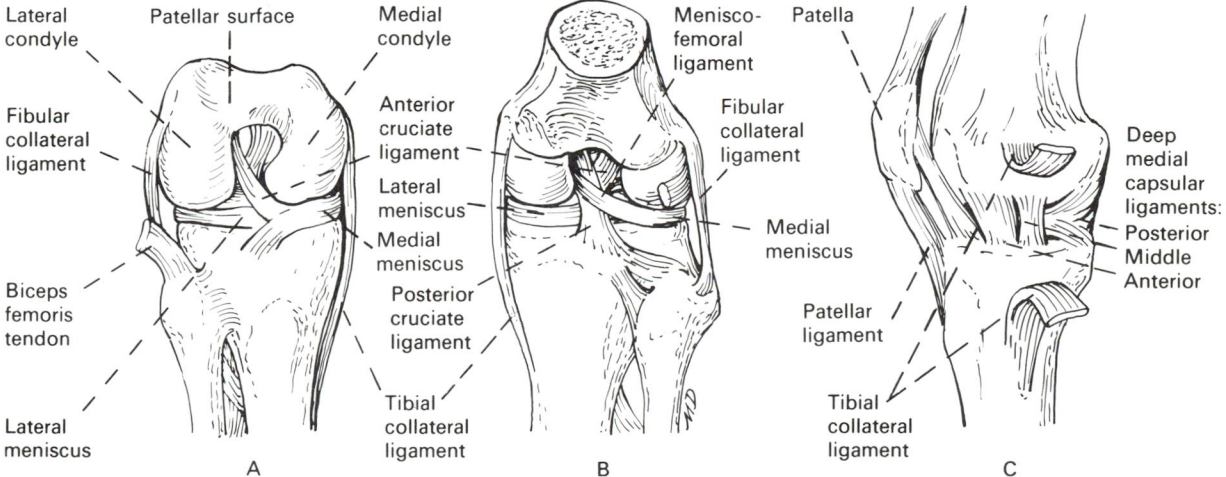

FIG. 75-8. Accessory ligaments and menisci of the knee joint. *A.* Anterior view. *B.* Posterior view. *C.* Medial view. The two collateral ligaments, the anterior and posterior cruciate ligaments, and the medial and lateral menisci are interposed between the two bones. In *C* the superficial portion of the medial collateral ligament has been cut and the ends reflected to show the deep section, which is composed of anterior, middle, and posterior ligaments. The anterior portion consists of parallel fibers that cover the anterior aspect of the joint, extend anteriorly into the extension mechanism, and attach loosely to the medial meniscus. These fibers are slightly relaxed during knee extension but tighten during flexion. The middle portion has distinct fibers and is comprised of superior and inferior divisions. The superior (meniscofemoral) segment is thicker and fixes the medial meniscus to the femur, while the inferior (meniscotibial) segment is looser and permits the tibia to move on the meniscus. The posterior ligament is comprised of thin, indistinct, and fan-shaped fibers that pass posteriorly to aid in the formation of the posterior popliteal capsule. They are attached to the posterior aspects of the medial meniscus and blend with the semimembranosus muscle. *A* and *B* modified from Clemente, C.D. (ed.): Gray's Anatomy of the Human Body. 30th Am. Ed. Philadelphia, Lea & Febiger, 1985; *C* modified from Cailliet, R.: Knee Pain and Disability. 2nd Ed. Philadelphia, F.A. Davis, 1983.

ACCESSORY LIGAMENTS. The major ligaments of the knee are independent of its capsule. One pair, the fibular and tibial collateral ligaments, is outside the knee joint, and the other pair, the cruciate ligaments, is inside the joint (3, 6).

The medial (tibial) collateral ligament is composed of superficial and deep sections. The superficial section is a broad flat band that extends from the medial epicondyle of the femur to the tibia, about 10 cm below the joint line. Along its posterior edge the superficial ligament fuses with the deep or capsular component of the collateral ligament. The medial meniscus is tethered to the tibial collateral ligament by this attachment (3). (The deep portion of the ligament is shown in Fig. 75-9C.)

The lateral (fibular) collateral ligament (Fig. 75-8A) is a cord-like structure that runs between the lateral femoral epicondyle and the tip of the fibula. It has no connections with either the deep capsular portion of the collateral ligament or the lateral meniscus. Both the tibial and fibular collateral ligaments become taut in full extension, in which their chief function is to provide side-to-side stability to the knee joint.

The cruciate ligaments, located inside the joint, run in a criss-cross fashion between the tibia and femur (Figs. 75-8 and 75-9). Their main function is to prevent anteroposterior displacement of the two bones on one or another (Fig. 75-10). Both cruciate ligaments are taut in full extension, and they also impart side-to-side stability to the knee (2, 3, 6).

MENISCI. The menisci are two fibrocartilaginous semilunar wedges that partially divide the joint cavity and deepen the shallow articular facets of the tibia. Their concave inner margins are markedly thinner than their convex peripheral rims, which fuse with the capsule. Both menisci are anchored by their anterior and posterior horns to the intercondylar eminence. The upper and lower surfaces of the menisci are in contact with the articular cartilage of the femoral and tibial condyles, respectively, and both surfaces are moistened by synovial fluid. Both menisci are anchored to the intercondylar eminence by their anterior and posterior horns.

The lateral meniscus becomes attached posteriorly to the medial condyle of the femur by the meniscofemoral ligament (of Wrisberg). Its movements are guided by the movements of the femur, and its mobility is enhanced by the popliteus muscle, which can pull the meniscus backward over the smooth edge of the lateral tibial condyle. The medial meniscus is less mobile, partly because it is attached to the tibial collateral

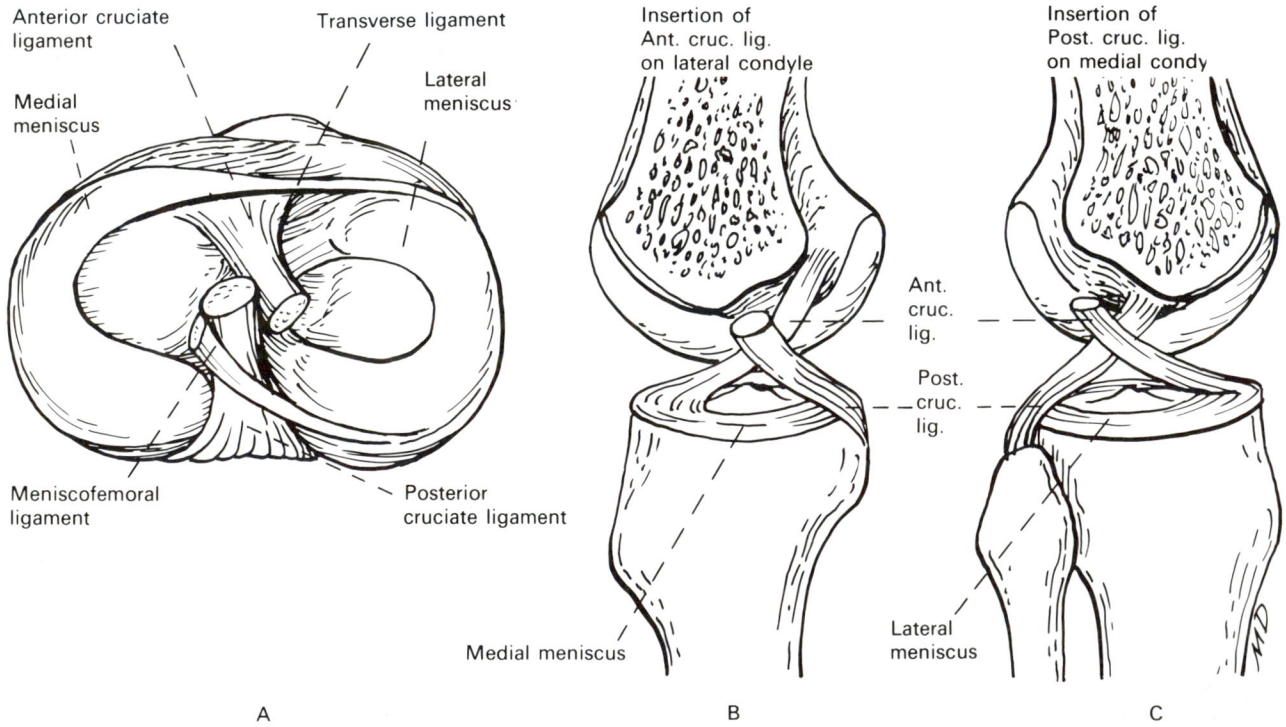

FIG. 75-9. Menisci and cruciate ligaments. **A.** Superior view of the top of the right tibia. The medial meniscus is about 10 mm wide, with its posterior horn wider than the middle portion and its curve wider than that of the lateral meniscus. The anterior horn of the medial meniscus connects to the anterior ridge of the tibia, the anterior intercondylar eminence, and the anterior cruciate ligament by fibrous ligamentous tissue and, by way of the transverse ligament, connects to the anterior horn of the lateral meniscus. The lateral meniscus is about 12 to 13 mm wide and its curvature is greater than the medial meniscus, causing it to resemble a closed ring. Both its anterior and posterior horns insert directly into the intercondylar eminence and connect to the posterior cruciate ligament by fibrous tissue. Most of the posterior horn inserts into the femoral intercondylar fossa by way of the meniscofemoral ligament (of Wrisberg), which proceeds superiorly and medially and blends with the posterior cruciate ligament. **B, C.** Medial and posterior views showing the cruciate ligaments. The anterior cruciate ligament is attached to the anterior part of the intercondylar eminence and passes posteriorly into the intercondylar fossa to attach to the medial side of the lateral condyle of the femur. The posterior cruciate ligament is attached to the posterior part of the intercondylar eminence and passes anteriorly in the intercondylar fossa to attach to the medial aspect of the medial condyle of the femur.

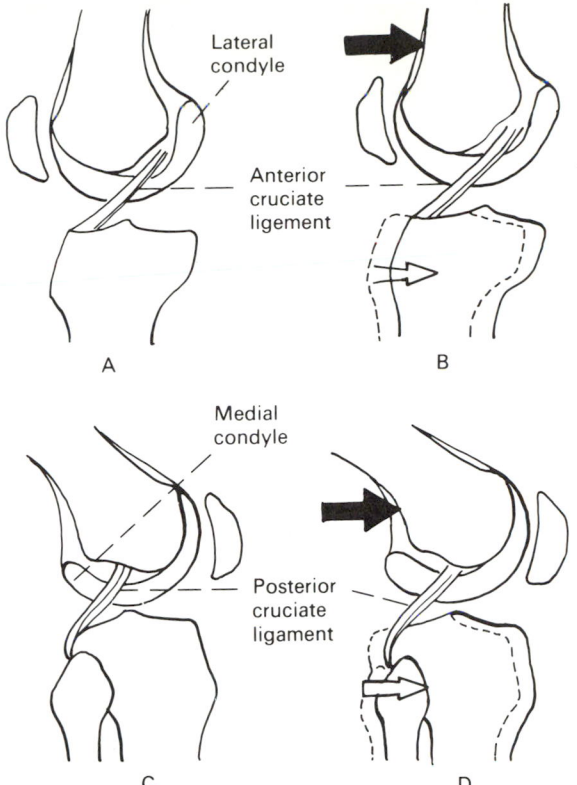

Lateral
condyle

Anterior
cruciate
ligament

A

B

Medial
condyle

Posterior
cruciate
ligament

C

D

Fig. 75-10. Function and restriction imposed by the cruciate ligament. *A.* Medial view of the right knee showing the attachment of the anterior cruciate ligament. *B.* Pressure on the lower part of the femur (*black arrow*), which tends to produce hyperextension, is prevented by the ligament. *C.* Lateral view of the right knee showing the attachment of the posterior cruciate ligament. *D.* Pressure posterior to the femur (*black arrow*), which would tend to displace the femur anteriorly, is prevented by the cruciate ligament. It also aids in normal knee flexion by acting as a drag force. Modified from Cailliet, R.: Knee Pain and Disability, 2nd Ed. Philadelphia, F.A. Davis, 1983.

ligament, which restricts its mobility, and it is more widely open than the lateral meniscus (3).

The menisci are penetrated by nerves derived from the capsular plexus but are avascular except for their most peripheral zone, which is fused with the capsule. Torn menisci result in much pain but no intra-articular hemorrhage; because of their avascularity they do not heal (4).

Synovial Membrane

The synovial membrane lines the inner surface of the capsule and covers all intra-articular structures except the menisci, with its attachment following the articular margins closely (Fig. 75-11). The cruciate ligaments, popliteus muscle, and a large fat pad behind the patellar ligament are therefore intracapsular but extrasynovial (Figs. 75-11 and 75-12). The synovial membrane projects from both medial and lateral borders of the articular surfaces of the patella as two fringe-like folds to the interior of the joint (2). These alar folds converge and continue as a single band, the infrapatellar synovial fold, attaching to the anterior aspect of the intercondylar fossa of the femur. At the

upper posterior aspect of the joint the synovial membrane forms true pouches or bursae which lie deep to the origin of the gastrocnemius muscle (Fig. 75-12B).

The synovial membrane passes downward from the femur on both sides of the joint lining the capsule at its points of attachment to the menisci. It then passes downward over the proximal surface of the menisci to their free borders, which are not covered by synovial membrane, and then along their distal surfaces. At the posterior part of the lateral meniscus the synovial membrane forms a small sac, the soft popliteal recess, between the groove on the surface of the meniscus and the tendon of the popliteus muscle. The membrane is then reflected anteriorly across the cruciate ligament (Fig. 75-12).

Bursae

A number of bursae are related to the knee joint. Anterior to the knee joint are four bursae: (a) the large subcutaneous prepatellar bursa, which is interposed between the patella and the skin; (b) the small deep infrapatellar bursa, which lies between the upper part of the tibia and the patellar ligament; (c) the superficial infrapatellar bursa, which is between the lower part of the tuberosity of the tibia and the skin; and (d) the suprapatellar bursa, which lies between the anterior surface of the lower part of the femur and the deep surface of the quadriceps femoris that usually communicates with the knee joint (Fig. 75-12C).

Lateral to the knee joint are also four bursae: (a) the lateral gastrocnemius bursa, which sometimes communicates with the joint between the lateral head of the gastrocnemius muscle and the capsule (Fig. 75-12B); (b) the inferior biceps femoral bursa, which is between the fibular collateral ligament and the tendon of the biceps femoris; (c) the popliteus bursa, which lies between the tendon of the popliteus muscle and the lateral condyle of the femur that is usually an extension from the synovial membrane of the joint; and (d) a bursa between the fibular collateral ligament and the tendon of the popliteus muscle.

Medial to the knee joint are five bursae: (a) the medial gastrocnemius bursa, which is between the medial head of the gastrocnemius and the capsule (Fig. 75-12B) and that sends a prolongation between the tendon of the medial head of the gastrocnemius and the tendon of the semimembranosus, and also communicates with the joint; (b) the anserine bursa, superficial to the tibial collateral ligament, which lies between it and the tendons of the sartorius, gracilis, and semitendinosus; (c) a bursa deep to the tibial collateral ligament, which is between it and the tendon of the semimembranosus; (d) a bursa between the tendon of the semimembranosus and medial condyle of the tibia; and (e) a bursa that is occasionally found between the tendons of the semitendinosus muscle.

Nerves and Blood Supply of the Knee Joint

Nerves. The knee joint is supplied by a fairly large number of articular twigs from muscular branches contributed by the femoral, obturator, tibial, and common peroneal nerves (Fig. 75-13). The articular branches of the femoral nerve to the knee joint arise from the saphenous nerve and from the nerves to the three vasti muscles. The branch from the saphenous nerve, which can contain some fibers from the anterior division of the obturator nerve (10), is distributed to the anteromedial part of the knee joint, while a branch from the nerve to the vastus medialis is distributed to the medial part of the joint. A branch from the nerve to the vastus intermedius is distributed to the suprapatellar part of

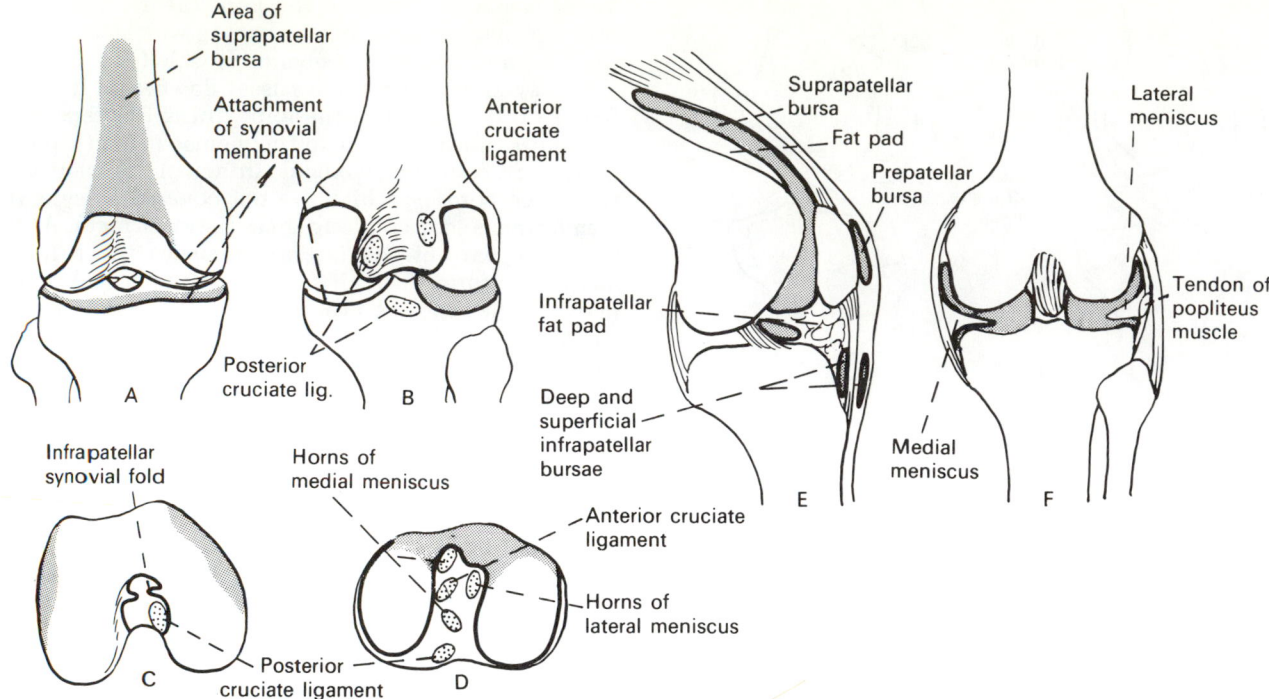

FIG. 75-11. Attachment of the synovial membrane and its reflection on the surface of the bone. **A.** Anterior view of the knee joint. **B.** Posterior view of the knee joint. **C.** Articular surface of the femur. **D.** Articular surface of the tibia. The thick black lines show the boundary of the synovial membrane while the gray areas indicate its reflection on the surface of the bones. **E.** Sagittal section. **F.** Frontal section showing the boundaries of the synovial membrane (*thick black lines*) and some of the bursae around the joint. Modified from Hollinshead, W.H.: Anatomy for Surgeons. 3rd Ed. Vol. 3, The Back and Limbs. Philadelphia, Harper & Row, 1982.

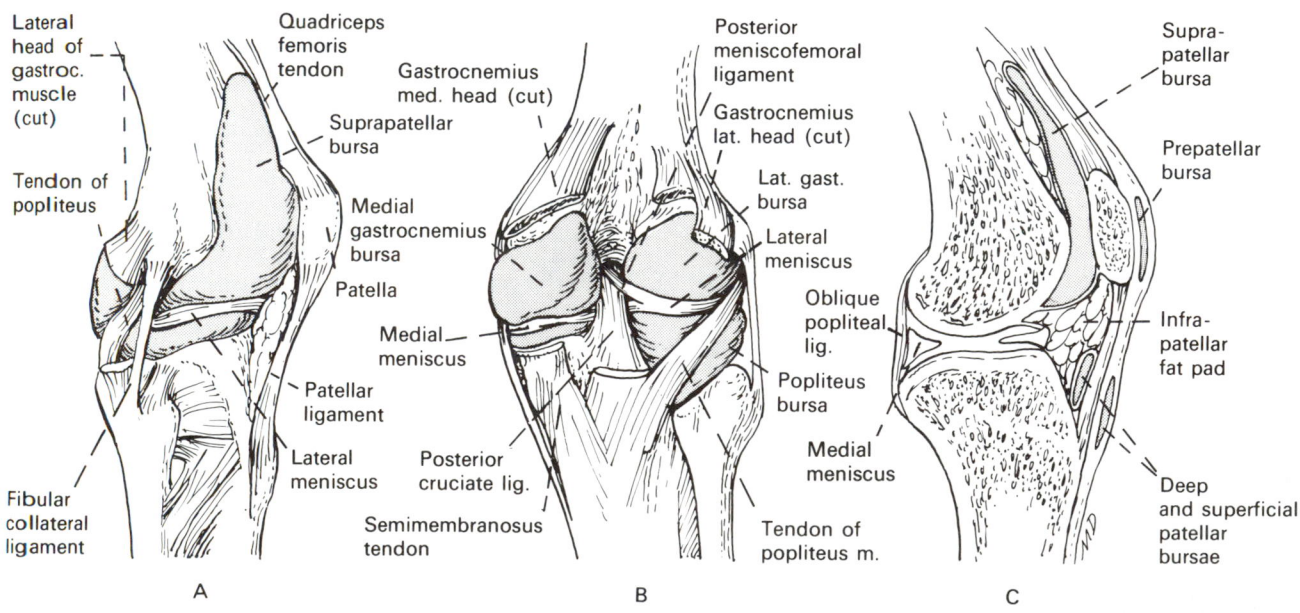

FIG. 75-12. Synovial membrane of the right knee joint. **A.** Lateral view. **B.** Posterior view showing the synovial membrane distended (*indicated in gray*). Posteriorly a smaller extension of the synovial cavity is interposed in the form of bursae between the popliteus muscle and the tibia as that muscle exits from the joint. The lateral gastrocnemius bursa lies between the lateral head of the gastrocnemius muscle and the capsule while the medial gastrocnemius bursa lies between the medial tendon of the gastrocnemius and the capsule. **C.** Sagittal section of the knee joint showing the synovial membrane and some of the bursae of the knee joint. As the membrane is draped over the fat it is raised up into an infrapatellar fold and forms a ridge over which the two limbs of the U-shaped synovial cavity communicate with each other. The anterior conjoined portion of the cavity of the synovial membrane sweeps upward from its femoral attachment to cover the anterior surface of the femur; then, about 7 to 8 cm above the patella, it reflects anteriorly onto the quadriceps tendon and attaches to the superior margin of the patella, thus producing the suprapatellar bursa or pouch. **A** and **B** modified from Clemente, C.D. (ed.): Gray's Anatomy of the Human Body. 30th Am. Ed. Philadelphia, Lea & Febiger, 1985; **C** modified from Rosse, C., and Clawson, D.K.: The Musculoskeletal System in Health and Disease. Hagerstown, MD, Harper & Row, 1980.

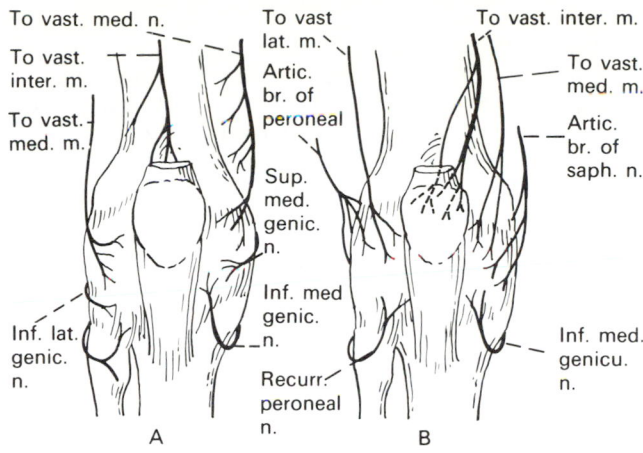

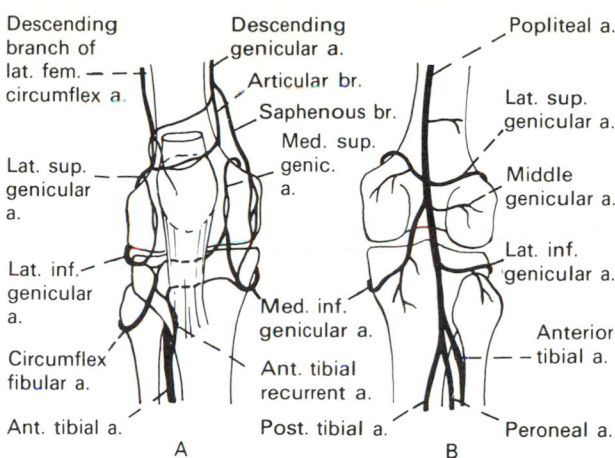

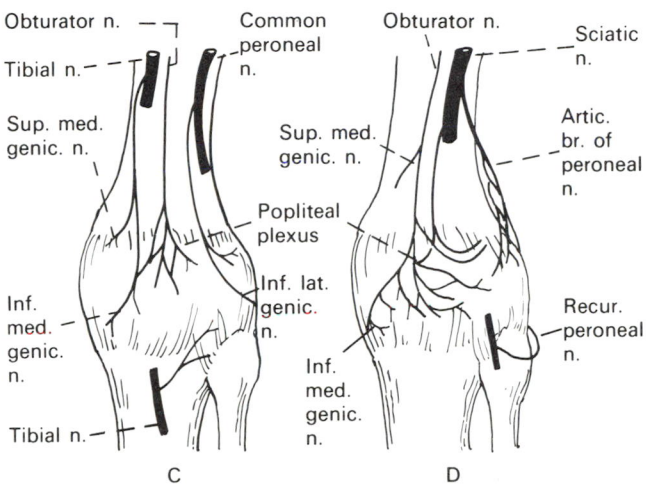

FIG. 75-13. Nerves that supply the knee joint. *A, B.* Anterior views. *C, D.* Posterior views. See text for details. Modified from Gardner, E.: The innervation of the knee joint. Anat. Rec., *101*:109, 1948.

FIG. 75-14. Blood supply of the knee joint. *A.* The arteries that supply the knee joint include the descending genicular branch of the femoral artery, which gives off saphenous and articular branches that supply the joint, the descending branch of the lateral femoral circumflex artery, which is a branch of the deep femoral artery, the lateral and medial superior genicular arteries and the lateral and medial inferior genicular arteries, which are branches of the popliteal artery, and the recurrent branch of the anterior tibial artery. Occasionally a posterior tibial recurrent artery is present, which helps to supply the joint. *B.* The fibrous capsule is perforated posteriorly by the middle genicular artery, which supplies particularly the tissue of the intercondylar region—that is, the cruciate ligaments and attachments of the menisci. The menisci have minimal vascularity at their extremities, while the rest of the menisci are avascular. Modified from Clemente, C.D. (ed.): Gray's Anatomy of the Human Body. 30th Am. Ed. Philadelphia, Lea & Febiger, 1985.

Movement and Stability of the Knee Joint

Movement

Movement of the knee joint is made possible by the muscles of the thigh and many of the muscles of the leg (Figs. 75-3 and 75-4) as well as those of the thigh. The function and nerve supply of the muscles responsible for movement of the knee and leg are listed in Table 75-3.

In the tibiofemoral joint the range of motion is the greatest in the sagittal plane, where the range from full extension to full flexion of the knee is from 0 to about 140° (16). Knee flexion and extension are accompanied by a gliding motion of the tibia on the femur, with simultaneous rotation—external rotation of the tibia on the femur occurs during knee extension, and internal rotation occurs during flexion. The first 20° of flexion causes a rocking motion, but after that flexion is composed of a gliding motion. After 20° of flexion the ligaments relax and permit both gliding and axial rotation (6).

In the transverse plane (rotation) the range of motion in the tibiofemoral joint increases from full extension of the knee up to 90° of flexion (16). In full extension almost no rotation is possible because of the interlocking of the femoral and tibial condyles, which occurs mainly because the medial femoral condyle is longer than the lateral femoral condyle (16). At 90° of flexion external rotation of the knee ranges from 0 to approximately 45° and internal rotation ranges from 0

the knee joint, and a branch from the nerve to the vastus lateralis is distributed to the anterolateral part of the joint. Gardner (15) found a significant amount of overlap, and anastomoses among these branches are often seen.

The branch from the obturator nerve is usually derived from its posterior division, follows the femoral and popliteal arteries to the knee joint, and is distributed especially to the posteromedial part of the capsule. The tibial nerve provides a single large branch that breaks up into subsidiary branches, which accompany various genicular vessels or run directly to the capsule to supply its posterior part. A single branch from the common peroneal nerve is distributed to the anterolateral part of the capsule.

The recurrent branch of the peroneal nerve arises at the point of division of the common peroneal into its superficial and deep branches, and is mainly distributed to the periosteum of the anterolateral surfaces of the tibia and the tibiofibular joint. In addition, some of its subsidiary branches follow blood vessels to the knee joint and supply the infrapatellar fat pad and adjacent capsule. The horns of the menisci, but not the body, are well innervated, as is the posterior meniscofemoral ligament (3).

BLOOD VESSELS. The arteries of the knee joint are branches of the vessels that enter into the anastomosis around the joint that receives contributions from the femoral, deep femoral, and popliteal arteries (Fig. 75-14).

TABLE 75-3. Function and Nerve Supply of Muscles Responsible for Movement of the Knee and Leg

Region/ Muscle Group/ Function	Peripheral Nerve Supply	Segmental Nerve Supply*
Extension		
Rectus femoris	Femoral	L2, 3, 4
Vastus medialis, intermedius and lateralis	Femoral	L2, 3, 4
Sartorius	Femoral	L2, 3, 4
Leg flexion		
Semitendinosus	Sciatic (tibial)	L5, S1, 2
Semimembranosus	Sciatic (tibial)	L5, S1
Biceps femoris (long head)	Sciatic (tibial)	L5, S1, 2
Gracilis	Obturator	L2, 3
Biceps femoris (short head)	Sciatic (peroneal)	S1, 2, 3
Gastrocnemius	Sciatic (tibial)	S1, 2
Medial rotators		
Semitendinosus	Sciatic (tibial)	L5, S1, 2
Semimembranosus	Sciatic (tibial)	L5, S1
Sartorius	Femoral	L2, 3, 4
Gracilis	Obturator	L2, *3, 4*, 5
Lateral rotators		
Biceps femoris		
Popliteus	Tibial	*L4, 5, S1*, 2, 3

*Italics indicate the primary roots supplying the muscles.

to about 30°. Beyond 90° of knee flexion the range of motion in the transverse plane decreases, primarily because of restriction by the ligaments and other soft tissues.

Nordin and Frankel (16) noted that a similar pattern is found in the frontal plane (abduction or adduction) because, when the knee is fully extended, almost no abduction or adduction is possible. When the knee is flexed up to 30°, motion in this plane increases, but even at a maximum it is flexed only a few degrees in passive abduction or passive adduction. Beyond 30° of flexion, motion in this plane decreases, again because of restriction by the ligaments and other soft tissues.

A full range of knee activity is needed for performing the various physical activities of daily life in a normal manner, and any restriction of knee motion is compensated for by increased motion in other joints. The range of motion of the tibiofemoral joint in the sagittal plane during level walking was measured by Murray and associates (17), who noted that during the entire gait cycle the knee was never fully extended by normal individuals. They found that the knee joint was at 5° of flexion, both at the beginning of the stance, at heel strike, and at the end of the stance phase just before toe-off, while 75° of flexion was observed during the middle of the swing phase.

Others have studied the range of tibiofemoral joint motion in the sagittal plane during common physical activities (18, 19). The range of motion from knee extension to knee flexion is 0 to 67° during walking, 0 to 83° during climbing stairs, 0 to 90° during descending stairs, 0 to 93° sitting, 0 to 106° tying a shoe, and 0 to 117° lifting an object.

Stability

Stability of the knee joint is crucial to proper function of the knee. Because the bony surfaces have a negligible influence on stability, the integrity of the ligaments and muscles is essential (3, 6). In relaxed standing the force of gravity maintains the knee in extension (Chapter 70). In this position the joint depends on its ligaments for stability, with the reinforced part of the capsule and the anterior cruciate ligament being the chief factors in checking hyperextension. The tension of all ligaments, however, is increased in this extended position (3).

Once the weight-bearing knee is flexed, action by the muscle is essential to stabilize the joint (3, 16). Even a few degrees of flexion are accompanied by contraction of the quadriceps, whose power can maintain stability in the knee despite considerable laxity of the ligaments. The quadriceps is important in stabilizing the patella. Because the femoral shaft articulates with the tibia at an angle, the pull of the quadriceps tends to displace the patella laterally. This is prevented by the prominent trochlea of the lateral femoral condyle or by the attachment of the vastus medialis into the medial border of the patella (3).

In the flexed position of the weight-bearing knee the femoral condyles have a tendency to slip anteriorly on the tibial plateau, but this is prevented by the anterior cruciate ligament and the popliteus muscle (Fig. 75-8). The iliotibial tract is also important in knee function, particularly when weight is borne on the flexed knee. Because it is attached to the anterior surface of the lateral tibial condyle the iliotibial tract can transmit forces to the knee from the gluteus maximus and tensor fasciae latae. The pelvis, with the femur, is balanced on the sloping tibial plateau by the gluteus maximus and tensor fasciae latae by way of the iliotibial tract (3).

Kinetics

Kinetic analysis is used in any situation, static or dynamic, to determine the magnitude of the forces on a joint that are produced by muscle, body weight, connective tissue, or externally applied loads. By kinetic analysis those situations that produce excessively high forces can be identified. Nordin and Frankel (16) have summarized a number of studies on the statics and dynamics of the tibiofemoral and patellofemoral joints.

During walking, just after heel strike, the joint reaction force ranges from two to three times body weight and is associated with contraction of the hamstring muscles (16). During knee flexion, at the beginning of the stance phase, the joint reaction force is approximately two times body weight and is associated with contraction of the quadriceps muscle, which acts to prevent buckling of the knee. The peak joint reaction force occurs during the late stance phase, just before toe-off, when it ranges from two to four times body weight and is associated with contraction of the gastrocnemius muscle.

During the gait cycle the joint reaction force shifts from the lateral to the medial tibial plateau, which sustains the peak force in the stance phase. In the swing phase, when the force is minimal, it is sustained primarily by the lateral plateau. The larger size and greater thickness of the medial plateau allows it to sustain the higher forces imposed on it during walking as well as during other activities. Although the tibial plateaus are the main load-bearing structures in the knee, the cartilage, menisci, and ligaments also bear loads. The menisci help to distribute the stresses imposed on the tibial plateau.

B. CLINICAL EVALUATION OF THE PATIENT

The thigh and knee are frequent sites of painful disorders. In addition to many mechanical injuries it can sustain, the knee is prone to almost every type of inflammatory and degenerative joint disease. Moreover, the metaphyseal regions of the femur and tibia at the knee are common sites of osteomyelitis and neoplasia. To make a correct diagnosis and carry out the appropriate therapeutic strategy, it is essential to evaluate the patient thoroughly (Chapters 31 and 70). Here those aspects of the history and physical examination that are relevant to painful disorders of the thigh and knee are reviewed (Table 75-4).

History

The history begins by obtaining detailed information about the pain and other symptoms and signs. This is important in the diagnosis of all diseases but is of particular significance in cases of injury. The mechanisms of injury provide important clues in regard to destructive damage. If the major presenting complaint is pain, information about it should be obtained, including its distribution, intensity, duration, and temporal characteristics, as well as what factors aggravate and relieve it. The patient must be asked to describe the characteristics of the pain as experienced at the time of onset, during the interval, and at the time of evaluation.

In nontraumatic cases, history of the pain can suggest a diagnosis and indicate whether the cause is likely to be in bone, muscle, or joint tissue. Local causes of thigh pain include osteomyelitis or neoplasm, whereas local causes of knee pain can almost always be diagnosed by physical examination. Pain in the knee can also be a referred phenomenon caused by pathology of the hip joint or lumbosacral spine (Chapters 70 and 74).

Other complaints can include weakness of the quadriceps, a clicking noise, stiffness, swelling, deformity, restricted movement, or locking of the joint. Weakness and wasting of the quadriceps consequent to prolonged immobilization predisposes to a feeling of insecurity or to an actual inability to stand up. With a weak quadriceps the knee feels insecure even if all ligaments have healed adequately (4).

Clicking of the knee occurs commonly in many normal joints, in which case no pain is associated, or it can be caused by lax ligaments in the knee or weak quadriceps. The sounds are generated in the patellofemoral joint or by the movement of the menisci (3). Painful grating or clicking sounds indicate degenerative joint disease or a damaged meniscus.

Stiffness associated with pain occurs with various types of arthritides. Stiffness also develops after periods of immobilization following knee surgery.

Locking of the knee joint in some degree of flexion occurs with meniscal tears and loose bodies (3). With meniscal tears extension is restricted but the knee can usually be flexed from the locked position. When a loose body is trapped between the condyles, movement is restricted in all directions. Pain and effusion (swelling) resulting in synovial irritation are usually present in both instances.

Physical Examination

Exposure of the lower part of the body is essential for a proper examination. Patients should be wearing shorts or a pelvic slip. Table 75-4 lists the sequence for routine clinical examination in patients complaining of painful disorders of the knee and thigh.

Inspection

The physical examination begins with inspection while the patient is standing in the anatomic position. It is important to note the alignment of the femur, tibia, and patella (Table 75-4). Mild degrees of genu valgum and genu varum are common in children and normal growth usually corrects the deformity unless it is excessive, in which case congenital rarifying disease of the bone must be considered. Hyperextension deformity (genu recurvatum) results from muscle imbalance, a growth abnormality, or an unhealed ligamentous injury, all of which distort the mechanics of the joint and displace the normal relation of the line of gravitational force to the knee.

The level of the two patellae and of the popliteal skin creases should be compared while the patient is in relaxed standing position. Note should be made as to whether both knees are straight when the soles of the feet are on the ground. The contour of the soft tissues in the thigh and around the knee should be noted, with special attention paid to the bulk of the quadriceps on both sides. The muscles should be compared relaxed and during active isometric contraction, keeping the

---

TABLE 75-4. Evaluation of the Patient with Knee Pain

I. History

A. Present history
1. Characteristics of the pain: Distribution, intensity, quality, temporal characteristics
2. Factors that aggravate, relieve, and have no effect on the pain

B. Past medical and family history

II. Physical examination

A. Inspection
1. Alignment of femur, tibia, and patella
2. Presence of genu: valgum, varum, recurvatum
3. Level of both patellae
4. Knees straight with feet flat on ground?
5. Soft tissue contour
6. Muscle girth
7. Color and texture of skin
8. Presence of scars or sinuses
9. Gait cycle

B. Palpation (bilateral); Patient recumbent
1. Tibial tuberosity, swelling, tenderness; tibiofemoral joint
2. Skin temperature, tenderness
3. Swelling: exostosis, fluid, thickening of synovial membrane
4. Side-to-side movement of patella—pain? tenderness? crepitus? grating?
5. Popliteal area: pulse, swelling, cyst?

C. Measurement of girth (diameter): 2, 8, and 15 cm above knee

D. Range of motion and muscle strength: flexion, extension, medial and lateral rotation

E. Sensory examination
1. Pain: pinprick, pinch
2. Temperature, touch, proprioception

F. Knee stability: medial and lateral ligaments; anterior and posterior cruciate ligaments

G. Other parts of physical examination: hip joint, low back, leg

III. Special tests

A. Radiography, radioisotope bone scan

B. Arthroscopy

knees extended. Atrophy of the quadriceps is a cardinal sign of a diseased knee.

The color of the skin should be noted. The knee should be inspected with the patient walking, with attention paid to the phases of the gait cycle.

Palpation

The skin temperature and texture should be palpated, being especially gentle over painful and swollen joints (3). All accessible anatomic structures should also be palpated, and any tenderness, swelling, or breach in continuity should be noted.

With the quadriceps relaxed, the relatively flat patello-femoral articular surfaces should permit manual side-to-side displacement of the patella. The patella and femoral surfaces of the joint are palpated. In children the tibial tuberosity might be tender, swollen, and hypertrophied because of trauma and inflammation of the epiphyseal cartilage (3). This must be distinguished from a tender metaphysis, which suggests osteomyelitis. The edges of the menisci should be palpated along the joint line slightly anteriorly on either side of the patellar ligament. Aggravation of pain and tenderness indicates a meniscal tear. Such symptoms must be distin-

guished from those resulting from partial tear of the collateral ligament.

Roughness of the articular surface should be tested by eliciting crepitus. This is done by passively moving the patella on the femur or the tibia on the femur, in the latter instance keeping one hand cupped over the patella. A grating sensation can be felt or heard; this is usually caused by degenerative joint disease, osteochondritis, chondromalacia, or loose bodies (3).

Areas of diffuse swelling should be carefully palpated. Malignant primary tumors around the knee or lower thigh and osteomyelitis of the femur or tibia usually present as a hot, diffuse, tender swelling.

Swelling around the knee joint has three basic causes: (a) thickening or enlargement of bone; (b) fluid within the joint; and (c) thickening of the synovial membrane (5, 6). Localized thickening of the bone, an exostosis, is easily palpated. More diffuse bone enlargement is caused by bone infection or by expansion of a bone tumor or cyst. A large effusion in the joint, which elevates the patella, obliterates the normal depressions that are visible on either side of the patella. This elevation can be confirmed by ballottement of the patella against the femoral condyles (Fig. 75-15). Effusion of blood, serous fluid, or pus can be distinguished by the history and physical examination and confirmed by aspiration and examination of the fluid.

Thickening of the synovial membrane is always a prominent feature of chronic inflammatory arthritis. The thickening is often more obvious above the patella, where the duplicated membrane forms the suprapatellar pouch.

Testing of Movement and Muscle Strength

Accurate assessment of the range of movement and of the strength of the thigh muscles is particularly important in the knee because even a slight impairment of movement is significant (5). If movement is painful, accompanied by crepitation, or both, this should be noted.

Flexion of the knee is normally limited by contact between the calf and thigh and varies with the build of the patient. A thin patient can flex more than a muscular or fat patient and can usually bring the heel in contact with the buttocks. The range of the contralateral normal knee must be taken as the normal range of movement for the individual. The strength of the flexor muscles can be tested by opposing knee flexion, which is best performed with the patient lying prone (Fig. 75-16A).

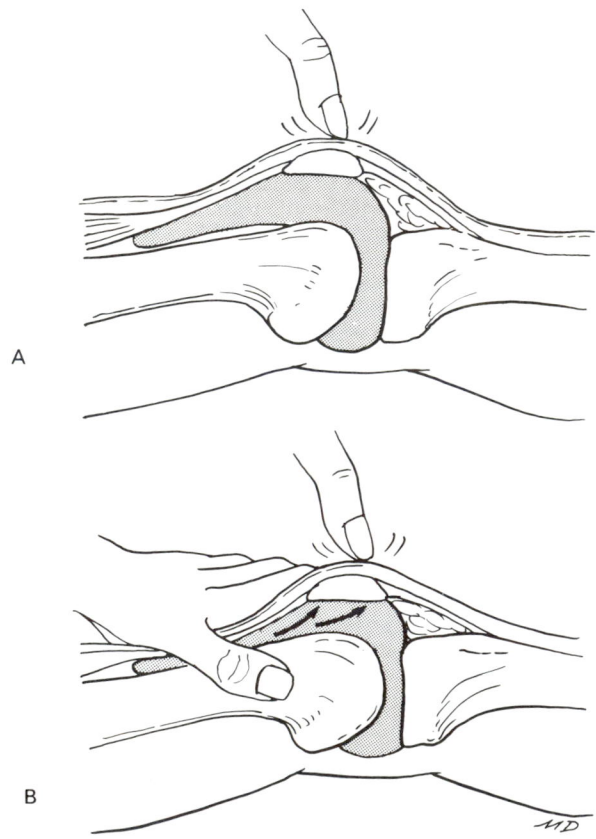

FIG. 75-15. Technique of ballottement of the patella and of testing for the presence of a large effusion into the joint. *A.* With a large effusion (shaded area) the patella is greatly elevated, making ballottement of the patella against the femoral condyle with the second finger possible. *B.* With moderate effusion (shaded area) the patella might not be elevated. Thus, fluid must be displaced from the suprapatellar pouch and the site of the joint cavity by compressing the region with the left hand. When the patella is elevated ballottement with the second finger of the right hand can be carried out. Modified from Rosse, C.: The Thigh and the Knee. *In* The Musculoskeletal System in Health and Disease. Edited by C. Rosse and D.K. Clawson. Hagerstown, MD, Harper & Row, 1980.

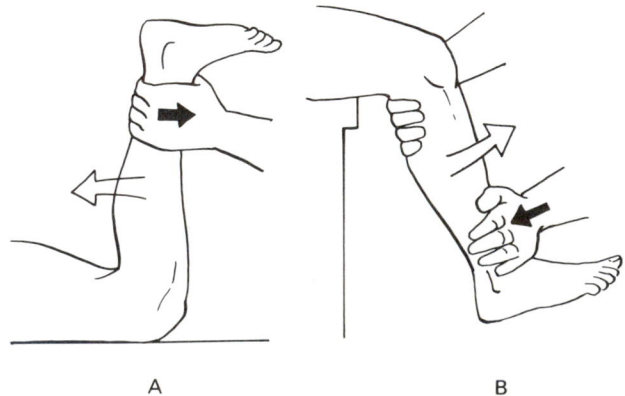

FIG. 75-16. Testing the strength of the muscles of the knee. *A.* The flexor muscles are tested with the patient lying prone and the leg partly flexed. The patient attemps to flex the leg on the thigh further against the resistance offered by the examiner. *B.* The extensor muscles are tested with the patient sitting at the edge of the examining table. The patient attempts to extend the knee against the resistance of the examiner.

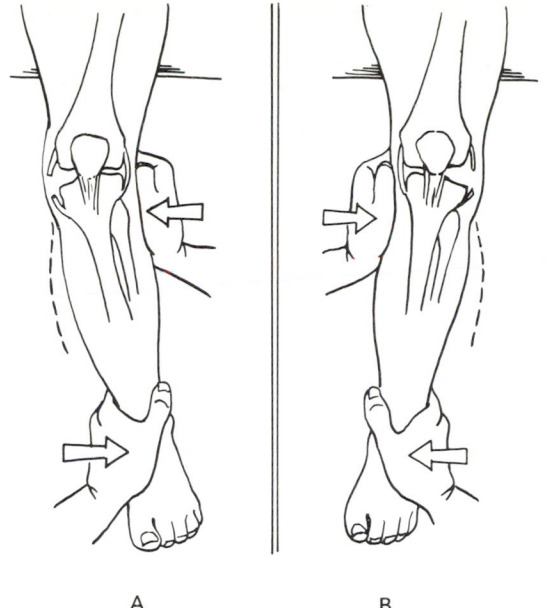

In full extension the angle between the tibia and femur is slightly greater than 180° in women and slightly less than 180° in men. It is important to detect even a slight impairment of knee extension, using the passive range of motion of the contralateral limb as the norm. The strength of the quadriceps and other extensors is assessed by having the patient sitting and attempting to extend the knee against the examiner's firm resistance on the leg (Fig. 75-16B).

Evaluation of Joint Stability

In addition to the function of the muscle it is essential to test both collateral (Fig. 75-17) and both cruciate (Fig. 75-18) ligaments. The muscles must be relaxed when assessing ligamentous integrity (3). The knee must be slightly flexed to test the collateral ligaments, thus eliminating the stabilizing effect of the cruciate ligaments on the extended knee.

Evaluation of Extrinsic Causes of Pain

Pain in the knee can be caused by diseases of the hip, such as arthritis and a slipped upper femoral epiphysis, or by lumbosacral disorders, such as prolapse of an intervertebral disk and occasionally spinal stenosis. It is therefore essential to examine these regions (Chapters 70 and 74), including a neurologic examination of the lower limbs and orthopedic and radiologic examinations of the lumbosacral spine and hip joints.

Imaging and Arthroscopic Evaluation

Imaging

Generally anteroposterior and lateral films of the femur and knee joint are sufficient. Part of the tibia and fibula should be included, in addition to a length of the femur. Tangential projections of femoral condyles with the knee flexed are sometimes helpful, especially when osteochondritis dissecans is suspected (5, 6). Tangential views of the patella might also be advisable. If physical examination suggests that the knee symptoms are referred phenomena from lesions of the hip or

FIG. 75-17. Testing the collateral ligaments of the knee. **A.** With the left knee slightly flexed to eliminate the stabilizing effect of the cruciate ligament on the extended knee, the tibial collateral ligament is tested by grasping the patient's ankle with one hand and using the other hand as a fulcrum at the knee. Abduction force is then applied at the ankle in an attempt to produce a valgus deformity of the knee. **B.** The lateral collateral ligament is tested by the examiner attempting to produce a varus deformity. Modified from Rosse, C.: The Thigh and the Knee. *In* The Musculoskeletal System in Health and Disease. Edited by C. Rosse and D.K. Clawson. Hagerstown, MD, Harper & Row, 1980.

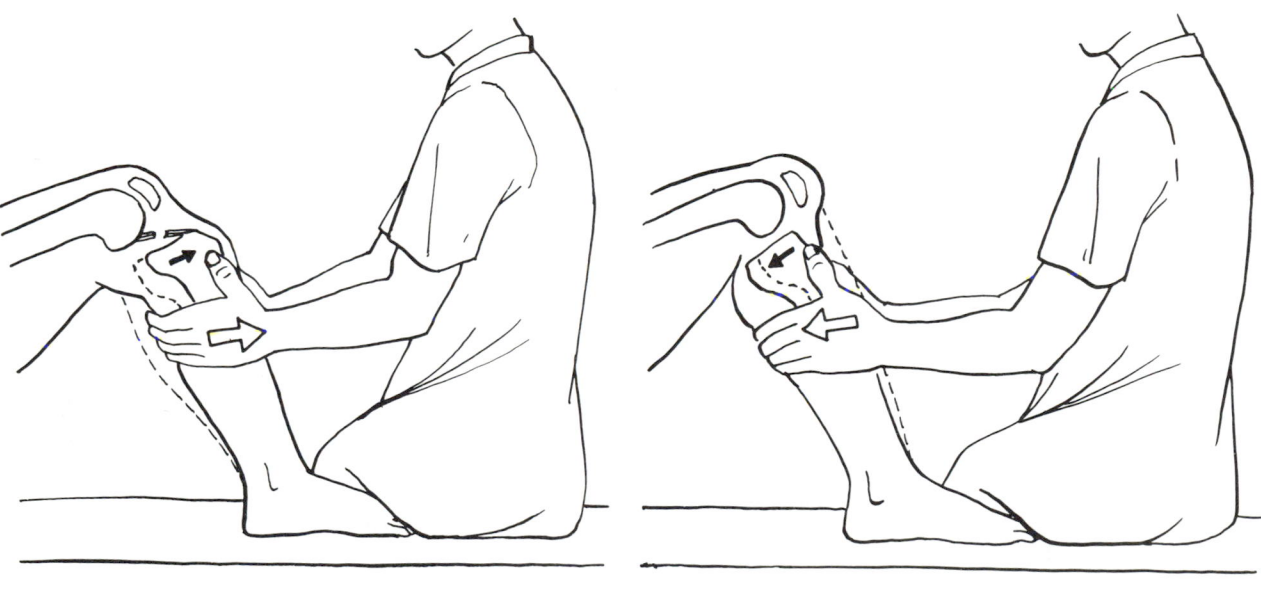

A   B

FIG. 75-18. Testing the cruciate ligaments of the knee. **A.** With the patient lying supine on the examining table, the knee flexed to about 120° and the foot stabilized, the examiner grasps the upper end of the tibia with both hands, with the fingers interlocked behind and the tip of each thumb placed on each tibial condyle. The anterior cruciate ligament is tested by attempting to displace the tibia anteriorly on the femur. If the ligament is torn, a forward displacement of the tibia occurs (anterior drawer sign). **B.** The integrity of the posterior cruciate ligament is tested in the same manner by attempting to produce posterior displacement of the tibia.

spine, appropriate radiographs of these regions should be obtained. Arthrography can be helpful in certain cases of internal derangement, and radioisotope bone scanning can be useful in the diagnosis of inflammatory or neoplastic lesions.

Arthroscopy

Arthroscopy has become an important adjunct to clinical and radiographic examination in the diagnosis of knee pathology. Recent advances in design and clarity of the telescope and refinements of fiberoptic illumination have greatly improved the usefulness of this method as a diagnostic procedure and as a therapeutic measure. For arthroscopy the knee region must be anesthetized either by local infiltration or, more preferably, by block of the sciatic, femoral, and obturator nerves, or by unilateral subarachnoid block.

C. PAINFUL DISORDERS OF THE THIGH

Traumatic Disorders

Fractures

Fractures of the upper part of the femur and acetabulum were discussed in Chapter 74. Here we consider fractures of the femoral shaft. As stated earlier in the chapter, in 1986 nearly 176,000 persons had fractures of the femur, causing about 2.9 million days of restricted activity, 1.6 million days of bed disability, and over 610,000 days of work lost (10, 11).

Symptoms and Signs

Fracture of the femur invariably causes continuous deep aching pain localized to the thigh. The intensity and duration of the pain vary with the type of fracture and whether it is associated with severe soft tissue injury. An undisplaced fracture produces mild to moderate pain whereas a compound fracture involving extensive soft tissue injury is likely to produce continuous, severe, deep, aching pain and also sharp well-localized superficial pain.

Because femoral shaft fractures are generally secondary to high-energy forces, they are frequently associated with life-threatening systemic complications. Hypovolemic shock and fat embolism syndrome can accompany both open and closed femur fractures. Moreover, some patients sustain injuries to other organs.

Diagnosis

The diagnosis is based on the history of injury and radiographic confirmation. Careful assessment of the patient's physical and psychologic status is essential prior to initiating treatment.

Treatment

The initial phases of treatment depend on the condition of patients. Aggressive resuscitative measures should be carried out on patients who manifest hypovolemic shock. Obviously, an initial phase of the treatment involves pain relief. Because pain control in patients with multiple trauma is discussed on page 371 and pain control in patients with fractures is considered on page 374, only brief comments are made here; these also apply to the management of severe pain resulting from other injuries of the thigh and knee.

PAIN CONTROL. The initial step in pain control involves the evaluation of the physical, psychologic, and mental condition of the patient and the determination of the status of circulatory, respiratory, and cerebral function and of the location, intensity, and possible mechanisms of the pain. It is also important to assess the degree of anxiety and apprehension and the roles these might have in the patient's pain behavior. Systemic analgesics and adjuvant drugs are the most practical methods of relieving severe pain at the site of injury and during transportation to the hospital. Other methods include the use of inhalation analgesia and of drugs such as ketamine (page 372).

Once the patient is in the hospital and a fracture or other severe injury is suspected, the physician should ensure that the patient continues to have effective pain relief with opioids, which can be administered even before radiographs are taken. In medical centers in which skilled personnel are available the pain is best managed with continuous epidural analgesia produced by an opioid combined with a dilute solution of a local anesthetic, given in sufficient amounts to produce analgesia of the site of injury (T10 to S5 for the femur and knee joint). In addition to producing complete preoperative pain relief this procedure can be used for orthopedic therapy—closed or open reduction—and this can be best achieved with maximal muscle relaxation.

Regional anesthesia, in addition to providing complete relaxation that is limited to the lower limbs, obviates the risk of vomiting or regurgitating and the consequent aspiration of gastric contents into the lungs that is inherent in the use of general anesthesia. It also prevents massive nociceptive input and the neuroendocrine response (pages 176 and 369; also see Chapter 91). Continuous analgesia with a dilute solution of a local anesthetic and an opioid should be continued postoperatively to provide effective pain relief, prevent the neuroendocrine response, and permit early motion and rehabilitation (20). Evidence of the superiority of this method over the standard management of patients with knee injuries is cited on pages 467, 472–476. An alternative method of anesthesia for the operation is sciatic-femoral-obturator nerve block with 0.5% bupivacaine and epinephrine (Chapter 94).

ORTHOPEDIC MANAGEMENT. The definitive orthopedic management of fracture of the femoral shaft depends on what Bucholz and Mooney (20) have called the patient-fracture-surgeon variables. Children can almost uniformly be treated successfully with traction and external mobilization. Early mobilization of adult polytrauma patients is desirable to avoid pulmonary and other complications of prolonged bed rest. Except in patients in whom emergency operative stabilization of long bone fractures is desirable, femoral nailing can be delayed until the general medical status is stable (21). Most authorities favor the use of percutaneous (closed) intramedullary nailing. Hansen and Winquist (22) have had outstanding success with closed intramedullary nailing of the femur, using the Kuntscher technique with reaming (Fig. 75-19).

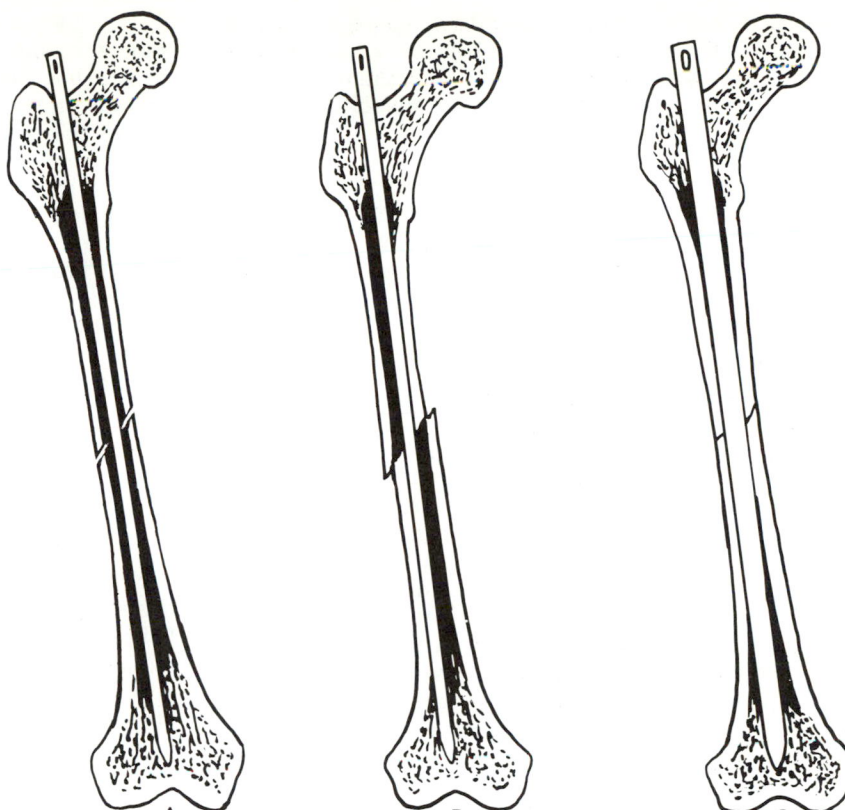

FIG. 75-19. *A.* Internal splinting of the shaft fracture with a narrow intramedullary rod. *B.* This often results in displacement and shortening. *C.* Intramedullary reaming and nailing with a large rod allows better cortical contact and stability, thus minimizing this complication. Modified from Bucholz, R.W., and Mooney V.: Fractures of the femoral shaft. *In* Surgery of the Musculoskeletal System, Vol. 3. Edited by C.M. Evarts. New York, Churchill Livingstone, 1983.

Contusion of the Quadriceps

The most common injury sustained by the quadriceps muscle is contusion, usually during an athletic activity. The contusion can be mild, moderate, or severe.

Symptoms and Signs

Mild contusion is associated with localized pain and tenderness with active flexion greater than 90° (7). A moderate degree of contusion is associated with localized pain and swelling of the thigh, which is tender to palpation, and flexion is limited to less than 90°. A limp is usually present and daily activities are restricted by the pain. Severe contusion is associated with continuous mild, moderate, or severe pain, gross swelling, and severe disability, and active flexion is less than 45°.

Diagnosis and Treatment

Diagnosis is based on the history and physical findings. Treatment can be divided into three phases. Initially the goal is minimizing hemorrhage with rest, elevation, compression, and ice packs. Isometric quadriceps exercises are permitted, but no other active or passive measures or physical therapy is used (7). This phase usually lasts 24 hours for mild cases and 48 hours for more severe cases. The goal of the second phase is restoration of movement, particularly extension. Flexion should be instituted slowly and at the patient's own pace. This is continued until 90° of flexion has been restored and crutches have been abandoned, with a normal gait achieved. The goal of

the third phase is restoration of the limb to normal function using progressive resistance exercises.

Rupture of the Quadriceps

Etiology and Pathophysiology

Rupture of a significant group of fibers of the rectus femoris can result from muscular violence alone or from the effect of a hard object, such as a kick with a boot or a head butt violently contacting the contracted quadriceps. Gross injuries occur when a heavy weight such as a beam or girder pins the limb against the ground and divides the muscle against the shaft of the femur (5, 7). Gross injuries of the vastus medialis can occur as a result of the limb being trapped, in which case the muscle fibers are divided, or as a result of an acute traumatic dislocation of the patella, when the rupture occurs close to the attachment of the bone. The vastus lateralis, which is seldom injured, appears to be protected by the powerful iliotibial tract. The vastus intermedius is most frequently damaged by hemorrhage that is produced by a kick or other form of direct violence.

Symptoms and Signs

With minor injuries of the rectus femoris patients complain of disabling pain on contracting the muscle. Examination reveals a small area of deep tenderness. With larger ruptures it might be possible to palpate a gap in the fibers, and this can be associated with discoloration of the skin. Frequently such patients are seen at a late stage, when they exhibit a swelling in the midline of the middle third of the thigh that consists of retractable muscle fibers above a shallow depression. This type of local rupture of the rectus femoris does not affect the strength of the quadriceps and seldom causes any real physical disability (7).

Diagnosis and Treatment

Diagnosis is made through the history and physical findings. Pain and tenderness can be relieved by injection of a dilute solution of local anesthetic (e.g., 0.125% bupivacaine) into the area, repeated at daily intervals. This usually permits immediate resumption of activities. Surgery can be done for cosmetic purposes but produces no effect on function (5, 7).

Reflex Spasm of the Quadriceps

Etiology

Various injuries and a few disease states can provoke bouts of reflex spasm of the quadriceps that can cause transient severe pain. The reflex spasm can be a result of impact injuries to the muscles or can be associated with acute or chronic diseases of the hip, and occasionally of the knee joint. My experience with 11 hip operations and observation of hundreds of patients who have undergone hip replacement or some other operative intervention on the hip suggest that bouts of severe reflex muscle spasm associated with excruciating pain are experienced by most patients. Surprisingly, these bouts of spasm occur on the second, third, or fourth postoperative day.

Pathophysiology

It has long been recognized that acute tissue damage caused by injury or visceral disease often provokes reflex spasm of the muscles that are supplied by the same and adjacent spinal cord segments as the site of injury. Whereas reflex spasm is intended to maintain homeostasis, often it produces complications (Chapter 25). Until recently it was believed that these reflexes were produced as a result of continuous nociceptive input from the site of injury, stimulating interneurons in the dorsal horn and motor neurons in the anterior horn, with a consequent increase in skeletal muscle tension and spasm. It has recently been shown that this massive nociceptive input not only stimulates various spinal cord neurons, the axons of which pass to the brain, but also sensitizes dorsal horn neurons, interneurons, and motor neurons, persisting for days and even for weeks or months (23). The increased sensitivity decreases the threshold of these cells, and as a result they can be activated by innocuous sensory stimulation such as light touch or proprioception (movement), which under normal conditions has no effect. This sensitization phenomenon is partly responsible for the production of hyperalgesia and allodynia in causalgia and other reflex sympathetic dystrophies, and for the abnormal motor response mentioned above. It explains why such spasm occurs days after the pain from the surgical wound has diminished.

Treatment

The usual intramuscular doses of potent opioids such as morphine are ineffective in preventing or relieving the intense reflex muscle spasm and the associated severe pain. Even patient-controlled analgesia, which produces a steady state of analgesia, does not provide sufficient relief. Intraspinal opioids dampen the reflex spasm, but only interruption of the afferent and efferent limbs of the reflexes with local anesthetic can relieve the spasm and prevent or eliminate the pain. This is best achieved by the administration of continuous epidural analgesia that extends from the T10 to the S2 segments, either through repeated boluses or by continuous infusion (Chapter 94). This blocks all nociceptive input from the hip joint, the area of the surgical incision, and the efferent somatomotor and sympathetic fibers to the quadriceps and other parts of the thigh. This method of postoperative pain relief not only completely relieves pain and prevents the reflex spasm but also permits earlier mobilization and reduces the length of hospitalization (20).

Infections

Osteomyelitis

Acute pyogenic osteomyelitis frequently involves the femur, which is one of the more commonly involved bones. The infection is carried to the femur through the bloodstream (hematogenous osteomyelitis) or is introduced through an external wound, especially in cases of compound fracture (5, 8). The lower end of the femur is affected more often than the upper end.

Chronic pyogenic osteomyelitis is almost always a sequel to acute infection that has been neglected or has responded poorly to treatment (5, 7). Although the lower end of the femur is usually affected more often than the upper end (as in acute cases), the infection often spreads to involve a large part of the femoral shaft.

Both acute and chronic osteomyelitis produce moderate to severe pain, fever, malaise, lethargy, and often vomiting. The clinical features of chronic osteomyelitis include local pain, draining sinuses, heat, swelling, tenderness, and erythema over the involved bone. A detailed discussion of the causes, pathophysiology, symptoms and signs, diagnosis, and treatment is found on pages 393 and 394.

Metabolic and Endocrine Disorders

The femur can be affected by various metabolic bone diseases, including osteoporosis, osteomalacia, osteitis fibrosa, and osteosclerosis. The femur is also one of the bones that can be affected by Paget's disease of bone, which is not a metabolic bone disorder. These conditions are discussed in detail in Chapter 23 (pages 395 and 398).

Neoplasms

The femur is one of the most common sites of benign and malignant tumors and of metastasis from other primary tumors.

Benign Tumors

The three most important benign tumors that involve the femur are osteoma, chondroma, and osteochondroma. Usually the first two produce little or no pain and require no therapy, except if their size indicates excision and curettage.

Primary Malignant Tumors

The femur is a common site of several types of primary malignant bone tumors—osteosarcoma, chondrosarcoma, fibrosarcoma, giant cell tumor, Ewing's tumor, and multiple myeloma (5, 8, 24–25). Osteosarcoma, next to multiple myeloma, is the most common primary malignant bone tumor, the majority occurring in and about the knee; the distal femur is the most common site and the proximal tibia is next in frequency. Osteosarcoma afflicts patients in the second decade of life. Chondrosarcoma, the second most common primary malignant bone tumor, involves the femur in 20% of such tumors; it occurs in the 4th, 5th, and 6th decades of life. Fibrosarcoma is also most frequently found in the distal femur and proximal tibia; in 50% of such lesions it occurs in the 3rd, 4th, and 5th decades of life. About 50% of all giant cell tumors arise in the region of the knee, half of them occurring in the distal femur and the other half in the proximal tibia. This tumor occurs in the 3rd and 4th decade of life (26). Multiple myeloma produces widespread osteolytic lesions throughout the skeleton, including parts of the femur and tibia; it afflicts persons between the ages of 50 and 70 (26). With all of these malignant tumors, moderate to severe pain in and around the knee joint is the most prominent symptom, often associated with swelling and tenderness. More details on these tumors are presented in the last subsection of this chapter.

Metastatic Neoplasms

The femur is commonly invaded by metastatic tumors, especially in its proximal half. Primary tumors that metastasize readily to the femur are carcinoma of the lungs, breast, prostate, kidneys, and thyroid (24). The bone structure is usually destroyed by the tumor and pathologic fractures are common. Pain is a predominant symptom and is especially severe with pathologic fractures.

Radiotherapy is often effective for a period of time and can promote union of a pathologic fracture. Metastasis from the thyroid can respond to radioactive iodine while metastasis from the breast, prostate, or thyroid can respond to hormone therapy, adrenalectomy, hypophysectomy, and other therapeutic modalities (Chapter 24). Most pathologic fractures of the femur are effectively managed by internal fixation with a nail plate or a long modified intramedullary nail, which decreases pain and facilitates nursing care.

D. PAINFUL DISORDERS OF THE KNEE JOINT

Traumatic Disorders

The knee is designed to be a shock-absorbing mechanism, and this can readily be appreciated when watching a skier traversing a mogul-dotted terrain. The major function of its muscle groups and ligamentous attachments, therefore, is to absorb the energy of the body as the foot is planted on the ground. Based on an individual's strength and the direction of the forces encountered, these forces either dissipate within these structures or exceed the ability of the knee to withstand them. An important characteristic of bone is that it is viscoelastic—that is, it is composed of both fluid and solid phases (26). This type of structure allows more energy to be dissipated and allows more variable loading rates than if the bone were comprised completely of the solid phase. Hence, the rate at which energy is applied results in a characteristic injury.

In general, a slower speed injury (i.e., occurring because of the leg twisting and turning with foot planted) results in damage to ligaments. As the fibrils of soft tissue are stretched they can no longer absorb energy; therefore, they are stretched beyond approximately 10% of their length and tear. In such cases a tear is a sprain or strain, as in the skier who catches a tip on a mogul. At high speeds, such as in automobile accidents, the soft tissues tear and the forces go on to be dissipated within the bony structure itself, causing fractures. Patellar fractures and dislocations are usually seen in association with these high-energy impact forces. In addition, the minor trauma of repeated low-energy stresses can cause overuse syndromes.

Fractures

Fractures in the region of the knee joint are frequent causes of pain and disability. Unless properly managed they can produce prolonged or even permanent impairment of joint function. Some of these fractures are complicated and difficult to manage; only an overview, however, is presented here.

Etiology and Pathophysiology

Fractures about the knee joint include fractures of the distal end of the femur, the proximal end of the tibia, and the patella (Fig. 75-20). Fractures of the distal end of the femur include supracondylar, intercondylar, and condylar fractures, and fractures of the tibial plateau include fractures involving the lateral or medial condyle with or without comminution or displacement, and with variable degree of depression (5–7). The patella can sustain a transverse or comminuted fracture. Injury is sometimes sustained by the cartilage, such as chondral fractures that involve the articular cartilage or osteochondral fractures that involve the articular cartilage and underlying subcondylar bone.

Fractures about the knee joint are generally the result of severe direct violence caused by a vehicular accident or a severe direct blow to the joint. They can also be torsion injuries, with a fixed foot internally or externally rotated in relation to the femur, or can be a result of cartilaginous damage secondary to subluxation of the patella.

Symptoms and Signs

Invariably, moderate to severe pain is experienced at the time of injury and remains a predominant symptom until healing occurs. The pain is usually a continuous, dull, aching discomfort associated with bouts of sharp pain. It is generally localized to the knee region but can spread to the lower thigh and upper leg. The continuous severe pain is unrelated to weight-bearing or movement, although these markedly aggravate it. Associated with the pain are exquisite tenderness

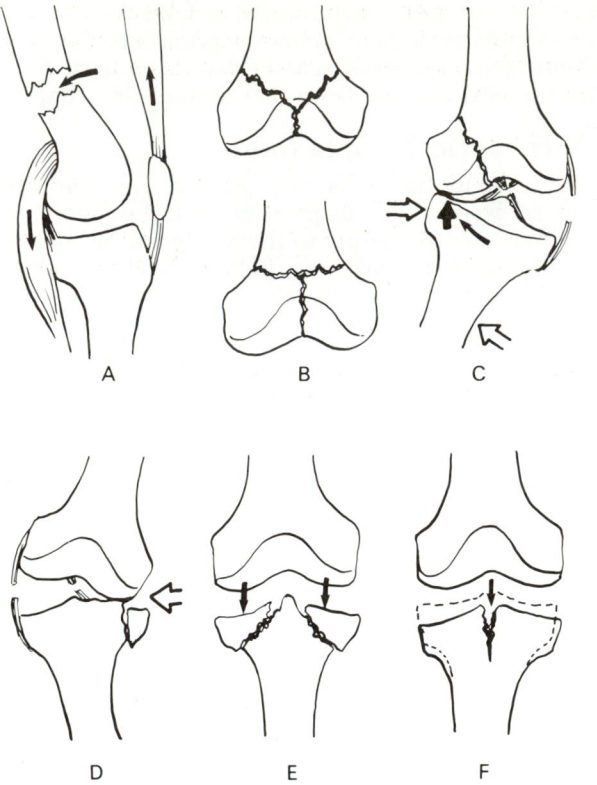

FIG. 75-20. Various types of fractures of the bones of the knee joint. **A.** Supracondylar fracture with the gastrocnemius pulling the distal fragments posteriorly into the popliteal fossa and the hamstring and quadriceps pulling to shorten the femur. **B.** Intercondylar fracture of the distal femur: Y fracture (*top*); T fracture (*bottom*). **C.** Condylar fracture from severe valgus (varus) stress. Force applied to the knee joint or laterally to the tibia (*arrows*) can cause fracture of the femoral condyle, tear of the opposite collateral ligament, and tear of either or both of the cruciate ligaments, with compression of the meniscus. **D.** Fracture of one tibial plateau. Direct trauma to the tibial plateau, such as a fall on extended legs, can cause a Y fracture (**E**) or a T fracture (**F**) of the plateau. Modified from Cailliet, R.: Knee Pain and Disability. 2nd Ed. Philadelphia, F.A. Davis, 1983.

localized to the area of injury, crepitation, effusion, usually caused by hemarthrosis, and disability that varies depending on the site and severity of the injury.

Diagnosis

The history of gross trauma together with the findings and inspection of the knee are usually sufficient to indicate fracture. In such circumstances it is important to avoid gross movements during the examination, and if the fracture is severe observation of the patient's gait is avoided. Radiographs are usually diagnostic but can be unrewarding in cases of chondral fracture (5, 6). Needle aspiration is performed under strict aseptic techniques using local infiltration analgesia in a patient with a large effusion. The aspiration of blood suggests an intra-articular fracture or fracture that is not detectable on plain radiographs.

Treatment

The treatment of fractures and other severe injuries has four objectives: effective pain relief, mobilization of the injured part, early motion, and rehabilitation and strengthening.

PAIN CONTROL. The relief of pain is discussed above in Section B. Briefly, opioids are used at the site of injury and while transporting the patient to the hospital but, once in the hospital, more effective measures for relieving the pain and suppressing abnormal reflex spasm should be used. These entail the use of continuous epidural analgesia achieved with dilute solutions of a local anesthetic and opioids during the preoperative period and epidural anesthesia with stronger solutions of local anesthetics for the operation (see pp. 374–375). Unfortunately, many orthopedic and general surgeons who manage patients with knee injuries are unaware of the use of these measures or skilled personnel are not available to carry them out. Consequently general anesthesia is often used. This entails not only the risk of pulmonary complications, but, unless muscle relaxants are given to the point of apnea, adequate relaxation of the affected muscle is not produced. Even worse is the fact that many physicians give adult patients 5 to 10 mg of diazepam (Valium) over 5 to 10 minutes and then attempt to reduce fractures. Some also administer 30 to 50 mg of meperidine or 2 to 4 mg of morphine IM and then attempt to reduce the fracture within the next 15 to 20 minutes. Diazepam has no analgesic action but is primarily an anxiolytic agent and produces only minimal relaxation of skeletal muscles, so it is totally inadequate for reduction of fractures. Opioids can relieve pain but IM doses require 45 minutes to produce their peak effect, with only partial relief of pain, and cause no relaxation of skeletal muscles.

ORTHOPEDIC MANAGEMENT. Management of fractures obviously depends on the exact mechanisms of the fracture, the alignment of the fragments, the articular integrity, and proper joint surface alignment (7). Basic principles that underlie all treatment include removal of fragments, removal of associated meniscus tears, replacement of fragments by internal fixation, and reconstruction of the extensor mechanisms involved (6). Many fractures of the knee can be treated by closed reduction but, in complicated cases, open reduction is necessary. The joint should be aspirated prior to an attempt at reduction, if it is distended with blood.

Closed reduction is usually carried out with skeletal traction to achieve alignment of the bones. Following reduction a plaster spica cast is applied and isometric exercises of the quadriceps are started immediately. Because of the critical role of the patella in the functioning of the knee joint, it is essential to try to preserve the patella when it has been fractured. Surgical removal of the patella should be considered only if it has been severely comminuted, leaving no single fragment large enough to be useful.

Dislocations

Complete dislocation of the knee joint, involving the lower end of the femur and the upper end of the tibia, is fortunately uncommon in relation to injuries of the joint in general (7). Dislocation of the superior tibiofibular joint is also an unusual injury. In contrast, dislocation of the patella is relatively frequent and is often followed by recurrent dislocation.

Etiology and Pathophysiology

Complete dislocation of the knee joint can occur only as a result of the most extreme direct violence applied to the lower end of the femur when the upper end of the tibia is firmly fixed, or to the upper end of the tibia when the femur is fixed (7). This can be classified according to the relations of the tibia to the femur as anterior, posterior, lateral, medial, or rotary. All types involve partial or complete rupture of the collateral and cruciate ligaments and injury of the popliteus, gastrocnemius, and vastus medialis muscles.

Dislocation of the superior tibiofibular joint usually presents in combination with fracture of the lateral condyle of the tibia or as an isolated injury.

Lateral dislocation or subluxation of the patella from its femoropatellar groove occurs when a violent force is directed against the medial aspect of the bone. Such an insult can occur as a result of a severe fall or an external injury such as an automobile accident or athletic injury, with violent lateral rotatory stress imposed on the knee of the weight-bearing leg (6, 7). In such circumstances not only are the medial capsule and adjacent attachments of the vastus medialis to the patella likely to be torn, but a medial tangential osteochondral fracture of the patella has probably been sustained. In rare instances the bone can be dislocated medially or inferiorly, or can be rotated on its axis.

Symptoms and Signs

At the time of dislocation, almost all patients experience severe, acute, and agonizing pain, usually localized to the site of injury. Those with complete anterior dislocation of the joint experience agonizing pain in the popliteal fossa. The pain is likely to continue as a result of injury to the ligaments, capsule, and muscles. The injury is soon followed by gross swelling. If anterior dislocation has occurred the popliteal artery might be damaged, whereas the common peroneal or tibial nerves can be damaged with medial and lateral dislocation, with consequent neurologic symptoms (5, 7).

Patients with dislocation of the superior tibiofibular joint experience pain and tenderness over the head of the fibula and lateral ligament, together with pain on attempting to adduct the joint. Movements of the knee are usually not markedly restricted and no general swelling or soft tissue or synovial effusion is present (7). Some patients incur damage to the common peroneal nerve.

Patients who sustain patellar dislocation and subluxation also experience severe pain. The knee has a tendency to buckle, causing patients to fall or lose their balance and to develop tenderness over the anterior knee area (6, 7). Effusion is frequent but not as severe as in an internal knee injury and it is usually difficult to extend the knee (7). Patients who have recurrent dislocation of the patella experience the same symptoms; in addition, if the knee is extended it attaches actively to the patella when it returns to its normal position. Examination for recurrent patellar dislocation usually reveals increased laxity of the extensor mechanism and excessive movements of the patella in the lateral direction. The vastus medialis can be atro-phied and crepitation can be felt and heard between the patella and its femoral groove. Radiographic studies in the adult can reveal a malformed patella or shallow femoral condyle.

Diagnosis

Diagnosis of dislocation around the knee joint is usually made from a detailed history, especially in regard to the mechanism of injury, and from inspection and palpation of the knee. Radiographic studies confirm the diagnosis.

Treatment

Patients with severe pain should be given an appropriate IV dose of opioid, repeated once or twice at intervals of 15 to 20 minutes. During this time patients are evaluated. For closed reduction of the dislocation, it is essential to have elimination of the pain and complete relaxation. Many orthopedic authorities (6, 7) have stated that reduction "is accomplished by manipulation under general anesthesia," but general anesthesia should be avoided because many patients have undigested food, entailing the risk of vomiting or regurgitation and aspiration of gastric contents. Therefore, regional anesthesia in the form of subarachnoid or continuous epidural block is preferable. The former has the advantage of rapid induction and thus might be more effective for patients who require urgent intervention because of damage to the popliteal artery. Regional anesthesia can be used not only for closed reduction but for any open operation that might be required. It is especially advantageous for those with circulatory insufficiency caused by popliteal arterial damage. Continuous epidural analgesia should be maintained in such patients during the postoperative period to provide not only pain relief but also vasomotor block, thus decreasing the risk of ischemia of the limb (Chapter 94).

Ligamentous and Capsular Injuries

Normally, ligaments about a joint prevent abnormal excessive motion of that joint. When an injury causes excessive joint motion, however, the ligament is injured, and this constitutes a sprain (5–7). Sprains can vary from complete tear of the ligament with or without avulsion of the fragment of bone to which it is attached to minor tearing of a few fibers without loss of integrity of the ligament. The tear can be longitudinal, transverse, or oblique, and can result in elongation of the remaining ligamentous fibers. "Strain" is the term used for a condition in which a physical force imposed on the ligamentous tissue possibly exceeds that produced by normal stress but does not cause deformation or damage to the ligament, and physiologic recovery usually follows (6). Sprains of the ligaments of the knee joint are frequent in individuals who are active in sports, but can also occur as a result of an accident.

Etiology and Pathophysiology

Injury to the ligaments and capsule of the knee joint are produced by abnormal motion, including excessive abduction or adduction of the extended knee, excessive rotation, severe hyperextension or hyperflexion, or a combination of these. Ligamentous injuries are generally classified as mild, moderate, or severe (5–7). In a mild injury a few fibers are torn but the integrity of the ligament is maintained and the joint remains stable. In moderate injuries the fibers are torn enough to decrease ligamentous function but still maintain joint stability. Some excessive joint motion is evident as compared to that of the other side. A severe injury entails complete tearing of fibers, with loss of integrity and evidence of joint instability.

Symptoms and Signs

The patient with a mild sprain can experience mild to moderate pain that is aggravated by palpation of the injured ligament or by stressing it. Associated with pain are tenderness and some local swelling, but no effusion or locking is present and the joint appears stable. Movements that stress the affected ligament can be painful. The patient with a moderate sprain has similar signs and symptoms but can also have locking of the joint if a concurrent meniscus injury has occurred, moderate joint effusion, or hemarthrosis. Some instability might also be present (5, 7).

A severe ligamentous sprain (Fig. 75-21) is characterized by tearing of the ligament through its substance and retraction from its attachment with or without avulsion of a piece of bone or cartilage, and causes immediate and severe pain and disability. Swelling, if it occurs, is immediate and usually marked, and locking can occur because of a concomitant tear in the meniscus or because of the severity of the effusion. Marked joint disability results.

Diagnosis

Early examination is of utmost importance before swelling, pain, and protective reflex muscle spasm obscure the clinical picture. Radiographs taken with valgus or varus stress reveal excessive motion of the joint. Tests for assessing the condition of the collateral and cruciate ligaments of the knee are shown in Figures 75-17 and 75-18.

Treatment

Treatment of ligamentous tear is discussed on page 381. In brief, treatment of mild strain consists of relief of pain by administration of NSAIDs, restriction of activities, and initial application of ice packs followed by heat. Cold and heat can be alternated, and a compression bandage can then be applied.

Treatment of moderate sprains consists of complete resting of the knee by bed rest or wheelchair, with the leg elevated, and application of ice packs, which are helpful for the first 48 to 72 hours. Ambulation for personal needs should be done with the aid of crutches but the involved limb should not bear weight. The joint should be aspirated if effusion is moderate or marked and should be repeated if it recurs. When pain and effusion cease heat can be applied (7).

Treatment of severe ligamentous tears and resulting instability can be managed by prolonged conservative treatment or by surgical intervention. In addition to the use of appropriate analgesics, ice packs, and immobilization, conservative treatment consists of re-education and redevelopment of the quadriceps muscle.

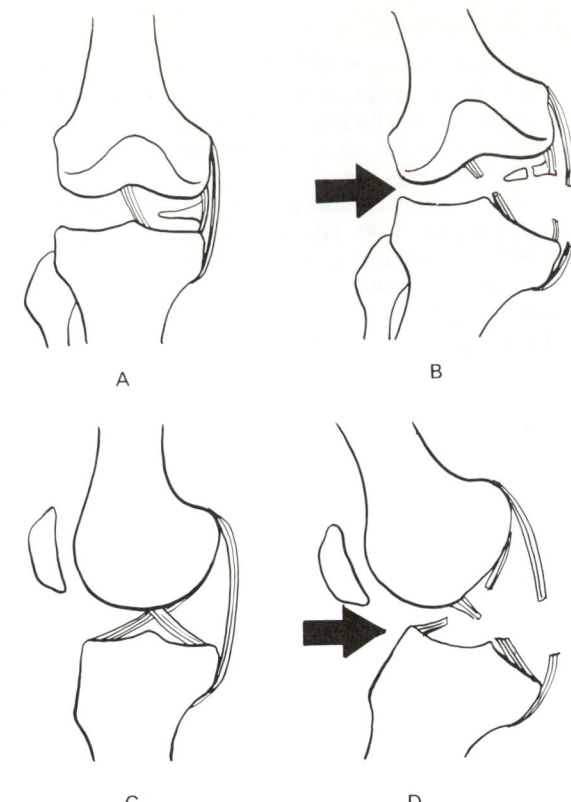

FIG. 75-21. Severe ligamentous sprain. **A.** Anterior view of a normal joint. **B.** Severe lateral stress disrupts the medial collateral ligaments, medial meniscus, and anterior cruciate ligament; this is known as the unhappy triad. **C.** Lateral view of normal joint. **D.** Severe anterior stress. This can produce hyperextension of the joint and disrupt both the anterior and posterior cruciate ligaments and the posterior capsule. Examination reveals a positive drawer sign. Modified from Cailliet, R.: Knee Pain and Disability. 2nd Ed. Philadelphia, F.A. Davis, 1983.

This must be done conscientiously and vigorously pursued for at least 3 months. Smillie (7) has suggested that no operative reconstruction of the medial ligaments can be expected to be effective in the absence of normal quadriceps control. Therefore, no surgery should be considered until nonweight-bearing exercises have been done for 3 months. Surgical intervention can be considered in carefully selected patients with tears of the medial or lateral collateral ligaments or of the anterior cruciate ligament.

Meniscal Injuries

Injuries to a meniscus invariably cause sudden severe pain and disability. The damage to the meniscus occurs as a result of compressive or traction forces or a combination of these. Injury results from bearing weight on the knee combined with faulty, forceful, or excessive motion, either in flexion-rotation or extension-rotation (6, 7). A combination of weight-bearing with rotatory stress during flexion and extension is an important cause of meniscus injury (see page 383 for a detailed discussion of the symptoms and signs of miniscal injuries).

Inflammatory and Degenerative Diseases

The knee joint is a common site of various arthritides and synovitis. All these conditions are manifested by pain, swelling, tenderness, and impairment or loss of function. Arthritides are discussed in Chapter 20, so here only a few comments relevant to the knee joint are made. Synovitis and bursitis are then discussed in more detail.

Arthritides

Pyogenic arthritis is more common in the knee joint than in most other joints (see pages 347 and 348), partly because the knee is exposed to injury and partly because of the close relationship of the joint cavity to the lower metaphysis of the femur, which is one of the common sites of acute osteomyelitis. The condition is usually acute or subacute in onset with moderate to severe pain, swelling, and loss of function. Radiography might not reveal any abnormality in the early stages. Treatment consists of immediate aspiration to determine the offending organism and consequent appropriate antibiotic therapy.

Rheumatoid arthritis often affects the knee joint and is thus a common cause of mild to moderate or severe pain, tenderness, stiffness, and swelling of the knee joint caused by synovial thickening (see pages 335 to 340). Palpation reveals that the region is warm but not hot. Movements are impaired and, if these are forced, they markedly aggravate the pain. Bowleg or knock-knee deformity can occur. The goal of treatment is to reduce pain and swelling to preserve joint function, so that activities of daily living are not restricted. Pain should be controlled by NSAIDs, given alone or with modest doses of weak opioids.

Hemophilic arthritis affects the knee more often than any other joint in the body (26). It is characterized by hemorrhage into the joint; with rest the blood is slowly reabsorbed, but further bleeding usually occurs (5, 27). With each episode of bleeding the knee becomes swollen, partly from contaminated blood and partly from synovial thickening. The overlying skin is abnormally warm and joint movements are restricted and painful. The condition can recur. Treatment includes control of pain and aspiration of the knee under the temporary cover of antihemophilic factor.

Formerly, tuberculous arthritis of the knee was often another cause of knee pain and impairment, usually in children or younger adults. Currently it is uncommon in industrialized and medically advanced countries. This and other less common forms of arthritides are discussed elsewhere (Chapter 20).

Osteoarthritis of the Knee

The knee is affected by osteoarthritis more often than any other joint (5). It is one of the most common afflictions seen in patients over the age of 60 (28).

Etiology and Pathophysiology

In most patients the cause of osteoarthritis of the knee is not known (28). It is not clear whether it is secondary to repeated traumatic episodes during the lifetime of the joint or is a programmed response secondary to aging. A predisposing factor is overweight. The result continues to be loss of cartilage, loss of lubricating qualities, increased osteophyte formation, and inflammatory changes, which produce pain. The osteophytes can expand the capsular structures and cause stretching of tendons over prominences about the knee, causing additional pain (9).

Symptoms and Signs

Early degenerative changes can be asymptomatic until synovitis develops, accompanied by effusion, stiffness, capsular thickening, and formation of large osteophytes (9). Inflammatory changes, osteophytes, and stretching of the tendons cause pain that is aggravated by activity. The pain is dull and aching and is usually poorly localized in and around the knee, or it can be localized to the medial or lateral aspect of the joint (28). Stiffness lasting less than 30 minutes is present in the morning or after prolonged rest during the day, but improves with activity. Atrophy and weakness of the quadriceps muscle develop with progression of the arthritis. Crepitus might be noted with flexion of the knee. The knee becomes unstable with loss of ligamentous and muscle support, and the patient might be hesitant to walk on uneven surfaces. On examination, the knee is found to be slightly thickened from hypertrophy of bone at the joint margin, where a rim of osteophytes might be palpable.

Diagnosis

Diagnosis is based on physical and radiographic findings. The first clear sign of osteoarthritis of the knee is sharpening or "spiking" of the joint margins, especially of the patella and tibia. Later, narrowing of the cartilaginous space is obvious. Osteophytes form at the joint margin and the subchondral bone can become sclerotic (5, 8). Special radiographic views and CT scans or MRI provide more specific information on the pathophysiology of osteoarthritis of the knee.

Treatment

The general treatment of osteoarthritis is discussed on page 335. Pain and inflammation are controlled by giving salicylates or other NSAIDs. Physical therapy includes the application of hot moist packs or some other form of heat and a supervised program of exercises, with emphasis on the quadriceps muscle. Overweight patients benefit from weight reduction programs.

In patients for whom conservative management is ineffective and who continue to have persistent severe pain associated with deformity, operative intervention is indicated. The most common procedures include removal of loose bodies, upper tibial osteotomy, excision of the patella, and arthroplasty that involves placement of a knee prosthesis (8). Arthrodesis can be the appropriate intervention in severe cases, especially when other operations have failed and when the other knee and hips are normal (5).

Bursitis

Any of the bursae around the knee (see above, Basic Considerations) can become swollen and asymptomatic or can become inflamed and swollen and cause pain and tenderness (8). The bursitis can be acute, chronic, or recurrent. Because they produce discomfort the bursae should be considered in the differential diagnosis of pain in the knee. The most important bursae are the prepatellar, infrapatellar or deep infrapatellar, gastrocnemius, semimembranosus, and posterior. Baker's cyst is a distension of the posterior bursa but is usually not painful. It is generally treated conservatively unless the enlargement impairs function of the knee and requires excision.

Etiology and Pathophysiology

The most frequent cause of prepatellar bursitis is chronic microtrauma in those accustomed to working on their knees or who are returning to work after a prolonged absence (8). Prolonged continuous or repeated pressure or microtrauma are important factors. The deep infrapatellar bursa is rarely affected by disease or injury but can be subjected to effusion as a result of a direct blow over the ligament.

Symptoms and Signs

Patients with acute or chronic bursitis experience pain caused by tension of the skin in extreme knee flexion or by direct pressure, local tenderness, swelling, and inflammation. The bursitis can be on one side or can occur bilaterally, depending on whether one or both knees experience the microtrauma. The swelling is readily distinguishable from that of intra-articular synovial effusion because it remains the same size and consistency on straight leg raising, showing that it is outside the joint.

Diagnosis and Treatment

Diagnosis is based on the history and on physical and radiographic findings. Treatment depends on whether the condition is acute or chronic and on the cause. An acute attack results from a single incident of trauma or unaccustomed kneeling. The condition usually resolves with aspiration of the fluid and the application of a compressive bandage; this is often curative because it keeps the opposing synovial surfaces in contact. If the history reveals that the swelling was not previously present but occurred within half an hour after some trivial injury, the effusion is likely to be blood (hemobursitis). Treatment consists of aspiration and elastic compression to bring the opposing surfaces into contact. In some cases the bursa and the fluid contained therein become infected, necessitating appropriate systemic antibiotics for treatment. Sometimes bursitis subsides with aspiration; a bursitis that fails to subside with aspiration frequently becomes chronically distended or is the subject of recurrent effusion, and requires total excision of the inflamed and thickened bursa (8).

Synovitis

Synovitis is a reaction of the synovial membrane to irritation, with consequent effusion into the membrane. In cases of acute synovitis pain and swelling are the predominant symptoms (8). Chronic synovitis can be asymptomatic in the early stages but eventually it produces pain, which prompts patients to consult a physician months after onset. Treatment of patients by bed rest with the knee flexed over a pillow until the effusion subsides is likely to cause wasting of the quadriceps muscle, which then adds to the initial injury and produces more effusion, thus maintaining a vicious cycle (8).

Etiology and Pathophysiology

Exogenous trauma is the most common cause of acute synovitis (8). This could be a single instance of a direct or twisting injury or could be the result of microtrauma caused by repeated stress of the knee joint associated with certain types of work. Another cause of "unrecognized trauma" is injury sustained in the course of surgery (8). This might cause persistent effusion, or patients could develop postoperative synovitis because of a premature return to weight-bearing without adequate quadriceps rehabilitation (7, 8). The trauma is sometimes endogenous in the form of microtrauma—for example certain joint configurations might be accepted as being within the limits of normality but could be mechanically unsound and fail to withstand prolonged activity (7, 8). Other causes of acute synovitis include synovial irritation by extra-articular foreign bodies such as shotgun pellets; or gout, pseudogout, or some other chronic condition involving the joint could be a causative factor. Chronic synovitis that lasts months and sometimes years can be associated with chronic rheumatic fever, infectious arthritis, ankylosing spondylitis, familial Mediterranean fever, and other systemic disorders (8).

Symptoms and Signs

In addition to the effusion, acute synovitis invariably produces continuous deep aching pain and tenderness, often limitation of motion and, if the condition is caused by factors other than trauma, manifestations of regional or systemic disease are also present. A serious byproduct of the condition is atrophy or wasting of the quadriceps muscle because of immobility.

Diagnosis

Diagnosis of trauma-induced synovitis is made through a detailed history, especially querying the patient about even mild trauma in the past and about any treatment that has been given. Synovitis resulting from endogenous trauma requires careful examination of the knee joint to detect any subtle abnormalities. Radiography is essential to demonstrate the presence of extra-articular foreign bodies or evidence of local pathology. If diagnostic doubt exists, arthroscopy is done.

Treatment

Treatment of acute synovitis of any cause consists of the application of a compression bandage, aspiration if the volume of fluid prevents complete extension, and varying degrees of rest, depending on the underlying pathology, and aggressive quadriceps exercises. If rest from weight-bearing is necessary, quadriceps exercises should not be postponed beyond the acute phase or longer than 4 days (3, 5, 8). Effective relief from mild to moderate pain can be achieved with appropriate doses of NSAIDs given alone or with moderate doses of codeine. If patients experience moderate to severe pain that inhibits or discourages them from carrying out the exercises, strong opioids given at regular intervals should be considered. For inpatients the pain is most effectively controlled with continuous intraspinal opioids or epidural analgesia, which has the advantages cited above.

Pigmented Villonodular Synovitis

Pigmented villonodular synovitis is a proliferation of synovial tissue with recurrent bloody effusion. The condition occurs in two forms, a circumscribed nodular or pedunculated form and a diffuse form (8).

The clinical features of the circumscribed form include small areas of local swelling, the presence of which might be unknown to the patient. The condition can cause a transient effusion. The diffuse form is characterized by widespread synovial thickening with voluminous swelling. These conditions can be differentiated from those caused by the presence of loose bodies in the joint.

Treatment of the circumscribed or pedunculated type consists of excision of part of the structure to which it is attached. Treatment of the diffuse type involves a complete synovectomy as the condition dictates and circumstances permit (8).

Other Painful Articular Disorders

This section reviews other painful disorders that involve bone, ligaments, and other soft tissues of the knee joint. These conditions include osteochondritis dissecans, loose bodies in the knee, chondromalacia patellae, apophysitis of the tibial tubercle, Pellegrini-Stieda disease, and neoplasms.

Osteochondritis Dissecans

Osteochondritis dissecans is a condition of unknown origin characterized by local necrosis of a segment of the articular surface of the bone and overlying articular cartilage, with eventual separation of the fragment to form an intra-articular loose body. The knee is affected more often than any other joint, with 85% of lesions appearing on the medial or central portion of the medial femoral condyle and 15% occurring laterally (8, 29, 30). The condition is more common in adolescents than young adults, less common in patients in their thirties and forties, and rare in the elderly. It occurs three times more often in males than in females (30).

Etiology and Pathophysiology

The cause is unknown, although injury is an important predisposing factor (30). The lesion has been reported as an autosomal dominant condition in families; it has been found to affect several members of a family or several joints in the same patient (31).

The lesion consists of an island or fragment of bone in the femoral condyle and consists of subchondral bone with its articular cartilage, which is usually 1 to 2 cm in diameter (30). The subchondral bone is avascular, and a clear line of demarcation forms between this segment and the surrounding normal bone and cartilage. After many months the fragment separates as one, two, or three loose bodies, leaving a shallow cavity in the articular surface that is ultimately filled with fibrocartilage. The damage to the joint surface predisposes the patient to the development of osteoarthritis years later (5, 8, 30).

Symptoms and Signs

The patient usually complains of pain in the knee after exercise, a feeling of insecurity in the knee, and intermittent swelling of the knee joint (8). With separation of the loose body within the joint, the predominant symptom is recurrent sudden locking. Examination reveals effusion of the joint, atrophy of the quadriceps, and impairment of movement.

Diagnosis

The diagnosis is suspected from the history and symptoms and signs and is confirmed by radiography, which shows a clear-cut defect of the bone at the articular surface of the medial or lateral femoral condyle. The lesion is best shown in the tangential posterior-anterior projection with the knee semiflexed (5).

Treatment

In the developmental stage treatment should be expectant and conservative (5, 8). The knee is supported with a bandage and strenuous activities are curtailed. In the early stages the lesion heals spontaneously, especially in younger adolescents. When a clear demarcation has been formed between the separating fragment and the surrounding normal bone, the loose piece(s) should be removed arthroscopically, especially if small. The shallow cavity that is left in the condyle gradually fills with fibrocartilage and adequate function is usually restored (5, 8).

Loose Bodies in the Knee

In addition to osteochondritis dissecans, the knee joint is most commonly affected by the formation of loose bodies in patients with osteoarthritis. Patients can have from 1 to 10 loose bodies and chip fracture of the joint surface. In cases of synovial chondromatosis, 50 to 500 loose bodies have been reported (5).

Symptoms and Signs

The most prominent symptom is recurrent locking of the joint caused by interposition of the loose piece between the joint surfaces, which usually occurs suddenly without warning and is accompanied by severe pain (5, 8). Patients can often disengage the loose bodies and free the joint by maneuvering the limb. The knee is subsequently found to be swollen with fluid. Because few patients are seen by the physician when the knee is locked, physical examination can be normal except for effusion of the joint. If the condition occurs frequently enough and patients decrease activity, some atrophy of the quadriceps muscle might occur. Sometimes a loose body can be palpated.

Diagnosis and Treatment

The diagnosis is suspected from the history and can be confirmed by radiography, which reveals the loose bodies; often they are in the suprapatellar pouch (5). If the loose body produces no locking or other symptoms or signs, the treatment should be expectant. On the other hand, if recurrent locking occurs, arthroscopic removal of the loose bodies is indicated, especially if the locking occurs frequently enough to affect the quadriceps muscle.

Spontaneous Osteonecrosis

Spontaneous osteonecrosis, also called osteochondritis dissecans of the elderly, involves the medial femoral condyle and affects women over the age of 60 (32).

Etiology and Pathophysiology

The cause of spontaneous osteonecrosis, like that of juvenile osteochondritis dissecans, is unknown. The lesion is in the weight-bearing area of the medial femoral condyle. It is characterized by the presence of a horizontal cleavage lesion with a displaced flap of meniscus (8). Microtrauma might be an important contributing factor to this condition.

Symptoms and Signs

The patient usually presents with a history of spontaneous and sudden onset of intense pain at the medial condyle of the femur (32). The pain decreases in intensity from severe to moderate and is associated with tenderness to deep pressure over the medial femoral condyle, with pain aggravated at the limit of forced flexion. Occasionally synovial effusion is present.

Diagnosis and Treatment

The history of sudden spontaneous pain, together with the physical findings, should be helpful in the diagnosis. Radiography done in the early stages shows a flattening of the articular cartilage of the condyle and later a zone of translucency surrounded by a halo of sclerosis with or without a nidus of dead subchondral bone (9). Strontium-85 scintigraphy shows values in the affected condyle that are five to ten times greater than those of the normal knee (8).

Treatment should be conservative, consisting of NSAIDs to control pain and the use of crutches to reduce the effect of weight-bearing. If clinical and radiologic evidence reveals that an osteocartilaginous loose body is separating, arthrotomy for the removal of the loose body is indicated.

Chondromalacia Patellae

Chondromalacia patellae is a morbid softening, fissuring, and degenerative process of the articular surface of the kneecap (30, 32, 34, 35).

Etiology and Pathophysiology

This condition can have many causes, such as excessive use and stress during athletic activity, disuse following prolonged traction or cast immobilization, direct injury such as a blow to the patella, impact of the knee on a car dashboard during an accident, an old patellar fracture with imperfect reduction, or continuous direct pressure caused by a long-leg plaster cast (8, 33, 34, 35). The condition can be classified into four grades, depending on the degree of swelling or fibrillation, the size of fissuring, and fragmentation. Grade 4 is characterized by erosion of the articular cartilage down to subchondral bone (8). In almost 75% of patients the lesion is located within an ellipse passing transversely across the central area of the patella, with the superior and inferior thirds of the articular surface nearly always being spared (8).

Symptoms and Signs

The most prominent symptom consists of pain or severe aching experienced in or under the patella and aggravated by movements that oppose the patella and femur under compression, as in ascending or descending stairs or rising from a chair (8, 30, 33). Localized aching also occurs after periods of immobility with the knee in the flexed position, such as prolonged periods of watching television or working at a desk. Associated with the pain are stiffness of the joint and impaired movement, and occasionally momentary locking. Crepitation and grinding, usually corresponding directly to the degree of surface cartilaginous disruption, can be sensed by the patient and easily palpated by the physician, who places the palm on the patella and has the patient actively flex and extend the knee (8).

Diagnosis

Diagnosis is suspected from the history and physical examination but can only be confirmed by arthroscopic visualization of the pathology of the patellofemoral joint.

Treatment

Patients should be reassured that no serious problem exists and that the pain is the worst feature of the condition. It is critical to monitor patients so that they exercise the quadriceps by straight leg raising and progressively loaded straight leg raising. Smillie has cautioned against using resistance exercises in which the patellofemoral joint is heavily loaded and has also warned against immobilization in any form (8). If symptoms and signs are associated with a severe grade of pathology, consideration should be given to repair of identifiable mechanical defects, such as malalignment of the extensor mechanism, lateral capsular release, and tibial tubercle elevation. Patellectomy should only be considered in patients with severe symptoms and signs in whom no other procedure has been successful, because patellectomy results in a 30 to 40% loss of quadriceps muscle power (30, 34).

Apophysitis of the Tibial Tubercle

Apophysitis of the tibial tubercle, also known as Osgood-Schlatter disease, is a childhood affliction in which the tibial tubercle becomes enlarged and temporarily painful. The condition constitutes a strain on the developing tibial tubercle caused by the pull of the patellar tendon (5–8). The condition usually occurs in children 10 to 14 years of age, and males are affected more frequently than females (5, 8).

Symptoms and Signs

The predominant symptom is pain in front of and below the knee that is aggravated by strenuous activity (8). On examination the tibial tubercles are unduly prominent and are tender on palpation. Pain is increased when the quadriceps is tensed as for straight leg raising against resistance. The knee joint itself is normal and the symptoms and signs are confined to the region of the tibial tubercle (5).

Diagnosis and Treatment

The diagnosis is made on the history and physical examination and is confirmed by radiography, which reveals enlargement and sometimes fragmentation of the tibial tubercle. The disorder is self-limiting and normal function is generally restored (5, 8). In many cases treatment is not required but, if local pain and tenderness are severe, the knee should be rested and a plaster cylinder extending from the groin to the malleoli should be applied.

Pellegrini-Stieda Disease

Pellegrini-Stieda disease is ossification in a subligamentous hematoma after partial avulsion of the medial ligament from the medial condyle of the femur (5). A related condition is calcified deposits within the medial or lateral ligament.

Symptoms and Signs

Patients with Pellegrini-Stieda disease complain of persistent pain and tenderness at the medial side of the knee after an injury to the medial ligament. Usually thickening and tenderness are found at the site of attachment of the ligament to the medial femoral condyle.

Diagnosis and Treatment

Radiography reveals a thin plaque of new bone close to the medial condyle and calcified deposits in the medial collateral ligament.

Treatment of Pellegrini-Stieda disease consists of active mobilization and muscle strengthening exercises. Patients with painful calcified ligaments, a lesion homologous to supraspinatus tendinitis, should have the calcified material removed by aspiration or surgery (5).

Neoplastic Diseases

Neoplastic lesions of the knee, of either the bone or soft tissues, must always be considered in the differential diagnosis. Because neoplasms that affect the lower end of the femur and upper tibia have been mentioned, here we will elaborate on two benign tumors and on the pathophysiology and treatment of malignant tumors.

Benign Tumors

Osteochondromatosis

Among the benign tumors, osteochondromatosis (synovial chondromatosis) is most common in the knee. It consists of numerous osteocartilaginous or cartilaginous loose bodies formed by abnormal synovial membrane (36). They develop as a result of metaplasia of the membrane and subsynovial connective tissue. They are usually regarded as benign, but malignant change to chondrosarcoma has been reported (25). The presenting complaint is likely to be pain that is progressive and is of long standing, accompanied by swelling, stiffness, and possibly locking incidents. On examination limitation of movement is found. Sometimes the loose bodies are palpable and their presence is known to the patient.

Diagnosis is made by radiography and arthroscopy. Treatment varies from simple removal of the loose bodies to local synovectomy and total anterior synovectomy, but the latter is associated with the risk of rotation of movement (5, 8, 36). In some patients removal of the loose bodies or subtotal synovectomy is followed by spontaneous regression of the disease.

Osteoid Osteoma

Osteoid osteoma is a benign neoplasm characterized by severe but poorly localized pain that is worse at night. It occurs more frequently in males than in females, in the 2nd decade of life (37). The pain is out of proportion to physical and radiologic findings, which might lead to misdiagnosis of the condition. Diagnosis is made by a radiographic feature of a zone of sclerotic bone that surrounds a small area of translucency in the center, usually in the medial epiphysis of the femur. Treatment is by excision of the block of bone that contains the lesion.

Malignant Tumors

As mentioned in Section C, the most important primary malignant tumors that affect the bones of the knee joint, i.e., the lower femur and upper tibia, are osteosarcoma, chondrosarcoma, fibrosarcoma, giant cell tumor, Ewing's tumor, and multiple myeloma (8, 26, 38–40).

Pathophysiology

The first four tumors mentioned above are spindle cell sarcomas, and Ewing's tumor is a small cell sarcoma. In addition to differences in the ages in which they occur, there are also differences regarding the propensity for invasion and ability to metastasize among these different neoplasms. Osteosarcoma is not only invasive locally, but it metastasizes to the lungs in 85 to 90% of the patients; it is a fast growing tumor (38–39). Low-grade chondrosarcoma and fibrosarcoma tend to be locally invasive, slow-growing, and do not metastasize, but very-high-grade lesions have a high frequency of metastasis, particularly to the lungs. Most common forms of giant cell tumors are of low-grade histology with little propensity to metastasize. Ewing's tumor, composed of a large number of round small cells that are quite anaplastic, tends to extend through the bony cortex into the soft tissue, where the lesion progresses to a large mass. Hematogenous spread to the lung is frequent.

Symptoms and Signs

All of these malignant tumors have pain as their most common presenting symptom. With osteosarcoma and Ewing's tumor the child usually complains of progressively increasing pain localized to the bone or to the knee joint associated with a progressively enlarging swelling and tenderness. With Ewing's tumor the pain is intense and is associated with fever, malaise, and luekocytosis. Because of their slow growth, chondrosarcoma and fibrosarcoma might be present for several years before the patient begins to have pain or swelling. Giant cell tumor usually presents with progressively increasing pain, swelling, and tenderness at the local site, or the patient might experience severe pain from a pathologic fracture consequent to the lesion. With multiple myeloma there can be insidious bone pain and tenderness, but there is no swelling.

Treatment

Osteosarcoma is usually treated with surgical excision and/or combination chemotherapy. The level of amputation of the extremity must be carefully selected after analysis of the standard radiographs and bone scan. In recent years combination chemotherapy has also been found useful as the sole therapy or as an adjuvant to surgical excision. Low-grade chondrosarcoma and fibrosarcoma can be treated by surgical control with adequate bone and soft tissue margins (26), but high-grade lesions require the latter plus the addition of systemic chemotherapy to prevent distant metastases. For giant cell tumor, good surgical control consisting of an en bloc excision of the entire tumor is recommended.

Formerly Ewing's sarcoma treated with either surgical excision or moderate doses of radiation produced long-term survival in fewer than 10% of the patients (25). Currently two forms of systemic treatment are being used, multiagent chemotherapy and megavoltage radiation therapy. The latter has produced excellent local control and good to excellent functional results in most patients (25).

Pain control is described in detail in Chapter 24. As mentioned there, children with severe pain due to lesions of the lower limbs are best managed with continuous caudal analgesia produced with a combination of a dilute solution of a local anesthetic and opioids.

REFERENCES

1. Clemente, C.D. (ed.): Gray's Anatomy of the Human Body. 30th Am. Ed. Philadelphia, Lea & Febiger, 1985, pp. 275–285, 397–408.
2. Hollinshead, W.H.: Anatomy for Surgeons. Vol. 3, The Back and Limbs. Philadelphia, Harper & Row, 1982, pp. 674–767.
3. Rosse, C.: The thigh and the knee. In The Musculoskeletal System in Health and Disease. Edited by C. Rosse and D.K. Clawson. Hagerstown, MD, Harper & Row, 1980, pp. 273–290.
4. Evarts, C.M. (ed.): Surgery of the Musculoskeletal System, Vol. 3. New York, Churchill Livingstone, 1983.
5. Adams, J.C.: Outline of Orthopaedics. 10th Ed. Edinburgh, Churchill Livingstone, 1986, pp. 376–415.
6. Cailliet, R.: Knee Pain and Disability. 2nd Ed. Philadelphia, F.A. Davis, 1983, pp. 1–142.
7. Smillie, I.S.: Injuries of the Knee Joint. 5th Ed. Edinburgh, Churchill Livingstone, 1978.
8. Smillie, I.S.: Diseases of the Knee Joint. 2nd Ed. Edinburgh, Churchill Livingstone, 1980.
9. Lockhart, R.D., Hamilton, G.F., and Fyfe, S.W.: Anatomy of the Human Body. Philadelphia, J.B. Lippincott, 1960, p. 291.
10. Holbrook, T.L., et al.: The Frequence of Occurrence, Impact and Cost of Selected Musculoskeletal Conditions in the United States. Chicago, American Academy of Orthopedic Surgeons, 1984.
11. National Center for Health Statistics: Current Estimates from National Health Interview Survey. United States, 1986. Series 10, # 164. DHHS Publ. No. (PHS) 87-1592. Hyattsville, MD, National Center for Health Statistics, 1987.
12. Koch, H.: The management of chronic pain in office-based ambulatory care: National Ambulatory Medical Care Survey. Advance Data from Vital and Health Statistics, # 123. DHHS Publ. No. (PHS) 86-1250. Hyattsville, MD, Public Health Service, 1986.
13. Knapp, D.A., and Koch, H.: The management of new pain in office-based ambulatory care. In National Ambulatory Medical Care Survey, 1980-81. Advance Data from Vital and Health Statistics, # 97. DHHS Publ. No. (PHS) 84-1250. Hyattsville, MD, National Center for Health Statistics, 1984.
14. National Center for Health Statistics: Utilization of Short Stay Hospitals, United States, 1985 Annual Summary. Data from the National Health Survey, Series 13, No 91. DHHS Publ. No. (PHS) 87-1752. Hyattsville, MD, National Center for Health Statistics, 1987.
15. Gardner, E.: The innervation of the knee joint. Anat. Rec., 101:109, 1948.
16. Nordin, M., and Frankel, V.H.: Basic Biomechanics of the Skeletal System. Edited by V.H. Frankel and M. Nordin. Philadelphia, Lea & Febiger, 1980, pp. 113–148.
17. Murray, M.P., Drought, A.B., and Kory, R.C.: Walking patterns of normal men. J. Bone Joint Surg. [Am.], 46:335, 1964.
18. Kettelkamp, D.B., et al.: An electrogoniometric study of knee motion in normal gait. J. Bone Joint Surg. [Am.], 52:775, 1970.
19. Laubenthal, K.N., Smidt, G.L., and Kettelkamp, D.B.: A quantitative analysis of knee motion duting activities of daily living. Phys. Ther., 52:34, 1972.
20. Pflug, A.E., et al.: The effects of postoperative peridural analgesia on pulmonary therapy and pulmonary complications. Anesthesiology, 41:8, 1974.
21. Bucholz, R.W., and Mooney, V.: Fractures of the femoral shaft. In Surgery of the Musculoskeletal System, Vol. 3. Edited by C.M. Evarts. New York, Churchill Livingstone, 1983, pp. 5:201–221.
22. Hansen, S., and Winquist, R.: Closed intramedullary nailing of the femur: Kuntscher technique with reaming. Clin. Orthop., 138:56, 1979.
23. Woolf, C.J., and Wall, P.D.: The relative effectiveness of C-primary afferents of different origins in evoking a prolonged facilitation on the flexor reflex in the rat. J. Neurosci., 6:1433, 1986.
24. Weiss, L., and Gilberts, H.A. (eds.): Bone Metastasis. Boston, G.K. Hall, 1981, pp. 54–63.
25. Rosenberg, S.A., et al.: Sarcomas of the soft tissue and bone. In Cancer: Principles and Practice of Oncology. Edited by V.T. DeVita, Jr., S. Hellman, and S.A. Rosenberg. Philadelphia, Lippincott, 1982, pp. 1067–1093.
26. Liotta, L.A., Lanzer, W.L., and Garbisa, S.: Identification of a type V collagenolytic enzyme. Biochem. Biophys. Res. Commun., 98:184, 1984.
27. Stuart, J., et al.: Haemorrhagic episodes in haemophilia: a five-year prospective study. Br. Med. J., 2:1, 624, 1966.
28. Moskowitz, R.W.: Clinical and laboratory findings in osteoarthritis. In Arthritis and Allied Conditions. 10th Ed. Edited by D.J. McCarthy. Philadelphia, Lea & Febiger, 1985, pp. 1408–1432.
29. Aichroth, P.: Osteochondritis dissecans of the knee: A clinical survey. J. Bone Joint Surg. [Am.], 53:440, 1971.
30. Johnson, R.P., and Brewer, B.J.: Mechanical disorders of the knee. In Arthritis and Allied Conditions. 10th Ed. Edited by D.J. McCarthy. Philadelphia, Lea & Febiger, 1985, pp. 1223–1234.
31. Stougaard, J.: Familial occurrence of osteochondritis dissecans. J. Bone Joint Surg. [Br.], 46:542, 1964.
32. Lotke, P.A., and Ecker, M.L.: Osteonecrosis-like syndrome of the medial tibial plateau. Clin. Orthop., 176:148, 1983.
33. Insall, J.: Current concepts review: Patellar pain. J. Bone Joint Surg. [Am.], 64:147, 1982.
34. Gruber, M.A.: The conservative treatment of chondromalacia patellae. In Symposium on Disorders of the Knee Joint. Orthop. Clin. North Am., 10:105, 1979.
35. Jackson, R.W.: Etiology of chondromalacia patellae. In AAOS Instructional Course Lectures, Vol. 25. St. Louis, C.V. Mosby, 1976, pp. 36–40.
36. Dunn, A.W., and Whisler, J.H.: Synovial chondromatosis of the knee with associated extracapsular chondroma. J. Bone Joint Surg. [Am.], 44:1747, 1973.
37. Micheli, L.J., and Jupiter, J.: Osteoid osteoma as a cause of knee pain in the young athlete. Am. J. Sports Med., 6:199, 1978.
38. Schajowicz, F.: Tumors and Tumor-Like Lesions of Bone and Joint. New York, Springer-Verlag, 1981.
39. Barnes, R., and Catto, M.: Chondrosarcoma of bone. J. Bone Joint Surg. [Br.], 48:729, 1966.
40. Jeffree, G.M., and Price, C.H.G.: Metastatic spread of fibrosarcoma of bone. J. Bone Joint Surg. [Br.], 58:418, 1976.

76 · PAIN IN THE LEG, ANKLE, AND FOOT

JOHN J. BONICA *and* FREDERICK G. LIPPERT III

PAINFUL disorders that afflict the leg, ankle, and foot rank only after backache and headache in accounting for visits to physicians (1, 2), and rank second to back pain in accounting for visits to orthopedic surgeons (3). It has been estimated that 40% of Americans have foot pain with some 25 million podiatrists in active practice. Contributing factors for such a high prevalence of pain in the lower limbs include heredity, posture or stress, poor footwear, trauma, infections, and arthritides. This constellation of disorders, together with the complex nature of the functional anatomy of the leg, ankle, and foot, poses a challenge to physicians and other health professionals to make a correct diagnosis and to carry out effective therapy for pain, and require a thorough knowledge of the anatomy, biomechanics, and function of these structures.

In this chapter we consider these issues and specific disorders. The material is presented in five major sections: A, Basic Considerations, including classification and epidemiology of pain in this region and a summary of the anatomy, function, and biomechanics of the leg, ankle, and foot; B, Evaluation of the Patient, which complements the information in Chapter 70 but gives more detail; C, Painful Disorders of the Leg; D, Painful Disorders of the Ankle and Heel; and E, Painful Conditions of the Foot. More detailed discussion can be found elsewhere (4–11).

A. BASIC CONSIDERATIONS

Etiology

Table 76-1 lists the most important painful disorders that affect the leg, ankle, and foot. In this chapter those listed in the first three major categories are discussed. Those in categories IV and V are considered in detail in Chapters 10–15, 21, 28, and 73; their relevance to the lower limbs is considered briefly in Chapter 77.

Epidemiology

Table 76-2 presents the 1986 estimates of the numbers and types of injuries and morbidity caused by various musculoskeletal disorders of the leg, ankle, and foot and the health services required by patients. Data from the National Ambulatory Medical Care Survey 1980–1981 (1) extrapolated for 1986 indicate that acute pain in the knee, leg, ankle, and foot

TABLE 76-1. Classification of Painful Disorders in the Leg, Ankle, and Foot

I. MUSCULOSKELETAL DISORDERS OF THE LEG
A. **Trauma:** fractures; dislocations; rupture of gastrocnemius, Achilles tendon, or other muscles or tendons; sprain of muscle or tendons; muscle spasm
B. **Infections:** acute or chronic osteomyelitis; other infections
C. **Tumors:** benign, malignant, metastatic

II. MUSCULOSKELETAL DISORDERS OF THE ANKLE
A. **Arthritides:** septic, rheumatoid, gouty, hemophilic, neuropathic; osteoarthritis
B. **Trauma:** fracture; dislocation or subluxation; recurrent subluxation; laxity; tendinitis
C. **Other diseases of bone:** benign or malignant tumor; osteochondritis ossificans

III. MUSCULOSKELETAL DISORDERS OF THE FOOT
A. **Hindfoot:** plantar fasciitis; tarsal coalition; Achilles tendinitis; heel pad deficiency; tarsal tunnel syndrome
B. **Midfoot:** medial arch strain; Lisfranc's joint instability; post-tib insufficiency; ganglion
C. **Forefoot:** stress effects; metatarsalgia; callosities
D. **Great toe:** hallux valgus (bunion); hallux rigidis; hypermobility; sesamoiditis; gout
E. **Small toes:** hammer toe; claw toe; soft or hard corns; neuroma; overlapping toes; bunionette; neuropathy; vascular problems

IV. OTHER PAINFUL DISORDERS THAT AFFECT THE LEG, FOOT, AND ANKLE
A. **Neuropathic painful disorders:** radiculalgia, neuralgia, causalgia; central nervous system disease; postamputation pain; entrapment syndromes
B. **Myofascial syndromes:** thigh muscle, leg muscle, or foot muscle involvement
C. **Peripheral vascular disease:** Acute arterial obstruction; arteriosclerosis obliterans; Buerger's disease; Raynaud's disease (phenomenon); other disorders of the microcirculation; cold injuries

V. REFERRED PAIN
A. **Pain referred from the pelvic viscera**
B. **Pain referred from the thigh**

prompted nearly 5 million visits to physicians. This number is second only to the number of physician visits caused by pain in the ear. Chronic painful conditions in these structures were responsible for nearly 4 million visits to physicians, representing 10% of all visits for chronic painful conditions (2).

Table 76-2 also lists the incidence of musculoskeletal injuries involving bones, joints, and soft tissues of the leg, ankle, and foot (12). These injuries, together with arthritis and other conditions affecting the leg, ankle, and foot, are among the most frequent causes of pain and disability in the United States and probably in most other industrialized nations. The economic impact of these injuries is also significant. Using the 1986 cost for workdays lost, visits to physicians and hospital stays can be estimated to have amounted to 2.4 billion dollars (13). To this figure can be added the economic impact of arthritis, infections, tumors, and other chronic painful conditions of the leg, ankle, or foot, or a combination of these. The total cost for 1986 was probably more than 8.5 billion dollars.

Anatomy and Function of the Leg, Ankle, and Foot

Rosse (8) has emphasized that whereas the leg, ankle, and foot are built on the same basic plan as the forearm, wrist, and hand, and are morphologically equivalent structures, significant differences do exist that reflect the different function and needs of these parts of the limbs. The distal part of the upper limb is structured for versatility and movement of the hand and freedom, but the lower limb is built for bearing weight and for propulsion to aid in locomotion. During development there is rotation and extension to position the lower limbs for bearing weight in the erect stance. Consequently, the flexor aspect of the leg faces posteriorly and its extensor aspect faces anteriorly while the sole of the foot faces backward and the palm of the hand faces forward, and the foot can assume a position at a right angle to the leg. Therefore, flexion of the foot is described as plantar flexion and extension is often referred to as dorsiflexion (8). In the anatomic position the thumb is on the lateral margin of the hand whereas the big toe is on the medial margin of the foot.

The ankle and foot are the focal points to which the total body weight is transmitted in ambulation and strenuous physical activity and are well suited for these functions. Thick heel and toe pads act as shock absorbers during walking and running, and the joints are capable of making adjustments necessary for fine balance on various terrains (14). In some forms of strenuous physical activity the ankle is subjected to up to five times the body weight.

Proper function involves the skeleton ligaments, and muscles of the leg, ankle, and foot. We will first consider the anatomy of the tibia and fibula and the muscles, nerves, and blood vessels of the leg. We will then discuss the anatomy of the skeleton and of the joints and muscles of the ankle and foot, after which we will discuss the movements and biomechanics of the ankle and foot.

Anatomy of the Skeleton, Joints, and Muscles of the Leg

Tibia and Fibula

The tibia and fibula, two parallel bones, constitute the skeleton of the leg that corresponds to the radius and ulna of the upper limb. Unlike the arrangements

TABLE 76-2. Musculoskeletal Injuries Involving the Leg, Ankle, and Foot*

Type of Injury	Morbidity				Health Services Required		
	Total Number	Restricted Activity (days)	Bed Disability (days)	Workdays Lost	Visits to Physicians	Hospital Discharges	Total Hospital Stay (days)
Fracture							
Tibia or fibula	212	8,056	3,138	3,201	578	108	1,026
Ankle or foot	900	13,860	2,700	4,500	978	36	342
Sprain							
Knee or leg	1,810	17,195	3,620	5,792	752	36	234
Ankle or foot	5,222	24,021	6,266	7,310	1,883	18	91
Dislocation	176	2,886	968	1,196	440	148	641
Open wound	3,500	11,550	3,150	4,900	1,820	43	172
All:	11,820	77,568	19,842	26,899	6,451	389	2,506

Data extrapolated from Holbrook, T.L., et al.: The Frequency of Occurrence, Impact, and Cost of Musculoskeletal Conditions in the United States. Chicago, American Academy of Orthopedic Surgeons, 1984; and from the National Center for Health Statistics: Current Estimates for the National Health Institute Survey, United States, 1982. Ser. 10, No. 150. Hyattsville, MD, DHHS, 1985, Publ. (PHS) 85-1578.
*1986 estimates of incidence, morbidity, and health services required (in thousands).

FIG. 76-1. Anatomy of the tibia and fibula showing the sites of origin (gray areas) and insertion (black areas) of the muscles that move the ankle and foot. **A.** Anterior view. **B.** Posterior view. The lateral condyle usually presents a raised area to which the strongest and most supportive part of the iliotibial tract is attached; the facet for articulation with the head of the fibula is on its curved inferior surface. A posteriorly placed deep transverse groove for the major part of the insertion of the semimembranosus muscle is on the medial condyle. The anterior border and medial surface of the tibia are largely subcutaneous. The posterior surface gives origin to the tibial portions of the soleus, tibialis posterior, and flexor digitorum longus muscles and receives the insertion of the popliteus and two muscles of the hamstring group. The lower end of the tibia bears the medial malleolus; its articular surface is continuous with that of the inferior surface, which enters with it into articulation with the trochlea of the talus bone. The fibular notch for articulation with the fibula is the lateral surface of the lower end of the tibia. The head of the fibula is subcutaneous and rises laterally to its apex; the facet for its articulation with the tibia is on its medial crest. The lateral malleolus is the expanded lower end of the fibula and, like the head, is subcutaneous. Its medial surface is largely occupied by the malleolar articular surface for the talus. Modified from Clemente, C.D. (ed.): Gray's Anatomy of the Human Body. 30th Am. Ed. Philadelphia, Lea & Febiger, 1985.

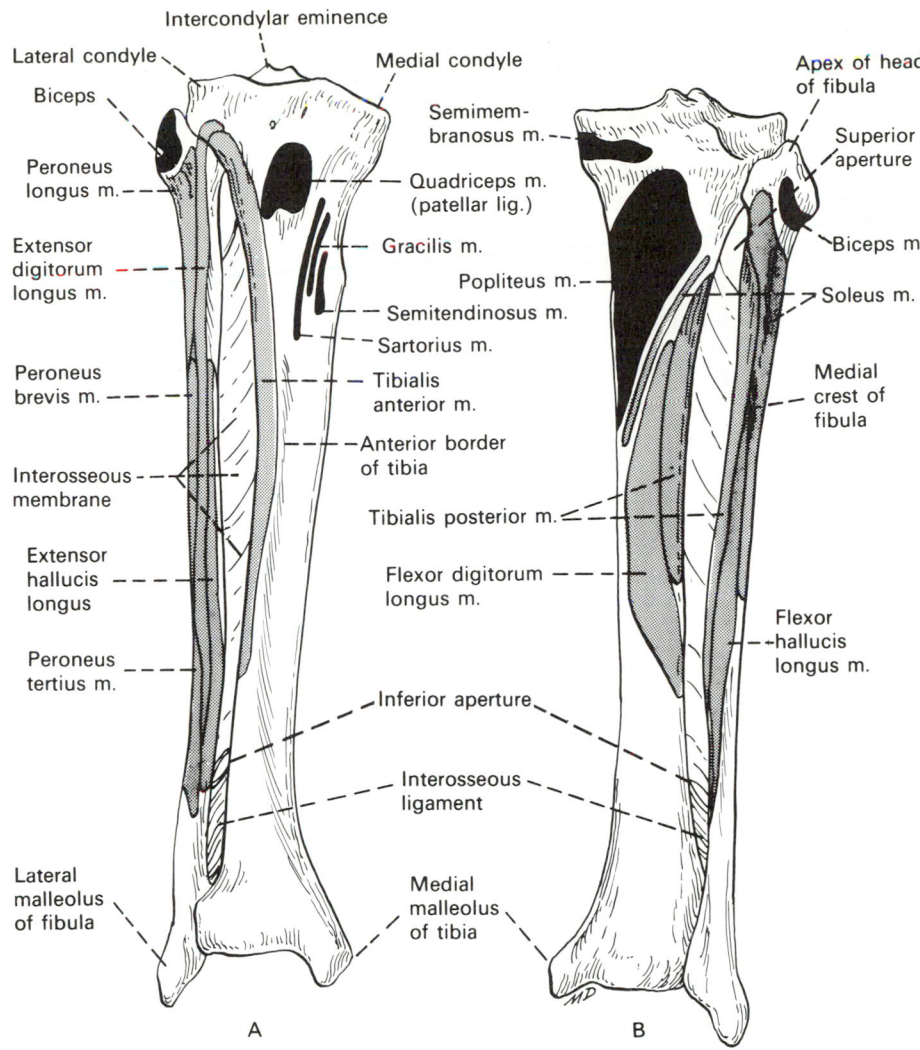

at the elbow and wrist, however, the fibula is excluded from the knee joint but forms an integral part of the mortise-like concave articular surface of the ankle joint (8). The anatomy of the tibia and fibula, including the sites of origin and insertion of muscles, is shown in Figure 76-1.

TIBIOFIBULAR JOINTS. The tibia and fibula are united to each other by the superior tibiofibular synovial joint, the interosseous membrane, and the inferior tibiofibular joint. *The superior tibiofibular synovial joint* lies between the head of the fibula and a posterolateral part of the lower surface of the lateral tibial condyle. The anterior and posterior ligaments of the head of the fibula run upward and medial to the tibia and strengthen its capsule (see Fig. 76-1). This joint is supplied by twigs from the common peroneal nerve and a twig from the nerve to the popliteus muscle, which is derived from the tibial nerve.

The interosseous membrane consists of thin but strong fibers that pass downward and laterally from the interosseous margin of the tibia to that of the fibula (Fig. 76-1). The membrane separates the muscles of the anterior compartment from those in the posterior compartment. Above the upper end of the

membrane, just below the superior tibiofibular joint, is a large oval aperture for passage of the anterior tibial vessels to the front of the leg. Close to its lower end (about 5 cm above the medial malleolus) is a smaller aperture for the perforating branch of the peroneal artery. Between the adjacent lower ends of the tibia and fibula the membrane is continuous with the crural tibiofibular interosseous ligament.

The *tibiofibular interosseous ligament* is composed of thick, short, strong fibers that run from the tibia to the fibula and stop short of the ankle joint near its articular margin (4, 8). The interosseous ligament should be distinguished from the interosseous membrane because it is much stronger; it is the key structure in preventing separation of the two bones by force applied to the lateral malleolus by way of the talus and calcaneus. Rosse (8) has pointed out that the ligament is so strong that, when these forces are excessive (e.g., in an eversion injury), the fibula fractures proximal to the ligament rather than the ligament rupturing. The tibiofibular interosseous ligament acts as a fulcrum between the two lever arms so that minor rotational displacement of the malleolus, the short arm of the lever, is magnified at the proximal end of the fibula (Fig. 76-1).

The inferior tibiofibular joint is the only syndesmosis in the entire appendicular skeleton. This fibrous joint acts to fix the distal end of the fibula in a groove on the lateral aspect of the tibia and is essential for the integrity of the ankle joint. The inferior tibiofibular joint is reinforced by the thinner and weaker anterior and posterior inferior tibiofibular ligaments, which are placed superficially on the front and back of the joint. The nerve supply of this joint is discussed in the next subsection.

Muscles of the Leg and Foot

Muscular Compartments of the Leg

Figure 76-2 illustrates the compartments of the leg at midcalf. The muscles within these compartments, which provide movement at the ankle and tarsus, are arranged in a manner similar to that of the prime movers of the wrist and carpals. These compartments, as in the forearm, contain long flexors and extensors of the toes, but the orientation of the compartments is reversed, with the flexors occupying the posterior compartment and the extensors located anteriorly (8). A third compartment is present laterally for which there is no counterpart in the forearm; this contains the peroneal muscles. Each compartment is supplied by its own nerve—the tibial nerve supplies the flexor compartment, the deep peroneal nerve supplies the extensors, and the superficial peroneal nerve supplies the long and short peroneal muscles. Table 76-3 lists the muscles of the leg and foot, their function, and their nerve supply. The segmental nerve supply to the skin, muscles, and bone is shown in Figure 70-30, and the peripheral nerve supply to these structures is shown in Figure 70-31.

Prime Movers of the Ankle

PLANTAR FLEXORS. Figure 76-3 depicts the muscles of the back of the leg, which include the primary plantar flexors, the gastrocnemius, the soleus, and the plantaris, which act together as the triceps surae. These three muscle bellies represent the most important motor unit that provides the impetus for propulsion (5, 8). Other muscles that pass behind the axis of the ankle can plantar flex the foot but, because they do not use the heel as a lever arm, they are less powerful and less effective (5, 8). These muscles include the tibialis posterior, the peroneus longus and brevis, the flexor hallucis longus, and the flexor digitorum longus.

PLANTAR DORSIFLEXORS. Primary dorsiflexors of the ankle include the tibialis anterior and peroneus tertius, but the joint can also be dorsiflexed by the extensor hallucis longus and extensor digitorum longus (Fig. 76-4). The tibialis anterior is the bulkiest muscle in the anterior compartment. The peroneus tertius is actually part of the muscle belly of the digital extensor but, because its tendon inserts into the base of the 5th metatarsal, its action is restricted to ankle dorsiflexion.

Extrinsic Flexors and Extensors of the Toes

FLEXORS. Because the superficial digital flexor represented by the soleus does not reach the digits only one common extrinsic digital flexor is found in the calf, the flexor digitorum longus (Fig. 76-3C); this corresponds to the flexor digitorum profundus in the forearm (8) (Fig. 76-4). Similarly, as in the forearm, the flexor hallucis longus is a separate muscle that corresponds to the flexor pollicis longus. The flexor digitorum longus arises from the tibia and the flexor

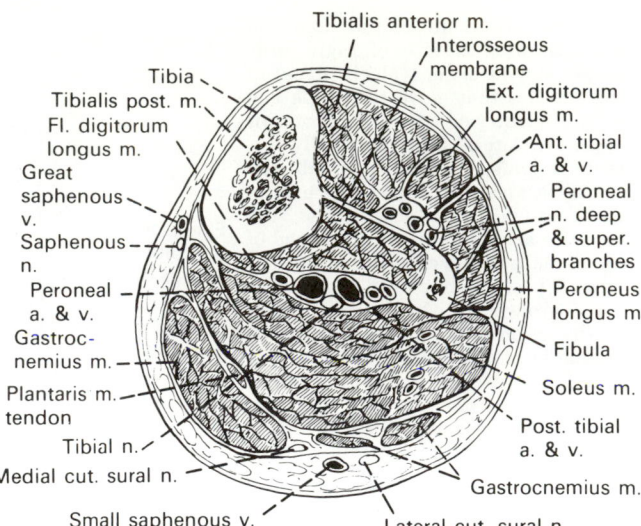

FIG. 76-2. Transverse section of the leg at midcalf showing the three major compartments covered by the deep fascia of the leg, which is also known as the crural fascia. The anterior compartment is separated from the posterior compartment by the interosseous membrane. The anterior and posterior crural intermuscular septa enclose the peroneus longus and brevis, which separate them from the muscles of the anterior and posterior crural region. Also note the location of the major vessels and nerves. Modified from Eycleshymer, A.C., and Schoemaker, D.M.: A Cross-Section Anatomy. New York, D. Appleton-Century, 1911, p. 96.

hallucis arises from the fibula (76-1B); the tendons pass on the medial side of the heel and enter the sole of the foot behind the malleolus (Fig. 76-4C). The tendons are invested in synovial sheaths and are retained in place by the flexor retinaculum, which is much thinner than the corresponding structure in the wrist (6, 10) (See Fig. 76-7). Tendons insert into the distal phalanges. The anatomic arrangement of synovial and fibrous flexor sheaths in the toes through which the tendons pass is similar to that of the fingers.

EXTENSORS. The extensor hallucis longus and extensor digitorum longus are located in the anterior compartment (Fig. 76-4). Both originate from the fibula and insert into the toes through the dorsal digital expansions, analogous to those in the fingers (Fig. 76-16). The tendons are held in place in front of the ankle by the superior and inferior extensor retinacula and are enclosed in a synovial membrane (see Fig. 76-6).

Inverters and Everters

The peroneus longus and peroneus brevis are the primary muscles that evert the foot (Fig. 76-5). Both arise from the tibia and pass behind the lateral malleolus. The brevis inserts into the base of the 5th metatarsal while the longus crosses the sole before it inserts into the base of the 1st metatarsal and the bones around it.

The tibialis posterior, the deepest muscle in the flexor compartment, is the principal inverter of the foot (Fig. 76-3). In this function it is substantially assisted by the tibialis anterior (Fig. 76-4). Figure 76-6 illustrates the synovial sheaths of the tendons and retinacula around the ankle joint.

Nerve and Blood Supply of the Leg

Figure 76-7 depicts the major arteries and nerves of the leg. The anatomy and distribution of the tibial and peroneal nerves are described in detail in Chapter 70.

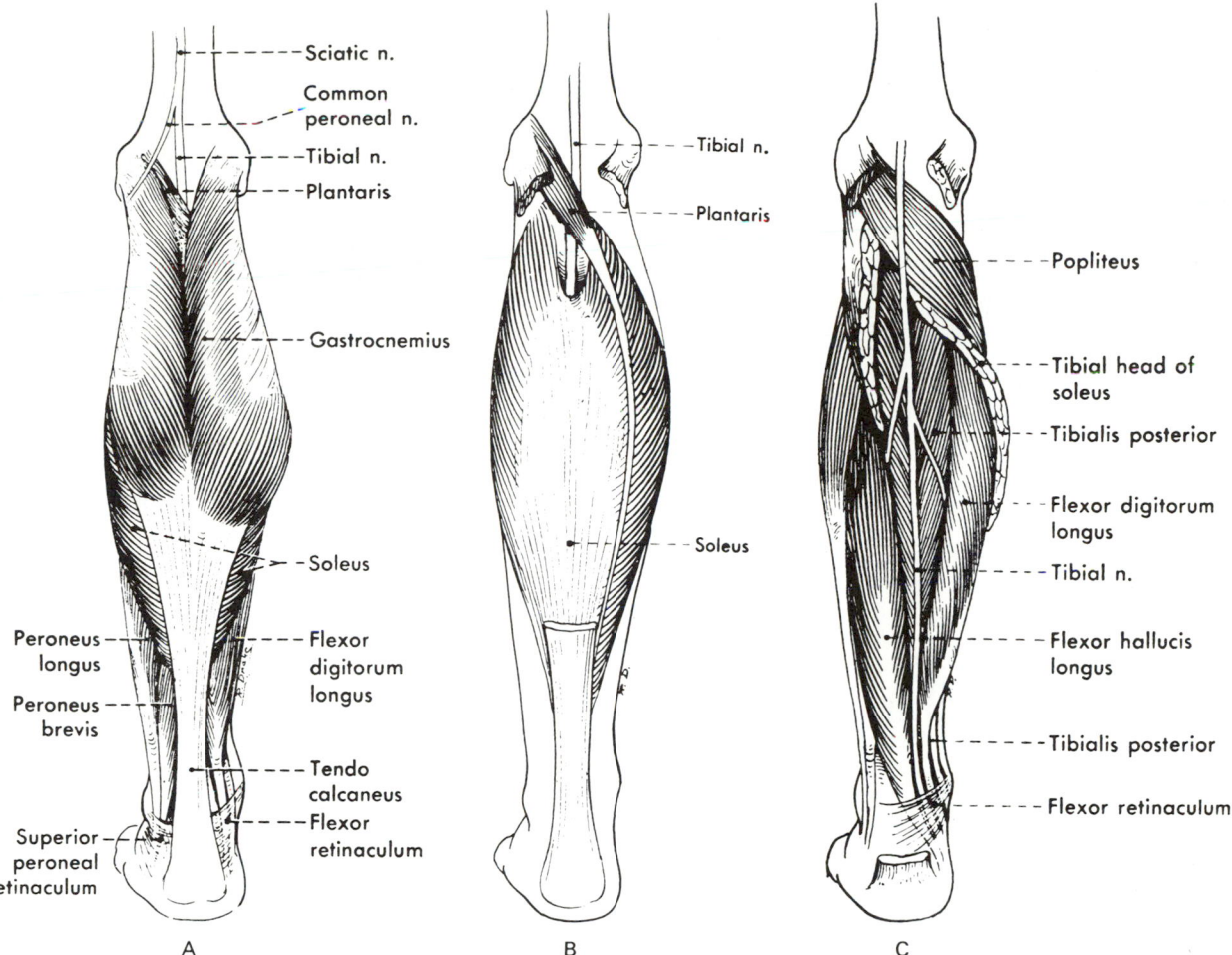

FIG. 76-3. Posterior muscles of the calf of the left leg. Most of these act as plantar flexors, while others act as flexors of the foot and toes. **A.** The superficial layer consists of the gastrocnemius muscle, which is composed of two heads that originate from the two femoral condyles. In the upper calf they fuse to form a common belly and the calcaneal (Achilles) tendon, which inserts into the posterior surface of the calcaneus. **B.** The second layer consists of the soleus and plantaris muscles. The soleus arises from two heads united by a tendinous arch from which additional fibers arise. Its muscular fibers end in a broad aponeurosis applied to the posterior surface of the muscle and adjacent to the aponeurosis of the gastrocnemius muscle on its anterior surface. The soleus narrows into a tendon that unites with the tendon of the gastrocnemius to form the tendo calcaneus. The plantaris arises from the lateral condyle of the femur, passes obliquely medially, and forms a thin tendon that inserts just medial to the tendo calcaneus on the calcaneus bone. **C.** Deep muscles of the calf showing the tibial nerve. The heads of the gastrocnemius and the tibial head of the soleus have been cut to show the deeper sections. The tibialis posterior, the deepest of the posterior muscles, arises from the interosseous membrane and, from the medial parts of the posterior surfaces of the tibia and fibula (Fig. 76-1B), passes downward and converges into a tendon that proceeds anterior or deep to the flexor digitorum longus, lying with it in a groove behind the medial malleolus but enclosed in a separate sheath. The tendon passes deep to the flexor retinaculum and superficial to the deltoid ligament, crosses the foot, and inserts into the tuberosity of the navicular bone (Fig. 76-15). This muscle, together with the tibialis anterior, inverts the foot. The flexor digitorum longus arises from the tibia and the flexor hallucis arises from the fibula. Both descend and converge into tendons that negotiate the heel on the medial side and enter the sole of the foot behind the medial malleolus, and both are invested in tendon sheaths. The common tendon of the flexor digitorum longus splits into four tendons with their own sheaths to insert into the base of the distal phalanges of the 2nd, 3rd, 4th, and 5th toes, and the flexor hallucis inserts into the base of the distal phalanx of the great toe. These muscles flex the toes by pulling on the distal phalanges (See Fig. 76-15 for insertions of these muscles). From Hollinshead, W.H.: Anatomy for Surgeons. 3rd Ed. Vol. 3, The Back and Limbs. Philadelphia, Harper & Row, 1982.

The leg and foot receive their arterial blood supply from the lower portion of the popliteal artery and its two major branches, the anterior tibial and posterior tibial arteries. The popliteal artery gives off lateral and medial inferior genicular arteries, which contribute to the circumpatellar anastomosis. The anterior tibial artery diverges from the posterior tibial artery by passing anteriorly through the superior aperture of the interosseous membrane and then descending to the ankle, where it terminates as the dorsalis pedis artery. Along its course it gives off (a) the fibular artery, which supplies the soleus and peroneus longus muscles; (b) the anterior tibial recurrent artery, which contributes to the formation of the patellar plexus; (c) numerous muscular branches that supply the muscles of the back of the leg; and (d) the anterior medial and lateral malleolar arteries, which supply the ankle joint. Along its course the dorsalis pedis artery gives off the lateral and medial tarsal arteries and the arcuate arteries (Fig. 47-7).

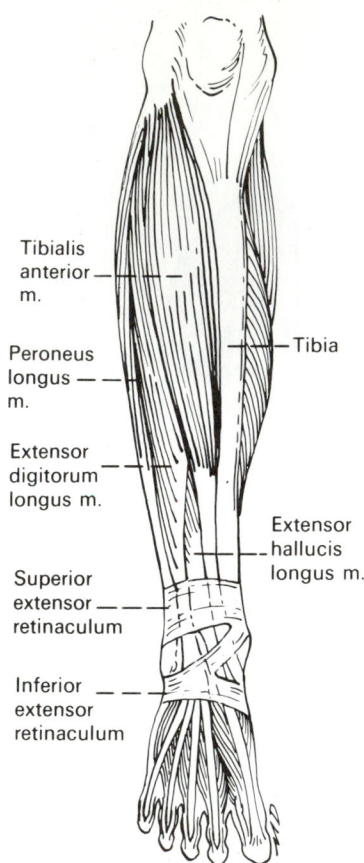

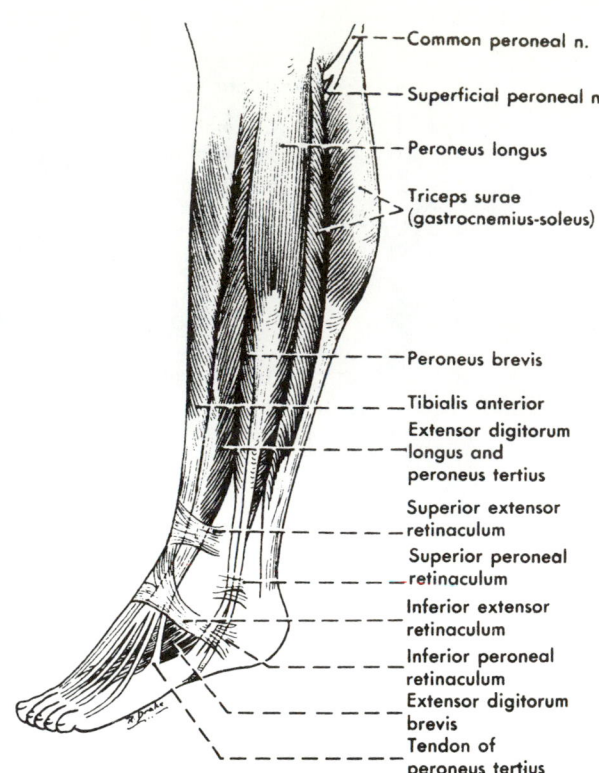

FIG. 76-5. Lateral muscles of the left leg. The two muscles in the anterolateral compartment of the leg are the peroneus longus and peroneus brevis, which arise from the head and upper two-thirds of the lateral surface of the tibia (Fig. 76-1A). Above the ankle they form two tendons that pass behind the lateral malleolus, lateral to the axis of the subtalar joint. The brevis inserts into the base of the 5th metatarsal and the longus enters the sole of the foot in a groove of the cuboid bone and crosses the sole before it inserts into the base of the 1st metatarsal and the bones around it (see Fig. 76-16 for the insertions of these muscles). These muscles evert the foot. From Hollinshead, W.H.: Anatomy for Surgeons. 3rd Ed. Vol. 3, The Back and Limbs. Philadelphia, Harper & Row, 1982.

FIG. 76-4. Anterior muscles of the leg. The tibialis anterior, the largest of the anterior leg muscles, arises from the inferior surface of the lateral condyle of the femur and the interosseous membrane and inserts into the medial cuneiform and base of the 1st metatarsal. The extensor digitorum longus and extensor hallucis longus arise from the anterior surface of the tibia and pass under the superior and inferior extensor retinacula, where the extensor digitorum longus divides into four separate tendons that insert into the middle phalanx of the four smaller toes and the extensor hallucis longus inserts into the distal phalanx of the great toe. The tibialis anterior acts as a dorsiflexor. In this function the muscle is supported by the peroneus tertius, which arises from a small area on the anterior surface of the lower part of the tibia and from the distal part of the interosseous membrane. This gives rise to a tendon that lies on the side of the tendon of the extensor digitorum longus, passes under the superior and inferior extensor retinacula in the same canal as the extensor digitorum longus, and inserts onto the dorsal surface of the base of the metatarsal of the 4th and 5th toes (see Figs. 76-15 and 76-16 for insertions of these muscles). Modified from Clemente, C.D. (ed.): Gray's Anatomy of the Human Body. 30th Am. Ed. Philadelphia, Lea & Febiger, 1985.

The posterior tibial artery descends in back of the leg as far as the ankle, where it divides into the medial and lateral plantar arteries. Along its course it gives off (a) the large peroneal artery, which gives off numerous muscular branches, nutrient arteries to the tibia and fibula, and perforating and communicating branches; (b) a large nutrient artery to the tibia; (c) muscular branches to the soleus and deep muscles in the back of the leg; (d) the posterior medial malleolar artery, which contributes to the malleolar arterial network, and several large medial calcaneal arteries.

Anatomy of the Ankle and Foot

Skeleton

The foot is an intricate structure composed of 26 articulating bones similar to the bones of the hand but modified because of the foot's weight-bearing function (Fig. 76-8). The bones of the ankle and foot are the tarsals, metatarsals, and phalanges. The tarsal bones differ from the carpal bones of the wrist but the metatarsals and phalanges are similar to the metacarpals and phalanges of the hand (7, 10). The tarsals differ from the carpals in shape, size, and arrangement. It is customary to refer to the three segments of the foot as the anterior portion or forefoot, the middle portion or midfoot, and the posterior portion or hindfoot. The hindfoot is composed of the talus and calcaneus, the midfoot is composed of the navicular, cuboid, and three cuneiform bones, and the forefoot is composed of the metatarsals and phalanges.

The talus has a body, neck, and head (Fig. 76-9). The superior and both sides of the body, the large trochlear tali,

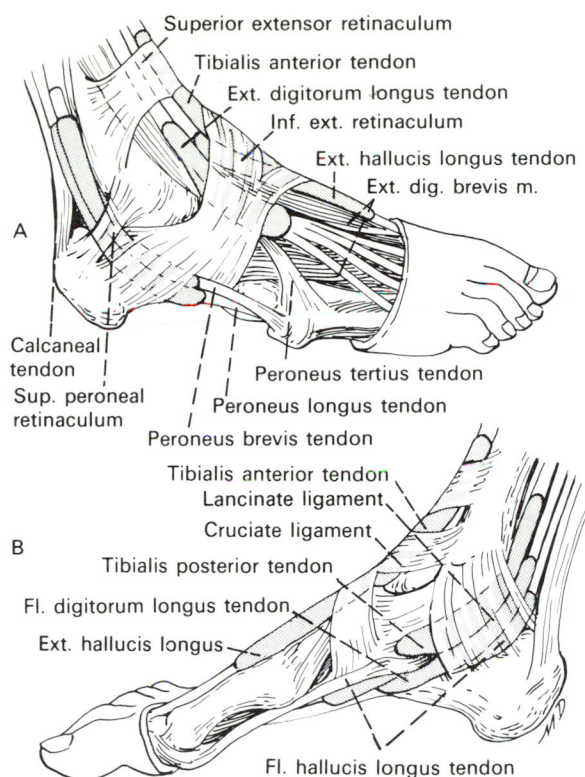

FIG. 76-6. Synovial sheaths of the tendons around the ankle. **A.** Anterolateral aspect showing the tendons and synovial sheaths of the tibialis anterior and extensor digitorum longus, which pass under the superior and inferior extensor retinacula. Beyond the sheath the extensor digitorum longus divides into four tendons that pass to the middle and distal phalanges of the four lesser toes while the extensor hallucis longus inserts into the base of the distal phalanx of the great toe. Note the insertion of the peroneus tertius onto the bases of the 4th and 5th metatarsals (Fig. 76-16B). The peroneus longus and brevis have individual synovial sheaths that pass under the peroneal retinaculum. **B.** Medial aspect showing the synovial sheaths of the tibialis posterior, flexor digitorum longus, and flexor hallucis longus, which pass behind the medial malleolus. These are covered by the flexor retinaculum, which also contains the end of the tibial nerve and the beginning of two plantar nerves. This is a site for entrapment of these nerves. Modified from Clemente, C.D. (ed.): Gray's Anatomy of the Human Body. 30th Am. Ed. Philadelphia, Lea & Febiger, 1985.

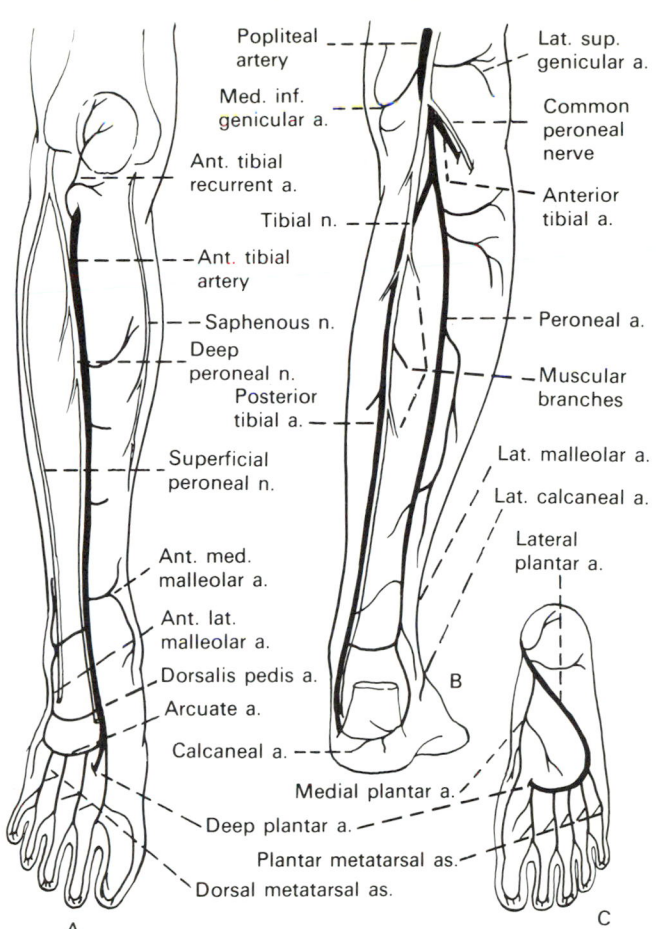

FIG. 76-7. Nerve and blood supply of the leg. **A.** Anterior view. **B.** Posterior view. **C.** Plantar surface of the foot. The anatomy of the nerves is described in Chapter 70. Modified from Clemente, C.D. (ed.): Gray's Anatomy of the Human Body. 30th Am. Ed. Philadelphia, Lea & Febiger, 1985.

articulate with the tibia and fibula, which unite to form the ankle mortise. Because of the malleoli the talus is hardly accessible to palpation. The calcaneus, the largest of the tarsal bones, represents a backward projecting heel that lies beneath the talus and supports it. Various parts of the calcaneus can be explored by palpation, including its surfaces and the sinus tarsi, which is the lateral aperture of the tarsal canal; this can be felt as a bony depression filled by soft tissue just inferior to the talar neck (8). The sustentaculum tali, a finger's breadth below the tip of the medial malleolus, supports the talus and can be identified as a buttress projecting medially from the calcaneus.

The navicular bone, identifiable by a tubercle that is 3.5 cm anterior to the medial malleolus, is level with the sustentaculum. The cuboid is palpable just proximal to the prominent tuberosity of the 5th metatarsal, which overlaps the cuboid as it projects backward from its base.

Joints

ANKLE JOINT. The ankle joint is principally uniaxial and is classified as a ginglymus, or hinge joint (4, 5, 8). It is formed above by the lower end of the tibia and its malleolus, the malleolus of the fibula, and the inferior transverse ligament. Together these form a deep cavity for the reception of the proximal convex surface of the talus and its flat medial and lateral facets, which constitute a mortise. A cast of this mortise duplicates all contours of the trochlea, with better congruence between the articular surfaces of the talocrural joint than any other joint in the body (8). This allows a good fit to be maintained throughout the whole range of plantar flexion and dorsiflexion; no lateral play or accessory movements are permitted in the mortise in any position. The distance between the malleoli does not increase when the ankle is dorsiflexed, although a small amount of lateral rotation of the fibular malleolus is permitted by the obliquity of the tibiofibular interosseous ligament.

The bones are connected by an articular capsule and by various ligaments that attach to the tip of each malleolus, with each component spanning not only

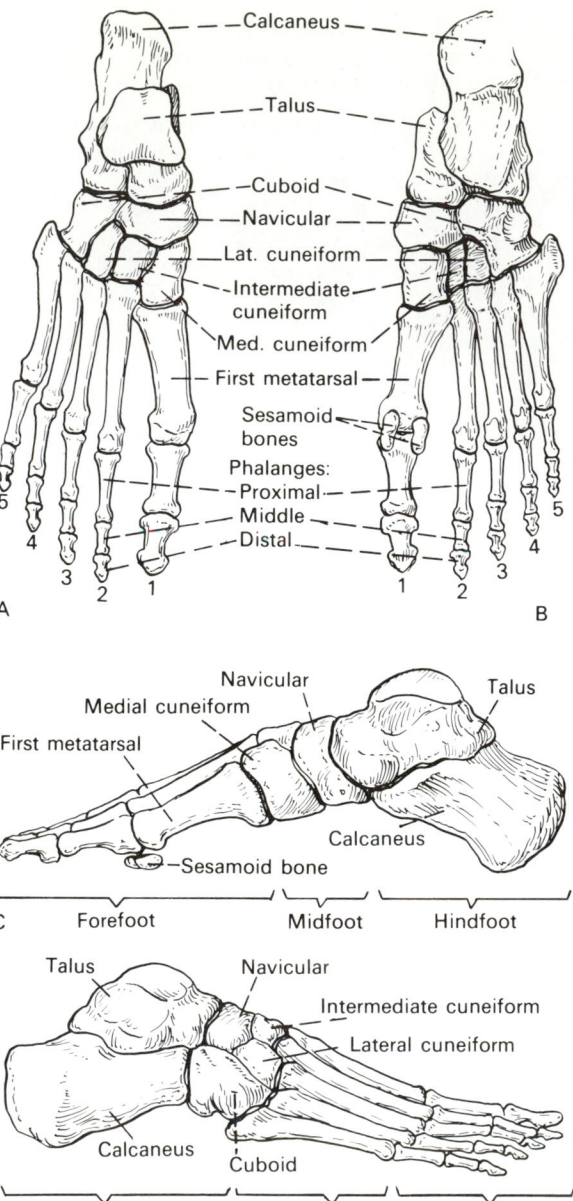

FIG. 76-8. Bones of the ankle and foot. **A.** Superior surface. **B.** Plantar surface. **C.** Medial view. **D.** Lateral view. The seven bones of the hindfoot and midfoot, which constitute the tarsus, are arranged in two rows, with one bone between them. In the posterior row the talus sits on the calcaneus and in the distal row the cuneiform and cuboid bones lie side by side, with the navicular bone between the two rows on the medial side. Only the talus enters into the articulation with the bones of the leg, and therefore all the weight on the foot is transmitted through this bone to the others and to the points of contact with the ground. Normally the calcaneus and the heads of the five metatarsals are the weight-bearing points of the foot (**C** and **D**). The skeleton of the foot is arched between these points with the arch being much higher on the medial side (**C**) than on the lateral side (**D**). The calcaneus, the largest and strongest bone of the foot, represents a backward projecting heel that lies beneath the talus and supports it. It transmits the weight of the body to the ground and provides a strong lever for the muscles of the calf. The navicular bone, identified by a tubercle that is 3.5 cm anterior to the medial malleolus, is on the medial side of the tarsus. Its posterior concave surface articulates with the head of the talus and its anterior or distal convex surface articulates with the three cuneiform bones. The cuboid is in line and articulates with the 4th and 5th metatarsals anteriorly, with the lateral cuneiform and navicular bones medially, and with the calcaneus posteriorly. The three cuneiforms, which together with the cuboid constitute the distal row of tarsal bones, are in line with the three medial rays of the foot and articulate with the corresponding metatarsals anteriorly. The arrangement of the metatarsals and phalanges is similar to that of the corresponding segments of the hand. Modified from Hollinshead, W.H.: Anatomy for Surgeons. 3rd Ed. Vol. 3, The Back and Limbs. Philadelphia, Harper & Row, 1982.

the ankle joint but also the talocalcaneal joint (Fig. 76-10). These bands stabilize both the ankle and talocalcaneal joints because of their calcaneal attachments, and help to integrate motion between the (10).

The articular capsule surrounds the joint and is attached above to the borders of the articular surface of the tibia and malleoli and below to the talus around its articular surface (Fig. 76-10A). Both its anterior and posterior parts are thin, with the anterior part being broad and the posterior part mainly consisting of transverse fibers.

The collateral ligaments provide side-to-side stability to the ankle joint and the tibiocalcaneal and calcaneofibular ligaments stabilize the talocalcaneal joints (Fig. 76-10B, C). Inversion and eversion injuries are likely to cause ruptures of the lateral or medial collateral ligament of the ankle or fracture of the

malleoli, especially the medial malleolus, which can sometimes be evulsed without rupture of the strong deltoid ligament (8). The crural interosseous ligament is also necessary for the integrity of the talocrural joint. The anterior and posterior ligaments of the arches prevent excessive plantar flexion or dorsiflexion (Fig. 76-10C, D).

INTERTARSAL JOINTS. Because movements at the ankle joint are limited almost strictly to plantar flexion and dorsiflexion, it is the intertarsal joints that add the additional mobility to the foot that allows it to be inverted and adducted (supinated) or everted and abducted (pronated) (7, 10). Moreover, because the foot is arched so that the weight transmitted to it is in turn transmitted to the calcaneus and forward to the heads of the metatarsals, most of the intertarsal joints are under particular strain during weight bearing and must be strongly braced if the arches of the foot are to function properly (8). The plantar surface of the foot is

FIG. 76-9. Anatomy of the right talus and calcaneus showing their relationship to the tibia and fibula, to other bones of the tarsus, and to the proximal ends of the metatarsals. *A.* Lateral view. *B.* Medial view. The talus has a body, a neck, and a head. *C.* The superior aspect and both sides of the body and the large trochlea tali articulate with the tibia and fibula, which unite to form the ankle mortise. The tibia contacts the entire superior aspect of the talus and is weight-bearing, with its medial malleolus extending one-third of the way down the medial aspect of the talus; the fibular malleolus covers the entire lateral aspect of the body of the talus. The rounded head of the talus fits into the concavity of the navicular bone and its inferior surface is composed of the oblique sulcus tali, which makes contact with the corresponding sulcus calcanei to form the tarsal canal. The tarsal canal separates the nonarticular portions of the talus and calcaneus. The talar neck is situated between the head and trochlea, and fits closely between the two malleoli. Note the axis of rotation of the mortise as the ankle plantar flexes and dorsiflexes. It passes through the fibula but below the tibia. *D.* Viewed from above the talus is wedge-shaped, with the anterior portion wider than the posterior portion. Because the tibia is anterior to the fibula, the longitudinal axis is perpendicular to the axis of the mortise and forms an external "toe-out" of 16°. *A* and *B* modified from Clemente, C.D. (ed.): Gray's Anatomy of the Human Body. 30th Am. Ed. Philadelphia, Lea & Febiger, 1985; *C* and *D* modified from Cailliet, R.: Foot and Ankle Pain. 2nd Ed. Philadelphia, F.A. Davis, 1983.

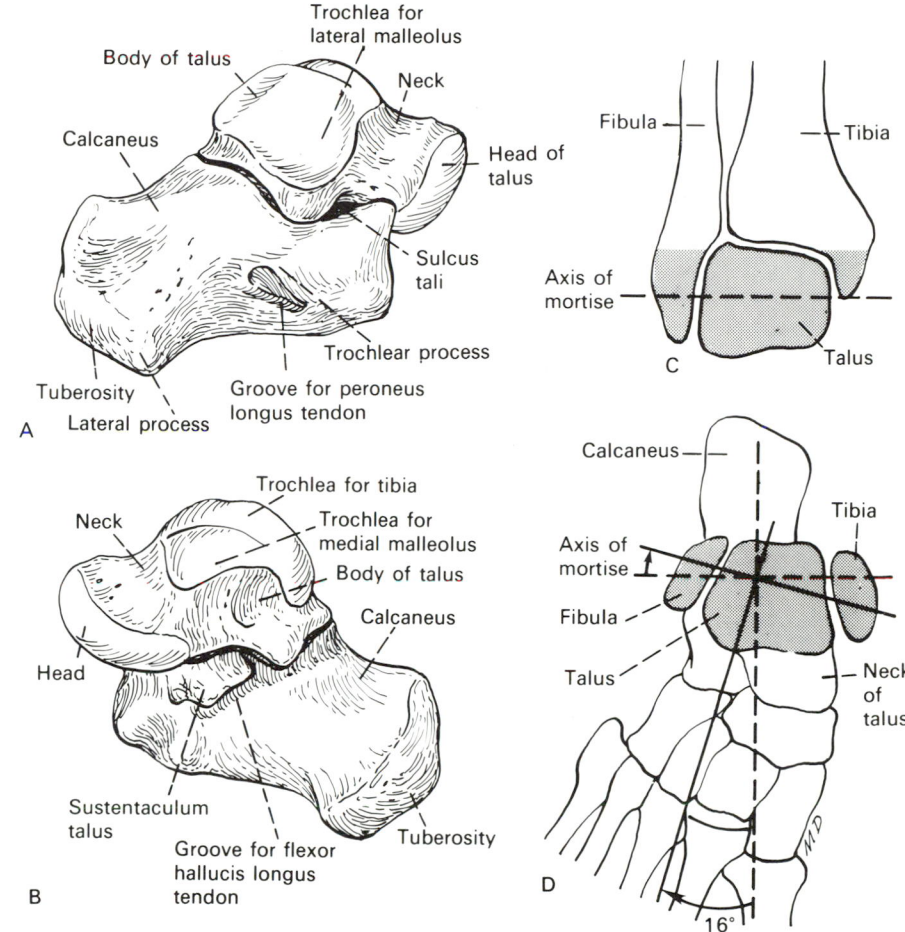

therefore provided with strong *intertarsal ligaments* that bind the bones together and help to prevent collapse of the arch. In addition, the short muscles of the foot, the plantar aponeurosis, and the long tendons passing into the sole of the foot from the leg all help to maintain the intertarsal joints in normal position (Fig. 76-11A).

The subtalar joint functions as a link between the talus and calcaneus, which permits inversion and eversion of the heel. The *transverse tarsal joint* links the hindfoot and midfoot and extends the range of movement of inversion-eversion produced by the subtalar joint (8). The transverse tarsal joint consists of two anatomically separate articulations, the talocalcaneonavicular and calcaneocuboid joints. Independent movements are not possible in any of these joints (8). The subtalar joint and the lateral and medial components of the transverse tarsal joint are enclosed by an independent fibrous capsule lined by synovial membrane (Fig. 76-11).

In addition to the spring ligament and the tibiocalcaneal and calcaneofibular portions of the collateral ligaments of the ankle, these intertarsal joints are strengthened further by the talocalcaneal interosseous, cervical, bifurcate, and short plantar ligaments (Fig. 76-11B). The talocalcaneal interosseous ligament occupies the tarsal canal and separates

the subtalar joint from the talocalcaneonavicular joint, reinforcing both structures. The cervical ligament is located in the sinus tarsi and is attached to the neck of the talus and the upper surface of the calcaneus (8). One limb of the bifurcate ligament, the dorsal calcaneonavicular ligament, which is found more anteriorly in the sinus, connects the calcaneus and navicular, and the other limb, the dorsal calcaneocuboid ligament, connects the calcaneus and cuboid bones. The plantar calcaneocuboid ligament, also known as the short plantar ligament, is more important than its dorsal counterpart.

The long plantar ligament (Fig. 76-11C), the longest of all the tarsal ligaments, is attached posteriorly to the plantar surface of the calcaneus in front of the calcaneal tuberosity. Anteriorly its deep fibers stretch to the tuberosity on the plantar surface of the cuboid wall and its most superficial fibers are continued distally to the bases of the 2nd, 3rd, 4th, and 5th metatarsal bones. These anteriorly extending fibers of the long plantar ligament convert the groove on the plantar surface of the cuboid into a canal for the tendon of the peroneus longus muscle. This ligament reinforces the lateral longitudinal arch and helps to prevent its flattening (4, 5, 8).

Other intertarsal joints are found between the navicular and cuneiform bones, the cuboid and cuneiform bones, and

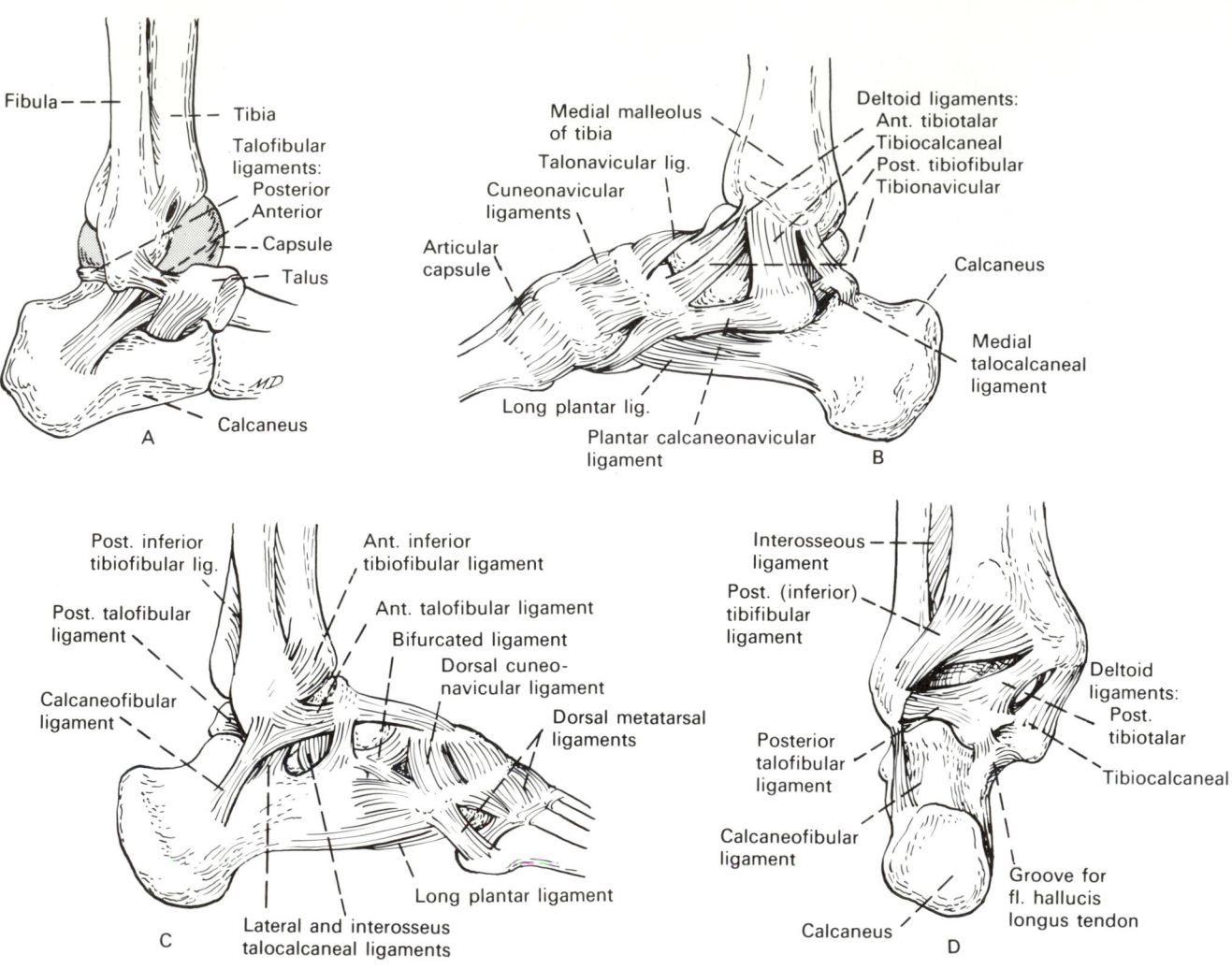

FIG. 76-10. Anatomy of the capsule and ligaments of the right ankle joint. **A.** Lateral view. The articular capsule surrounds the joint and is attached above to the borders of the articular surface of the tibia and malleoli and below to the talus around its articular surface. **B.** Medial view. The medial collateral ligament is known as the deltoid ligament because it fans out in a triangular shape from the margins of the tibial malleolus to attach in continuity to the navicular anteriorly and to the calcaneus and talus posteriorly. The deltoid ligament consists of superficial and deep portions. The superficial portion is made up of the tibionavicular or anterior portion, which passes anteriorly and inserts into the tuberosity of the navicular bone, and the tibiocalcaneal portion, which descends almost perpendicularly and inserts into the whole length of the sustentaculum tali of the calcaneus. The posterior or tibiotalar fibers pass posteriorly and laterally and are attached to the inner surface of the talus. The deep fibers are the anterior tibiotalar ligament, which attaches to the tip of the medial malleolus above and to the medial surface of the talus below. The deltoid ligament is covered by the tendons of the tibialis posterior and flexor digitorum longus. **C.** Lateral view. The lateral collateral ligament consists of three discrete bands. The anterior talofibular ligament, the shortest of the three, is attached posteriorly to the anterior margin of the fibular malleolus and anteriorly and medially to the talus in front of its lateral articular surface. The posterior talofibular ligament, stronger and deeper than the anterior ligament, runs almost horizontally from the depression at the medial and back part of the fibular malleolus to a prominent tubercle on the posterior surface of the talus, immediately lateral to the groove for the tendon of the flexor hallucis longus. The calcaneofibular ligament, the strongest of the three, is a narrow rounded cord that passes from the apex of the fibular malleolus downward and slightly posteriorly to a tubercle on the lateral surface of the calcaneus. **D.** Posterior view of the ankle joint showing the posterior inferior tibiofibular, posterior talofibular, posterior tibiotalar, and tibiocalcaneal ligaments as well as the interosseous ligament. Modified from Clemente, C.D. (ed.): Gray's Anatomy of the Human Body. 30th Am. Ed. Philadelphia, Lea & Febiger, 1985.

among the cuneiforms (6). These can all form one continuous joint cavity, the cuneonavicular, or the cuneocuboid can be separate. These joints are supported by the dorsal and plantar cuneonavicular, the dorsal and plantar cuboideonavicular, and the cuboideonavicular interosseous ligaments. The cuneiforms are supported by the weak transverse dorsal intercuneiform ligaments and by the stronger plantar intercuneiform ligaments.

JOINTS OF THE MIDFOOT AND FOREFOOT. The tarsometatarsal gliding joints are between the medial, intermediate, and lateral cuneiforms and cuboid bones, and between the bases of the five metatarsal bones. These joints are strengthened by the dorsal and plantar tarsometatarsal liga-

ments and by the interosseous cuneometatarsal ligaments (Fig. 76-11B).

The bases of the metatarsal bones are connected by the dorsal plantar and interosseous intermetatarsal ligaments. The heads of the metatarsal bones are interconnected on their plantar aspects by the deep transverse metatarsal ligament. Some fibers of this ligament attach to the base of the proximal phalanx and the metatarsal heads. The range of extension is greater in these joints than the range of flexion.

The metatarsophalangeal (MP) joints are strengthened by the plantar and collateral ligaments. The anatomy of the interphalangeal joint corresponds to that in the hand (5, 8).

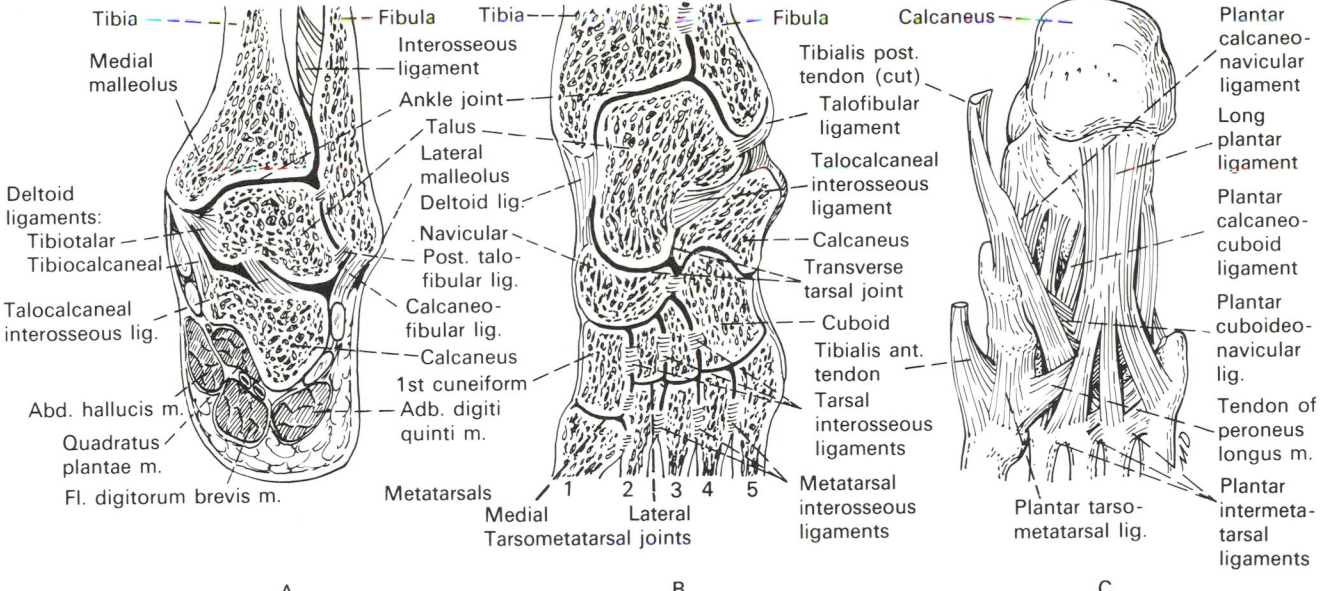

Tibia -- -- -- -- -- -- **Fibula** Tibia -- -- -- -- **Fibula** **Calcaneus** -- -- -- -- -- **Plantar calcaneo-navicular ligament**

Medial malleolus — **Interosseous ligament** — **Ankle joint** — **Talus** — **Lateral malleolus** — **Deltoid lig.** — **Navicular** — **Post. talo-fibular lig.** — **Calcaneo-fibular lig.** — **Calcaneus** — **1st cuneiform** — **Adb. digiti quinti m.**

Deltoid ligaments: Tibiotalar — **Tibiocalcaneal**

Talocalcaneal interosseous lig.

Abd. hallucis m.
Quadratus plantae m.
Fl. digitorum brevis m.

Metatarsals / 1 2 | 3 4 5
Medial **Lateral**
Tarsometatarsal joints

Tibialis post. tendon (cut) — **Talofibular ligament** — **Talocalcaneal interosseous ligament** — **Calcaneus** — **Transverse tarsal joint** — **Cuboid** — **Tibialis ant. tendon** — **Tarsal interosseous ligaments** — **Metatarsal interosseous ligaments**

Long plantar ligament — **Plantar calcaneo-cuboid ligament** — **Plantar cuboideo-navicular lig.** — **Tendon of peroneus longus m.** — **Plantar intermeta-tarsal ligaments**

Plantar tarso-metatarsal lig.

A   B   C

FIG. 76-11. Ligaments of the internal part of the ankle and foot and of the sole. **A.** Crural section through the right ankle (talocrural joint) and the talocalcaneal joints showing the talocalcaneal interosseous ligament, the deep portion of the deltoid ligament, some of the tendons and muscles in back of the heel, and the relationship of structures coursing beneath the malleoli. **B.** Oblique view of the ankle, subtalar, and transverse talar joints, and of the tarsometatarsal joints. **C.** Ligaments of the sole of the foot with the tendons of the peroneus longus and the tibialis posterior and anterior muscles. The long plantar ligament is attached posteriorly to the plantar surface of the calcaneus in front of the calcaneal tuberosity and passes anteriorly in a fanwise fashion with its deep fibers stretching to the tuberosity on the plantar surface of the cuboid bone; the most superficial fibers are connected distally to the bases of the 2nd, 3rd, 4th, and 5th metatarsal bones. The plantar calcaneocuboid ligament, also known as the short plantar ligament, is deep to the long plantar ligament, from which it is separated by a little areolar tissue. It is a short wide band of great strength that extends from the plantar aspect of the anterior tubercle of the calcaneous to the plantar surface of the cuboid behind the peroneal groove. The plantar calcaneonavicular ligament, also called the spring ligament, is a broad band of fibers that connects these two bones. Modified from Clemente, C.D. (ed.): Gray's Anatomy of the Human Body. 30th Am. Ed. Philadelphia, Lea & Febiger, 1985.

Nerve and Blood Supply of the Joints of the Ankle and Foot

Figure 76-12 depicts the nerve supply to the ankle joints, intertarsal joints, and joints of the midfoot and forefoot. The ankle joint is supplied chiefly by twigs from the deep peroneal and tibial nerves and also by the saphenous nerve (5, 14). The dorsal aspects of the intertarsal joints are supplied chiefly by branches from both the superficial and deep peroneal nerves (15). The saphenous nerve helps to supply the joints at the medial border of the foot. The lateral and medial plantar nerves send twigs to the plantar aspects of the joints.

The blood vessels supplying the ankle joints consist of the malleolar branches of the anterior tibial and peroneal arteries. Blood is supplied to the other joints of the foot from the dorsalis pedis and its branches, the medial and lateral plantar arteries, and the plantar arch.

Fascia and Intrinsic Muscles of the Foot

PLANTAR APONEUROSIS AND PLANTAR FASCIA. The superficial fascia forms a tough thick padding over the sole of the foot but is bare on the dorsum (4, 5, 8). The plantar aponeurosis is attached posteriorly to the calcaneus and proceeds anteriorly in a fanwise

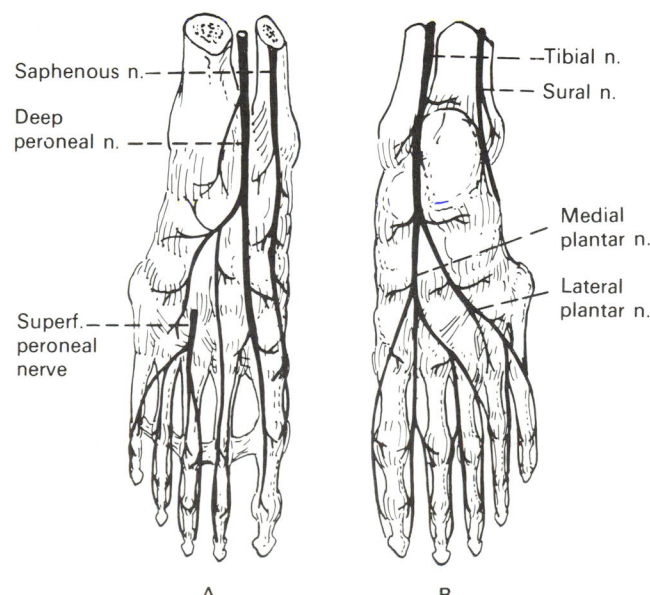

Saphenous n. —
Deep peroneal n. — —
Superf. peroneal nerve — —

Tibial n.
Sural n.
Medial plantar n.
Lateral plantar n.

A   B

FIG. 76-12. Nerve supply of the ankle joints and joints of the foot. **A.** Dorsal view. **B.** Plantar view. Many fibers supply the ankle joint superiorly and inferiorly and on both sides. See text for details.

fashion toward the toes (Fig. 76-13). Throughout the sole of the foot it sends fiber bundles to the skin and septa into the depth of the sole (4, 5, 8). Each side of the aponeurosis gives off an intermuscular septum that demarcates the intrinsic muscles of the 1st and 5th digits from a central compartment, which is occupied by the flexor tendons and the lumbricals. Additional sagittal septa over the ball of the foot connect the plantar aponeurosis to the fascia that covers the interosseous muscles and the deep transverse metatarsal ligament, thus forming tunnels that transmit the flexor tendons, lumbricals, and some of the digital nerves. These structures are protected from compression by the ball of the foot being sustained during the heel-off to toe-off phases of the gait cycle by cushions of connective tissue that sprout from the sagittal septa and fat pads.

INTRINSIC MUSCLES. Figure 76-14 depicts the intrinsic muscles of the plantar aspect of the foot, and Figure 76-15 is a plantar view of the bones of the foot, indicating the origins of the intrinsic muscles and the insertions of the intrinsic and extrinsic muscles. Figure 76-16 illustrates the muscles of the dorsum of the foot and the bones that give origin to the intrinsic

muscles, and shows the insertions of the extrinsic and intrinsic muscles that move the foot.

Nerve and Blood Supply of the Foot

Figure 76-17 depicts the nerve supply of the foot. The skin and sole of the foot are supplied by the medial and lateral plantar nerves and by the medial calcaneal branch of the tibial nerve. A strip of the lateral side of the foot is supplied by the lateral dorsal cutaneous branch of the sural nerve, which is also a branch of the tibial nerve. The saphenous nerve supplies a thin part of the skin and fascia on the medial aspect of the midfoot. Motor innervation of the intrinsic muscles is primarily from the L5 and S1 segments (Table 76-3). The cutaneous innervation of the dorsum of the foot is chiefly from the superficial peroneal nerve, which breaks up into medial and lateral branches. A twig from the deep peroneal nerve supplies adjacent sides of the 1st interdigital cleft, the saphenous nerve supplies the skin along the medial side of the foot, and the sural nerve supplies the lateral edge of the foot. (The segmental nerve supply to the skin, muscles, and bones of the foot is depicted in Figure 70-30, and the peripheral nerve supply is shown in Figure 70-31).

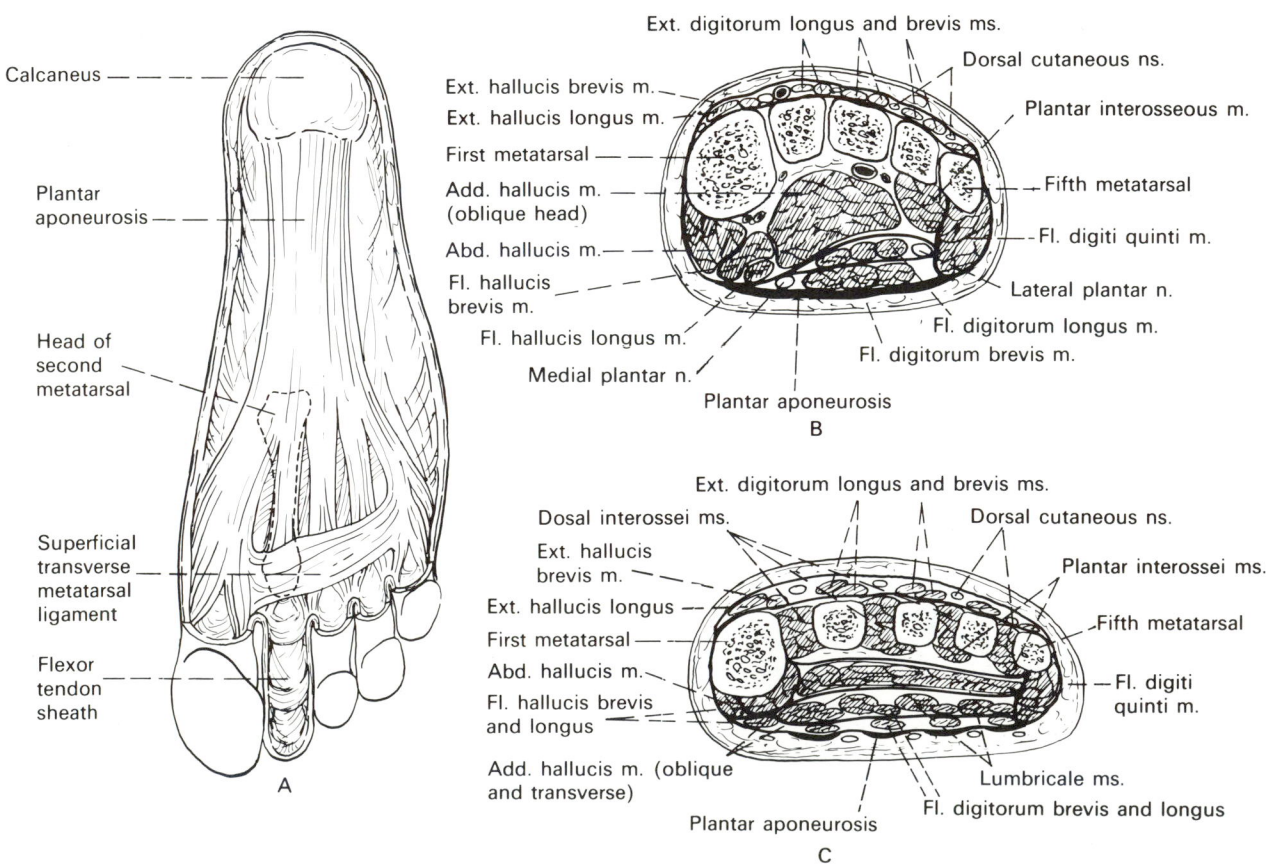

FIG. 76-13. Plantar aponeurosis and bones and muscles of the right foot. A. Inferior view. The plantar aponeurosis extends forward from its attachment to the posterior aspect of the calcaneus as a strong narrow band that divides at about the middle of the foot into digitation for the five toes. B. Cross section through the posterior metatarsal arch showing the fascial compartment and the relationship between the bones and supporting ligaments and muscles. The plantar aponeurosis and associated fascia are shown in black. The aponeurosis is thick on the plantar surface and rather thin on the lateral and dorsal aspects of the foot. C. Cross section at the anterior metatarsal arch. The bones are barely elevated. A modified from Hollinshead, W.H.: Anatomy for Surgeons. 3rd Ed. Vol. 3, The Back and Limbs. Philadelphia, Harper & Row, 1982. B and C modified from Eycleshymer, A.C., and Schoemaker, D.M.: A Cross-Section Anatomy. New York, D. Appleton-Century, 1911, p. 159.

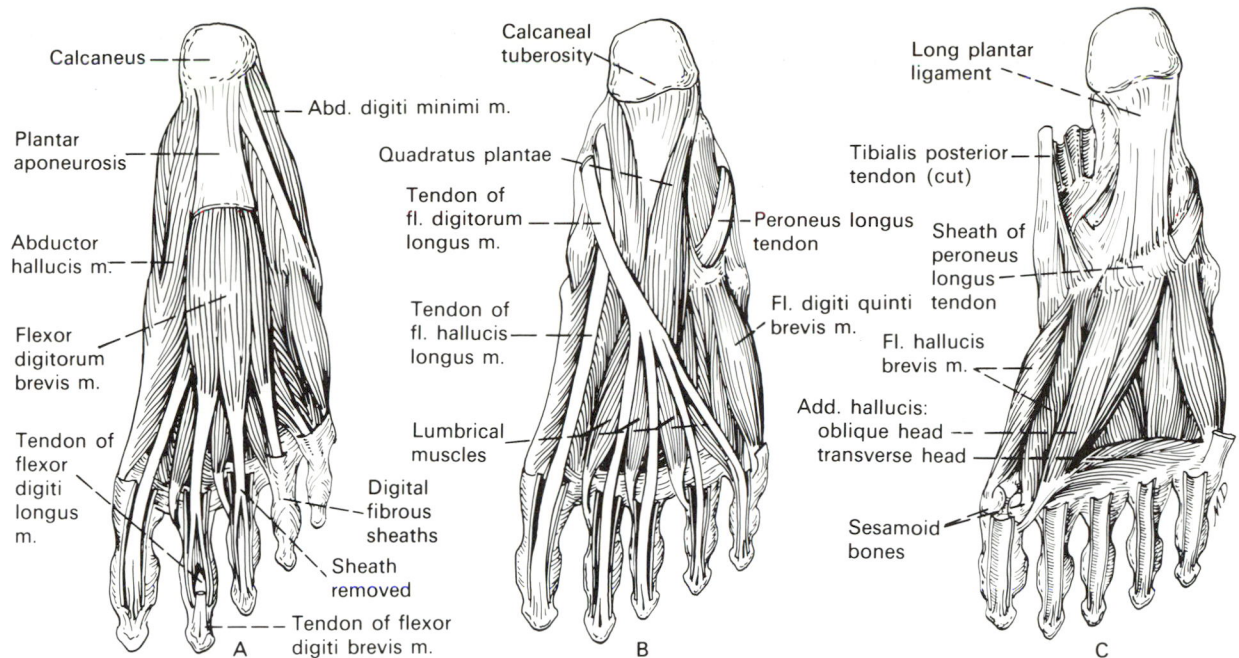

FIG. 76-14. Plantar muscles of the right foot. **A.** The first layer consists of the abductor hallucis, flexor digitorum brevis, and abductor digiti minimi. **B.** The second layer consists of the quadratus plantae and lumbrical muscles. The tendons of the flexor digitorum longus and flexor hallucis longus lie over these muscles. **C.** The third layer consists of the flexor hallucis brevis, adductor hallucis (composed of an oblique head and a transverse head), and flexor digiti minimi brevis. The fourth layer consists of the plantar and dorsal interossei (not shown). Modified from Clemente, C.D. (ed.): Gray's Anatomy of the Human Body. 30th Am. Ed. Philadelphia, Lea & Febiger, 1985.

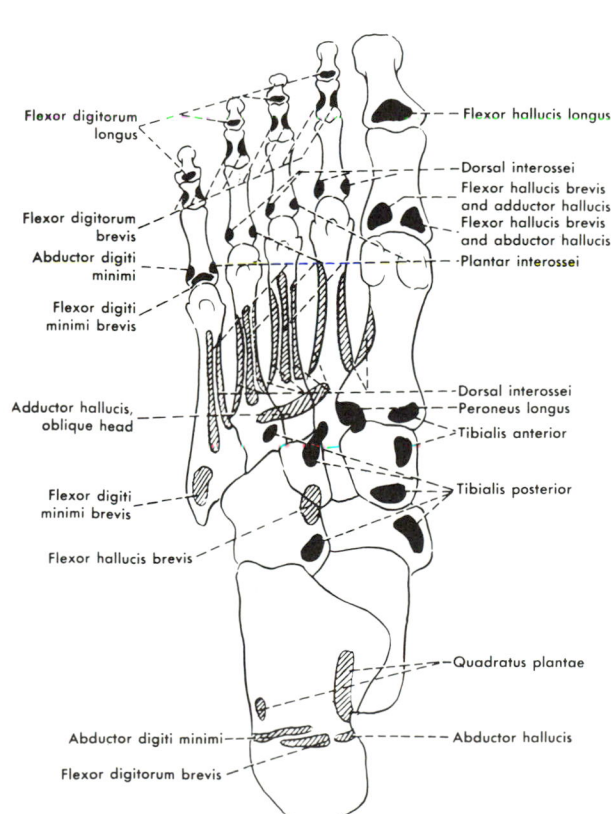

FIG. 76-15. Plantar view of the bones of the right foot showing the origins of the intrinsic muscles (*striped*) and the insertions of the extrinsic and intrinsic muscles (*black*). From Hollinshead, W.H.: Anatomy for Surgeons. 3rd Ed. Vol. 3, The Back and Limbs. Philadelphia, Harper & Row, 1982.

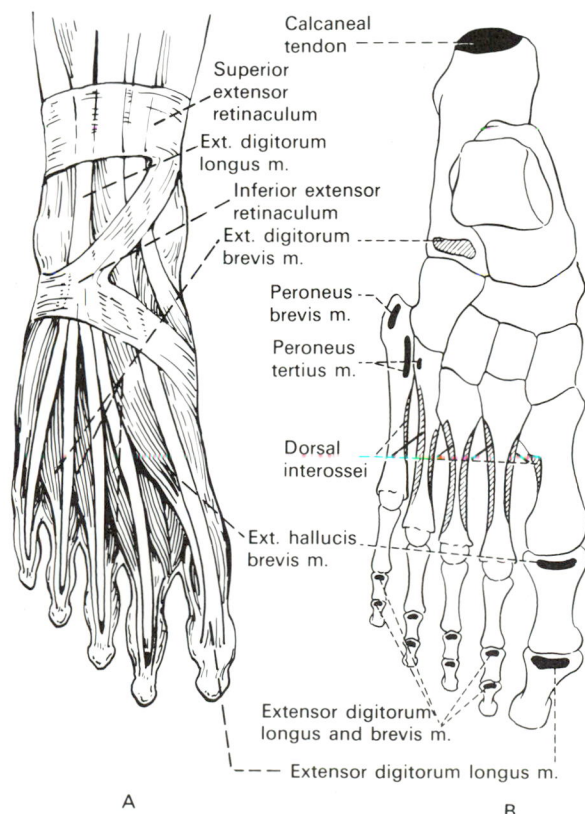

FIG. 76-16. **A.** Muscles of the dorsal surface of the right foot. **B.** Dorsal view of the bones of the foot showing the origins of the intrinsic muscles (*striped*) and the insertions of the intrinsic and extrinsic muscles (*black*). Modified from Hollinshead, W.H.: Anatomy for Surgeons. 3rd Ed. Vol. 3, The Back and Limbs. Philadelphia, Harper & Row, 1982.

Pain in the Leg, Ankle, and Foot **1597**

TABLE 76-3. Muscles of the Leg, Ankle, and Foot and their Nerve Supply

Region/Muscle Group/Function	Peripheral Nerve Supply	Segmental Nerve Supply*
Ankle and foot motion		
Dorsiflexion		
Tibialis anterior	Deep peroneal	L4, *5*, S1
Peroneus longus and brevis	Superficial peroneal	L4, *5*, S1
Plantar flexion		
Gastrocnemius	Tibial	*S1*, 2
Soleus	Tibial	*S1*, 2
Plantaris	Tibial	*S1*, 2
Eversion: peroneus longus and brevis	Superficial peroneal	L4, *5*, S1
Inversion		
Tibialis anterior	Deep peroneal	L4, *5*, S1
Tibialis posterior	Tibial	*L5*, S1
Toes		
Flexion		
Flexor digitorum longus and brevis	Tibial (brevis-medius plantaris)	*L5*, S1,
Flexor hallucis longus and brevis	Tibial (brevis-medius plantaris)	*L5*, S1
Extension		
Extensor hallucis longus	Tibial	*L5*, S1
Extensor digitorum longus and brevis	Deep peroneal	*L5*, S1
Abduction		
Abductor hallucis	Medial plantar	*L5*, S1
Abductor digiti minimi	Lateral plantar	*S1*, 2
Abductor of first toe: abductor hallucis	Lateral plantar	*S1*, 2
Other foot muscles		
Quadratus plantae—flexor terminal phalanx	Lateral plantar	*S1*, 2
Flexor digiti minimi—flexor proximal phalanx	Lateral plantar	*S1*, 2
1st lumbrical—flexor proximal phalanx of 2nd toe	Medial plantar	*L5*, *S1*
2nd, 3rd lumbricals—extend two distal phalanges of 3rd, 4th, 5th toes	Lateral plantar	*S1*, 2
Dorsal interossei (abduct 2nd, 3rd, 4th toes)	Lateral plantar	*S1*, 2
Plantar interossei (adduct 3rd, 4th, 5th toes)	Lateral plantar	*S1*, 2

*Italics indicate the main roots.

Blood is supplied to the foot by the terminal branches of the anterior and posterior tibial arteries, which anastomose with one another freely through the 1st intermetatarsal space (See Fig. 76-7). The top of the foot is supplied by the dorsalis pedis artery and its branches, which are derived from the anterior tibial artery, while the plantar surface is supplied by the medial and lateral plantar arteries, which are derived from the posterior tibial artery. As shown in Figure 76-7, the dorsalis pedis artery gives off medial and lateral metatarsal arteries, which supply the front part of the ankle joint, the first tarsal and deep plantar arteries, and the arcuate artery, which gives off the first metatarsal artery, and the plantar arch (derived from the lateral plantar artery) gives off the 2nd, 3rd, 4th, and 5th plantar metatarsals. These arteries supply the anterior tarsal joint and the tarsometatarsal and metatarsophalangeal joints on the dorsal and plantar side of the foot. Moreover, each plantar metatarsal artery gives off two digital arteries, which supply the dorsal and plantar aspects of the joints of adjacent toes.

Arches of the Foot

The foot has four arches, two longitudinal arches and two transverse arches. The medial and lateral longitudinal arches are formed by the union of specifi-

cally shaped bones, which together with the ligamentous support maintain the arches. The most important ligaments are shown in Figure 76-18. The plantar aponeurosis acts as a bowstring, as do the long and short plantar and spring ligaments. The medial arch is dome-shaped and is higher than the lateral arch, which is lower and flatter (Fig. 76-8). The posterior transverse or midtarsal arch is formed by the navicular, the three cuneiforms, the cuboid, and the bases of the metatarsal bones, and is maintained more by the ligaments and tendons that bind the bases of the metatarsals than by the structure of these bones (4). The anterior metatarsal arch, formed by the heads of the metatarsal bones, is shallow but complete on each foot, and is maintained by the deep transverse metatarsal ligaments. The degree of this arch depends on the pronation or supination of the forefoot and on the abduction and adduction of this anterior segment. The supinated foot usually has a higher anterior metatarsal arch whereas the pronated foot tends to flatten, almost eliminating any arching.

Movement and Biomechanics of the Foot

Movement

In the neutral or anatomic position the foot makes a 90° angle with the tibia (7, 10, 15, 16). Plantar flexion

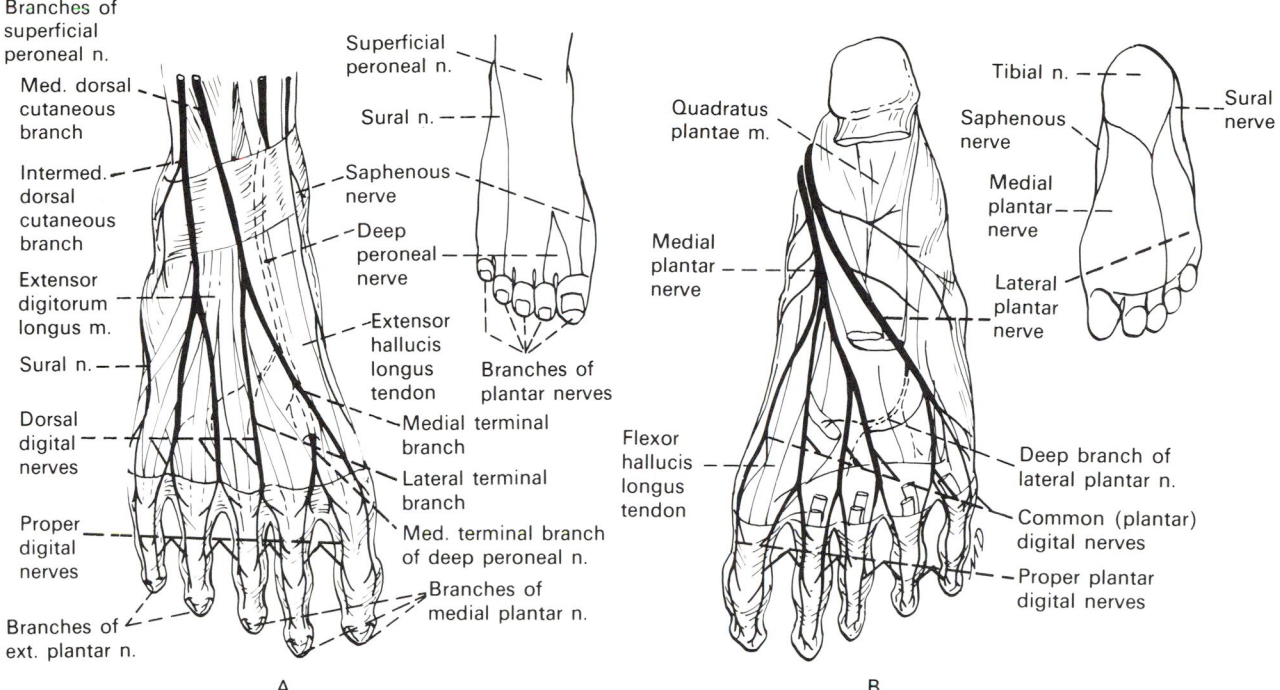

FIG. 76-17. Nerves of the foot. **A.** Dorsal view. **B.** Plantar view. See text for details. Modified from Goss, C.M. (ed.): Gray's Anatomy of the Human Body. 29th Am. Ed. Philadelphia, Lea & Febiger, 1959.

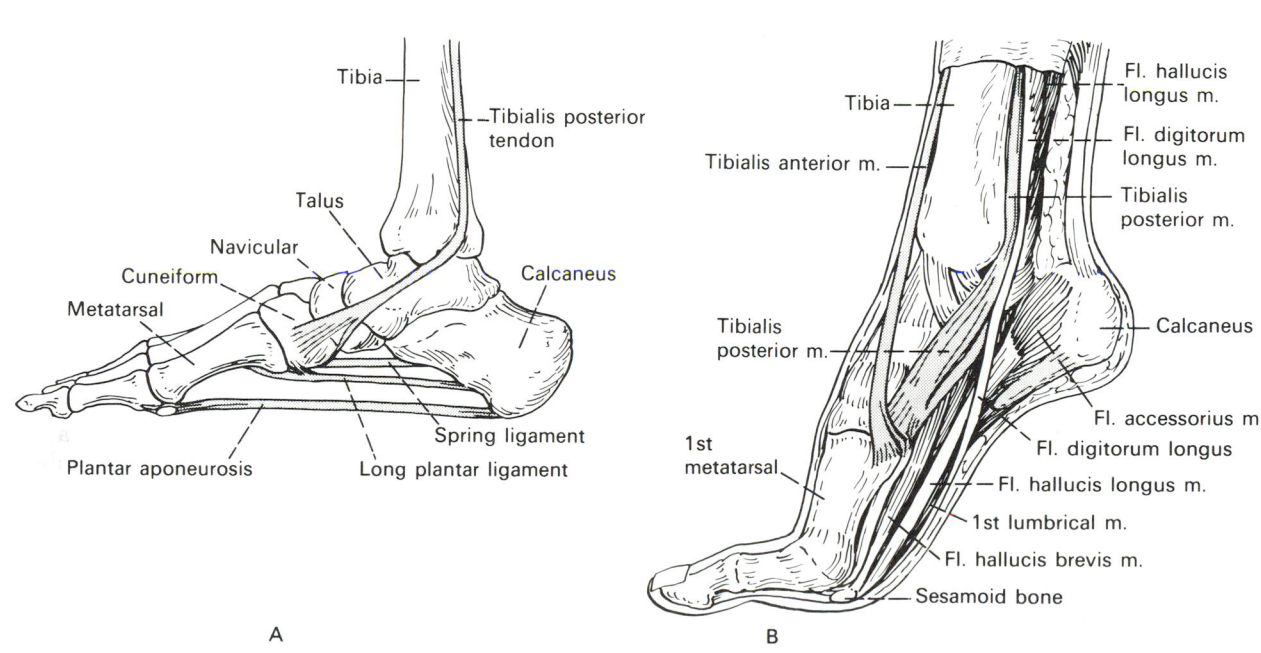

FIG. 76-18. **A.** Most important structures for maintenance of the longitudinal arches of the foot. For the sake of simplicity all ligaments are shown in the same sagittal plane and are seen from the same side. **B.** Dynamic stabilization of the medial arch. With the foot raised, as in walking, the heel is raised and the toes remain applied to the ground. The sesamoid bones and the flexor hallucis brevis tendons act as a cushioned support for the 1st metatarsal and give it increased height. The quadratus plantae lines the hollow between the flexor hallucis longus tendon and the heel. The tibialis posterior provides dynamic support in this stance.

increases and dorsiflexion decreases this angle; these motions occur principally at the ankle joint, with the axis passing through the tips of the two malleoli. The total range of motion of the ankle joint in the sagittal plane is approximately 45° but can vary widely among individuals and with age (15–17). Ten to 20° of this range of motion is in dorsiflexion and the remaining 25 to 35° is in plantar flexion. As a result of the different levels of these bony points, the axis slopes posteriorly, downward, and laterally (6, 8, 16, 17). Because of this deviation from the horizontal the foot deviates from the sagittal plane during plantar flexion and is associated with some toeing in, while during dorsiflexion some toeing out occurs. Toeing in and out can also be produced by tibial rotation or fixed tibial torsion but not by abduction or adduction at the ankle, because the talocrural joint permits only flexion and extension (10, 16) (Fig. 76-19).

Inversion and eversions are movements that turn the sole of the foot inward and outward, respectively (8, 16, 17). This side-to-side rotation of the foot occurs at the subtalar and transverse tarsal joints around an anterior posterior axis, which deviates slightly from the sagittal plane. During inversion the heel deviates medially and during eversion it deviates laterally from its neutral position, with the calcaneus vertically aligned with the midline of the tibia (Fig. 76-19A). In addition to the heel this motion involves the forefoot, and its deviation is gauged by the line of the 2nd metatarsal in relation to the tibia (Fib. 76-19B). In addition to rotation, because the axis of inversion and eversion is not strictly in the sagittal plane, the foot is adducted during inversion and abducted during eversion, a movement that occurs chiefly at the transverse tarsal joint.

These movements result from displacement of the metatarsals in relation to one another and involve the transverse tarsal joint and the joints distal to it (8, 16). The foot cannot actively adduct independently of inversion, nor can it abduct independently of eversion. In the neutral position the heads of the metatarsals are in the same horizontal plane that is in contact with the ground. Adduction associated with inversion elevates the head of the 1st metatarsal and depresses the head of the 5th metatarsal, while abduction associated with eversion has the opposite effect (Fig. 76-20).

Biomechanics

The foot is a weight-bearing structure used exclusively for locomotion. It adapts to uneven ground and allows the center of gravity of the body to be positioned over the center of support. The fit and construction of shoes affect shock absorption and the support afforded to the foot. Footwear available today is designed specifically for such activities as sports, aerobics, walking, running, and dancing, and provide the support, fit, control, shock absorption and, in some cases, splinting necessary for the specific activity. Wearing a shoe that is not designed for a vigorous form of activity can in itself be a source of pain (see below).

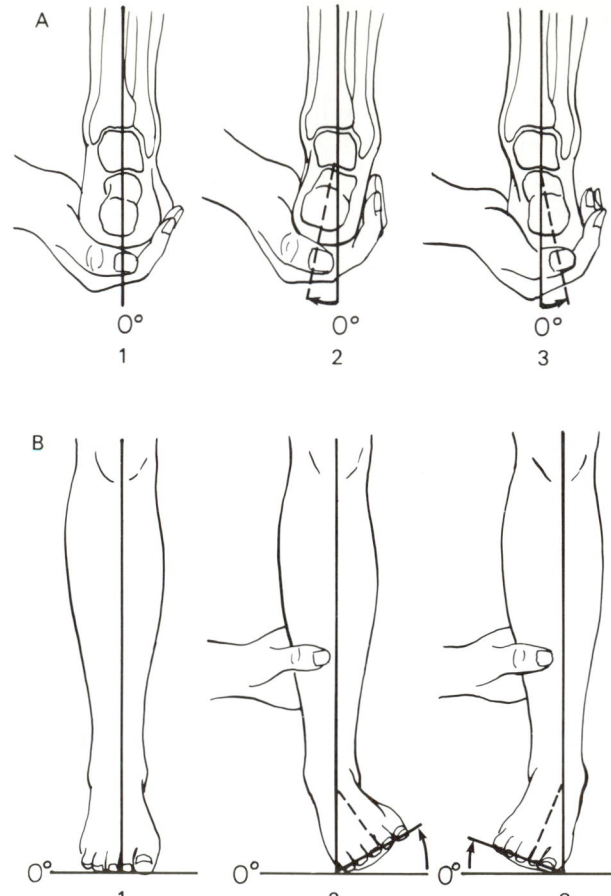

FIG. 76-19. Inversion and eversion. **A.** Movements at the heel showing inversion and eversion. In the neutral position the vertical axis of the heel is aligned with the longitudinal axis of the tibia (1). By grasping the calcaneus with the hand the entire heel can be moved inward (inversion) (2) or outward (eversion) (3) about 5°. Excessive inversion indicates laxity or tear of the calcaneofibular ligament and excessive eversion indicates tear or laxity of the deltoid ligament. **B.** Inversion and eversion of the forefoot. In the neutral position the line of the 2nd metatarsal is aligned with the midline of the tibia (1). Inversion is associated with adduction (2) and eversion is associated with abduction of the forefoot (3). Modified from the American Academy of Orthopedic Surgeons: Joint Motion: Method of Measuring and Recording. Chicago, American Academy of Orthopedic Surgeons, 1965.

Foot biomechanics deals with the alignment of and forces acting on the foot, which is composed of 26 bones, 19 muscles, and 107 ligaments that form 4 arches (medial and lateral longitudinal and posterior and anterior transverse). The shape of the foot is related to the supporting ligaments and musculotendinous units, in addition to the loading environment. Foot alignment during weight bearing determines the loading environment to which the foot is subjected. The alignment of the foot is determined by the shape of bony structures, ligamentous tension, coordination of the musculotendinous units, and alignment of the leg in general.

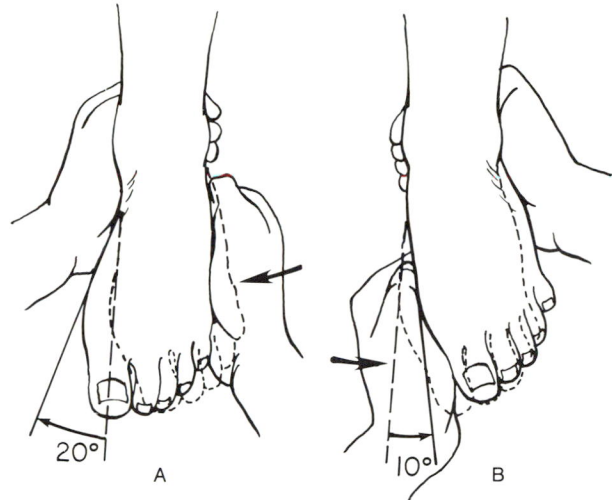

FIG. 76-20. Testing for adduction (*A*) or abduction (*B*) of the forefoot. This takes place primarily at the transverse tarsal joint and at joints distal to it. The examiner holds the patient's foot at the calcaneus. One hand stabilizes the heel in a neutral position during the test and the other moves the forefoot medially and laterally. Under normal circumstances adduction invariably accompanies inversion and abduction accompanies eversion. Modified from Hoppenfeld, S.: Physical Examination of the Spine and Extremities. New York, Apple-Century-Crofts, 1976.

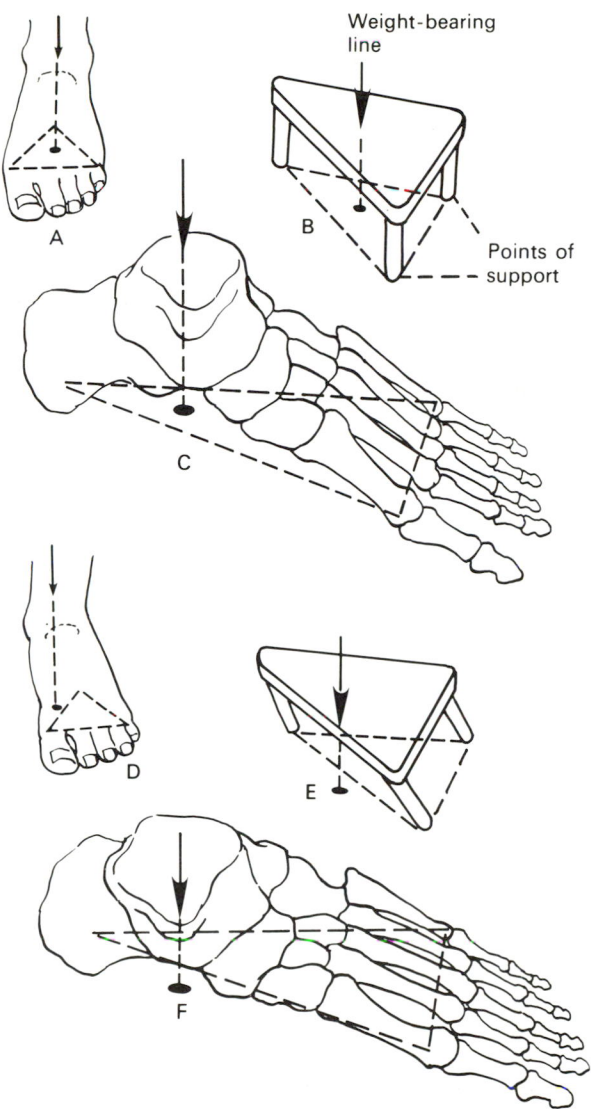

FIG. 76-21. Weight-bearing alignment of the foot. This can be conceptualized as a tripod formed by the heads of the 1st and 5th metatarsals anteriorly and the calcaneus posteriorly. *A, B, C.* The normal weight-bearing line should fall within the center of the tripod. *D, E.* The weight-bearing line falls medially in a pronated foot. *F.* The foot rolls inward and the structures on the medial side of the foot are placed under tension, eventually causing deformation of the foot.

The foot can be thought of as a tripod, with the os calcis providing one point of support and the heads of the 5th and 1st metatarsals providing the other two points of support (Fig. 76-21). The weight-bearing line normally passes through the ankle joint into this tripod area. If the weight-bearing line passes outside the area, strain problems arise. For example, in a pronated foot, the weight-bearing line falls medially, the foot rolls inward, and structures on the medial side of the foot are placed in tension. If the weight-bearing line falls laterally in a supinated foot the foot rolls outward and overloads the lateral border of the foot. In addition a varus thrust occurs at the knee, which can cause medial knee pain. Thus, abnormal foot biomechanics in an active individual can eventually lead to local and even widespread discomfort (6, 11, 16, 17).

B. EVALUATION OF THE PATIENT

The epidemiologic data cited above emphasize that a large segment of the population seeks health care because of pain in the foot, ankle, and leg. Comfortable feet are usually taken for granted but the smallest problem can quickly dominate a person's sense of well-being. Not all feet are created equal, nor are they treated equally by their owners. Variations in size, shape, posture, soft tissue tone, and strength are significant in the development of foot pain syndromes. To these anatomic variables can be added the daily wear and tear on the feet by shoes that are often designed more for fashion than for fit, support, and comfort. The leg, foot, and ankle are also subjected to diseases that affect the musculoskeletal system elsewhere, including inflammatory joint disease, degenerative joint disease and infection, trauma, and various systemic disorders.

Pain in the foot, ankle, and leg of any degree, even in sedentary persons, becomes an urgent matter. Fortunately, simple therapeutic measures can greatly relieve pain in the foot. A patient with a painful ingrown nail is just as grateful for the relief provided by cotton placed between the nail and the nail fold as the arthritic who has just undergone successful total hip arthroplasty. Physicians can do a great service to a patient by being aware of and using the general

TABLE 76-4. Evaluation of the Patient with Pain in the Leg, Ankle, and Foot

---

I. HISTORY
  A. Characteristics of the pain: location and distribution; intensity, quality, temporal characteristics; factors that aggravate and relieve pain
  B. Associated symptoms and signs: numbness, paresthesia, swelling, cramping, deformities, ulcerations
  C. General medical and family history

II. PHYSICAL EXAMINATION
  A. Inspection
    1. Bony contours and alignment: patella with 1st interdigital space; valgus or varus?
    2. Soft tissue contours: medial arch, atrophy of muscles, swelling of joints, deformity
    3. All five toes straight?—overriding, clawing, valgus or varus deviation?
    4. Color of skin: cyanosis, pallor, redness on dependence
    5. Texture of skin and hair: atrophy of skin? coarseness of hair?
    6. Scarring, sinuses, ulceration of skin
  B. Inspection with patient standing on both feet
    1. Medial arch of both feet
    2. Alignment of vertical axis of heel with calcaneus; flat feet?
    3. Is angle between two feet 30° with toeing out? center of gravity?
    4. Standing on tips of all toes
    5. Standing on one foot with other foot off ground:
      a. Normally results in pronation
      b. Rotation of body to one side and the other while on one foot—medial rotation of tibia produces pronation (abduction), lateral rotation produces supernation (adduction)
  C. Palpation
    1. Skin temperature; local tenderness; bone and soft tissue contours
    2. Ankle and foot
      a. Calcaneus tendon—swelling, integrity?
      b. Pressure on tendon and calcaneus: tenderness, spurs
      c. Medial arch: tenderness, strain of plantar aponeurosis
      d. Palpation of calcaneus tuberosity; strain of ligament
      e. Ball of the foot: pressure on metatarsal heads, tenderness, callouses, fusiform swelling (neuroma)
  D. State of peripheral circulation, palpation of pulses: femoral, popliteal, dorsalis pedis, posterior tibial
  E. Range of muscle and muscle strength
    1. At ankle: plantar flexion
    2. At subtalar joint: inversion-adduction, eversion-abduction
    3. At midtarsal joint: inversion-adduction, eversion-abduction
    4. At the toes: flexion, extension
  F. Stability: ankle joint, lateral and medial ligaments; subtarsal, midtarsal joints; tarsophalangeal joint
  G. Gait: observation of gait, footwear trial
  H. Examination of lower back, hip, and thigh; general survey of other parts of body

III. NEUROLOGIC EXAMINATION
  Sensory changes
  Motor changes
  Reflex changes

IV. Radiographic and other special examinations: see Table 76-5

---

principles for treating pain in this part of the limb described in this chapter.

Evaluation of the patient with pain in the leg, ankle, or foot, or in a combination of these, should be carried out similarly to that described in Chapters 31 and 70. Table 76-4 summarizes the major points of the history and clinical examination of a patient suspected of having a painful disorder of the leg, ankle, or foot. Because the anatomy of the leg and foot render them so accessible to examination, a diagnosis can almost always be made based on the history and physical examination (8, 10, 15, 18). Because pain in the leg and foot can be caused by systemic disease or pain can be referred from disorders of the low back or the vascular system, a general history and physical examination should be carried out when so indicated. The following discussion concentrates on pain confined to the leg and foot and presents a routine for evaluation of the functional anatomy of the region. The leg and foot must

also be examined as a dynamic unit because they are important components of the locomotor system (8).

History

The clinical evaluation of the patient with pain in the foot, ankle, or leg begins by taking a detailed history and then proceeding methodically through the features and characteristics of the pain. If feasible, the patient should be given a questionnaire to fill out prior to examination because this helps to create a more reflective mindset and to elicit more accurate information.

The patient should be asked specifically when and under what circumstances the pain was first experienced, and the time course of the onset of pain. Pain of acute onset can usually be traced to specific events such as traumatic episodes, overuse, or an unusual activity such as standing on a ladder all weekend while painting the house. A sedentary person who begins an aerobic dance course can be expected to have pain in the leg, ankle, and foot. Gradual or insidious development of pain without a precipitating event might reflect a systemic problem or structural abnormality that the person has had for many years, and that is just becoming symptomatic.

The characteristics of the pain, including location, intensity, quality, temporal profile, and aggravating and relieving factors, should be elicited. The patient should be asked to point exactly to where the pain is located and to trace the distribution of any radiation. Pain aggravated by walking or running and relieved by rest can be caused by circulatory insufficiency of the leg or by a stress fracture of the ankle or foot. Some measure of the intensity of the pain should be used, such as the 1 to 10 intensity scale (0 being no pain and 10 being the most severe pain imaginable). Any relationship of the pain to weather (e.g., arthritis), other joint involvement (e.g., systemic disease), or to a general illness from which the current symptoms might stem should be ascertained.

The quality of the pain does much to help with the differential diagnosis. Local pathology can usually be found with sharp well-localized discomfort. More diffuse aching about the leg or whole foot can be caused by systemic disease or by a collapsed foot or foot strain, and might not be associated with other physical findings. The temporal profile of the pain should be elicited. Is the pain intermittent or continuous? Is the overall trend one of improvement, worsening, or no change since onset?

In inquiring about the functional disability, pain intensity levels can be correlated with actual disability, such as during activities of daily living, work-related activities, and recreational activities. In each category the physician should ask enough questions to develop a clear picture of the type of loading environment and degree of physical stress that the foot, ankle, and leg must absorb during a typical day and the duration of exposure before symptoms appear. This is particularly important in patients suspected of having calf pain caused by peripheral vascular disease, and in patients with pain in the ankle and foot caused by bone or joint pathology.

Patients who complain of foot pain should be asked about the type of footwear they wear because this type of pain is often caused or at least aggravated by inappropriate footwear. Although the public is growing more knowledgeable about footwear many patients are unaware of the relationship of their shoes to their foot pain. Ideally, the physician should see the type of shoes worn by patients for recreational and work-related activities. If the feet hurt in shoes but patients are comfortable barefoot, improper fit of shoes should immediately be suspected.

Physical Examination

The leg, foot, and ankle are visible and readily available for detailed examination. The patient should be suitably undressed to allow examination from the waist down.

Inspection

The physical examination begins with observation of the patient, who first sits on the edge of the examination table, then stands on both feet, and then on one foot, and then assumes a prone position. The patient sits on the edge of the examination table with the legs and feet well lit, hanging free in front of the examiner, who sits comfortably to make the following observations. The patella should be in vertical alignment with the 1st interosseous or interdigital space. Significant deviation of the foot axis from the sagittal plane suggests tibial torsion of valgus or varus deformity of the forefoot (8, 15, 18). The relaxed foot should hang in slight plantar flexion unless there is bony deformity, contracture, or muscle spasm in the leg. The medial longitudinal arch should be recognizable. All five toes should be straight or only slightly bent, with no overriding clawing valgus or varus deviation. Abnormal signs include local areas of increased or decreased temperature, presence of hair on the small toes, abnormal coloration (e.g., blanching, blotching, or cyanosis, as seen in peripheral vascular disease), or localized areas of redness from shoe pressure. Ingrown nail problems that are painfully disabling can be avoided by cutting the nails squarely and beyond the nail fold.

Next, the patient should stand, preferably on a platform, the medial arch should be inspected in relation to the weight-bearing feet, and the alignment of the vertical axis of the heel with the calcaneus tendon should be noted (10, 18). If the foot is flat it is important to observe whether the heel is everted. The patient is asked to stand on tiptoes, which should produce inversion of the heel and an increase in the longitudinal arch. This is followed by asking the patient to stand on one weight-bearing foot while the opposite leg is lifted—in the normal foot this results in pronation. The patient is requested to rotate the body from side to side while standing on one leg. The medial and lateral rotation of the tibia during this movement produces alternating pronation and supination of the normal foot.

The heel and sole of the foot are examined with the patient prone. Subtle differences, such as swelling about the origin of the plantar fascia, are best appreciated by comparing one side to the other in good light and with the patient properly positioned (18).

Many diagnostic signs in the foot are caused by changes in the biomechanics of standing and walking. A foot with an abnormal arch lacks normal motion; in the standing position excessive varus or valgus or adduction or abduction can produce asymmetric pressure areas and overuse of joints. Inspection of the foot for callosities, corns, areas of redness, and increased skin thickening indicates where pressure is being concentrated. Skin and nails should be inspected for hair, color, and temperature. The skin's texture should be examined along with the presence of excessive or diminished sweating. These functions are altered with peripheral vascular disease, reflex sympathetic dystrophy, and peripheral neuropathies.

Shoe wear patterns provide helpful clues. Normal wear at the heel is slightly lateral to the midline. Excessive wear at the heel or sole associated with medial or lateral drift of the upper surface of the shoe indicates abnormal foot posture and dynamics. The interior of the shoe, particularly the toe box, should be inspected for signs of toe pressure.

Palpation

As noted in Table 76-4, palpation of the heel region includes grasping the calcaneus or Achilles tendon (Fig. 76-22A). Tenderness of the tendon can result from minor tears caused by overuse, or the connective tissue around it can be inflamed. Palpation of a gap in the tendon usually indicates rupture. Tenderness at the insertion of the tendon on the back of the heel can be caused by bursitis (Fig. 76-22B), and tenderness on the plantar surface of the calcaneus can be caused by palpable bony spurs or by strain and inflammation in the plantar aponeurosis and its calcaneal attachment (Fig. 76-22C).

Palpation of the hollow of the sole of the foot can elicit tenderness caused by strain of the plantar aponeurosis (Fig. 76-22D). Tenderness immediately proximal to the tuberosity of the navicular suggests a strained spring ligament. Tenderness elicited by pressure on the metatarsal heads suggests neuroma of the digital nerves or calluses (Fig. 76-22E). Usually the head of the 2nd metatarsal is the most painful in metatarsalgia. Careful palpation can reveal a fusiform swelling, which suggests the presence of neuroma.

Determining the state of the peripheral circulation is an essential part of the examination of the leg, foot, and ankle that is often forgotten (7). A reasonably accurate assessment can be made by feeling the skin temperature and texture, by verifying the presence of the pulses in the dorsalis pedis and posterior tibial arteries at the ankle, the posterior tibial pulse in back of the knee, and the femoral pulse below the inguinal ligament, and by determining the rate of capillary filling. The texture of the skin and nails should be carefully observed and palpated. Arterial insufficiency of the leg and foot causes loss of hair, which also becomes thin and elastic, the nails become coarse, thickened, and irregular, and the tips of the toes become ulcerated (Chapters 11 and 28). If a peripheral vascular disease is suspected, special studies should be carried out, including ankle pressure recordings, Doppler ultrasound analysis, and other tests (Chapter 28).

Range of Motion

In examining the active and passive ranges of motion, it should be determined whether pain is a limiting factor. Movement should be separately tested at the ankle, subtalar, transverse, tarsal, and metatarsophalangeal joints. This is most easily done with the patient in the sitting position. The examiner should look especially for restriction at the subtalar joint, which is a sign of tarsal coalition. Loss of motion at the metatarsophalangeal joint of the toe indicates hallux rigidus. Excessive laxity at the 1st tarsometatarsal joint can decrease the weight borne by the hallux and transfer more weight to the 2nd metatarsal head.

Figure 76-23 depicts the method of examining movement at the ankle and midtarsal joints and toe movements. To test the range of plantar flexion and dorsiflexion the examiner grasps the heel with one hand and stabilizes the foot with the other. Although considerable variation exists, at least 15 to 20° should be in dorsiflexion and 20 to 25° in plantar flexion. The two sides should be compared.

Tests for active range of motion and strength are shown in Figure 76-24. The results of these tests also provide an indication of the muscle power in the various functional units.

Joint Stability

The collateral and anterior tibiofibular ligaments should be palpated for tenderness. To test the stability of the ankle the leg should be grasped with one hand and the heel with the other and moved posteriorly or anteriorly. If the foot can be pushed forward in the ankle mortise (anterior drawer sign), this suggests that the anterior talofibular, or tibionavicular ligament, or both, is torn (Fig. 22-4). Figure 76-19 illustrates tests for eversion and inversion. Excessive inversion or eversion indicates tears in the calcaneofibular or deltoid ligaments, respectively (5, 8, 15, 18). Figure 76-20 illustrates tests for adduction and abduction (14).

Gait

While the patient walks back and forth in the corridor the examiner notes any antalgia and observes the position of the toes during the foot-flat, toe-off, and swing phases of the gait. Toes that lie in a normal position during stance can assume a claw toe or hammertoe configuration during swing-through or push-off. These dynamic postures lead to callosities and contractures. A medial or lateral thrust at the ankle causes strain of the muscle tendon groups—for example, the posterior tibial tendon medially and the peronei laterally. With the patient standing next to the shoes the degree of splaying or speading of the forefoot and of shoe fit should be noted. Excessive supination, cavus or high arch pattern, and the presence of excessive pronation are noted.

Neurologic Examination

Although having the patient walk on the toes, heels, and lateral and medial edges of the foot provides a rough estimation of muscle strength, the strength of each muscle should be tested individually. The power of the triceps surae can be tested by opposing plantar flexion or by observing elevation of the heel while the patient attempts to stand on tiptoe. The

ankle jerk test also objectively reveals the integrity of the muscle and the nerve pathway. The dorsiflexors of the ankle can be tested by opposing dorsiflexion. Similarly, the power of the extrinsic flexors and extensors of the toes can be evaluated by opposing their action.

A neurologic examination should include elicitation of the ankle jerk reflex while the foot is in slight passive dorsiflexion. Sensory examination should include pinprick, pin scratch, tactile, and proprioceptive tests (Chapter 31). Painful areas should be evaluated for the presence of neuroma by gentle tapping (Tinel's test). Foot trauma often produces injury to the sensory nerves, either by contusion or by stretching.

Diminished strength, as noted by isometric testing, can reflect incompetency of the musculotendinous unit caused by overstretching, tendon ruptures, degenerative changes within the tendon or associated muscle groups, and neurologic disease. The calf circumference should be measured. Any decrease of more than 2 cm is objective evidence of muscle atrophy, which is most often a sign of peripheral neuropathy or disease atrophy resulting from pain. Focal areas of increased warmth, swelling, and tenderness indicate inflammation, which then must be localized to a particular joint, tendon, or tendon sheath complex. Crepitation over a tendon sheath during active motion is pathognomonic of acute tenosynovitis.

Radiographic Examination

The radiographic examination includes routine radiographs, special views, and stress radiographs of the leg, ankle, or foot, whichever is indicated. When possible, weight-bearing radiographs should be obtained, including anteroposterior (AP), lateral, and oblique views of the foot and ankle. Care should be taken to note abnormalities in the structural alignment of the foot, condition of the joints, mineralization, and any overlying soft tissue abnormalities. Special views show the sesamoids (Fig. 76-25) and the tarsal coalitions (19).

When laxity is suspected stress radiographs are performed, usually by the orthopedic surgeon. Anteroposterior and lateral stress radiographs of the ankle should be taken on both the affected and normal sides. The views are then compared to note any joint subluxation. A similar stress series is done with inversion and eversion stress applied. Midfoot discomfort related to an old Lisfranc's injury can be caused by residual joint laxity. Abduction, adduction, and hyperflexion stresses are applied to both feet, noting any increased motion on the abnormal side.

Footwear Trial

When strain, overuse, or overload syndromes are suspected, a trial of supportive footwear provides a good diagnostic test. We use a special test shoe that can be made to simulate various footwear corrections. The patient's feedback helps to determine the best shoe orthotic correction and prescription (20, 21) (Figs. 76-26 and 76-27).

Special Examinations

Arthrography, tomography, and arthroscopy provide specific information about joints. Ankle and subtalar arthrography are used to evaluate capsular laxity and integrity, irregular joint surfaces, and the presence of loose bodies. Tomography and CT scanning are useful for evaluating the subtalar area for tarsal coalitions. Arthroscopy of the ankle, which enables the orthopedic surgeon to inspect chondral lesions and to do limited shaving of chondromalacia, is still being perfected. Arthroscopy is facilitated by an external fixation technique that distracts the ankle (22). CT scanning, magnetic resonance imaging (MRI), and ultrasonography have special applicability to the foot. Soft tissue tumors are particularly amenable to these procedures because they can

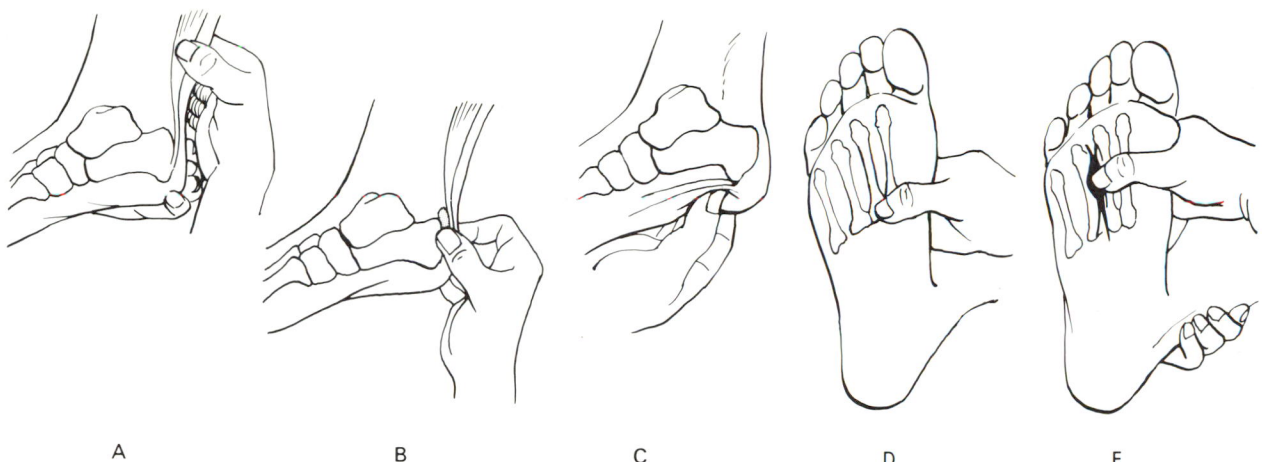

A   B   C   D   E

FIG. 76-22. Elicitation of pain of various causes by palpation of the heel and the sole surface of the foot. *A.* Palpation of the Achilles tendon. *B.* Palpation of the calcaneal bursa. *C.* Palpation of the undersurface of the calcaneus at the point of attachment of the plantar fascia can elicit pain caused by plantar fasciitis. *D.* Palpation of the heads of the metatarsals can cause pain. *E.* Palpation of an interdigital neuroma can produce sharp shooting pain. See text for details.

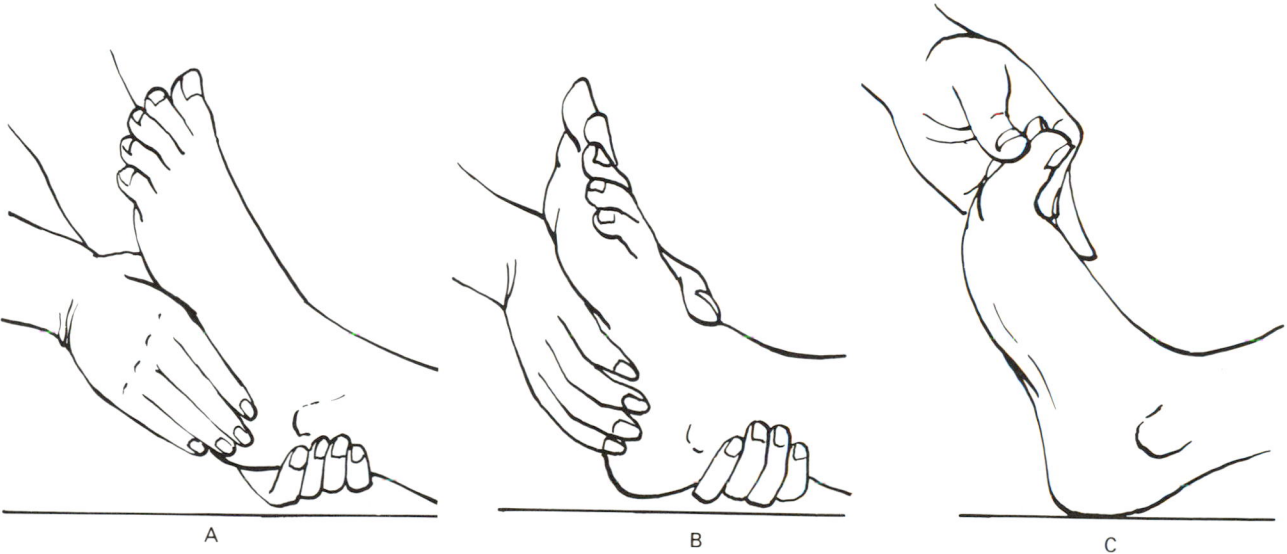

A   B   C

FIG. 76-23. Maneuvers for examining movements at the ankle, midtarsal joint, and metatarsophalangeal joint of the big toe. *A.* Examination of ankle movement. The examiner's hand grips the hindfoot and tendocalcaneus rather than the forefoot so that the movements of the subtalar and metatarsal joints are eliminated. The normal range of ankle movement varies, but in the average normal foot it is 20 to 25° for dorsal flexion and 25 to 35° for plantar flexion. *B.* Examination of metatarsal movement. The examiner grasps the tendocalcaneus firmly so that the subtalar movement is eliminated. The other hand lightly grasps the midfoot near the bases of the metatarsals and the patient is asked to twist the foot alternately inward and outward into inversion and eversion. Normal rotation should be 15 to 20° on each side of neutral. *C.* Examination of the normal range of motion at the metatarsophalangeal joint of the big toe. This should be nearly 90°; less than 60° of dorsal flexion is considered abnormal. Modified from Adams, J.C.: Outline of Orthopedics. 10th Ed. Edinburgh, Churchill Livingstone, 1986.

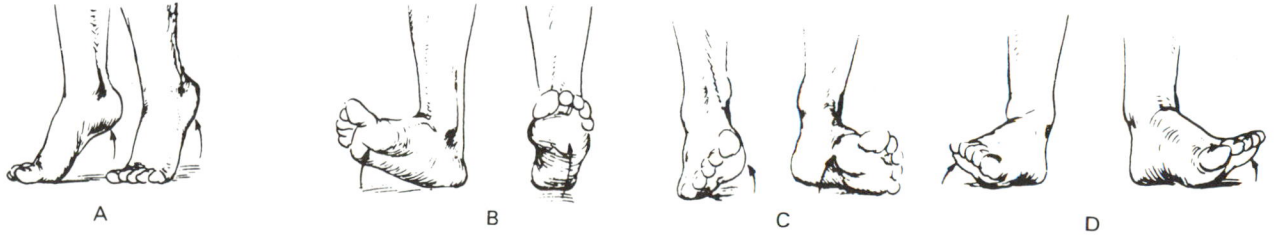

A   B   C   D

FIG. 76-24. Rapid method of testing active range of motion and the strength of the muscles that control movement of the ankle and foot. *A.* Test of plantar flexion and toe motion. The patient is asked to walk on the toes. *B.* Test of dorsiflexion. The patient is asked to walk on the heel. *C.* Test of inversion. The patient is asked to walk on the lateral borders of the feet. *D.* Test of eversion. The patient is asked to walk on the medial borders of the feet. From Hoppenfeld, S.: Physical Examination of the Spine and Extremities. New York, Apple-Century-Crofts, 1976.

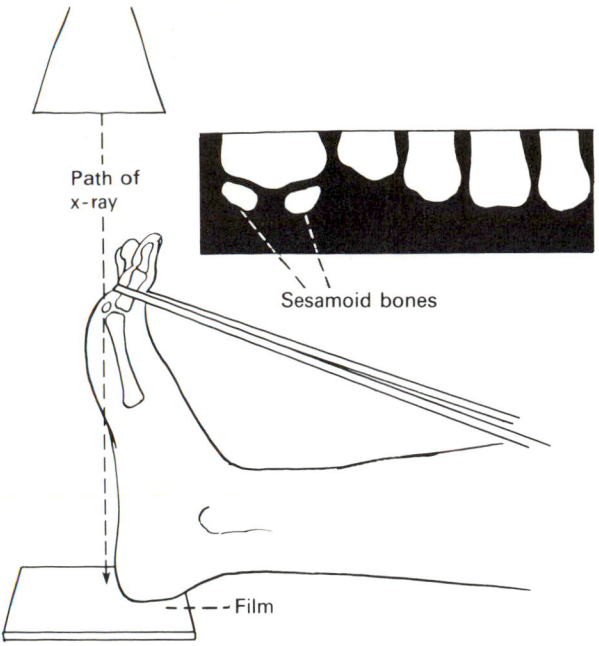

FIG. 76-25. Special method for obtaining radiographs to assess the joint surfaces and sesamoid alignment of the foot.

help to locate the extent of infiltration and to determine whether the tumor is solid or cystic (23, 24). Electromyography and nerve conduction velocity testing, particularly across the tarsal canal, help to evaluate the tarsal tunnel for entrapment. Doppler testing provides useful information about the adequacy of circulation to the digit level.

Diagnostic Blocks

When a particular joint is suspected to be the painful source or the integrity of an old fusion site is questioned, injection of a low concentration of a local anesthetic (e.g., 0.5% lidocaine or 0.25% bupivacaine) into the joint can help to localize the source of pain. For example, an injection made between the metatarsal heads can help to distinguish between Morton's neuroma and metatarsalgia. When the pain follows peripheral nerve patterns a localized entrapment neuropathy should be suspected.

Laboratory Tests

Diagnostic tests for foot problems include joint fluid analysis and joint biopsy. Joint aspiration, particularly of the MP joints, ankle, and subtalar joints, is easily performed. Joint fluid is typically sent for cell count differential, culture, and sensitivity testing and for the presence of uric acid or calcium pyrophosphate crystals. When osteomyelitis is suspected, needle or open biopsy of the small joints can be done for pathologic analysis. Table 76-5 summarizes physical findings and diagnostic tests for painful foot and ankle conditions.

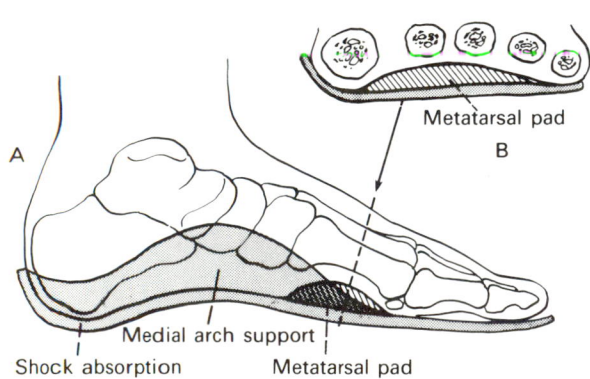

FIG. 76-26. Two commonly used orthotics. **A.** Medial arch support. This provides support and control of the medial and longitudinal arches. **B.** Metatarsal pad. This relieves stress from weight-bearing forces under the metatarsal heads.

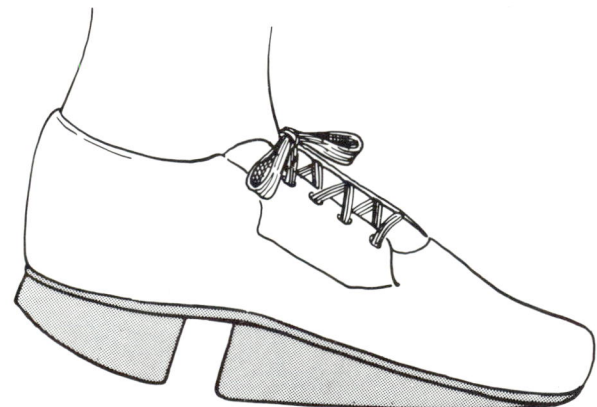

FIG. 76-27. Shoe with rocker bottom heel and sole. This helps to produce a smooth rolling motion during gait that reduces forces on the metatarsal heads.

C. PAINFUL DISORDERS OF THE LEG

Fractures

The tibia and fibula are two of the most frequently fractured long bones in the body. In this age of vehicular accidents the tibia and fibula are frequently subjected to high-energy trauma. The tibia has little soft tissue coverage and a poor blood supply (25). Because of these factors severe injury, particularly when combined with inadequate or inappropriate treatment, can lead to complications and major disability. The following incidence of complications has been noted after open fracture has been diagnosed: chronic infection, 10%; nonunion, 15%; and amputation, 5% (25) (Fig. 76-28).

Symptoms and Signs

Pain is the predominant symptom of fracture of the leg. Depending on whether the fracture is open or closed, associated signs such as swelling and bleeding are noted. Unless early restoration of function is carried out, muscle atrophy, loss of joint motion, osteoporosis, and dystrophy of prolonged disuse can occur.

Treatment

The treatment of the pain of fracture is discussed in Chapter 23. Most patients have sufficient pain to require opioids given intramuscularly or, preferably, by

TABLE 76-5. Diagnostic Tests for Ankle and Foot Pain

Painful Condition	Imaging Tests								Special Tests						
	Ultrasonography	MRI	CT scanning	Arthrography	Tomography	Stress radiography	Plain radiography	Bone scanning	Generic shoe	Walking cast	Arthroscopy	Injection	Doppler	Nerve conduction	Electromyography
Ankle															
Arthritis							X	X			X	X			
Laxity				X	X	X	X								
Tendinitis							X		X	X					
Osteochondral diseases			X	X	X		X				X				
Hindfoot															
Plantar fasciitis									X						
Tarsal coalition			X		X		X	X				X			
Achilles tendinitis	X								X						
Heel pad deficiency									X						
Tarsal tunnel entrapment														X	X
Midfoot															
Medial arch strain							X		X						
Lisfranc's joint instability						X	X	X				X			
Post. tib. tendon insufficiency	X						X		X						
Ganglion		X													
Forefoot															
Stress effects							X	X							
Metatarsalgia									X			X			
Callosities									X						
Great toe															
Hallux valgus (bunion)							X		X						
Hallux rigidis							X		X						
Hypermobility							X		X						
Sesamoiditis							X	X	X	X					
Gout							X								
Small toes															
Hammertoes							X								
Claw toes							X								
Soft corns							X								
Hard corns							X								
Neuroma									X			X			
Toe overlap							X								
Bunionette							X								
Neuropathy														X	X

the use of patient-controlled analgesia. An alternative is the use of intraspinal opioids or continuous epidural analgesia, which can be started prior to radiography and orthopedic therapy (closed or open). Excellent results have been cited by Chapman (25) using non-surgical and surgical methods.

Acute Rupture of the Gastrocnemius Muscle

Rupture of the gastrocnemius muscle is usually the result of a vigorous contracture of the muscle, in which the knee fails to flex and the foot is dorsiflexed (26). Occasionally the rupture is caused by a direct blow from a sharp object on the muscle while it is in active contraction. The rupture usually occurs in the substance of the medial head of the gastrocnemius or at the musculoaponeurotic junction.

Signs and Symptoms

The rupture is characterized by sudden pain and a snapping sensation in the calf, and often occurs while the patient is playing tennis (tennis leg) (9, 26). The

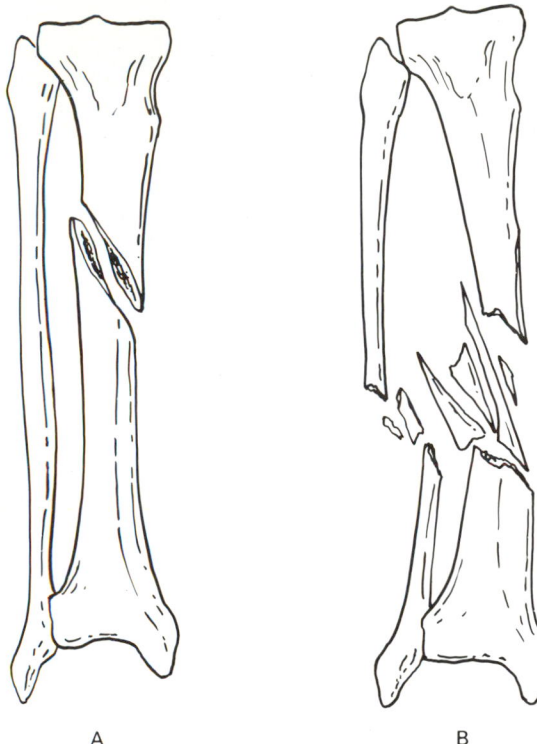

FIG. 76-28. Fracture of the tibia. *A.* Long spiral fracture. This is typical of a low-energy torsion injury, such as commonly seen in association with skiing. *B.* Comminuted fracture of the tibia with wide displacement of the tibia from the fibula. This indicates severe soft tissue trauma characteristic of a high-energy fracture commonly associated with motor vehicle accidents. Modified from Chapman, M.W.: Fractures of the tibial and fibular shafts. *In* Surgery of the Musculoskeletal System. Edited by C.W. Evarts. New York, Churchill Livingstone, 1983.

sudden pain is associated with local tenderness on the medial aspect of the muscle, and the patient cannot walk without a limp or crutches. Examination reveals a palpable gap in the muscle. In most severe cases the course of the rupture can be complicated by the formation of a large dense hematoma under the crural fascia and by increasing pain, particularly when the patient attempts to dorsiflex the ankle. Signs of muscle ischemia in the posterior superficial compartment of the leg can develop as a result of the hematoma.

Diagnosis and Treatment

The diagnosis is made through the history and physical examination. The control of pain is similar to that for rupture of the Achilles tendon (see below). A partial tear is treated with a short leg cast with the foot in slight equinus. A built-up heel is used for 3 to 4 weeks to allow the patient to bear weight without crutches (9, 26). Alternatively the patient can start ambulation with crutches and bear partial weight with a built-up heel after 10 to 14 days. If partial ischemia is present, surgical evacuation of the hematoma is indicated.

Rupture of the Calcaneal Tendon

According to Adams (9), rupture of the calcaneal (Achilles) tendon is often overlooked because the symptoms are wrongly ascribed to strain or to rupture of the plantaris tendon.

Etiology and Pathophysiology

Rupture of the tendon is usually caused by excessive stress of the muscle while running or jumping. It can also occur as a result of external trauma. The rupture is nearly always complete and is usually found about 5 cm above the insertion of the tendon (7). If left untreated, the tendon unites spontaneously by lengthening (7, 26).

Symptoms and Signs

The main feature of a ruptured Achilles tendon is sudden agonizing pain in the back of the ankle that can be attributed to external trauma, even when it occurs during running or jumping. The patient usually can walk, but with a limp (26). On examination tenderness is noted at the site of rupture, with general thickening from effusion of blood and edema, and a gap can usually be palpated in the course of the tendon. The power of plantar flexion at the ankle is greatly decreased, but some strength remains through the action of the tibialis posterior, the peronei, and the toe flexors (9).

Diagnosis

The retention of some power of plantar flexion can cause the unwary physician to make an incorrect diagnosis (9). It is a crucial test to ask the patient to lift the heel from the ground while standing only on the affected leg. Another test is to squeeze the calf of the affected leg, which normally provokes plantar flexion. If the Achilles tendon is ruptured, motion is markedly decreased or absent (15, 26).

Treatment

In the event pain is moderate in severity, non-opioid analgesics are sufficient, but in many, if not most patients, the pain is severe and it is generally necessary to use strong opioid analgesics. Patient-controlled analgesia, intraspinal opioids, and epidural analgesia can be used (see above).

Rupture of the Achilles tendon can be treated by immobilization in plaster for 5 weeks with the foot in slight equinus to relax the tendon and to help prevent lengthening (26). Surgery entails repair of the tendon, preferably by sutures or stainless steel wire. Tension on the suture line is relaxed by immobilizing the limb in 90° knee flexion and moderate ankle plantar flexion for 2 weeks followed by a below-knee plaster with the ankle at a 90° angle for 4 weeks (26). The operation should be done with continuous epidural anesthesia to prevent the neuroendocrine stress response, and the anesthesia should be continued for 24 to 48 hours to provide postoperative pain relief.

Rupture of the Anterior Tibialis Tendon

Acute and chronic rupture of the anterior tibialis tendon usually occurs between the extensor retinaculum and the insertion of the tendon (26). The patient has a feeling of instability of the ankle, weakness, and limitation of dorsal flexion, and the gait is of the foot-drop type. Pain is usually present. Operative repair is the procedure of choice (26).

Rupture of the Posterior Tibialis Tendon

Etiology and Pathophysiology

Rupture of the posterior tibialis tendon can occur acutely as a result of an injury or can occur spontaneously in patients with chronic tenosynovitis. Occasionally it occurs with periosteal new bone formation as the result of infection, rheumatoid arthritis, or pigmented villonodular synovitis (26, 27).

Symptoms and Signs

Acute rupture is associated with the sudden onset of pain in the medial aspect of the ankle and with valgus instability that is associated with a painful flat foot (26, 27). Examination reveals exquisite tenderness just behind the medial malleolus.

Diagnosis and Treatment

Diagnosis is made from the history and physical examination. Early surgical treatment is essential because late repair is difficult and often unsatisfactory as a result of retraction of the tendon (26, 27). Nonsurgical treatment with an arch support and a medial heel wedge and flare is not as effective. If the posterior tibial tendon is irreparable and symptoms warrant it, a tendon graft and transfer or a triple arthrodesis might be necessary. While awaiting surgery pain is controlled by NSAIDs alone or in combination with opioids, or continuous epidural analgesia is initiated and used for the operation and for postoperative pain relief (see Chapter 94).

Shin Splints

Shin splint is a lay term used to describe pain along the anterior or posterior part of the tibia. The pain can be caused by a tibial stress fracture or more frequently by strain of the anterior or posterior tibial muscles resulting from overuse of the lower extremities, as from running, aerobic dancing, or skating. The condition is described in detail on page 380.

Infections of Bone

The tibia is one of the most common sites of hematogenous osteomyelitis (9). Because of its susceptibility to sustaining compound fractures, the tibia is also the most common site of osteomyelitis from direct contamination. The fibula is less often affected. Chronic osteomyelitis in the lower leg, as elsewhere, is nearly always the sequel of acute osteomyelitis and can follow other sources of infection. Clinical aspects and therapy of this condition are discussed in Chapter 23.

Syphilitic infection of bone is now rare in Western countries. When it does occur, however, the tibia is often the bone affected (9). The infection can take the form of localized gumma or diffuse osteoperiostitis and is characterized by gradually enlarging swelling and moderate to severe pain. Adams (9) has noted that the possibility of syphilis should be borne in mind because the swelling is easily mistaken for tumor.

Bone Tumors

The upper end of the tibia or fibula, like the lower end of the femur, is a common site for giant cell tumor. It usually occurs in young adults, expanding the bone and extending to within a short distance of the articular surface, and causing pain and swelling. Treatment of these tumors includes complete excision of the upper end of the tibia to sacrifice the knee joint, bridging the gap with bone graft and providing stability by means of a long intramedullary nail, or by the use of a custom-made prosthesis to replace the knee joint and the upper half of the tibia (9). If the fibula is involved the entire affected end of the bone should be excised together with an adequate margin of healthy bone.

The tibia, like the femur, is a common site for primary malignant tumors, especially osteosarcoma and Ewing's tumor, both of which usually affect children or young adults (9). Both are highly malignant and have a high mortality rate. Treatment of pain is discussed in Chapter 24. Because Ewing's tumor is radiosensitive, treatment by radiotherapy supplemented by chemotherapy can be effective, thus avoiding amputation (9).

Other Painful Disorders

Other painful disorders of the leg (Table 76-1) are discussed elsewhere. Intermittent claudication pain in the calf caused by arterial insufficiency in the lower limb as a result of peripheral vascular disease is discussed in Chapter 28. Myofascial pain syndromes with trigger areas frequently involve the calf or anterior leg muscles and cause pain (Chapters 21 and 77).

D. PAINFUL DISORDERS OF THE ANKLE AND HEEL

Post-Traumatic Pain

Pain caused by acute injuries can result from fracture or dislocation of the bones of the ankle joint or from tear or actual rupture of the surrounding ligaments. In all these conditions the pain is acute, usually moderate to severe, and requires management with a combination of NSAIDs and strong opioids (Chapter 23). Stress fracture of the bones of the ankle occurs when the activity level increases so quickly that the ratio of bone deposition to resorption decreases, so that no new trabeculae are deposited along the line of stress. Stress fractures are characterized by moderate to severe aching pain that is greatly aggravated by weight bearing. Typically stress fractures are initially manifested as pain during vigorous activity. If the patient nevertheless persists in the activity the pain generally worsens and is present even during nonathletic activities of daily living. Treatment requires rest of the injured part and avoidance of significant stress on the bone during the time required for healing, usually 4 to 6 weeks (see Table 22-4).

Ankle Sprains

Ligamentous sprains most commonly occur in the ankle, especially during basketball or volleyball, or can occur as a result of a fall. They constitute a frequent cause of pain and disability. Most such injuries occur on the lateral side of the ankle and can be treated nonsurgically (28). Although isolated ligamentous injuries are uncommon, they are usually associated with fracture of the distal fibula or with tibiofibular interosseous ligamentous tears. Total disruption of the medial and lateral ligamentous complexes is rare, but can occur with a subluxation or dislocation of the talus and go unrecognized because of spontaneous reduction of the talus into the ankle mortise.

Symptoms and Signs

Ankle sprains are characterized by sudden sharp pain and are usually followed by dysfunction such as the inability to walk or run. Swelling becomes marked within 6 to 12 hours of injury, and the patient cannot bear full weight on the injured leg. Examination reveals the swelling together with tenderness to palpation of the injured ligament (6–8). Ecchymosis is present in the foot and the lower leg.

Diagnosis and Treatment

The diagnosis and treatment of ankle sprains are discussed on pages 381 and 382.

Ankle Laxity

Ankle laxity following numerous ankle sprains leads to chronic swelling and discomfort. Initial treatment consists of ankle strengthening exercises, ankle restraints such as elastic corsets, and shoe modification designed to eliminate inversion of the ankle. Occasionally a clamshell-type foot or ankle orthosis is necessary for ambulatory stability. If these measures fail surgical reconstruction of the lateral ligaments of the ankle is indicated using a portion of the peroneus brevis tendon or, if possible, the ligaments are repaired directly.

Ankle Fractures

Etiology and Pathophysiology

Ankle fractures are common injuries that can vary in severity from an undisplaced incomplete fracture of the malleolus to a severely comminuted injury involving the weight-bearing surface of the tibia, with ligament disruption (29). In contrast to long bone injuries severe comminution or displacement is not always associated with high-energy trauma but usually occurs as a result of rotational stresses, with the weight of the body acting as the causative force because the ankle bears up to five times the body weight (29). Figure 76-29 shows several types of fractures of the ankle, which usually involve the malleoli or the lower part of the fibula. Like other similar injuries to bone, ankle fractures are characterized by sudden severe pain aggravated by weight bearing and are associated with swelling, ecchymosis, and inability to ambulate.

Treatment

The goal in the treatment of ankle fracture is anatomic reduction, so that normal function can be restored (29). Although opinion differs regarding the best method of treatment, excellent long-term results are obtained only when an anatomic reduction is achieved (29). Any residual displacement or instability predisposes to late degenerative changes.

Ankle fractures can be treated either by manipulation and immobilization or by open reduction and internal fixation. Closed reduction and plaster immobilization should be reserved for stable fractures, whereas unstable fractures are best treated by open reduction and internal fixation. This is best done with regional anesthesia for the operation and continued for 48 to 72 hours for postoperative pain relief. More detailed discussion of the management of pain caused by these fractures is contained in Chapter 23.

Arthritides of the Ankle

Various arthritides can affect the ankle joint (Table 76-1). Pyogenic arthritis of the ankle is uncommon whereas rheumatoid arthritis often affects one or both ankles, in common with other joints (24). Gouty arthritis usually affects the great toe but can develop in the ankle and in other peripheral joints. Hemophilic arthritis and neuropathic arthritis are uncommon. Most patients who have arthritides experience pain in the joint, which requires effective management. These and other aspects of arthritides are discussed in Chapter 20.

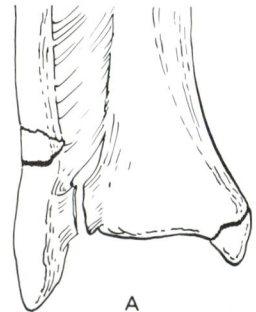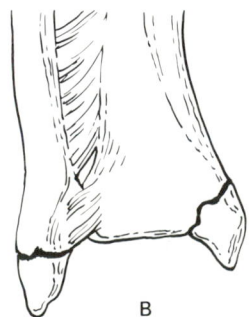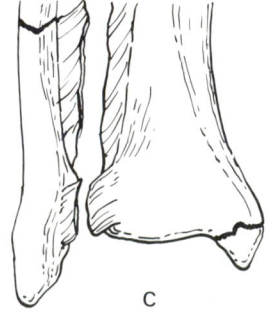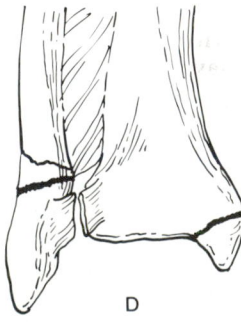

FIG. 76-29. Types of ankle fractures. **A.** Supination-eversion injury (Launge-Hansen classification). **B.** Supination-adduction injury. **C.** Pronation-eversion fracture. **D.** Pronation-abduction fracture. Modified from Yablon, I.G., and Segal, D.: Ankle fractures. *In* Surgery of the Musculoskeletal System. Edited by C.W. Evarts. New York, Churchill Livingstone, 1983.

Osteoarthritis of the Ankle Joint

Degenerative destruction of articular cartilage is less common in the ankle than in the knee and hip. A known predisposing factor that causes the ankle to wear out prematurely is always present. The most common factor is irregularity or malalignment of the joint surface after a fracture but, in some cases, another articular disease such as previous rheumatoid arthritis is a primary factor.

The most common symptom is pain, which slowly increases over months or years and is associated with limp. On examination the joint is found to be slightly thickened from the marginal bony hypertrophy and movements are limited somewhat or severely according to the degree of the arthritis. Radiography reveals the typical features of osteoarthritis consistent with narrowing of the cartilage space, a tendency to sclerosis of the bone adjacent to the joint, and hypertrophy or osteophyte formation at the joint margins.

Treatment of osteoarthritis is discussed in Chapter 21.

Dislocation of the Peroneal Tendon

Etiology and Pathophysiology

Dislocation of the peroneal tendon is a condition that resembles but is more severe than sprain of the lateral collateral ligaments (6, 7). The peroneal tendon passes behind the lateral malleolus and is held there by the overlying retinaculum. Forceful dorsiflexion with simultaneous peroneal contraction can rupture the retinaculum and dislocate the tendon. This can occur during athletic activities, especially in those who are untrained.

Symptoms and Signs

At the time of dislocation sharp moderate to severe pain is felt in the lateral aspect of the ankle and is accompanied by some difficulty in walking. Examination reveals tenderness at the lateral malleolus, and palpation of the subluxating tendon reveals that it is dislocated.

Diagnosis and Treatment

Early diagnosis permits surgical repair of the retinaculum. While the patient is awaiting surgery the pain is managed with NSAIDs alone or in combination with a mild or strong opioid. If surgical repair is delayed the tissues atrophy rapidly and cannot be repaired and other corrective surgical procedures are necessary to minimize the pain, dislocation, and stability (6).

Posterior Calcaneal Bursitis

Etiology and Pathophysiology

Inflammation of the bursa between the Achilles tendon and skin is usually caused by friction from ill-fitting shoes and is prevalent in women who wear high-heeled shoes (8, 30). Chronic irritation thickens the walls of the bursa and the overlying skin.

Symptoms and Signs

Exquisite pain and tenderness over the posterior aspect of the heel and under the skin are common features and are aggravated by direct palpation and pressure. The bursa is usually visibly inflamed and is often distended with fluid. With chronic bursitis the walls of the bursa and the overlying skin are thickened.

Diagnosis and Treatment

Diagnosis is made through the history and physical examination, including careful evaluation of the fitting of the shoe. Treatment begins with proper-fitting shoes with moderately low heels. The moderate to severe pain of acute bursitis is relieved by the application of ice and NSAIDs (9). In acute bursitis associated with severe pain, the swollen bursa is drained by needle aspiration followed by injection of a local anesthetic and steroid into the bursa (9, 30). Moleskin placed over the thickened skin prevents further friction but in some cases it is necessary to cut out the back of the shoe or raise the heel inside the shoe. Surgical excision of the bursa is rarely if ever indicated (8, 30).

Osteochondritis Dissecans

Etiology and Pathophysiology

Osteochondritis dissecans is characterized by a small osteochondral defect that often follows one or more ankle sprains. It involves the talar dome anterolaterally on the lateral side and posteromedially on the medial side (31). The right ankle is involved with slightly greater frequency than the left. Although a talar lesion can occur at any age it most often affects adolescents and young adults, with a peak influence in the third decade (31). Although this condition also occasionally develops spontaneously, usually the role of trauma as a causative factor is established. Berndt and Harty (32) produced impressive experimental evidence of the traumatic origin of this condition, which they termed "transchondral talar fracture," and classified it according to severity (Fig. 76-30).

Symptoms and Signs

Initially the patient can experience mild to moderate ankle pain, with some "catching" with motion that the patient frequently attributes to "mild ankle sprain" (31). When the bone lesion loosens it mechanically abrades the joint, producing intermittent locking, chronic pain, and swelling on the side of the involvement and a feeling of instability.

Diagnosis

Many osteochondral talar fractures are missed at first presentation, either because radiographs of a routine ankle sprain are not taken or because the talar fracture is overlooked (31). Therefore, all ankle sprains deserve thorough radiographic evaluation. Because anteroposterior and lateral films might only show subtle findings, an oblique radiograph is necessary (31). These are followed by tomographs of the talus to demonstrate the location and extent of the lesion.

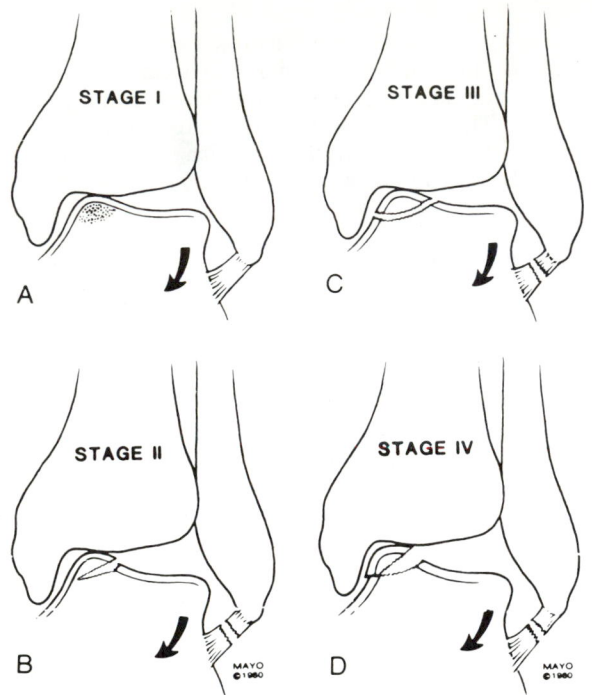

FIG. 76-30. Classification of osteochondral fracture of the talus (according to Berndt and Harty). *A.* Stage I: cyclic compression fracture of the talar dome; lateral ligaments remain intact. Articular cartilage remains intact and viable while underlying trabecular bone becomes necrotic. *B.* Stage II: incomplete fracture of the bone and cartilage with rupture of lateral ligaments. *C.* Stage III: complete osteochondral fracture with the fragment undisplaced from its bed. *D.* Stage IV: complete osteochondral fracture with displacement of fragment within the ankle joint. From Stauffer, R.N.: Intra-articular ankle problems. *In* Surgery of the Musculoskeletal System. Edited by C.W. Evarts. New York, Churchill Livingstone, 1983.

Treatment

If the condition is diagnosed early a conservative or nonsurgical approach can be considered, but patients in the later stages of the disease require surgical treatment. This consists of curettage of the lesion to remove all loose cartilage followed by drilling of the subchondral bone to promote ingrowth of new fibrocartilage. Even though a large area might be affected, the new surface created by the fibrocartilage appears to hold up well. Pain is usually relieved, allowing full activities to be resumed (32).

Calcaneal Paratendinitis

Etiology and Pathophysiology

Inflammation of the paratendinous tissues in the posterior aspect of the heel in the region of the calcaneal (Achilles) tendon insertion causes pain in the posterior aspect of the heel (8, 9, 12). The term "tenosynovitis" is a misnomer when applied to this condition because this tendon has no synovial tendon sheath (9). The inflammation occurs in the loose connective tissue around the tendon that is known as the paratendon. The condition is usually caused by overuse, repeated microtrauma, or gross trauma to the tendon. In some patients it can reflect underlying inflammatory disease such as rheumatoid arthritis, in which case the tendon can rupture spontaneously.

Symptoms and Signs

Pain in the region of the calcaneal tendon is worsened by activity such as running or dancing. Examination by palpation between the finger and thumb deep to the tendon, reveals tenderness with slight local thickening (Fig. 76-22B). Occasionally the area is swollen and distended and exhibits crepitation during motion. The pain is markedly aggravated by jumping or dancing or by other activity that stretches the tendon (8, 9).

Diagnosis and Treatment

Diagnosis is made through the history and physical examination. Treatment must be started promptly. Pain is usually controlled with NSAIDs but, if the pain is severe, injections of a local anesthetic and steroids deep to the tendon provide relief (9, 33). The tendon itself must *not* be injected to prevent it from being weakened. Definitive treatment measures include a heel lift to reduce tension and stretching if the heel cord is found to be tight. If simple measures fail the ankle should be immobilized in a below-the-knee plaster cast for 4 weeks (8, 9). In rare cases surgical excision of the inflamed connective tissue or the inflamed bursa might be necessary (8, 9).

Sometimes patients with chronic paratendinitis develop a degenerative core within the tendon that must be removed surgically for symptomatic relief (8, 9). Calcaneal exostoses (pump bumps) can cause an overlying bursitis in the vicinity of the tendon that can become intractable (30). Unfortunately, excision of the exostoses often leads to intractable tendinitis.

E. PAINFUL CONDITIONS OF THE FOOT

Arthritides

The joints of the foot can be affected by pyogenic arthritis, rheumatoid arthritis, gouty arthritis, and osteoarthritis or degenerative joint disease. Although gouty arthritis is most common in the joint of the great toe it can also occur in other joints. Here the two most common types of arthritis that affect the joints of the foot are considered: degenerative arthritis and inflammatory rheumatoid arthritis.

Degenerative Arthritis

Symptoms and Signs

Degenerative arthritis is characterized by aching, boring, and intense pain localized to the involved joint that persists both day and night. The pain is aggravated by inclement weather and weight bearing and worsens as the day progresses. The pain is relieved by rest, limitation of motion, increased shock absorption, and decreased weight bearing. Signs include joint enlargement, decreased range of motion, deformity (including subluxation) and crepitation with motion. Radiography reveals hypertrophic changes about the articular margins such as beaking, osteophytes, sclerosis, and cysts.

Treatment

Osteoarthritis or degenerative joint disease of the foot is initially treated nonoperatively by splinting of affected joints and increased shock absorption. The foot can be splinted by wearing a shoe with a stiff shank and a rocker bottom sole (See Fig. 76-27). Forefoot and toe motion during push-off are reduced. Foam, leather, and other materials are used to make removable shoe inserts, which increase shock absorption. An NSAID to reduce inflammation and pain can be used; the standard dose of ibuprofen is 600 mg tid with meals for 2 to 3 weeks. If no relief is obtained a trial with another NSAID is worthwhile. If still unsuccessful, additional NSAIDs are probably going to be ineffective. Other medical therapies are discussed elsewhere (page 332).

When pain persists despite conservative treatment, several operative options are available. Bony osteophytes, which decrease motion and cause impingement pain at the ankle and at the metatarsophalangeal joint of the big toe, can be excised. Diffuse involvement of those joints not responding to conservative treatment requires arthrodesis (8, 9). If the joint is fused in a plantigrade position, pain can be relieved and function restored. The long-term effect of fusing joints in the foot is the development of arthritic changes in adjacent joints, which must compensate for the loss of motion.

Inflammatory Arthritis

Symptoms and Signs

Inflammatory arthritis is characterized by exquisite pain localized to involved joints. It is accompanied by stiffness after sitting or rest and is aggravated by inactivity. Some relief is achieved with heat, splinting, and limitation of the range of motion. Associated signs include increased warmth, joint effusion, capsular thickening about the joint, increased laxity, and progressive subluxation, particularly about the ankle, subtalar, and metatarsophalangeal (MP) joints. Motion is progressively lost.

Inflammatory joint disease of the foot produces joint laxity and osteoporosis. Specific deformity includes valgus of the hindfoot, pronation of the midfoot, supination of the forefoot, and clawing of the small toes, leading to metatarsalgia.

Treatment

In addition to medical treatment of the underlying inflammatory disease, comfort and function of the foot can be improved by wearing accommodative shoes to provide support, total contact, and extra toe room. Surgery is directed at relieving deformities that predispose to pressure problems and at restoring the foot to a plantigrade position. Ankle fusion, triple arthrodeses, and selected fusion of the small bones

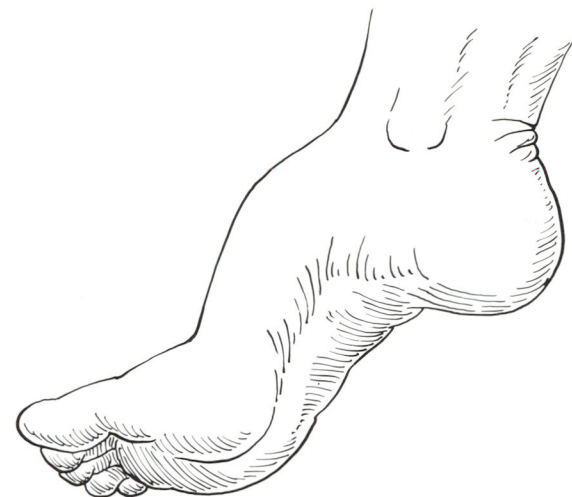

FIG. 76-31. Pes cavus. The high arched foot is rigid. This limits shock absorption so that weight-bearing forces become concentrated on the metatarsal heads and the heel. Underlying neurologic disease should be considered in such patients.

of the midfoot are all helpful, with few complications. Prominent metatarsal heads cause intractable keratoses and metatarsalgia. A proximal oblique osteotomy of the metatarsal shaft allows the head to ride upward and restores comfort and function (24).

Pes Cavus

In pes cavus, or hollow foot, the longitudinal arch of the foot is accentuated (Fig. 76-31). The deformity can have a congenital basis or an underlying neurologic disorder can cause muscle imbalance. The metatarsal heads are lowered in relation to the hind part of the foot, with consequent exaggeration of the longitudinal arch (11). The soft tissues in the sole are abnormally short and eventually the bones themselves alter their shape, perpetuating the deformity. Clawing of the toes, which are hyperextended at the MP joints and are flexed at the proximal and distal interphalangeal joints, is often seen. The toes therefore become almost functionless and cannot take their normal share in weight bearing. As a result excessive weight falls on the metatarsal heads.

In many patients specific treatment is not required. Mild symptoms can often be relieved by using a sponge rubber pad beneath the metatarsal heads to distribute the weight more widely. It is best to prescribe shoes made especially to fit the altered shape of the feet. If symptoms are severe surgery might be required.

Pain in the Hindfoot

Plantar Fasciitis

Etiology and Pathophysiology

Pain under the heel is most frequently caused by a plantar fasciitis, which is believed to be an inflammatory condition beneath the anterior part of the calcaneus (8, 9). The condition can be part of a more widespread inflammatory condition, such as Reiter's disease (9). It is common in those in occupations that entail excessive standing or walking, especially when the individual is unaccustomed to such activity. It is more common in a pronated foot that has a flattened longitudinal arch and frequently occurs after a period of bed rest. Men are more susceptible than women (8). A bony prominence or spur can develop at the attachment of the plantar fascia to the calcaneus. This bony prominence can extend transversely across the entire plantar surface of the bone and is considered to be ossification and calcification resulting from traction of the plantar fascia on the periosteum.

Symptoms and Signs

Moderate to severe pain and tenderness beneath the anterior portion of the heel, often radiating into the sole of the foot, is the presenting complaint. Examination reveals a point of exquisite deep tenderness at the anteromedial area of the calcaneus, the point of attachment of the plantar fascia (Fig. 76-22C).

Diagnosis and Treatment

Diagnosis is made through the history and physical examination. Radiography reveals nothing or shows a typical spur arising from the calcaneus. Because spurs are often found in asymptomatic feet, however, and are not found in patients with symptoms, this finding might be coincidental. Other conditions that cause pain in this region include infracalcaneal bursitis under the fascial attachment, atraumatic periostitis, and tearing of some of the fibers attached to the bone.

Initial treatment consists of preventing hyperpronation of the foot by the patient wearing well-constructed shoes with a medial arch support. Alternatively a sponge rubber cushion with its center removed can be used under the heel. Pain is usually effectively relieved by NSAIDs. If the pain is persistent and severe, injection of a mixture of a local anesthetic and steroid into the painful region can be considered. The injection can be made directly into the area through the pedal pad or by entering the heel from either the medial or lateral approach, but it is important to inject the solution at the site of maximum tenderness (8). It is rarely necessary to use more than three weekly injections for persistent relief. If these are ineffective a walking cast is necessary for 1 to 2 weeks to control the pain. Release of the plantar fascia is sometimes necessary for chronic cases, but generally this condition responds to nonoperative treatment (33).

Tarsal Coalition

Pathophysiology and Symptoms and Signs

Congenital fibrous union or fusion between the bones of the hindfoot and midfoot can remain undetected throughout life. The condition can lead to subtalar arthritis or to arthritis of other joints in the midfoot, particularly with prolonged standing or walking on uneven surfaces. Inflammation of the joint is likely to cause pain, as can motion of the subtalar joint. Crepitation can be elicited by motion of the joint, and tenderness can be produced by pressure over the sinus tarsi in front of the lateral malleolus. Weight bearing is usually painful and rest affords relief.

Diagnosis and Treatment

History of the pain and a lack of subtalar motion are diagnostic. Treatment consists of diminishing subtalar motion by the use of supportive shoes and a medial arch insert to provide increased shock absorption. A trial of supervised conservative treatment is mandatory before considering surgery. Most patients usually respond to these measures (33, 34). Surgery involves fusing the area of fibrous coalition or taking down the coalition when the joint surfaces are compatible with normal movement.

Heel Pad Deficiency

Etiology and Pathophysiology

Generalized pain over the entire calcaneal fat pad (painful heel pad) occurs when the heel pad is deficient or is subjected to unusual stress (6). The heel pad is normally composed of fatty tissue and elastic fibrous tissue enclosed within the compartment formed by the fibrous septa. Normally this tissue has an elasticity that acts as a shock absorber, but its elasticity decreases with age and the weight of the body must be borne by the unpadded calcaneus. Persistent stress on the fat pad can also cause this deficiency. Cavus feet are prone to this problem.

Symptoms and Signs

Pain develops when repeated stress must be borne by the unpadded calcaneus. In contrast to plantar fasciitis, which involves localized pain, the pain of a deficient heel pad is generalized over the entire calcaneal pad. If the condition remains untreated it results in scar formation and calcification of the calcaneus. Acute stress on the pad can rupture or strain the compartments and cause temporary loss of compressibility.

Diagnosis and Treatment

Diagnosis is made through the history and physical examination and by the results of various imaging tests (Table 76-5). The pain is effectively controlled by NSAIDs but, if the pain is severe, infiltration of 5 ml of a dilute solution of a long-acting local anesthetic (e.g., 0.25% bupivacaine) relieves pain for 8 to 10 hours. Definitive treatment of the condition involves addition of a shock-absorbing insert to the shoe and ensuring that the heel is supported by a firm center (35).

Tarsal Tunnel Syndrome

Etiology and Pathophysiology

Entrapment of the medial and lateral plantar nerves within the tarsal tunnel can cause pain and paresthesia and weakness of the intrinsic flexors of the foot (6, 36). The posterior tibial nerve descends to the ankle along the medial margin of the calcaneal tendon and ends between the heel and medial malleolus deep to the flexor retinaculum (also called the laciniate ligament), where it divides into the medial and lateral plantar nerves. The flexor retinaculum is a strong fibrous band that extends from the medial malleolus proximally to the margin of the calcaneus distally, where it converts a series of bony grooves into canals for passage of the tendons of the flexor muscles, the posterior tibial vessels, and the tibial nerves. The ligament can cause the tibial nerve to become trapped within the tunnel, with resulting edema and scar formation that limit blood supply and inhibit the full elongation (uncoiling) of the nerve between joint movements. Pathophysiology eventually leads to axonal and then to wallerian degeneration (see Chapters 10 and 73 for details).

Symptoms and Signs

Entrapment of the plantar nerves causes pain that is nocturnal, a paresthetic burning sensation or numbness, or a combination of these (6, 36). The symptoms can be felt when the patient is standing or reclining. Distribution of these symptoms depends on which nerve branch is most affected: with involvement of both plantar nerves the symptoms extend from behind the malleolus over the plantar surface of the foot and the dorsum of the distal part of the toes. Sometimes the medial calcaneal branch of the tibia, which perforates the flexor retinaculum and is distributed to the skin of the heel and medial side of the sole of the foot, is trapped and causes pain and other symptoms localized to these areas. Tenderness can usually be elicited over the nerve behind the medial malleolus, and a positive Tinel's sign can be elicited by tapping the nerve at that site.

Diagnosis and Treatment

Entrapment of the medial and lateral plantar branches of the tibial nerve presents a challenging diagnosis. Because the condition can coexist with peripheral neuropathies it is necessary to decide whether the pain and other symptoms and signs are caused by the neuropathy itself or by tarsal tunnel compression. Electromyographic and nerve conduction velocity studies can be helpful.

An attempt should be made to treat the condition conservatively. Injection of local anesthetic and steroids into the tarsal tunnel can be helpful, as can NSAIDs (9). Transcutaneous electrical nerve stimulation should also be tried. If the patient experiences lancinating pain, tricyclic antidepressants such as amitriptyline should be given (Chapter 73).

If the symptoms persist after a few weeks of conservative management, surgical decompression is justified. Surgery consists of dividing the proximal ridge of the abductor hallucis, often a site of compression, and releasing the tunnel. Varicose veins and ganglions are frequent sources of compression within the tunnel. These patients should be checked to see that their foot is not hyperpronating, because this increases tension on the plantar nerves and aggravates symptoms (7, 36).

Painful Conditions of the Midfoot

Medial Arch Strain

Medial arch strain can occur in normal feet from prolonged standing on hard surfaces, particularly when the foot is not well supported. Treatment consists of activity modification and wearing of shoes that support the heel and arch and provide good shock absorption. Any hyperpronation with footwear should be corrected, because this predisposes to medial arch strain.

Lisfranc's Joint Instability

Etiology and Symptoms and Signs

A twisting injury to the midfoot such as severe inversion or a plantar flexion injury of the forefoot leads to injury of Lisfranc's (metatarsal cuneiform) joint. Pain and swelling that persist long after soft tissue healing should have occurred should help to increase the index of suspicion. Palpation usually reveals tenderness of the affected joint.

Diagnosis

The history and findings of the physical examination should lead to the diagnosis. Whereas Lisfranc's fractures are detectable by radiography, joint subluxations and sprains are difficult to demonstrate by this method. Stress radiographs taken with the foot plantar flexed and inverted and bone scans of the foot are helpful.

Treatment

When recognized early, support of the foot either by a cast or a well-fitted shoe promotes healing of the ligaments. If seen 3 to 4 months later a chronic condition can have developed that might require selective fusion of the painful joints, particularly the metatarsal cuneiform joints. Overweight patients usually have the poorest results, either with conservative or surgical treatment (33, 37).

Posterior Tibial Tendon Insufficiency

Etiology and Pathophysiology

The posterior tibial tendon is the main dynamic support of the medial arch. Whenever this tendon is congenitally situated in a mechanically deficient way, such as to an accessory navicular, or is injured, the arch eventually collapses. A tight heel cord aggravates the situation by holding the heel in valgus. The tendon can be torn, sprained, or stretched with eversion-type injuries (38). Over time the foot assumes a pronated posture that is asymmetric to the opposite foot. The patient cannot rise up on that foot or invert the heel. Rheumatoid arthritis produces degenerative changes in the tendon and can lead to silent rupture.

Symptoms and Signs

The major problem with posterior tibial tendon insufficiency is that it causes progressive breakdown and destruction of the midfoot. The patient experiences persistent dull aching pain associated with tenderness, and occasionally swelling is present. Eventually the patient experiences difficulty in standing and walking.

Diagnosis and Treatment

Diagnosis is made through the history and physical examination and by the results of special tests (Table 76-5), including ultrasound and plain radiography. Early treatment consists of the wearing of supportive shoes to correct and control pronation. Later, when the condition has been established and collapse has already started, augmentation of the posterior tibial tendon helps to restore dynamic support of the arch. Augmentation is usually accomplished using the extensor digitorum longus or extensor hallucis longus and with direct repair of the posterior tibial tendon. In cases of severe deformity, or when degenerative changes have occurred in the midfoot, a triple arthrodesis *to restore the normal position of the foot* is required (6, 26).

Ganglion

Etiology and Symptoms and Signs

A ganglion is a mucus-filled cyst that usually arises from a joint or tendon sheath from continued stress (6, 7, 38). The condition is particularly uncomfortable in the foot because of shoe pressure. Motion of the foot during weight bearing tends to pump fluid into the ganglion. The condition causes pain and some tenderness on palpation that are aggravated by pressure and ambulation.

Treatment

Nonoperative treatment is usually unsuccessful. Aspiration and installation of steroids sometimes help, but in Lippert's experience (20) these are rarely successful. Definitive treatment requires excision of the ganglion down to its origin. The neck of the ganglion can be tied off or excised completely so that the ball valve effect is eliminated. Patients should be protected in a walking cast for 10 to 14 days to allow the soft tissues to heal and the source of the ganglion to be obliterated by scar.

Painful Disorders of the Forefoot

Stress Fracture

Sedentary individuals and those who begin a new activity that requires running or prolonged walking tend to develop a stress fracture (march fracture) in the neck of the metatarsal bones. Although any bone of the foot can be involved, stress fracture of the 2nd metatarsal occurs as a consequence of running or dancing on hard surfaces. Sometimes bone scans are necessary for the diagnosis, although radiographic changes are usually evident about 10 to 14 days after fracture. Treatment consists of the use of a walking cast until healing occurs, which might require 4 to 6 weeks. If the cast is removed too soon the stress fracture tends to become chronic and more difficult to treat. The treatment indicated here is different than that discussed on page 379.

Metatarsalgia

Metatarsalgia refers to pain under the heads of the metatarsals that bear a disproportionate amount of the body weight during the static stance phase of walking, when the 1st metatarsal carries two-sixths of the body weight and the other one-sixth (7).

Etiology and Pathophysiology

In a pronated or splayed foot the balance of weight bearing is upset. The transverse arch is depressed and greater weight is borne on the 2nd, 3rd, and 4th metatarsal heads. The interosseous ligaments that support the arch are stretched, permitting the forefoot to broaden and splay out (7).

The condition is more common in cavus and rheumatoid feet, in which claw toes have pushed the metatarsal heads downward and displaced the protective padding distally. Women who wear high-heeled shoes are more prone to metatarsalgia as a result of the position of the foot, which concentrates the weight-bearing forces on the metatarsal heads.

Symptoms and Signs

Initially patients experience tenderness of the metatarsal head, which has been described as "walking with a pebble in the shoe" (6, 7, 38). Later a callus forms over the 2nd or 3rd metatarsal head, which itself is painful and causes further irritation by increasing the weight bearing on the metatarsal head. The tenderness is aggravated when the examiner squeezes the metatarsal head between the thumb and index finger. The examiner should compress each metatarsal head individually and must not compress the tissues between the heads (ligaments and interdigital nerves), because this could cause pain and tenderness and confuse the diagnosis.

Diagnosis and Treatment

The diagnosis is made through the history and careful physical examination and by the results of plain radiography and bone scanning (see Table 76-5). Most individuals obtain relief with the use of a metatarsal pad placed in the shoe or as a removable insert (Fig. 76-26). The device redistributes the weight-bearing forces away from the metatarsal heads into the arch region. Occasionally patients present with metatarsalgia under one or two heads secondary to a previous fracture or to some other structural abnormality. Selective padding is usually effective. When an intractable keratosis occurs under one of the metatarsal heads and does not respond to padding, pressure can be reduced by performing an osteotomy of the metatarsal shaft or by excising the condyles of the metatarsal head. The goal of surgery is to equalize weight bearing under the metatarsal heads. Failure to accomplish this results in a painful transfer keratosis (7, 9, 11).

Painful Conditions of the Great Toe

Hallux Valgus

Etiology and Pathophysiology

Hallux valgus is a bunion of the great toe. It is more common in women, especially those past middle age. Although the underlying cause can be congenital, ill-fitting shoes with a narrow toe are the single most significant factor in the progression of this condition (7, 9, 10, 39). The wearing of high heels favors the development of hallux valgus because the forefoot is forced into the narrow pointed part of the shoe.

Outward deviation of the big toe is the most obvious feature of the deformity. An additional feature that is almost always found is deviation of the 1st metatarsal

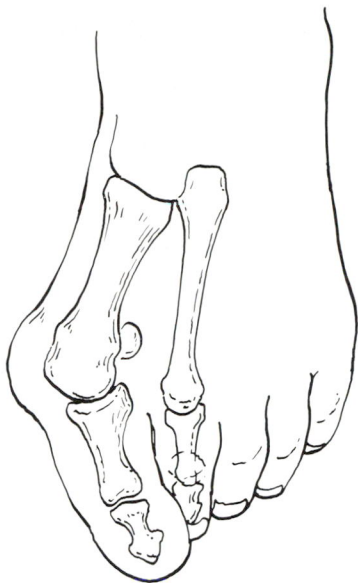

FIG. 76-32. Hallux valgus. See text for details

medially, so that the gap between the head of the 1st and 2nd metatarsals is unduly wide. After several years two secondary changes occur: formation of a thick-walled bursa (bunion) of the medial prominence and the metatarsal head, which becomes inflamed and occasionally separates and, later, osteoarthritis of the MP joint develops, resulting from malalignment (Fig. 76-32).

Symptoms and Signs

Early symptoms arise from tenderness over the bunion from pressure against the shoe, and the patient encounters difficulty in obtaining comfortable footwear. Additional symptoms later arise from osteoarthritis of the MP joint and from flattening of the transverse arch (anterior flatfoot), which is a common associated deformity. On examination the deformity is obvious and the skin over the prominent joint is hard, red, and tender. Early in the condition the MP joint opens freely and painlessly, but in severe cases of many years' duration the secondary osteoarthritis makes movement limited and painful. In late stages the forefoot is often flat and splayed and the toes can be severely curved (6, 7).

Treatment

Nonoperative treatment consists of wearing extra-wide shoes and inserts to prevent pronation. Walking with the foot pronated causes further deformation forces to be applied by the floor. The goal of surgery is to reduce the 1st intermetatarsal angle to 0° by an appropriate osteotomy. Contractures around the metatarsal head must be released to reposition the 1st metatarsal head close to its neighbor. Treatment is usually successful in relieving the pain and deformity provided that the 1st metatarsal is not excessively shortened and is not allowed to progress into an elevated position. Some recurrence of the deformity is typical but is not associated with recurrence of pain.

Postoperatively patients must wear shoes that accommodate their feet comfortably to enjoy the best results (9, 39).

Hallux Rigidus

Etiology and Pathophysiology

Hallux rigidus is osteoarthritis of the first MP joint characterized by lack of motion of the joint and impingement pain at push-off (Fig. 76-33). Again, although the condition might involve a congenital abnormality of the joint, improper shoes (especially those causing hyperextension of the joint), abnormal gait, obesity, and trauma to the joint are contributing factors (44).

Symptoms and Signs

Almost all patients present with symptoms of pain and restriction of motion in the 1st MP joint. These are usually of gradual onset and patients might give a history that indicates no possible cause (30). A specific characteristic of pain in hallux rigidus is that it is present with any walking, whereas patients with hallux valgus complain of pain only when walking while wearing shoes (40, 41). During the initial phase the motion most severely restricted is dorsiflexion while plantar flexion can be unaffected. Many patients, however, present with some restriction of almost all motions. Palpation usually elicits considerable tenderness, and any forceful motion, especially dorsiflexion, causes pain. These patients have a particularly difficult time finding any shoe that allows more comfortable walking.

Diagnosis and Treatment

The diagnosis is made through the history and physical and radiographic examination (see Table 76-5). Nonoperative treatment consists of splinting the joint through the use of a stiff-soled shoe with a rocker bottom sole (Fig. 76-27). Frequently these measures and the use of NSAIDs are all that is required. Operative treatment consists of improving the range of motion by excising osteophytes and freeing up the sesamoid complex. At least 30 to 40° of dorsiflexion at

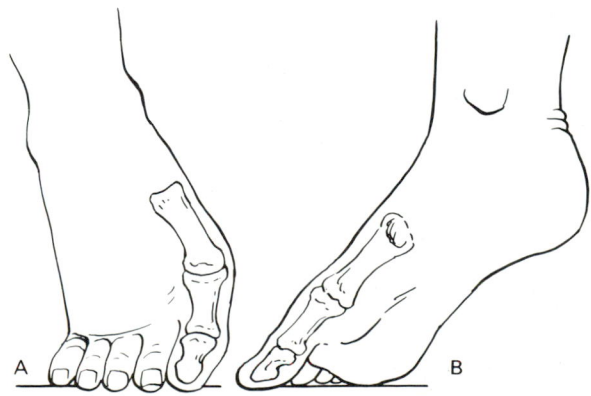

FIG. 76-33. Hallux rigidus. **A.** Anterior view. **B.** Medial view. Arthritis of the metatarsophalangeal joint reduces motion, especially in dorsiflexion. Toe push-off is painful.

surgery is required for pain relief. Advanced changes in the joint require metatarsophalangeal fusion with the toe in 20 to 30° of dorsiflexion. The best position is determined by having patients stand in their shoes and taking a lateral radiograph. Silastic implants can be used but remain controversial because of their uncertain life expectancy and the tendency of these implants to break down and become infected.

Hypermobility of the 1st Ray

Hypermobility of the 1st ray leads to diminished weight bearing on the 1st ray, resulting in pain and intractable keratosis under the head of the 2nd metatarsal. Treatment consists of transferring more weight to the 1st ray. This can be accomplished by having the patient use a shoe insert that is built up selectively under the 1st metatarsal head. In some cases fusing the tarsal or metatarsal joint is required to increase the weight-bearing capability of the 1st ray.

Intractable Keratosis

Intractable keratosis refers to hard calluses located under one or more of the metatarsal heads and often associated with aching pain. Despite conscientious attempts of the patient to reduce the thickness of these lesions by paring and grinding, daily weight-bearing forces encourage the formation of deeply penetrating indurated lesions. When local measures fail the pressure on the metatarsal head must be reduced surgically. These options are described above; care must be taken to avoid uneven weight-bearing forces that could transfer the keratoses to adjacent metatarsal heads (42).

Sesamoiditis

Sesamoiditis, which must be distinguished from metatarsalgia, is an inflammation involving the sesamoid–metatarsal head complex. The presenting picture is one of localized swelling and pain aggravated by dorsiflexion of the MP joint.

Treatment consists of eliminating weight from the area until the inflammatory reaction subsides. A walking cast is often necessary in addition to the use of NSAIDs. The temptation to remove the sesamoids surgically should be resisted, especially the lateral sesamoid, because this often causes hallux varus.

Gout

Acute gouty arthritis of the first MP joint causes severe pain of the utmost urgency to the patient. Anti-inflammatories help to control the overall reaction while splinting the toe in a bunion shoe allows the patient to walk. The diagnosis is established by aspirating the joint to test for uric acid crystals and by determining the serum uric acid level. The condition usually responds to treatment measures within 24 hours. Surgery is rarely indicated unless advanced degenerative changes have taken place, in which case the treatment for hallux ridigus applies (see Chapter 20 for a detailed discussion).

Painful Disorders of the Small Toes
Interdigital Neuroma

Interdigital neuroma, also known as Morton's neuroma and Morton's metatarsalgia, is characterized typically by metatarsal pain combined with radiating and lancinating pain in the 3rd and 4th toes (8, 9, 43).

Etiology and Pathophysiology

The pain and characteristic neurologic symptoms and signs are caused by the neuroma, which is a fibrous thickening of the digital nerve of the cleft between the 3rd and 4th metatarsals just proximal to where the nerve divides into its terminal digital branches. The neuroma takes the form of a fusiform swelling, usually about 1 cm long, that surrounds the nerve as it lies in the space between the heads of the 3rd and 4th metatarsals. The cause of the fibrous thickening is uncertain.

Symptoms and Signs

This condition involves middle-aged women more often than younger women and men. The condition is characterized by pain in the forefoot on standing or walking (9). The pain starts in the metatarsal region and radiates forward into the contiguous side of the 3rd and 4th toes or to the 4th toe alone. Like neuralgia in general the pain is sharp, burning, and piercing in character and is often associated with bouts of lancinating pain. Patients often state that they can relieve the pain by taking the shoe off and squeezing or manipulating the forefoot (9, 10, 43). On physical examination the forefoot is often splayed, as in anterior flatfoot. Moving the metatarsal head from side to side and applying pressure to the sole of the foot between the 3rd and 4th metatarsal heads elicits pain and is often associated with a clicking sound.

Diagnosis and Treatment

Interdigital neuroma is often diagnosed but inadequately resected. Patients should be followed to ensure that the symptoms are consistent and also that any conservative measures used are not related to discomfort.

Conservative measures include wearing shoes with extra-wide toe boxes, pads between the metatarsal heads to separate the involved toes and metatarsal pads to relieve pressure on the metatarsal heads. Steroids injected into the web space are sometimes helpful, but injury to the affected digital nerve from the injection can aggravate the condition. Surgical treatment consists of dividing the transverse metatarsal ligament, which allows the toes to spread apart, or of excising the neuroma itself. In the latter case all branches that extend to and from the neuroma into the toe must be divided or the problem can recur. The main complications of neuroma surgery are missing the neuroma and incomplete resection (43).

Hammer Toes and Claw Toes

Hammertoes and claw toes are deformities caused by a combination of neurologic imbalance, anatomic predisposition, activity level, and shoe wear. They

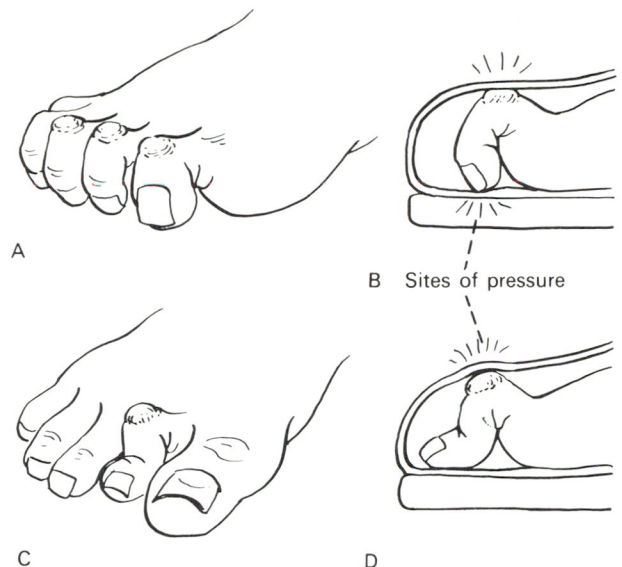

B Sites of pressure

C   D

FIG. 76-34. Typical small toe deformities. Claw toe (*A*, *B*) and hammer toe (*C*, *D*) deformities often cause corns and calluses when standard footwear is worn. Extra deep shoes avoid these problems.

cause painful corns and callosities and interfere with their shared weight-bearing distribution on the metatarsal heads (Fig. 76-34). When seen early the use of metatarsal pads and extra toe room stretched into the shoes are usually sufficient to relieve pressure points. Later, with more severe deformity, an intractable keratosis develops underneath the metatarsal head of the involved toe. The treatment of both deformities is the same—that is, correcting the deformity while restoring some weight-bearing function. The long flexor tendon is transferred to the dorsum of the proximal phalanx by the surgeon, who performs an interphalangeal fusion after resecting sufficient bone to correct the deformity. Dorsal capsular release of the MP joint is also done if contracture is present. The toe is stabilized with an intramedullary pin for about 3 weeks while tissue healing takes place. The result is a straight toe that contacts the floor and has active flexion and extension and some weight-bearing function (44).

Soft Corns

Soft corns occur between toes. The term "soft" refers to a tendency to macerate in the moist interdigital environment. They are caused by ill-fitting shoes that squeeze the toes together. The typical soft corn results from skin pressure between the condyle of one phalanx and the phalangeal shaft of its neighbor. Conservative treatment involves wearing wider shoes and using web space pads made of a soft material to separate the toes. Occasionally it becomes necessary to remove the bony prominences surgically.

REFERENCES

1. Knapp, D.A., and Koch, H.: The management of new pain in office-based ambulatory care: National Ambulatory Medical Care Survey, 1980–81. National Center for Health Statistics Advanced Data, *97*:1, DHHS Publ. No. (PHS) 84-1240, 1984.

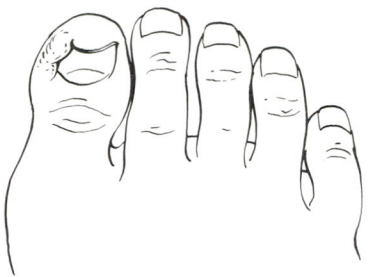

FIG. 76-35. Ingrown toenail. This is often caused by improper nail cutting techniques or by wearing poorly fitting footwear, which can create pressure against the lateral nail fold and produce exquisite pain and tenderness.

Hard Corns

Hard corns occur over the interphalangeal (IP) joints of hammer toes and claw toes and the dorsum of the 5th toes, particularly on overlapping or inward-curling toes. A resistant corn is located at the lateral nail border of the 5th toe and is caused by the toe contacting the floor or shoe at that point. Corns on the IP joints of hammer toes or claw toes can be treated by correcting the underlying deformity, as described above. Small toe corns might require a terminal Syme's amputation to provide a soft tissue surface for floor contact (44).

Overlapping Toes

Overlapping toes cause intractable corns, either from floor contact or impingement against the shoe. Whereas conservative measures described for hammer toes and claw toes should be considered, this condition often requires surgical correction of the deformity. The approach is the same as that used for hammer toes and claw toes.

Ingrown Toenails

An ingrown toenail can be exquisitely painful, particularly when aggravated by pressure from the shoe (Fig. 76-35). Causes include improper nail trimming (cutting the nails back at the nail margins), incurvation of the nail plate, and hypertrophied ungualabia. Preventive measures consist of proper nail trimming and wearing shoes with an adequate toe box.

Once established, and if in an early phase, packing cotton underneath the nail pushes the nail fold away and helps the inflammation to subside. Once the condition has become chronic, with hypertrophy of the nail fold, surgical measures are required. A simple medial or lateral border nail plate resection decompresses the area of inflammation and allows the tissues to heal. Often a new nail grows in without problems in the absence of nail bed deformity. When the nail bed is incurved, conservative measures usually fail once the inflammatory process has become established. A complete nail bed excision and matrixectomy constitute the recommended approach (45).

2. Koch, H.: The management of chronic pain in office-based ambulatory care: National Ambulatory Medical Care Survey. National Center for Health Statistics Advanced Data, NIH 123, DHHS Publ. No. (PHS) 86-150, 1986.
3. Holbrook, T.L., et al.: The Frequency of Occurrence, Impact, and Cost of Musculoskeletal Conditions in the United

States. Chicago, American Academy of Orthopedic Surgeons, 1984.

4. National Center for Health Statistics: Current Estimates from the National Health Institute Survey, United States, 1982. Ser. 10, No. 150. Hyattsville, MD, DHHS, 1985, Publ. No. (PHS) 85-1578.

5. Gould, A., et al.: Epidemiological survey of foot problems in the continental United States, 1978 to 1979. Foot Ankle, *1*:8, 1980.

6. Clemente, C.D. (ed.): Gray's Anatomy of the Human Body. 30th Am. Ed. Philadelphia, Lea & Febiger, 1985, pp. 284–300, 408–424, 573–590.

7. Hollinshead, W.H.: Anatomy for Surgeons. 3rd Ed. Vol. 3, The Back and Limbs. Philadelphia, Harper & Row, 1982, pp. 733–859.

8. Cailliet, R.: Foot and Ankle Pain. 2nd Ed. Philadelphia, F.A. Davis, 1983.

9. Adams, J.C.: Outline of Orthopedics. 10th Ed. Edinburgh, Churchill Livingstone, 1986, pp. 416–467.

10. Rosse, C.: The leg, ankle and foot. *In* The Musculoskeletal System in Health and Disease. Edited by C. Rosse and D.K. Clawson. Hagerstown, MD, Harper & Row, 1980, pp. 291–313.

11. Mann, R.A.: Surgery of the Foot. 5th Ed. St. Louis, C.V. Mosby, 1986.

12. Jahss, M.H.: Disorders of the Foot. Philadelphia, W.B. Saunders, 1982.

13. Giannestras, N.J.: Foot Disorders—Medical and Surgical Management. Philadelphia, Lea & Febiger, 1973.

14. Gardner, E., and Gray, D.: The innervation of the joints of the foot. Anat. Rec., *161*:141, 1968.

15. Hoppenfeld, S.: Physical Examination of the Spine and Extremities. New York, Appleton-Century-Crofts, 1976, pp. 197–235.

16. Frankel, V.H., and Nordin, M.: Biomechanics of the ankle. *In* Basic Biomechanics of the Skeletal System. Edited by V.H. Frankel and M. Nordin. Philadelphia, Lea & Febiger, 1980, pp. 179–191.

17. Sarrafian, S.K.: Functional characteristics of the foot and plantar aponeurosis under tibiotalar loading. Foot Ankle, *8*:4, 1987.

18. Smith, R.W.: Evaluation of the adult forefoot. Clin. Orthop., *142*:19, 1979.

19. Gould, A.: Graphing the adult foot and ankle. Foot Ankle, *2*:213, 1982.

20. Lippert, F.G.: The Generic Shoe—A Diagnostic Tool. Presented at the Foot and Ankle Society Meeting, Santa Fe, July 1987.

21. Camper, P.: Dissertation on the best form of shoe. Clin. Orthop., *110*:2 1975.

22. Parisien, S.J.: Arthroscopy of the ankle—state of the art. Contemp. Orthop., *5*:21, 1982.

23. Sartoras, D.J., and Resnick, D.: Pictorial review: Cross-sectional imaging of the foot and ankle. Foot Ankle, *8*:59, 1987.

24. Rodman, G.P. and Schumacher, H.R., (eds.): Primer on Rheumatic Diseases, 8th Ed. Atlanta, Arthritis Foundation, 1983.

25. Chapman, M.W.: Fractures of the tibial and fibular shafts. *In* Surgery of the Musculoskeletal System. Edited by C.W. Evarts. New York, Churchill Livingston, 1983, pp. 8:5–62.

26. Elstrom, J.A., and Pankovich, A.M.: Muscle and tendon surgery of the leg. *In* Surgery of the Musculoskeletal System. Edited by C.W. Evarts. New York, Churchill Livingstone, 1983, pp. 8:171–205.

27. Norris, S.H., and Mankin, H.J.: Chronic tenosynovitis of the posterior tibial tendon with new bone formation. J. Bone Joint Surg. [Br.], *60*:523, 1978.

28. Leach, R.E., and Schepsis, A.A.: Acute injuries to ligaments of the ankle. *In* Surgery of the Musculoskeletal System. Edited by C.W. Evarts. New York, Churchill Livingstone, 1983, pp. 8:143–170.

29. Yablon, I.G., and Segal, D.: Ankle fracture. *In* Surgery of the Musculoskeletal System. Edited by C.W. Evarts. New York, Churchill Livingstone, 1983, pp. 8:87–114.

30. Keck, S.W., and Kelly, P.J.: Bursitis of posterior part of the heel. J. Bone Joint Surg. [Am.], *47*:267, 1965.

31. Stauffer, R.N.: Intra-articular ankle problems. *In* Surgery of the Musculoskeletal System. Edited by C.W. Evarts. New York, Churchill Livingstone, 1983, pp. 8:115–142.

32. Berndt, A.L., and Harty, M.: Transchondral fractures (osteochondritis dissecans) of the talus. J. Bone Joint Surg. [Am.], *41*:988, 1959.

33. D'Ambrosia, R.D.: Conservative management of the metatarsal and heel pain in the adult foot. Orthopedics, *10*:137, 1987.

34. Jayakumar, S., and Cowell, H.R.: Rigid flat foot. Clin. Orthop., *122*:77, 1977.

35. Baxter, D.E., and Thigpen, M.: Heel pain, operative results. Foot Ankle, *5*:16, 1984.

36. Mann, R.A.: The tarsal tunnel syndrome. Clin. Orthop., *181*:167, 1983.

37. Graham, J., and Waddell, J.P.: Tarsometatarsal dislocation. J. Bone Joint Surg. [Br.], *55*:666, 1973.

38. Johnson, J.T.H.: Neuropathic fractures and joint injuries. Pathogenesis and rationale of prevention and treatment. J. Bone Joint Surg. [Am.], *49*:1, 1967.

39. Lapidus, T.W.: The author's bunion operation from 1931 to 1959. Clin. Orthop., *16*:119, 1960.

40. Cracchiolo, A., III: Hallux rigidus. *In* Surgery of the Musculoskeletal System. Edited by C.W. Evarts. New York, Churchill Livingstone, 1983, pp. 9:121–130.

41. Milgram, J.E.: Office measures for relief of the painful foot. J. Bone Joint Surg. [Am.] *46*:1095, 1964.

42. Mann, R.A., et al.: Intractable plantar keratoses. Orthop. Clin. North Am., *4*:67, 1973.

43. Mann, R.A., and Reynolds, J.C.: Interdigital neuroma—a critical analysis. Foot Ankle, *3*:238, 1984.

44. Coughlin, M.J.: Lesser toe deformities. Orthopedics, 10:63, 1987.

45. Lanthrop, R.G.: Ingrowing nails, causes and treatment. Cutis, *20*:119, 1977.

77 • OTHER PAINFUL DISORDERS OF THE LOWER LIMBS

JOHN J. BONICA

with contributions by
ANDERS E. SOLA

THIS chapter contains a brief discussion of painful disorders affecting the hip and lower limbs not included in Chapters 74, 75, and 76. In addition, the chapter includes discussion of some of the neuropathic disorders considered in Chapter 73 in somewhat different aspect. The information is presented in five parts: A, pain syndromes due to dysfunction of muscles, B, neuropathic painful disorders including causalgia and other reflex sympathetic dystrophy and postamputation pain, C, peripheral vascular disease, D, referred pain to the limb from disorders of the low back and pelvis, and E, pain in the lower limbs predominantly of psychologic origin. Because all of these pain syndromes are discussed in detail in Part II and other sections of Part IV of this book, only comments relevant to the lower limb are included in this chapter. Table 77-1 contains a list of the conditions that are considered. Sola helped in the development of some of the illustrations depicting the pattern of pain produced by myofascial syndrome with trigger points.

A. PAIN SYNDROMES DUE TO MUSCLE DYSFUNCTION

Kraus (1–3), a pioneer and world-renowned authority on the treatment of muscle pain, has repeatedly emphasized that in order to effectively treat the pain due to muscle dysfunction, it is necessary to differentiate among the different types of conditions that cause pain. These include (a) muscle spasm, (b) muscle tension, (c) muscle deficiency, (d) myofascial syndrome with trigger points, and (e) myofascial syndromes due to endocrine disorders. Gunn (4) has also emphasized the role of radiculopathy in causing muscular contractures, as discussed in Chapters 23 and 90. Others have emphasized the important role of fibromyalgia (pp. 388, 389), which is still another cause of pain due to muscle dysfunction. Skeletal muscle spasm, tension, and deficiency usually produce acute transient pain, although in some cases untreated skeletal muscle spasm causes persistent pain. Myofascial pain syndromes with trigger points, muscle contractures, and fibromyalgia usually produce persistent chronic pain because they frequently are not properly diagnosed and treated soon after onset. I will first consider the first three disorders together and then discuss myofascial pain syndromes with trigger points that develop in the thigh, calf, and foot.

Pain Due to Increased Skeletal Muscle Tension, Spasm, and Deficiency

Spasms of the skeletal muscles of the thigh, calf, and foot are frequent causes of pain. Depending on the cause and rapidity of onset, the pain can be sharp, severe, and well localized or dull and aching in quality, mild to moderate in severity, and somewhat more diffuse. The pain is always aggravated by increased activity of affected muscles. It is associated with deep and often cutaneous tenderness and frequently with autonomic manifestations.

Muscle Spasm

Etiology and Pathophysiology

Spasm of striated muscle can be caused by acute macrotrauma, chronic microtrauma, excessive tension, or pathologic processes in the muscle-nerve complex (1). In addition, increased tension or spasm of the skeletal muscle can be a reflex manifestation of neurologic, deep somatic, visceral, and/or psychologic disorder. Moreover, paraplegia often produces extreme spasticity of the lower limbs that often causes severe pain and interferes with nourishment, nursing care, and rehabilitation. Because these conditions are discussed in detail on pages 387 and 388 and in other chapters of Part IV of the book, here I will merely make additional comments about therapy.

Symptoms and Signs

Because untreated skeletal muscle spasm locks the patient into a vicious cycle of pain that causes increased contraction and, in turn, increases pain and severely limits movements, the patient tends to assume and maintain whatever position feels most comfortable and to exert the least possible strain on the affected muscle (1). Although it is generally believed that such spasm has a "protective" role, there is impressive evidence that the aforementioned vicious circle can lead to nonuse of the limb and cause muscle deficiency (1–3, 5).

Treatment

It is essential to relieve the pain promptly and initiate what Kraus (1–3) and others (5) have called "immediate controlled mobilization" as soon as the pain is relieved by one of the methods discussed on page 388 or by the use of ethyl chloride spray over the area of pain. Controlled mobilization should be promptly followed by exercises to restore elasticity and increase the length and relaxation of the muscle. Kraus (1) also

TABLE 77-1. Other Painful Disorders of the Hips and Lower Limbs

I. PAIN DUE TO MUSCLE DYSFUNCTION
  A. Skeletal muscle spasm
  B. Postoperative painful muscle spasm
  C. Skeletal muscle tension
  D. Skeletal muscle deficiency (nonuse)
  E. Myofascial pain syndrome with trigger points
  F. Fibromyalgia

II. PAIN DUE TO NEUROPATHIC DISORDERS
  A. Causalgia and other reflex sympathetic dystrophy
  B. Postamputation pain
  C. Painful legs and moving toes

III. PAIN DUE TO PERIPHERAL VASCULAR DISEASE
  A. Arterial Occlusive Disease
    1. Arteriosclerosis obliterans
    2. Thromboangiitis obliterans
    3. Acute arterial occlusion
  B. Disease of the microcirculation
    1. Raynaud's disease
    2. Raynaud's phenomenon
    3. Cold injuries
      a. Pernio syndrome
      b. Trench/immersion foot
      c. Frostbite
    4. Acrocyanosis
    5. Livedo reticularis
    6. Erythromelalgia
  C. Diseases of peripheral veins
    1. Acute venous occlusion
    2. Chronic venous occlusion

IV. REFERRED PAIN
  A. Pain referred from disorders of the low back
  B. Pain referred from disorders of the abdomen and pelvis

V. PAIN OF PSYCHOLOGIC ORIGIN
  A. Delusional or hallucinatory pain
  B. Hysterical or hypochondriac pain

---

reports the use of tetanizing and sinusoidal currents to relieve the muscle spasm. He suggests placing the electrode over the painful area and turning up the tetanizing current gradually until the affected muscle contracts adequately, but without discomfort, for a period of 10 minutes, after which it is turned off. Then, with the electrodes remaining in the same position, the sinusoidal current is gradually applied until muscle contraction is produced; this is continued for 10 minutes. He believes that the combination of these therapies followed by ethyl chloride spray and exercise is the most effective method of relieving painful spasm.

For sprains of the lower limbs he suggests applying the electrodes to antagonistic muscles to produce gentle joint movement. For example, electrodes should be applied to the soleus–anterior tibialis or vastus medialis–popliteus because the current helps relieve swelling prior to active exercise following application of ethyl chloride. He strongly urges not to use tetanizing currents when treating spasm in the extremities.

Other methods for relieving the spasm include the application of ice or coolant sprays like fluoromethane, as advocated by Travell and Simons (6). On the basis of his extensive experience, Kraus (1) firmly believes that ethyl chloride spray is more effective than either of

these methods. It is my own belief that the most effective way of relieving severe excruciating pain due to frequent bouts of persistent muscle spasm not relieved by more conservative measures is infiltration of a dilute solution of local anesthetic into the muscles or block of the nerve supplying the affected muscle. Although some believe that local anesthetics produce adverse aftereffects, this is not the case when dilute solutions of local anesthetic (e.g., 0.125% bupivacaine) are injected into the muscle mass.

Postoperative Muscle Spasm

In Chapters 25, 69, and 73, mention is made of the severe excruciating pain that follows operations on the back and major joints. In this section I will discuss the reflex spasm that follows certain operations on the hip, knee, and ankle. Most patients who have major hip surgery (especially arthroplasty) done with general anesthesia experience unexpected bouts of severe spasm of the quadriceps muscles that produce excruciating pain. Of 11 hip operations I underwent between 1970 and 1981, eight were carried out with regional anesthesia, which was continued for 48 to 72 hours postoperatively; the last three were done with general anesthesia, and postoperatively I was prescribed and administered 50 to 75 mg of meperidine. After the first eight operations I had an uneventful postoperative course, but after the last three I experienced frequent, totally unexpected bouts of severe reflex spasm of the ipsilateral quadriceps muscles that produced excruciating pain that lasted 3 to 10 minutes. The bouts began to occur on the second postoperative day and occurred at irregular intervals during the day and night and seemed to be provoked by slight movement of the affected limb or my pelvis. The 3 months of hospitalization following the ninth and tenth operations and the $1\frac{1}{2}$ months of hospitalization that followed the last surgery were spent in a hospital wing with private and semiprivate rooms that were occupied wholly by patients who had had arthroplasty of the hip. During these periods I heard screams from various other patients, and on investigation through the efforts of the orthopedic and anesthesiology staff I learned that these patients experienced similar bouts of painful reflex spasm. During the subsequent 6 years I interviewed dozens of patients who had had the operation and learned that those who had been managed with general anesthesia had a high incidence of painful spasm. Some patients experienced spasm of the adductors, but none of the patients had spasm of the abductors or hamstring muscle.

Major operations on the knee, especially arthroplasty, can cause similar spasm in the quadriceps or in the muscles of the calf, and surgery of the ankle can cause severe spasm of the intrinsic muscles of the foot. Rather perplexingly, the reflex muscle spasm does not occur during the first postoperative day but begins as soon as the patient begins to ambulate, often with crutches.

The mechanisms of such abnormal reflex responses are unknown, but data from animal experiments suggest that during operation carried out with general anesthesia the massive nociceptive input from noxious stimulation of nociceptive afferents, particularly C-fibers that supply the periosteum, the richly innervated joints, and the muscles and structures around them, apparently produces sensitization not only of the peripheral nociceptors, but also of dorsal horn neurons, interneurons, and anterior motor neurons (7–9). These effects of increased excitability in the spinal cord are particularly strong and prolonged, and consequently non-nociceptive input (e.g., proprioception, touch) triggers the increased reflex excitability with consequent spasm of the muscles supplied by the same and adjacent segments that supply the joint and surrounding structures. With regional anesthesia, whether it is achieved by subarachnoid or epidural block or block of peripheral nerves, the massive afferent nociceptive input is blocked at the site of the injection of the local anesthetic and consequently these and other reflex responses (discussed in detail in Chapter 7) do not occur.

Therapy of the painful reflex spasm is directed to decreasing the hyper-reflexia with pharmacologic agents or with regional analgesia. Diazepam given in doses of 10 mg every 4 hours has proven highly effective in terminating spasm associated with pain. Similarly, continuous epidural analgesia with infusion will also terminate the spasm and the associated pain (Chapter 94).

Increased Muscle Tension

Increased muscle tension caused by prolonged contraction of a muscle or muscle groups beyond functional postural needs is another cause of muscle pain. In the majority of cases this is due to emotional factors which, through psychophysiologic mechanisms, produce persistent increased tension of the muscles. In addition to being painful, muscle tension is often a precursor of muscle spasm. As mentioned on page 388, this type of muscle pain is best treated by biofeedback, relaxation, and other psychologic techniques described in Section B of Part V of this book.

Muscle Strain (Muscle Deficiency)

Etiology and Pathophysiology

Unusual or sustained intense exercise can cause pain, tenderness, and swelling of the muscles of the calf or the anterior compartment. This may progress to a genuine anterior compartment syndrome discussed on page 380. Thus a tennis player who has not played for months and then plays three sets of singles is likely to develop a painful muscle spasm in the calf, the so-called charley horse, during the game or to feel pain and tenderness after several hours or the next day. Another cause of this type of pain, which Kraus (1) calls "muscle deficiency" pain, is sitting for a protracted period of time without moving about as occurs during a long automobile ride or a long air flight trip. Sitting causes the hamstring muscles to become tight and produce pain soon after the person begins to walk about.

These and many other examples of this type of pain are more likely to occur in individuals who are sedentary and rarely exercise. In such persons, momentary undue stretching of the quadriceps or the calf muscles can and frequently does provoke excruciating painful spasm of the muscle that fortunately only lasts a minute or two, although occasionally there is residual soreness for several days.

Treatment

Muscle deficiency pain can be prevented by exercise programs to provide adequate muscular fitness. The therapeutic exercise must be properly prescribed, that is, directed to individual needs in proper dosage and form (3). If the pain is moderate and persists, it can be relieved by nonsteroidal anti-inflammatory drugs (NSAIDs).

Myofascial Pain Syndromes with Trigger Points

Myofascial pain syndromes with trigger points are associated with abnormal muscle sensitivity secondary to higher levels of sympathetic excitation. The results are localized biochemical changes and other, as yet unknown pathophysiologic disorders that produce both local and referred pain that follow predictable patterns (6, 10–13). As in other regions of the body, myofascial pain syndromes with trigger points are common causes of pain in the thigh, leg, and foot. Because these conditions are discussed in detail in Chapter 21, only brief comments relevant to these conditions in this part of the body will be made here.

Etiology and Pathophysiology

Trigger points (TPs) are little, tender nodules of degenerated muscle tissue caused by major trauma or persistent mechanical stress with consequent microtrauma caused by repetitive or continuous use of one or more muscles during work or certain athletic exercise. They can also result from poor posture, degenerative joint disease, emotional stress, and endocrine imbalance (1). Sola (11, 12) has postulated that sympathetic hyperactivity provokes local biochemical changes that result in vasoconstriction with consequent histologic and histochemical changes in muscle fibers. This hypothesis has recently found support from the controlled study by Bengtsson and Bengtsson (14) that demonstrated that regional sympathetic blockade (which produces vasodilation) eliminated a number of tender or trigger points. How these tender points cause pain is unknown, but it is likely that they initiate and sustain nociceptive impulses that bombard the central nervous system to produce local and referred pain and a number of associated symptoms (see Chapter 21 for details).

Symptoms and Signs

The pain of myofascial syndrome in the lower limb varies from slight to severe, unrelenting, and disabling discomfort. The pain can be either sharp or dull and can be located around the trigger area or referred to distant parts. Trigger point hypersensitivity in the quadriceps or calf muscles can cause pain and limited range of motion in the knee or ankle and foot. Some patients experience vague numbness in the limb, particularly in the morning, together with aching, tingling, or a cool foot as well as other manifestations of autonomic disturbances.

In the absence of specific clinical findings in patients who complain of pain in the thigh, leg, or foot, the muscles of that part should be examined carefully for hyperactive tender points. The clinician should also keep in mind that TPs are likely to be activated as a secondary cause of pain in association with any injury or strain and that failure to diagnose and treat hyperactive trigger points will intensify the pain, delay healing, and make rehabilitation more difficult (6, 10–13).

Diagnosis

Screening of myofascial pain syndromes should include a complete history and thorough physical examination as discussed in Chapters 21 and 31. Disorders that must be ruled out include a variety of musculoskeletal conditions discussed in the preceding three chapters. A thorough assessment of neuromuscular function should be undertaken, including passive and active range of motion of muscles in the thigh, leg, and foot.

To identify TPs of specific muscles, the physician systematically palpates the suspected muscle or muscles with a finger or a blunt object and compares the particular muscle with the contralateral muscle. It is important to note signs of local and/or ipsilateral hand coolness, sweating, edema, and piloerection. For location of trigger points, the patient should be positioned so that the muscles of the thigh, calf, and knee are relaxed. If the muscles seem to tighten under the palpating finger, the examiner can relax the pressure and then quickly probe again as the muscle "gives" (1). If the patient is very muscular or has a thick layer of fat, it might be necessary to place the fingers of one hand on top of the other and combine the pressure of both hands. Once a trigger point is located, it is useful to employ Fisher's pressure gauge described in Chapter 21. The gauge is pressed gently and steadily after instructing the patient to inform the examiner when the pressure becomes painful. The pain threshold value of one side should be compared with that of the corresponding area of the other side. In addition to examining the muscles of the limbs, it is important to palpate the muscles of the buttocks and low back, which frequently have trigger points that cause spillover pain to the thigh and even the leg. Indeed, Sola (11) has noted that trigger points in the gluteus medius and low back muscles are frequent and activate latent TPs in other parts of the body.

Treatment

The need for a comprehensive approach in managing patients with myofascial syndrome with TPs is duly emphasized in Chapter 21, where such a program is discussed in detail. I prefer penetration and injection of TPs with a dilute solution of a long-acting local anesthetic such as 0.125 to 0.25% bupivacaine. I agree with Kraus (1) that although injection of saline solution or even dry needling can be used effectively, both produce postinjection pain, whereas injection of the aforementioned local anesthetic will provide relief for 4 to 6 hours or longer. Usually 1 to 2 ml of solution is injected into the TP so as to rupture it. When the TP is penetrated the clinician can actually feel the tight muscle "grab" the needle point, and after the injection one can feel the muscle relax and release the needle dramatically. If the patient develops spasm of the muscle after penetration of the TP, Kraus (1) suggests

that sinusoidal current, ethyl chloride spray, and gentle limbering movement be used on three successive days after all myofascial TP injections.

After injection the patient is maintained in a comfortable position and observed for 15 to 20 minutes. The treated muscles should be guarded against overuse for several days because they are susceptible to the reactivation of TPs. When TPs are located in muscle near a joint or the joint itself is involved, bupivacaine treatment can be used in combination with injection of steroids and physical therapy. An important part of treatment is a progressive exercise program, particularly when muscles that are critically important to function of joints are involved.

Specific Syndromes of the Thigh

Figures 77-1 to 77-6 depict the most important myofascial syndromes with TPs in muscles of the thigh. The gluteus maximus and gluteus medius produce spillover pain in the upper posterior thigh, but because the most intense pain (essential zone) is in the low back this is described in Chapter 73. The descriptions that follow are based on personal observations (13) and those of Sola (11, 12) and especially those of Simons and Travell (10). As in the upper limb, the syndromes are grouped according to the part of the thigh or leg in which the pain is located.

POSTERIOR THIGH SYNDROMES. Figures 77-1 and 77-2 depict four myofascial pain syndromes that produce pain most prominently in back of the thigh.

The gluteus minimus can develop TPs in its anterior or posterior parts, thus producing two distinctly different pain patterns. Figure 77-1A shows a TP in the posterior part of the gluteus minimus that produces pain that has a somewhat sciatic distribution,

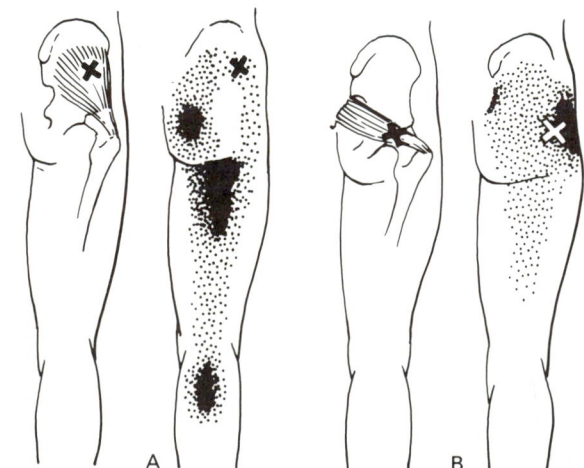

FIG. 77-1. Myofascial syndromes that produce pain predominantly in the posterior aspect of the thigh. **A.** Pain pattern provoked by a trigger point in the posterior part of the gluteus minimus. **B.** Piriformis syndrome. In this and all of the other figures that follow, the figure on the reader's left shows the muscle and location of the TP marked with an X. The figure on the right shows the pain pattern; the black area indicates the "essential" zone where pain is felt most intensely and by most patients, and the stippled area represents the "spillover" zone where the referred pain is milder and is experienced by only some patients.

concentrating with most intense pain in the posterior upper thigh and upper calf and the lower part of the buttock. This syndrome is often mistaken for an S1 radiculopathy and diagnosed as sciatica. The differential diagnosis is easily done because the myofascial syndrome is not accompanied by change in reflex, sensory or motor function. Injection of the TP requires a long needle because of the deeply situated muscle. For stretch and spray, the spray should begin at the posterior portion of the gluteus minimus and continue along the crest of the ilium and downward over the posterior thigh and calf (10).

The piriformis syndrome is depicted in Figure 77-1B. It produces pain in the posterior and lateral aspects of the gluteal region and the posterior aspect of the thigh. An active TP in the piriformis restricts the combination of adduction and internal rotation of the thigh at the hip. If the condition is associated with severe spasm of the piriformis muscle, it can cause compression of the sciatic nerve and thus produce a piriformis entrapment syndrome (Chapter 73). The TP can be best palpated with the patient lying on the side with the affected side up, hip flexed, the femur adducted and the knee flexed resting on the plinth (1). This position rotates the femur slightly inward, making the piriformis muscle available for palpation, which can be done by rectum or by palpating externally (10).

The vastus lateralis is another muscle that develops TPs in two different parts. Figure 77-2A depicts the pain pattern provoked by a TP in the posterior part of the muscle. As can be noted, the pain is located in the posterolateral part of the middle portion of the thigh.

The biceps femoris, among the hamstring group of muscles, usually develops a TP in its lower third that provokes pain that is most intense in the back of the knee with spillover over the upper calf and lower part of the thigh (Fig. 77-2B). This syndrome is a common source of restricted flexion of the hip with a positive straight-leg-raising test. Penetration of the muscle and injection of local anesthetics usually can be achieved

with a 5-cm 25-gauge needle. If spray and stretch is used, the spray is applied from hip to ankle while the hamstring muscles are gently stretched by elevating the leg with knee straight in a position of abduction (10).

LATERAL THIGH PAIN. Figures 77-3 and 77-4 depict four myofascial syndromes that produce pain predominantly on the lateral aspects of the thigh. Figure 77-4A depicts a TP in the *anterior portion of the gluteus minimus* that produces pain primarily along the lateral thigh that usually extends to the lateral aspect of the leg as far as the ankle with the most intense pain in the thigh. Again, injection of the TP requires a long needle because of the deeply situated muscle. If stretch and spray is used, the sweep of spray is applied along the anterior portion of the muscle belly and downward over the lateral thigh and leg to the ankle (10).

The vastus lateralis, with TPs in the lower anterior part of the muscle, (Fig. 77-3B) provokes pain along the length of the muscle with some spillover on the lateral aspect of the glutei around the TP, which can be easily located. If stretch and spray is used, the spray is initiated on the upper part of the lateral aspect of the thigh and then continued downward to the lateral part of the knee (10).

The tensor fasciae latae can develop TPs in its upper or middle part. Figure 77-4B shows the pattern of pain produced by the lower TP. The pain extends along the lateral aspect of the leg as far as the ankle, with the most intense pain in the thigh. Figure 77-4C shows the pattern of pain produced by a TP in the upper part of the muscle, which is limited to the lateral aspect of the thigh.

ANTERIOR THIGH PAIN. Figures 77-5 and 77-6 depict the myofascial syndromes that produce pain predominantly on the anterior part of the thigh. Figure 77-5A depicts the pattern of pain produced by a TP in the *adductor longus*. The pain is usually located in the

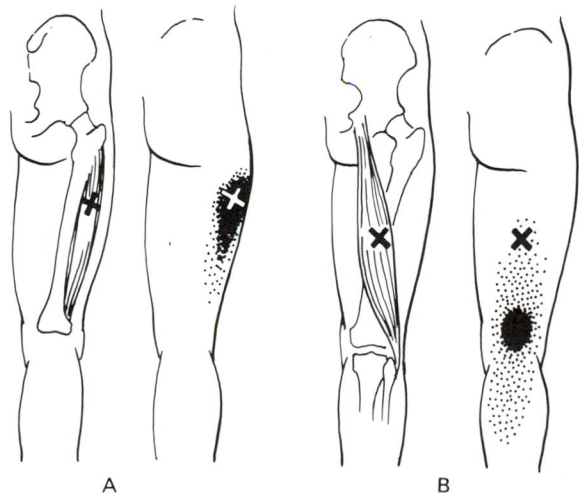

FIG. 77-2. Other myofascial syndromes that produce pain predominantly in the posterior aspect of the thigh. **A.** Vastus lateralis syndrome. **B.** Biceps femoris syndrome. See Figure 77-1 for explanation.

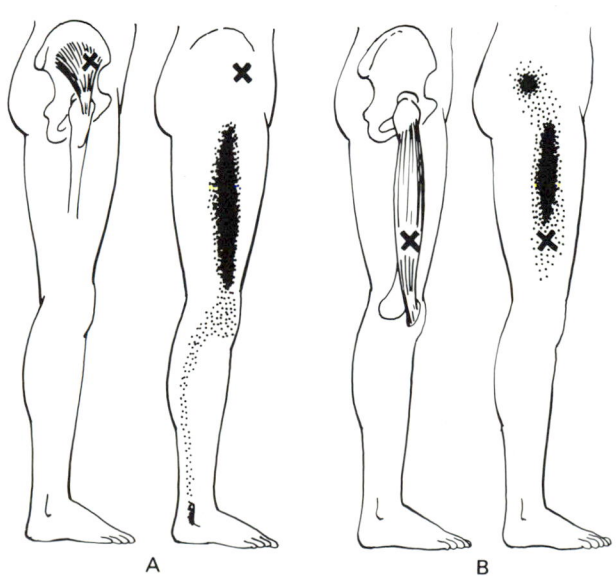

FIG. 77-3. Myofascial syndromes that produce pain predominantly in the lateral aspect of the thigh. **A.** Myofascial pain syndrome produced by a TP in the anterior aspect of the gluteus minimus. **B.** The vastus lateralis syndrome. See Figure 77-1 for explanation.

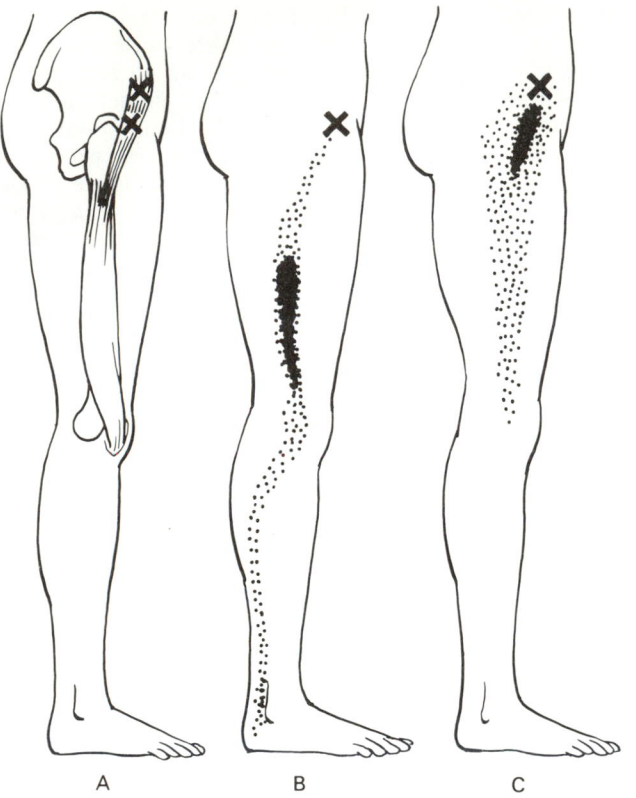

FIG. 77-4. Myofascial syndromes produced by TPs in the tensor fasciae latae. See text for details and Figure 77-1 for explanation of the figure.

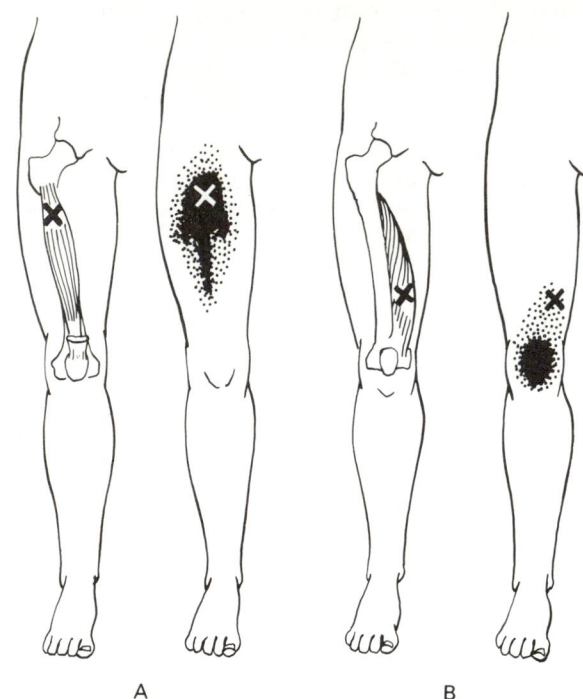

FIG. 77-6. Myofascial syndromes that produce pain primarily in the anterior part of the thigh. **A.** Vastus intermedius syndrome. **B.** Vastus medialis syndrome. See Figure 77-1 for explanation.

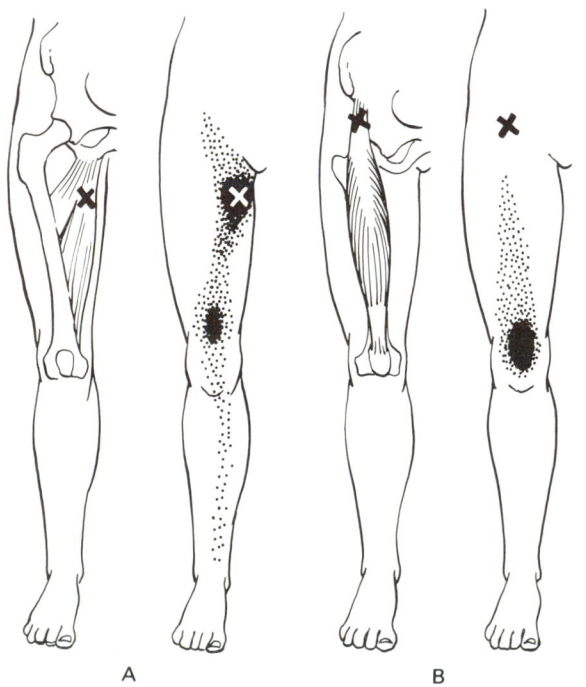

FIG. 77-5. Myofascial syndromes that produce pain primarily in the anterior part of the thigh. **A.** Adductor longus syndrome. **B.** Rectus femoris syndrome. See Figure 77-1 for explanation.

anteromedial part of the thigh and upward in the groin with spillover over the anteromedial part of the leg. Active TPs in this muscle markedly restrict abduction of the thigh and are a common source of groin and distal anterior thigh pain above the knee. Injection of the TP should be carried out with special care because of the proximity of the femoral vein and its many branches which cover the muscle. For stretch and spray therapy the muscle is covered with a sweep of vapocoolant while the leg is slowly abducted to stretch the muscles. The spray is continued upward over the inguinal painful region and then downward over the thigh, knee, and the anteromedial part of the leg where the spillover zone exists (10).

The rectus femoris pain syndrome usually develops near the origin of the muscle, just below the inguinal ligament. In this case the pain is referred mostly to the kneecap and the lower part of the anterior thigh (Fig. 77-5B). Injection requires a 5-cm 25-gauge needle, or a 22-gauge needle for muscular individuals. For stretch and spray the spray is begun in the inguinal region and then across the anterior thigh as far as the knee (10).

The vastus intermedius develops TPs that are deeper than, and distal to, the rectus femoris TP and provoke intense pain locally around the TP and over the upper part of the thigh (Fig. 77-6A). Care must be exercised in injecting a TP because of the proximity of the femoral vessels in the femoral triangle.

The vastus medialis usually develops TPs just above the knee and produces pain in the anterior part of the knee and lower part of the thigh (Fig. 77-6B).

Myofascial Syndromes in Leg and Foot

POSTERIOR LEG AND FOOT PAIN. Figure 77-7 depicts the two myofascial syndromes that produce pain predominantly in back of the leg and plantar aspect of the foot.

The gastrocnemius muscle usually develops TPs along either the medial or lateral border of the muscle at the level of the junction of the upper third with the middle third of the leg (Fig. 77-7A). These TPs usually produce pain referred to the back of the leg extending from the back of the knee to the ankle and also in the instep of the foot. Patients with this syndrome have difficulty in walking uphill and often experience nocturnal calf cramps. Penetration of the trigger area requires only a short, thin needle. If spray and stretch is used the patient is taught to stretch the muscle by standing with the involved leg behind the other and leading the body forward, keeping the knee straight and the heel solidly on the floor. Coolant spray is applied before pain occurs from the stretch (10).

The soleus muscle can develop TPs anywhere, but the most frequent site is just above the point where the muscle converges into its tendon (Fig. 77-7B). This syndrome is a frequent cause of pain and tenderness in the heel that is erroneously diagnosed as being due to a bony spur on the calcaneus. Injection of the TP can be achieved with a 3-cm or 5-cm 25-gauge needle. For stretch and spray the patient is placed in the prone position with the leg flexed to 90°, so that the foot projects upward. The operator applies one or two sweeps of the vapocoolant spray over the calf and presses down on the ball of foot to dorsiflex the ankle and stretch the soleus muscles while gently maintaining the pressure (10).

ANTERIOR LEG AND FOOT PAIN. Figure 77-8 depicts two muscles that can develop TPs that provoke pain in the anterior part of the leg and dorsal part of the foot.

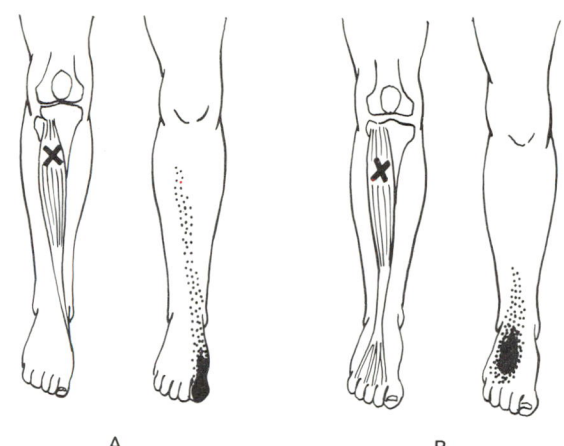

A   B

FIG. 77-8. Myofascial syndromes that produce pain in the anterior aspect of the leg and dorsal aspect of the foot. *A.* Tibialis anterior syndrome. *B.* Extensor digitorum longus syndrome. A similar pattern of pain is produced by TPs in the hallucis longus. See Figure 77-1 for explanation.

The tibialis anterior muscle usually develops TPs in the upper part of the muscle just lateral to the tubercle of the tibia, to which the patellar ligament is attached. Figure 77-8B shows the pattern of pain, which is distributed from the trigger area down the anterior part of the leg and anteromedial part of the foot, with the most intense pain in the great toe. Injection requires only a short, thin needle; stretch and spray is done from the site of the trigger area toward the foot while at the same time everting the foot (10).

The extensor digitorum longus and hallucis longus usually develop TPs in the upper part of the muscles just below the knee and produce pain in the dorsum of

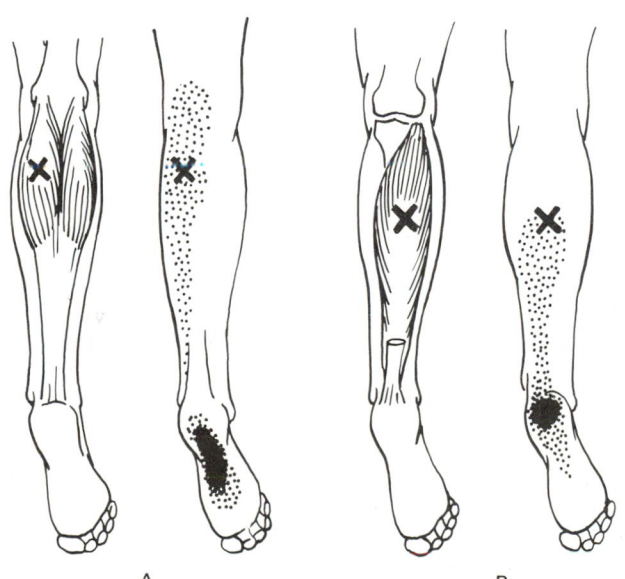

A   B

FIG. 77-7. Myofascial syndromes that produce pain in the back of the leg and the plantar aspect of the foot. *A.* Gastrocnemius syndrome. *B.* Soleus syndrome. See Figure 77-1 for explanation.

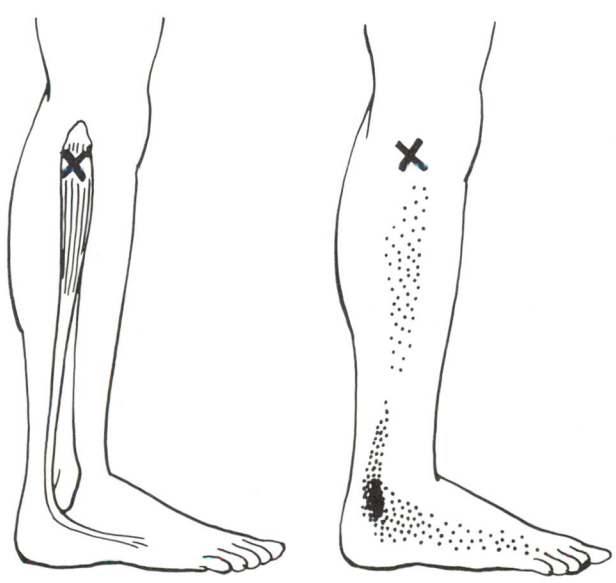

FIG. 77-9. The peroneus longus myofascial syndrome. The TP (X) is usually located in the upper part of the muscle, and it produces pain in the lateral aspect of the leg and foot. See Figure 77-1 for explanation.

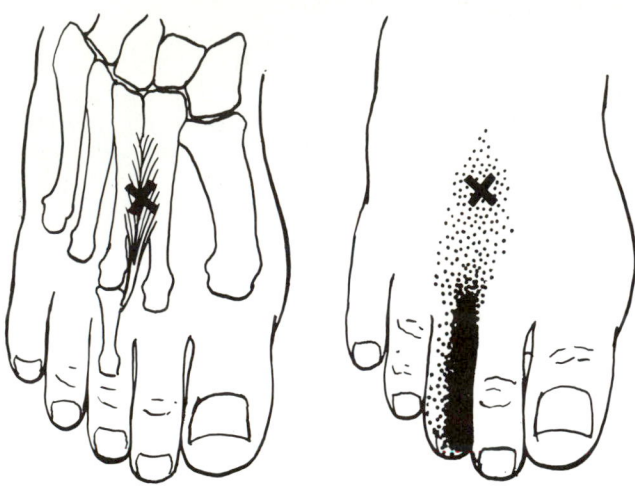

Fig. 77-10. Myofascial pain syndrome produced by a TP (X) in the second dorsal interosseus muscle. See Figure 77-1 for explanation.

the foot and toe with some spillover in the lower anterior part of the leg (Fig. 77-8B). The technique of injection and spray and stretch is similar to that for the tibialis anterior syndrome except that the foot is plantar flexed during the spray (10).

LATERAL LEG AND FOOT PAIN. Figure 77-9 depicts a myofascial pain syndrome that produces pain in the lateral aspect of the leg and foot and in the dorsal part of the foot. The *peroneus longus* develops TPs that are usually located in the upper part of the muscle. The syndrome is characterized by mild to moderate pain in the anterolateral aspect of the leg, lateral side of the ankle, and the dorsolateral part of the foot.

The dorsal interossei can develop TPs that cause pain along the side of the digit to which the muscle is attached. Figure 77-10 shows the TP pattern in the third dorsal interosseus muscle. Treatment is by injection or stretch and spray.

Fibromyalgia

Primary fibromyalgia (PFS) is a diffuse myofascial pain syndrome that is also known as "fibrositis," articular rheumatism, fibromyalgia, and fibromyositis. It is said to be a frequent cause of pain in the body, including the lower limb. The condition is characterized by diffuse aching musculoskeletal pain associated with multiple discrete predictable tender points and stiffness (14, 15) (Fig. 72-17).

The most important feature of fibromyalgia is widespread aching pain of more than 3 months' duration that is poorly circumscribed and perceived as deep, usually referred to muscle or bony prominences (15). Although pain in the trunk and proximal girdle is aching in character, distal limb pain is often perceived as associated with fatigue, swelling, numbness, and stiffness. The pain is usually continuous, but there can be day-to-day fluctuation.

Treatment is said to consist of psychologic support and symptomatic treatment with heat, massage, and low-dose amitriptyline or cyclobenzaprine. Strenuous physical exercise has also been reported to modify manifestation of PFS, and sympathetic block reduces the number of tender points (14).

B. PAIN OF NEUROPATHIC ORIGIN

Causalgia and Other Reflex Sympathetic Dystrophy

Causalgia

Causalgia involves the lower limbs somewhat less frequently than the upper limbs. As discussed in detail in Chapter 11, this condition is usually seen during wartime. In most patients the condition is due to lesions of major nerves, most frequently the sciatic, less frequently the branches of the sciatic, e.g., the peroneal or tibial nerves or both. The condition is sometimes due to involvement of the obturator, femoral, or saphenous nerve. It is characterized by burning pain, allodynia, hyperpathia, vasomotor and sudomotor disturbances, and trophic changes if the condition is not treated promptly.

Reflex Sympathetic Dystrophy

Reflex sympathetic dystrophy (RSD) (or sympathetically maintained pain), in contrast to causalgia, is a common clinical problem that unfortunately is often misdiagnosed and improperly treated. Causes, symptoms, diagnosis, and treatment are discussed in detail in Chapter 11.

As in the upper limb, RSD in the lower extremity can be caused by trauma to small nerves, ligamentous tears, particularly of the ankle and knee, damage to the soft tissue of the foot, ankle, or leg resulting from sprain, dislocation, or fracture of bones, crush injuries of the toes and ankle, and laceration of open wounds. Usually there is no correlation between severity of the injury and the incidence, severity, and course of the subsequent RSD.

The most frequent iatrogenic cause of RSD in the lower limb is tight casts, although RSD also develops in patients who have had surgical amputation of the toes, feet, or leg, excision of small ganglia, and injection of the sciatic nerve with either analgesics or antibiotics.

Reflex sympathetic dystrophy also occurs as a complication of visceral and neurologic disease of the central nervous system (16–18). Vasomotor and sudomotor disturbances, edema, and trophic changes in lower limbs after cerebrovascular accidents were described over 12 decades ago, but it was not until the 1940s that deTakats (16) and others emphasized the relationship between hemiplegia and the signs and symptoms of the shoulder-hand syndrome. More recently Nathan and colleagues (17, 18) have discussed reflex sympathetic dystrophy involving the lower limbs as a result of other lesions of the CNS.

Lumbar sympathetic block or intravenous regional sympathetic block with guanethidine, used early, is usually highly effective in relieving the pain and other symptoms and in reversing any vasomotor and sudomotor disturbances and early trophic changes. To obtain optimal results it is essential to combine sympathetic interruption with active exercise and other rehabilitation procedures. These are especially important in patients who have advanced to the second stage of the disease, when trophic changes are more advanced and require aggressive multimodal rehabilitation programs.

Painful Legs and Moving Toes

Spillane, Nathan, and their colleagues (19) in 1971 published the first report on the rather perplexing condition of painful legs and moving toes. Subsequently they provided evidence that the condition was due to disease of the spinal cord or the peripheral nervous system or both (20). More recently, Montagna and associates (21) reported cases associated with polyneuropathy. This condition is characterized by deep, often gnawing, twisting, or aching pain in the legs with involuntary movements of the limbs, especially the digits. The pain is most intense in the lower leg and foot and occasionally the great toe. The pain is usually severe, deep, and poorly localized and is more severe in the leg than in the periphery. Sometimes the pain is relieved by activity, although it can be aggravated by exercise. The condition can be unilateral or bilateral, or it can begin unilaterally and spread to the other limb.

The movements of the toe may be florid or almost imperceptible; in the latter case the patient might never have noticed them. They consist of irregular, involuntary, sometimes writhing movements of the toes that cannot be imitated voluntarily but can be suppressed for a minute or two by voluntary effort. They recur when the patient no longer tends to them. In addition to the toes, movements can involve the feet. There is usually no relation between the pain and the movements.

The condition continues indefinitely, and to date no consistently effective measures have been reported (20).

Postamputation Pain

The lower limb is amputated more frequently than the upper limb. Virtually all patients describe phantom limb sensation, and a significant percentage develop phantom limb pain or stump pain or both. Because this subject is discussed in detail in Chapter 12, only brief comments will be made here about the possibility of preventing or at least reducing the incidence of postamputation pain in patients who have moderate to severe pain prior to operation.

Bach and associates (22) recently evaluated the efficacy of preoperative analgesia on the incidence of postamputation phantom limb pain and phantom sensation. They studied 25 patients with severe preoperative limb pain due to occlusive arterial disease complicated by diabetes mellitus in 44%. The pain had persisted from 1 to 6 months in 23 patients and over 6 months in 2 and who were scheduled to undergo amputation. One group of 11 patients received a continuous lumbar epidural blockade with bupivacaine or morphine or a combination of these to achieve complete pain relief for 72 hours prior to amputation. A control group of 14 patients who also had persistent constant severe limb pain were treated with nonopioid and opioid analgesics administered by standard methods for the same period. All 25 patients received epidural or spinal anesthesia for the amputation procedure and opioids and nonopioid analgesia after the procedure. Seven days after surgery, 3 patients (27%) in the group that received preoperative regional analgesia had phantom limb pain compared with 9 patients (64%) in the control group (P < 0.01) (Fig. 77-11). Six months after the surgery, all 10 patients in the blockade group were pain-free whereas 5 of 13 patients (38%) in the control group had phantom limb pain (P < 0.05). Follow-up 1 year after surgery revealed that all patients in the blockade group were still pain-free, but 3 of 11 patients (27%) in the control group had phantom limb pain. Moreover, none of the treated group had phantom sensation, but in the control group 1 had phantom limb sensation at 6 months and 2 at 1 year (Fig. 77-11). If these results are replicated by

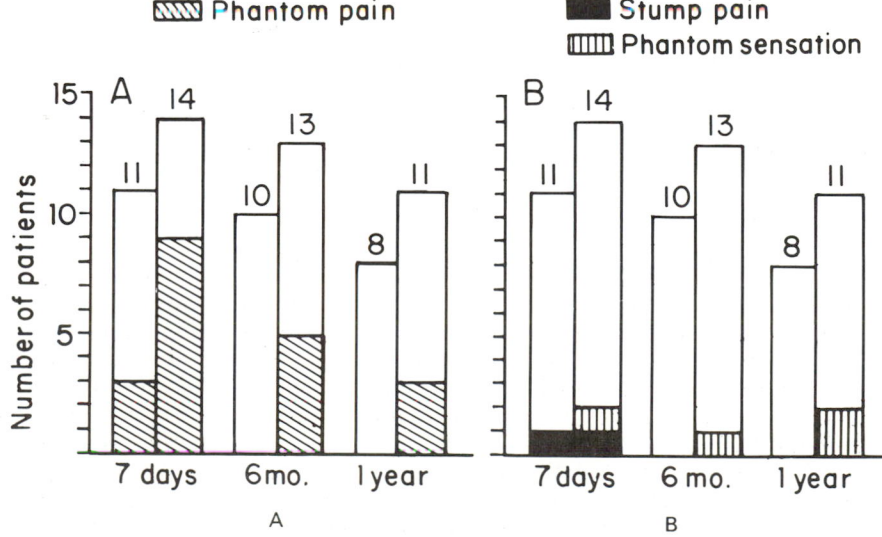

☒ Phantom pain   ■ Stump pain   ▥ Phantom sensation

FIG. 77-11. Bar graph showing the incidence of postamputation phantom limb pain (**A**) and postamputation stump pain and painless phantom sensation (**B**). The group of patients who received complete pain relief with continuous epidural analgesia prior to the operation (N = 11) is shown on the left, and the control group (N = 14) is shown on the right of each double column. One patient in each group died within 6 months, and another 2 patients in each group died within 1 year, thus explaining the lower numbers at these follow-up periods. Modified from Bach, S., et al.: Phantom limb pain in amputees during their first 12 months following limb amputation after preoperative lumbar epidural blockade. Pain, 33:299, 1988.

other groups, regional analgesia should be seriously considered to provide both preoperative pain relief and anesthesia for surgery in order to prevent or reduce the risk of postamputation pain.

The possible mechanisms of prevention of postamputation pain with preoperative analgesia are discussed in Chapters 7, 25, and 94. To recapitulate, animal experimental studies have shown that during operations carried out with the patient receiving light balanced general anesthesia, the spinal cord receives a massive afferent barrage produced by surgery, particularly when peripheral nerves are sectioned, whereas under regional analgesia the cord receives no afferent signals set off during surgery (23). It has been shown that the arrival of a volley of nerve impulses in unmyelinated C fibers sets off a prolonged, widespread increase of reflex excitability (24, 25) and of interneuron excitability (26), which is particulary strong and prolonged if the stimulation is applied to deep tissues such as muscle or joints rather than skin (8, 9). When peripheral nerves are cut, a brief but maximal injury discharge is generated that triggers prolonged spinal cord excitability (8, 25) and even postsynaptic spinal cord morphologic changes (27). By using regional analgesia preoperatively and during the operation, one prevents the bombardment of the CNS, thus obviating these spinal cord changes (23).

C. PERIPHERAL VASCULAR DISEASE

In the lower limb, disease of the peripheral arteries, and to a lesser extent the veins, are among the most common causes of pain. Although these conditions are discussed in detail in Chapter 28, here I wish to summarize some of the most important points in regard to etiology, symptoms and signs, and particularly treatment.

Arteriosclerosis Obliterans (XV-1, XV-2)

Arteriosclerosis obliterans (ASO) is a peripheral manifestation of generalized atherosclerosis most commonly found in the lower abdominal aorta, the iliac artery, and its branches in the lower limb. Plaques and thrombosis are particularly common in the femoral artery in Hunter's canal and in the popliteal artery just above the knee joint (28). The anterior and posterior tibial arteries are frequently occluded together in the leg, but are occluded at different sites around the ankle—the posterior where it rounds the medial malleolus and the anterior where it is superficial and becomes the dorsalis pedis artery. The peroneal artery, which is well imbedded in muscle, escapes when other major vessels are included, and it may be the main blood supply to the extremity (29) (Fig. 28-2). The exception to this rule is patients who have ASO and diabetes, in whom the peroneal arteries are frequently involved. ASO is responsible for 95% of the cases of chronic occlusive arterial disease and involves the arteries of the lower limbs much more frequently than those of the upper limbs (28).

Etiology and Pathophysiology

Despite numerous studies, no single factor has been identified as the specific cause of ASO, but risk factors include age, sex, and diabetes. Smoking, hyperlipidemia, and hypertension clearly accelerate the progression of ASO. The influence of other factors and the pathophysiology of ASO are discussed on page 506.

Symptoms and Signs

The earliest symptom of ASO is intermittent claudication—a condition characterized by extreme fatigue, cramping, and tightening of muscle that progresses to a sharp pain, and occasionally numbness brought on by walking and relieved within a few minutes by rest. It is not necessary to sit down to obtain relief, but merely to stop walking (28). The distance the patient can walk varies with the degree and extent of arterial occlusion but remains constant for a given time. With mild degrees of occlusion the patient can walk several blocks, but as the disease progresses there is a decrease in distance traversed before claudication occurs. The pain is more severe and occurs earlier when the patient walks rapidly or uphill (30). Arcangeli et al. (31) found that in most patients with ASO trigger points are present in the myofascial structures of the calf, thigh, buttock, or even in the foot. These points are sites of spontaneous pain and can be intensified by firm digital pressure.

The location of the intermittent claudication depends on the muscle group most severely affected by the arterial insufficiency. Because the femoral-popliteal artery segment is most often involved in ASO, intermittent claudication occurs most often in the calf muscles. The close correlation between the site of intermittent claudication and location of the occlusive disease is characteristic of ASO (see Fig. 28-4). Thus, aortoiliac disease causes intermittent claudication in the buttocks, hips, thighs, and calf (the Leriche syndrome). The pain is usually severe and disabling. Some patients who have involvement of the popliteal-tibial segment and the arteries of the foot develop intermittent claudication involving the muscles below the knee and in the foot (32). When the disease is confined to the tibial arteries or the peroneal artery it does not produce claudication, and occlusion of the popliteal and superficial femoral arteries produces only mild calf claudication.

Rest pain develops if the disease progresses to involve multiple levels of occlusion including the collateral vessels. The condition becomes so extensive that the arterial pressure and flow to the distal limb and foot are insufficient. Rest pain also has the following distinguishing characteristic features (32): (a) it always involves the toes and distal foot; (b) the pain is frequently burning in quality, constant and severe, initially worse at night when the patient is in bed because of the loss of beneficial effects of gravity in carrying out the blood distally, but eventually is experienced during the day as well; (c) it can be partially or completely relieved by dependency and aggravated by elevating the foot; (d) it is frequently associated with trophic changes in the foot and toes and with ulceration or gangrene; and (e) it rarely improves spontaneously unless blood perfusion to the ischemic area can be increased. At this stage of severe ischemia, ischemic neuropathy can develop and produce severe lancinating, shooting, or sharp pain in the leg and foot. This pain is also most distressing during recumbency and can be relieved by keeping the involved extremity dependent.

Diminished or absent pulses in the affected extremity are the most important physical sign of ASO, and the site of absent pulses indicates the site of occlusion. Color changes that occur when the foot is elevated or dependent are a confirmatory physical sign of arterial insufficiency. Pain referred to the thigh, knee, calf, ankle, and foot can be caused by visceral disease of the lower abdomen and pelvis and diseases of the low back. These are discussed in detail in Chapters 66, 67, 68, 71, and 72.

Treatment

In patients with mild to moderate rest pain, the discomfort can be controlled with NSAIDs, such as aspirin or acetaminophen, combined with codeine. The dose of the NSAID can be gradually increased to 1 g q4h, and codeine can be increased to 128 mg q4h. This combination can be used for long periods of time with insignificant risk of physical dependence and no risk of addiction or tolerance. Side effects of both drugs should be treated (see Chapter 78).

Chemical sympathectomy with alcohol and phenol is an extremely effective procedure and should be considered for all patients who have severe rest pain, especially those who are debilitated or suffering from severe cardiac or respiratory disease, for whom anesthesia and surgical intervention carry significant risks. This procedure can be administered on an outpatient basis, it reduces postoperative morbidity, especially the risk of thrombosis associated with the surgical operation and bedrest, and it drastically reduces the cost to the patient. The results cited on pages 512–514 indicate that chemical sympathectomy produces complete or good pain relief in some 70 to 80% of patients and relief of intermittent claudication in 25 to 30%. The relief lasted some 6 months, after which the process was repeated with similar results. Another benefit of sympathectomy is that it shortens the time to a clear demarcation area of the amputation level and improves the vascular supply of the stump. Moreover, sympathectomy for pain relief performed a month before amputation can prevent postamputation pain. This is suggested by the fact that none of the patients treated in this fashion developed severe phantom limb pain.

Another exciting development related to this issue of amputation in patients with peripheral vascular disease is the study recently carried out by Bach and associates (22), discussed in Section B (Postamputation Pain). As mentioned there, they used regional analgesia in patients with ASO to prevent postamputation phantom limb pain. Because the data and the possible mechanisms are discussed in the subsection on amputation, this discussion will not be repeated here except to re-emphasize that patients with severe pain due to peripheral vascular disease that involves the tissues such as muscles and joints continue to have massive nociceptive barrage preoperatively and intraoperatively, especially from unmyelinated C fibers. These fibers set off a prolonged widespread increase in reflex excitability (8, 24) and of the excitability of dorsal horn neurons, interneurons, and often motor neurons (24). By using regional analgesia preoperatively and during the operation, bombardment of the CNS is prevented, thus obviating these changes.

Thromboangiitis Obliterans (XIV-2)

Thromboangiitis obliterans (TAO), also known as Buerger's disease (33), is an occlusive disease of medium-sized and small arteries and veins, affecting chiefly the distal parts (primarily of the lower limbs) in young adult male smokers (34, 35).

Etiology and Pathophysiology

The cause of thromboangiitis obliterans is not known, but it is known that it occurs nearly exclusively in young males who are cigarette smokers, and a striking relationship has been noted between exacerbations and continued use of tobacco and between remissions and cessations of smoking (36). The acute pathologic lesions consist of segmental inflammation of all layers of the walls of medium-sized and small arteries and veins, although the architecture of the wall is preserved. The arteries most commonly involved are the posterior tibial, anterior tibial, plantar, and digital (36). Large arteries such as the femoral are affected only later and only when the disease is severe and progressive. Thrombosis occurs in the inflamed segment, producing occlusion of the lumen. Other pathophysiologic changes are discussed in detail on page 514.

Symptoms and Signs

In addition to the fact that it occurs in young male cigarette smokers, the following are other distinguishing clinical features of TAO: (a) there is usually bilateral symmetrical involvement; (b) the distal location of the occlusion in the leg leads to development of instep claudication, a unique feature of the disease; and (c) cold sensitivity of the Raynaud's type is present in at least half of the patients (36).

The most common and most bothersome pain problems are intermittent claudication and ischemic rest pain. The intermittent claudication might be an ache, a sense of fatigue or a persistent cramp, or a severe aching, squeezing pain that is typical in its relationship to the walk-pain-rest-relief cycle. The ischemic rest pain usually involves the toes and feet, is often very severe, has a burning quality, is unrelenting, is aggravated by elevation of the extremity, and might not be relieved by dependency. Late in the course of progressive TAO with severe ischemia, the patient might experience pain of ischemic neuropathy, which is severe and widespread in the extremity.

Diagnosis

The diagnosis of TAO is readily made on the history and physical examination, particularly from measurement of pulses in distal parts of the limbs. The posterior tibial or dorsalis pedis pulsations, or both, can be greatly diminished or absent. Special tests discussed in Chapter 28 can also be used to confirm the diagnosis.

Treatment

The cornerstone of therapy of TAO is complete and permanent avoidance of tobacco in any form (36, 37). Long-term anticoagulant therapies, adrenocortical steroids, vasodilating drugs, alcohol intake by mouth, and a variety of other agents have been tried with varying degrees of success. In the early stages of the disease, prescribing vasodilating drugs or alcohol by mouth can increase blood flow to the skin of the foot. Regional sympathetic block using a long-lasting local anesthetic should be used as a diagnostic procedure to determine the degree of reflex vasospasm associated with TIA and also to predict the effects of permanent interruption (28, 37). This and other therapy are discussed in detail on page 515.

Acute Arterial Occlusion

The medium-sized arteries of the lower limbs are the most frequently acutely occluded vessels. The three most important etiologic factors are thrombosis, embolism, and direct injury to the vessel (38). Another cause is the development of acute compartmental syndrome with consequent acute occlusion of the posterior tibial artery with compression of the nerve (see page 380 for details).

Symptoms and Signs

The degree of occlusion, the extent of collateral blood flow, the site of occlusion, and the duration of the ischemia all affect the severity and extent of symptoms and the outcome of therapy. With mild occlusion there are transient periods of dull ache localized to the site of occlusion. Severe obstruction of blood flow to an extremity is generally heralded by the well-recognized complex of the five Ps: pain, pallor, loss of pulses, paresthesia, and paralysis (37). In more than half of the patients the pain is generally rapid in onset, reaching peak severity in minutes to hours. Associated with the pain are pallor and loss of pulses; these signs are followed rapidly by loss of motor function and complete loss of all sensation. If the circulation is not restored within 6 to 8 hours of onset of paresthesia, the chance of salvage of the extremity is greatly diminished (38).

Treatment

Treatment is of course to restore normal blood flow. In the case of embolism, treatment consists of embolectomy, which in most cases can be done by using the Fogarty catheter, anticoagulant therapy, and concomitant sympathetic interruption to relieve reflex vasospasm (37, 38). Patients who develop arterial thrombosis usually can be treated by gently passing a Fogarty catheter from the proximal portion of the artery beyond the occluded segment so as to withdraw the obstructing thrombus. Patients who have laceration require surgical repair. If an epidural catheter can be inserted one-half hour before anticoagulant therapy is initiated, this should be done, and a long-acting local anesthetic should be injected to provide pain relief prior to surgery and anesthesia for the operation. If this is not possible, sympathetic interruption is carried out by regional intravenous sympathetic block using guanethidine.

Diseases of the Microcirculation

Although Raynaud's disease and Raynaud's phenomenon occur more frequently in the upper limb, they also affect the digits of the lower limb.

Raynaud's Disease

Raynaud's disease is characterized by symmetrical impairment of the circulation of the digits and phasic color changes, which often progress to ulceration of the fingertips and even gangrene. The larger arteries are not occluded. The criteria for establishing a diagnosis of this disease are given in Chapter 28, in which the pathophysiology is also discussed.

The characteristic sign of Raynaud's disease is that the fingers turn white on exposure to cold, then blue, and finally red during the rewarming process, the so-called triphasic color change (39). At first, only the tips of the digits are involved, but later the proximal parts of the toes are involved. In later stages of the disease, color changes can extend back to the rest of the foot. In advanced stages of Raynaud's disease the attacks become so severe and so frequent as to be disabling.

Therapy for Raynaud's disease depends on the severity of the signs and symptoms. In milder cases, certain general measures are sufficient; in moderate cases, vasodilators are usually beneficial. Surgical sympathectomy should be considered in patients with moderate or severe disease. Sympathetic interruption with a local anesthetic should be used to predict the effect of surgical sympathectomy (39).

Raynaud's Phenomenon

Raynaud's phenomenon by definition is secondary to other pathologic processes (p. 528). The condition occurs more frequently in the upper limb than in the lower limb, although it can involve this region. Therapy for this condition is directed toward eliminating its causes and mechanisms.

Cold Injuries

Exposure to cold temperatures can produce lesions that involve cells and extravascular fluid (direct effects) and that disrupt the integrity of peripheral circulation and the function of organized tissues (indirect effects) (40). The mildest form of cold injury is called frostnip and tends to occur in organs farthest away from the core of the body, such as the fingers, toes, hands, and feet. More severe cold injury can be divided into freezing injuries such as frostbite and nonfreezing injuries such as immersion foot and pernio.

Pernio or *chilblain* is the mildest form of the various disorders due to local cold injuries. *Immersion foot* and *trench foot* are similar entities observed during wartime in personnel whose feet have been wet but not freezing cold for a prolonged period of time. These conditions can be managed conservatively as discussed on page 522.

Frostbite of the feet occurs when limbs are exposed to freezing conditions. The pathophysiology involves two major mechanisms: (a) vasoconstriction with subsequent stasis and thrombus formation and (b) formation of ice crystals in the extracellular fluids (40, 41). Classically the condition is divided into four degrees; the 3rd and 4th degrees are the most serious and can cause loss of digits. The sequelae of moderate to severe frostbite include (a) persistent hypersensitivity to cold, (b) pain at rest and in phantom limb if spontaneous amputation has occurred, (c) hypesthesia and subjective numbness alone or in combination with hyperesthesia and allodynia, (d) hyperhidrosis and decrease in hair, (e) persistent skin changes, and (f) such signs of reflex sympathetic dystrophy as osteoporosis and rigid nails (see Chapter 11). The symptoms are generally worse in the winter and after exposure to cold.

Most instances of frostbite can be prevented by adequate prophylactic measures. When it occurs it should be considered a vascular emergency. The therapy for this condition is discussed in detail on page 524.

Other Disorders of the Microcirculation

Acrocyanosis

Acrocyanosis is a vasospastic disorder manifested by persistent coldness, intense cyanosis, and frequently edema and hyperhidrosis. Symptoms are most marked during the winter. Although it is frequently confused with Raynaud's disease, the symptoms are sufficiently different to make it a separate entity (42).

Treatment is conservative in mild conditions. The patient should be informed about the benign nature of the disease, instructed to avoid exposure to cold, and advised to move to a warm climate. If patients are extremely disabled, a trial of vasodilators can be given. Regional sympathetic denervation achieved with long-acting local anesthetic or intravenous guanethidine can be tried.

Livedo Reticularis

Livedo reticularis (LR) is characterized by a local and prominent mottling and blotchy or reticular ("fishnet") reddish-blue discoloration of the skin of the extremities (42). The cause of the condition is unknown, although there is unquestionably some inherent vasomotor instability in these patients, most of whom are women.

Treatment is usually conservative. When patients are distressed by the cosmetic effects, a trial of vasodilators should be carried out. If ulceration is present and cannot be managed by conservative measures, sympathetic denervation should be considered.

Erythromelalgia

Erythromelalgia is almost the exact antithesis of Raynaud's disease and acrocyanosis. It is characterized by redness and burning pain in the extremities due to abnormal vasodilation. Spittel (42) reported that as little as 650 mg of aspirin produces striking and persistent relief for as long as several days. Others use methysergide, a serotonin-blocking agent, with the claim that it provides dramatic relief of primary erythromelalgia (see 42 for references).

Diseases of the Peripheral Veins

Thrombophlebitis

Thrombophlebitis consists of partial or complete occlusion of a vein by thrombus, associated with inflammatory changes in the vein and adjacent structures. The inflammatory reaction promotes adherence of the thrombus to the venous walls, so migration of the thrombus occurs infrequently (32).

The symptoms and signs of superficial thrombophlebitis include pain and exquisite tenderness along the region of the involved vein, perivenous erythema and edema, and, in many instances, edema involving the lower part of the limb. Patients with deep thrombophlebitis manifest moderate to severe calf pain, exquisite tenderness, Homan's sign (calf pain on dorsiflexion of the foot), dilated superficial veins, and diffuse edema and pallor of the involved extremity.

The therapy for thrombophlebitis is largely supportive, with application of heat, elevation of the foot, anti-inflammatory drugs such as indomethacin, antibiotics, and heparin (32). The pain is controlled with aspirin or other types of nonsteroidal anti-inflammatory agents; if these prove ineffective, potent opioids are given by mouth.

Acute Deep Venous Thrombosis

Deep venous thrombosis is one of the most frequent of painful disorders. Together with its sequelae, it is associated with significant morbidity and mortality, often prolonged hospitalization, decreased productivity, and lifelong disability that not only decreases the quality of life of millions of Americans but costs the nation in excess of a billion dollars annually (43).

The usual signs and symptoms of deep venous thrombosis of the lower extremity include pain and exquisite tenderness of the calf, increased tissue turgor (or resistance, particularly in the calf), edema, and increased skin temperature of the affected limb (due to diversion of blood to superficial veins).

The goals of therapy are to (a) abort ongoing thrombotic process, (b) restore venous patency, (c) prevent pulmonary embolism, and (d) minimize the sequelae of peripheral venous hypertension (32, 43). All patients should be hospitalized and placed at bed rest with elevation of the involved extremity above the level of the right atrium. Pain should be controlled with systemic analgesics in the form of anti-inflammatory agents, but patients who experience severe pain should be given opioids, preferably by mouth, at fixed intervals.

D. REFERRED PAIN

Pain in the thigh, leg, and foot can be referred from the low back, abdomen, and pelvis. Various abdominal conditions that can cause referred pain to the thigh and knee are discussed in Section E of Part II.

Referred pain from pelvic disorders is discussed in various chapters in Section E of Part IV, and pain caused by disorders of the low back is considered in Chapter 71.

E. PAIN OF PSYCHOLOGIC ORIGIN

In addition to pain due to increased muscle tension caused by emotional stress and other psychologic problems, pain in the lower limb can be caused by psychiatric disorders, which are classified as delusional or hallucinatory and hysterical or hypochondriac. Merskey discusses these psychiatric disorders in detail in Chapter 19; he believes that they are rarely a cause of regional pain.

REFERENCES

1. Kraus, H.: Diagnosis and treatment of muscle pain. Chicago, Quintessence Publishing, 1988, pp. 11–50.
2. Kraus, H.: Therapeutic Exercise. Springfield, IL, Charles C Thomas, 1949, pp. 33–34.
3. Kraus, H., Mahoney, J., and Weber, S.: Immediate mobilization of certain ligamentous injuries of the knee. Gen. Pract., 24:126, 1961.
4. Gunn, C.C.: Neuropathic pain—a new theory for chronic pain of intrinsic origin. Ann. R. Coll. Phys. Surg. Canada, 22:327, 1989.
5. Korcok, M.: Motion, not immobility, advocated for healing synovial joints. JAMA, 246:2005, 1981.
6. Travell, J., and Simons, D.: Myofascial Pain and Dysfunction: The Triggerpoint Manual. Baltimore, Williams & Wilkins, 1983.
7. Woolf, C.J., and Wall, P.D.: A dissociation between the analgesic and antinociceptive effects of morphine. Neurosci. Lett., 64:238, 1986.
8. Wall, P.D., and Woolf, C.J.: Muscle but not cutaneous C-afferent input produces prolonged increases in the excitability of the flexion reflex in the rat. J. Physiol. (Lond.), 356:443, 1984.
9. Woolf, C.J., and Wall, P.D.: The brief and the prolonged facilitatory effects of unmyelinated afferent input on the rat spinal cord are independently influenced by peripheral nerve injury. Neuroscience, 17:1199, 1986.
10. Simons, D.G., and Travell, J.G.: Myofascial origins of low back pain. 3. Pelvic and lower extremity muscles. Postgrad. Med., 73:99, 1983.
11. Sola, A.E.: Treatment of myofascial pain syndromes. In Recent Advances in Pain Research and Therapy. Vol. 7. Edited by C. Benedetti et al. New York, Raven Press, 1984, pp. 467–485.
12. Sola, A.E.: Trigger point therapy. In Clinical Procedures in Emergency Medicine. Edited by J.R. Roberts and J.R. Hedges. Philadelphia, W.B. Saunders, 1985, pp. 674–686.
13. Bonica, J.J.: Management of myofascial pain syndromes in general practice. JAMA, 164:732, 1957.
14. Bengtsson, A., and Bengtsson, M.: Regional sympathetic blockade in primary fibromyalgia. Pain, 33:161, 1988.
15. McCain, G.A., and Scudds, R.A.: The concept of primary fibromyalgia (fibrositis): Clinical value relation and significance to other chronic musculoskeletal pain syndromes. Pain, 33:273, 1988.
16. deTakats, G.: Causalgic states in peace and war. JAMA, 128:699, 1945.
17. Loh, L., Nathan, P.W., and Schott, G.D.: Pain due to lesions of the central nervous system removed by sympathetic block. Br. Med. J., 282:1026, 1981.
18. Nathan, P.W.: Involvement of the sympathetic nervous system. In Pain and Society. Edited by H.W. Kosterlitz and L.Y. Terenius. Weinheim, Verlag Chemie, 1980, pp. 311–324.
19. Spillane, J.D., et al.: Painful legs and moving toes. Brain, 94:541, 1971.
20. Nathan, P.W.: Painful legs and moving toes: Evidence on the site of the lesion. J. Neurol. Neurosurg. Psychiatry, 41:934, 1978.
21. Montagna, P., et al.: Painful legs and moving toes: Associated with polyneuropathy. J. Neurol. Neurosurg. Psychiatry, 46:399, 1983.
22. Bach, S., Noreng, M.F., and Tjellden, N.U.: Phantom limb pain in amputees during the first 12 months following limb amputation, after preoperative lumbar epidural blockade. Pain, 33:297, 1988.
23. Wall, P.D.: Editorial: The prevention of postoperative pain. Pain, 33:289, 1988.
24. Woolf, C.J.: Evidence for a central component of post-injury pain hypersensitivity. Nature, 306:686, 1983.
25. Wall, P.D., et al: Slow changes in the flexion reflex following arthritis of tenotomy. Brain Res., 1988, 447:215, 1988.
26. Cook, A.J., et al.: Expansion of cutaneous receptive fields of dorsal horn neurones following C-primary afferent fibre inputs. Nature, 325:151, 1987.
27. Sugimoto, T., et al.: Rapid transneuronal destruction following peripheral nerve transection. Pain, 30:385, 1987.
28. deWolfe, V.G.: Chronic occlusive arterial disease of the lower extremities. In Clinical Vascular Disease. Edited by J.A. Spittell, Jr. Philadelphia, F.A. Davis, 1983, pp. 15–35.
29. Bierman, E.L.: Atherosclerosis and other forms of arteriosclerosis. In Harrison's Principles of Internal Medicine. Edited by R.G. Petersdorf. New York, McGraw-Hill, 1983, pp. 1465–1474.
30. Coffman, J.D.: Principles of conservative treatment of occlusive arterial disease. In Clinical Vascular Disease. Edited by J.A. Spittell, Jr., Philadelphia, F.A. Davis, 1983.
31. Arcangeli, P., et al.: Mechanisms of ischemic pain in peripheral occlusive arterial disease. In Advances in Pain Research and Therapy. Vol. 1. Edited by J.J. Bonica and D. Albe-Fessard. New York, Raven Press, 1976, pp. 965–973.
32. Strandness, D.E.: Vascular disease of the extremities. In Harrison's Textbook of Medicine, 10th Ed. Edited by R.G. Petersdorf et al. New York, McGraw-Hill, 1983, pp. 1491–1498.
33. Buerger, L.: Thromboangiitis obliterans: A study of the vascular lesions leading to presenile spontaneous gangrene. Am. J. Med. Sci., 136:567, 1908.
34. Strandness, D.E., Jr.: Thromboangiitis obliterans: Fact or fiction. In Peripheral Arterial Disease: A Physiologic Approach. Edited by D.E. Strandness, Jr. Boston, Little, Brown, 1969, pp. 253–264.
35. McKusick, D.A., et al.: Buerger's disease: A distinct clinical and pathologic entity. JAMA, 181:5, 1962.
36. Juergens, J.L.: Thromboangiitis obliterans. In Peripheral Vascular Disease. Edited by J.L. Juergens, J.A. Spittell, Jr., and J.F. Fairbairn II. Philadelphia, F.A. Davis, 1983, pp. 469–491.
37. Perry, M.O.: Management of acute arterial insufficiency. In Vascular Surgery. 2nd Ed. Edited by R.B. Ruthford. Philadelphia, W.B. Saunders, 1984, pp. 440–448.
38. Hollier, L.H.: Acute arterial occlusion. In Clinical Vascular Disease. Edited by J.A. Spittell, Jr. Philadelphia, F.A. Davis, 1983, pp. 49–57.
39. Spittell, J.A., Jr.: Raynaud's phenomenon and allied vasospastic disorders. In Peripheral Vascular Disease. 5th Ed. Edited by J.L. Juergens, J.A. Spittell, Jr., and J.F. Fairbairn. Philadelphia, W.B. Saunders, 1980, pp. 555–583.
40. Petersdorf, R.G.: Disturbances of heat regulations. In Harrison's Textbook of Medicine. 10th Ed. Edited by R.G. Petersdorf et al. New York, McGraw-Hill, 1983, pp. 50–56.
41. Gage, A.M., and Gage, A.A.: Frostbite: Trauma and emergency medicine. Comp. Ther., 7:25, 1981.
42. Spittell, J.A., Jr.: Vasospastic disorders. In Clinical Vascular Disease. Edited by J.A. Spittell, Jr. Philadelphia, F.A. Davis, 1983, pp. 75–86.
43. Silver, D., and Stubbs, D.H.: Venous thrombosis, pulmonary embolism, and the post-phlebitic syndrome. In Diagnosis and Management of Peripheral Vascular Disease. Edited by D.C. Miller and A.J. Roon. Menlo Park, CA, Addison-Wesley, 1982, pp. 270–290.

Methods, Procedures, and Techniques for the Symptomatic Control of Pain

INTRODUCTION
JOHN J. BONICA

This last part of the book is composed of seven sections, each of which has chapters that describe specific therapeutic modalities for the symptomatic control of acute and chronic pain. The word symptomatic is intended to convey the fact that most of these therapies are not intended to eliminate the cause of the pain but rather to reduce or eliminate the pain itself. Methods to eliminate the cause of the pain (when this is possible) are discussed in various chapters of Part IV dealing with various diseases associated with acute or chronic pain. The therapeutic modalities are presented in descending order of frequency and practicability of use by all health professionals and also whether or not they are invasive or noninvasive. Thus, sections A and B discuss procedures that are noninvasive, section E and F discuss invasive techniques, and sections C, D, and G contain both noninvasive and invasive procedures.

Section A presents a chapter on the nonopioid and opioid analgesics, one on psychotropic drugs, and one on the critically important role of nurses in managing patients with pain. Section B contains six chapters in what I arbitrarily call "psychologic and psychosocial" techniques, including contingency management, cognitive-behavioral therapy, biofeedback, hypnosis, relaxation, and psychotherapy. Section C contains discussions of physical and surgical therapy including operative and nonoperative orthopedic procedures; physical therapy and rehabilitation medicine; radiation therapy, chemotherapy, hormone therapy, and surgery for cancer pain; and a chapter on acupuncture and one on nutritional therapy. Section D describes methods of neuroaugmentative techniques involving electrical stimulation of the skin (TENS), nerves, spinal cord, and brain. Section E contains three chapters describing regional analgesia with local anesthetics, regional analgesia with intraspinal narcotics, and regional analgesia with neurolytic agents intended to prolong the interruption of nociceptive pathways. Section F has three chapters on ablative neurosurgical procedures. and section G discusses the multidisciplinary, multimodal approach to complex chronic pain problems.

Each section is preceded by a brief historical perspective of the methods, and in some sections, guidelines for their use. Each chapter follows a somewhat uniform format. It begins with an introduction that assesses the current status of the therapy in managing pain, the contents of the chapter, and a list of references to books or review articles. This is followed by a subsection on "basic considerations," which includes the pharmacologic, physiologic, psychologic, anatomic, or physical bases for the use of the procedures and their indications. For example, Chapter 78 discusses the chemistry and clinical pharmacology—including the pharmacokinetics and pharmacodynamics—of various nonopioid and opioid systemic analgesics. Chapters in section B provide the psychologic and psychosocial basis of the various therapies. In each chapter, this subsection is followed by a description of the technique and the results obtained as well as the side effects and complications that can occur, and their incidence and treatment.

Description of the technique of application varies according to the procedure. Some simple techniques and procedures that can be done by family physicians or specialists, such as drug regimens or simple regional blocks, TENS, certain physical therapies, and certain psychologic techniques, are described in sufficient detail to permit either the generalist or the specialist to learn how to do them and apply them. Descriptions of complicated regional analgesia procedures and neurosurgical operations are brief; in the case of regional analgesia it usually comprises an illustration and legend. These descriptions are not intended to be used as the sole basis for learning and applying these techniques, because the acquisition of proficiency in any of these procedures requires apprenticeship under the supervision of an experienced anesthesiologist or neurosurgeon who can teach the basic aspects of the technique and then supervise the student in carrying out the procedure so as to gain experience and skill. Rather, the primary objective of presenting these complex techniques is to provide readers who do *not* practice them with some idea of what the procedures entail as well as a discussion of their indications, advantages, disadvantages, and complications. This is in accordance of with my long-held conviction that anyone managing patients with pain should be acquainted with all currently available therapeutic procedures. Only with such knowledge and a broad perspective can the physician inform and guide the patient as to what therapy (or combination of therapies) is suitable for each particular pain problem.

Finally, in discussing results obtained with each of the procedures, there is some duplication with data presented in various chapters contained in Parts II and IV of the book. However, the data on results and complications presented in sections D, E, and F of this part of the book are more comprehensive and include not only those obtained by the author(s), but a summary of those data contained in important published reports. As indicated in the preface, it is hoped that this section provides the reader with a comprehensive overview of the various therapeutic modalities available to treat patients with various types of pain.

INTRODUCTION

CONSTANTINO BENEDETTI and STEPHEN H. BUTLER

Over the course of human history pain has been treated by psychologic techniques, physical methods (e.g., surgical intervention, electrical stimulation, pressure, cold, heat, counterirritation, acupuncture), and by drugs, especially analgesics. The physical methods presently used for the treatment of pain are described elsewhere in this book. In the first chapter of this section the use of medications for the relief of pain is discussed. The analgesics that were mostly used in the past (the derivatives of which are still being used) are the extracts of opium and of willow bark, wintergreen leaves, and Spiraea (1, 2). Chapter 79 describes the use of psychotropic drugs, and the last chapter of this section discusses the role that nurses have in pain management.

HISTORICAL PERSPECTIVES

Opioids

Extracts of Papaver somniferum, the oriental poppy, have been used over centuries by many cultures for their analgesic and other properties. This was known 5000 years ago, when the Sumerians mentioned the extracts obtained from *Hu gil*, the plant of joy, in an ancient pharmacopeia. The Greek Theophrastus, in the third century B.C., called the juice of the poppy plant *opus*, from which we derived the name "opium." Greek and Roman physicians used opium-containing preparations to treat arthritic pain, chest pain, and cough and to induce sedation. The ancient Hebrews employed opium in potions for analgesia and sleep during surgery and for condemned criminals to alleviate the pain of death. Arabian physicians were familiar with the medicinal properties of the oriental poppy, and Arab traders introduced it to the Orient. Opium was used extensively to treat the symptoms of dysentery in epidemics in Europe and the Middle East prior to 1000 A.D. It was described, united with other plant extracts, for surgical analgesia in the medical school of Salerno in the ninth century A.D. and of Bologna in the thirteenth century A.D. (3). Toxicity problems caused by this potent mixture, a familiar spector, restricted its use to a few centers of learning and led to unpopularity in Europe, but it was reintroduced, in a much less potent and more controlled solution, by Paracelsus in the sixteenth century.

A young German pharmacist, Friedrich A.W. Sertürner, extracted an alkaloid from opium in 1803 that he called *morphium*, from the Greek god of dreams. This was then abbreviated to "morphia" and "morphine." We now know that over 25 alkaloids can be extracted from the juice of Papaver somniferum (4, 5). The most important are morphine (4 to 21%), codeine (0.8 to 2.5%), papaverine (0.5 to 2.5%), and thebaine (0.5 to 2%) (6). The isolation of the pure alkaloids introduced the era of scientific pharmacology that used the active ingredients produced by the poppy. The understanding of the mode of action of opioids has been gradually evolving, but great advances were made only during the last 35 years (7). An interaction of opioids with specific receptors was hypothesized in the 1960s (8), but it was not until opiate receptors were first demonstrated in the nervous system (9–11) and endogenous opioids were discovered (12–17) that important advances were made in the understanding of the complex modes of action of this group of drugs. Despite these advances we still cannot clearly understand the intrinsic mechanism of action of either endogenous or exogenous opioids (18–19).

Nonsteroidal Agents

Extracts of willow bark, wintergreen leaves, and Spiraea have been used for medicinal purposes by many cultures over centuries. Willow bark extract was first noted in the medical literature for the treatment of fever or "ague" by Edmund Stone in England in the nineteenth century. Isolation of "salicin" from willow bark occurred in the early 1800s, a compound that yielded salicylic acid. Salicylic acid was also produced from the other plants mentioned above. Initially only its antipyretic effects were appreciated but, by the end of the nineteenth century, its analgesic, anti-inflammatory, and uricosuric properties were also identified.

At this time other compounds from the para-aminophenol family, such as phenacetin, were found to have antipyretic and analgesic effects. A veritable explosion of compounds with analgesic, antipyretic, anti-inflammatory, and uricosuric effects has occurred, increasing the number of nonsteroidal anti-inflammatory drugs (NSAIDs) available. They are similar in their ability to treat pain, inflammation, fever, and gout, and are used more frequently than any other group of pharmacologic compounds (20).

Psychotropic Agents

Mind- and consciousness-altering drugs have been a part of human life since earliest times, as evidenced by the use of drugs such as alcohol in the form of beer from cereal, wine from fruits and berries, and mead from honey (21). Rauwolfia serpentina extracts were reported in Indian medical literature describing sedating and hypotensive properties with a long history of use (21). Although phenothiazines (active derivatives of Rauwolfia) were independently synthesized as part of the development of aniline dyes in the 1800s, their medicinal use was not explored until the 1940s (22). As outlined by Monks (Chapter 79), chlorpromazine was introduced in 1955 and its analgesic and analgesic-potentiating properties were discovered later.

The tricyclic antidepressants were derived from a random production of compounds synthesized from iminodibenzyl in the 1940s. This process was an effort by Hafliger and associates to discover novel phenothiazine-like agents. Imiprimine was felt to be a promising sedative in animal studies, and subsequent human experiments in mental patients by Kuhn serendipitously indicated antidepressant activities (23). Again, as indicated by Monks (Chapter 79), it took until the 1950s for possible analgesic properties to be reported (24, 25).

The lithium salts have been in use for a variety of medical problems such as gout, for sedation, and as anticonvulsants. Fortuitous animal use led to their testing in mania in the late 1940s, but it was not until the 1970s that lithium was used in cluster headache (26, 27).

The Human Factor

As previously mentioned, pain management embodies not only the use of medications but also psychological and different physical methods. Therefore the human factor has always been an essential aspect of pain management. In prehistoric time, the medicine man, the shaman, and the elderly women of the tribe were often the healers of primitive society. In Western civilization, the vestals during the Roman empire and afterward the men and women belonging to various religious denominations dedicated their time to the care of the ill. The development of the nursing profession during the last century brought order to this vocation. Of the members of the modern health care team, nurses spend the most time with patients. Nurses

therefore can have an enormous impact on the management of pain patients. Considering the significant role that anxiety has on the overall pain experience, the ability of a nurse to achieve rapport with the patient is extremely important (Chapter 80).

Properly trained nurses are the major resources for the various methods used to alleviate pain. Massage, application of heat or cold, and the use of transcutaneous nerve stimulation all contribute to improve the comfort of the suffering patient.

In the past, because of limited knowledge of algology and pharmacology, nurses have been responsible, like most health care personnel, for improperly treating pain patients (28). Nurses' education must therefore evolve, and deeply established misconceptions must be reversed. They must learn the clear distinction that exists between acute pain, cancer pain, and chronic pain from either obvious or elusive organic causes. The pharmacology of analgesics should be an important part of the nursing curriculum. Recent scientific information should be used to resolve the exaggerated fear of respiratory depression and psychologic dependence caused by opioids, which is responsible for the widespread underuse of these medications and therefore for the continued suffering of patients in pain (29).

The role of nurses in the field of algology is rapidly evolving. Until recently their major efforts were restricted to the hospital setting, but now nurses are assuming an ever-expanding role in the treatment of patients in pain clinics, hospices, extended care facilities, and homecare settings. They are also serving as consultants in both acute and chronic pain. In hospitals where acute pain services have been established a nurse consultant can be of great assistance in training other nurses who take care of patients on a daily basis.

REFERENCES

1. Haas, H.: History of antipyretic analgesic therapy (symposium). Am. J. Med., 75(5A):1, 1983.
2. Tainter, M.L., and Ferris, A.J.: History. In Aspirin in Modern Therapy. New York, Bayer, 1969, pp. 1–3.
3. Benedetti, C.: Intraspinal analgesia: An historical overview. Acta Anaesthesiol. Scand. [Suppl. 85], 31:17, 1987.
4. Fulop-Miller, R.: Triumph Over Pain. New York, Literary Guild of America, 1938.
5. Jaffe, J.H., and Martin, W.R.: Opioid analgesics and antagonists. In The Pharmacological Basis of Therapeutics. Edited by L.S. Goodman, et al. New York, Macmillan, 1985, pp. 491–531.
6. Lewis, W.H., and Elvin-Lewis, M.P.F. (Eds): Medical Botany: Plants Affecting Man's Health. New York, John Wiley & Sons, 1977.
7. Way, L.E.: Review and overview of four decades of opiate research. In Neurochemical Mechanisms of Opiates and Endorphins. Advances in Biochemistry and Psychopharmacology. Edited by H.H. Loh and D.H. Ross. Vol. 20. New York, Raven Press, 1979, pp. 3–27.
8. Portoghese, P.S.: A new concept on the mode of interaction of narcotic analgesics with receptors. J. Med. Chem., 8:60, 1965.
9. Goldstein, A., Lowney, L.I., and Pal, P.K.: Stereospecific and nonspecific interactions of the morphine congener levorphanol in subcellular fractions of interactions of the mouse brain. Proc. Natl. Acad. Sci. U.S.A., 68:1742, 1971.
10. Pert, C., and Snyder, S.: Opiate receptor: Demonstration in nervous tissue. Science, 179:1011, 1973.

11. Kuhar, M.H., Pert, C.B., and Snyder, S.H.: Regional distribution of opiate receptor binding in monkey and human brain. Nature, 245:447, 1973.
12. Terenius, L., and Wahlström, A.: Search for an endogenous ligand for opiate receptor. Acta Physiol. Scand., 94:74, 1975.
13. Hughes, J.: Isolation of an endogenous compound from the brain with pharmacological properties similar to morphine. Brain Res., 88:295, 1975.
14. Pasternak, G.W., and Snyder, S.H.: Identification of novel high affinity opiate receptor binding in rat brain. Nature, 253:563, 1975.
15. Hughes, J., et al.: Purification and properties of enkephalin, the possible endogenous ligand for the morphine receptor. Life Sci., 16:1753, 1975.
16. Hughes, J., et al.: Identification of two related pentapeptides from the brain with potent opiate agonist activity. Nature, 258:577, 1975.
17. Benedetti, C.: Neuroanatomy and biochemistry of antinociception. In Advances in Pain Research and Therapy. Vol 2. Edited by J.J. Bonica and V. Ventafridda. New York, Raven Press, 1979, pp. 31–44.
18. Kosterlitz, H.W.: Opioid peptides and their receptors. The Wellcome Foundation Lecture, 1982. Proc. R. Soc. Lond. [Biol.], 255:27, 1985.
19. Kosterlitz, H.W., and Paterson, S.J.: Opioid receptors and mechanisms of opioid analgesia. In Advances in Pain Research and Therapy, Vol. 14. Edited by C. Benedetti, C.R. Chapman and G. Giron. New York, Raven Press, 1989, pp. 37–43.
20. Flower, R.J., Moncada, S., and Vane, J.R.: Analgesic-antipyretics and anti-inflammatory agents: Drugs employed

in the treatment of gout. *In* The Pharmacological Basis of Therapeutics. Edited by L.S. Goodman, et al. New York, Macmillan, 1985, pp. 682–713.

21. Lewis, W.H., and Elvin-Lewis, M.P.F. (Eds.): Depressants. *In* Medical Botany: Plants Affecting Man's Health. New York, John Wiley & Sons, 1977, pp. 432–448.

22. Siddiqui, S., and Siddiqui, R.H.: Chemical examination of the roots of *Rauwolfia serpentina* Benth. J. Ind. Chem. Soc., *8*:667, 1932.

23. Kuhn, R.: The treatment of depressant states with 622355 (imipramine hydrochloride). Am. J. Psychiatry, *115*:459, 464, 1958.

24. Saunders, C.: The treatment of intractable pain in terminal cancer. Proc. R. Soc. Med., *56*:195, 1963.

25. Lee, R., and Spencer, P.S.J.: Antidepressants and pain: A review of the pharmacological data supporting the use of certain tricyclics in chronic pain. J. Int. Med. Res., *5*:146, 1977.

26. Kudrow, L.: Lithium prophylaxis for chronic cluster headache. Headache, *17*:15, 1977.

27. Mathew, N.T.: Clinical subtypes of cluster headache and response to lithium therapy. Headache, *18*:26, 1978.

28. Marks, R.M., and Sachar, E.F.: Undertreatment of medical inpatients with narcotic analgesics. Ann. Intern. Med., *78*:173, 1973.

29. Porter, J., and Jick, H.: Addiction rare in patients treated with narcotics. N. Engl. J. Med., *302*:123, 1980.

78 · SYSTEMIC ANALGESICS

Costantino Benedetti and Stephen H. Butler

THIS chapter discusses the pharmacology and clinical application of systemic analgesics, which include opioid (narcotic) drugs, nonopioid (non-narcotic) analgesics, and a heterogeneous group of agents used for pain control. For many decades, these drugs, given alone or as part of a multimodal program, have constituted the most frequently used method of pain control. The reason for their popularity and widespread use is that in most countries of the world they are readily available and inexpensive, and, when properly administered, provide effective pain relief (1–8). Recently great advances have been made in our knowledge of pain and its mechanisms and in the pharmacokinetics, pharmacodynamics, and general pharmacology of systemic analgesics, accompanied by a marked improvement in delivery systems.

Despite these advantages and recent advances, which permit the selection of the optimal drug, dose, and route for providing pain relief, this is often not done. Bonica indicates in Chapters 1, 24, and 25 that formerly, and even today, most patients with acute pain, cancer pain, and chronic nonmalignant pain are not adequately relieved. This situation exists because students of medicine, nursing, dentistry, and other health professions are not given adequate information about the clinical pharmacology of these drugs. Consequently, many practitioners underestimate the dosage range and overestimate the duration of action of systemic analgesics and have irrational fears of producing addiction (psychologic dependence), physical dependence, and respiratory depression.

This chapter intends to help rectify these deficiencies. We present an overview of the pharmacology and clinical application of systemic analgesics in four major sections: A, Basic Considerations, which includes a review of the general principles of pharmacokinetics and pharmacodynamics; B, Opioid Analgesics; C, Nonopioid (Non-Narcotic) Analgesics, all but one of which are nonsteroidal anti-inflammatory drugs (NSAIDs); and D, General Principles of Application of Analgesics. More detailed information is presented elsewhere (8–20).

A. BASIC CONSIDERATIONS

General Pharmacologic Principles

Pharmacology refers to all available information about a drug, including its history, source, production, and physical and chemical properties (as a chemical or compound), in addition to information related to its interaction with the recipient organism, usually humans, in regard to absorption, distribution, biotransformation, excretion, biochemical and biological effects, mechanism of action, and therapeutic effects and uses. *Pharmacokinetics* is the study of the uptake or absorption, distribution, biotransformation, and excretion of pharmacologic agents. *Pharmacodynamics* is the study of the biochemical effects of drugs and their mechanisms of action.

Pharmacokinetics

Absorption

Absorption depends primarily on the physical characteristics of the drug and on the physicochemical properties of the membranes it must cross. Molecular size and shape, solubility, ionization constant, and relative lipid solubility of a drug's ionized and unionized forms are important factors affecting absorption.

DRUG SOLUBILITY. Drug solubility, specifically in water for most drugs given orally, must be considered.

CONCENTRATION. The concentration of the form administered, especially injectables, is an important factor. A high concentration of drug in a small volume of solute leads to faster absorption, and a low concentration of drug in a large volume leads to slow absorption. Rates of absorption can therefore be controlled to some extent by changing concentration, as indicated for the drug and clinical situation.

AREA AND PERFUSION OF ABSORPTION SITE. Modification of the area and perfusion of the absorption site can influence drug levels at the site of action, and thus are relevant factors (e.g., intracutaneous versus subcutaneous versus intramuscular depot).

ROUTE OF ADMINISTRATION. The route of administration of a drug is important for ease of administration and desired therapeutic effect, among other considerations. *Oral administration* is the most common route and suffices in patients who can take oral preparations and do not need immediate analgesia. *Subcutaneous administration* obviates the need for normal gastrointestinal function and is somewhat faster for some analgesics; this route has variable uptake times, however, depending on the exact placement of the needle and on patients' adiposity. The *intramuscular route* is less variable for most compounds but absorption is not rapid. The *intravenous route* is most efficient for an immediate effect with bolus administration and also helps to maintain a steady state by continuous infusion. Unfortunately, use of this route is limited to situations in which patients can be closely observed, and is usually not appropriate except over the short term for hospitalized patients. The *rectal route* is appropriate for all medications absorbed well by the gut and, indeed, most oral medications come in suppository form. It can often be used when gastrointestinal upset or the need to avoid oral intake precludes the use of the oral route. *Sublingual administration* is possible only with selected drugs that pass the mucosal barrier quickly. This route is preferable for patients with gastrointestinal upset to avoid injection, which usually necessitates the presence of health care personnel.

Distribution

After drugs are absorbed or injected into the circulation they are distributed throughout various areas of the body, including the compartment of their site of action. Activity is based on the concentration of the drug at the site of action and is influenced by distribution effects to various body compartments. Distribution occurs in two separate phases: an early phase through the bloodstream to highly perfused organs such as the heart, liver, kidney, and brain, which is related directly to cardiac output and regional flow; and a second phase of slow diffusion into less well-perfused areas, such as the viscera, skin, muscle, fat, and bone. For some drugs pharmacokinetic data allow this slow phase to be split further, and various artificial volumes of distribution have been defined (20).

Obviously, blood flow to various organs is important in defining distribution, especially in terms of effect. A highly diffusible drug such as sodium thiopental (Pentothal), which acts on the brain, a highly perfused organ, has a rapid effect, whereas a drug such as amphotericin given systemically to treat a cutaneous fungal infection has a slow effect.

The distribution of drugs is influenced by their binding to plasma protein. Highly bound drugs have a low volume of distribution and have little access to cellular sites of action. The metabolism and excretion of drugs, either directly or in metabolized forms, are also limited by high plasma protein binding.

Lipid solubility has various effects on distribution. Lipid-insoluble drugs do not cross tissue barriers readily and have a small volume of distribution but, more importantly, have limited access to sites of action. Highly lipid-soluble drugs diffuse rapidly to potential sites of action but also accumulate in body fat and thus are slowly excreted.

The volume of distribution is referred to frequently in discussions of drug pharmacokinetics. It reflects the extent to which a drug is distributed within the body at a given time. It can be defined as the amount of drug in the body divided by the plasma concentration. The volume of distribution might be greater than the volume of body fluids for some drugs at steady state but, for others (e.g., those that are highly plasma protein bound), it can be close to the plasma volume.

Biotransformation

Biotransformation refers to the structural change of a drug through enzymatic transformation in various organs of the body. This activity occurs primarily in the liver and to a lesser extent in the kidney and other organs for some compounds. It is principally a metabolic activity that facilitates elimination. In a few

specific cases, however, it transforms an inactive compound, or pro-drug, into an active form (e.g., Sulindac to its active sulfate form) (Table 78-8).

LIVER. The primary site of biotransformation of drugs is the liver. The processes involve nonsynthetic reactions (e.g., oxidation, reduction, hydrolysis) and synthetic reactions (e.g., conjugation) primarily caused by activity of microsomal enzyme systems. These have various rates of activity depending on genetic factors and on the influence of other compounds or chemicals, which can cause systems to produce faster rates of metabolism.

Glucuronide synthesis is the main conjugation reaction in the detoxification process. The glucuronide compounds are generally inactive and are easily excreted. Other conjugation reactions produce acetylated compounds, glycines, and sulfates, but to a lesser extent. Again, these compounds are inactive and are readily excreted, primarily in the urine but also in the feces through the biliary system.

Hydrolysis is the process for deactivation of esters and amides (e.g., local anesthetics). Reduction detoxification has two pathways, one for azo compounds $(RN=NR')$ and another for nitro compounds (RNO_2).

Oxidative reactions are more varied and include dealkylation, aliphatic and aromatic hydroxylation, N-oxidation, N-hydroxylation, sulfoxide formation, deamination, and desulfuration.

Other Sites: Biotransformation reactions occur in sites other than the liver, although to a much lesser extent. These include the kidneys, lungs, gastrointestinal tract, and plasma.

Elimination

The usual deactivation processes also facilitate drug excretion. Many drugs are excreted unchanged (e.g., some inhalation anesthetics). Elimination is primarily through renal excretion by glomerular filtration and active tubular secretion. Many drug metabolites formed in the liver are added to bile and excreted by the gastrointestinal tract, although usually these metabolites are found in the bloodstream and urine. Minor sites of elimination include sweat, tears, and saliva.

Pharmacodynamics

Mechanisms of Drug Action

RECEPTOR BINDING. Cell proteins (e.g., enzymes, receptors, and proteins involved in transport processes) are the primary sites of drug action. Receptor-drug interaction is currently of most interest. This is important for the opioids but not for the nonopioid analgesics, which appear to interact mainly with enzymes. Obviously, the structure of a specific drug is the most important indicator of activity. Changes in molecular structure can increase potency but these same changes tend to increase toxicity. Specific molecular changes are increasingly allowing for sophisticated structural alterations to match desired functional effects.

NONCELLULAR ACTIONS. Some drugs interact with ions to produce an effect (e.g., antacids). Others are

TABLE 78-1. Major Routes of Drug Metabolism

Type	Equation	Examples of Drug

FUNCTIONALIZATION REACTIONS

Oxidation

Aliphatic hydroxylation

$R \cdot OCH_2R' \longrightarrow R \cdot CHOH \cdot R'$
(alcohol)

Thiopentone, methohexitone, pentazocine, pethidine, glutethimide, doxapram

Aromatic hydroxylation

$R \cdot C_6H_5 \longrightarrow R \cdot C_6H_4 \cdot OH$
(phenol)

Chlorpromazine, lignocaine, bupivacaine, mepivacaine, pethidine, phenobarbitone, glutethimide

O-Dealkylation

$R \cdot O \cdot CH_2R' \longrightarrow [R \cdot O \cdot CHOH \cdot R'] \longrightarrow R \cdot OH + R' \cdot CHO$
(ether)   (alcohol)   (aldehyde)

Phenacetin, codeine, methoxyflurane, fluroxene

N-Dealkylation

$R \cdot NHCH_2R' \longrightarrow [R \cdot NHCHOH \cdot R'] \longrightarrow R \cdot NH_2 + R' \cdot CHO$
(2° amine)   (1° amine)   (aldehyde)

Ephedrine, isoprenaline (isoproterenol)

$R_2N \cdot CH_2R' \longrightarrow [R_2N \cdot CHOH \cdot R'] \longrightarrow R_2NH + R' \cdot CHO$
(3° amine)   (2° amine)   (aldehyde)

Lignocaine, mepivacaine, bupivacaine, etidocaine, pethidine, chlorpromazine, ketamine, fentanyl, morphine, codeine, atropine, methadone, propoxyphene, diazepam (ring amide)

S-Dealkylation

$R \cdot S \cdot CH_2R' \longrightarrow [R \cdot S \cdot CHOH \cdot R'] \longrightarrow R \cdot SH + R' \cdot CHO$
(sulfide)   (thiol)   (aldehyde)

Methitural

N-Oxidation

$R \cdot NH_2 \longrightarrow R \cdot NHOH$
(1° amine)   (hydroxylamine)

Norpethidine

$R_3 \cdot N \longrightarrow R_3N \longrightarrow O$
(3° amine)   (amine oxide)

Chlorpromazine, tetracaine, morphine, pethidine

S-Oxidation

$$R \cdot S \cdot R' \longrightarrow R \overset{\overset{\text{O}}{\|}}{\cdot} S \cdot R'$$
(sulfide)   (sulfoxide)

Chlorpromazine

Deamination (equivalent to N-dealkylation)

$R_2CH \cdot NHR' \longrightarrow [R_2CHOH \cdot NHR'] \longrightarrow R_2CO + R' \cdot NH_2$
(amine)   (carbinolamine)   (aldehyde   (amine or or ketone)   ammonia)

Amphetamine

Desulfuration

$R_2C{=}NOH$
(oxime)

$$R \overset{\overset{\text{S}}{\|}}{\cdot} C \cdot R \longrightarrow \left[R \overset{\overset{\text{S} \cdot \text{OH}}{\|}}{\cdot} C \cdot R' \right] \longrightarrow R \overset{\overset{\text{O}}{\|}}{\cdot} C \cdot R'$$
(thioketone)   (ketone)

Thiobarbiturates

Dehalogenation (X = Cl or Br)

$$R \cdot CH(X)_2 \longrightarrow \left[R \overset{\overset{\text{OH}}{|}}{\cdot} C(X)_2 \right] \longrightarrow R \cdot COOH$$
(alkylidene halide)   (carboxylic acid)

Halothane, methoxyflurane, enflurane

Reduction

Azo reduction

$R \cdot N{=}N \cdot R' \longrightarrow R \cdot NH_2 + R' \cdot NH_2$
(1° amine)

Fazadinium

Nitro reduction

$R \cdot NO_2 \longrightarrow R \cdot NH_2$
(1° amine)

Nitrazepam

Carbonyl reduction

$R \cdot CO \cdot R' \longrightarrow R \cdot CHOH \cdot R'$
(ketone)   (alcohol)

Prednisone

Alcohol dehydrogenase

$R \cdot CH_2OH \longrightarrow R \cdot CHO$
(aldehyde)

Ethanol

$R \cdot CH(OH)_2 \longrightarrow R \cdot CH_2OH$
(alcohol)

Chloral hydrate

Hydrolysis

Ester hydrolysis

$R \cdot COOR' \longrightarrow R \cdot COOH + R'OH$
(carboxylic acid)   (alcohol)

Acetylsalicylic acid, procaine, chloroprocaine, tetracaine, cocaine, suxamethonium, propanidid, pethidine, etomidate, pancuronium (equivalent to deacetylation)

TABLE 78-1. (Cont.)

Type	Equation	Examples of Drug
Amide hydrolysis	$R \cdot CONHR' \longrightarrow R \cdot COOH + R'NH_2$ (carboxylic acid) (amine)	Prilocaine, lignocaine, etidocaine, fentanyl

CONJUGATION REACTIONS*

Type	Equation	Examples of Drug
Glucuronides O-Glucuronides	$R \cdot OH$ (alcohol) $R \cdot C_6H_4OH$ (phenol) $+ UDPGA \xrightarrow{\text{UDP-glucuronyl transferase}}$ $R \cdot O$ glucuronide $R \cdot C_6H_4O$ glucuronide $+ UDP$	Oxazepam, paracetamol, morphine, codeine, nalorphine, naloxone
N-Glucuronides	$R \cdot C_6H_4 \cdot NH_2$ (amine) $R \cdot SO_2NH \cdot R'$ (sulfonamide) $+ UDPGA \xrightarrow{\text{UDP-glucuronyl transferase}}$ $R \cdot C_6H_4NH$ glucuronide $R \cdot SO_2NR'$ | glucuronide $+ UDP$	
Sulfates	$R \cdot OH$ (alcohol) $R \cdot C_6H_4OH$ (phenol) $+ PAPS \xrightarrow{\text{Sulfokinase}}$ $R \cdot OS_2H$ $R \cdot C_6H_4O \cdot SO_3H$ $+ ADP$	Paracetamol, morphine, isoprenaline (isoproterenol)
Acetylation	$R \cdot C_6H_4 \cdot NH_2$ (amine) $R \cdot SO_2NHR'$ (sulfonamide) $\xrightarrow{\text{ATP/Co-A}}$ $R \cdot C_6H_4 \cdot NHCOCH_3$ $R \cdot SO_2NR'$ | $COCH_3$	Procainamide
Methylation	$R \cdot C_6H_4OH$ (phenol) $R \cdot NH_2$ (amine) $+ SAM \xrightarrow{\text{Methyltransferase}}$ $R \cdot C_6H_4OCH_3$ $R \cdot NHCH_3$	Morphine Noradrenaline
Conjugation with amino acids	$R \cdot C_6H_4 \cdot COOH + glycine \longrightarrow R \cdot C_6H_4 \cdot CONHCH_2COOH$ (carboxylic acid) (hippuric acid)	Salicylic acid
Conjugation with glutathione	$R \cdot C_6H_5 + GSH \longrightarrow R \cdot C_6H_4 \cdot S \cdot CH_2CH(COOH) \cdot NHCOCH_3$ (mercapturic acid)	Paracetamol

*Cofactors: UDPGA, uridine diphosphate glucuronic acid; PAPS, adenosine-3'-phosphate-5'-phosphosulfate; GSH, glutathione; SAM, S-adenosylmethionine; ATP/Co-A, adenosine triphosphate/acetyl coenzyme A.

substituted by the body for cellular substrates, thus changing cell function. Others act by somewhat ill-defined physicochemical mechanisms that are not specifically related to structure.

Analgesic Effect

The analgesic effect is the relief of pain induced by a drug. The opioid drugs generally act at receptor sites, mimicking the actions of endogenous transmitters. The nonopioid drugs, specifically the NSAIDs, inhibit specific enzymes in the prostaglandin cascade. These mechanisms are discussed in greater detail below.

Basic Concepts

POTENCY. Potency refers to the intensity of effect for a given dose of drug. It is a relatively unimportant factor despite its use by pharmaceutical firms as a selling point. For therapeutic applications potency is stated in dosage units.

EQUIANALGESIA. Equianalgesia indicates that the same degree of pain relief is obtained from two specified medications at given doses (e.g., the analgesic effect of morphine 10 mg IM equals that of meperidine 75 mg IM).

THERAPEUTIC INDEX. The therapeutic index is an indication of the safety of a given drug, also called margin of safety or selectivity. It is defined as the ratio of the median toxic dose to the median effective dose ($TD_{50}:ED_{50}$).

RELATIVE TOXICITY RATIO. The relative toxicity ratio is a comparison of the toxic effects of two given drugs with the same desired clinical effect. For example, if pentobarbital and phenobarbital are given for seizure control, the toxicity ratio with respect to respiratory depression is 10:3 because phenobarbital has approximately a threefold advantage over pentobarbital as an antiseizure drug but an equal sedating effect.

Drug-Drug Interaction

Drugs can interact with each other to produce potentiation, additive effects, or antipotentiation. *Potentiation* is said to occur when the net effect of two drugs used together is greater than the sum of their individual effects. This can be seen particularly when an opioid analgesic is given with a nonopioid analgesic.

Additive effects are noted when the net effect of two drugs used together is equal to the sum of their original effects. *Antipotentiation* occurs when the net effect of two drugs used together is less than the sum of their individual effects, as when an NSAID is given with another NSAID.

Clinical Pharmacology

Relation Between Dose and Effect

At low doses a graded response in terms of a specific effect is seen with incremental dosing. For most drugs, including analgesics, a maximum "ceiling" analgesic effect is reached, which cannot be elevated with increased doses. Plotting dose versus effect yields a linear, concave upward, concave downward, or sigmoid curve, which might or might not correspond to the drug-receptor interaction curve if more than one receptor type is responsible for the effect. Therefore, do not expect a simple relationship to exist between dose and effect, especially in a large population in whom individual differences in response further complicate the issue.

Factors in Dose Adjustment

BIOAVAILABILITY. Absolute bioavailability refers to the fraction of a given dose of drug that reaches the general circulation as compared to the same dose given intravenously. Relative bioavailability compares the absolute bioavailability of two different dosage forms. Physiologic bioavailability is a measure of the effect of the administered drug. Variables start at the manufacturing level—biologic nonequivalence has been seen with drug preparations from several companies (21). Bioavailability is affected by such factors as the form of administration (e.g., tablet or liquid) and the site (e.g., oral or intramuscular). The rate of absorption from the site of administration (e.g., full stomach or empty stomach) is important. The binding to plasma protein can also influence bioavailability and varies with different plasma protein levels because of diet, disease states, and hepatic function (22, 23). The rate of clearance from the circulation can be modified to a significant extent by the competence of renal or hepatic function or both.

CLEARANCE. Clearance is defined as the rate of elimination by all routes divided by the concentration of the drug, usually in blood or plasma. It is an important factor, because dosing and accumulation of a given drug are closely related when selecting the doses and times of administration necessary to reach a steady state (see below). Variations in clearance might mean modifying the dose, dosing interval, or both.

VOLUME OF DISTRIBUTION. The volume of distribution is equal to the amount of drug in the body divided by the blood or plasma concentration, as previously defined.

HALF-LIFE. The half-life of a drug is a measure of how rapidly its concentration changes. It is inversely related to clearance and is directly related to the volume of distribution. It is defined as the time taken for the concentration of a drug (e.g., in blood or plasma) to decrease by a factor of two following administration (Fig. 78-1).

STEADY STATE. A steady state level of a drug refers to the accumulation of a drug in the body compartment under consideration, so that relatively little change in concentration is seen over time. This is a concentration plateau and depends on the rates of administration and clearance from the phase in which it is active. Thus, when the rate of administration to a compartment equals the rate of clearance from a compartment a steady state is reached. The rate of decrease from a steady state depends on the half-life of the drug.

For example, the accumulation of nitrous oxide has a fast phase (3.5-minute half-life) and a slow phase (30-minute half-life). The rapid rise in its arterial concentration occurs during the fast phase because redistribution is minimal, but true steady state is prolonged because the terminal phase of accumulation depends on many factors. For clinical purposes a steady state is said to be reached after 5 to 6 half-lives (i.e., 96.9% and 98.4% of maximum concentration, respectively). For nitrous oxide this would be about 3×5, or 15 minutes.

Diazepam, on the other hand, has a redistribution half-life of 1 hour and a terminal half-life of 30 hours. Accumulation is slower and a steady state would not be reached for 506 hours with continuous infusion (analogous to breathing nitrous oxide). It is therefore given in bolus, and a steady state is not necessary or desirable for its clinical effectiveness.

Dosing of Drugs

The way in which a drug is administered—by a single dose, by an intermittent dose, or by continuous dosing—is determined by the clinical pharmacology of the drug and by the clinical situation for which it is

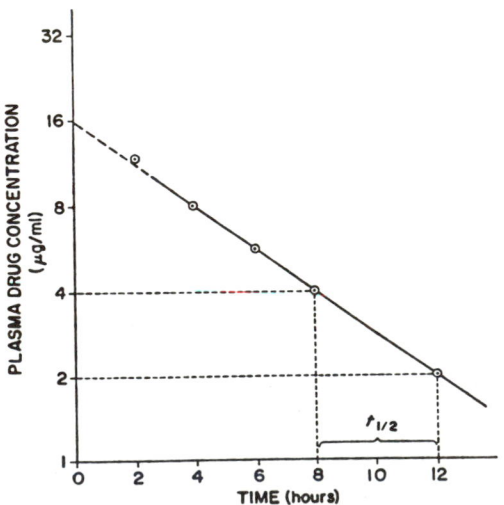

FIG. 78-1. Graphic depiction of determination of half-life ($t_{1/2}$) of a drug. In this example $t_{1/2} = 4$ hours, as seen from the change in plasma concentration from 16 to 8, 8 to 4, and 4 to 2 μg/ml on the plasma decay curve. Modified from Benet, L.Z. and Sheiner, L.B.: Pharmacokinetics: the dynamics of drug absorption, distribution, and elimination. *In* The Pharmacological Basis of Therapeutics, 7th ed. Edited by A.G. Gilman, L.S. Goodman, T.W. Rall and F. Murad. New York, MacMillan Publishing Company, 1985, pp. 3–34.

used. A single dose of an analgesic with a long half-life for a relatively short pain experience is appropriate. Recently, the use of methadone by IV bolus intraoperatively has been proposed to provide postoperative pain relief (24). For some procedures, such as herniorrhaphy, the long half-life of methadone (24 to 36 hours) can provide most of the postoperative analgesia with a single large dose so that NSAIDs might be all that are necessary for pain relief beyond its effective duration. Intermittent dosing with opioids of intermediate half-lives (e.g., morphine or meperidine) is commonly used for the relief of longer-lasting postoperative pain, as with a thoracotomy.

Continuous dosing by IV drip allows blood concentration closer to a steady state to be controlled, and is especially appropriate for drugs with a short half-life. Some interest in this method for relieving postoperative pain using fentanyl or sufentanyl has been manifested (20).

A *loading dose* is an initial large bolus given to produce a rapid increase in the therapeutic blood level of a drug and can be maintained by giving intermittent smaller doses or by continuous infusion. A *maintenance dose* is the amount of drug necessary to maintain a steady state when given intermittently or by continuous infusion.

More detailed discussion of this topic is presented elsewhere (9–20).

Therapeutic Monitoring

To use analgesics effectively, the dose of a given drug must be matched to the requirements of a given patient and the timing must be such that blood levels remain at or above the minimum effective analgesic concentration (MEAC). The balance must be maintained while the patient is monitored for overdose and significant side effects. This might sound complicated but, unfortunately, analgesics are usually given by rote without consideration for the volume of distribution, for individual variations in absorption, metabolism, and clearance, or for the clinical state. In the hospital monitoring is the primary responsibility of the nurses and physicians. Meticulous pharmacokinetic calculations and frequent measurement of blood levels would be ideal but are not practical in most institutions at present, and are a secondary consideration for the clinical response. The effects of the first few doses are critically important so that an accurate estimate of maintenance dose and dosing time can be made.

In some cases, especially with the terminally ill who are treated at home, the family might have to be responsible for monitoring the patient. This requires the family to be knowledgeable about the medication and its pharmacology as well as to be in close communication with treating physicians and nurses to optimize care. If the appropriate drug is given in the wrong dose and at the wrong interval, then the health care system has failed. Unfortunately this can be the case when analgesia is desired, and lack of careful therapeutic monitoring is usually the cause.

In the last 10 years remarkable and rapid advances have been made in several fields pertinent to the treatment of pain. More information is available about the physiology of pain and its psychologic effects on the individual, the interaction of pain and the personality, and emotional and psychologic reactions and their modification by social and environmental factors. Knowledge of the pharmacology, pharmacokinetics, and toxicology of the rapidly expanding number of analgesics is becoming increasingly sophisticated and complex. Despite all this, treatment of pain is often inadequate and medications used for pain relief are often a source of abuse. This can lead to the development of tolerance and physical dependence fostered unwittingly by both the patient and treating physician, or can lead the patient to develop side effects, some of which are potentially lethal. Therefore, in approaching the control of pain, a few simple guidelines must be followed.

EVALUATION OF PAIN. The source and cause of pain and its severity should be analyzed not only from a nociceptive viewpoint but also from a psychologic-behavioral perspective.

USE OF OPTIMAL DRUG AND OPTIMAL DOSE. The most appropriate medication for the problem should be selected for each individual patient in an optimal dosage in terms of amount and frequency. *Optimal dosage* is the minimum amount of a drug repeated at appropriate intervals to give the desired therapeutic effect with a minimum of side effects. Appropriate monitoring of the patient by personal observation, and in some cases by blood studies, is necessary to follow compliance to dosage regimens, to assess the therapeutic effects, and to identify untoward side effects or toxicity of the medications prescribed. The interaction of the drug and patient is highly dynamic. For example, pathologic alterations of hepatic or renal function, or both, can drastically decrease the metabolism and excretion of morphine to the extent that a properly tailored analgesic dose can become a lethal overdose.

TYPE OF PAIN. As discussed repeatedly in this book, it is important to distinguish between acute pain, pain associated with cancer, and chronic nonmalignant pain when choosing a therapeutic approach involving systemic analgesics for patient treatment. Generally the approaches to the treatment of acute pain problems and pain associated with cancer are somewhat similar, whereas the therapeutic approach to chronic nonmalignant pain is quite different. Opioid analgesics in adequate doses, given at appropriate intervals, as a continuous infusion, or as an infusion with a patient-controlled analgesia (PCA) unit, constitute the primary approach to most acute pain problems and to most pain associated with cancer. Opioids are generally contraindicated for chronic continuous pain whereas, if properly prescribed, they can be useful in chronic recurrent or cyclical pain states of non-neoplastic origin. Treatment must be individually tailored because of wide variation in response to medication. The requirements, side effects, and toxicity of drugs vary widely among patients with similar clinical problems. In one study of postoperative pain, a four- to fivefold difference in requirements for opioids was seen after major laparotomies (25). In monitoring the responses of a homogeneous group of rheumatic patients to NSAIDs a marked variation in suitability of different drugs was noted that could not be explained by the clinical picture (26).

Not all pain associated with cancer responds equally to the same analgesic. Pain associated with bone metastases responds well to NSAIDs (27). In a recent study in which epidural morphine was used for the treatment of cancer-related pain, it was found that this form of treatment best relieved continuous somatic pain while it was not effective in treating neuropathic or cutaneous pain (28). This underscores the need to monitor patients and drug effects carefully, to individualize treatment, and to optimize effectiveness. Standard orders for analgesic administration do a great disservice to most patients receiving care.

Recent Advances in Pharmacologic Therapy

Prompted by the introduction of the Melzack and Wall (29) gate theory of pain over two decades ago, by the International Association for the Study of Pain, and by others (Chapter 1), exciting new results in the field of pain research have advanced the sophistication of applied pharmacology to the treatment of pain. Knowledge of the neurophysiology and biochemistry of pain transmission and modulation systems (30), of drug receptors and their influences within these systems, and of changes in these systems produced by acute and chronic pain is continually increasing (31, 32). More information is available about drugs long used for analgesia and about promising new drugs designed to be more specific for pain modulation. Drug delivery itself is becoming more specific in regard to the agents being administered and to the problems for which they are being given. A brief review is important here so that practitioners can be aware of more sophisticated approaches that can enhance pain relief and reduce side effects.

CLINICAL TRIALS. By using controlled clinical trials with and without placebo, as proposed by Beecher (33) and Houde (34), among others, newer drugs of the opioid and nonopioid classes can be compared not only to placebos but also to standards of their class, such as morphine for the opioids and aspirin for the nonopioids. This has led to a re-evaluation of the effectiveness of some older drugs as well as of the availability of new drugs to the clinician. Close scrutiny of analgesic effects, side effects, and toxic effects using such trials in both humans and animals (35) has resulted in safer and more effective clinical care.

PAIN MEASUREMENT. Combined with the methodology of controlled clinical trials, newer techniques of pain measurement, both objective and subjective, have allowed more accurate evaluation of the effectiveness of analgesic medications in animals, in normal human subjects (36), and in those suffering from acute or chronic pain (35) (Chapter 32). Increasing interest in pain measurement has been applied to the psychology of pain as well, allowing peripheral and central effects of pharmacologic intervention and the use of drugs other than analgesics to be evaluated. Pain measurement is still in its infancy despite more recent experience, and a "pain thermometer" has yet to be found that would allow an accurate objective measure

of pain and suffering. The search for this elusive tool promises to expand our knowledge of pain and to improve research and treatment strategies.

ANALYTIC TECHNIQUES. Analytic chemistry has become a much more sophisticated science. Minute quantities of chemicals (including analgesics) in blood and in many other body fluids and tissues can be analyzed (35, 36). The in vivo release of neurotransmitters and its modification by different drugs in animal models can be monitored (37). New imaging techniques (e.g., PET scanning, MRI) allow the metabolism of the human brain to be observed and recorded and expand the prospects of more specific pain research in the future.

PHARMACOKINETIC STUDIES. The increasing accuracy of analytic chemical methods now allows the pharmacokinetics of opioids and nonopioids in tissue compartments of the body to be followed—for example, in plasma and also in target structures, such as the nervous and integumentary systems. This allows prediction of dose and correct dosing interval for these drugs so that adequate blood and tissue levels can be maintained for better pain control. These techniques are becoming more available and promise to be a future check on clinical monitoring. Analytic studies have also shown wide variations among patients in regard to plasma drug concentration (38–44). Such results are often ignored, however—many physicians still maintain fixed routine doses and intervals of dosing in patients with both acute and chronic pain, frequently resulting in inadequate analgesia.

MATHEMATICAL MODELS. As a direct result of pharmacokinetic studies, mathematical models of drug distribution have been determined that are used to predict more appropriate prescribing practices (45). These models have also explained redistribution patterns within the body, suggesting unrecognized sites of action and explaining some peculiarities in response with prolonged administration. Again, this has enlarged our knowledge of pharmacokinetics so as to provide better patient care.

NOVEL DRUG DELIVERY SYSTEMS. Nowhere have so many changes occurred so widely as in the area of drug delivery systems. An early modification was enteric-coated aspirin, which allowed the aspirin to be passed into the small gut before absorption, thus reducing gastric irritation. This technique has now also been applied to other NSAIDs. Coating morphine granules with varying thicknesses of wax in a single dose has allowed this relatively short-acting drug to be given in a slow-release form, resulting in less frequent dosing and more stable blood levels. Other encapsulated drug forms rely on absorption of water for dissolving the medication to allow gradual release as the capsule passes through the digestive system. Some opioids and other nonanalgesic drugs are available in sublingual forms that are useful and indeed necessary for those with difficulty in swallowing. This type of delivery also prevents extraction of large quantities of drug from the blood by first pass through the liver, thus allowing higher blood levels with lower doses of drug.

Opioids are being delivered in other ingenious ways. Catheters placed in the epidural or subarachnoid space allow for delivery of a restricted amount of drug to affect the nociceptive system, primarily at the spinal cord level (46, 47). Central catheter placement near the periaquaductal gray is also used for opioid administration (48). The use of internal and external pumps permits continuous delivery of small doses of drug to sustain an analgesic effect at a predictably constant level. These pumps are also used to deliver opioids intravenously and subcutaneously, producing more effective analgesia for the control of postoperative pain and pain associated with cancer.

Thus, changes in the pharmacologic approach to analgesia, when used properly, can now tailor treatment to individual patients and their problems. Knowledge of these techniques is increasing and hopefully they will be more often applied in the clinical situation.

B. OPIOID ANALGESICS

This section describes the general pharmacology of opioids, including the mechanism of analgesia, other therapeutic effects, and the undesirable effects and complications induced by this group of drugs. This is followed by a discussion of the most important opioid analgesics.

General Principles of Pharmacology

Opioids have widespread pharmacologic effects on almost every organ and function in the human body (30). Some of these effects are beneficial and some are not. The most important targets are the central nervous system and the gastrointestinal system. The effects on the central nervous system are remarkably diverse and include analgesia, changes in mood, sedation, drowsiness, and clouding of the sensorium; the limbic system, hypothalamus, brain stem centers of respiration, cardiac and vasomotor function, and the respiratory system are also affected. Different opioids act on various organ systems in similar ways but with different intensities (Tables 78-2 and 78-3).

Site and Mechanism of Analgesia

Unlike the NSAIDs, which have a ceiling effect for analgesia, opioids act in a dose-dependent manner and usually can control all types of pain up to the induction of surgical anesthesia. The major drawbacks are the side effects, which increase proportionately with dose. Systemic opioids induce analgesia by acting at different levels of the central nervous system (49). At the spinal cord level they impair or inhibit the transmission of nociceptive input from the periphery to the central nervous system in a dose-related manner. At the level of the basal ganglia opioids activate a descending inhibitory system that modulates peripheral nociceptive input at the spinal cord level. By acting on the limbic system opioids alter the emotional response to pain, thus making it much more bearable (31). Therapeutic analgesic doses of opioids control dull, prolonged, aching pain better than sharp colicky pain. At high doses (e.g., 2 to 3 mg morphine/kg body weight), however, they induce a state of analgesia, with obliteration of autonomic responses to the most intense nociceptive stimuli (50).

Although great advances have been made in elucidating the opioid system our knowledge is far from complete, and a detailed and clear understanding of the intrinsic mechanism of action of opioids is still lacking. Several factors prevent the elucidation of this mechanism:

a. The multiplicity of opioid substances, each of which interacts with more than one site of the macromolecules that form the opiate receptors (51, 52).

b. The ability of one substance to act as an agonist in one animal tissue and as an antagonist in another, adding further confusion (53).

c. The difficulty of finding not only agonists that bind to one type of opioid receptor but also of finding antagonists that are receptor-specific. Naloxone, for instance, is a mu antagonist at low doses (up to 15 nM) but at higher doses antagonizes also sigma and kappa agonists (51).

d. The recent discovery (but lack of physiologic significance) that animal tissues can transform the nonpeptide, nonmorphinan reticuline to morphine and codeine, and that these substances are present in low doses in animals (54–57).

Despite these difficulties, we now have a great deal of information regarding this complex system. Opioid agonists, either exogenous or endogenous, produce analgesia and other central effects by dynamically binding to specific receptors in the encephalon and spinal cord. Once opioids have interacted with the receptor site, either stimulation or depression of different neuronal populations is initiated. For instance, in most animal species, opioids stimulate the Edinger-Westphal nucleus of the oculomotor nerve to produce miosis and the chemoreceptor trigger zone in the area postrema to decrease the threshold of nausea and vomiting, whereas they depress the respiratory centers.

Recent evidence indicates that the descending antinociceptive system, activated mainly by the interaction of opioids with receptors in the periaqueductal gray of the brain stem, requires a much lower concentration of these drugs to produce analgesia than the analgesia elicited strictly by the activation of the receptors of the substantia gelatinosa of the spinal cord (46). Therefore, opioids at low cerebrospinal fluid (CSF) concentrations, such as those obtainable after oral, intramuscular, or intravenous administration, act mostly through the descending antinociceptive system. After intraspinal administration, in which high CSF concentrations are produced, the activation of opioid receptors in the substantia gelatinosa constitutes the major mechanism of analgesia (46).

Several opiate receptors are now known, each with more or less different functions and drug affinities (30, 51, 52, 58). Five receptors have been identified: mu, kappa, delta, sigma, and epsilon (51, 52, 58) (Tables 78-4 and 78-5). In brief, the mu receptors

TABLE 78-2. Pharmacokinetic and Pharmacodynamic Data of Opioid Analgesics Used for Moderate to Severe Pain

Class; Generic Name; Proprietary Name	Route*	Equi-Analgesic Dose (mg)†	Peak (h)‡	Duration (h)‡	Half-Life (h)	Comments	Precautions
AGONISTS							
Naturally occurring opium derivatives							
Morphine	IM§	10–15	0.5–1	3–5	2–3.5‖	Standard of comparison for opioid-type analgesics	Impaired ventilation; bronchial asthma; increased intracranial pressure; liver failure; renal failure
	PO§	30–60†	1.5–2	4			
Codeine	IM	120	0.5–1	4–6	3	Less potent than morphine; excellent oral potency	Like morphine
	PO	30–200		3–4			
Partially synthetic derivatives of morphine							
Hydromorphone (Dilaudid)	IM	1–2	0.5–1	3–4	2–3	Like heroin	Like morphine
	PO	2–4	1.5–2	4–6			
Oxymorphone (Numorphan)	IM	1–1.5	0.5–1	3–5	NA*	Like morphine	Like morphine
Heroin	IM	4	0.5–1	3–4	2–3	Slightly shorter acting	Like morphine
	PO	4–8	1.5–2	3–4			
Oxycodone	PO	30	1	4–6	NA	Available only (5-mg doses) in combination with acetaminophen (Percocet) or aspirin (Percodan), which limits dose escalation	Like morphine
Synthetic compounds							
Morphonans							
Levorphanol (Levo-Dromoran)	IM	2	0.5–1	5–8	12–16	Like methadone	Like methadone
	PO	4	1.5–2				
Phenylheptylamines							
Methadone (Dolophine)	IM	8–10	0.5–1	4–8	15–30	Good oral potency; long plasma half-life	Like morphine, cumulative with repeated doses
	PO	10	1.5–2	4–12			
Propoxyphene HCl (Darvon)	PO	32–65		4–6	3.5	"Weak" opioid, often used in combination with nonopioid analgesics	Cumulative with repeated doses; convulsions with overdose
Phenylpiperidines							
Meperidine (Demerol)	IM	75–100	0.5–1	2–3		Shorter acting and about 10% as potent as morphine; has mild atropine-like antispasmodic effects	Normeperidine accumulates with repetitive dosing, causing CNS excitation; not for patients with impaired renal function or for those receiving monoamine oxidase inhibitors
	PO	200–300	1–2	2–3			
Alphaprodine (Nisentil)	IM	40		1.5–2		Similar to meperidine but shorter acting; low placental transfer	Like meperidine

TABLE 78-2. (Cont.)

Class; Generic Name; Proprietary Name	Route*	Equi-Analgesic Dose (mg)†	Peak (h)‡	Duration (h)‡	Half-Life (h)	Comments	Precautions
Fentanyl	IV	50–100 µg		0.75–1		Short-acting potent opioid; mostly used in anesthesia or continuous infusion	More severe side effects than morphine
AGONIST-ANTAGONISTS							
Buprenorphine (Temgesic)	IM SL	0.3–0.6 0.4–0.8	0.5–1 2–3	6–8 6–8	NA	Partial agonist of the morphine type, less abuse liability than morphine	Can precipitate withdrawal in narcotic-dependent patients
Butorphanol (Stadol)	IM	2	0.5–1	4	2.5–3.5	Like nalbuphine	Like pentazocine
Pentazocine (Talwin)	IM PO	40–60 50–200	0.5–1 1.5–2	3–4 3–4	2–3	Mixed agonist-antagonist; less abuse liability than morphine; included in Schedule IV of Controlled Substances Act	Can cause psychotomimetic effects; might precipitate withdrawal in narcotic-dependent patients; not for those with myocardial infarction
Nalbuphine (Nubain)	IM	10–20	0.5–1	4–6	5	Mu-antagonist and kappa-agonist. Possible mild sigma-agonist; not scheduled	Incidence of psychotomimetic effects lower than with pentazocine

*IM, intramuscular; PO, oral; SL sublingual; NA, not available.
†These doses are recommended starting doses from which the optimal dose for each patient is determined by titration and the maximal dose is limited by adverse effects.
‡Peak time and duration of analgesia are based on mean values and refer to the stated equianalgesic doses.
§For single oral dose the ratio of intramuscular:oral is 1:6; for repeated doses the ratio is closer to 1:3.
‖Plasma half-life at least for morphine is age-dependent; it increases with age.

Adapted from Inturrisi, C.E., and Foley, K.M.: Narcotic analgesics in the management of pain. *In* Analgesics: Neurochemical, Behavioral, and Chemical Perspectives. Edited by M. Kuhar and G.W. Pasternak. New York, Raven Press, 1984, pp. 257–288.

mediate supraspinal analgesia, euphoria, respiratory depression, and physical dependence; the kappa receptors mediate spinal analgesia, miosis, and sedation; and the delta receptors mediate analgesia, show little or no cross tolerance with mu agonists and, when partially activated by a subanalgesic dose of delta agonists, greatly potentiate morphine analgesia. The sigma receptors mediate dysphoria, hallucination, and stimulation of respiratory and vasomotor centers. Recent findings suggest that sigma receptor agonists, which include ketamine and phencyclidine (PCP, "angel dust"), are potent agonists of excitatory transmitters at the spinal cord level and are not reversed by naloxone. These characteristics suggest that the sigma receptor might not belong to the family of opiate receptors (58). The identity and existence of the epsilon receptor are also in question (51).

Recent clinical observations indicate that agonists for different opiate receptors might relieve different types of pain syndromes. For instance, pancreatic pain is poorly relieved by average doses of morphine but is well controlled by standard doses of buprenorphine (Staffan Arnér, personal communication, 1987).

Other Central Nervous System Effects

Different opioids act on various organ systems in similar ways but with different intensities (Table 78-3). High doses of opioids injected intravenously at a fast rate can induce muscular rigidity associated with a decrease in chest compliance that could progress to the inability to ventilate. This occurs not only in humans but also in rats and other experimental animals. The precise mechanism of this effect is not known but it is probably caused by the interaction of opioids with receptors located in the substantia nigra and striatum (59).

Limbic System

The detailed neural mechanisms by which opioids produce euphoria and tranquility have not been completely elucidated. Microinjections of an opioid in the nucleus accumbens, which forms the floor of the anterior horn of the lateral ventricle, induces the experimental animal to seek reinjection of this substance. This is interpreted as an indication of the euphoric or pleasurable effect induced by opioids. The

TABLE 78-3. Systemic Pharmacologic and Toxicologic Effects of Opioid Analgesics Used for Moderate to Severe Pain*

Class; Generic Name	Central Nervous System						Cardiovascular System		Gastro-intestinal Peristalsis	Biliary Common Duct Pressure	Bronchial Constriction	Genitourinary System		Histamine Release
	Analgesia	Mood	Sedation	Emetic Center	Cough Center	Respiratory Center	Cardiac Rate	Blood Pressure				Ureter Tone	Bladder Tone	
Agonists														
Morphine	↑↑↑↑	↑=↓	↑↑↑	↑↑↑	↓↓↓	↓↓↓	=↓	=↓	↓↓↓	↑↑	↑↑↑	↑↑	↑↑↑	↑↑↑↑
Codeine	↑↑	=↑	↑	↑	↓↓↓	↓	NA†	↓↓↓↓ (if given IV)	↓	↑	NA	NA	NA	↑↑↑↑
Hydromorphone	LM†	LM	↑↑	LM	LM	LM	LM	LM	LM	LM	LM	LM	LM	NA
Oxymorphone	LM	LM	LM	LM	LM	LM	LM	LM	LM	LM	LM	LM	LM	NA
Heroin	LM	=↓	LM	LM	LM	LM	LM	LM	LM	LM	LM	LM	LM	LM
Oxicodone	↑↑↑	=↑	LM	LM	LM	LM	LM	LM	LM	LM	LM	LM	LM	LM
Morphonans	↑↑↑	=	↑	↑	↓↓↓	↓↓↓	LM	LM	LM	LM	LM	LM	LM	↑
Phenylheptamines	↑	NA	↑↑	↑↑		↓↓	↑↑↑		↓↓	NA	NA	NA	NA	
Meperidine	↑↑↑	↑↑	↑↑	↑↑	↓↓	↓↓↓↓	=or↑	↓↓↓	↓↓	↑↑↑	NA	↑	↑	
Alphaprodine	LM	LM	LM	LM	LM	LM	LM	LM	LM	LM	LM	LM	LM	NA
Fentanyl	↑↑↑↑		↑↑↑	↑↑↑↑	↓↓↓	↓↓↓↓	↓↓↓	↓↓↓	↓↓↓	↑↑↑↑	NA		=	
Agonist-antagonists														
Buprenorphine	↑↑↑	↑ or ↓	↑↑↑	↑↑↑		↓↓↓	LM	LM	↓↓	↑↑	NA	NA	NA	NA
Butorphanol	↑↑	=	↑↑↑↑	↑↑↑	NA	↓↓↓	↑↑↑	↑↑↑	↓↓	↑	NA	NA	NA	NA
Pentazocine	↑	↓↓↓	↑↑↑↑	↓↑		↓↓↓	↑↑↑	↑↑↑	↓↓	↑	NA	NA	NA	NA
Nalbuphine	↑↑	↓↓	↑↑↑↑	↓↓	NA	↓↓	=↓	↑=↓	↓	NA	NA	NA	NA	NA

*Some toxic effects are quite different among opioids. For example, fentanyl increases common bile duct pressure 99% above the predrug level while pentazocine only increases it by 15%; IV morphine causes a wide variation in histamine release while fentanyl does not. In other cases, the toxic effect of an opioid might be statistically identical to morphine but on an individual basis considerable difference might be present that warrant change of an opioid if some side effects are particularly intense with one specific drug.

†LM, like morphine; NA, not available; ↑ increased; ↓ decreased; = remains unchanged. Intensity of effect: ↑ or ↓ mild; ↑↑ or ↓↓ moderate; ↑↑↑ or ↓↓↓ strong; ↑↑↑↑ or ↓↓↓↓ very strong.

locus ceruleus, located on the floor of the fourth ventricle, is endowed with a large number of opioid receptors and is believed to play a major role in the production of feelings of alarm, anxiety, and fear. The activity of these neurons is inhibited by the opioids (60).

Hypothalamus and Pituitary

In general, opioids decrease the response of the hypothalamus to afferent stimulation. This is apparently an indirect response, because the effect of electrical stimulation of the hypothalamus is not altered by the administration of opioids. The hypothalamus is involved in the maintenance of body temperature and contains autonomic centers that control sympathetic and parasympathetic systems (Chapter 6). A single dose of morphine slightly lowers body temperature in humans while the chronic use of high-dose opioids seems to increase body temperature.

The administration of opioids in the usual therapeutic dose causes a slight decrease in pituitary hormone levels. The acute administration of large doses of opioids is followed by a decrease in the concentration of luteinizing hormone, follicle-stimulating hormone, ACTH, and beta-endorphins. This is a result of a decreased release of gonadotropin-releasing hormone and corticotropin-releasing factor from the hypothalamus (9). Tolerance, however, soon develops, and

TABLE 78-4. Opiate Receptor Effects

mu₁	mu₂	kappa	sigma (?)	delta
Morphine; β-endorphin		Bremazocine; dynorphin	N-allylcyclazocine	Morphine; leu-enkephalin
Analgesia	No analgesia	Analgesia; excessive heat	No analgesia	No analgesia
Apnea, ?	Apnea	Apnea, ?	Tachypnea	Apnea, +
Indifference	Sedation	Sedation	Delirium	
Miosis		Miosis	Mydriasis	
Nausea and vomiting				Nausea and vomiting
Constipation				
Urine retention		Diuresis		
Pruritus				Pruritus
Temperature increase		No change	No change	
Tolerance +; delta cross tolerance		Little tolerance; No mu cross tolerance		Tolerance; mu cross tolerance

? possible, + marked.

TABLE 78-5. Opiate Receptor Interactions

Drug	Receptor				
	mu	kappa	sigma	delta	epsilon
Exogenous					
Morphine	+ + +	+		+ +	
Fentanyl	+ + + +			+	
Alfentanil	+ + +			?	
Sufentanil	+ + + +			+	
Lofentanil	+ + +			?	
Meperidine	+ +			+ +	
Hydromorphone	+ + +			+ +	
Methadone	+ + +			+ +	
Naloxone	− − −	−	−	−	
Naloxazone	− − − −				
Naloxonazine	− − − −				
Nalbuphine	− − −	+ + +	+		
Pentazocine	−	+ + +	+ +	?	− −
Bremazocine		+ + +			
Ketocyclazocine		+ + +			
Butorphanol		+ +	+ +		
Phencyclidine			+ + +		
Endogenous					
β-endorphin	+ + +			+ +	+ + +
DADL				+ + +	
Leu-enkephalin	+			+ + +	+ +
Met-enkephalin	+ + +			+ + +	
Dynorphin (small)		+ + + +			
Dynorphin (large)		+ + +			
α-Neoendorphin		+ + +			

Pluses indicate an agonist effect: + mild; + + moderate; + + + strong; + + + + very strong. Minuses indicate an antagonist effect: − mild; − − moderate; − − − strong; − − − − very strong.
DADL = Tyr-DAla-Gly-Phe-DLeu.

patients receiving opioids chronically are found to have normal concentrations of circulating cortisol, luteinizing hormone, and testosterone (9).

The systemic administration of the opioid antagonist naloxone effects the release of several hypophyseal hormones. It increases the concentration of luteinizing hormone and follicle-stimulating hormone while it decreases those of prolactin and growth hormone. Thus, it could be deduced that endogenous opioid peptide might regulate, in part, the secretion of some pituitary hormones (61).

Interpretation of the effect of opioids on antidiuretic hormone is controversial. Some studies have shown that the plasma concentration of this hormone increases with opioid administration and decreases with naloxone (62). Other authors, however, believe that the increase in diuresis is caused by hemodynamic or renal effects of opioids and not by the alterations of antidiuretic hormone concentration in the plasma (9).

Psychomimesis

Convulsions can be caused by some opioids, and seizures with different characteristics are caused by different opioids. Morphine, methadone, and *d*-propoxyphene, when given in high doses, cause convulsions that are reversible with naloxone. Alternatively, meperidine, its metabolite normeperidine, and thebaine produce convulsions that are not reversed by naloxone (63). These seizures, at times, are not even reversible with anticonvulsive agents. In humans, however, opioids induce convulsions and seizures at doses that are much higher than those required for analgesia.

Brain Stem and Medullary Centers

Opioids, in particular the mu receptor agonist, depress respiration. This is noticeable even at therapeutic doses of morphine and increases progressively with higher doses. The effect of opioids on respiration is multifaceted: they depress both respiratory rate and tidal volume and, as a consequence, decrease minute ventilation. The major effect is a decrease in responsiveness of the medullary respiratory centers to carbon dioxide tension. Pain counteracts some of this depression.

Depression of the cough reflex is also caused by opioids. This does not parallel the effect on respiratory centers, as demonstrated by the fact that opioids have been developed that effectively suppress cough without significantly impairing ventilation.

The chemoreceptor trigger zone for emesis is located in the area postrema of the medulla, and opioids cause direct stimulation of this area. This effect is antagonized by certain substances (e.g., chlorpromazine) with potent dopamine blocking effects. This adverse effect of opioids does not occur in all patients and it is much more frequent in ambulatory patients.

Other Effects

Cardiovascular System

Therapeutic doses of opioids do not have a significant effect on the myocardium of healthy individuals. In patients with coronary heart disease, though, therapeutic doses of morphine cause a decrease in oxygen consumption, cardiac work, left ventricular pressure, and diastolic pressure (9). Thus, large doses of opioids are used to induce anesthesia in cardiac cripples. Morphine and morphine-like opioids have a vasodilating effect on the peripheral vasculature, as a result of peripheral arteriolar and venous dilatation caused by various mechanisms. Morphine causes release of histamine (64), but histamine blocking agents only partially reverse the hypotension that instead is completely reversed by naloxone. Because of the vasodilating effect of morphine it should be used with caution in hypovolemic patients because it can aggravate the hypotension and occasionally induces hypovolemic shock. Equally important, morphine should be used with great care in patients with cor pulmonale because sudden death has been reported (9). The minor cardiovascular effect observed with the use of opioids can reflect a stimulating and depressing effect of this substance on different parts of the central nervous system involved with cardiovascular regulation. During shock caused by sepsis, hypovolemia, or spinal cord injury, the administration of opioids worsens the clinical picture, whereas improvement has been noted with the administration of large doses of naloxone (9).

Pulmonary System

It has been reported that high doses of meperidine or morphine can cause constriction of the bronchi; this is rarely seen with usual analgesic doses. During an asthmatic attack opioids should not be used because their depressive action on the respiratory center, release of histamine, drying of secretions, and decrease of the cough reflex, might worsen the clinical picture by decreasing respiratory drive and increasing airway resistance.

Gastrointestinal System

Opioids have a generalized depressant effect on the motility of the gastrointestinal tract (9).

STOMACH. Opioids cause a slight decrease in secretion of hydrochloric acid, increase antral tone, and decrease gastric motility, resulting in an increased time for gastric emptying (up to 12 hours) and consequent poor absorption of other oral medication.

SMALL INTESTINE. Digestion of food in the small intestine is decreased, along with biliary and pancreatic secretion. Smooth muscle tone increases and propulsive peristaltic contractions decrease markedly. The duodenum is more affected by opioids than the ileum. More water is absorbed and the viscosity of the chyme is increased because of the prolonged time that chyme is in the small intestine.

LARGE INTESTINE. Propulsive contractions of the colon are greatly diminished or completely abolished by opioids. Tone can increase to the point of spasm; this further delays the transit of the gastrointestinal contents. The feces lose a considerable amount of water and become dry and compacted, which causes constipation. The mechanism of action seems to be both at the level of the gastrointestinal tract and the level of the central nervous system. Tolerance to the constipating effect of opioids does not develop to a great extent and most patients on chronic opioid therapy suffer from constipation.

BILIARY TRACT. Therapeutic doses of opioids cause marked spasm of the biliary tract, especially of the sphincter of Oddi, thus increasing pressure in the common duct. This increased pressure can last 2 to 12 hours after administration of a therapeutic dose. The effect can be reversed by naloxone, smooth muscle relaxants such as nitroglycerin, 0.6 mg sublingually, or amyl nitrate. Equianalgesic doses of fentanyl, meperidine, morphine, and pentazocine increase the pressure in the common bile duct of 99, 61, 53, and 15%, respectively, above baseline (65). This increase in pressure can cause epigastric distress, which can be relieved by small amounts of naloxone.

Genitourinary Tract

URETER AND BLADDER. Opioids tend to increase the tone and amplitude of contraction of the ureter, but this response varies in humans (19). They can also produce urinary urgency by increasing the tone of the detrusor muscle of the urinary bladder; the increased tone of the sphincter vesicae makes urination difficult to the point of requiring catheterization, even following therapeutic doses of morphine. This has been observed particularly in a large percentage of male patients receiving intraspinal opioids (66). Naloxone antagonizes this action.

UTERUS. Therapeutic doses of opioids decrease uterine contractions and can prolong labor (67). Large doses of opioids should not be used during labor, not only because of this effect on the mother, but also because they can cross the placenta and reach the central nervous system of the fetus. Their effects can persist in the neonate, who is particularly sensitive to the respiratory depressant effect of opioids. Uterine hyperactivity, however, is decreased by morphine, which tends to return contractility to normal. In this particular situation the duration of labor and delivery can be shortened by morphine.

Immune System

Individuals who abuse narcotics suffer from an increased incidence of infections (68). This effect could have multiple explanations: abusers could be exposed to more infective pathogens, their immune systems could be depressed by malnutrition and increased stress factors, or the opioids could have a depressive effect on the immune response (quite likely all the above factors are responsible for the increased susceptibility to infections of these individuals). To test the opioid hypothesis numerous animal and in vitro experiments have been performed since 1980. The results have been contradictory, indicating that the system, as should be expected, is very complex (69, 70). One line of research implicates the opioids as having a suppressing effect on a particular immune response. Some types of inescapable stress induce the release of opioid peptides that depress the natural killer (NK) cells, a subpopulation of lymphocytes that recognize and destroy certain tumor cells. In animals this effect is also induced by very high doses of systemic morphine, and it is blocked by opioid antagonists (71). This immunosuppressive effect shows development of tolerance when induced by morphine, but tolerance does not develop when the immunosuppressive effect is caused by opioid-peptides-releasing stress. In several highly selective experiments with rats, this immunosuppresive effect was responsible for the increased development of an experimental mammary ascitis tumor (72). Although not conclusive, these findings indicate that some endogenous and, in high doses, exogenous opioids can downregulate the immune response in a complex, not yet clearly understood manner.

Adverse Side Effects

Clinical trials have shown that potent opioids, administered in equianalgesic doses to the general population, produce a similar statistical incidence and degree of effects; depending on the particular circumstance these are either welcomed or undesired. Certain patients experience one or more of these effects to a greater degree than the general population, and these effects vary with different opioids. Thus, all patients receiving opioid therapy should be closely monitored for adverse side effects and complications; if particularly intense, other opioids should be tried at equianalgesic doses.

Central Nervous System

Euphoria, which at times can be desirable, is a frequently occurring side effect of opioid therapy, but some patients experience unpleasant dysphoria. Suppression of the cough reflex can be beneficial in patients with persistent cough but is undesirable in patients in whom any depression of the ability to expectorate can prove deleterious. Excessive sedation, drowsiness, confusion, dizziness, and unsteadiness can develop during the first few days of opioid therapy but usually clear in 3 to 5 days. Persistent sedation and drowsiness can be ameliorated by the concomitant use of amphetamines (73), by reducing the dose and increasing the frequency of the opioid administration to ensure sustained analgesia, or by both. This is appropriate for relatively short-term therapy and for patients with terminal cancer.

Multifocal myoclonic seizures can occur in patients who erroneously receive chronic meperidine therapy. These result from the accumulation of its active metabolite, normeperidine, which produces central nervous system hyperexcitability and lowers the seizure threshold (8). This hyperirritability is not reversed by naloxone but can be suppressed by the administration of intravenous anticonvulsants and by switching to another opioid.

Constipation

This is the most frequent and most uncomfortable side effect of opioids and, as mentioned above, tolerance does not develop. Therefore, with the onset of opioid therapy, measures should be instituted to ensure a regular bowel regimen by administering cathartics, stool softeners, and fluids to avoid constipation, which can lead to frank bowel obstruction.

Opioids also produce biliary spasm and urinary retention. These side effects should be considered when prescribing opioids to patients with pathologic changes involving these specific organs.

Nausea and Vomiting

Nausea and vomiting are common and highly disliked side effects of opioid therapy. Patients will refuse these analgesics if the emesis is not treated. This effect is potentiated by vestibular stimulation; ambulatory patients suffer more emesis than supine patients. Nausea and vomiting can be prevented or effectively treated. Nausea can be prevented by the concomitant use of hydroxyzine, by giving a reduced dose of opioids (74), or by the concomitant use of perchlorperazine or haloperidol. Transdermal scopolamine (Transderm Scōp), commonly used to prevent emesis associated with motion sickness, is also an effective treatment of opioid-induced nausea and vomiting (personal observation by C.B.). If the patient is vomiting the antiemetic drug should be given intramuscularly or rectally. Moreover, it might be desirable to switch to rectal administration of opioids (morphine and dihydromorphinone are available in suppository form). In patients for whom opioids are prescribed for home care, it is often advisable to issue a week's supply of an antiemetic drug to be used prophylactically to avoid nausea and vomiting.

Pruritus

Pruritus is mostly limited to the face, alae of the nose, the palate, and the torso. This side effect is much more evident with intraspinal opioids (66). Its mechanism of action is not known but it appears to be centrally mediated. It is controlled by small, carefully titrated doses of naloxone. Recent reports that nalbuphine, a mu antagonist–kappa agonist, reverses the pruritus caused by intraspinal morphine imply that this side effect is mu-mediated (75, 76).

Tolerance

Tolerance is a normal pharmacologic response to chronic opioid therapy. It is characterized by the development of decreasing analgesic effects and other actions of a drug. Tolerance develops at different rates for various effects. For example, tolerance to the analgesic and euphoric effects of morphine develops much more rapidly than tolerance to its constipating effects. Tolerance develops faster when opioids are administered intravenously or intramuscularly than when given orally or rectally.

The earliest sign of tolerance is the patient's complaint that the duration or degree of analgesia, or both, has decreased, although no increase is seen in the nociceptive input. This is treated by increasing the frequency or dose of the drug, or both. Although cross tolerance among opioids occurs it is not complete; therefore, switching to an alternative opioid often results in adequate pain relief. The alternative opioid is given in equianalgesic doses, the patient is carefully monitored, and the dose, time interval, or both, is either increased or reduced according to individual needs.

Physical Dependence

Physical dependence is another physiologic response to the pharmacologic effects of chronic opioid use. It is characterized by the development of the abstinence syndrome on abrupt withdrawal of the drug. The syndrome consists of yawning, lacrimation, frequent sneezing, agitation, tremors, insomnia, fever, tachycardia, and other signs of hyperexcitability of the sympathetic nervous system. The time of onset and the characteristics of the abstinence syndrome vary. It can be prevented by slowly tapering the dose of the opioid at a rate of 15 to 20% daily and it can be effectively treated by reinstituting the drug in doses of about 25 to 40% of the previous daily dose (77).

Severe Complications

Respiratory Depression

Provided that the opioid is titrated to achieve adequate pain relief, clinically significant respiratory depression usually does not occur, because pain is a powerful respiratory stimulant and counteracts the opioid-induced depression. On the other hand, this complication occurs if the drug is given in excessive doses or if adequate doses are administered too frequently. For example, severe depression can develop in debilitated patients who are given methadone too often with consequent rapid build-up of plasma levels and perhaps accumulation of metabolites that are not analgesic but that still depress medullary centers. Sudden deterioration of hepatic and renal functions decreases the elimination of an opioid and causes it to accumulate.

Respiratory depression or even arrest can occur in patients on opioid therapy who undergo a neurosurgical operation or nerve block that abruptly eliminates the pain and its respiratory stimulating effects. It is especially important to watch such patients closely during and after these procedures (77).

Mild respiratory depression can be terminated by reducing the drug dosage, whereas moderate or severe depression should be treated with naloxone given in doses of 0.1 to 0.4 mg IV. Because naloxone is a fast-but short-acting agent, repeated administration or an IV drip might be necessary to prevent severe respiratory depression or arrest from recurring in patients on long-acting opioids. For patients who have been on chronic opioid therapy it is important to administer the naloxone slowly, or it could precipitate severe withdrawal symptoms. Physicians should also be aware that naloxone has, on rare occasions, produced severe pulmonary edema (78).

Psychologic Dependence

Psychologic dependence, often referred to as addiction, is characterized by an abnormal behavior pattern of drug use, by craving of a drug for effects other than pain relief, by becoming overwhelmingly involved in the procurement and use of the drug, and by the tendency to relapse after withdrawal (79). Fear of addiction has been an important factor in the under-dosing of opioids in patients with cancer pain and other severe pain, but opioid addiction rarely occurs in patients receiving opioids for medical purposes. In a study of nearly 40,000 hospitalized medical patients who were monitored for psychologic dependence Porter and Jick (80) found that, among the nearly 12,000 patients who received one or more doses of opioids, only four cases of psychological dependence in patients who had no previous history of addiction were documented. In another study of cancer patients receiving chronic opioid therapy, Kanner and Foley (81) found that drug abuse and psychologic dependence did not occur in this population. These and other data suggest that the medical use of opioids is rarely associated with development of addiction. Moreover, in patients with severe pain caused by recurrent or metastatic advanced cancer who are likely to require opioid therapy until death, addiction and physical dependence should not be considered as criteria for not giving opioids in adequate doses. Therefore, patients with cancer pain who are to be managed with opioids should be given ample doses for effective pain relief for as long as necessary.

Pharmacokinetics and Pharmacodynamics

After IV injection or absorption into the vascular system, an opioid is immediately affected by plasma pH and by its propensity to bind to various circulating elements (e.g., red blood cells, plasma proteins). The substance must leave the plasma to trigger its pharmacologic action, diffuse into the tissues, and reach the receptors. Several factors favor movement of the drug to its sites of action: lower protein binding; lower ionization; and higher lipid solubility.

In plasma only the unbound and nonionized portion of the drug, the diffusible fraction, is free to leave the vasculature. The diffusible fraction determines the initial concentration gradient and therefore the rate of diffusion. The other factor in determining the rate of movement of the drug from plasma to tissues is lipid solubility. For rapid access to the CNS, an opioid must have both a high diffusible fraction in plasma and a high lipid solubility. Lipid solubility is an important property of intraspinal opioids, and influences their onset of action, duration, diffusion, and side effects (Chapter 95).

The product of the diffusible fraction and the lipid solubility of an opioid is known as the "diffusion potential" into the CNS. The ratio of the diffusion potential of an opioid compared to that of morphine is called the lipid diffusion index, or LDI. Thus, the LDI of morphine = 1, of meperidine = 14, and of fentanyl = 160.

After an IV bolus of fentanyl the opioid enters the brain rapidly because of its high diffusion potential. As the plasma concentration falls as a result of removal of the drug by tissues and biotransformation, the gradient reverses and fentanyl leaves the brain equally rapidly. Meperidine follows the same process of forward and then reverse transfer to and from the brain, but more slowly because of its lower diffusion potential. Morphine has the lowest diffusion potential of all the common opioids, resulting in considerable delay between IV morphine injection and development of maximal brain concentration (and onset of maximal effect). Morphine leaves plasma so slowly that biotransformation or elimination lowers plasma concentration and further decreases the "driving concentration" during the onset period, causing a further reduction in its rate of diffusion into the CNS. Because of its low lipid solubility, however, less drug is nonspecifically bound by brain lipids and less is needed in the CNS to exert the same effects. This low lipid solubility is responsible for a slow dynamic interaction between the plasma and the CNS. Once morphine has penetrated the CNS tissue the diffusion back to the plasma is slow. In 1979 Nishitateno (82) elegantly demonstrated that the plasma concentration of morphine does not parallel the brain concentration of the drug. As clearly demonstrated in Figure 78-2 (82), the brain concentration remains at higher levels compared to the decreasing plasma concentration over time.

Once a specific plasma concentration of opioid has been reached, the final effect is not equal for every individual. This varied response is best illustrated by considering the wide range that exists among patients in regard to the minimal effective analgesic concentration (MEAC) for each specific opioid. The MEAC is the minimal plasma level of an opioid that can control severe pain in a particular patient. For example, while a patient with a plasma concentration of meperidine (pethidine) of 410 ng/ml might still experience severe pain, the pain is relieved when a concentration of 460 ng/ml has been reached. Therefore, this is the MEAC for meperidine for that patient (44). Although the MEAC is fairly consistent for each individual patient (Mather et al. [42] found at most a twofold

TABLE 78-6. Minimum Effective Analgesic Plasma Concentrations (Median)

Analgesic	Minimum Effective Analgesic Concentration (MEAC), ng/ml, mean ± SD (range)
Hydrocodone	6
Ketobemidone	25 ± 11
(n = 15)	(10–51)
Morphine	16 ± 9
(n = 10)	(6–33)
Pethidine	455 ± 174
(n = 20)	(94–754)
Fentanyl	1
Alfentanil	10

From Lehmann, K.A.: The pharmacokinetics of opioid analgesics, with special reference to patient-controlled administration. *In* Patient-Controlled Analgesia. Edited by M. Harmer, M. Rosen, and M.D. Vickers. Oxford, Blackwell Scientific Publications, 1985, pp. 18–29.

intrasubject variation), a great intersubject variation has been noted. Austin and colleagues (44) found that, in six patients, the intersubject MEAC varied from 270 to 700 ng/ml for meperidine, while Tamsen et al. (83) found a similar variation, ranging from 94 to 754 ng/ml. In practical terms this represents an eightfold difference in intersubject requirements for meperidine, confirming empiric clinical observations of a seven- to eightfold difference in opioid requirements. Morphine has a mean MEAC of 16 ng/ml, with a range of 6 to 33 ng/ml (Table 78-6) (84). Thus, it is clear that the optimal control of pain is achieved by maintaining the plasma concentration of the opioid at a constant value just above the MEAC for specific patients. All this underscores the necessity of individualizing opioid dosage according to the responses and needs of individual patients.

Specific Opioids

Opioids have been classified in different ways (Table 78-7). One system subdivides them into weak opioids with low addiction potential and stronger opioids with higher addiction potential. Another system considers opioids for their agonist, partial agonist, and agonist-antagonist activities. Opioids can also be divided into naturally occurring, semisynthetic, and synthetic groups. The naturally occurring opioids are the alkaloids of opium, and are comprised of two chemical classes. Those of one class contain the three-ringed phenanthrene nucleus and include morphine, codeine, and thebaine. The other class consists of the benzylisoquinoline alkaloids, which lack any analgesic activity; examples of this group are papaverine and noscapine. The semisynthetic opioids are obtained by simple modification of a naturally occurring alkaloid; for instance, heroin is derived from morphine and etorphine is synthesized from thebaine. Synthetic opioids contain the phenanthrene nucleus of morphine but are completely synthesized. The synthetic opioids are further subdivided into several groups based on their chemical structure (e.g., morphinans, phenylheptylamines, phenylpiperidines).

The most useful opioids are described in some detail in this section. Tables 78-2 and 78-3 contain data for

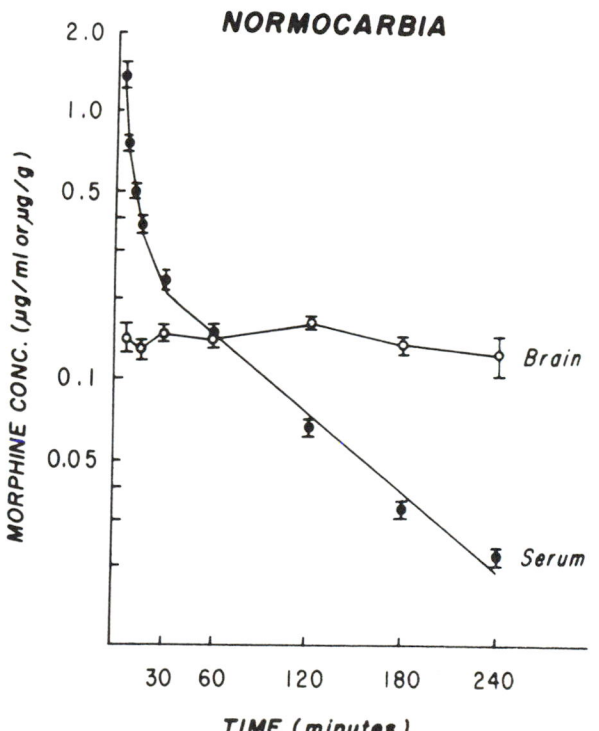

FIG. 78-2. Serum and brain decrement curves in normocarbic dogs showing relationship of brain morphine concentration to that in serum. Note intersections of serum and brain morphine decrement curves at approximately 1 hour. (*Vertical bars*, SE; n = 7.) From Nishitateno, K., et al.: Pharmacokinetics of morphine: Concentrations in the serum and brain of the dog during hyperventilation. Anesthesiology, *50*:520, 1979.

TABLE 78-7. Different Classification Systems for Opioids

Weak or Strong Opioids	Opium and its Derivatives	Agonists and Antagonists
Weak	Natural opium alkaloids	Agonists
Codeine	Phenanthrene derivatives	Alfentanil
Propoxyphene (Darvon)	Morphine	Aphaprodine
	Codeine	Codeine
Strong	Thebaine (nonanalgesic)	Diacetylmorphine
Alfentanil (Alfenta)		Dihydromorphinone
Alphaprodine (Nisentil)	Benylisoquinoline derivatives	Dihydrohydroxymorphinone
Buprenorphine (Bupronex, Temgesic)	(nonanalgesic)	Etorphine
Butorphanol (Stadol, Dorphanol)	Papaverine	Fentanyl
Cholecystokinin	Noscapine	Levorphanol
Diacetylmorphine (heroin)		Meperidine
Dihydromorphinone, hydromorphone (Dilaudid)	Semisynthetic derivatives of	Methadone
Dihydrohydroxymorphinone, oxymorphone	opium alkaloids	Morphine
(Numorphan)		Oxycodone
Etorphine	Morphine derivatives	Propoxyphene
Fentanyl (Sublimaze)	Diacetylmorphine	Sufentanil
Levorphanol (Levo-Dromoran)	Dihydromorphinone	
Meperidine (Demerol)	Dihydrohydroxymorphinone	Partial agonists, agonist-antagonists
Methadone (Dolophine)		Buprenorphine
Morphine	Thebaine derivatives	Butorphanol
Nalbuphine (Nubain)	Buprenorphine	Nalbuphine
Naloxone (Narcan)	Oxycodone	Pentazocine
Naltrexone (Trexan)		
Oxycodone (Percocet, Tylox)	Synthetic compounds	Antagonists
Pentazocine (Talwin)	Morphinans	Cholecystokinin
Sufentanil (Sufenta)	Levorphanol	Naloxone
	Nalbuphine	Naltrexone
	Naloxone	
	Naltrexone	
	Phenylheptylamines	
	Methadone	
	Propoxyphene	
	Phenylpiperidine	
	Alfentanil	
	Alphaprodine	
	Fentanyl	
	Meperidine	
	Sufentanil	

comparison. As mentioned several times, because of great intersubject variability, the dosages indicated after each drug are only given for orientation and represent the average dose required to control moderate to severe pain in adult patients. In the clinical setting the dose for each individual must be titrated with regard to amount, frequency, and the specific need for adequate pain control.

Agonist Opioids

The binding of an agonist to stereospecific receptors causes its pharmacologic effects. Agonist opioids include morphine, codeine, meperidine, dihydromorphinone, and methadone.

Naturally Occurring Opium Alkaloids

MORPHINE. Morphine is the reference standard for all the potent opioid analgesics. It is generally administered by the IM or IV route for the treatment of acute severe pain in which a definite end to the episode is anticipated. Oral preparations diluted in fluid are available and have been used widely for the relief of cancer pain.

The newly developed controlled-release preparation MS Contin offers great advantages for long-term therapy in patients with terminal cancer pain because it provides constant plasma levels for long periods of time. The dose must be adjusted because tolerance develops and the possible increase in nociceptive input from spreading cancer increases requirements. Side effects associated with the use of morphine have been noted above. Tolerance and physical dependence develop when this drug is given for a period of several weeks to months. In conclusion, morphine remains the major drug used for the treatment of acute pain and of advanced or terminal cancer pain (Chapter 24). Since 1979 morphine has been used extensively by the intraspinal route to induce intensive and prolonged analgesia (Chapter 95).

CODEINE. Except for aspirin, codeine is probably the most widely used analgesic and the most commonly used prescription opioid in the world. This is because of its high oral efficacy and its low incidence and degree of physical dependence in most of those given the drug for prolonged periods. Tolerance can develop, necessitating an increase in dosage, frequency of administration, or both. Its mechanism of action is similar to that of all opioids and its side effects are similar but less intense. These include nausea, vomiting, sedation, dizziness, and constipation. Addition of a NSAID produces increased analgesic activity, which makes codeine even more useful in the clinical setting. The major disadvantage of the use of codeine is that it is not as effective in treating severe pain, so stronger opioids must be used in such cases.

Partially Synthetic Morphine Derivatives

DIHYDROMORPHINONE. Hydromorphone (Dilaudid) is a semisynthetic derivative of morphine that is approximately 6 to 8 times as potent; compared to 10 mg of morphine its equianalgesic dose is 1.5 mg. It is easily absorbed by the gastrointestinal tract and is thus effective after oral and rectal administration. The analgesic effect appears approximately 15 minutes after parenteral administration and 30 minutes after oral administration. Because this drug induces fewer bothersome side effects than morphine it is often preferred by patients, and it is more likely to produce psychologic dependence.

DIHYDROHYDROXYMORPHINONE. Also called oxymorphone (Numorphan), this parenteral opioid has a potency 7 to 10 times that of morphine and pharmacologic effects quite similar to those of morphine. A rectal suppository preparation containing 5 mg of oxymorphone is available.

DIACETYLMORPHINE. Diacetylmorphine—heroin—is not available for clinical use in the United States. It is used in many other parts of the world, however, especially for the treatment of terminal cancer pain. Intramuscular heroin is approximately twice as potent as morphine. It has a slightly faster onset of action but shorter duration than morphine (85). Heroin is readily absorbed by the oral, nasal, and gastrointestinal routes. Oral heroin is rapidly metabolized to morphine during its first pass through the liver, i.e., before it enters the CNS, in which its pharmacologic effects are mediated. Therefore, equal milligram doses of morphine produce slightly higher blood morphine levels than heroin (86). Several studies have failed to show the advantage of the use of this drug over morphine when used at equipotent dosages, by oral or other routes (87).

Synthetic Compounds

Synthetic opioids include morphinan (used clinically as levorphanol), phenylheptylamines, which include methadone and propoxyphene, and phenylpiperidines, which include meperidine, alphaprodine, and fentanyl.

LEVORPHANOL. Levorphanol (Levo-Dromoran) is a synthetic opioid with a potency approximately four times that of morphine. Its side effects and mechanism of action are similar to those of morphine, but perhaps with less nausea and vomiting. It is quite ineffective when given orally and is usually not used by this route.

METHADONE. Methadone (Dolophine) is a synthetic opioid that is slightly more potent but less dependence-producing than morphine. Methadone produces less euphoria and less sedation than many other opioids. The central mechanism of action is similar to that of morphine. It is well absorbed when taken orally so it is of little advantage to administer it parenterally. Methadone has a long half-life and consequently a longer duration of action than any of the aforementioned opioids, which makes it ideal for long-term administration. Therefore, it is commonly used in addiction rehabilitation programs and is useful in managing pain problems that require prolonged treatment with opioids. Its longer duration of action occurs primarily because most of the drug is protein-bound and slowly released. To reach a steady state, however, it must be administered for several days. During the first 2 to 3 days, therefore, methadone should be given every 4 to 6 hours and thereafter every 6, 12, and even 24 hours. The range of dosage and frequency varies according to the severity of the pain and the patient's tolerance. Oral doses of 5 to 10 mg q6h or q8h are often prescribed. Doses of up to 20 to 30 mg q4h have been given, however, without ill effects in terminal cancer patients.

Its efficacy has been proven in the management of terminal cancer patients with pain, and it has been given for up to 2 years without any significant abuse manifestation. Less clear are indications for its long-term use in chronic nonmalignant pain problems; in general, long-term opioid administration should be avoided in such cases. Patients with chronic pain, though, such as low back pain, with cyclic variations of intensity and severe time-limited bouts of pain, can certainly be treated with methadone (or with any other long-acting opioid) on a recurrent basis.

PROPOXYPHENE. Propoxyphene (Darvon) was first introduced with the premise that it had the same analgesic potential as codeine but without the dependence liability or side effects. Several clinical trials have shown, however, that 90 to 120 mg orally is equipotent to 60 mg of codeine and doses of 60 mg are no more effective than 600 mg of aspirin. Doses of 32 mg or lower are no more efficacious than placebo (88). From clinical experience propoxyphene appears to have an abuse potential but it is not certain whether this is physiologic or psychologic. It is often compounded with other medications, such as acetylsalicylic acid or acetaminophen. Unless the drug has been used at high dosages, such as 800 to 1200 mg per day, it is not clear that withdrawal reactions ensue after abrupt cessation of the drug. Thus, propoxyphene appears to be less effective as an analgesic than codeine and has enjoyed some popularity because of its alleged lower dependence potential, a property not observed in practice. In addition to being less potent, its higher cost should discourage clinicians from prescribing it as a substitute for codeine.

MEPERIDINE. Meperidine (pethidine; Demerol) is a synthetic phenylpiperidine opioid analgesic often used interchangeably with morphine. It produces less smooth muscle contraction than morphine (65). In equianalgesic doses it appears to have the same central side effects and its mechanism of action appears to be the same. Meperidine is absorbed by the gastrointestinal tract but the oral dose is about 50% less effective than when given intramuscularly. Its major disadvantage is that its duration of action is shorter than morphine, a factor often overlooked by physicians. The drug is usually given every 4 to 6 hours; this produces unacceptable analgesia, especially in the postoperative period. Chronic administration of meperidine has been associated with seizures caused by accumulation of its metabolite, normeperidine, which lowers the seizure threshold and causes CNS hyperirritability. Meperidine given at a dose of 15 to 25 mg IV prevents or controls the shivering associated with volatile anesthetics, subarachnoid or epidural block, and chemotherapy.

ALPHAPRODINE. Alphaprodine (Nisentil) is another derivative of phenylpiperidine and is similar to meperidine but approximately twice as potent as an analgesic, with an even shorter duration of action. Because of this latter property it has been used frequently for analgesia during the early phases of labor when epidural block is not available to the patient. It is no longer available in the United States.

FENTANYL. Fentanyl is a synthetic opioid related to phenylpiperidine. It is approximately 80 to 100 times as potent as morphine. It is generally used for anesthesia in combination with other anesthetic agents. Recently it has been found to be effective for the management of acute pain, such as postoperative and traumatic pain, when administered transdermally (89) and epidurally (90). Because it is highly lipophilic, fentanyl does not accumulate in the cerebrospinal fluid, and intraspinal fentanyl has not been reported to induce respiratory depression (Chapter 95).

Theoretically, the new drug sufentanil, which is 5 to 10 times as potent as fentanyl, and alfentanil, which is about 10 times less potent than fentanyl, should offer even greater advantages over this opioid when given intraspinally because of their higher lipophilic properties.

Agonist-Antagonist Derivatives

Agonist-antagonist opioids are less efficacious than the pure agonists but they can produce analgesia with less respiratory depression and have a lower abuse potential. A ceiling effect on respiratory depression as well as on analgesia has been noted with this class of opioids. Recently, in an attempt to isolate a drug with high analgesic activity and a low incidence of side effects, several drugs with agonist-antagonist activity, or with partial agonistic activity, have been introduced to clinical practice.

BUPRENORPHINE. Buprenorphine (Buprenex; Temgesic) is a semisynthetic derivative of thebaine; it is highly lipophilic and binds strongly to the mu-class opiate receptor. Buprenorphine is about 20 to 30 times more potent than morphine when given intramuscularly, and therefore its equianalgesic dose is 0.3 mg. It is easily absorbed from the oral mucosa and a sublingual preparation has been developed and is used in most parts of the world. Buprenorphine produces its analgesic effect 45 to 60 minutes after parenteral administration. Its duration of action varies from 3 to 14 hours after a single dose. Data from over 9000 patients indicate that the mean duration of action is a little over 8 hours (91). The drug has proved effective in postoperative (92) and myocardial infarction pain,

pain of neoplastic and orthopedic origin, labor pain, and as an adjunct to anesthesia. The side effects are similar to those of morphine, but euphoria seems to be less frequent while sedation is more evident (91).

Chronic pain patients were given sublingual buprenorphine for several months without the need to increase the dosage, indicating that the development of tolerance to its analgesic effect might be slower than with other opioids (93). Some patients chose to discontinue the drug because of side effects, especially sedation and nausea, rather than failure to obtain analgesia. Abrupt withdrawal of buprenorphine in dependent patients causes a mild to moderate abstinence syndrome that is much less severe than after morphine withdrawal. The abstinence syndrome peaks approximately 2 weeks after discontinuation of buprenorphine and lasts for over 1 week.

The side effects are mostly sedation, nausea and vomiting, constipation, diaphoresis, and some respiratory depression. Patients using other opioids should not be abruptly switched to buprenorphine because this could precipitate an abstinence syndrome.

BUTORPHANOL. Butorphanol (Stadol; Dorphanol) is a morphinan with characteristics similar to those of pentazocine but with greater analgesic efficacy and fewer side effects. Its parenteral use is associated with significant sedation even though patients remain responsive (9). It produces approximately 50% less nausea and vomiting than morphine, and side effects such as constipation and urinary retention are less frequent after chronic administration than with morphine if used at therapeutic doses. This drug has been available for over 10 years and few cases of drug abuse have been reported. A transnasal preparation of the drug has been developed for the treatment of acute pain (94).

NALBUPHINE. Nalbuphine (Nubain) is an analgesic derivative of the agonist oxymorphone and the antagonist naloxone. It apparently is a kappa and sigma agonist and a moderately potent mu antagonist. Nalbuphine is well absorbed after oral, intramuscular, or subcutaneous administration, but the oral form is not presently marketed. The analgesic effect after intramuscular administration appears after 45 to 60 minutes and has a duration of action slightly longer than that of morphine. When used in equipotent dosage the respiratory depression is similar to that produced by morphine. No further increase in respiratory depression has been noted with doses of nalbuphine above 30 mg (9).

The drug has been successfully used in the management of cancer patients and seems to act like morphine (95). Euphoria is observed after administration of 8 mg of nalbuphine IM and dysphoria and psychotomimetic reactions are not problematic until 70 mg have been given. A primary side effect is sedation, which is similar to that induced by butorphanol. The plasma half-life of nalbuphine is approximately 5 hours and it is metabolized mainly in the liver. Tolerance and physical dependence have been described. High doses of the drug tend to produce irritability, inability to concentrate, depression, and headaches after approximately 1 week. Because nalbuphine is a mu antagonist it can precipitate an abstinence syndrome in patients taking large doses of morphine over time; therefore these patients should not be switched to nalbuphine abruptly.

PENTAZOCINE. Pentazocine (Talwin) is a benzomorphine derivative that has both opioid agonist and antagonist properties. It was first introduced with the claim that it was an effective opioid with no dependence potential. Its mechanism of action is similar to that of other opioids, and it has the advantage that it can be administered both parenterally and orally. Pentazocine has the same side effects as other opioids, including respiratory depression, somnolence, decreased cough reflex, nausea and, in many patients, unpleasant hallucinations. Abrupt discontinuation of the drug after prolonged use causes a severe abstinence syndrome that is often worse than that caused by morphine or other opioids (96).

Another problem is that some physicians administer opioids on a rotating weekly basis, using three or four different opioids alternately, mistakenly assuming that this decreases the possibility and incidence of dependence and tolerance. The alternate use of an agonist with an agonist-antagonist can cause severe problems, both in the management of pain and in the appearance of abstinence symptoms. The use of pentazocine after a pure agonist can reverse the analgesic effect by its antagonistic action.

Opioid Antagonists

In 1915 Pohl produced the first opioid antagonist by making a minor change in the structure of the codeine molecule (66). Minor changes of other opioid agonists have produced substances that bind to one or more opioid receptor and have no pharmacologic effect. These can displace or, more probably, replace an opioid agonist from the receptor, therefore reducing or abolishing the pharmacologic effect caused by the opioid agonist in a dose-dependent fashion. Naloxone, the (N-allyl) derivative of oxymorphone, and naltrexone are two opioid antagonists. They both have a high affinity for mu receptors but can also interact with delta and kappa receptors to some degree. High doses of naloxone must be used to antagonize the effect of delta and kappa ligands.

NALOXONE. Naloxone is often used to reverse the respiratory depression induced by an overdose of opioids. It is administered IV at a dose of 1 to 5 μg/kg. The effect is rapid and the respiratory depression is promptly corrected. IV naloxone, carefully titrated, is often used after administration of intraspinal opioids to abolish unwanted side effects such as pruritus, urinary retention, nausea, and vomiting without significantly affecting the analgesics (Chapter 95). If used judiciously it does not cause significant reversal of the analgesia. Naloxone is a short-acting medication (30 to 45 minutes) and supplemental doses might be needed in patients with respiratory depression induced by long-acting opioids. Intramuscular injections of twice the initial IV dose can provide therapeutic plasma levels of longer duration (97). Alternatively, a continuous infusion of 5 μg/kg/hour of naloxone can be used for long-term treatment of respiratory depression, such as that induced by a high dose of intraspinal opioid.

A rapid injection of IV naloxone can cause nausea and vomiting, which can be mostly prevented by giving the therapeutic dose over 2 or 3 minutes. Cardiovascular stimulation has occurred following administration of opioid antagonists. Tachycardia, hypertension, pulmonary edema, and cardiac dysrhythmia up to ventricular fibrillation have occurred following the administration of naloxone. These effects are attributed to a sudden increase in sympathetic nervous system activity.

NALTREXONE. Naltrexone also acts predominantly as a mu antagonist. In contrast to naloxone, however, it is quite active after oral administration, and its effect is sustained for up to 24 hours (19).

CHOLECYSTOKININ. The duodenal mucosa secretes an octapeptide, cholecystokinin, which increases the contractility of the gallbladder and relaxes the sphincter of Oddi. When administered in the central nervous system it antagonizes the analgesic effect of opioids. It has been suggested that cholecystokinin might be an endogenous opioid antagonist. This hypothesis is further substantiated by the fact that proglumide, a cholecystokinin antagonist, potentiates opioid analgesia in animals (98).

Analgesic Combinations

Several combinations of opioids and NSAIDs are manufactured. Codeine has been combined with aspirin or acetaminophen. Percodan and Percocet contain oxycodone plus aspirin and acetaminophen, respectively. Oxycodone is a semisynthetic codeine analogue derived from the opium alkaloid thebaine. It is only available in the United States as part of one of the above-mentioned combinations. Oxycodone is effective orally. Its analgesic action and dependence liability are greater than those of codeine on a milligram-to-milligram basis.

Analgesic combinations are effective in relieving moderate pain but can cause problems because of their dependence-producing potential. They are often prescribed too freely and for too long by unwary physicians for the relief of nonmalignant chronic pain. As a consequence they can cause both psychologic and physical dependence that are often difficult to correct without treatment at a detoxification center.

The combination of opioids and anxiolytics or amphetamines has been shown to increase analgesic effects while decreasing some side effects of opioids. Hydroxyzine, 25 to 100 mg PO or IM, increases the analgesic effect of morphine by at least 50% and decreases the anxiety associated with acute pain. The antiemetic action decreases the incidence of and can abolish the nausea and vomiting induced by opioids. At high doses this drug can produce sedation and dryness of the mouth (74).

Dextroamphetamine in a dose of 5 to 10 mg, especially given in the morning (it can cause insomnia when used later in the day), increases the analgesic effect of morphine by 50 to 100% and decreases the respiratory depression and sedation induced by opioids. It has been used advantageously both for postoperative pain control (73) and for prolonged treatment of terminal cancer pain (1). It should be used with caution in patients with known cardiac problems and urinary retention, however, because it can aggravate these conditions.

C. NONOPIOID (NON-NARCOTIC) ANALGESICS

The nonopioid analgesics discussed here are phenacetin and a large group of compounds generally referred to as nonsteroidal anti-inflammatory drugs (NSAIDs). They are usually considered to be peripherally acting analgesics (16, 99) but have various clinical effects, including not only analgesic but also antipyretic and anti-inflammatory actions (100, 101) (Tables 78-8 and 78-9).

A peculiar finding related to the clinical use of all NSAIDs is the unpredictable individual variation in response (26). Rheumatologists are aware of this and institute therapeutic trials on all patients to determine the most effective agent on an individual basis. The differences in response seem to be associated with the body's reaction to a particular disease state. The metabolic pathway stimulated can be significantly

TABLE 78-8. Classification, Pharmacokinetics, and Pharmacology of Nonopioid Analgesics

Class; generic name; proprietary name	Dosage (in mg, PO)	Pharmacologic Properties			Therapeutic Effects		
		Peak Effect (h)	Duration (h)	Half-Life (h)	Analgesic	Anti-inflammatory	Anti-pyretic
Salicylates							
Acetylsalicylic acid, aspirin	325–1,000 q4–6h	2	4–6	0.25	+ + +	+ + +	+ + +
Choline salicylate (Trilisate)	870–1,740 q3–4h	0.5–1	>12	(2–30 for salicylate met)	+ + +	+ + +	+ + +
Diflunisal (Dolobid; Dolobis)	200–500 q12h	1–2	12+	8–20	+ + +	+ +	+
Para-aminophenols							
Acetaminophen, paracetamol (Tylenol; Datril; Panadol)	325–1,000 q4–6h	0.5–1	4–6	1–4	+ + +	0	+ + +
Indoleacetic acid derivatives							
Indomethacin (Indocid; Indocin; Indomethine)	25–75 q6h	2	6–8	2–3	+ + +	+ + +	+ + +
Sulindac (Clinoril; Arthrobid)	150–200 q12h	1–2	12	7–18	+ + +	+ + +	+ + +
Zomepirac (Zomax)	100 q6h		4–6		+ + +	+	+ +
Pyrazole derivatives							
Phenylbutazone (Butazolidin; Antadol; Phebuzine)	100–200 q6h	2	6–8	50–100	+ +	+ + + +	+ +
Oxyphenbutazone (Tanderil; Rapostan, Rheumapax; Oxalid; Tandearil)	100–200 q6h	2		Days	+ +	+ + +	+ +
Azapropazone (Apazone; Rheumox)	600 q8–12h	2		Days	+ +	+ + +	+ +
Fenmates							
Mefanamic acid (Ponstel; Ponstan; Ponstil; Namphen)	500 q6–8h	2		3–4	+ +	+ +	+
Pyrroleacetic acid derivatives							
Tolmetin (Tolectin)	200–400 q6–8h	0.5–1		1–3	+ +	+ + +	+ +
Propionic acid derivatives							
Ibuprofen (Motrin; Advil; Nuprin; Brufen)	200–800 q8–12h	1–2	4–6	2	+ + +	+ + +	+ +
Neproxin (Naprosyn; Naprosine; Naprnx; Proxen)	250–500 q8–12h	2	8–12	12–15	+ + +	+ + +	+ +
Fenoprofen (Nalfon; Fenopran; Nalgesic; Progesic)	300–600 q6–8h	2			+ +	+ + +	+
Ketoprofen (Orudis; Alrheumat)	50–100 q6–8h	1–2	6	1–35*	+ +	+ + +	+
Suprofen (Suprol)	200 q4–6h	0.5–1	4	2	+ + +	+ +	+
Benzothiazine derivatives							
Piroxican (Feldene)	20 q12–24h	2–4	24+	45	+ + +	+ + +	+
Phenothiazines							
Methotrimeprazine (Levoprome; Nozinan; Neozine; Nirvan)	10–20 q4–6h	0.5–1.5	4	15–30	+ + +	0	0

*0 no effect; + minimal effect; + + moderate effect; + + + strong effect; + + + + maximum effect.

TABLE 78-9. Adverse (Toxic) and Other Physiologic Effects of Nonopioid Analgesics

Class; Generic Name	Gastrointestinal System		Hemopoiesis	Renal toxicity	Hepatic toxicity	Allergy	Hypersensitivity	CNS Side effects
	Dyspepsia	Bleeding						
Salicylates								
Acetylsalicylic acid	+ + +	+ + +	Platelet cohesiveness	+	+ +	+ + +	+ + +	Tinnitus in overdose
Choline salicylate	+	+	Little effect in clinical doses	+	+ +	+ + +	+ + +	Tinnitus in overdose
Diflunisal	+	0	Platelets	+ +	+ + +	+		0
Para-aminophenols								
Acetaminophen	0	0	Little effect	+ +	+ + +	0	0	
Indoleacetic acid derivatives								
Indomethacin	+ + +	+ +	Platelets (pancytopenia)	+ +	+ +	+	+ +	Headache, psychosis
Sulindac	+ +	+	Platelet function	+	+	+ +	+	Psychosis headache
Zomepirac	+	+	Little	+	+	+ + + +	+ + +	Drowsiness, headache
Pyrazole derivatives								
Phenylbutazone	+ + +	+ + +	Aplastic anemia	+ +	+ +	+	+ + +	Vertigo, insomnia, blurred vision, euphoria
Oxyphenbutazone	+ +	+ +	Marrow depression	+ +	+ +	+	+ + +	Mild
Azapropazone	+ +	+ +	Marrow depression	+	+	+	+ +	Minimal
Fenamates								
Mefanamic acid	+ + +	+ +	Hemolytic anemia	+ +	+	+	+	Headache, dizziness
Pyrroleacetic acid derivatives								
Tolmetin	+ + +	+ +	Platelet cohesiveness	+	+	+	+	Nervousness, insomnia, drowsiness
Propionic acid derivatives								
Ibuprofen	+ +	+	Platelet cohesiveness	+	+	+	+	Headache, dizziness, toxic amblyopia
Naproxin	+ + +	+ +	Platelet cohesiveness	+	+	+	+	Drowsiness, headache, dizziness, fatigue, toxicity
Fenoprofen	+	+	Platelet cohesiveness	+	+	+	+ +	Tinnitus, dizziness, lassitude
Ketoprofen	+	+	Platelet cohesiveness	+	+ +	+	+	Headache, dizziness, drowsiness
Suprofen	+ +	+	Platelet cohesiveness	+	+	+	+	Headache, dizziness, drowsiness, depression
Benzothiazine derivatives								
Piroxicam	+ +	+	Platelet cohesiveness; anemia	+	+	+	+	Insomnia
Phenothiazines								
Methotrimeprazine	+ +	0	Agranulocytosis with long use	0	0	+	+	Significant sedation and amnesia, confusion in elderly

*0 no effect; + minimal effect; + + moderate effect; + + + strong effect; + + + + maximum effect.

different in patients diagnosed as having the same problem, such as rheumatoid arthritis (102).

General Principles of Pharmacology
Mechanism of Analgesic Action

NSAIDs have both central and peripheral sites of action in the body (16, 99–101). It seems that the analgesic effect is a peripheral one that acts primarily on the synthesis of prostaglandins at the site of inflammation (102). The antipyretic effects are thought to be caused by a central mechanism, again possibly as a result of inhibition of prostaglandin synthesis. This rather vague invocation of prostaglandin synthesis inhibition does not consider the complicated mechanisms of prostaglandin production and release from damaged tissues, nor does it consider the different actions of separate types of prostaglandins, both centrally and peripherally.

The inflammatory response at the cellular and subcellular levels is responsible for the production of prostaglandins. With cell wall breakdown, primarily of white cells leaking from capillaries in response to the inflammatory stimulus, arachidonic acid is released. Prostaglandin synthetase acts on this compound to produce a cascade of compounds that end in various forms of prostaglandins. Prostaglandin E_2 stimulates nociceptors, either directly or by sensitizing them to the action of other algogenic agents such as bradykinin, which is released from the interior of the cells at the time of membrane rupture (as above).

Early evidence showed that the analgesic action of aspirin-like agents was at least partly a result of their ability to inhibit prostaglandin synthesis (103). It is now known that the specific activity of NSAIDs on the arachidonic acid cascade is at the initial stage of production of prostaglandin precursors (Fig. 4-1). The enzyme cyclo-oxygenase, which is necessary for this conversion, is antagonized by all classes of drugs with anti-inflammatory effects, including NSAIDs (17). Other activities at a peripheral level have not been demonstrated.

Much new research has been done on the presence of arachidonic acid metabolites in the central nervous system of mammals. Despite much conjecture, the precise role of the prostaglandins in normal and pathologic central functions has not been clarified. On a basic level, it was found that prostaglandins of the D and E series potentiate opioids centrally while those of the F series inhibit this action (101). This mechanism occurs through facilitation of brain serotonergic activity by prostaglandins of the E and D series and through attenuation of this activity by those of the F series. It appears that the effect of NSAIDs on central pain depends on their relative impact on various types of prostaglandins. This information is also significant in assessing the effects of combinations of NSAIDs and opioids.

Other Effects

Of primary interest is the antipyretic effect produced by all these agents through an interaction, not yet well detailed, with prostaglandin systems in the CNS (100). Historically, the early nonopioid analgesics were developed as antipyretics, with analgesia being discovered as a side effect. Many NSAIDs are not approved for sale as analgesics or antipyretics but are marketed because of their anti-inflammatory properties. Their interaction with the prostaglandin system as described above is responsible for this effect. Because acetaminophen lacks this anti-inflammatory property it cannot be included in the category of NSAIDs.

Fluid Retention and Vasodilation

NSAIDs can cause fluid retention that is usually mild. It can be significant, however, in those with an altered cardiac reserve, who might show signs of cardiac failure with continued use (104).

Some mild vasodilation can be seen with high doses of nonopioid analgesics but is rarely significant (104).

Allergy and Hypersensitivity

Other than acetaminophen, NSAIDs can all be allergenic. Severe manifestations, including anaphylaxis, have occurred with the use of some agents (104). Cross sensitivity can occur with this allergenic response,

and a careful history of allergy to aspirin or to other NSAIDs should be obtained before administration of these medications.

Renal Dysfunction

All NSAIDs have a variable propensity for producing papillary necrosis, and can cause renal failure. Many nonopioid analgesics should not be used, or should be used with extreme caution, in individuals who have a history of decreased renal reserve. The syndrome of analgesic nephropathy initially ascribed to phenacetin is also seen with many of the newer agents (105).

Gastric Irritation

Peptic ulcer and gastric bleeding have been variously reported with the use of most NSAIDs. The ulcers and bleeding can be a result of direct irritation of the gastric mucosa by the drugs when taken orally, which allows further tissue erosion by gastric secretions. An indirect effect can be seen with oral administration but also after administration by other routes. The inhibition of prostaglandin synthesis affects prostaglandins produced in the stomach. These inhibit gastric acid production and promote production of an acid-resistant mucosal coating. By stopping this process the gastric mucosa is more prone to acid damage (106).

Coagulation

Inhibition of platelet aggregation is another effect produced by most nonopioid analgesics. Aspirin causes the most such inhibition of all drugs of this class. Prolonged bleeding times are seen and their use immediately prior to trauma and surgery might cause some coagulation problems. On the other hand, there is now evidence that aspirin-induced inhibition of platelet aggregation decreases the risk of coronary thrombosis.

Hepatic Dysfunction

Mild abnormalities of hepatic function can occur but are usually not significant. Some caution must be used in their prescription to those with a history of hepatic dysfunction. Overdose can lead to frank liver failure, especially with phenacetin and acetaminophen.

Uricosuria

Most NSAIDs increase the urinary excretion of urates and many, such as salicylates, have been used to treat acute and chronic gout. This effect is dose-dependent, with low doses actually inhibiting urate excretion and high doses being necessary for gout treatment.

Central Nervous System

Many NSAIDs cause CNS side effects, including headache, dizziness, and confusion. These can be severe enough to cause patients, especially the elderly, to discontinue treatment.

Tocolytic Properties

Prostaglandins of the E and F series seem to be necessary for the uterus to initiate labor and potentiate uterine contractile forces. It is thought that inhibition of prostaglandin products can postpone labor in both animals and humans, as well as prolong its course (107).

Pharmacokinetics and Pharmacodynamics

Absorption

All NSAIDs and acetaminophen are readily absorbed from the upper intestinal tract and are generally given as oral preparations. Some absorption can also occur from the stomach, particularly if the pH is low. These drugs are also absorbed through any mucous membrane, so acetaminophen, aspirin, and many other NSAIDs can be given in suppository form, although this is done primarily for their antipyretic effect with acetaminophen and aspirin. The plasma concentration following oral administration reflects adequate oral dosage within 30 minutes and reaches a peak in approximately 2 hours. It gradually declines thereafter, depending on the half-life of the agent.

Because these drugs generally irritate the gastric mucosa, various formulations have been devised to reduce this side effect (see above).

Biotransformation

The nonopioid analgesics generally are strongly plasma protein bound (16). They are metabolized primarily through hepatic conjugation to sulfuric or glucuronic compounds that return to the plasma. Small amounts of drug can be conjugated in other body tissues as well, but these amounts are insignificant.

Distribution

The nonopioid analgesics are rapidly distributed throughout all body tissues and cell membranes by a passive process. Because they are highly plasma protein bound, the plasma concentrations are much higher than in other tissues. They bypass the blood-brain barrier, and leave the CNS by passive transport and also by active transport across the choroid plexus.

Excretion

All nonopioid analgesics are excreted primarily in the urine. They appear both in the free form and in conjugated form in the liver. The relative concentrations of the free and conjugated forms vary with the pH of the urine, with higher concentrations of the acidic agents being found in alkalinized urine. Small amounts of these drugs are found in the bile and thus pass into the intestine to be excreted in the feces.

Pharmacology of Individual Drugs

Salicylates

Aspirin

Aspirin is reviewed in detail here as the prototypic compound, but individual characteristics of other drugs of this class are also discussed. Tables 78-8 and 78-9 outline their classification, pharmacokinetics, pharmacology, and adverse effects.

PHARMACOLOGY. Aspirin is probably the most widely used analgesic. It has strong antipyretic and anti-inflammatory properties in addition to its analgesic effects. These are all based on central and peripheral inhibition of prostaglandin production. The analgesic effect is primarily a peripheral effect caused by a decrease in inflammation, although a central action has also been noted. Analgesia is most effective for mild to moderate pain arising from integumental structures rather than from the viscera. Aspirin is also effective in relieving moderate to severe bone pain.

Aspirin is absorbed rapidly from the stomach and upper small intestine when taken orally, with peak plasma levels being reached in about 2 hours, gradually declining thereafter. This compound is distributed throughout most body tissues by a passive process. Metabolism occurs primarily in the liver and excretion is through the kidneys and the feces in conjugated forms. The plasma half-life for aspirin is approximately 15 minutes. For salicylate, one of its metabolites, it is 2 to 3 hours for low doses and up to 30 hours for high doses (108).

SIDE EFFECTS. The primary side effect of salicylate ingestion is epigastric distress, nausea, and vomiting. All salicylates can produce gastrointestinal hemorrhage, exacerbation of peptic ulcer disease, and erosive gastritis (109). Gastrointestinal problems are usually dose-related but can be seen as a hypersensitivity response at low doses. Chronic aspirin ingestion can produce iron deficiency anemia through blood loss from the gastrointestinal tract. Self-limiting and reversible changes of liver function can occur with high doses of aspirin (110). Bleeding time is prolonged with even small doses, and a single dose of aspirin can double the bleeding time for up to 1 week. Aspirin should therefore be avoided in patients with liver damage, hypoprothrombinemia, vitamin K deficiency, or hemophilia. The toxic effects of aspirin can be related to high-dose therapy or to hypersensitivity. Salicylate intoxication is marked by CNS disturbances and significant alterations in acid-base balance, and can be fatal.

Another complication of aspirin therapy is hypersensitivity response, which is usually present in adults and is rare in children. A previous history of hypersensitivity to other chemicals and the presence of asthma and nasal polyps are warning signs. An acute anaphylactoid response, which can be fatal, can be seen with small doses of aspirin.

In conclusion, aspirin is an effective analgesic for certain types of mild to moderate pain, such as headache, arthritis, dysmenorrhea, neuralgia, and myalgia, for the moderate or severe pain of bone cancer, and to decrease the risk of coronary disease. The spectrum of side effects seen with aspirin is characteristic of all NSAIDs and must be considered when any of these medications is prescribed for the treatment of pain, inflammation, or fever.

Choline Magnesium Trisalicylate

PHARMACOLOGY. Choline magnesium trisalicylate is a mixture of choline salicylate and magnesium salicylate. Its analgesic, antipyretic, and anti-inflammatory properties are similar to those of aspirin. It does have some different properties, however, which can recommend its use over the more commonly used aspirin. It is water-soluble and thus is available in both tablet and liquid forms, making it more convenient for pediatric use. This property also can account for significantly less irritation of the gastric mucosa, so it is often tolerated by those for whom gastric irritation precludes their taking aspirin. It has a much longer half-life than aspirin and can be prescribed on a once- to twice-daily basis, resulting in better compliance with the therapeutic course.

SIDE EFFECTS. Choline magnesium trisalicylate, at therapeutic doses, does not demonstrate significant inhibition of platelet aggregation and can be used in circumstances in which the bleeding potential of aspirin is a problem—for example, in patients with a bleeding diathesis or in those in the perioperative period.

Diflunisal

PHARMACOLOGY. Diflunisal is a difluorophenyl derivative of salicylic acid recently marketed primarily as an analgesic (111). It has a long half-life but also shows a gradual increase in drug levels over time (cumulative effect). This means that dosing is necessary only twice a day, but that a loading dose is necessary to reach effective plasma concentrations.

SIDE EFFECTS. Diflunisal is less irritating to the gastrointestinal tract than aspirin and also has a much lower effect on platelet aggregation, the effects being readily reversible on discontinuation of the medication. One disadvantage over aspirin is that it is much less antipyretic because it does not cross the blood-brain barrier readily.

Para-Aminophenol Derivatives

Acetanilid, a parent compound of these drugs, was introduced as an antipyretic in 1886. Derivatives were synthesized because of its toxicity, and phenacetin was ultimately introduced as an analgesic-antipyretic. It was found that acetaminophen (paracetamol) was the active metabolite in humans, and it is now the most common derivative of para-aminophenol in use. Phenacetin was removed from the market because of the high correlation that was found between nephrotoxicity and the use of this compound.

Acetaminophen

PHARMACOLOGY. Acetaminophen (and phenacetin) have analgesic and antipyretic effects similar to those of aspirin. Acetaminophen appears to act as a prostaglandin biosynthesis inhibitor, but it seems that its effect is more pronounced centrally than peripherally (18). Perhaps this is why it is more specifically antipyretic than anti-inflammatory, and suggests that the analgesic activity of all NSAIDs is related to central activity as well as to peripheral anti-inflammatory effects.

SIDE EFFECTS. Toxic effects are rarely seen in individuals who adhere to recommended therapeutic doses. When phenacetin was available, toxic effects from therapeutic doses appeared in individuals who could not metabolize the compound through normal pathways with acetaminophen being the first metabolic byproduct. Nephrotoxicity, thrombocytopenia, and hepatic toxicity are the primary toxic side effects of acute or chronic overdose. Methemoglobinemia and hemolytic anemia, although common with phenacetin, are rarely seen with acetaminophen.

This mild systemic analgesic is often combined with weak opioids in compounds for the relief of mild to moderate pain. It is recommended as an antipyretic and can be used for those sensitive to aspirin and for children and adolescents, in whom the association of Reye's syndrome with aspirin treatment for fever has been found (112).

Indoleacetic Acid Derivatives

Indoleacetic acid derivatives were synthesized after a search for drugs with anti-inflammatory properties. The initial product was indomethacin, introduced to clinical care in 1963 specifically for the treatment of rheumatoid arthritis. Other compounds with less toxicity than indomethacin have been found, and it can be assumed that this group of medications will yield more compounds in the future (113).

Indomethacin

PHARMACOLOGY. Indomethacin has prominent analgesic, anti-inflammatory, and antipyretic properties, similar to those of aspirin. Because it is one of the most potent inhibitors of cyclo-oxygenase it is used primarily for its anti-inflammatory properties in the treatment of rheumatologic disease. After aspirin it is the analgesic drug of choice for the initial treatment of pain associated with metastatic disease of bone (114). Once control of such pain has been attained with indomethacin, a less toxic NSAID can be substituted.

SIDE EFFECTS. A high incidence of untoward side effects has been noted with the use of indomethacin (115), and approximately 20% of patients are intolerant of this medication. Gastrointestinal complaints, including nausea, anorexia, and abdominal pain, are common. Ulceration can occur anywhere in the upper gastrointestinal tract, with perforation and hemorrhage. Acute pancreatitis has been reported and, rarely, fatal hepatitis and jaundice have been seen (116). Indomethacin can produce severe headache and has also been implicated in the production of depression, psychosis, hallucinations, and suicide. Bone marrow depression and, rarely, aplastic anemia, can occur with long-term administration. A hypersensitivity reaction similar to that noted with aspirin can occur, and some cross sensitivity can be present. Because of the severity of some of these side effects it is recommended that indomethacin be used as tolerated over a limited period of time (e.g., 2 weeks), and other less toxic compounds can be substituted when the pain, inflammatory process, or both, is under control.

Sulindac

PHARMACOLOGY. Sulindac is closely related to indomethacin and was produced as an alternative with less toxic side effects (113). It acts as a pro-drug (i.e., an inactive chemical changed to an active compound through a metabolic transformation within the body) and is converted to a sulfide metabolite, which is a potent inhibitor of cyclo-oxygenase. This probably accounts for its low production of gastrointestinal symptoms and signs, because the active drug does not appear in the gastrointestinal tract.

SIDE EFFECTS. Toxic effects are primarily gastrointestinal but are not severe and are restricted mostly to abdominal pain, nausea, and constipation. Drowsiness, dizziness, and headache can also occur. Skin rash and pruritus have also been reported with this drug. Some cross sensitivity to aspirin allergy can occur, with possible similar manifestations.

Sulindac is used primarily for the treatment of rheumatologic problems.

Zomepirac

PHARMACOLOGY. Zomepirac was produced from the indoleacetic acid molecule and is primarily an analgesic agent (113, 117). It has anti-inflammatory and antipyretic properties but these, especially the former, are not pronounced; the anti-inflammatory effects are far weaker than other compounds of this class.

SIDE EFFECTS. Zomepirac displays a low tendency to produce gastrointestinal and hemopoietic side effects. It has been discontinued in North America, however, because of a relatively high incidence of fatal allergic responses associated with its use.

Pyrazole Derivatives

Pyrazole derivatives were introduced originally as antipyretics in the late nineteenth century but were found to have analgesic and anti-inflammatory properties, and were used for these as well. The two most common forms, antipyrine and aminopyrine, were used extensively and appeared in many over-the-counter medications until it was discovered that aminopyrine caused severe bone marrow toxicity. In 1938 aminopyrine was prohibited for use in the United States. This class of medications also interferes with prostaglandin synthesis; this appears to be the basis for the triple actions of antipyresis, analgesia, and anti-inflammatory effects. They do cause induction of hepatic microsomal enzyme systems and thus increase biotransformation of many other drugs.

Phenylbutazone

The introduction of phenylbutazone was somewhat accidental. It is a congener of antipyrine and aminopyrine and was used originally as a solubilizing agent for aminopyrine. When these compounds were withdrawn from clinical use, a search for pharmacologic relatives yielded phenylbutazone as a possible therapeutic agent.

PHARMACOLOGY. Phenylbutazone, like aspirin, has analgesic, anti-inflammatory, and antipyretic properties. Similarly, it inhibits the biosynthesis of prostaglandins but also inhibits the biosynthesis of mucopolysaccharide sulfates in cartilage and uncouples oxidative phosphorylation. These actions provide the basis for its anti-inflammatory and probably also its antipyretic and analgesic effects. It is more effective than aspirin as an anti-inflammatory agent but less effective as an analgesic (118).

SIDE EFFECTS. Although its primary untoward effects are gastrointestinal, CNS effects are seen in a small number of individuals. The most important adverse effects appear as primary or activated ulcer disease, serum sickness–type hypersensitivity, hepatitis, nephritis, and various forms of bone marrow depression, which can lead to aplastic anemia and agranulocytosis. These toxic reactions are more often seen in elderly individuals and thus phenylbutazone should not be used in this population.

Phenylbutazone is used for the short-term treatment of rheumatoid arthritis, primarily as an anti-inflammatory agent. It has been used over the short term for its analgesic properties in these patients and in postsurgical patients but is not recommended for the latter because of its high incidence of toxic reactions.

Oxyphenbutazone

PHARMACOLOGY. Oxyphenbutazone is a normal metabolite of phenylbutazone and has the same properties, primarily anti-inflammatory, as well as analgesic and antipyretic effects. It is more highly protein-bound than its parent compound and has a plasma half-life of up to several days. This gives it some possible advantages in that effective serum concentrations can easily be maintained.

SIDE EFFECTS. Oxyphenbutazone tends to have less gastric irritation than phenylbutazone and is more readily tolerated by some individuals. It is not used primarily as an analgesic but is used for its anti-inflammatory effects.

Azapropazone

PHARMACOLOGY. Azapropazone is another derivative of phenylbutazone and has similar activity to the parent compound. Its pharmacokinetics are similar to those of phenylbutazone. It is not used as an analgesic but is used primarily for the treatment of rheumatic conditions. It has a potent uricosuric effect, so it is useful for treating acute gout.

SIDE EFFECTS. Azapropazone has significantly fewer side effects than phenylbutazone and has a low toxicity. The overall incidence of untoward reactions is probably lower than 10%. No cases of agranulocytosis have been reported to be associated with its use.

Fenamates

The fenamates were discovered because of the continual search for "a better aspirin." The amine analog of salicylic acid and anthranilic acid was investigated and a number of compounds derived from it were studied as analgesics, anti-inflammatory agents, and antipyretics. Because of the toxicity of most of these compounds, few are now available for clinical use.

Mefanamic Acid

PHARMACOLOGY. Mefanamic acid is an inhibitor of cyclo-oxygenase and alters the prostaglandin cascade, thus accounting for its effects. It can also antagonize certain effects of prostaglandins, a property that many nonopioid analgesics do not possess. It has been proposed for use primarily for its analgesic properties in rheumatic diseases, but can also be helpful in soft tissue injuries, other painful musculoskeletal conditions, and dysmenorrhea (119).

SIDE EFFECTS. In addition to a significant number of gastrointestinal adverse effects, isolated cases of hemolytic anemia that might be of autoimmune origin have also been reported with the use of mefanamic acid. It appears that its toxicity limits its usefulness; use of this drug offers no advantage over other available agents, and thus it should not be used.

Pyrroleacetic Acid Derivatives

The search for yet another effective anti-inflammatory analgesic agent led to the introduction of tolmetin sodium in the mid-1970s (120). Elaboration on pyrroleacetic acid led to this discovery in a search for a molecule that would maintain therapeutic efficiency but have fewer side effects than found in anti-inflammatory and analgesic agents already available. As with most other families of compounds produced, clinical effectiveness is present only with similarities in side effects and toxicity.

Tolmetin

PHARMACOLOGY. Tolmetin has anti-inflammatory effects, somewhere between those of aspirin and phenylbutazone (120). It also appears to interfere with the prostaglandin cascade to produce its anti-inflammatory effects and has good antipyretic and analgesic actions, although it is not primarily prescribed as an analgesic. Its main use as an anti-inflammatory agent has been for rheumatoid arthritis, osteoarthritis, and ankylosing spondylitis.

SIDE EFFECTS. Overall, in clinically effective doses, the incidence of side effects is slightly lower than those of aspirin and significantly lower than those of phenylbutazone.

Alclofenac

Alclofenac is a new compound that is similar to tolmetin but is slightly less effective in terms of its anti-inflammatory effects. It is not presently available in North America.

Propionic Acid Derivatives

The search for new aspirin-like compounds has been most successful in finding compounds of the propionic acid family, which offer advantages over the use of many older anti-inflammatory analgesic compounds. In fact some of these agents, such as ibuprofen and suprofen, are now marketed primarily as analgesics. They were introduced in the early 1970s and newer compounds of the group continue to appear. This causes some difficulty for the practitioner because heavy promotion by pharmaceutical firms makes it difficult to identify the drugs that are more beneficial than other nonopioid analgesics available.

Propionic acid derivatives all have effective anti-inflammatory, analgesic, and antipyretic activity. As would be expected, they produce gastrointestinal side effects and cause gastrointestinal erosion. They act by inhibiting cyclo-oxygenase and interfering with the biosynthesis of prostaglandins. A wide variation in potency from one agent to the other has been found.

They all alter platelet function and produce prolonged bleeding times.

Ibuprofen

PHARMACOLOGY. Ibuprofen is the most widely used of this class of compounds and is now available as an over-the-counter preparation in North America (e.g., Nuprin, Datril, Advil). Ibuprofen is rapidly absorbed from the upper gastrointestinal tract and is also available in suppository form—it is well absorbed rectally but at a slower rate. It is 99% plasma protein bound and passes slowly through the synovium, where it is of greatest use for the treatment of rheumatologic diseases. It is used equally as an analgesic and anti-inflammatory and, although not advertised as such, also has antipyretic properties (121).

SIDE EFFECTS. Ibuprofen has been approved for cautious administration in people with peptic ulcer disease, but its use is not advised when active untreated ulcers are present. A low incidence of other side effects is associated with its use.

Naproxen

PHARMACOLOGY. Naproxen is readily absorbed from the gastrointestinal tract when taken either orally or rectally (suppository). Uptake is rapid but can be slowed with concomitant ingestion of food. Sodium bicarbonate aids absorption whereas aluminum hydroxide or magnesium oxide reduces the rate of absorption. This drug has a long half-life in plasma, 12 to 15 hours; this accounts for its popularity because it can be given in a bid dosage.

SIDE EFFECTS. Naproxen is somewhat more toxic than ibuprofen, having gastrointestinal and CNS effects (122).

Fenoprofen

Fenoprofen is more often used for rheumatologic problems than as an analgesic (123). It is extremely well tolerated as compared to other nonopioid analgesics.

Ketoprofen

Ketoprofen is used primarily as an anti-inflammatory agent in the treatment of rheumatic disease. Side effects, primarily gastrointestinal disturbance, occur in about 15% of patients, a third of these being significant enough to cause discontinuation of the medication.

Suprofen

Suprofen is the first of the propionic acid derivatives to be presented primarily as an analgesic, although it shares anti-inflammatory and antipyretic properties with others of its group of compounds (124). Its use has been associated with flank pain thought to be caused by uricosuric activity, and recently the drug was removed from the North American market.

Benzothiazine Derivatives

The benzothiazine derivatives are the latest class of chemical compounds to be studied for their combined analgesic, anti-inflammatory, and antipyretic effects. They were introduced to the North American market in 1982 (125).

Piroxicam

PHARMACOLOGY. Piroxicam is completely absorbed when given orally, and concomitant ingestion of food and antacids does not affect absorption. It is used primarily for arthritis and acute musculoskeletal injuries because of its combined analgesic and anti-inflammatory effects. It has the advantage of having a long half-life, so patient compliance is high with a dosage of once or twice daily.

SIDE EFFECTS. Up to 40% of patients experience gastrointestinal side effects. These are only severe enough, however, in approximately 10% of patients so as to cause them to discontinue the medication.

Phenothiazine Derivatives

Phenothiazines generally are not considered as analgesics despite having been used extensively with opioid analgesics as potentiators. One member of the class has specifically been isolated as having analgesic properties.

Methotrimeprazine

PHARMACOLOGY. Methotrimeprazine is used in an IM form only, with analgesia usually developing between 20 to 40 minutes later because peak plasma levels occur 30 to 90 minutes following IM injection. The serum half-life is 15 to 30 hours and the duration of significant analgesia is 4 hours. Traces of the unmetabolized drug are excreted in the urine and feces but it is primarily conjugated to sulfoxide and glucuronide forms in the liver and then excreted in the urine. As with most phenothiazines, methotrimeprazine is a potent CNS depressant, suppressing sensory and motor functions, and leading to sedation, amnesia, and analgesia. The actual site of action in the nociceptive system is not known. Analgesia is the equivalent of that produced with morphine and meperidine (126). Little respiratory depression is associated with analgesia but significant sedation occurs. No addiction or withdrawal symptoms are noted, even when used over a long period. It has antihistaminic, anticholinergic, and antiadrenergic properties, as do other phenothiazines.

SIDE EFFECTS. Following acute injection the primary side effects are those of the other phenothiazines

(Table 78-9). This drug can produce orthostatic hypotension and fainting. Sedation can be a problem if patients are ambulatory. The side effects of methotrimeprazine are particularly noted in the elderly or in those with cardiac disease. Abdominal discomfort, nausea and vomiting, and urinary retention are seen in some. Long-term therapy has been associated with both agranulocytosis and jaundice. Care must be taken when this drug is given in combination with opioids, barbiturates, or tranquilizers, because its sedative effects are synergistic with those of these compounds.

Other Agents Used for Painful Conditions

The first edition of this text listed a wide variety of medications as skeletal muscle relaxants (e.g., curare), antispasmodics (e.g., atropine, nitrates, xanthines), vasodilators (e.g., tetraethyl ammonium chloride, priscoline, papaverine, histamine), and vasoconstrictors (e.g., ergotamine) (1). With the exception of ergotamine for the prevention of vascular headache, these drugs are no longer used for pain.

Other vasoactive agents, both dilators and constrictors, are used in the treatment of vascular headaches (Chapter 39). Various medications are used for the treatment of muscle spasm associated with pain and appear to have little long-term effect in terms of muscle relaxation but some effectiveness for the relief of muscle spasm associated with acute injury. Their mechanism of action is unclear; because they have no direct analgesic effect they are not described further here.

Sedatives, tranquilizers, and hypnotics are often given for treatment of acute and chronic pain despite their lack of analgesic effect. The barbiturates and benzodiazepines are most commonly used, especially for headache. Their long-term use is to be condemned because of the habituation and dysphoria that accompany this practice. Withdrawal seizures are a potentially lethal side effect that is not well recognized.

NSAIDs all have a uricosuric effect. The use of specific medications for the treatment of gout is discussed in detail in Chapter 20.

D. GENERAL PRINCIPLES OF APPLICATION OF ANALGESICS

An enormous amount of information is available about the pharmacokinetics of analgesic medications. Even with this knowledge, however, providing a patient with the most effective analgesia and precise dosing schedule for a specific pain problem is difficult and time-consuming. These difficulties are encountered mainly as a result of the paucity of pharmacodynamic information about the analgesic and toxic effects of these drugs, and because of the wide individual variations in drug requirements that, at present, do not seem to follow any specific pattern. Several steps should thus be taken before prescribing analgesics.

Formulating a Treatment Plan

To reach a therapeutic plan for individual patients, great care should be taken in obtaining a detailed history and performing a complete physical examination. The management of pain patients requires a long time commitment on the part of the physician. Three phases or periods of the painful symptoms and signs should be considered: the onset, the evolution, and the present status (Chapter 31). Also, accurate notes should be made of the location, distribution, quality, and intensity of the pain, both at the time of onset and at the time of examination. The patient should be questioned about the circumstances or activities that worsen the pain, what relieves it, and whether the pain has a significant emotional impact and restrictive effect on the patient's activities. A detailed drug history, former and current, should be obtained, both by subjective information from the patient and by clinical observation (Chapter 31).

After the diagnosis has been established and the mechanism of the pain determined, other factors should be taken into account before formulating a therapeutic plan. These include the nature of the disease causing the pain, the patient's age, physical and nutritional status, renal and hepatic function, mental status, support from the family, and ability and willingness to follow medical directions. In general the patient, and always the family, should be made aware of the planned form of therapy. Often systemic analgesics are just part of a larger therapeutic plan that includes other components for managing the patient's illness.

Most patients who experience severe chronic pain require strong psychologic support. This is often accomplished by the attitude of the physician, which should be reassuring, cheerful, sympathetic, and understanding. Most patients are quick to sense an attitude of hopelessness or lack of interest on the part of the physician. Therefore, the physician should do everything possible to provide a sense of security and to assure patients that attempts will be made to relieve their suffering by all available means.

Pain Management

In formulating effective analgesic therapy all the abovementioned factors should be taken into consideration. The basic rule is to use the most effective drug or combination of drugs for relief of a specific pain state that produces the least serious or distressful side effects. Close follow-up of the patient permits modification of the pain treatment to parallel the evolution of its underlying cause(s).

Mild to Moderate Pain

Nonopioid analgesics are effective in relieving mild to moderate pain. Pain arising primarily from integumental structures such as cephalalgia, arthralgia, and myalgia are successfully treated with NSAIDs. Obviously, pain from acute inflammation is responsive to these drugs (other than acetaminophen), and they are often used in the treatment of inflammatory arthritides. It would appear that they are now underused for the relief of pain related to tissue trauma, especially for postoperative pain, in which they might prove to be significant adjuncts to opioid analgesics.

The nonopioid analgesics are often forgotten when treating pain in cancer patients but should constitute the first line of approach. They are particularly effective in relieving the moderate to severe pain associated with bony metastases (114) but are also effective in relieving pain caused by mechanical compression of integumental structures or by mechanical distension of subcutaneous tissue and in inflammation myalgia or arthralgia that can result from antitumor therapy, especially in irradiation (27, 77).

The choice of which drug to use in any particular situation cannot be dictated by the clinical picture alone. Acetylsalicylic acid is the usual initial choice for many patients and physicians, but a significant individual variation in response to the NSAIDs exists: individuals with identical clinical problems often do not respond the same way to the same drugs. Therefore, it is necessary to search by trial and error for the most beneficial drug for a particular patient with a specific clinical pain problem (26). An adequate trial of a drug is dependent on its use over time at a maximum dosage.

All these agents have a ceiling effect in terms of analgesia beyond which further dosage increases produce no improvement (17). These ceilings have not been precisely determined for all the medications discussed because of toxicity problems that interfere with clinical trials.

These agents share many common effects. Of concern is a small patient population with bronchial asthma and nasal polyps that might have a severe response to these drugs, presenting with urticaria and bronchospasm related to prostaglandin synthesis inhibition. This is classically seen with acetylsalicylic acid but, in these individuals, it is provoked equally by any of the NSAIDs (127). This is a potentially life-threatening situation and, prior to initiation of treatment with any of these drugs, a history of problems should be elicited.

Because of the gastrointestinal irritation associated with all NSAIDs except acetaminophen, patients with active peptic ulcer disease or symptoms of esophagitis should not be given these medications (128). If the disease processes are inactive some of these medications (e.g., ibuprofen) can be used cautiously, together with antiulcer therapy.

Patients with a bleeding disorder, either congenital or acquired, should be treated cautiously with nonopioid analgesics. This is particularly true of aspirin but applies to all NSAIDs. It is also advisable to stop them at least 1 week prior to elective surgery. For most agents other than aspirin the effects on platelet aggregation are easily reversible, and 1 week of abstinence might not be necessary.

Because of prostaglandin synthesis inhibition any of these agents can prolong labor, and the coagulopathy can also cause some problems in pregnant women. Therefore, these drugs should be avoided near term (17, 107).

Acute Moderate to Severe Pain

Acute moderate to severe pain is generally associated with a pathologic process, and it is usually treated effectively with opioid analgesics. The most important function of pain is as an indicator of threatened or ongoing tissue damage, causing the individual to seek medical aid, diagnosis, and treatment. Once this has been accomplished, however, the patient should be promptly relieved of pain, not only for humanitarian reasons but also because pain is now recognized as a fundamental cause of morbidity and mortality and should thus be considered and treated as aggressively as any pathogen (129–134).

During the last several years great advances have been made in the management of acute pain, mostly traumatic and postoperative pain. Whenever professional expertise and proper monitoring are available, epidural opioids offer excellent analgesia with a low degree of sedation and mental clouding and allow early ambulation and activity of the injured area (for a more detailed description of this technique see Chapter 95). Another excellent method for the control of severe acute pain is the use of patient-controlled analgesia.

Patient-Controlled Analgesia

In the early 1970s the first reports of a new method for the administration of analgesics to patients with acute and cancer pain appeared (135–137). Patient-controlled analgesia (PCA) was developed to help solve the problem of inadequate analgesia being given to hospitalized patients. It consists of the self-administration of analgesics intravenously by an infusion pump that delivers a predetermined bolus dose whenever activated by the patient. During the past several years the use of PCA has become popular in many medical centers around the world, and more patients and medical personnel are accepting it as a satisfactory method of pain control (94, 138–142). It is becoming apparent that 85% of patients treated with this method obtain good to excellent analgesia, 10% fail to understand how to use the PCA pump, and 5% state that they prefer the attention of the nurse to the self-administration of analgesics.

When properly used, PCA is a great technique for providing analgesia because it bypasses the complexities of individual pharmacokinetics and pharmacodynamics that are responsible for the enormous interpatient variation in drug requirement, and provides a clear profile of doses needed for comfort. Because the ideal opioid does not exist—all have more or less severe and annoying side effects—we are seeing that patients tend to reach a level of comfort that usually is a balance between acceptable pain and minimal side effects. With PCA, patients can maintain a plasma concentration of opioids close to their MEAC

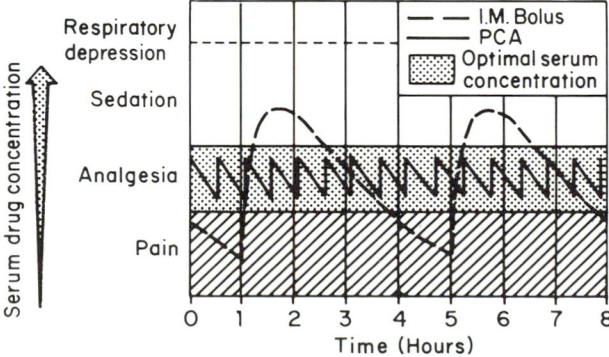

FIG. 78-3. Theoretical relationship between dosing interval, analgesic drug concentration, and clinical effects when comparing a patient-controlled analgesia (PCA) system (*solid line*) with conventional intramuscular therapy (*dashed line*). Modified from Bennett, R.L., and Griffen, W.: Contemp. Surg., *23*:63, 1983.

(Fig. 78-3) that indirectly and approximately reflects the concentration of drug at the receptor site (139).

Special PCA pumps are required for the application of this technique (Fig. 78-4). Several PCA pumps are now available with different features (Table 78-10). We believe that the minimal requirement for a PCA pump is the ability to provide boluses on demand over a baseline continuous infusion. Obviously, the parameters and limits are set by the physician. The availability of these pumps implies an initial capital investment on the part of the hospital. This cost is offset by the time saved by nursing personnel, who do not have to administer drugs on a routine basis, and by more effective analgesia, an important factor in preventing postoperative or post-traumatic complications (133, 134) and thus decreasing time and cost of hospitalization (132, 134). Morphine is commonly used for PCA, but other opioids have been used; a recent study analyzed the analgesia provided by the most frequently used opioids versus side effects and patient acceptance (Table 78-11) (143).

The most effective protocol for the use of PCA for acute pain is to begin with an IV bolus of morphine, starting with 4 mg for a 70-kg adult, and then to titrate slowly enough IV morphine to have the patient comfortable within the next 20 to 30 minutes. At this point the parameters of the PCA pump are set to deliver a 1- or 2-mg bolus of morphine with each request and a lockout period of 10 to 15 minutes. The lockout period prevents redosing before the drug has time to take effect.

After an 8-hour period the total use of morphine is calculated and the comfort of the patient is assessed. A comfortable nonsedated patient indicates proper use of the PCA. The pump is then set to deliver a continuous infusion of morphine with an hourly rate of one-eighth of the total dose used during the preceding 8 hours, and the patient is still allowed to use the PCA feature of the pump if pain reoccurs.

Re-evaluation every 24 hours of the patient's comfort, sedation, and usage of the drug permit adjustments of the continuous infusion to the patient's requirements. This technique provides good analgesia and has an advantage over single PCA boluses because the patient's plasma level of opiate does not fall much below the MEAC, especially during sleep. PCA pumps should soon be available that allow the patient not only to administer boluses but also to decrease the rate of the continuous infusion if the side effects become too bothersome.

Although intraspinal opioids and PCA provide the best and most satisfactory analgesia for the control of acute pain, they are not available in all medical centers. Effective pain relief can still be provided with a continuous infusion of opioids or, even more simply, with intramuscular opioids, provided that these are carefully titrated to the individual's need and a "cookbook" approach to pain management is avoided.

Continuous Infusion

Acute pain can be effectively treated with continuous infusions of opioids, but the patient must be carefully monitored because of the possibility of overdosing. The infusion rate should be constantly

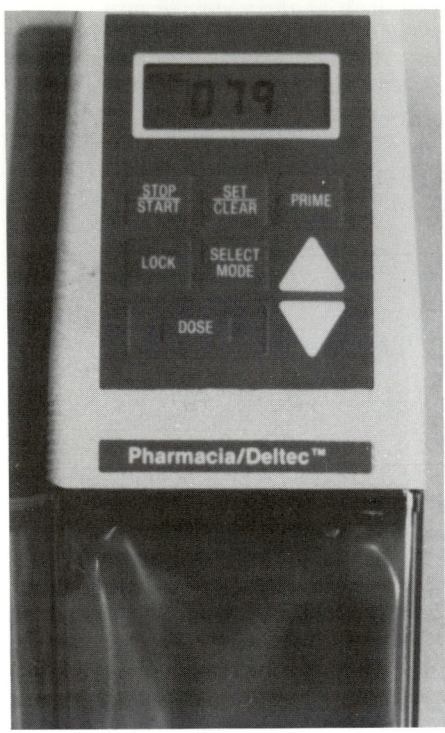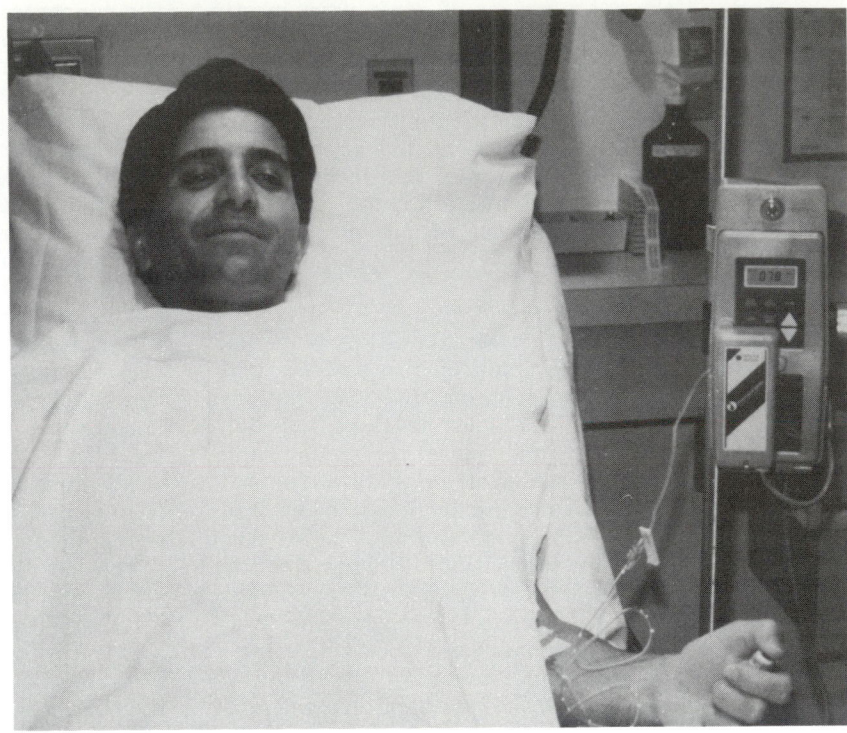

FIG. 78-4. *A*. Patient-controlled analgesia (PCA) pump. This model uses not only the features of PCA and continuous infusion, either singly or combined, but can also be converted from a portable to a stationary pump. *B*. PCA pump in use. (Courtesy of Pharmacia-Deltec.)

TABLE 78-10. Patient-Controlled Analgesia Pumps

Feature	Model						
	Pharmacia-Deltec	Prominject	Harvard PCA 4000	Abbott Lifecare PCA Infusor	ODAC	Cardiff Palliator	Palliator MS 402
Incremental dose*	Variable in mg	Variable in units of mass (e.g., mg, μg)	Variable in ml	Variable in ml	Variable in ml	Variable in ml	Variable in mg
Background infusion mode available	Yes	Yes	No	Yes	Yes	No	Yes
Concentration setting	Six preset concentrations	Variable in units of mass/L	No	No; prepacked drugs in special syringes used	Yes; results in printer output in mg	Set as dilution from 1–400 μl/mg	Variable from 1–99 mg/ml
Lockout time*	Variable from 5–199 min	Variable from 5–999 min	Variable from 3–60 min	Variable from 5–99 min	Variable from 1–99 min	Variable from 1–99 min	Variable from 1–30 min
Infusion rate or infusion time	1 min/bolus	1 min for bolus dose, 1 hour for optional follow-up infusion	Bolus dose 2.5 ml/min	Fixed, 4 ml/min	Background variable in ml/min 0.01–0.99	Variable from 1–99 ml/hour	Variable from 3–15 min
Cumulative dose display	Yes	Yes	Yes	Yes	On printer	Yes	Yes
Patient demand signal	Single press	Two presses/1 sec	Single press	Single press	Two presses/1 sec	Two presses 1 sec	Two presses 2 sec
Printer	No	Yes	Yes	Interface	Yes	No	Interface
Battery power	Yes	Yes	Yes	Yes	Yes	No	Yes
Manufacturer	Pharmacia-Deltec	Pharmacia AB, Sweden	C.R. Bard, Inc., United States	Abbott Laboratories, United States	Janssen Scientific, Belgium	Graseby Medical Ltd., U.K.	Graseby Medical Ltd., U.K.

*A combination of *dose* setting and *lockout time* setting gives a maximum *dose*/hour for all machines, but this is not a preset feature.
Adapted from Lammer, P., Bullingham, R.E.S., and Jacobs, O.L.R.: The PRODAC demand analgesia computer. *In* Patient-Controlled Analgesia. Edited by M. Harmer, M. Rosen, and M.D. Vickers. Oxford, Blackwell Scientific Publications, 1985, pp. 106–107.

TABLE 78-11. Postoperative Intravenous On-Demand Analgesia*

Analgesic	Pain Score	Emesis (%)	Patient's Evaluation (%)			Preferred by Nurse (%)
			+	=	−	
Fentanyl	1.07	32.5	81.0	19.1	0.0	17.5
Alfentanil	1.37	10.0	80.0	13.3	6.7	15.0
Piritramide	1.42	17.5	73.3	15.4	15.4	17.5
Buprenorphine	1.57	10.0	92.9	7.1	0.0	5.0
Pentazocine	1.60	15.0	68.4	15.8	15.8	5.0
Morphine (n = 21)	1.95	4.8	81.8	9.1	9.1	9.5
Pethidine	2.22	7.5	47.1	35.3	17.7	5.0
Tramadol	2.27	7.5	36.0	24.0	40.0	20.0
Nefopam	2.90	2.5	46.2	7.7	46.2	15.0
Metamizole	3.02	22.5	11.1	37.0	51.9	22.5

*Forty patients per group. + positive response; = indifferent; − negative.
From Lehmann K.A.: Practical experience with demand analgesia for postoperative pain. *In* Patient-Controlled Analgesia. Edited by M. Harmer, M. Rosen, and M.D. Vickers. Oxford, Blackwell Scientific Publications, 1985, pp. 134–139.

modified in response to the patient's comfort and presence of side effects. The most effective way of using this technique is to give an initial loading dose of the chosen opioid so that the MEAC is rapidly achieved. One way of accomplishing this in a 70-kg adult patient is to give IV 5 mg of morphine, 50 mg of meperidine, or 1 mg of dihydromorphinone slowly (1 to 2 minutes), followed by a continuous infusion of 2 to 3 mg of morphine, 20 to 30 mg of meperidine, or 0.5 to 1 mg of dihydromorphinone per hour. Another equal bolus might have to be given 30 minutes later if the desired analgesia is not obtained. Patients must be carefully monitored to observe any signs of drug accumulation and toxicity.

Intramuscular Administration

The most frequent route of administration of opioids in the postoperative period is still IM injection because of its relative ease of administration. Several studies and clinical observations indicate that it provides variable results from the point of view of time of onset, intensity, and duration of analgesia. Austin and colleagues (44) have shown that the IM administration of 100 mg meperidine produces a peak meperidine concentration (PMC) that varies fivefold in different patients, and that any one patient given meperidine at different times of the day can show a twofold difference in PMC. The study also showed that pain control was poor during the first 4-hour dosing interval and effective analgesia did not occur until the third or fourth dose. Even with later doses effective relief was achieved in about 45 minutes, lasted only 75 to 90 minutes, and then pain increased steadily to severe levels by the fourth hour.

It is difficult to explain all the factors that can influence the plasma level and onset of analgesia, but certainly an important one is the site of the IM injection. Injection into a well-perfused muscle such as the deltoid provides a faster and higher plasma level than an injection into a less well-perfused muscle or even into adipose tissue. This can occur when the injection is done in the gluteal region and certainly influences the uptake of the drugs into the vascular system (144). The patient still must be carefully followed, the analgesia evaluated, and the dosage regimen revised so that the proper amount is given at regular intervals 20

to 30 minutes shorter than the duration of the analgesia provided by that particular drug to that particular patient.

Other Routes of Administration

During the early postoperative period, oral intake is often curtailed. Oral opioids are therefore not used but other routes of administration are presently available, and new ones are being developed. In several countries rectal opioids are used, often with success and with good patient compliance (145). Sublingual buprenorphine is used extensively where available, providing effective long-lasting analgesia in most patients who use it properly (92, 93). The tablets must be allowed to dissolve sublingually and be absorbed by the oral mucosa to provide the desired effect.

Transdermal fentanyl is just being developed (89) and tested, as is transnasal butorphanol (94). Only time and extensive clinical trials can properly evaluate the effectiveness of these novel modes of administration.

Chronic Pain

If the basic knowledge of pharmacology is properly applied, most types of acute pain can be treated easily and successfully. Chronic pain is much more difficult to treat, and improperly prescribed medications often lead to ineffective pain control and to psychologic and physical dependence. Many patients with chronic pain have medication difficulties because of treatment by several physicians who have prescribed different analgesics and sedatives that are often incompatible with one another (e.g., meperidine and pentazocine simultaneously). This can lead to inadequate analgesia, depressive states, lethargy, and dysphoria. These patients often indulge in self-administration of large doses of ethanol to decrease their suffering and to obtain its supposed analgesic effect (146). One should always inquire about ethanol use and account for it when devising an alternative form of therapy to avoid withdrawal symptoms.

If a severe drug problem is suspected, hospitalization is necessary for the patient to be treated in a formal detoxification program. The procedure is usually as follows:

a. The patient is informed thoroughly about the treatment, and all drugs the patient might possess must be removed from the patient's room.

b. For the initial 48 hours of hospitalization the patient is allowed to request and have any analgesic and sedative that he or she feels is necessary to be comfortable. (The nursing personnel should carefully record the drug, the amount, and the time it is given.)

c. The patient should be observed closely for signs of sedation or nervousness, which indicate either overdosing or underdosing.

After 48 hours, the types and amounts of drugs given are calculated. The average consumption for each drug is computed and, using conversion tables (Tables 78-12 and 78-13) (147), all opioids are converted to an equianalgesic dose of methadone and all sedatives are converted to an equivalent dose of phenobarbital. The doses are divided into four equal amounts and given to the patient every 6 hours in a liquid medium that usually contains a masking flavor. Hydroxyzine 25 to 50 mg and acetaminophen 325 to 650 mg are often added to the solution to increase its effect. This mixture is referred to as a pain cocktail (147). To detoxify the patient the methadone is decreased by 10 to 20% each day and the phenobarbital is decreased by 5 to 10% each day. Once the patient has been detoxified the pain can be more clearly evaluated and the patient started on proper reactivation therapy and other appropriate treatment (page 1707).

Despite detoxification, behavioral modification, and proper physical therapy, many patients with chronic nonmalignant pain, especially those with recurrent severe lumbosacral pain, postamputation pain, and myofascial pain syndrome, continue to experience debilitating pain several times during the course of

TABLE 78-12. Equivalent Analgesic Doses of Narcotics

Drug	Dose (mg) Equal to 1 Narcotic Equivalent*	
	Oral	IM
Alphaprodine (Nisentil)		45.0
Anileridine (Leritine)		35.0
Codeine	200.0	130.0
Diacetylmorphine (heroin)		3.0
Fentanyl (Sublimaze)		0.1
Hydromorphone (Dilaudid)	7.5	1.5
Meperidine (Demerol)	400.0	100.0
Methadone		8.0
Morphine	60.0	10.0
Oxycodone (Percodan)	30.0	15.0
Oxymorphone (Numorphan)		1.5
Pentazocine (Talwin)	180.0	60.0

*1 narcotic equivalent = 10 mg oral methadone.
From Ready, L.B., Sarkis, E., and Turner, J.A.: Self-reported vs. actual use of medications in chronic pain patients. Pain, *12*:285, 1982.

TABLE 78-13. Equivalent Doses of Sedatives, Hypnotics, and Tranquilizers

Drug	Oral dose (mg) Equal to 1 Sedative Equivalent*
Secobarbital (Seconal)	100
Pentobarbital (Nembutal)	100
Chlordiazepoxide (Librium)	25
Diazepam (Valium)	10
Flurazepam (Dalmane)	30
Methaqualone (Quaalude)	300
Glutethimide (Doriden)	500
Ethchlorvynol (Placidyl)	750
Chloral hydrate	1000
Hydroxyzine (Vistaril)	50–100
Diphenhydramine (Benadryl)	50–100
Meprobamate	400
Whiskey (110-proof)	90 ml (3 oz)

*1 sedative equivalent = 30 mg of phenobarbital.
From Ready, L.B., Sarkis, E., and Turner, J.A.: Self-reported vs. actual use of medications in chronic pain patients. Pain, *12*:285, 1982.

the year. We have successfully treated these patients using different analgesic techniques, including transcutaneous nerve stimulation (Chapter 92), repeated trigger point injections (Chapter 21), and even long-term use of an opioid-containing pain cocktail. If the pain cocktail has been used long term we are particularly careful to vary the dose of the active drugs with the fluctuation of the pain. In this manner we have been able to treat patients for many years with low doses of opioids and prevent the development of significant tolerance. This form of therapy can only work if patients are closely followed by the physician and the pain re-evaluated frequently.

The outcome has been encouraging. A great majority of patients have showed significant improvement in their life-styles, social interactions, and even job performance. Many treated patients were spared further debilitating surgical procedures, which often aggravated the pre-existing pain syndrome. Whenever the intensity of pain was decreased, so was the use of opioids. Only a small percentage of patients (less than 6%) treated with chronic opioid therapy showed a pathologic opioid-seeking behavior. This was noted almost exclusively in individuals with a previous history of substance abuse of any type. Taub (148) has presented more extensive observations on this subject, and also includes data on 313 patients treated with long-term opioid therapy. Portenoy and Foley (149) reported similar findings in the 38 patients that they studied.

Cancer Pain

Chapter 24 presents a detailed discussion of the management of cancer pain.

REFERENCES

1. Bonica, J.J.: The Management of Pain. Philadelphia, Lea & Febiger, 1953.
2. Bonica, J.J., and Ventafridda, V. (eds.): Advances in Pain Research and Therapy, Vol. 2. New York, Raven Press, 1979.
3. Twycross, R.G.: Controlling pain in cancer patients. Mod. Med., (Lond.), *8*:2, 1982.
4. Arnër, S., et al.: Narcotic analgesics in the treatment of cancer and postoperative pain. Acta Anaesthesiol. Scand. [Suppl. 74], *26*:1, 1982.
5. Twycross, R.G., and Ventafridda, V.: The Continuing Care

of Terminal Cancer Patients. New York, Pergamon Press, 1980.

6. Foley, K.M.: The management of pain of malignant origin. *In* Current Neurology, Vol. 2, Chap. 18. Edited by H.R. Tyler and D.M. Dawson. Boston, Houghton Mifflin, 1979, pp. 279–302.

7. Daut, R.L., and Cleeland, C.S.: The prevalence and severity of pain in cancer. Cancer, *50*:1913, 1982.

8. Halpern, L.M., and Bonica, J.J.: Analgesics. *In* Drugs of Choice. Edited by W. Modell. St Louis, C.V. Mosby, 1984, pp. 207–247.

9. Jaffe, J.H., and Martin, W.R.: Opioid analgesics and antagonists. *In* The Pharmacological Basis of Therapeutics. Edited by L.S. Goodman, et al. New York, Macmillan, 1985, pp. 491–531.

10. Mather, L.E., and Denson, D.D.: Pharmacokinetic considerations for drug dosing. *In* Practical Management of Pain. Edited by P. Raj. Chicago, Year Book Medical Publishers, 1986, pp. 489–502.

11. Benet, L.Z., and Sheiner, L.B.: Pharmacokinetics: The dynamics of drug absorption, distribution, and elimination. *In* The Pharmacological Basis of Therapeutics. 7th Ed. Edited by L.S. Goodman, et al. New York, Macmillan, 1985, pp. 3–34.

12. Ross, E.M., and Gilman, A.G.: Pharmacodynamics: Mechanisms of drug action and the relationship between drug concentration and effect. *In* The Pharmacological Basis of Therapeutics. 7th Ed. Edited by L.S. Goodman, et al. New York, Macmillan, 1985, pp. 35–48.

13. Blashke, T.F., Nies, A.S., and Mamelok, R.D.: Principles of therapeutics. *In* The Pharmacological Basis of Therapeutics. 7th Ed. Edited by L.S. Goodman. New York, Macmillan, 1985, pp. 49–65.

14. Foley, K.M., and Inturrisi, C.E. (eds.): Advances in Pain Research and Therapy, Vol. 8. New York, Raven Press, 1986.

15. Day, R.O., et al.: Clinical pharmacology of non-steroidal anti-inflammatory drugs. Pharmacol. Ther., *33*:383, 1987.

16. Flower, R.J.: Drugs which inhibit prostaglandins biosynthesis. Pharmacol. Rev., *26*:33, 1974.

17. Brune, K., and Lanz, R.: Nonopioid analgesics. *In* Analgesics: Neurochemical, Behavioural and Clinical Perspectives. Edited by M. Kuhar and G. Pasternak. New York, Raven Press, 1984, pp. 149–173.

18. Flower, R.J., Moncada, S., and Vane, J.R.: Analgesic-antipyretics and anti-inflammatory agents: Drugs employed in the treatment of gout. *In* The Pharmacological Basis of Therapeutics. 7th Ed. Edited by L.S. Goodman, et al. New York, Macmillan, 1985, pp. 674–715.

19. Stoelting, R.K.: Pharmacology and Physiology in Anesthetic Practice. Philadelphia, J.B. Lippincott, 1987.

20. Hull, C.J.: Pharmacokinetics and pharmacodynamics. Br. J. Anaesthesiol., *51*:579, 1979.

21. Strom, B.L.: Generic drug substitution revisited. N. Engl. J. Med., *23*:1456, 1987.

22. Krishnaswamy, K., Ushasri, V., Naidu, A.N.: The effect of malnutrition on the pharmacokinetics of phenylbutazone. Clin. Pharmacokinet, *6*:152, 1981.

23. Kinniburgh, D.W., and Boyd, N.O.: Isolation of peptides from uremic plasma that inhibit phenytoin binding to normal plasma proteins. Clin. Pharmacol. Ther., *30*:276, 1981.

24. Gourlay, G.K., Wilson, R.R., and Glynn, C.J.: Methadone produces prolonged post-operative analgesia. Br. Med. J., *284*:630, 1982.

25. Tamsen, A.: Patient characteristics influencing pain relief. *In* Patient-Controlled Analgesia. Edited by M. Harmer, M. Rosen, and M.D. Vickers. Oxford, Blackwell Scientific Publications, 1985, pp. 30–37.

26. Huskisson, L.C., Woolf, D.L., and Bawe, H.: Four new anti-inflammatory drugs: Responses and variations. Br. Med. J., *1*:1048, 1976.

27. Ventafridda, V., et al.: Use of non-steroidal anti-inflammatory drugs in the treatment of pain in cancer. Br. J. Clin. Pharmacol., *10*:343, 1980.

28. Arnër, S., and Arnër, B.: Differential effects of epidural morphine in the treatment of cancer-related pain. Acta Anaesthesiol. Scand., *29*:32, 1985.

29. Melzack, R., and Wall, P.D.: Pain mechanisms: A new theory. Science, *150*:971, 1965.

30. Akil, H., et al.: Endogenous opioids: Biology and function. Ann. Rev. Neurosci., *7*:223, 1984.

31. Benedetti, C.: Neuroanatomy and biochemistry of antinociception. *In* Advances in Pain Research and Therapy, Vol. 2. Edited by J.J. Bonica and V. Ventafridda. New York, Raven Press, 1979, pp. 31–44.

32. Zimmermann, M.: Neurophysiology of nociception, pain, and pain therapy. *In* Advances in Pain Research and Therapy, Vol. 2. Edited by J.J. Bonica and V. Ventafridda. New York, Raven Press, 1979, pp. 13–29.

33. Beecher, H.K.: Measurement of Subjective Responses. New York, Oxford University Press, 1959.

34. Houde, R.W.: Methods for measuring clinical pain in humans. Acta Anaesthesiol. Scand. [Suppl. 74], *26*:25, 1982.

35. Payne, R., and Foley, K.M.: Advances in the management of cancer pain. Cancer Treat. Rep. *68*:173, 1984.

36. Umans, J.G., et al.: Determination of heroin and its metabolites by high-performance liquid chromatography. J. Chromatogr., *233*:213, 1982.

37. Justice, J.B. (ed.): Voltammetry in the Neurosciences. Clifton, NJ, Humana Press, 1987.

38. Austin, K.L., Stapleton, J.V., and Mather, L.E.: Relationship of meperidine concentration and analgesic response. A preliminary report. Anesthesiology, *53*:460, 1980.

39. Pazlow, L.K.: Pharmacokinetic aspects of optimal pain treatment. Acta Anaesthesiol. Scand. [Suppl. 74], *26*:43, 1982.

40. Graves, D.A., et al.: Patient-controlled analgesia. Ann. Intern. Med., *99*:360, 1983.

41. Dahlström, B.E., et al.: Relation between morphine pharmacokinetics and analgesia. J. Pharmacokinet. Biopharmacol., *6*:41, 1978.

42. Mather, L.E., et al.: Pethidine revisited: Plasma concentration and effects after intramuscular injection. Br. J. Anaesthesiol., *47*:1269, 1975.

43. Kaiko, R.F., et al.: Clinical analgesic studies and sources of variation in analgesic responses to morphine. *In* Advances in Pain Research and Therapy, Vol. 8. Edited by K.M. Foley and C.E. Inturrisi. New York, Raven Press, 1986, pp. 13–23.

44. Austin, K.L., Stapleton, J.V., and Mather, L.E.: Multiple intramuscular injections: A major source of variability in analgesic response to meperidine. Pain, *8*:47, 1980.

45. Hull, C.J.: Opioid infusions for the management of postoperative pain. *In* Acute Pain. Edited by G. Smith and B.G. Covino. Borough Green, Butterworth, 1985, pp. 155–179.

46. Nordberg, G.: Pharmacokinetic aspects of spinal morphine analgesia. Acta Anaesthesiol. Scand. [Suppl. 79], *28*:1, 1984.

47. Cherry, D.A.: Drug delivery systems for epidural administration of opioids. Acta Anaesthesiol. Scand. [Suppl. 85], *31*:54, 1987.

48. Lobato, R.D., et al.: Intraventricular morphine for intractable cancer pain: Rationale, methods, clinical results. Acta Anaesthesiol. Scand. [Suppl. 85], *31*:68, 1987.

49. Duggan, A.W., and North, R.A.: Electrophysiology of opioids. Pharmacol. Rev., *35*:219, 1983.

50. Lowenstein, E.: Morphine "anesthesia"—a perspective. Anesthesiology, *35*:563, 1971.

51. Kosterlitz, H.W.: Opioid peptides and their receptors. The Wellcome Foundation Lecture, 1982. Proc. R. Soc. Lond. [Biol.], *225*:27, 1985.

52. Kosterlitz, H.W., and Paterson, S.J.: Types of opioid receptors: Relation to antinociception. Philos. Trans. R. Soc. Lond. [Biol.], *308*:291, 1985.

53. Kosterlitz, H.W., and Paterson, S.J.: Opioid receptors and mechanisms of opioid analgesia. *In* Advances in Pain Research and Therapy, Vol. 14. Edited by C. Benedetti, C.R. Chapman, and G. Giron. New York, Raven Press, 1989, pp. 37–43.

54. Donnerer, J., et al.: Chemical characterization and regulation of endogenous morphine and codeine in the rat. J. Pharmacol. Exp. Ther., *242*:583, 1987.

55. Donnerer, J. et al.: Presence and formation of codeine and morphine in the rat. Proc. Natl. Acad. Sci. U.S.A., *83*:4566, 1986.

56. Weitz, C.J., Faull, K.F., and Goldstein, A.: Synthesis of the skeleton of the morphine molecule by mammalian liver. Nature, *330*:674, 1987.

57. Weitz, C.J., et al.: Morphine and codeine from mammalian brain. Proc. Natl. Acad. Sci. U.S.A., *83*:9784, 1986.

58. Neil, A., and Terenius L.: Receptor mechanisms for nociception. In Regional Opioids in Anesthesiology and Pain Management. Edited by U.H. Sjostrand and N. Rawal. Boston, Little, Brown & Co., 1986, pp. 1–15.

59. Portoghese, P.S.: A new concept on the mode of interactions of narcotic analgesics with receptors. J. Med. Chem., *8*:60, 1965.

60. Redmond, D.E., Jr., and Krystal, J.H.: Multiple mechanisms of withdrawal from opioid drugs. Annu. Rev. Neurosci., *7*:443, 1984.

61. Beaumont, A., and Hughes, J.: Biology of opioid peptides. Annu. Rev. Pharmacol. Toxicol., *19*:245, 1979.

62. Papper, S., and Papper, E.M.: The effects of pre-anesthetics, anesthetic, and post-operative drugs on renal function. Clin. Pharmacol. Ther., 5:205, 1964.
63. Martin, W.R.: Pharmacology of opioids. Pharmacol. Rev., 35:283, 1983.
64. Rosow, C.E., et al.: Histamine release during morphine and fentanyl anesthesia. Anesthesiology, 56:93, 1982.
65. Radnay, P.A., et al.: The effect of equianalgesic doses of fentanyl, morphine, meperidine, and pentazocine on common bile duct pressure. Anaesthesist, 29:26, 1980.
66. Benedetti, C.: Intraspinal analgesia: An historical overview. Acta Anaesthesiol. Scand. [Suppl. 85], 31:17, 1987.
67. Campbell, C., Phillips, O.C., and Frazier, T.M.: Analgesia during labor: A comparison of pentobarbital, meperidine, and morphine. Obstet. Gynecol., 17:714, 1961.
68. Greening, A.P.: Opiates, opioid peptides, and immunity. Lancet, 1:774, 1984.
69. Ader, R.: Psychoneuroimmunology. New York, Academic Press, 1981.
70. Sklar, L.S., and Anisman, H.: Stress and cancer. Psychol. Bull., 89:369, 1981.
71. Shavit, Y., et al.: Opioid peptides mediate the suppresive effect of stress on natural killer cell cytotoxicity. Science, 223:188, 1984.
72. Shavit, Y., et al.: Stress, opioid peptides, the immune system, and cancer. J. Immunol., 135:834, 1985.
73. Forrest, W.H., et al.: Dextroamphetamine with morphine for the treatment of postoperative pain. N. Engl. J. Med., 296:712, 1977.
74. Beaver, W.T.: Comparison of analgesic effects of morphine sulfate, hydroxyzine and other combinations in patients with postoperative pain. In Advances in Pain Research and Therapy. Edited by J.J. Bonica and V. Ventafridda. New York, Raven Press, 1976, pp. 553–557.
75. Wakefield, R.D., and Mesaros, M.: Reversal of pruritus, secondary to epidural morphine, with the narcotic agonist/antagonist nalbuphine (Nubain) (Abst.). Anesthesiology, 63:A255, 1985.
76. Henderson, S.K., and Cohen, H.: Nalbuphine augmentation of analgesia and reversal of side effects following epidural hydromorphone. Anesthesiology, 65:216, 1986.
77. Bonica, J.J., and Benedetti, C.: Management of cancer pain. In Comprehensive Textbook of Oncology, Chap. 45. Edited by A.R. Moossa, M.C. Robson, and S.C. Schimpff. Baltimore, Williams & Wilkins, 1985, pp. 443–477.
78. Flacke, J.W., Flacke, W.E., and Williams, G.D.: Acute pulmonary edema following naloxone reversal of high-dose morphine anesthesia. Anesthesiology, 47:376, 1977.
79. WHO Expert Committee on Addiction Producing Drug: WHO TECH. Rep. Ser. 407:6, 1967.
80. Porter, J., and Jick, H.: Addiction rare in patients treated with narcotics. N. Engl. J. Med., 302:123, 1980.
81. Kanner, R.F., and Foley, K.M.: Patterns of narcotic drug use in a cancer pain clinic. Ann. N.Y. Acad. Sci., 362:162, 1980.
82. Nishitateno, K., et al.: Pharmacokinetics of morphine: Concentrations in the serum and brain of the dog during hyperventilation. Anesthesiology, 50:520, 1979.
83. Tamsen, A., et al.: Patient-controlled analgesic therapy part two: Individual analgesic demand and analgesic plasma concentrations of pethidine in postoperative pain. Clin. Pharmacokinet., 7:252, 1982.
84. Dahlström, B., et al.: Patient-controlled analgesic therapy, part IV: Pharmacokinetics and analgesic plasma concentrations of morphine. Clin. Pharmacokinet. 7:266, 1982.
85. Kaiko, R.F., et al.: Clinical analgesic studies of intramuscular heroin and morphine in postoperative and chronic pain. In Advances in Pain Research and Therapy, Vol. 8. Edited by K.M. Foley and C.E. Inturrisi. New York, Raven Press, 1986, pp. 107–116.
86. Inturrisi, C.E.: Pharmacokinetics of oral, intravenous, and continuous infusions of heroin. In Advances in Pain Research and Therapy, Vol. 8. Edited by K.M. Foley and C.E. Inturrisi. New York, Raven Press, 1986, pp. 117–127.
87. Inturrisi, C.E., et al.: Heroin: Disposition in cancer patients. Clin. Pharmacol. Ther., 31:235, 1982.
88. Beaver, W.T.: Mild analgesics, a review of their clinical pharmacology (Part II). Am. J. Med. Sci., 251:576, 1966.
89. Caplan, R.A., and Southam M.: Transdermal drug delivery and its application to pain control. In Advances in Pain Research and Therapy, Vol. 14. Edited by C. Benedetti, C.R. Chapman, and G. Giron. New York, Raven Press, 1989, pp. 241–258.
90. Wolfe, M.J., and Davies, G.K.: Analgesic action of extradural fentanyl. Br. J. Anaesthesiol., 52:357, 1980.
91. Lewis, J.W., Rance, M.J., and Sanger, D.J.: The pharmacology and abuse potential of buprenorphine: A new antagonist analgesic. Adv. Substance Abuse, 3:103, 1983.
92. Bullingham, R.E.S., et al.: Sublingual buprenorphine used postoperatively: Ten-hour plasma drug concentration analysis. Br. J. Clin. Pharmacol., 13:665, 1982.
93. Ventafridda, V., et al.: Chronic analgesic study on buprenorphine action in cancer pain—comparison with pentazocine. Drug Res., 4:587, 1983.
94. Cool, W.M., Kurtz, N.M., and Chu, G.: Transnasal delivery of systemic drugs. In Advances in Pain Research and Therapy, Vol. 14. Edited by C. Benedetti, C.R. Chapman, and G. Giron. New York, Raven Press, 1989, pp. 233–240.
95. Wallenstein, S.L., et al. Nalbuphine: Clinical analgesic studies. In Advances in Pain Research and Therapy, Vol. 8. Edited by K.M. Foley and C.E. Inturrisi. New York, Raven Press, 1986, pp. 247–252.
96. Jasinski, D.R., Martin, W.R., and Hoeldtke R.D.: Effects of short- and long-term administration of pentazocine in man. Clin. Pharmacol. Ther., 11:385, 1970.
97. Heisterkamp, D.V., and Cohen, P.J.: The use of naloxone to antagonize large doses of opiates administered during nitrous oxide anesthesia. Anesth. Analg., 53:12, 1974.
98. Price, D.D., et al.: Potentiation of systemic morphine analgesia in humans by proglumide, a cholecystokinin antagonist. Anesth. Analg., 64:801, 1985.
99. Ferreira, S.H., and Vane, J.R.: New aspects of the mode of action of nonsteroid anti-inflammatory drugs. Annu. Rev. Pharmacol., 14:57, 1974.
100. Feldberg, W.: Fever, prostaglandins and antipyretics. In Prostaglandin Synthetase Inhibitors. Edited by J.J. Robinson and J.R. Vane. New York, Raven Press, 1974, pp. 197–203.
101. Bhattacharya, S.K.: Prostaglandins and central serotonergic activity in the rat. Pharm. Res., pp. 195, 198, 1985.
102. Baber, N., Halliday, D.C., and Van Den Neuvel, W.J.A.: Indomethacin in rheumatoid arthritis. Clinical effects, pharmacokinetics and platelet studies in responders and nonresponders. Ann. Rheum. Dis., 38:128, 1979.
103. Ferreira, S.H.: Prostaglandins, aspirin-like drugs and analgesia. Nature, 240:200, 1975.
104. Kantor, T.F.: Peripherally-acting analgesics. In Analgesics: Neurochemical, Behavioural and Clinical Perspectives. Edited by M. Kuhar and G. Pasternak. New York, Raven Press, 1984, pp. 289–312.
105. Adams, D.H., et al.: Non-steroidal anti-inflammatory drugs and renal failure. Lancet, 1:57, 1986.
106. Whittle, B.J.R., and Vane, J.R.: Prostacyclin, thromboxanes, and prostaglandins—actions and roles in the gastrointestinal tract. In Progress in Gastroenterology. Edited by G.B. Jerzy Glass and P. Sherlock. New York, Grune & Stratton, 1983, pp. 97–115.
107. Rall, T.W., and Schleifer, L.S.: Oxytocin, prostaglandins, ergot alkaloids, and other drugs: Tocolytic agents. In The Pharmacological Basis of Therapeutics. 7th Ed. Edited by L.S. Goodman, et al. New York, Macmillan, 1985, pp. 926–945.
108. Davison, C.: Salicylate metabolism in man. Ann. N.Y. Acad. Sci., 179:249, 1971.
109. Baskin, W.N., Ivey, K.J., and Krause, W.J.: Aspirin-induced ultrastructural changes in human gastric mucosa. Correlation with potential differences. Ann. Intern. Med., 5:299, 303, 1976.
110. Halla, J.T.: Aspirin, liver and rheumatic diseases. J. Med. Assoc. State Ala., 46:23, 1976.
111. Forbes, J.A., Calderazzo, J.P., and Fowser, M.W.: A 12-hour evaluation of the analgesic efficacy of diflunisal, aspirin and placebo in postoperative dental pain. J. Clin. Pharmacol., 22:89, 1982.
112. Committee on Infectious Diseases: Aspirin and Reye's syndrome. Pediatrics, 69:310, 1982.
113. Shen, T.Y., and Winter, C.A.: Chemical and biological studies on indomethacin, sulindac and their analogues. Adv. Drug Res., 12:90, 1977.
114. Benedetti, C., Chiesi, P., and Lorenzon, I.: Meglumine indomethacin in the treatment of cancer pain. Proceedings of the Fifth World Congress of Anesthesiologists, Kyoto, Japan, 1972. Amsterdam, Excerpta Medica, 1973, pp. 297–299.
115. Boardman, P.L., and Hart, E.D.: Side-effects of indomethacin. Ann. Rheum. Dis., 26:127, 1967.

116. Cuthbert, M.F.: Adverse reactions to non-steroidal anti-rheumatic drugs. Curr. Med. Res. Opin., *2*:600, 1974.
117. Forrest, S.H., Jr.: Orally administered zomepirac and parenterally administered morphine. JAMA, *244*:2298, 1980.
118. Symposium: Rheumatology Workshop. A modern review of Geigy Pyrazoles. J. Int. Med. Res., *5* (Suppl. 2):2, 1977.
119. Kendall, P.H. (ed.): Symposium: Fenamates In Medicine. London, Bailliere, Tindall & Cassell, 1966.
120. Wong, W.: Chemistry and pharmacology of tolmetin. *In* Tolmetin—A New Non-Steroidal Anti-Inflammatory Agent. Edited by J.R. Ward. Amsterdam, Excerpta Medica, 1975.
121. Adams, S.S., and Buckler, J.W.: Ibuprofen and flurbiprofen. Clin. Rheum. Dis., *5*:359, 1979.
122. Brogden, R.N., et al.: Naproxen: A review of its pharmacological properties and therapeutic efficacy and use. Drugs, *9*:326, 1975.
123. Brogden, R.N., et al.: Fenoprofen: A review of its pharmacological properties and therapeutic efficacy in rheumatic diseases. Drugs, *13*:241, 1977.
124. Clinical experiences with Suprol (suprofen) capsules. *In* Postgraduate Medicine: Custom Communications. New York, McGraw-Hill, 1986.
125. Symposium: Pharmacology, efficacy, and safety of a new class of anti-inflammatory agents: A review of piroxican. Am. J. Med., *72*:1, 1982.
126. Lasagna, L., and Dekornfeld, T.J.: Methotrimeprazine: A new phenothiazine with analgesic properties. JAMA, *178*:887, 1961.
127. Szczeklik, A., Gryglewski, R.J., and Czerniawska-Mysik, G.: Relationship of inhibition of prostaglandin biosynthesis by analgesics to asthma attacks in aspirin-sensitive patients. Br. Med. J., *1*:67, 1975.
128. Paulus, H.E., and Whitehouse, M.W.: Nonsteroid anti-inflammatory agents. Annu. Rev. Pharmacol., *13*:107, 1973.
129. Bonica, J.J., and Benedetti, C.: Postoperative pain. *In* Surgical Care: A Physiologic Approach to Clinical Management. Edited by R.E. Condon and J.J. De Cosse. Philadelphia, Lea & Febiger, 1980, pp. 394–415.
130. Benedetti, C.: The role of pain in the development of respiratory insufficiency. Le Insufficienze Respiratorie, Parte I. Edited by R. Cuocolo and A. Blasi. Napoli, Francesco Giannini & Figli, 1981, pp. 93–111.
131. Benedetti, C., Bonica, J.J., and Bellucci, G.: Pathophysiology and therapy of postoperative pain: A review. *In* Advances in Pain Research and Therapy, Vol. 7. Edited by C. Benedetti, et al. New York, Raven Press, 1984, pp. 373–407.
132. Yeager, M.P., et al.: Epidural anesthesia and analgesia in high-risk surgical patients. Anesthesiology, *66*:729, 1987.
133. Anand, K.J.S., Sippell, W.G., and Aynsley-Green, A.: Randomised trial of fentanyl anesthesia in preterm babies undergoing surgery: Effects on the stress response. Lancet, *1*:243, 1987.
134. Anand, K.J.S., Phil, D., and Hickey, P.R.: Pain and its effects in the human neonate and fetus. N. Engl. J. Med., *317*:1321, 1987.
135. Forrest, W.H., Smethurst, P.W.R., and Kienetz, M.E.: Self-administration of intravenous analgesics. Anesthesiology, *33*:363, 1970.
136. Keeri-Szanto, M.: Apparatus for demand analgesia. Can. Anaesth. Soc. J., *18*:581, 1971.
137. Sechzer, P.H.: Studies in pain with the analgesic demand system. Anaesth. Analg., *50*:1, 1971.
138. Keeri-Szanto, M.: Demand analgesia. J. Med., *13*:241, 1982.
139. Tamsen, A., et al.: Patient-controlled analgesic therapy, part one: Pharmacokinetics of pethidine in the perioperative and postoperative periods. Clin. Pharmacokinet., 7:149, 1982.
140. Rosen, M., Slattery, P., and Vickers, M.D.: Cardiff palliator. Br. J. Anaesthesiol., *55*:9, 1983.
141. Lehmann, K.A.: Autoregulation de l'analgésie postoperatoire. Cah. Anesthesiol., *33*:119, 1985.
142. Tamsen, A., Sjoestroem, S., and Hartvig, P.: The Uppsala experience of patient-controlled analgesia. *In* Advances in Pain Research and Therapy, Vol. 8. Edited by K.M. Foley and C.E. Inturrisi. New York, Raven Press, 1986, pp. 325–332.
143. Lehmann, K.A.: Practical experience with demand analgesia for postoperative pain. *In* Patient-Controlled Analgesia. Edited by M. Harmer, M. Rosen, and M.D. Vickers. Oxford, Blackwell Scientific Publications, 1985, pp. 134–139.
144. Grabinski, P.Y., et al.: Plasma levels and analgesia following deltoid and gluteal injections of methadone and morphine. J. Clin. Pharmacol., *23*:48, 1983.
145. Hanning, C.D.: Non-parenteral techniques. *In* Acute Pain. Edited by G. Smith and B. Covino. London, Butterworth, 1985, pp. 180–204.
146. Benedetti, C., et al.: Effects of ethanol on evoked potentials elicited by painful dental stimuli. Pain, *20*:S162, 1984.
147. Ready, L.B., Sarkis, E., and Turner, J.A.: Self-reported vs. actual use of medications in chronic pain patients. Pain, *12*:285, 1982.
148. Taub, A.: Opioid analgesics in the treatment of chronic intractable pain of non-neoplastic origin. *In* Narcotic Analgesics in Anesthesiology. Edited by L.M. Kitahata and J.G. Collins. Baltimore, Williams & Wilkins, 1982, pp. 199–208.
149. Portenoy, R.K., and Foley, K.M.: Chronic use of opioid analgesics in non-malignant pain: Report of 38 cases. Pain, *25*:171, 1986.

79 · PSYCHOTROPIC DRUGS

RICHARD MONKS

ANTIDEPRESSANTS, neuroleptics, and lithium carbonate have been found useful in treating some types of acute and chronic pain (1, 2). Antianxiety drugs, of which only the benzodiazepines (BDZs) will be considered here, can be helpful in some acute painful conditions but are of questionable value in chronic pain. Psychostimulants can have a limited role in the treatment of cancer and other chronic pain problems. Other psychotropic drugs have not been found effective in pain management and will not be discussed.

The analgesic properties of psychotropics were reported shortly after their introduction into psychiatric practice (2). In 1955 chlorpromazine, a phenothiazine neuroleptic developed to potentiate anesthesia, was found to have analgesic effects in acute and chronic neurologic pain. In 1960 imipramine, a heterocyclic antidepressant (HCAD), was noted to decrease pain and depression in some patients with chronic pain. In 1974 lithium was first reported to alleviate chronic and episodic cluster headache.

Psychotropic drugs have been reported to have analgesic effects for those pain syndromes listed in Table 79-1. Pain of psychologic origin, noted in the table, refers to disorders in which structural damage was not found and in which anxiety and depression were obvious, antedating or coinciding with the onset of atypical pain. Neuroleptics may be indicated in acute severe pain in which respiratory depression, CNS depression, drug dependency, or analgesic hypersensitivity precludes adequate narcotic or BDZ use (e.g., migraine, myocardial infarction, or postsurgical and labor pain (3–5). Combined antidepressant-neuroleptic treatment has been increasingly used for chronic pain not responsive to either type of drug alone (2, 6). A similar indication may obtain for combined antidepressant-anticonvulsant (carbamazepine, clonazepam, or diphenylhydantoin) therapy for intractable chronic neuralgia (2, 7, 8).

In general medical and surgical practice, psychotropic use is largely confined to prescribing benzodiazepines, especially diazepam (Valium) and flurazepam (Dalmane), for insomnia, nausea, emotional distress, and occasionally for pain. It has been repeatedly noted that physicians lack knowledge and confidence in prescribing antidepressants and neuroleptics. However, antidepressants and neuroleptics are commonly used in specialized pain treatment settings (pain centers) as part of a comprehensive approach to treating chronic pain. It has been estimated that up to half of the chronic pain patients in pain centers are dependent on benzodiazepines and/or narcotics (9).

The general principles of psychotropic use have been well described (10). The following points are worth emphasizing:

1. There must be an adequate indication for psychotropic use. Moreover, control of symptoms with psychotropics must not delay the identification of treatable causes of pain.
2. A collaborative relationship with the patient, family, and other health providers is best. Indications, goals, methods, and potential hazards of treatment should be explained in a clear manner.
3. Time permitting, therapy should begin with the most benign and efficacious intervention and be changed to a more hazardous regimen only if treatment fails (e.g., TENS → antidepressant → antidepressant-neuroleptic therapy).
4. Adequate therapeutic trials (dose, duration) are essential.
5. Other drugs should be reduced or eliminated, if possible, before or soon after psychotropics are started. If analgesics are to be retained, a timetabled schedule is best.
6. The physician must be available during initiation of therapy and during any major change in regimen.
7. Doses of psychotropics for the elderly are usually one-third to one-half of those for healthy younger adults. Because of pharmacokinetic changes with age, steady-state blood levels and maximum side effects might not be reached for weeks.

In this chapter, information about each group of psychotropic drugs is presented in two major parts: (a) physiologic and pharmacologic effects; and (b) clinical considerations including indications, technique of administration, efficacy, and side effects and complications. A more detailed consideration of certain aspects of this subject can be found elsewhere (1, 2, 11, 12).

TABLE 79-1. Possible Indications for Psychotropic Drugs

Psychotropic Category	Specific Pain Syndrome Indications
Antidepressant Heterocyclics	Cancer pain, chronic arthritic pain, chronic benign pain, diabetic neuropathy, low back pain, migraine, myofascial dysfunction syndrome, pain of psychologic origin, perineal neuralgia, phantom pain, postherpetic neuralgia, tension headache, trigeminal neuralgia
Monoamine oxidase inhibitors	Atypical facial pain, migraine
Neuroleptics	Cancer pain, causalgia, chronic arthritis pain, fibromyositis, herpes zoster pain, labor pain, migraine, myocardial infarction, phantom limb pain, postoperative pain, postherpetic neuralgia, thalamic pain, traumatic neuropathy pain
Lithium salts	Chronic and episodic cluster headache, painful shoulder syndrome

ANTIDEPRESSANTS

Mechanism of Action

Although the physiologic and pharmacologic basis of antidepressant analgesia is unknown, several mechanisms have been suggested and will be discussed briefly here.

ANTIDEPRESSANT EFFECT. The majority of individuals with chronic pain are depressed (11), and frequently both disorders respond to antidepressant drug therapy (2, 13, 14). Nonmalignant chronic pain can be a manifestation of a primary depressive disorder (15, 16), and analgesic effects of antidepressant drugs are more likely when depressive symptoms began before the onset of pain (14).

It has been hypothesized that antidepressant drugs alleviate depression by correcting relative or absolute deficiencies of monoamine (MA) neurotransmitters such as serotonin (5-HT), norepinephrine (NE), and dopamine (DA) in brain areas governing mood (17). Within hours to days after administration various antidepressants act on MA neurons to block monoamine reuptake from the synaptic cleft, increase its presynaptic release, or decrease presynaptic receptor inhibition of MA release. Monoamine oxidase inhibitors (MAOIs) decrease intraneuronal presynaptic MA degradation with similar enhancement of MA neurotransmission. The acute MA effects of antidepressants used in pain treatment are listed in Tables 79-2 and 79-3. Chronic adaptive changes in MA receptor functioning occur within weeks, probably stabilizing acute changes (18).

INDEPENDENT ANALGESIC EFFECTS. Heterocyclic antidepressants and monoamine oxidase inhibitors appear to have analgesic properties that are independent of their antidepressant effects. These drugs may relieve chronic pain in the absence of detectable depression or of improvement in coexisting depression (2). Also, analgesic responses frequently occur more rapidly and at lower doses of antidepressant drugs than do typical responses in depressive disorders (2).

Analgesic properties of antidepressants have been attributed to nonspecific physiologic effects such as diminished arousal, muscle relaxation, and restored sleep cycles. These mechanisms are unlikely to explain the superiority of heterocyclic antidepressants over benzodiazepines and placebos in relieving chronic pain.

NEUROTRANSMITTER AND OPIATE EFFECTS. Antidepressant drugs might relieve pain by altering MA components in the endorphin-mediated analgesia system (EMAS), the major known descending antinociceptive pathway (19). In animals, antidepressants that enhance 5-HT neurotransmission augment stimulation-produced analgesia and morphine analgesia, whereas those with predominant NE effects have the opposite effect. In human chronic pain, direct comparisons of various HCADs showed superior analgesic effects in those with stronger 5-HT properties (24, 25). Other studies, however, have indicated that the less-serotonergic antidepressants imipramine and desipramine are as effective.

Endorphins might play a role in HCAD analgesia. In animals, HCADs bind rather weakly to opiate receptors, and endorphins seem to enhance HCAD postsynaptic receptor effects (11). However, monoamines seem to be more directly involved in HCAD analgesia than do endorphins (26). In chronic pain patients treated with zimelidine, an HCAD with selective 5-HT effects, analgesic responses were correlated with decreased endorphin and 5-hydroxyindoleacetic acid (the major metabolite of brain 5-HT) in cerebrospinal fluid (27).

Clinical Considerations

Indications

In addition to their use for specific pain syndromes (Table 79-1), psychotropics are prescribed to alleviate distressing target symptoms that undermine the patient's coping skills, motivation, and compliance.

Typically, antidepressants are used to treat depression, insomnia, and anxiety, especially during detoxification from alcohol, narcotics, and antianxiety drugs (9). Indications for a trial of antidepressant therapy are further strengthened by a history of depression preceding or coinciding with pain onset (14); a past favorable response of depression or pain to antidepressants; and a current episode of depression with endogenous symptoms (insidious onset, anorexia, early morning awakening, psychomotor changes, and anhedonia). Biologic markers of depression such as dexamethasone nonsuppression, shortened REM sleep latency, and level of urinary 3-methoxy-4-hydroxyphenethylene glycol (MHPG) can predict pain relief with heterocyclic antidepressants (13, 16, 17, 28).

Technique of Administration

Heterocyclic Antidepressants

The generic names and dosages of HCADs used for management of chronic pain are listed in Table 79-3.

TABLE 79-2. Biogenic Amine and Anticholinergic Effects of Antidepressants Used in Pain Management

Drug	Biogenic Amine Effect*†		Anticholinergic Effect*‡
	5-HT	NE	
Heterocyclics			
A. Tricyclics			
Amitriptyline	+ + + +	+ +	+ + + +
Clomipramine	+ + + +	+ +	+ + +
Desipramine	+ +	+ + + +	+
Doxepin	+ +	+	+ + +
Imipramine	+ + +	+ + + +	+ +
Nortriptyline	+ +	+ + +	+ +
Trimipramine	+	+	+ +
B. Second-generation drugs			
Maprotiline	+	+ +	+
Trazodone	+ +	+	−
Monoamine oxidase inhibitor			
Phenelzine	+	+	+

*Value of effects: + + + + marked; + + + moderate; + + mild; + minimal; − absent. Only values in a vertical column should be compared.
†Data from refs. 1, 12, 18, 19.
‡Data from refs. 1, 12, 19–21.

TABLE 79-3. Dosages and Effects of Antidepressants Used in Pain Management

Drug	Initial Dosage*	Maintenance Dosage*	Efficacy in Depression†‡	Adverse and Side Effects†§	
				Orthostatic Hypotension	Sedation
Heterocyclics					
A. Tricyclics					
Amitriptyline	10–300	10–150	+ + + +	+ +	+ + +
Clomipramine	20–200	20–150	+ + + +	+ +	+ +
Desipramine	75–300	75–100	+ + + +	+ +	−
Doxepin	30–300	30–200	+ + + +	+ +	+ + + +
Imipramine	20–300	20–150	+ + + +	+ + +	+
Nortriptyline	50–150	50–150	+ + + +	+	+
Trimipramine	50–225	75–150	+ + + +	+ +	+ + +
B. Second-generation drugs					
Maprotiline	75–300	75–125	+ + + +	+	+ +
Trazodone	50–600	100–300	+ + + ?	+ +	+ + +
Monoamine oxidase inhibitor					
Phenelzine	45–90	45–75	+ +	+ + +	−

*Antidepressant dose reflects material from the clinical literature cited in this chapter and the author's personal experience.
†Value of effects: + + + + marked; + + + moderate; + + mild; + minimal; − absent; ? questionable (data inadequate). Only values in a vertical column should be compared.
‡Data from Refs. 1, 10, 12.
§Data from Refs. 10, 20, 93.

PRECAUTIONS. Baseline laboratory tests should include liver function tests if there is a suggestion of liver disease. An ECG is done if high doses of HCAD or combined therapy are to be used and for males over 30 and women over 40 with no ECG in the previous year. Other tests are performed only if clinically indicated.

CHOICE OF DRUGS. There is little evidence to recommend the use of one HCAD over another for depression or for pain. The strongest indication for using a specific HCAD would be a history of favorable response to that drug in the patient or a close blood relative. A history of therapeutic failure or adverse effects with a particular HCAD should be thoroughly investigated. Inadequate trials, noncompliance, and minor adverse effects are the usual reasons for not determining the true potential of a particular drug. If the drug history is unhelpful, there may be an advantage in using a drug with strong 5-HT effects or one that has been shown to be effective in the pain disorder being treated. Drug side effects can be exploited (e.g., using a more sedating HCAD for patients with marked sleep disturbance, agitation, or anxiety). Often an HCAD must be chosen to avoid potentially severe adverse effects.

INITIAL ADMINISTRATION. More cautious regimens decrease alarming side effects and improve compliance. For example, it is usual to begin amitriptyline with 25 mg orally 1 to 2 hours before bedtime to enhance sleep. The dosage is increased by 25 mg each day and given in 2 or 3 divided doses with the greatest part taken in the evening. This is continued until a therapeutic response is obtained or a total dose of 150 mg/day is reached. If intolerable side effects occur, the dosage is temporarily lowered to the last tolerable level and increased again in 2 days or when adaptation occurs. If there is no response at 150 mg/day for 1 week, the dosage may be increased by 25 mg/day to the maximum initial dosage (Table 79-3). If there is no therapeutic effect after 2 weeks and compliance is not a problem, further response is unlikely; in this case, the dosage should be decreased by 25 mg each day and the drug discontinued.

Most analgesic effects occur at dosages equivalent to 75 to 150 mg/day of amitriptyline, but exceptions are not unusual. For example, head pain (migraine, face and head pain of psychologic origin, and chronic tension headaches) may be relieved at levels equivalent to 25 to 75 mg of amitriptyline (2, 29–31).

Some European authors have suggested initiating HCAD therapy for inpatients with intravenous infusion (e.g., clomipramine at 25 to 50 mg/day for 3 to 5 days) followed by the usual oral doses, but convincing evidence of the efficacy of this technique is not available (2).

MAINTENANCE ADMINISTRATION. Maintenance therapy for chronic pain or depression might be necessary for months or even years. After 1 month of stable maximum therapeutic effect at the initial dosage of an HCAD, it is usually possible to slowly (10 to 25 mg every 1 to 2 weeks) decrease the dosage to a lower maintenance dosage (Table 79-3). During the maintenance phase, the drug can be prescribed in a single daily dose, usually in the evening, in order to improve compliance. After 3 to 6 months of sustained remission, an attempt should be made to discontinue drug therapy by decreasing the daily dose by 10 to 25 mg every 2 to 3 weeks. If the drug must be continued, similar attempts to discontinue its usage should be made every 6 months.

NONRESPONSE OR RELAPSE. If the first HCAD tried is ineffective despite an adequate trial, three options are available. If the patient is tolerating the drug adequately, a plasma level can be obtained; if it is low, the dose can be increased. About two-thirds of "refractory" depressions occur with subtherapeutic plasma levels (32). In the obviously depressed patient, especially if depression is thought to be the primary disorder, a switch to another HCAD with different MA effects (Table 79-2) is indicated. For example, if clomipramine fails, a drug with a stronger NE effect, such as imipramine, would be substituted and a second adequate trial instituted.

The third option in the case of nonresponse is to add a neuroleptic to the HCAD regimen. This choice is rational for patients with milder depressive symptoms that started after the onset of pain. In order to minimize adverse effects, oral doses of high-potency neuroleptics such as haloperidol (0.5 to 5 mg/day), fluphenazine (0.5 to 5 mg/day), flupenthixol (0.5 to 3 mg/day), or perphenazine (4 to 64 mg/day) are used. If one of these drugs is ineffective, or if more sedation is required, a low-potency neuroleptic such as methotrimeprazine (15 to 100 mg/day), chlorpromazine (25 to 100 mg/day), or pericyazine (5 to 100 mg/day) can be used. The neuroleptic is started at the lowest dose listed above and increased by increments of this dose each day until a therapeutic effect or the maximum recommended dose is reached. If no therapeutic response is noted by 2 weeks, the neuroleptic and then the HCAD are discontinued. If the combination is effective, an attempt should be made to discontinue the HCAD because the neuroleptic alone might be adequate. Maintenance dosage guidelines are the same as those given in Tables 79-3 and 79-5 for each drug given alone. Additional information on combined therapy is presented later in this chapter.

Monoamine Oxidase Inhibitors

Dosages for phenelzine, a common MAOI antidepressant, are given in Table 79-3.

PRECAUTIONS. Because of potential adverse reactions, MAOIs are usually reserved for HCAD-resistant disorders. Patients must be capable of complying with dietary, beverage, and drug restrictions and must be instructed on how to handle hypertensive crises.

INITIAL ADMINISTRATION. Phenelzine is started at 15 mg/day on awakening, and 15 mg is added each day until a total daily dosage of 60 mg is reached, given in 2 divided morning doses to prevent insomnia. If there is no response after 2 weeks, the dosage may be increased each 3 days by 15 mg/day to a total dosage of 90 mg/day. If no response is obtained after 2 weeks, the dosage is tapered off and the drug discontinued.

MAINTENANCE ADMINISTRATION. Guidelines for maintenance use and for discontinuing phenelzine are similar to those for heterocyclic antidepressants.

NONRESPONSE OR RELAPSE. Measures of platelet MAO inhibition can be used to determine adequate dosage and compliance problems (1). L-Tryptophan, neuroleptics, benzodiazepines, and lithium have been used with MAOIs to obtain increased efficacy in depression, but little is known about any improvement in analgesic response (33).

Efficacy

Heterocyclic Antidepressants

Table 79-4 summarizes the results of clinical trials with heterocyclic antidepressants that were judged to meet minimum standards for adequate, controlled, double-blind studies (29–44). All reported on chronic pain. Antidepressant therapy was associated with important antidepressant and analgesic effects that were superior to those observed with placebo or BDZ controls. Two exceptions were noted. In one trial (39) imipramine at a rather low dose (75 mg/day) and placebo were equally effective in chronic low back pain. In the other trial (43), amitriptyline and placebo were equally ineffective for atypical pains. The patients in this trial were not significantly depressed, in contrast to those in three other trials that indicated antidepressants were effective for similar pains (29, 35).

Data from available antidepressant trials are summarized in Table 79-4. More than half of the patients obtained moderate to total pain relief in 47 of the 54 trials giving this information. Analgesic use was significantly diminished in a small number of studies with adequate data. Compliance was acceptable (<12% of patients discontinued medications, and blood levels, where measured, were within expectable limits). The majority of patients studied had pain refractory to multiple previous therapies. Unfortunately, most of these trials lasted only 3 months or less. However, 1 study of 104 patients with chronic benign pain included a 21- to 28-month follow-up (45). At this time, about one-third of all patients reported moderate to total pain relief, and the majority of these still required maintenance doses of antidepressants.

Seven controlled trials compared analgesic effects of one HCAD with another in chronic pain. Significant differences were only noted in three trials. Clomipramine was superior to amitriptyline for trigeminal neuralgia (25). Later, in an expanded study, doxepin and desipramine were reported to have equivalent effects (46). Doxepin was preferable to desipramine for depressed patients with low back pain (46) and to amitriptyline for pain of psychologic origin (29).

Monamine Oxidase Inhibitors

One adequate, controlled double-blind trial (33) and two uncontrolled single-group outcome studies of MAOIs were found (33, 47). In all three, important analgesic effects of phenelzine in chronic pain were found, and this effect was clinically and statistically superior to that of placebo in the controlled study. The majority of patients continued to experience moderate or total relief on phenelzine for up to 7 months.

Side Effects and Complications

Side effects, adverse effects, and contraindications to the use of psychotropics are described in detail elsewhere (1, 10, 48).

Heterocyclic Antidepressants

Anticholinergic effects of heterocyclic antidepressants are due to muscarinic receptor stimulation and vary in intensity depending on the drug used (Table

TABLE 79-4. Results of Controlled Clinical Trials with Antidepressants (AD) for Chronic Pain

Disorder	Drug	Outcome*			Source
		AD Superior to Placebo	AD Equal to Placebo	No Analgesia	
Arthritis	Dibenzepin	+			Thorpe and Marchant-Williams (34)
	Imipramine	+			Gingras (35)
	Imipramine	+			McDonald Scott (36)
Diabetic neuropathy	Amitriptyline	+			Kvinesdal et al. (37)
	Imipramine	+			Turkington (38)
	Imipramine	+			Jenkins et al. (39)
Low back pain	Imipramine		+		Jenkins et al. (39)
Migraine	Amitriptyline	+			Couch et al. (40)
	Amitriptyline	+			Gomersall and Stuart (41)
Cancer pain	Imipramine	+			Fiorentino (42)
Psychologic origin pain	Amitriptyline	+			Okasha et al. (29)
	Amitriptyline			+	Pilowsky et al. (43)
	Doxepin	+			Okasha et al. (29)
	Phenelzine†	+			Lascelles (33)
Postherpetic neuralgia	Amitriptyline	+			Watson et al. (44)
Tension headache	Amitriptyline	+			Diamond and Baltes (30)
	Amitriptyline	+			Lance and Curran (31)

* + indicates conclusion supported by evidence in the trial. No analgesia column indicates neither drug nor placebo demonstrated analgesic properties.
†This is the only monoamine oxidase trial in this table.
Modified from Monks and Merskey (2).

79-2), the dose used, the presence of other anticholinergic drugs (neuroleptics, antihistaminics, antiparkinsonian drugs), and the vulnerability of the patient to these effects. Milder, often transient effects include dry mouth, palpitations, blurred vision, constipation, and edema. More serious adverse effects include aggravation of narrow-angle glaucoma, impotence, and, especially in the elderly, urinary retention and delirium. Bethanecol can be used to decrease urine retention if antidepressant doses cannot be lowered without loss of therapeutic efficacy. If an HCAD must be used in patients at risk, drugs such as desipramine or trazodone are preferable, because these exhibit little anticholinergic effect.

Allergic hypersensitivy reactions such as cholestatic jaundice, skin reactions, and agranulocytosis are relatively uncommon. A history of this type of reaction to an antidepressant or neuroleptic necessitates extreme caution. If alternative nondrug therapy is not feasible, a drug with a different chemical structure should be chosen (e.g., maprotiline or trazodone if a reaction occurs to one of the older drugs).

Anticholinergic and quinidine-like cardiac effects of heterocyclic antidepressants are seldom a problem clinically, except in overdoses and in patients with preexisting conduction disorders. All available tricyclic antidepressants have these effects. The "second-generation" antidepressants have been reported to have some arrhythmogenic properties. Lower doses of doxepin, desipramine, or maprotiline might be considered if drug therapy is essential.

Central nervous system (CNS) side effects are quite common with heterocyclic antidepressants. Sedation, hypotension, weight gain, and potentiation of CNS depressants are probably the result of H_1 histamic receptor blockade. Frequently two forms of sedation are seen: a more severe transient (<72 hours) form and a milder persisting form. Patients should be told about the transient form and instructed to contact their physician if the sedative effect does not decrease within 72 hours. This transient sedation might occur only with the initial doses. The various HCADs differ in their sedative effects (Table 79-3). Agitation, insomnia, and exacerbation of mania or schizophrenia can occur; careful history taking can help alert the clinician to the need for caution in predisposed patients. In known epileptics, slow initial administration and the use of doxepin or trazodone is recommended. Maprotiline in high doses should be avoided.

Orthostatic hypotension is common with HCADs that block adrenergic receptors (Table 79-3). HCADs like imipramine can be particularly hazardous for the elderly and others vulnerable to falls or hypotension. Patients with pretreatment hypotension are at particular risk. Safer drugs should be chosen for these vulnerable individuals and orthostatic blood pressure changes noted twice weekly in the initial 2 weeks of therapy. Helpful interventions include patient education, use of a bedside commode and night light, and surgical support stockings. Improvement is often seen with an increase in sodium and fluid intake and, in patients treated for hypertension, a reduction in antihypertensive medication. In severe cases, 9-alpha-fluorhydrocortisone (0.025 to 0.050 mg twice per day orally) is recommended.

Heterocyclic antidepressants interact with other drugs, potentiating CNS depressants (alcohol, antianxiety sedatives, narcotics), antagonizing some antihypertensives (methyldopa, guanethidine), and producing hypertensive episodes with monamine oxidase inhibitors.

Overdoses of an HCAD can be lethal. Patients with suicidal ideas should be referred for psychiatric assessment. Prescriptions for depressed patients should not exceed the lethal dose (about 1-week supply of most HCADs).

Mild withdrawal reactions (headache, diarrhea, vivid dreams) can occur if HCADs are stopped abruptly, even after short-term use. If possible, these drugs should be tapered off over a period of 3 to 4 weeks. Fortunately, more severe reactions are rare and occur only with high doses.

Second-generation HCADs were introduced with the claim that their more selective brain receptor activities would prevent the adverse effects associated with older drugs, but recent reports suggest that this might not be so. In fact, certain second-generation drugs appear to have specific adverse effects qualitatively or quantitatively unique among the HCADs. Trazodone use has been associated with irreversible priapism in males. Maprotiline is associated with an increased incidence of seizures, especially at higher doses (over 200 mg) and in individuals predisposed to this problem. Amoxapine has neuroleptic properties and can induce a variety of extrapyramidal syndromes including tardive dyskinesia (49).

The safety of any heterocyclic antidepressant during pregnancy or lactation has not been established.

In the pain trials reviewed for this chapter, HCAD use was relatively safe. Drowsiness (3 to 23% of patients) and delirium (3 to 13% of patients) were the most frequently reported adverse effects and were usually associated with high doses or drug combinations (HCAD with a neuroleptic or anticonvulsant) in the elderly. A total of 2 deaths occurred in all trials (myocardial infarction, suicide), both in patients with advanced neoplasms. Long-term use of tricyclic antidepressants in pain patients and in depressed patients has not been associated with serious medical, intellectual, or social impairment.

Monoamine Oxidase Inhibitors

Monoamine oxidase inhibitors (MAOIs) can cause ejaculatory and orgasmic difficulties, orthostatic hypotension, peripheral neuropathy, rare parenchymal hepatotoxic reactions, urinary retention, and various CNS side effects (insomnia, agitation, exacerbation of mania and schizophrenia).

Monoamine oxidase inhibitors interact with various sympathomimetic substances, producing a syndrome varying in severity from headaches to hypertensive crisis and, rarely, intracranial bleeding. These severe reactions are almost entirely preventable if intake of certain medications, foods, and beverages is avoided (1, 10). Hypertensive reactions are treated by phentolamine (2 to 5 mg intravenously) or chlorpromazine (50 to 100 mg intramuscularly). Patients may carry 100 to 200 mg of oral chlorpromazine to use should a physician's care be unavailable. Monoamine oxidase inhibitors exhibited no long-term complications in a limited number of trials with chronic pain and with anxiety disorders.

NEUROLEPTICS

Physiologic and Pharmacologic Basis

Mechanisms underlying neuroleptic analgesia are unknown, but several explanations have been offered.

ANTIPSYCHOTIC ACTION. The vast majority of pains responsive to neuroleptics are not associated with any psychotic phenomena and do not have delusional qualities.

PHYSIOLOGIC ACTION. Single-dose analgesic effects of more sedating neuroleptics might be the result of decreased arousal. However, high-potency alerting neuroleptics have analgesic properties in chronic pain, often when more potent anxiolytics like the benzodiazepines have failed. Neuroleptics can cause local anesthesic effects in spinal nerves, and skeletal muscle relaxation can be induced in certain spastic conditions (1), but it is unlikely these effects are of importance at usual clinical doses.

NEUROTRANSMITTER ACTIONS. Neuroleptics bind and block postsynaptic dopamine receptor sites in the brain. Their effect on the endorphin-mediated analgesia system is not known. Neither adrenergic nor muscarinic-blocking effects seem to correlate with

analgesic effectiveness of particular neuroleptics. The chemical structure of neuroleptics and opiates is similar. Some neuroleptics bind to opiate receptors, and many block naloxone binding (50).

Clinical Considerations

Indications

Neuroleptics are indicated to treat delusional pain and other manifestations of psychotic disorders, such as schizophrenia, psychotic depressions, monosymptomatic hypochondriacal psychosis (51), and various organic mental disorders. Overwhelming pain with anxiety, psychomotor agitation, and insomnia that is not responsive to benzodiazepines in acute pain or to heterocyclic antidepressants in chronic pain can be treated by neuroleptics. In oncology settings, neuroleptics are indicated for nausea, vomiting, bladder or rectal tenesmus, and ureteral spasm (3).

Technique of Administration

The generic names and dosages of neuroleptics used in pain management are listed in Table 79-5.

TABLE 79-5. Dosages and Side Effects of Neuroleptics Used for Pain Management

Drug	Initial Dosage* (mg/day, orally)	Maintenance Dosage† (mg/day, orally)	Side and Adverse Effects‡			
			Anticholinergic	Autonomic (Hypotension)	Extrapyramidal	Sedative
Phenothiazines						
Chlorpromazine	75–500	25–150	+ + +	+ + +	+	+ + +
Fluphenazine	1–10	1–3	+	+	+ + +	+
Methotrimeprazine	5–100	15–50	+ + +	+ + +	+ +	+ + +
Pericyazine	5–200	5–100	+ + +	+ + +	+	+ + +
Perphenazine	8–64	4–16	+ +	+ +	+ +	+ +
Thioridazine	10–200	25–75	+ + +	+ + +	+	+ + +
Trifluoperazine	3–20	3–10	+	+	+ + +	+
Thioxanthenes						
Chlorprothixene	50–200	50–150	+ + +	+ + +	+	+ + +
Flupenthixol	0.5–2	0.5–1	+	−	+ + +	−
Miscellaneous						
Haloperidol	0.5–30	0.5–10	+	+	+ + +	+ +

*Neuroleptic doses reflect material from the clinical material cited in this chapter and the author's personal experience.

†Modified from Baldessarini, R.J.: Drugs and the treatment of psychiatric disorders. *In* The Pharmacological Basis of Therapeutics. 7th Ed. Edited by A.G. Gilman et al. New York, Macmillan, 1985.

‡Value of effects: + + + moderate; + + mild; + minimal; − absent. Only values in a vertical column should be compared.

PRECAUTIONS. Baseline tests are identical to those with HCAD therapy. A written informed consent is advisable, especially regarding the risk of tardive dyskinesia (52).

INITIAL ADMINISTRATION. High-potency neuroleptics such as haloperidol or fluphenazine are started with a 1-mg oral test dose (0.25 to 0.50 mg in the elderly); if tolerated, the dosage is increased by 1 mg/day to the usual effective dose of 3 to 5 mg/day (0.5 to 2 mg/day in the elderly). If there is no response after 1 week, the dosage is further increased by 1 mg/day, as tolerated, to the effective or maximum dosage.

Low-potency neuroleptics may be preferable if agitation and insomnia are severe and if autonomic or anticholinergic side effects are not a contraindication. Methotrimeprazine can be started at 10 to 15 mg 2 to 3 hours before bedtime and increased by 2.5 to 10 mg/day, given in 3 divided doses with the largest portion in the evening, until the effective or maximum dosage is achieved. With high- or low-potency neuroleptics, a therapeutic response should be seen within 2 weeks after the maximum tolerable dosage is achieved or the drug should be tapered off and discontinued.

MAINTENANCE ADMINISTRATION. Guidelines for neuroleptic maintenance resemble those for HCADs.

Usual dosages are listed in Table 79-5. Frequent attempts should be made to find the lowest possible effective dose in view of the risk of tardive dyskinesia (53–57). A careful clinical examination and chart notation regarding involuntary movements should be routine at each follow-up visit.

Efficacy

Of 31 trials reviewed in which neuroleptics were used for acute or chronic pain, only the five listed in Table 79-6 were adequate, controlled, double-blind studies. In all five studies the analgesic effects of single doses of neuroleptic were compared with the effects of a narcotic analgesic or placebo or both. In 3 of these studies, a dose of 15 mg of methotrimeprazine was found to be equivalent to 8 to 10 mg morphine for patients with chronic pain for 3 to 6 hours after administration of the drugs. In 1 other of these adequate trials, 5 or 10 mg oral haloperidol had significant antiemetic effects but any analgesic effect was equal to that of the saline control (57). Only one adequate controlled trial of ongoing neuroleptic therapy was found in the literature. Fluphenazine 1 mg orally per day was clinically effective and clearly superior to

TABLE 79-6. Results of Controlled Clinical Trials with Neuroleptics for Pain Management

Type of Pain	Drug	Relative Analgesic Effect*	Source
Cancer	Methotrimeprazine	15 mg drug equals 8 mg morphine	Beaver et al. (53)
Mixed chronic	Methotrimeprazine	15 mg drug equals 10 mg morphine	Bloomfield et al. (54)
Mixed chronic	Methotrimeprazine	15 mg drug equals 15 mg morphine	Kast (55)
Myocardial infarction	Methotrimeprazine	12.5 mg drug equals 50 mg meperidine	Davidson et al. (56)
Postoperative pain	Haloperidol	5 or 10 mg drug equals saline	Judkins and Harmer (57)

*Interpretation of effect is limited to first 3 to 6 hours following single parenteral dose of neuroleptic or control (narcotic or saline).

placebo for high-frequency chronic tension headache in a 2-month blind crossover study (58).

Preliminary reports of two placebo-controlled crossover trials of flupenthixol for severe cancer pain and for chronic osteoarthritic hip pain suggest that this neuroleptic possesses significant analgesic and antidepressant properties (59, 60).

Important analgesic effects were reported in 84% of all neuroleptic trials. A number of single-patient experiments and single-group outcome studies of patients with neoplastic pain, postherpetic neuralgia, and thalamic pain provide strong support for the existence of neuroleptic-induced analgesia (2). Patients with very chronic unremitting pain refractory to multiple previous therapies responded rapidly (4 days or less) to neuroleptic therapy, frequently experienced total pain relief, and suffered relapse rapidly when a placebo was substituted or the neuroleptic was stopped. Outcome depended on the use of adequate neuroleptic dose (2, 61) and on the chronicity of the disorder treated; for example, postherpetic neuralgia was totally relieved in 90% of patients if less than 3 months in duration but improved in only 20% if present for a longer time (61). Compliance was an issue in only 1 study using moderate doses (75 to 100 mg/day) of chlorprothixene (61). Follow-up data were limited to 3 months in most neuroleptic trials. The importance of longer trials is underscored by 2 trials in which initial impressive relief disappeared after 6 months despite continued neuroleptic use (62).

Except for some combined neuroleptic-antidepressant trials, no direct comparisons of neuroleptics with other psychotropics or neuroleptics were found. In one study haloperidol was found to permit successful relaxation training in patients with chronic facial pain previously resistant to this and other forms of behavior therapy (62).

Side Effects and Complications

Like heterocyclic antidepressants, neuroleptics can cause anticholinergic effects, orthostatic hypotension, quinidine-like cardiac effects, and sedation (Table 79-5). These side effects are more prominent in the low-potency phenothiazines and thiothixenes than in high-potency neuroleptics. Acute extrapyramidal syndromes (parkinsonism, akathisia, and dystonias) also occur early in treatment, especially with high-potency drugs (Table 79-5).

Late-appearing neurologic syndromes include perioral tremor (relatively benign, responsive to antiparkinsonian drugs) and tardive dyskinesia (TD). The latter usually appears when the neuroleptic is decreased or stopped and, in adults, presents as an oral-facial dyskinesia with or without choreoathetosis (51). Although TD is more common in older females on high dosages after prolonged neuroleptic use, it occurs infrequently even in patients on low dosages after several months. Tardive dyskinesia can resist treatment and persist for years in an appreciable number of patients. Short-term low-dose neuroleptic use is preferable, and the drug should be stopped at the first signs of TD (52). Routine use of antiparkinsonian drugs increases the risk of TD and is best avoided.

Other adverse effects of neuroleptics include weight gain and sexual dysfunction (not uncommon with low-potency drugs), endocrine disorders, exacerbation of epileptic disorders, hypersensitivity reactions, neuroleptic malignant syndrome, and various ocular and dermatologic manifestations. They can also increase the effects of CNS depressants and block the action of guanethidine.

In chronic pain trials, the commonest problems were somnolence and delirium, usually occurring with high-dose methotrimeprazine or thiothixene therapy. In these predominantly short-term trials, only one patient was noted to develop TD.

COMBINED THERAPY

Combined Antidepressant-Neuroleptic Therapy

In one double-blind placebo-controlled crossover study a combination of 60 mg nortriptyline and 3 mg fluphenazine orally each day was superior to placebo and provided at least a 50% reduction in pain and paresthesia in 15 of 18 patients with chronic pain of diabetic neuropathy (63). None of the other 14 trials of combined antidepressant-neuroleptic therapy for chronic pain was controlled. However, more than half of all patients treated reported total pain relief, often after failures with many other therapies. The best results were obtained with arthritic pain, diabetic neuropathy, postherpetic neuralgia, and other neurologic pain disorders (2, 6, 64). Compliance was a problem only when sedating phenothiazines with hypotensive adverse effects were used with an antidepressant. Follow-up lasted more than 6 months in most studies, with continued remission being dependent on maintenance doses of the drugs.

Antidepressant-neuroleptic combined therapy resulted in more frequent analgesic effects and fewer dropouts than neuroleptic therapy alone in one open trial (65).

Combined Antidepressant-Anticonvulsant Therapy

For neuralgia resistant to HCADs or HCAD-neuroleptic combinations, an anticonvulsant may be added to an adequate HCAD regimen (e.g., daily oral doses of amitriptyline or clomipramine at 10 to 150 mg with carbamazepine at 150 to 1000 mg or valproic acid at 250 to 750 mg). Because of frequent adverse effects, hospitalization and close monitoring of the blood levels of both drugs are advisable in the elderly (2, 7). No controlled trials of antidepressant-anticonvulsant combined therapy were found. Encouraging results in 2 uncontrolled trials (2, 7, 66) were tempered by a high dropout rate in one (7).

Complex Techniques

Certain psychotropic treatments are usually carried out in psychiatric or specialized pain treatment settings.

Biologic markers possibly predict antidepressant effects with heterocyclic antidepressants and may prove useful in chronic pain (16, 17, 28). Dexamethasone nonsuppression (plasma cortisol ≥ 5 g/dl at 4 p.m. or 10 p.m. the day following an 11:00 p.m. oral dose of 1 mg of dexamethasone) and a positive dextroamphetamine challenge test (improvement in depressed mood and/or psychomotor retardation 2 hours after a 30-mg oral dose) can predict a response to an HCAD with NE properties such as imipramine (17, 28).

Plasma HCAD levels can be used to monitor compliance, decrease adverse drug effects, and determine the impact of drug interactions (37, 43, 44). Optimal levels for analgesic effect of HCADs have yet to be identified.

More vigorous treatment of depression is available for patients with an obvious depressive disorder refractory to adequate trials of two different HCADs. In outpatients, triodothyronine, lithium, L-tryptophan, or L-dopa may be added to increase the efficacy of an HCAD. It is also possible to switch to a second-generation HCAD, which may have different monoamine properties (Table 79-2). If there is no response to HCAD therapy, a switch to a MAOI such as phenelzine is indicated after a 2-week washout period. Finally, HCAD-MAOI combined treatment or electroconvulsive therapy (67) may be considered in highly resistant disorders.

Heterocyclic antidepressants (e.g., 50 to 75 mg doxepin at bedtime) are used in substitution-detoxification programs for those patients dependent on antianxiety sedatives, alcohol, or narcotics (9). The course of HCAD use is frequently of short duration (1 to 2 months).

LITHIUM SALTS

Physiologic and Pharmacologic Basis

The analgesic effect of lithium in episodic and chronic cluster headache does not appear to depend on mood-stabilizing or antidepressant effects (68, 69). Although the responsible physiologic and pharmacologic mechanisms are unknown, lithium does alter many neurotransmitter activities, which may have a role in pain. For example, it enhances 5-HT availability in the brain; diminishes catecholamine neuron activity; alters adrenergic, dopamine, gamma-aminobutyric acid (GABA), opiate, and benzodiazepine receptor activity; and stabilizes prostaglandin E_1 synthesis.

Clinical Considerations

Indications

Lithium salts are given for acute and chronic cluster headache, painful shoulder syndrome, and pain of psychologic origin associated with certain primary affective disorders (mania, some recurrent depressions).

Technique of Administration

Lithium salts are given orally, usually as lithium carbonate.

PRECAUTIONS. Lithium use for pain is contraindicated in the presence of certain medical conditions (renal tubular disease, myocardial infarction, myasthenia gravis, and cardiac conduction defects) and in early pregnancy (10). Patients must be willing to have regular blood tests and be capable of recognizing early signs of intoxication. Baseline investigations include serum creatinine and electrolytes, thyroid tests, hemogram, pregnancy test, urinalysis, and ECG. Close monitoring of serum levels is necessary when using drugs that increase lithium levels (e.g., diuretics, carbamazepine and nonsteroidal anti-inflammatory drugs).

INITIAL ADMINISTRATION. In cluster headaches, lithium carbonate 300 mg is given orally the first day and increased to 300 mg 3 times per day by the end of the first week (2, 70, 71). The dosage is adjusted according to clinical response and severity of side effects; weekly serum lithium levels should be kept at 0.4 to 1.2 mEq/L.

MAINTENANCE ADMINISTRATION. A gradual reduction in lithium dosage can be tried after 1 to 2 months of stable improvement. Usual maintenance serum lithium levels are 0.4 to 0.8 mEq/L. Once maintenance dosage is achieved, lithium determinations may be performed less frequently (monthly, then every 3 months). Serum creatinine and thyroid-stimulating hormone levels are determined every 6 months. Other tests are performed only if clinically indicated (72). After a 3- to 6-month symptom-free interval, lithium dosage may be tapered off and an attempt made to discontinue the drug.

Efficacy

None of 11 trials of lithium use in acute or chronic pain that were reviewed was controlled and blind (2, 68–70). About one-third of 69 patients with episodic cluster headache experienced good to total control of pain in a 1-month treatment period. More than two-thirds of 98 patients with chronic cluster headache obtained good to total pain relief for periods of 6 months or longer. In one open controlled trial, lithium was strikingly superior to methylsergide and to prednisone for chronic cluster headache pain (71).

In an uncontrolled trial of lithium and amitriptyline for painful shoulder syndrome, an increased range of motion of the joint and complete relief from pain were experienced by 40% of patients, and resolution of radiographic abnormalities occurred in a significant number (72). Compliance in all lithium studies was adequate.

Side Effects and Complications

Untoward lithium effects include acute intoxication, birth defects, and cardiac, dermatologic, epileptic, neuromuscular, neurotoxic, renal, and thyroid disorders

(1, 48). Careful monitoring of clinical symptoms and serum lithium levels render short-term lithium use relatively safe. In a minority of patients, long-term lithium treatment causes tubulo-interstitial morphologic kidney changes and a partly irreversible reduction in tubular function (48). Preventive measures include using the lowest effective dose of lithium for the least time possible and monitoring renal function. Lithium-induced goiter and hypothyroidism usually respond to thyroid hormone. In patients with cluster headaches, the commonest treatable symptom was tremor, which was manageable by decreasing the dose or treating with propranol.

ANTIANXIETY DRUGS

Benzodiazepines (BDZs) that have been used in the treatment of pain are listed in Table 79-7.

Physiologic/Pharmacologic Basis

Analgesic effects of BDZs in acute pain have been attributed to reduction in anxiety, muscle tension, and insomnia. One BDZ, alprazolam, appears to have clinically important antidepressant properties (75). Stimulation of BDZ receptors affects norepinephrine, serotonin (5-HT), dopamine, and gamma-aminobutyric acid neurotransmission (76), possibly influencing the endorphin-mediated analgesia system. This possibility is supported by studies in which diazepam analgesia was partially antagonized by naloxone in animals and humans (77, 78). However, more prolonged BDZ use can decrease 5-HT release and induce BDZ receptor subsensitivity, potentially reversing the analgesic effects of these and other drugs (2).

Clinical Considerations

Indications

The benzodiazepines are used for short-term (4 weeks or less) treatment of acute pain associated with obvious anxiety, muscle spasm, or insomnia (e.g., myocardial infarction, anxiety-related gastrointestinal disorders, and vertebral disk pain). Intermittent use for similar acute exacerbations during chronic pain disorders might be indicated if nondrug treatment is unsuccessful or unavailable. Clonazepam, a BDZ with sedative and anticonvulsant properties, has shown some promise in treating neuralgias associated with lancinating pain (8).

Technique of Administration

The generic names, dosages, half-lives, and main indications for benzodiazepines are listed in Table 79.7.

PRECAUTIONS. From the onset the patient should be educated to expect only short-term BDZ use. Alternative therapies for anxiety and muscle tension should be arranged as soon as possible. A BDZ should not be used with known alcohol or other drug abusers. Baseline tests are only performed if clinically indicated (79).

INITIAL ADMINISTRATION. Benzodiazepine choice, dose, and administration schedules are those used in the treatment of anxiety and are well described elsewhere (1, 80). Doses in excess of 10 to 15 mg/day oral diazepam (or its equivalent) are seldom indicated.

After 3 to 4 weeks of BDZ therapy, the drug is tapered and withdrawn over 1 week. Further brief, intermittent periods of BDZ therapy can be used for exacerbations in pain disorders.

Efficacy

Two flawed double-blind placebo-controlled trials suggest that diazepam and chlorazepate can be useful in decreasing severe chest pain immediately after myocardial infarction or up to 12 weeks thereafter (4).

Three adequate double-blind studies compared BDZs with placebo and one or more HCADs in chronic pain. The analgesic effects of BDZs in head pain of psychologic origin (29) and chronic tension headache (30) were significantly inferior to at least one HCAD control drug. Furthermore, BDZs were without effect in pain of diabetic neuropathy, despite excellent responses with an HCAD (38). Compliance was probably adequate, but follow-up was limited in these studies.

Side Effects and Complications

Physical dependency and withdrawal reactions occur rarely following prolonged (more than 6 weeks) moderate or high-dose BDZ use (81). Impaired attention, coordination, intellect, judgment, and memory are probably quite common with prolonged use

TABLE 79-7. Dosages and Indications for Benzodiazepines Used in Treatment of Pain

Drug	Dosage Range (mg/day, oral)	Average Dosage (mg/day, oral)	Half-Life (hours)*	Main Indications
Alprazolam	0.75–4	1.5	12–15	Panics, anxiety-depression
Chlordiazepoxide	10–100	30	7–46	Anxiety
Clonazepam	2–10	8	18–50	Panics, seizures, neuralgias
Clorazepate	7.5–60	30	30–100	Anxiety
Diazepam	4–40	15	26–53	Anxiety, muscle spasm
Lorazepam	1–6	3	10–20	Anxiety
Oxazepam	30–120	60	5–15	Anxiety

*From refs. 73, 74.

of therapeutic doses of BDZs (82, 83). The elderly, brain-damaged, and those on other psychoactive drugs are particularly vulnerable. Other reported adverse effects include depression, suicidal thoughts, impulsivity, and rebound insomnia.

In the short-term BDZ pain trials reviewed, no untoward effects were noted. However, studies of patients treated in pain centers suggest that global and specific neuropsychologic test impairments and EEG abnormalities occur more often in those patients on BDZs than in comparable controls (82, 83).

In the general population, 15% of all BDZ users continue these drugs on a daily long-term basis. Most claim continued benefit without tolerance to the drug. Similar results were found in one study of patients on diazepam up to 16 years for treatment of chronic pain and muscle spasm (84). Unfortunately, neuropsychological testing was not reported.

PSYCHOSTIMULANTS

The psychostimulants are a group of indirectly acting sympathomimetic drugs with powerful central nervous system stimulating effects and variable peripheral adrenergic actions. Drugs in this group that have been used in the treatment of acute and chronic pain include dextroamphetamine, methylphenidate, and cocaine.

Physiologic and Pharmacologic Basis

Psychostimulants have euphoriant and antidepressant properties, which might alter pain perception, but such changes do not appear to be necessary for analgesic effect, at least in acute experimental pain (85).

Cocaine has a local anesthetic action, which may be important when the drug is given intranasally for pain attributable to sphenopalatine ganglion dysfunction (86). The significance of specific central binding sites for (^{3}H)-cocaine is unknown (87).

It is not known which neurotransmitter mechanisms are associated with psychostimulant-induced analgesia. Most evidence is from animal experiments with acute pain in which dextroamphetamine demonstrated antinociceptive properties when used alone, with monoamine oxidase inhibitors, or with morphine (88, 89). Dextroamphetamine is thought to exert noradrenergic and dopaminergic effects at lower doses and to release and act as an agonist for serotonin (5-HT) at higher doses (1, 88). In single-dose experiments in mice, dextroamphetamine analgesia was inhibited by apomorphine (DA agonist), reserpine (depletes NE, DA, and 5-HT), p-chlorophenylalanine (inhibits 5-HT synthesis), and naloxone but enhanced by haloperidol (DA blocker) (89). These results suggest that dextroamphetamine analgesia involves 5-HT, DA, and endogenous opioid peptide activity.

Clinical Considerations

Indications

Psychostimulants are most commonly prescribed to alleviate persistent troublesome drowsiness due to narcotic administration for pain of advanced malignant disease (1, 90). A short-term or more prolonged course of psychostimulant drugs is occasionally useful to improve mood, energy initiative, and social involvement in depressed patients when conventional antidepressant measures have not helped (91).

Psychostimulants may be indicated to provide analgesia in certain pain disorders. Dextroamphetamine has been used for spasmodic torticollis (1) and combined with morphine for severe postoperative pain (92). Dextroamphetamine and methylphenidate are said to be indicated for patients thought to have excessive 5-HT activity in their central and peripheral autonomic systems and presenting with one or more of the following: depression, early morning awakening, spastic colon, gallbladder hypokinesia, menstrual pain, and headaches (88). Cocaine has been used intranasally for head, neck, and shoulder pain attributed to splenopalatine ganglion and nasal sympathetic system dysfunction (86).

Techniques of Administration

PRECAUTIONS. Use of psychostimulant drugs is inadvisable for those with a history of anxiety disorders, substance abuse, paranoid disorders, or schizophrenia. Medical contraindications include the presence of hyperthyroidism, seizure disorders, cardiac arrhythmias, or uncontrollable hypertension (1, 10). A baseline ECG, hemogram, and platelet count should be repeated periodically.

INITIAL ADMINISTRATION. In one study of acute postoperative pain, 5 or 10 mg of dextroamphetamine was combined with 3 to 12 mg of morphine in one intramuscular dose; the results of this treatment lasted 4 to 5 hours (92).

For more prolonged therapy, the oral route is used. For example, a 2.5-mg test dose of dextroamphetamine could be given. If there is no contraindication, the drug is started at an oral dosage of 5 to 10 mg per day in two or three divided doses not given later than mid-afternoon. The dosage is then rapidly increased to achieve optimal effect, with the recommended range being 5 to 20 mg/day (1, 10). In the case of methylphenidate, daily oral dosages start at 10 to 40 mg and usually are maintained at 10 to 30 mg (10). One regimen used with reported success for facial pain secondary to advanced head and neck cancer started at a daily oral dosage of 5 mg methadone and 10 mg dextroamphetamine; this was increased over a period of 2 to 3 days to a daily maintenance dosage of 20 to 30 mg methadone and 20 mg dextroamphetamine (93).

Intranasal doses of cocaine for acute pain are usually given using a 10% aqueous solution and range from 0.2 to 2 mg/kg (85).

Efficacy

There have been notably few clinical trials of psychostimulant use in human pain. Two adequate controlled trials of psychostimulant use for acute pain were reviewed. In one, a double-blind single-dose study, the effects of various doses of morphine alone were compared with the effects of the same doses of morphine combined with two different doses of dextroamphetamine in patients with severe postoperative pain. Analgesic properties of combinations containing 5 mg or 10 mg dextroamphetamine were one and one-half and two times as potent as morphine alone, respectively. Subjective sleepiness was decreased and various performance tasks were significantly improved in the dextroamphetamine groups (92). In another double-blind single-dose trial 30 mg intranasal cocaine was statistically but not strikingly superior to saline placebo in reducing ischemic tourniquet pain in volunteers, without detectable change in mood or state of consciousness (85).

One single-dose double-blind crossover trial compared 15 mg dextroamphetamine with 40 mg fenfluramine (a specific release of 5-HT) and placebo for acute experimental pain (ice water) and chronic low back pain. Dextroamphetamine was effective for both acute and chronic pain while fenfluramine was only effective for chronic pain (94). Two double-blind crossover trials examined the use of cocaine in morphine or diamorphine elixir given to terminal cancer patients with pain (95, 96). Cocaine at 10 mg orally per dose of elixir produced no clinical or statistical difference in pain, nausea, or confusion. In one study cocaine was thought to produce a small but transient increase in alertness (95).

Side Effects and Complications

Important adverse effects of psychostimulants are unusual in dosages lower than the equivalent of 15 mg/day oral dextroamphetamine, but idiosyncratic reactions can occur at dosages as low as 2 mg (1, 10). Adverse effects on the central nervous system include restlessness, anxiety, insomnia, delirium, visual disturbances, seizures, and exacerbation of pre-existing schizophrenia. Chronic use of higher dosages can lead to personality changes, paranoid psychosis, psychologic dependency, and a withdrawal syndrome marked by fatigue and depression. Cardiovascular adverse effects are headache, palpitations, hypertension, hypotension, angina, cardiac arrhythmias, and circulatory collapse. Gastrointestinal problems include anorexia, nausea, diarrhea, and abdominal cramps. Hypersensitivity reactions sometimes occur (arthralgias, exfoliative dermatitis, erythema multiforme, fever, thrombocytopenic purpura). Sweating, dizziness, and nausea were the most common adverse effects of acute psychostimulant administration in the one trial giving adequate information (92).

Drug interactions can lead to important complications. Psychostimulants increase the hypotensive effects of guanethidine; decrease the metabolism of anticoagulants, anticonvulsants, and heterocyclic antidepressants; and cause hypertensive crises when given to patients on monamine oxidase inhibitors.

SUMMARY

On the basis of available evidence, suggested psychotropic regimens for some specific pain disorders are listed in Table 79-8. General principles, precautions, administration technique, and suggested progression from basic to more complex techniques have been discussed.

Additional adequate clinical trials are required to establish the efficacy of psychotropics in most pain disorders. Existing trials have important limitations in one or more key parameters such as design, study population(s), diagnostic procedures, therapeutic regimen, compliance, outcome measures, and statistical analyses employed. Psychotropics have yet to be compared with or combined with other forms of therapy such as acupuncture, biofeedback, psychologic or milieu therapies, and nerve blocks. Newer heterocyclic antidepressants and neuroleptics with more selective pharmacologic actions might be more helpful in elucidating mechanisms underlying pain and analgesia.

Notwithstanding these reservations, the following conclusions can be drawn:

1. Antidepressant drugs are efficacious in alleviating depression, and frequently pain, in patients with primary depressive disorders. They can be useful in relieving pain-related problems such as anxiety, depression secondary to pain, and insomnia. They probably have an analgesic effect in specific chronic pain conditions such as chronic osteoarthritis and rheumatoid arthritis, diabetic neuropathy, migraine, head and face

TABLE 79-8. Suggested Psychotropic Treatment of Specific Pain Syndromes

Pain Syndrome	Suggested Regimen*
Acute pain	
Delusional pain	Neuroleptic → add antidepressant or electroconvulsive therapy
Cluster headaches	Lithium carbonate prophylaxis
Herpes zoster	Neuroleptics (short-term)†
Myocardial infarction	Diazepam (1–2 weeks)
Chronic pain	
Arthritis	Imipramine → clomipramine → add neuroleptic
Cancer	Clomipramine → add neuroleptic
Cluster headache	Lithium carbonate → add amitriptyline
Diabetic neuropathy	Imipramine → amitriptyline → add neuroleptic
Migraine	Amitriptyline → washout → phenelzine
Neuralgias	Clomipramine → amitriptyline → add neuroleptic → amitriptyline/anticonvulsant
Psychologic origin	Doxepin → amitriptyline → washout → phenelzine
Tension headache	Amitriptyline → doxepin
Various neurologic	Same as for neuralgias

*Initial choice is listed first followed by alternatives to be tried with nonresponders (→).

†This suggestion should be regarded as controversial pending further studies to replicate trials discussed in this chapter.

pain of psychologic origin, postherpetic neuralgia, and tension headache.

2. Neuroleptics are the treatment of choice for delusional pain. They may be efficacious alone or in combination with an HCAD for some types of otherwise treatment-resistant chronic pain (arthritic pain, causalgias, neuralgias, neuropathies, phantom pain, and thalamic pain).

3. Lithium carbonate seems to be efficacious in relieving chronic cluster headache and in preventing episodic cluster headache.

4. Benzodiazepines can be useful in short-term management of acute anxiety-related pain. Their continuous use in chronic pain cannot be recommended at this time.

5. The use of psychostimulants in acute and chronic pain is based on clinical utility rather than any substantial evidence. They can be helpful in a small number of patients with persistent sedation from narcotics or with intractable depression and pain.

6. Psychotropic treatment of pain, as described in this chapter, seems to be feasible and relatively free of important undesirable effects.

REFERENCES

1. Baldessarini, R.J.: Drugs and the treatment of psychiatric disorders. In The Pharmacological Basis of Therapeutics. 7th Ed. Edited by A.G. Gilman, L.S. Goodman, T.W. Rall, and F. Murad. New York, Macmillan, 1985.
2. Monks, R., and Merskey, H.: Psychotropic drugs. In Textbook of Pain. 2nd Ed. Edited by P.D. Wall and R. Melzack. London, Churchill Livingstone, 1989, pp. 702–721.
3. Twycross, R.G.: Non narcotic, corticosteroid and psychotropic drugs. In The Continuing Care of Terminal Cancer Patients. Edited by R.G. Twycross and V. Ventafridda. Oxford, Pergamon, 1979.
4. Monks, R.C.: Psychopharmacological management of post myocardial infarction depression and anxiety. Can. Fam. Physician, 27:1117, 1981.
5. Clark, R.B., and Seifen, A.B.: Systemic medication during labor and delivery. In Obstetrics and Gynecology Annual. Edited by R.M. Wynn. Norwalk, CT, Appleton-Century-Crofts, 1982.
6. Kocher, R.: Use of psychotropic drugs for treatment of chronic severe pain. In Advances in Pain Research and Therapy. Edited by J.J. Bonica and D. Albe Fessard. New York, Raven Press, 1976.
7. Gerson, G.R., Jones, R.B., and Luscombe, D.K.: Studies on the concomitant use of carbamazepine and clomipramine for the relief of post herpetic neuraliga. Postgrad. Med. J., 53(Suppl. 4):104, 1977.
8. Swerdlow, M., and Cundill, J.G.: Anticonvulsant drugs used in the treatment of lancinating pain. A comparison. Anaesthesia, 36:1129, 1981.
9. Halpern, L.: Substitution-detoxification and its role in the management of chronic benign pain. J. Clin. Psychiatry, 43:10, 1982.
10. Klein, D.F., Gittleman, R., Quitkin, F., and Rifkin, A.: Diagnosis and Drug Treatment of Psychiatric Disorders: Adults and Children. Baltimore, Williams & Wilkins, 1980.
11. Walsh, T.D.: Antidepressants in chronic pain. Clin. Neuropharmacol., 6:271, 1983.
12. Feighner, J.P.: The new generation of antidepressants. J. Clin. Psychiatry, 44:49, 1983.
13. Ward, N.G., Bloom, V.L., Fawcett, J., and Friedel, R.P.: Urinary 3-methoxy-4-hydroxyphenethylene glycol in the prediction of pain and depression relief with doxepin: Preliminary findings. J. Nerv. Ment. Dis., 171:55, 1983.
14. Bradley, J.J.: Severe localized pain associated with the depressive syndrome. Br. J. Psychiatry, 109:741, 1963.
15. Blumer, D., and Heilbronn, M.: Chronic pain as a variant of depressive disease. The pain-prone disorder. J. Nerv. Ment. Dis., 170:381, 1982.
16. Blumer, D., Zorick, F., Heilbronn, M., and Roth, T.: Biological markers for depression in chronic pain. J. Nerv. Ment. Dis., 170:425, 1982.
17. Baldessarini, R.J.: A summary of biomedical aspects of mood disorders. McLean Hosp. J., 6:1, 1981.
18. Maas, J.W.: Biogenic amines and depression: Biochemical and pharmacological separation of two types of depression. Arch. Gen. Psychiatry, 32:1357, 1975.
19. Richelson, E., and Nelson, A.: Antagonism by antidepressants of neurotransmitter receptors of normal human brain in vitro. J. Pharm. Exp. Ther., 230:94, 1984.
20. Richelson, E.: Tricyclic antidepressants: Interactions with histamine and muscarinic acetylcholine receptors. In Antidepressants: Neurochemical Behavioral and Clinical Perspectives. Edited by S.J. Enna, J.B. Malick, and E. Richelson. New York, Raven Press, 1981.
21. Synder, S.H., and Yamamura, H.I.: Antidepressants and the muscarinic acetylcholine receptor. Arch. Gen. Psychiatry, 34:236, 1977.
22. Sugrue, M.F.: Chronic antidepressant therapy and associated changes in central monoaminergic receptor functioning. Pharmacol. Ther., 21:1, 1983.
23. Basbaum, A.I., and Fields, H.L.: Endogenous pain control mechanisms: Review and hypothesis. Ann. Neurol., 4:451, 1978.
24. Sternbach, R.A., Janowsky, D.S., Huey, I.Y., and Segal, D.S.: Effects of altering brain serotonin activity on human chronic pain. In Advances in Pain Research and Therapy. Edited by J.J. Bonica and D. Albe Fessard. New York, Raven Press, 1976.
25. Carasso, R.L., Yehuda, S., and Streifler, M.: Clomipramine and amitriptyline in the treatment of severe pain. Int. J. Neurosci., 9:191, 1979.
26. Spiegel, K., Kalb, R., and Pasternak, G.W.: Analgesic activity of tricyclic antidepressants. Ann. Neurol., 13:462, 1983.
27. Johansson, F., Von Knorring, L., Sedvall, G., and Terenius, L.: Changes in endorphins and 5-hydroxyindoleacetic acid in cerebrospinal fluid as a result of treatment with a serotonin reuptake inhibitor (zimelidine) in chronic pain patients. Psychiatry. Res., 2:167, 1980.
28. Taska, R., and Brodie, H.: New trends in the diagnosis and treatment of depression. J. Clin. Psychiatry, 44(Sec. 2):11, 1983.
29. Okasha, A., Ghaleb, H.A., and Sadek, A.: A double blind trial for the clinical management of psychogenic headache. Br. J. Psychiatry, 122:181, 1973.
30. Diamond, S., and Baltes, B.J.: Chronic tension headache: Treatment with amiptyline—a double blind study. Headache, 11:110, 1971.
31. Lance, J.W., and Curran, D.A.: Treatment of chronic tension headache. Lancet, 1:1236, 1964.
32. Keller, M.B., et al.: Treatment received by depressed patients. JAMA, 248:1848, 1982.
33. Lascelles, R.G.: Atypical facial pain and depression. Br. J. Psychiatry, 122:651, 1966.
34. Thorpe, P., and Marchant-Williams, R.: The role of an antidepressant, dibenzepin (Noveril), in the relief of pain in chronic arthritic states. Med. J. Aust., 1:264, 1974.
35. Gingras, M.: A clinical trial of Tofranil in rheumatic pain in general practice. J. Int. Med. Res., 4(Suppl. 2):41, 1976.
36. McDonald Scott, W.A.: The relief of pain with an antidepressant in arthritis. Practitioner, 202:802, 1969.
37. Kvinesdal, B., Molin, J., Frøland, A., and Gram, L.F.: Imipramine treatment of painful diabetic neuropathy. JAMA, 251:1727, 1984.
38. Turkington, R.W.: Depression masquerading as diabetic neuropathy. JAMA, 243:1147, 1980.
39. Jenkins, D.G., Ebbutt, A.F., and Evans, C.D.: Imipramine in treatment of low back pain. J. Int. Med. Res., 4(Suppl. 2):28, 1976.
40. Couch, J.R., Ziegler, D.K., and Hassanein, R.: Amitriptyline in the prophylaxis of migraine. Effectiveness and relationship of antimigraine and antidepressant effects. Neurology, 26:121, 1976.
41. Gomersall, J.D., and Stuart, A.: Amitriptyline in migraine prophylaxis: Changes in pattern of attacks during a controlled clinical trial. J. Neurol. Neurosurg. Psychiatry, 36:684, 1973.
42. Fiorentino, M.: Sperimentazione controllara dell' Imipramina come analgesico maggiore in oncologia. Riv. Med. Trentina, 5:387, 1967.

43. Pilowsky, I., et al.: A controlled study of amitriptyline in the treatment of chronic pain. Pain, *14*:169, 1982.
44. Watson, C.P.N., et al.: Amitriptyline versus placebo in post herpetic neuralgia. Neurology, *32*:671, 1982.
45. Blumer, D., and Heilbronn, M.: Second year follow-up study on systematic treatment of chronic pain with antidepressants. Henry Ford Hosp. Med. J., *29*:67, 1981.
46. Ward, N.G.: Tricyclic antidepressants for chronic low-back pain: Mechanisms of action and predictors of response. Spine, *11*:661, 1986.
47. Anthony, M.: Monoamine oxidase inhibition in the treatment of migraine. Arch. Neurol., *21*:263, 1969.
48. Bendz, H.: Kidney function in lithium-treated patients. Acta Psychiatr. Scand., *68*:303, 1983.
49. Coccaro, E.F., and Siever, L.J.: Second generation antidepressants: A comparative review. J. Clin. Pharmacol., *25*:241, 1985.
50. Creuse, I., Feinberg, A.P., and Snyder, S.H.: Butyrophenone influences on the opiate receptor. Eur. J. Pharmacol., *36*:231, 1976.
51. Munro, A., and Chmara, J.: Monosymptomatic hypochondriacal psychosis. A diagnosis checklist based on 50 cases of the disorder. Can. J. Psychiatry, *27*:374, 1982.
52. The Task Force on Late Neurological Effects of Antipsychotic Drugs: Tardive Dyskinesia: Summary of a Task Force Report of the American Psychiatric Association. Am. J. Psychiatry, *137*:1163, 1980.
53. Beaver, W.T., et al.: A comparison of the analgesic effect of methotrimeprazine and morphine in patients with cancer. Clin. Pharmacol. Ther., 7:436, 1966.
54. Bloomfield, S., et al.: Comparative analgesic activity of levomepromazine and morphine in patients with chronic pain. Can. Med. Assoc. J., *90*:1156, 1964.
55. Kast, E.C.: An understanding of pain and its measurement. Med. Times, *94*:1501, 1966.
56. Davidson, O., et al.: Analgesic treatment with levomepromazine in acute myocardial infarction. A randomized clinical trial. Acta. Med. Scand., *205*:191, 1979.
57. Judkins, K.C., and Harmer, M.: Haloperidol as an adjunct analgesia in the management of post operative pain. Anesthesia, *37*:1118, 1982.
58. Hakkarainen, H.: Fluphenazine for tension headache: Double blind study. Headache, *17*:216, 1977.
59. Landa, L., et al.: Beneficial effects of flupenthixol in cancer pain patients. Pain (Suppl.), *2*:252, 1984.
60. Breivik, H., and Slødahl, J.: Beneficial effects of flupenthixol for osteoarthritis pain of the hip: A double blind crossover comparison with placebo. Pain (Suppl.), *2*:254, 1984.
61. Nathan, P.W.: Chlorprothixene (Taractan) in post herpetic neuralgia and other severe chronic pain. Pain, *5*:367, 1978.
62. Raft, D., Toomey, T., and Greff, J.M.: Behavior modification and haloperidol in chronic facial pain. South. Med. J., *72*:155, 1979.
63. Gomez-Perez, F.J., et al.: Nortriptyline and fluphenazine in the symptomatic treatment of diabetic neuropathy: A double-blind cross-over study. Pain, *23*:395, 1985.
64. Sherwin, D.: A new method for treating "headaches." Am. J. Psychiatry, *136*:1181, 1979.
65. Langhor, H.D., Stöhr, M., and Petruch, F.: An open and double-blind crossover study on the efficacy of clomipramine (Anafranil) in patients with painful mono- and polyneuropathies. Eur. Neurol., *21*:309, 1982.
66. Raferty, H.: The management of post herpetic pain using sodium valproate and amitriptyline. J. Irish Med. Assoc., *72*:399, 1979.
67. Mandel, M.R.: Electroconvulsive therapy for chronic pain associated with depression. Am. J. Psychiatry, *132*:632, 1975.
68. Kudrow, L.: Lithium prophylaxis for chronic cluster headache. Headache, *17*:15, 1977.
69. Mathew, N.T.: Clinical subtypes of cluster headache and response to lithium therapy. Headache, *18*:26, 1978.
70. Ekbom, K.: Lithium for cluster headache: Review of the literature and preliminary results of long-term treatment. Headache, *21*:132, 1981.
71. Kudrow, K.L.: Comparative results of prednisone, methysergide and lithium therapy in cluster headache. *In* Current Concepts in Migraine Research. Edited by R. Greene. New York, Raven Press, 1978.
72. Tyber, M.A.: Treatment of the painful shoulder syndrome with amitriptyline and lithium carbonate. Can. Med. Assoc. J., *111*:137, 1974.
73. Cooper, A.J.: Benzodiazepine update: A guide to rational prescribing. Mod. Med. Canada, *38*:209, 1983.
74. Hollister, L.E.: Principles of therapeutic applications of benzodiazepines. J. Psychoactive Drugs, *15*:41, 1983.
75. Dawson, G.W., Jue, S.G., and Brogden, R.N.: Alprozolam. A review of its pharmacodynamic properties and efficacy in the treatment of anxiety and depression. Drugs, *27*:132, 1974.
76. Hamlin, C., and Gold, M.S.: Anxiolytics: Predicting response/maximizing efficacy. *In* Advances in Psychopharmacology: Predicting and Improving Treatment Response. Edited by M.S. Gold, R.B. Lydiard, and J.S. Carman. Boca Raton, FL, CRC Press, 1984.
77. Wuster, M., Duka, T., and Herz, A.: Diazepam—induced release of opioid activity in the rat brain. Neurosci. Lett., *16*:335, 1980.
78. Haas, S., Emrich, H.M., and Beckmann, H.: Analgesic and euphoric effects of high dose diazepam in schizophrenia. Neuropsychobiology, *8*:123, 1982.
79. Laboratory tests for patients taking psychotropic drugs. Biol. Therapies in Psychiatry, *6*:5, 1983.
80. Greenblatt, D.J., Shader, R.I., and Abernathy, D.R.: Current status of benzodiazepines. Parts I and II. N. Engl. J. Med., *309*:354 and 410, 1983.
81. Marks, J.: The benzodiazepines—use and abuse. Arzneimittel-Forsch. Drug Res., *30*(5a):898, 1980.
82. Hendler, N., Cimini, A., Terence, M.A., and Long, D.: A comparison of cognitive impairment due to benzodiazepines and to narcotics. Am. J. Psychiatry, *137*:828, 1980.
83. McNairy, S.L., et al.: Prescription medication dependence and neuropsychologic function. Pain, *18*:169, 1984.
84. Hollister, L.E., Conley, F.K., Britt, R.H., and Shuer, L.: Long-term use of diazepam. JAMA, *246*:1568, 1981.
85. Yang, J.C., et al.: Effect of intranasal cocaine on experimental pain in man. Anesth. Analg., *61*:358, 1982.
86. Ruskin, A.P.: Sphenopalatine ganglion: Remote effects including "psychosomatic" symptoms. Rage reaction, pain and spasms. Arch. Phys. Med. Rehabil., *60*:353, 1979.
87. Reith, M.G.A., Sershen, H., and Lajtha, A.: Saturable (^{3}H)-cocaine binding in central nervous system of mouse. Life Sci., *27*:1055, 1980.
88. Lechin, F., and vander Dijs, B.: Physiological, clinical and therapeutical basis of a new hypothesis for headache. Headache, *20*:77, 1980.
89. Kubola, K., et al.: Characteristics of analgesia induced by noncatecholic phenylethylamines in mice. Life Sci., *31*:1221, 1982.
90. Gourlay, G.K., and Cousins, M.J.: Strong analgesia in severe pain. Drugs, *28*:79, 1984.
91. Kaufmann, M.W., and Murray, G.B.: The use of *d*-amphetamine in radically ill depressed patients. J. Clin. Psychiatry, *43*:463, 1982.
92. Forrest, W.H., et al.: Dextroamphetamine with morphine for the treatment of post operative pain. N. Engl. J. Med., *296*:712, 1977.
93. Shapshay, S.M., Scott, R.M., McCann, C.F., and Stoelting, I.: Pain control in advanced and recurrent head and neck cancer. Otolaryngol. Clin. North Am., *13*:551, 1980.
94. Ward, N.G., et al.: Differential effects of fenfluramine and dextroamphetamine on acute and chronic pain. Pain (Suppl. 2):252, 1984.
95. Twycross, R.G.: The Brompton Cocktail. *In* Advances in Pain Research and Therapy. Vol. 2. Edited by J.J. Bonica and V. Ventafridda, New York, Raven Press, 1979.
96. Melzack, R., Mount, B.M., and Gordon, J.M.: The Brompton mixture versus morphine solution given orally: Effects on pain. Can. Med. Assoc. J., *12*:435, 1979.

JOSIE HOWARD-RUBEN *and* LORA McGUIRE

EFFECTIVE pain management depends on the collaboration of diverse health care specialists working as a multidisciplinary team. Each professional discipline contributes a unique blend of knowledge and clinical expertise to the care of the patient in pain. Teamwork, excellent communication skills, and compassion are clinical imperatives in the management of pain. By virtue of their constant presence in the clinical setting as well as their unique biopsychosocial perspective, professional nurses play a vital role in pain care.

A nurse has the opportunity to provide pain relief by simply saying to a patient, "I believe you are in pain, and I will do all I can to help relieve your pain." This simple statement greatly diminishes a patient's anxiety level. A major goal of nursing is to establish trust and rapport with the patient, and statements of belief such as the above are extremely important in achieving this goal. For too long, patients have been trying with imagination but little success to prove to nurses and physicians that they are in pain, often by displaying certain stereotypical behaviors. The patient's statements of pain should be all that is necessary for pain intervention to begin (1).

Twycross and Lack (2) suggest these ways in which nurses can participate in pain management:

Give the patient an opportunity to express anxieties and fears

Encourage the patient by quietly emphasizing that his pain will soon be controlled better

Support the patient through the period of initial side effects that are commonly seen with morphine-like drugs

Advise the patient on when to increase the dose of analgesic

Contact the doctor rather than wait for the next visit or round if the patient becomes less well when a new treatment is started

Contact the doctor if the patient fails to get a good night's sleep

Monitor bowel function

Advise the patient on diet and fluid intake

To this list we add the additional objectives of educating patients about pain therapies, displaying integrity by being available to patients and honoring commitments made to them, and acting as change agents in health care settings by stimulating a constant evaluation of pain management strategies. Table 80-1 provides an example of nursing activities related to pain management with cancer patients (3).

Meinhart and McCaffery (4) believe that "the failure to treat pain is inhumane and constitutes professional negligence." Professionals committed to the relief of pain actively pursue pain relief therapies for patients. Often it is the professional nurse who is most engaged in caring for the patient with pain. In fact, the basic goals of nursing care correlate exactly with the goals of the entire health care team in relation to pain management. Nursing assists each patient to achieve the highest level of functioning possible via wellness promotion and illness prevention.

The material in this chapter is presented in three major parts: A, overview of the nursing process, especially in relation to patients experiencing pain; B, preparation of nurses for pain management; and C, clinical role of nurses in managing patients with pain in the hospital, in the home, in the pain clinic, in a hospice, in an extended health care facility, and as a consultant.

THE NURSING PROCESS

The role of the professional nurse in pain care is both independent and interdependent. Nurses systematically assess a clinical situation through the *nursing process*, which offers a framework for the logical integration of data, the formulation of impressions, the development and execution of a nursing care plan, and ultimate evaluation of the effectiveness of the therapeutic plan. This dynamic process is interactional, scientific, purposeful, and systematic. It includes the following steps (3):

Assessment. Collecting subjective and objective data relevant to nursing care

Data analysis. Formulating impressions or nursing diagnoses that are relevant to nursing care

Planning. Establishing priorities, patient outcomes, and specific nursing interventions

Implementation. Carrying out interventions

Evaluation. Determining the extent to which nursing goals have been achieved and establishing the need for alternative nursing actions

Assessment

Depending on the clinical setting in which a nurse practices, the specific framework for assessment and data collection will vary. For example, a nurse working primarily with ambulatory patients with low back pain needs to gather data very different from those required by a nurse practicing in a hospice setting. Whatever

TABLE 80-1. Typical Nursing Interventions for Cancer Patients Experiencing Pain

I. Restoring optimum level of health

Administers narcotics, nonopiates, and/or nonsteroidal anti-inflammatory drugs (NSAIDs)

Observes patient for alterations in elimination, respiratory depression, and gastrointestinal bleeding

Assists patient to identify times when drugs should be administered

Monitors bowel status and oxygenation

Assists patient with bath, meals, and other activities, gradually coaching patient to be as independent as possible

Creates a safe environment through use of commode, trapeze, egg crate mattress, etc.

Advises and counsels patient on reporting symptoms of pain

Teaches patient to use walker, trapeze, or other devices

II. Maintaining optimum level of health

Interviews patient about significant clinical findings

Teaches patient and family that pain caused by metastatic disease requires reporting of any exacerbation of pain, sensory or motor changes, and changes in appearance of painful area

Counsels on ambulation, positioning, and use of comfort devices (e.g., heating pad)

Advises on need to monitor for occult blood in stool with NSAIDs and to implement a bowel program with narcotic

Reviews purpose of narcotic and NSAIDs and explains importance of taking medications on schedule

Provides written drug cards

Ascertains that local pharmacies stock prescribed drugs

Reinforces importance of returning for medical follow-up and treatment

Adapted from Long, B., and Phipps, W. (eds.): Essentials of Medical-Surgical Nursing: A Nursing Process Approach. St. Louis, C.V. Mosby, 1985.

the setting, both subjective and objective data are considered. Donovan (5) stated that pain assessment is the first step toward understanding pain as the patient experiences it and provides the framework for a positive patient-nurse alliance.

Generally, an initial assessment is made when a patient first enters the health care system. The patient interview, interaction with the patient and family, review of health care records and reports, and dialogues with other health care providers are all part of the data collection process. Although baseline assessments, often called a nursing data base, are vitally important, the assessment process is continuous and ongoing. Integral to the process of data collection is the recording (documentation) of pertinent information. Again, each setting demands different methods of record-keeping. The important point is that pertinent data must be recorded accurately and must be accessible to all members of the health care team caring for the patient.

The assessment process in pain cases is difficult, often painstaking. Because the pain experience is so highly subjective, the nurse must be a consummate practitioner of the art of assessment. In contrast to hypertension or infection, for example, pain often lacks physiologic or behavioral correlates that establish its existence. McCaffery (1) defines pain as "whatever the person experiencing it says it is, existing whenever

* Reprinted with permission from Copp, L.A.: The spectrum of suffering. Am. J. Nurs., 74(3):491, 1974.

they say it does." Successful pain assessment depends on nurses' accepting this definition. As Graffam (6) aptly states, "Patients should be assessed, not judged."

Nursing pain assessment, in conjunction with medical diagnosis, provides the basis for planning patient care. The purposes of assessment are to assist the nurse in establishing a nursing diagnosis; to assist in evaluation and planning of nursing care measures prescribed for pain relief; to help the individual with pain develop positive adaptation mechanisms; and to aid in establishing the degree of relief experienced by the patient with pain (7).

A great shortcoming of professional nursing in pain care has been its failure to accurately document all aspects of the patient's reported pain experience. Because nurses are available to and accountable for patients throughout the day and night, they have access to a wide range of patient experiences and behaviors. A patient can successfully convey a particular image to a physician for a brief period each day, but it is difficult to maintain a facade with care-givers who are present throughout the day. Because they are likely to have a unique impression of a patient's pain experience, nurses owe a careful documentary of that experience to the entire health care team.

Components of Pain Assessment

Many pain assessment tools have been promulgated, each having its own benefits and advantages. Several broad parameters, however, must form the cornerstone of pain assessment in all settings.

LOCATION. If possible, the exact site of pain should be described. The patient might find it helpful to point to or to trace the area(s) of pain on a silhouette of a human figure. Whether the pain is deep or superficial, constant, or migratory should be consistently noted by the professional nurse.

INTENSITY. Many descriptors can be employed to document pain intensity. In addition to common adjectives, we recommend the use of a visual analog scale ranging from 0 to 10 (0 = no pain and 10 = the worst pain imaginable). Continuous documentation of pain ratings is possible with such a scale, which provides a standard language for evaluating pain therapies and gauging pain relief, with the patient serving as his own control. Confidence in care-givers is augmented when a consistent method of reporting pain is employed. The patient sees tangible evidence of the multidisciplinary team concept in action on his behalf.

QUALITY. Descriptions of the quality of pain represent another facet of the assessment of pain. These allow the patient to share his own unique perception of his pain. The patient should be encouraged to use his own words to fully describe the pain he is experiencing.

In a study of 148 patients in pain, Copp (8) reported that they used the following words to describe their pain (listed in order of frequency mentioned):*

1. Treacherous
2. Mean
3. Hateful
4. Detestable
5. Sneaky
6. Intense
7. Dark
8. Hidden
9. Obnoxious
10. Faceless

11. Degrading	23. Deceitful
12. Cruel	24. Dominating
13. Inconsiderate	25. Loud
14. Invading	26. Vulgar
15. Variety of words meaning satanic	27. Wicked
16. Nasty	28. Persevering
17. Sharp	29. Testing
18. Cunning	30. Tempting
19. Nervous	31. Ill-tempered
20. Persistent	32. Nagging
21. Sly	33. Mysterious
22. Strong	34. Clawing
	35. Probing

The mystical, evil quality of pain experienced by these patients is captured in these descriptors. These subjective patient impressions are a unique, personal aspect of the pain experience and should be recorded so that they are accessible to all care providers.

CHRONOLOGY. The quality and quantity of pain over time should also be documented. Is pain constant or intermittent? At what times does it occur? Patterns of pain occurrence serve to assist in the establishment of an appropriate plan of care.

PAST PAIN EXPERIENCE. An opportunity for the patient to relate those actions that have given him pain relief in the past is an important part of assessment. Health care providers might view noninvasive pain relief measures such as distraction, massage, or even eating specific foods as trivial. This attitude, however, does little to serve the patient in pain. The health care team, and nurses in particular, must go to great lengths to incorporate the patient's own pain-relieving techniques into an overall plan of care as long as they cause no harm.

Copp (8) provides a detailed list of self-care behaviors directed toward pain relief as reported by patients. These include heat, cold, relaxation, posturing, rest, strenuous activity, verbalization of certain words, diversion, ritualistic behaviors, rubbing, pacing, pounding, rocking, biting, clenching, counting, imagery, prayer, projection into the past or future, conversation, self-hypnosis, medications, and separation from body. The individual's own resources and coping mechanisms should be respected and cultivated rather than denied in a pain relief program.

Summary of Data Collected

The preceding discussion has described some important aspects of the assessment process. The following summary outlines in more detail the various types of information and data that should be collected in a nursing assessment of a pain patient:

Pain characteristics
1. Precipitating factors and onset
2. Intensity, duration, location, and quality
3. Aggravating and ameliorating factors

Physiologic parameters
1. Changes in vital signs
2. Alteration in pupil size
3. Presence of diaphoresis, nausea, vomiting, muscle

guarding, muscle tension, and overt pain behaviors (absence of physiologic signs *does not* indicate absence of pain)

Fatigue threshold
1. Sleep patterns
2. Activity level
3. Irritability
4. Rate and tone of voice
5. Level of social interaction
6. Ability to eat and drink adequate amounts of food and fluid

Environmental factors
1. Level of stimulation (noise, light, odor, temperature, and movement)
2. Physical location of facilities (bathroom, night table, etc.)
3. Patient preferences

Psychosocial factors
1. Age and gender
2. Cultural background and religious/spiritual beliefs
3. Presence of family and friends; interaction with significant others
4. Presence and level of anxiety or depression
5. Ability to verbalize needs and feelings
6. Mood and affect
7. Pain history

Patient's view of pain
1. Patient's understanding of reason for pain and description of how much pain is acceptable
2. Patient's feelings about meaning of pain, effect of pain on his activities, and any useful purposes that pain serves
3. Priority of pain relief for patient

Patient's past experience with pain and pain relief measures
1. Presence of pain in the past and comparison with current pain
2. Chronology of pain onset
3. Measures that have afforded pain relief in the past including their duration and level of relief
4. Measures that have been found ineffective in relieving pain in the past
5. Patient's suggestions about what will reduce or relieve current pain

Patient's coping mechanisms
1. Usual coping styles
2. Effectiveness at present
3. Level of need for information about condition
4. Patient's expectations of staff and family

As noted already, continuous assessment and re-evaluation of the pain experience is necessary. McGuire (9) has developed a useful pain assessment tool. A more detailed discussion of pain assessment is presented in Chapter 32.

Data Analysis

Based on analysis of the data collected, two broad conclusions—that a need is being met or that it is not—

can be determined. Needs that are either not being met or that present potential nursing care problems can be formulated into statements called *nursing diagnoses*. Such diagnoses serve as indicators of the need for nursing care. All patients with a medical diagnosis have accompanying nursing diagnoses related to their medical problem, but the purposes and scope of medical and nursing diagnoses differ. For example, a patient with a medical diagnosis of rheumatoid arthritis might have the following nursing diagnoses: (a) pain related to rheumatoid arthritis, (b) self-care deficit due to stiffness in hands, and (c) impaired physical mobility due to lower extremity pain. Each of these diagnoses suggests particular nursing interventions, and they are considered in planning nursing care.

Planning, Implementation, and Evaluation

Based on the priority of a particular problem, establishment of nurse-patient goals in observable patient-outcome terms is the next step in the nursing process. Generally, both short- and long-term goals are specified. Action plans for nursing care are then formulated to meet these goals.

In the inpatient setting, nurses are available on an around-the-clock basis. Therefore they can continually observe the patient's symptoms and responses to pain treatment and make valuable assessments of the patient's overall therapeutic plan. In the outpatient setting, the nurse is available by phone and often can evaluate the patient's pain problems and refer the patient for medical attention when necessary.

PREPARATION OF NURSES FOR PAIN CARE

Patient Advocacy

In all areas of health care, nurses advocate for patients by clarifying information, answering questions, allaying concerns, assisting in negotiation of the complex health care system, and supporting the patient's choices. Effective patient advocacy requires time, patience, and courage on the part of the nurse. Advocacy is a critical component in pain management. Several guiding principles provide the philosophic framework for the nurse engaged in pain care. Of fundamental importance is the nurse's conviction that every patient has a right to pain relief. Alleviation of pain and suffering, regardless of its cause, must be the foundation on which the knowledge and attitudes of pain management nurses is established.

It follows then that pain management nurses should refrain from being judgmental and labeling patients as "addicted," "malingering," or "manipulative." Such labeling impedes effective pain management and historically has contributed to a lack of understanding of the patient with pain in many health care settings. Unfortunately, many health care providers, including many nurses, receive little education on pain and its management. To a large extent, they incorporate outdated beliefs and attitudes from the nurses (and other health team members) preceding them. The misconceptions and biases of health care professionals about patients in pain are discussed fully in a later section.

Nursing Education

Nursing curricula traditionally have offered minimal information on any aspect of pain management aside from the acute pain model. Most nurses, and physicians as well, were taught to assess patients according to the acute pain framework. This model holds that all patients in pain have observable signs and symptoms such as pallor, restlessness, grimacing, and rapid heart rate. No doubt, many readers can recall the grimacing sketch of the patient in pain as portrayed in many textbooks. Little wonder that practitioners so educated have difficulty believing that patients who are not exhibiting such behaviors can truly be in pain. Obviously, aggressive reform is necessary in such educational programs. Some recent nursing texts (10, 11), particularly in the fields of cancer nursing and hospice care, reflect the most current knowledge of pain management, but many others still in common use, especially in more general nursing areas, do not. Furthermore, nurses who were trained some years ago need additional education about current principles and practices of pain management.

A recent telephone survey of 12 oncology nurses with a pain specialty revealed that their preparation consisted primarily of clinical experience and self-directed learning. The respondents concurred that baccalaureate programs rarely provided adequate coverage of pain management and that, in some situations, more formal exposure to pain care and theory occurred at the master's level. Several had pursued concentrated study of pain management issues at the master's and doctoral level or in independent research projects (12).

McCaffery and Beebe (13) have made an excellent contribution to the nursing literature with the text *Pain: Clinical Manual for Nursing Practices*. A wide range of relevant material is presented in this one-volume text, making it a valuable addition to the library of any health care provider involved in pain management. Cancer and hospice nursing, as well as other nursing subspecialties, have made great strides in recent years in the development of standards of practice: Pain and comfort standards now address the high priority of pain relief (14). The greatest nursing education need now exists for nurses who have not previously studied such specialty nursing knowledge. Because of their previous socialization to antiquated attitudes and norms, practicing nurses and physicians are a prime target for re-education and exposure to more appropriate attitudes and knowledge. Meinhart and McCaffery (4) state that "the failure to treat pain is inhumane and constitutes professional negligence." Nurses committed to the relief of pain believe that every person has a right to freedom from pain and that in clinical practice everything possible should be done to help solve a patient's pain problem.

For the reasons already stated, the continuing education of nurses regarding pain warrants great attention.

As nurses are hired into positions, in-service training on pain management should be included in orientation programs. Regardless of the setting of care, pain management should be considered as a high nursing priority. Traditionally, such topics as emergency care, infection control, and diabetic instruction have been addressed in such orientations. Pain management also deserves this degree of attention, thus immediately establishing the priority with which nursing administrators view pain care. In addition, greater emphasis should be placed on upgrading the knowledge of practicing nurses. They should be given release time to attend conferences and should be required to share their new knowledge with colleagues so that new information is rapidly disseminated among staff members. Nursing journals in all areas, both specialty and general care, should publish more articles on pain management. Innovative approaches as well as basic principles require coverage. Nursing administrators and clinical specialists should encourage staff to incorporate these findings into their practice base.

Misconceptions and Biases about Pain

Inadequate training is not the only cause of the average nurse's inability to effectively care for patients in pain. Another cause is that many nurses, like many other health professionals, often cling to outdated beliefs, misconceptions, and biases about patients in pain. McCaffery (1) describes several misconceptions that hamper the care of patients in pain (Table 80-2). Many factors contribute to these incorrect attitudes: exaggerated fear of addiction and of respiratory depression, denial of pain and its severity, lack of knowledge about the pharmacology of drugs, and unawareness of other treatment modalities. Nursing pain specialists can help to erase these misconceptions and the lack of knowledge that fuels them by demonstrating appropriate actions in practice (15). In addition, nursing studies in pain management are needed to dispel misconceptions and to contribute to nursing science and practice in a relevant fashion (16).

The classic study by Marks and Sachar (17) revealed that physicians often underprescribe narcotics and nurses often undermedicate patients. Cases were highlighted by the authors providing evidence of the irrational treatment of pain with analgesics. For example, because the pharmacologic properties of meperidine were not well understood by the house physicians, they underprescribed this drug. The nursing staff exacerbated the problem further by decreasing medication dosages and by increasing intervals between subsequent dosages. Charap (18) focused on the care received by terminally ill patients. A multiple-choice, true-false survey was used to examine the knowledge, attitudes, and experience of medical personnel treating pain in such patients. The results again documented a serious lack of knowledge of both pain management techniques and of the basic tenets of analgesic therapy. Risks of physical dependence and addiction were overestimated and the subjects (surgical residents, oncology fellows, and senior nursing staff) believed that patients generally were overmedicated. Howard-Ruben and Wickham (19) surveyed a group of registered nurses and medical residents about their knowledge of

TABLE 80-2. Misconceptions that Hamper Assessment of Patients with Pain

Misconceptions	Correct View
Health team members are the authorities on the existence and nature of the patient's pain	The patient is the authority on his pain. Pain is whatever the experiencing person says it is, existing whenever he says it does. The patient is believed
The patient who uses his pain to obtain benefits or preferential treatment does not hurt as much as he says and may not hurt at all	The patient who uses his pain to his own advantage may still hurt as much as he says he does
The patient's pain can always be verified by the presence of certain behavioral and/or physiological expressions of pain	Physiological and behavioral adaptation occurs, leading to periods of little or no signs of pain. Lack of pain expression does not mean lack of pain
All "real" pain has an identifiable physical cause	Not all physical causes of pain can be identified. All pain is real, regardless of its cause. Calling pain imaginary does not make it go away
Psychogenic pain does not really hurt and is almost the same as malingering	A localized sensation does exist in psychogenic pain
The severity and duration of pain can be predicted accurately on the basis of the stimuli for pain	There is no direct and invariant relationship between any stimulus and the perception of pain
All patients can and should be encouraged to have a high tolerance for pain	Pain tolerance is the individual's unique response, varying between patients and in the same patient from one situation to another
Health team members tend to make accurate inferences about the severity and existence of the patient's pain	Health team members tend to infer less pain than the patient experiences

From McCaffrey, M.: Nursing Management of the Patient in Pain. Philadelphia, J.B. Lippincott, 1979. Reprinted with permission.

pain management in cancer patients. An open-ended question about concerns in pain management care revealed a lack of pain management expertise and many unwarranted concerns.

In spite of the ever-increasing volume and quality of professional resources devoted to pain management, deficient knowledge bases and harmful attitudes still prevail well into the 1980s. The authors challenge readers to review their own biases, attitudes, and shortcomings of knowledge in caring for the patient in pain. Graffam (6) summarized nurses' attitudes towards patients in pain as follows: (a) Nurses often believe that the pain reported by patients is "not real" or is exaggerated; (b) many nurses fear addicting patients; and (c) nurses sometimes consider patients who complain of pain as weak. In addition, Graffam found that nurses generally possess an inadequate knowledge base about pain.

Strauss et al. (20) suggested that failure to relieve pain often occurs because no one member of the health care team is held totally accountable for the relief of pain. This situation must be changed, as all aspects of the process are important. However, administrative priorities historically have not included pain.

As stated earlier, professionals' fear of addiction is a major reason why patients in pain are often undertreated with narcotics. Although the incidence of addiction in patients receiving narcotics for medical purposes is estimated to be less than 1% (21) the average nurse still fears "addicting" patients. This fear can be traced to confusion regarding four frequently misused terms, which are correctly defined here (1):

Drug abuse. Voluntary behavioral response in which a person uses drugs in a culturally unacceptable manner

Drug addiction. Voluntary, overwhelming involvement with obtaining and using drugs for psychic effects, rather than for medical reasons

Drug tolerance. An involuntary physiologic condition occurring after repeated administration of a drug (especially a narcotic) when a given dosage begins to lose its effectiveness (i.e., decreased duration of action and then decreased analgesic effect occurs)

Physical dependence. An involuntary physiologic condition that occurs after repeated administration of a narcotic for several weeks and is accompanied by withdrawal (abstinence) symptoms when the drug is abruptly stopped

A patient is done a great disservice when he is physically dependent on a narcotic but is labeled "an addict." As patient advocates, every nurse has a responsibility to educate her colleagues to distinguish these conditions.

Another factor that often causes nurses to undertreat with narcotics is an exaggerated fear of respiratory depression, even though it has been shown that respiratory depression rarely occurs in patients taking narcotics for chronic pain (1). Houde (22) reported that as patients become tolerant to their narcotics, they develop a tolerance to respiratory depression effects as well. Walsh (23) conducted a prospective trial of advanced cancer patients receiving narcotics in order to assess their respiratory function. He concluded that "chronic ventilatory failure appears to be neither common or severe when oral morphine is used to treat chronic severe pain in advanced cancer—even in the presence of pre-existing respiratory disease." Further clinical trials such as this one should be replicated and the results disseminated widely in order to dispel common but often erroneous beliefs about respiratory depression.

A modern, patient-centered approach to pain management requires eradication of irrational fears about narcotic use. Hence the urgency of improving the education of practicing nurses and other health care professionals. The result of these changes will be appropriate drug use and *not* an increase in drug abuse (24).

CLINICAL ROLES OF NURSES IN PAIN CARE

Because pain care is delivered in a multitude of settings, generalizations about the role of nursing are complicated. However, in the following sections, an overview of the role of the nurse in specific settings is considered. Each section provides a framework for development of a nursing role in each care setting. Unique constraints and opportunities within each setting will dictate particular role functions. For instance, in some settings, nurses fulfill primarily a technical role (12), whereas in others nurses participate as full members of the multidisciplinary health care team. The latter situation is preferable as it affords the greatest opportunity for full utilization of the skills of the professional nurse in pain care.

In Hospitals

Most nurses are employed in acute care settings where they have daily contact with patients in pain. However, as discussed earlier, too many nurses still do not consider pain management a high priority. In the hospital, more than in any other care setting, nurses are accustomed to life-threatening conditions. Thus, the patient in pain has low priority, since he is not usually critically ill.

If nurses are to truly function as patient advocates, they must be responsible for contributing to pain relief for all patients. Many people believe that in a hospital a patients's pain will be controlled, but this notion is not always accurate. A recent study found that of 353 adult medical-surgical hospitalized patients, 58% said they had excruciating or horrible pain at some time while hospitalized (25). In their clinical practice, the authors have found failure to adequately control pain a common occurrence. The literature supports these observations. For example, a report based on a large research project illustrates the general attitudes of staff toward patients in pain. In the discussion of "cooperative" and "uncooperative" patients, the definition of cooperative implies that patients in this category are maximally passive (26). Further, a patient's *endurance* and *expression* of pain significantly influence the staff's determination of the legitimacy of the patient's experience of pain. Individual differences in pain etiology, signs or visibility of pain, response to relief procedures, and endurance all merge to create a milieu in which the patients' credibility is continually tested (26). Another study addressed patients' attitudes toward relief of postoperative pain. Despite a general consensus by patients that they were satisfied by postoperative pain relief, approximately 25% of the sample described their pain as moderate, severe, or unbearable (27). Even children are subject to less than optimal pain care because of misconceptions that napping, refusal of injections, and other behaviors indicate that pain does not exist (28).

The common causes of inadequate pain control in hospitals have already been discussed: lack of understanding of the pain process, inadequate knowledge of the pharmacology of analgesics, and exaggerated fears of untoward side effects and addiction (17–19, 29–31).

Inadequate staffing in hospitals also contributes to poor care for patients in pain. Nurses, for example, usually complain that they have little time to assess pain or to apply noninvasive pain relief techniques. Another reason that pain is not controlled adequately is that nurses in acute care settings have little access to pain experts and resources. Hospitals should have a multidisciplinary pain team and a pain clinical nurse specialist to oversee the pain treatment for any patient with a pain problem.

Medications are the most common form of pain control. If used correctly, they can relieve pain effectively and safely. Nurses play a valuable role in the administration of medications for pain relief. Since they spend more time with patients than almost any other health professional, nurses often have valuable insight into which medications will provide the best relief for particular patients. Nurses should share these assessments with physicians and recommend drug dosages, intervals, and routes when appropriate.

A critical task of nurses in hospitals is to document the effectiveness of prescribed interventions and to inform physicians when they are ineffective in providing pain relief. A vexing problem for the nurse is the "I'm fine, Doctor" patient syndrome. For several reasons, patients generally develop closer and more familiar relationships with their nurses than with physicians. Consequently, it is common for a patient to complain of pain to a nurse but profess to be free of pain in response to the physician's query, "How are you feeling?" In such a situation, the physician is likely to discount the nurse's contention that the patient has complained of pain and needs orders written for pain relief. The authors of this chapter sincerely hope that physicians will recognize this type of situation, appreciate the difficult position of the nurse, and give more credence to the nurse's truthful report and chart documentation that the patient has, indeed, stated he was in pain.

A preventive approach is best in the timing of analgesics. Clinical experience has shown that pain is better controlled when an analgesic is given on an around-the-clock schedule rather than on a prn basis. The advantages of scheduled versus prn administration of analgesics have been discussed elsewhere (2, 32). The major reasons for the advantages of scheduled analgesics are as follows:

Analgesics are most effective if given before the pain occurs or becomes severe

Blood levels of the analgesic will always be in an effective range

Anxiety about pain medication will be decreased (anxiety may increase the perception of pain)

Giving an analgesic prn puts the patient in a dependent position of having to request pain medication *after* the pain has occurred

A negative behavior—pain—is reinforced by prn timing. If a hospital patient knows he will get his analgesic regularly, just as he is given his antibiotic or insulin, he will be less anxious, and his pain will decrease. This same patient will most likely be able to manage his own medications without difficulty when at home.

If the physician will not order an analgesic around-the-clock, it is the nurse's responsibility to teach the patient to request the medication before the pain becomes severe. The nurse should offer the analgesic as often as it can be administered and attempt to administer it on a regular basis. In the hospital, patients are not accustomed to asking for medications, they receive antibiotics, insulin, cardiac drugs, and many other medications whenever they are scheduled to be given. It often takes considerable effort to convince patients that when medication is ordered prn, they must *request* it. Competent nurses must explain this to their patients and encourage them to ask for an analgesic in a timely fashion. They also should recommend around-the-clock administration when this is more appropriate.

Many times nurses do not accurately follow a physician's order for around-the-clock analgesic. It is unacceptable for a nurse not to administer an analgesic (even though it is ordered) because the patient does not request it or "appear" to be in pain. This happens most often when a patient is sleeping. A nurse may assume that a patient is not in pain if he is sleeping or that he might be difficult to wake to administer an analgesic. However, this same nurse does not hesitate to arouse a sleeping patient no matter what time of day or night to administer antibiotic or cardiac medication. This inconsistency stems from the fact that pain is not perceived to be a serious problem. Howard-Ruben et al. (11) suggested placing a brightly colored card stating "Please wake patient for nighttime doses of analgesic—per patient request" in the medication kardex. This clearly communicates a simple nursing practice, which may contribute to enhanced pain control.

Another important function of the hospital nurse is to coordinate the health care team and supervise the activities of nursing assistants and orderlies. It is crucial for these team members to understand the concepts of pain management. They must not ignore patients' requests for pain relief and they should respond quickly. They, too, must be familiar with treatment modalities, so they can enhance rather than impede the intervention. In pain management, as in all aspects of health care, nurses need to have cooperative working relationships with physicians. Nurses also should work with patients and families and organize team conferences to discuss pain management issues.

Development of Nursing Care Plans

Another important function of hospital nurses is preparation of written nursing care plans for their patients. In a pain management case, this plan (a) describes the pain problem based on a careful assessment of the patient; (b) lists appropriate and specific interventions for achieving specified outcomes; and (c) provides for evaluation of the effectiveness of interventions and formulation of new plans as needed. The most common desired outcome with a patient in pain is for the patient to indicate verbally or by other means that his pain is reduced and his comfort and activity are increased. The patient might specify other goals as well—for example, to sleep for a period of four hours without breakthrough pain. The various components of the assessment process were discussed earlier in this chapter and will not be repeated. Note, however, that assessment should be conducted not only when the patient initially enters the hospital but also at repeated intervals.

Numerous interventions are available to nurses working with patients in pain. The following summary is an example of the kinds of interventions that might be specified in a nursing care plan:

Employ psychosocial relief measures
1. Honor commitments made to patients about pain control
2. Assure patient that you will not abandon him or the efforts to relieve his pain
3. Believe the patient's report of pain
4. Project a positive attitude that pain relief measures will prove helpful
5. "Be present" to patient, spending significant time to assess response to therapy
6. Enhance patient's control over situation by encouraging use of self-care methods that have relieved pain (e.g., prayer, massage)
7. Allow patient some control in planning timing of interventions (document specifics here; for example, premedicate patient with narcotic 20 min prior to transporting to radiation therapy)
8. Assist in treatment for underlying anxiety and/or depression if it coexists with pain
9. Teach patient and significant others about pain control plan and techniques (include specifics)

Administer analgesics as ordered by physician
1. Evaluate patient response to medication; assess its appropriateness and adequacy of dosage
2. Administer medication at first sign of pain
3. Schedule medication, according to its pharmacologic action and patient response, on an around-the-clock basis. NEVER PRN!
4. Refer to equianalgesic tables when changing drug or its route, conferring with physician, pain clinical nurse specialist and pharmacist, when available
5. Assess and manage side effects of analgesics such as nausea and vomiting, constipation, drowsiness, dry mouth, and dizziness (indicate specifics)

Enhance physical comfort of patient
1. Reposition patient; provide extra pillows
2. Give backrub and massage
3. Control temperature, odor, light, noise, and other environmental factors
4. Arrange for physical therapy
5. Equipment and devices (e.g., walker, commode)

Use nondrug pain relief measures
1. Demonstrate relaxation and breathing techniques
2. Provide distractions (e.g., imagery, reading, television, music)
3. Give massage
4. Apply heat or cold
5. Apply cutaneous stimulation

In Home Care Settings

As health care funding patterns change, more patients are receiving health care services outside of hospitals. In particular, home care has flourished in the last few years. For example, antibiotics and morphine infusions often are administered in the home setting; even ventilator-dependent patients function in their own homes. This development has contributed to a crisis of sorts in professional nursing. Earlier hospital discharges, increasing sophistication of health care technologies, regional nursing shortages, and an overall increase in the number of home care patients and the seriousness of their diagnoses have mandated rapid evolution in home care nursing. In response, home care agencies have proliferated.

Home care nurses play a pivotal role in managing pain patients at home. Often, such patients require sophisticated technologies to manage pain, environmental assessment and restructuring, physical therapy, psychosocial support, and symptom management. Assessment of problems and early intervention can be enhanced by astute home care nurses. Today, health care providers can structure therapies for home care that might have previously been ruled out because adequate support services were not available.

Ambulatory infusion pumps or implanted devices, managed by a home care or oncology nurse, provide patients with the freedom to receive parenteral or intrathecal narcotics at home, if this is the best form of therapy. Telephone follow-up and close monitoring by a nurse affords early identification of problems and rapid problem solving should it be necessary (33–35). Virtually all pain therapies can be efficiently managed in a patient's home under *skilled nursing supervision*. This, of course, is the key condition. In order for any plan to be implemented effectively, nurses with the appropriate skills and knowledge must be available. Given adequate patient education and appropriate equipment and resources, the nurse is the central figure in management of patients at home. The professional interactions of nurses with other health care providers, their knowledge of health care systems and technologies, and their ability to negotiate for equipment and resources make nurses a valuable and essential component of home health care.

In Pain Clinics

The role of the nurse in a pain clinic varies depending upon the setting and the clinic's scope of care delivery. Clinics may focus on particular modalities of treatment or particular disease syndromes, or they may offer comprehensive programs, which often include research efforts (12). In most clinics, nurses are active members of the multidisciplinary team. Their functions generally include taking patient histories and keeping accurate records on continuing assessments and progress.

Ideally, the pain clinic nurse should be responsible for patient screening and assessment, coordination of clinical care, patient treatment, and education. This nurse generally would interact with all team members, set up meetings and patient conferences, and be responsible for making sure the management program for each patient is followed.

Nurses employed in pain clinics must be knowledgeable about all treatment modalities and procedures because they will explain and reinforce these treatments, as well as clarify physicians' instructions. Such nurses can work with patients on behavior modification techniques and share this information during scheduled team conferences.

Pain clinic nurses should be involved in few non-nursing duties (filing, making appointments, etc.). The job description for a pain clinic nurse should be designed for maximum involvement with patients. These nurses must be able to establish rapport with patients and their family, as counseling is a major component of their job. Since patients usually are more willing to open up to nurses, they can significantly improve communication of patients' needs to other team members. Pain clinic nurses also refer patients for appropriate services and provide follow-up care through phone calls and visits.

In Hospices

The term *hospice* refers to a program combining skilled palliative care and support services for family units experiencing terminal illness. While all health care disciplines and volunteers are vital to the hospice concept, the major responsibility for the coordination of care is assumed by nursing. Hospice nursing emphasizes symptom control and comfort, and involves family members as part of the patient care team (36).

The goals of hospice care are thoroughly outlined in Chapter 24. Walborn (37) has delineated the specific attitudes, knowledge, and skills required by individual nurses in order to provide effective hospice nursing care (Table 80-3).

In Extended Care Facilities

The care of patients in an extended care facility is similar to that required in hospitals. However, because of the relatively low staff:patient ratios, the overall patient mix, and the large proportion of staff members with minimal levels of training, provision of optimal pain care is a challenge in extended care facilities. Creative approaches to nursing care, including employment of nurse consultants on a case-by-case basis, can improve the quality of care delivered to patients with specific problems. In-service education, role modeling, and administrative emphasis on effective pain management must form the basis for the provision of care in these facilities.

Because many patients in extended care facilities are aged, principles of geriatric care are implemented in these settings. The aging process is unique for each patient, a factor that contributes to the variability of the geriatric population. Because drug pharmacokinetics are altered and safety concerns are heightened in elderly patients, consultation with geriatric nurse specialists is appropriate in many cases.

As Consultants

Consultation is a process whereby professionals confer in an attempt to generate clarification, diagnosis, and potential solutions to a work-related problem (38). In the case of the nursing pain consultant, the specialist is the consultant while the consultee is the professional (i.e., staff nurse or attending physician) who has initiated the consultation. Several consultative processes have been described in the literature (39), but two are most common to nursing practice.

In a *client-centered case consultation*, emphasis is on assessment of the patient's problems (i.e., nursing diagnosis) and development of a plan of nursing care tailored to address those problems. Throughout the consultative process, the nurse consultant (often a clinical nurse specialist) endeavors not only to improve the patient's care but also to develop the skill and knowledge development of the consultee.

The focus of *consultee-centered case consultation* is primarily on the consultee's identified lack of knowledge or particular skill. The consultant's major goal is to improve the consultee's skill, rather than to provide patient care or education herself.

The authors' own considerable experience as nursing pain consultants in a variety of settings indicates that inadequate control of pain in clinical practice often occurs for the following reasons:

Failure to administer narcotics on an around-the-clock basis due to fear of incurring addiction or respiratory depression

Failure to perform systematic pain assessment

Failure to use narcotics if patient does not appear close to death

Lack of knowledge about drug pharmacology, resulting in inappropriate selection of medication, dosages, and scheduling intervals

Lack of knowledge about "titration to effect" concept

Failure to manage side effects

TABLE 80-3. Required Attitudes, Knowledge, and Skills of Hospice Nurses

Attitudes	Knowledge	Skills
Receptive to working with the dying and their families as part of health care team	Death and dying process	Crisis intervention
	Stages of grief	Problem solving
Allows client to determine goals and outcome of self-care practices	Concepts of separation	Communication
	Family theory	Assisting
Promotes independence, not dependence, in clients	Crisis intervention theory	Nursing process
	Normal growth and development	Basic nursing techniques
	Maslow's hierarchy	Integrating volunteer groups into the team
	Teaching and learning principles	Using community resources
	Basic nursing care	
	Community resources	

Adapted with permission from Walborn, K.: A nursing model for the hospice: Primary and self-care nursing. Nurs. Clin. North Am., *15*(1):205, 1980.

Poor communication among disciplines and nursing staff

Feelings of helplessness and inadequacy

Fear of creating dissension if a pain plan is not effective

This list is not exhaustive and other problems occur in the clinical setting. However, this list constitutes ample evidence that most settings of care would benefit from the involvement of a nursing pain consutltant in patient care.

REFERENCES

1. McCaffery, M.: Nursing Management of the Patient in Pain. Philadelphia, J.B. Lippincott, 1979.
2. Twycross, R., and Lack, S.: Therapeutics in Terminal Care. London, Pittmann Publishing, 1984.
3. Long, B., and Phipps, W. (eds.): Essential of Medical-Surgical Nursing: A Nursing Process Approach. St. Louis, C.V. Mosby, 1985.
4. Meinhart, N.T., and McCaffery, M.: Pain: A Nursing Approach to Assessment and Analysis. New York, Appleton-Century-Crofts, 1983.
5. Donovan, M.I.: Nursing assessment of cancer pain. Semin. Oncol. Nurs., 1(2):109, 1985.
6. Graffam, S.: Nurse response to patients in pain: An analysis and imperative for action. Nurs. Leadership, 2(3):23, 1979.
7. Johnson, M.: Assessment of clinical pain. In Pain: A Source Book for Nurses and Other Health Care Professionals. Edited by A. Jacox. Boston, Little, Brown, 1977.
8. Copp, L.A.: The spectrum of suffering. Am. J. Nurs., 74(3):491, 1974.
9. McGuire, L.: A short, simple tool for assessing your patient's pain. Nursing 81, 11(3):48, 1981.
10. Willoughby, S.: Alteration in comfort: Pain. In Guidelines for Cancer Nursing Practice. Edited by J. McNally, J. Stair, and E. Somerville. Orlando, FL, Grune and Stratton, 1985, pp. 78–84.
11. Howard-Ruben, J., McGuire, L., and Groenwald, S. Pain. In Cancer Nursing: Principles and Practice. Edited by S. Groenwald. Boston, Jones and Bartlett, 1987, pp. 171–220.
12. Mioduszewski, J., and McCray, N.: The evolving role of the oncology nurse in managing cancer pain. Semin. Oncol. Nurs., 1:123, 1985.
13. McCaffery, M., and Beele, A.: Pain: Clinical Manual for Nursing Practice. St. Louis, C. V. Mosby, 1989.
14. Oncology Nursing Society and American Nurses' Association. Outcome Standards for Cancer Nursing Practice. Kansas City, MO, American Nurses' Association, 1979.
15. Spross, J.: Cancer pain and suffering: Life, legend and literature. Oncol. Nurs. Forum, 12:23, 1985.
16. Bagley, C.S., Falinski, E., Garnizo, N., and Hooker, L.: Pain management: A pilot project. Cancer Nurs., 5(3):191, 1982.
17. Marks, R., and Sachar, E.: Undertreatment of medical inpatients with narcotic analgesics. Am. J. Internal Med., 78(2):173, 1973.
18. Charap, A.D.: The knowledge, attitudes and experience of medical personnel treating pain in the terminally ill. Mt. Sinai J. Med. (NY), 45(4):561, 1978.
19. Howard-Ruben, J., and Wickham, R.: Measurement of the knowledge and attitudes of staff nurses and medical residents of cancer pain in the hospitalized oncology patient. Proceedings of the Oncology Nursing Society 11th Annual Congress. Oncol. Nurs. Forum, 13(Suppl.):84, 1986.
20. Strauss, A.L., et al.: Pain: An interorganizational work-interactional perspective. Nurs. Outlook, 22:560, 1974.
21. Porter, J., and Jick, H.: Addiction rare in patients treated with narcotics. Letters to the editor. N. Engl. J. Med., 302:133, 1980.
22. Houde, R.W.: The use and misuse of narcotics in the treatment of chronic pain. Adv. Neurol., 4:527, 1974.
23. Walsh, T.D.: Opiates and respiratory function in advanced cancer. Recent Results Cancer Res. 89:115, 1984.
24. Angarola, R.T. (ed.): Narcotic analgesias: Fears and responsibilities. J. Pain & Symptom Manag., 1(2):77, 1986.
25. Donovan, M.I., Dillon, P., and McGuire, L.: Incidence and characteristics of pain in a sample of medical-surgical inpatients. Pain, 30:69, 1987.
26. Wiener, C.: Pain assessment on an orthopedic ward. Nurs. Outlook, 23(8):508, 1975.
27. Donovan, B.D.: Patient attitudes to postoperative pain relief. Anaesth. Intensive Care, 11(2):125, 1983.
28. Hawley, D.D.: Postoperative pain in children: Misconception, descriptions and interventions. Pediatr. Nurs., 10(1):20, 1984.
29. Weis, O.F., Sriwatantkul, K., Alloza, J., Weinthaub, M., and Lasagna, L.: Attitudes of patients, housestaff, and nurses toward postoperative analgesic care. Anesth. Analg., 60:70, 1983.
30. Myers, J.: Cancer pain: Assessment of nurses' knowledge and attitudes. Oncol. Nurs. Forum, 12(4):62, 1985.
31. Fox, L.: Pain management in the terminally ill cancer patient: An investigation of nurses' attitudes, knowledge, and clinical practice. Milit. Med., 147:455, 1982.
32. Twycross, R., and Lack, S.: Symptom Control in Far Advanced Cancer: Pain Relief. London, Pittman Publishing, 1983.
33. Coyle, N., Mauskop, A., Maggard, J., and Foley, K.: Continuous subcutaneous infusions of opiates in cancer patients with pain. Oncol. Nurs. Forum, 13(4):53, 1986.
34. Paice, J.A.: Intrathecal morphine infusion for intractable cancer pain: A new use for implanted pumps. Oncol. Nurs. Forum, 13(3):41, 1986.
35. Rohr, V.: Giving intrathecal drugs. Am. J. Nurs., 86(7):829, 1986.
36. Hongladarom, G., and Porter, S.: What is Hospice? 2nd Ed. Seattle, Fred Hutchinson Cancer Research Center Cancer Control Program, 1981.
37. Walborn, K.: A nursing model for the hospice: Primary and self-care nursing. Nurs. Clin. North Am., 15(1):205, 1980.
38. Keithly, J., Shelly, S., and Benner, J.: Nurse consultant. Nursing 79, 9(11):105, 1979.
39. Caplan, G. The Theory and Practice of Mental Health Consultation. New York, Basic Books, 1970.

INTRODUCTION
C. RICHARD CHAPMAN

Psychologic approaches to pain control are among the oldest and are an intrinsic part of medical practice in every culture; current methods have evolved from a rich and varied medical tradition. Although the technical refinements of modern medicine are spectacular, the basic strategies of symptomatic pain control have not changed over the centuries. These are (a) attenuation or blockade of nociception through intervention at the periphery; (b) activation of inhibitory processes that gate nociception at the spinal cord or brain stem; and (c) interference with the perception of pain, alteration of the meaning of the pain, alteration of the affect associated with the pain, and/or modification of pain behavior or pain expression.

Although some therapies for pain may involve all three strategies of pain control, most can be ascribed to one. For example, aspirin and other nonsteroidal anti-inflammatory drugs (NSAIDs), physical and related therapeutic modalities, peripheral neural augmentation techniques, regional analgesia, and peripheral neural ablative procedures are representative of the first category of interventions. Pharmacologic interventions involving opioids activate nociception-inhibiting neural circuits and therefore are categorized as the second type of intervention. All psychologic interventions are directed at brain processes or the interface between the individual and the environment and are therefore assigned to the third category.

In medicine, psychologic interventions sometimes are viewed as alternatives to conventional, more invasive procedures, but it is important to appreciate that they are often integrated with somatic interventions in multidisciplinary practice. Patient-controlled analgesia techniques in which patients administer opioids to themselves via computer-controlled infusion pumps are an example of combined pharmacologic and psychologic intervention. A comprehensive, and typically multidisciplinary, approach to the systematic control of pain involves using two or more of the three strategies in combination. The suitability of any one strategy or any combination strategy for the individual case depends on whether the pain is acute or chronic, the risks posed by the intervention or combination of interventions to the patient, and the probability of long-term success. Psychologic techniques, as opposed to formal psychotherapies (e.g., hypnosis), also can be applied in nonpsychotherapy settings and sometimes are integrated with somatically focused interventions.

The chapters in this section provide a comprehensive overview of the major methods for psychologic pain control, including discussion of the advantages and limitations of each of the approaches. The methods described represent the most common psychologic and psychiatric approaches to pain control, but other approaches will be encountered by interested readers who undertake a comprehensive literature search. The fundamental principles of most major psychologic interventions are presented in the chapters that follow.

The reader should not expect to find a single psychotherapy for pain; it would be as unlikely as a single pharmacologic or surgical pain therapy. Pain problems are extremely complex, and the patients who have them vary not only in their psychologic and organic pathology but also in their ability to benefit from one or another treatment option. Moreover, chronic behavioral pain problems are often intimately interlinked with the patient's family or other parts of his or her social environment. The physician interested in psychologic interventions may occasionally observe tensions among psychiatric and psychologic practitioners and arguments about the merits of one approach versus another. These differ little from arguments among physicians or surgeons about therapeutic efficacy (e.g., which pharmacologic approach is best for managing cancer pain or which surgery is best for tic douloureux) and should not be cause for concern.

The choice of psychologic interventions must depend on both the nature of each case and the therapeutic skills of the behavioral clinicians in a given multidisciplinary team. Moreover, some interventions are better suited than others for certain patient populations, and some practitioners are more committed than others to certain of the philosophic or theoretical underpinnings or principles associated with the different types of psychotherapies. From a practical viewpoint the issue of matching the patient to the therapy is no different for psychologic interventions than for the other types of treatment.

The methods discussed in this section have three characteristics in common: (a) they are comparatively noninvasive and therefore involve minimal risk; (b) they are more time-consuming for both the care giver and the patient than the other types of treatment; and (c) they require the patient to take an active rather than a passive role in his or her own pain relief. In psychologic and psychosocial interventions, negotiation between the patient and the care giver is formal and structured; in the other types of interventions, such negotiation is comparatively incidental and informal.

Chapter 81 by Fordyce introduces contingency management for chronic pain, an approach based on the principles derived from behaviorism. The theoretical basis of this approach is relatively simple and is concerned with what patients do. The behavioral psychotherapist addresses only those phenomena that can be directly observed and measured, namely actions. Thoughts, feelings, emotions, and hypothetical constructs like the unconscious are not considered; anything that cannot be observed and measured does not belong in the process of evaluation and intervention. In this framework, pain is viewed as a pattern of behavior sensitive to reward from the environment, which can shape it, and chronicity is defined in terms of learning. Affective states such as depression are observed behaviorally and related to behavioral variables such as a deprivation of adequate rewards. In recent years this approach has gained a wide following. It is suitable neither to all patient populations nor to all pain problems, but it provides a direct approach to the rehabilitation of certain types of chronic pain patients.

Chapter 82 by Turner and Romano also is based on a behavioral perspective, but the cognitive-behavioral approach combines behaviorism with cognitive psychology. Thought processes are assumed to play a powerful role in determining behavior in this approach; therefore, therapy is targeted in part at correcting negative distortions in patients' beliefs and attitudes about themselves, their physical capabilities, and their roles as sick persons in society. Whereas the strict behaviorist seeks to shape activity level and behavior through contingency management, the congnitive-behavioral therapist teaches the patient skills that help him or her identify and cope with or alter negative, self-defeating thoughts that degrade affect and suppress healthy behaviors. These methods have application to both acute and chronic pain. In other contexts this approach may be identified as coping skills training.

Blanchard and Ahles discuss a technologic method of psychotherapy—biofeedback—in Chapter 83. This method is suitable when a specific pain problem is targeted and the goal for the patient is to achieve control of that problem (e.g., recurrent headache). The patient must master a specific skill for a clearly delimited problem. Electronic instrumentation that can detect, amplify, and monitor biologic signals and a suitable facility for extended uninterrupted practice are needed for biofeedback therapy. Typically, biofeedback therapy is used only for chronic pain problems because therapeutic success is equated with mastery, which requires extended practice.

The use of hypnosis for pain control is discussed by Barber in Chapter 84. Hypnotic pain control is a recognized phenomenon, but it is poorly documented in controlled research and its basic mechanisms remain speculative at best. Its potential uses in acute, cancer, and possible chronic pain cases are probably far from being fully realized. Like other psychologic interventions, hypnosis requires the patient to take an active role in his or her own therapy. The patient does not enter into a state of total passivity but rather seems to achieve a heightened capability to work together with the therapist to achieve certain goals. Hypnotic methods are particularly well suited for acute pain patients even though there is an element of mastery in hypnotic pain control.

Relaxation is often a key element in cognitive-behavioral therapy and hypnosis, and it is the most common goal of biofeedback. Relaxation training can also stand alone, however, as a psychotherapeutic intervention for acute or chronic pain. In Chapter 85 Syrjala presents the principles of relaxation therapy and describes how it is undertaken. This method, like biofeedback, can be used to directly address discrete, well-defined problems. It requires no special equipment, however, and can be done in almost any clinical setting. Although patients often benefit from immediate intervention by a therapist trained in relaxation induction, mastery of relaxation is crucial for long-range therapeutic benefit. The skills needed for such therapy can be learned by nonpsychiatrically trained physicians and nonphysician health care providers. Relaxation training is a basic element in virtually every multidisciplinary pain control center.

Finally, Chapter 86 by Tunks and Merskey addresses the use of classic psychotherapy for pain control. Unlike the chapters that precede it, this chapter focuses on the role of traditional psychiatric psychotherapy in pain control. This approach concentrates on the emotional problems of patients rather than their behaviors, thought patterns, or specific symptoms. Psychotherapy is better suited than other approaches for dealing with cases in which the pain seems to follow from a psychiatric disorder and environmental contingencies cannot be demonstrated. In addition, this approach is less concerned than the others with the symptomatic relief of pain; rather the goal is to achieve a major adjustment in relationships, personality, and/or life goals. This is the only chapter to emphasize the role of the psychotherapist in providing psychologic support to patients under stress.

81 • CONTINGENCY MANAGEMENT

WILBERT E. FORDYCE

THIS chapter concerns the use of contingency management procedures in the treatment of chronic pain. It builds on the overlapping topics discussed in Chapter 82, Cognitive-Behavioral Therapy, Chapter 16, Learned Pain: Pain as Behavior, and Chapter 100, Multidisciplinary, Multimodal Management of Chronic Pain. The term "contingency management" refers to a set of methods for helping patients to change behavior. Though the terms contingency management and operant conditioning are essentially interchangeable, the former is more precise and so is used here. It is a method not for treating pain per se but rather for helping patients to modify pain behaviors and related activities or actions. Contingency management can also be viewed as a method for rehabilitating pain patients by increasing functional performance in daily life (1).

The behavioral perspective, which underlies contingency management, has been described by Brady (2) as follows:

... health related processes interact in profound and enduring ways with environmental circumstances and behavioral activities.... Conceptually, the roots of this behavioral perspective ... can be identified with the fundamentals of environmentalism, which has two main features. The first of these is that knowledge comes from experience rather than from innate ideas, divine revelation, or any other obscure source. And the second holds that action is governed primarily by consequences rather than by instinct, reason, will, cognitions, beliefs, attitudes, or any of the myriad explanatory fictions that appear to have been created out of whole cloth by the magic of the human language (p. 31).

OVERVIEW AND RELATION TO OTHER METHODS

Optimal treatment of chronic pain is a multimodal process. No single narrowly based intervention is likely to bring about comprehensive and lasting change in long-established pain problems. This holds true whether the therapy involves surgery, medication, or such noninvasive modalities as ultrasound, traction, massage, contingency management, or cognitive-behavioral methods. The application of contingency management techniques to the modification of pain behavior and other associated behaviors should almost always be done in conjunction with other modalities. In particular, the effects of these procedures can be enhanced by addressing the often profound misunderstandings patients have about the nature of pain, the healing process, the adverse effects of disuse, and the adverse effects of prolonged use of analgesics.

There is a synergistic relationship between contingency management methods and didactic sessions, properly termed *cognitive* (informational). This point will be developed only briefly here because it forms an important part of Chapter 82. The essence of the matter is that in chronic soft-tissue injury pain, and some other pain problems, the symptom, pain behavior, has become the problem: disability. Contingency management is a technology for changing pain behavior; that is, changing disability. The behaviors targeted for change are themselves influenced by what the patient anticipates. Anticipations can be viewed as meanings attached to cues or stimuli the patient encounters (i.e., the events he expects will follow the cues or stimuli perceived). If, for whatever reason, a patient anticipates adverse or painful consequences whenever he uses a body part or assumes a particular body position, pain behaviors are more likely to occur, either before the action is undertaken, as a means of forestalling anticipated suffering, or shortly thereafter. Moreover,

as developed in Chapter 16, such pain behaviors may be effectively reinforced in a variety of ways, the most important of which is that they successfully avoid an anticipated adverse consequence. Thus, any intervention that helps modify anticipations is relevant.

Information about pain, healing, and the effects of disuse is likely to influence what the patient anticipates. Information by itself, however, is not a powerful way to change established behaviors. If it were, simply providing chronic pain patients with brochures or other materials that clearly explain the rapid nature of the healing process, the adverse effects of disuse, and how properly designed motion can promote healing would be sufficient to change pain behavior. Of course, such an approach does not work, any more than providing inveterate smokers with information about the adverse effects of smoking results in cessation of smoking. Relevant information, however, can promote a readiness to undertake reactivation trials. Since pain behaviors related to body action are altered by the successful undertaking and expansion of activity, cognitive components to treatment can facilitate change of pain behaviors but, in the case of chronic pain, are unlikely to suffice by themselves. Conversely, the effectiveness of contingency management methods for altering behavior may be lessened considerably if the patient's readiness to participate is hampered by anticipating adverse consequences to reactivation.

Contingency management is indicated as a treatment for chronic pain patients who are (a) receiving excessive pain-related medications; (b) too deactivated or engaging in too much guarding behavior; (c) not engaging in normal physical activities (deactivation); (d) displaying poor pacing behaviors (e.g., doing too much and then too little); (e) displaying excessive concern about the pain problem; and (f) engaging in excessive health care utilization. Additional information regarding the indications and contraindications for contingency management is presented in Chapter 16. This chapter focuses on how to use the methods.

Contingency management involves the use of environmental consequences in a studied way to help a person to modify behavior. It includes analyzing which environmental consequences explain some of the strength or weakness of the behavior of interest and then changing those consequences to others that will support a different behavior or different pattern of behavior (3). Cognitive-behavioral methods, while implicitly and often explicitly using systematic environmental contingencies as part of a treatment strategy, focus more on helping to modify the patient's perception or labeling of sensations and, as a result, the behaviors linked to those perceptions. Both approaches strive to teach patients and their families that hurt and harm are not the same (i.e., that once healing time has passed, moving and doing things with painful body parts is the way to make them better). As noted already, this is accomplished not only by providing patients with information but also by providing for learning by doing.

Contingency management and cognitive-behavioral methods clearly overlap and sometimes are indistinguishable. Contingency management methods rely more heavily on modifying environmental contingencies, whereas the cognitive aspects of cognitive-behavioral methods focus primarily on how the patient understands or thinks about his pain problem and associated events (i.e., the focus is on processes determining how the problem is labeled). The assumption is made that cognitive labeling itself significantly influences pain behavior and the willingness to engage in treatment activities designed to modify that behavior. In the case of behaviors that have only recently emerged, as in acute pain, the impact of labeling is relatively great and the need to modify environmental contingencies correspondingly less. In the case of chronic pain, reliance on relabeling as the only means to bring about behavior change is unlikely to succeed (3).

TERMINOLOGY AND PRINCIPLES

The underlying principle of contingency management is that behavior is sensitive to consequences. Contingency management strategies are simply methods for applying that basic principle to help persons to modify sick and well behaviors pertinent to their pain problems. In this section, the terminology and principles of contingency management are presented. More detailed accounts of the methods are available elsewhere (4–6).

A *behavior* is a specific action or pattern of activity elicited by a discrete stimulus or by a stimulus constellation such as a specific social setting. Behavior occurs, or stops occurring, in response to environmental cues, which indicate the time and place of the reinforcement, punishment, or extinction (absence of reinforcement) contingencies. The emphasis should be on specific, not general, behaviors. For example, acting honestly is a general behavior, whereas answering a particular question truthfully is a specific honest behavior. In the context of clinical pain, simply saying that a patient manifests pain behaviors is too broad and too vague. Instead, specific behaviors (e.g., walking with a limp, moaning when flexing forward, or asking for analgesics) should be described.

Behavioral problems, including pain behavior, should first be analyzed into which behaviors are occurring too frequently (e.g., reclining, taking medications, limping), too infrequently (e.g., walking, working, gardening), or not at all. This analysis must be detailed and specific. For example, noting that a patient is "not moving enough" is too general; the movement should be specified (walking, flexing forward, etc.).

A behavior is described as strong if it has a high probability of occurring. The *strength* (probability of occurring) of a behavior increases when it is followed rapidly, contingently, and systematically by a *reinforcing consequence*. For example, chronic pain patients may come to limp or to grimace more consistently if such behavioral displays are followed by special attention or supportive actions from others. This is particularly likely to occur if such attention and supportive actions generally occur only when pain behaviors are emitted (i.e., attention or support is pain behavior contingent).

The strength of a behavior decreases when it is followed by an *aversive consequence* or when previously reinforcing consequences are withdrawn. For example, when a spouse, for whatever reason, ceases directing special attention or supportive actions in response to a patient's expressions of pain, the strength of this pain behavior is likely to diminish. Such reduction in strength of pain behaviors is usually not immediate. Initially, when reinforcing responses to pain behaviors are terminated, the pain behaviors tend to increase (accelerate), just as hunger increases when one first begins dieting. However, consistent withdrawal of reinforcement to a behavior can be expected to lead eventually to a reduction in the strength or frequency of that behavior.

The strength (frequency) of a behavior also tends to diminish if effective reinforcement becomes contingent upon occurrence of a behavior incompatible with the one to be reduced. The difference between this approach and that of withdrawing a reinforcing consequence is illustrated by two widely different methods for reducing excessive reclining or sitting behavior in a pain patient. Suppose, for example, that a patient's spouse is attentive whenever the patient reclines at a time when, were there no pain problem, the person likely would be active. The spouse thereby tends to reinforce reclining behavior. In an effort to reduce reclining, the withdrawal approach would have the spouse cease being attentive when the patient reclines; that is, reclining behavior is discouraged by being ignored. An alternative, and one that offers a number of advantages, is for spouse attention to become *contingent* on the patient's arising to move around. Reclining is ignored, but more importantly, walking is reinforced. Since accelerating a behavior generally is easier than decelerating one, this strategy is preferred (6). Reinforcement (in this example, attention) is made contingent upon—one could say "attached to"—walking rather than reclining.

Which consequences function as *reinforcers* depends on the experience of the individual. Extreme illustrations will clarify this point. Some persons, because of earlier learning or conditioning experiences, find physical punishment pleasurable or reinforcing. Such masochistic individuals are likely to engage in behaviors that lead to physical punishment or abuse (i.e., these behaviors are strong). Such cases are rare. Of course, most persons experience punishment or physical abuse as aversive and tend to avoid behaviors likely to lead to punishment. To illustrate in the context of clinical pain, some patients find immobilization highly aversive and activity and movement reinforcing; such patients tend to resist prescriptions of rest. In contrast, patients who find activity aversive and rest reinforcing are likely to welcome prescriptions of rest. The central point here is that one cannot assume a given consequence will be reinforcing or aversive: It will depend on the past experience of the person. To determine whether a particular consequence is reinforcing—or aversive—requires detailed observation of each patient.

Observation of which behaviors occur frequently in a person is the easiest way to determine what is reinforcing for that person. This is the Premack principle (7). Rest is almost certainly a potent reinforcer for a person who frequently reclines, whereas for a person who paces and moves restlessly, rest is unlikely to be reinforcing, though activity or movement probably will be.

To be effective, a reinforcer must occur promptly and be contingent on completion of the behavior it is designed to reinforce. Furthermore, successful behavior change requires precise definition of the behavior to be changed and the units by which it is to be measured. Units of behavior are best thought of as *movement cycles*. A movement cycle is a repeatable part of a specific behavior. For example, stepping forward with the left foot is not a movement cycle for walking, stepping with the left and then the right foot is, for completion of the cycle makes repetition possible.

Punishment is rarely an expeditious or appropriate way to help a person to change behavior for two major reasons. First, rather than leading to a decrease in a target behavior, punishment, if severe enough, often results in behavior being displaced in time and occurring with undiminished frequency in other settings. Second, the treatment relationship and the readiness of a patient to respond to therapist direction often are compromised if the therapist is a frequent source of aversive or punishing stimuli.

As noted already, accelerating (increasing) a behavior is easier to accomplish than decelerating (decreasing) one. Therefore, efforts to increase a behavior incompatible with the target behavior, which is occurring too frequently, generally are more effective than direct efforts to reduce the target behavior. For example, excessive reclining behavior in a chronic pain patient is treated more effectively by increasing walking and other "uptime" activities than by trying to decrease reclining. The concept of *incompatible response* and its use is also illustrated by excessive limping. Speed walking, which is described in detail later, is an effective way of diminishing a limp when that limp is occurring either from disuse or from overguarding against a defect that no longer exists. In this example, limping markedly and walking rapidly are the incompatible behaviors. It is easier to accelerate the rate of walking than to decelerate a limp.

Contingency management methods are not a substitute for a treatment relationship. The treatment relationship, including full informed consent and consensus as to objectives, is a prerequisite of all behavior change methods. During treatment, therapists must behave in ways which encourage patients to undertake some behaviors they believe will be harmful or, at the least, painful. If patients do not believe that compliance with therapist instructions and directions will lead to beneficial effects, patient performance almost certainly will suffer. Because initially patients are unlikely to know that beneficial effects will follow treatment effort, they must view their therapists positively and have trust in them. Establishing patient trust and confidence in the therapist is what the treatment relationship is all about.

BEHAVIORAL EVALUATION OF PAIN

Proper evaluation of chronic pain requires a coordinated medical science–behavioral science approach. The components of a behavioral evaluation of clinical pain are essentially the same whether the pain problem is in the low back or in other parts of the body. More detailed descriptions of evaluation methods can be found in Fordyce (8) and Heaton et al. (9).

Diagnosis requires analysis of the relationships between pain behaviors and environmental consequences. Information about these relationships can, in turn, best be obtained by (a) a prescreening questionnaire; (b) interviews with the patient and, separately, the spouse; (c) psychological tests, particularly the Minnesota Multiphasic Personality Inventory (MMPI); and (d) diary forms completed by the patient to portray the time distribution of body position and social and physical activities. These methods of data collection, the subsequent data analysis, and the possible indications and contraindications are discussed in the following sections.

Data Collection

Prescreening Questionnaire

Much routine information can be obtained by use of a questionnaire completed by the patient before being interviewed. Data about age, education, family structure, patient and spouse vocations, and sources of family income usually can readily be obtained in this manner. Brief descriptions of any prior treatment for pain and of the location of pain (by shading in on an outline of the human figure) can also be obtained.

Patient and Spouse Interviews

The patient and his spouse (or significant other) should be interviewed in some depth. Interviewing them separately is generally preferable, although joint interviews can be effective (see Chapter 33).

Although no set pattern of questions to be asked can be suggested, clinical experience has shown the types of information that are important. The precise wording of questions to derive that information will depend upon the nature and site of the pain problem and the interviewer's skills. Care should be exercised to avoid suggesting in the questions which responses are good/bad, expected/unexpected, or diagnostic of operant/nonoperant pain. In general, questions should avoid mentioning the word pain. This helps to avoid cueing the patient to respond in certain ways; for example, if asked how often pain causes one to awaken, a positive response may be encouraged in some patients.

Minnesota Multiphasic Personality Inventory and Other Psychologic Tests

The MMPI is the best-developed, best-standardized, best-validated measure of a patient's behavioral repertoire relevant to issues of chronic pain. Innumerable reports have been published on the effectiveness of the MMPI for making useful discriminations in the context of clinical pain (10–14). The results of such studies have often been conflicting. The problem of assessing the effectiveness of the MMPI and similar devices is complicated by differences in classifying subjects in a study, measuring or identifying treatment outcomes, methods for analyzing the data, and conceptualization of the questions or hypotheses of the studies.

As yet, there are no validated procedures for making critical clinical decisions about pain patients solely on the basis of MMPI data. Nonetheless, the MMPI can play a major role in assessment of clinical pain. Computer-based memory banks are available from which experience data can be drawn in the preparation of MMPI reports (15). If MMPI data are interpreted individually, the skill of the interpreter is a significant variable.

Several alternative tests or measuring devices also can prove helpful in the assessment of pain. The essential objective of such tests is to predict the probable high- and low-frequency behaviors of a person (i.e., what he does often or rarely). Such data indicate the readiness of the person to communicate to others that he is suffering body distress. Readiness to do that usually indicates more likelihood that body sensations—intense or weak, painful or only ambiguous—will be labeled as painful. As noted previously, once a sensation is labeled as painful, pain behaviors are more likely to be emitted and those around the patient are more likely to reinforce those behaviors.

Tests can also assess the extent to which the patient is presently coping with daily living demands. The more life's problems seem to be overwhelming or aversive, the more likely conditioning effects are to play a role in perpetuation of pain behaviors. Tests can also assess level of emotional distress. Patients who present with many pain complaints but with little concern about them are more likely to have pain behaviors controlled by the environment.

Information useful in predicting behavior patterns can also be obtained by intensive interview assessment, though usually not as efficiently as with the MMPI. At the present time, the MMPI is generally the most cost-effective source for such information. In addition, there are far more empirical studies demonstrating relationships between MMPI measures and a variety of factors pertinent to clinical pain than is true of any other measuring device.

Patient Diaries

Having patients keep diaries for a period of time before workup provides information that supplements the patient interview and MMPI data. Such diaries record how much or little—and when—a patient sits, stands, walks, or reclines, subjective pain levels, and medication intake. Of course, patient-recorded diary data cannot be assumed to be valid and accurate. Significant discrepancies have been found between diary-reported activity levels and more direct observations (16, 17). Diaries can provide a rough approximation of the amount of reclining time, the extent of interruption of nighttime reclining, and the level of daytime resting. Diary-recorded medication consumption provides a rough estimate of possible toxicity or addiction. Patient diaries are a useful and cost-effective assessment tool; however, it must be clearly understood that, by themselves, they often do not give an accurate account of present patient functioning.

Analysis of Data

Interpretation of the data obtained in a pain assessment is critical for reaching valid and useful conclusions. More detailed discussion of this topic is presented in reference 8.

Type of Activity

The distinction between effort-dependent and effort-independent activities should be kept clearly in mind in interpreting responses to interview questions. For example, when patients are asked which activities are limited by pain, responses pertaining to autonomically mediated body functions (e.g., micturition) should be interpreted differently from those relating to activities solely involving operants (i.e., body movements subject to voluntary control). In the former case, pain and the associated effort-independent activity (e.g., bladder accidents) are only minimally subject to influence from learning or conditioning effects from environmental contingencies. In the latter case, however, operants are involved and the activities (e.g., lifting or bending) are effort-dependent. Performance or nonperformance of such activities can be influenced by a host of factors independent of nociception.

Time Patterns

The time pattern of certain behaviors provides insight into the nature of the pain problem and the possible effectiveness of contingency management therapy. In particular, whether a patient falls asleep easily (with or without medications), the extent of nighttime awakening, and the degree to which nighttime sleep is compromised by daytime sleep should be determined. How frequently a patient wakens during the night and what he does on awakening (take pain-alleviating action, relieve bladder urgency or thirst, etc.) also should be probed. The core issue here is that pain behaviors controlled by nociception are likely to lead to greater subjective distress and sleep disruption when environmental stimuli are reduced by retiring to bed and darkness. The lack of such disruption or increased nighttime suffering suggests that the pain problem is somewhat more likely to be controlled by environmental contingencies.

A second time-pattern issue concerns episodic versus continuous pain. Episodic pain with intervals between episodes of several days or weeks, or more, generally is not operant in nature unless the episodes coincide with specific environmental consequences that also occur episodically. For example, were special attention from a spouse to be exerting significant influence on the persistence of pain behaviors, that attention is not likely to vary markedly in large blocks of time (e.g., two weeks of attention and three weeks without it). If, however, the spouse is absent during the week while traveling as part of employment but is home on weekends, the occurrence of pain behavior might systematically reflect the presence or absence of the spouse.

Pain-Activity Relationships

Information about which activities (e.g., lifting, standing, driving a car, walking) increase or decrease pain also provides clues about the nature of the pain. Typical questions are "Which activities, when you do them, may bring on the pain or make it worse?" and "What do you not do because of pain that you otherwise would?" Watch for discrepancies in patients' responses. If a person reports that sitting increases pain but riding a motorcycle or sitting through a long movie does not, operant factors are probably present. One also looks for evidence that the relinquished activities were valued. For example, a patient who describes herself as a meticulous housekeeper, particularly if that picture is also conveyed by the spouse, and who no longer can keep up her house because of reported pain is almost certainly being forced to give up a highly valued activity. For such a person, limitation in housekeeping behavior is likely to be aversive, not reinforcing, and thus the pain probably is not operant in nature.

Patterns of sexual activity often are useful in assessing chronic pain. A major reduction in the frequency of sexual activity that coincides with onset of the pain problem and is not accounted for by heavy medication intake is likely to indicate either that nociception is considerable or that sexual activity was aversive before onset of the pain problem. Conversely, little change in the frequency of sexual activity when the physical demands of such activity are likely to be influenced by the pain problem may well indicate operant factors are present.

Spouse and Family Responses

Pain behaviors that consistently elicit highly supportive behavior (e.g., assistance with chores, attention, protection from responsibility) from the spouse or significant others are likely to become conditioned. Detailed information about which pain behaviors elicit supportive responses and the nature of those responses can be useful in planning contingency management therapy.

Indications and Contraindications

Chronic pain problems that are reported to be steadily improving are almost certainly *not* problems of operant pain. This is so because logically environmental contingencies cannot be sustaining pain behaviors that, in the absence of significant environmental changes, are diminishing in frequency or scope.

The most common indications that operant pain is present and that contingency management treatment is appropriate are the following:

1. Pain behaviors occur in the absence of supporting physical findings or appear much in excess relative to those findings.
2. Pain behaviors are a product of disuse, overguarding or overanticipation of painful effects, or systematic reinforcement in the patient's immediate environment, or they serve to yield "time out" from activities that the patient finds aversive irrespective of pain.

The following kinds of evidence, on the other hand, suggest that a pain problem is not operant in nature and thus contraindicate contingency management treatment or that though the problem is largely operant, behavioral treatment is unlikely to succeed.

1. Pain behaviors seem directly linked to and proportional to physical findings.
2. There is no evidence of systematic reinforcement of pain behaviors or of indirect reinforcement by the patient gaining "time out" from aversive activities.
3. There is no evidence of excessive deactivation or overguarding behavior.
4. The evidence indicates that were pain behaviors reduced and activity level increased, the patient's environment would not support that change and/or that work or recreational opportunities that would serve to reinforce well behavior would not exist.
5. There is mental/emotional disturbance too severe to permit the patient to become effectively engaged in retraining or to relate to the treatment team.

Vascular or migraine headache problems do not often respond to contingency management methods, unless there appear to be systematic relationships between onset of headaches and environmental events. Those eliciting events may be in the form of stressors. Alternatively, they may be discriminated stimuli, which evoke a phobia-like headache response; that is, the symptoms are under stimulus control, and the stimuli are in the social environment.

The site of the originating pain problem is rarely of great significance.

TREATMENT

Application of contingency management procedures to problems of chronic pain typically targets some combination of the following problem behaviors:

Overmedication: decreasing consumption of analgesic and other palliative medications

Reduced activity level: increasing the scope and frequency of body movement in patients who are deactivated or have long been guarding against certain body movements

Excessive pain behaviors: reducing verbal and body language behaviors that cause others to identify patients as suffering

Deficits in well behavior: anticipating and encouraging activities patients will engage in following treatment, including vocational, daily living, and avocational activities

Inappropriate responses to pain behavior: modifying the responses of family members and others to patient pain and activity behavior

Overmedication

The pain cocktail strategy (4, 18) is an effective way of helping persons with high intakes of analgesic, muscle relaxant, or tranquilizing medications to reduce their reliance on drugs.

When overmedication is a presenting problem, one must distinguish between *detoxification* and *deconditioning*. The former refers to rapidly lowering narcotic intake so that impaired thought processes can become clearer and a more precise definition of the pain problem can be made. This can usually be achieved by reducing the active ingredients in the pain cocktail by 10 or 20% per day. Often such rapid reduction leads to an increase in pain behaviors when low drug levels are reached. At that point, the patient's mental functioning probably has improved enough that a precise picture of the pain problem can be obtained. One can then incrementally change dosage levels of active ingredients. Care should be exercised to look for any adverse side effects from too rapid withdrawal.

Some patients who have long been on high levels of narcotics do not fare well with rapid detoxification. An important element of drug withdrawal is a concomitant increase in exercise and activity level and a pairing of reductions in medications with increasing reliance on alternative methods for coping with suffering. In patients with long-established narcotic habits, the reduction in drug consumption may have to occur relatively slowly (e.g., a 20% reduction per week). Linking detoxification to a reactivation program (e.g., physical therapy exercise, psychological support, and vocational or social post-treatment planning) will facilitate the process.

Procedure

Patients coming with high levels of analgesic intake almost certainly will require detoxification and/or deconditioning on an inpatient basis, at least until intake levels have reached modest proportions.

The procedures should be explained fully to the patient before proceeding. Informed consent is essential not only for obvious ethical and legal reasons but because candor often lays to rest patient doubts about whether treatment is being fully explained and openly carried out. As a *chronic* pain patient, he will likely have undergone repeated treatment failures. In addition, it is commonplace for the patient to feel that his physician doubts whether he is really suffering. Instead "it is all in the head" is the message perceived, whether intended or not. Therefore, special efforts should be made to spell out all details regarding the pain cocktail strategy and to make clear that it is *not* a placebo procedure.

1. For 2 days, provide free access to whatever analgesics the patient has been using. This provides a baseline *drug profile*. Nursing staff must keep careful record of which medications are taken, in what quantities, and how often. If the patient has been on injectables, switch immediately to oral ingestion; this change may require an increase in consumption over preadmission levels. The reason for switching to oral ingestion is that both detoxification and relearning are involved. The ultimate goal is either no analgesics or a minimum, taken orally. Injection of medications provides a more intense learning experience than oral ingestion and hence carries greater risk of the patient becoming habituated to the procedure. Shifting to oral intake eliminates one of the more potent learning conditions that can serve to intensify the patient's habituation.

2. Convert narcotic intake to equivalent amounts of methadone. Convert sedative hypnotics to equivalent amounts of phenobarbital. Discontinue tranquilizers and other pain-related medications (Tables 78-12 and 78-13, p. 1672).

3. Place the analgesic and sedative equivalents in a color- and taste-masking vehicle such as cherry syrup. This is the pain cocktail. The total volume of each dose is 10 cc, delivered every 4 or 6 hours, such that 24-hour total ingestion matches or slightly exceeds the drug profile level. After a day or so of stabilization and dosage adjustment, begin to taper the active ingredients at 20% per day for narcotics and 10% per day for sedatives.

4. If the patient reports a marked increase in pain or displays a sharp increase in pain behavior during reduction, wait a day or two and then retreat to a higher level of analgesia and resume fading. When zero levels are attained, as they usually are, wait 2 to 3 days and then inform the patient of his achievement.

5. If zero levels are not achieved, fading can be continued in a follow-up regimen, but it is prudent to slow the rate of reduction to, for example, 10% per 2-week period or per month.

Reduced Activity Level

Reactivation is the key element in almost all treatment regimens for chronic pain. More detailed review of the effects of exercise and how to program it can be found elsewhere (19–22). Disuse, the conviction that to use a painful part is to risk further damage and/or an increase in the pain problem, depression, limping without structural defect, and decreased confidence in the safety of moving and self-efficacy are all pain-related problems for which exercise and reactivation are likely to be helpful. The situation is, of course, quite different in acute pain. During healing, rest and suitable amounts of activity limitation are often quite appropriate. After healing, however, if chronic pain emerges, rest rapidly becomes counterproductive.

Procedure

Patients should be given sheets of graph paper, a folder in which to carry them, instruction in how to make bar graphs or histograms of exercise performance and incrementing achievement quotas.

1. Select exercises consistent with the site and nature of the pain problem. Walking measured laps should be included, irrespective of the site of pain, unless specifically contraindicated.
2. Schedule daily exercise sessions, two to three sessions per day is ideal.
3. Initially instruct the patient about how to do each exercise and direct him to do each exercise "until pain, weakness, or fatigue cause you to want to stop. You decide when to stop." The therapist records precisely how much is done; these are baseline trials. Approximately four baseline trials usually suffice to indicate the patient's current level for each exercise.
4. Use the baseline level for each exercise to set an initial quota for the patient to meet. Each quota should be the highest value that, when increased by one repetition per session, ensures the patient will be able to succeed for a minimum of four sessions. Typically, the starting quota is set at about two-thirds of the average baseline level. Although an increment rate of one repetition per session is common, the therapist should adjust the rate higher or lower to assure that the patient advances as rapidly as possible consistent with therapist confidence that increments can be met. A ceiling should also be set at whatever constitutes a medically prudent activity level, considering all exercises prescribed and the patient's physical status. Finally, the "trajectory" of incrementing sufficient to reach the ceiling in the time available for treatment should be set.

Quota failures are rare. Unless they occur repeatedly, they can usually be ignored, while the patient continues with the previously set increment rate. If quota failures persist (e.g., in three consecutive trials), the therapist should review the problem with the patient. The perspective should be maintained that it is *not* the responsibility of the treatment team to get the patient to meet quotas but of the patient to decide whether he is going to use the treatment opportunity to get better. If some adjustment seems indicated, quotas can be lowered to modestly below the amount last successfully achieved and increments reinstituted. Alternatively, a slower increment rate can be applied.

Persistent quota failures, when one is satisfied there is no reason other than the patient's report of increased pain, particularly when failures occur at levels lower than attained during baseline trials, usually indicate patient desire to maintain the sick role. In the face of such a situation, the therapist usually meets with the patient and spouse, reviews exercise performance and treatment objectives, and assigns to the patient and spouse the task of deciding whether to continue or terminate. Continuation of treatment should be contingent on achieving exercise quotas.

Speed walking is a very useful exercise for reactivation. This exercise consists of walking a fixed distance (e.g., 50 m) in gradually decreasing elapsed times (22). Speed walking has several functions. Mainly, it helps patients to appreciate fully that it is safe to move freely; that is, activity will not worsen their condition. Pronounced limping, distorted gait, or knee buckling often can be remedied by including speed walking in the exercise set. Because of the diminishing time quotas built into the exercise, walking speed must be increased, which sets up a classical incompatible response situation, as discussed earlier. The body automatically strives for economy of motion. To walk with a limp or in a guarded fashion in order to protect against anticipated or feared knee buckling is laborious and requires extra energy expenditure; it also interferes with rapid walking. Because one cannot limp or walk guardedly and move very rapidly, speed walking often is an effective way of causing a limp or guarded walking to disappear, assuming, of course, that structural mechanisms are intact. In addition, overprotective or overly concerned family members can hardly fail to be impressed at seeing the formerly impaired and gingerly moving patient walking at the very brisk pace of 22 s for 50 m.

The procedure is first to time the patient walking a 50-m lap. Next, set a speed goal in elapsed seconds based on age, sex, and general health. Usually a speed of 20 to 24 s for males and 22 to 26 s for females is an appropriate target. Lowering the speed target is rarely indicated. Cardiac status, compromised knee function, etc., may be reasons for raising the elapsed time target. Next, on a sheet of graph paper (which can be kept with the other exercise bar graphs), with seconds on the vertical and trial numbers on the horizontal axis, draw a sloping line from the point on the vertical axis that is 1 to 2 s above the baseline elapsed time to the target elapsed time at the number of trials judged at the outset to be appropriate. Assuming two trials per day, 25 to 30 trials is usually an appropriate number. Performance in elapsed seconds for each trial should be plotted against the corresponding trial number. Generally, the plotted "score" will be below the sloping line. If it is not, a second trial can be required, but that is not often needed.

Aerobic exercise also is a useful adjunct to other exercises when there are no medical contraindications.

Excessive Pain Behaviors

In the case of pain behaviors, treatment seeks to modify the public communication of pain by altering social contingencies to its expression (2, 18). The underlying principle is that communication of suffering by word or action to others tends to result in overprotective behaviors and social reinforcement from those around the patient; those consequences then tend to support pain behaviors and inhibit alternative well behaviors. The goal of treatment is *extinction*, or reduction, of a too frequently occurring behavior. For extinction to be achieved, the behavior to be changed must occur and must not be reinforced, alternative behaviors must be available, and those alternatives must be reinforced.

Programs that directly attempt to prohibit talking about pain are counterproductive because they fail to permit the behavior to be extinguished to occur, and thus inhibit extinction. Let the person talk about pain to staff. Be sure, however, that staff attention and immediate social responsiveness is minimal. For example, when the patient moans, grimaces, rubs the involved body part, or limps, staff should not seek to reassure or to change the subject, but should maintain eye contact, thereby acknowledging the person as a person. The essence of staff response should be in the theme: "I recognize you as a person and I am aware of how you are feeling. But I do not worry about it and I shall direct my special attention to what you do to get better, not how much you hurt." On the other hand, patient performance of activity and exercise, particularly when not accompanied by pain behavior, should receive attention and approval.

Deficits in Well Behavior

In chronic illness, including chronic pain, one cannot assume the reduction of symptoms will automatically be followed by resumption of effective well behavior. Persons who have been "sick" a long time may not know how to be well; they may have had major defects in their well behavior repertoire for an extended period. Consequently, the evaluation and treatment of chronic pain requires integrated and synergistic medical and behavioral expertise. Problems likely to impair the patient's ability to be well and to resume and to maintain effective functioning, if they exist, must be identified at the outset. This implies that one dimension of evaluation is identification of treatment goals. The treatment program must address any problems that threaten to compromise treatment goals. If that is not done, treatment failures or short-lived successes will inevitably be numerous.

Selection of treatment goals should be based, in part, on consideration of what the patient would be doing

were treatment successful. Next, the limitations in achieving those post-treatment target activities, in addition to those occurring because of pain, must be considered. These target activities can be grouped into social/familial/leisure and vocational. Each needs to be assessed. The remedial steps, if any, needed to ensure optimal outcome must be identified.

In the case of social/familial/leisure activities, it is usually best to work with the patient and spouse together to identify problems and goals in this area. In the case of vocational matters, treatment programs should have, as an integral part of their resources, vocational counseling and appraisal. Those working on vocational matters should be integral members of the treatment team and not simply "on-call" consultants. Close contact with vocational personnel of referring agencies whose objectives concern patient return to employment is also important.

Such issues as stress or anger management, marital counseling, sexual dysfunction, and goal-setting skills may make up a part of the total treatment package. These are dealt with in the next chapter. The techniques by which they are addressed may include contingency management methods, but rarely are they dealt with solely by such methods.

Inappropriate Responses to Pain Behaviors

The essentials of this component of treatment are similar to those described in the earlier section on excessive pain behavior. Spouses and significant others should be involved in both evaluation and treatment. If there is no spouse or significant other, pain behaviors obviously cannot have been influenced significantly by such a person; hence, there is no need to address the matter. That situation is rare.

Spouses or significant others should receive instruction in how to respond to sick and well behavior. Often it is helpful to provide guided rehearsal for them. It is also helpful to provide opportunity for spouses and significant others to observe speed walking and other exercise performance in the later stages of treatment when substantial progress has occurred.

REFERENCES

1. Roberts, A.H.: The behavioral treatment of pain. *In* The Comprehensive Handbook of Behavioral Medicine. Vol. 2. Syndromes and Special Areas. Edited by J.M. Ferguson and C.B. Taylor. Jamaica, NY, Spectrum, 1981, pp. 171–189.
2. Brady, J.B.: A behavioral perspective on child health. *In* Child Health Behavior: A Behavioral Pediatrics Perspective. Edited by N. Krasnegor, J. Arasteh, and M. Cataldo. New York, John Wiley and Sons, 1986, p. 31.
3. Baer, D.M.: Advances and gaps in a behavioral methodology of pediatric medicine. *In* Child Health Behavior: A Behavioral Pediatric Perspective. Edited by N. Krasnegor, J. Arasteh, and M. Cataldo. New York, John Wiley and Sons, 1986, pp. 54–69.
4. Fordyce, W.E.: Behavioral Methods for Chronic Pain and Illness. St. Louis, C.V. Mosby, 1976.
5. Berni, R., and Fordyce, W.: Behavior Modification and the Nursing Process, 2nd Ed. St. Louis, C.V. Mosby, 1977.
6. Wahler, R.G., and Hann, D.M.: A behavioral perspective in childhood psychopathology: Expanding the three-term operant contingency. *In* Child Health Behavior: A Behavioral Pediatrics Perspective. Edited by N. Krasnegor, J. Arasteh, and M. Cataldo. New York, John Wiley and Sons, 1986, pp. 146–167.
7. Premack, D.: Toward empirical behavior laws: I. Positive reinforcement. Psychol. Rev., *66*:219, 1959.
8. Fordyce, W.E.: Behavioral concepts in chronic pain and illness. *In* The Behavioral Management of Anxiety, Depression, and Pain. Edited by P.O. Davidson. New York, Brunner/Mazel, 1976, pp. 147–188.
9. Heaton, R. et al.: A standardized evaluation of psychosocial factors in chronic pain. Pain, *12*:165, 1982.
10. Fordyce, W.: Use of the MMPI in the assessment of chronic pain. *In* Clinical Notes on the MMPI. No. 3. Edited by J. Butcher, G. Dahlstrom, M. Gynther, and W. Schofield. Nutley, New Jersey, Hoffmann-LaRoche, 1979.
11. Bradley, L., Prokop, C., Margolis, R., and Gentry, D.: Multivariate analyses of low back pain patients. J. Behav. Med., *1*(3):253, 1978.
12. Prokop, C.K.: Hysteria scale elevations in low back pain patients: A risk factor for misdiagnosis? J. Consult. Clin. Psychol., *54*:558, 1986.
13. Cox, G., Chapman, C., and Black, R.: The MMPI and chronic pain: The diagnosis of psychogenic pain. J. Behav. Med., *1*(4):437, 1978.
14. Rosen, J., Frymoyer, J., and Clements, J.: A further look at validity of the MMPI with low back patients. J. Clin. Psychol., *36*:994, 1980.

15. Butcher, J.N.: The Minnesota Report. Minneapolis, Interpretive Scoring Systems, 1985.
16. Sanders, S.: Toward a practical instrument system for the automatic measurement of "uptime" in chronic pain patients. Pain, *9*:103, 1980.
17. Linton, S.: Controlling pain reports through operant conditioning: A laboratory demonstration. Percept. Mot. Skills, *60*:427, 1985.
18. Loeser, J., and Fordyce, W.: Chronic pain. *In* Behavioral Science in the Practice of Medicine. Edited by J. Carr and H. Dengerink. New York, Elsevier, 1983, pp. 331–345.
19. Cairns, D., and Pasino, J.: Comparison of verbal reinforcement and feedback in the operant treatment of disability due to chronic low back pain. Pain, *2*:301, 1976.
20. Doleys, D., Crocker, M., and Patton, D.: Responses of patients with chronic pain to exercise quotas. Am. J. Phys. Ther. Assoc., *62*:1111, 1982.
21. Fordyce, W., Roberts, A., and Sternbach, R.: The behavioral management of chronic pain: A response to critics. Pain, *22*:113, 1985.
22. Fordyce, W., Shelton, J., and Dundore, D.: The modification of avoidance learning in pain behaviors. J. Behav. Med., *5*:405, 1982.

82 · COGNITIVE-BEHAVIORAL THERAPY

JUDITH A. TURNER *and* JOAN M. ROMANO

ALTHOUGH cognitive-behavioral therapies reflect a relatively new development in the field of psychotherapy and have been applied to the treatment of pain even more recently, preliminary research suggests that they hold promise for a diverse array of clinical pain syndromes. There has been growing interest in the use of cognitive-behavioral procedures to prepare patients for acute pain such as that associated with childbirth and many medical and surgical procedures. Cognitive-behavioral methods are now used frequently to help manage chronic nonmalignant pain problems and also to reduce pain and discomfort associated with cancer and its treatment.

Cognitive-behavioral therapies have been developed and refined primarily in the past decade, as behavioral scientists increasingly questioned the adequacy of simple learning theory models in explaining human behavior and began to explore the importance of patients' thoughts, attributions, appraisals, and images in affecting emotions and behavior. In recent years, the popularity of this approach has increased, and a variety of cognitive-behavioral therapies have been developed for different patient populations. Beck and his colleagues (1, 2), for example, designed a cognitive therapy for depression that emphasized the identification and correction of negative distortions in patients' views of themselves and their experiences; this has been adapted for use with anxiety, anger, and other problems. For such diverse conditions as anxiety, psychosis, and learning disorders, Meichenbaum (3) described the application of techniques aimed at modifying patients' thoughts and images in combination with more traditional behavior therapy procedures such as relaxation. Meichenbaum and others emphasize a coping skills model, that is, teaching patients a variety of methods that can be applied across problems and situations.

Paralleling this increasing interest on the part of behavioral scientists in the cognitive aspects of behavior and behavior change, health care providers and researchers have begun to recognize the role that cognitive, emotional, and behavioral factors play in the experience of pain. With this recognition has come an appreciation of the importance of examining the impact of psychologic factors (e.g., the meaning of the pain for the individual, anxiety, depression) on an individual's pain experience and the potential for altering pain and associated responses through psychologic techniques (e.g., distraction, relaxation). The rationale for applying cognitive-behavioral treatment strategies to both acute and chronic pain problems is that learning new cognitive and behavioral responses to pain and stress can give the individual a sense of control over pain and decrease negative emotions, thoughts, and judgments related to the pain; this, in turn, may reduce pain, suffering, and pain behavior. These cognitive-behavioral techniques are typically incorporated as part of a broader, comprehensive pain management approach.

In this chapter, we first briefly review the fundamental principles underlying cognitive-behavioral treatments and then describe representative controlled studies and summarize findings related to the efficacy of these methods for clinical pain. A description of various specific techniques and factors in influencing their efficacy follows. A more detailed examination of cognitive-behavioral techniques for pain can be found in *Pain and Behavioral Medicine: A Cognitive-Behavioral Perspective* (4) and in critical reviews by Turner and Chapman (5), Turner and Romano (6), Pearce (7), and Tan (8). The reader interested in an overview of the historical development of cognitive theory and cognitive-behavioral therapies in the field of psychotherapy is referred to Mahoney and Arnkoff (9).

FUNDAMENTAL PRINCIPLES

Because striking differences exist among interventions labeled cognitive-behavioral, generalizations regarding fundamental characteristics and procedural details are difficult to make. Turk et al. (4) noted that these dissimilarities related to (a) theoretical underpinnings; (b) aspects of cognition targeted for change; (c) therapist styles; (d) inclusion of behavior therapy procedures; and (e) particular strategies or techniques employed. Nonetheless, the following characteristics are common to all cognitive-behavioral therapies: (a) the assumption that emotions and

behaviors are greatly influenced by cognitions; (b) an emphasis on using active, structured techniques aimed at modifying patients' cognitions, feelings, and behaviors; (c) a focus on helping patients acquire skills in using such techniques on their own; and (d) a time-limited therapeutic framework.

The cognitive-behavioral therapist works from the premise that patients must be actively involved in learning to manage their own problems, including pain. Patients must have a clear rationale for the use of cognitive-behavioral techniques in dealing with their pain and be receptive to trying them. Many patients initially tend to disbelieve that a psychologic treatment could be helpful in decreasing pain; such a proposition is sometimes viewed, especially by chronic pain patients, as implying that their pain is purely psychologic in origin or is otherwise "not real" or legitimate. It is important that patients view the therapist as someone who accepts the reality of their pain problems and has some useful tools to offer in managing them. This can usually be facilitated by educating patients about the complex nature of pain, stressing the interrelationships among cognitive, affective, behavioral, and sensory components. Therapist and patient typically work as collaborators, with the aim of having the patient acquire effective skills that increase self-control and independence from the therapist.

Mahoney and Arnkoff (9) described three major types of cognitive therapy: (a) cognitive restructuring; (b) coping skills training; and (c) problem-solving. The first two approaches are summarized briefly in Table 82-1; the third has not been studied with pain problems.

TABLE 82-1. Major Types of Cognitive-Behavioral Therapies for Pain

Type	Description
Cognitive restructuring	Patients are taught to monitor and evaluate negative thoughts and to generate more accurate and adaptive cognitions. *Example*: A chronic pain patient who responds to increased pain by thinking "I can't take this anymore" is taught to examine such thoughts and develop more accurate and adaptive ones; for example, "Is it really true that I can't deal with this? No. It may be difficult, but I've done it before and can again."
Coping skills training	Patients are provided a rationale for the use of techniques and then taught various skills for managing pain and stress.
Relaxation	*Example*: Physical and/or mental relaxation methods
Imagery	*Example*: Imagining pleasant scenes
Coping self-statements	*Examples*: "Relax." "I can cope." "Focus on what you have to do."

EFFICACY FOR CLINICAL PAIN

The efficacy of cognitive-behavioral therapies for several types of acute clinical pain (postoperative pain, pain associated with medical procedures and treatment of burns, and childbirth) has been evaluated. A variety of chronic pain syndromes have also been the target of study. Unfortunately, the systematic investigation of the efficacy of cognitive-behavioral techniques for treatment of pain problems is still in its infancy, as evidenced by the paucity of controlled studies.

Acute Pain

Postoperative Pain

Preoperative interventions involving instruction in cognitive-behavioral strategies have been reported generally to have positive effects, including reduction in pain ratings and analgesic medication requests. A number of investigators have examined the effects of preparing patients by providing information about the surgery (procedural information) and the sensations the patient will experience afterwards (sensory information); these are not considered to be cognitive-behavioral treatments unless additional training in some type of coping skill is provided. The question of whether cognitive-behavioral training produces greater effects than information provision alone has not yet been resolved. Table 82-2 summarizes representative studies. Not only have there been relatively few controlled studies of cognitive-behavioral interventions for postoperative pain, but even fewer have

TABLE 82-2. Effects of Preoperative Cognitive-Behavioral Interventions on Postoperative Pain

Source	No. of Patients	Techniques Compared	Results
Langer et al. (10)	60	(a) Instruction in generating positive views of hospital experience (b) (a) Plus procedural and sensory information (c) Procedural and sensory information only (d) Therapist contact only	Patients in (d) made more medication requests after surgery than patients in (a), (b), and (c). More patients in (a) and (b) requested no medication
Wells (11)	12	(a) Instruction in muscle relaxation and breathing techniques to decrease distracting thoughts (b) Sensory and procedural information	Group (a) patients rated distress (but not pain) postoperatively as lower than group (b)
Pickett and Clum (12)	59	(a) Cognitive distraction training (different imagined surgery scenes followed by pleasant images) (b) Relaxation training (c) "Relaxation information" (d) No treatment control	Group (a) had lower "worst pain" and anxiety ratings compared with no treatment control, but no differences found in medication use and McGill Pain Questionnaire scores

employed self-report measures of pain per se, as opposed to ratings of anxiety or distress. Studies that have included measures of pain have yielded mixed results.

One problem in evaluating the research data in this area stems from the lack of details in published reports about the content of the interventions, especially what rationale and instructions were given to patients. This makes it difficult to evaluate the adequacy of the treatments and to compare results across studies. The frequent use of only one session to provide the intervention also raises the question of whether this is sufficient time for an adequate trial of the treatment.

Painful Medical Procedures

Mixed results regarding the benefits of cognitive-behavioral techniques with painful medical procedures have been reported. Representative studies are summarized in Table 82-3. The few published controlled studies generally have not found cognitive-behavioral interventions to affect pain felt during the procedure, although there may be other benefits, such as decreased anxiety. In the case of dressing changes and bathing in the treatment of burns, pain tolerance may be increased and medication requests decreased by cognitive-behavioral strategies (13).

Childbirth

Reviews by Tan (8), Turk et al. (4), and Reading (16) concluded that prepared childbirth techniques—including relaxation, attention focusing, distraction, controlled breathing, and education (information provision)—generally are associated with increased maternal cooperation with the physician during labor and delivery, decreased use of analgesics and anesthetics, and increased maternal satisfaction with the childbirth experience. Whether or not childbirth preparation training reduces pain is unclear. Although some investigators have reported that parturients who received such training rated their labor pain much less (17) and some slightly less (18, 19) than those who had not received training, other studies (20, 21) have found no such relationship (Table 82-4).

A number of caveats must be applied to the interpretation of such studies. Most importantly, these and other similar studies lack adequate controls; thus, definitive statements about the relationship of specific antenatal interventions to childbirth experiences cannot be formulated. For example, the finding that mothers trained in such techniques receive less anesthesia and analgesic medication may be due to self-selection (i.e., mothers who participate in childbirth preparation classes may be more motivated to give birth without medication) and may reflect a number of factors not related to pain experience.

Chronic Nonmalignant Pain

Cognitive-behavioral strategies have been applied to a number of different chronic pain problems, most commonly headache. Table 82-5 lists representative studies. The techniques employed most frequently in controlled treatment studies of headache have been some variants of stress management and coping skills training. These typically involve teaching patients to identify stressful situations and their associated reactions, then to substitute more adaptive responses. Studies generally have found that cognitive-behavioral interventions decrease headache frequency, duration, and intensity, and that these improvements are maintained after treatment. However, the small number of

TABLE 82-3. Effects of Cognitive-Behavioral Treatments for Painful Medical Procedures

Source	No. of Patients	Medical Procedure	Techniques Compared	Results
Wernick et al. (13)	16	Burns (dressing changes and bathing)	(a) Education about stress and pain, breathing, relaxation, attention diversion, and cognitive restructuring (b) No treatment control	Group (a) had significant improvement in anxiety, number of pain medication requests, patient and staff ratings of pain tolerance during dressing changes, and treatment compliance. Group (b) had little significant improvement
Kendall et al. (14)	44	Cardiac catheterization	(a) Cognitive-behavioral treatment (application of coping strategies and positive coping statements in response to anxiety-arousing stimuli) (b) Procedural information provision (c) Attention placebo control (d) Standard treatment control	Group (a) patients rated by physicians and technicians as best adjusted during catheterization. Patient-rated anxiety lower in (a) and (b). No differences in pain ratings between various groups
Tan and Poser (15)	36	Knee arthrogram	(a) Procedural information provision (b) No intervention (c) Cognitive-behavioral skills training	No group differences on ratings of pain, fear, and discomfort

TABLE 82-4. Effects of Prepared Childbirth Training*

Source	No. of Subjects	Type of Training	Results
Norr et al. (17)	249	Lamaze preparation (information about childbirth, instruction in breathing exercises)	Women who had Lamaze preparation rated labor pain somewhat lower than did women who did not attend Lamaze classes
Melzack et al. (18)	240	Prepared childbirth training (instruction in obstetric physiology, breathing, and relaxation techniques)	Women who elected childbirth training rated labor pain lower than those who did not
Melzack et al. (19)	141	Prepared childbirth training	Primiparas who elected childbirth training rated labor pain slightly lower than those who did not. No difference in pain ratings between trained and untrained multiparas
Davenport-Slack and Boylan (20)	75	Prepared childbirth training	Training did not affect labor pain ratings
Nettelbladt et al. (21)	78	Antenatal training program of information and relaxation exercises	Training did not affect labor pain ratings

*All studies were uncontrolled.

well-controlled investigations precludes drawing conclusions about the effective components of such interventions.

Even fewer controlled studies of cognitive-behavioral approaches have been conducted with chronic pain problems other than headache. As shown in Table 82-6, these have generally found positive effects for cognitive-behavioral interventions in decreasing both patient self-report of pain and pain behaviors. Turner's (30) finding of continued improvement in chronic low back pain patients following cognitive-behavioral treatment supports the contention of some that cognitive-behavioral treatments, with their emphasis on fostering patients' acquisition and independent utilization of skills, may have greater potential for long-term maintenance of gains than do traditional therapies.

Cancer Pain

Pain associated with cancer represents a major clinical problem, affecting about half of all patients with the intermediate stages of the disease (31, 32) and about 70% of those with advanced/terminal cancer (32). Despite its prevalence, cancer pain is an undeveloped area in terms of systematic research aimed at defining its parameters and effective treatments. Increasing recognition of the role that cognitive and emotional factors

TABLE 82-5. Effects of Cognitive-Behavioral Treatments for Chronic Headache

Source	No. of Patients	Techniques Compared	Results
Anderson et al. (22)	14	(a) Autogenic relaxation (b) Cognitive coping skills training (c) Combination of (a) and (b)*	All conditions resulted in approximately equal reductions in headache activity
Bakal et al. (23)	45	Coping skills training plus EMG biofeedback plus relaxation (uncontrolled study)	Significant improvement in duration, intensity of headaches, and medication use; gains maintained at follow-up
Holroyd and Andrasik (24)	19	(a) Stress coping training (b) EMG biofeedback	Group (a) maintained significant reduction in headache activity. Significantly superior to group (b) at 2-year follow-up
Kremsdorf et al. (25)	2	(a) Coping skills training (b) EMG biofeedback (c) Combination of (a) and (b)*	Decrease in headache activity occurred primarily in coping condition
Mitchell and White (26)	12	(a) Self-recording headache frequency (b) (a) Plus recording antecedent stress (c) (a) and (b) Plus relaxation training and instructions to relax under stress (d) All of the above plus additional stress management training	73% reduction in headache frequency in group (d); 45% reduction in group (c); no decrease in groups (a) and (b). At follow-up, 83% reduction from baseline in group (d), 55% in group (c)

*Techniques compared within subjects. Subjects served as own controls.

TABLE 82-6. Effects of Cognitive-Behavioral Treatments for Chronic Pain Problems Other than Headache

Source	No. of Patients	Type of Pain	Techniques Compared	Results
Engstrom (27)	32	Low back	(a) Cognitive-behavioral training including relaxation, imagery, self-instruction, charting of progress, and development of coping strategies as well as education about chronic pain (b) Placebo medication control	Group (a) improved significantly compared with group (b) on measures of pain and beliefs concerning ability to control pain post-treatment and at 3-week follow-up
Khatami and Rush (28)	5	Head, rectal, low back	(a) Relaxation training, EMG biofeedback, self-hypnosis (b) Cognitive stress management training (c) Family intervention*	Decreased pain, medication use, and depression post-treatment and at follow-up
Moore and Chaney (29)	43	Low back	(a) Cognitive-behavioral group treatment including relaxation training, cognitive stress management, goal setting, and education about chronic pain (b) (a) Plus spouses attend group treatment sessions (c) Waiting list control	Both groups (a) and (b) significantly improved in pain, disability, and health care utilization compared with (c). Treatment gains were maintained at 3- to 7-month follow-up
Turner (30)	36	Low back	(a) Cognitive-behavioral therapy including relaxation, imagery, coping skills training, and goal setting (b) Relaxation only (c) Attention/waiting list control	Both groups (a) and (b) significantly improved in pain and disability post-treatment compared with controls. Group (a) more improved than group (b) in pain tolerance and activity self-ratings at 1-month follow-up. At 1½- to 2-year follow-up, health care use markedly decreased in both groups

*Uncontrolled study in which all patients received all treatments.

play in the experience of cancer pain and distress (33) has fostered interest in the application of psychologically based treatments for these problems.

Hypnosis (34), biofeedback (35), and imagery (36) have been applied to cancer pain with some promising results, but controlled studies generally have not been conducted and are needed to assess the efficacy of such approaches. Although controlled studies have been conducted of cognitive-behavioral techniques aimed at decreasing nausea, vomiting, and emotional distress associated with chemotherapy, these have not focused on pain per se. For example, Lyles et al. (37) found that a combination of imagery and relaxation resulted in significantly lowered anxiety, nausea, and physiologic arousal during chemotherapy and significantly less nausea afterwards than either therapist contact with no training or no intervention. Such encouraging results from this and other studies support the potential of cognitive-behavioral treatments for increasing the comfort and sense of well-being of patients with malignant disease and highlight the need for similar investigations targeted at pain reduction (see Chapter 24 for detailed discussion of cancer pain).

Summary of Efficacy Research

Positive effects have been found to be associated with training in various cognitive-behavioral procedures before surgery, painful medical procedures, and childbirth; however, it is not clear whether such training is more beneficial than education (information provision) only. Preliminary research suggests that cognitive-behavioral interventions may be more effective in improving anxiety, distress, and compliance in acute pain situations than in reducing pain per se. Cognitive-behavioral treatments have been demonstrated more clearly to decrease self-reported pain in chronic pain syndromes. A number of factors may account for this difference. For one thing, more extensive treatment is usually provided for chronic pain patients. Chronic pain problems also are typically far more complex than acute pain problems and are more susceptible to influence by psychologic and behavioral processes. Pain ratings by chronic pain patients may improve after cognitive-behavioral treatment to the extent that they are influenced by such variables. This explanation is consistent with the suggestion that cognitive-behavioral techniques have greater effects on affective, cognitive, and behavioral factors than on sensory pain perception.

The paucity of well-designed and well-controlled studies prevents us from drawing any definitive conclusions about the efficacy of specific cognitive-behavioral techniques in decreasing pain or pain-related behaviors associated with particular procedures or syndromes. The relative efficacy of different cognitive-behavioral techniques, as well as their utility when compared with other psychologic treatments (e.g., relaxation alone), for different pain syndromes remains unclear. A recent review (38) of the effects of distraction techniques suggested that these procedures may be more helpful in alleviating mild pain than severe pain.

This question warrants additional research, as does the larger question of which cognitive-behavioral treatments are indicated in particular pain problems and for particular patients.

DESCRIPTION OF TECHNIQUES

Cognitive-behavioral interventions for clinical pain typically include educational and training components. In most treatments, the first step involves educating patients about the role of cognitions and emotions in pain and the interrelationships among stress, tension, and pain. Patients are told that they have the potential to cope more effectively with pain and anxiety by using the cognitive and behavioral techniques that are taught. Cognitive-behavioral interventions for acute pain associated with medical procedures and childbirth also usually include the provision of preparatory information about the procedure and the sensations patients will experience during and afterwards.

Cognitive-behavioral treatments are more likely to be successful if certain guidelines are followed (4, 39). These include the following:

1. Organizing and presenting information in logical categories (e.g., diagnosis, treatment, expected results)
2. Providing details of the treatment both verbally and in written form
3. Tailoring instructions for each patient
4. Presenting information gradually to avoid overwhelming patients
5. Emphasizing the "how" rather than the "why" of the treatment
6. Assessing patients' understanding by asking them to describe what they will do after the session
7. Providing a method by which patients can assess their performance of homework assignments
8. Including patients' families in the treatment program
9. Following up with patients to make sure they remember and understand the techniques

As noted earlier, cognitive-behavioral treatments for pain can be classified into two categories: cognitive restructuring procedures and coping skills training (Table 82-1). However, these two types of interventions overlap considerably; in practice, they reflect different emphases rather than completely different therapeutic modalities.

Cognitive Restructuring

Cognitive restructuring is typified by Ellis' rational-emotive therapy (40), Meichenbaum's self-instructional training (3), and Beck's cognitive therapy (2). Although there are some differences among these approaches in theory and application, they share the following common fundamental assumptions:

1. One's thoughts, beliefs, and interpretations (cognitions) related to a situation in large part determine one's emotional and behavioral responses to it.

2. Negative feelings and emotional distress are often caused by maladaptive or negatively distorted cognitions.
3. One can become aware of one's cognitions and learn to examine the extent to which they are rational, adaptive, and justified by evidence.
4. One can learn to substitute more adaptive, rational, and accurate cognitions for ones that are maladaptive or distorted, and this will result in decreased negative feelings and increased adaptive behaviors.

The term *restructuring* does not imply a literal change in any internal structure or process. However, it does serve to indicate that what is being learned is a generalizable method for examining and modifying one's thoughts about experiences and events. Because of this emphasis on learning a skill generalizable to use in a number of situations, cognitive restructuring techniques have been used more frequently in treatments for chronic pain than in treatments for acute pain. A somewhat similar approach, use of coping self-statements, has been more widely applied to acute pain problems and will be discussed in a later section.

Education of the Patient

In cases of chronic pain, cognitive restructuring training begins with educating patients about the close interrelationships among pain, thoughts, and emotions. In using cognitive-behavioral techniques with chronic pain patients, establishing a plausible rationale for these interventions is critical, as many of these patients tend to reject psychologic approaches to their problems, believing that such methods are irrelevant or imply that their pain problems are not "real." We have found that a simplified explanation of the gate control theory of pain provides an excellent way to begin introducing the notion that psychologic as well as physiologic factors may play a role in determining how pain is experienced. This concept can be made personally relevant to patients if the therapist helps them to identify factors that increase or decrease their experience of pain, discussing these in terms of opening or closing the "pain gate." These factors may be classified as physical, emotional, and cognitive, as shown in Table 82-7.

It is important that patients come to accept that pain is not simply a physical sensation, signaling tissue damage, but also a subjective experience influenced by thoughts and feelings. They should be taught that chronic pain does not serve a useful function as a warning signal and that, regardless of the physical modalities being used to treat the pain and/or its organic causes, the addition of interventions targeted at

TABLE 82-7. Examples of Influences on the Pain Gate

Type of Influence	Open Gate	Close Gate
Physical	Overexertion Muscle tension	Muscle relaxation Counter-stimulation Heat or ice Medication Regular exercise
Emotional	Anxiety Depression	Happiness Mental relaxation
Cognitive	Worry Increased attention to pain Catastrophizing	Attention focus on something other than pain Coping self-statements

modifying negative emotions and cognitions related to the pain may be of considerable help.

Role of Cognitions

In explaining to patients the role that cognitions play in increasing or decreasing pain, we have found the following model helpful:

Event ⟶ Cognitions (interpretations of event) ⟶

Consequences (emotional reactions to event)

Patients usually need a number of examples to understand this model. For example, suppose a patient experiences increased pain after walking some distance (the event) and then thinks to himself, "I know something is wrong that the doctors haven't found. This is going to get worse and I'll be crippled." The usual consequence of such cognitions is anxiety, fear, and worry. The consequences will be much less negative, however, if the patient thinks, "I walked much farther than usual today. I'll remember to pace myself better next time. Meanwhile I'll rest a little, and this pain will get better."

As a second example of this model, suppose that a patient has increased pain after entertaining friends. Negative cognitions (e.g., "I can't stand this pain. I can't do anything anymore. I'll never be able to lead a normal life again") are likely to result in anger and depression. On the other hand, if the patient interprets the experience more positively, he is likely to feel much less angry and depressed (e.g., "My friends and I enjoyed this evening. I'll take a hot bath and an aspirin now, and the pain will be better soon. I can cope with this pain, and I'm able to do most things that I want to").

The major point to be learned from such a model is that one's emotional reactions to and behaviors after an event depend to a large extent on one's thoughts. Patients sometimes question this concept, believing that it implies they are responsible for producing all of their own distress or pain. The therapist should emphasize that although we often cannot control or avoid distressing life events, we almost always can exert some control over how much suffering and life disruption such events produce. Once patients understand these connections between thoughts and feelings, they

are trained to identify their negative "automatic thoughts," evaluate the accuracy of these thoughts, and counter with more positive or realistic cognitions. Many chronic pain patients find it very difficult to recognize their negative automatic thoughts in response to increased pain or stress, and a number of sessions may be needed to develop this skill. It is often helpful to have patients "relive" a recent situation in which there was much pain, stress, anxiety, or depression, relating step by step what happened when, how they were feeling, and what they were thinking.

Examining Thoughts and Feelings

Patients typically need much help in fully describing their thoughts and feelings. They may say they simply felt anxious and had only one thought in a particular situation, when careful questioning may reveal several important additional feelings and thoughts. Each feeling described should be explainable by at least one thought. For example, if a patient says he felt angry in a certain situation, but can give no thoughts that would lead to feelings of anger, the therapist should help the patient to reconstruct what thought was associated with that feeling. Similarly, if a patient describes a thought (e.g., "That was unfair") that would be associated with anger in most people but does not list that feeling, the therapist might point out that most people would feel angry if they thought that, and ask if the patient might not have felt somewhat angry at that time.

Between sessions, it is extremely useful to have patients record their thoughts and feelings during or immediately following situations in which they experience increased pain or stress. These records can be used during the following therapy session to provide examples for continued learning and practice of skills. It is important that patients learn to distinguish events, thoughts, and feelings. Many patients at first incorrectly record thoughts as events or feelings, feelings as thoughts, etc.

Only when patients can readily identify automatic thoughts and feelings should the therapist move on to instructing them in evaluating the accuracy of negative thoughts and generating alternative thoughts. In this process, the therapist and patient work together to examine whether negative thoughts are realistic and whether there may be other possible interpretations of the event or situation. The goal is not to persuade patients that their thinking is "wrong" but to help them examine the extent to which negative automatic thoughts are supported by evidence. For example, if a patient's automatic thought is "I can't do anything any more because of this pain," the therapist might ask, "Is it true that you can't do anything? Is there anything you can do despite the pain?" The therapist and patient might then go on to list what the patient is able to do, as well as what the patient can no longer do. They might also discuss the importance of activities that the patient cannot do, and whether there are any ways the patient might be able to accomplish some of these activities despite the pain. Finally, the patient and therapist might design a homework assignment to test the patient's thoughts and assumptions, and provide additional information for further discussion.

To summarize, the therapist aims to teach patients how to identify negative distorted thoughts, examine the accuracy of these thoughts, and generate more realistic and more positive ones. Thus, the focus is not on solving a particular problem but rather on learning a cognitive skill for dealing with negative emotions that are excessively distressing or dysfunctional. The goal is not to eliminate negative emotions, which are recognized to be a normal part of life, but rather to reduce the intensity of negative emotions that result from distorted cognitions about events and situations. Such negative beliefs and emotions are thought to cause increased pain, suffering, and functional disability, although studies are needed to confirm this.

Coping Skills Treatments

Coping skills therapies aim to help patients develop a repertoire of skills for managing pain and stress. Although these skills often include cognitive restructuring, they also encompass numerous other techniques, such as relaxation and distraction. Most reported applications of cognitive-behavioral techniques to acute and chronic pain fall within this division, as can be seen by the descriptions of research studies provided earlier in this chapter. Of the various specific coping procedures that have been taught in therapeutic situations, relaxation, imagery, and the generation of positive coping self-statements seem to be the most commonly employed.

Relaxation and Attention Diversion Techniques

Many different methods of relaxation exist. Some entail progressively tensing then relaxing different muscle groups; others emphasize passive muscle relaxation without tensing; and still others focus on deep, slow breathing. As with instruction in any cognitive or behavioral technique, the therapist should explain to patients why and how the procedure helps relieve pain, and emphasize the necessity of regular practice to develop skills and realize maximum benefits.

Patients can be told that pain and other physical and psychologic stressors often result in increased muscle tension. Muscle tension tends to spread to adjacent muscle groups and has the effect of further increasing pain. To illustrate this, patients may be instructed to clench their fists and observe the impact on other muscles in their arms, shoulders, and jaws. The therapist then explains that relaxation is a very effective means of reducing the muscle tension and mental stress and anxiety that make pain worse, thus breaking up the vicious cycle of pain and tension.

Relaxation and imagery methods are also helpful in diverting attention from pain, improving sleep (often disrupted in chronic pain syndromes), and giving patients a sense of control over pain. Further, patients learn to monitor muscle tension in their bodies and to decrease tension before it mounts. Mentioning the effective use of relaxation and breathing techniques for childbirth pain may help enhance the credibility of this technique for patients.

Relaxation must be taught over a number of sessions—in our experience, at least six—for a patient to become proficient in its application. Ideally the patient and therapist meet once or twice a week, and the patient practices relaxation daily at home between sessions. The therapist watches the patient closely during the sessions to see how relaxed the patient is able to become and what body areas he has difficulty in relaxing. During each session some time should be spent discussing problems the patient has had in doing the home practice and in generating possible solutions. Typical problems include not being able to find time to practice and distracting thoughts.

In our experience, there is no "right" protocol that patients must follow in order to relax fully; rather, the therapist and each patient should work together to develop a method tailored to each individual. After patients become proficient at being able to relax in a quiet, comfortable place, the therapist helps them learn to relax in any situation. A combination of breathing and muscle relaxation techniques can be used to relax in any body position and in most daily situations.

Many techniques are helpful for enhancing relaxation: saying a word such as "calm," "relax," or "one" silently to oneself; focusing on a pleasant image; and listening to music. Mental imagery can be used with muscle relaxation techniques as a procedure for decreasing pain. Again, numerous types of imagery have been described (41). Pain can be imagined as an object that can be manipulated to decrease discomfort or the patient can imagine being in a pleasant place such as a meadow or a beach, to give just two examples. It is very important that the patient find an image that is highly involving, if possible using all five senses. Many patients are best able to work with images of actual situations they have experienced.

All of these strategies involve diverting attention from the pain, the rationale being that patients cannot attend as much to pain when they are focusing on something else. Other attention diversion techniques are available: (a) focusing in detail on physical surroundings (e.g., counting floor or ceiling tiles); (b) remembering the words to a song; and (c) counting backwards (4). Generally, however, these types of attention diversion techniques are more appropriate for acute pain and are not found useful by chronic pain patients. Techniques of relaxation and imagery are discussed in greater detail in Chapter 85.

Positive Coping Self-Statements

The use of positive self-statements is another coping skill frequently taught. This involves instructing patients to substitute positive thoughts for such negative ones as "I can't stand this" or "How much longer will this go on?" Examples of coping statements are "I can deal with this," "Focus on relaxing," and "This tension is a cue to use my coping skills." Although this technique is similar to the cognitive restructuring approaches described already, less emphasis is placed on acquiring a general method of examining and modifying cognitive processes than on learning a set of particular coping self-statements to be used in situations of pain and stress.

In training patients to use these techniques in anticipation of a painful event such as childbirth or a painful medical procedure, the patient is first given information about the sequence of upcoming events and the sensations that may be experienced at different times. The patient is then told that anxiety and tension can increase discomfort, and that the level of anxiety experienced is strongly influenced by what one says to oneself about the experience. Examples are useful in illustrating these points. Most patients can understand that certain thoughts (e.g., "I can't take this"; "This is unbearable") produce increased anxiety and focus on pain and suffering. A useful way to decrease this anxiety and tension is to respond to negative thoughts by substituting or countering with thoughts emphasizing the patient's ability to cope.

Once the rationale has been established and the method demonstrated, it is useful to have the patient rehearse these techniques when imagining himself in the painful situation. The therapist can coach the patient through imagining each step of a painful medical procedure, in terms of what he will observe happening, what physical sensations he will experience, and what thoughts and emotions he might have. The patient is instructed to recognize the natural reactions of anxiety, muscular tension, and negative thoughts (e.g., "This is horrible"; "I can't stand this") and to then counter these thoughts with more positive ones (e.g., "This won't last long. I can handle it. Just relax").

Coping statements may be used in four different phases of coping with pain (4). In the first phase—preparing for the pain—such statements as "Think about what you can do to deal with this. Stop worrying" are used. In the second phase—confronting and handling the sensations—such statements as "Use the tension as a cue to relax. Don't think about the pain" are helpful as the pain begins to increase. The third phase—critical moments—involves feelings of intense pain and/or beliefs that one cannot deal with the pain. Statements such as "Just focus on a strategy for dealing with the pain. Stop the negative thoughts. I'll get through this" are helpful in countering negative thoughts about one's ability to cope. In the final phase—reflections on how one did—the patient praises himself for coping with the pain with statements such as "I handled that pretty well." This breakdown into phases is particularly applicable to acute pain associated with childbirth or medical procedures. However, chronic pain patients may also adapt it to their individual situations and characteristic pain problems (e.g., in dealing with discomfort associated with specific body movements or exercises).

Stress Inoculation

One of the most common coping skills interventions reported in the pain literature is *stress inoculation*, which is a treatment package of cognitive-behavioral techniques developed by Meichenbaum (42). Originally conceived as a flexible approach for the management of stress-related problems, this intervention incorporates a number of the techniques described already. It has been demonstrated helpful in the treatment of anger and anxiety; Meichenbaum and Turk (43) subsequently adapted this comprehensive approach for use with experimental and clinical pain. Three major phases constitute the intervention: education (providing a rationale for the use of coping skills), training, and rehearsal of skill usage. Diverse strategies, including relaxation, attention diversion, and positive coping statements are taught, with the goal of providing the patient with a repertoire of skills for coping with pain.

Published reports on stress inoculation and other cognitive-behavioral interventions vary in the relative emphasis on the patient learning specific techniques under study versus utilizing individual coping strategies the patient has used and found effective in the past. Kendall et al. (14) took the latter approach. In their study on preparation for cardiac catheterization, the therapist worked with the patient first to identify those aspects of the upcoming procedure the patient perceived to be stressful (e.g., the "machinery"). The therapist and the patient then identified stress reduction techniques the patient had found helpful in past stressful circumstances. Finally, the patient was instructed to use these strategies, to reassure himself that he could cope with the stress of the catheterization, and to rehearse this process in advance.

FACTORS AFFECTING EFFICACY OF TREATMENTS

Compliance with Homework Assignments

Homework is usually required of patients in cognitive-behavioral treatment. This may consist of recording pain and mood ratings, thoughts and feelings in different situations, and practicing new techniques and behaviors. Noncompliance with such assignments frequently occurs. Therapists can use the following strategies to help reduce noncompliance:

1. Enlist the patient as a collaborator in setting up the assignment, incorporating his suggestions rather than telling the patient what to do.
2. Start out with a very simple, easy assignment that the therapist and patient feel confident the patient can do; then progress gradually to more difficult and complex assignments.
3. Suggest that the patient enlist the assistance of a spouse or family member. For example, the patient could ask his spouse to help prevent interruptions during his relaxation practice.
4. Make sure the patient understands the homework assignment (what is to be done and the rationale) and believes it to be useful.
5. Ask the patient what problems he anticipates might interfere with successfully completing the assignment, then generate ways of coping with such problems.
6. Reinforce completion of homework assignments by attention and interest. If an assignment is not completed, work with the patient to understand why. Did the patient forget? Did the assignment seem too difficult? Once the reasons for not completing the assignment are understood, assignments may be modified to enhance the chances of successful completion in the future.

Preparing for Setbacks

An important component of treatment with chronic pain patients is dealing with the issue of future setbacks. Several things may be done before setbacks occur to minimize the probability of their occurring and their negative impact. Discussing the patient's expectations of treatment, what it can and cannot do, and the time frame for change is very important. Many patients have unrealistic hopes for rapid, complete pain relief, but they may not disclose these beliefs.

The therapist should tell patients, early in treatment, that setbacks (e.g., decreased rate of progress, periods of increased pain or depression, etc.) are quite likely to occur, both during treatment and afterwards. Patients should be assured that setbacks during treatment can be very useful in providing information as well as an opportunity to practice newly learned coping skills. The therapist should encourage patients to share their negative thoughts about the treatment and to discuss setbacks, so that the reasons for them and various ways of handling them can be explored. Before the end of treatment, discussing possible future setbacks and rehearsing how to deal with them can reduce post-treatment setbacks.

Therapist Characteristics

Although many of the procedures described in this chapter appear relatively straightforward, therapists must be trained in their appropriate application. Complex issues often arise during treatment, which require considerable skill on the part of the therapist. These may include the emergence of symptoms of major psychopathology, significant marital or family distress, issues related to dying (in the case of cancer pain), and persistent somatic focus and resistance to the use of psychologic techniques (in the case of chronic pain syndromes). Whether or not such issues are salient, the importance of therapist style characteristics cannot be overemphasized. As with any psychotherapy, therapist warmth, empathy, respect for the patient, and attentiveness to the patient are important to the success of the treatment.

Patient Characteristics

A number of patient characteristics and situational factors may be important in influencing response to cognitive-behavioral treatment. Work by Wilson (44) and others suggests that patient differences in level of anxiety and typical coping style influence response to presurgical interventions, and Blanchard et al. (45) found that various indicators of psychologic disturbance predicted outcome following behavioral treatments for headache.

Several other factors are likely to influence treatment success, particularly in chronic pain problems, and are worthy of empirical investigation. Patients who present to a pain clinic only because they were requested to do so by an agency such as Worker's Compensation, or because of pressure from family or physician, will almost certainly be less receptive to any psychologic treatment than patients who refer themselves for a behaviorally oriented program. Also, willingness to comply with and participate fully in a psychologic treatment is likely to be minimal in patients who are convinced they have an organically-based problem not influenced significantly by psychologic factors. Attitudes of family members are also very important. Spouses who believe patients' pain is caused totally by organic factors and that psychologic treatments are not relevant are unlikely to support treatment efforts and may undermine patient progress. Finally, the availability of personal, social, and environmental resources that can support treatment gains may well be critical in determining the long-term outcome.

Limitations and Contraindications

Data are generally unavailable on particular factors that would predict positive or negative response to cognitive-behavioral treatments for pain. A potential limitation in cases of acute pain is suggested by preliminary studies showing that cognitive-behavioral strategies may be more effective in reducing anxiety than in decreasing pain per se, but clarification of this issue awaits further research. In chronic pain problems complicated by factors such as drug dependence, deactivation, or potent environmental reinforcers of pain behaviors, cognitive-behavioral techniques alone may be insufficient to produce changes in these patterns. However, they may be useful as part of a more comprehensive multimodal treatment program.

Adverse effects of cognitive-behavioral therapies appear to be rare but have been reported. For example, some patients describe increased anxiety associated with the use of relaxation (46). However, since these treatments carry few if any serious risks, chronic pain patients who fail to respond initially to a particular technique may be given trials of other cognitive-behavioral strategies.

In sum, because cognitive-behavioral therapy for pain is such a new field, little is known about any limitations and contraindications. We anticipate that increased empirical study of these methods will provide data for specifying when these techniques are most appropriate and likely to be effective.

REFERENCES

1. Beck, A.T.: Cognitive Therapy and the Emotional Disorders. New York, International Universities Press, 1976.
2. Beck, A.T., Rush, A.J., Shaw, B.R., and Emery, G.: Cognitive Therapy of Depression. New York, Guilford Press, 1979.
3. Meichenbaum, D.H.: Cognitive-Behavior Modification: An Integrative Approach. New York, Plenum, 1977.
4. Turk, D.C., Meichenbaum, D., and Genest, M.: Pain and Behavioral Medicine: A Cognitive-Behavioral Perspective. New York, Guilford Press, 1983.
5. Turner, J.A., and Chapman, C.R.: Psychological interventions for chronic pain: a critical review. II. Operant conditioning, hypnosis, and cognitive-behavioral therapy. Pain, 12:23, 1982.
6. Turner, J.A., and Romano, J.M.: Evaluating psychological interventions for chronic pain: Issues and recent developments. In Advances in Pain Research and Therapy. Vol. 7. Edited by C. Benedetti, C.R. Chapman, and G. Moricca. New York, Raven Press, 1984, pp. 257–296.
7. Pearce, S.: A review of cognitive-behavioral methods for the treatment of chronic pain. J. Psychosom. Res., 27:431, 1983.

8. Tan, S.: Cognitive and cognitive-behavioral methods for pain control: A selective review. Pain, *12*:201, 1982.
9. Mahoney, M.J., and Arnkoff, D.: Cognitive and self-control therapies. *In* Handbook of Psychotherapy and Behavior Change: An Empirical Analysis. Edited by S.L. Garfield and A.E. Bergin. New York, John Wiley and Sons, 1978, pp. 689–722.
10. Langer, E.J., Janis, I.L., and Wolfer, J.A.: Reduction of psychological stress in surgical patients. J. Exp. Soc. Psychol., *1*:155, 1975.
11. Wells, N.: The effect of relaxation on postoperative muscle tension and pain. Nurs. Res., *31*:236, 1982.
12. Pickett, C., and Clum, G.A.: Comparative treatment strategies and their interaction with locus of control in the reduction of postsurgical pain and anxiety. J. Consult. Clin. Psychol., *50*:439, 1982.
13. Wernick, R.L., Jaremko, M.E., and Taylor, P.W.: Pain management in severely burned adults: A test of stress inoculation. J. Behav. Med., *4*:103, 1981.
14. Kendall, P.C., et al.: Cognitive-behavioral and patient education interventions in cardiac catheterization procedures: The Palo Alto medical psychology project. J. Consult. Clin. Psychol., *47*:49, 1979.
15. Tan, S., and Poser, E.G.: Acute pain in a clinical setting: Effects of cognitive-behavioral skills training. Behav. Res. Ther., *20*:535, 1982.
16. Reading, A.E.: The short term effects of psychological preparation for surgery. Soc. Sci. Med., *13A*:641, 1979.
17. Norr, K.L., et al.: Explaining pain and enjoyment in childbirth. J. Health Soc. Behav., *18*:260, 1977.
18. Melzack, R., Taenzer, P., Feldman, P., and Kinch, R.: Labour is still painful after prepared childbirth training. Can. Med. Assoc. J., *125*:357, 1981.
19. Melzack, R., et al.: Severity of labour pain: Influence of physical as well as psychologic variables. Can. Med. Assoc. J., *130*:579, 1984.
20. Davenport-Slack, B., and Boylan, C.H.: Psychologic correlates of childbirth pain. Psychosom. Med., *36*:215, 1974.
21. Nettelbladt, P., Fagerstrom, C., and Uddenberg, N.: The significance of reported childbirth pain. J. Psychosom. Res., *20*:215, 1976.
22. Anderson, N.B., Lawrence, P.S., and Olson, T.W.: Within-subject analysis of autogenic training and cognitive coping training in the treatment of tension headache pain. J. Behav. Ther. Exp. Psychiatry, *12*:219, 1981.
23. Bakal, D.A., Demjan, S., and Kaganov, J.A.: Cognitive-behavioral treatment of chronic headache. Headache, *21*:81, 1981.
24. Holroyd, K.A., and Andrasik, F.: Do the effects of cognitive therapy endure? A two-year follow-up of tension headache sufferers treated with cognitive therapy or biofeedback. Cog. Ther. Res., *6*:325, 1982.
25. Kremsdorf, R.B., Kochanowicz, N.A., and Costell, S.: Cognitive skills training versus EMG biofeedback in the treatment of tension headaches. Biofeedback Self Regul., *6*:93, 1981.
26. Mitchell, K.R., and White, R.G.: Behavioral self-management: An application to the problem of migraine headaches. Behav. Ther., *8*:213, 1977.
27. Engstrom, D.: Cognitive behavioral therapy methods in chronic pain treatment. *In* Advances in Pain Research and Therapy. Vol. 5. Edited by J.J. Bonica, U. Lindblom, A. Iggo, L.E. Jones, and C. Benedetti. New York, Raven Press, 1983, pp. 829–838.
28. Khatami, M., and Rush, A.J.: A pilot study of the treatment of outpatients with chronic pain: Symptom control, stimulus control and social system intervention. Pain, *5*:163, 1978.
29. Moore, J.E., and Chaney, E.F.: Outpatient group treatment of chronic pain: Effects of spouse involvement. J. Consult. Clin. Psychol., *53*:326, 1985.
30. Turner, J.A.: Comparison of group progressive-relaxation training and cognitive-behavioral group therapy for chronic low back pain. J. Consult. Clin. Psychol., *50*:757, 1982.
31. Daut, R.L., and Cleeland, C.S.: The prevalence and severity of pain in cancer. Cancer, *50*:1913, 1982.
32. Bonica, J.J.: Treatment of cancer pain: Current status and future needs. *In* Advances in Pain Research and Therapy. Vol. 9. Edited by H.L. Fields, R. Dubner, and F. Cervero. New York, Raven Press, 1985, pp. 589–616.
33. Ahles, T.A., Blanchard, E.B., and Ruckdeschel, J.C.: The multidimensional nature of cancer-related pain. Pain, *17*:277, 1983.
34. Finer, B.: Hypnotherapy in pain of advanced cancer. *In* Advances in Pain Research and Therapy. Vol. 2, Edited by J.J. Bonica and V. Ventafridda. New York, Raven Press, 1979, pp. 223–229.
35. Fotopoulos, S.S., Graham, C., and Cook, M.R.: Psychophysiologic control of cancer pain. *In* Advances in Pain Research and Therapy. Vol. 2. Edited by J.J. Bonica and V. Ventafridda. New York, Raven Press, 1979, pp. 231–243.
36. Simonton, O.C., Matthews-Simonton, S., and Sparks, T.F.: Psychological intervention in the treatment of cancer. Psychosomatics, *21*:226, 1980.
36. Simonton, O.C., Matthews-Simonton, S., and Sparks, T.F.: Psychological intervention in the treatment of cancer. Psychosomatics, *21*:226, 1980.
37. Lyles, J.N., Burish, T.G., Krozely, M.G., and Oldham, R.K.: Efficacy of relaxation training and guided imagery in reducing the aversiveness of cancer chemotherapy. J. Consult. Clin. Psychol., *50*:509, 1982.
38. McCaul, K.D., and Malott, J.M.: Distraction and coping with pain. Psychol. Bull., *95*:516, 1984.
39. Dunbar, J.: Adhering to medical advice: A review. Int. J. Ment. Health, *9*:70, 1980.
40. Ellis, A.: Reason and Emotion in Psychotherapy. New York, Lyle Stuart, 1962.
41. Bresler, D.E.: Free Yourself from Pain. New York, Simon and Schuster, 1979.
42. Meichenbaum, D.: A self-instructional approach to stress management: A proposal for stress inoculation training. *In* Stress and Anxiety. Vol. 1. Edited by I. Sarason and D.C. Spielberger. New York, John Wiley and Sons, 1975, pp. 227–263.
43. Meichenbaum, D., and Turk, D.: The cognitive-behavioral management of anxiety, anger, and pain. *In* The Behavioral Management of Anxiety, Depression, and Pain. Edited by P.O. Davidson. New York, Brunner/Mazel, 1976, pp. 1–34.
44. Wilson, J.F.: Behavioral preparation for surgery: Benefit or harm? J. Behav. Med., *4*:79, 1981.
45. Blanchard, E.B., et al.: Biofeedback and relaxation training with three kinds of headache: Treatment effects and their prediction. J. Consult. Clin. Psychol., *50*:562, 1982.
46. Heide, F.J., and Borkovec, T.D.: Relaxation-induced anxiety: Paradoxical anxiety enhancement due to relaxation training. J. Consult. Clin. Psychol., *51*:171, 1983.

83 · BIOFEEDBACK THERAPY

Edward B. Blanchard *and* Tim A. Ahles

BIOFEEDBACK, a relatively new psychosocial treatment for pain, which was first reported in the literature around 1970 (1), has been defined as "a process in which a person learns to reliably influence physiological responses of two kinds: either responses which are not ordinarily under voluntary control or responses which ordinarily are easily regulated but for which regulation has broken down due to trauma or disease" (2). This process requires special electronic devices that (a) detect and amplify various biologic responses and (b) convert these amplified responses into information that is easy to process (Fig. 83-1).

Biofeedback has been used for a wide variety of pain problems; however, both the largest number of published studies, and the best, in terms of data from controlled evaluations of efficacy, are concerned with either tension or vascular (migrainous) headache. The use of biofeedback training for both tension headache (3) and migraine headache (4) has been endorsed by the Biofeedback Society of America (BSA) and by the American Association for the Study of Headache (5). The American Psychiatric Association (6) has given limited endorsement to the use of biofeedback for these two types of headache in the context of comprehensive psychologic or psychiatric care.

In view of these considerations, the bulk of this chapter is devoted to biofeedback treatment of headache with the remainder devoted to the numerous other pain problems for which biofeedback has been used. Several comprehensive reviews of the literature on the use of biofeedback for pain (7–9) and for headache (10–12) are available.

BIOFEEDBACK TREATMENT OF CHRONIC HEADACHE

Tension (Muscle Contraction) Headache

The phenomenology and pathophysiology of tension (muscle contraction) headache were described by Olesen and Bonica in Chapter 39 and will not be repeated.

Frontal EMG Biofeedback

The initial report on biofeedback treatment of tension headache (1) described the procedure for frontal EMG biofeedback, which is still the standard one (3). This procedure consists of measuring the electromyogram (EMG) from electrodes attached to the forehead and then, with appropriate electronic processing of the signal, providing the patient with information on the change in electrical activity on a moment by moment basis so that the patient can learn to relax the musculature of the face and scalp and also learn to detect early symptoms of increased muscle tension. The feedback signal to the patient is almost always auditory and may consist of a tone that varies in pitch, a series of clicks that vary in frequency, or other appropriate indicators of variation.

Before the electrodes are attached, the skin surface beneath the electrodes should be cleaned with a mild abrasive, followed by alcohol. The electrodes are attached with double-sided adhesive collars, paper tape, or Velcro bands.

Treatment sessions usually last 30 to 60 min; 15 to 45 min of each session is devoted to the actual feedback training. We have typically used the following format for biofeedback training sessions:

1. Attachment of electrodes and initial adaptation: 10 min.

2. In-session baseline: Patient sits quietly with eyes closed for 5 min.

3. Self-control 1: Patient is asked to control response in absence of feedback signal for 5 min.

4. Feedback training with feedback signal available: 20 min.

5. Self-control 2: Patient is asked to continue to control response in absence of feedback signal for 5 min.

Published reports have used from about 5 or 6 up to 16 treatment sessions. We recommend planning at least 10 to 12 sessions on a once or twice per week basis.

ELECTRODE PLACEMENT. Although the vast majority of published reports and the accepted standard from the BSA is a frontal or forehead electrode placement, there is some controversy about this point. In the standard placement, the active electrodes are centered above each eye, approximately $2\frac{1}{2}$ cm above the eyebrow. A ground electrode is typically placed midway between them, as shown in Figure 83-2. With this very wide placement, muscle activity is detected not only in the forehead, but probably also from the rest of the face, scalp, and neck, down to the clavicles (13).

Some writers (14, 15) have advocated attaching electrodes to other sites, such as the back of the neck or temporalis area, especially if the patient localizes his pain there. However, two studies (16, 17) that compared biofeedback training from different sites found *no* advantage for one site over the other.

RELAXATION TRAINING AS AN ADJUNCT. The initial reports of the use of frontal EMG biofeedback training for tension headache included formal training in relaxation techniques and instructions for the patient to practice these relaxation techniques at home

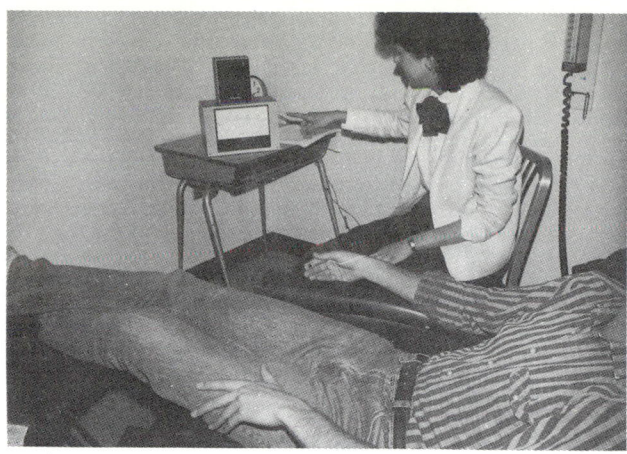

FIG. 83-1. Therapist calls patient's attention to visual feedback meter in biofeedback treatment for migraine headache.

on a regular basis (1, 18). Use of relaxation training as an adjunct to EMG biofeedback training continues to be the usual clinical practice.

As discussed in the next section, several studies have compared the efficacy of EMG biofeedback training and relaxation training for headache reduction. The major conclusion to be drawn from these studies is that the two techniques are equally effective.

REVIEW OF CURRENT LITERATURE. Part A of Table 83-1 contains a summary of the treatment conditions, number of patients, and duration of treatment from numerous published studies on frontal EMG biofeedback therapy for tension headache. The results of these studies are discussed in this section.

Small-scale controlled studies have shown that frontal EMG biofeedback, either with or without adjunctive relaxation training, is superior to a no-treatment

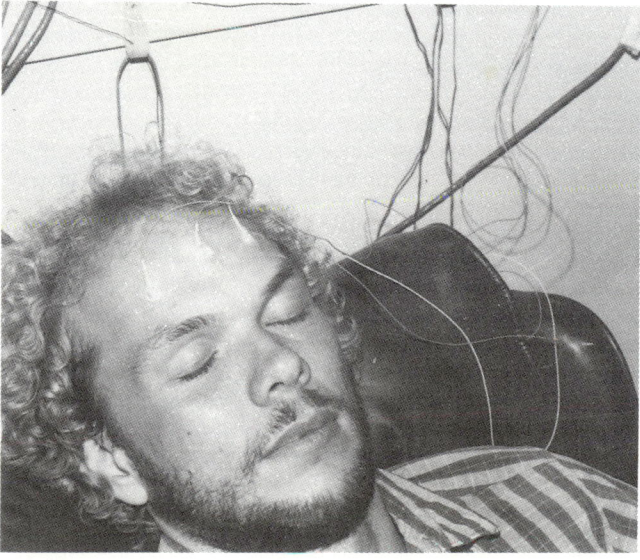

FIG. 83-2. Electrode placement for frontal EMG biofeedback. Active electrodes are placed approximately 2.5 cm. above the eyebrow, centered on each eye; the ground electrode is centered between them.

condition in which patients merely monitor headache activity (16, 18–20, 23). This conclusion was confirmed in a critical analysis of the literature by Blanchard et al. (39).

Four controlled studies (18, 20, 21, 24) have shown frontal EMG biofeedback training to be superior to psychologic or pharmacologic placebo.

Several controlled studies have compared frontal EMG biofeedback with some form of relaxation training. Of these, one found biofeedback training superior (22), one found relaxation superior (23), and the others found no difference (16, 19, 21). This same finding emerged in the analysis by Blanchard et al. (39). In a sequential comparison, we found that approximately 45% of tension headache patients who did *not* have a successful response to relaxation training were much improved after a course of EMG biofeedback training (25, 40).

Two studies have compared EMG biofeedback with drug treatment for tension headache. Bruhn et al. (26) found EMG biofeedback superior to the "most suitable available therapy" (i.e., combination of drugs and physical therapy). Paiva et al. (27) reported that EMG biofeedback and diazepam were equally effective at the end of treatment but that biofeedback training was more effective during a 4-week follow-up after the drug was discontinued.

Several studies (25, 40, 41) have focused on predicting treatment outcome with frontal EMG biofeedback therapy. The most reliable finding seems to be that patients who are depressed (score about 8 on the Beck Depression Inventory or above 70 on scale 2 [Depression] of the MMPI) tend to do markedly poorer than nondepressed patients.

The conclusion that can be drawn from these studies is that frontal EMG biofeedback, either alone or with adjunctive relaxation training, is more effective for treatment of tension headache than placebo and at least as effective as drug treatment or other active psychologic treatment. One-year follow-up data reported by Andrasik et al. (42) demonstrated excellent maintenance of short-term treatment effects. In fact, patients were more improved at 1 year than they had been at the end of treatment.

Migraine Headache

Thermal Biofeedback

Sargent et al. (43) first described a procedure for biofeedback treatment of migraine headache. In this procedure, which probably is the standard one now, the temperature of the ventral surface of the fingertip (usually the index finger of the nondominant hand) is measured and information on it is made immediately available to the patient by means of auditory or visual signals (Fig. 83-3). We have found that over 80% of vascular headache patients prefer visual rather than auditory feedback. Within this feedback loop the patient is asked to warm his hands.

AUTOGENIC TRAINING AS AN ADJUNCT. In the procedure of Sargent et al. (43), patients are given some training in the use of so-called *autogenic phrases* (44) and asked to practice these at home and use them as a way of influencing hand temperature. Research reports

TABLE 83-1. Biofeedback Therapy for Headache

Source	Treatments*	No. of Patients	Duration of Therapy	Results — At end of Treatment	Results — Follow-up	Comment
A. TENSION (MUSCLE CONTRACTION) HEADACHE						
Budzynski et al. (18)	EMG + R PP MON	18	16 sessions over 8 weeks	EMG + R > PP = MON	3 months, EMG + R > PP	
Haynes et al. (19)	EMG R MON	21	6 sessions over 3 weeks	EMG = R > MON	6 months, EMG = R > MON	
Holroyd et al. (20)	EMG PP MON	31	7 sessions over 4 weeks	EMG > PP = MON	None	
Cox et al. (21)	EMG + R R DP	27	8 sessions over 4 weeks	EMG + R = R > DP	4 months, EMG + R = R > MON	
Hutchings & Reinking (22)	EMG + R R EMG	18	10 sessions over 10 weeks	EMG + R = EMG > R	1 year, no difference	
Chesney & Shelton (23)	EMG + R R EMG MON	24	8 sessions over 2 weeks	EMG + R = R > MON = EMG	None	
Martin & Mathews (16)	EMG R	24	14 sessions over 14 weeks	EMG = R	3 months, EMG = R	
Philips (24)	EMG PP	15	12 sessions over 6 weeks	EMG > PP	2 months, EMG > PP	
Blanchard et al. (25)	R R then EMG	33	10 sessions of R, 12 sessions of EMG over 8–16 weeks	EMG > R	1 year, same results	EMG used only with R failures
Bruhn et al. (26)	EMG D + PT	23	16 sessions over 8 weeks	EMG > D + PT	3 months, EMG only	
Paiva et al. (27)	EMG D (diazepam)	32	12 sessions over 4 weeks	D > EMG	1 month, EMG = D	
B. MIGRAINE HEADACHE						
Blanchard et al. (28)	TBF + AT R MON	30	12 sessions over 6 weeks	TBF + AT = R > MON	12 months, TBF + AT = R	
Sargent et al. (29)	TBF + AT EMG + AT AT MON	136	8 sessions over 8 weeks	TBF + AT = EMG + AT = AT > MON	6 months, TBD + AT = EMG + AT = AT	
Kewman & Roberts (30)	TBF PP MON	34	10 sessions over 9 weeks	TBF = PP = MON	None	
Lake et al. (31)	TBF EMG TBF + PSY MON	24	8 sessions over 4 weeks	EMG > MON EMG = TBF = TBF + PSY TBF = TBF + PSY = MON	3 months, same results	
Largen et al. (32)	TBF + AT PP	11	12–16 sessions over 5 weeks	TBF + AT = PP	None	
Blanchard et al. (25)	R R then TBF + AT	30	10 sessions of R, 12 sessions of TBF + AT over 8–16 weeks	TBF + AT > R	12 months, same results	TBF used only with R failures
Cohen et al. (33)	TBF EMG CVM EEG	42	24 sessions over 8 weeks	TBF = EMG = CVM = EEG	8 months, same results	Nonsignificant decrease in headache
Mullinix et al. (34)	TBF + AT PP	11	9 sessions over 9 weeks	TBF + AT = PP	None	
Sovak et al. (35)	TBF + AT D (propranolol)	48	8–10 sessions over 3 months	TBF + AT = D	None	
Mathew (36)	BF D-1 (ergot) D-2 (propranolol) D-3 (amitriptyline)	142	10 sessions over 10 weeks	D-2 > D-3 > BF > D-1	3 months	
Bild & Adams (37)	CVM EMG MON	21	10 sessions over 4–6 weeks	CVM = EMG EMG = MON CVM > MON	None	
Friar & Beatty (38)	CVM PP	18	8 sessions over 3 weeks	CVM > PP	None	

*AT = autogenic training; BF = thermal biofeedback plus frontal EMG biofeedback; CVM = cephalic vasomotor biofeedback; D = drug treatment; DP = drug placebo; EEG = EEG alpha biofeedback; EMG = frontal EMG biofeedback; MON = headache monitoring; PP = psychological placebo; PSY = psychotherapy; PT = physical therapy; R = relaxation training; and TBF = thermal biofeedback.

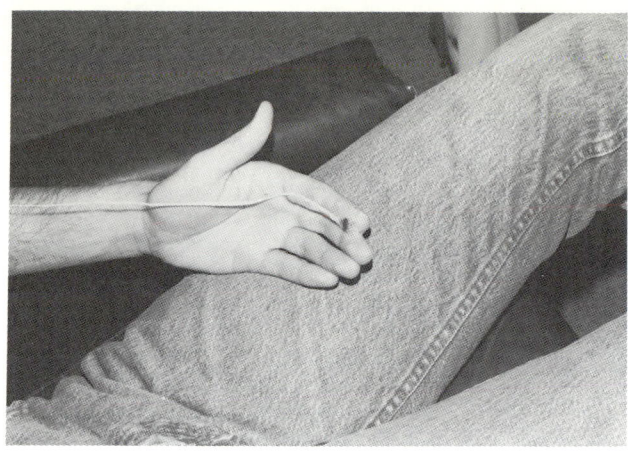

FIG. 83-3. Thermistor placement for thermal biofeedback. Care should be taken not to cut off circulation to the fingertip.

are about evenly divided between those using thermal biofeedback alone and those combining autogenic phrases with thermal biofeedback (which we call *autogenic feedback training*). Although no direct controlled comparisons have been made of the two variants, a meta-analytic comparison (12) showed an advantage for the combined procedure over thermal biofeedback alone.

We recommend the same temporal format for thermal biofeedback training sessions as described earlier for frontal EMG biofeedback. Although the number of sessions reported in the literature ranges from 6 to 20, we recommend at least 10 to 12 sessions.

REVIEW OF THE CURRENT LITERATURE. Summaries of studies on thermal biofeedback therapy for migraine headache are presented in part B of Table 83-1.

Two controlled studies (28, 29) have found autogenic feedback training superior to headache monitoring (no treatment). However, two other studies of thermal biofeedback alone did *not* find it superior to headache monitoring (30, 31).

Among the studies that have compared either thermal biofeedback or autogenic feedback with psychologic placebo conditions for relief of migraine headache, none has shown active treatment to be superior to a psychologic placebo (30, 32, 34).

Several researchers have reported comparisons of either thermal biofeedback or autogenic feedback training with other active psychologic therapies such as relaxation training (28, 29) and frontal EMG biofeedback. None of these studies has shown thermal biofeedback treatment to be superior to other active treatment. In our laboratory (25, 40), however, we have found that significant numbers of migraine patients who fail to respond to relaxation training do respond well to subsequent thermal biofeedback.

Mathew (36) reported that a combination of thermal and EMG biofeedback was superior to ergotamine and analgesics but inferior to either propranolol or amitriptyline. Sovak et al. (35) found autogenic feedback training and propranolol equally effective.

One large-scale (45) uncontrolled trial and two controlled trials (46, 47) have found thermal biofeedback to be very effective with childhood migraine. Over 80% of patients seem to show clinically significant improvement in the short term.

Both data from our laboratory (25, 40) and the work of others (48) have shown that migraine patients with marked elevations on scales 1 and 3 of the MMPI do not respond as well as other migraine patients to biofeedback training.

Although autogenic feedback training is superior to headache monitoring and probably to routine drug therapy with ergotamines and analgesics in migraine patients, neither it nor thermal biofeedback alone has been shown conclusively to be superior to other psychologic treatments, prophylactic drug treatments, or psychologic placebos. One-year follow-up data (42, 49) show good maintenance of headache reductions.

Frontal EMG Biofeedback

At least four reports have been published on the use of frontal EMG biofeedback for the treatment of migraine (29, 31, 33, 37). These reports indicate EMG biofeedback is about as effective as thermal biofeedback or autogenic biofeedback training.

Cephalic Vasomotor Biofeedback

An alternative form of biofeedback training for migraine headache has been described in several reports. In this procedure, called *cephalic vasomotor biofeedback*, the vasomotor response of the temporal artery is measured using some form of photoplethysmograph. The patient is then taught with the assistance of feedback to voluntarily constrict this artery. Although one controlled study (37) found this form of biofeedback to be superior to headache monitoring and another (38) found it superior to placebo, it has not been found consistently superior to any of the other forms of biofeedback training. Cephalic vasomotor biofeedback should probably still be considered experimental at this point.

Combined Migraine and Tension Headache

A fairly extensive literature exists on the biofeedback treatment of pure migraine headache and pure tension headache, but there are only a few studies on the treatment of patients who have combined migraine and tension headache. In one large uncontrolled study of such patients, 60 of 134 were moderately improved or better at a 2-year follow-up after a treatment regimen combining frontal EMG and thermal biofeedback and several kinds of relaxation (50).

Mathew (36) reported that a similar combined biofeedback and relaxation treatment regimen was superior to ergotamines and analgesics, but not as good as either propranolol or amitriptyline. Finally, in a quasi-controlled comparison of autogenic feedback training with relaxation training, we (25) found biofeedback significantly better. Our own experience leads us to recommend combining thermal biofeedback with progressive relaxation training in the treatment of patients with both tension and migraine headache.

Cluster Headache

Even less information has been published on biofeedback treatment of cluster headache than on that of combined headache. In the only sizable uncontrolled series we know of, 3 of 11 patients (27%) were helped somewhat by a lengthy treatment regimen consisting of 10 sessions of relaxation training followed by 12 sessions of thermal biofeedback (51). At a 30-month follow-up, the 3 patients continued to report somewhat less intense headaches and somewhat shorter cluster bouts. At this time, biofeedback does not seem to be a strong choice for treatment of cluster headache.

Side Effects and Complications of Biofeedback

To the best of our knowledge, there have been no reports of untoward side effects from biofeedback training. In fact, the side effects are usually positive, patients reporting improved sleep and relief of other problems (28).

Complications could arise for diabetic patients on regular doses of insulin and for hypertensive patients on regular doses of antihypertensive medications. If such patients become proficient at the self-regulatory procedures and practice them regularly, the required insulin or drug dosage may need to be reduced. Suitable precautions should be taken to monitor other chronic drug use in headache patients receiving biofeedback training so that appropriate adjustments can be made.

Conclusions

We conclude that for tension headache, frontal EMG biofeedback is superior to headache monitoring and to psychologic placebos and is as effective as relaxation training or drug therapy. For migraine headache, the biofeedback treatment of choice seems to be the combination of thermal biofeedback and autogenic training (i.e., autogenic feedback training). Whereas this treatment is superior to headache monitoring, it has not been found consistently superior to psychologic placebo or to other forms of biofeedback training or relaxation training. It also has not been found superior to drug treatment for prophylaxis. Despite this, we recommend autogenic feedback therapy for migraine patients, especially children.

Although the evidence is limited, autogenic feedback training combined with relaxation appears to be effective in the treatment of combined migraine and tension headache for many patients. For cluster headache, however, biofeedback training is not indicated.

BIOFEEDBACK TRAINING FOR BACK PAIN

Low Back Pain

Low back pain is a complex clinical pain syndrome, which has been treated with a number of modalities (Chapter 71). Biofeedback treatment is based on the premise that patients with low back pain have elevated levels of muscular tension, particularly in the paraspinal musculature (52). Only EMG biofeedback has been used with this population, and the training procedures are similar to those described for treatment of tension headache. Typically, paraspinal electrode placements have been used but frontalis placements have also been used (53, 54).

Although biofeedback is used extensively in comprehensive pain treatment programs (55, 56), few studies have examined the efficacy of biofeedback alone in the treatment of low back pain. In this section, we review only those studies that used biofeedback as the primary mode of treatment (Table 83-2, part A).

In one series of single-case studies (57) and two relatively small single-group outcome studies (52, 54), EMG biofeedback was shown to be effective in reducing EMG levels and subjective reports of pain and tension. The efficacy of EMG biofeedback was also supported in a larger ($N = 111$) single-group outcome study (53). This program consisted primarily of biofeedback and relaxation training but patients were also treated with physical therapy and psychotropic medications when appropriate.

Two studies compared the effectiveness of EMG biofeedback for low back pain with no-treatment control groups. The first study (58) supported the efficacy of biofeedback, whereas no differences in reported pain were found between the biofeedback and no-treatment control group in the second study (59). In this study, biofeedback training was conducted while the patients were standing rather than in a supine position, as in the other studies described. Nouwen (59) hypothesized that the prolonged standing (30 min with two 2.5 min breaks) could have caused protracted ligamentous strain that interfered with the biofeedback training and led to the negative study results.

Only one study, by Keefe et al. (53), examined patient characteristics that might predict treatment outcome. These investigators found that the patients with the best outcomes initially rated their pain as more severe, had fewer years of continuous pain, were less likely to be receiving disability payments, and had fewer surgical procedures. In contrast to headache patients, the MMPI was not found to predict treatment outcome in patients with low back pain.

Low Back, Neck, and Shoulder Pain

Several studies have examined the efficacy of EMG biofeedback in patients with multiple pain sites or used heterogeneous populations, i.e., a mixture of patients with localized low back, upper back, neck, or shoulder pain. These studies reviewed here are summarized in part B of Table 83-2.

In an early single-group outcome study (60) of EMG biofeedback therapy for patients suffering from shoulder and back pain, only one of eight patients obtained significant relief. A subsequent case study (61) and a single-group outcome study (62), however, reported significant improvement in patients' subjective pain reports.

Large and Lamb (63) used a within-subject control design to compare a waiting list period, control period (sitting in the biofeedback laboratory, but receiving no feedback), and EMG biofeedback. They found that EMG biofeedback was superior in training relaxation, but not in reducing pain levels. Caution must be

TABLE 83-2. EMG Biofeedback (BF) Therapy for Back Pain

Source	Study Design	No. of Patients	Duration of Therapy	Results Short term	Results Long term	Comments
A. Low Back Pain						
Nigal & Fischer-Williams (57)	Multiple single cases	4	10–24 sessions	Decrease in EMG levels, pain, and medication use	—	—
Freeman et al. (52)	Single-group outcome	8	10 sessions	4/8 pts had significant reductions in EMG levels and pain reports	—	4/8 pts dropped out prior to completion of the project
Keefe et al. (54)	Single-group outcome	18	Minimum of 6 sessions	Decrease in EMG levels and ratings of tension; 15/18 pts had decreased pain following home practice	9/13 pts maintained initial gains at 1 year	—
Keefe et al. (53)	Single-group outcome	111	Average of 10 sessions	Decreased pain in 29%; decreased drug use in 49.2%; increased activity level in 63.2%; significant decrease in EMG levels	—	Treatment included physical therapy & psychotropic drugs
Nouwen & Solinger (58)	Treatment vs. no treatment	Treatment = 19 No treatment = 7	20 sessions	Significantly lower EMG and pain levels in treatment group	Pain reports remained low but EMG levels returned to baseline at 3 mo	—
Nouwen (59)	Treatment vs. no treatment	10/group	15 sessions	Decrease in EMG levels but not in pain reports in treatment group	—	Treatment was done in a standing position rather than the standard supine position
B. Low Back, Neck, and Shoulder Pain						
Peck & Kraft (60)	Single-group outcome	8	6 sessions	1/8 pts improved	—	—
Belar & Cohen (61)	Single case	1	17 sessions	Decreased EMG and pain levels; increased activity	Results maintained at 12 weeks	—
Hendler et al. (62)	Single-group outcome	13	5 sessions	6/13 pts had lower pain; no decrease in EMG levels	—	No statistical presentation of data
Large & Lamb (63)	BF, no BF, and waiting list (with-in-subject control)	18	6 sessions	BF better than no BF and waiting list in reducing EMG but not pain levels	—	Division of pts into groups resulted in a relatively small no./group for statistical analysis
Flor et al. (64)	BF vs. pseudotherapy vs. conventional medical treatment	8/group	12 sessions	BF better than pseudotherapy and conventional medical treatment in reducing pain and EMG levels	Improvement maintained at 4 mo	—

exercised in interpreting these results, however, because of the relatively small number of patients in each group.

Flor et al. (64) compared the efficacy of EMG biofeedback, pseudotherapy (false feedback), and conventional medical treatment in a group of patients with chronic rheumatic back pain. The pain was localized in either the lumbosacral or neck-shoulder area. These investigators found that biofeedback was superior to pseudotherapy or conventional medical treatment in reducing the duration and intensity of pain as well as EMG levels.

Conclusions

Biofeedback appears to hold promise as a clinically useful technique in the treatment of patients with back pain, but four of the studies reviewed (53, 54, 57, 61) included explicit training in relaxation in addition to EMG biofeedback and no direct comparisons of biofeedback and relaxation training have been reported. Additionally, only one study reported 1-year follow-up results (54). Although patients in this study continued to improve, more large-scale follow-up studies are clearly needed.

The following types of studies are needed before firm conclusions concerning the efficacy of EMG biofeedback for back pain are possible: (a) comparisons of biofeedback with other treatment methods, such as relaxation training; (b) further comparisons of biofeedback with appropriate control groups; (c) large-scale control-group outcome studies; (d) longer follow-up evaluations; (e) evaluations of treatment outcome based on the cause of the pain (e.g., rheumatic conditions, trauma, no obvious cause); (f) evaluations of various treatment procedures (e.g., paraspinal or frontalis electrode placements and training while supine or standing); and (g) further evaluations of patient characteristics predictive of outcome. Finally, a major question in this area is whether biofeedback is sufficiently efficacious to be used alone in the treatment of back pain, or whether it is best used within the context of a comprehensive pain management program.

BIOFEEDBACK TREATMENT OF TEMPOROMANDIBULAR JOINT SYNDROME

Temporomandibular joint (TMJ) syndrome, also known as myofascial pain dysfunction syndrome, is seen by a number of authorities (65) as the result of hyperactivity of the masticatory muscles (see Chapter 40). Although disagreement exists as to the cause of the hyperactivity (e.g., occlusal problems vs. psychologic stress), several researchers have examined the use of EMG biofeedback as a treatment, which can provide relief by teaching patients to relax the muscles of the jaw. Consistent with the logic of this approach, the most common electrode placement is on the masseter muscle, although temporalis placements have also been used.

A summary of the current literature on biofeedback therapy for TMJ syndrome is presented in Table 83-3. Three systematic case studies (66–68) and three single-group outcome studies (69–71) have all supported the efficacy of EMG biofeedback in the treatment of TMJ syndrome. One series of case studies (60), however, found only minimal improvement with biofeedback. In

TABLE 83-3. Biofeedback (BF) for Therapy for Temporomandibular Joint Syndrome

Source	Study Design	No. of Patients	Duration of Therapy	Results		Comments
				Short term	Long term	
Carlsson et al. (66)	Single case	1	18 sessions	Pt pain free	Pain free at 6 mo	—
Carlsson & Gale (67)	Single case	1	9 sessions	Pt symptom free	Symptom free at 1 yr	—
Peck & Kraft (60)	Multiple single cases	6	6 sessions	2/6 pts showed slight improvement	—	—
Clarke & Kardachi (68)	Multiple single cases	7	?	6/7 pts improved	—	BF training was done during sleep
Gessel (69)	Single-group outcome	23	3–14 sessions	15/23 pts improved	—	Criteria of improvement are unclear
Carlsson & Gale (70)	Single-group outcome	11	6–18 sessions	—	8/11 pts symptom free or significantly improved at 4–15 mo	—
Principato & Barwell (71)	Single-group outcome	25	6–10 sessions	84% of pts were symptom free	—	—
Dohrmann & Laskin (72)	Treatment vs. no treatment	Treatment = 16 No treatment = 8	12 sessions	Treatment better than no treatment in reducing pain and EMG levels and increasing incisal opening without discomfort	9/16 treatment pts symptom free at 1 year; 3 had a recurrence of mild symptoms	—
Dahlstrom et al. (73)	BF vs. occlusal splint therapy	15/group	3–6 sessions	Both groups showed significant but equal improvement	—	—
Trott & Goss (74)	BF vs. physical therapy (PT)	BF = 24 PT = 10	BF = 6 sessions max PT = 9 sessions max	Both groups showed significant but equal improvement	—	—
Moss et al. (75)	Multiple-baseline single cases alternating BF and relaxation training	5	Variable	3/5 pts improved with no advantage to the addition of BF over relaxation training	—	—
Stenn et al. (76)	Relaxation, cognitive behavior therapy, and BF (group 1) vs. relaxation and cognitive behavior therapy (group 2)	Group 1 = 6 Group 2 = 5	8 sessions	Both groups improved but group 1 showed significantly greater improvement	Improvement was maintained at 3 mo	—

the single-group outcome studies, the percentages of patients demonstrating a significant improvement were 65%, 73%, and 84%. Biofeedback training was provided using procedures similar to those described earlier in all but one of these studies. In this study, Clarke and Kardachi (68) instructed patients to wear the EMG electrodes during sleep in an attempt to reduce bruxing, which might contribute to the TMJ syndrome. Although this is an innovative technique, the authors provided no data concerning patients' ability to reduce EMG levels during sleep or the difficulties encountered (e.g., disruption of sleep).

Dohrmann and Laskin (72) compared biofeedback with a control condition in which patients merely rested comfortably in the treatment room. The biofeedback group demonstrated significant reduction in pain and increased incisal opening without discomfort compared with the control group.

The study by Gessel (69) is the only one that examined patient characteristics associated with treatment outcome. The results suggested that patients with higher levels of depression were less likely to be helped with biofeedback and more likely to improve with antidepressant medications. Unfortunately, the criteria used for establishing the presence of depression were not clearly presented.

Comparisons with Other Treatments

Biofeedback was shown to be equally as effective as occlusal splint therapy (73) and a physical therapy protocol, which included passive mobilization and ultrasound (74). Dahlstrom et al. (73) suggested that occlusal splint therapy is more time and cost efficient than biofeedback and may therefore be the treatment of choice. They suggested, however, that certain patients will respond to one modality rather than another. Further research in this area is clearly necessary.

In a series of single-case studies using a multiple-baseline design, Moss et al. (75) found that EMG biofeedback provided no significant improvement over that achieved with progressive relaxation alone. In a study of two treatment approaches, however, Stenn et al. (76) found support for biofeedback over relaxation training. In this study, all patients received relaxation training and cognitive behavior modification; one group also received a concurrent trial of EMG biofeedback. The results suggested that inclusion of EMG biofeedback led to greater levels of improvement.

Conclusions

We conclude that EMG biofeedback is a clinically useful technique in the treatment of TMJ syndrome. Biofeedback appears to produce improvement in a significant number of patients and is at least as effective as occlusal splint therapy and physiotherapy. Unfortunately, studies examining the relative efficacy of biofeedback versus relaxation training are equivocal. In the studies reviewed, follow-up periods ranged from 1 month to 1 year, but the beneficial effects of biofeedback generally were maintained. Deficiencies in the research on biofeedback therapy for TMJ syndrome are similar to those discussed in the section on back pain. A particularly important research area is the comparison of biofeedback with credible placebo groups, because several recent studies suggest that 52 to 64% of patients with TMJ syndrome obtain relief from credible placebo treatments (65).

BIOFEEDBACK TREATMENT OF OTHER CHRONIC PAIN DISORDERS

Biofeedback has been used with several other chronic pain syndromes. Most of these reports are single-case studies, and no attempt will be made to evaluate them. A summary of these studies is presented in Table 83-4. They include the following treatments: EMG biofeedback for the treatment of pain secondary to rheumatoid arthritis (77); thermal biofeedback for the treatment of pain due to causalgia (78), painful restless leg syndrome (79), electrical burn pain (80), and arthritic pain secondary to hemophilia (81); respiratory biofeedback for the treatment of Tietze's syndrome pain (82); and EMG and electrodermal biofeedback for the treatment of cancer pain (83).

EMG BIOFEEDBACK DURING MOVEMENT

The EMG procedures described thus far have involved training the person while in a static, usually supine position, with the goal of reducing the absolute level of EMG activity. Wolf and his associates (84–86), however, have proposed an alternative approach based on changing abnormal EMG patterns identified during dynamic movement. The logic of this approach grew from studies demonstrating that although some low back pain patients may not have elevated EMG levels during resting, abnormalities can occur during movements such as extension, flexion, and rotation of the trunk (84). These investigators have reported two case studies (85, 86) in which EMG biofeedback during dynamic movement was successfully used to correct EMG abnormalities and reduce low back pain. Similar procedures were effectively used to reduce excessive EMG activity of the trapezium in a muscle contraction headache patient while he walked on a treadmill (87) and to retrain the vastus medialis of a patient with arthritic knee pain who rode an ergometer (88). In both cases, EMG abnormalities were corrected and significant reductions in pain were reported.

The potential advantage of such an approach is that treatment can be tailored to correcting the specific EMG abnormalities identified in the patient. Nevertheless, large-scale studies are necessary to establish normative physiologic data. Such data would allow the

TABLE 83-4. Biofeedback Therapy for Other Chronic Pain Disorders

Technique	Source	Study Design	No. of Patients	Duration of Therapy	Results		Comments
					Short term	Long term	
A. RHEUMATOID ARTHRITIS PAIN							
EMG biofeedback	Wickramasekera et al. (77)	Single case	2	22 sessions (pt 1) 24 sessions (pt 2)	Decreased pain & increased activity	—	Autogenic relaxation included
B. CAUSALGIA							
Thermal biofeedback	Blanchard (78)	Single case	1	18 sessions	Decreased pain & increased hand temperature	Improvement maintained at 1 year	—
C. PAINFUL RESTLESS LEG SYDROME							
Thermal biofeedback	Ahles & Shariff (79)	Single case	1	14 sessions	Decreased pain & medication intake; increased foot temperature	Improvement maintained at 6 mo	Autogenic relaxation included
D. ELECTRICAL BURN							
Thermal biofeedback	Bird & Colborne (80)	Single case	1	14 sessions	Decreased pain & increased hand temperature	—	—
E. ARTHRITIC PAIN SECONDARY TO HEMOPHILIA							
Thermal biofeedback	Varni (81)	Single case	1	8 sessions	Decrease in arthritic pain but not in acute pain secondary to a bleed	Improvement maintained at 8 mo	Progressive relaxation, imagery, and meditative breathing were included
F. TIETZE'S SYNDROME PAIN							
Respiratory biofeedback	Jones & Evans (82)	Single case	1	5 sessions	Decreased pain & increased activity; regulated breathing	Improvement maintained at 2 & 5 mo	—
G. CANCER PAIN							
EMG & electrodermal biofeedback	Fotopoulos et al. (83)	Single-group outcome	12	11 sessions	Decreased pain for 3/5 pts within session and 2/5 at home	—	6 pts died or became too ill to participate

therapist to identify EMG abnormalities and establish realistic treatment goals (86). Although EMG biofeedback during dynamic movement appears to be a promising approach, much more research is clearly necessary.

REFERENCES

1. Budzynski, T., Stoyva, J., and Adler, C.: Feedback induced muscle relaxation: Application to tension headache. J. Behav. Ther. Exp. Psychiatry, 1:205, 1970.
2. Blanchard, E.B., and Epstein, L.H.: A Biofeedback Primer. Reading, MA, Addison-Wesley, 1978.
3. Budzynski, T.: Biofeedback in the treatment of muscle-contraction (tension) headache. Biofeedback Self Regul., 3:408, 1978.
4. Diamond, S., Diamond-Falk, Jr., and DeVeno, T.: Biofeedback in the treatment of vascular headache. Biofeedback Self Regul., 3:385, 1978.
5. Board of Directors, American Association for the Study of Headache: Biofeedback therapy. Headache, 18:107, 1978.
6. Task Force on Biofeedback of the American Psychiatric Association (Martin T. Orne, Chairman): Task Force Report 19: Biofeedback. Washington, DC, American Psychiatric Assoc., 1980.
7. Turk, D.C., Meichenbaum, D.H., and Berman, W.H.: Application of biofeedback for the regulation of pain: A critical review. Psychol. Bull., 86:1322, 1979.
8. Turner, J.A., and Chapman, C.R.: Psychological interventions for chronic pain: A critical review. I. Relaxation training and biofeedback. Pain, 12:1, 1982.
9. Jessup, B.A., Neufeld, R.W.J., and Merskey, H.: Biofeedback therapy for headache and other pain: An evaluating review. Pain, 7:225, 1979.
10. Adams, H.E., Feuerstein, M., and Fowler, J.L.: Migraine headache: Review of parameters, etiology, and intervention. Psychol. Bull., 87:217, 1980.
11. Blanchard, E.B., Ahles, T.A., and Shaw, E.R.: Behavioral treatment of headaches. Prog. Behav. Modif., 8:207, 1979.
12. Blanchard, E.B., and Andrasik, F.: Psychological assessment and treatment of headache: Recent developments and emerging issues. J. Consult. Clin. Psychol., 50:859, 1982.
13. Basmajian, J.V.: Facts vs. myths in EMG biofeedback. Biofeedback Self Regul., 1:369, 1976.

14. Belar, C.D.: A comment on Silver and Blanchard's (1978) review of the treatment of tension headaches by EMG feedback and relaxation training. J. Behav. Med., 2:215, 1979.

15. Hudzinski, L.G.: Neck musculature and EMG biofeedback in the treatment of muscle contraction headache. Headache, 23:86, 1983.

16. Martin, P.R., and Mathews, A.M.: Tension headaches: Psychophysiological investigation and treatment. J. Psychosom. Res., 22:389, 1978.

17. Hart, J.D., and Cichanski, K.A.: A comparison of frontal EMG biofeedback and neck EMG biofeedback in the treatment of muscle-contraction headache. Biofeedback Self Regul., 6:63, 1981.

18. Budzynski, T.H., Stoyva, J.M., Adler, C.S., and Mullaney, D.J.: EMG biofeedback and tension headache: A controlled outcome study. Psychosom. Med., 6:509, 1973.

19. Haynes, S.N., Griffin, P., Mooney, D., and Parise, M.: Electromyographic biofeedback and relaxation instructions in the treatment of muscle contraction headaches. Behav. Ther., 6:672, 1975.

20. Holroyd, K.A., Andrasik, F., and Noble, J.: Comparison of EMG biofeedback and a credible pseudotherapy in treating tension headache. J. Behav. Med., 3:29, 1980.

21. Cox, D.J., Freundlich, A., and Meyer, R.G.: Differential effectiveness of electromyographic feedback, verbal relaxation instructions, and medication placebo with tension headaches. J. Consult. Clin. Psychol., 43:892, 1975.

22. Hutchings, D.F., and Reinking, R.H.: Tension headaches: What form of therapy is most effective? Biofeedback Self Regul., 1:183, 1976.

23. Chesney, M.A., and Shelton, J.L.: A comparison of muscle relaxation and electromyogram biofeedback treatments for muscle contraction headache. J. Behav. Ther. Exp. Psychiatry, 7:221, 1976.

24. Philips, C.: The modification of tension headache pain using EMG biofeedback. Behav. Res. Ther., 15:119, 1977.

25. Blanchard, E.B., et al.: Biofeedback and relaxation training with three kinds of headache: Treatment effects and their prediction. J. Consult. Clin. Psychol., 50:562, 1982.

26. Bruhn, P., Olesen, J., and Melgaard, B.: Controlled trial of EMG feedback and muscle-contraction headache. Ann. Neurol., 6:34, 1979.

27. Paiva, T., et al.: The effects of frontalis EMG biofeedback and diazepam in the treatment of tension headache. Headache, 22:216, 1982.

28. Blanchard, E.B., et al.: Temperature biofeedback in the treatment of migraine headaches. Arch. Gen. Psychiatry, 35:581, 1978.

29. Sargent, J., et al.: Results of a controlled, experimental, outcome study of non-drug treatment for the control of migraine headaches. J. Behav. Med., 9:291, 1986.

30. Kewman, D., and Roberts, A.H.: Skin temperature biofeedback and migraine headache: A double-blind study. Biofeedback Self Regul., 5:327, 1980.

31. Lake, A., Raney, J., and Papsdorf, J.D.: Biofeedback and rational-emotive therapy in the management of migraine headache. J. Appl. Behav. Anal., 12:127, 1979.

32. Largen, J.W., Mathew, R.J., Dobbins, K., and Claghorn, J.L.: Specific and non-specific effects of skin temperature control and migraine management. Headache, 21:36, 1981.

33. Cohen, M.J., McArthur, D.L., and Rickles, W.H.: Comparison of four biofeedback treatments for migraine headache: Physiological and headache variables. Psychosom. Med., 42:463, 1980.

34. Mullinix, J., Norton, B., Hack, S., and Fishman, M.: Skin temperature biofeedback and migraine. Headache, 17:242, 1978.

35. Sovak, N., Kunzel, M., Sternback, R.A., and Dalessio, D.J.: Mechanism of the biofeedback therapy of migraine: Volitional manipulation of the psychophysiological background. Headache, 21:89, 1982.

36. Mathew, N.T.: Prophylaxis of migraine and mixed headache. A randomized controlled study. Headache, 21:105, 1982.

37. Bild, R., and Adams, H.E.: Modification of migraine headaches by cephalic blood volume pulse and EMG biofeedback. J. Consult. Clin. Psychol., 48:51, 1980.

38. Friar, L.R., and Beatty, J.: Migraine: Management by trained control of vasoconstriction. J. Consult. Clin. Psychol., 44:46, 1976.

39. Blanchard, E.B., et al.: Migraine and tension headache: A meta-analytic review. Behav. Ther., 11:613, 1980.

40. Blanchard, E.G., et al.: Sequential comparisons of relaxation training and biofeedback in the treatment of three kinds of chronic headache or, the machines may be necessary some of the time. Behav. Res. Ther., 20:469, 1982.

41. Blanchard, E.B., et al.: Prediction of outcome from the non-pharmacological treatment of chronic headache. Neurology, 33:1596, 1983.

42. Andrasik, F., Blanchard, E.B., Neff, D.F., and Rodichok, L.D.: Biofeedback and relaxation training for chronic headache: A controlled comparison of booster treatments and regular contacts for long-term maintenance. J. Consult. Clin. Psychol., 52:609, 1984.

43. Sargent, J.D., Green, E.E., and Walters, E.D.: Preliminary report on the use of autogenic feedback training in the treatment of migraine and tension headaches. Psychosom. Med., 35:129, 1973.

44. Schultz, J.H., and Luthe, U.: Autogenic Training. Vol. 1. New York, Grune and Stratton, 1969.

45. Diamond, S., and Franklin, M.: Autogenic training with biofeedback in the treatment of children with migraine. In Therapy of Psychosomatic Medicine. Rome, Edizioni Luigi Pozzi, 1975, pp. 190–192.

46. Labbe, E.L., and Williamson, D.A.: Treatment of childhood migraine using autogenic feedback training. J. Consult. Clin. Psychol., 52:968, 1984.

47. Andrasik, F., Blanchard, E.B., Edlund, S.R., and Rosenblum, D.L.: Autogenic feedback in the treatment of two children with migraine headache. Child. Fam. Behav. Ther., 4:13, 1982.

48. Werder, D.S., Sargent, J.D., and Coyne, L.: MMPI profiles of headache patients using self-regulation to control headache activity. Paper presented at the annual meeting of the American Association of Biofeedback Clinicians, October 31, 1981, Kansas City.

49. Silver, B.V., et al.: Temperature biofeedback and relaxation training in the treatment of migraine headaches: One year follow-up. Biofeedback Self Regul., 4:359, 1979.

50. Stroebel, C.F., Ford, N.R., Strong, P., and Szarek, B.L.: Quieting response training: Five-year evaluation of a clinical biofeedback practice. In Proceedings of the Biofeedback Society of America 12th Annual Meeting, March 1981, Louisville, KY, pp. 78–81.

51. Blanchard, E.B., Andrasik, F., Jurish, S.E., and Teders, S.J.: The treatment of cluster headache with relaxation and thermal biofeedback. Biofeedback Self Regul., 7:185, 1982.

52. Freeman, C.W., Calsyn, D.A., Paige, A.B., and Halar, E.M.: Biofeedback with low back pain patients. Am. J. Clin. Biofeedback, 3:118, 1980.

53. Keefe, F.J., Block, A.R., Williams, R.B., and Surwit, R.S.: Behavioral treatment of chronic low back pain: Clinical outcome and individual differences in pain relief. Pain, 11:221, 1981.

54. Keefe, F.J., et al.: EMG-assisted relaxation training in the management of chronic low back pain. Am. J. Clin. Biofeedback, 4:93, 1981.

55. Gottlieb, H., et al.: Comprehensive rehabilitation of patients having chronic low back pain. Arch. Phys. Med. Rehabil., 58:101, 1977.

56. Chapman, S.L., Brena, S.F., and Bradford, L.A.: Treatment outcome in a chronic pain rehabilitation program. Pain, 11:255, 1981.

57. Nigal, A.J., and Fischer-Williams, M.: Treatment of low back strain with electromyographic biofeedback and relaxation training. Psychosomatics, 21:495, 1980.

58. Nouwen, A., and Solinger, J.W.: The effectiveness of EMG biofeedback training in low back pain. Biofeedback Self Regul., 4:103, 1979.

59. Nouwen, A.: EMG biofeedback used to reduce standing levels of paraspinal muscle tension in chronic low back pain. Pain, 17:353, 1983.

60. Peck, C.L., and Kraft, G.H.: Electromyographic biofeedback for pain related to muscle tension. Arch. Surg., 112:889, 1977.

61. Belar, C.D., and Cohen, J.L.: The use of EMG feedback and progressive relaxation in the treatment of a woman with chronic back pain. Biofeedback Self Regul., 4:345, 1979.

62. Hendler, N., Derogatis, L., Avella, J., and Long, D.: EMG biofeedback in patients with chronic pain. Dis. Nerv. Syst., 38:505, 1977.

63. Large, R.G., and Lamb, A.M.: Electromyographic (EMG) feedback in chronic musculoskeletal pain: A controlled trial. Pain, 17:167, 1983.

64. Flor, H., Haag, G., Turk, D.C., and Koehler, H.: Efficacy of EMG biofeedback, pseudotherapy, and conventional medical treatment for chronic rheumatic back pain. Pain, *17*:21, 1983.
65. Scott, D.S., and Gregg, J.M.: Myofascial pain of the temporomandibular joint: A review of the behavioral-relaxation therapies. Pain, *9*:231, 1980.
66. Carlsson, S.G., Gale, E.N., and Ohman, A.: Treatment of temporomandibular joint syndrome with biofeedback training. J. Am. Dent. Assoc., *91*:602, 1975.
67. Carlsson, S.G., and Gale, E.N.: Biofeedback treatment for muscle pain associated with the temporomandibular joint. J. Behav. Ther. Exp. Psychiatry, 7:383, 1976.
68. Clarke, N.G., and Kardachi, B.J.: The treatment of myofascial pain-dysfunction syndrome using the biofeedback principle. J. Periodontol., *48*:643, 1977.
69. Gessel, A.H.: Electromyographic biofeedback and tricyclic antidepressants in myofascial pain-dysfunction syndrome: Psychological predictors of outcome. J. Am. Dent. Assoc., *91*:1048, 1975.
70. Carlsson, S.G., and Gale, E.N.: Biofeedback in the treatment of long-term temporomandibular joint pain: An outcome study. Biofeedback Self Regul., *2*:161, 1977.
71. Principato, J.J., and Barwell, D.R.: Biofeedback training and relaxation exercises for treatment of temporomandibular joint dysfunction. Otolaryngology, *86*:766, 1978.
72. Dohrmann, R.J., and Laskin, D.M.: An evaluation of electromyographic biofeedback in the treatment of myofascial pain-dysfunction syndrome. J. Am. Dent. Assoc., *96*:656, 1978.
73. Dahlstrom, L., Carlsson, G.E., and Carlsson, S.G.: Comparison of effects of electromyographic biofeedback and occlusal splint therapy on mandibular function. Scand. J. Dent. Res., *90*:151, 1982.
74. Trott, P.H., and Goss, A.N.: Physiotherapy in diagnosis and treatment of the myofascial pain dysfunction syndrome. Int. J. Oral. Surg., 7:360, 1978.
75. Moss, R.A., Wedding, D., and Sanders, S.H.: The comparative efficacy of relaxation training and masseter EMG feedback in the treatment of TMJ dysfunction. J. Oral Rehabil., *10*:9, 1983.
76. Stenn, P.G., Mothersill, K.J., and Brooke, R.I.: Biofeedback and a cognitive behavioral approach to treatment of myofascial pain dysfunction syndrome. Behav. Ther., *10*:29, 1979.
77. Wickramasekera, I., Truong, X.T., Bush, M., and Orr, C.: The management of rheumatoid arthritic pain: Preliminary observations. *In* Biofeedback, Behavior Therapy, and Hypnosis. Edited by I. Wickramasekera. Chicago, Nelson-Hall, 1976.
78. Blanchard, E.G.: The use of temperature biofeedback in the treatment of pain due to causalgia. Biofeedback Self Regul., *4*:183, 1979.
79. Ahles, T.A., and Shariff, M.: Temperature biofeedback and autogenic relaxation training in the treatment of restless leg syndrome. Paper presented at meeting of the Association for Advancement of Behavior Therapy, 1983, Washington, DC.
80. Bird, E.I., and Colborne, G.R.: Rehabilitation of an electrical burn patient through thermal biofeedback. Biofeedback Self Regul., *5*:283, 1980.
81. Varni, J.W.: Behavioral medicine in hemophilia arthritic pain management: Two case studies. Arch. Phys. Med. Rehab., *62*:183, 1981.
82. Jones, G.E., and Evans, P.A.: Treatment of Tietze's syndrome pain through paced respiration. Biofeedback Self Regul., *5*:295, 1980.
83. Fotopoulos, S.S., et al.: Cancer pain: Evaluation of electromyographic and electrodermal feedback. Prog. Clin. Biol. Res., *132D*:33, 1983.
84. Wolf, S.L., Basmajian, J.V., Russe, T.C., and Kutner, M.: Normative data on low back mobility and activity levels. Am. J. Phys. Med., *58*:217, 1979.
85. Jones, A.L., and Wolf, S.L.: Treating chronic low back pain: EMG biofeedback training during movement. Phys. Ther., *60*:58, 1980.
86. Wolf, S.L., Nacht, M., and Kelly, J.L.: EMG feedback training during dynamic movement for low back pain patients. Behav. Ther., *13*:395, 1982.
87. Ahles, T.A., King, A., and Martin, J.E.: EMG biofeedback during dynamic movement as a treatment for tension headache. Headache, *24*:41, 1984.
88. King, A.C., Ahles, T.A., Martin, J.E., and White, R.: EMG biofeedback-controlled exercise for a person with chronic arthritic knee pain. Arch. Phys. Med. Rehabil., *65*:341, 1984.

84 • HYPNOSIS

JOSEPH BARBER

HYPNOSIS can dramatically alter an individual's perception of pain, and its value as a clinical technique has been well documented. This chapter focuses on hypnotic analgesia and anesthesia and how they are used in the clinical management of pain. The material is presented in three parts: A, Basic Considerations, including a brief historical overview of the mechanism of hypnosis and other relevant basic issues; B, Technical Considerations, with brief discussion of the most common techniques used; and C, Clinical Applications, including a brief summary of results obtained in various acute and chronic pain problems. For more detailed accounts of research on and clinical application of hypnosis, the reader should consult the books by Barber and Adrian (1), Crasilneck and Hall (2), Gardner and Olness (3), Haley (4), Hilgard and Hilgard (5), and Hilgard and LeBaron (6).

A. BASIC CONSIDERATIONS

Historical Development

Treatment of physical conditions by suggestion has a long prescientific history, encumbered by superstitious beliefs. The man regarded as the "father of hypnosis" was an Austrian physician, Franz Anton Mesmer, who bridged the transition from supernatural to natural explanations of what we now call hypnosis. He was the first modern scientific investigator of hypnosis, although he is often mistakenly regarded as a supernaturalist (7). Mesmer was able to successfully treat physical conditions (many of which are now understood to be psychogenic) with what amounted to suggestion, but which he explained, using the most popular scientific constructs of his day, as "animal magnetism." His was the first known attempt to understand and explain the phenomenon of suggestion by reference to contemporary scientific concepts. Although we now think of Mesmer as unscientific, he was, in fact, a voice of empiricism and reason amid widespread religious superstition. Mesmer's clinical accomplishments caught the attention of medical practitioners throughout Europe, and the modern use of hypnosis was carried on by them.

Perhaps the most remarkable example of hypnotic control of pain is the use of hypnotic anesthesia during surgery. As early as 1846, James Esdaile, an English surgeon working in India, reported successfully using hypnoanesthesia for a variety of major surgeries (8). Ether anesthesia was introduced that same year, and chloroform the next. Because mesmerism (as the phenomenon came to be called) was perceived as less scientific than pharmacologic agents, its use as a surgical anesthetic ended when chemoanesthesia became more readily accessible.

James Braid, an English physician, investigated mesmerism and further refined the explanation of its action by reference to contemporary understandings of the nervous system. He believed the phenomenon was related to sleep, and was the first to use the term *hypnosis* (5). The clinical use of hypnosis evolved with an uneven progress, encountering intense opposition from the medical and scientific communities throughout the years. Even so, hypnosis has continued to be experimentally investigated and applied clinically; numerous accounts now exist of surgery performed with hypnosis or self-hypnosis (9) as the sole anesthetic.

In the 1950s, both the British and the American medical associations approved the use of hypnosis in clinical treatment, and specialty boards in hypnosis were created. The current clinical and scientific respectability of hypnosis is largely due to the intrepid efforts of clinicians such as Braid and Esdaile (and more recently, Erickson) and of scientists such as Clark Hull and Ernest and Josephine Hilgard. In recent years, hypnosis has been increasingly employed in the treatment of a multitude of pain problems and psychophysiologic disorders, including acute pain associated with burns, surgery, and malignancy, as well as chronic pain syndromes such as trigeminal neuralgia, peripheral neuropathies, and thalamic pain syndrome.

Mechanisms of Hypnosis

Neither gender nor intelligence is relevant to the development of the hypnotic state (5). Nor is age a factor; much work has been done with the hypnotic treatment of children in pain (10–14). The clinical usefulness of hypnosis has long been recognized, but only recently have sophisticated scientific explanations been attempted. Although the actual neurophysiologic or even psychologic mechanism of hypnosis has not yet been elucidated (contributing to skepticism about the validity of hypnosis), modern researchers have clarified the issues pertinent to understanding the mechanism and have offered some useful theoretical explanations.

The two fundamental approaches to understanding hypnotic phenomena are usually referred to as *state* and *nonstate* theories. State theorists reason that the characteristics of a hypnotized person are a function of a dramatic alteration in cognitive functioning (e.g., shifts in perceptual and conceptual processing and memory functions) due to a change in state of consciousness (15, 16). Orne (16) and, more recently, Sheehan and McConkey (17) have provided different and useful paradigms for examining demonstrable alterations in consciousness created by hypnotic suggestion. For nonstate theorists, on the other hand, hypnotic phenomena are explainable by reference to situational factors (18–20). They argue that hypnotized individuals behave as they do because of a complex determination by social variables (expectancy, compliance, etc.), not because of any alterations of consciousness.

Sternbach (21) suggested that the identification of physiologic substrates of hypnotic phenomena would provide a means for understanding the nature of hypnosis, and thus lay to rest the state-nonstate controversy. To date such investigations have not been very informative, however. Three studies (22–24) concluded that hypnotic analgesia is not subserved by release of endorphins. It may well be, however, that hypnosis is such a complex cognitive phenomenon that identification of specific neurohumoral or other physiologic substrates is not likely, and that even if such identifications are made, they will not be particularly helpful in understanding the psychologic nature of hypnosis.

One of the most fully developed theories of hypnosis has been advanced by E. R. Hilgard. His investigation of the "hidden observer" phenomenon led to his "neodissociation theory" of hypnosis. Briefly, this theory proposes that hypnotic analgesia can be explained as a rearrangement of the hierarchy of cognitive controls and assumes that at least two such control systems function simultaneously in human consciousness (5, 15).

A descriptive definition of hypnosis depends upon one's point of view in the state-nonstate controversy. Hypnosis is an experience or condition (probably an altered state of consciousness) characterized by a markedly increased receptivity to suggestion, the capacity for alteration of perception and memory, and the capacity for voluntary control of a variety of usually involuntary physiologic functions. All of these features of altered cognitive functioning can be useful in the control of pain, but clearly the most important are the alterations of perception and of physical functioning. With respect to alteration in perception, hypnotized individuals can experience both positive and negative hallucination. Positive hallucination refers to perceiving something that one would not otherwise perceive; negative hallucination refers to not perceiving something that one otherwise would perceive. Such hallucinations can occur in any sensory modality. As will be illustrated later, it is the capacity for such perceptual alteration that allows the development of hypnotic analgesia or anesthesia. Accumulating evidence suggests that alteration of affect is also crucial in the hypnotic management of pain.

Hypnosis can also be used to effect control over a wide variety of physiologic functions, including control over autonomic activity in general. This control might account for the success of hypnosis in alleviating the physical symptoms of psychosomatic syndromes such as some conditions of dermatitis, hypertension, Raynaud's syndrome, and asthma. In this chapter, however, the focus is on hypnotic analgesia and anesthesia and how they are used in the clinical management of pain.

Hypnotic Responsiveness

In the past, many thought that hypnotic treatment could be effective for only the small minority of individuals who are highly hypnotizable. Some suggested that only weak-minded individuals (those whose minds are easily influenced by others), hysterics, or the unintelligent could benefit (5). Over the past 25 years, however, meticulous research has demonstrated that such a characterization is false. Although response to hypnosis is variable, it is not correlated with intelligence or personality style (25). In fact, the only psychologic characteristic that has been found to covary with hypnotizability is *imaginative absorption*—that is, the capacity of an individual to become absorbed by the process of his or her imagination (25). Although all individuals possess this capacity to varying degrees, some people are particularly able to become totally immersed in the process of their cognitions. Such individuals tend to be more readily responsive than others. Individuals who do not have much awareness of their inner life, are unable to articulate their inner experience, and have little capacity for being highly absorbed by their own experience by and large tend to be less responsive (25).

Hypnotic responsiveness (also called *hypnotic susceptibility* or *hypnotizability*) can be determined by standardized tests. The most widely known of such tests is the Stanford Hypnotic Susceptibility Scale (26). To measure responsiveness, an individual is first given a standardized hypnotic induction. Such an induction is begun by having the individual stare fixedly at a point (such as a dot on a wall) while the hypnotist suggests relaxation, drowsiness, and finally an involuntary closure of the eyes. Once the subject's eyes have closed (and the subject is, presumably, lightly hypnotized), further suggestions are then given to "deepen" the hypnotic experience. Suggestions are then given to produce a variety of phenomena that hypnotized individuals are known to be capable of experiencing (e.g., immobility of a limb, inability to speak, auditory hallucination, age regression, response to posthypnotic suggestion, and amnesia). It is responsiveness to these suggestions that determines the subject's hypnotizability score. (The Stanford scale, for instance, has a range of 0 to 12 because there are 12 items to which the subject can respond.) The testing of thousands of individuals suggests that hypnotic responsiveness is a widespread characteristic and, in fact, is normally distributed throughout the population. A few individuals are unresponsive, most respond moderately, and a few respond quite fully. Response to such scales is quite stable. Test-retest reliability over a 10-year period is approximately 0.60 (5).

Such tests are most often used in experimental investigations of hypnosis, but some clinicans use them as a means of screening patients before attemptimg treatment with hypnosis. They believe that an individual is likely to benefit from the clinical use of hypnosis only if he or she is highly responsive, as measured by a standard test (5, 25, 27). Others (28–34) believe that hypnotic responsiveness, as measured by such standard tests, does not reflect an individual's potential for benefit from hypnotic treatment. For instance, in an experimental setting a significant correlation often exists between hypnotic responsiveness scores and the ability to control pain (5), but such a correlation may not obtain if a different type of hypnotic technique is used (28–31, 33, 34). In clinical situations, patients whose response to hypnotizability tests is poor sometimes respond adequately to hypnotic techniques designed to produce pain control (28, 30). Perhaps the most compelling evidence in this regard is Esdaile's (8) successful induction of hypnotic anesthesia for surgery in more than 300 serial cases, even though only a few of those patients were likely to be highly responsive. In a clinical context, most individuals probably can benefit from hypnosis, independent of their hypnotizability scores (30, 34), though some will benefit more readily than others.

The treatment of pain patients raises particular issues with respect to hypnotic responsiveness. Some have argued that patients' responsiveness should be measured before attempting treatment (5). However, I believe that such testing should be done only under very carefully considered circumstances because of the potentially discouraging effects of hypnotizability testing and because low hypnotizables can achieve hypnotic pain reduction. If a patient performs poorly on a hypnotizability test, this knowledge in itself can negatively affect both the clinician's and the patient's confidence in further hypnotic treatment. The possibility of clinical benefit will become apparent quickly enough without such measurement. An opposing view is articulated by Frederick Frankel in *Hypnosis: Trance as a Coping Mechanism* (New York, Plenum, 1976).

Efficacy of Hypnosis in Treatment of Pain

Research over the past 30 years has demonstrated that hypnotized individuals (including college students, children, and the general population) are able to reduce or eliminate a variety of experimentally induced pain, including ischemic, cold-pressor, electric, and thermal. Careful investigation has established that pain control achieved by hypnosis is superior to that achieved by other psychologic means, such as biofeedback or distraction (2, 5). For a full account of such research, see Hilgard and Hilgard (5).

Most of the clinical literature shows hypnosis to be even more effective for pain control (and more frequently so) than experimental reports suggest (5, 35, 36). An experimental study by Price and Barber (31) suggests two possible ways to account for the differences obtained in laboratory and clinical hypnosis. In this study, subjects were asked to measure (using a visual analog scale) heat pain on both sensory and affective dimensions, both during a baseline and a hypnotic condition. Hypnosis was induced using nontraditional methods. (Nontraditional refers to what are sometimes called Ericksonian or naturalistic methods, which do not rely on standardized induction techniques but instead use the setting and the subject's or patient's particular needs at the time in the formulation of suggestions (28–31, 33). Analgesic suggestions were similarly nontraditional. Low-hypnotizable subjects were able to reduce affective pain as well as highly hypnotiz-able subjects, but highly hypnotizable subjects were somewhat better able to reduce sensory pain.

Although hypnosis can reduce both components of pain, in clinical work it is really only necessary for a patient to reduce the affective component in order to relieve his or her suffering. The results of this study (31) suggest that the affective component is readily affected by hypnosis. Perhaps the well-known disparity between clinical and experimental effects of hypnosis is at least partly a function of the greater effect on the affective component. This explanation is offered in addition to that of Orne (27), who suggested that contextual effects of the clinical situation, both direct and indirect, must account for at least a part of what would otherwise be taken to be the hypnotic effect. For instance, the motivation of patients clearly differs from that of experimental subjects; and the meaning of the clinician's attention is very different from that of the experimenter's. Whatever the explanation, it is clear from experimental investigations and clinical experience that hypnosis in the clinical context can be effective for managing pain of any kind or intensity with a wide range of patients.

Potential Adverse Effects of Hypnosis

Because hypnosis can cause radical alterations in cognitions and behavior—with a concomitant appearance of nonvolitionality—some have been concerned that hypnosis could be harmful. Much effort has been made to settle the question of whether hypnosis can cause an individual to behave in ways one would normally find morally offensive or injurious to self. Although no instance of harm coming to an individual specifically through the agency of hypnosis has been reliably documented (27), this concern is raised often because of the bizarre and foolish antics performed by subjects at the hands of nightclub hypnotists. The behavior demonstrated in such nightclub acts can be explained without reference to hypnosis (e.g., compliance with demand characteristics). Nonetheless, the psychologic changes that can be produced by hypnosis are sufficiently powerful to warrant its use only by trained clinicians. Hypnosis, like any other clinical tool, can be misused. This is an argument for the careful training of clinicians, however, not for avoiding the use of a powerful clinical tool.

Even though the experience of being hypnotized is generally innocuous and often pleasant, hypnosis should only be undertaken by someone with sufficient clinical skills. Because hypnosis can be used in several clinical areas, a clinician trained in one area sometimes is tempted to use hypnotherapy to treat a patient whose problem would otherwise lie outside the clinician's training. For example, a psychologist might be well trained to treat a patient's pain, so long as the patient has already been examined by a competent physician and so long as the psychologist is mindful of the medical aspects of the patient's condition. It would not be appropriate for the psychologist to treat a patient's pain without proper medical collaboration. Similarly, a gynecologist might be properly trained to treat a patient's pelvic pain with hypnosis, but it would be inappropriate, without further training, to treat the patient's psychosexual dysfunction with hypnotherapy.

Further, if the patient's pelvic pain is psychogenic, it should be treated by someone with appropriate training. One should only treat a problem one is trained to treat; if one is also trained in the use of hypnosis for such a problem, hypnosis will probably make treatment more effective. Training in hypnosis, however, is not an alternative for adequate clinical training in general.

B. TECHNICAL CONSIDERATIONS

A number of hypnotic techniques, capable of altering either the sensory or the affective dimensions of pain, are available; these may be helpful, depending upon the circumstances. Selecting a particular technique in any given situation is a clinical judgment that should be based on what will best meet the needs of the patient. The experienced clinician is not limited by the techniques described here, of course. Erickson (37), for instance, reported a variety of unorthodox but remarkably effective hypnotic treatments for pain.

Requisites for Optimal Results

Whether or not the hypnotic responsiveness of a patient is measured, other aspects of each case should be evaluated before initiating hypnosis. Such evaluation includes the same medical evaluation that is standard practice before initiating any other treatment for pain. Just as one would not prescribe a pharmacologic analgesic for a patient presenting with headache in the absence of an adequate workup, so one would not use hypnosis to treat a pain complaint without proper evaluation of the nature of the pain. Additionally, the patient needs to be evaluated with respect to his or her motivation, treatment goals, and expectations of treatment outcome.

To a greater extent than with other clinical procedures, treatment with hypnosis requires development of good rapport with patients. Patients are not infrequently wary of being hypnotized, partly for erroneous reasons (e.g., concern that hypnosis involves giving up one's will) and partly for correct reasons (e.g., a sense that the experience could increase awareness of chronic anxiety). Such wariness can detract from the effectiveness of hypnosis. Discussing with patients their past experience with hypnosis, beliefs about hypnosis, and concerns about the experience can provide significant relief from such concern. Even brief, but attentive, discussion with a patient can also reveal the patient's own style of cognition (which information can be used when creating an induction technique); whether or not fantasy is a comfortable experience (again, this information can aid in a determination of the kind of induction to be used, as well as the kinds of therapeutic suggestions to offer); and how the patient understands the potential for relief through hypnosis. The more fully the clinician understands the importance of active participation by the patient in the process of hypnosis, and engages that participation, the more likely hypnosis will be effective (38).

Specific Techniques

Five techniques that can be used to create hypnotic analgesia are hallucination of anesthesia, direct diminution of pain, sensory substitution, displacement of pain, and dissociation. It is important to note that in hypnotic treatment, multiple suggestions for comfort generally are given; the specific suggestions described in the following sections are only illustrative of the types that are used.

Hallucination of Anesthesia

Hypnosis can create a hallucination of anesthesia that renders a body area insensitive to pain. In such a case, the patient is actually unable to feel the pain and instead feels numbness—just as if a local anesthetic had been injected. In fact, a patient's familiarity with the experience of anesthetic numbness can be helpful in recreating that feeling.

A childhood experience of mine illustrates this technique. When I was about nine years old, I had an unpleasant and painful series of experiences with one dentist and so was taken to see another dentist. He told me something new—that I could imagine that my arm and hand were like a sponge, and that this could absorb all the feelings from my mouth, leaving my mouth feeling only numbness. I don't recall just how much he told me about it—it seemed like a natural and brief prologue to the operative procedure. But he was right. I recall now the odd numbness I felt in my mouth and the relief that my subsequent dental experiences would be more pleasant.

Anesthesia can also be suggested by referring to a patient's past experience with an anesthetic; for example, "It can begin to feel as if an anesthetic salve has been applied to [the painful area], and [the painful area] is becoming numb, with almost no sensation at all . . . perhaps just a bit of tingling." The hallucination of numbness is, in my clinical experience, a relatively more difficult phenomenon to achieve than others.

Diminution of Pain

Direct diminution of pain is a simple technique that seeks to accomplish the reduction of sensory pain. The following suggestion might be made, for example: "You can continue to enjoy feeling increasingly well, with each breath you take . . . almost as if the discomfort is somehow gradually going away." Hypnosis can create a sense of diminution of the intensity of pain, as if the "volume" of the pain were turned down. In fact, such metaphors as "turning down the volume" can be effective hypnotic suggestions. (Metaphors for turning down volume, dimming brightness, cooling heat, etc. are most effective when matched to the patient's own phenomenology of pain intensity or quality.)

Sensory Substitution

Hypnosis can create sensory substitution. For example, a sensation of intolerable burning can be replaced unconsciously by another sensation, not necessarily pleasant, such as itching, coldness, or tingling. Such a substitute feeling has several virtues. First, it allows the patient to know the pain is still there. Thus, a cancer patient, for example, does not have to be concerned that he or she will forget the cancer still persists, and thereby is reassured about continued medical attention. Second, a substitute feeling, especially if not particularly pleasant, is more plausible than, say, a sensation of "no feeling" or of pleasure. A third advantage for the patient is that many secondary gains associated with pain can still be obtained without suffering. A clinician might temporarily use this as part of the clinical strategy, while working toward eventually diminishing debilitating secondary gains.

Sensory substitution might be accomplished with the following kind of suggestion, which was successfully used with a 42-year-old paraplegic woman suffering burning dysesthesia in the legs: "The feelings that you describe as hot needles stabbing you can begin, oddly enough, to seem as if the needles are becoming more and more blunt and soft, almost as if they have become tiny, massaging fingers. What an interesting sensation you can begin to have . . . thousands of warm fingers buzzing, massaging your legs. Not entirely pleasant, but perhaps a welcome relief."

Pain Displacement

Displacement of pain from one area of the body to another can be accomplished in patients with well-localized pain that is primarily disabling because of its location (e.g., abdominal pain is less tolerable and more disabling than limb pain). Because moving pain is sometimes easier than eliminating it, pain displacement can be a valuable temporizing technique that can serve to increase the confidence of patients who are pessimistic about their hypnotic abilities. A typical suggestion for creating displacement is, "You may have already noticed that the pain moves, ever so slightly, and you can begin to notice that the movement seems to be in an outwardly spiraling circular direction. As you continue to attend to that movement, you may not notice until sometime later that the pain has somehow moved out of your abdomen and seems to be staying in your left hand."

Dissociation

Aside from creating the kinds of sensory alterations just described, hypnotic suggestions can also create a dissociation from pain. In such a case, the patient is able to accurately describe the still persisting pain—but with a sense of distance and with no affective involvement. That is, the pain is still perceived, but the patient no longer suffers from it. Dissociation is often useful when the patient is relatively immobile (e.g., during surgery or some other painful procedure, or when bedridden).

A suggestion to create dissociation might begin as follows: "It is unnecessary for you to have to stay here, in bed, conscious of all the routine that occurs. I wonder if you might prefer to enjoy a kind of vacation from this room. You might like to imagine yourself, for instance, stepping out of the room, moving down the hall, and settling nicely into the solarium. Or, later today you might prefer to feel as if you are enjoying a lovely sunny afternoon resting on the beach. Your body can remain here, in bed, in order that all the routine things can be done for you, but your mind can take you far away, and you can enjoy whatever you'd like, with nothing to bother you, with no need to be aware of the hospital."

Extending Pain Relief

In general, one can expect that patients will be comfortable during the hypnotic treatment itself. This has limited usefulness, however, when the objective is to activate and rehabilitate patients beyond the period taken up with the hypnotic process. In this situation, the use of posthypnotic suggestions or self-hypnosis can extend the pain relief.

Posthypnotic Suggestion

A posthypnotic suggestion is one that is intended to have effect after the hypnotic state has ended and the patient has regained normal waking consciousness. In general posthypnotic suggestions include a cue that initiates the suggested experience (or behavior). For instance, I could suggest, "Whenever I lift your arm, you will discover, at that moment, how really comfortable you feel." If effective, this suggestion would create analgesia whenever I lifted the patient's arm. Although this strategy might have instructive value, it is not a practical solution to the patient's pain problem, because I will not always be present to lift the arm.

The cue could be a function of context, however. For example, a clinician might say, "Whenever you need to feel relief from this pain, you'll suddenly notice that in fact you are feeling better than you were. And you can be suprised, throughout the day, to notice that somehow you continue to feel better than you thought you would." In this way, the patient's own recognition of the need for comfort is the cue, and no behavior on the clinician's part is necessary. In general, one can expect that hypnotic relief achieved by posthypnotic suggestion initially will extend throughout a day, possibly longer.

Self-Hypnotic Management

The most effective means for creating both independence for the patient and long-lasting pain relief is through self-hypnosis. Most patients can learn self-hypnosis quite readily and can learn to apply their skills to the development of analgesia over increasingly greater lengths of time (27, 32). Patients' interest in learning and willingness to use self-hypnosis is a valuable index of their motivation and capacity for recovery and rehabilitation (as well as a means of assessing broader psychologic issues).

As patients become more and more independent of the clinician and increase their mastery of self-hypnotic skills, follow-up becomes increasingly important. Patients need to know that help is available in the future, however infrequently they might need it. Sometimes many months go by during which a patient successfully uses self-hypnotic management of pain, and then, for a variety of reasons (including intensification of enviromental stressors), finds increasing difficulty in managing the pain. At such a time, a "booster" treatment might be all that is necessary to return the patient to independent functioning.

Clinical Training in Hypnosis

Most medical schools, dental schools, and clinical psychology training programs provide training in the use of hypnosis. For the postgraduate, training in clinical hypnosis is available through many continuing medical and education programs and through professional hypnosis societies. In the United States there are two such societies, whose membership is limited to health care providers: The American Society of Clinical Hypnosis and The Society for Clinical and Experimental Hypnosis. The International Hypnosis Society also provides training in hypnosis. The American Psychological Association, through its Division 30: Psychological Hypnosis, also provides information and training in hypnosis to psychologists. For information about training in hypnosis, one can communicate with a local university or medical school, or with one of these societies.

Although learning hypnosis techniques requires time and energy, this cognitive tool can be a welcome relief for clinicians frustrated by their inability to help patients who need pain relief that is beyond the reach of medicine.

C. CLINICAL APPLICATIONS

Although hypnosis is often regarded as a technique that is *applied to* a patient, without the patient's active cooperation, this is certainly not so in a clinical context. The clinical efficacy of hypnosis relies heavily on the active cooperation of the patient.

Because hypnosis affects pain and suffering at a very high level of neural organization—consciousness itself—its effect is apparently not a function of the source or kind of pain involved. Any pain, whether it is peripheral or central, lancinating or dull, burning or cold, resulting from injury or disease, benign or malignant, acute or chronic, can be reinterpreted by consciousness so that it no longer is painful or causes suffering.

Acute Pain

Hypnosis is valuable in the relief of acute pain when analgesics are not available or are contraindicated; it can also be used to potentiate the effects of analgesics. Hypnosis can be induced to create pain relief for a victim at the site of an accident or in an emergency room, as well as for a patient in a postsurgical or burn ward (11, 13, 35). In such cases, the analgesic effect of hypnosis is variable, ranging from only partial to complete reduction of discomfort, for a few minutes to an entire day. In most cases, one could expect the duration of effectiveness in a new patient to be at least an hour.

In the case of acute pain, the usual hypnotic effect is like the effect of an analgesic in combination with an anxiolytic agent. Consequently, adjunctive hypnotic treatment may greatly aid concurrent medical care, for example, by improving a burn patient's comfort and appetite (11, 13, 35). Patients suffering acute pain feel comfortable and quiescent following successful hypnotic treatment, as if they had been given a narcotic. It is difficult to describe the psychologic benefit to patients of experiencing comfort through hypnotic means without sounding unduly enthusiastic. Indeed, many patients benefit well beyond what would be expected from taking a narcotic for comfort. When a clinician takes the time and attention to speak calmingly and comfortingly to a patient, in addition to comforting the patient he or she greatly improves the patient's confidence for recovery and cooperation in other treatments. Some of the benign effects of hypnosis are similar to a narcotic in this situation, and so are the side effects. For example, a patient might not respond normally to a physical examination while under the effect of hypnotic analgesia, and this needs to be taken into account when further assessment is to be made.

Although clinical experience has demonstrated the value of hypnosis in reducing acute pain in many situations, there are few systematic studies of this effect. A brief review of the literature on hypnotic diminution of acute pain follows.

Postoperative Pain

Since Esdaile's report (8) of over 300 surgical operations done under hypnotic anesthesia, a number of single-case reports have ben published. With the advent of modern chemoanesthesia, the need for hypnosis in the operating room normally obtains only for patients at risk for the use of chemoanesthesia. At the 1985 International Congress on Hypnosis and Psychosomatic Medicine, a series of 23 major surgeries done with hypnosis as the sole anesthetic was described by Alexander Levitan, M.D.

A number of clinical reports demonstrate that hypnosis is an effective treatment, both adjunctive to pharmaceutical analgesics and as the sole analgesic, for postoperative pain. Few reports, however, document the sytematic use of hypnosis over a number of cases. Koulouch (39) reported the effects on 254 patients of preoperative hypnotic treatment to reduce postoperative pain. These patients required less postoperative analgesia and tended to have shorter postoperative hospital stays than patients who did not undergo hypnotic treatment. Other investigators have reported similar effects of employing suggestion during the surgical procedure itself (40).

Postburn Pain

A number of factors hinder recovery of the severely burned patient: constant pain, loss of appetite, the requirement for repeated painful procedures, contractures resulting from failure to do painful exercises, and depression (2). Crasilneck et al. (41) were the first to present a clinical report of successful hypnotic treatment of burn pain. Finer and Nylen (42) described the unique value of hypnosis in burn pain when chemoanesthesia was contraindicated. Hypnosis has also been used in the treatment of children suffering from burn pain (43). Wakeman and Kaplan (13) investigated two groups of burn patients: those with up to 30% total body burns ($N = 24$) and those with 31 to 60% body burns ($N = 18$). Hypnosis produced significant reductions in pain in both groups. Interestingly, there was a slightly greater degree of reduction in adolescent patients than in adults. Schafer (11) investigated 20 patients on a burn ward; 14 experienced significant reduction in pain following hypnosis.

Dental Pain

Throughout this century, dentistry, more than any other health specialty, has maintained a high level of interest in the pain-relieving qualities of hypnosis. As already discussed, hypnosis is an effective alternative to chemoanesthetics for producing comfort during operative procedures. Gottfredson (44), in an elegant clinical experiment, reported on the effectiveness of hypnosis as the sole anesthetic in 25 patients. He found that 75% of the high-hypnotizable patients and 38% of the low-hypnotizable patients completed dental treatment without requesting a chemoanesthetic. Barber (34) reported a clinical series of 100 dental patients, among whom only one was unable to successfully undergo dental operative treatment with hypnosis as the sole anesthetic.

Labor Pain

There are numerous anecdotal reports of hypnosis used to reduce the pain of childbirth. The clinician using hypnosis in obstetrical cases "may incorporate any or all of the techniques used in 'natural childbirth' and 'psychoprophylaxis' and may develop techniques of his own appropriate to his abilities and to the characteristics of his practice" (5, p. 107). Davidson (45) studied 210 women undergoing childbirth. Compared with a no-treatment control group and a group taught relaxation and controlled breathing, the hypnosis group reported significantly lower pain levels. In another study (46), 22 hypnotized patients had significantly more comfortable labor and deliveries than a comparable nonhypnotic control group. The analgesic effect of hypnosis appears to be significantly greater than that of natural childbirth (5).

Acute Pain from Other Medical Procedures

An excellent description of hypnotic treatment (and other psychologic interventions) for iatrogenic pain in children and adolescents is offered by J. R. Hilgard and LeBaron (6). They investigated 63 pediatric patients undergoing bone marrow aspiration procedures. Of these, 24 agreed to attempt hypnosis and of these, 15 experienced significantly reduced pain. The remaining 9 patients experienced reduced anxiety, which enabled them to tolerate the experience better. Kellerman et al. (12) investigated 18 pediatric patients undergoing bone marrow aspirations. Of the 16 who participated in hypnosis, all were said to have reduced "distress." (The disparity in results in these two studies might largely reflect differences in measuring the dependent variable; Kellerman et al. [12] combined anxiety and pain in defining "distress," whereas J. R. Hilgard and LeBaron (6) assessed them separately).

Zeltzer and LeBaron (47) compared hypnosis with nonhypnotic techniques (e.g., deep breathing, distraction, and the usual things done for such a patient) for reduction of pain and anxiety during painful procedures in children and adolescents with cancer. Only hypnosis was effective in reducing pain.

Chronic Pain

When a surgical or pharmacologic approach to persistent pain is not successful, or is contraindicated in a particular case, hypnosis can offer dramatic benefit. Hypnosis is not an automatic solution to a complex pain problem, however. The very chronicity of suffering from pain syndromes creates complex changes in a patient's behavior and personality. As a consequence, the treatment of chronic pain generally requires multiple interventions and often requires an interdisciplinary team aproach. Hypnosis can be of great value *if* it is properly integrated into such a treatment plan.

Hypnosis often is an important early *part* of the total treatment of such patients (34). Temporary relief of pain can be an important motivation for patients and can inspire them to initiate new behavior. Even a patient who has conscious or unconscious reservations about long-term relief of pain (and destruction of secondary gain) might easily be persuaded to experience temporary relief. Once experienced, such relief can be a powerful motivator, which the treatment team can use as leverage to encourage the patient to cooperate with other treatments. A second important role for hypnosis in chronic pain management is in the patient's self-care (discussed earlier under Self-Hypnotic Management).

Cancer Pain

Sometimes cancer patients fear that a loss of pain perception will lead them to forget they are still ill (and will lead to diminished resistance to their disease). This and other fears of cancer patients can be dealt with by the attentive clinician, however, and hypnosis can be effectively used to significantly increase the comfort of such patients.

In one of the few systematic reports available, Olness (48) investigated 25 children and adolescents undergoing treatment for cancer; of 21 patients who agreed to use hypnosis, 19 showed significant reduction in pain.

Headache

Although it is widely reported that hypnosis can be used as an effective treatment for headache there are few systematic studies of its use. Drummond (49) summarized a number of single-case reports demonstrating the efficacy of hypnosis in treating a variety of headaches. Cedercreutz et al. (50) studied 155 patients who suffered headache secondary to head injury and found hypnosis effective in significantly reducing pain. Cedercreutz (51) reported successful hypnotic treatment of 100 migraine patients. In another migraine study, Olness and McDonald (52) treated 15 children and adolescents with refractory migraine headaches and found that all 15 were able to control migraines with self-hypnosis. Whereas hypnosis is ordinarily used as an analgesic in other pain syndromes, it can be useful in actually preventing migraine headache (by the development of increased control of cephalic vasomotor activity by the patient) and in reducing muscle contracture headache (by inducing muscular relaxation).

Low Back Pain

Numerous single-case reports of the successful use of hypnosis for low back pain are available. However, few systematic studies of its effectiveness have been reported. Crasilneck (53) reported that 20 of 24 patients with low back pain were able to significantly reduce their pain using hypnosis. McCauley et al. (54) investigated 17 patients whom they treated with hypnosis and relaxation. They found that both techniques were effective in significantly reducing pain. Sachs et al. (36) treated 8 patients with low back and lower limb pain and found that all patients were able to significantly reduce their pain.

Phantom Limb Pain

Although phantom limb pain represents a sometimes intractable clinical picture, hypnosis can sometimes create complete freedom from pain. Cedercreutz (55) treated phantom pain with hypnosis in amputees. He reported that pain was relieved in 22% of the patients and was significantly reduced in another 13%.

Sickle Cell Anemia Pain

Zeltzer et al. (10) studied two adolescents who were successfully treated with hypnosis to reduce the frequency and intensity of pain crises.

Chronic Pain of Psychologic Origin

In general, hypnosis is *not* effective in the treatment of psychogenic pain syndromes. Such syndromes require more complex psychotherapeutic treatment. In additon, certain psychologic syndromes (e.g., personality disorders) can make the use of hypnosis more problematic. Such disorders do not automatically contraindicate the use of hypnosis, but their presence does indicate the need for careful clinical application of hypnosis in treatment (and certainly indicates the need for psychotherapeutic consultation if the treating clinician is not a psychologist or psychiatrist).

SUMMARY

Many studies suggest that the more hypnotically responsiveness a person is, the more likely will be successful hypnotic analgesia, but this issue is still an open question. Recent research has suggested that virtually any motivated patient can gain at least some relief from pain through hypnotic treatment. Pain reduction can involve a change in either the sensory-discriminative component or the motivational-affective component. Hypnosis can certainly contribute an anxiolytic effect, but hypnotic analgesia is independent of this effect.

Hypnotic treatment for pain can be effective for a wide variety of painful conditions. Because the effect is at the highest level of neural organization, the nature or location of pain is not an essential determinant of success (as it would be, say, with local anesthetic acting on the peripheral nerves). Hypnotic treatment techniques are evolving with an increasing understanding of human psychology. Greater emphasis is being placed on active participation by the patient, primarily through greater utilization of self-hypnosis. As these techniques evolve, the authoritarian approach characteristic of past hypnotic techniques is being abandoned. A more contemporary, humanistic approach on the part of the clinician is more likely to be encountered by patients today.

ACKNOWLEDGMENT. I thank Cheri Adrian for her generous attention to this manuscript.

REFERENCES

1. Barber, J., and Adrian, C. (eds.): Psychological Approaches to the Management of Pain. New York, Brunner/Mazel, 1982.
2. Crasilneck, H.B., and Hall, J.A.: Clinical Hypnosis: Principles and Applications. New York, Grune and Stratton, 1975.
3. Gardner, G.G., and Olness, K.: Hypnosis and Hypnotherapy in Children. New York, Grune and Stratton, 1981.
4. Haley, J. (ed.): Advanced Techniques of Hypnosis and Therapy. (Selected papers of Milton H. Erickson.) New York, Grune and Stratton, 1967.
5. Hilgard, E.R., and Hilgard, J.R.: Hypnosis in the Relief of Pain. 2nd Ed. Los Altos, CA, William Kaufmann, 1983.
6. Hilgard, J.R., and LeBaron, S.: Hypnotherapy of Pain in Children with Cancer. Los Altos, CA, William Kaufmann, 1984.
7. Mesmer, F.A.: Mesmerism: A Translation of the Original Medical and Scientific Writing of F. A. Mesmer, M.D. (Compiled and translated by George J. Bloch, Ph.D.; introduction by Ernest R. Hilgard Ph.D.) Los Altos, CA, William Kaufmann, 1980.
8. Esdaile, J.: Hypnosis in Medicine and Surgery. (Introduction and supplementary reports by W. S. Kroger.) New York, Julian, 1957.
9. Rausch, V.: Cholecystectomy with self-hypnosis. Int. J. Clin. Exp. Hypn., 22:124, 1980.
10. Zelzter, L. Dash, J., and Holland, J.: Hypnotically induced pain control in sickle cell anemia. Pediatrics, 64:533, 1979.
11. Schafer, D.W.: Hypnosis use on a burn unit. Int. J. Clin. Exp. Hypn., 23:1, 1975.
12. Kellerman, J., Zeltzer, L., Ellenberg, L., and Dash, J.: Adolescents with cancer. J. Adolesc. Health Care, 4:76, 1983.
13. Wakeman, R.J., and Kaplan, J.Z.: An experimental study of hypnosis in painful burns. Am. J. Clin. Hypn., 21:3, 1978.
14. Hilgard, J.R., and LeBaron, S.: Relief of anxiety and pain in children and adolescents with cancer: Quantitative measures and clinical observations. Int. J. Clin. Exp. Hypn., 30:417, 1982.
15. Hilgard, E.R.: Divided Consciousness: Multiple Controls in Human Thought and Action. New York, John Wiley and Sons, 1977.
16. Orne, M.T.: The nature of hypnosis: Artifact and essence. J. Abnorm. Soc. Psychol., 58:277, 1959.
17. Sheehan, P.W., and McConkey, K.M.: Hypnosis and Experience: The Exploration of Phenomena and Process. Hillsdale, NJ, Lawrence Erlbaum Associates, 1982.
18. Barber, T.X.: Hypnosis: A Scientific Approach. New York, Van Nostrand, 1969.
19. Sarbin, T.R., and Coe, W.C.: Hypnosis: A Social Psychological Analysis of Influence Communication. New York, Holt, Rinehart & Winston, 1972.
20. Sarbin, T.R., and Coe, W.C.: Hypnosis and psychopathology: Replacing old myths with fresh metaphors. J. Abnorm. Psychol., 88:506, 1979.
21. Sternbach, R.A.: On strategies for identifying neurochemical correlates of hypnotic analgesia. Int. J. Clin. Exp. Hypn., 30:251, 1982.
22. Barber, J., and Mayer, D.: An investigation of the efficacy and neural mechanism of a hypnotic analgesia procedure in experimental and clinical dental pain. Pain, 4:41, 1977.

23. Finer, B., and Terenius, L.: Endorphin involvements during hypnotic analgesia in chronic pain patients. Paper presented at the Third World Congress on Pain of the International Association for the Study of Pain, Sept. 4–11, 1981. Edinburgh, Scotland.
24. Goldstein, A., and Hilgard, E.R.: Failure of the opiate antagonist naloxone to modify hypotic analgesia. Proc. Natl. Acad. Sci. USA, *72*:2041, 1975.
25. Hilgard, J.R.: Personality and Hypnosis: A Study of Imaginative Involvement. Chicago, Univ. of Chicago Press, 1970.
26. Weitzenhoffer, A.M., and Hilgard, E.R.: Stanford Hypnotic Susceptibility Scale, Forms A and B. Palo Alto, CA, Consulting Psychologists Press, 1959.
27. Orne, M.T.: Hypnotic control of pain: Toward a clarification of the different psychological processes involved. *In* Pain. Edited by J.J. Bonica. New York, Raven Press, 1980.
28. Barber, J: Hypnosis and the unhypnotizable. Am. J. Clin. Hypn., *23*:4, 1980.
29. Fricton, J.R., and Roth, P.: The effects of direct and indirect hypnotic suggestions for analgesia in high and low susceptible subjects. Am. J. Clin. Hypn., *27*:226, 1985.
30. Gillett, P.L., and Coe, W.C.: The effects of rapid induction analgesia (R.I.A.), hypnotic susceptibility, and the severity of discomfort on the reduction of dental pain. Am. J. Clin. Hypn., *19*:81, 1984.
31. Price, D.D., and Barber, J.: A quantitative analysis of the efficacy of hypnotic analgesia. J. Abnorm. Psychol., *96*:46, 1987.
32. Schafer, D.W., and Hernandez, A.: Hypnosis, pain and the context of therapy. Int. J. Clin. Exp. Hypn., *3*:145, 1978.
33. Barber, J.: Rapid induction analgesia: A clinical report. Am. J. Clin. Hypn., *19*:138, 1977.
34. Barber, J.: Incorporating hypnosis in the management of chronic pain. *In* Psychological Approaches to the Management of Pain. Edited by J. Barber and C. Adrian. New York, Brunner/Mazel, 1982.
35. Turner, J.A., and Chapman, C.R.: Psychological interventions for chronic pain: A critical review. II.: Operant conditioning, hypnosis, and cognitive-behavioral therapy. Pain, *1*:23, 1982.
36. Sachs, L.B., Feuerstein, M., and Vitale, J.H.: Hypnotic self-regulation of chronic pain. Am. J. Clin. Hypn., *20*:106, 1977.
37. Erickson, M.H.: The interspersal hypnotic technique for symptom correction and pain control. *In* Psychological Approaches to the Management of Pain. Edited by J. Barber and C. Adrian. New York, Brunner/Mazel, 1982.
38. Diamond, M.J.: It takes two to tango: Some thoughts on the neglected importance of the hypnotist in an interactive hypnotherapeutic relationship. Am. J. Clin. Hypn., *27*:3 1984.
39. Koulouch, F.T.: Hypnosis and surgical convalescence: A study of subjective factors in postoperative recovery. Am. J. Clin. Hypn., *7*:120, 1964.
40. Pearson, R.E.: Responses to suggestions given under general anesthesia. Am. J. Clin. Hypn., *4*:106, 1961.
41. Crasilneck, H.B., Stirman, J.A., and Wilson, B.J.: Use of hypnosis in the management of patients with burns. JAMA, *158*:103, 1955.
42. Finer, B.L., and Nylen, B.O.: Cardiac arrest in the treatment of burns and report on hypnosis as a substitute for anesthesia. Plast. Reconst. Surg., *27*:49, 1961.
43. LaBaw, W.L.: Adjunctive trance therapy with severely burned children. Int. J. Child. Psychol., *2*:80, 1973.
44. Gottfredson, D.K.: Hypnosis as an anesthetic in dentistry. Diss. Abstr. Int. B, *33*(7):3303, 1973.
45. Davidson, J.A.: Assessment of the value of hypnosis in pregnancy and labor. Br. Med. J., *2*:951, 1962.
46. Rock, N., Shipley, T., and Campbell, C.: Hypnosis with untrained, nonvolunteer patients in labor. Int. J. Clin. Exp. Hypn., *17*:25, 1969.
47. Zeltzer, L., and LeBaron, S.: Hypnosis and nonhypnotic techniques for reduction of pain and anxiety during painful procedures in children and adolescents with cancer. J. Pediatr., *101*:1032, 1982.
48. Olness, K.: Imagery (self-hypnosis) as an adjunct therapy in childhood cancer: Clinical experience with 25 patients. Am. J. Pediatr. Hematol. Oncol., *3*:313, 1981.
49. Drummond, F.E.: Hypnosis in the treatment of headache: A review of the last ten years. J. Am. Soc. Psychosom. Dent. Med., *28*:87, 1981.
50. Cedercreutz, C., Lahteenmaki, R., and Tulikoura, J: Hypnotic treatment of headache and vertigo in skull injured patients. Int. J. Clin. Exp. Hypn., *24*:195, 1976.
51. Cedercreutz, C.: Hypnotic treatment of 100 cases of migraine. *In* Hypnosis at its Bicentennial. Edited by F.H. Frankel and H.S. Zamansky. New York, Plenum Press, 1978.
52. Olness, K., and McDonald, J.: Self-hypnosis and biofeedback in the management of juvenile migraine. Dev. Behav. Pediatr., *2*:168, 1981.
53. Crasilneck, H.B.: Hypnosis in the control of chronic low back pain. Am. J. Clin. Hypn., *22*:71, 1979.
54. McCauley, J.D., et al.: Hypnosis compared to relaxation in the outpatient management of chronic low back pain. Arch. Phys. Med. Rehabil., *64*:547, 1983.
55. Cedercreutz, C.: Hypnosis in surgery. Int. J. Clin. Exp. Hypn., *9*:93, 1961.

85 · RELAXATION TECHNIQUES

KAREN L. SYRJALA

ALTHOUGH relaxation techniques are rarely used on their own in the treatment of pain, they are a component of most psychology-based pain programs. Within such programs, relaxation is commonly used to disrupt the pain-dysfunction feedback loop by increasing patient control over general well-being, thereby decreasing the focus on pain, as well as the tension, anxiety, or depression related to pain. Relaxation has been effectively combined with other cognitive-behavior strategies, particularly distraction, in the treatment of chronic low back pain, cancer pain, rheumatoid arthritis, childbirth, and acutely painful procedures. Headache and temporomandibular joint (TMJ) pain have been treated successfully with relaxation alone.

Relaxation has three primary advantages over the similar but more complex techniques of biofeedback and hypnosis: (a) patients can be trained in the use of relaxation skills with relative ease; (b) no special equipment or extensive training of the therapist is required; and (c) patients readily accept relaxation techniques, whereas they are more likely to reject hypnosis (1).

In this chapter, I first discuss some basic considerations including a historical perspective of relaxation techniques, their physiologic effects, indications for use, and efficacy compared with hypnosis and biofeedback. Details on the implementation of the techniques are then presented, as well as possible complications that should be kept in mind. The final section is a brief review of the application and efficacy of relaxation techniques for specific pain syndromes. For further details on the application of specific approaches, the reader is referred to several textbooks (2–8). In addition, Bernstein and Borkovec (9) have written a manual for training professionals in progressive relaxation. A how-to handbook written for patients to use on their own is available (10) and can be used as a learning and guidance tool for practitioners as well. For more extensive reviews of research on relaxation with various pain problems, see the reviews by Turner and Romano (11) and Turner and Chapman (12).

BASIC CONSIDERATIONS

Historical Perspectives

Relaxation was conceived of in the 1930s as a technique for reducing tension and anxiety. Progressive muscle relaxation (PMR) was first introduced by Jacobson (2), who found that by extensive practice with systematic tensing and releasing of muscle groups, anxious patients could learn to discriminate the resulting sensations and produce an experience of deep relaxation. Wolpe (3) modified the procedure into a program that could be completed in six 20-min training sessions with twice daily home practice. He then incorporated relaxation into his systematic desensitization therapy for phobias, reasoning that relaxation would provide a response incompatible with fear. The relaxed state was paired with gradual exposure to the feared stimulus.

Autogenic training (AT) originated with a Berlin psychiatrist, Johannes H. Schultz, and was popularized in North America by Luthe (4). AT does not require tensing of muscles but instead consists of turning attention to each muscle group in turn, suggesting sensations of heaviness and warmth.

After progression through the muscle groups, attention is turned to slowing the heart rate, developing a regular respiration pattern, and finally regulating the viscera and cooling the forehead. The objective of AT is autonomic regulation as well as muscle relaxation. In its passive concentration, AT resembles meditation; in its use of suggestion, it resembles hypnosis without the hypnotherapist.

Benson (5) has described the relaxation response as a form of meditation without the religious or lifestyle connotations of transcendental meditation, Zen, or yoga. In the two most tested meditation strategies, the relaxation response and mindfulness meditation, patients are taught to empty the mind of extraneous thoughts and focus on a phrase or on a detached observation (6, 7).

Although relaxation began as a treatment for anxiety, from the time that behavioral and cognitive-behavioral psychologists began working with pain patients, relaxation techniques have been a key element of standard treatment (8). A sequential combination of PMR and AT is most frequently taught, with some use of deep breathing and guided imagery. Although not technically included in any of the original versions of relaxation already mentioned, deep breathing can be the first step toward helping patients focus attention before proceeding with further relaxation. Guided imagery, which serves as an effective distraction technique, can be critical to the success of relaxation as a pain relief tool.

Physiologic Responses

The mechanisms through which relaxation reduces pain are still under debate, except for consensus on the obvious mechanism of tension relief. Very little is known about brain physiologic changes in response to relaxation, but more is known about peripheral physiologic change. Even brief PMR training has produced significant reductions in heart rate, respiratory rate, and EMG forearm muscle tension (13). Furthermore, during relaxation, changes have been greater than those during hypnosis for systems not under voluntary control (e.g., heart rate and tonic muscle tension). Other documented physiologic responses to relaxation include decreases in oxygen consumption, blood pressure, and serum lactic acid levels, increases in skin resistance, and alterations in blood flow (14). Plasma norepinephrine levels have been found to either increase or not change following relaxation (15). These peripheral changes, which indicate a generalized decreased arousal of the sympathetic nervous system, have been hypothesized to be related to a decreased end-organ responsiveness to norepinephrine (14).

Increased electroencephalogram alpha and theta waves have been reported (14), but few other brain activity changes have been confirmed as responses to relaxation. One theory holds that relaxation and meditation result in a shift in hemispheric dominance with greater activation of centers in the right hemisphere (14).

Reduced sympathetic activity following relaxation does not fully explain the pain reductions found in a substantial number of conditions (11, 12, 16, 17). The reduction in reported pain appears directly due to muscle relaxation effects and decreased sympathetic arousal in tension headaches and TMJ pain, but altered blood flow may account for the effect with migraines, and cognitive distraction or hemispheric dominance changes may account for some of the pain relief reported for other acute and chronic pain conditions. A further, unproven hypothesis speculates that pain relief is a function of changes in catecholamines or endorphins.

Indications for Use

Relaxation is recommended in any condition where tension is the cause of pain or tension and fear may be augmenting the pain problem. In acute pain situations such as childbirth, trauma, or procedural pain, relaxation may be combined with medication and other distraction strategies (e.g., imagery or tasks requiring concentration). Relaxation is clearly indicated in the treatment of tension, migraine, and cluster headaches

and in TMJ pain. In other chronic conditions, meditation has been demonstrated to reduce pain (16). Turner (18) compared relaxation alone to relaxation plus other cognitive-behavioral therapy for chronic low back pain. Both groups of patients improved in pain levels. The cognitive-behavioral group improved somewhat more than the relaxation-alone group at 1 month but not at 2-year follow-up. Other studies support the use of relaxation as one component of effective cognitive-behavioral treatment for chronic pain (11, 17, 19).

Efficacy

Comparisons have been made between relaxation strategies and hypnosis or biofeedback, as well as between different relaxation techniques. Each of these techniques, including hypnosis and biofeedback, elicits similar physiologic responses and subjective reductions in pain when compared to no treatment (11, 12, 14, 17). In general, research results indicate that hypnosis, biofeedback, and audiotaped relaxation are less effective than live PMR in achieving reductions in sympathetic arousal (13, 20). An exception is frontalis EMG levels, which show greater reductions with autogenic relaxation than with tense-release relaxation although both approaches produce some decrease in EMG (21). This may be of some interest to practitioners choosing between relaxation techniques for the treatment of tension headache.

Much of the research on the effectiveness of relaxation training for pain reduction has been conducted with tension headache patients. This research supports the finding that relaxation is effective and that results are maintained at follow-up (11). Relaxation training alone appears to be a reasonable first step for headache sufferers, with the addition of biofeedback for those patients who are unsuccessful with relaxation alone (22). Similarly, research with TMJ pain patients suggests that many patients can be treated successfully with relaxation alone, although some may benefit from the addition of biofeedback (23). With other conditions, relaxation is best implemented as a component of a cognitive-behavioral treatment package. Further discussion of the efficacy of relaxation with specific conditions is presented in the "Clinical Applications" section later in this chapter.

SPECIFIC TECHNIQUES AND COMPLICATIONS

Preparation of the Patient

Relaxation may be learned and practiced by virtually anyone. The techniques can be taught after relatively limited training, but practitioners should be aware of and prepared to handle possible complications. Before relaxation training is begun, the practitioner should explain to pain patients the rationale for the particular procedure being used. Many patients view relaxation as irrelevant to their pain problem or even as an indication that the doctor thinks the pain is just tension or "all in my head." A brief discussion of the feedback loop between pain and tension or fear is helpful. Patients can also be told that relaxation training is harmless and, if nothing else, will leave the patient feel-

ing relaxed. The practitioner can then suggest that the procedure be tried as an "experiment," with nothing to lose. This approach is preferable to promising patients dramatic pain relief, since this rarely occurs initially. Patients also need to understand that the benefits of relaxation take time to reach their peak and that daily home practice is necessary to become adept at the procedure and to maintain benefits. Home practice is usually supported by use of audio tapes.

To prevent surprises and help patients feel secure, the practitioner should describe the basic steps involved in the technique and estimate the length of time required to complete it. Although increased comfort can be achieved in as little as 5 min, deep relaxation requires at least 20 min and may continue for up to 45 min. Patients ought to be advised that they will be asked to close their eyes, although this is not mandatory, and that they are free to move at any time to make themselves more comfortable. Use of a reclining chair with a head rest is desirable, but patients should not lie on a bed, because they are likely to fall asleep, unless the goal is rest for a sleep-deprived patient in pain.

Training Procedures

Deep breathing is the most rapidly learned of the relaxation techniques. Very little training is needed to obtain benefits. For patients in intense acute pain, deep breathing may be the most that they can accomplish. It also can be quite effective in capturing and holding a very distressed patient's attention and may be the first step toward using imagery to further distract the patient from the distress of the moment. No reports exist on the usefulness of deep breathing in isolation from other strategies for pain control, although it is a component of many relaxation procedures that have been researched. It is commonly used in childbirth preparation (19). Instructions for deep breathing are given in Table 85-1.

Progressive muscle relaxation is the most routine of the techniques. Since it requires the patient to tense and release muscle groups, it provides the most feedback to the practitioner (as well as the patient) on the participation of the patient. The tense–release format provides momentum from which the patient can achieve relaxation well below usual levels of tension relief. Table 85-2 provides an outline of PMR. Before implementing this technique with a patient, the practitioner is urged to read the manual by Bernstein and Borkovec (9) from which Table 85-2 is adapted.

Autogenic relaxation is similar to progressive muscle relaxation in that it progresses through the body, focusing attention on relaxing each area of the body in turn. Autogenics, however, does not require tensing muscles first. The focus is on imagining a feeling of warmth and heaviness in each area. Imagery may be inserted after completion of the relaxation phase or may be combined with the relaxation phrases. The training procedure is detailed in Table 85-3. This technique is useful with patients who are quite fatigued and in general discomfort (e.g., cancer patients). The imagery component may relate only to feelings of warmth, heaviness, and sensations that accompany relaxation or be augmented at length depending on the will and interest of patient and practitioner.

Imagery creates distraction as well as hypnosis-like experiences of comfort, well-being, and mastery of a problem. For instance, a patient can be asked to choose a place where he has felt relaxed and comfortable at a time when he was pain-free. As the patient recaptures the familiar experience of this place with all of the senses (sight, hearing, taste, smell, touch), he also recaptures the feeling of comfort. The practitioner then suggests to the patient that by imagining himself in that place, he can once again be comfortable and in control of his experience. An alternative imagery strategy is more akin to meditation. This approach involves focusing on the pain rather than away from it, and picturing details of the pain location (24). There is some indication that for more extreme, unremitting types of pain such as with terminal cancer, focusing on the pain rather than away from it is more effective in achieving pain reduction (25).

In execution, meditation most resembles deep breathing. Instead of focusing sequentially on each part of the body, meditation requires a cultivated "detached

TABLE 85-1. Instructions for Deep Breathing

I. Perform the following steps in sequence:*
   A. Deep breathing may be done in any position. If possible, sit, lie or stand comfortably, with a straight spine.
   B. Inhale through your nose while counting slowly to four.
   C. As you inhale,
      1. First fill the lower section of your lungs. Your diaphragm will push your abdomen outward to make room for the air.
      2. Second, fill the middle part of your lungs as your lower ribs and chest move forward to accomodate the air.
      3. Third, fill the upper part of your lungs as you raise your chest and shoulders slightly and draw your abdomen in a little to support your lungs.
      4. With practice, these three steps can be performed in one smooth, continuous inhalation.
   D. Hold your breath for a slow count of three.
   E. Exhale through your mouth, making a relaxing, whooshing sound like the wind as you blow out to a slow count of four.
   F. As you exhale, follow the same order as the inhalation:
      1. First, pull your abdomen in.
      2. Next, exhale from your middle chest.
      3. Finally, exhale from your upper chest as you allow your shoulders to sink and relax and your abdomen to puff out again slightly.

II. As the pattern becomes automatic, scan your body for other areas of tension, then return to the sound and feeling of breathing as you become more and more relaxed.

III. Continue deep breathing for 5 to 10 minutes at a time. If you become lightheaded at any point, alternate six regular breaths with six deep breaths.

IV. When you have learned to relax yourself using deep breathing, practice it whenever and wherever you feel yourself getting tense.

---

*Following the instructions provided results in the most complete relaxation, but the various steps can be shortened or adapted depending on the clinical situation.
Adapted from Davis, M., Eshelman, E.F., and McKay, M.: The Relaxation and Stress Reduction Workbook. Oakland, New Harbinger Publications, 1982.

TABLE 85-2. Progressive Muscle Relaxation Training Procedure

I. **Sequence of events**
   A. Attention is focused on each muscle group in turn.
   B. At a predetermined signal from the therapist, the muscle group is tensed.
   C. Tension is maintained for 5 to 7 seconds (this duration is shorter in the case of the feet).
   D. At a predetermined cue, the muscle group is released.
   E. Attention is maintained upon the muscle group as it relaxes.

II. **Introduction to the patient**
   Progressive relaxation training consists of learning to tense and release various muscle groups throughout the body. Learning relaxation skills is like learning other motor skills. I will not be doing anything to you; you will simply be learning a technique. We employ tension in order to ultimately produce relaxation. Strong tension is noticeable and you will learn to attend to these feelings. The initial production of tension gives us some "momentum" so that, when we release the tension, deep relaxation is the result.

III. **Tensing sequence and instructions**
   Sixteen muscle groups initially are tensed and relaxed. As the patient's skill develops, the number of groups is reduced. Before starting, determine which side is dominant. Instruct the patient to release tension immediately upon cue rather than gradually and to remove constraining items (e.g., watch, rings, eyeglasses, contact lenses, shoes). After the sequence is completed, respond to any questions and comments. Be sure to determine alternative tensing strategies when necessary.
   A. Arms and hands
      1. Dominant hand and lower arm (make a tight fist)
      2. Dominant biceps (push elbow down against chair)
      3. Nondominant hand and lower arm
      4. Nondominant biceps.
   B. Face and neck (model face-making to put patient at ease)
      1. Forehead (lift eyebrows as high as possible)
      2. Central section (squint and wrinkle nose)
      3. Lower face and jaw (bite hard and pull back corners of mouth)
      4. Neck (pull chin toward chest and keep it from touching chest)
   C. Chest and abdomen
      1. Chest, shoulders, and upper back (pull shoulder blades together)
      2. Abdomen (make stomach hard)
   D. Legs and feet
      1. Dominant upper leg (counterpose top and bottom muscles)
      2. Dominant calf (pull toes toward head)
      3. Dominant foot (point and curl toes, turning foot inward)
      4. Nondominant upper leg
      5. Nondominant calf
      6. Nondominant foot

IV. **Relaxation patter**
   Various statements may be inserted during the relaxation phase of the tense–release cycle to encourage relaxation. Vary the combination employed after each cycle, so that the patter does not become routine and predictable. The following are typical comments:
      . . . and relax, letting all the tension go
      . . . focusing on these muscles as they just relax completely, noticing what it feels like as the muscles become more and more relaxed
      . . . focusing all your attention on the feelings associated with relaxation flowing into these muscles
      . . . just enjoying the pleasant feelings of relaxation, as the muscles go on relaxing more and more deeply, more and more completely
      . . . nothing for you to do but focus your attention on the very pleasant feelings of relaxation flowing into this area, noticing what it's like as the muscles become more and more deeply relaxed
      . . . enjoying the feelings in the muscles as they loosen up, smooth out, unwind, and relax more and more deeply
      . . . letting those muscles go and noticing how they feel now as compared to before
      . . . notice how those muscles feel when so completely relaxed
      . . . pay attention only to the sensations of relaxation as the relaxation process takes place
      . . . calm, peaceful and relaxed

Adapted from Bernstein, D.A., and Borkovec, T.D.: Progressive Relaxation Training: A Manual for the Helping Professions. Champaign, Illinois, Research Press, 1973. Reprinted with permission.

observation" (16). Two similar approaches to meditation have been useful in medical settings. One involves repeating a phrase or word to oneself and is referred to as the *relaxation response* (5); the other is called *mindfulness meditation* (7). Mindfulness meditation is similar to the imagery approaches that focuses on the pain (24). Attention is focused not on changing pain perception but on insight developed from distinguishing the sensations as they occur moment by moment.

Thoughts about pain are also observed from the position of a neutral observer. Although relaxation response training is easy to implement, few data exist on its effectiveness as a pain reduction method. Mindfulness meditation has been shown to reduce pain in chronic pain patients (7, 16), but an experienced practitioner is recommended as a trainer. Instructions for relaxation response meditation are given in Table 85-4.

TABLE 85-3. Autogenic Training Procedure

I. **Posture instructions** (patient should assume one of three possible postures.)
    A. Sit in an armchair with your head, back, and extremities comfortably supported.
    B. Sit on a stool, chair, or the floor, slightly stooped over, with your arms resting on your thighs and your hands draped on or between your knees.
    C. Lie down with your head and body supported, your legs about 8 inches apart and your arms resting comfortably at your sides without touching them.
    D. Scan your body to be sure that the position you choose is tension free. In particular, look for overextension of limbs such as unsupported arms, head, or legs, tightening of the limbs at the joints, or crooked spine.

II. **Reassurance comments**
    A. You will not be able to maintain perfect passive concentration at first. Your mind will wander. That's okay. When you find this happening, just get back to the verbal formula as soon as possible.
    B. You may experience some initial symptoms described as "autogenic discharges." These are normal but distracting. These discharges are usually in the form of sensations, which may be pleasant or unpleasant. Remember that they are transitory and will pass as you continue with the exercise.

III. **Use of verbal formulas**
    A. General instructions
      1. Repeat the verbal formulas for 10 to 30 minutes a day. The pace should be slow and regular with pauses to allow time to notice changes in sensation or to follow images.
      2. To give added sensation of heaviness, you might imagine weights attached to your arms and legs, gently pulling them down.
      3. To imagine warmth, visualize yourself in a warm bath or shower, feeling the warmth of the water all around you. If you prefer, see yourself in the sunshine, feeling the warmth of the sun being absorbed into your skin and relaxing your entire body.
      4. Repeat the verbal statements several times before moving on to further imagery.
    B. Sample statements
      1. My right arm is heavy and warm.
      2. My left arm is heavy and warm.
      3. Both of my arms are heavy and warm. I can feel the warmth of the sun (water) on them.
      4. My right leg is heavy and warm
      5. My left leg is heavy and warm.
      6. Both of my legs are heavy and warm.
      7. I can feel the warmth of the sun (water) being absorbed into them.
      8. My arms and legs are heavy and warm.
      9. My heartbeat is calm and regular.
     10. It breathes me.
     11. I feel quiet.
     12. My whole body feels quiet, heavy, comfortable and relaxed.
     13. My mind is quiet. Deep in my mind I can visualize and experience myself as relaxed, comfortable, and still.

IV. **Imagery instructions**
    A. Imagine yourself in the place you would most enjoy being right now. This may be a place where you feel most comfortable and relaxed; it may even include an activity you enjoy doing; if you like, it may be a place in your imagination. Picture yourself in that place.
    B. Concentrate on the details of sight. What are the shapes around you? What are the colors? Notice the different shades of color.
    C. Notice the temperature. Does it feel warm against your skin? Continue to absorb that feeling of warmth, letting yourself soak up that warmth as you relax more and more.
    D. Perhaps you would like to reach out and touch something in that place, just observing how it feels in your hand, whether it is smooth and soft, curved, rough; just notice the texture and feel of it.
    E. Notice as much as you can about the place that you are in. You may even find a few surprises. Notice if there is any movement. Is anyone else in that place with you? Just observe and listen; notice the sounds.
    F. At any time, if there is anything you would like to change, you can do that too. Just observe, and if you would like to change anything, go ahead. Do whatever you would like to help yourself be as comfortable and relaxed as you would like right now.
    G. Observe yourself in that place, feeling comfortable and relaxed.

V. **Concluding instructions**
    A. Continue at your own pace, with as much repetition and imagery as you like.
    B. When you are ready to stop, say to yourself, "When I open my eyes, I will feel refreshed and alert." Then open your eyes; breathe a few deep breaths as you stretch and flex your arms and shoulders.
    C. Be sure that you are fully alert and attentive to your environment before you go on to your regular activities.

Adapted from Davis, M., Eshelman, E.F., and McKay, M.: The Relaxation and Stress Reduction Workbook. Oakland, New Harbinger Publications, 1982.

Complications

Minor Problems

One of the advantages of relaxation techniques in comparison with more invasive therapies is the lack of lasting adverse side effects. Most complications are rare, harmless, and can be handled with quick, matter-of-fact resolution of the problem. Muscle cramps can develop with PMR, in which case the patient can be asked to generate less tension in problem areas for shorter periods of time. If necessary, a pause can be taken while cramped muscles are massaged by the patient. Movements are not uncommon but are generally discouraged unless they involve brief shifts to a more comfortable position. Talking or laughter can usually be stopped by simply ignoring it. Unless the patient comments, spasms should simply be ignored. Patients can be reassured that muscle spasms are common when

TABLE 85-4. Instructions for Relaxation Response Meditation

1. Pick a focus word or phrase that is rooted in your personal belief system.
2. Sit quietly in a comfortable position.
3. Close your eyes.
4. Relax your muscles.
5. Become aware of your breathing, and breathe very slowly and naturally. Simultaneously, repeat your focus word or phrase as you exhale. Use one word or phrase during your sessions so that you'll automatically come to associate it with the calming effect of the relaxation response.
6. Assume a passive attitude, and if other thoughts intrude in your mind, gently disregard them.
7. Continue for 10 to 20 minutes.
8. Practice the technique once or twice daily.

From Benson, H., and Proctor, W.: Beyond the Relaxation Response: How to Harness the Healing Power of Your Personal Beliefs. New York, New York Times Book Co., 1984.

people relax and occur in many people when they fall asleep. Because some patients experience intrusive thoughts as disruptive, they should be told ahead of time that such thoughts are to be expected. Suggesting that attention be gently returned to the relaxation or meditation is usually adequate. If a patient falls asleep, the therapist might need to speak in a progressively louder voice until the patient is again awake. Patients who report falling asleep regularly during home practice should be instructed to practice earlier in the day and in a sitting position.

When only very brief training is possible before a medical procedure such as surgery, some have recommended that relaxation be used only with patients who have "sensitizing" coping styles, that is, those who prefer information (26, 27). Avoiders appear to make less successful use of the techniques for pain relief; avoiders do not report negative effects but merely fewer positive effects.

Problems Requiring Attention

Problems toward which the therapist must be more careful and attentive are infrequently reported. For certain patients, tension or pain can be localized in an area not sufficiently covered by the standard procedures. If residual tension remains, it is acceptable to develop a tension or relaxation strategy that specifically targets the localized area. Pain patients commonly have an initially greater awareness of the pain as attention is focused on internal states. In this case, patients can be instructed either to observe the pain in a detached manner (usually the intensity will lessen) or to move attention to another part of the body.

Patients who have been particularly out of touch with body sensations can suddenly become aware of any number or type of strange, unfamiliar sensations while relaxing and focusing on the body. Patients might feel like they are floating and disoriented to such an extent that they must open their eyes until they once again feel comfortable. If this sensation or others are frightening, the practitioner will need to respond with reassurance. Other discomforting sensations can include tingling, nausea, lightheadedness, or a sense of losing control. Caution and a slower progression in learning should be exercised with patients who report fear of losing control. Sexual arousal can also occur from the relaxation and perceived seduction of the setting. If treated matter-of-factly as similar to other normal intrusive thoughts, this usually resolves (9).

An increase in anxiety has been reported in some patients learning relaxation (28). Switching to a different relaxation that more fully occupies the patient's attention may help reduce such anxiety. Discussion of the nature of the anxiety may reveal an alternative set of thoughts or images that can provide a more neutral focal point for the patient.

Failure to practice is by far the most common problem encountered in relaxation training. The practitioner can remind the patient of other learning experiences such as reading or swimming in which practice led to mastery. Discussion of changes in the home environment that would assist practice may also be helpful. Above all, the practitioner must insist that practice is an important element of learning and using any relaxation technique successfully.

CLINICAL APPLICATIONS

Chronic Conditions

Even though relaxation is most often used as one element in a set of cognitive-behavioral treatments for chronic pain rather than as an independent pain control technique, research indicates that it can contribute to reduced pain levels and medication use as well as increased functioning in a number of chronic conditions. A thorough review of the effectiveness of cognitive-behavioral strategies that include relaxation is presented by Turner and Romano (11) and in Chapter 82 of this book.

Kabat-Zinn (7, 16) used mindfulness meditation to successfully treat a variety of chronic problems including pain located in the low back, neck, shoulder, arm, leg, face, head, chest, peripheral nerves, and multiple sites. Of the 80 to 90% of patients willing to enter the training program, 80 to 90% completed the program. A majority (72%) of the patients were able to reduce their pain by 33% or more. In addition, improvement was noted in body image, activity, mood disturbance, and medication use. Compliance both during and after participation in the program was reported to be high. These results support the contention that meditation may have a generalized beneficial effect for chronic pain patients. Although Benson (5) proposed a single mechanism of effect for all the relaxation techniques, which he calls the relaxation response, it is useful to look at the effect of individual approaches with different pain syndromes.

Headache

By far the largest body of research on relaxation has focused on headache. Tension headache research dominates the literature and generally reveals relaxation to be as effective or more effective than biofeedback (11, 12, 29, 31). The same results have been found with migraine headache, although fewer studies are available. The most careful explorations into the relative roles of relaxation and biofeedback in relieving headache have been reported by Blanchard et al. (22, 29, 30) and Andrasik et al. (33). In terms of both cost-effectiveness and success, the optimal therapy for tension, migraine, or mixed tension and migraine pain appears to be a two-step treatment beginning with PMR. For those patients who do not show substantial reduction in headache activity with PMR, the second step is instituted. For vascular headache patients, the second step is thermal biofeedback; for tension headache patients, frontalis EMG biofeedback is the second step. Blanchard et al. (32) found that with this two-step therapy 73% of tension headache patients and 52% of vascular headache patients were much improved. All groups improved with relaxation, with the tension headache patients improving the most. Among those patients who received biofeedback, the vascular headache patients responded most favorably.

Philips and Hunter (34) tested the effects of PMR versus PMR with calming imagery for tension headache patients. The two groups showed similar improvements in pain. The authors suggested that the addition of imagery produced a larger improvement in pain based on several outcome measures even though no individual measure showed significant superior effects.

The superiority or equivalence of relaxation and biofeedback has not been supported by all research. LaCroix et al. (35), for instance, found that thermal biofeedback was superior to frontalis EMG feedback and relaxation for migraine patients although all groups improved. In regard to home practice, Andrasik et al. (33) reported that post-treatment practice was unrelated to maintenance of effects; it should be noted, however, that all patients in this study were provided with regular contact.

Temporomandibular Joint Pain

The rather limited research on relaxation for TMJ pain supports the conclusion that relaxation is effective in reducing pain and is at least as successful as biofeedback, the most commonly compared treatment. Funch and Gale (23) reported that biofeedback and audiotaped relaxation training were equally effective in reducing TMJ pain. Patients who were more successful with relaxation were generally younger, had experienced TMJ pain for a shorter period of time, and reported other psychophysiologic disorders. Patients who were more successful with biofeedback tended to be older, married, and had experienced pain for a longer period of time. The differential effect of relaxation and biofeedback with different patients also was found in a single-subject, multiple-baseline study by Moss et al. (36). In this study, relaxation with EMG feedback was most effective for three out of four patients tested.

Low Back Pain

The few studies available comparing relaxation with other techniques for low back pain indicate that relaxation is an effective treatment but that combining relaxation with other cognitive-behavioral strategies may be advantageous. Turner (18) compared PMR treatment with PMR plus additional cognitive-behavioral therapy or no treatment. The two treatment groups both reported reduced pain intensity and disability immediately following treatment and at 1.5- and 2-year follow-up. The cognitive-behavioral group, however, showed some superiority in maintaining treatment gains and in hours worked per week. McCauley et al. (37) compared PMR with hypnosis in the treatment of low back pain and found that both treatments were similarly effective and superior to a placebo EMG treatment. Sanders (38) compared single sessions of PMR, assertion training, reinforcement of activity, and "functional pain-behavioral analysis training" in four low back pain patients. With the exception of functional analysis, each treatment differentially affected medication use, pain ratings, and uptime.

More research is needed on the relationship of component interventions to specific outcomes in the low back pain patient, even though these studies suggest that relaxation makes some contribution to favorable outcomes.

Cancer Pain

Cancer patients may experience acute procedure-related pain or chronic tumor-related pain. The chronic pain may be stable (e.g., postmastectomy pain) or progressive (e.g., tumor invasion pain). Successful treatment depends to some extent on tailoring therapy to the type of pain. In clinical reports, relaxation with guided imagery, sometimes called hypnosis, is touted (39, 40). However, there is little controlled research on the efficacy of relaxation and imagery with adult cancer patients. As noted by Jay et al. (41), research on adult cancer patients has focused on chronic pain, while research on children with cancer has focused on acute procedural pain. Although most imagery interventions can be considered either relaxation with imagery or hypnosis, most researchers have chosen to call their interventions hypnosis. This may change in view of recent research demonstrating that patients are less fearful and more willing to participate in the same treatment when it is called relaxation than when it is called hypnosis (1).

Spiegel and Bloom (42) provided group self-hypnosis training to breast cancer patients and reported an additive analgesic effect of hypnosis, with smaller increases in pain and suffering over time. Syrjala et al. (43) provided three groups of bone marrow transplant patients with training in relaxation and imagery (termed hypnosis), cognitive-behavioral training including PMR, or support with no training. The group receiving imagery reported lower average levels of oral pain following chemoradiotherapy than the other two groups. The limited data currently available suggest both the need for further controlled research and the possible important role of imagery in helping cancer patients cope with pain.

Acute Conditions

Childbirth

Preparation for childbirth, which is now quite common, usually includes breathing exercises with a visual focus and sometimes includes formal relaxation training. As Tan (19) noted in his review, studies on the effectiveness of these strategies in reducing pain in childbirth are supportive but not unequivocal. Many of these studies do not include actual measures of pain levels in reporting favorable outcomes. Laboratory research has suggested that the attention-focusing component of preparation is more effective in reducing pain than is relaxation training (44), and that sensory transformation coping strategies are more effective than relaxation (45). Despite the equivocal data on pain reduction associated with childbirth preparation, the reduced distress resulting from such programs probably supports their continued use.

Acute Traumatic, Procedural, and Postoperative Pain

A number of sources confirm the benefits of relaxation training before various procedures and surgery. Only anecdotal evidence was found for the use of deep breathing, relaxation, and imagery during acute trauma. This is a difficult area to research because of the unpredictable availability of subjects and the wide variety of possible injuries. Thus, support for the use of these strategies in trauma situations must be extrapolated from research on other acute pain conditions

Relaxation training before stressful procedures has been shown to be effective in reducing a number of measures of pain and distress. For example, patients trained in PMR and deep breathing before sigmoidoscopy rated themselves as less anxious and made fewer requests to stop the procedure than patients who were not trained in relaxation (46). Both relaxation and information have been reported to reduce heart rate and observer ratings of distress during endoscopy; only relaxation also increased positive mood (27).

Laboratory and clinical studies have found that the effectiveness of relaxation training in acute situations may depend on the coping style of the patient. In the laboratory, it has been reported that patients who were more external in their "locus of control" were better able to use relaxation training than were patients who were more internal, that is, saw themselves as the agent of control (47). During procedural discomfort, patients who reported that they preferred to avoid thinking about unpleasant things were helped more by relaxation than by information, whereas the reverse was true of the nonavoiders (27). In addition, patients who indicated that they were less independent benefited from both relaxation and information, while those who were more independent benefited from neither. Relaxation and information were not demonstrated to be harmful to patients who were not matched on intervention and coping style. Finally, with postoperative patients, Scott and Clum (26) found that brief relaxation training was profitable for those who had "sensitizing" coping styles, but not for those who were avoiders.

Applications with Children

Research on the use of relaxation techniques with children is far less extensive and well controlled than the research with adults. A review of painful pediatric conditions and the interventions that have been successful is provided by Lavigne et al. (48). The terminology used in much of the published research is inconsistent. For example, treatments that include active fantasy, guided imagery, breathing, and relaxation are interchangeably defined as "hypnosis," "relaxation," or "imagery."

With pediatric cancer patients, interventions for pain have focused on procedure-related distress. Effective treatments have included breathing and imagery, sometimes incorporated into a cognitive-behavioral package (41). Distraction and breathing exercises have received some support as useful techniques for relieving pain during debridement for pediatric burn patients (48). A number of case studies suggest that relaxation, particularly if coupled with imagery, can be effective in treating other pediatric pain problems. For instance, Varni et al. (49) reported the successful use of relaxation and breathing to increase pain control in a 9-year-old child with hemophilia. As with research involving adults, controlled relaxation studies involving children are mostly concerned with headache. Unlike relaxation research with adults, which has focused on tension headache, child research has focused on autogenic relaxation for migraine. This research clearly supports the use of autogenics for relief of migraine in younger populations (48).

Since children are usually easily engaged in active imagery, this component can be successfully introduced into most interventions with children in pain. Clinicians interested in the use of imagery are referred to the literature on hypnosis, as most researchers using imagery with children have termed their interventions "hypnosis."

SUMMARY

In conclusion, relaxation techniques—including progressive muscle relaxation, autogenic training, deep breathing, and meditation—can be valuable in the treatment of both acute and chronic pain syndromes. The advantages of relaxation include its relative cost-effectiveness and lack of lasting harmful side effects. Although the specific physiologic mechanisms through which relaxation reduces pain have not been proven, relaxation reduces muscle tension, quiets the sympathetic nervous system, and provides a cognitive distraction from distress.

For headache and TMJ pain, relaxation appears to be the first treatment of choice, with biofeedback instituted for those patients who do not benefit from relaxation. For other chronic conditions, relaxation seems to be as effective as biofeedback. Similarly, relaxation with imagery is difficult to distinguish from hypnosis either in procedure or in effect. With acute pain, relaxation is reported to be as effective as other cognitive-behavioral approaches that have been studied. With chronic pain, there is evidence that relaxation diminishes pain, but a package of cognitive-behavioral training that includes relaxation may be more effective. For children, relaxation with imagery has been shown to be very effective in reducing pain and distress, particularly in acute conditions. Further research is needed into the effectiveness of relaxation techniques with adults in acute pain and with children in chronic pain.

REFERENCES

1. Hendler, C.S., and Redd, W.H.: Fear of hypnosis: The role of labeling in patient's acceptance of behavioral interventions. Behav. Ther., 17:2, 1986.
2. Jacobson, E.: Progressive Relaxation. Chicago, Univ. of Chicago Press, Midway Reprint, 1974.
3. Wolpe, J.: The Practice of Behavior Therapy. New York, Pergamon, 1969.
4. Luthe, W.: Autogenic training: Method, research and application in medicine. Am. J. Psychother., 17:174, 1963.
5. Benson, H.: The Relaxation Response. New York, Academic Press, 1975.
6. Benson, H., and Proctor, W.: Beyond the Relaxation Response: How to Harness the Healing Power of Your Personal Beliefs. New York, New York Times Book Co., 1984.
7. Kabat-Zinn, J.: An outpatient program in behavioral medicine for chronic pain patients based on the practice of mindfulness meditation: Theoretical considerations and preliminary results. Gen. Hosp. Psychiatry., 4:33, 1982.
8. Turk, D.C., Meichenbaum, D., and Genest, M.: Pain and Behavioral Medicine: A Cognitive Behavioral Perspective. New York, Guilford Press, 1983.
9. Bernstein, D.A., and Borkovec, T.D.: Progressive Relaxation Training: A Manual for the Helping Professions. Champaign, IL, Research Press, 1973.
10. Davis, M., Eshelman, E.F., and McKay, M.: The Relaxation and Stress Reduction Workbook. Oakland, New Harbinger Pub., 1982.
11. Turner, J.A., and Romano, J.M.: Evaluating psychological interventions for chronic pain: Issues and recent developments. In Advances in Pain Research and Therapy. Vol. 7. Edited by C. Benedetti, C.R. Chapman, and G. Moricca. New York, Raven Press, 1984.
12. Turner, J.A., and Chapman, C.R.: Psychological interventions for chronic pain: A critical review. I. Relaxation training and biofeedback. Pain, 12:1, 1982.
13. Paul, G.L.: Physiological effects of relaxation training and hypnotic suggestion. J. Abnorm. Psychol., 74:425, 1969.
14. Kutz, I., Borysenko, J.Z., and Benson, H.: Meditation and psychotherapy: A rationale for the integration of dynamic psychotherapy, the relaxation response, and mindfulness meditation. Am. J. Psychiatry, 142:1, 1985.
15. Hoffman, J.W., et al.: Reduced sympathetic nervous system responsivity associated with the relaxation response. Science, 215:190, 1982.
16. Kabat-Zinn, J., Lipworth, L., and Burney, R.: The clinical use of mindfulness meditation for the self-regulation of chronic pain. J. Behav. Med., 8:163, 1985.
17. Turner, J.A., and Chapman, C.R.: Psychological interventions for chronic pain: A critical review. II. Operant conditioning, hypnosis, and cognitive-behavioral therapy. Pain, 12:23, 1982.
18. Turner, J.A.: Comparison of group progressive-relaxation training and cognitive-behavioral group therapy for chronic low back pain. J. Consult. Clin. Psychol., 50:757, 1982.
19. Tan, S.: Cognitive and cognitive-behavioral methods for pain control: A selected review. Pain, 12:201, 1982.
20. Lehrer, P.M.: How to relax and how not to relax: A re-evaluation of the work of Edmund Jacobson—I. Behav. Res. Ther., 20:417, 1982.
21. Haynes, S., Mosely, D., and McGowan, W.: Relaxation and biofeedback training in the reduction of frontalis muscle tension. Psychophysiology, 12:547, 1975b.
22. Blanchard, E.B., et al.: Sequential comparisons of relaxation training and biofeedback in the treatment of three kinds of chronic headache or, the machines may be necessary some of the time. Behav. Res. Ther., 20:469, 1982.
23. Funch, D.P., and Gale, E.N.: Biofeedback and relaxation therapy for chronic temporomandibular joint pain: Predicting successful outcomes. J. Consult. Clin. Psychol., 52:928, 1984.
24. Levine, S.: Who Dies? An Investigation of Conscious Living and Conscious Dying. Garden City, Anchor Press, 1982.
25. McCaul, K.D., and Malott, J.M.: Distraction and coping with pain. Psychol. Bull., 95:516, 1984.
26. Scott, L.E., and Clum, G.A.: Examining the interaction effects of coping style and brief interventions in the treatment of postsurgical pain. Pain, 20:279, 1984.
27. Wilson, J.F., Moore, R.W., Randolph, S., and Hanson, B.J.: Behavioral preparation of patients for gastrointestinal endoscopy: Information, relaxation, and coping style. J. Human Stress, 8:13, 1982.
28. Heide, F.J., and Borkovec, T.D.: Relaxation-induced anxiety: Paradoxical anxiety enhancement due to relaxation training. J. Consult. Clin. Psychol., 51:171, 1983.
29. Blanchard, E.B., et al.: Migraine and tension headache: A meta-analytic review. Behav. Ther., 11:613, 1980.
30. Blanchard, E.B., Andrasik, F., and Silver, V.B.: Biofeedback and relaxation in the treatment of tension headaches: A reply to Belar. J. Behav. Med., 3:22, 1980.
31. Blanchard, E.B., and Andrasik, F.: Psychological assessment and treatment of headache: Recent developments and emerging issues. J. Consult. Clin. Psychol., 50:859, 1982.
32. Blanchard, E.B., et al.: Biofeedback and relaxation training with three kinds of headache: Treatment effects and their prediction. J. Consult. Clin. Psychol., 50:562, 1982.
33. Andrasik, F., Blanchard, E.B., and Neff, D.F.: Biofeedback and relaxation training for chronic headache: A controlled comparison of booster treatments and regular contacts for long-term maintenance. J. Consult. Clin. Psychol., 52:609, 1984.
34. Philips, C., and Hunter, M.: The treatment of tension headache. II. EMG "normality" and relaxation. Behav. Res. Ther., 19:499, 1981.
35. LaCroix, J.M., et al.: Biofeedback and relaxation in the treatment of migraine headaches: Comparative effectiveness and physiological correlates. J. Neurol. Neurosurg. Psychiatry, 46:525, 1983.
36. Moss, R.A., Wedding, D., and Sanders, S.H.: The comparative efficacy of relaxation training and masseter EMG feedback in the treatment of TMJ dysfunction. J. Oral Rehabil., 10:9, 1983.
37. McCauley, J.D., et al.: Hypnosis compared to relaxation in the outpatient management of chronic low back pain. Arch. Phys. Med. Rehabil., 64:548, 1983.
38. Sanders, S.H.: A component analysis of behavioral methods used in the treatment of chronic pain patients. Poster session presented at annual meeting of Assoc. Adv. Behav. Ther., 1982, Los Angeles.
39. Margolis, C.G.: Hypnotic imagery with cancer patients. Am. J. Clin. Hypn., 25:128, 1982.
40. Donovan, M.I.: Relaxation with guided imagery: A useful technique. Cancer Nurs. (February):27, 1980.
41. Jay, S.M., Elliot, C., and Varni, J.W.: Acute and chronic pain in adults and children with cancer. J. Consult. Clin. Psychol., 54:601, 1986.
42. Spiegel, D., and Bloom, J.R.: Group therapy and hypnosis reduce metastatic breast carcinoma pain. Psychosom. Med., 45:333, 1983.
43. Syrjala, K.L., Cummings, C., Donaldson, G., and Chapman, C.R.: Hypnosis for oral pain following chemotherapy and irradiation. Paper presented at the 5th World Congress of the Int. Assoc. for the Study of Pain, August, 1987, Hamburg, Germany.
44. Wideman, M.V., and Singer, J.E.: The role of psychological mechanisms in preparation for childbirth. Am. Psychol., 39:1357, 1984.
45. Geden, E., Beck, N., Hauge, G., and Pohlman, S.: Self-report and psychophysiological effects of five pain-coping strategies. Nurs. Res., 33:260, 1984.
46. Kaplan, R.M., Atkins, C.J., and Lenhard, L.: Coping with a stressful sigmoidoscopy: Evaluation of cognitive and relaxation preparations. J. Behav. Med., 5:67, 1982.
47. Clum, G.A., Luscomb, R.L., and Scott, L.: Relaxation training and cognitive redirection strategies in the treatment of acute pain. Pain, 12:175, 1982.
48. Lavigne, J.V., Schulein, M.J., and Hahn, Y.S.: Psychological aspects of painful medical conditions in children. II. Personality factors, family characteristics and treatment. Pain, 27:147, 1986.
49. Varni, J.W., Gilbert, A., and Dietrich, S.L.: Behavioral medicine in pain and analgesia management for the hemophiliac child with factor VIII inhibitor. Pain, 11:121, 1981.

86 · PSYCHOTHERAPY IN THE MANAGEMENT OF CHRONIC PAIN

ELDON R. TUNKS *and* HAROLD MERSKEY

PSYCHOTHERAPY has been defined as any form of treatment for mental illness, behavioral maladaptations, and other problems assumed to be of an emotional nature in which a therapist deliberately establishes a professional relationship with a patient for the purposes of removing, modifying, or retarding existing symptoms, or attenuating or reversing disturbed patterns of behavior, and of promoting positive personality growth and development (1). The relationship between the therapist and patient is an essential component of psychotherapy and can be summed up as follows (2, p. 28):

1. The doctor or therapist is concerned with the emotional problems of the patient.
2. He or she is able to relinquish the doctor's traditional controlling role.

3. He or she has the capacity to reflect upon the emotional interaction between the patient and himself or herself and the courage to comment on it in order to promote insight and change.

The material in this chapter is presented in two major sections: A, Basic Considerations, including a brief overview of the effectiveness of various psychotherapies, indications for their use with chronic pain patients, and factors influencing their success, and B, Clinical Applications. This section describes and evaluates the main types of psychotherapy used in the management of patients with chronic pain. These include supportive, dynamic, family, and group psychotherapy. More detailed discussion of these and other topics related to psychotherapy can be found in several books on the subject (3–8).

A. BASIC CONSIDERATIONS

Efficacy of Psychotherapy

Although an extensive literature exists concerning psychotherapy and its effectiveness, assessing the efficacy of psychotherapy is difficult because of the plethora of psychotherapies and theoretical models and the large "relationship aspect" of the psychotherapeutic situation. The most extensive review available of the methodologic and efficacy issues in psychotherapy (9) noted that the problem of defining and measuring effectiveness in psychotherapy plagues all schools of psychologic treatment, whether they be behavioral, dynamic, group, milieu, or any other type. What can be demonstrated is that different psychotherapies appear to be effective for different purposes, and that psychotherapy is clearly better than no psychotherapy or placebo treatment. The most significant problems in evaluating psychotherapeutic efficacy relate to three major issues:

1. Outcome measures are usually not built in to the therapeutic technique, with the exception of some of the newer behavioral and cognitive-behavioral therapies.
2. The treatment relationship is fundamental and not easily quantified either in its degree of formation or in its impact.
3. Therapeutic outcome involves intangible variables, including improvement in sense of self, satisfaction, and reduction in subjective distress, that are very difficult to measure and even more difficult to compare.

Each of the two major types of psychologic treatment—behavioral therapy and insight-oriented psychotherapy—deals with an essential part of the individual. Behavioral therapies focus on an individual's actions, including his adaptive and healthy behaviors as well as those that relate to his illness and maintain his distress. It is reasonable to believe that a change in behavior will affect the experience of self and of illness. On the other hand, insight psychotherapy is valued by persons who experience subjective distress (e.g., anxiety, depression, insecurity, and worry about troubled relationships) and who perceive themselves as "ill." They want to have these feelings recognized and, at times, need to work with the therapist specifically on their understanding of meaningfulness, on attitudes, relationships, and goals, as a springboard to making change. To help patients in a truly compassionate way, the therapist must consider both behavior and feelings. Therefore, neither the behavioral therapies nor the psychotherapies can stand completely on their own. Each is complementary to the whole business of helping, and in fact, good psychotherapists and good behavioral therapists resemble each other in the actual way that they carry on their work, whatever their theoretical leaning.

Indications for Psychotherapy with Pain Patients

The use of psychotherapy with chronic pain patients must be assessed with care. A psychotherapeutic approach that may be quite suitable and helpful for neurotic outpatients in a psychiatry department may be totally inappropriate and unworkable with patients with chronic pain. One of the special features of pain patients is that they suffer from a subjective state, which has been defined as "an unpleasant sensory and emotional experience associated with actual or potential tissue damage or described in terms of such damage" (10). Chronic pain is probably the outstanding example of such a subjective condition, which can result either from physical or from psychologic causes or from both. In theory, any treatment that might improve the subjective state could be considered for a patient in pain, whatever the initial cause. In practice, psychotherapy for pain is indicated in three situations or conditions:

1. Psychotherapy is appropriate when much or all of the pain seems to follow from a psychologic disorder without a major physical contribution. Not many such cases, however, are susceptible to symptom relief through psychotherapy alone. Indeed, in many cases of pain associated with depression, antidepressant medication is more effective than psychotherapy.

There is clear evidence that chronic pain patients who attend clinics have a higher loading of psychosocial risk factors (e.g., litigation, emotional impairment, poor work history, interference with daily activity by the pain problem, and an increased tendency to use health care resources) than others (11, 12). In these patients, the medical disorder is not the sole issue; they also have significant problems of dissatisfaction and emotional adjustment, for which psychotherapy is potentially relevant. With such patients, psychotherapy may not provide significant symptomatic relief for the pain itself, but it aids the individual in adjusting his human relationships, aims, sense of self, and goals.

2. Patients with prolonged and severe physical illness, but without evidence of premorbid predisposition to psychologic illness, may develop emotional changes in response to suffering. For them, too, some forms of psychotherapy can be a useful part of treatment. (See "Supportive Psychotherapy" discussed later).

3. Psychotherapy has long been recognized as a tool for helping people to make adjustments in their lives as well as to relieve them of symptoms. Where the goal is to alter human relationships and behaviors, either psychotherapy or behavior therapy, or both, may make a contribution. Where the aim is primarily to change subjective distress related to relationships, conflicts, and the sense of self, psychotherapy is the treatment of choice.

Factors Affecting Psychotherapeutic Outcome

In psychotherapy for people with chronic pain, the requisites for success include certain nonspecific factors found in any psychologically oriented therapy and other factors that specifically relate to the chronic pain condition.

Nonspecific Factors

The nonspecific factors essential for success with any type of psychologic therapy include the following:

1. The therapist and patient must be in therapeutic contact.
2. A consistent therapeutic rationale must unite patient and therapist.
3. Mutually agreed-upon therapeutic goals must be established.
4. There is an agreed focus for treatment.
5. Structured therapeutic exercises that provide opportunities for new learning are provided.
6. There must be active participation by the motivated patient.
7. Successful experiences leading to a sense of mastery are promoted.
8. Opportunities for application of the new learning to problem areas are created.
9. A therapeutic relationship that acts as the context for this process exists.

For additional discussion, see Rogers (13), Marmor (14), and Frank et al. (15).

Factors Specific to Chronic Pain Patients

In dealing with chronic pain patients, the psychotherapist must be aware of several other requisites for success:

1. The need to deal with a multidisciplinary setting and to appreciate the problems of colleagues who are not psychiatrists or psychologists in handling patients who have a combination of physical and psychologic disorders.
2. The need to look not only at the patient but also at the significance of his or her symptoms in his or her environment, whether at home or at work.
3. The need for an extra degree of tolerance for negative attitudes of patients who are not "psychologically minded" or willing to look at their symptoms and difficulties in terms of emotional issues.
4. A greater need for flexibility in therapeutic methods.
5. A readiness to discover and accept the patient's goals and needs.
6. A willingness to assume the role of tutor or guide or even broker rather than the more traditional role of impartial therapist.
7. The need for clearly defined goal-oriented methods in therapy.

In terms of the last requirement, much can be learned from behaviorists. Their approach involves offering clear definitions of therapeutic steps and clear descriptions of how those steps will be measured, and placing responsibility on patients for measuring their own progress consistently toward that outcome.

B. CLINICAL APPLICATIONS

In this section, we discuss the major psychotherapies that have been used in the clinical management of chronic pain patients. These are supportive, dynamic, family, and group psychotherapy.

Supportive Psychotherapy

The most important and widespread form of psychotherapy—supportive—is knowingly and unknowingly used by specialists in psychologic methods and by other health professionals. The trusting relationship with the physician, therapist, or clergy is the paradigm of this approach, which extends into every nook and cranny of professional work. One example is the trust that patients develop for their favorite doctor ("He listens and he takes the time to explain things"). Another example is the reliance on a social worker for help in filling in an application form for benefits, which then leads to attachment to that worker and to the advice provided. At a minimal level, supportive psychotherapy gives a patient the feeling that there is one other person who shares at least some of his or her concerns, is sympathetic to him or her, and will be happy when he or she feels better, or disappointed or sad when there are reverses. At the very least, supportive psychotherapy provides companionship for the lonely and empathy for the isolated.

The theoretical basis for supportive psychotherapy emphasizes reality and the possibility and importance of making choices. Notwithstanding pain and adverse circumstances, it is possible to reduce impairment and to increase the sense of well-being by drawing on one's own skills, available aid, and expert advice. Although the theory is not psychologically esoteric, and the practice is within the competence of most healthcare workers, formal psychologic training improves one's skill to provide supportive therapy. It is a professional activity, and more than mere handholding because beneficial change, and not just maintenance of the status quo, is expected. Supportive psychotherapy can be carried out knowledgeably and effectively, or badly.

Treatment Strategy

The style of the therapist is that of both broker and expert. Sometimes the task is to listen and help the patient achieve his or her own stated goals; at other times, to provide information and advice. Therapeutic sessions are not rigidly prescribed but are offered while educating the patient to be prepared to generate his or her own objectives. Sessions may last from one-half hour to one hour, at intervals of every few days to every few weeks, depending on the patient's need. Termination of therapy depends on several factors, including the end of formal pain clinic treatment, the resolution of certain important psychologic or social problems, or the desire to "try it on one's own."

Supportive psychotherapy should be inherent in the management of every patient in an organized pain therapy program. The provision of a patient manager (16), the practice of comprehensive evaluation and discussion in which patients are made to feel that their total situation is being examined and assisted, and the concentration of personal interest on patients, all provide a structure of support and encouragement for them. The most important motivator for change is the opinion and attitude of someone who is respected and liked. This is often taken to be a placebo response but strictly speaking, that is not the case. The placebo response is based upon faith alone in the efficacy of a particular measure, usually a drug. Competent supportive psychotherapy, however, provides more than the incidental benefits of concern, expectation, and resourceful management. In its complete form, it begins with an assessment, operates with a clearly defined rationale, weighs up the personality structure and strengths of the individual, and evaluates the "defenses of the ego." The latter is the way in which the individual preserves his or her psychologic integrity and responsibilities in the face of emotional distress, conflict, and adversity.

Supportive psychotherapy also considers patients' style of problem-solving, which may be supported and facilitated by the therapist, or assistance may be given in developing other methods of coping. The life situation and problems of patients must be taken into account. The primary objective of supportive psychotherapy is to shore up patients' ability to cope and assist them to reorganize their coping skills in the most adaptive and economical direction.

The following case description illustrates the use of supportive psychotherapy, including assessment, rationale, and technique:

AB was a 25-year-old single man who had complained of pain in his neck since a hockey injury at age 16. He was withdrawn, socially isolated, very hypochondriacal, and demanding surgery. The assessment by the therapist, in this case a psychiatrist in the pain clinic, revealed that patient believed the pain was due to "degeneration of the bones," although review of clinical investigations showed that increased muscle tension was the only finding. The current level of functioning was very poor; the patient spent most of his time in his room listening to music or playing his guitar. His previous functioning and strengths were considered, in terms of his minimal school achievement and lack of occupational experience and knowledge, as providing a poor foundation for adaptation, but he did admit a belief that he was no longer physically fit and that he would probably feel better if he were. The survey of social resources (including job, family, social involvements, and professional agencies) showed that he had lived with his mother since his parents had separated many years before and that he had virtually no friends. Moreover, agency assistance was precluded by his constant preoccupation about his health, which served as an excuse for not keeping appointments or even leaving the house.

Based on the impression that AB's illness behavior and withdrawal expressed a poor self-esteem and depression, and provided a refuge under his mother's protection, the therapist suggested to him that he had allowed his life to stop at 16 and that continuing as he was for the rest of his life would be intolerable. The patient accepted this. During the clinical investigation, which demonstrated no lesion, the therapist acted as a translator of medical results, seeing the patient every few weeks for a half-hour conversation. When it became clear that the most appropriate treatment would be a program of work adjustment training, the therapist assumed the key task of persuading AB to undertake this course of action. The therapist offered continued contact and support *if* AB would make a commitment to actively begin to pursue a program leading to social involvement and work.

Thereafter, the therapist saw AB weekly, throughout the course of rehabilitation, helping him to plan, one step at a time, a program of work training and of social interaction, and reviewing his progress regularly. This was accomplished in part by making obvious to AB the therapist's association with the pain team and by having the patient define for himself a series of clear goals for change (e.g., beginning a regular exercise program, being on time for scheduled programs, going for job interviews, learning bus routes). During each supportive psychotherapy session, lasting about one hour, the progress toward the goals was discussed, and lack of progress was confronted.

The unifying rationale acceptable to AB was that he was terribly out of shape and could never expect himself to work or have fun unless he improved his fitness and developed self-confidence by practice. A meeting was also held between the therapist, AB, and his mother to agree on new norms for living at home, including being out of his room and helping himself more. As a result of therapy, AB's depression and hypochondriacal behavior were diminished markedly and his self-esteem was improved. Discharge from the pain clinic and supportive psychotherapy were agreed upon after referral to a work readiness training program in the community.

Dynamic Psychotherapy

Dynamic psychotherapy, based on concepts drawn from the original psychoanalytic frameworks, involves the analysis and reorganization of thoughts and feelings through insights gained in the psychotherapeutic relationship. This approach assumes that the reality of the patient's inner world and unconscious processes are determinants of human behavior. Some central concepts of dynamic psychotherapy include the following:

1. Certain properties of the mind, such as drive, need for mastery, conscience, and perception of the self, exist, behave in lawful ways, and are subject to modification.

2. Patterns of feeling and behaving in response to current problems reflect solutions to problems that the individual has learned in the past.

3. Psychologic equilibrium, includes the psychologic energy and mechanisms to maintain this stability,

4. Each individual acquires by experiences during maturation a repertoire of patterns of feeling, believing, and behaving. These patterns are fundamental to both healthy (adaptive) and also neurotic (maladaptive) styles of adjustment and characterize personality.

Further descriptions of the psychodynamic perspective with respect to chronic pain can be found elsewhere (4, 17, 18).

Dynamic psychotherapy alone is not the most appropriate treatment for the majority of chronic pain sufferers, although one might get that impression from some classic papers that deal with pain from a psychodynamics viewpoint (19–21). This treatment, however, is likely to give good results when combined with other pain treatment modalities (22). The patients for whom dynamic insight-oriented psychotherapy is the best treatment usually (a) suffer a sense of psychologic discomfort, (b) experience distress with regard to their key relationships, (c) perceive themselves as having changed for the worse, (d) are perplexed by their own impulses or attitudes, (e) experience difficulties because of "transference relationships" in which they recreate within new relationships the conflicts that they have previously experienced during their maturation, and (f) demonstrate resistance to therapeutic progress because of hidden motives that they themselves fail to perceive.

Treatment Strategy

With chronic pain patients, dynamic psychotherapy is usually short-term (perhaps 10 to 20 sessions) and focused on a few specific psychologic issues, rather than on major personality reconstruction. Sessions are usually an hour long and held at regular intervals. Although sessions could be as often as twice per week, weekly or semimonthly sessions are more common. In the majority of cases, this method of psychotherapy is one of several treatment approaches that are offered concurrently, including even other psychologic approaches. Dynamic psychotherapy is not, for example, incompatible with behavioral therapies, vocational counseling, or medical treatments for pain.

The following case study illustrates the use of dynamic psychotherapy in a pain clinic setting:

CD was referred for headaches, which he had suffered for 30 of his 41 years. Attacks occurred daily, sometimes with migraine and sometimes with tension features. Besides prescribed propranolol, he was consuming handfuls of analgesics containing aspirin, codeine, and caffeine. He readily admitted that his headaches were worse when he felt stressed, that his family background had been unhappy, that he was worried about his marriage, since he had only recently reunited with his wife after a separation, and that they were attending a human sexuality clinic for counseling regarding long-term sexual difficulties. The psychiatrist suggested to CD that part of his headache problem was due to his sense of anxiety and loss of control, of which the medication abuse was a symptom, and that his emotional distress arose from emotional conflicts involving his family.

The treatment program involved discontinuing use of analgesics, adjusting the dose of propranolol, and participation in a relaxation therapy class. CD also agreed to psychotherapy, which was held in hourly sessions every 2 weeks. The therapist chose a psychodynamic model because (a) CD recognized and sought relief from emotional distress, (b) he had had previously positive experiences with counseling and was motivated to engage in psychotherapy, and (c) he attributed his main difficulties (pain and medication abuse) at least partly to psychologic problems.

In the psychotherapy sessions, the therapist had CD recount events and emotional feelings of his childhood, comparing them with the family events and feelings he was now experiencing and helping him to recognize his patterns of feeling, thinking, and reacting. His father had been a ne'er-do-well, constantly fighting with his mother, and showing favoritism to CD's brother, of whom CD felt extremely jealous. Although CD had always stubbornly and unsuccessfully tried to win his father's favor by being at his parents' beck and call, his brother took little responsibility for the parents and yet continued to enjoy father's favor. The pattern of trying hard to please, feeling unappreciated, and reacting with frustration and self pity was paralleled in CD's relationship with his wife. Although the headaches often seemed to arise from emotional stress, they also served the purpose of allowing CD to receive attention and concern from his wife, deflect criticism, and sometimes delay the responsibilities he had assumed. He gained insight into these patterns and into how he had tended to perpetuate them. As his self-esteem grew, he became more assertive with his family and suffered fewer headaches.

Family Therapy

Chronic pain is such a disruptive problem that it is bound to affect a patient's family. Accordingly, it is prudent to involve family members right from the beginning of pain treatment programs. In some cases, psychotherapy of the marital or family unit is indicated as part of chronic pain management. The importance of the family perspective in chronic pain has been discussed in numerous reports (4, 25–30).

The intent of family therapy is not merely to search for conflict (as some families initially fear) but rather to consider both the assets and liabilities in a family's function, in an effort to help the family organize its coping in the most satisfactory way.

Certain family factors are especially important in cases of chronic pain. These include the role of family members as agents of pain behavior reinforcement (28, 31), the value placed by the family on illness-related communications, and the degree of stability with which the family has absorbed the sick role (25).

Common indications for family therapy include the following:

1. The family is motivated to accept a family therapy approach.
2. Illness in a family member is reflected in disturbances in family function.
3. There is reason to believe that family dynamics may contribute to or perpetuate the problem.
4. The family is overwhelmed by multiple problems, in addition to having a member with chronic pain.
5. The identified patient is a child.
6. There are indications that the family can be mobilized therapeutically to influence the pain behavior.

Treatment Strategy

Whereas dynamic psychotherapy focuses on cause and the past in understanding the present, family therapy is oriented to the here-and-now, considers the whole family as the "patient," concentrates on communication rather than on introspection, and is active in style. Family therapy, also, usually lasts a shorter period of time, is more demanding, and is more intensive than individual psychotherapy. A course of family therapy with chronic pain patients commonly consists of 3 to 20 sessions; 5 or 6 sessions probably is most typical.

The following case example illustrates some of the indications for family therapy and a typical treatment approach:

CD (mentioned in the previous section) brought his wife ED, age 36, to an interview. Each seemed cautious of offending the other, and ED appeared both protective of her husband and afraid of his temper. Besides the problem of sexual dysfunction, they revealed a history of his physical aggression against her. Her family background was very similar to his in that she had an older brother who seemed the family favorite, while she was the one the parents called if they needed anything. Strong parallels were discovered in their ways of handling emotional distress. He would retreat to bed with a headache; she would withdraw with depression. Either might provoke a fight with the other, allowing blame for the problem to be placed on the spouse. Either one might secretly buy an expensive object as a way of dealing with the sense of feeling cheated. (Unfortunately, this was causing financial embarrassment.)

In hourly sessions conducted at intervals of two per week during times of crisis, and two per month on the average, they gained insight into these patterns, set limits on their style of relating to their respective families, and developed a more mature way of relating to each other as spouses.

Group Therapy

Numerous types of group therapy have been developed, including groups, marital couples' groups, therapeutic milieu, and cognitive-behavioral groups in pain clinics. Thorough discussions of group approaches for chronic pain patients have been presented by others (32–37). Three important advantages of group therapy are that it (a) economizes therapist time (by allowing several patients to be treated simultaneously); (b) allows for the therapeutic influence of one patient on another; and (c) permits a forum for an educational component of therapy.

Briefly stated, the theoretical rationale of this approach is that people recreate their interpersonal conflicts and demonstrate their assumptions when they are in the context of a group. The group, furthermore, has a modulating influence on the behavior of each member, which the therapist can direct therapeutically.

The common reasons for referring pain patients for group therapy are (a) to provide a vehicle for the educative component of a pain management program, usually in the form of classes; (b) to increase patients' awareness of key psychologic factors in their treatment; (c) to promote informed and motivated participation in the treatment, especially in the case of a comprehensive or inpatient pain management program; and (d) to provide a context for the normalizing effect of a peer group and modeling by other patients of healthier ways of coping.

Treatment Strategy

The following are general guidelines for conducting effective group therapy:

1. A group, to be effective and manageable, should consist of at least 4 and not more than 12 members.
2. Generally, psychiatric patients and chronic pain patients should not be included in the same group.
3. New patients should be admitted to a group all at one time and only at specific intervals to avoid the disruptive effect that an uninitiated and anxious new group member may have on the rest of an established group.
4. The group should be structured to be relevant to the problems of chronic pain patients. In group therapy with psychiatric patients it may be acceptable for the therapist to give little information beyond the initial introduction and to concentrate instead on group dynamics as they appear spontaneously. In pain clinic practice, however, a didactic component usually is necessary to resolve misconceptions and fears that pain patients have and to deal with practical issues related to living with chronic pain.

5. An explicit set of norms usually is expected. These typically include not abusing medication or alcohol, learning to be more appropriately assertive, and minimizing illness benavior.

6. Practical methods for pain control (for example, relaxation exercises, cognitive techniques for pain control such as imagery, or active therapeutic exercises such as role playing) are often helpful and included in some sessions.

7. Opportunities should be provided for discussion and interpretation of emotional and adjustment issues that affect the whole group.

8. For the most part, resistance in group members can be worked through using group therapy methods, but a member who is consistently disruptive and unwilling to abide by group norms may have to be discharged.

An inpatient pain clinic program usually has daily group sessions for the duration of the treatment program, often 3 to 8 weeks. In an outpatient program, its groups typically meet once or twice weekly, for a total of perhaps 6 to 20 meetings. Each group session should last at least 1 hour to be effective; care, however, must be taken to accommodate for the fact that some pain patients have limited sitting tolerance.

The combination of cognitive input and examples of new coping strategies, either by direct teaching or through observation of others, improves group members' socialization and self-confidence and reduces their sense of isolation, with beneficial effects in reducing abnormal illness behavior.

Summary

The psychologic dimension is always important in cases of chronic pain. However, no one psychologic method can possibly address the full spectrum of therapeutic need. A variety of psychotherapeutic methods ought to be available: supportive psychotherapy always and often other approaches such as dynamic, family, and group therapies, as well as various behavioral approaches. Such a flexible approach permits each patient's needs to be considered individually.

REFERENCES

1. OHIP Schedule of Benefits. Physicians' Services: Ontario, Ministry of Health, 1984.
2. Merskey, H.: Psychiatric Illness. 3rd Ed. London, Baillière & Tindall, 1980.
3. Roy, R., and Tunks, E.: Chronic Pain: Psychosocial Factors in Rehabilitation. Baltimore, Williams & Wilkins, 1982.
4. Bellissimo, A., and Tunks, E.: Chronic Pain: The Psychotherapeutic Spectrum. New York, Praeger, 1984.
5. Fordyce, W.: Behavioral Methods for Chronic Pain and Illness. St. Louis, C.V. Mosby, 1976.
6. Sternbach, R.A. (ed.): The Psychology of Pain. 2nd Ed. New York, Raven Press, 1986.
7. Barber, J., and Adrian, C. (eds.): Psychological Approaches to the Management of Pain. New York, Brunner/Mazel, 1982.
8. Turk, D.C., Meichenbaum, D., and Genest, M.: Pain and Behavioral Medicine: A Cognitive-Bahavioral Perspective. New York, Guilford, 1983.
9. APA Commission on Psychotherapies (Chairman, T.B. Karasu): Psychotherapy Research: Methodological and Efficacy Issues. American Psychiatric Association, 1982.
10. Subcommittee on Taxonomy, Int. Assoc. for the Study of Pain (Chairman, H. Merskey): Pain terms: A list with definitions and notes on usage. Pain, 6:249, 1979.
11. Crook, J., Rideout, E., and Browne, G.: The prevalence of pain complaints in a general population. Pain, 18:299, 1984.
12. Crook, J., and Tunks, E.: Defining the "chronic pain syndrome": An epidemiological method. In Advances in Pain Research and Therapy. Vol. 9. Edited by H.L. Fields, R. Dubner, and F. Cervero. New York, Raven Press, 1985, pp. 871–877.
13. Rogers, C.R.: The necessary and sufficient conditions of therapeutic personality change. J. Consult. Psychol., 21:95, 1957.
14. Marmor, J.: Dynamic psychotherapy and behavioral therapy: Are they irreconcilable? Arch. Gen. Psychiatry, 24:22, 1971.
15. Frank, J.D., et al.: Effective Ingredients of Successful Psychotherapy New York, Brunner/Mazel, 1978.
16. Bonica, J.J.: Organization and function of a pain clinic. In Advances in Neurology. Vol. 4. Pain. Edited by J.J. Bonica. New York, Raven Press, 1974, pp. 433–443.
17. Pilowsky, I.: Psychodynamic aspects of the pain experience. In The Psychology of Pain. Edited by R.A. Sternbach. New York, Raven Press, 1978, pp. 203–217.
18. Pilowsky, I., and Bassett, D.: Individual dynamic psychotherapy for chronic pain. In Chronic Pain: Psychosocial Factors in Rehabilitation. Edited by R. Roy and E. Tunks. Baltimore, Williams & Wilkins, 1982, pp. 107–124.

19. Szasz, T.S.: The nature of pain. Arch. Neurol. Psychiatry, 74:174, 1955.
20. Engel, G.L.: Psychogenic pain and the pain-prone patient. Amer. J. Med., 26:899, 1959.
21. Walters, A.: Psychogenic regional sensory and motor disorders, alias hysteria. Can. Psychiat. Assoc. J., 14:573, 1969.
22. Sarno, J.E.: Chronic back pain and psychic conflict. Scand. J. Rehabil. Med., 8:143, 1976.
23. Liebman, R., Honig, P., and Berger, H.: An integrated treatment program for psychogenic pain. Family Process, 15:397, 1976.
24. Khatami, M., and Rush, A.J.: A pilot study of the treatment of outpatients with chronic pain: Symptom control, stimulus control, and social system intervention. Pain, 5:163, 1978.
25. Mohamed, S.N., Weisz, G.M., and Waring, E.M.: The relationship of chronic pain to depression, marital adjustment, and family dynamics. Pain, 5:285, 1978.
26. Hudgens, A.J.: Family oriented treatment of chronic pain. J. Marital Fam. Ther., (Oct.):67, 1979.
27. Shanfield, S.B., Heiman, E.M., Cope, N., and Jones, J.R.: Pain and the marital relationship: Psychiatric distress. Pain, 7:343, 1979.
28. Block, A.R., Kremer, E.F., and Gaylor, M.: Behavioral treatment of chronic pain: The spouse as a discriminative cue for pain behavior. Pain, 9:243, 1980.
29. Waring, E.M.: Conjoint marital and family therapy. In Chronic Pain: Psychosocial Factors in Rehabilitation. Edited by R. Roy and E. Tunks. Baltimore, Williams & Wilkins, 1982, pp. 151–165.
30. Violon, A., and Giurgea, D.: Familial models for chronic pain. Pain, 18:199, 1984.
31. Liberman, R.: Behavioral approaches to family and couple therapy. Am. J. Orthopsychiatry, 40:106, 1970.
32. Greenhoot, J.H., and Sternbach, R.A.: Conjoint treatment of chronic pain. In Advances in Neurology. Vol. 4. Pain. Edited by J.J. Bonica. New York, Raven Press, 1974, pp. 595–603.
33. Newman, R.I., Painter, J.R., and Seres, J.L.: A therapeutic milieu for chronic pain patients. J. Human Stress, 4:8, 1978.
34. Pinsky, J.J.: Chronic, intractable, benign pain: A syndrome and its treatment with intensive short-term group psychotherapy. J. Human Stress, 4:17, 1978.
35. Wilson, R.R., and Aronoff, G.M.: The therapeutic community in the treatment of chronic pain. J. Chronic Dis., 32:477, 1979.
36. Baptiste, S., and Herman, E.: Group therapy: a specific model. In Chronic Pain: Psychosocial Factors in Rehabilitation. Edited by R. Roy and E. Tunks. Baltimore, Williams & Wilkins, 1982, pp. 166–178.
37. Moore, M.E., Berk, S.N., and Nypaver, A.: Chronic pain: Inpatient treatment with small group effects. Arch. Phys. Med. Rehabil., 65:356, 1984.

INTRODUCTION

JOHN J. BONICA

This section contains five chapters dealing with subjects that have been arbitrarily labeled physical modalities. The first chapter, written by Frederick Matsen and myself, deals with orthopedic nonsurgical and surgical procedures for treating musculoskeletal disorders, one of the primary objectives of these procedures being the relief of pain. It contains concise descriptions of the procedures intended to relieve acute and chronic pain and the bases of these procedures. It also contains a small section on the use of orthopedic operations for patients with cancer-related pain.

Chapter 88, written by Mathew Lee and his colleagues, provides an overview of various modalities used in physical medicine and rehabilitation for patients with acute and chronic pain. After briefly reviewing the history and development of these modalities, these authors discuss in a concise fashion the physiologic bases, indications, side effects, and contraindication of each of the many types of thermotherapy, cryotherapy, electrotherapy, mechanotherapy, therapeutic exercises, traction, manipulation, immobilization, and laser therapy. In the latter part of the chapter they discuss the clinical applications of the various modalities.

Chapter 89, the third in this section, written by four authors, presents an overview of various modalities used for treatment of patients with cancer-related pain and is a more detailed discussion of information summarized in Chapter 24. The first section, on radiation therapy, provides an overview of the various radiation modalities in common use, physical principles of radiation therapy, factors that affect cellular response to radiation, and clinical applications of local radiation therapy and systemic radiation therapy including hemibody and total body irradiation. In addition to providing information about results, they also discuss the short-term and long-term toxicity of radiation

therapy. The second section deals with chemotherapy and the third section with endocrine therapy, with a discussion of the indications, efficacy, and side effects. The final section deals with palliative surgery, intended primarily for the relief of pain and other symptoms.

Chapter 90 discusses acupuncture for the management of patients with acute and chronic pain. C. Richard Chapman provides a comprehensive and fair critical review of the methods, indications, side effects, and complications of classical acupuncture as practiced by Oriental practitioners, and modern techniques used in various parts of the world, including electroacupuncture. He then reviews the scientific knowledge base derived from animal studies, human laboratory studies, and clinical studies with a summary of the efficacy of acupuncture in management of patients with acute and chronic pain. In the second part of the chapter, C. Chan Gunn, a physiatrist of Oriental origin educated in England, discusses the clinical application of acupuncture used as motor-point or trigger-point therapy in patients with chronic musculoskeletal problems. He discusses the hypothetical conceptualization of the therapy, the approach to diagnosis, and the general principles of treatment, including the technique of solid acupuncture needle penetration of motor points or trigger points.

Chapter 91, written by myself with contributions by Giuseppe Maggio, deals with nutrition and pain. This chapter provides a brief review of the role of nutrition in patients with postoperative pain and other acute pain problems, in patients with cancer pain, and particularly the role of nutrition therapy in management of patients with nonmalignant chronic pain. The chapter cites various nutritional diets that have been suggested not only to improve the physical condition of the patient but also to decrease pain.

87 · ORTHOPEDIC MANAGEMENT OF PAIN

FREDERICK A. MATSEN III *and* JOHN J. BONICA

MUSCULOSKELETAL disorders constitute the most frequent cause of pain, suffering, and disability (described elsewhere in this book; see Parts II and IV). Various orthopedic therapies are currently used, not only to correct the pathopysiologic process but also to relieve the associated pain. Often the sole treatment of minor musculoskeletal disorders is encouragement and reassurance to the patient. As Adams (1) has emphasized, many patients only consult a physician because of their fear that they might have cancer or some other serious disease. Reassurance that serious pathology is not evident is often sufficient to make patients feel better, thereby reducing their pain and suffering.

Active orthopedic treatment in the management of patients with chronic pain falls into three major categories: A, nonoperative (noninvasive) procedures; B, operative interventions for the relief of pain caused by nonmalignant disease; and C, palliative surgical procedures for the relief of advanced cancer pain. This chapter presents a concise discussion of the indications and an overview of the techniques being used for these purposes. This material is intended for physicians who manage patients with pain and who are not orthopedic surgeons. A more detailed discussion can be found elsewhere (1–6).

A. NONSURGICAL THERAPIES

Nonoperative procedures used by orthopedic surgeons to relieve pain include rest, support, physical therapy, local injection of local anesthetics and other compounds, systemic drugs, and manipulation. These measures are discussed briefly here to place them in proper perspective from the viewpoint of orthopedic management.

Rest

For centuries rest has been used as a therapeutic agent for various disease processes, especially musculoskeletal disorders. In 1871 Hilton (7) published a book on the value of rest and H.O. Thomas of Liverpool, one of the pioneers of British orthopedic surgery (1), emphasized its value in the treatment of diseases of the spine and limbs. Subsequently rest became one of the mainstays of orthopedic treatment. Complete rest demands recumbency in bed or immobilization of the diseased part in plaster. When orthopedic surgeons use the word "rest," however, they do not necessarily mean complete inactivity or immobility but rather "relative rest," which implies simply a reduction of wonted activity and avoidance of strain for a limited period of time. Indeed, complete rest is enjoined much less today than in the past because of the deleterious effects that physical inactivity and immobility have on the entire organism. It has now been impressively shown that bed rest of more than a few days duration is associated with a progressive shortening of muscle fibers and the developement of muscle atrophy, as well as with deleterious effects on bone and joints.

Postoperative pain that leads to prolonged bed rest is usually associated with a high risk of thromboembolism, pulmonary complications, and impaired metabolism of muscle (Chapter 25). Prolonged bed rest in patients with acute back pain also has deleterious effects (Chapter 71). In such cases bed rest for more than 2 or 3 days invariably leads to rapid deterioration of function of muscles, bones, and joints, and thus initiates a vicious circle that invariably leads to chronic back pain. It is therefore essential that patients with musculoskeletal disorders be encouraged to resume activity as soon as possible, even if the activity aggravates the pain. Therefore it is important to help patients resume activity by providing pain relief with systemic analgesics, especially in the form of nonsteroidal anti-inflammatory drugs. If necessary, appropriate doses of codeine or of even stronger opioids can be added for a few days. An alternative measure which is now being used more frequently in many medical centers is the use of intraspinal opioids (Chapter 95) or regional analgesia (Chapter 94). Properly carried out, these techniques not only provide effective pain relief and permit patients to resume activity, but also increase regional blood flow and decrease the neuroendocrine response and consequent metabolic and biochemical disturbances provoked by a pain-induced injury (Chapter 7).

Support

Support of an injured limb or spine can be required in the form of casts, splints, braces, slings, or bandages. Although rest and support are often used together, support but not rest is often required— for example, to stabilize a joint rendered insecure by muscle paralysis or to prevent the development of deformity (1). Temporary support can be provided by a cast or splint made from plaster of Paris or from one of the newer strengthening materials. For example, a Velpeau dressing is used for the first postoperative days after arthrodesis of the shoulder until the postoperative pain has subsided. A Velpeau dressing is also useful in immobilizing fractures of the scapula, certain fractures of the upper humerus, dislocation of the shoulder, and soft tissue injuries of the upper extremity. It is considered to be an excellent support for minimizing pain after operation on the shoulder.

Slings provide rest for many conditions of the upper limbs, such as fractures with or without casts, sprains of the shoulder, elbow, or wrist, lateral epicondylitis, acute arthritis, and other injuries. Overuse of the sling should be avoided, however, because of the insidious development of a frozen shoulder or of reflex sympathetic dystrophy. Regional analgesia aids in overcoming this danger by permitting painless motion earlier and by decreasing the patient's fear of painful motion.

When support is to be prolonged or permanent an individually made surgical appliance or arthrosis is required. Such appliances include steel-reinforced lumbar corsets, spinal braces, cervical collars, lift supports, walking calipers, a below-knee steel with ankle straps, and devices to control foot drop. Braces and splints immobilize like casts but have the advantage of sturdiness with less bulk, durability for prolonged use, flexibility of joints when necessary, and ready removal and reapplication. Splints are useful for preventing and correcting the painful contractures associated with soft tissue injuries of the forearm and hand. The ischial weight-bearing caliper allows walking by transferring body weight from the lower extremity to the ischium, making early ambulation possible in patients with certain fractures of the hip, femur, knee, and fibula. Long leg braces permit ambulation in those with knee ligament sprains and provide stimulation of bone growth in cases of stable delayed union or non-union of the tibia. Shoe lifts or other appliances can help to provide pain relief for patients with inequality of leg length, pelvic tilt, or other problems (Chapters 71 and 76).

Physiotherapy

Physiotherapy in its various forms is important in the nonoperative and postoperative management of patients with musculoskeletal disorders. Although it was formerly prescribed empirically by physicians, today orthopedic surgeons, physiatrists, and physiotherapists are knowledgeable and well trained, so that in most medical centers physiotherapy is appropriately applied. The most important forms used in patients with musculoskeletal disorders include the following: (a) exercise, (b) passive joint movement, and (c) application of heat or cold, ultrasound therapy, massage, and electrical stimulation of muscles. Because most of these are discussed in detail elsewhere (Chapter 88), discussion here is limited to a few comments on electrical stimulation.

Electrical stimulation of muscles can be used in conjunction with exercise for patients who have muscle impairment but an intact nerve supply or in those whose muscles are denervated (1, 8). In regard to the former, electrical muscle stimulation can be used for improving the function of the intrinsic muscles of the foot, for re-education following a tendon transfer operation, and for restoring activity to a quadriceps muscle that has been inhibited after surgery on the knee. Because the nerve supply is intact the muscle can be stimulated through its motor nerve by faradism or by an electrical stimulator. If a muscle has been denervated because of a peripheral nerve injury, it can be stimulated electrically while recovery of nerve function is awaited. This procedure retards the process of atrophy and fibrosis that can occur in any denervated muscle after about 2 years. The muscle is stimulated by galvanism, in which shocks of relatively long duration stimulate the muscle fibers directly. Direct current increases blood and lymph flow and tissue metabolism and thus relieves pain and decreases sclerosis of areolar tissue (8).

Local Injections and Regional Analgesia

Local infiltration of a local anesthetic into a joint, alone or combined with a steroid, can be useful in those with osteoarthritis, rheumatoid arthritis, and other arthritides. Some orthopedic surgeons inject extra-articular lesions, such as tendinitis of the shoulder, lateral or medial epicondylitis, and other periarticular disorders. Injection of a local anesthetic or dry needling is also widely used for the treatment of myofascial pain syndromes. These and other indications for local injection therapy are described elsewhere (Chapters 20, 21, 50, 72, and 94).

Regional analgesia by injection of a long-lasting local anesthetic such as bupivacaine on the nerves that supply an entire limb or part of the limb provides effective pain relief and thus permits painless active motion of an injured part. Continuous lumbar epidural analgesia is also indicated for relief in patients who develop severe pain caused by regional reflex skeletal muscle spasm following injury or who have severe pain associated with a herniated intervertebral disk or some other orthopedic pathologic process. In addition to providing complete pain relief (much more relief than with a systemic analgesic), regional analgesia eliminates the reflex responses provoked by acute injury (Chapter 7). The use of regional analgesia for managing pain of musculoskeletal (and other) origin is described elsewhere (Chapter 94).

Pharmacologic Therapy

Various groups of drugs have a minor but important role in the orthopedic management of pain. These include antibacterial agents for treating infection, especially acute osteomyelitis and acute pyogenic arthritis, systemic opioid analgesics, which should be prescribed only for a short period to control severe pain, and sedatives to promote sleep. Anti-inflammatory drugs such as cortisone, prednisone, and their analogs are used to treat excessive inflammatory responses that might occur, especially in those with rheumatoid arthritis and related disorders. Nonsteroidal anti-inflammatory drugs (NSAIDs), such as aspirin, indomethacin, and ibuprofen, are the mainstays of treatment of pain resulting from inflammatory conditions such as rheumatoid arthritis. Specific drugs are used to treat specific diseases, such as cytotoxic agents for chemotherapy and hormone-like drugs for hormone-dependent neoplasms.

Manipulation

Technique

JOINT STIFFNESS. Closed manipulation can be useful for joints that are stiff and refractory to a concerted attempt at physical therapy and, properly done, respond to close manipulation with the region anesthetized (Fig. 87-1). This procedure, which is intended to break up adhesions and manage contractures, can be helpful but carries the risk of injury to certain structures, such as the joint surface, tendons, ligaments, and even the bone itself. Excessive force should be avoided because of the danger of bone fracture, which could cause fresh bleeding within the joint and thereby aggravate the stiffness. It is better to use moderate force, obtain slight improvement, and then repeat the manipulation after a while. An alternative therapy that could be considered in such circumstances is an open release, wherein the structures limiting joint motion can be safely and selectively divided.

DISLOCATION. Closed manipulation of a joint dislocation is commonly carried out. Analgesia or anesthesia is used to make the patient more comfortable and to encourage relaxation of muscles in spasm, thereby lessening the forces necessary to achieve reduction. Dislocation of each type of joint has techniques described for relocation. Just as with the closed manipulation of a stiff joint (see above), care must be exercised to avoid additional injury—for example, converting a shoulder dislocation in an older patient into a fracture dislocation. Adequate prereduction assessment of the injury and adequate muscle relaxation minimize the risk of such procedures.

FRACTURE. Closed reduction of fractures is commonly used to restore alignment after a fracture (5, 6). As with closed manipulation of joints, good analgesia and muscle relaxation are essential for minimizing muscle spasm and achieving adequate reduction. The reduction maneuver might require unlocking of fracture fragments followed by traction, bending, and rotation to restore normal alignment. Postreduction roentgenograms are required to document the position and stability of the reduction. Some fractures can be reduced by traction but go on to redisplacement after the traction is removed. If the amount of redisplacement is unacceptable, postreduction stabilization by skin or skeletal traction or by external pin fixation might be required. Stable reductions are managed by splinting or casting until skeletal stability is restored by locking of fragments or early healing. In such cases open reduction might be required. Complications of closed reduction can include additional comminution of the fracture and neurovascular injury.

Anesthesia

To achieve maximum benefits from manipulation, it is essential to have the patient feel no pain during the procedure and to have the muscles adjacent to the joint or fracture site completely relaxed—that is, paralyzed. This is best achieved with regional anesthesia using a long-acting local anesthetic, such as bupivacaine with epinephrine. Thus, for manipulation of the shoulder joint or reduction of fracture of the humerus, a supraclavicular brachial plexus block or interscalene brachial plexus block (see Figs. 94-16 and 94-17) achieved with 0.5% bupivacaine with epinephrine provides complete muscular paralysis and anesthesia that lasts 5 to 8 hours or longer. Axillary plexus block is sufficient for manipulation of the elbow, wrist joint, or fracture in the lower arm, forearm, or hand. For manipulation of the hip or knee joint, either a subarachnoid or continuous epidural block is

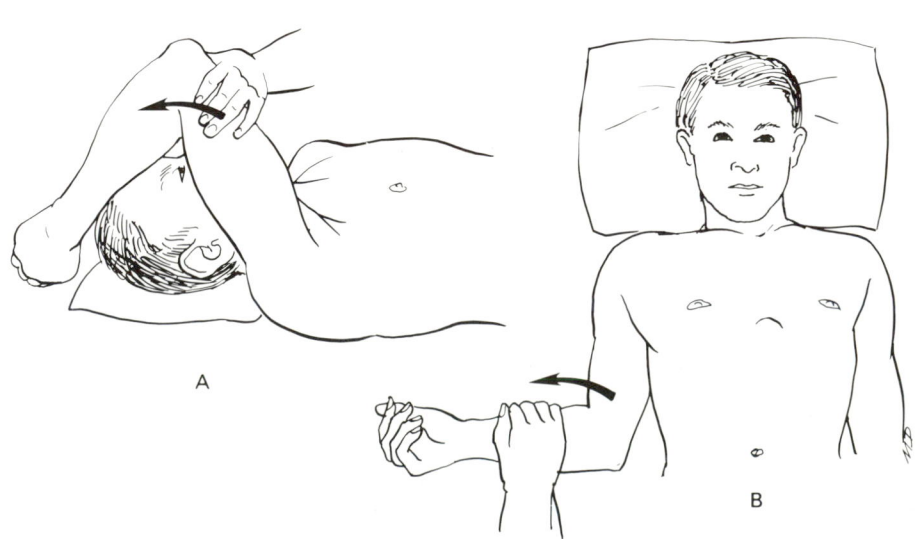

FIG. 87-1. Closed manipulation of a painful stiff shoulder under regional anesthesia. In the vast majority of cases the stiffness can be resolved by a gentle, frequent stretching program that gradually elongates tightened tissues and resolves adhesions. In selected refractory cases it can be useful to examine the patient's shoulder, preferably under regional anesthesia, gently pushing the arm into forward flexion (*A*) and into external rotation (*B*) to determine the range of motion with the muscles relaxed. Occasionally on this maneuver some (soft) adhesions can be ruptured, which then allow the patient more comfort and freedom of motion. This procedure must be carried out with great gentleness because it is possible to injure the joint surface, the periarticular tissues, or even the humerus with vigorous shoulder manipulation. Moreover, rough manipulation also produces a painful shoulder after the effects of the anesthetic have worn off, leaving the patient more prone to stiffness than before the procedure.

sufficient. Segmental epidural block is the procedure of choice for manipulation of joints in the low back. In addition to providing complete pain relief and muscle relaxation, regional anesthesia has the advantages of producing sympathetic interruption and consequently increasing blood flow to the limb for about 10 to 15 hours, thus enhancing the healing process. If general anesthesia needs to be used, it is essential to use tracheal intubation and a potent skeletal muscle relaxant.

B. OPEN SURGICAL THERAPY

Orthopedic operative procedures that are commonly used to reduce or eliminate pain and its associated pathophysiology include soft tissue excision, bone excision, osteotomy, open reduction, arthrodesis or arthroplasty, ligament reconstruction, tendon surgery, nerve surgery, fasciotomy, amputation, bone grafting, releases, and arthroscopy. For optimal results it is essential to select patients carefully for the most appropriate operation, carry out the procedure skillfully, and provide patients with optimal surgical care. As with some other chapters in this part of the book, each technique is not described in detail but is depicted in the corresponding figure.

Bone Excision

Bone excision is indicated for various clinical circumstances, ranging from benign lesions to malignant tumors. The procedure is particularly useful for relieving pain caused by bony prominences that impinge or block range of motion, for removing devitalized and devascularized bone resulting from chronic osteomyelitis, and for managing severe fractures.

Technique

BONY PROMINENCES. Bony prominences can cause pain by impinging on, or blocking of, the range of motion. Pain in the lumbar spine can arise from the "kissing " of lumbar spinous processes. Pain in the shoulder can arise from the impingement of the acromion on the rotator cuff (Fig. 87-2). In the forearm, bone from fracture callus can impede the movements of pronation and supination. A prominent olecranon process can prevent full extension of the elbow. Heterotopic bone in the forearm, about the hip, in the shoulder, or elsewhere can interfere with or prevent motion of the involved joint. The following are principles for the excision of bone to relieve pain caused by these conditions:

a. Determine that bone impingement is the cause of the pain problem. This is done by using radiographs in various positions to document the impingement and by demonstrating relief of pain by injecting a local anesthetic into the impingement zone.

b. Ensure an adequate resection, so that scarring in the area does not recreate the impingement problem.

c. Avoid complications of bone excision, such as weakening of the structure, excision of important attachment sites, or compromise of joint surfaces.

CHRONIC OSTEOMYELITIS. Bone excision is frequently indicated for the management of chronic osteomyelitis. Devitalized and devascularized bone can harbor organisms out of the reach of systemically administered antibiotics and prevent resolution of the infection. Generally, bone must be excised back to healthy tissue. This can leave a substantial bony defect that might require limb shortening, bone grafting, or some other special technique to restore structure and function.

FRACTURES. Bone excision and replacement by autograft, allograft, or prosthesis is also indicated for the management of severe fractures (e.g., of the spine, humeral head, or femoral head) (5, 6) and of benign and malignant bone tumors. Each of these cases should involve careful consideration in regard to the extent of the resection and the nature of the reconstruction. The timing of these procedures is also important. For example, a badly comminuted fracture of the radial head that prevents pronation and supination might require early excision so that these motions are not permanently lost. A femoral neck fracture in an elderly woman frequently requires excision and replacement by a prosthesis to avoid the complications of immobility. Other bone resections, on the other hand, might require extensive preoperative analysis. For example, a chondrosarcoma of the pelvis or an osteogenic sarcoma of the distal femur must be carefully staged preoperatively to understand the compartments involved, the extent of bony involvement, the proximity of neurovascular structures, and the presence or absence of metastases before appropriate excision therapy can be planned.

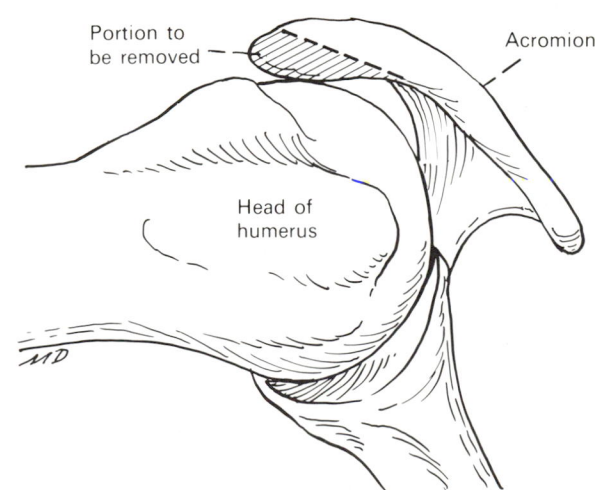

FIG. 87-2. Acromioplasty. A principal cause of shoulder tendinitis is rubbing on the rotator cuff by the anteroinferior surface of the acromion. This condition is managed by resection of this anteroinferior surface of the acromion, allowing free passage of the head of the humerus and of the attached rotator cuff beneath the acromion.

Results

The results of bony excision depend on the process being treated, the adequacy of the excision, and the adequacy of the reconstruction. A vigorous excision for tibial osteomyelitis can produce a bad result if the bone goes on to a pathologic fracture. Excision of bone for acromial impingement or even malignant tumor can have outstanding results if the painful problem is eliminated and the structure is well reconstructed.

Osteotomy

Osteotomy, or cutting and realignment of the bone, is often carried out to reconstruct a congenital, post-traumatic, or degenerative deformity (2, 5). An acetabulum, poorly formed as part of a congenital hip dysplasia, can produce painful hip subluxation in a child. An innominate osteotomy can help to restore a more normal acetabulum configuration and hip joint stability, with return of comfort and function (9). A femoral fracture can heal bent inward and rotated internally, with functional shortening, muscle imbalance, and malposition of the lower extremity. Osteotomy at the fracture site with restoration of alignment and length, followed by stable fixation during the healing process, can be most successful. This type of procedure, however, requires careful preoperative assessment of the particular deformity, so that complete correction and stable fixation can be achieved.

Degenerative osteoarthritis of the knee frequently affects only the medial compartments. A high tibial osteotomy can realign the resulting varus configuration, shifting the load to the relatively unaffected lateral compartment. This type of reconstruction can restore comfort and function to the knee and avoid the potential problems of prosthetic arthroplasty (Fig. 87-3).

Osteotomy of the spine is of major value in restoring comfort and function to those with certain developmental, traumatic, or degenerative disorders (9, 10). For example, ankylosing spondylitis can produce such severe cervical and thoracic kyphosis that patients cannot look ahead to see where they are going. An extension osteotomy can restore their ability to see the horizon without trying to assume some painful compensating position.

Soft Tissue Excision

KNEE CARTILAGE. Certain musculoskeletal soft tissues (e.g., the semilunar cartilages or menisci of the knee joint) are predisposed to injury and, when damaged, might require excision. These cartilages can be damaged by compressional or rotational loads across the knee, catching and tearing their substance. Torn and displaced meniscal fragments can cause pain and interfere with normal joint motion by catching between the femur and the tibia. Degenerative tears can also arise from wear and tear on the joint surface. Resection of the torn meniscus fragments can relieve the "catching" and pain but does not, however, restore normal function of the meniscus, so substantial efforts are now being directed toward meniscus repair in young active individuals. Currently, most meniscus surgery procedures are carried out arthroscopically to minimize attendant damage to the knee joint, and the painful symptoms caused by the displaced meniscus fragments are usually relieved. The contribution of meniscectomy to the subsequent development of degenerative joint disease of the affected joint is also of concern.

DISKECTOMY. A vertebral diskectomy is another type of soft tissue excision. It was formerly believed that ruptured disks were a frequent cause of low back pain and that disk excision was indicated when disk

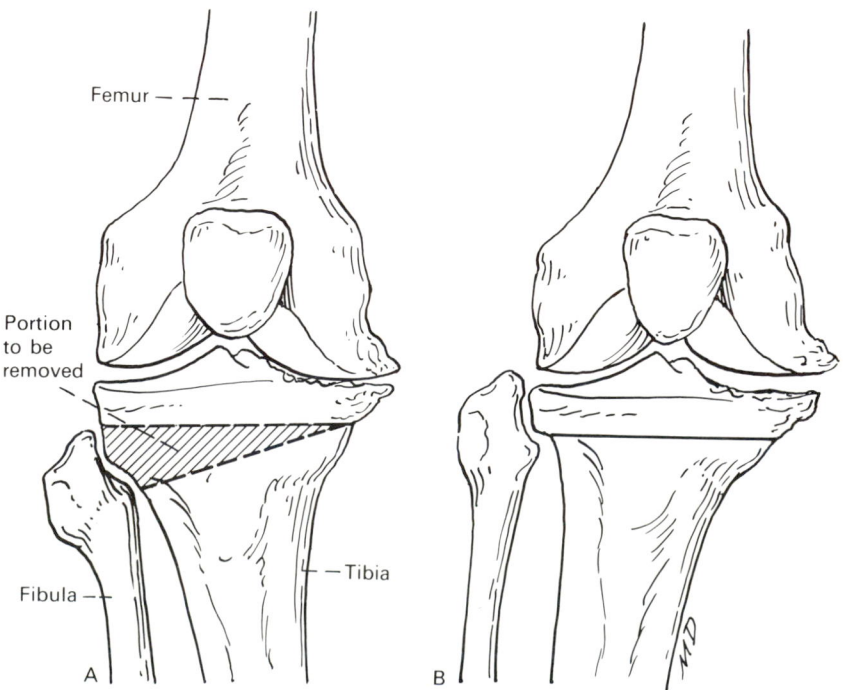

FIG. 87-3. High tibial valgus osteotomy. **A.** Frequently osteoarthritis selectively involves the medial compartment of the knee joint, which produces a progressive varus or bow-legged deformity of the leg in which the load is concentrated on the damaged medial side. A high tibial valgus osteotomy achieved by section of a laterally based wedge of the upper tibia can be a helpful therapeutic measure in this situation. **B.** When this wedge is removed and the dissection is closed the varus deformity is eliminated and the load is transferred toward the relatively unscathed lateral compartment.

Femur

Portion to be removed

Fibula

Tibia

abnormalities were identified. It is now being increasingly shown that disk excision does not beneficially alter the course of degenerative disease of the lumbar spine unless it is accompanied by progressive neurologic involvement (9). The results of early mobilization and exercise are being compared to those of diskectomy and diskectomy and fusion, and the indications for surgery are coming under progressively greater scrutiny. Most authorities now agree that a progressive neurologic deficit, particularly one that affects multiple nerve roots, is an indication for disk excision after myelographic, CT, MRI, or electrodiagnostic confirmation of the location of the lesion. Although it has been demostrated that chemonucleolysis can dissolve the lesion, the indications for diskectomy have yet to be determined precisely.

Combined soft tissue and bony excision might be indicated in the presence of spinal stenosis, in which the space available for the spinal cord, spinal nerve roots, or both, is inadequate (9). The resulting neurogenic claudication is painful and functionally limiting. If electrodiagnostic tests such as somatosensory evoked potentials and CT scanning or myelography document the presence and location of the stenosis, excellent relief can be obtained by extensive decompression of the spinal canal in the affected areas.

SYNOVECTOMY. A third type of soft tissue excision is synovectomy. Rheumatoid arthritis, pseudogout, hemophilia, and chronic infections can induce a major proliferative reaction by the synovium and can produce pain, limited range of motion, and joint destruction. Open surgical synovectomy has been the standard approach. The surgical trauma of this procedure, however, and the difficulty of accomplishing visualization of the entire joint make it less than optimal. Arthroscopic synovectomy is widely used for the knee joint. Radiation synovectomy is currently being evaluated. Although these procedures undoubtedly can reduce the volume of synovium within the joint, their effectiveness in relieving the patient's symptoms in the short run and in changing the long-term course of the disease are still uncertain. Figure 87-4 depicts synovectomy of the elbow joint to relieve pain caused by swelling and progressive joint destruction as a result of rheumatiod arthritis.

Open Reduction

Open reduction of fractures and dislocations is often indicated when closed manipulation is either too hazardous or unsuccessful. At the time of open reduction the bone fragments are directly manipulated by the surgeon after any interfering or interposed structures are removed. At times a stable configuration can be achieved by the open reduction, and no additional surgery is required. On other occasions repair of ligaments, tendons, and associated fractures can be indicated in association with open reduction of dislocations. After open reduction of fracture, internal fixation with wire, screws, plates, or nails, or a combination of these, is frequently done to restore integrity of the bone so that early resumption of function can be achieved (Fig. 87-5). Open reduction and internal fixation of fractures can be supplemented by bone grafting to optimize the chances of prompt union.

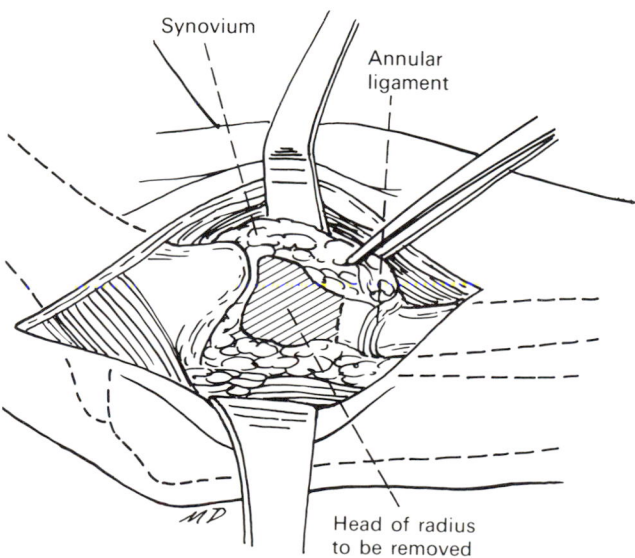

FIG. 87-4. Synovectomy for rheumatoid arthritis of the elbow joint. Hypertrophic synovial tissue can produce chronic pain, swelling, and progressive joint destruction. Resection of the hypertrophic synovium in the elbow, along with radial head resection, can be useful for reducing swelling and increasing the comfort on pronation and supination if the radiohumeral joint has been irreversibly damaged.

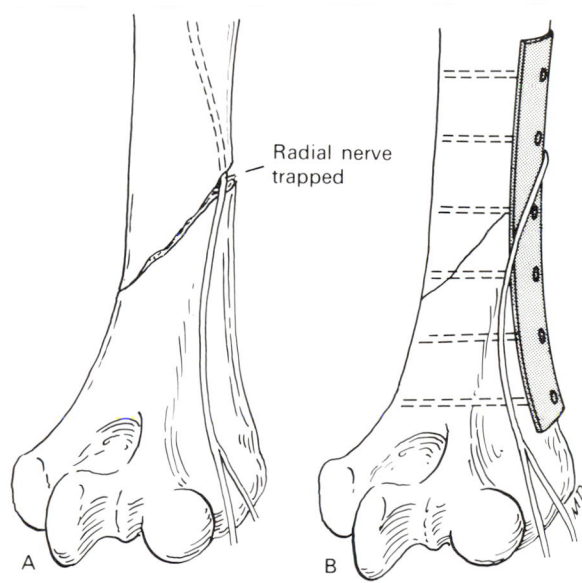

FIG. 87-5. Open reduction and internal rotation of a distal humeral shaft fracture. Fractures of the distal humerus are not infrequently associated with radial nerve lesions. When the radial nerve is injured at the time of the fracture it is prudent to wait 6 to 12 weeks for nerve recovery. When the nerve is initially intact and then subsequently loses function during the process of reduction, however, it is possible that the nerve is trapped within the fracture. If radial nerve function is acutely lost, open reduction and extraction of the nerve by internal fixation of the fracture, using a plate, is effective for protecting the nerve and permitting earlier return to function of the arm.

These open procedures are usually beneficial to the patient. Complications can occur from the surgical procedure (e.g., neurovascular damage, infection) or from failure to achieve a secure fixation (e.g., redisplacement) or healing (e.g., recurrent dislocation, fracture nonunion).

Arthrodesis

Arthrodesis, or joint fusion, is a common procedure for stopping the motion at a joint because it has become destroyed, unstable, or unusable as a result of lack of motor power. Disabling pain often occurs, along with danger of complications. For example, C1 and C2 vertebrae can become unstable because of rupture of the transverse ligament of the atlas in a patient with arthritis, jeopardizing the cervical cord at this level. Arthrodesis of these two vertebrae is the most effective way of preventing neurologic problems resulting from instability at this level. A shoulder that has become unstable from brachial plexus injury can be flail and render the rest of the upper extremity relatively useless (12). In such situations function can be enhanced by fusing the humerus to the scapula in a position that favors use of the elbow, wrist, and hand (Fig. 87-6).

The hip of a young patient deprived of its articular cartilage because of septic arthritis presents an indication for hip fusion rather than arthroplasty, which is relatively contraindicated in a young person after a septic process. Although the arthrodesis carries no hope of normal function, it does provide stability, strength, and comfort in the hip area.

Arthrodesis can be accomplished by various techniques, including internal fixation with plates, screws, or rods, bone grafting to increase the chances of union, and postoperative mobilization. Complications

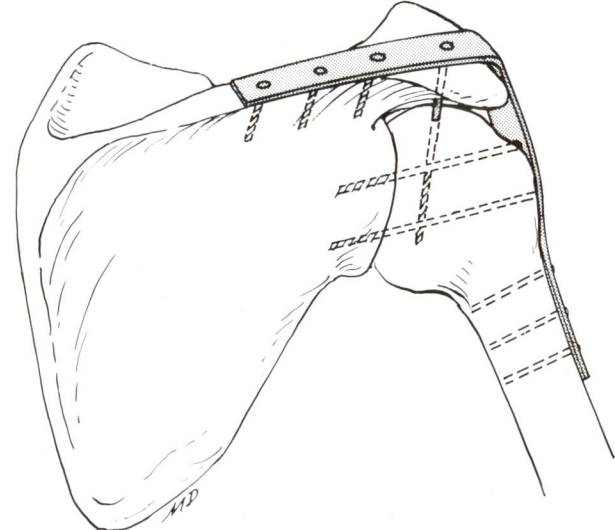

Fig. 87-6. Arthrodesis of the shoulder joint. When the joint surface of the shoulder and the major muscles of the shoulder (the detoid and rotator cuff) are substantially damaged, comfort and some function can be restored by fusing the humeral head to the scapula. Here a contoured plate and screws are used to provide internal stability to the shoulder fusion. The shoulder is fused in a position that allows the hand to reach the front pocket, opposite axilla, and forehead.

include failure to achieve union and those related to lack of mobility at the joint, such as problems at the spine, knees, and contralateral hip after a hip fusion or loss of internal rotation after a shoulder fusion.

Arthroplasty

Destruction of joint surfaces caused by degenerative, traumatic, or postrheumatic arthritis is often managed by arthroplasty (13), or joint reconstruction, which can be biologic or prosthetic. Biologic arthroplasty procedures include resurfacing of the bone ends with fascia or dermis or a distraction-resection type of arthroplasty that allows the body to regenerate a new bearing surface. Resection arthroplasty is effective in certain circumstances, such as when the radiocapitellar joint is involved in rheumatoid arthritis of the elbow. Proximal row carpectomy of the wrist is another example. Resection arthroplasty is not commonly used with the major joints, however, unless all other options have been exhausted, such as with multiple septic failures of a hip arthroplasty; in such a case joint excision is the remaining alternative.

In the last two decades a great deal of interest has arisen in regard to the use of prosthetic arthroplasty, which involves the replacement of the damaged joint surfaces with Silastic or metal on polyethylene (13). Common examples include total arthroplasties of the hip, knee, shoulder, elbow, ankle, wrist, and fingers (Fig. 87-7). These new joint surfaces are anchored into position either by biologic fixation (e.g., press fit, with or without tissue ingrowth) or by fixation enhancement with methylmethacrylate. These procedures, by definition, eliminate the pain caused by rubbing of abnormal joint surfaces. Prosthetic arthroplasty is often of great benefit to the patient, but the procedure can fail because of infection, loosening, fracture, instability, or abnormal joint mechanics.

Ligament Reconstruction

Supportive ligaments of joints are susceptible to certain traumatic or degenerative disruptions. The shoulder ligaments can be disrupted and can result in shoulder dislocations, which are frequently associated with bouts of severe acute pain. Disruption of the anterior cruciate and medial collateral ligaments of the knee produces instability and pain, particularly during athletic activities. Symptomatic ligament instability requires reconstruction, usually by repair. Figure 87-8 illustrates rupture and repair of the acromioclavicular and coracoclavicular ligaments caused by a fall on the shoulder during an athletic activity.

Reconstruction of ligaments can also be done by biologic replacement, such as the use of semitendinosus graft for anterior cruciate ligament instability, or by prosthetic replacement, such as the use of a Gore-Tex graft for anterior cruciate insufficiency.

Ligament repairs and reconstruction challenge the surgeon's ability to restore normal stability and motion to the joint. These procedures are frequently indicated, but the result is rarely a completely normal joint. Delayed ligament reconstruction is usually considered when bracing and muscle rehabilitation have been impractical or ineffective.

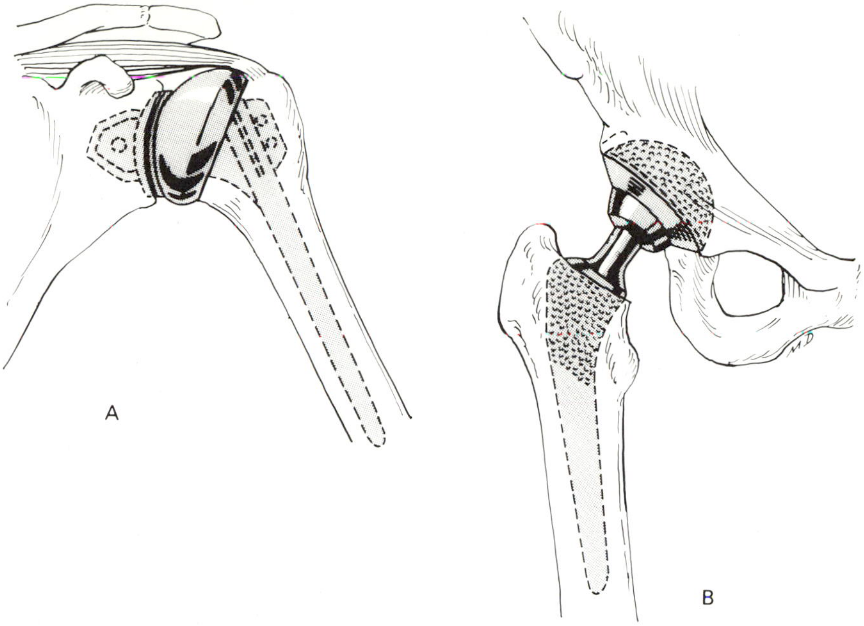

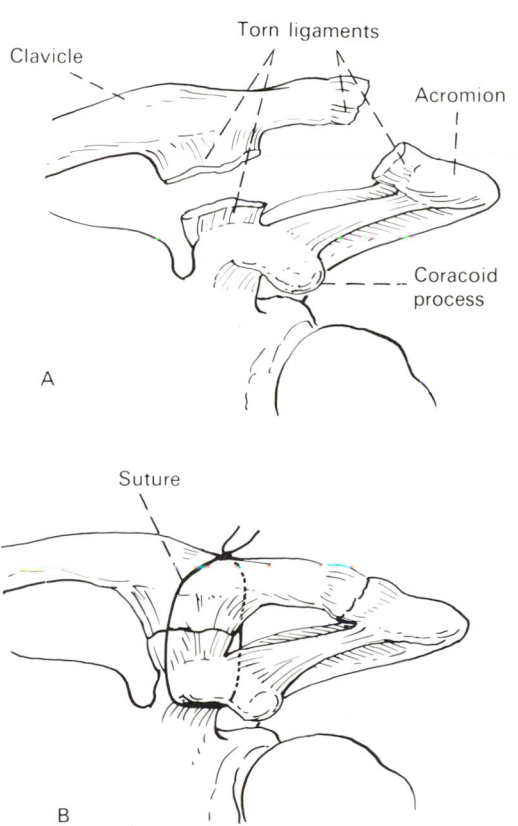

FIG. 87-7. Joint replacement. **A.** Total shoulder arthoplasty **B.** Total hip arthroplasty. In a shoulder replacement it is actually the articulating surfaces of the joints that are replaced. Stability and motion of the joint still depend on capsule ligaments and muscle, as in the physiologic joint. Key elements in these procedures include accurate alignment of compartments, secure fixation of the components in the bone, and careful balancing of the ligaments and muscles about the joint.

Clavicle

Torn ligaments

Acromion

Coracoid process

A

Suture

B

FIG. 87-8. Ligament reconstruction. **A.** Third-degree acromioclavicular separation. In this injury, often sustained in landing on the shoulder after a fall while biking, skiing, playing football, or wrestling, the acromioclavicular and coracoclavicular ligaments can be torn. **B.** When substantial instability results, the torn ligaments are reconstructed by passing secure suture around the coracoid process and the clavicle. The bones are held in proximity while healing occurs.

Tendon Surgery

Essentially, the function of a tendon can be adversely affected in one of three ways: (a) it can become stuck; (b) the myotendinous unit can be contracted; and (c) it can rupture. Injuries in the area of tendons or tendon surgery, or infections around the tendons, can produce adhesions that limit tendon movement, thereby restricting the range of active and passive motion and frequently causing moderate to severe pain. If physical therapy is ineffective in restoring normal flexibility and pull through of the tendon, tenolysis might be required. In this procedure the adhesions are sharply divided and the tendon is started on early motion to prevent restricting adhesions from reforming.

Contracture of the myotendinous unit can result from muscle ischemia, immobilization, or spastic disorders of muscle. The contracture can cause pain and limited range of motion and function. A typical example is a heel cord contracture after a stroke or ischemic contracture of the finger flexors. Tendon lengthening can be accomplished by creating a step cut in the tendon, by a tenotomy (or tendon section), or by tendon excision.

Tendon ruptures can be treated by tendon repair, tendon advancement into bone, tendon grafting, or tenodesis. Figure 87-9 depicts repair of a ruptured rotator cuff tendon. Tendon repair is often used to manage lacerations or ruptures in the tendon midsubstance, such as a flexor tendon laceration at the wrist or an Achilles tendon rupture. Tendon advancement into bone is used when the tendon defect occurs in close proximity to its insertion into the bone—for example, when a flexor digitorum profundus tendon is ruptured near its attachment to the distal phalanx or when the rotator cuff is ruptured near the greater tuberosity. Tendon grafting is used with major tendon loss or when it is undesirable to have a tendon suture

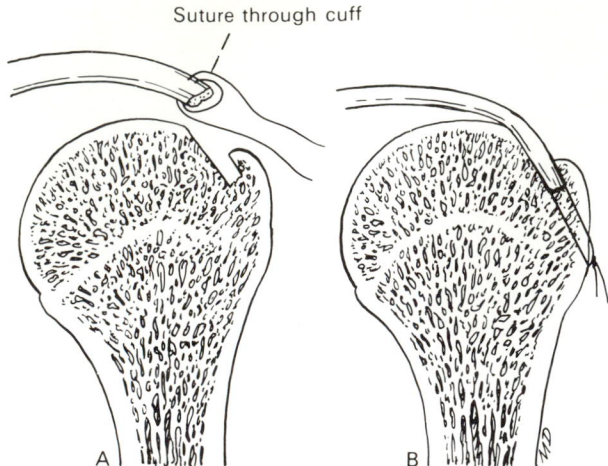

FIG. 87-9. Repair of a ruptured rotator cuff tendon. This is one of the most common tendon ruptures that is seen in orthopedic fractures. Often misdiagnosed as "bursitis" or tendinitis, this condition can involve part or all of the musculotendinous cuff that is so important to shoulder function. *A.* When the tendons are lost from the greater tuberosity, repair can often be accomplished by creating a bony trough in the tuberosity, pulling the tendon through the trough, and suturing it in place. *B.* Drilling holes in bone enable the tendon to be pulled into the trough, which is made in cancellous bone, and secured into position during healing.

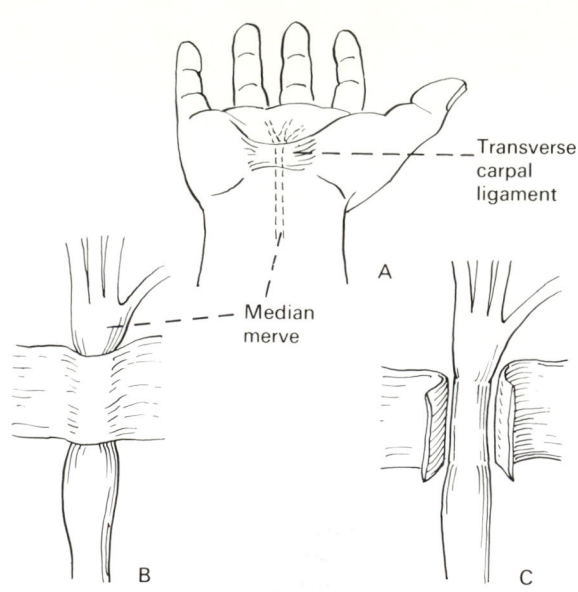

FIG. 87-10. Nerve surgery for the relief of carpal tunnel syndrome. *A, B.* The median nerve is compressed at the wrist, by the transverse carpal ligament, producing pain, hypesthesia in the thumb, index, and long fingers, and weakness of the thenar muscles. *C.* Once the diagnosis has been established, symptoms can usually be dramatically ameliorated by section of the transverse carpal ligament.

line within a certain area, such as in the flexor sheath of the fingers. Finally, tenodesis can be used when it is difficult to restore normal tendon integrity; function can be at least partially restored by securing the ruptured end of the tendon. A classic example is tenodesis of the long head of the biceps to the proximal humerus after an intra-articular rupture.

Nerve Surgery

Nerves can be adversely affected by compression, scarring, or severance. Nerve compression syndromes are usually treated by surgical decompression (14), such as section of the transverse carpal ligament in a carpal tunnel syndrome (Fig. 87-10) or ulnar nerve transfer for ulnar nerve compression at the elbow.

Scarring of nerve after an injury or infection can require a surgical neurolysis. An external neurolysis surgically frees the nerve from a surrounding scar, whereas an internal neurolysis attempts to free the axons from an internal scar. Nerves that are divided can be repaired by direct suture if the ends are fresh and clean, by nerve shortening if a small amount of nerve is damaged, or by nerve grafting if a larger amount of nerve is irrevocably damaged.

Many factors influence the result of nerve surgery. A carpal tunnel decompression, for example, usually brings about a dramatic improvement in the patient's comfort and function, whereas long cable grafting of nerves can produce minimal return of motor function and only protective sensation.

An additional nerve procedure that might be required is the excision of a neuroma. This painful ball of nerve scar can be exquisitely sensitive to applied pressure or can be spontaneously painful. The neuroma can occur after a definite episode of trauma or with repeated microtrauma (e.g., Morton's neuroma at the junction of the medial and lateral plantar nerves). Neuromas usually respond to excision, leaving the resected ends buried deep in bone or soft tissue so that they cannot be stimulated mechanically.

Fasciotomy

Increased tissue pressure from any cause can produce ischemia, with resulting pain and loss of function. This condition, known as compartmental syndrome, requires immediate surgical decompression through a skin incision and fasciotomy to preserve neuromuscular viability (15). The results of this procedure are directly related to the timeliness of the decompression (ideally within 4 hours after onset of the condition) and to the completeness of the decompression (see Fig. 22-3 p. 380).

Fasciotomy can also be indicated in the palm for treating Dupuytren's contracture, in which the extension of the fingers is limited by contracture of the palmar fascia. Surgical release is helpful in restoring comfort and range of motion to the hand. Potential problems include recurrence and the formation of palmar hematoma.

Amputation

Indications for amputation of all or part of an extremity include malignant tumor, refractory infection, nonhealing ulcer, or untreatable ischemia (16). At times amputation is indicated because of total loss of function of a part—for example, in a severe brachial plexus injury resulting in a flail arm below the shoulder. Amputations usually heal, provided they are performed technically well and the flaps have adequate vascularity. Amputations are often not successful in the management of those with chronic pain; in these situations phantom pain develops in some patients (see Chapter 12).

Release of Tight Structures

Occasionally indications arise for the release of structures that have become excessively tight to the point that they are interfering with function or causing pain. One example is lateral retinacular release of knee, which is indicated when a tight lateral retinaculum is pulling the patella eccentrically to the lateral side. Another release is quadricepsplasty, which is indicated when the quadriceps muscle is stuck to the tumor and prevents normal motion and comfort.

Arthroscopy

Looking within a joint by endoscopy or arthroscopy is a widely used procedure in orthopedics. It can be diagnostic (e.g., trying to find out why a knee catches or is painful) or therapeutic (e.g., guiding the reconstruction of the anterior cruciate ligament or managing a meniscus tear).

C. ORTHOPEDIC SURGERY FOR CONTROL OF CANCER PAIN

In many patients with cancer, the pain is caused by primary or metastatic tumors of bone (Chapter 24). Orthopedic surgery is indicated for a significant percentage of these patients as part of a multimodal and interdisciplinary therapy program. In this section we briefly discuss the orthopedic management of pain caused by primary benign and malignant tumors and by metastatic bone lesions. A more detailed discussion of this subject can be found elsewhere (17–21).

Primary Bone Tumors

Benign Primary Bone Tumors

INTRAOSSEOUS BENIGN TUMORS. Intraosseous benign tumor growth is often associated with pain and requires marginal excision to remove the tumor and the cause of the pain. Osteoid osteoma, a benign osteoblastic lesion with a typical well-demarcated nidus, undergoes intraosseous growth with a special pattern of pain that occurs mainly at night and can be temporarily relieved by the use of NSAIDs. For permanent relief of pain, however, it is essential to excise the nidus surgically; it must be completely removed to avoid a recurrence. The characteristic pain disappears promptly after operation.

EXTRAOSSEOUS TUMOR GROWTH. A benign bone tumor with expansive extraosseous growth should be removed surgically if it causes pain or if its benign nature cannot be verified. A good example of this is a large osteochondroma that causes extraosseous expansion and consequent pressure and irritation of periosteal nociceptors. If the tumor involves the femur the pain is aggravated when the patient is sitting. Osteochondroma of the lumbar spine is frequently associated with low back pain that becomes progressively worse. As the tumor grows it compresses the sacral plexus or the sciatic nerve, causing severe pain that requires surgical excision.

Malignant Primary Bone Tumors

Malignant primary bone tumors that may indicate early surgical therapy include chondrosarcoma, fibrosarcoma, giant cell tumor, osteosarcoma, and malignant fibrous histiocytoma. The first three are usually low-grade tumors that tend to be locally invasive, are slow-growing, and have little propensity to metastasize, but all of them produce progressively more severe pain as they enlarge and stretch the periosteum and also encroach on soft tissue around them. Thus a tumor of the head and neck of the humerus produces continuous pain in the shoulder, tumors of the femoral head and neck produce steady severe hip pain, and tumors of the lower femur and upper tibia produce severe knee pain. These low-grade malignant tumors can be treated by wide en bloc resection of the entire tumor. In some instances, orthopedic surgeons curette giant cell tumors, removing all of the tumor tissue and then filling the cavity with cancellous bone fixed with a fiber adhesion system to promote a new growth of granulation tissue and to keep the bone chips temporarily immobile so that they do not fall into the joint (18). The operation results in relief of pain, but a slight limitation of hip movement can occur. Others (21) use curettage and laser to evacuate the tumor. In any case, with removal of the tumor the pain is eliminated.

Some primary malignant bone tumors that are sensitive to chemotherapy, including osteogenic sarcoma and Ewing's sarcoma, are treated by aggressive multiagent chemotherapy. Often such therapy reduces, eliminates, or prevents macroscopic occult metastasis and can even decrease the size of the tumor and thus eliminate or reduce the pain (Chapter 89). Combined aggressive chemotherapy and surgery have lowered the mortality rate from osteogenic sarcomas by approximately 50% in comparison with radical surgery alone in a 5-year followup (18). Good results have been obtained in the treatment of Ewing's tumor and osteosarcoma with aggressive combined chemotherapy (21).

Depending on the age of the patient and on the sensitivity of the tumor to chemotherapy, three surgical procedures for the treatment of the pain of a malignant primary bone tumor can be done. First, the limb can be amputated, which removes the cause of the pain from the primary tumor but can be followed by phantom or stump pain or both. Second, resection-plasty can be used for surgical treatment of osteogenic sarcomas of the distal femur (20). With this method the tumor is resected along with two-thirds of the femur, including the knee joint, but the sciatic nerve, femoral artery, and two veins are preserved to guarantee nerve and blood supply to the leg. This usually produces relief of pain without the risk of phantom or stump pain developing. Finally, an endoprosthetic replacement can be done, a procedure that is carried out for lesions of the hip, knee, or shoulder joint if radical tumor resection is possible. This method has the advantage of eliminating the primary tumor and consequently the cause of pain, without the risk of phantom or stump pain. Great caution must be exercised to avoid infection and to prevent loosening of the endoprosthetic replacement.

Metastatic Bone Tumors

Metastases of primary tumors of bone occur more often than primary bone tumors, particulary in patients with breast, prostate, thyroid, kidney, and lung cancer and other types of malignant tumors (Chapters 24 and 57). Invariably such tumors are painful because of osteolytic or osteoblastic bone destruction, expansive tumor growth, and consequent pathologic fractures. These tumors are usually treated with radiotherapy alone or combined with chemotherapy, but frequently orthopedic surgery in the form of bracing or metal plates is required. Indeed, fracture of the long bones that is causing severe pain might require orthopedic intervention as the primary therapy for relieving the pain.

The following are indications for orthopedic surgery in cases of skeletal metastasis (17):

a. The tumor shows little or no sensitivity to radiotherapy, chemotherapy, or both.

b. The maximum dose of radiation is applied and moderate to severe pain and instability are still present.

c. Pathologic fractures, particularly in the lower extremities, are causing severe pain and instability.

d. It is hoped that pain can be relieved and the quality of life can be improved, resulting in early mobilization and rehabilitation.

Surgery can be done provided the general condition of the patient, prognosis, and operability of the tumor have been considered and the advantages, disadvantages, limitations, and intra- and postoperative complications have been discussed with the patient.

Surgical treatment entails resection or excochleation of the metastatic tumor for implantation of an endoprosthetic replacement or combined osteosynthesis with polymethylmethacrylate and metallic implants. Generally, metastatic lesions in the spine are treated with radiotherapy, orthotic bracing, and chemotherapy. Exceptions to this are those with solitary nonradiosensitive metastatic destruction to vertebrae, with initial paraplegia, severe pain, or both (17).

REFERENCES

1. Adam, J.C.: Outline of Orthopaedics. 10th Ed. Baltimore, Williams & Wilkins, 1986, pp. 24–40.
2. Evarts, C.M.: Surgery of the Musculoskeletal System. New York, Churchill Livingstone, 1983, pp. 3-3–3-273, 6-3–6-173.
3. Speed, J.S., and Knight, R.A.: Campbell's Operative Orthopaedics. St. Louis, C.V. Mosby, 1951.
4. Matsen, F.A.: Glenohumeral instability. In Surgery of the Musculoskeletal System. Edited by C.M. Evarts. New York, Churchill Livingstone, 1983, pp. 3-49–3-75.
5. Rang, M.: Children's Fractures. Philadelphia, J.B. Lippincott, 1974.
6. Rockwood, C.A., and Green, D.P.: Fractures. Philadelphia, J.B. Lippincott, 1975.
7. Hilton, J.: Rest and pain (1871). Reprint edited by E.W. Walls and E.E. Phillip. Philadelphia, J.V. Lippincott, 1950.
8. Stillwell, G.K.: Clinical electric stimulation. In Therapeutic Electricity and Ultraviolet Radiation. 2nd Ed. Edited by S. Licht. New Haven, CT, Elizabeth Licht, Publisher, 1967, pp. 105–155.
9. Fortune, W.P.: Hip osteotomies. In Surgery of the Musculoskeletal System. Edited by C.M. Evarts. New York, Churchill Livingstone, 1983, pp. 6-31–6-56.
10. Whitesides, T.: The spine. In Surgery of the Musculoskeletal System. Edited by C.M. Evarts. New York, Churchill Livingstone, 1983, pp. 4-3–4-310.
11. Wiesel, S.W., and Rothman, R.H.: Lumbar disc disease and spinal stenosis. In Surgery of the Musculoskeletal System. Edited by C.M. Evarts. New York, Churchill Livingstone, 1983, pp. 4-57–4-84.
12. Cofield, R.H.: Arthrodesis and resection arthroplasty of the shoulder. In Surgery of the Musculoskeletal System. Edited by C.M. Evarts. New York, Churchill Livingstone, 1983, pp. 3-125–3-144.
13. Stinchfield, F.E.: Total hip replacement: An overview. In Surgery of the Musculoskeletal System. Edited by C.M. Evarts. New York, Churchill Livingstone, 1983, pp. 6-157–6-171.
14. Jabaley, M.E.: Peripheral nerve injuries. In Surgery of the Musculoskeletal System. Edited by C.M. Evarts. New York, Churchill Livingstone, 1983, pp. 1-107–1-144.
15. Matsen, F.A.: Compartmental Syndromes. New York, Grune & Stratton, 1980.
16. Epps, C.H.: Amputations. In Surgery of the Musculoskeletal System. Edited by C.M. Evarts. New York, Churchill Livingstone, 1983, pp. 12-3–12-154.
17. Mankin, H.J.: Bone and soft tissue tumors. In Surgery of the Musculoskeletal System. Edited by C.M. Evarts. New York, Churchill Livingstone, 1983, pp. 11-3–11-402.
18. Braun, A., and Rohe, K.: Orthopedic surgery for management of tumor pain. In Pain in the Cancer Patient. Edited by M. Zimmermann, P. Drings, and G. Wagner. Heidelberg, Springer-Verlag, 1984, pp. 157–170.
19. Enneking, W.F.: Musculoskeletal Tumor Surgery. New York, Churchill Livingstone, 1983.
20. Salzer, M., et al.: Treatment of osteosarcoma of the distal femur by rotation-plasty. Arch. Orthop. Trauma. Surg., 99:131, 1981.
21. Rosenberg, S.A., et al.: Sarcomas of the soft tissue and bone. In Cancer: Principles and Practice of Oncology. Edited by V.T. DeVita, Jr., S. Hellman, and S.A. Rosenberg. Philadelphia, J.B. Lippincott, 1982, pp. 1067–1093.

88 · PHYSICAL THERAPY AND REHABILITATION MEDICINE

Mathew H.M. Lee, Masayoshi Itoh, Gai-Fu William Yang, *and* Alice L. Eason

THE use of physical agents or methods in the relief of pain can be traced back to the dawn of civilization. When primitive man hurt or felt discomfort, he instinctively rubbed the area. He crawled into the sunshine to receive the benefits of its warmth. Later he might learn to apply snow or a hot stone over the affected area to soothe the painful sensation. Ancient physicians in Egypt and Greece employed electricity in the form of shocks from torpus and catfish for the treatment of certain diseases, including pain.

The Romans and Greeks, who practiced various forms of hydrotherapy, massage, exercise, and thermotherapy, influenced the development of many modern pain control techniques. Numerous scientists and physicians have contributed to our understanding of the mechanisms involved in various physical modalities for pain, and many well-documented experiments are described in Morowitz (1) and Licht (2).

Physical medicine is the treatment of disabilities, including pain due to disease, injury, or loss of a body part, with various physical modalities. Treatment of chronic pain, in particular, requires a team approach. Generally, the team would consist of a physiatrist (a physician specializing in physical medicine and rehabilitation), a neurologist, an orthopedist, a physical therapist trained to administer various modalities, and an occupational therapist (OT), who also performs various exercises but generally applies them as a part of a functional activity. The OT's most important contribution to pain management is instructing patients how to perform the activities of daily living in an energy-efficient and pain-avoiding manner. A social worker's assessment of a patient's home situation, support system, and job situation is also essential in the care of a patient as a whole person.

Yeh et al. (3) defined three goals of physical therapy in pain control:

1. To determine the most effective means of decreasing or controlling the patient's pain.
2. To correct as much as possible the dysfunctions identified on the initial evaluation.
3. To restore the patient's confidence in the ability to move and enjoy physical activity by reducing fear of further injury or pain.

This chapter is divided into three main sections. In the first, we briefly discuss some fundamental aspects of physical modalities in the management of pain. The second section contains a brief description of each modality, including its indications, physiologic effects, and technique of administration. The major modalities discussed are thermotherapy (heat), cryotherapy (cold), electrotherapy, mechanotherapy (exercise, massage, traction), and laser. Full details of the techniques involved in using each modality can be found in several rehabilitation medicine textbooks (2, 4–9). In the third section, clinical applications of various modalities in the treatment of specific conditions are discussed.

GENERAL CONSIDERATIONS

Physical modalities, when properly used, can decrease acute pain and relieve subacute or chronic pain for an extended period. Prescribing physicians need not know all the details of each modality, but before prescribing any physical modality, a physician should know its indications, contraindications, precautions, and principles of application, as well as its availability. A referral or prescription for any physical therapy should include the patient's name, sex, age, diagnosis, precautions, modality to be used, area(s) to be treated, frequency of treatment, and any other special instructions.

As with other pain control methods, the use of physical therapy does not guarantee the elimination or minimization of pain in part because perception of pain differs greatly from one person to another. Before prescribing physical modalities, the physician must be well aware of the cause, diagnosis, prognosis, nature, and duration of pain; the patient's emotional, social, and economic status; and his coping skills. Learning about the total patient, "his psyche as well as his physical" part, through an in-depth history and physical examination is essential in developing a successful pain management strategy, since each influences the outcome of the treatment (10).

The effect of each physical modality is different. Some modalities, such as hydrocollator packs, may provide almost instantaneous relief of pain, but after a certain period of time, pain may recur. Others, such as ultrasound, may produce a slow but cumulative effect. At times, pain relief may last for a long time, and complete relief of pain sometimes occurs. Although total elimination of pain is ideal, this goal is not always obtainable, particularly with chronic pain. Even when there is residual discomfort (i.e., pain exists but is bearable), therapeutic regimes are considered successful if patients can engage in daily living activities or function relatively well in work activities.

One may question the rationale of using physical modalities that have only short-lasting effects, but such modalities have their place in the comprehensive approach to pain control. Even temporary relief of pain is welcomed by persons suffering from chronic pain. Furthermore, during the pain-free period, other rehabilitation regimes that are beneficial for further decrease of pain (e.g., stretching or strengthening exercises) may be applied.

Several reasons can account for no change in the level of pain after a series of treatments with various modalities: the patient's pain perception; the selection of an inappropriate modality; or the pain mechanism may be such that physical treatments have no impact. Regardless of the reason, the development of a new treatment plan is warranted.

Just as a person who is suffering from chronic pain and is receiving drug therapy may develop drug dependency, a person may develop a dependency on physical modalities. Therefore, prolonged application of a modality sometimes is harmful. If this situation occurs, the physician should explain the problem to the patient and the modality should be tapered, altered, or discontinued.

SPECIFIC PHYSICAL THERAPIES

Thermotherapy

Historically, heat and cold have been used more often than other modalities in the relief of pain because of their special properties and physiologic effects. Heat therapy provides analgesic, decongestive, antispasmodic, and sedative effects.

PHYSIOLOGIC EFFECTS. Physiologic reactions to elevated tissue temperature resulting from heat therapy include decreased vasomotor tone, increased tissue metabolism, and increased blood flow (10, 11). The increased blood flow aids in restoring proper nutrition and elimination of waste products. Heat also raises the threshold of sensory nerve endings (12) and may break the pain/spasm/pain cycle by influencing the muscle spindles and gamma system (13). If a muscle is heated, the desirable range is 42 to 43° C; a temperature exceeding 46° C will result in a burn. Heat also alters the viscoelastic properties of connective tissue and is, therefore, usually followed by massage and stretching to regain the length of muscles and tendons, thereby reducing pain. In addition, heat has also been reported to assist in diminishing chronic inflammatory processes (14, 15).

SIDE EFFECTS AND CONTRAINDICATIONS. Elevation of tissue temperature increases the activity of proteolytic enzymes in rheumatoid arthritis and can accelerate the destructive process in the joints despite symptomatic improvement (16). Heat induces capillary dilatation and increases local blood flow as well as edema. Therefore, heat should be avoided in acute inflammation or trauma until the initial process has subsided. When extensive areas of the body are heated, a generalized increase in cardiac output occurs. This can be dangerous in patients with cardiovascular and respiratory insufficiency or failure.

Local heat increases the metabolic demand of the tissue and, if there is circulatory compromise in that area, may precipitate ischemia and gangrene. Extreme caution should be taken when treating patients with bleeding diathesis or those who are on anticoagulants because the increased blood flow and vascularity may lead to complications. Thus, heat is absolutely contraindicated in a hemorrhage site. When a patient has a sensation impairment or is obtunded, heat is relatively contraindicated, because of the loss of the protective axon reflex. Increasing body temperature may result in neurologic deterioration in patients with multiple sclerosis. Heat is generally not indicated for patients with malignancy, since it may accelerate cancerous cell growth and metastasis (17). The exception to this is the use of local hyperthermia in conjunction with ionizing radiation for treatment of certain tumors. If heat therapy is used with very young, elderly, psychotic, or retarded patients, or persons with sensory impairment, extreme caution must be taken, because their perception of heat may be altered and they may be unable to alert the care provider of a burning sensation (18, 19). Constant inspection of the treated area is mandatory to prevent burn.

Thermotherapy can be subdivided into modalities that heat the superficial layers of tissue and those that heat the deeper structures. They can also be subdivided according to the primary mode of heat transfer into the tissues: conduction, convection, and the conversion of other forms of energy into heat by absorption (Table 88-1).

Conduction Heat

Hot Packs

The heat from hot packs penetrates the skin only superficially; the subcutaneous fat and musculature are not heated significantly (20). The amount of heat conducted from a pack to the skin is directly proportional to the duration and temperature gradient and inversely proportional to the thickness of the layer of towels between the skin and pack.

A common device for providing conduction heat is the hydrocollator pack. These packs contain silica gel, enclosed within a cotton bag, which absorbs hot water and retains heat for about 30 min. These packs are

TABLE 88-1. Therapeutic Heating Modalities

Primary Mode of Heat Transfer	Modality	Depth
Conduction	Hot packs	Superficial heat
	Paraffin bath	Superficial heat
Convection	Hydrotherapy	Superficial heat
	Fluidotherapy	Superficial heat
Conversion	Infrared	Superficial heat
	Shortwaves	Deep heat
	Microwaves	Deep heat
	Ultrasound	Deep heat

heated in a thermostatically controlled water container. The temperature of the pack, when applied, is about 71 to 79° C. The pack is applied to the treatment area in a drip-dry fashion over layers of terry cloth for 20 to 30 min. Hydrocollator packs are available in various sizes (regular, cervical, knee, eye, back, and shoulder) for use on different areas (Fig. 88-1).

Other devices that provide conduction heat include the hot water bottle, electric heating pad, and commercially available chemical packs. These heat packs are effective in relieving pain from various sources such as muscle spasm, tendinitis, and bursitis. Because of their flexibility, ease of placement over multiple sites, and simple, rapid application, they are the most commonly used modalities in pain management.

Hot packs have no major contraindications other than those mentioned previously. Hydrocollator packs are bulky and heavy and may not be suitable for tender areas. An electric heating pad is dangerous unless the manual turn-off mechanism is attached and the person must depress the device to keep the heat on.

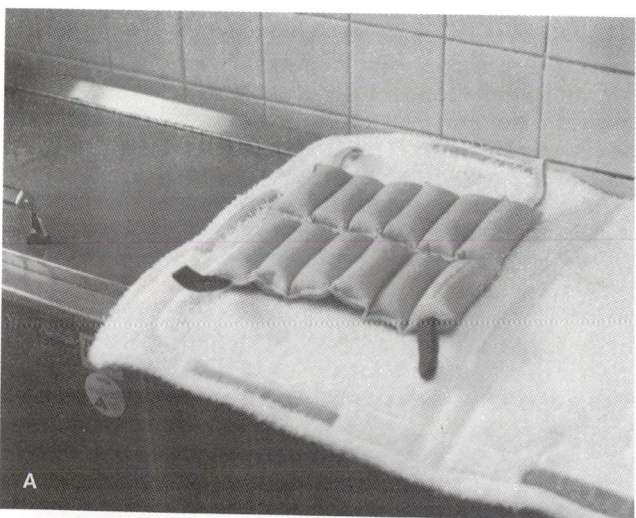

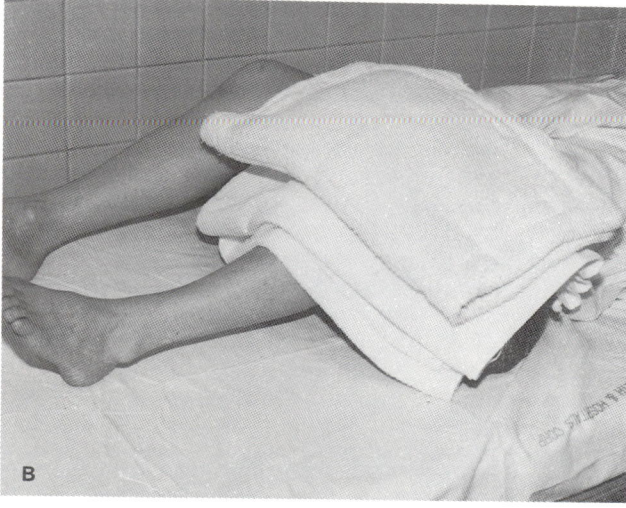

FIG. 88-1. *A.* Hot pack being prepared for application. The pack is wrapped in commercially available terry cloth covers with Velcro closure for application. *B.* Pack in place.

Paraffin Bath

Another way to provide conduction heat is by use of a paraffin bath. This is prepared by placing four to six parts paraffin wax and one part mineral oil in a thermostatically controlled stainless steel unit, which maintains the mixture in a liquid state at a temperature of 51.7 to 54.4° C. The temperature should not be higher than 53.3° C for the general population. The heating effect is primarily due to the latent heat during solidification and the specific heat of the wax.

The area to be treated should be washed, cleaned, and dried. Paraffin can be applied either by dipping the extremity rapidly into the container (Fig. 88-2) or by painting the treatment area 6 to 8 times with a brush until the wax forms a coating. After 20 to 30 min, the wax can be easily peeled off and may be reused. The skin becomes soft, pliable, and red, ready for massage or exercise (21).

Paraffin treatment produces a marked increase in the tissue temperature up to 46° C on the surface of the skin and a rapid decrease in the temperature of subcutaneous tissue (22). Paraffin therapy is of special advantage for arthritis of the small joints of the hands and feet, as the heated wax coating around the joint provides optimal heat effects. It is contraindicated where there is a skin cut, rash, local infection, or dermatitis.

Convection Heat

Hydrotherapy

Convection heat is provided by hot or warm water. The most common water temperature is 36.6 to 43° C. If an extremity is involved, a whirlpool at a temperature up to 45° C often is used. If total body immersion is necessary, a hot tub, Hubbard tank, or pool with a temperature of 36.7 to 37.7° C can be used. The maximum temperature for half the body is 40° C, and the

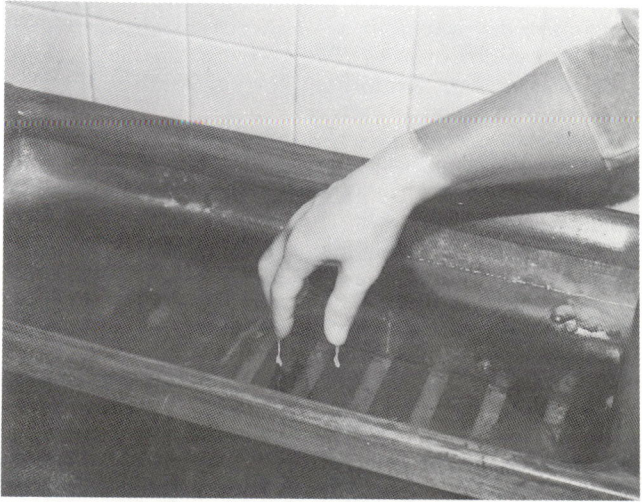

FIG. 88-2. The hand is rapidly immersed into a paraffin bath six to eight times, creating a thick coating of wax, which looks like a glove.

maximum for the hands or feet is 43.3° C. The duration of treatment is 20 to 30 min.

Agitation enhances the benefits of heated water through its massage-like effect. In addition to debridement of necrotic tissue, agitation also keeps the water temperature uniform all over the skin. After the layer of water surrounding the skin has cooled, agitation brings another layer of higher-temperature water to the area being treated. Therefore, the primary heat transfer process is convection, and the degree of heat transfer is determined by the water temperature. An additional benefit of hydrotherapy is the buoyancy of the water, which eliminates gravity stress pain to the joints and permits exercise of weakened patients.

CLINICAL ASPECTS. Convection heat is very superficial and most of the temperature elevation is limited to the area within the skin layers. However, if the total body is immersed in water over 37.7° C, core temperature may be elevated, creating an artificial fever (23); in this situation, the patient would become exhausted and the heat-regulatory mechanism might be impaired. Therefore, it is dangerous to use Hubbard tank therapy with a patient with cardiovascular disease, adrenal suppression, systemic lupus erythematosus (24), or multiple sclerosis. Hubbard tank or pool therapy should be used with caution in pregnancy, since developmental abnormalities apparently evolve during the first trimester if body temperature is increased to or above 38.9° C irrespective of the fever's origin (25). If total body immersion hydrotherapy is applied, oral temperature should be monitored and maintained below 37.7° C.

Hubbard tank or pool therapy is usually indicated for a patient with multiple joint pain, as the large pool allows ambulation training with elimination of gravity. Other forms of hydrotherapy include moist air, cabinet, contrast bath, and hot sitz bath.

Fluidotherapy

Used as an alternative to whirlpool therapy, fluidotherapy employs a container of glass beads with an average diameter of 0.419 mm at a density of 71 kg/m³ through which thermostatically controlled streams of dry warm air are blown to produce a warm, semifluid mixture (26). The part of the body to be treated is immersed and heat is transferred to the skin superficially through convection.

Borrel et al. (27) measured the increase in the temperature of small joints in the hands and feet and of the hand muscles after fluidotherapy at 47.8° C, immersion in paraffin bath, and immersion in a water bath at 38.9° C. They reported that fluidotherapy transmitted more heat to the treated area than the other two modalities. However, this finding is misleading, since the temperature in all three modalities was not the same.

The indications and contraindications for fluidotherapy are the same as those for paraffin therapy.

Conversion Heat

When infrared radiation, shortwaves, microwaves, or ultrasound interacts with tissues, some energy is converted into heat. This heat, like that generated by other means, can have therapeutic effects.

Infrared Radiation

Infrared radiation is emitted by luminous sources (bulbs of various wattages) and nonluminous sources (heating elements of resistant material). Since skin is a poor heat conductor, the radiation penetrates the skin surface less than 10 mm before being absorbed by the tissues and converted to heat energy. A rise in skin temperature over 42.8° C rapidly produces arteriolar flare and wheal. The patient feels the heat instantly (28, 29) if the lamp is warmed up for 10 min before applying it to the area. Currently, infrared therapy is seldom used because it provides less relief of pain than treatment with paraffin or hot packs.

CLINICAL ASPECTS. The lamp should be centered over the treatment area at a distance of approximately 25 to 61 cm and at a right angle for maximum benefit (Fig. 88-3). The duration of treatment is usually 20 to 30 min. All metal-containing objects should be removed from the area to prevent burns, since metals easily absorb infrared radiation. A wet compress pad should be placed over any scar tissues and abrasions, and the eyes if treatment is to the face (30, 31).

Infrared is commonly used for relaxation-inducing relief of pain from muscle spasm or tension, myofibrositis, and rheumatic joints. It has also been used to dry the skin over the inguinal and perineal areas and gluteal fold to prevent bedsores. It should not be used if the patient is sensitive to light. Reactions such as heat-induced urticaria have been observed (32).

Shortwave Diathermy

In shortwave diathermy, a patient is placed within an electromagnetic field created by a high-frequency alternating current. The patient's impedance forms a part of the secondary circuit of a high-frequency generator; heat results from the tissue resistance to the passage of the electrical current. The patient's circuitry must be in resonance with the oscillating circuit of the machine. The frequencies specified by the Federal Communications Commission for shortwave operations are 13.66, 27.33, and 40.98 MHz (33).

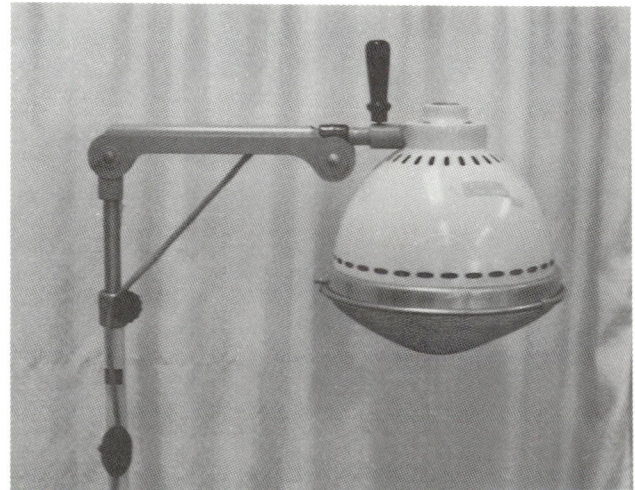

FIG. 88-3. Infrared lamp used for superficial heating. Arm of lamp is adjustable for maintaining precise, safe distance from area to be treated.

CLINCAL ASPECTS. The dosage is determined by the patient's heat tolerance, since it is not practical to measure the high-frequency current flow through the body tissue. The greatest heating effect occurs in the top 1 to 2 cm of the subcutaneous tissues and superficial musculature (34). Lehmann et al. (35) reported that the temperature reached 40 to 45° C in the human thigh after 20-min exposure to a shortwave helical coil at 27.12 MHz.

Heat is transmitted to the treated area by capacitive coupling (Fig. 88-4) using a pair of condensor plates, by an inductive applicator with various configurations of coils, or by other means, such as internal vaginal and rectal electrodes. The choice of applicator depends mostly upon the area to be treated. The treatment area should be covered with a single layer of towel to absorb perspiration in order to prevent concentration of electric energy. Metal objects (e.g., metal chair, bed, jewelry, safety pins, watch) should be removed from the electromagnetic field, because heat accumulation on the metal will cause a skin burn. The duration of treatment is usually 20 min (36, 37).

Common indications for heat therapy are applicable to shortwave diathermy. This modality is particularly useful in the relief of pain associated with muscle spasm, since the heat penetrates the superficial musculature. For pain from rheumatic diseases, shortwave diathermy should be used only after the inflammatory process subsides otherwise potential damage may occur from increased collagenase activity (38).

In addition to the contraindications for heat therapy described previously, shortwave diathermy should not be considered for patients with superficial metal implants of any type, such as a cardiac pacemaker, electronic control brace (39), or intrauterine devices with copper or other metals, because metals absorb heat easily and create a burn. When there are deep-seated metal implants, such as cup or total arthroplasties of the hip, shortwave diathermy can be used, but extreme caution must be exercised. During their menstrual period, women should avoid shortwave diathermy to the low back because it increases menstrual flow (39). Pregnant women should not be treated with vaginal diathermy because of possible damage to the fetus (35). Some authors state that shortwave diathermy should not be applied to the growth zones of children's bones because it disturbs growth (15, 40).

Microwave Diathermy

Two frequencies of microwave radiation, 2456 and 915 MHz, are approved for medical use (41). Recent data, however, suggest that the optimal frequency to minimize the heating effect in subcutaneous tissues and to maximize it in underlying tissues is 900 MHz or below (42).

Microwave energy is absorbed in the body and raises the tissue temperature. With approved frequencies, the highest temperature reflections are found at the interface between fat and muscle, and a large amount of energy is converted into heat in the subcutaneous tissue (43).

CLINICAL ASPECTS. Microwave diathermy is no more effective than shortwave diathermy when heating is desired in deep tissue. However, microwave diathermy is easier to apply, provides deep heating without undue heating of the skin, and produces a more localized deep heat than the widespread heat from shortwave diathermy (44–46).

Microwaves are applied through directors varying in size, diameter, or rectangular length, depending upon the part of the body to be treated. A spacer attached to the director is used to determine the proper distance of the microwave source from the body surface. No towel is used between the skin and director, and treatment is given for 20 to 30 min.

The contraindications for microwave diathermy are essentially the same as those for shortwave diathermy.

Ultrasound

Ultrasound therapy provides deep, localized, penetrating heat. Ultrasound consists of sound waves at frequencies above those heard by the human ear (16,000 to 20,000 cycles per second). High-frequency ultrasound (800,000 to 1,000,000 cps) is now also available for therapeutic use. Ultrasound waves can be produced by a quartz or barium titanate crystal placed between two electrodes, which emits mechanical vibrations by reversal of the piezoelectric effect (47).

PHYSIOLOGIC ASPECTS. The effect of the ultrasound waves is mechanical, producing heat and chemical reactions. Heat is generated by collisions of particles with different masses and energy states. A higher energy level can be obtained when different particles collide and an interface reaction is produced. The waves will be reflected because they are smaller than many crystal particles. The amount of reflection depends on the mismatch of acoustic impedance. Lehmann and Johnson (48) demonstrated that 30% of energy may be reflected at a soft tissue–bone interface. Thus, it is possible to heat the capsule of the hip joint selectively.

Ultrasound is propagated in the form of longitudinal compression waves. The mechanical reaction occurring within an ultrasonic beam is created by the particle movement as a result of this wave propagation. The movement may induce a secondary reaction, cavitation, because dissolved gases are always present in tissues. Gas-filled cavities may form in the body fluid

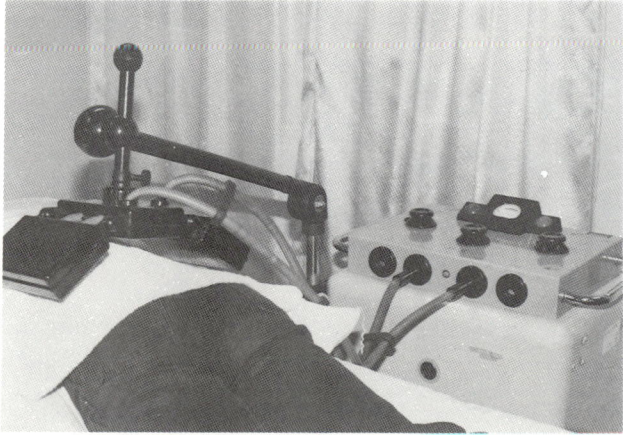

FIG. 88-4. Patient receiving shortwave diathermy to low back. Heat is transmitted through hinged-type drums. A single layer of Turkish towel is applied to the treatment area.

during the rarefaction phase of sound wave propagation. During the following compression phase, cavities may collapse as gas moves to the surrounding fluid. Cavities will expand during the next rarefaction phase as gas moves into them (49). After this repetitive cycle, the cavities will grow. Mechanical destruction is produced when the cavities collapse or when gas bubbles grow large enough to vibrate in resonance with the sound waves (50). A chemical reaction from altering the membrane or cellular functions has been described as a result of this cavitation process.

The most important physiologic and therapeutic effect of the application of ultrasound is heating. A small amount of energy is converted into heat in the skin and subcutaneous fat, and very little in the musculature (51). Ultrasound penetrates muscles quite satisfactorily, and one-half of the energy intensity is still available at about 3 cm. Most of the energy is converted to heat at the bone interface (39, 52). This heating effect increases blood flow, elevates pain threshold, enhances capillary permeability and tissue metabolism, facilitates fibrous extensibility, and alters the neuromuscular activity that leads to muscle relaxation (53–55).

APPLICATION TECHNIQUE.　To ensure the effectiveness of ultrasound therapy, the body part to be treated is cleaned with water or alcohol, and then a coupling agent is applied over the skin area. The coupling agent assures efficient energy transmission to the tissue from the piezoelectric applicator. There is no significant difference in energy transmission between different coupling agents, which include water, Soni-gel, Aquasonic, Ultra-phonic, Medco, and mineral oil (56). The agent should not contain any gas bubbles because these dissipate the energy, reflect and scatter ultrasound, and decrease its effectiveness (56). Some ultrasound machines have a built-in sensor and make a bell sound when the contact between the skin and applicator is less than two-thirds or one-half of the surface area of the applicator.

Because of variability in the acoustic field, possible standing wave formation, and cavitation, the applicator should be passed slowly in circular or parallel overlapping back-and-forth strokes for 5 to 10 min per treatment area (Fig. 88-5A). A stationary technique can be used with machines that have a pulsed, intermittent output control. In the underwater technique, the body part to be treated and the transducer applicator are immersed in a water bath (Fig. 88-5B). The applicator is kept at a distance of 1 to 2.5 cm from the body part and held at a right angle to it.

The incident energy intensity with these techniques ranges from 0.5 to 4.0 watts/cm^2. The patient should feel only slightly warm and pleasant sensations. If prickly pain is felt, the intensity should be decreased because such pain indicates the periosteum temperature is reaching 46° C or above. As tolerance increases during the course of treatment, greater intensities may become necessary. If the patient complains of pain during treatment, the intensity should be reduced or the applicator should be moved slightly faster. An overdosage of ultrasound can cause pain and damage tissues (52, 57, 58). The patient must be instructed to inform the therapist if pain occurs. Pain, not a sense of warmth, is the best indicator of an intensity that is too high or inappropriate application.

INDICATIONS.　Because of its deep heat penetration, ultrasound has proven to be effective, especially when it is used in conjunction with stretching or therapeutic exercises, for bursitis (59, 60), calcified bursitis (61, 62), tendinitis, joint contracture (63), and periarthritic conditions (64, 65). Other conditions in which ultrasound has been found helpful include scarring from injury, burn, or diseases such as scleroderma (66, 67); relief of pain from postoperative neuroma following amputation (68, 69); chronic ulcerations (70); pain from sprains for a short period after onset (71); myofascial syndrome (72, 73); and plantar warts (74).

PRECAUTIONS AND CONTRAINDICATIONS.　Under certain circumstances, ultrasound produces "standing waves" in blood vessels, with "banding" and stasis of red cells, which are potentially dangerous. The heart should not be exposed directly to ultrasound because its action potentials and contractile and conduction properties could be changed (75). Ultrasound should not be applied to an eye, even in a therapeutic dose, because the fluid media in the eyes can easily form cavitation from ultrasonic waves and irreversible damage

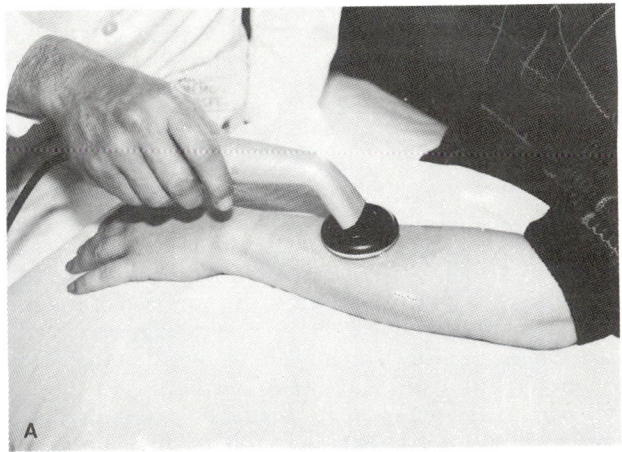

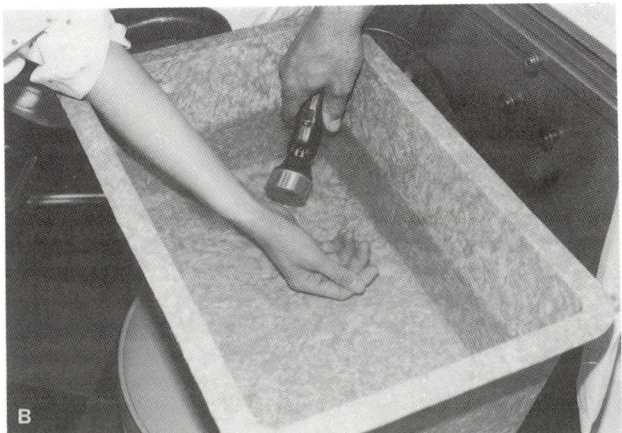

FIG. 88-5. A. Direct technique of treatment with ultrasound. A commercially available gel, applied to the body part, acts as a coupling agent through which ultrasound waves pass. B. Underwater technique of applying ultrasound. Transducer head should be 1 to 2 cm from part being treated.

may result. The same situation occurs in amniotic fluid with possible fetal malformation due to thermal damage (25).

The spinal cord, after laminectomy, should not be treated with ultrasound, even at lower dosages, because the spinal cord may receive higher energy levels due to the absence of the facet joints and surrounding tissues. Joints that have been replaced with methyl methacrylate and high-density polyethylene material also should not be exposed to ultrasound, because selective absorption of heat by these materials may produce overheating of the area. All metallic implants, are good heat conductors, and their presence is a contraindication for ultrasound treatment because they transmit the heat rapidly away from the treated area. Other common contraindications are conditions that can be aggravated by ultrasound such as malignant tumor and peripheral vascular insufficiency. All general contraindications to heat treatment also are applicable to ultrasound therapy.

RELATED THERAPIES. The combination of ultrasound and electric stimulation is a common practice today; in this technique the ultrasound applicator is also an electrode. No reputable studies, however, have demonstrated that this combination therapy is superior to either modality used alone or consecutively. In phonophoresis, ultrasound is used to drive ions or medications to the affected area, where the pain or a decubitus ulcer may occur. Although this technique has received some attention, research is needed to establish its efficacy.

Cryotherapy

No consensus exists on the effectiveness of cold over heat for pain control. Review of the literature and clinical impressions indicate that these two extremes of the temperature spectrum have similar effects in many areas. The pain threshold can be elevated as a direct effect of heat or cold on the free nerve endings, C fibers, and receptors by blocking pain transmission. Muscle spasm due to joint or skeletal pathology can be reduced by either heat or cold. Spasticity, one of the symptoms of upper motor neuron disease, is controlled very effectively by cold therapy, breaking the vicious cycle of painful spasm, provided the muscle is actually cooled. Cold produces longer-lasting effects than heat, since blood flow is decreased with cold; a reactive hyperthermia may be induced, however, when cold is removed. Heat can also reduce spasticity, and when heat is removed from the treated area, the muscle tone returns to its original state very rapidly. Edema, swelling, or tissue damage is aggravated by heat but reduced by cold. On the other hand, the joint stiffness symptom is decreased by heat and increased by cold.

PHYSIOLOGIC EFFECTS AND INDICATIONS. Cryotherapy, the application of cold to a local area, has several beneficial therapeutic effects, including analgesia, anti-inflammation, retardation of neuromuscular transmission, and antipyrexia.

Analgesia is produced by vasoconstriction and decreased nerve conduction velocity (76, 77). These two factors reduce the amount of noxious stimuli transmitted into the dorsal horn from the painful area. There-fore, the "gate of pain" cannot be opened to send pain stimuli to the higher center. The initial extreme cold is followed by a burning sensation (78), which acts as a counterirritant and thus activates the brain stem to exert inhibitory influences on the noxious input, thereby closing the gate of pain (79). This counterirritation may also stimulate the brain to secrete endorphins. The long-lasting pain relief following cryotherapy may be due to disruption of the self-sustaining neural loops (80).

The anti-inflammatory effects of cold are derived primarily from vasoconstriction (followed by periodic vasodilation to maintain tissue viability) and from a decreased metabolic rate, histamine release, lymph production, and capillary permeability. Vasoconstriction is produced reflexly via sympathetic fibers and by the direct effect of cold on blood vessels (81). The decreased blood flow leads to diminishing edema, bleeding, leukocytosis, and proteolytic enzyme activity in cooled tissues (82, 83). Because of these effects, cryotherapy has been used routinely for acute injury or trauma.

Other physiologic effects of cold include decreased activity of the muscle spindle (84–86), neuromuscular junction (87), and peripheral nerve (88, 89). These effects are the theoretical basis for reduction of spasticity, muscle spasm, and muscle tone and are perhaps the basis for utilizing cold in muscle re-education or facilitation techniques (90). These techniques use ice massage of the skin over the muscle whose function should be enhanced as a part of the rehabilitation program. The decrease in muscle spasm often observed after cryotherapy may also be due to the analgesic effect of the treatment; that is, protective muscle splinting would diminish when pain subsides, thus disrupting the pain-spasm-pain cycle. This sequence possibly explains the long-term pain relief obtained from cold treatment. Although cold increases muscle viscosity and then increases muscle stiffness, this effect can be minimized by therapeutic exercises immediately after cryotherapy while the analgesic effect is still present.

Contraindications to cryotherapy are vascular insufficiency with inadequate transport of metabolites to and from the tissue, anesthetic area, cold sensitivity or intolerance with uticaria/purpura, indolent wounds, Raynaud's phenomenon, cryoglobulinemia, and paroxysmal cold hemoglobinuria (91). For psychologic reasons, some patients cannot accept this type of therapy.

Cold Packs

Cold packs are available in different sizes and shapes. Commercially available cold packs are made of a soft, supple, pliable gel that is enclosed in a thin rubber plastic pouch (Fig. 88-6). Packs are stored in a special cold pack machine or freezer until ready for use. Packs remain cold for up to one-half hour after removal from a freezer. The area to be treated should be exposed and covered with four to six layers of Turkish toweling depending on the patient's tolerance. The cold pack is applied on the towels for 20 to 30 min or until anesthesia of the area is attained. Prolonged application can cause freezing of the skin and frostbite (92–95).

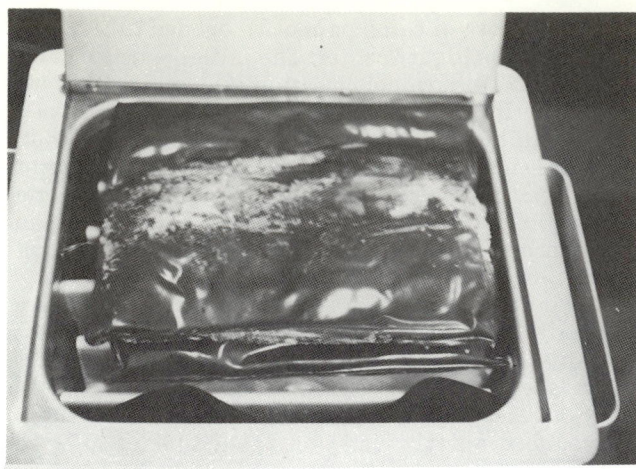

FIG. 88-6. Cold pack enclosed in rubber plastic pouch.

Vapocoolant Sprays

Fluorimethane and ethyl chloride sprays are commercially available and can be used to relieve pain secondary to irritable trigger points or muscle spasm. With the spray container held at a 35° angle and 46 cm from the treated area, a jet stream of fluorimethane is directed at the origin of the muscle down to the insertion, with three or four back and forth sweeps at 10-sec intervals, followed by a gentle muscle stretch or deep tissue massage. The number of sweeps depends on the size of the muscle or area being treated (96–99). Overchilling of the muscle can cause an increase in spasm and reverse the objective of the treatment.

Ice Water

A mixture of ice and water is a good and inexpensive agent for cryotherapy. The temperature of the mixture should be 0° C. The part of the body to be treated should be immersed in the ice water. This may be painful at first, and the body part should be withdrawn after 20 to 30 sec of immersion. This action is repeated several times over a period of 5 min. Another method is wrapping the treated area with Turkish towels that have been dipped in water with shaved ice at a temperature of 14.4° C or lower. The treatment period is approximately 30 min. A cold shower or a brisk swim in cold water can be stimulating and invigorating, and beneficial when a person is depressed or lethargic.

Ice Stick or Block

Usually used for ice massage, this technique involves moving a block or stick of ice over the surface to be cooled. It takes at least 10 min to observe cooling effects on the muscle in a thin individual and one-half hour in an obese person (10). The therapeutic effect is obtained when the clonus or the tendon jerk is abolished or when resistance to rapid motion is decreased.

Electrotherapy

The development of electrotherapy for pain management has evolved from centuries of experimental research on electricity. During the last century, the stimulation of muscle by using galvanic (direct) and faradic (alternating) current was developed. Therapeutic electricity is still in use to stimulate both denervated and innervated muscles.

Direct (Galvanic) Current

Direct current is steady, continuous, unidirectional, and it can cause muscle contraction in a denervated state. Consequently, the galvanic current is used mainly to produce muscular contraction in order to retard the progression of atrophy (100). Because denervated muscle fatigues rapidly, only 25 to 50 strong contractions can be obtained at one session. A strong contraction against resistance may be more beneficial. Animal studies have shown that 1 to 2 hours per session and three or four sessions a day are required to retard muscle atrophy. The physiologic effects of direct current include an increase in blood and lymph flow and tissue metabolism, thus relieving pain, and a decrease in intrafascicular/interfascicular agglutination and sclerosis of the areolar tissue.

Recently, several high-voltage galvanic stimulators have gained attention in pain treatment. They produce a sharp rise and decline of electrical impulses with the high voltage generator. The advantages are deeper penetration and less pain to the skin over the treated area, resulting in more comfort to the patient.

APPLICATION TECHNIQUE. The current must enter and leave the body through two wet electrodes with the proper polarity. In most instances, the active electrode, either cathode or anode, should give the desired reaction. The size of the dispersive or indifferent electrode should be equal to or larger than the active electrode to complete the circuit for current conduction. The positive and the negative electrode have different chemical reactions, as shown in Table 88-2 (101).

For machines that are poorly labeled or in need of checking, there are two methods to determine polarity—a litmus paper test and water test. An acid reaction under the positive pole and an alkaline reaction on the side of the negative pole can be detected with a piece of litmus paper. The water test shows more bubbles around the negative pole.

TABLE 88-2. Chemical Reactions at Positive and Negative Electrodes

Positive Pole (Anode)	Negative Pole (Cathode)
Attracts oxygen	Attracts hydrogen
Acid	Alkaline
Dehydrates tissues	Liquifies tissues
Vasoconstrictor	Vasodilator
Causes ischemia	Causes hyperemia
Stops bleeding	Causes bleeding
More germicidal	Less germicidal
Sedative	Stimulant
Repels bases, metals, and alkaloids	Repels acids, acid radicals, and halogens
Corrodes metals by oxidation	Does not corrode metals
Relieves pain in congestion	Causes pain (except in cases in which there is ischemia)

From Shestack, R.: Electrical current. In Handbook of Physical Therapy. 3rd Ed. New York, Springer, 1977.

It is advisable to switch polarity every 15 min by using the control installed in the apparatus or to change placement of the electrodes to prevent undesired chemical irritation. Since a denervated muscle does not have a motor point, the active electrode may be placed at the point where the best response is obtained or over each end of the muscle to induce a good contraction in the whole muscle.

Iontophoresis

Another useful application of direct current is iontophoresis, or ion transfer. In this technique, an electrical current of low intensity is applied to the tissue as an electromotive force to induce chemical changes, causing an increase in blood flow, and to introduce substances such as zinc oxide into decubitus ulcers in order to accentuate the healing process. Positive ions (zinc, copper) and alkaloids (e.g., histamine) are driven into the skin at the anode; negative ions and acidoids (salicylic acid) are driven into the skin at the cathode (102).

CLINICAL ASPECTS. The active electrode should be covered with absorptive material thick enough to hold the solution containing the ion or substance to be transferred. Most ions or substances are moved into the area where the skin is broken, or along the sweat glands and hair follicles. Ions diffuse to the circulatory system after penetrating the skin. The treatment current is 0.1 to 0.5 mamp/cm^2 of surface of the active electrode; the duration is 15 to 30 min depending on the medium being used.

For pain relief, lidocaine, cocaine, or Nupercaine (liquid or solution less than 1%) is a good agent to be driven into the skin and then to the painful tissue through circulation to produce anesthesia. Very good results have been claimed with the use of procaine iontophoresis, followed by active exercise, in the treatment of sprains, bursitis, low back pain, sciatica, chronic shoulder spasm, and other spasms of muscular origin (see Chapter 94).

Alternating Current

With an alternating current, the direction of electron flow changes constantly; therefore polarity is not important. There are two basic types of alternating current for medical use—faradic current and sinusoidal-wave current. Faradic current consists of two pulses in opposite directions that follow each other closely. One is a high-intensity/short-duration pulse; the other is a low-intensity/long-duration pulse.

Only innervated muscle responds to faradic stimulation; therefore, this current is mainly indicated to stimulate muscle via its nerve supply. An innervated muscle is easily stimulated by impulses as brief as 0.1 msec. The repetitive stimulation produces relaxation of a muscle in spasm. For spastic paraplegia after spinal cord injury, the application of faradic current to appropriate muscles may reduce spasticity.

Sinusoidal-wave current is a uniform, continuous alternating current with sinusoidal cycles. Each cycle has an equal amount of positive and negative electricity, so the chemical reaction is neutral. This current creates a muscular contraction with each impulse and may be rapid or slow. The applications of sinusoidal-wave current are almost identical to those of faradic current.

For quite some time, interferential therapy has been used for pain control and muscle stimulation. In this technique, two pairs of electrodes are placed perpendicular to each other. This therapeutic modality requires less frequency at each pair of electrodes but produces a modulated (higher) frequency at the cross point of the two currents. The cross point of the currents is located at the point of pain by adjustment of the placement and size of the four electrodes. The patient's maximum comfort is obtained by effectively stimulating specific trigger points deep in the tissue and, at the same time, minimizing stimulation of the pain receptors.

The use of electricity for pain management could be abused by the medical professional and patient. Although transcutaneous electrical nerve stimulation (TENS) is used with varying degrees of success in pain relief (see Chapter 92), it is overprescribed by physicians.

Mechanotherapy

Massage

Massage plays a very important role in pain management and may be the earliest and most primitive pain remedy. Instinctively, human beings will rub or squeeze a sore muscle, cold foot, or aching shoulder with their own hands.

The primary physiologic effect of massage is regulation of muscle tone through reflex and mechanical actions. The reflex effect is the result of stimulation of peripheral receptors in the skin produced by irritative and repetitive movements of the therapist's hands or devices. This stimulation transmits impulses to the higher central nerve center and produces sensations of psychologic pleasure or well-being (5). Therefore, massage has a positive influence on the human psyche. Peripherally, this stimulation induces muscle relaxation and arteriole dilation or constriction. Its mechanical actions increase local blood circulation, enhance the flexibility of the muscle, intensify the movement of lymph, and loosen scar tissue or adherent connective tissue bands.

Massage cannot strengthen weak muscles and, therefore, should not be used as a substitute for active or resistive exercises. Massage, however, does prepare the body for strengthening exercises and facilitates better performance.

CLINICAL ASPECTS. The common techniques of massage are effleurage (stroking), petrissage (kneading), tapotement (percussion), and friction (rubbing). The fundamental technique of massage involves movement of the therapist's hands in a centripetal direction in a rhythmic fashion (fast or slow according to the technique being used), to aid the venous and lymphatic flow, with exertion of the proper amount of pressure depending on the degree of muscle relaxation (lighter pressure for more relaxed areas). A mild medium such as mineral oil or powder may be used. The patient is placed in a comfortable position in a nonstressful environment with the area to be treated exposed.

Massage is indicated for conditions in which relief of pain, reduction of swelling, or mobilization of adhesive tissues is desired. Some of these conditions are arthritis, fibrositis, sprain, strain, contusion, bursitis, and muscle spasm.

The major contraindications include presence of an acute inflammatory process in the area to be treated, thrombophlebitis or lymphangitis, acute burn, dermatitis, malignancy, advanced arteriosclerosis, nephritis, and severe debilitation.

Therapeutic Exercise

Exercise therapy is the cornerstone treatment for subacute and chronic pain (103). During acute pain, exercise generally is contraindicated except for maintaining self-administered passive range of motion (ROM) of all extremities and the trunk.

CLINICAL ASPECTS. Subacute pain is less intense and is often intermittent in nature; therefore, therapeutic exercise is highly desirable and realistic for restoration of function to the affected area through an intensive outpatient program. During rehabilitation in the subacute phase, the emphasis should be placed on teaching the patient how to handle recurring pain. Even after pain is eliminated or decreased to the bearable level by heat, cold, or other modalities, pain is likely to recur if a patient has muscles that are too weak to maintain good posture, accompanied by varying degrees of incoordination and poor endurance.

During the chronic phase of pain, a patient may have had a prolonged period of decreased activity, leading to weakened muscles and contracted joints, which may cause increased pain. Therefore, a therapeutic exercise program that increases range of motion and elasticity of soft tissues by decreasing tension, spasm, and contracture—followed by a program that emphasizes increasing strength and endurance (i.e., progressive resistive exercises)—may be the most rational regime

for a patient to gain his or her maximum functional level. If a patient has too much pain to institute this exercise regime, heat, cold, or hydrotherapy may be applied to prepare the patient for exercise.

In general, strenuous exercises should be avoided or should be performed with extreme caution by patients with cardiopulmonary dysfunction, malignancy, recent or nonunited fracture, acute inflammation, or osteoporosis.

PHYSIOLOGIC EFFECTS. Exercise has a local effect on the muscles and joints being treated. In general, it strengthens weak muscles and mobilizes stiff joints, reestablishes neuromuscular balance and coordination, and increases endurance and speed. In addition, it preserves muscle activity and range of motion of joints during immobilization. Physiologically, exercise increases blood flow, cardiac output, and respiratory reserve and produces transient increases in albumin, sugar, nitrogen, and chlorides in the urine. It also has a general effect on the various systems of the body as well as altering the metabolism (104, 105). The scientific literature is extensive concerning the effects of exercise on cardiovascular (106), metabolic (107), nutritional (108), respiratory (109), blood flow, and heat regulatory (110) systems.

Basically, there are three types of exercise: isotonic, isometric, and isokinetic. The techniques of each are discussed in the following sections. Figures 88-7 and 88-8 illustrate common therapeutic exercises.

Isotonic Exercise

Isotonic exercises are performed against a steady load with joint movement. Tension within the muscles does not change greatly during isotonic exercise. It is often used to build up muscle power after an injury or pain attack by applying a preset weight, according to different criteria, and requiring a patient to perform predetermined repetitions. DeLorme (111) claimed that

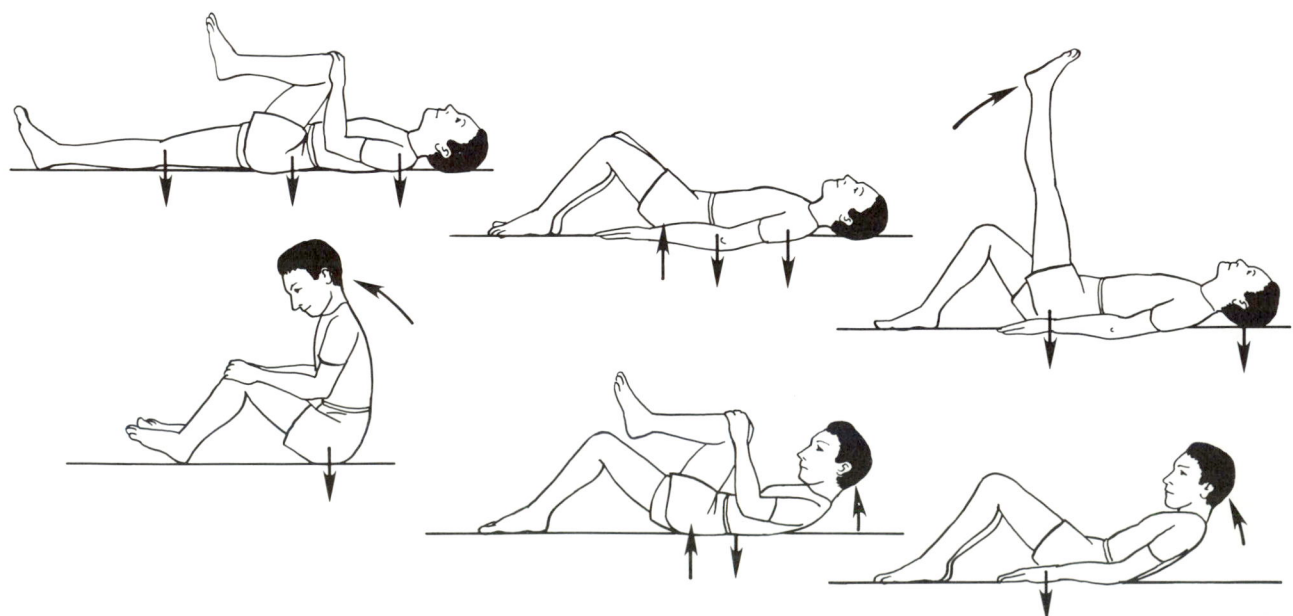

FIG. 88-7. Low back exercises that emphasize pelvic tilting and aid in reducing low back pain.

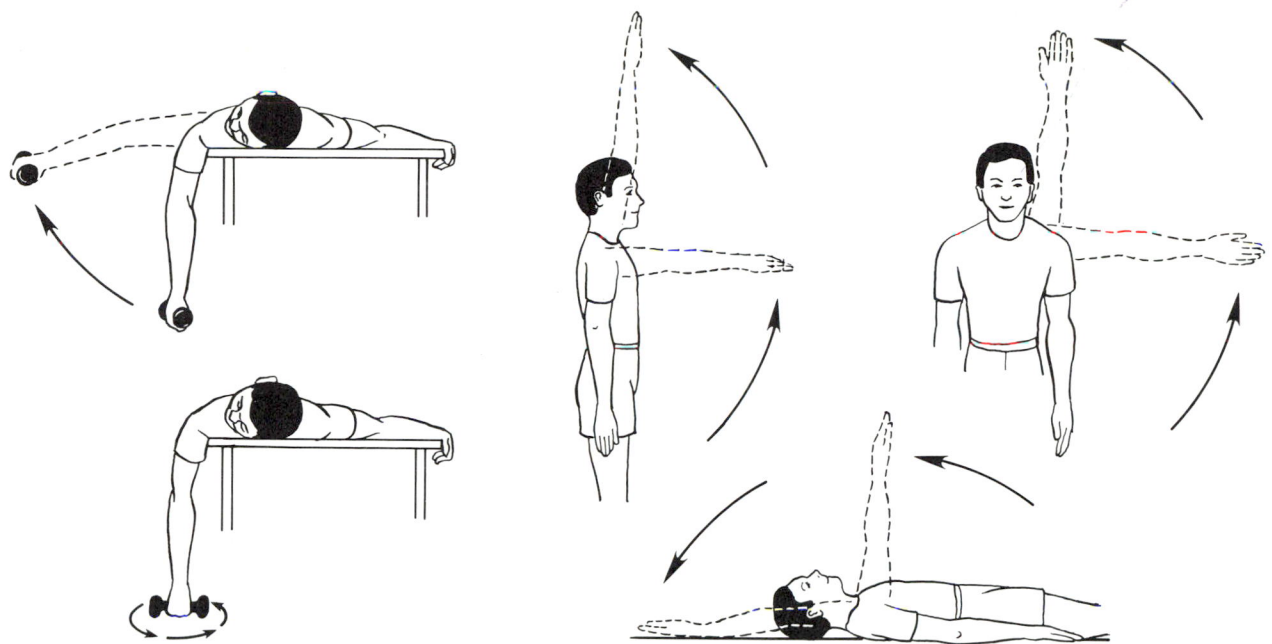

FIG. 88-8. Active exercises to increase mobility for the shoulder. These can be easily performed by a patient once instructions have been given by the physical therapist.

in order to rebuild strength, a weekly series of 10 repetition maximum (RM) each against a resistance of 25%, 50%, 75%, and 100% of the patient's maximum capacity is required. This type of regime is called progressive resistance exercise (PRE). De Lateur et al. (112) performed numerous tests of the DeLorme axiom and concluded that it is correct in extreme cases but may not be applicable to the average patient.

The Oxford technique (113) is a modified PRE regime done in a reverse manner; that is, the weight is decreased with 10 RM each at 100%, 75%, 50%, and 25% of maximum capacity. This method, designed to avoid fatigue during and after training, was found to be less effective in obtaining maximum strengthening. Hellebrandt and Houtz (114) stated that work capacity can be increased by either PRE or progressively increasing the rate of repetition with a steady load.

Many other types of isotonic exercise have been used, but PRE is widely accepted. When a patient is in pain and cannot perform PRE, then other forms of exercises (e.g., active, active assistive, or passive) should be considered. Active exercise is the movement of a body part against gravity by a patient without any assistance. Active assistive exercise is performed by a patient with various amounts of assistance from a therapist to achieve full range of motion. Passive exercise is carried out by a therapist for a patient, who does not take any active role in the movement of the extremity or body part. A forceful passive exercise is called stretching, mobilization, or manipulation depending upon the degree of force exerted by the therapist. A combination of each of these exercises enhances circulation, decreases joint stiffness, increases neuromusculoskeletal functions, and eliminates pain if pain is due to any of these causes.

Isometric Exercise

Isometric exercise is performed against resistance without joint movement. The length of the muscle remains the same during the exercise. A strain gauge is used to provide instant feedback of the force exerted. Brief isometric exercises have been studied by Liberson and Asa (115) and Rose et al. (116). Liberson and Asa recommended that brief isometric exercises be performed for 5 to 6 sec with an interval of 20 sec between repetitions to achieve maximum results.

Isometric exercise increases isometric strength effectively. It consumes less time and is more convenient to perform than isotonic exercise for both patients and therapists. Although isometric exercises increase performance endurance to a higher level than isotonic resistive exercises (117) it places undue stress on the heart and circulation due to the unpredictable rise of blood pressure and heart rate (118, 119). In addition, since most activities of daily living require dynamic movement of the joints, a patient with pain should not rely totally on isometric exercise to achieve independence in these activities.

Isometric exercises are indicated in a patient with acute painful joints, a cast or immobilizer for fracture, or during the postoperative period of orthopedic procedures. Because this type of exercise involves no movement of the joint, it is especially useful for a patient in acute pain to maintain muscle volume or to increase muscle strength. Isometric exercises are relatively contraindicated for a patient with cardiovascular disease and hypertension for reasons described previously. It is not recommended for those who cannot learn the isometric technique.

Isokinetic Exercise

The concept of isokinetic exercise was developed during the early 1960s and was first reported by Hislop and Perrine (120). This type of exercise is performed against a variable resistance with joint movement occurring and muscles exerting maximal force throughout the range of movement. The angular speed of movement is predetermined by an electromechanical device, and the resistance is automatically adjusted to the exerted force. Any effort applied is countered by an equal amount of force.

Isokinetic exercise can be used as an investigational tool to study torque, work, range of motion, power, speed, and motor skill (121). It can also be used to determine the severity of disability of the muscle groups or joint functions and provides simple diagrammatic evidence of such disability (122). At present, isokinetic exercise is used primarily for diagnosing the extent of injuries and determining when an athlete can return to competition. In this application, the strength of the injured limb is compared with that of the unaffected one, and the length of time necessary for rehabilitation can be predicted.

Isokinetic exercise can allow a pain-free and safe ROM exercise after the postoperative period or injury. In a chronic pain situation, isokinetic exercise may be superior for building strength and endurance, since it elicits significantly greater muscle potential, as determined by electromyography, than either isotonic or isometric exercise (123).

Traction

Traction is the technique of applying a pulling force produced by a machine, device, or human to a part of the body in order to stretch soft tissues and to separate joint surfaces or bone fragments. It has been used to reduce fracture or dislocation since the beginning of recorded history. Later, it came to be used as a means of pain control. When applied properly to the injured part, traction can relieve pain, secure rest, overcome painful muscle spasm, and prevent adhesion formation (6) as well as maintain anatomic alignment and prevent or correct a deformity. Unfortunately, it has been one of the most overused and poorly prescribed physical modalities, the force or weight being inadequate most of the time.

APPLICATION TECHNIQUE. A generally accepted rule is that the weight of traction must exceed the weight of the treated part to produce a distracting effect on the part. Therefore, cervical traction should initially employ a weight in the range of 11 kg (124) and increase gradually to 18 to 23 kg. Pelvic traction should use 34 to 45 kg at the beginning and increase to 91 to 136 kg or even more to be effective (125). The traction weight for disk herniation frequently is not enough to separate the disk space and/or neural foramina. However, if the purpose of traction is to reduce muscle spasm and provide a chance for bedrest, the weight can be less; otherwise, overstretching of the soft tissue may exacerbate the patient's pain, particularly when trigger points are present in the area to be pulled.

Other common errors in the use of traction are an improper direction and angle of pull. Generally, cervical traction should not be applied in the extension direction. Even though the illustration on self-administered cervical traction kits often shows a person with the neck pulled in extension, extension of the back aggravates lumbosacral strain and sprain and extension of the neck also exacerbates cervical spondylosis with radiculopathy. The angle of pull should be about 20 to 30° of flexion to achieve the full effectiveness of cervical traction (126). For lumbar traction, the angle of pull is approximately 18° flexion of the pelvis to flatten the lumbar spine (127).

The force of traction can be applied constantly or intermittently by a motorized machine or manually. Cervical traction can be applied in the sitting or supine position using a head halter with a chin and occiput strap, which is attached to a crossbar overhead (Fig. 88-9). Pelvic traction is applied, most of the time, in the supine position with a belt or harness placed around the patient's waist and extended over the end of the bed to exert traction by a weight or machine pulling. Sometimes another belt is placed over the lower chest and high abdomen to provide a counter or stabilizing force. Treatment duration varies from 30 min to 24 hours a day depending upon the patient's tolerance and the purpose of traction.

THERAPEUTIC EFFECTS. Studies show a separation at the level of C2 to C7 of 3 to 14 mm with traction weight of 20 kg (124) and a significant widening of the lumbar intervertebral spaces with traction weight of 91 to 136 kg (128). Christie (129) found that traction

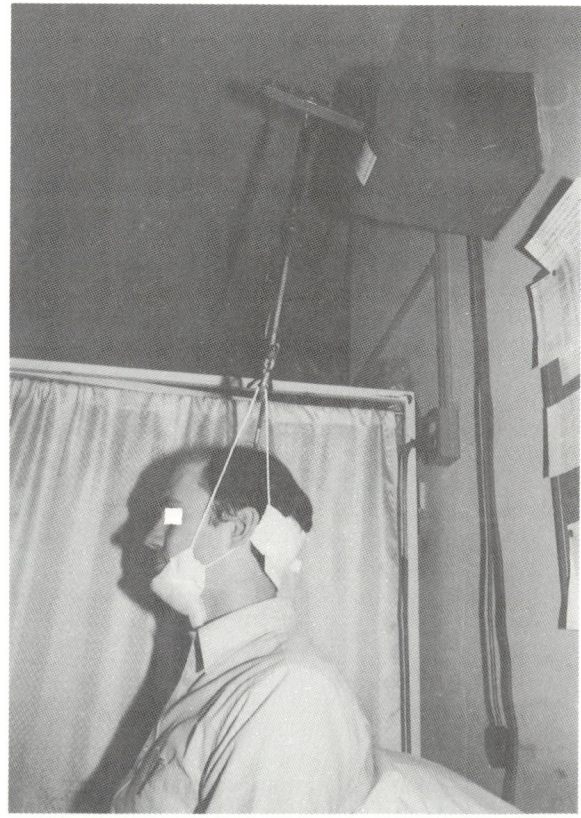

FIG. 88-9. Seated patient in cervical traction with head halter. Neck is in slightly flexed position.

improved only 30% of patients with chronic low back pain; in patients with acute lumbar pain, no difference was found between traction and a bland pill. Weber (130) observed no significant difference in pain, mobility of lumbar spine, or presence of neurologic signs in a double-blind control study on 72 patients with sciatica due to prolapsed disk. Mathews and Hickling (131) reported almost the same findings as Weber.

Traction, however, can be valuable in the management of painful disorders of the neck and back. When used judiciously, beneficial results include distracting vertebral bodies while enlarging neural foramina, stretching muscles and ligaments, separating apophysial joints, and keeping the patient in bedrest.

Contraindications for traction include malignancy, cord compression, infectious spine, osteoporosis, cardiovascular condition, rheumatoid arthritis due to instability and subluxation of the joints, active peptic ulcer, hiatus hernia, aortic aneursym, and gross hemorrhoids (132).

Manipulation

Manipulation is surrounded by many unanswered questions, and it is difficult to confirm its effectiveness scientifically. Manipulation is a forceful passive movement that stretches the tissue of periarticular or intraarticular adhesion and helps to restore range of motion. One applies manual pressure, then counterpressure; sometimes a "click" sound or "snap" sensation is noted. Manipulation differs from regular stretching and traction in that it involves a brief, quick maneuver that goes beyond the usual range of motion of the treated part. This technique sometimes is referred to as *mobilization* in the literature.

When performed precisely, manipulation usually relieves pain or other symptoms instantaneously. Forceful manipulation followed by a sustained force of equal or less pressure can result in an increased ROM. The skill to apply the proper amount of force to the tissue requires considerable practice, sensitivity, and coordination of body movement.

The characteristic snap or cracking noise usually occurs when manipulation is carried beyond the point of limit or "tension" by a sudden slight and very short thrust to obtain a supplementary movement. The snap sound may represent a vacuum phenomenon secondary to an altered tissue resistance, thus gaining a few degrees of ROM. The thrust must be very small; if violent, it can be painful and dangerous (133). Manipulation should be entirely painless if at all possible. Maigne (133) suggests that the noise is caused by cavitation from negative pressure in the synovial fluid during the thrust movement. When the dissolved gas in the synovial fluid is released, it produces the cracking sound. Subsequently, this sound can be produced again, 15 to 30 min later, after the released gas has been completely redissolved in the synovial fluid. Therefore, the occurrence of this sound does not guarantee that manipulation was successful.

CLINICAL ASPECTS. Manipulation should be preceded by a heat modality to relax soft tissues around the area; this is followed by passive exercise to the joint, then a gliding (Fig. 88-10) or thrust movement to further the range of the joint. Some patients may expe-

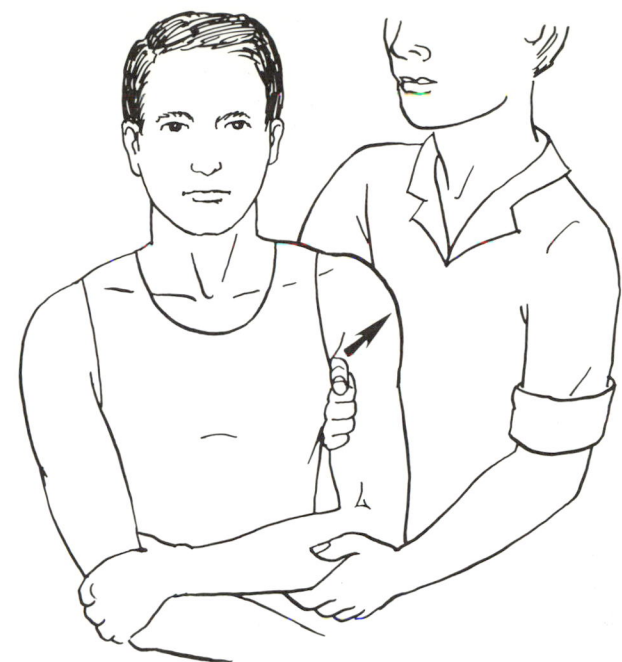

FIG. 88-10. Position of hands for manipulation of the glenohumeral joint.

rience slight discomfort a few hours after the treatment, but it will gradually subside. This discomfort is less following the second and third sessions. After each session, if there is no improvement of the treated condition, the treatment should be discontinued and a review of the diagnosis and techniques used undertaken. As a rule, re-evaluation before and after each treatment is the only way to achieve successful manipulation.

When pain in the spine or joints is due to a structure fault, manipulation is useful, but it is absolutely essential to assess the part to be treated clinically and radiologically. The presence of infection, inflammation, tumor, fracture, osteoporosis, or instability of joint structure contraindicates this treatment. Manipulation should be avoided in patients with a massive disk herniation, confirmed motor weakness, and reflex arterial spasm.

Other Modalities

Immobilization (Rest)

Immobilization—the restriction of movement of a part of the body or joint—is one of the most primitive, yet effective modalities for pain relief. It is almost mandatory for management of all acute pain caused by musculoskeletal conditions, from spasm to fracture. Technically, the muscle spasm caused by pain is nature's immobilization—a self-defensive mechanism or Payr's defense reflex (67). The injured part is protected from movement by the natural immobilization resulting from pain. However, prolonged immobilization can lead to joint contracture and ankylosis, muscle atrophy, weakness, osteoporosis, pneumonia, and cardiovascular deconditioning. In addition, it alters blood chemistry and metabolic requirements (66). Therefore,

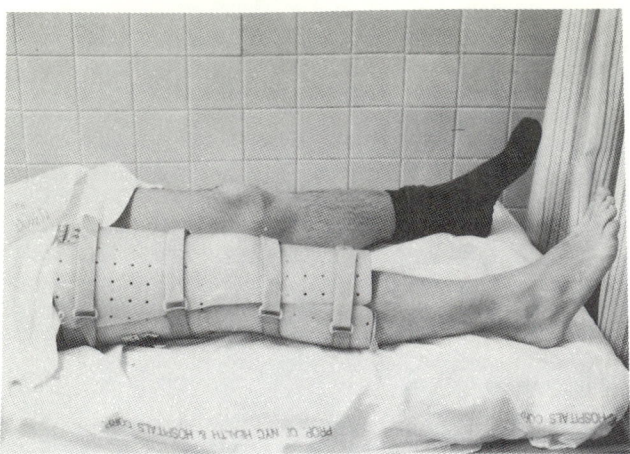

FIG. 88-11. Rigid plastic lower extremity splint provides immobilization of limb.

immobilization should continue only as long as clinically necessary.

Bedrest is the most common method of immobilization of the entire body. Immobilization of a part can be accomplished by means of an elastic bandage, splint (Fig. 88-11), sling, orthosis, or plaster of Paris. When immobilization is necessary, the position of the body part, particularly joints that must be included, has to be carefully determined. Unless it is indicated, no joint should be immobilized at its maximum range of motion (i.e., in the fully extended or flexed position). The immobilization angle is 5 to 10° of flexion for the knee and 0 to 90° for the ankle. When a joint is immobilized at the proper angle, the body part can be restored faster, easier, and with less pain after the immobilizing device is removed.

Supporting Devices

Supporting devices, such as an orthosis, crutch, cane, collar, or even wheelchair, are often beneficial for pain control. These devices, however, should be prescribed with a clear understanding of their biomechanical functions. For example, a lumbar orthosis or abdominal binder compresses the abdomen, increases the intra-abdominal pressure, decreases lumbar lordosis and stress to the spine, and finally relieves low back pain. This orthosis also restricts body movement and leads to muscle weakening. Its prolonged use may create new disability and pain. Therefore, use of a supportive device should be re-evaluated periodically to ensure that its benefits outweigh the side effects.

Cold (Low-Energy) Irradiation

High-power lasers of 10 to over 100 watts (W) have been used successfully for surgical procedures and hemostasis. In recent years, cold lasers of approximately 1 mW have been used increasingly in a variety of analgesic and wound-healing procedures (134).

While the first lasers for medical applications used a ruby rod producing only a red light, current devices can produce both fixed and variable frequencies at different wavelengths and power (135, 136). In the United States, the most frequently used low-power lasers are the infrared gallium-aluminum-arsenide laser and the visible helium-neon laser. A common biostimulation unit provides a high-quality, pulse-modulated or continuous coherent light at 632.8 nm obtained from a helium-neon source or gallium arsenide at 904 nm from a gallium-arsenide source.

At these energy levels, no appreciable temperature changes are produced in the treated tissues; therefore, any effects have been attributed to nonthermal mechanisms. Some have postulated that effects result from properties unique to lasers such as minimal beam divergence, coherence (wavelengths in phase), and monochromaticity (single wavelength). Biologically, low-power lasers impact upon the membrane transport system, autonomic nervous system, prostaglandin chemistry, and platelet aggregation.

INDICATIONS AND CONTRAINDICATIONS. Successful treatment of tension and vascular headaches and a variety of musculoskeletal, neurologic, and rheumatic conditions with low-energy lasers have been reported (137–139). Kroetlinger (140) even used an acupuncture approach, applying laser to acupuncture sites (141). Most investigators have reported relief of symptoms in 80% of patients treated. Although many studies report pain alleviation, medical applications of cold laser remain controversial. The quality of the investigations, number of subjects, and varied techniques preclude statistical verification of its efficacy (142). Further clinical evaluation of laser therapy is warranted.

Side effects of laser therapy, except in the case of prolonged, direct eye exposure, are minimal, and cell culture studies show little or no mutagenic effects (143). Contraindications include pregnancy, fontanelles of growing children, photosensitive individuals, and cancer patients.

CLINICAL APPLICATIONS

A summary of the physical modalities indicated in various painful conditions is presented in Table 88-3.

Arthritis

During the acute inflammatory stage of arthritis, immobilization of the joint in a proper position is important. Isometric exercise is useful for prevention of muscle atrophy. During this phase, neither thermotherapy nor cryotherapy is beneficial.

When the acute phase is over, joint contractures due to shortening of the capsular or periarticular tissues, thickening and scarring of the synovium, and ligamentous and capsular tightness due to prolonged immobilization may be treated with appropriate thermotherapy (34), followed by therapeutic exercises, for lasting control of pain or discomfort. The choice of particular heat modalities depends largely on the joint to be treated. Small joints may be effectively treated in a

TABLE 88-3. Indications for Use of Physical Therapy Modalities

Indication	Modality
Arthritis	Infrared, hot packs, paraffin, microwaves, hydrotherapy, therapeutic exercise, massage, mobilization, traction, and cold laser
Low back pain	Hot packs, cold packs, therapeutic exercise, cold laser, TENS, ultrasound, massage, infrared, shortwaves, and hydrotherapy
Burns	Hydrotherapy and cold laser
Bursitis	Shortwaves, microwaves, ultrasound, cold laser, TENS, and ice packs
Contusions	Infrared, cold packs, ultrasound, and shortwaves
Herniated disk	Microwave, traction, ultrasound, cold packs, and therapeutic exercise
Injuries (immediately after)	Immobilization
Myositis	Hot packs, ultrasound, and microwaves
Muscle spasm	Massage, vapocoolent spray, cold packs, and therapeutic exercise
Neuromas	Ultrasound
Painful stiff shoulder	Hot packs, cold packs, infrared, immobilization, ultrasound, and therapeutic exercise
Postimmobilization	Vapocoolent spray, hydrotherapy, and therapeutic exercise
Painful joints with minimal restriction of motion	Mobilization and ultrasound
Radiculoneuropathy	Traction
Sprains, strains	Paraffin, shortwaves, microwaves, ice packs, ultrasound, therapeutic exercise, immobilization, and hydrotherapy
Sciatica	Infrared, therapeutic exercise, ultrasound, shortwaves and TENS
Scar tissue	Cold laser
Stasis ulcer	Cold laser
Shoulder–hand syndrome	Hot packs and therapeutic exercise
Tenosynovitis	Hot packs, shortwaves, paraffin, ultrasound, immobilization, cold packs, and therapeutic exercise
Torticolis	Ultrasound and cold packs
Tennis elbow	Vapocoolent spray, hydrotherapy, and therapeutic exercise
Tears of the rotator cuff	Microwaves, immobilization, and therapeutic exercise
Whiplash	Hot packs, microwaves, immobilization, and therapeutic exercise

paraffin bath or whirlpool or by infrared radiation. Shortwave diathermy, microwave diathermy, and ultrasound can be used to increase the temperature of deep tissues in large joints such as the ankle, knee, hip, or shoulder. Some studies suggest that ultrasound is superior to microwaves or infrared radiation for joint contractures (63, 144, 145). When multiple joints are involved, hydrotherapy with total immersion of the body is the preferred heat therapy. Patients with painful weight-bearing joint(s) need ambulation exercises in a therapeutic pool until the pain becomes tolerable.

Simultaneously with or immediately after the application of heat, during a period of no pain or minimum pain, stretching, range of motion exercises, or other mobilization modalities should be given to increase joint mobility.

Stiffness and discomfort in joints of the hands and feet, especially in the morning, can be treated effectively with contrast bath (146). Contrasts baths involve the sudden, alternate immersion of the extremities, first in hot, then in cold, water. One large water container is filled with 38–40° C hot water; the other is filled with 10–16° C cold water. For 4 to 6 minutes the extremities are first placed in the hot water; followed immediately by immersion in the cold water for one or two minutes. The last immersion takes place in the hot water.

Application of cryotherapy to arthritic joints was advocated by Harris and McCroskery (147) based on the theory that cold reduces the activity of destructive enzymes such as collagenase, but this theory has not been proven (148). Other studies (149, 150), however, have concluded that cold increases joint stiffness.

Muscle Spasm

Muscle spasm, an extremely painful condition, is often associated with neuromuscular or skeletal impairment. It is considered a defense reflex, and generally, no pathology exists in the muscle itself at its onset. Muscle spasm may eventually lead to atrophy and weakness of muscles. Thus, management of painful muscle spasm is almost always symptomatic and must be instituted promptly in order to prevent secondary disabilities.

The basic principle behind the treatment strategy is to reduce spindle sensitivity. The choice of physical modalities depends mainly upon the muscle to be treated and the underlying pathology. Muscle spasm due to intervertebral disk herniation without radiculopathy has been successfully treated with shortwave diathermy or superficial heat (e.g., hot pack or infrared radiation). These superficial heat modalities elevate skin temperature and thereby attain muscle relaxation reflexly.

Clinical observations by Landon (151) indicates that although both heat and cold can reduce muscle spasm, heat is more effective in the acute phase, whereas cold seems to be the treatment of choice for the chronic stage. Brief applications of cold pack or ice massage are useless because they facilitate alpha motor neuron discharges. Therefore, such cryotherapy must be applied for at least 10 min in order for the muscle to be sufficiently cooled.

Once spasm is controlled and the muscle relaxes, gentle isotonic exercise and massage further enhance muscle relaxation. When muscle spasm is associated with rheumatoid arthritis, the choice of heat modalities must be carefully made so that the treatment does not aggravate inflammation.

Spasticity

Spasticity is usually defined as increased muscle tone due to upper motor neuron disease and is a disabling, often painful condition. Similar to muscle spasm, spasticity may be reduced by decreasing the sensitivity of muscle spindles.

Knutsoon (152) reported that application of cold reduced clonus, enhancing and strengthening the protagonist's power because of reduced spasticity of the antagonist in 50% of test subjects. Miglietta (153) and Hartviksen (154) made similar observations, finding that the effect of cold on suppression of spasticity lasted for a long period.

The muscle must be sufficiently cooled to gain a therapeutic effect. During the period when spasticity is reduced, various exercises can be instituted to increase the protagonist's strength and muscle re-education techniques may be employed. Although heat can reduce spasticity, clinical experience shows that the effect of heat is very transient.

Myofascial Pain Syndromes

Myofascial pain syndromes constitute a group of disorders characterized by the presence of extremely sensitive small areas, called trigger points. Trigger points are small circumscribed hypersensitive areas in muscles, ligaments, joint capsules, tendons, etc. (73, 155, 156). The appearance of trigger points seems to be related to various inflammatory or traumatic conditions.

Trigger points can cause muscle spasm, which should be treated accordingly. Depending on their location, trigger points can be treated with an evaporative cooling spray, microwave diathermy, ultrasound, or interferential therapy, but other treatment methods such as acupuncture (Chapter 91), cold laser, and injection of a local anesthetic (157) are more effective. In addition, various therapeutic exercises and massage are essential ingredients for management of myofascial pain syndromes.

Tenosynovitis and Painful Stiff Shoulder

Tenosynovitis, caused by trauma, rheumatoid arthritis, osteoarthritis, or other diseases, is a painful condition usually associated with movement of the affected part of the body segment. Immobilization with a splint or Ace bandage during the acute phase is invaluable. Application of heat or cold is indicated during the recovery state after a period of immobilization.

So-called painful stiff shoulder may have a single cause or be due to a combination of calcified bursitis involving the subdeltoid or subacrominal bursa, tendinitis of the biceps, and supraspinatus with or without calcific deposits and capsulitis. Painful stiff shoulder is characterized by severe limitation in the range of motion, the degree of which depends upon the localized pathology and aching at rest. Thus, when a patient attempts to make a certain movement, pain becomes excruciating, accompanied by a considerable amount of muscle spasm. Unless treated promptly, "frozen shoulder" may develop.

There is no patent treatment regime for this condition. The fundamental principle of treatment is the relief of pain and the restoration of normal shoulder function. Before treatment is started, a thorough examination, including electromyography, must be conducted in order to rule out an irritable cervical root lesion. In the acute early phase, the majority of patients prefer cryotherapy. However, some obtain pain relief with some form of thermotherapy.

Immobilization of the shoulder using a sling often provides satisfactory results. However, the patient must perform passive range of motion exercises several times a day, which should not produce pain. The basis of physical therapy lies in a judicious combination of rest and exercise within the painless range (158).

Since passive exercise, stretching, or manipulation is always painful, heat, ice, or the injection of hydrocortisone or a local anesthetic should precede it. McGee and Freshman (159) developed a special technique of stretching the shoulder immediately after ultrasound application. Manipulation with or without any form of analgesic procedure may be continued if less pain accompanies active exercise while achieving a wider range of motion.

Sprains and Strains

Sprain of a joint and strain of a muscle are the most common forms of sports injuries; they also occur in everyday life as well as in the work place. Sprains and strains are characterized by the acute onset of severe pain and loss of function of the injured part of the body. The purposes of first aid are prevention of extravasation with edema, elimination of pain by reducing Payr's defense reflex and Leriche's sympathetic reflex, and enhancement of healing and rehabilitation (160).

Immediate immobilization with a splint, elevation of the injured part, and application of cryotherapy in the form of a cold pack or even ice reduce muscle spasm.

Compression of the sprained joint with an elastic bandage for at least 20 to 30 min immediately after the injury minimizes edema and, thus, pain. Compression can be continued for several days, but the tourniquet effect must be avoided. In strains, compression application is difficult. Cryotherapy should be continued for 24 to 72 hours.

Severe pain experienced at the onset of an injury gradually subsides in 48 to 72 hours. At this point, residual pain may be minimized by thermotherapy. The most commonly used heat modality is a hot pack, such as hydrocollator, but immersion in paraffin or hydrotherapy can be an effective alternative. If a strain involves deep muscles, other heat modalities, such as shortwave or microwave diathermy, can be used. These heat modalities directly or indirectly reduce muscle spindle activity and decrease edema by increasing blood circulation indirectly.

Active exercise should be started 48 to 72 hours after an injury. Isotonic exercise may be instituted if active exercise does not increase pain. These exercises increase blood circulation in the injured area and further minimize pain as well as enhance the restoration of function.

Low Back Pain

Low back pain is the most common musculoskeletal disorder seen in the physical medicine clinic and physician's office, and yet the most difficult to treat (see Chapter 71). Regardless of treatment, surgical or conservative, the prognosis is not promising. The cause of the pain and its mechanism must be identified through a careful review of the patient's history, detailed clinical examination, and specific laboratory testing before any physical therapy is instituted, since the treatment method differs according to the cause of pain.

A common approach to low back pain due to structural abnormalities, such as spondylolisthesis or spondylosis, is the reduction of excessive lordosis to decrease the sacral angle (161). Posture exercises, stretching exercises for the low back, and isometric exercises of the abdominal muscles are physical modalities said to be useful, but this is disputed (see p. 1474).

Most cases of kinetic low back pain are probably caused by poorly coordinated and/or faulty biomechanical movements. Treatment of acute kinetic low back pain requires bedrest with semiflexion of the pelvis if well tolerated. The use of traction by itself may have disappointing results. Since a major portion of pain is due to muscle spasm, it is essential to induce muscle relaxation. Some claim that muscle relaxation can be obtained by application of shortwave diathermy for 20 to 30 min (39). The frequent application of cryotherapy, in the form of a cold pack, is far more effective than heat therapy. Alternate applications of cryotherapy and thermotherapy have been utilized frequently with good results.

After the acute pain subsides, gentle trunk exercise and careful ambulation exercise can further decrease muscle spasm. At times, hydrotherapy may be useful for trunk exercises. If pain persists in spite of a period of bedrest and physical therapy, a supportive device such as a back brace or corset may be necessary.

SUMMARY AND CONCLUSIONS

Numerous investigations of heat therapy have confirmed that the therapeutic effects of heat are the consequence of elevated tissue temperature. Many heat modalities are available; the temperature distribution and the maximum tolerance level associated with each modality differ significantly. Lehmann et al. (15) stated that the skin and superficial subcutaneous tissue are selectively heated by infrared, hydrocollator packs, paraffin, fluidotherapy, and hydrotherapy. The deeper subcutaneous tissue and superficial musculature can be selectively heated by shortwaves with capacitor plates or by microwaves at a frequency of 2,456 MHz. The superficial musculature is best heated by shortwaves at 27 MHz applied with an induction coil; the entire muscle is selectively heated by exposure to microwaves at 915 MHz. Deep tissue such as joints, ligaments, fibrous scars, myofascial interfaces, nerve trunks, tendons, and tendon sheaths can only be selectively heated by ultrasound at 0.8 to 1.0 MHz. Pelvic tissue can be selectively heated by shortwave with an internal or vaginal applicator at a frequency of 27 MHz. These findings make it easier for the clinician to select a modality according to the depth of the tissue to be treated.

Cold, which produces vasoconstriction, followed by reflex vasodilatation, is most useful in acute injuries. It is highly effective for chronic spasm and pain (89, 90). Electrotherapy is effective in decreasing muscle spasm, thus decreasing pain, and has been widely used as an adjunct to ultrasound therapy.

The usefulness of massage in pain reduction is well recognized. Traction, when it is properly applied, can decrease muscle tension or even relieve the pressure on painful nerve root entrapment. Immobilization and supportive devices are indispensable means for control of acute pain. Therapeutic exercise is a very important modality for strengthening weak muscles and helping patients to regain or maintain ability to engage in a meaningful life and employment.

All of these therapeutic physical modalities can be used singularly or in combination to obtain pain relief. The choice depends largely on which tissue is to be treated, the patient's preference and tolerance, and the physician's knowledge and experience. Accurate diagnosis, a goal-oriented treatment plan, use of appropriate physical modalities in conjunction with nonphysical measures, and frequent monitoring and assessment are essential ingredients for successful treatment outcome.

In this chapter we have described a variety of physical modalities that are currently in use. There is, however, no set routine procedure or order for utilizing various modalities in the treatment of specific painful conditions. Each case must be decided individually. In some case, the prescribing physician must choose from a number of equally effective modalities. Thus, this chapter has conscientiously avoided being a recipe for physical medicine.

Pain can be caused by primary disease entities or can be secondary to psychologic and environmental factors. Many treatment techniques are available in physical medicine, but generally the efficacy of these physical modalities has been demonstrated only empirically. In the absence of a universally accepted method to quantify the severity of pain, any scientific study that claims one modality is far superior to another in providing pain relief in a given painful condition always becomes the subject of controversy. The modality acclaimed for its effectiveness in pain control today may become obsolete tomorrow.

The physiologic mechanisms underlying the effects of various physical modalities are not well understood; nor are the mechanism of formation of the pain stimulus, its transmission to the cerebral centers, or the mode of interpretation of incoming stimuli at the center. As noted already, the absence of standard methods for quantifying pain presents various difficulties in pain research. Physical modalities of one form or another have played and will continue to play a significant role in pain rehabilitation programs. Research to increase our understanding of the causes, mechanisms, and measurement of pain should eventually enhance the therapeutic effectiveness of such programs and of individual physical modalities.

REFERENCES

1. Morowitz, H.J.: The physics of heat. In Therapeutic Heat and Cold. 2nd Ed. Edited by S. Licht. Baltimore, Waverly Press, 1965, pp. 1–23.
2. Licht, S.: History of electrotherapy. In Therapeutic Electricity and Ultraviolet Radiation. 2nd Ed. Edited by S. Licht. Baltimore, Waverly Press, 1967, pp. 1–70.
3. Yeh, C., et al.: Physical therapy: evaluation and treatment of chronic pain. In Evaluation and Treatment of Chronic Pain. Edited by G.M. Aronoff. Baltimore, Urban & Schwarzenberg, 1985, pp. 251–261.
4. Aronoff, G.M.: Evaluation and Treatment of Chronic Pain. Baltimore, Urban & Schwarzenberg, 1985.
5. Kottke, F.J., et al. (eds.): Krusen's Handbook of Physical Medicine and Rehabilitation. 3rd Ed. Philadelphia, W.B. Saunders, 1982.
6. Griffin, J.E., and Karselis, T.C.: Physical Agents for Physical Therapists. 2nd Ed. Springfield, IL, Charles C Thomas, 1982.
7. Shestack, R.: Handbook of Physical Therapy. 3rd Ed. New York, Springer Verlag, 1977.
8. Ruskin, A.P.: Current Therapy in Physiatry, Physical Medicine and Rehabilitation. Philadelphia, W.B. Saunders, 1984.
9. Licht, S. (ed.): Therapeutic Heat and Cold. 2nd Ed. Baltimore, Waverly Press, 1965.
10. Abramson, D., et al.: Changes in blood flow, oxygen uptake, and tissue temperatures produced by therapeutic physical agents: 2° effects of SWD. Am. J. Phys. Med., 39:87, 1960.
11. Brown, M., and Baker, R.D.: Effect of pulsed SWD on skeletal muscle injury in rabbits. J. Am. Phys. Ther. Assoc., 67:208, 1987.
12. Lehmann, J.F., Brunner, A.D., and Stowe, R.W.: Pain threshold measurements after therapeutic application of ultrasound, microwaves, and infrared. Arch. Phys. Med. Rehabil., 39:560, 1958.
13. Fischer, E., and Solomon, S.: Physiological responses to heat and cold. In Therapeutic Heat and Cold. 2nd Ed. Edited by S. Licht. Baltimore, Waverly Press, 1965.
14. de Lateur, B.J.: Spectrum of physical treatment measures. In Medical Rehabilitation. Edited by J. V. Basmajian and R. L. Kirby. Baltimore, Williams & Wilkins, 1984.
15. Lehmann, J.F. (ed.): Therapeutic Heat and Cold. 3rd Ed. Baltimore, Williams & Wilkins, 1982.
16. Reischer, M.A., and Spindler, H.A.: The use of physical medicine and rehabilitation in the management of pain. In Diagnosis and Treatment of Chronic Pain. Edited by N.H. Hendler, D.M. Long, and T.N. Wise. Boston, John Wright, PSG, Inc., 1982.
17. Hayashi, S.: Der Einfluss del Ultraschallwellen und Utrakurtzwellen auf den malignen Tumor. J. Med. Sci. Biophy. (Japan), 6:138, 1940.
18. Cordray, Y.M., and Krusen, E.M. Jr.: Use of hydrocollator packs in the treatment of neck and shoulder pains. Arch. Phys. Med. 40:105, 1959.
19. Edholm, O.G., Fox, R.H., and MacPherson, R.K. The effect of body heating on the circulation in skin and muscle. J. Physiol. 134:612, 1956.
20. Lehmann, J.H., et al.: Temperature distributions in the human thigh produced by infrared, hot pack and microwave applications. Arch. Phys. Med. Rehabil., 47:291, 1966.
21. Millard, J.B.: Paraffin-wax baths in the treatment of rheumatoid arthritis. Ann. Dis., 14:278, 1955.
22. Abramson, D.I., et al.: Effect of paraffin bath and hot formentations on local tissue temperature. Arch. Phys. Med. Rehabil., 45:87, 1964.
23. Krusen, F.H., and Elkins, E.C.: Investigation in fever therapy. Arch. Phys. Ther., 20:77, 1939.
24. Dubois, E.L.: Management of systemic lupus erythematosus. Mod. Treatment, 3:1245, 1969.
25. Smith, D.W., Clarren, S.K., and Harvey, M.A.S.: Hyperthermia as a possible teratogenic agent. J. Pediatr., 92:878, 1978.
26. Borrell, R.M., et al.: Fluidotherapy: Evaluation of a new heat modality. Arch. Phys. Med. Rehabil., 58:69, 1977.
27. Borrell, R.M., et al.: Comparison of in vivo temperatures produced by hydrotherapy, paraffin wax treatment, and fluidotherapy. Phys. Ther., 60:1273, 1980.
28. Benedict, A.A.: Infrared absorption studies of fowl and mammalian erythrocytes. J. Exp. Cell Res., 7:565, 1954.
29. Florence, R., and Shelley, W.: Compact high-intensity radiant heat unit for clinical use. J. Invest. Dermatol., 36:241, 1961.
30. Shriber, W.J.: A Manual of Electrotherapy. 4th Ed. Philadelphia, Lea & Febiger, 1975.
31. Stone, E.K.: Luminous and infrared heating. In Therapeutic Heat and Cold. 2nd Ed. Edited by S. Licht. Baltimore, Waverly Press, 1965. pp. 52–64.
32. Weiss, N.S., Dodell, P., and Brown, H.E.: Thermal urticaria: An unusual case. Ann. Allergy, 37:55, 1976.
33. FCC: Rules and Regulations. Vol. 2, Subpart A, Section 18:13. Washington, DC, Federal Communications Commission, 1964.
34. Lehmann, J.F., Warren, C.G., and Scham, S.M.: Therapeutic heat and cold. Clin. Orthop., 99:207, 1974.
35. Lehmann, J.F., de Lateur, B.J., and Stonebridge, J.B.: Selective heating by shortwave diatherapy with a helical coil Arch. Phys. Med. Rehabil., 50:117, 1969.
36. Etter, H.S., Pudenz, R.H., and Gersh, I.: The effect of diathermy on tissues contiguous to implanted surgical metals. Arch. Phys. Med. Rehabil., 28:333, 1947.
37. Downey, J.A., et al.: Vascular response in the forearm to heating by shortwave diathermy. Arch. Phys. Med. Rehabil., 51:354, 1970.
38. Harris, R.: The effect of various forms of physical therapy on radiosodium clearance from the normal and arthritic knee joint. Ann. Phys. Med., 3:1, 1963.
39. Lehmann, J.F.: Diathermy. In Handbook of Physical Medicine and Rehabilitation. 2nd Ed. Edited by F.H. Krusen, F.J. Kottke, and P.M. Ellwood, Jr. Philadelphia, W.B. Saunders, 1971.
40. Michaelson, S.M.: Bioeffects of high-frequency currents and electromagnetic radiation. In Therapeutic Heat and Cold. 3rd Ed. Edited by J.F. Lehmann. Baltimore, Williams & Wilkins, 1982, pp. 278–352.
41. Food and Drug Administration. Performance standard for microwave diathermy products. Fed. Reg., 40:23877, 1975.
42. Schwan, H.P.: Survey of microwave absorption characteristics of body tissues. In Proc. Second Tri-Serv. Conf. Biol. Effects of Microwave Energy, 1958.
43. Lehmann, J.F., et al.: Comparison of relative heating patterns produced in tissues by exposure to microwave energy at

frequencies of 2450 and 900 megacycles. Arch. Phys. Med. Rehabil., *43*:69, 1962.

44. Worden, R.E., et al.: The heating effects of microwave diathermy with and without ischemia. Arch. Phys. Med. Rehabil., *29*:751, 1948.

45. Hall, E.L.: Diathermy generators. Arch. Phys. Med. Rehabil., *33*:28, 1952.

46. Moor, F.B.: Microwave diathermy. *In* Therapeutic Heat and Cold. 2nd Ed. Edited by S. Licht. Baltimore, Waverly Press, 1965, pp. 310–320.

47. Bergmann, L.: Der Ultraschall und seine Anwendung in Wissenshaft und Technik. Stuttgart, S. Hirzel, Verlag, 1949.

48. Lehmann, J.F., and Johnson, E.W.: Some factors influencing the temperature distribution in thighs exposed to ultrasound. Arch. Phys. Med. Rehabil., *39*:347, 1958.

49. Gould, R.K.: Rectified diffusion in the presence of, and absence of, acoustic streaming. J. Acoust. Soc. Am., *56*:1740, 1974.

50. Williams, A.R., and Miller, D.L.: Photometric detection of ATP release from human erythrocytes exposed to ultrasonically activated gas-filled pores. Ultrasound Med. Biol., *6*:251, 1980.

51. Chan, A.K., Sigelmann, R.A., and Guy, A.W.: Calculations of therapeutic heat generated by ultrasound in fat-muscle-bone layers. IEEE Trans. Biomed. Eng., *21*:280, 1973.

52. Lehmann, J.F., DeLateur, B.J., Warren, C.G., and Stonebridge, J.B.: Heating of joint structures by ultrasound. Arch. Phys. Med. Rehabil., *49*:29, 1968.

53. Szumski, A.J.: Mechanisms of pain relief as a result of therapeutic application of ultrasound. Phys. Ther. Rev., *40*:116, 1960.

54. Lehmann, J., Warren, G., and Guy, A.: Therapy with continuous wave ultrasound. *In* Ultrasound: Its Applications in Medicine and Biology. Edited by F. Fry. Amsterdam, Elsevier Science, 1978, pp. 566–585.

55. Lehmann, J. Warren, G., and Scham, S.: Therapeutic heat and cold. Clin. Orthop., *99*:207, 1974.

56. Warren, C.G., Koblanski, J.N., and Sigelmann, R.A.: Ultrasound coupling media: Their relative transmisivity. Arch. Phys. Med. Rehabil., *57*:218, 1976.

57. Gersten, J.W.: Effect of metallic objects on temperature rises produced in tissue by ultrasound. Am. J. Phys. Med., *37*:75, 1958.

58. Malensen, P.W., and Gersten, J.W.: The effect of ultrasound on peripheral nerve. Arch. Phys. Med. Rehabil., *42*:645, 1961.

59. Aldes, J.H., Jadeson, W.J., and Grabinski, S.A.: A new approach to the treatment of subdeltoid bursitis. Am. J. Phys. Med., *33*:79, 1954.

60. Bearzy, H.J.: Clinical applications of ultrasonic energy in the treatment of acute and chronic subacromial bursitis. Arch. Phys. Med. Rehabil., *34*:228, 1953.

61. Aldes, J.H., and Klaras, T.: Use of ultrasonic radiation in the treatment of subdeltoid bursitis with and without calcareous deposits. West. J. Surg., *62*:369, 1954.

62. Flax, H.J.: Ultrasound treatment of peritendinitis calcarea of the shoulder. Am. J. Phys. Med., *43*:117, 1964.

63. Lehmann, J.F., et al.: Clinical evaluation of a new approach in the treatment of contracture associated with hip fracture after internal fixation. Arch. Phys. Med. Rehabil., *42*:95, 1961.

64. Friedland, F.: Ultrasonic therapy in rheumatic diseases. JAMA, *163*:799, 1957.

65. DePreux, T.: Ultrasonic wave therapy of osteoarthritis hip joint. Br. J. Phys. Med., *15*:14, 1952.

66. Uchman, L.S.: Role of ultrasound in scleroderma. A preliminary report of two cases. Am. J. Phys. Med., *35*:118, 1956.

67. Bierman, W.: Ultrasound in the treatment of scars. Arch. Phys. Med. Rehabil., *35*:209, 1954.

68. Tepperberg, I., and Marjey, E.: Ultrasound therapy of painful postoperative neurofibromas. Am. J. Phys. Med., *32*:27, 1953.

69. Rubin, D., and Kuitert, J.: Use of ultrasonic vibration in the treatment of pain arising from phantom limbs, scars and neuromas. Arch. Phys. Med., Rehabil., *35*:225, 1955.

70. Paul B.J., et al.: Use of ultrasound in the treatment of pressure sores in patients with spinal cord injury. Arch. Phys. Med. Rehabil., *41*:438, 1960.

71. Coventry, M.B.: Problem of painful shoulder. JAMA, *151*:177, 1953.

72. Bonica, J.J.: Management of myofascial pain syndromes in general practice. JAMA, *164*:732, 1957.

73. Travell, J., and Rinzler, S.H.: The myofascial genesis of pain. Postgrad. Med., *11*:425, 1952.

74. Kent, H.: Plantar warts: Treatment with ultrasound. Arch. Phys. Med. Rehabil., *40*:15, 1959.

75. Mortimer, A.J., et al.: The effects of ultrasound on the mechanical properties of rat cardiac muscle. Ultrasonics, *16*:179, 1978.

76. Lee, J.M., Warren, M.P., and Mason, S.M.: Effects of ice on nerve conduction velocity. Phys. Ther., *64*:2, 1978.

77. Waylonis, G.W.: The physiological effects of ice massage. Arch. Phys. Med. Rehabil., *48*:37, 1967.

78. Downer, A.H.: Physical Therapy Procedures. Springfield, IL, Charles C Thomas, 1970.

79. Melzack, R., and Wall, P.D.: Pain mechanisms: A new theory. Science, *150*:971, 1965.

80. Melzack, R., Guite, S., and Gonshor, A.: Relief of dental pain by ice massage of the hand. Can. Med. Assoc. J., *122*:189, 1980.

81. Perkins, J.F., et al.: Sudden vasoconstriction in denervated or sympathectomized paws exposed to cold. Am. J. Physiol., *155*:165, 1948.

82. Olson, J.E., and Stravino, V.D.: A review of cryotherapy. Phys. Ther., *52*:840, 1972.

83. Schmidt, K.L., et al.: Heat, cold and inflammation. Rheumatology, *38*:391, 1979.

84. Eldred, E., Lindsley, D.E., and Buchwald, J.S.: The effect of cooling on mammalian muscle spindle. Exp. Neurol., *2*:144, 1960.

85. Lippold, O.C.J., Nicholls, J.G., and Redfearn, J.W.T.: A study of the afferent discharge produced by cooling a mammalian muscle spindle. J. Physiol., *153*:218, 1960.

86. Ottoson, D.: The effects of temperature on the isolated muscle spindle. J. Physiol., *180*:636, 1965.

87. Li, C.L.: Effect of cooling on neuromuscular transmission in the rat. Am. J. Physiol., *194*:200, 1958.

88. Douglas, W.W., and Malcolm, J.L.: The effect of localized cooling on conduction in cat nerves. J. Physiol., *130*:53, 1955.

89. Chatfield, P.O.: Hypothermia and its effects on the sensory and peripheral motor systems. Ann. NY Acad. Sci., *80*:445, 1959.

90. Clendenin, M.A., and Szumski, A.J.: Influence of cutaneous ice application on single motor units in humans. Phys. Ther., *57*:166, 1971.

91. Rusk, H.A.: Principles of physical medicine. *In* Rehabilitation Medicine. 4th Ed. St. Louis, C.V. Mosby, 1977.

92. Beirman, W.: Therapeutic use of cold. JAMA, *157*:189, 1955.

93. Mercomber, S., and Herman, R.: Effects of local hypothermia on reflex and voluntary activity. Phys. Ther., *51*:271, 1971.

94. Wolf, S.L., and Basmajian J.V.: Intramuscular temperatures deep to localized cold stimulation. Phys. Ther., *53*:1284, 1973.

95. Grant, A.E.: Massage with ice (cryokinetics) and treatment of painful conditions of the musculoskeletal system. Arch. Phys. Med. Rehabil., *45*:233, 1964.

96. Glick, E.N., and Lucas, M.: Ice therapy. Ann. Phys. Med., *10*:70, 1969.

97. Travell, J.G.: Ethyl chloride spray for painful muscle spasm. Arch. Phys. Med. Rehabil., *33*:291, 1952.

98. Kraus, H.: The use of surface anesthesia in the treatment of painful motion. JAMA, *116*:2582, 1941.

99. Zohn, D.A., and Mennell, J. McM: Musculoskeletal Pain: Diagnosis and Physical Treatment. Boston, Little Brown, 1976.

100. Stillwell, G.K.: Clinical electric stimulation. *In* Therapeutic Electricity and Ultraviolet Radiation. 2nd Ed. Edited by S. Licht. Baltimore, Waverley Press, 1967, pp. 105–155.

101. Shestack, R.: Electrical current. *In* Handbook of Physical Therapy. 3rd Ed. New York, Springer, 1977, pp. 23–45.

102. Gangarosa, L.P., et al.: Conductivity of drugs used for iontophoresis. J. Pharm. Sci., *67*:1439, 1978.

103. Grabois, M.: Treatment of pain syndromes through exercise. *In* Therapeutics Through Exercise. Edited by D.T. Lowenthal, K. Bharadwaja, and W.W. Oaks. New York, Grune & Stratton, 1979, pp. 181–185.

104. Licht, S. (ed.): Therapeutic Exercise. 2nd Ed. Baltimore, Waverly Press, 1965.

105. Cailliet, R.: Low Back Pain: Correction of Faulty Mechanics in Therapeutic Approach to Low Back Pain. Philadelphia, F.A. Davis, 1968.

106. Andersen, K.L.: The cardiovascular system in exercises. *In* Exercise Physiology. Edited by H.B. Falls. New York. Academic Press, 1968, pp. 79–128.

107. Mottram, R.F.: Metabolism of exercising muscle. *In* Frontiers of Fitness. Edited by J. Shepherd. Springfield, IL, Charles C Thomas, 1971, pp. 61–78.

108. Simonson, E.: Nutrition and work performance. *In* Physiology of Work Capacity and Fatigue. Edited by E. Simonson. Springfield, IL, Charles C Thomas, 1971, pp. 348–405.

109. Dejours, P.: Control of respiration in muscular exercises. *In* Handbook of Physiology, Section 3, Respiration: Vol. 1. Edited by W.O. Fenn, and H. Rahn. Washington, DC, American Physiological Society, 1964, pp. 631–648.

110. Asmussen, E.: Muscular exercise. *In* Handbook of Physiology, Section 3, Respiration: Vol. 2. Edited by W.O. Fenn, and H. Rahn. Washington, DC, American Physiological Society, 1964, pp. 939–978.

111. DeLorme, T.L.: Restoration of muscle power by heavy-resistance exercises. J. Bone Joint Surg., *27*:645, 1945.

112. de Lateur, B.J., Lehmann, J.F., and Fordyle, W.E.: A test of the De Lorme axion. Arch. Phys. Med. Rehabil., *49*:245, 1968.

113. Zinovieff, A.N.: Heavy-resistance exercise: "Oxford technique." Br. J. Phys. Med., *14*:129, 1951.

114. Hellebrandt, F.A.Q., and Houtz, S.J.: Methods of muscle training: Influence of pacing. Phys. Ther. Rev., *38*:319, 1958.

115. Liberson, W.T., and Asa, M.M.: Further studies of brief isometric exercises. Arch. Phys. Med. Rehabil., *40*:330, 1959.

116. Rose, D.L., Radzyminski, S.F.G., and Beatty, R.R.: Effect of brief maximal exercises on strength of quadriceps femoris. Arch. Phys. Med. Rehabil., *38*:157, 1957.

117. Liverson, W.T.: Brief isometric exercises. *In* Therapeutic Exercise. 3rd Ed. Edited by J.B. Basamajin. Baltimore, Williams & Wilkins, 1980, pp. 201–219.

118. Lind, A.R., and McNichol, G.W.: Cardiovascular responses to holding and carrying weights by hand and shoulder harness. J. Appl. Physiol., *25*:262, 1968.

119. Ramos, M.V., et al.: Cardiovascular effects of spread of excitation during prolonged isometric exercises. Arch. Phys. Med. Rehabil., *54*:496, 1973.

120. Hislop, H.J., and Perrine, J.J.: The isokinetics concepts of exercise. Phys. Ther., *47*:114, 1967.

121. Moffroid, M., et al.: A study of isokinetic exercise. Phys. Ther., *49*:735, 1969.

122. Simmons, J., Roth, D., and Merta, R.: Calculation of disability using the Cybex II System. Orthopedics, *5*:181, 1982.

123. Rosentwig, J., and Ghinson, M.M.: Comparison of isometric, isotonic and isokinetic exercises by electromyography. Arch. Phys. Med. Rehabil., *53*:249, 1972.

124. Judovich, B.D.: Herniated cervical disc; a new form of traction therapy. Am. J. Surg., *84*:646, 1952.

125. Cyriax, J.H.: Discussion on the treatment of backache by traction. Proc. R. Soc. Med., *45*:808, 1955.

126. Crue, B.: Importance of flexion in cervical halter traction. Bull. Los Angeles Neurol. Soc., *30*:95, 1965.

127. Colachis, S.C., Jr., and Strohm, B.R.: Effects of intermittent traction on separation of lumbar vertebrae. Arch. Phys. Med. Rehabil., *50*:215, 1969.

128. Lehmann, J.F., and Brunner, G.D.: A device for the application of heavy lumbar traction: Its mechanical effects. Arch. Phys. Med. Rehabil., *39*:696, 1958.

129. Christie, B.G.B.: Discussion on the treatment of backache by traction. Proc. R. Soc. Med., *48*:811, 1955.

130. Weber, H.: Traction therapy in sciatica due to disc prolapse. J. Oslo City Hosp., *23*:167, 1973.

131. Mathews J.A., and Hickling, J.: Lumbar traction: A double-blind controlled study for sciatica. Rheumatol. Rehabil., *14*:222, 1975.

132. Hinterbuchner, C.: Traction. *In* Manipulation, Traction and Massage. Edited by J.B. Rogoff. Baltimore, Williams & Wilkins, 1980, pp. 184–210.

133. Maigne, R.: Manipulation of the spine. *In* Manipulation, Traction and Massage. Edited by J.B. Rogoff. Baltimore, Williams & Wilkins, 1980, pp. 59–120.

134. Goldman, L., and Rockwell, R.J., Jr.: Lasers in Medicine. New York, Gordon and Breach, 1971.

135. Goldman, L. (ed.): The Biomedical Laser: Technology and Clinical Applications. New York, Springer-Verlag, 1981.

136. Willet, C.S.: Introduction to Gas Lasers: Population Inversion Mechanism. Oxford, Pergamon, 1974.

137. Calderhead, G., et al.: The Nd YAG and GA Al As lasers: A comparative analysis in pain therapy. Laser Acupunct., *21*:1, 1982.

138. Oyamada, Y., and Izu, S.: Application of low energy laser in chronic rheumatic arthritis and related rheumatoid diseases (abstract). *In* Proceedings of the 6th Congress of the International Society for Laser Surgery and Medicine, 1985, p. 80.

139. Castel, J.C.: Pain management with acupuncture and transcutaneous electrical nerve stimulation techniques and photostimulation (laser). 18A–18E, Neuromedtronics, Chicago, Illinois, 1982.

140. Kroetlinger, M.: On the use of the laser in acupuncture. Int. J. Acupunct. Electrother. Res., *5*:297, 1980.

141. Barnes, J.F.: Electronic acupuncture and cold laser therapy adjuncts to pain treatment. J. Craniomandibular Practice *2*:151, 1984.

142. Basford, J.R.: Low energy laser treatment of pain and wounds: Hype, hope or hokum. Mayo Clinic Proc., *61*:671, 1986.

143. Apfelberg, D.B., Mittelman, H., and Chadi, B.: Carcinogenic potential of in vitro carbon dioxide laser exposure of fibroblast. Obstet. Gynecol., *61*:493, 1983.

144. Lehmann, J.F., Erickson, D.J., Martin, G.M., and Krusen F.H.: Comparison of ultrasound and microwave diathermy in the physical treatment of periarthritis of the shoulder. Arch. Phys. Med. Rehabil., *35*:627, 1954.

145. Hinzelman, U.: Ultraschalltherapie rheumatischer Erkrankugen. Dtsch. Med. Wochenschr., *74*:869, 1949.

146. Martin, G.M., et al.: Cutaneous temperature of the extremities of normal subjects and of patients with rheumatoid arthritis. Arch. Phys. Med., *27*:665, 1946.

147. Harris, E., Jr., and McCroskery, P.A.: The influence of temperature and fibril stability on degeneration of cartilage collagen by rheumatoid synovial collagenase. N. Engl. J. Med., *290*:1, 1974.

148. Pegg, S.M.H., Little, T.R., and Littler, E.N.: A trial of ice therapy and exercise in chronic arthritis. Physiotherapy, *55*:51, 1969.

149. Johns, R.J., and Wright, V.: Relative importance of various tissues in joint stiffness. J. Appl. Physiol., *17*:824, 1962.

150. Backlund, L., and Tiselius, P.: Objective measurement of joint stiffness in rheumatoid arthritis. Acta Rheum. Scand., *13*:275, 1967.

151. Landon, B.R.: Heat or cold for the relief of low back pain? Phys. Ther., *47*:1126, 1967.

152. Knutsoon, E.: Topical cyrotherapy in spasticity. Scand. J. Rehabil. Med., *2*:159, 1970.

153. Miglietta, O.: Action of cold on spasticity. Am. J. Phys. Med., *52*:198, 1973.

154. Hartviksen, K.: Ice therapy in spasticity. Acta Neurol. Scand., *38*(Suppl. 3):79, 1962.

155. Kraus, H.: Clinical Treatment of Back and Neck Pain. New York, McGraw-Hill, 1970.

156. Simons, D.G.: Muscle pain syndrome—Parts I and II. Am. J. Phys. Med., *54*:289, 1975; *55*:15, 1976.

157. Fischer, A.A.: Diagnosis and management of chronic pain in physical medicine and rehabilitation. *In* Current Therapy in Physiatry. Edited by A.P. Ruskin. Philadelphia, W.B. Saunders, 1980, pp. 123–149.

158. Nichols, P.J.R.: Pain in the neck and shoulder. *In* Rehabilitation Medicine: The Management of Physical Disabilities. 2nd Ed. Edited by P.J.R. Nichols. London, Butterworths, 1980, pp. 79–82.

159. McGee, M., and Freshman, S.: Ultrasound and stretch: A decreased range of motion. A slide-tape presentation. Seattle Health Sciences Learning Resource Center, Univ. of Washington, 1978.

160. Smodlaka, V.N.: Sports medicine. *In* Current Therapy in Physiatry: Physical Medicine and Rehabilitation. Edited by A.P. Ruskin. Philadelphia, W.B. Saunders 1984, pp. 366–376.

161. Cailliet, R.: Spine: disorder and deformities. *In* Handbook of Physical Medicine and Rehabilitation. 3rd Ed. Edited by F.J. Kottke, G.K. Stillwell, and J.F. Lehmann. Philadelphia, W.B. Saunders, 1982, pp. 707–723.

89 · RADIATION THERAPY, CHEMOTHERAPY, HORMONE THERAPY, AND SURGERY FOR PAIN RELATED TO CANCER

ROGER J. BERRY, JOHN J. BONICA, ANNE NAYSMITH,
and ARMANDO SANTORO

THIS chapter contains a discussion of the bases and clinical applications of radiation therapy, chemotherapy, hormone therapy, and surgery primarily for the control of cancer-related pain. Although these anticancer modalities are briefly commented on in Chapters 24, 45, and 57 and in other chapters of Part IV of the book, they are considered in detail in this chapter to provide readers who are not oncologists with an understanding of their role in managing patients with cancer-related pain. Rational use of these therapies requires knowledge of tumor biology, the physical principles of radiation therapy, the pharmacokinetics of chemotherapy and hormone therapy, and their mechanisms of action, side effects, and complications.

Each of these therapies can be used either separately as a primary form of treatment or in combination with other methods. Selection of the agent or agents depends on the therapeutic intent—cure or palliation—which, in turn, is determined by the histologic type and site of the tumor, the clinical stage of the disease, the physical and psychologic condition of the patient, and, most important, the resources available in the institution. Because none of these therapies is tumor-specific all have side effects and complications.

The material is presented in three major sections: A, Radiation Therapy, written by Berry, Bonica, and Naysmith; B, Chemotherapy and Hormone Therapy, written by Santoro and Bonica; and C, Surgical Therapy, written by Bonica and Santoro on the basis of information provided by Gennari (1) and other sources.

A. RADIATION THERAPY

Radiotherapy, like surgery, is a localized or regional form of treatment and cannot be considered curative for disseminated disease. The choice of radical radiotherapy is determined by the histology and accessibility of the tumor, its intrinsic radiosensitivity, the clinical stage and operability of the lesion, the tolerance of adjacent tissues and the patient's physical condition, and morbidity that may be associated with a particular mode of treatment. Radiotherapy can be used alone or in combination with either surgery or chemotherapy. The role of radiotherapy in overall cancer treatment is beyond the scope of this section, which is devoted to the use of this modality for the relief of cancer pain.

Palliative treatment for cancer pain forms a large part of the work of most radiotherapists. As discussed in Chapter 24, about three-quarters of the patients with cancer have significant pain (see Table 24-1), and about 50% of those in the early and intermediate stages of the disease have pain (2). Bonica (2) has estimated that, in 1987, 1.13 million Americans and 8.8 million people worldwide had cancer related pain. Table 24-5 contains a summary of the pain syndromes in cancer patients; as noted, in most patients the pain is due to direct tumor involvement of bones, nerves, or soft tissue. Worthwhile pain relief is likely to be achieved in 65 to 90% of the irradiated sites (3). Indeed, so routine has such treatment become that little of it is subjected to controlled trials and recent literature is scanty.

This section discusses the use of radiation therapy in the context of managing patients with cancer pain and outlines the main indications for the use of radiation treatment and the treatment methods available. Doses and fractionation schedules currently employed are reviewed, the immediate and delayed complications of irradiation are discussed, and possible interactions with other forms of anticancer treatments are mentioned. Before proceeding with the clinical aspects of radiation therapy, we present a brief discussion of the physical principles underlying this form of therapy.

Basic Considerations

Radiation Modalities

Radiation can be administered via an external beam, by intracavitary placement, by interstitial implantation of radioactive sources, or by systemic administration of radioisotopes (4). For purposes of our discussion regarding pain control, external beam therapy is the modality most frequently used (5). The equipment to administer external beam therapy includes the "deep x-ray" machines operated in the 200- to 300-kV range, referred to as the super-kilovoltage range; machines operated in the more modern supervoltage energy range, generally taken to be between 2 and 10 megavolts (MeV); and machines operated in the megavoltage energies that provide radiation above 10 MeV (4, 5).

Deep x-ray machines operating at voltages of 200 to 300 kV have used since the 1920s for the treatment of cancer pain and still have a role in the relief of pain from bony metastases. Now, however, megavoltage equipment, which has been available since the late 1950s, is used more commonly to deliver radiotherapy. Cobalt-60 teletherapy sources have a gamma-ray energy of approximately 1.3 MeV, are robust and economical, and give physical sparing of the skin, but the most widely used machine is the electron linear accelerator, producing x-ray beams with energies of 5 to 10 MeV. These produce a stable beam, with skin sparing and sharply defined beam edges, and the depth of penetration of the beam can be varied (within limits) for different applications. Treatment times are short, on the order of a few minutes per fraction, for most treatment schedules. A similar device, the betatron, accelerates electrons magnetically in a circular path within a vacuum tube.

Physical Principles of Radiation Therapy

Two ionizing radiations, x rays and gamma rays, are of importance in external beam irradiation. X rays, or roentgen rays, are electromagnetic, nonparticulate ionizing radiations created through interaction of electrons in human-made machines; gamma (γ) rays, on the other hand, originate in the atomic nucleus during radioactive decay of naturally occurring or artificially produced radioactive elements such as radium or cobalt-60 (4).

These radiations have short wavelengths and have extremely high penetrating power in materials of low atomic number such as water and tissue, but they are stopped efficiently in material of high atomic number such as lead (4, 5).

Irradiation of cells causes a series of complex radiochemical events that lead to the production of free radicals in the water molecules of the cells' microenvironment (5). These free radicals are highly reactive abnormal ions, and, together with oxidizing agents, they interact with DNA molecules and produce a variety of DNA disruption and damage. Such damage will prevent or delay mitosis. Once alterations in the nucleotide sequence occur, a change in transcription or defective repair results, leading to death of the affected cells.

Basis Definitions

The roentgen, the basic unit of radiation exposure, is defined as follows. $X = \Delta q / \Delta m$, where X is the exposure in roentgens, Δq is the sum of all the electric charges on all ions of one sign (positive or negative) produced in air when irradiated by photons (γ rays or x rays), and Δm is the mass of air that is irradiated by the photons (4). Using this definition, 1 roentgen = 2.58×10^{-14} coulomb/kg of air.

The rad, the unit of radiation absorbed dose, is defined as the absorption of 100 ergs/per gram of irradiated matter (4, 5). *The gray* (Gy) (1 joule/kg) is the international unit of absorbed dose, which is becoming the established unit for reporting radiation dosage. One Gy = 100 rad.

Radiation quality is a term used to indicate the ability of radiation to penetrate matter below the surface. When considering radiotherapy doses, it is important to know the depth/dose characteristics of the treatment beam (4). As the energy of the incident radiation beam changes, the depth/dose characteristics of the beam also change: the higher the energy of the beam, the more penetrating it is.

Factors That Affect Cellular Response to Radiation

Many factors affect the response of cells to radiation, including radiation sensitivity, cellular repair capacity, and the size of the cell population (4).

Cell Stage

The response of cells to radiation depends in part on the position of cells in the cell cycle. Cells in mitosis are more sensitive to radiation damage then cells in interphase. Response can be enhanced by irradiating when the majority of cells are in the radiation-sensitive phase—a condition that can be brought about with drugs that synchronize phases in the cell cycle.

The response of cells to radiation also varies as a function of cell turnover: very rapidly dividing cells respond more quickly than slowly dividing cells.

Cell Oxygenation

Oxygen can enhance the radiosensitivity of cells (4, 5). Oxygen is a potent radiation sensitizer presumably because of its high electronegativity and its ability to scavenge and interact with free radicals. Cells that are well oxygenated are killed by a much lower dose than hypoxic cells. This increased response may be due to the ability of oxygen to attach to DNA strand breaks, preventing repair.

The effect of oxygen on cellular response can be quantified. The oxygen enhancement ratio (OER) is the ratio of the dose for hypoxic cells to the dose for oxygenated cells to achieve the same biologic affect. For x rays the OER is 2.5 to 3, indicating that the dose of radiation needed to achieve the same effect is 2.5 to 3 times greater for hypoxic cells than for oxgenated cells (4).

The oxygen enhancement ratio has important clinical implications for irradiation of tumors and the effect that the radiation may have on the surrounding normal tissue. Within the tumor, a number of necrotic cells are usually present in the center because the tumor has outgrown its blood supplies. Adjacent to the necrotic zone is a zone of hypoxia in which cells are alive but compromised in oxygen supply. Toward the periphery of the tumor there are areas of well-oxygenated cells close to the vascular network supplying that particular region. The tissue surrounding the tumor has a good vascular network and consequently is well oxygenated. Radiation will cause different cellular effects within this composite of necrotic, hypoxic, and well-oxygenated tissues. Well-oxygenated tumor cells respond to radiation and die, but the hypoxic region of the tumor is less radioresponsive than the surrounding normal tissue. To eliminate this differential response of hypoxic tumor cells and surrounding normal cells, radiotherapists exploit the reoxygenation that occurs in tumors in response to fractionated doses of radiation.

This process proceeds in the following fashion: In response to a dose of radiation, well-oxygenated cells at the periphery of a tumor die in greater percentages than the internal hypoxic cells (4). As a result, oxygen is now free to diffuse further into the tumor so that previously hypoxic cells become better oxygenated. Consequently, in response to the next dose of radiation, the cells are more radiosensitive than during the first radiation dose. This response to oxygenation occurs after each dose (4). Standard radiotherapy protocols call for a prescribed dose over a given period of time, usually in five increments weekly. When radiation is used in this manner, the inherent differential between hypoxic tumor cells and surrounding normal tissue is continually reduced because of reoxygenation, thus allowing a greater response than would be possible with single-dose irradiation. Hyperbaric oxygen has also been used to improve the cell kill of hypoxic cells (5).

Other Factors

Other factors that influence the cellular response to irradiation include the linear energy transfer (LET) of the radiation and the use of drugs that sensitize hypoxic cells. LET is defined as the density of ionizing events resulting from a specific radiation. In general, particle beams (neutrons, protons, stripped nuclei) have higher LET than photons (x rays). Ionizing events resulting from the passage of particles through tissues are closer together than photons; therefore, more energy is deposited per unit length of path. Because of this higher level of energy transfer, cells are more damaged than they would be from the passage of lower-LET photons (4).

Of various compounds that have been tested as sensitizers of hypoxic cells, the nitroimidazoles appear to have the greatest potential because of pharmacologic processes that promote distribution of the drug to the central portion of the tumor in spite of poor blood supply (5). Among these, metronidazole (Flagyl) has been active in animal model systems that are now in use in several countries (5). These compounds act by mimicking oxygen in fixing DNA damage caused by radiation. They increase the radiosensitivity of hypoxic cells but do not sensitize normal oxic cells to radiation and therefore exert a selective effect between tumors and normal tissue. Obviously, hypoxic radio-sensitizers have the potential of enhancing the usefulness of photon radiotherapy by maximizing the tumor cell kill with doses well within the range tolerated by normal tissue (5).

Clinical Considerations

To obtain optimal results in radiation therapy, it is essential that one be familiar with all of the basic principles discussed in Chapter 24 in the section "Evaluation of the Patient and the Pain." In addition to evaluation of the patient, it is essential to carefully identify the cause and mechanisms of the pain. Moreover, it is essential to understand the personality and emotional and psychologic status of the patient. If anxiety and depression are present, these should be managed. Chemical abnormalities, particularly hypercalcemia, appear clinically to increase the patient's sensitivity to pain and should be corrected. As emphasized in Chapter 24, the most common causes of pain in cancer patients are malignant disease of bone, nerve infiltration and compression by tumors, and invasion of soft tissue and hollow viscera.

Important Causes of Cancer Pain

Malignant Disease of Bone

Primary bone tumors, while painful, are rare. Secondary involvement of bone, however, can occur in up to 80% of cancer patients, depending on the primary site of disease (3). Chronic unremitting pain, often exacerbated by movement or weight bearing and accompanied by local tenderness, is the predominant symptom.

Pain can be due to one of three processes: (a) expanding lesions elevate and stretch the periosteum, giving rise to pain; (b) local chemical mediators, thought to be principally prostaglandin E_2, are involved in osteolysis by tumors and exacerbate pain (6); and (c) bone destruction can exacerbate pain. When more than half of the cortex has been destroyed, deformity occurs during weight bearing and causes pain (7). Pathologic fracture causes immediate severe pain, which can usually only be relieved adequately by surgical fixation or replacement arthroplasty followed by radiotherapy.

Infiltration and Compression of Nerves

Primary or secondary malignancies can give rise to pain of neuropathic origin either by direct invasion of nerves or nerve plexuses or by compression of adjacent structures. (a) Peripheral nerves may be directly invaded by tumor. (b) Nerve plexus involvement commonly gives rise to intractable pain in addition to the neurologic signs of involvement of either the brachial or lumbosacral plexus. (c) Spinal cord or nerve root compression is usually caused by an epidural tumor mass, often associated with vertebral metastases. Back pain, usually severe, commonly precedes paraplegia (see Chapter 57).

Stretch of Sensitive Membranes

Expansion of an organ by metastatic tumor, often increased by accompanying edema, can cause pain when it occurs rapidly. Cerebral metastases giving rise to raised intracranial pressure are associated with severe headache. Visceral metastases, particularly intrahepatic secondary tumors, can enlarge the organ rapidly enough for severe pain to be experienced from the visceral peritoneum. Other mechanisms include obstruction of a hollow viscus or a large artery or vein (see Table 24-5).

Pain Not of Malignant Origin

About 20 to 30% of patients with advanced cancer have pain not directly related to the malignant process (2). This can coexist with pain caused directly by the cancer, or it can be the only cause of pain. Previous treatment, such as surgery, radiation therapy, or chemotherapy, accounts for 25% of pain in cancer patients. Moreover, common painful conditions such as osteoarthrosis can exist concomitantly with the malignancy.

It is vital to distinguish pain of nonmalignant origin. Correct explanation might reassure the patient to the extent that the pain is no longer a problem. More important, inappropriate treatment, such as irradiation, can be avoided.

Radiotherapy in Control of Cancer Pain

Pain caused by cancer is effectively controlled by cytoreductive therapy, where such therapy can be given with a high probability of success. Successful chemotherapy for a lymphoma, or hormonal management of disseminated breast or prostatic cancer, will relieve malignant pain at all the affected sites. Many patients, however, have tumors for which no effective anti-tumor therapy is available, or have relapsed after such therapy, and require local palliation of their pain.

In general, radiotherapy as a method of pain control is most likely to be effective where a tumor has involved bone, less so where nerve invasion has taken place, and least effective when a soft tissue mass is the source of pain. The probability of pain relief depends also on the effective radiation dose that can be delivered (i.e., the tolerance of normal tissue at the painful site) and the radiosensitivity of the tumor. The clinical radiosensitivity of various tumors is shown in the following list:

Radiosensitive tumors (rapid shrinkage can be expected after radiotherapy)
  Leukemia
  Lymphoma
  Small-cell carcinoma of the bronchus
  Seminoma
  Myeloma
Moderately radiosensitive tumors (tumor shrinkage can usually be expected after radiotherapy)
  Nonsemiomatous germ cell tumors
  Squamous carcinoma in most sites
  Adenocarcinoma of the breast
  Bony metastasis from adenocarcinoma arising in most primary sites
Poorly radiosensitive tumors (tumor shrinkage after radiotherapy might be limited or slow)
  Adenocarcinoma, most sites
  Malignant melanoma
  Sarcoma of bone and soft tissue

It is common for radiotherapy to relieve pain successfully at one site, only to have the patient develop severe pain elsewhere. There are several reasons for this. One particularly painful area is likely to occupy the patient's conscious attention; when that pain improves, discomfort from other sites is more clearly perceived. Also, pain from involved bones is largely precipitated by movement and weight bearing; the improvement in mobility produced by radiotherapy to the most severely affected area might exacerbate pain elsewhere. Further, the underlying disease is usually a progressive one. Radiotherapy should therefore be planned as part of the overall management of the symptoms of advanced cancer, with a view to the future development of the disease, to allow retreatment of troublesome areas wherever possible, make it easy to match fields to adjacent sites, and minimize the amount of time the patient spends receiving treatment.

Local Radiation Therapy

The term *local radiation therapy* is used for radiation to treatment volumes that are smaller than half of the trunk; it covers the majority of radiation given for the control of pain.

Local Treatment of Bone Metastases

The sites involved and the patient's general health determine the selection of areas to be irradiated. Pain at a single site occurs in a minority of cancer patients. Local irradiation usually reduces or eliminates such pain, producing less patient morbidity than high doses of potent opioid analgesics. Bone pain on weight bearing can be difficult to control, but radiotherapy to the painful lesion is frequently effective in improving mobility and reducing analgesic requirements.

Multiple sites of bone pain constitute a common problem. To treat each site separately can involve the patient in time-consuming radiation treatment, and other methods of delivering radiotherapy to large areas are worth considering. Systemic nonopioid or opioid analgesics, or a combination of these, often control most of the pain, leaving a few particularly painful sites. Local radiotherapy of these areas is a useful alternative to a further increase in analgesic dosage. In such cases, radiotherapy is a localized analgesic to be combined with systemic analgesics in the same way as a nerve block procedure.

Radiotherapy has traditionally been delivered in daily fractions of 1.8 to 3 Gy to total doses of 30 to 40 Gy over 3 to 4 weeks. More recent work has demonstrated, however, that larger fractions can be given safely, allowing palliative treatment to be delivered more quickly (3, 7–11). A variety of schedules has been reported (Table 89-1). For lesions of long bones and ribs, 30 Gy in 6–10 fractions over 2 weeks, 20 Gy in 5 fractions over 1 week, and single fractions of 8 to 15 Gy appear equally effective and safe. Large single fractions are seldom given to the spine or pelvis because of the risk of producing neurologic problems or diarrhea, or to large areas because of unacceptably severe early "radiation sickness" with nausea and vomiting. If the initial dose is less than 15 Gy in a single fraction, or 20 Gy in 1 week, the same area can usually be retreated once if pain recurs.

Two recent randomized studies have confirmed that there is no advantage in increasing the dose or the number of fractions above the minimum required to relieve symptoms. The Radiation Therapy Oncology Group compared short low-dose treatment (15 Gy in 1 week) with higher-dose treatment (20–25 Gy in 1 week) and more protracted treatment (30 Gy in 2 weeks or 40.5 Gy in 3 weeks) in 1016 patients (3). Almost 90% of patients experienced worthwhile improvement, and 54% achieved complete pain relief, with no differences among any of the treatment schedules. A much smaller study, randomizing 57 patients with isolated bone deposits between 24 Gy in 6 fractions over 3 weeks and 20 Gy in 2 fractions over 1 week, again demonstrated identical rates of pain relief with either schedule (11). There is therefore no indication for protracted treatment schedules for palliative radiotherapy for the relief of bone pain.

TABLE 89-1. Radiotherapy Schedules and Response Rates for Bone Metastases

Source	Number of Patients Evaluated	Schedule	Response Rate (Percent)
Allen et al. (12)	110	5 Gy × 2 2.5 Gy × 8 4 Gy × 8	77
		2 Gy × 20 5 Gy × 4 2.5 Gy × 16	78
		4 Gy × 8 6 Gy × 5 4 Gy × 10	80
Hendrickson et al. (7)	86	9 Gy × 1 6 Gy × 2 3 Gy × 5	88
		2 Gy × 10 4 Gy × 5 3 Gy × 10	84
Penn (8)	144	8–15 Gy × 1 3 Gy × 10	89 94
Gilbert et al. (9)	120	2 Gy × 15 2 Gy × 20 4 Gy × 5 6.5 Gy × 2	73
Katz (10)	32	2.67 Gy × 15 3 Gy × 10 4 Gy × 5	74
		5 Gy × 6 6 Gy × 6 7.5 Gy × 2 8 Gy × 3 10 Gy × 2	79
Tong et al. (3)	759	2.7 Gy × 15 3 Gy × 5 3 Gy × 10 4 Gy × 5 5 Gy × 5	83
Madsen (11)	57	4 Gy × 6 10 Gy × 2	47 48

Although pain relief is achieved rather rapidly, it is seldom immediate. There have been claims that large fraction sizes produce more rapid relief (3), but this is difficult to demonstrate. Of those who will eventually benefit, 80 to 90% will demonstrate improvement within 2 to 4 weeks of treatment (12), and 50% will have complete pain relief, but improvement continues for up to 20 weeks (3).

The survival of patients with bone metastases is related more to the site of the primary tumor than to the extent of bone disease; patients with breast and prostatic cancer survive longer than those with bronchogenic primary tumors. In bone metastases from breast cancer the median duration of pain relief after radiotherapy is around 12 months in surviving patients (13), 50% of patients remaining pain free until death (9).

Local Treatment of Nonosseous Lesions

Radiotherapy is used less often, and on the whole is less successful, in relieving pain fron nonosseous lesions. *Headache from cerebral metastases*, however, is well relieved by radiotherapy to the whole brain in doses such as 20 Gy in 5 fractions over 1 week or 25 to 30 Gy in 10 fractions over 2 weeks together with corticosteroids. *Painful epidural metastases* from radiosensitive tumors respond moderately well to more prolonged treatment, such as 40 Gy in 20 fractions over 4 weeks.

Plexus invasion, whether of the brachial plexus by a bronchogenic tumor or of the lumbosacral plexus by recurrent tumor in the pelvis, responds poorly to radiotherapy. Back pain caused by enlarged para-aortic lymph nodes can be successfully treated provided the tumor is radiosensitive.

Carcinoma of the pancreas usually causes severe pain. Small numbers of patients have been successfully treated using high-dose radiotherapy (14). Localization of the lesion using CT scanning allows accurate delivery of the radiation. In this situation, however, neurolytic celiac plexus or splanchnic block is probably to be preferred (see Chapter 96). *Pain from a soft tissue mass*, a common problem in the chest or pelvis, might not respond to radiotherapy.

Toxicity of Local Radiation Therapy

Short-Term Toxicity

Short-term toxicity arises during treatment and subsides within 2 to 3 weeks. Skin reactions are slight, usually limited to mild erythema.

GASTROINTESTINAL DISORDERS. Gastrointestinal nausea is related to site and size of the irradiated field. It is common if the upper abdomen is irradiated and also seen when a large field is used, e.g., the hemipelvis. It is usually mild. Pharyngitis and esophagitis might be seen during irradiation of the chest or cervical or dorsal spine, but they are uncommon at low doses. Monilial infection of the mouth can develop and should be treated appropriately. Diarrhea can result from irradiation of the lower lumbar spine or pelvis. It usually responds to a low-residue diet and antidiarrheal agents.

PATHOLOGIC FRACTURES. Pathologic fractures have been ascribed to radiotherapy given to a bone metastasis. This ascription is difficult to confirm or deny. Radiotherapy is commonly given to lytic metastases in long bones, where fractures are also common. When more than 75% of the cortex of a long bone is destroyed there is a high chance of spontaneous fracture (15), a risk that can increase if pain relief allows greater mobilization, whether or not radiotherapy has also increased osteoporosis. Prophylactic fixation is indicated in lesions at high risk of fracture if the patient's general condition is good (15).

PSYCHOLOGIC PROBLEMS. Psychologic problems must not be underestimated. Even low-dose irradiation can cause general tiredness, which the patient might misinterpret as indicating progression of the cancer. The patient can be exhausted by multiple visits to have radiotherapy, and demoralized if new painful lesions develop before the initial treatment course is finished. For many patients, radiotherapy is a frightening event. Clear explanations, counseling, emotional support, and, if necessary, formal teaching of relaxation techniques can all help to minimize the patient's distress. It is important that the course of radiotherapy be kept as brief as possible.

Delayed Toxicity

Few patients receiving palliative radiation for cancer pain will survive to develop late radiation damage, but it is impossible to predict which patient will live for extended periods.

RADIATION MYELOPATHY. Radiation myelopathy can cause paraplegia. The tolerance of the spinal cord can be exceeded if a painful area is retreated with a high total dose or given large single fractions. Radiation myelopathy is rare if the total dose is below 40 Gy and the daily fraction size below 29 Gy. Radiation-induced spinal cord pathology usually takes two forms, transient myelopathy and chronic progressive myelopathy (16, 17). Transient myelopathy is most frequently seen about 4 months after external radiation therapy to the upper respiratory tract in which the cervical spinal cord is included in the portal. This type usually produces electric shock-like sensation precipitated by neck flexion, but no neurologic signs of myelopathy, and the symptoms gradually abate over 2 to 36 weeks (16). Chronic progressive myelopathy can develop after radiation therapy to the head and neck area, mediastinum, and cervical/superclavicular and axillary nodes (17). These patients typically present 5 to 30 months after irradiation (average 14 months) with paresthesia and spastic motor weakness and a Brown-Sequard syndrome. Pain is an early symptom and can become very severe. Paraplegia has developed immediately after a single large fraction to the lumbar spine (11).

RADIATION PLEXOPATHY. Pain in the distribution of the brachial plexus after radiation therapy is caused by fibrosis of the surrounding connective tissues and secondary injury to nerves. It can appear as early as 6 months, or as late as 20 years, after radiation treatment. It is often difficult to differentiate between radiation plexopathy and recurrent tumor (18, 19). The clinical symptoms include complaints of numbness or paresthesia in the hand, usually with a C5–C6 distribution. Pain occurs late in the course of the clinical entity and is often characterized as diffuse arm pain, and this is often associated with lymphedema in the arm, skin changes, and induration of the supraclavicular and axillary areas.

Radiation fibrosis of the lumbosacral plexus is much less common that that involving the brachial plexus (18, 19). The lower incidence appears to be related to the types of tumor and shortened survival time compared to that of carcinoma of the breast. Patients develop pain that progresses, leading to disability and dysfunction associated with progressive motor and sensory dysfunction of the leg and monoparesis.

RADIATION-INDUCED PERIPHERAL NERVE TUMORS. Foley and associates (20) have reported on a series of 9 patients who developed radiation-induced nerve tumors, 5 presenting with pain, progressive neurologic deficit, and palpable mass involving either the brachial or lumbar plexus. These tumors usually develop 4 to 20 years after radiation therapy, when patients have been cured of their original tumors.

VISCERAL DAMAGE. Damage to bladder and bowel occurs progressively after high-dose irradiation. If the tissue tolerance is exceeded, bladder irritation (frequency, urgency, and hematuria) can progress to fibrosis. Acute bowel damage (diarrhea, proctitis) is succeeded by small vessel arteritis in the bowel wall. Bowel surgery can precipitate necrosis of the ischemic segment. Retreatment to a painful pelvic recurrence might have to be limited in dose in order to avoid these problems.

CARCINOGENESIS. Carcinogenesis is a feared late complication of radiation therapy, but it is not relevant to the relief of pain in the cancer patient. The interval between irradiation and the development of a second, radiation-induced tumor can be more than 20 years. Even when extensive high-dose radiotherapy is superimposed on alkylating agent chemotherapy, the latency of second-tumor production is measured in years, considerably longer than the life expectancy of this group of patients.

Systemic Radiation Therapy

Large areas of the body can be irradiated either by external beams or by the administration of radioisotopes.

Hemibody Irradiation

When there are widespread bone metastases affecting a large part of the skeleton, multiple local treatments can impose a heavy burden on the patient. In this situation there is increasing interest in the use of radiation to half of the body as a single fraction, followed if necessary by radiation to the other half in 4 to 6 weeks (21–26). If the whole body is irradiated simultaneously, the dose that can be tolerated is severely limited by bone marrow suppression. If only half the body is irradiated, the affected marrow is recolonized by stem cells from the unirradiated area. When this process has reconstituted the marrow, the second half can be safely treated.

Employing a linear accelerator, treatment is delivered using opposed portals with the patient more than 200 cm from the radiation source. Dose rates are kept low, usually 0.3 to 0.4 Gy/minute, to a total of 7 or 8 Gy as a single fraction to the upper half, and up to 10 Gy to the lower half of the body. If a cobalt-60 machine is used, the dose to the upper half of the body has to be reduced or lung shielding introduced to compensate for higher absorption by the lung (21).

Patients likely to benefit from this technique are those with widespread bone metastases from carcinoma of the breast, bronchus, or prostate, and myeloma unresponsive to chemotherapy. There is insufficient reported experience to assess the usefulness of the technique with other primary tumors.

TOXICITY OF HEMIBODY IRRADIATION. There is appreciable toxicity from upper half-body irradiation. The acute reaction includes nausea, vomiting, pyrexia, tachycardia, and hypotension. This can be reduced by adequately premedicating the patient with corticosteroids and antiemetics; intravenous fluids are sometimes given. If the salivary glands, eyes, and scalp are irradiated, a dry mouth, conjunctivitis, and alopecia can develop.

The most serious problem is radiation pneumonitis, which can progress to fatal fibrosis (23). The incidence is dose-related, and it is increased in patients who have previous or subsequent mediastinal or lung irradiation or radiosensitizing chemotherapy. It is minimized by restricting the dose to 6 or 7 Gy and possibly by using low dose rates (22, 23).

The acute reaction to lower half-body irradiation is milder. Diarrhea is common; nausea and vomiting can occur. Severe and prolonged marrow suppression has been a problem in patients receiving both upper and lower half-body irradiation, particularly if there is pre-existing marrow depletion due to chemotherapy or extensive tumor involvement.

Despite the toxicity, encouraging results have been reported with this technique (21, 22, 24–27). Pain relief is achieved within 24 to 72 hours in 60 to 80% of patients (21) and is as prolonged as with localized radiotherapy. In addition, tumor control can correct hypercalcemia in patients with myeloma.

Total Body Irradiation Using Strontium

A new technique for irradiating all areas where new bone is being made is the administration of strontium. Following confirmation by conventional nuclear medicine bone scan techniques that the painful lesions concentrate bone-seeking isotopes, a single intravenous injection of up to 3.7 MBq/kg (100 μCi/kg) of strontium is given. Hematologic toxicity limits the use of higher doses. Some encouraging preliminary results have been achieved in the treatment of bone metastases from carcinoma of the prostate, but the technique is only likely to be useful where the painful metastatic disease shows active osteoblastic activity.

Interactions between Radiation Therapy and Drug Therapy

Interactions between radiation therapy and drug therapy fall into two classes: necessary adjustments in analgesic dosage as radiation becomes effective, and an increase in toxicity to certain organs when radiation and chemotherapy are superimposed. Analgesic requirements are likely to fall as radiation becomes effective. Appropriate adjustments should be made to avoid doses that are higher than needed. Irradiation should not be regarded as a failure if the analgesic dose cannot be reduced. It might be that the patient has better pain control on the same analgesics, or has the same amount of pain but greatly increased mobility.

Chemotherapy interactions are less important in this group of patients than in those likely to have a normal life expectancy. Prior treatment with L-phenylalanine mustard (L-PAM), bleomycin, or high-dose cyclophosphamide has been associated with increased pulmonary damage from subsequent irradiation; this may lead to radiation pneumonitis after whole lung or upper half-body irradiation. Chemotherapy with doxorubicin, methotrexate, or bleomycin intensifies the normal tissue reaction to radiotherapy. The cardiotoxicity of anthracyclines is increased by mediastinal irradiation, making cardiac failure more common. Hepatic toxicity has been reported after combined radiotherapy and either actinomycin D or doxorubicin. The possibility of such interactions should not prevent a patient with advanced cancer being given radiotherapy if that is the best way of relieving his pain, although doses may need to be reduced.

Radiotherapy for Nonmalignant Painful Conditions

For ankylosing spondylitis, the traditional treatment has been an applied dose of 20 Gy in 20 fractions over 4 weeks given with 200- to 300-Kv x rays to the entire axial skeleton from occiput to sacroilliac joints. Although this treatment is undeniably effective in achieving pain relief and allows greater mobility and decreased deformity it is accompanied by an increased risk of leukemia and solid tumors which is considered unacceptable (28). Even today, for patients who fail to respond to aggressive conventional rheumatologic methods, radiotherapy to affected joints using similar doses but minimal treatment volumes remains effective and may well be justified. This should only be done after informed discussion with patients of the likely benefits and risks.

More experimentally, irradiation of all lymphoid areas (total nodal irradiation) is being used for treatment of patients with severe, advanced rheumatoid arthritis that fails to respond to conventional management (29). Such irradiation is undoubtedly capable of producing prolonged lymphopenia and resultant immune suppression that could modify the course of the disease, but the long-term results and risks have not been evaluated.

Conclusions

Radiotherapy to relieve cancer pain is successful if the symptoms can be alleviated without burdening the patient by the treatment itself, either because of the time it takes or because of its toxicity. Close cooperation is essential between the radiotherapist and the doctor caring for the patient. Radiotherapy should be planned as part of the overall management of the patient in pain from cancer.

B. CHEMOTHERAPY AND HORMONE THERAPY

In recent years, the medical treatment for various forms of neoplastic disease has markedly improved in terms of strategy, number of effective drugs, and incidence of favorable responses (5, 30–33). Consequently, the medical approach to cancer can now be regarded as an established method of therapy with either curative or palliative purposes, depending on the histology and stage of the neoplasm. Despite these advances, a considerable number of cancer patients still suffer from poorly controlled pain due to progressive disease. Moreover, the specific impact of medical treatment of the pain produced by advanced cancer has not yet been fully analyzed, because the response to anticancer drugs has been considered significant only when documented by an objective regression of metastatic parameters (32–34). Because of the frequent concomitant supportive measures, subjective improvement alone, including pain relief, in the past was almost never regarded as a meaningful response to anticancer therapy. Nevertheless, any treatment that can reduce the size of tumor theoretically should lead to relief of cancer pain. On the other hand, antimitotic drugs are often highly toxic, particularly in patients with low performance status either as a result of disease or previous treatments. Consequently, it is important to properly balance the expected advantages of cancer chemotherapy with the risk of toxic manifestations (32).

Today a large number of anticancer drugs and other agents are available for curative and palliative purposes (5, 30, 32–36). All of these agents can be categorized into six major classes: (a) alkylating agents, (b) antimetabolites, (c) plant alkaloids, (d) antitumor antibiotics, (e) endocrine agents, and (f) a "miscellaneous" group. We first discuss the cytotoxic chemotherapeutic drugs that make up the first four classes and the miscellaneous group. The issue of hormonal manipulation as antitumor modality is considered in the second part of this section.

Chemotherapy

The most important chemotherapeutic agents, their dosages, usual routes of administration, side effects, and indications are listed in Table 89-2. All of these cytotoxic drugs interfere with cell division, some by disturbing mitotic spindle formation, some by specific enzyme inhibition, some by cross-linkage of DNA or RNA, and some by several actions simultaneously at different sites of the cell. Precise mechanism of action varies with each drug, and this variation is reflected in different patterns of normal tissue toxicity.

In some patients chemotherapy is used as an adjuvant to radiation therapy or surgery or a combination of these that are considered the primary treatment, and in other patients it is used as the primary therapy. Adjuvant chemotherapy is used in patients who appear cured but are suspected of having residual disease or micrometastasis; or it may be used in patients with advanced cancer. Chemotherapy is the primary method of effectively treating a variety of neoplasms and has advantages over radical surgery or high-voltage radiation therapy because the complications inherent in these methods are avoided. Regardless of the objectives of application, it is now clear that single-drug chemotherapy is generally less effective than combination chemotherapy in ensuring tumor cell destruction with an acceptable toxicity to patients.

On the basis of an extensive review of in vivo and in vitro laboratory research and clinical experiences acquired during the 1950s and 1960s, DeVita and Schien (36) developed a set of basic principles of combination chemotherapy for cancer patients. Among the most important of these are the following: (a) all of the component drugs in a combination must have activity against the neoplasm being treated; (b) drugs must be administered at dosages close to the minimum effec-

tive dosage for each drug as a single agent, or beyond if possible (the higher the dosage of each drug is raised the more likely that beneficial results will be obtained); (c) drugs that interrupt the synthesis of cellular macromolecules at several sites can be combined for additive or synergistic effects on the various synthetic pathways (the different mechanisms of cytotoxic action have been categorized by pattern of inhibitory actions—see ref. 36); (d) drugs in combination should have as little cross toxicity as possible; and (e) mechanism of tumor cell resistance in two agents in combination must not be similar.

Clinical Applications

Anticancer therapy must be started with those types of cancer for which chemotherapeutic regimens have proven effective. Conventionally, a complete response (CR) represents total disappearance of all observable disease for a variable period of time, which is usually from 1 to 3 months, depending on the criteria used (5, 30–32). A partial response (PR) represents a decrease in measurable tumor size of 50% or more. Table 24-9 (p. 419) indicates that, irrespective of drug combination used, many forms of solid tumors are now showing objective response to specific chemotherapy. Although cure of most forms of cancer is still an elusive objective, it cannot be denied that available drug treatments are currently able to produce good partial remission and even complete remission in some cancers for which two decades ago only supportive therapy was available. As a general rule, the achievement of significant response (CR + PR) is almost always translated into an improved survival of responders compared with nonresponders, and is also translated into relief of pain related to the tumor mass. Furthermore, in a fraction of patients with specific forms of cancer, such as pediatric tumors, lymphomas, testicular cancer, and ovarian cancer, complete remission of the neoplastic disease is followed by prolonged disease-free survival compatible with cure (32).

Highly Responsive Tumors

In Hodgkin's disease, treatment with effective polychemotherapy such as MOPP (mechlorethamine, vincristine [Oncovin], procarbazine, and prednisone) or ABVD (Adriamycin, bleomycin, vinblastine, and decarbazine), alone or in combination, produces a remission rate that varies from 60 to 90% without recurrence and a life expectancy of 5 to 10 years in 60 to 80% of patients. The therapeutic effect of this strategy is rapid, even in advanced cases, producing rapid pain relief in those patients with pain, and resolution of other symptoms and signs. Analogous but slightly inferior results can be obtained in non-Hodgkin lymphomas with such combinations as BACOP (bleomycin, Adriamycin, cyclophosphamide, vincristine, and prednisone) or CHOP (cyclophosphamide, Adriamycin, vincristine, and prednisone). Similar results are also obtained, with various chemotherapeutic regimens, in carcinoma of the testicle with PVB (platinum, vinblastine, and bleomycin), in Wilm's tumor, and in the leukemias (especially the lymphoblastic types).

TABLE 89-2. Commonly Used Cytotoxic Anticancer Agents

Class (Drug)*	Optimal Dose when Used Alone (mg/m²), Route, and Schedule†	Toxicities†			Indications
		Bone Marrow Suppr.	Nausea, Vomiting	Other Toxicity	
A. ALKYLATING AGENTS					
Mechlorethamine (Mustargen)	4 IV bolus q̄ 3–4 wk	4+	3+	Vesicant to skin, phlebitis	Hodgkin's disease, non-Hodgkin's lymphoma, lung cancer
Cyclophosphamide (Cytoxan)	400 in 20-ml SW IV bolus q̄d × 5 100 PO qd × 14	3+	2+	Alopecia and cystitis	Lymphomas; breast, lung, and ovarian cancer; myeloma; leukemias; head and neck cancer
Melphalan (Alkeran)	4 PO q̄d cont. 8 IV in 200-ml DxW infusion over 45 min qd × 5	3+	1+	Persistent thrombocytopenia on long use	Breast and ovarian cancer, myeloma
Busulfan (Myeleran)	2–6 PO qd cont.	3+	1+	Pigmentation, pulmonary fibrosis	Pre-bone marrow transplantation, chronic myelogenous leukemia
Chlorambucil (Leukeran)	1–3 PO qd cont.	3+	0	Pancytopenia with long-term use	Chronic lymphocytic leukemia, nodular lymphomas
CCNU (Lomustine)	100–150 PO q̄ 6 wk	4+	2+	Cumulative marrow suppression, chronic renal failure	Brain tumors, lung and colon cancer, lymphomas
BCNU (Carmustine)	200–225 in 2–3 ml DxW IV infusion (30 min) q̄ 6 wk	4+	4+	Chronic renal failure, pulmonary fibrosis, tanning of skin	Hodgkin's disease, non-Hodgkin's lymphoma, myeloma, brain tumors
MeCCNU (Semustine)	100–150 PO q̄ 6 wk	4+	2+	Pronounced thrombocytopenia, chronic renal failure	Colon and gastric cancer, brain tumors, lymphomas
Streptozocin (streptozotocin, Zanosar)	500 in 5-ml DxW infusion (6h) qd × 5, q̄ 3–4 wk	0	2+	Hepatotoxicity, renal tubular acidosis, renal failure	Islet cell tumors of pancreas, Hodgkin's disease, carcinoid tumors
Cisplain (cis-platinum, Platinol)	50–100 in liter NS IV infusion (6h) q̄ 3–4 wk	1+	3+	Nephrotoxicity, ototoxicity, peripheral neuropathy	Testicular tumors, ovarian and lung cancer, lymphomas
B. ANTIMETABOLITES					
Methotrexate: high dose with rescue	1500 in 100-ml NS IV infusion (10 min) q̄ 3 wk	1+	2+		
Methotrexate: no rescue	25 in 25-ml NS IV bolus twice weekly	4+	1+	Fatigue, buccal ulcerations	Breast, lung, cervical, and head and neck cancers, sarcomas, acute lymphocytic leukemia, meningeal leukemia, carcinomatosis
	12 IT in 10 ml Elliot's B solution q̄ 4 d	1+	0		
5-Fluorouracil (5-FU)	500 IV bolus q̄ wk or q̄ wk × 5 800–1200 IA infusion over 24h qd × 2–3 wk	3+	2+	Mucositis, diarrhea, photophobia, alopecia, cerebellar ataxia	Colon, breast, ovarian, gastric, and pancreatic cancer
6-Mercaptopurine (Purinethol)	100 PO qd × 5	2+	1+	Hepatotoxicity	For maintenance phase of acute lymphocytic leukemia
6-Thioguanine	100 in 15 ml IV bolus qd × 5	2+	1+	Cholestasis	Acute myelogenous leukemia
Cytarabine (cytosine arabinoside, Cytosar-U)	100 in 20 ml IV bolus (20 min) q̄ 12h × 5–10 d	4+	2+	Mucositis, alopecia, hepatotoxicity	Acute myelogenous leukemia, non-Hodgkin's lymphoma, meningeal leukemia, carcinomatosis

TABLE 89-2. (Cont.)

Class (Drug)*	Optimal Dose when Used Alone (mg/m²), Route, and Schedule†	Toxicities‡			Indications
		Bone Marrow Suppr.	Nausea, Vomiting	Other Toxicity	
Hydroxyurea	1000–1500 in 10–15 ml SW IV infusion (1–5 min) qd × 5 100 PO qd cont.	3+	1+	None	Alternate to busulfan for chronic myelogenous leukemia, rapid reduction of high WBC in acute or chronic myelogenous leukemia
C. PLANT ALKALOIDS					
Vinblastine (Velban)	4 in 10-ml NS IV infusion (1–5 min) q̄ wk	3+	1+	Mild peripheral neuropathy	Hodgkin's disease, head and neck tumors, testicular tumors
Vincristine (Oncovin)	1 in 10-ml NS IV infusion (1–5 min) q̄ wk	1+	1+	Local necrosis, peripheral neuropathy (paresthesias, etc.), alopecia, ileus, motor weakness	Lymphomas, acute lymphocytic leukemia, childhood sarcomas
Etoposide (VP-16)	85 in 20-ml NS IV infusion (1–5 min) q̄ wk 200 PO 2 d q̄ wk	1–2+	1+	Mucositis, bronchospasm, hypotension with rapid IV infusion	Small cell lung cancer, breast cancer, lymphomas (relapsed)
D. ANTIBIOTICS					
Doxorubicin (Adriamycin)	75 in 15-ml SW IV infusion (1–5 min) q̄ 3 wk	4+	2+	Mucositis, alopecia, myocardiopathy	Breast, lung, ovarian, pancreatic, gastric, and thyroid cancer, leukemia and lymphomas, sarcomas
Bleomycin (Blenoxane)	10 IV q̄ wk	1+	1+	Pneumonitis, muscositis, pulmonary fibrosis, alopecia, skin changes	Head and neck tumors, cervical carcinoma, lymphoma
Dactinomycin (Cosmegen)	0.6 in SW IV bolus (1–5 min) qd × 5, q̄ mo	3+	2+	Mucositis, phlebitis, diarrhea, alopecia, skin changes	Wilm's tumor, gestational, trophoblastic neoplasia, soft tissue sarcoma, childhood solid tumor
Daunorubicin (Cerubidine)	30 in 30-ml SW IV infusion (30 min) qod to toxicity	4+	2+	Mucositis, hepatotoxicity, myocardiopathy	Acute nonlymphatic and lymphatic leukemias, childhood solid tumors
Mithramycin (Mithracin)	1.75 in 100-ml DxW IV infusion (15–30 min) qod to toxicity	3+	3+	Hemorrhage, skin flushing, thrombocytopenia, hypocalcemia	Malignant hypercalcemia, testicular tumor (salvage therapy)
Mitomycin C (Mutamycin)	2 in 4-ml SW IV bolus (1–5 min) qd × 3, q̄ 3 wk	3+	2+	Mucositis, pneumonitis, renal failure	Breast, lung, colon, gastric, pancreatic, and bladder carcinoma
E. MISCELLANEOUS					
Procarbaxine (Matulane)	100–200 d PO cont.	3+	2+	Side effects of monoamine oxidase inhibitors, skin rash	Lung and testicular cancer, brain tumors, lymphomas
L-Asparaginase (Elspar)	200 units/kilo IV d 2–4 wk	0	2+	Pancreatitis, CNS toxicity, hypofibrinogenemia	Acute myelogenous leukemia, T-cell lymphoma
Hexamethylmelamine	480 PO qd × 21	1+	3+	Anorexia, central and peripheral neuropathy	Ovarian and small cell lung carcinoma

*The names of drugs in parentheses represent proprietary names and in some instances other generic names.
†Suggested range of doses from starting to maintenance dose in previously untreated patients. The doses and intervals between doses of all myelosuppressive agents should be continuously adjusted by monitoring WBC and platelet counts. Doses differ when used in combinations and are reduced in previously treated patients with compromised bone marrow.
NS normal saline; SW sterile water; DxW dextrose in water; IV intravenous; PO by mouth; IT intrathecal; IA intra-arterial; min minutes; qd every day; qod every other day.
‡Degree of toxicity: 4+ marked, 3+ severe, 2+ moderate, 1+ minimal or mild, 0 none.
Modified from Chabner, B.A., and Myers, C.E.: Clinical pharmacology of cancer chemotherapy. In Cancer: Principles and Practice of Oncology. 2nd Ed. Edited by V.T. DeVita, S. Hellman, and S.A. Rosenberg. Philadelphia, Lippincott, 1985, pp. 287–328, and Riggs, C.: Clinical pharmacology of individual antineoplastic agents. In Comprehensive Textbook of Oncology. Edited by A.R. Moossa, M.C. Robson, and S.C. Schimpff. Baltimore, Williams & Wilkins, 1986, pp. 210–234.

Moderately Responsive Tumors

In moderately chemosensitive tumors (see Table 24-9), the results obtained with the various chemotherapeutic combinations are less favorable (30 to 60% success), and in general the therapeutic effect is slower in onset. For example, in breast cancer with localized secondary bone mestastasis, the combination of chemotherapy together with radiation therapy directed to the bone lesion might produce improved results. The same can be said about soft tissue sarcoma, especially in the presence of large abdominal masses; a favorable therapeutic result is observed only in 25 to 40% of the cases and generally after 4 or 5 cycles of chemotherapy.

Poorly Responsive Tumors

In tumors with poor radiosensitivity such as adenocarcinoma, malignant melanoma, and sarcoma of bone and soft tissue, favorable results are rarely obtained with chemotherapeutic drugs. In this group of tumors, anticancer modalities are rarely effective in reducing the size of the tumor and the associated pain and other symptoms and signs. Unfortunately, many factors are often responsible for the limited efficacy of anticancer drugs alone. First, solid tumors that often produce pain usually do not respond well to current drug regimens. In fact, complete remission occurs in fewer than one-third of patients, and in the large majority of cases it is short-lived. Pain is often produced by large tumor masses, the size of which is inversely related to the incidence of a satisfactory drug response. Furthermore, because pain usually develops in late stages of the disease, second- or third-line drug treatments yield a minimal response rate. Finally, in certain target sites (e.g., head and neck, pelvis) prior radical surgery and especially prior radiation therapy negatively affect the vascular supply in almost every patient, thus preventing an effective drug concentration from reaching and remaining in the target site for a long enough time.

Analgesic Efficiency

Despite the aforementioned limitations, effective first-line drug therapy does produce pain relief along with objective tumor regression as reflected by the examples listed in Table 89-3. For instance, advanced local breast cancer may be painful when inflammatory reaction distends the breast, when local extensive infiltration of the chest wall occurs, and when the tumor ulcerates. In all these situations, medical therapy (chemotherapy and/or endocrine therapy) produces complete or partial remission in 50 to 70% of patients, and the objective response is almost always associated with marked regression and even disappearance of pain.

In contrast, in the presence of skeletal metastasis, tumor response to drugs is usually slow, and pain control is best achieved by combining drugs with radiotherapy. Radiation therapy is always the treatment of first choice when supraclavicular adenopathy in breast cancer produces compression of the brachial plexus and lymphedema of the arm. On the other hand, in prostate cancer, endocrine therapy (orchiectomy, estrogen) produces a high and prompt response rate. Therefore, palliative radiation therapy is used only in the late stages of the disease.

TABLE 89-3. Efficacy of Chemotherapy in Relieving Pain*

Primary Cancer	Source or Site of Pain	Degree of Pain Relief*
Breast	Tumor ulceration	+++
	Chest wall infiltration	+++
	Bone metastasis	++
	Lymphedema of arm	+
Prostate	Bone metastases	+++
Lymphomas	Para-aortic adenopathy → back pain	++++
	Superior vena cave obstruction	+++
	Spinal cord compression	+++
Leukemia } Myeloma }	Periosteal irration/invasion	+++
	Medullary pressure	+++
Testicle	Para-aortic adenopathy → back pain	++
Oral/ Pharyngeal }	Tumor ulceration	++
	Invasion of nerves	++
Lung	Pancoast syndrome	+
Colorectal } Cervical } Bladder }	Low abdominal } Perineal } pain Low back }	+
Intracranial Tumors	Increaded CF pressure → severe headache	
	(a) with corticosteroids	+++
	(b) without corticosteroids	+

*++++ complete relief; +++ very good, but incomplete relief; ++ moderate relief; + little or no relief.
From Bonadonna, G., and Molinari, R.: Role and limits of anticancer drugs in the treatment of advanced cancer pain. In Advances in Pain Research and Therapy. Vol. 2. Edited by J.J. Bonica and V. Ventafridda. New York, Raven Press, 1979, pp. 131–144.

Back pain produced by large retroperitoneal adenopathies is promptly and well controlled by anticancer drugs in all types of malignant lymphomas but less well in testicular cancer. A similar prompt relief of symptoms and pain related to either superior vena cava obstruction or spinal cord compression in malignant lymphoma is achieved with combination chemotherapy. The tumors of the thoracic inlet, called superior sulcus or Pancoast tumor, involve the nerves of the brachial plexus and the sympathetic chain and are characterized by severe shoulder and arm pain. Although combination chemotherapy can produce a fairly prompt objective remission in about 50% of patients, the degree of tumor regression is usually not sufficient to achieve satisfactory pain control. Therefore it is always advisable to combine chemotherapy with radiation therapy. This strategy should also be applied to intracranial tumors (either primary or metastatic) when not resectable. In fact, available drugs do not induce a satisfactory remission rate which could relieve a severe and persistent headache.

Recurrence of various types of tumors in the low abdomen, pelvis, and the pharyngeal and cervical regions often produces pain that is difficult to control by means of anticancer drugs. In these clinical situations in which severe and protracted pain is caused by infiltration of nervous structures, conventional analgesics, nerve blocks, and/or neurosurgical procedures must be considered the treatments of choice, rather than waiting for the response of a second- or third-line chemotherapy.

Termination of Chemotherapy

An important step in the medical treatment of patients with advanced cancer is deciding when to stop anticancer chemotherapy. Many factors can influence this decision. The rationale in favor of continuing anticancer therapy is not only the possible achievement of an objective response, but also the fact that the patient feels the difference between anticancer therapy and terminal care. On the other hand, the tendency toward an aggressive approach should be tempered by consideration of both the toxic manifestation of chemotherapy and other factors. These include tumor resistance to chemotherapy, short life expectancy, important organ failure, and lack of patient and family cooperation. The risk/benefit ratio should receive careful consideration, and further anticancer treatment must be dismissed when the possibility of inducing an objective response becomes negligible.

Side Effects and Complications

Side effects and complications of each of the various drugs are indicated in Table 89-2. As stated in Chapter 24, chemotherapeutic agents can also produce a toxic peripheral neuropathy manifested as painful paresthesia, hyporeflexia, and less frequently sensory or motor loss or autonomic dysfunction (37). The drugs most commonly associated with this complication are the vinca alkaloids, especially vincristine, as well as cisplatin, procarbazine, and less frequently misoniadazole and hexamethylmelamine (38). Acute herpes zoster and postherpetic neuralgia occur with increased frequently in patients with cancer and especially in those receiving chemotherapy or

TABLE 89-4. Hormonal Agents Used for Cancer Therapy

Drugs	Dose, Route, and Other Administration	Adverse Side Effects	Indications
Androgens			
Testosterone propionate*	50–100 mg 3 × weekly IM	Fluid retention, masculinization	Breast cancer, pre- and post-menopausal women with ER (+) tumors; stimulation of erythropoiesis
Fluoxymesterone*	10–20 mg/day PO	Fluid retention, occasional hypercalcemia	Breast cancer, pre- and post-menopausal women with ER(+) tumors; stimulation of erythropoiesis
Estrogens			
Diethylstilbestrol (DES)	1–15 mg/day† PO	Nausea, vomiting, urinary incontinence, feminization, increased mortality from heart disease in males, hypercalcemia	Prostate cancer, breast cancer‡
Ethinyl estradiol	0.1–3 mg/day† PO	Uterine bleeding	Breast cancer; postmenopausal women with ER(+) tumors
Antiestrogens			
Tamoxifen	10–40 mg/day PO	Mild nausea, mild fluid retention, hot flashes	ER(+) breast cancer
Progestins			
6-Methylhydroxyprogesterone (MAP)	100–200 mg/day PO or 200–600 mg 2 × weekly IM	Mild fluid retention, occasional hypercalemia, thrombocytosis	Endometrial carcinoma, renal-cell carcinoma, ovarian carcinoma
Hydroxyprogesterone	1 mg 2 × weekly IM		
Thyroid Hormones			
Thyroxin	To tolerance PO	Hyperthyroidism, arrhythmias, angina	Papillary adenocarcinoma of thyroids§
Adrenal Cortical Compounds			
Prednisone	40 mg/m²/day PO	Hyperglycemia, euphoria, fluid retention, immunosuppression, osteoporosis, hypertension, hypokalemic alkalosis	Lymphomas; leukemias; and multiple myeloma in combination with other drugs; CNS metastases and spinal cord compression to reduce swelling (high-dose dexamethasone)
Dexamethasone	0.5–16 mg/day PO		
Methylprednisone sodium succinate	10–125 mg/day IM or IV		
Hydroxycortisone sodium succinate	100–500 mg/day IV		

*Six to 12 weeks required for full effect
†For prostate cancer, dosage should not exceed 1 mg of DES or 0.1 mg ethinyl estradiol/day.
‡Of those with prostate cancer treated with DES, 70%, respond with prolongation of life.
§Positive response rate 70%; many remain disease-free more than 10 years.
Modified from DeVita, V.T.: Principles of cancer therapy. In Harrison's Principles of Internal Medicine, 10th Ed. Edited by R.G. Petersdorf et al. New York, McGraw-Hill, 1983, p. 772.

immunosuppressive drugs. Chronic steroid therapy sometimes causes necrosis of the femoral and humeral heads (39), whereas withdrawal of these drugs can cause steroid pseudorheumatism (40). The management of these is discussed in Chapter 24 and other parts of the book.

Endocrine Therapy

In the 1890s, Beatson (41) was the first to demonstrate hormonal control of breast cancer when he induced regression of metastatic tumor by ovariectomy. In 1941, Huggins and Hodges (42) reported the successful use of exogenous estrogen administration for prostatic carcinoma. Since then, several other tumors have been shown to respond to hormonal manipulation, which is achieved either by oblating endocrine glands or by administration of an exogenous hormone or hormone antagonist.

Mechanism of Action

The mechanism of action of these agents has become clarified with the demonstration that receptors that bind with estrogen exist in the cytosol of normal and malignant cells (5). Hormones bind to receptors in the cytoplasm and sterically alter the shape of the receptive protein itself, which, after transport to the cell nucleus, interacts with DNA, and this results in altered messenger RNA production and protein synthesis (5). Following this interaction, cytoplasmic receptor concentration is restored and the cycle can be repeated. Estrogen receptors (ER) can be quantitated as 8-S and 4-S proteins (5). Primary tumors in humans have ER values that range from zero to almost 1,000 fmol/mg cytosol protein. Receptors also exist for progesterones and androgens, and receptors for corticosteriods have been identified in the cytosol of leukemic cells (5).

Hormonal ablation can be achieved by surgical means, as occurs with oophorectomy, adrenalectomy, and hypophysiectomy, or by irradiation of the ovaries or ablating the pituitary gland with the various radioactive compounds, or by injecting alcohol, as discussed in Chapter 96. Medical adrenalectomy can be achieved by administering aminoglutethamide, a potent inhibitor of the conversion of cholesterol to

TABLE 89-5. Results with Hormonal Therapy in Advanced Cancer

Agent or Technique, by Type of Tumor	No. of Reports	Tumor Remission (% of Tumors)		Pain Relief (% of Patients)
		Objective	Subjective	
Breast				
Androgens	7	14	37	44
Antiestrogens	2	24	43	33
Progestines (other than MAP)	3	32	50	44
MAP-LD*	4	28	51	21
MAP-HD†	4	45	ND†	83
Corticosteroids	2	4	16	12
L-DOPA	1	33	33	33
Hypophysectomy				
Surgical	4	30	42	82
Chemical (alcohol injection)	2	30	ND	90
Adrenalectomy	2	36	41	44
Prostate				
Estrogens (DES-P)§	3	42	76	81
Cyproterone Acetate (CP)	2	80	ND	80
MAP-LD	1	ND	ND	75
MAP-HD	2	ND	100	100
Surgical hypophysectomy	3	ND	35	71
Adrenalectomy	3	20	ND	71
Orchidectomy	1	ND	71	ND
Clear-Cell Renal Cancer				
Progestins (other than MAP)	2	8	53	ND
Androgens	1	ND	100	ND
MAP-LD	2	8	53	75
MAP-HD	2	ND	100	86
Corticosteroids	1	ND	100	ND
Endometrial				
MAP-LD	2	35	75	ND
17 Hydroxyprogesterone	2	33	70	ND

*MAP = medroxyprogesterone acetate; LD = low dose (<500 mg/day)
†HD = high dose (1000–1500 mg/day)
‡ND = no data available
§DES-P = diethylstilvesterol diphasphate

Modified from Pannuti, F., et al.: The role of endocrine therapy for relief of pain due to advanced cancer. *In* Advances in Pain Research and Therapy. Vol. 2. Edited by J.J. Bonica and V. Ventafridda. New York, Raven Press, 1979, pp. 145–166, and from Pannuti, F.: Hormonal treatment. *In* The Continuing Care of Terminal Cancer Patients. Edited by R.F. Twycross and V. Ventafridda. New York, Pergamon Press, 1980, pp. 79–89.

pregnanelone in the adrenal gland (5). Hormone additive therapy is achieved by the administration of estrogens, progestins, androgens, antiestrogens, corticosteroids, and thyroid hormones. Table 89-4 lists the hormonal agents used in the treatment of various cancers, their dosage ranges, and side effects. The dosages used generally produce plasma levels that are substantially higher than physiologic levels. Such hormone changes can cause complex endocrine effects, such as pituitary inhibition of luteinizing hormone (LH), follicle-stimulating hormone (FSH), and prolactin, as well as changes in endogenous steroid hormone production (5).

Endocrine Therapy for Relief of Cancer Pain

Pannuti and associates (43, 44) were among the first to point out that most reports containing results of anticancer treatment in patients with advanced malignant neoplasm are usually concerned only with measuring volume-reduction of the tumor masses. Most writers have neglected, and often deliberately excluded the assessment of subjective response, including that related to pain, because this factor was not thought to be a reliable measure of the efficacy of treatment. Pannuti and colleagues further pointed out that there was no universally accepted rating system or qualification of pain relief on the part of oncologists, and this obviously led to heterogeneous results that could not be compared.

At the First International Symposium on Cancer Pain (43) and at another symposium held subsequently (44), Pannuti and colleagues presented a comprehensive summary of the results reported by a number of oncologists. Table 89-5 contains mean data presented by Pannuti et al. (43, 44) that provide an overview of the response of patients with four types of cancers to hormonal therapy. These reports were one of the first in which the efficacy of hormonal therapy on pain relief was correlated with the efficacy of these agents on tumor remission. Unfortunately, a significant number of reports had no data on the degrees of pain relief.

As can be noted in Table 89-5 Pannuti et al. (43) gave progentin therapy in the form of high doses of injectable medroxyprogesterone acetate (MAP-HD) and noted pain relief in 83% of breast cancer patients with predominantly bone metastasis, although only 45% had objective evidence of tumor remission. In view of the corticosteroid-like side effects from these large doses of MAP, it is possible that much of the subjective response was due to nonspecific steroid action. It was also noted that hypophysectomy provides a high degree of pain relief.

In regard to advanced cancer of the prostate, MAP-HD and hypophysectomy produced the highest degree of pain relief. For hypophysectomy, pain relief was twice as good as subjective tumor remission. In regard to renal carcinoma, androgens and progestins (particularly in the form of MAP-HD) provide pain relief and a subjective tumor remission in about 40% of the patients.

Although ovarian carcinoma contains steroid receptors, very little objective response to hormone has been demonstrated (43). Subjective response to the tumor occurred in some patients with progestin therapy, but no information is available concerning pain relief.

Well-differentiated papillary thyroid carcinoma, found particularly in women below the age of 40, is likely to be dependent on TSH, and pituitary TSH secretion can be suppressed by thyroxine administration. Over 50% of the subgroup of viral cancer will respond objectively, but no data are available concerning pain relief.

Side Effects

Endocrine therapy is generally much better tolerated than chemotherapy. None of these agents produces marrow suppression. Corticosteroids and high doses of MPA, given for long periods of time, are associated with classical cushingoid side effects, and parental MPA can cause gluteal abscess (43).

Sex hormones, particularly estrogens, can cause intermittent uterine bleeding, which can be upsetting, especially for postmenopausal women. Androgens cause virilization and increased libido in some women. Estrogen given to males causes alopecia, testicular atrophy, gynecomastia, loss of libido, and impotence. Their long-continued administration is also associated with high mortality from cardiac and cerebrovascular disease. Adrenalectomy causes side effects similar to those of estrogens with the exception of the excess cardiovascular complications. Surgical adrenalectomy and hypophysectomy are both major operative procedures and carry a small but significant mortality risk. As discussed in Chapter 94, however, neuroadenolysis of the pituitary with alcohol produces high incidences of pain relief with much less morbidity and virtually no mortality, although hormone replacement is required.

C. SURGICAL THERAPY

Surgery is the oldest method of treating patients with cancer; it dates back to ancient Egypt. Its use was sporadic, however, until the advent of surgical anesthesia and antisepsis. Currently, surgery can be used for prevention, diagnosis, and cure of cancer, as part of a multimodal therapy, and as a palliative measure in patients with advanced cancer. Regardless of the objective, it is essential that sound surgical principles be scrupulously followed because the consequence of the disease itself may have compromised the patient's ability to cope with the added impact of surgical trauma (45–49). Detailed discussion of surgical therapy is beyond the scope of this book and can be found elsewhere (45–49).

Preventive, Diagnostic, and Curative Surgery

Prevention

A variety of underlying conditions or congenital or genetic traits are associated with an extremely high incidence of subsequent cancer. These include familial polyposis of the colon, familial colon cancer, ulcerative colitis, leukoplakia of buccal mucosa, carcinoma in situ of the cervix, familial breast or ovarian cancer, and cryptorchidism (45, 46). The important decision in these and other premalignant conditions is when to use prophylactic removal of the offending organ to prevent subsequent malignancy. Once diagnosis is confirmed, early removal of the tumor is generally desirable.

Diagnosis

The role of surgery in the diagnosis of cancer is well established because, with few exceptions, cancer diagnosis is based on histologic interpretation of tissue removed by operation. The variety of techniques that are used include aspiration biopsy, needle biopsy, incisional biopsy, and excisional biopsy. In general, excisional, rather than incisional biopsies of primary tumor are to be preferred whenever possible because removing the lesion in toto not only ensures an adequate amount of tissue for examination but allows microscopic visualization of the interface between the tumor and the host and minimizes the risk of dissemination of tumor cells (45, 46).

Curative Operations

A significant number of common cancers, especially solid tumors confined to the anatomic site of origin, can be cured by surgical removal of the lesion. Unfortunately, when patients with these tumors present to the physician for the first time, about 70% already have micrometastasis beyond the primary site. The extension of the surgical resection to include areas of regional lymph vessels and their accompanying nodes can cure some of these patients (46). All of the tissue should be removed en bloc to prevent mechanical seeding of tumor cells by keeping manipulation of the cancer to a minimum during the course of dissection and exerting care that instruments do not come into direct contact with viable cancer cells. Examples of curative surgery include the wide excision of primary melanoma in the skin, which can be cured locally by surgery alone in about 90% of cases, and resection of colon cancer with a 5-cm margin from the tumor cells, which results in a recurrence rate of less than 5% (46). In many other cancers, however, it is essential to integrate surgery with radiation therapy or chemotherapy or a combination of these.

Palliative Surgery

Treatment of advanced cancer almost always involves the use of chemotherapy or radiation therapy or a combination of these, together with surgery. In recent years, palliative surgery has been used more and more to relieve pain or functional abnormalities caused by the cancer and thus improve the quality of life of these patients. The following summary is derived from Gennari (1) and other sources (45–49).

Urgent Palliative Surgery

Urgent palliative surgery means the surgical practice necessitated by emergency conditions, such as intestinal perforation or serious bleeding (1). Tumors of the gastrointestinal tract frequently cause heavy bleeding owing to the neoplastic erosion of a blood vessel. In these cases it is almost impossible to employ a raphe because of weak tissue, and it is thus essential to do a resection that might not always be carried out according to oncologic criteria of radicality. In this situation the surgeon is more concerned with resolving the emergency than removing all of the clearly metastatic lymph nodes. In the same way, a colostomy is required for a closed stenosis at the rectal-sigmoid junction, or, if the neoplasm is not resectable, Hartman's or Mukuliecz's operations are necessary when peritoneal or hepatic metastases are present (1).

Experience has demonstrated that, regardless of association with chemotherapy and/or radiotherapy, the survival of these patients is improved, both in duration and in quality of life, because pain, caused by local inflammatory events, is decreased by the absence of fecal passage.

Reductive Palliative Surgery

Reductive palliative surgery is so defined because, at the end of the surgical treatment, a notable reduction in the tumor mass is obtained. The result of such a treatment is that the radiologist and/or chemotherapist has the opportunity to devise a therapeutic scheme that, even though it has no curative purpose, allows, in many cases, a recovery of the patient's general conditions, a restoration of some compromised functional capacities, and thus not only an extended survival but, more important, an improvement of the quality of life. Experience at the National Cancer Institute in Milan has shown that, whereas palliative surgery or radiotherapy alone resulted in a 30% 1-year survival and 0% at 3 years, association of the two types of treatment gave 100% survival at 1 year and 20% at 5 years (1). Such data corroborate the fact that palliative surgery as the only therapeutic treatment is extremely limited, but that it has a wider application when used as part of the multidisciplinary approach.

Surgery of Metastases

Some tumors have a rather restricted activity that is expressed by a late, sometimes single metastasis and by a relatively slow local progression. In these cases, which are represented by bone metastases from thyroid or renal carcinomas, a surgical treatment, aggressive and conservative at the same time, is well justified. At the National Cancer Institute in Milan this approach has produced fairly good results (1).

Ablative Surgery

Ablative surgery, which has been referred to as indirect palliative surgery, entails the removal of organs whose functional activities have an effect on the development of the neoplastic disease. This includes ovariectomy, adrenalectomy or hypophysectomy for metastatic breast cancer with positive estrogen and progesterone receptors, and castration for metastatic prostatic cancer. Of all the forms of palliative surgery, this type has given the best results in terms of response, both subjective (decrease of pain and recovery of muscle function) and objective (regression of pathologic parameters). Ablative surgery for ovarian cancer is particularly indicated for younger or pre-menopausal patients.

Orthopedic Surgery

Orthopedic surgery is important in the management of patients with severe cancer pain caused by primary or metastatic bone tumors. Prosthetic replacement of the hip, knee, or shoulder joint should be considered if radical tumor resection is possible. In such cases, salvage of the limb and prompt relief of pain significantly improve the patient's quality of life. The subject is discussed in Chapter 87.

REFERENCES

1. Gennari, L.: Palliative surgery. *In* Advances in Pain Research and Therapy. Vol. 2. Edited by J.J. Bonica and V. Ventafridda. New York, Raven Press, 1979.
2. Bonica, J.J.: Treatment of cancer pain: Current status and future needs. *In* Advances in Pain Research and Therapy. Vol. 9. Edited by H.L. Fields, R. Dubner, and F. Cervero. New York, Raven Press, 1985, pp. 589–628.
3. Tong, D., Gillick, L., and Hendrickson, F.R.: The palliation of symptomatic osseous metastases: Final results of the study by the Radiation Therapy Oncology Group. Cancer, *50*:893, 1982.
4. Ahja, R.K., Milligan, A., and Dobelbower, R.R.: Radiation therapy in cancer management: Principles and complications. *In* Comprehensive Textbook of Oncology. Edited by A.R. Moossa, M.C. Robson, and S.C. Schimpff. Baltimore, Williams & Wilkins, 1986, pp. 257–288.
5. DeVita, V.T.: Principles of cancer therapy. *In* Harrison's Principles of Internal Medicine. 10th Ed. Edited by R.G. Petersdorf et al. New York, McGraw-Hill, 1983, pp. 765–787.
6. Ferreira, S.H.: Prostaglandins, aspirin-like drugs and analgesia. Nature New Biology, *240*:200, 1972.
7. Hendrickson, F.R., Shehata, W.M., and Kirchner, A.B.: Radiation therapy for osseous metastases. Int. J. Rad. Oncol. Biol. Phys., *1*:275, 1976.
8. Penn, C.R.H.: Single dose and fractionated palliative irradiation for osseous metastases. Clin. Radiol., *27*:405, 1976.
9. Gilbert, H.A., et al.: Evaluation of radiation therapy for bone metastases: Pain relief and quality of life. Am. J. Roentgenol., *129*:1095, 1977.
10. Katz, H.R.: The results of different fractionation schemes in the palliative irradiation of metastatic melanoma. Int. J. Rad. Oncol. Biol. Phys., 7:907, 1981.
11. Madsen, E.L.: Painful bone metastasis: Efficacy of radiotherapy assessed by the patients: A randomised trial comparing 4 Gy × 6 versus 10 Gy × 2. Int. J. Rad. Oncol. Biol. Phys., *9*:1775, 1983.
12. Allen, K.L., Johnson, T.W., and Hibbs, G.G.: Effective bone palliation as related to various treatment regimens. Cancer, *37*:984, 1976.
13. Garmatis, C.J., and Chu, F.C.H.: The effectiveness of radiation therapy in the treatment of bone metastases from breast cancer. Radiology, *126*:235, 1978.
14. Green, N., Beron, E., Melbye, R.W., and George, F.W.: Carcinoma of pancreas—palliative radiotherapy. Am. J. Roentgenol., *117*:620, 1973.
15. Fidler, M.: Internal fixation of secondary neoplastic deposits in long bones. Br. Med. J., *1*:341, 1973.
16. Palmer, J.J.: Radiation myelopathy. Brain, *95*:109, 1972.
17. Jellinger, K., and Sturm, K.W.: Delayed radiation myelopathy in man. J. Neurol. Sci., *14*:389, 1971.
18. Kori, F., Foley, K.M., and Posner, J.D.: Brachial plexus lesions in patients with cancer: Clinical findings in 100 cases. Neurology, *31*:45, 1981.
19. Thomas, J.E., Cascino, T.E., and Earle, J.D.: Differential diagnosis between radiation and tumor plexopathy of the pelvis. Neurology, *35*:1, 1985.
20. Foley, K.M., et al.: Radiation-induced malignant and atypical peripheral nerve sheath tumors. Ann. Neurol., *7*:311, 1980.
21. Salazar, O.M., Rubin, P., Keller, B., and Scarantino, C.: Systemic (half body) radiation therapy: Response and toxicity. Int. J. Rad. Oncol. Biol. Phys., *4*:937, 1978.
22. Qasim, M.M.: Half-body irradiation (HBI) in metastatic carcinomas. Clin. Radiol., *32*:215, 1981.
23. Fryer, C.J.H., Fitzpatrick, P.J., Rider, W.D., and Poon, P.: Radiation pneumonitis: Experience following a large single dose of radiation. Int. J. Rad. Oncol. Biol. Phys., *4*:931, 1978.
24. Rowland, C.G., Bullimore, J.A., Smith, P.J.B., and Roberts, J.B.M.: Half-body irradiation in the treatment of metastatic prostatic carcinoma. Br. J. Urol., *53*:628, 1981.
25. Rowland, C.G., Garrett, M.J., and Crowley, F.A.: Half-body radiation in plasma cell myeloma. Clin. Radio., *34*:507, 1983.
26. Rostom, A.Y., O'Cathail, S.M., and Folkes, A.: Systemic irradiation in multiple myeloma. Brt. J. Haematol., *58*:423, 1984.
27. Tobias, J.S., et al.: Hemibody irradiation in multiple myeloma. Rad. Oncol., *3*:11, 1985.
28. Smith, P.G., and Doll. R.: Mortality among patients with ankylosing spondylitis after a single treatment course with x-rays. Br. Med. J., *284*:449, 1982.
29. Calin, A.: X-radiation in the management of rheumatoid disease. Br. J. Hosp. Med., *33*:261, 1985.
30. DeVita, V.T.: Principles of chemotherapy. *In* Cancer: Principles and Practices of Oncology. 2nd Ed. Edited by V.T. DeVita, S. Helman, and S.A. Rosenburg. Philadelphia, Lippincott, 1985, pp. 257–285.
31. Chabner, B.A., and Myers, C.E.: Clinical pharmacology of cancer chemotherapy. *In* Cancer: Principle and Practice of Oncology. 2nd Ed. Edited by V.T. DeVita, S. Helman, and S.A. Rosenburg. Philadelphia, Lippincott, 1985, pp. 287–328.
32. Bonadonna, G., and Molinari, R.: Role and limits of anti-cancer drugs in the treatment of advanced cancer pain. *In* Advances in Pain Research and Therapy. Vol. 2. Edited by J.J. Bonica and V. Ventafridda. New York, Raven Press, 1979.
33. Brule, G.: Role and limits of oncologic chemotherapy of advanced cancer pain. *In* Advances in Pain Research and Therapy. Vol. 2. Edited by J.J. Bonica and V. Ventafridda. New York, Raven Press, 1979.
34. Riggs, C.E.: Clinical oncology of individual antineoplastic agents. *In* Comprehensive Textbook of Oncology. Edited by A.R. Moossa, M.C. Robson, and F.C. Schimpff. Baltimore, Williams & Wilkins, 1986, pp. 210–234.
35. Riggs, C.E.: Combination chemotherapy. *In* Comprehensive Textbook of Oncology. Edited by A.R. Moossa, M.C. Robson, and F.C. Schimpff. Baltimore, Williams & Wilkins, 1986, pp. 235–243.
36. DeVita, V.T., and Schein, P.S.: The use of drugs in combination for the treatment of cancer: Rationale and results. N. Engl. J. Med., *288*:998, 1973.
37. Perry, M.C.: Chemotherapy, toxicity, and the clinician. Semin. Oncol., *9*:1, 1982.
38. Young, D.F., and Posner, J.D.: Nervous system toxicity of chemotherapeutic agents. *In* Handbook of Clinical Neurology. Edited by T.J. Vinken and G.W. Bruyn. Amsterdam, North Holland, 1980, pp. 91–129.
39. Solomon, L.: Drug-induced arthropathy and necrosis of the femoral head. J. Bone Joint Surg., *55*:246, 1973.
40. Rotstein, J., and Good, R.A.: Steroid pseudorheumatism. Arch. Intern. Med., *99*:545, 1957.
41. Beatson, G.T.: On the treatment of inoperable cases of carcinoma of the mammae: Suggestions for a new method of treatment with illustrative cases. Lancet, *2*:104, 1896.
42. Huggins, C., and Hodges, V.C.: Studies on prostatic cancer. Cancer Res., *1*:293, 1941.
43. Pannuti, F., et al.: The role of endocrine therapy for relief of pain due to advanced cancer. *In* Advances in Pain Research and Therapy. Vol. 2. Edited by J.J. Bonica and V. Ventafridda. New York, Raven Press, 1979, pp. 145–166.
44. Pannuti, F.: Hormonal treatment. *In* The Continuing Care of Terminal Cancer Patients. Edited by R.F. Twycross and V. Ventafridda. New York, Pergamon Press, 1980, pp. 79–89.
45. Cole, J.W.: Principles and complication of surgical therapy. *In* Comprehensive Textbook of Oncology. Edited by A.R. Moossa, M.C. Robson, and S.C. Schimpff. Baltimore, Williams & Wilkins, 1986, pp. 269–271.
46. Rosenberg, S.A.: Principles of surgical oncology. *In* Cancer: Principles and Practice of Oncology. 2nd edition. Edited by V.T. DeVita, Jr., S. Hellman, and S.A. Rosenberg. Philadelphia, Lippincott, 1985, pp. 215–225.
47. Pilch. Y.H.: Surgical Oncology. New York, McGraw-Hill, 1984.

90 · ACUPUNCTURE

C. RICHARD CHAPMAN *and* C. CHAN GUNN

ACUPUNCTURE is a therapeutic procedure in which small, solid needles are inserted into the skin at varying depths, typically penetrating the underlying musculature. This method, derived from practices in ancient Oriental medicine, was essentially unknown to most physicians in the United States when the first edition of this book was written. Bonica (1) mentioned acupuncture as a form of local therapy and cited its use by Osler for treating various painful conditions during the latter part of the nineteenth century. Because of the publicity given to Chinese demonstrations of acupuncture pain control for surgery in the 1970s, acupuncture has since become familiar both to the medical community and to the lay public. Its practice remains controversial, and in some states nonphysician acupuncturists have won the right to practice their trade either independently or under the auspices of a licensed physician.

Acupuncture is of interest to physicians concerned with pain management in day-to-day practice for two reasons: (a) it offers a comparatively safe alternative to the prescription of medication for pain problems; and (b) patients often ask their primary care physicians for advice on whether they should engage the services of an acupuncturist or for referral to an acupuncturist. It is therefore worthwhile to have a working knowledge of acupuncture techniques, the potential of this approach for pain management, the issues surrounding its putative mechanisms, and its limitations.

This chapter is intended to provide an overview of the current clinical and scientific knowledge base on acupuncture for pain therapy. It consists of two parts, a critical review of current knowledge in the field and a description of a Western approach to acupuncture

therapy for musculoskeletal pain. We discuss the use of acupuncture for the control of acute and chronic pain rather than its possible use for the prevention of pain during surgery. Acupuncture pain control in the surgical setting, although now recognized as a valid phenomenon, is of no practical importance in Western medical practice and its adoption in the West is no longer at issue. Bonica (2) has written a definitive report on the use of acupuncture for surgery. Surgical use is of interest only to the extent that it sheds light on the mechanism(s) of acupuncture therapy for pain prevention or relief.

In addressing acupunctural pain therapy, which is practiced widely in the United States, this chapter draws heavily on the research produced in this area since 1980, but, where appropriate, earlier studies are also considered. Ancient Chinese medicine is noted only briefly, because this information is of little relevance and is available in copious detail elsewhere (3–8). The purpose of this chapter is to provide interested physicians with a working knowledge of the field so that they can judge the potential of acupuncture techniques for specific pain management problems.

The material is presented in two major sections: A, Basic Considerations, including the three basic types of acupunctural therapy for pain and the indications for these therapies, a brief description of how acupuncture is performed, a broad review and evaluation of the scientific base for the use of acupuncture for managing pain, and a summary of the current state of knowledge in this field; and B, Acupuncture for Trigger Point Therapy, including clinical uses and a brief guideline for its application to chronic musculoskeletal problems. Chapman wrote Section A, and Gunn wrote Section B.

A. BASIC CONSIDERATIONS

Types of Acupunctural Therapy

Review of the current medical literature reveals that the term "acupuncture" can refer to at least three different interventions: classic acupuncture based on Chinese medicine, acupuncture as a form of trigger point therapy, and acupuncture as a procedure for electric stimulation. These are distinctly different therapies and each must be considered separately.

Classic Acupuncture

The first and best known form of acupuncture is the practice of traditional methods according to the principles of ancient Chinese medicine (8, 9). Taoist doctrine saw human health as existing within the tensions created by opposing forces in nature, the *yin* (dark, female) and the *yang* (light, male). Medical intervention carried out within this tradition was undertaken

to balance opposing energy forces considered to be out of harmony. A concept of energy flow that combined circulation and neurologic function was fundamental to the practice of classic acupuncture. Vital life energy was thought to flow through a set of interconnected channels, called meridians, that followed a circadian rhythm.

One of the internal organs was thought to be associated with each meridian, and the meridians are named according to organs. For example, the meridian for the gallbladder runs from the external canthus of the eye, back and forth along the skull, and down to the shoulders, from which it descends along the side of the body and ends at the fourth toe. It is a yang meridian—its function is balanced against that of its yin counterpart, the liver meridian. The latter runs from the great toe to the groin and into the chest, where it is said to disappear from the map of meridians because it courses deep into the body and has no surface representation. Diseases and discomforts such as pain were classified according to the meridians they involved and according to whether they had a yin (cold, hypofunctional) or yang (hot, hyperfunctional) nature.

The meridians were said to be interconnected with the vital life energy, *chi*, flowing through them. Excesses or deficiencies in the flow of energy were said to cause pain, discomfort, hypo- or hyperfunction and, with time, trophic changes. By inserting the needles strategically along individual meridians or at their junctures, the acupuncturist attempted to balance the flow of energy throughout the body.

Numerous variations on classic acupuncture exist. Among them is a system of ear acupuncture based on the belief that the pinna contains a map of acupuncture points representing the entire human body. Research on this type of diagnosis and therapy is limited, but controlled trials have failed to yield supporting evidence (10). The many embellishments of classic acupuncture are outside the scope of this chapter.

Today in the Orient many practitioners still employ classic Oriental medicine principles in the treatment of pain and disease states, which are also popular in many parts of Europe. When Western physicians practice traditional acupuncture it is often based on a "cookbook" approach in which a routine set of meridian points is used to treat each type of pain problem (3, 4). This is neither bona fide Western nor Oriental medicine because classic practice in its pure form emphasizes the unique individual diagnosis of each patient.

Although these and other concepts of ancient medicine were exceptionally enlightened for their time (e.g., they conceived of circulation and certain basic principles of neurology), they are now history. It is hardly surprising that much of the ancient folk medicine cannot be validated by modern science. For example, one organ postulated by the ancient Chinese to affect energy flow, the triple heater, is nonexistent. Similarly, meridians exist neither as anatomic structures nor as patterns of neurologic response. Whereas contemporary studies have shown that acupuncture points are often characterized by low skin resistance and tenderness to palpation, these are also the characteristics of trigger points (Chapter 21). Correspondence between meridian pathways and patterns of referred pain or sensation produced by finger pressure at tender points overlying muscle is not surprising or unknown to Western medicine (11–13). Such correspondences help to confirm that ancient Oriental therapists identified and treated conditions that are still observed and often undertreated today. They do not validate the notion that acupuncture has some special or mysterious origin that gives it an advantage over comtemporary, scientifically based practices.

Variations of traditional medicine exist in a revised form in contemporary medicine in the Far East. For example, Japanese Ryodoraku treatment maintains most of the basic tenets of classic acupuncture, but the mechanism underlying treatment is considered to be the autonomic nervous system (14, 15). Therapists attempt to balance sympathetic and parasympathetic functions of the autonomic nervous system and rely heavily on readings of electric skin resistance at traditional meridian points for diagnosis. Meridians are considered to be patterns of autonomic activation. This and other hybrid therapies offer bridges between classic Oriental and modern science. Unfortunately, such possibilities remain in the realm of conjecture for want of scientific data to support basic hypotheses.

It is difficult to justify the perpetuation of ancient folk medicine concepts, at least in their pure form, in contemporary medical practice, but the romance of the ancient knowledge has gained a strong following among lay practitioners of folk medicine and among some physicians. It is strongly rooted in the culture of several major nations, and in some industrialized countries, including Japan, Chinese medicine is taught in degree-granting institutions. Approximately one-sixth of the world's population relies occasionally on Chinese medicine.

Trigger Point Therapy

The second application of acupuncture is essentially neurologic. Degenerative changes in neural function related to stress, prior injury, and aging can upset the normal properties of skeletal muscle, as well as those of other tissues and organs, in subtle ways that might not be evident on conventional neurologic examination. Abnormal areas of skeletal musculature can be felt as tender, ropy strands or points that are associated with signs of excessive sympathetic activity (e.g., coldness, mild edema), pain on palpation, and general fatigue. Such points have been identified by Bonica (1, 11), Travell and Simons (12), Sola (13), and others as "tender points" or "trigger points" that can be effectively treated by stimulation to achieve relief of persistent pain. Chapters 21, 45, 52, 58, and 77 describe trigger points, their associated myofascial pain syndromes, and treatment of these syndromes.

When acupuncture needles are used to treat the tender points in muscle associated with chronic pain, acupuncture is nearly indistinguishable from trigger point therapy. The close relationship of trigger points as defined by Western medicine and acupuncture points as identified by ancient texts of Oriental medicine has been addressed by Melzack (16) and by Gunn and colleagues (17). Although many trigger point therapists choose to inject local anesthetic or normal saline solution into tender areas, some use stimulation with an acupuncture needle at the same site. Many, like Sola, believe that trigger points are associated with sympathetic hyperactivity and that local chemical blockade of the trigger point eliminates the basic pathophysiology.

The possible mechanisms underlying trigger point therapy have been reviewed in depth by Travell and Simons (12) and by Sola (13, 18). We postulate that such treatment reverses the effects of chronic nerve damage, such as radiculopathy, on skeletal muscle (see below). Pain of this type is almost invariably accompanied by muscle contractures, and pain relief is predicated on the release of painful contractures.

Electric Stimulation Therapy

Electric stimulation for pain relief might be as old as acupuncture itself. Records from the ancient Greeks and Romans indicated that fish that could produce an electric discharge were used to treat patients with pain. During prolonged surgeries in the early 1970s Chinese acupuncturists found extended manual twirling with needles inefficient (and perhaps monotonous as well) and replaced this practice with electric stimulation. In parallel, Western practitioners, inspired by the gate control theory of Melzack and Wall (19), began to develop electric stimulation therapies for pain control. This has led to the widespread use of transcutaneous electrical nerve stimulation (TENS) and the development of an industry in the United States that manufactures TENS units. (TENS therapy for pain is reviewed in Chapter 92).

Little difference in the practice of pain control with TENS methods and with acupuncture has been noted, and research in one area contributes information to the other. The two approaches have in common three sets of parameters for electric therapy: (a) high-frequency, low-intensity stimulation (generally delivered at the area of painful focus); (b) low-frequency, high-intensity stimulation (typically delivered distal to the area of pain, perhaps at a classic acupuncture point); and (c) burst mode stimulation, in which brief bursts of high-frequency stimulation are given. These methods appear to have different effects in different situations. More detailed information on the parameters of choice for electric therapy and the differential application of the three sets of parameters for selective pain problems is presented in Chapter 92.

Acupuncturists differ from TENS therapists in the use of needles rather than broad electrodes and in a general tendency to use electric therapy for systemic rather than local effects, although prominent exceptions to this rule are found. Because needles penetrate the skin and underlying muscle, some therapists combine electric and trigger point therapy.

Procedure

Classic Methods

The insertion of acupuncture needles is not technically demanding, but a surprising variety of techniques exists. Many claims have been made—but with no actual evidence—that different procedures of needle insertion produce different therapeutic results, and acupuncturists do not agree among themselves about optimal needle technique. Many classic therapists think it important to slant the needle either in the direction of assumed energy flow in the treated meridian or against the energy flow, and some use gold and silver needles for special purposes. In some cases mugwort is pressed into a ball and attached to the top of the needle. The acupuncturist lights the herb after needle insertion, and the smoldering material gently heats the inserted needle. These concerns and other exotic refinements related to classic theory are of no practical importance for medical application.

Modern Methods

Figure 90-1 demonstrates a typical procedure used by classic therapists for needle insertion. Individual therapists vary considerably in the way they manipu-

late the needle during insertion. Some use a lifting-and-twisting-motion, others quickly insert it without rotation, and still others slowly penetrate the skin and underlying tissue. A few therapists penetrate only the skin and contend that no benefit is obtained by stimulating deeper tissues. Others argue that superficial and deep penetration are appropriate for different types of disorders. No "right" way exists, however, and patient comfort is perhaps the most important criterion. Even this would be argued by the few acupuncturists who believe that stimulation of deep muscle and periosteum is of therapeutic benefit.

Students of acupuncture in China typically learn by inserting needles in themselves. This type of practice helps to ensure a technique that is minimally distressing to patients. Some physicians prefer to use needle guide tubes or devices that mount the needle in a guide cylinder equipped with a piston that taps the needle into place at the touch of a finger. Such methods help to minimize the distress of treatment and to maintain sterility. Figure 90-2 illustrates a Japanese needle system. Such equipment lends itself well to Western trigger point therapy; we advocate the use of this type of instrument in the second part of this chapter.

Chinese therapists emphasize the importance of *te chi* at the site of insertion: the underlying muscle appears to grab the needle and hold it firmly. The patient reports a concomitant feeling of heaviness or pressure at the needle. Trigger point therapists such as Sola (13) and Gunn (see below and ref. 72) have noted that the insertion of needles in muscle tissue that is not associated with a trigger point does not produce this response. In most classic practice the therapist does not remove the needle until the *te chi* has dissipated and the needle can be lifted from the tissue without effort.

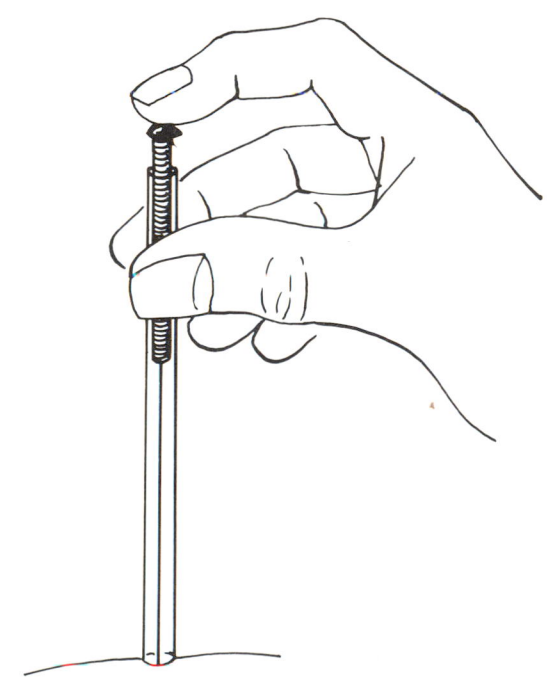

FIG. 90-1. Classic acupuncture needle insertion techniques: The tapping method.

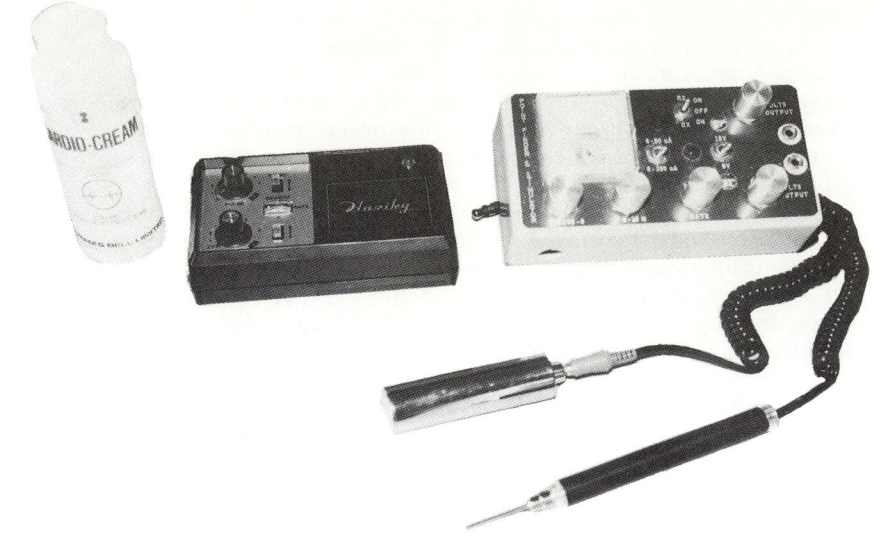

A

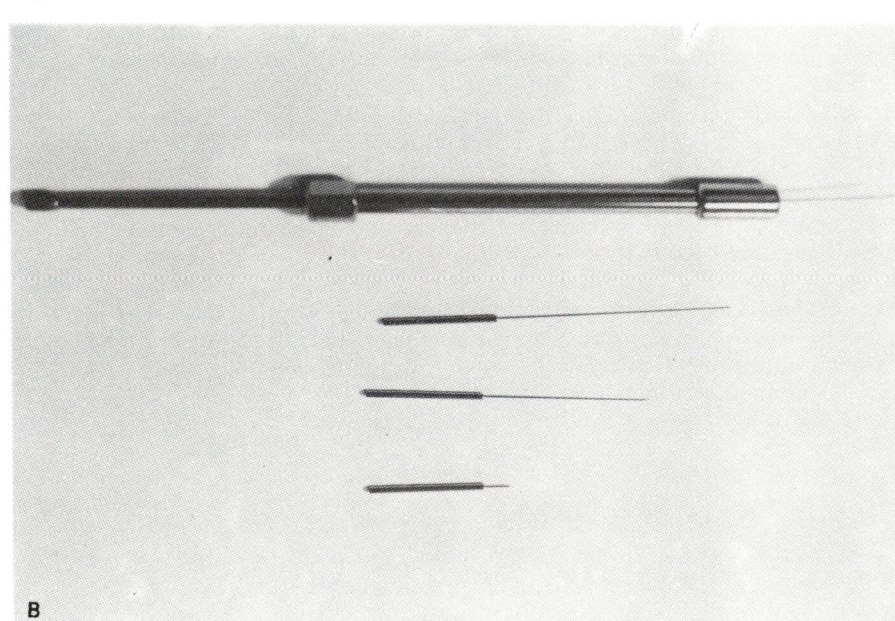

B

FIG. 90-2. A needle system developed in Japan for acupuncture that is uniquely suited for trigger point therapy. **A.** Equipment to search for acupuncture points. From left to right: plastic container containing conducting cream, a battery pack, and a resistance meter with one lead (heavy upper) held by the patient and the other lead ending as a pencil point probe to detect acupuncture points. **B.** Three disposable acupuncture needles and a needle holder/plunger to assist in needle placement.

The technique used by trigger point therapists for needle insertion has been borrowed from traditional acupuncture. Stainless steel acupuncture needles of three lengths (3, 5, and 6 cm) are commonly employed. The length of the needle is dictated by the location of the point to be treated; deeper and thicker muscles require longer needles. A fine gauge needle—30-gauge or less—with a pointed tip is believed to be less traumatic than the beveled cutting edge of a hollow needle. The fine, flexible needle transmits the nature and consistency of tissues penetrated.

The direction of needle insertion is generally perpendicular to the skin so as to penetrate the muscle zone of innervation. Tubular guides are used to facilitate skin penetration and to avoid touching the needle. We have used multiple needles for the several motor bands within a myotome belonging to both anterior and posterior primary rami that require treatment, but we now prefer the convenient use of only one needle in the plunger-type needle holder, which allows the same needle to be used at multiple loci (Fig. 90-2).

Side Effects and Complications
Potential Complications

As noted above, acupuncture is a potential source of infection if sterile precautions are not taken. If an old, worn needle is employed it can be broken during insertion and require surgical removal. In addition, improper needle insertion can cause pneumothorax. The literature reveals a few cases in which patients have harmed themselves by inserting needles improperly, but few complications of acupuncture when performed by a trained physician have been noted. The safety of the technique compares favorably with the use of prescription medications, trigger point injections, and TENS.

The practice of acupuncture by nonphysicians is a growing concern among physicians as the use of acupuncture spreads. Most nonphysician practitioners are skilled and safe, but the possibility that serious problems might remain undiagnosed in patients under the care of nonphysicians is disquieting. Acupuncture can alleviate or mask symptoms that are of medical importance. Therefore the physician who has a patient who is also being seen by an acupuncturist should be certain that the patient has a proper and thorough medical evaluation and should be alert to the fact that concomitant acupuncture treatment can affect or even suppress the symptoms with which the patient would normally present.

Precautions

It is essential to sterilize acupuncture needles with autoclave or gas because they could transmit hepatitis or other viral disease. The skin should be cleansed with alcohol at the site of treatment. The dangers of acupuncture therapy are minimal when sterile precautions are used. It is important to guard against pneumothorax when placing needles in the chest and shoulder areas, particularly when treating the parascapular and intercostal muscles. Treatment of the trapezius muscle requires particular caution because the patient might flinch with needle insertion, leading to inadvertent puncture of the apical pleura. When treating the lumbar muscles, care should be taken to avoid deep penetration that could injure the underlying kidney. Vasovagal syncope responses are sometimes seen, typically when needles are inserted in the region of the brachial plexus, and it is good practice to have the patient lie down or sit in a supported position. The guidelines offered by Sola and Bonica in Chapter 21 and by Travell and Simons (12) for trigger point therapy are equally suitable for acupuncture.

Scientific Basis: Problems in Scientific Development

Traditional acupuncture is without a scientific basis of any sort (16). Modern research on acupuncture is a formidable undertaking, and work to date has been problematic at both the basic science and the clinical levels because scientific inquiry has not followed a logical progression. Just when the scientific community took interest in acupuncture in the mid-1970s, the raphe-spinal structures were identified as the mechanism subserving opioid analgesia and the enkephalins and endorphins were discovered. Many investigators rushed to hypothesize that endogenous opioids must be the mechanism of acupuncture pain control, and acupuncture research became caught up in the enthusiasm of endorphin researchers for linking all sorts of hitherto unexplainable phenomena to endogenous opioids (20–23). This in turn led the scientific and clinical communities to engage for a time in backward reasoning: acupuncture must be effective because so much work is being done to elucidate its mechanism. Proponents of acupuncture therapy have pointed proudly to animal studies that show links between acupuncture and endorphins, enkephalins, or dynorphins. Whether acupuncture analgesia in humans can be related meaningfully to that in animals has not been considered. This unfortunate unsystematic progression has produced a knowledge base of limited value. To be fair, however, the problem of bias in research is not limited to the acupuncture field—it is well known in the philosophy of science. The tendency to be biased in interpreting scientific data that bear on clinical issues has been described (24), and "confirmation bias" of the sort demonstrated by some acupuncture researchers has been discussed by Greenwald and colleagues (25).

Unfortunately, despite more than a decade of study, the fundamental clinical research questions of whether acupuncture treatment can prevent or relieve acute and chronic pain are still inconclusively answered. Indeed, many of the most basic questions remain unasked. As the review below demonstrates, the literature is far from proving that acupuncture is effective in pain control. The American Medical Association reviewed this issue at its 1981 meeting and decided that insufficient evidence exists to conclude that acupuncture has any more effect on pain than a placebo or sham acupuncture (26). Sweet (27) was less kind, attacking acupuncture as essentially worthless. Clinical efficacy studies have, for the most part, been weak in design, measurement technology, and long-term follow-up. Consequently, it is still not known which acute and chronic pain problems, if any, can or cannot be helped by acupuncture.

Animal, human laboratory, and clinical research studies are reviewed broadly in the remainder of this section. The purpose of these overviews is to encapsulate the scientific knowledge base.

Animal Studies

A comprehensive review of the large literature on animals cannot be undertaken here, and its relevance for the clinician concerned with pain patients is moot. It is important, however, that the clinician not be misled by claims of acupuncture zealots based on data from animal researchers. Although valuable, animal studies shed little light on the value of acupuncture for patient care for the reasons to be described.

Many animal investigations of acupuncture analgesia have been done, mainly with small animals, but a few have used dogs or horses (28–30). Measurement of pain has mostly been restricted to reflex responses or to simple behavioral indicators, such as escape from a stimulus. Only a few studies have tried to define the nature of acupuncture analgesia in a controlled fashion; most have attempted to identify a mechanism. In general, investigators have inappropriately made strong and direct generalizations to humans from animal data without regard to species differences and to the limited relationship of animal laboratory algesimetry models to human chronic pain as seen in the clinical setting.

The results of animal studies are inconclusive as evidence for human study, in part because parallel findings have emerged in the animal literature concerned with acupuncture analgesia and with stress-induced analgesia (31, 32). These findings indicate species-specific responses to acupuncture. When animals are subjected to intensive stress, such as cold water immersion, fright, or painful stimulation, a major hypothalamic–pituitary axis response is produced that includes liberation of cortisols, ACTH, and beta-endorphin, among other substances. Consequently, stress as a physiologic response is characterized by reduced sensitivity to injury or other pain challenge. Such analgesia is typically reversed by the opioid antagonist naloxone (31). In small mammals, such as rabbits, response to a stressor can take extreme forms, which include total immobility.

Frightening a small animal can induce a state popularly called "animal hypnosis" (having nothing to do with human hypnosis), in which the animal is quickly rendered unconscious and insensible (33–35). The more severe the stress, the longer the immobility of the animal, and fear potentiates this immobility response. In nature such animals are often carried off by a predator and left near its den for a later meal. The putative hypnotic state gives them a chance to feign death, effect a recovery, and escape at a later time. This can be demonstrated in the laboratory by simply throwing a rabbit onto its back; one can then carry out an apparently painless laparotomy (34).

Under certain stressful and threatening circumstances, animals in a laboratory setting can go in and out of a putative hypnotic state (35). Because acupuncture is not understood by animal subjects to be benign, the process of handling and painful stimulation with needles can induce a stress response unique to certain species. Support for this possibility was provided by Galeano and associates (36), who performed acupuncture in rabbits while taking care not to induce stress. Under these conditions acupuncture analgesia could not be induced. Thus, animals might not be suitable models for human acupuncture analgesia.

Failure to acknowledge the parallels in animal hypnosis and acupuncture analgesia in animals has led to the emergence of a literature that is difficult to interpret. Nineteen of 22 abstracted articles on acupuncture analgesia mechanisms identified through computer search for the period 1979 to 1983 supported the hypothesis that acupuncture analgesia in animals is mediated by endorphins. In contrast, none of the human research studies addressing the endorphin hypothesis during this period provided positive outcomes.

Human Laboratory Studies

The effects of acupuncture (usually electric) on pain sensibility in normal human subjects has been studied in various laboratory settings. In general, human studies differ substantially from animal work for three reasons: (a) volunteers are not stressed during testing, and every effort is made to ensure their comfort and satisfaction with the experiment; (b) the subjects understand the purpose of the experiment and appreciate the safety precautions taken on their behalf; and (c) more complex measures of pain are employed. Pain threshold, pain tolerance, psychophysical stimulus-matching techniques, visual analog judgments, performance in a sensory decision theory stimulus-judgment task, and brain-evoked potentials have all been used to evaluate the efficacy of acupuncture as an analgesic intervention. Pain has been induced in the laboratory by stimulating teeth or skin electrically, heating skin, immersing limbs in ice water, and applying a tourniquet.

The literature on human studies is less extensive than that on animals but is of sufficient size and complexity to present a full review here. The areas in which the studies have yielded consensus merit comment, however, as does the experience of our laboratory in a long-term research program on acupuncture analgesia. Chapman and colleagues (37–42) stimulated the teeth of study subjects in repeated studies to create safe but noteworthy experimental pain and measured the effects of acupuncture on pain perception using both sensory decision theory techniques and brain-evoked potentials. Consistent observations by Chapman and others include the following findings.

First, outcomes were generally positive although some investigators could not demonstrate alteration of pain perception with acupunctural stimulation (43). Although most studies controlled appropriately for expectancy and placebo effects, it was found that belief in the efficacy of acupuncture can play a role in the subjects' ratings of acupuncture pain control in the laboratory (44). In our laboratory we could observe reliable positive outcomes in a series of four sensory decision theory studies and four evoked-potential studies carried out over a period of several years (37–39, 44). The effect was not seen in every subject, but was typically clear in about 75% of the volunteers in any given experiment.

Second, the effect obtained, although statistically significant, is typically small or even minor from a clinical perspective. In one study we observed that acupuncture analgesia was approximately equal to the effects of inhaling 33% nitrous oxide in oxygen (37). In another study we found that the effects of acupuncture were no stronger than those of TENS delivered at the same sites in the same way (38). Only in rare cases did we see a subject who appeared to become totally insensitive to laboratory pain during electric acupuncture. Other investigators have reported similar findings (44, 45). These results are strikingly inconsistent with the demonstrations of apparently total pain control in the surgical setting in China. They are similarly problematic for the hypothesis that endorphins mediate acupuncture analgesia, because the effect is small. If such stimulation produces an endorphin-mediated response of sufficient strength to permit surgery without pain, it should appear more formidably in the laboratory.

Third, in accordance with observations of Chinese surgeries, laboratory investigators found that the analgesia can be elicited either by stimulating the subject within the same dermatome used for the delivery of the painful stimulus or by stimulating a meridian point (39, 46). The importance of piercing the acupuncture point with precision remains a moot issue. We found that successful demonstration of acupuncture analgesia for dental pain requires exacting care in placement of the needle at the *hoku* point in the hands (located between the thumb and the first finger), but others disagree that this is critical (17).

Finally, electric acupuncture requires low-frequency intense electrical stimulation and appears to be an all-or-none phenomenon. Andersson and colleagues (48) observed that the dental pain threshold could be altered only when the intensity of low-frequency electric stimulation was strong enough to elicit a pounding or throbbing sensation. We found that the evoked potential elicited by painful dental stimulation is reduced only when the acupunctural stimulation is at a level just below the subject's tolerance (40). It was not possible to demonstrate a dose-response effect by varying the intensity of acupunctural stimulation.

Two studies that have contributed uniquely to the laboratory literature merit comment. Chapman and colleagues (41) addressed the question of whether culture affects the response to acupuncture stimulation. Three groups of subjects were studied—non-Oriental Americans, second-generation Japanese-Americans, and Japanese living in Japan. Subjects were required to discriminate several levels of painful dental stimulation in a sensory decision theory task. Detection, discrimination ability, and response bias were measured both in control conditions and during electric acupuncture. Acupuncture yielded small but significant analgesia in all three groups, and neither race nor culture significantly affected the amount of pain control observed.

Price and associates (46) examined the effects of acupuncture on patients with chronic low back pain using a laboratory paradigm. They attempted to bridge laboratory experimentation and clinical pain control by testing patients with an experimental pain stimulus. A hand-held contact thermode was applied to the back and volar forearm of the subjects to deliver noxious heat stimuli. Patients rated both clinical pain and experimental pain under baseline conditions and again after acupuncture. Regardless of whether acupuncture was performed in the dermatomes involved in the back pain or at distant meridian points, both the clinical and experimental pains were reduced 1 to 2 hours after treatment for many patients. When patients were tested again several days after treatment, the therapeutic effect of the treatment on back pain remained but the effect on experimental pain was gone. This study needs to be replicated and extended before firm conclusions can be drawn about the use of experimental laboratory methods with patients, but it suggests that laboratory findings can provide valid evidence for the clinical application of acupuncture.

Whether human acupuncture analgesia is mediated by endorphins has been hotly contested (21, 42). Some investigators have attempted to resolve the issue by measuring plasma endorphins in association with acupuncture therapy, but plasma-borne endorphins cannot cross the blood-brain barrier and therefore are not "functional" in opiate receptor pharmacology. The existence of significant parallels between peripheral and central endorphin changes is still uncertain (23). It is difficult to reach firm conclusions from the evidence on either side of this issue at present; it can be confidently stated, however, that the mechanisms of acupuncture appear to be neither singular nor simple. The complexity increases when these questions are raised at the clinical level. For example, we cannot be confident that the neuropharmacology of the chronic pain patient is the same as that of the normal person or of the elective surgery patient who might respond well when given acupuncture for surgical pain control. Endorphin levels in plasma or cerebrospinal fluid might simply be one part of a larger constellation of neuropharmacologic response to disease, to chronic pain, or to its treatment; they do not necessarily offer the ultimate explanation for pain control during acupuncture.

Clinical Studies

Clinical investigation in the field of acupuncture has been undertaken primarily in the area of chronic pain, with few exceptions (e.g., the study of its effects on postoperative dental pain) (49). Such research has been extremely difficult to carry out effectively for several reasons:

(a) Chronic pain is a complex problem that often has psychologic dimensions as well as organic pathology.

(b) Chronic pain syndromes are sometimes complicated by previous surgeries, other failed therapies, or prescription drug abuse or dependency.

(c) Selection of reliable and valid outcome criteria is difficult, and outcomes are meaningful only when long-term follow-up is undertaken.

(d) No standards are available for correct acupuncture therapy for a given problem, such as back pain.

The last point is particularly problematic. If a cookbook set of acupuncture treatment points is chosen arbitrarily for the target pain syndrome to conduct the study in a systematic fashion, the principles of Oriental medicine are immediately violated. On the other hand, allowing acupuncturists to diagnose and treat each case individually produces a data set that is not amenable to rigorous analysis.

When these major obstacles have been overcome, the investigator must decide whether to use intrasegmental or extrasegmental (meridian) treatment strategies, whether to use electric stimulation and, if so, what parameters, whether to use controls, such as treating patients at the "wrong" points, and how many treatments should be given. A more detailed discussion of these and other design issues in acupuncture research has been provided by Vincent and Richardson (8).

Two types of errors threaten the integrity of any treatment outcome study. The first produces a positive outcome when no real treatment effect exists in nature. Failure to control for placebo effects, unreliable measures, and failure to undertake long-term follow-up can produce such outcomes. The second type is the failure to detect a treatment effect when one has occurred. Too few treatments, too small a sample size to achieve reasonable statistical power, inappropriate or insensitive measurement techniques, and failure to use a homogeneous group of patients can produce misleading negative data. An overview of the large and growing literature in this area reveals that all these errors have been made repeatedly (50). Lewith and Machin (51) have formally addressed the problem of insufficient sample size in the literature. Firm conclusions are therefore difficult to attain. It is clear, however, that acupuncture is not a panacea of sufficient strength to overcome all these problems and to demonstrate consistent and powerful effects on chronic pain.

In addition to small sample size, poor pain measurement has plagued studies of acupuncture therapy. The complexity of clinical pain measurement problems was discussed in detail by Syrjala and Chapman (52) and in Chapter 32. When pain is chronic it is necessary to use both subjective and behavioral outcome indexes tailored to the clinical problem in question, and long-term follow-up must be carried out to determine whether lasting benefits have been obtained. The chances of spontaneous recovery from chronic pain are small by definition, but chronic pain patients can leave any given physician with the polite impression that they have been helped significantly and then go on to another in the never-ending search for a cure. When follow-up procedures such as postal or telephone inquiries about satisfaction with outcome are used, few data of value can be obtained. A rigorous review would dismiss most of the published reports on the basis of these criteria alone.

The earliest clinical studies were largely uncontrolled investigations of mixed groups of chronic pain patients (53). Some early studies used no pain management at all. The data consisted of scaled judgments by the therapists themselves. With time, study designs improved and more suitable but still insufficient pain measurement methods were introduced. The most thoroughly studied clinical problems have been headache and back pain.

A brief review of the field prior to 1976 was provided by Mendelson (53), and more recent reviews have been offered by Lewith and Machin (51) and by Lewith (50). Richardson and Vincent (54) have provided the most comprehensive review to date, with particular emphasis on back pain and headache. They evaluated each of the studies critically on the basis of controls, measurement technology, and follow-up. All of the above investigators deserve credit for their attempts to extract information in a critical fashion from a weak and problematic body of literature. In addition, a few negative reports have been helpful in delimiting the range of effects of acupuncture. For example, Lewith and colleagues (55) concluded that acupuncture is ineffective for postherpetic neuralgia.

What conclusions, if any, can be drawn from the literature? In their review of the overall efficacy of acupuncture therapy, Lewith and Machin (51) concluded that a positive response is given by about 70% of chronic pain patients with the use of real acupuncture, whereas the positive rate for sham acupuncture controls is about 50% and for placebo about 30%. Lewith (50) reviewed the following in detail: six studies that compared acupuncture with conventional medical therapy; ten studies that compared acupuncture with random injection of needles; and two studies that compared acupuncture with placebo treatment. He concluded that acupuncture works to some degree in about 60% of patients with chronic pain, that the effects of acupuncture are greater than those of random needling or placebo treatment, and that acupuncture is as effective for musculoskeletal pain as other treatments such as physiotherapy or drugs. Lewith (50) noted that acupuncture causes fewer adverse reactions than the use of opioid analgesics and anti-inflammatory medications. Richardson and Vincent (54) found good evidence from controlled studies that acupuncture can provide effective short-term pain relief; the figures for effective relief range from 50 to 80% for both acute and chronic conditions. Long-range follow-up data are lacking, however, so little evidence has been found for the long-range benefits of acupuncture. Despite their positive broad conclusions, Richardson and Vincent (54) cautioned that the "placebogenic" qualities of acupuncture treatment might be greater than those of placebo treatments matched to drugs: acupuncture in some cases might simply function as a more effective placebo than its so-called placebo control.

Overall, given the above reviews, acupuncture appears to have positive therapeutic benefit, but it falls far short of the claims of its zealous advocates who believe it to be uniquely powerful. How important is the lack of a rigorous scientific data base? Most therapies in modern medicine, including many common surgical procedures, would appear weak if evaluated rigorously on the basis of the supporting literature— most medical practice is not derived from a systematic program of scientific research. Much has been demanded of acupuncture because it is basically a folk medicine and because strong claims have been made by its advocates.

B. ACUPUNCTURE AS TRIGGER POINT THERAPY

This part of the chapter introduces a Western approach to acupuncture that illustrates how acupunctural procedures can be employed in conventional medicine. It is derived from my extensive clinical experience with treatment of musculoskeletal pain. The therapeutic techniques introduced follow from my theory about the origins of chronic musculoskeletal pain, which is that such pain, when chronic, often results from peripheral neuropathy secondary to age-related degenerative changes or former injuries. Many problems seemingly localized to specific body areas are postulated to originate in subtle spondylotic radiculopathy. My therapy for such problems targets chronic

skeletal muscle contracture and is thought to work primarily through somatic and sympathetic spinal reflexes. This theory is not the only conceivable basis for performing acupuncture in Western medicine, but it provides a clear and practical demonstration of how the principles of ancient Chinese medicine and contemporary medicine can be reconciled.

Origin of Musculoskeletal Pain

Musculoskeletal pain that often arises and persists indefinitely in the absence of a detectable permanent injury or inflammation is the most common type of chronic pain; fortunately, it is also the most amenable to trigger point therapy. This type of pain is poorly understood, difficult to diagnose, and rarely treated successfully by other interventions. Muscle contracture is a fundamental component of such pain. When a nerve is injured or irritated, pain persists beyond healing only if the nerve has had pre-existing chronic damage (56). Spondylotic radiculopathy can be a cause of chronic nerve damage and a little-acknowledged source of musculoskeletal pain (13, 57).

Radiculopathy can cause pain by any of three possible mechanisms: (a) it can result in disuse supersensitivity in nerves and muscles and cause them to generate anomalous impulses that then proceed along conventional pathways to evoke abnormal sensorimotor activity, which can include pain (58–60); (b) muscle contractures can occur and cause pain by squeezing intramuscular nociceptors—when paraspinal contractures compress nerve roots, they can create a vicious circle of pain; (c) sustained contractures can lead to degeneration and secondary pain at activity-stressed parts of the body already weakened by radiculopathy-induced collagen degradation (61). According to this model, conditions such as tendinitis, epicondylitis, spondylosis, discogenic disease, and osteoarthritis are conventionally regarded as primary conditions but are sometimes secondary to a neuropathic process in which muscle contracture is a critical factor. This postulate is difficult to prove, but it provides a useful working hypothesis for patient examination and therapy.

Diagnosis

The varied presentations of acute pain and the gradual onset of radiculopathic pain can be confusing. When pain is produced by acute trauma or by a rapidly expanding space-occupying lesion, some degree of denervation is usually present; onset and diagnosis are therefore usually clear-cut (e.g., herniated intervertebral disk). Spondylotic radiculopathy generally follows a gradual, relapsing, and remitting course, however, which is silent unless pain is precipitated by an accident (often so minor that it can pass unnoticed by the patient). Because symptoms and signs of subtle neuropathy (as distinct from those of denervation) are less well known, the diagnosis is frequently missed, and involvement of the nerve root might not even be suspected (62) (Table 90-1). The origin of the pain is still more baffling when it is not the radiculopathic pain per se that manifests itself but secondary pain caused by neuropathy-related muscle shortening or contractures. For example, segmental pain from the cervical spine referred to the elbow is almost always diagnosed as "lateral epicondylitis" or "tennis elbow" and is commonly taken for a local condition (63) (Fig. 90-3).

The causes of subtle peripheral neuropathy are as many as those of nerve damage (e.g., neoplasm, toxicity, trauma, inflammation, infections). However, because the pathology of neuropathy is limited to axonal degeneration and segmental demyelination (with variable degrees of damage and reversibility), clinical manifestations are relatively few. These might or might not include pain: some neuropathies are asymptomatic, because pain occurs only when nociceptive

TABLE 90-1. Some Clinical Manifestations of Radiculopathy*

Affected Area	Manifestations
Dermatome	Vasomotor: skin is cooler, mottling; sudomotor: increased sweating; pilomotor: goose bumps, cutaneous hyperesthesia; trophedema or neurogenic edema, alteration in texture of skin and subcutaneous tissue; trophic changes in skin and nails, hair loss
Myotome	Myalgic hyperalgesia, tenderness over motor points; increased muscle tone, spasm (and reduced joint ranges)
Sclerotome	Periosteal and joint tenderness, swelling and effusion; enthesopathy (thickening in tendons attached to joints)

*Neuropathy can cause sensory, motor, or autonomic dysfunctions, or a combination of these, in the corresponding dermatome, myotome, and sclerotome. These areas do not necessarily coincide spatially, and the resulting multiphasic picture can be confusing.

pathways are involved (e.g., Raynaud's phenomenon, idiopathic hyperhidrosis) (64, 65).

The clinical manifestations of radiculopathy—mixed sensorimotor and autonomic disturbances—are diffuse and usually symmetric; even when symptoms are unilateral, latent signs are generally noted on the contralateral side. This observation is contrary to conventional neurologic principles. Autonomic nerves are involved in the overall pattern of neuropathy and can contribute to these peculiar pain patterns through

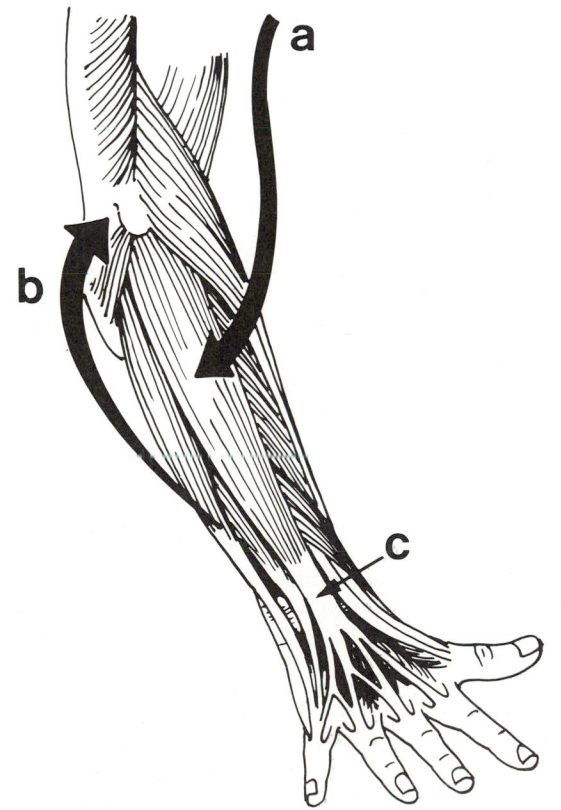

FIG. 90-3. Tennis elbow as seen from the viewpoint of spondylotic radiculopathy: (a) tenderness over a motor point; (b) pain and tenderness in lateral epicondyle; (c) contracture of the tendon of the extensor digitorum communis.

several mechanisms. Vasomotor, sudomotor, and pilomotor changes are commonly seen, and vasoconstriction gives neuropathic pain a cardinal feature that differentiates it from inflammatory pain—affected parts are perceptibly colder.

Laboratory, radiologic, and other tests are usually unhelpful. Radiologic findings only demonstrate late, secondary changes in joints. Routine electrodiagnostic tests are also unrevealing; nerve conduction velocities usually remain within normal ranges but F-wave latencies can be prolonged. Electromyography might only show increased and prolonged insertion activity (Chapter 35).

Although diagnosis depends almost entirely on the examiner's acumen and experience, the characteristic patterns of myofascial disorders are soon appreciated. Many syndromes are now clinically recognized although they are considered to be local conditions (Table 90-1). Because pain is primarily related to muscle, however, signs in muscles are the most consistent and relevant; these include increased muscle tone (62), tenderness over motor points (66), and tender, palpable contractures, which lead to restricted joint range (66, 67). In radiculopathy, signs are present in the territories of both primary rami. It is common knowledge that sciatic leg pain originates from the low back and the latter is always examined, but it is less well known that many other musculoskeletal pain syndromes also originate from the spine. Therefore, when pain presents in structures supplied by the anterior primary division of the spinal nerve (e.g., pain in the elbow or shoulder), structures supplied by the posterior primary division (i.e., the neck) must also be examined.

Once signs of neuropathy have been found, a knowledge of the nerve supply origins of muscles helps to identify the segmental nature of the pain and the levels of spinal involvement. For example, in chondromalacia patellae, crepitus and pain might be focused under the patella and in the knee, but careful examination reveals signs of radiculopathy (e.g., tenderness over muscle motor points and painful contractures) in the muscles that extend the knee through the patella (the quadriceps femoris muscles, L2–L4). Signs in the paraspinal muscles at the same levels then confirm the segmental levels of radiculopathy (66). Each muscle must be palpated. Because many deep paraspinal muscles explored by needling for contractures extend throughout most of the length of the spine (e.g., the longissimus), the entire spine must be examined even when symptoms are localized to one region (67). For example, low back pain is most common at the L5 to S1 levels but higher segmental levels are involved more often than not, frequently reaching lower dorsal levels.

General Principles of Treatment and Technical Considerations

Treatment for radiculopathic pain depends on the degree and reversibility of radiculopathy. Because these can vary considerably, the variety of treatment methods is extensive. Treatment goals are release of contractures, promotion of healing, and removal of the source of irritation. Most injuries to nerves are minor, and the neuropathy is minimal and transient. Pain therefore resolves spontaneously with time and the temporary relief of pain (e.g., with analgesics or the application of simple physical therapies such as heat or massage) might be all that is necessary while the nerve heals (usually within days or, at the most, weeks). When such measures fail treatment might require more effective therapies.

Musculoskeletal pain of radiculopathic origin is usually accompanied by contractures, and pain is usually relieved when these contractures are released. This suggests that contractures are an inherent component of this type of pain and that their release forms an important part of treatment. When simple methods fail to release contractures, more effective methods, such as stretching contractures and cooling them with fluorimethane sprays (12), intense focal pressure over acupuncture points (acupressure), or transcutaneous neural stimulation, can prove effective. When painful contractures do not respond to such measures, injection methods might be useful. Local anesthetics are commonly employed, but normal physiologic saline solution has also been used with good results (13) (Chapter 21). Benefits of injection methods are that they temporarily eliminate the primary focus of intense nociceptive input into the neuraxis and eliminate the secondary focus from local inflammation created by the needle. Dry-needle stimulation alters the trigger point and produces inflammation, and thus is also effective.

Physical therapies probably relieve neuropathic pain by reflex stimulation of the deprived (and supersensitive) muscle through its nerve (Chapter 23), but such stimulation is ordinarily brief. By contrast, dry needling or acupuncture can produce prolonged stimulation through the generation of a current of injury that lasts for days (67). Needle therapy might also have a unique beneficial feature; it is speculated that it promotes healing by the local release of the platelet-derived growth factor (68).

Theoretically, sustained shortening in paraspinal muscles acting across an intervertebral disk space can increase pressure on facet joints (i.e., facet-joint syndrome) as well as compress the disk, contributing to its eventual loss of height and to narrowing of the intervertebral foramina. Paraspinal contractures can thus irritate nerve roots indirectly (e.g., through pressure of a bulging disk) and cause radiculopathic manifestations that present some distance away in the territory of the neurotome. A vicious circle can arise and perpetuate segmental pain: pressure on a nerve root → radiculopathy → pain and contractures → further compression of the nerve root. Treatment of this predicament by the release of paraspinal muscle spasm is therefore indicated.

Selection of Points

Treatment sites are chosen on a neurophysiologic basis and in accordance with the segmental level of injury. The most effective sites for releasing contractures are at muscle motor points and musculotendinous junctions; these generally correspond to traditional acupuncture points (69, 70). A motor point is the skin region at which an innervated muscle is most accessible to percutaneous electric excitation at the lowest intensity. This point generally overlies the muscle motor band of innervation. Points belonging to the affected myotome(s) are chosen for treatment. For example, in treating an injury between the L3 and L4 vertebrae affecting the L4 nerve root, points in muscles belonging to the L4 myotome would be treated. Emphasis is placed on muscles that show palpable spasm and myalgic hyperalgesia (Chapter 21).

Location of Treatment Sites

The exact location of a motor point can vary slightly from patient to patient, but the relative position follows a fairly fixed pattern. Musculotendinous junctions are easily located by palpation and can be thickened (enthesopathic) in chronic musculoskeletal pain.

Recently an electric point finder, the neurometer, has been adopted by some for motor point location. The principle of the neurometer is similar to that of a standard calibration-stable stimulator with variable output control used to evoke muscle twitches in response to minimal electric stimulation. During stimulation the skin over motor points has the least resistance to the current because terminal branches of the muscle nerve there lie closest to the skin; a muscle twitch is produced with completion (or breaking) of the electric current between the electrodes by the patient's body.

The neurometer is powered by dry cells, generally 9 to 21 V (58), and consists of a milliammeter with a probe and ground or indifferent electrode. The indifferent electrode is held in the hand of the patient while the probe explores the body surface for areas where resistance to direct current is lowest. When the probe contacts such a point, the neurometer emits an audible signal and the milliammeter shows a reading. Unlike the standard calibration-stable stimulator, with visible muscle contraction as the indicator, the neurometer is not specific; it indicates a skin point that has low electric resistance, but not all such points are necessarily over motor bands. The accuracy of a neurometer has been criticized because skin resistance to direct current can vary according to room humidity, skin temperature, sudomotor activity, voltage, and other factors. In any individual under any given set of conditions, however, there is a definite relative difference in skin resistance over a motor point as compared with surrounding skin (69).

I do not use the neurometer because motor bands are known anatomic entities at fixed anatomic sites that vary only slightly from one person to another. Moreover, bands that require attention are frequently palpable or tender and thus are easily found. Charts showing the distribution of motor points are available. The earliest was prepared by the neurologist Wilhelm Erb in 1882, and anatomic guides for the electromyographer are available. A comparison of a traditional acupuncture chart with a chart of motor points shows many similarities (16).

Contracture Release by Electric Stimulation

A low-intensity current can be used to promote release of contractures involved in chronic pain syndromes. Electric stimulation can be in the form of a low-voltage (9 V) interrupted direct current administered for a few seconds to each inserted needle with a neurometer point-finder probe, or a phasic current can be applied through pairs of electrode leads to inserted needles for approximately 15 minutes. Visible muscle contractions usually indicate proper needle placement. Release of contractures occurs best when the stimulation frequency allows the muscle to relax between contractions and not summate to produce tetanic contraction. The summation frequency (about 30 to 100 Hz) varies from muscle to muscle—for example, that of the soleus, at about 30 Hz/s, is much lower than that of the tibialis anterior. Electric stimulation has little advantage over mechanical agitation when the needle has been accurately placed.

When the several most painful contractures in a muscle have been needled, the entire muscle relaxes within minutes and, when the several most painful muscles in a painful region have been treated, pain is relieved in the treated region. Muscle relaxation and pain relief in one region can spread to the contralateral side, to paraspinal muscles, and to the entire segment. These considerations suggest a reflex neural mechanism that might involve spinal modulatory systems.

Relaxation also involves smooth muscle, and it can spread to the entire segment, thus releasing vasospasm and constriction of lymphatics (71). The sympatholytic effect improves blood flow to the painful part and encourages lymph drainage. Painful joints can be treated by releasing contractures in all the muscles acting on the joint. This can be followed by subjective pain relief, sometimes within minutes, and confirmed by objective improvement in the range of motion of the joint.

Treatment of Fibrotic Contractures

It is theoretically possible for contractures to become chronic, eventually fibrotic, and painful (fibrositis or fibromyositis). When fibrosis has become a feature of contractures, response to treatment is modest. Treatment of extensively fibrotic contractures necessitates more frequent and extensive needling because part of the muscle shortening is maintained by fibrosis rather than by contracture. Release is often limited only to the individual muscle bands that are specifically treated—to relieve pain in such a muscle, all tender bands require needling. This implies more needle insertions per session, or more sessions with the same number of insertions. For significant, long-lasting pain relief and restoration of function, several treatments separated by days are usually necessary (72).

The progressive nature of symptomatic relief, substantiated by the gradual amelioration of objective clinical findings, suggests that a healing process is involved. The condition can be considered to be reversed when symptoms and signs are eliminated and do not recur. Acupuncture therefore does not relieve pain primarily by analgesia as it is traditionally defined (e.g., in a normal nervous system subjected to noxious afferent input) but rather by moderation of the manifestations of a neuropathic, supersensitive nervous system (e.g., releasing painful muscle contracture and vasoconstriction). Unlike other physical remedies, acupuncture may well promote healing.

Treatment of Specific Problems

The following are general guidelines for treating some common pain syndromes. In practice the sites for treatment are found by palpating muscle for tight contracture bands. Charts of points can be useful, but they do not indicate the depth that the needle has to penetrate.

Headache

Headaches of intracranial origin are rare (e.g., space-occupying tumors, cerebral hemorrhage, hypertension) but have to be excluded (Chapter 39). Acupuncture is effective in treating the following: (a) headaches of musculoskeletal origin related to muscular contraction occurring about the head and neck—these are usually secondary to cervical spondylosis and are probably the most common form of headache; and (b) headaches of vascular origin (e.g., migraine and cluster headaches; Chapter 39).

Commonly used points are in the head, neck, and upper shoulders. Points in the neck and upper shoulders are treated initially, and this can provide relief. Points in the head and hand can be added in later sessions if the pain persists. These include the following muscles:

In the head. Temporalis, corrugator supercilii, frontalis, masseter, levator labii superioris
In the neck. Splenius capitis and cervicis, semispinalis capitis, scalenus anterior, medius, and posterior, sternomastoid (Fig. 90-4).
In the shoulder. The upper trapezius is probably the most effective point for headache (but extreme care should be taken to avoid penetrating the lung), supraspinatus, infraspinatus, levator scapulae.
In the hand. The motor point of the first dorsal interosseous muscle between the thumb and index finger is a popular traditional point (known as the *ho-ku*) that is effective for headache and pain in the upper extremity. This small muscle might seem trivial, but it has the highest concentration of muscle spindles in the body and the hand has a large representation in both motor and sensory areas of the cerebral cortex.

Neck Pain (Including "Whiplash") and Upper Extremity Pain

Pain from the cervical spine is discussed together with pain in the upper extremity because the upper limb, having been derived in the developing human embryo from the upper extremity bud, is effectually an extension of the neck. Tender muscle points seldom occur in one part without being present in the other, and frequently both must be treated.

For treatment purposes, neck pain is discussed as upper, middle, and lower cervical spine pain:

Upper cervical spondylosis. Pain in C1, C2, and C3 often presents as occipital headache affecting muscles that insert at the occiput, or as pain in the neck muscles. Sometimes pain is referred to the jaw.
Middle cervical spondylosis. Pain in C4, C5, and C6 can present as headache, neck ache, or, commonly, as pain in the shoulder and upper arm.

Lower cervical spondylosis. Pain in C7, C8, and T1 can present as headache or neck ache but, more frequently, occurs as pain in the elbow (lateral epicondylitis, C6 and C7), wrist, and hand (C7, C8, T1). It is not unusual for pain to occur in the arm without apparent neck involvement. For example, in carpal tunnel syndrome, the symptoms are generally confined to the hand, but examination of the forearm and neck almost always discloses spasm and tenderness in the wrist flexors and extensors and in the paraspinal muscles of the same segments.

Acupuncture treatment of these conditions is generally effective for pain relief and function can be largely restored, but late changes following denervation, such as muscle wasting, are irreversible. Even surgical release of a carpal tunnel compression cannot reverse such changes. Treatment points are located in the neck, shoulder, elbow, and wrist:

Treatment points in the neck. The superficial neck muscles mentioned above for headache are used as well as deep paraspinal muscles at affected spinal levels: semispinalis capitis, semispinalis cervicis, spinalis cervicis, and multifidus.
Treatment points in the shoulder. The location of symptoms and therefore the primary points for treatment in the shoulder and arm depend on the spinal level(s) affected by spondylosis. Generally, more than one segmental level is affected.
For C3 and C4 the scapula is pulled upward by contractures in the trapezius and levator scapulae muscles. For C4 to C6 pain can occur during the initiation of abduction, primarily involving the rotator cuff muscles (i.e., rotator cuff tendinitis): the supraspinatus, infraspinatus, teres minor, and subscapularis, but the latter is not easily accessed for treatment. Pain and limitation of the first 60° of abduction (pain arc) can be present when the deltoid muscle (C5, C6) is involved. (Pain and tenderness at the mid-deltoid motor point is commonly labeled as bursitis. The scapula can be pulled medially by the rhomboideus major and minor (C5). Pain and limitation of forward extension and abduction are usually associated with limitation of the glenohumoral range caused by spasm in the infraspinatus (C4–C6) and teres muscles (C5–C7).
For C7 and C8 pain and limitation of internal posterior rotation is primarily associated with spasm in the pectoralis major (C7, C8) and pectoralis minor (C8, T1).
Occasionally spondylosis affects several levels and almost every muscle that activates the shoulder (C3–C8) is implicated to a greater or lesser degree. A "frozen shoulder" occurs when there are contractures in all the muscles that act on the shoulder. This condition, which usually resists all other physical measures, responds well to acupuncture.
Acromioclavicular joint pain usually responds to treatment of the pectoralis major (clavicular head), anterior deltoid, and upper trapezius muscles.
Treatment points in the elbow and wrist. Pain occurs more commonly on the lateral aspect of the elbow (lateral epicondylitis or tennis elbow), where the following muscles must be treated: biceps, brachialis, brachioradialis (C5, C6), extensor carpi radialis longus and

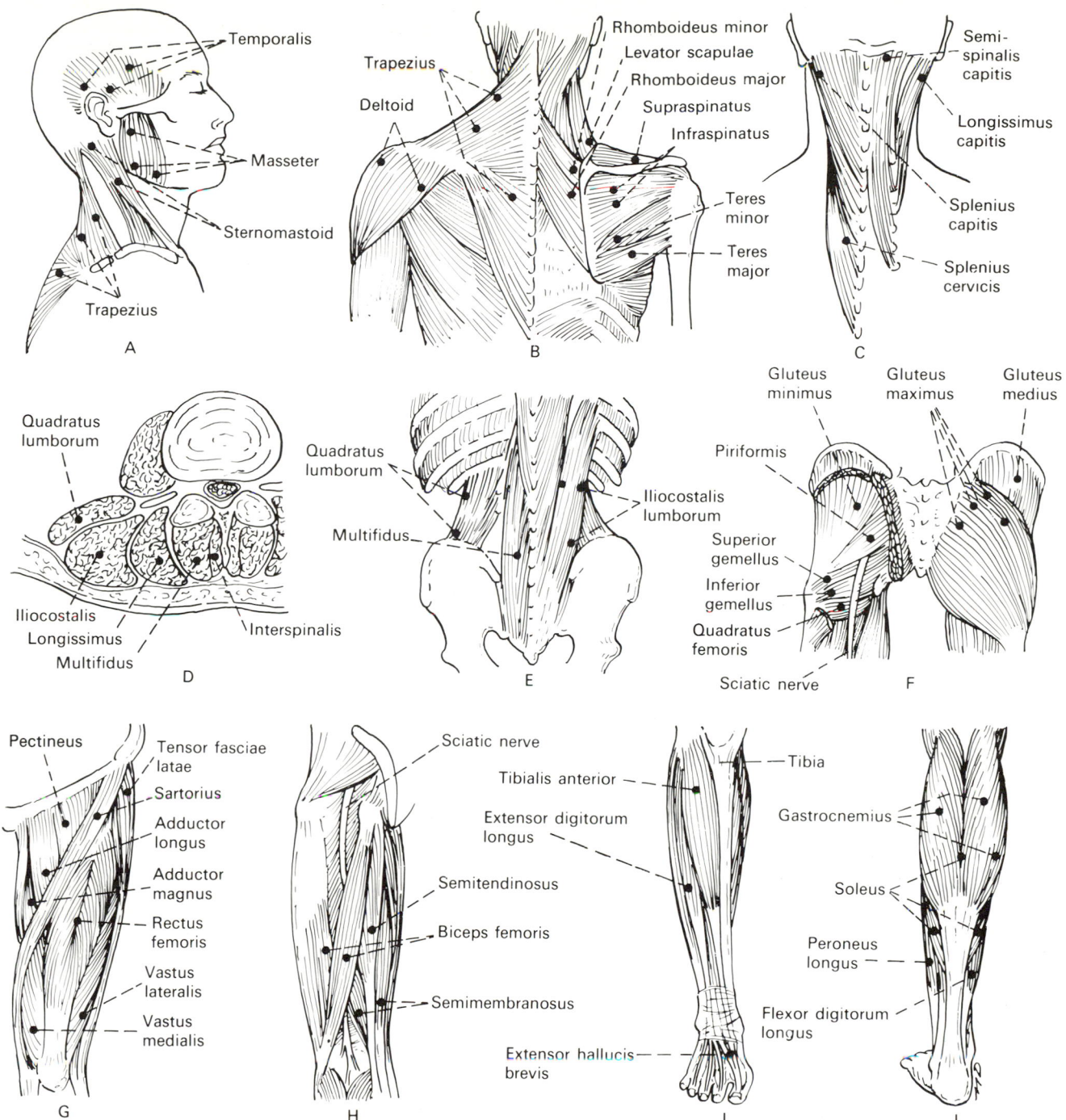

FIG. 90-4. Commonly used trigger points in various parts of the body.

brevis, anconeus, extensor digitorum, extensor carpi ulnaris (C6, C7), and supinator (C6). When pain is on the medial aspect of the elbow (golfer's elbow), the following muscles are treated: pronator teres, flexor carpi radialis and ulnaris, and triceps (C6–C8). The palmaris longus is the prime muscle treated in early Dupuytren's contracture (C7, C8).

For pain in the wrist, the above two groups of muscles are treated. For carpal tunnel syndrome, the thenar muscles (supplied by the median nerve) are added.

Low Back Pain and Lower Extremity Pain

Just as the neck and upper extremity must be considered together, the leg is considered to be an extension of the lumbar back, having been derived in the developing human embryo from the lower extremity bud. As in neck and upper limb pain, the therapy of low back pain and leg pain is usually a single process. When pain is of purely musculoskeletal origin, response to this treatment can be rewarding. Early discogenic pain is included in this category because spasm in the deep paravertebral muscles can cause strong compression of the disk. Unless impingement of the nerve root by irreversible structural changes is present, which is rare, the release of the muscles can provide relief and surgery can be avoided. Patients with discogenic disease proven by myelography and EMG studies have responded to this treatment with no recurrence of pain after several years' follow-up.

Examination of the lumbar back must go beyond the standard examination for signs of denervation (e.g., straight leg raising, Lasègue's test, attenuated reflexes, sensation loss, muscle wasting). In most back pain patients with early neuropathy, these signs are generally negative and the examiner must search for more subtle signs (e.g., trophedema, tenderness at motor points, increased muscle tone, autonomic signs). Careful examination for these signs demonstrates that, even if symptoms appear to be at one level, several segmental levels are usually involved. The key to successful treatment of persistent low back pain of musculoskeletal origin is that the entire lumbar back (often as high as lower dorsal levels) must be treated as well as the lower extremities (which might not necessarily be in pain). Treatment points are located in the lumbar back, buttock, thigh, hamstrings, calf, and anterior leg:

Treatment points in the lumbar back. Treatment points in the lower back include the quadratus lumborum, erector spinae, iliocostalis lumborum, iliocostalis thoracis, longissimus, and multifidus muscles (all lumbar segments). When the needle is inserted it serves as a useful and unique diagnostic tool for revealing the presence of any deep muscle spasm.

Treatment points in the buttock. Treatment points in the buttock include the gluteus maximus (L5, S1, S2), medius, and minimus (L4–S1); sometimes diagnosed as hip bursitis, superior (L5–S2) and inferior gemellus (L4–S1), piriformis (S1, S2; piriformis syndrome), and quadratus femoris (L4–S1) muscles. These points, especially in the glutei muscles, should be treated with a needle at least 3 inches long.

Treatment points in the thigh. Treatment points in the thigh include the rectus femoris, vastus lateralis, medialis, and intermedius, and tensor fascia latae (trochanteric bursitis). These points are needled particularly when pain originates from L2 to L4 segments. They are also the points to be used for knee pain. It can be most rewarding, in one session of treatment, to return full extension to the knee when an extension lag has resisted all forms of physical therapy. When pain is on the medial aspect of the knee the semimembranosus, semitendinosus, gracilis, and sartorius (pes anserinus) are treated. Even when mild effusion from a minor meniscus tear is present, but without the knee locking, the condition can be treated.

Treatment points on the medial aspect of the thigh. The adductor muscles, magnus, longus, and brevis (L3–L5), are treated when there is limitation of hip *F*lexion, *ab*duction, and *e*xtension and *r*otation (i.e., when the Faber test is positive).

Treatment points in the hamstring. Treatment points in the hamstrings include the semimembranosus, semitendinosus (L5–S1), and biceps femoris (L5–S2). These muscles are almost always involved in low back pain. Limitation of straight leg raising can often improve dramatically following treatment of these muscles.

Treatment points in the calf. Treatment points in the calf include the tibialis posterior (L5–S1), gastrocnemius, and soleus (L5–S2). These muscles are always involved in low back pain. Because they provide the major force in supporting the longitudinal arch of the foot, they are important points for pain in the heel and sole of the foot. For "metatarsalgia" the flexor digitorum in the sole is also needled.

Treatment points on the anterior leg. Two important muscles are used as treatment points on the anterior leg, the tibialis anterior (L4, L5) and extensor digitorum longus (L4, L5, S1). Treatment of these can relieve shin splints and pain in the ankle. When the extensor hallucis longus and brevis muscles are also needled, early hallux vulgus and bunion of the big toe can be corrected.

Autonomic Dysfunction

The autonomic nervous system is a division of the peripheral nervous system that is distributed to smooth muscles and glands throughout the body. It is entirely an efferent system, and it is vegetative in the sense that most of its functions are carried out below consciousness. It is, however, highly integrated in function with the rest of the nervous system. By treating striated muscles belonging to the same segments, the acupuncturist can treat spasm in smooth muscles and hyperactive glands that are inaccessible to needling. Some common conditions that respond to treatment are the following:

Vasomotor hyperactivity. When pain is associated with increased sympathetic activity (sympathetic maintained pain syndromes, such as Raynaud's disease and causalgia), it can be treated as for upper or lower limb pain, as appropriate.

Sudomotor hyperactivity. This can be treated as for upper or lower limb pain, as appropriate (e.g., idiopathic hyperhidrosis).

Smooth muscle spasm. Treatable conditions include asthma (trapezius and accessory muscles of respiration, paraspinal muscles in the dorsal back), visceral pain, colic, such as biliary (T5–T8), intestinal (T10–T12), and vermicular (T12–L5) (traditional acupuncture favors the points on the front of the leg, and the tibialis anterior motor point is known as "stomach 36"), and dysmenorrhea (L5–S2).

Glandular hyperactivity. Pain of gastric and peptic origin responds to treatment of paraspinal muscles (T5–T12).

C. SUMMARY AND CONCLUSIONS

More than a decade after its introduction on a large scale in the West, acupuncture remains a mystery and a point of controversy. It seems clear from the results of animal, human laboratory, and clinical studies that acupunctural stimulation (particularly electric stimulation) can alter pain perception and relieve pains of clinical origin. The human laboratory and clinical studies are consistent, however, in showing that acupunctural stimulation offers no panacea. The effects seen are inevitably modest when large groups of subjects or patients are examined, and the collective outcomes of the last decade clearly fail to support the exaggerated claims of many of the advocates of acupuncture made in the early 1970s. When the overlap of acupunctural therapy with trigger point treatment and electric stimulation therapy is considered, it becomes questionable whether acupuncture merits its own identity as a therapeutic procedure in Western medical practice and research. This situation suggests a pragmatic solution to the question of how acupuncture should be regarded by the physician concerned with pain management. The following three principles are offered as guidelines.

First, acupuncture should be addressed, considered, and scientifically investigated as a method for hyperstimulation therapy, as advocated by Melzack and Wall (47) or, more specifically, as a treatment for conditions of neural degeneration or neuropathy (as proposed here) and not as a form of Chinese medicine. The practice of classical Chinese medicine is without a scientific foundation in Western medical practice, but acupunctural techniques can be beneficially employed for the practice of electric stimulation therapy or trigger point therapy, or for both. Viewed in this framework, such techniques draw on a scientific rationale and on clinical data bases in two or more areas. Acupuncture techniques, stripped of their mystique, offer a safe and inexpensive therapeutic alternative to writing prescriptions. They need to be regarded as an alternative form of medicine only when practiced by nonphysicians.

Practitioners interested in acupuncture therapy should broaden their focus to include TENS and trigger point therapy. TENS is more expensive than acupuncture for the patient because a TENS unit needs to be purchased, but control over the therapy is largely in the hands of the patient rather than the doctor. Trigger point therapy differs little from acupuncture when a dry needle technique or saline injection is used, and it is slightly more expensive than acupuncture because it involves needles that cannot be reused. Because the tips of acupuncture needles are not beveled like those of injection needles, acupuncture is less traumatic to tissue, causes less minor bleeding, and is somewhat less painful.

Second, the possibility that acupunctural stimulation might be related to an alteration of endorphin levels should be de-emphasized in discussing such methods with patients and in considering whether a therapeutic trial with acupuncture is indicated for a given patient. The animal literature clearly shows an association of acupunctural stimulation to endorphins, but advocates of acupuncture appear to be confusing stress-induced analgesia in animals with the (hopefully) stress-reducing therapy performed in a physician's office. The link of endorphin levels to chronic pain states is as yet uncertain and controversial, and it is not known whether any long-term benefit of treatment would accrue to a patient with chronic pain even if acupuncture treatment resulted in endorphin release for a short period of time. Future findings could have a great impact on this conclusion.

Third, despite the problems and limitations of the clinical literature, it is clear that acupuncture offers little hope for a "miracle" cure for chronic pain problems. It is appropriate to advise patients that controlled outcome studies, although favorable, show limited and modest positive benefit of treatment overall and that insufficient information has been obtained to determine whether positive gains are lasting when pain is chronic. The literature does support claims that acupuncture is a low-risk treatment when properly performed; the cost of such treatment can be of greater concern to patients than safety. Physicians should be alert to the possible suppression of important symptoms of disease when patients undergo acupuncture therapy for pain.

It is most unfortunate that, after a decade of research in this area, the literature does not permit firm conclusions to be reached about therapeutic efficacy that could be summarized in a book such as this for clinical referral guidelines. It seems clear that classically performed acupuncture remains an experimental therapy. The clinical problems for which it is and is not appropriate have only begun to be defined. It is unsettling that no consensus has emerged in regard to how acupuncture should be practiced, who are fitting patients, and how many treatments are needed. The old truism remains, however: the absence of evidence is not equivalent to the evidence of absence. Broadly speaking, acupuncture appears to help patients suffering with chronic pain and to do so at a rate greater than that of control treatments. Care must be taken when patients engage the services of nonphysician acupuncturists because symptoms of clinically significant disease might not be brought to proper medical attention. When properly practiced, acupuncture is quite safe, and it offers an alternative to the conventional, often ineffectual, prescription of analgesic medication for patients with persisting pain.

REFERENCES

1. Bonica, J.J.: The Management of Pain. Philadelphia, Lea & Febiger, 1953.

2. Bonica, J.J.: Therapeutic acupuncture in the People's Republic of China: Implications for American medicine. JAMA, 228:1544, 1974.

3. Duke, M.: Acupuncture. New York, Pyramid House, 1972.

4. Kao, F.F.: Acupuncture Therapeutics: An Introductory Text. Garden City, NY, Triple Oak Publishing, 1973.

5. Tan, L.T., Tan, M.Y.C., and Veith, I. (eds.): Acupuncture Therapy. Philadelphia, Temple University Press, 1973.

6. Kaptchuk, T.J.: The Web That Has No Weaver: Understanding Chinese Medicine. New York, Cogdon and Weed, 1983.

7. MacDonald, A.: Acupuncture: From Ancient Art to Modern Medicine. London, Unwin, 1984.
8. Vincent, C., and Richardson, P.H.: The evaluation of therapeutic acupuncture: Concepts and methods. Pain, 24:1, 1986.
9. Steiner, R.P.: Acupuncture—cultural perspectives. 1. The Western view. Postgrad. Med., 74:60, 1983.
10. Melzack, R., and Katz, K.: Auriculotherapy fails to relieve chronic pain. A controlled crossover study. JAMA, 251:1041, 1984.
11. Bonica, J.J.: Management of myofascial pain syndromes in general practice. JAMA, 165:732, 1957.
12. Travell, J., and Simons, D.: Myofascial Pain and Dysfunction: The Trigger Point Manual. Baltimore, Williams & Wilkins, 1983.
13. Sola, A.E.: Treatment of myofascial pain syndromes. In Advances in Pain Research and Therapy, Vol. 7. Edited by C. Benedetti, C.R., Chapman, and G. Moricca. New York, Raven Press, 1984, pp. 467–485.
14. Hyodo, M.: An Objective Approach to Acupuncture. Osaka, Japan, Ryodoraku, Autonomic Nerve Society, 1975.
15. Hyodo, M.: Modern scientific acupuncture, as practiced in Japan. In Persistent Pain. Edited by S. Lipton and J. Miles. Orlando, Grune & Stratton, 1985, pp. 129–156.
16. Melzack, R.: Myofascial trigger points: Relation to acupuncture and mechanism of pain. Arch. Phys. Med. Rehabil., 62:114, 1981.
17. Gunn, C.C.: Neuropathic pain—a new theory for chronic pain of intrinsic origin. Ann. R. Coll. Phys. Surg. Can., 22:327, 1989.
18. Sola, A.E.: Trigger point therapy. In Clinical Procedures in Emergency Medicine. Edited by J.R. Roberts and J.R. Hedges. Philadelphia, W.B. Saunders, 1985, pp. 674–686.
19. Melzack, R., and Wall, P.D.: Pain mechanisms: A new theory. Science, 150:971, 1965.
20. Fields, H.L.: Pain II: New approaches to management. Ann. Neurol., 9:101, 1981.
21. Watkins, L.R., and Mayer, D.J.: Organization of endogenous opiate and nonopiate pain control systems. Science, 216:1158, 1982.
22. Copolov, D.L., and Helme, R.D.: Enkephalins and endorphins. Clinical, pharmacological and therapeutic implications. Drugs, 26:503, 1983.
23. Bloom, F.E.: The endorphins: A growing family of pharmacologically pertinent peptides. Ann. Rev. Pharmacol. Toxicol., 23:151, 1983.
24. Kleinmuts, B.: The scientific study of clinical judgment in psychology and medicine. Clin. Psychol. Rev., 4:111, 1984.
25. Greenwald, A.G., et al.: Under what conditions does theory obstruct research progress? Psychol. Rev., 93:216, 1986.
26. Annual Meeting Report: Acupuncture. J. Tenn. Med. Assoc., 75:202, 1981.
27. Sweet, W.H.: Some current problems in pain research and therapy (including needle puncture, "acupuncture"). Pain, 10:297, 1981.
28. Wright, M., and McGrath, C.J.: Physiologic and analgesic effects of acupuncture in the dog. J. Am. Vet. Med. Assoc., 178:502, 1981.
29. Klide, A.M.: Acupuncture for treatment of chronic back pain in the horse. Acupunct. Electrother. Res., 9:57, 1984.
30. Bosset, D.F., Page, E.H., and Stromberg, M.W.: Production of cutaneous analgesia by electroacupuncture in horses: Variations dependent on sex of subject and locus of stimulation. Am. J. Vet. Res., 45:620, 1984.
31. Bodnar, R.J., et al.: Dose-dependent reductions by naloxone of analgesia induced by cold-water stress. Pharmacol. Biochem. Behav., 8:667, 1978.
32. Maier, S.F.: The opioid/non-opioid nature of stress-induced analgesia and learned helplessness. J. Exp. Psychol. [Anim. Behav.], 9:80, 1983.
33. Gilman, T.T., and Marcuse, F.L.: Animal hypnosis. Psychol. Bull., 46:151, 1949.
34. Carli, G., Farabollini, F., and Fontani, G.: Effects of pain, morphine and naloxone on the duration of animal hypnosis. Behav. Brain. Res., 2:373, 1981.
35. Gallup, G.G.: Animal hypnosis: Factual status of a fictional concept. Psychol. Bull., 81:836, 1974.
36. Galeano, C., et al.: Acupuncture analgesia in rabbits. Pain, 6:71, 1979.
37. Chapman, C.R., Gehrig, J.D., and Wilson, M.E.: Acupuncture compared with 33 percent nitrous oxide for dental analgesia. Anesthesiology, 42:532, 1975.
38. Chapman, C.R., Wilson, M.E., and Gehrig, J.D.: Comparative effects of acupuncture and transcutaneous stimulation on the perception of painful dental stimuli. Pain, 2:265, 1976.
39. Chapman, C.R., Chen, A.C., and Bonica, J.J.: Effects of intrasegmental acupuncture on dental pain: Evaluation by threshold estimation and sensory decision theory. Pain, 3:213, 1977.
40. Schimek, F., et al.: Vary electrical acupuncture stimulation intensity: Effects on dental pain-evoked potentials. Anesth. Analg., 61:449, 1982.
41. Chapman, C.R., et al.: Comparative effects of acupuncture in Japan and the United States on dental pain perception. Pain, 12:319, 1982.
42. Chapman, C.R., et al.: Naloxone fails to reverse pain thresholds elevated by acupuncture: Acupuncture analgesia reconsidered. Pain, 16:13, 1983.
43. Clark, W.C., and Yang, J.C.: Acupunctural analgesia? Evaluation by signal detection theory. Science, 184:1096, 1974.
44. Norton, G.R., et al.: The effects of belief on acupuncture analgesia. Can. J. Behav. Sci./Rev. Can. Sci. Comp., 16:22, 1984.
45. Melzack, R., and Jeans, M.: Acupuncture analgesia. Minn. Med., 57:161, 1974.
46. Price, D.D., et al.: A psychophysical analysis of acupuncture analgesia. Pain, 19:27, 1984.
47. Melzack, R., and Wall, P.D.: The Challenge of Pain. New York, Basic Books, 1983.
48. Andersson, S.A., et al.: Electro-acupuncture. Effect on pain threshold measured with electrical stimulation of teeth. Brain Res., 63:393, 1973.
49. Sung, Y.F., et al.: Comparison of the effects of acupuncture and codeine on post-operative dental pain. Anesth. Analg. Curr. Res., 56:473, 1977.
50. Lewith, G.T.: How effective is acupuncture in the management of pain? J.R. Coll. Gen. Pract., 34:275, 278, 1984.
51. Lewith, G.T., and Machin, D.: On the evaluation of the clinical effects of acupuncture. Pain, 16:111, 1983.
52. Syrjala, K.L., and Chapman, C.R.: Measurement of clinical pain: A review and integration of research findings. In Advances in Pain Research and Therapy, Vol. 7. Edited by C. Benedetti, C.R. Chapman, and G. Moricca. New York, Raven Press, 1984, pp. 71–101.
53. Mendelson, G.: Acupuncture analgesia. I. Review of clinical studies. Aust. N.Z. J. Med., 7:642, 1977.
54. Richardson, P.H., and Vincent, C.: Acupuncture for the treatment of pain: A review of evaluative research. Pain, 24:15, 1986.
55. Lewith, G.T., Fields, J., and Machin, D.: Acupuncture compared with placebo in post-herpetic pain. Pain, 17:261, 1983.
56. Dyck, P.J., Lambert, E.H., and O'Brien, P.C.: Pain in peripheral neuropathy related to rate and kind of fiber degeneration. Neurology, 26:466, 1976.
57. Wilkinson, J.: Cervical Spondylosis: Its Early Diagnosis and Treatment. Philadelphia, W.B. Saunders, 1971.
58. Sharpless, S.K.: Supersensitivity-like phenomena in the central nervous system. Fed. Proc., 34:1990, 1975.
59. Thesleff, S., and Sellin, L.C.: Denervation supersensitivity. Trends Neurol. Sci., TINS, 3:122, 1980.
60. Willison, R.G.: Spontaneous discharges in motor nerve fibers. In Abnormal Nerves and Muscles Impulse Generators. Edited by W.J. Culp and J. Ochoa. New York, Oxford University Press, 1982, pp. 383–392.
61. Klein, L., Dawson, M.H., and Heiple, K.G.: Turnover of collagen in the adult rat after denervation. J. Bone Joint Surg. [Am.], 59:1065, 1977.
62. Gunn, C.C., and Milbrandt, W.E.: Early and subtle signs in low back sprain. Spine, 3:267, 1978.
63. Gunn, C.C., and Milbrandt, W.E.: Tennis elbow and the cervical spine. Can. Med. Assoc. J., 114:803, 1976.
64. Bradley, W.G.: Disorders of Peripheral Nerves. Oxford, Blackwell Scientific Publications, 1974.
65. Thomas, P.K.: Symptomatology and differential diagnosis of peripheral neuropathy: Clinical features and differential diagnosis. In Peripheral Neuropathy, Vol. 2. Edited by P.J. Dyck, et al. Philadelphia, W.B. Saunders, 1984, pp. 1169–1190.
66. Gunn, C.C., and Milbrandt, W.E.: Tenderness at motor points—a diagnostic and prognostic aid for low back injury. J. Bone Joint Surg. [Am.], 58:815, 1976.
67. Gunn, C.C.: Transcutaneous neural stimulation, acupuncture and the current of injury. Am. J. Acupunct., 6:191, 1978.

68. Ross, R. and Vogel, A.: The platelet-derived growth factor. Cell, *14*:203, 1978.
69. Gunn, C.C., and Milbrandt, W.E.: Acupuncture loci: A proposal for their classification according to their relationship to known neural structures. Am. J. Chin. Med., *4*:183, 1976.
70. Melzack, R., Stillwell, D.M., and Fox, E.J.: Trigger points and acupuncture points for pain: Correlations and implications. Pain, *3*:3, 1977.
71. Ernest, M., and Lee, M.H.M.: Sympathetic vasomotor changes induced by manual and electrical acupuncture of the Hoku Point visualized by thermography. Pain, *21*:25, 1985.
72. Gunn, C.C., and Milbrandt, W.E.: Dry needling of muscle motor points for chronic low-back pain; a randomized clinical trial with long-term follow-up. Spine, *5*:279, 1980.

91 · NUTRITION AND PAIN

JOHN J. BONICA

with contributions by

GIUSEPPE MAGGIO

THIS chapter discusses the relationship between diet, nutrition, health, disease, and pain. Nutrition can be defined as the sum of the processes concerned in growth, maintenance, and repair of the living body as a whole or its constituent parts (1). Malnutrition results when any component process—dietary intake, digestion, absorption, assimilation, metabolism, or excretion—is interfered with to such an extent that the physical and emotional well-being of the person are altered and replaced by illness or ill-being. Equally important is that malnutrition can be the consequence of a disease that interferes with one or more of these processes. In addition, pain, the most common phenomenon associated with disease, can and often does interfere with nutrition by provoking affective (mood) and physical alterations that decrease or eliminate appetite and alter the functions of the gastrointestinal tract and of metabolism. In such circumstances, effective relief of pain contributes to the overall care of the patient and helps to promote well-being.

This relationship between nutrition, health, and disease was a pre-eminent concept of the ancient Greek, Egyptian, Indian, Chinese, and Hebrew physicians. The strict dietary laws of the ancient Hebrews were intended to prevent disease, and when patients suffered from painful disorders special diets were prescribed. Hippocrates firmly believed, taught, and practiced this concept, because he repeatedly stated that "your medicine shall be your food and your food shall be your medicine" (2). The *Corpus Hippocraticum*, which reflects the medical spirit and methods of this venerated physician, contains specific diets for particular illnesses, including those with pain as a predominant symptom. Diet for the treatment of specific diseases continued to be important for treating painful disorders during medieval times and the renaissance.

With the advent of physiology as an experimental science at the beginning of the nineteenth century, there began a systematic study of the physiology of digestion, absorption, assimilation, and metabolism of food. During the ensuing century the study of nutrition progressed, albeit slowly. Advances in science and technology have been applied to the study of nutrition at the molecular level in the last 35 years (1). Conse-quently, a vast amount of new information has been acquired about the biologic, biochemical, and physiologic aspects of nutrition in those who are well, and also about the pathophysiologic and biochemical alterations that occur in those with various physical and mental disorders. In this chapter no attempt is made to discuss the basic and clinical aspects of these various disease states; these are described elsewhere (1).

Surprisingly, the subject of this chapter has been relatively neglected. Search of the literature reveals few published studies on the effect of pain on the nutritional status of patients who have undergone surgery or have been subjected to serious external injuries, and on those who have an acute or chronic painful visceral disease. Patients with cancer-related pain suffer from serious nutritional problems, but effect of pain on their nutritional status has not been defined. Similarly, patients with persistent nonmalignant chronic pain undergo progressive physical deterioration, in part as a result of nutritional problems, and the influence of the pain has also not been defined. Moreover, little is known about how diet and malnutrition produce painful disorders.

In this chapter I attempt to summarize the available information on this subject and to extrapolate it to support recommendations for the relief of pain as part of the overall therapeutic strategy. The material is presented in five major sections: A, Acute Pain and Nutrition, which describes the relationship of acute pain caused by surgery, trauma, and visceral disease to the alteration of nutrition in these patients and provides suggestions regarding methods of relieving the pain; B, Nutrition and Pain in Cancer Patients; C, Nutrition and Chronic Nonmalignant Pain, which describes such disorders as arthritis, headache, myofascial syndromes, some chronic visceral diseases, and neurologic disorders; and D, Nutritional Manipulation of Brain Neuroregulators for Treating Chronic Pain. Although I wrote the entire chapter, my friend Maggio, a full-time algologist practicing in Lugano, Switzerland, provided a comprehensive review of the literature and his own data on the role of nutrition as part of an integrated treatment program for patients with various nonmalignant chronic pain syndromes.

A. ACUTE PAIN AND NUTRITION

Trauma-Induced Acute Pain

The response of the human body to injury is summarized in Table 7-2 (page 177) and discussed on pages 176–177, 369–371, and 463–465. Noxious stimulation that produces tissue destruction, whether caused by surgery or injury (e.g., crush injury, fracture, burns), results in a local inflammatory reaction that is considered to be useful for healing. This reaction is a defense against infection and provokes a general response in the form of endocrine and metabolic activation, leading to hypermetabolism and an acceleration of most biochemical reactions, including substrate mobilization. The endocrine and metabolic changes produced by neurophysiologic segmental and suprasegmental reflexes (3–6) help to mobilize substrate from storage to central organs and traumatized tissues, resulting in a catabolic state and negative nitrogen balance. The degree and duration of these endocrine and metabolic changes are related to the degree and duration of tissue damage, and many biochemical changes last for days and sometimes weeks (4–7). Cortical responses include the perception of pain as an unpleasant sensation and a negative emotion and also the initiation of the psychodynamic mechanisms of anxiety, apprehension, and fear. These, in turn, greatly enhance the hypothalamic responses and produce cortically mediated increases in blood viscosity, clotting time, fibrinolysis, and platelet aggregation (see Chapter 7 for refs.). Cortisol and catecholamine responses to anxiety usually exceed the hypothalamic response that is provoked directly by nociceptive impulses reaching the hypothalamus (page 176).

The release mechanisms of the stress response involve afferent nociceptive input into the neuraxis through somatosensory and sympathetic afferent pathways, which produce the segmental and suprasegmental responses and efferent impulses from the hypothalamus and spinal cord that pass peripherally through efferent sympathetic pathways (Chapters 7, 22, and 25). Somatomotor efferent impulses are the result of segmental reflexes and produce increased skeletal muscle tension that progresses to spasm. In addition to nociceptive input, other factors that can enhance or amplify the stress response include hemorrhage, even of small magnitude and unaccompanied by hypotension, which activates atrial receptors (4), and acidosis, hypoxia, heat loss and, importantly, such psychologic factors as anxiety, apprehension, and fear (see above).

Pain and the neuroendocrine responses produced by tissue injury are responsible for alterations in the mechanisms of nutrition and in nutritional requirements during and after surgery or accidental trauma. Pain and reflex responses cause a decrease or loss of appetite, a marked decrease or inhibition of gastrointestinal function, with a consequent marked delay in gastric emptying, an increase in total colonic transit time, and an increase in the accumulation of nitrogen. Pain also decreases appetite and, if severe, can cause nausea and even vomiting, thus impairing oral intake. Moreover, the combined effects of increases in the epinephrine, glucagon, cortisol, growth hormone, and free fatty acid levels and of a concomitant decrease in the insulin level cause hepatic glycogenolysis and gluconeogenesis, resulting in hyperglycemia, glucose intolerance, and insulin resistance. Major trauma is accompanied by the release of cortisol, epinephrine, glucagon, and interleukin, which causes muscle protein catabolism with increased protein turnover and increased protein breakdown that exceeds protein synthesis. Increased secretion of catecholamines, cortisol, glucagon, and growth hormone causes increased lipolysis, lipid turnover, and

oxidation. Concomitantly, various catabolic hormones and other factors cause retention of water and sodium, increased secretion of potassium, and decreased fraction of extracellular fluid, which shifts to intracellular compartments. Most parameters of specific and nonspecific immunofunction also decrease in activity.

Other deleterious effects of pain and the neuroendocrine reflex response that complicate the nutritional status indirectly include pulmonary complications, cardiovascular disturbances, prolonged bed rest as a result of persistent pain, and a decrease of food or fluid intake, or of both, either consequent to the effects on the gastrointestinal tract or as prescribed by the surgeon or physician for patients with dysfunction of the gastrointestinal tract. All these effects prolong convalescence and hospitalization. Further discussion of the details of these neuroendocrine responses can be found elsewhere (pages 176–177, 369–371, and 463–465).

Pain and Nutrition in the Surgical Patient

The neuroendocrine and metabolic responses described above and in Chapter 25 occur in all surgical patients, but their magnitude and duration are to a large extent determined by the preoperative condition of the patient, the degree and duration of surgical trauma, the type, quality, and extent of anesthesiologic management, and the postoperative care (Chapter 25).

Phases of Surgical Convalescence

All surgical patients experience four stages of postoperative convalescence (4, 8). The first period, consisting of catabolism initiated by the physical insult induced by the operation, inadequate nutrition, and alteration of the hormonal environment, was termed the "adrenergic-corticoid phase" by Moore (8). This period is followed by a brief period of anabolism, which occurs at a variable time during convalescence. In general, in the absence of postoperative complications, this phase is said to start 3 to 6 days after an abdominal operation such as gastrectomy, often concomitant with the commencement of oral feeding (4). This "turning point" from catabolism to anabolism, referred to as the "corticoid-withdrawal phase" because it is characterized by spontaneous sodium and free water diuresis, a positive potassium balance, and a reduction in nitrogen excretion, is a short transitional phase that lasts only 1 to 2 days.

The third phase consists of a prolonged period of early anabolism characterized by positive nitrogen balance and weight gain. Protein synthesis is increased as a result of sustained enteral feedings and is related to the return of lean body mass and muscular strength. The positive nitrogen balance is usually in the range of 2 to 4 g of nitrogen/day, representing a daily gain of 60 to 120 g of lean tissue. The total amount of nitrogen ultimately gained equals the amount lost, but the rate of gain is much slower than the rate of initial loss. The fourth and final phase of surgical convalescence is late anabolism, characterized by much slower weight gain. During this period the patient is in nitrogen equilibrium but in positive carbon balance, which results from the deposition of body fat.

Role of the Metabolic Response

Early investigators who studied the catabolic response to surgery concluded that negative nitrogen balance was an "obligatory" and irreversible consequence of the metabolic response to injury. Studies that began about 40 years ago, however, have shown that nitrogen balance can be achieved, even in malnourished patients, by providing preoperative or postoperative nutritional support (9). These results spurred numerous laboratory and clinical studies that led to the remarkable current advances in the nutritional support of hospitalized patients. As emphasized by Souba and Wilmore (4), hospitalized patients who 20 years ago might have died from malnutrition, sepsis, and multiple system organ failure because parenteral feedings were not possible or were inadequate can now survive major surgical procedures, multiple trauma, and severe debilitating diseases because of recent advances in nutrition. Almost all hospitalized patients can now be fed safely and with varying degrees of effectiveness as a result of three developments: (a) the technique of central venous cannulation and infusion with hypertonic nutrient solutions directly into the superior vena cava; (b) the introduction of specific enteral formula diets, which can usually be delivered by a feeding tube; and (c) the availability of fat emulsions for safe intravenous administration. These advances, together with improvements in anesthesia, ventilatory support, and intensive care, the development of new antibiotics, and the preservation and administration of blood and blood products, have drastically reduced surgical morbidity and mortality rates.

These recent developments and new information about surgery and anesthesia suggest that the long-held concept that intraoperative and postoperative biochemical changes caused by surgical injury need *not* necessarily be considered to be a homeostatic response important for survival and for restitution of the patient to preoperative status (5, 6). Kehlet (5, 6, 10) has stated that modern surgery and anesthesia can prevent physiologic disturbances or, if they do occur, they can be repeatedly and successfully treated because substrates, blood, and other fluids are now readily available. The emphasis has thus been shifted to concern about the detrimental effects of surgery and anesthesia, such as increased demand on various organs, pulmonary complications, thromboembolism, myocardial infarction, fatigue and weakness that prolong convalescence, hospitalization, and delayed return to work. These deleterious effects, which were previously considered (justly or unjustly) to be caused by surgical imperfections or less than optimal anesthesia, or both, are the consequences of the pain and the associated stress response, and have led to studies of effective methods of modulating the response to surgical and accidental trauma. Kehlet (5, 6, 10) has suggested that, with the availability of current therapy, the stress response might have become maladaptive. The above-mentioned morbidity in high-risk surgical patients might therefore be reduced by inhibiting the surgically induced endocrine response, hypermetabolism, and resulting increased demands on body mass and physiologic reserves (6, 10).

Modification of Stress Metabolic Response

Recent studies have shown that the neuroendocrine response to surgery and to other trauma can be blunted or eliminated by neural blockade with a local anesthetic. This confirms the hypothesis of anociassociation proposed some 80 years ago by Crile (11), who suggested that nociceptive impulses provoked by operation could be blocked by prior infiltration of the site of the surgical incision with a local anesthetic, thus preventing the impulses from reaching the neuraxis and avoiding some of the harmful effects of surgery. Crile suggested that, if the patient required general anesthesia, infiltration of the operative site with a local anesthetic after the patient was unconscious would prevent shock. In contrast, Cannon (12) demonstrated the importance of the sympathetic nervous system in maintaining homeostasis in response to various stresses, such as hemorrhage, cold, and fluid deprivation. Crile's theory was supported by subsequent experimental studies in animals, however, which showed that induction of spinal anesthesia prior to application of blunt trauma to the hindlimb reduced shock and death (13).

In the 1st edition of this book I cited over 50 studies (14) on the use of various forms of regional anesthesia to prevent nociceptive input during and after surgical operations, thus avoiding some of the complications caused by the segmental and suprasegmental reflex responses. In Chapter 25 I cite recent reports pertaining to the use of various techniques of regional anesthesia with a local anesthetic, especially continuous epidural analgesia in the management of intraoperative and postoperative pain. This method markedly reduces or completely eliminates the neuroendocrine response, provided that the afferent and efferent neural pathways supplying the operative regions are interrupted. Thus, a regional blockade of T4 to S5 prevents changes in most of the catabolic hormones and in metabolic responses in patients undergoing abdominal hysterectomy, prostatectomy, hip replacement, or surgery of the lower limbs (see ref. 6). The addition of celiac plexus block, using a sufficient volume of a dilute solution of local anesthetic to block the phrenic plexus, to continuous epidural block of T4 to S5 inclusive produces beneficial effects in patients undergoing upper abdominal surgery (15).

Other reports support the results of the studies cited in Chapter 25 pertaining to the beneficial effects of regional anesthesia and analgesia on the neuroendocrine response during and after surgery, and on the incidence of postoperative complications as compared to those that occur with the use of general anesthesia (10, 16–21). Only a few examples pertaining to different techniques and operations are presented here.

Teasdale and associates (17) carried out a randomized control trial to compare local anesthesia (LA) to general anesthesia (GA) for short-stay inguinal hernia repair patients and noted that postoperatively those in the LA group could walk, eat, and pass urine much earlier than those in the GA group. The GA group of patients experienced a three- to five-fold increase in sore throat, vomiting, and headache and a two-fold increase in nausea as compared with those in the LA group at 6 and at 24 hours postoperatively.

In a prospective study to compare three postanalgesic regimens in 75 patients who underwent cholecystectomy with general anesthesia, Cuschieri and co-workers (18) randomly allocated 25 patients to be given continuous epidural analgesia (CEA) for 24 hours, 25 patients to be given intermittent intramuscular morphine (IIM), and 25 patients to be given continuous intravenous infusion of morphine (CIIM). Patients receiving CEA had more effective analgesia than patients receiving IIM or CIIM ($p < 0.0001$). Moreover, Pa_{O_2} values were also significantly higher in those in the CEA group for the first three postoperative days than in those in the CIIM and IIM groups ($p < 0.05$). In the IIM group the incidence of atelectasis was 40% and the incidence of pulmonary infection was 24%, for a total of 64% with pulmonary complications. In the CII group the rates were 28, 20, and 48% respectively, and in the CEA group the rates were 20, 1, and 21% respectively. Epidural analgesia for 12 hours has a profound and long-lasting effect on pulmonary function and on decreasing the incidence of postoperative pulmonary complications. Presumably the ability to breathe deeply and cough during the immediate postoperative period reduces small airway closure and atelectasis and helps to prevent the subsequent development of chest infection.

TABLE 91-1. Comparison of Continuous Epidural Anesthesia and Analgesia (CEAA) and General Anesthesia (GA) in High-Risk Surgical Patients

Parameter	CEAA (28 patients)*	GA (25 patients)*
Patient characteristics (preoperative)		
ASA physical status	2.8 ± 0.6	2.8 ± 0.8
Goldman index	9.1 ± 7	7.3 ± 4
Age (years)	71.2 ± 10	71.5 ± 8
Type of operation:		
Intra-abdominal	13	11
Intrathoracic	5	2
Major vascular	10	12
Baseline cortisol excretion: (μg/h)	10.3 ± 6	21.6 ± 11
Duration of CEAA	31	
Postoperative course		
Cortisol urinary excretion (μg/h) during 1st 24 h	37.2 ± 27	73.8 ± 62
Mortality	0	4
Morbidity (total no. in group)		
Cardiovascular failure	4	13
Respiratory failure	3†	8
Renal failure	1	3
Hepatic failure	1	2
GI failure	0	1
Major infections	2	10
Complication rate		
No. of patients with 1 or more complications	9	19
Percent of patient group	32	76
Economic impact		
ICU (days)	2.5	5.7
Intubation (h)	7.1	81.8
Hospital costs ($)	11,218	20,380
Physician costs ($)	3,801	5,134

*Figures rounded to nearest unit or decimal.
†Two of the 3 patients had a nonfunctioning epidural catheter.
Data from Yeager, M.P., et al.: Epidural anesthesia and analgesia in high-risk surgical patients. Anesthesiology, 66:729, 1987.

Perhaps one of the most important studies published recently was that by Yeager and associates (19), who conducted a randomized controlled clinical trial to evaluate the effects of continuous epidural anesthesia for surgery and analgesia for postoperative pain relief (CEAA) and general anesthesia (GA) on postoperative morbidity rates in a group of high-risk surgical patients. Of a total of 53 patients admitted to the study, 28 received CEAA and 25 received standard GA and standard analgesia during the postoperative period. This high-risk group consisted of patients scheduled for intrathoracic, intra-abdominal, or major vascular surgery whose preoperative evaluation by the surgical staff indicated that they would require intensive care because of the severity of pre-existing disease, magnitude of the anticipated surgical procedure, or both. Table 91-1 compares patient characteristics, postoperative course, complication rates, and economic impact for those in both groups. The CEAA patients received uninterrupted analgesia for an average of 31 hours. Cortisol levels during surgery and in the immediate postoperative period, as well as during the first 24 hours, were significantly lower in the CEAA group than in the GA group. Thus, epidural analgesia markedly minimizes one of the parameters of the neuroendocrine response during the operation and for the first operative day and has even longer lasting effects on the lungs and other organs. Moreover, there was significantly less morbidity and mortality in CEAA patients than in GA patients. The total hospital costs for those in the CEAA group were 55% of those in the control group, and the cost of physicians' services of the CEAA group was 74% of the control group. Notwithstanding the small number of cases, these important data provide evidence of the advantages of regional anesthesia for certain high-risk patients.

Postoperative Analgesia and Nutrition

The results of studies by Yeager and associates (19) and by others (Chapter 25) show that regional analgesia with local anesthetic is highly effective in controlling postoperative pain and reducing postoperative neuroendocrine and metabolic responses. Figures 91-1 and 91-2 illustrate the beneficial effects of continuous epidural analgesia for only 24 hours postoperatively on three parameters of the postoperative neuroendocrine response (in addition to those in Chapter 25). Blockade during surgery and for the ensuing 24 hours produces beneficial effects that lasted 5 to 7 days, which shows the importance of interrupting the input during this critical period to produce longer lasting benefits.

Although patient-controlled analgesia (PCA) and continuous epidural opioid analgesia (CEOA) are now being used more frequently than regional analgesia with a local anesthetic during the postoperative period, the latter is more effective in reducing the postoperative neuroendocrine and metabolic responses than PCA and CEOA (Fig. 25-9, page 743). Regional analgesia is more effective than epidural opioids in relieving the excruciating pain associated with reflex muscle spasm that occurs frequently after major joint surgery and laminectomy (Chapters 72 and 74). Regional anesthesia can relieve pain prior to amputation and reduce or eliminate the incidence of phantom limb pain

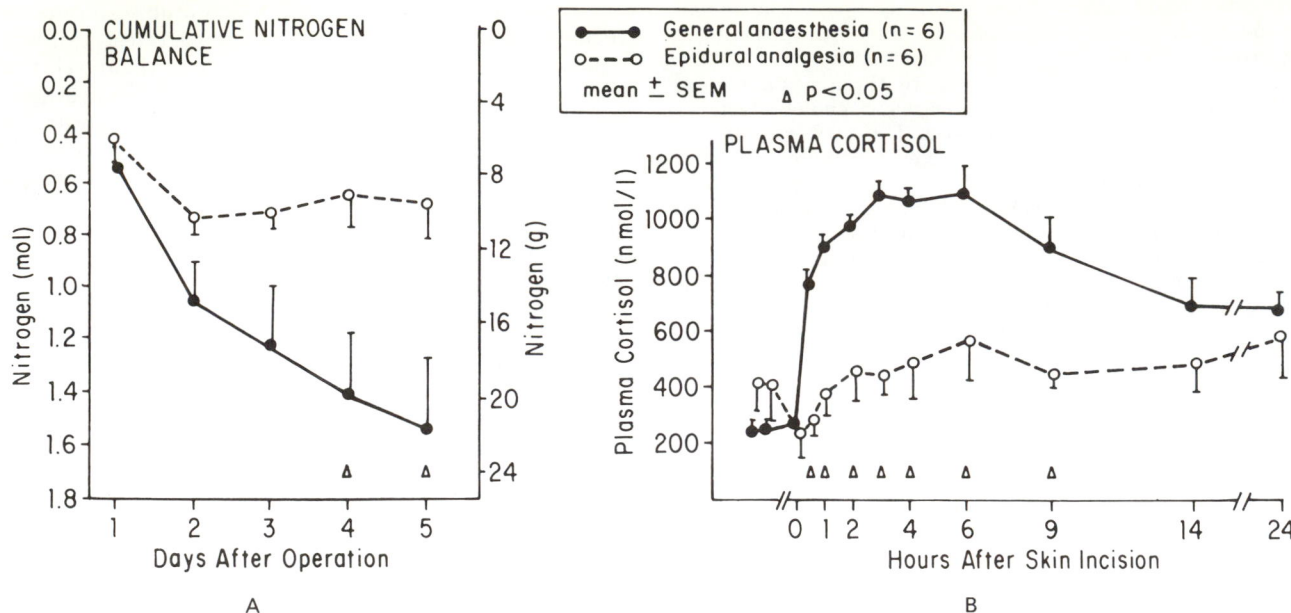

FIG. 91-1. Comparison of the influence of general anesthesia with halothane to that of continuous epidural anesthesia or analgesia on postoperative nitrogen balance in 12 women undergoing elective abdominal hysterectomy. The epidural anesthesia given to half of the patients was achieved by injection of 0.5% bupivacaine, which produced analgesia at the T4–S5 level inclusive that continued for the 24 hours following the operation. During this first day patients received only isotonic saline solution intravenously and tap water orally while, during the ensuing 4 days they were given oral nutrition that provided 20 g of nitrogen and about 2,900 calories. **A.** Cumulative nitrogen balance in the 12 patients. Patients who had epidural analgesia were in nitrogen balance from the second day after the operation, whereas those who had general anesthesia showed a negative balance throughout the study. This provided impressive evidence that blockade for 24 hours has a lasting effect on urinary nitrogen excretion. **B.** The plasma cortisol level increased in all patients with general anesthesia after the skin incision, whereas no significant changes were observed in patients receiving continuous epidural analgesia. Epidural analgesia also produced no intraoperative or postoperative increase in the glucose concentration. From Brandt, M.R., et al.: Epidural analgesia improves postoperative nitrogen balance. Br. Med. J., *1*:1106, 1978.

(Chapter 94). Other studies have also shown that the administration of local or regional anesthesia to those patients who require general anesthesia delays the onset of postoperative pain 8 to 10 hours after surgery, compared to 2 hours when only general anesthesia is used (Chapters 25 and 94). Modig (20) compared the CEAA and general anesthesia on patients undergoing total hip replacement and noted a much lower incidence of thromboembolism.

Because regional analgesia produces effective pain relief, does not cause nausea and vomiting, reduces or prevents the reflex-induced inhibition of the gastrointestinal tract that occurs with the use of systemic opioids, and permits early oral feeding and early ambulation, a shorter convalescent and hospital stay result. Pflug and associates (21), while in my department, compared continuous epidural analgesia with morphine analgesia in 16 patients who had major hip surgery and found that those in the regional analgesia group had a more benign postoperative course. This was manifested by earlier ambulation and earlier return of appetite. The mean hospital stay was 4.7 days for these patients as compared to 8.9 days for those managed with systemic analgesics. Kehlet (10) cited other studies showing that neural blockade reduced the duration of hospitalization.

Postoperative Nutritional Support

The type of surgery is most important in determining and evaluating nutritional needs, nutritional sup-port, and their relation to postoperative pain for patients undergoing elective surgery. These can be separated into four categories: (a) those who have surgery involving the alimentary tract (mouth, pharynx, esophagus, and gastrointestinal tract); (b) those who undergo intra-abdominal surgery that does not involve the gastrointestinal tract; (c) those who have intrathoracic and major back surgery; and (d) those who have superficial operations on the neck, body, and extremities. Patients in the first three groups have a higher incidence of severe pain than those in the last category, especially with movement, and parenteral opioids as usually administered rarely provide complete relief. Surgery on the gastrointestinal tract mandates that oral feeding be withheld for a number of days; in addition, these patients and those in the second category usually develop loss of gastrointestinal tone that progresses to varying degrees of ileus as a result of the intraoperative surgical manipulation. This is enhanced by the sympathetic hyperactivity that is part of the postoperative neuroencodrine response provoked by the surgical wound.

All these factors play a role in the production of a catabolic state, negative nitrogen balance, loss of protein, decrease in muscle mass, and consequently in delayed ambulation and prolonged convalescence and hospitalization. Many of these effects can be minimized, however, by using regional analgesia with local anesthetic for 2 to 3 days postoperatively.

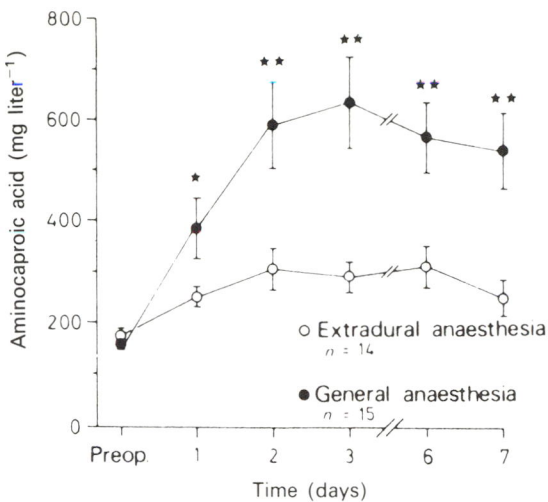

FIG. 91-2. Fibrinolysis inhibition activity (expressed as dilution of aminocaproic acid) in patients undergoing hip replacement under general anesthesia with nitrous oxide/oxygen and fentanyl or with continuous epidural analgesia with intermittent injections of 0.5% bupivacaine with adrenalin for 24 hours. The increase in fibrinolysis inhibition activity in serum was avoided by the use of epidural analgesia. At the same time the patients receiving epidural analgesia also showed higher concentrations of plasminogen activators and increased capacity for release of plasminogen activators; the capacity for activation of factor VIII was significantly reduced. Thus, fibrinolytic function was improved by epidural analgesia. From Modig, J., et al.: Role of extradural and of general anaesthesia in fibrinolysis and coagulation after total hip replacement. Br. J. Anaesth., *55*:625, 1983.

This is now possible because of the recent development of continuous techniques that can provide blockade and analgesia for several days. Such methods have been developed not only for continuous catheter epidural block, but also for intrapleural, intercostal, and brachial plexus blocks, and for blocks of most nerves that contain nociceptive and/or efferent sympathetic pathways, (Chapter 94).

Unfortunately, this form of postoperative pain management to help decrease the catabolic state is not available to most patients, who are usually managed by intramuscular opioids. Moreover, many patients who are well nourished preoperatively and undergo elective intra-abdominal operation do not receive supplemental nutrition to help decrease the catabolic response postoperatively. Usually dextrose solutions are given in sufficient quantities to provide adequate calories that can prevent detrimental losses of endogenous body proteins until patients begin to eat, usually on day 5, 6, or 7 after intra-abdominal surgery. Souba and Wilmore (4) have shown that parenteral intravenous nutrition markedly reduces the degree of negative nitrogen balance (Fig. 91-3). Even though they admitted that a balanced nutrient intake in the postoperative period reduces the negative nitrogen balance associated with elective surgery and helps to maintain body weight, they believe that

this approach is unwarranted in most patients undergoing elective operations [because] such feedings have not improved recovery rates or diminished postoperative complica-

tions in this particular group of patients. Therefore, the increased cost of feeding and the potential complications associated with intravenous nutrition cannot be justified (4).

In addition to their own experiences, they supported this position by citing two reports published in the 1970s. Figure 91-4 shows that the negative nitrogen balance can be reduced by 50% in patients managed with regional analgesia but not given nutrition. The combination of regional analgesia and nutritional support produces a positive nitrogen balance and shortens the hospitalization period.

In contrast, other studies have shown that nutritional support should be given to eliminate the catabolic state and thus permit patients to be discharged 2 to 4 days after major surgery. Moss and collaborators (22–24), as a result of well-controlled animal studies and clinical observations on patients requiring cholecystectomy or other intra-abdominal operations, have shown that total nutritional support results in the enhancement of DNA and protein synthesis in plasma and at the site of the wound, increases the insulin level, produces a positive nitrogen balance, and accelerates wound healing. In their clinical studies surgery was performed using general anesthesia and a triple-lumen nasogastric tube (Fig. 91-5). One lumen was used to aspirate both the esophagus and stomach, another to inflate a 30- to 40-mm balloon placed in the cardia to prevent swallowing of air, and the third lumen, passed through the pylorus into the duodenum, to permit enteral feeding of Vivonex HN.

Moss and associates (22–25) and others (26, 27) have demonstrated that efficient gastric decompression and postoperative nutritional support not only prevent a catabolic state, but reduce the occurrence of complications. In one study by Moss and colleagues (24), 43 consecutive well-instructed patients who underwent cholecystectomy were compared with a control group of 86 patients treated by the usual standard of care in the same community. Among the 43 patients, 35 (81%) requested no analgesics, whereas the other 8 patients received meperidine (mean, 17 mg) during the initial 24 hours; 40 of the 43 (93%) were discharged within 24 hours of surgery. Patients in a control group required a mean of 4.4 ± 0.3 doses of meperidine (290 ± 25 mg) or its equivalent during their first postoperative day and were discharged in 6.5 ± 0.7 days, with none discharged in less than 3 days.

Moss (25) summarized the procedure that permitted him to discharge 100 patients who underwent elective cholecystectomy within 24 hours of surgery. In addition to the aforementioned procedures, 40 to 50 ml of 0.5% bupivacaine was infiltrated into the cut surface of the peritoneum, fascia, subcutaneous tissue, and skin closure of the abdominal wall. Soon after arrival in the recovery room, a diluted elemental diet (Vivonex HN or TEN), 2,400 to 3,600 kcal/day, was administered through the duodenal tube and 600 kcal/day of glucose was given intravenously, for a total daily intake of 3,000 to 4,200 kcal. To prevent nausea and vomiting and to enhance gastric emptying, 10 mg of metoclopramide (Reglan) was given intravenously every 4 hours until 30 minutes before the nasogastric tube was removed the next morning, after which a general diet was tolerated. Patients were discharged soon thereafter. Among those in this group, 85% received no systemic analgesics, whereas 15% received an oral combination of propoxyphene and acetaminophen (Darvocet-N 100) that was effective. None of the patients discharged within 1 day of surgery developed serious

Fig. 91-3. Metabolic response of a previously healthy subject to an elective colectomy for multiple polyps. The intake is plotted upward from zero, and the output is plotted downward from the top of the intake line. *A.* The patient was given general anesthesia and was hydrated postoperatively with 5% dextrose with appropriate electrolytes, which totaled 3 L/day. On postoperative day (POD) 1 he had a urinary output of 1200 ml, 400 ml of fluid was obtained from the nasogastric tube, and a 2-kg weight gain from fluid retention. On POD 3 he spontaneously diuresed 2800 ml of urine. By POD 5 the nasogastric tube was removed and the patient was started on clear liquids by mouth. PODs 1 to 5 had a 4-day negative nitrogen balance of 54 g. During the 5-day period the patient had a 0 nitrogen intake and received approximately 600 kcal glucose/day. On POD 5 he had lost about 2 kg, half of which was lean body tissue. The patient was discharged on POD 7. *B.* Metabolic response of the same patient in *A* managed the same postoperatively except that he received 3 L of parenteral solution that provided maintenance calories of 2200 kcal/day and 12 g nitrogen/day as a balanced amino acid mixture. From PODs 1 to 5 he had a cumulative loss of 67 g of nitrogen, so that the net balance for the 5 days was −7 g. He lost no weight during his hospital course. Note also the difference in the sodium and potassium balances between *A* and *B*. (Negative balance, *solid black*; positive balance, *dashed area*; oral intake, *white area surrounded by solid line.* From Souba, W.W., and Wilmore, D.W.: Diet and nutrition in the care of the patient with surgery, trauma and sepsis. *In* Modern Nutrition in Health and Disease. 7th Ed. Edited by M.E. Shils and V.R. Young. Philadelphia, Lea & Febiger, 1988.

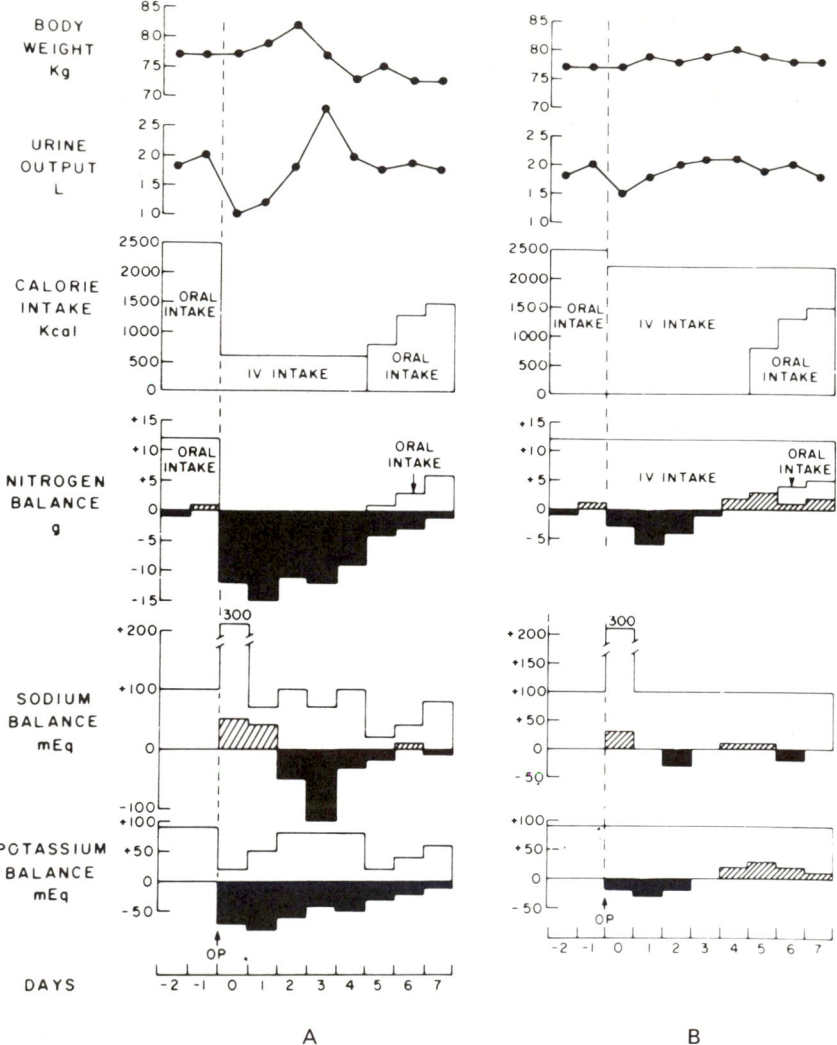

A   B

postoperative complications, and no deaths occurred. Bures-Forsthoefel and associates (26) used the Moss nasoesophagogastroduodenal catheter to provide prompt postoperative supplemental nutrition to 35 patients undergoing abdominal hysterectomy. This group was compared with 35 similar patients who were managed in the usual fashion and did not receive supplemental nutrition. In the first 24 hours after surgery those in the treated group had a positive nitrogen balance of 6.91 g, whereas those in the control group had a negative nitrogen balance of 8.33 g. In addition, the treated patients were discharged earlier than those in the control group.

Moss and others (22–27) have reported that early nutritional support results in a shortened hospital stay without an increase in complications. If their results can be replicated by other trials the procedure should be widely used, because it is not only beneficial to the patient in decreasing convalescence and providing an earlier return to normal function, but is cost-effective (the current rate for a hospital room in the

United States is $400 to $700/day). The advent of the Diagnostic Related Grouping (DRG) program has been the primary factor responsible for the development and proliferation of 1-day ambulatory surgery programs, even for patients requiring major surgery. Most such patients are given regional anesthesia for the procedure, and this produces postoperative pain relief for 6 to 8 hours.

Nutritional Support for High-Risk Patients

Although disagreement apparently exists in regard to providing nutritional support for the well-nourished patient, it is agreed that patients who are preoperatively malnourished or undernourished secondary to intestinal disease (e.g., short bowel syndrome, inflammatory bowel disease, or slow-growing malignant tumors), who have a loss of weight greater than 10%, and who require surgery, should be given preoperative nutritional support (3). Other patients who require postoperative nutritional support are those who are

FIG. 91-4. ***A.*** Metabolic response of a patient who underwent a similar operation to the patient shown in Figure 91-3A managed as described in the legend, with a negative nitrogen balance of 54 g. ***B.*** Metabolic response of patient managed the same as in ***A*** except that he was given continuous epidural anesthesia (T4–S5) for the operation and for postoperative days (PODs 1 and 2). The block of nociceptive afferents and of the sympathetic efferents markedly reduced or abolished the operation-induced neuroendocrine response, particularly the catecholamine, cortisol, ACTH, ADH, aldosterone, and rennin levels, and resulted in a decrease in the insulin level. This resulted in a marked decrease in muscle protein catabolism, hyperglycemia, retention of water and sodium, increased excretion of potassium, and prevention of the usual postoperative shift in amino acid composition in muscle. Because the regional analgesia blocked the sympathetic supply to the gastrointestinal tract during the postoperative period, gastric emptying was not delayed (as with pain and opioid medication), as evidenced by the fact that less than 100 ml of fluid was lost through the nasogastric tube. This, together with the absence of nausea, allowed removal of the nasogastric tube on the morning of the POD 3 and allowed oral intake to begin and to increase rapidly. The urinary output did not decrease during POD 1 as in the patient managed as described in Figure 91-3***A*** and ***B***. Moreover, there was no change in body weight because the usual stress-induced fluid retention did not occur. The degree of negative nitrogen balance was less than half that in ***A*** and, because of the earlier oral intake, the patient had positive nitrogen balance on the POD 3 and on subsequent PODs. Moreover, the sodium and potassium balances were also half those in ***A*** and became positive on POD 4 and 5 respectively. Because the patient could ambulate on the morning of POD 1, he had a more rapid convalescence and was discharged on POD 6. (Negative balance *solid black*, positive balance *stippled areas*, oral intake *dashed areas*.) ***A*** from Souba, W.W., and Wilmore, D.W.: Diet and nutrition in the care of the patient with surgery, trauma and sepsis. *In* Modern Nutrition in Health and Disease. 7th Ed. Edited by M.E. Shils and V.R. Young. Philadelphia, Lea & Febiger, 1988. ***B.*** Theoretical assumptions based on data by Kehlet (10), Brandt et al. (16), and personal observations (unpublished).

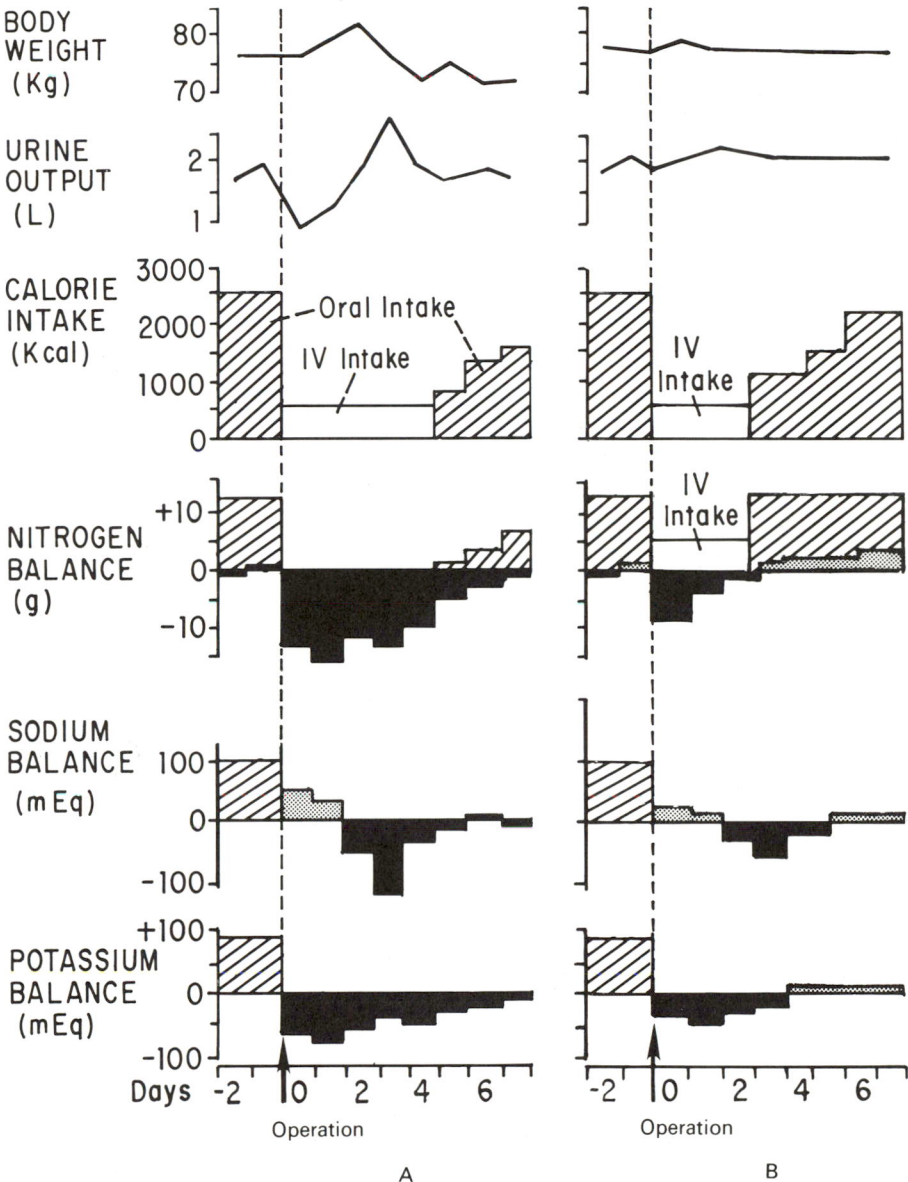

well nourished preoperatively but who develop serious complications following operation, such as prolonged postoperative ileus (3). An even greater number of patients who require postoperative nutritional support are those at increased operative risk or those known to abuse drugs or alcohol (3). Based on the results reported by Yeager and associates (19) and others (17, 18), expertly administered regional analgesia used alone or in combination with light balanced general anesthesia should be used to reduce neuroendocrine and metabolic responses to surgery.

Post-Traumatic Pain

Chapter 22 describes the pathophysiology of major and minor trauma, including neuroendocrine and metabolic responses to accidental injury. Accidental

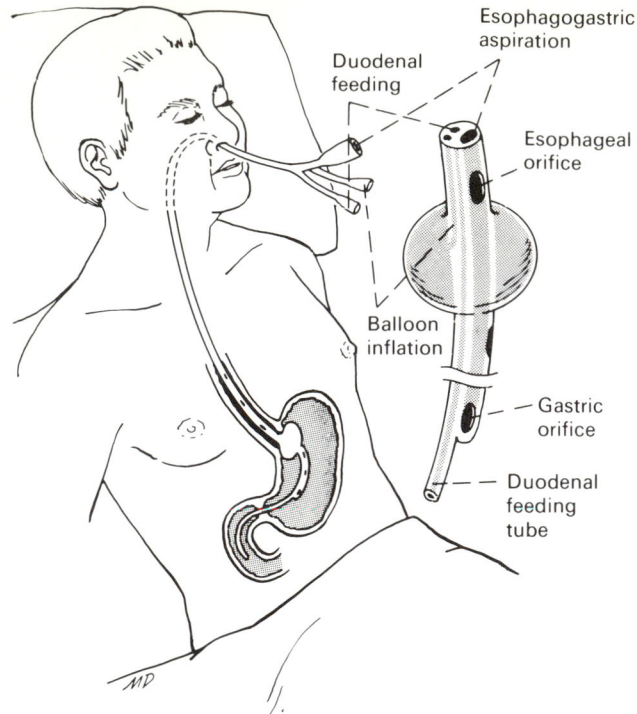

Fig. 91-5. Moss nasoesophagogastroduodenal tube with the balloon in the cardia without tension and the duodenal feeding lumen passed through the pylorus at the time of surgery. The inset depicts an enlargement of the distal part of the tube with the balloon inflated to prevent swallowing of air and showing the three lumina of the tube (the large openings on the side) for aspirating the esophagus and stomach and the duodenal feeding tube (cut). Modified from Moss, G., et al.: Postoperative metabolic patterns following immediate total nutritional support: Hormone levels, DNA synthesis, nitrogen balance, and accelerated wound healing. J. Surg. Res., *21*:383, 1976.

injury is a major cause of death and disability and is the leading cause of death in persons between 5 and 35 years of age in the United States, potentially the most productive segment of the population. Optimal care of the injured patient is often intensive and prolonged, and survival can be followed by years of rehabilitation. Metabolic and nutritional support is an important component of the overall care.

Although altered responses following injury were first described in the 1860s, it was not until the 1930s that careful studies of changes caused by injuries and the integrated response patterns were described by Cuthbertson (28). He divided the time course for most of these post-traumatic responses into two distinct periods, an early "ebb phase" and a subsequent "flow phase." The ebb or shock phase is usually brief (12 to 24 hours), develops immediately following injury, and is manifested by reduced cardiac output, blood pressure, body temperature, and oxygen consumption. These events are often associated with hemorrhage and result in hypoperfusion of tissues and lactic acidosis.

During the flow phase the responses to accidental injury are similar to those described for elective surgical patients, except that the responses are much stronger and extend over a longer period. Figure 91-6 indicates that metabolic rate and nitrogen excretion

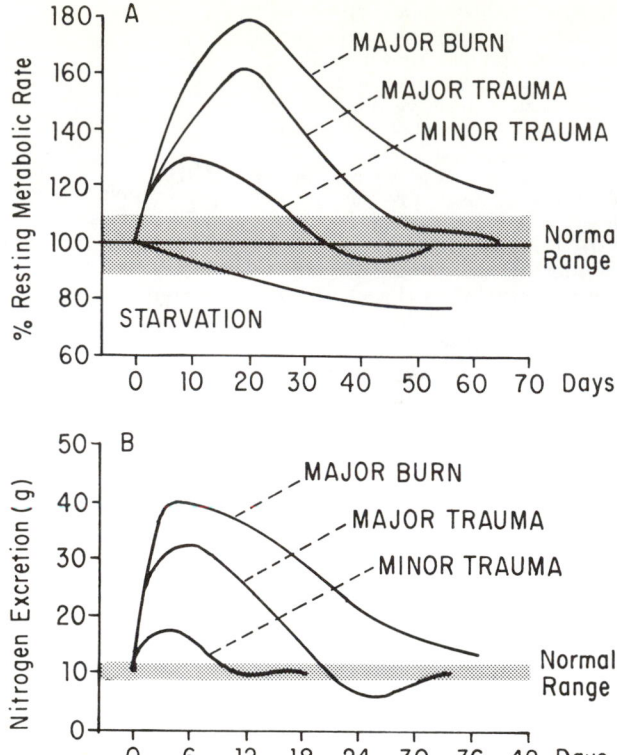

Fig. 91-6. Metabolic rate (**A**) and nitrogen excretion (**B**) are related to the extent of injury. The two responses generally parallel each other. These patients received 12 g of nitrogen/day. From Wilmore, D.W.: The Metabolic Management of the Critically Ill. New York, Plenum Medical Books, 1977.

are related to the extent of injury, with the two responses generally paralleling each other. The increases in metabolism above the basal metabolic rate (BMR) in glucose metabolism, and especially in protein metabolism, have profound effects on the body, and such patients require intensive nutritional support.

HYPERMETABOLISM. The degree of hypermetabolism (defined as an increase in the BMR above that predicted on the basis of age, sex, and body size) is generally related to the severity of injury. Patients with long bone fractures usually develop a 15 to 25% increase in the BMR, those with multiple injuries can have a 50% increase, and those with severe burns (over more than 50% of the body surface area) can have a 200% increase in the BMR (29). Usually concomitant with the development of hypermetabolism, patients develop 1 to 2°C increase in body temperature, a well-recognized component of the injury response that represents an upward shift in the thermoregulatory set point of the hypothalamus.

ALTERED GLUCOSE METABOLISM. Hyperglycemia commonly occurs following trauma, and the elevation of fasting blood sugar levels generally parallels the severity of the stress in the ebb phase (4). During the ebb phase insulin levels are low and glucose production is only slightly elevated. Later, during the flow phase, insulin concentrations are normal or elevated, but hyperglycemia persists; this represents an alteration in the relationship between insulin sensitivity and glucose disposal (4). Hepatic glucose production is increased, and the accelerated gluconeogenesis is generally related to the extent of injury. Much of the new glucose generated by the liver arises from 3-carbon precursors (e.g., lactate, pyruvate, amino acids, and glycerol) released from peripheral tissues (4).

Souba and Wilmore (4) have emphasized that these changes in glucose metabolism have a profound impact on the handling of exogenously administered glucose contained in enteral or parenteral feedings. Whereas administration of glucose increases the rate of glucose disposal in normal individuals, injured patients maintain a constant disposal rate. Moreover, the insulin elaborated by injured patients rises, but this fails to increase glucose clearance. Other studies have shown that glucose loading or insulin infusion, which in normal persons inhibits hepatic glucose production, only partially reduces endogenous production of glucose in trauma patients (see 4 for references). These and other studies indicate that profound insulin insensitivity occurs in injured patients (29).

ALTERED PROTEIN METABOLISM. Extensive urinary nitrogen loss occurs following major trauma, the degree of which depends on the extent of trauma, on nutritional status, and on age and sex, because these factors help to determine the muscle mass (29). In normal subjects nitrogen equilibrium is maintained by a careful balance between the rates of protein synthesis and the rates of degradation, whereas in patients with major trauma the increase in catabolic rate is marked but the increase in synthesis is slight. Because the rate of catabolism exceeds that of synthesis patients develop a negative nitrogen balance, even though they might be receiving a standard infusion of dextrose and water, thus indicating a significant acceleration of nitrogen turnover.

ALTERED FAT METABOLISM. To support hypermetabolism, increased gluconeogenesis, and interorgan substrate flux, stored triglyceride is mobilized and oxidized at an accelerated rate (4). The accelerated rates of lipolysis and oxidation are provoked by increases in catecholamine, cortisol, glucagon, and growth hormone levels, part of the hormonal response to injury. This response can be reduced by regional analgesia for pain relief. If severely injured patients remain unfed they rapidly deplete their fat and protein stores, resulting in a malnutrition that increases their susceptibility to the added stresses of hemorrhage, surgery, and infection, and possibly contributing to organ system failure, sepsis, and death.

Management of Patients with Major Trauma

The care of patients with major multisystem trauma can be divided into three phases: (a) emergency cardiopulmonary resuscitation at the site of injury and during transport to the hospital; (b) advanced life support consisting of treatment of traumatic shock and emergency (resuscitative) surgery, usually beginning in the emergency room and continuing in the operating room; and (c) prolonged life support or intensive therapy. Management during these three phases is discussed in detail in Chapter 22. Expertly administered regional anesthesia (RA), given alone or in combination with general anesthesia, should be used for the initial and subsequent surgical procedures. For reasons given above, RA should be continued during the postoperative intensive care period to provide continuous pain relief and to help reduce hypermetabolism. This is especially important in treating high-risk elderly patients with fracture of the lower or upper limbs and fracture of the pelvis. Obviously, extensive continuous epidural blockade with local anesthetic for surgery of the upper abdomen or chest should *not* be undertaken until hemodynamic stabilization has been accomplished. Alternatively,

intercostal block can be administered by a skilled anesthesiologist or local infiltration of the injured area can be done by the surgeon to decrease the neuroendocrine and metabolic stress responses initiated by the afferent input from the injured area (also see Chapters 22, 25, and 94).

Nutritional Support

Although surgeons disagree as to whether to provide nutritional support to patients who are well nourished prior to elective surgery, it is agreed that all patients who are well nourished at the time of injury should receive nutritional support if they sustain major trauma (4, 29). Obviously this is even more important in patients who are elderly, undernourished, or are at risk because of other disease states. Whereas elective surgical patients managed with insufficient food intake can tolerate a mild catabolic response following surgery, trauma patients cannot because of the accelerated tissue catabolism. Although nutritional support does not appreciably affect the hypermetabolic response associated with severe trauma, the provision of adequate calories and amino acids does reduce the magnitude of net lipogenesis, skeletal muscle proteolysis, and negative nitrogen balance.

After such trauma as fractures, once the wound has been closed and the fracture stabilized, the "obligatory" nitrogen loss can be partly reversed by nutritional means. Figure 91-7 shows the probable (theoretical) clinical course of a 57-year-old male in fairly good health prior to a fall that caused intracapsular fracture of the neck of the femur and managed in 3 different ways. These theoretical assumptions are based on extensive scientific data regarding management without parenteral nutritional support (A), with parenteral nutritional support (B), and with a combination of parenteral nutritional support and the use of continuous epidural analgesia for the operation and for the first 3 postoperative days to provide continuous pain relief and help decrease the hypermetabolic state and loss of nitrogen (C). Note the marked difference in the amount of negative nitrogen balance and weight loss between A and B. By using continuous epidural analgesia for the operation and postoperative pain relief (C), the ileus was obviated, the patient was able to take fluids and later food by mouth, and positive nitrogen balance was restored much earlier than with the management described for A or B.

Combined with other improvements in intensive care, parenteral nutritional support has been shown to reduce mortality and morbidity rates of patients with extensive injuries (4, 29). Nutritional support counteracts protein metabolism and negative nitrogen balance, optimizes wound healing and recovery by increasing synthesis of proteins, and—most important—aids host defenses (4). The development of techniques for intravenous administration of hypertonic nutrient solution, the use of peripheral venous feeding with fat emulsion, and the availability of specific enteral diets have made it possible for virtually all injured patients to receive safe and effective nutritional support (4, 28) (Fig. 91-8).

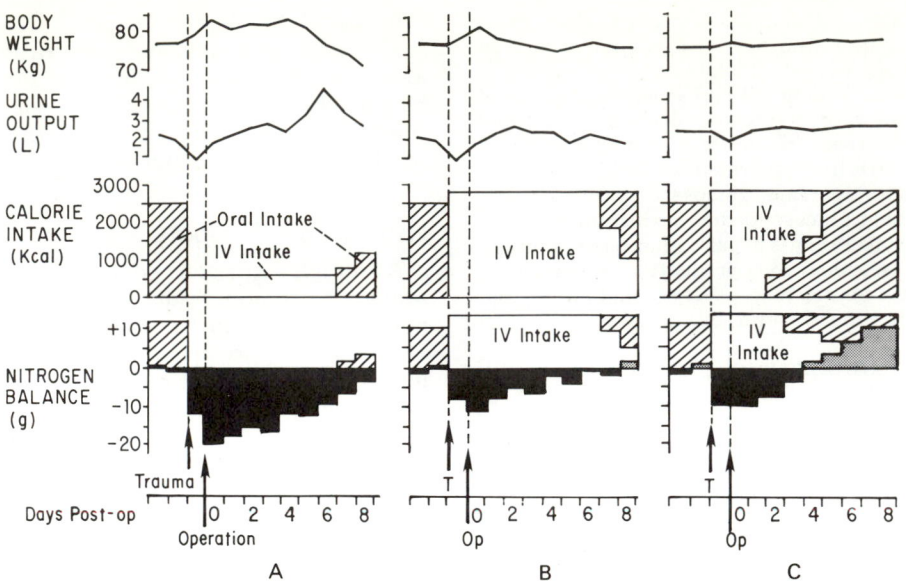

FIG. 91-7. Theoretical metabolic response of a 57-year-old man (76 kg, BSA 1.9 m²) who sustained a fracture of the neck of the femur consequent to a fall from a platform 9 feet above the ground managed in 3 different ways. Active resuscitation with intravenous fluid and blood products was started on admission to the emergency room and the patient was given 10 mg of morphine intramuscularly for the relief of pain. *A.* He was then transferred to the intensive care unit and a nasogastric tube was inserted; by 18 hours after the injury his blood volume was restored. The patient continued to receive an intravenous infusion of 5% dextrose and appropriate electrolytes at a rate of 120 ml/hour (2.9 L/day). He was taken to the operating room for open reduction and fixation under general anesthesia. One hour after surgery the patient complained of moderate to severe pain and was given intramuscular morphine prn while maintained on the intravenous infusion. His urine output during postoperative day (POD) 1 was 1500 ml and he gained 4 kg following fluid retention and resuscitation. The following morning he manifested signs of ileus, which persisted, and consequently was not fed but continued to receive intravenous fluids. On POD 6 the ileus resolved, spontaneous diuresis of 3000 ml ensued, and the patient began to take clear fluids that were gradually advanced to a regular diet over the next 5 days. Nitrogen balance studies from hospital days 1 to 7 revealed a cumulative 7-day nitrogen loss of 121 g. During this 7-day period the patient had 0 nitrogen intake and received 600 kcal glucose/day. By hospital day 8 the patient had lost 4 kg, half of which represented loss of lean body mass. The patient was discharged from the hospital 5 weeks after admission, at which time he had regained his initial body weight. *B.* Same patient as in *A* managed with parenteral nutrition consisting of all essential nutrients and provided by central venous infusion. The 3-L solution delivered 2600 calories/day plus 15 g of nitrogen/day as a balanced amino acid mixture. Nitrogen balance studies showed cumulative losses of 130 g from hospital days 1 through day 7, so that the patient's net nitrogen loss for the 7 days was 30 g. The patient lost 1 kg of body weight during this period. *C.* Same patient as in *A* managed with a combination of continuous epidural analgesia and parenteral nutrition. At the point when the patient's blood volume was considered to have been restored (18 hours postinjury), a catheter was inserted into the lumbar epidural space with its tip at L3 and 15 ml of 0.5% bupivacaine with 1:200,000 epinephrine was injected. This produced anesthesia that extended from the T6 to S5 dermatomes inclusive, with consequent complete pain relief and a mild degree of hypotension (15 mm Hg) that remained stable for 1 hour. Another bolus of 17 ml of bupivacaine with epinephrine was injected 15 minutes before surgery, which produced good anesthesia for the operation. Epidural analgesia was maintained with intermittent injections of bupivacaine at the T6–S5 level for the first 24 hours and the dose was subsequently reduced to provide analgesia from T9–S5, which provided complete pain relief. On the morning of postoperative day (POD) 2 the patient began oral intake with fluids. This was gradually advanced to a regular diet over the next 3 days, at which point the parenteral solution was decreased and then terminated on POD 5. The urinary output was maintained within normal limits because the blockade almost eliminated fluid retention and consequently no increase in body weight occurred as in *A* and *B.* Moreover, a positive nitrogen balance was noted on POD 4, which increased to normal values by POD 8. (Theoretical assumptions of *A* and *B* based on data published by Souba and Wilmore (4) and *C* based on data published by Kehlet (10), Brandt et al. (16), and personal observations (unpublished).)

The goals of nutritional support are the maintenance of body cell mass and the limitation of weight loss to less than 10% of preinjury weight (4). For optimal care it is necessary to evaluate the patient's nutritional status requirements, type of monitoring needed, routes of administration, and specific formulas. This is best achieved by the collaboration of a nutritionist with the surgeon and other members of the surgical team. A detailed description of the various aspects of nutritional management is beyond the scope of this book; further discussion can be found elsewhere (1, 29, 30). Part of the integrated management of these patients is adequate pain relief, by continuous regional analgesia with local anesthetics or by intraspinal opioids or a combination of these.

Acute Pain in Visceral Disease

The pain associated with acute visceral disease in the chest, abdomen, and pelvis is considered in detail in sections C, D, and E of Part IV. Except for acute pancreatitis, most other acute conditions do not incur alteration of nutritional balance of sufficient magnitude to warrant discussion here.

Acute pancreatitis produces severe excruciating pain and massive nociceptive input that provokes the neuroendocrine and metabolic response discussed above in connection with trauma. The reflex muscle spasm and ileus that invariably develop in patients with acute pancreatitis impair ventilation that can advance to progressive respiratory failure and death. Significant nutritional depletion similar to that of other severe gastrointestinal disease occurs, except that specific amino acid deprivation and malnutrition can exacerbate the pancreatic inflammatory process (31).

Pain is most effectively relieved by continuous segmental epidural analgesia with a local anesthetic (Chapter 94). This produces complete pain relief, eliminates reflex skeletal muscle spasm and reflex ileus, and improves ventilation. Nutritional support by the enteral route is contraindicated because ordinary food or even complete oral (full-protein) liquid diets can stimulate the pancreas; together with the concomitant gastrointestinal dysfunction the pathophysiology can be aggravated. Although elemental diets administered through a jejunostomy can provide nutritional support, they do not rest the pancreas completely and require a longer period to restore the lean body mass. In contrast, intravenous nutrition does not stimulate the pancreas, and lean body mass can be restored more rapidly than by the use of the elemental route (31). The combination of prompt institution of continuous epidural analgesia, initial fluid replacement therapy, intravenous nutrition, and other supportive measures can reduce the necessity for surgical intervention and lower the mortality rate. One group reported that, in the course of 6 years, the immediate use of continuous epidural analgesia and nutritional support reduced the need for surgery from 45 to 4% and the mortality rate from 14% to 4% (32).

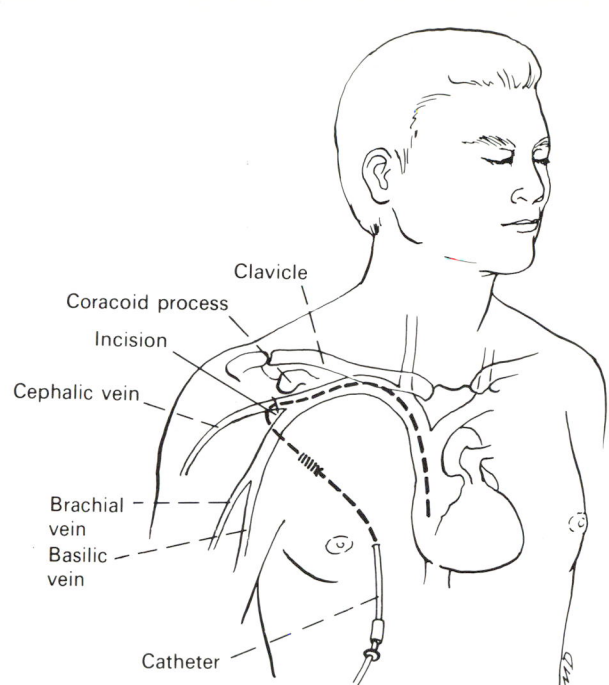

FIG. 91-8. Technique of parenteral infusion in the superior vena cava by the Scribner technique. The catheter is placed into the cephalic vein and its distal end is threaded through the subclavian and superior vena cava through an incision made in the skin. The proximal end of the catheter is tunneled subcutaneously to make its exit in the lower anterior chest. The catheter is then connected with the reservoir for infusion. Modified from Riella, M.C., and Scribner, B.H.: Five years' experience with a right atrial catheter for prolonged parenteral nutrition at home. Surg. Gynecol. Obstet., *143*:205, 1976.

B. NUTRITION AND PAIN IN CANCER PATIENTS

The incidence, severity, and other aspects of cancer-related pain and its treatment are discussed in detail elsewhere (Chapters 24, 45, 52, 57). This section attempts to describe the interrelationship between pain and nutrition in patients with neoplasms. The physical deterioration of cancer patients consequent to malnutrition has been emphasized and is well known (33–38). Little has been written, however, about how pain can contribute to the inadequate nutrition and how different therapeutic modalities for pain relief can affect nutrition.

Etiology of Malnutrition

The most important causes of malnutrition in cancer patients are presented in Table 91-2. No attempt is made here to present a detailed discussion of all the factors that lead to decreased nutrient intake, malabsorption, and increased caloric consumption, but some causes of anorexia, nausea and vomiting, and increased metabolism are reviewed, emphasizing the influence of pain and pain medication.

Decreased Nutrient Intake

ANOREXIA. Although anorexia is recognized as one of the most frequent symptoms in cancer patients (33–37), its causes are not definitely established. Anorexia is manifested most noticeably in patients with cancer in one or more areas of the alimentary tract, especially the liver, stomach, and pancreas, and in patients with widely disseminated disease. It is not present with all types of malignant neoplasms. Thus, women with cancer of the breast are usually not anorexic, even though they might have bone metastasis, but anorexia occurs in such women when the liver becomes involved (34). Its onset is usually insidious and is often unaccompanied by other manifestations of the disease, except progressive weight loss—hence, in patients with unexplained weight loss the physician should search for a neoplasm (33).

Minna and Bunn (35) have theorized that the combination of anorexia, cachexia, asthenia, loss of body tissue, and inability to conserve normal regulatory function of metabolism constitutes a paraneoplastic syndrome. This syndrome bears no correlation to the amount, type, or site of neoplastic tissue, can occur as an early symptom of the disease, or can appear in the presence of bulk neoplasm. The best evidence of the paraneoplastic nature of anorexia syndrome is its appearance before the malignancy is discovered and its disappearance with the resection or control of the tumor.

Although cachexia can result from decreased caloric intake caused by anorexia and tissue change, malabsorption, or a change in body metabolism, experimental evidence suggests that malnutrition alone cannot explain the cachexia in malignancy (38). Thus, in cachexia in patients with cancer, the caloric expenditure remains high and the basal metabolic

TABLE 91-2. Causes of Malnutrition in Cancer Patients

I. Decreased nutrient intake
  A. Anorexia
    1. Systemic effects of tumors
    2. Paraneoplastic syndromes
    3. Changes in taste and smell
    4. Anticancer therapy (surgery, radiation, chemotherapy)
    5. Pain, anxiety, and fear
    6. Depression
  B. Nausea and vomiting
    1. Effect of tumor
    2. Effect of chemotherapy, radiation therapy
    3. Effect of pain medication
    4. Gastrointestinal dysfunction
      a. Ileus
      b. Obstruction
  C. Other possible factors
    1. Decreased zinc level
    2. Naturally occurring and ectopic hormones

II. Malabsorption
  A. Pathology of alimentary tract
    1. Deficiency of pancreatic enzymes, bile salts
    2. Fistula
    3. Blind loop
  B. Effect of radiation, chemotherapy, surgery
  C. Severe malnutrition → villous hypoplasia

III. Increased caloric consumption
  A. Consumption by tumor
    1. 1.5 g tumor requires 153 g glucose/day
    2. Limb with sarcoma requires 500 g glucose/day
  B. Hypermetabolism
    1. Abnormal metabolic pathways—the Cori cycle
    2. Ectopic hormone products
    3. Catabolic effects of therapy
  C. Catabolic cell-derived factors
    1. Cachectin-tumor necrosis factor (TNA)
    2. Interleukin-1
  D. Increased protein kinetics
    1. Increased protein flux, synthesis, breakdown
    2. Anemia and chronic infection

IV. Effects of pain and pain medication

TABLE 91-3. Symptoms of 722 Cancer Patients on Admission to St. Christopher's Hospice in 1985

Symptom	Total (%)	Men (%)	Women (%)
Weakness	91	93	90
Anorexia	76	78	74
Pain	62	61	64
Dyspnea	51	58	47
Constipation	51	56	47
Cough	45	60	33
Nausea, vomiting	44	42	47
Dysphagia	25	28	22
Insomnia	24	25	24

From Baines, M.: Nausea and vomiting in patients with advanced cancer. J. Pain Symptom Management, *3*:81, 1988. Copyright by the U.S. Cancer Pain Relief Committee. Reprinted by permission of Elsevier Science Publishing Co., Inc.

therapy. Anticancer therapies (e.g., surgery, radiation to the abdomen, and chemotherapy) also play a major role in anorexia (33–35).

NAUSEA AND VOMITING. Next to weakness, anorexia, pain, dyspnea and constipation, nausea and vomiting are the most frequent symptoms seen in cancer patients (37) (Table 91-3). Usually nausea and vomiting are caused by chemotherapy, radiation therapy, and gastrointestinal dysfunction, such as ileus and obstruction. Opioids can also contribute to the problem (see below). Each of these factors produces nausea and vomiting by different mechanisms, and the mechanisms are of different types. Acute chemotherapy-induced emesis is the most common type and is seen with almost all the commonly used chemotherapeutic agents (37). Anticipatory emesis is caused by previous experience with the effects of a chemotherapeutic agent and occurs when patients are scheduled to receive a treatment. Delayed emesis is a poorly understood phenomenon in which emesis can begin 1 to 4 days after chemotherapy, even in patients in whom the emesis was well controlled on the day of treatment.

Malabsorption

Malabsorption is a major cause of malnutrition in patients who suffer from pathology of the alimentary tract, such as deficiency of pancreatic enzyme or bile salts, fistulas or blind loop, or as a result of irradiation, chemotherapy, or surgery. Severe malnutrition can produce villous hypoplasia and consequently impair the absorption process.

Increased Caloric Consumption

Tumor consumes glucose and other nutrients. It has been estimated that a 1.5-kg tumor, which represents 2.5% of the usual body weight, consumes 153 g of glucose/day (34). A large sarcoma of the limb can consume 500 g of glucose/day (41). Other causes of increased caloric consumption are listed in Table 91-2.

Bruera and MacDonald (42), in a review article, stated that probably the most important cause of increased consumption of energy is the misuse of metabolic pathways by the tumor through the Cori cycle. The tumor uses glucose from the diet and that produced by gluconeogenesis and from amino acids. The tumor then transforms glucose into lactate that must be reconstituted by the liver at the cost of a large expenditure of energy. This is known as the Cori cycle and has been shown to be significantly increased in patients with advanced cancer (43).

The wasting of cancer patients as a result of the loss of lean body mass and the body's apparent inability to adapt metabolically to impaired intake has been the subject of a number of studies that have shown an increase in protein flux, synthesis, and breakdown (33). Results have indicated that some but not all cancer patients have protein kinetics similar to those of patients whose catabolism has been

rate is increased (in some but not all cancer patients) despite the reduced dietary intake, indicating a derangement of host metabolism. These findings contrast with the lower metabolic rate of normal subjects following starvation. Thus, whereas with starvation in normal subjects the caloric expenditure is lowered, amino acids cease being used for gluconeogenesis, and exogenous glucose is readily oxidized, with malignancy they are not (35). Protein synthesis is maintained in malignancies rather than reduced, as in starvation.

Alterations of taste and perhaps of smell, with consequent aversion to food, have been incriminated as a cause of anorexia (39, 40). If this were the sole cause or even an important factor, however, it could be overcome by conventional methods of enteral or parenteral nutritional support. Changes in taste appear to be factors in anorexia that are associated with more fundamental metabolic changes initiated by tumors and are influenced to some extent by psychologic factors (39, 40).

Theologides (38) has suggested a role for neurotransmitter abnormalities produced by the tumor, which impinge on one or more of the regulatory mechanisms of hunger, satiety, metabolism, or taste and cause disruption of these patterns, thus producing a metabolic "chaotic" state. A related problem is food aversion caused by the tumor (39) or by its treatment (40), or as a learned phenomenon resulting from psychologic processes, especially in children exposed to certain foods in association with unpleasant systemic reactions such as nausea and vomiting consequent to chemo-

affected by severe trauma, sepsis, or chronic infection. When the catabolic rate persistently exceeds the synthetic rate, depletion of body protein occurs in accordance with the degree of discrepancy.

Other studies have suggested that "ectopic" hormones and ectopic peptide production caused by differentiation of malignant cells can produce metabolic, nutritional, electrolyte, and other clinical problems (33). Other factors that might be responsible for a hypermetabolic state include so-called "catabolic cell-derived factors." The cachectin-tumor necrosis factor (TNF), produced by normal macrophages in response to the presence of the tumor, and interleukin-1, produced by monocytes, particularly in patients with Hodgkin's disease and renal cell carcinoma, are the most important of these (33, 44, 45). The cachectin-TNF has been shown to induce a severe decrease in total body fat by inhibiting lipoprotein lipase and therefore the deposition of fat. In addition, it has direct effects on the tumor, including hemorrhage, necrosis, and changes in blood vessels, synovial surfaces, and kidneys, and could be one of the primary mediators of septic shock syndrome (42). The increased production of interleukin-1 in amounts not sufficient to cause fever but enough to cause an increase in the synthesis of protein, increased breakdown of protein, and decreased synthesis of albumin might be responsible for some of the metabolic abnormalities seen in these patients (46).

Influence of Pain and Pain Medication

The deleterious effects of pain, the anxiety often associated with it, and their effects on malnutrition in high-risk surgical and trauma patients suggest that these factors can also affect malnutrition in cancer patients with pain. Whereas the other factors listed in Table 91-2 and less important ones that might influence malnutrition have been studied intensively, I could find no reports of well-controlled studies that define the influence of pain on malnutrition in cancer patients. Two reports suggested that pain might be a factor, but provided no data (47, 48). The only study with possible relevance to this issue was that of Woodforde and Fielding (49), who studied cancer patients with and without pain. They found that patients with pain were significantly more emotionally disturbed than those without pain, and that they responded less well to treatment and died sooner. Evidence has shown that depression in cancer patients, which is often associated with pain, contributes to a decrease in caloric intake. My observations over the past 40 years and those of others (Ventafridda, personal communication, 1988) indicate that severe cancer pain decreases appetite, but that this can be improved with complete relief of the pain with regional anesthesia or neurosurgery. This is particularly important in patients who have pain that interferes with chewing and swallowing. Moreover, because the pain and nociceptive input cause a decrease or complete inhibition of gastrointestinal function, with a consequent delay in gastric emptying, it is likely that this is another factor that contributes to malnutrition. Extrapolation of data from well-controlled studies in surgical and obstetric patients suggests that pain significantly delays gastric emptying and digestion by the small intestine (50, 51) and that complete relief of pain with regional analgesia reverses this effect almost completely (51).

Another issue is the deleterious influence of medication given to relieve pain. Most patients with moderate or severe cancer-related pain are managed with opioids given alone or in combination with nonsteroidal anti-inflammatory drugs (NSAIDs) and adjunctive drugs, and this probably contributes to a decrease in nutrient intake and absorption. Morphine and other strong opioids decrease the secretion of hydrochloric acid in the stomach and decrease its motility; these effects are associated with an increase in tone of the antral portion of the stomach (51, 52). Together with an increase in tone of the first part of the duodenum the passage of gastric contents through the duodenum is delayed for as long as 12 hours, and therapeutic intubation for enteral feeding becomes exceedingly difficult (52). Both biliary and pancreatic secretions are diminished and consequently the digestion of food in the small intestine is delayed. In addition, propulsive contractions are decreased and the tone of the ileocecal valve is enhanced. Following morphine administration propulsive peristaltic waves in the colon are diminished or abolished, the tone of the musculature of the large bowel is increased to the point of spasm, and the tone of the anal sphincter is greatly augmented. All these factors not only impair digestion but cause chronic constipation—a major problem in patients with cancer who are receiving opioids (see Chapter 78).

In view of these considerations and those discussed in the preceding two sections it should prove helpful to give cancer patients with moderate to severe pain, who have malnutrition because of inadequate nutrient intake and perhaps malabsorption, a 1-week trial of regional analgesia achieved with a local anesthetic. This should help to determine its efficacy in relieving the pain and in decreasing the augmented sympathetic action on the gastrointestinal tract that might be responsible for the ileus and for the consequent delay in gastric emptying and impairment of digestion. Techniques are now available that can produce continuous regional analgesia with a local anesthetic for 1 week to control pain in almost any part of the body (Chapter 94). If regional analgesia proves effective, a neurolytic block or an ablative neurosurgical operation should be considered.

If such a trial is undertaken on a patient who has been on opioid analgesics for a prolonged period, induction and maintenance of the procedure require close monitoring of the patient for two problems that could develop. Because regional analgesia promptly removes the pain-induced stimulation of the respiratory center, the patient might develop respiratory depression from the residual effects of the narcotic that were given prior to induction of the regional analgesia. This can be easily managed with naloxone therapy. The second problem is the physical dependence that might have developed. This can be managed by gradually decreasing the dose of the narcotic over several days to prevent development of a withdrawal syndrome.

Treatment of Malnutrition

Goals

Cancer patients who have malnutrition have a reduced response to antineoplastic agents, diminished tolerance to the effects of radiation and chemotherapy, and a higher incidence of infection and other complications from surgical therapy (36, 47, 53, 54). Most of these patients have a high degree of physical and mental fatigue and decreased activity (42). These and other factors contribute to a significant decrease in survival. The obvious goals of successful treatment of malnutrition are improvement in the quality of life and an increased life expectancy.

Indications for Nutritional Support

Nutritional support can be instituted if it can be shown that the metabolic and nutritional defects of the cancer patient are amenable to reversal by such treatment (34). These include restoration of weight loss, which is a known prognostic factor in disease outcome. Clinical and biochemical parameters that suggest the use of or need for nutritional support in any patient whose hospital stay is expected to exceed 15 days and who cannot ingest at least 100 calories daily include the following: (a) weight loss in excess of 10% of pre-illness weight; (b) decrease in serum albumin concentration (less than 3.5 g%); (c) abnormalities in anthropometric indexes, which include triceps skin fold and arm muscular circumference, diminished transferrin and plasma vitamin levels, trace mineral deficiencies, and creatinine:height ratio less than 80% of predicted value; and (d) demonstrated immune incompetence (34, 55). Unfortunately, these parameters are imprecise in individual patients and can be altered by a number of variables, including the degree of hydration (34). Moreover, studies have shown that good correlation between these objective measures and clinical assessment by history and physical examination make these objective tests unnecessary in most of the obvious cases, but they can provide important information in regard to patient follow-up and should be included in research protocols (42).

Patients who are to undergo therapeutically effective anticancer therapy, who have a weight loss of 6% of pre-illness body weight or more, and who have demonstrated deficiency states should be considered for nutritional support (34). Certainly, patients with a weight loss of 15% or more of pre-illness body weight and functional deficits such as decreased energy and impaired wound healing, for whom anticancer therapy is being planned, are definite candidates for nutritional support. Once the decision has been made, two options are available, enteral and parenteral nutrition (Table 91-4).

ENTERAL NUTRITION. Patients who can eat and ingest normally and have a functional gastrointestinal tract should be managed by manipulating food according to need and their choice, and this can be highly effective. This requires a great deal of time and effort, however, on the part of patients and their family (34). Appetite stimulants are useful for patients in whom decreased caloric intake is the principal mechanism of malnutrition. Four agents that are useful for stimulating appetite are metoclopramide, methylprednisolone, cyproheptadine, and progesterone hormones (42).

Metoclopramide, an antidopaminergic drug, is an effective appetite stimulant and is probably the best agent for treating chemotherapy-induced emesis (56), and it significantly enhances gastric emptying. It is especially indicated for patients who have advanced cancer with anorexia or chronic

TABLE 91-4. Options for Nutritional Support in the Cancer Patient

Techniques	Options
Enteral	
Increased oral feeding	Involve the family
Specific digestive problems	Liquid supplements
	Patient preferences
	Multiple small meals
	Pancreatic enzymes
	Elemental diets
	Liquid formulas
Tube feeding	Soft small-bore weighted feeding tube
Parenteral	
Central TPN	Nonfunctional GI tract
	High energy and protein demand
Peripheral IV nutritional support	Poorly functional GI tract
	Low caloric need

From Brennan, M.F.: Supportive care of the cancer patient: Nutritional support. *In* Cancer: Principles and Practice of Oncology. Edited by V.T. DeVita, Jr., S. Hellman, and S.A. Rosenberg. Philadelphia, J.B. Lippincott, 1985.

nausea and delayed gastric emptying. Methylprednisolone has also been shown to increase appetite and food intake (42), but one study showed no change in nutritional status, and the effect on appetite and food intake disappeared after 3 weeks of treatment (54). Moreover, the effects of corticoid on blocking protein synthesis might counteract the benefits of increased appetite (42). Cyproheptadine, an antiserotonergic drug, has been found to induce weight gain in children and adults, but no controlled studies of its action have been reported. Progestational hormones such as medroxyprogesterone and megestrol acetate, which are used in the management of breast, prostate, and endometrial cancers, have been reported to increase appetite, produce a subjective sensation of increased energy, and cause weight gain (57), but no controlled trials have been reported.

In patients for whom oral ingestion of adequate nutrients is impossible, either because of the neoplasm or the therapy, but who have a functional gastrointestinal tract and no ileus, a small pediatric feeding tube can be placed into the stomach or duodenum (34) (Table 91-5). A complete nonprocessed liquid formula can be administered with the tube in the stomach. Many nutritionally complete liquid diets are now available and, although comparative studies have not been done, Shils and associates (58) published a summary of such formulas. Patients require about 1500 to 2000 ml of a liquid formula to meet the recommended daily requirements for protein, fat, carbohydrates, vitamins, and minerals. In most patients it should be progressively increased up to 3000 calories (34).

The nasogastric tube has two disadvantages—patients become intolerant of the tube and, more important, aspiration pneumonia is possible. The latter can be minimized by frequent aspiration of the tube to rule out stasis of the liquid in the stomach. If stasis occurs, metoclopramide should be used to enhance gastric emptying. An alternative is to advance the tube into the duodenum. If the patient becomes intolerant of the tube, jejunostomy feeding can be tried.

TABLE 91-5. Options for Enteral Feeding

Option	Route	Comments
Supplementary feeding	Oral	Multiple small feedings
Complete formula defined	Oral or nasogastric tube	Multiple small feedings
	Gastrostomy	Use small-bore 8F pediatric feeding tube, continuous infusion
Complete formula	Nasogastric tube	Start slowly with dilute solutions
Protein hydrolysates	Jejunal or gastrostomy tube, occasionally oral	Multiple small feedings or continuous infusion
Defined formulas for organ failure	Nasogastric tube	Of only occasional value because of other organ failure

From Brennan, M.F.: Supportive care of the cancer patient: Nutritional support. *In* Cancer: Principles and Practice of Oncology. Edited by V.T. DeVita, Jr., S. Hellman, and S.A. Rosenberg. Philadelphia, J.B. Lippincott, 1985.

Enteral nutrition has been found to be beneficial in patients with head and neck tumors who are undergoing aggressive combined therapy (e.g., chemotherapy, radiation therapy, surgery) and in patients receiving aggressive chemotherapy for potentially curable tumors who continue to lose weight after nutritional counseling (42).

TOTAL PARENTERAL NUTRITION. In cancer patients who cannot ingest, digest, or absorb nutrients through the gastrointestinal tract, total parenteral nutrition (TPN) given intravenously is the only alternative (34). Even if patients have a functional gastrointestinal tract, many physicians prefer to move directly to the IV route for those who need aggressive nutrition. Table 91-6 lists options for the administration of TNP; the desired metabolic consequences of TNP in cancer patients include the following (34):

Weight gain
Improved serum albumin level
Improved nitrogen retention (nitrogen balance)
Restoration of deficiency states (e.g., vitamins, trace metals)
Increase in subcutaneous fat (anthropometrics)
Increased lean tissue (^{40}K)*
Increase in whole body protein synthesis (^{15}N-glycine)*
Suppression of gluconeogenesis from alanine (^{14}C-alanine)*
Increase in quantitative glucose recycling (^{3}H-glucose, ^{14}C-glucose)*

*Isotopes in parentheses indicate what substances are measured in labeling studies.

Numerous studies have shown that weight gain can be achieved with nutritional support by the enteral or parenteral route (34, 59, 60). Although some have expressed concern that the weight gain might reflect more fat than lean tissue restoration (42), Brennan (34) has shown that, in some patients who have responded to anticancer therapy, lean tissues can be restored, as measured by a total body potassium determination or by nitrogen balance and nitrogen flux studies. Because cachexia in cancer patients can be a result of increased energy requirements, nutritional support can readily match these increased needs for many patients (34). Moreover, deficiencies of trace metals and electrolytes can readily be reversed. Nutritional support has also been shown to depress "obligatory gluconeogenesis," which if allowed to progress, results in rapid lean tissue mass dissolution and subsequent death from starvation.

Brennan (34) stated that the use of total parenteral nutrition in malnourished cancer patients undergoing effective antineoplastic therapy can be one of the most gratifying supportive measures. Patients can demonstrate major positive changes in well-being, growth, and restoration of multiple nutritional deficits, and in the functional ability to withstand further nonneoplastic injury. Metabolic changes in cancer patients have been shown to be reversed in ideal circumstances (see list, at left). Brennan (34) emphasized that most studies showing improvement were performed in situations in which patients responded to the antineoplastic therapy; the analogy of regrowing the normal malnourished adult is more appropriate. Brennan (34) pointed out that perhaps those most likely to benefit from TPN are patients undergoing

TABLE 91-6. Options in the Administration of Total Parenteral Nutrition

Route	Catheter Type	Comments
Percutaneous subclavian or jugular puncture	Polyvinychloride—intracath*	Preferred approach
	Silicone—Centrasil†	Undergoing evaluation but occasionally migrates
Peripheral insertion to superior vena cava	Silicone—Intrasil†	Peripheral access is often not available and phlebitis incidence is high
Surgically placed tunneled, cuffed catheter	Silicone—Hickman or Broviac type‡	Used extensively for home TPN and long-term venous access

From Brennan, M.F.: Supportive care of the cancer patient: Nutritional support. *In* Cancer: Principles and Practice of Oncology. Edited by V.T. DeVita, Jr., S. Hellman, and S.A. Rosenberg. Philadelphia, J.B. Lippincott, 1985.
*Becton Dickinson, #3162, Sandy, Utah.
†Vicra, Travenol Laboratories, Inc., Dallas, Texas.
‡Evermed, Medina, Washington.

resectional surgery for gastrointestinal cancer; randomized studies have shown improvement in nutritional indexes seen postoperatively, with a small but real decrease in surgical morbidity and mortality rates (59, 60).

Conclusion

Although aggressive nutritional support is helpful for patients who respond to antineoplastic therapy, the data on its use in advanced and terminal cancer patients are controversial. Brennan (34) pointed out that, in situations in which antineoplastic therapy is ineffective, routine TPN cannot be advocated; in patients without weight loss it might even decrease survival. Bruera and MacDonald (42) and others (61, 62) noted that aggressive nutritional therapy given to patients with advanced malignancy is also of questionable value and therefore used it in only a small percentage of patients. Koretz (61) reviewed a large number of controlled studies in patients with advanced cancer and found no significant impact of nutritional support on tumor response to radiation or chemotherapy (1 of 17 studies) or on improvement in survival (1 of 14 studies). Another study by a cooperative group also noted that aggressive nutrition has no influence on survival or tumor response (62). Surprisingly, studies that assessed the efficacy of parenteral or oral nutrition did not measure the influence on the quality of life, as indicated by performance status, strength, emotional well-being, and other parameters.

Bruera and MacDonald (42) pointed out that parenteral nutrition has not demonstrated any benefit over enteral nutrition in patients with a functional bowel. Given its morbidity rate (15%), high cost, and the concern that aggressive nutrition might stimulate tumor growth, parenteral nutrition is clearly indicated only in unusual cases of patients undergoing aggressive treatment for potentially curable tumors and in those who would obviously die of starvation because of slow-growing masses that cause bowel obstruction (42). They admitted that their opinion is not uniformly accepted, because one-third of patients receiving TPN in the United States have a diagnosis of cancer (63).

Unproven Diet and Nutrition Claims

Cancer is probably one of the foremost diseases in which food fads, "special" diets, and other methods of treatment, which either have never been demonstrated to be effective in scientifically accepted clinical trials or have failed such trials, have been and continue to be used widely. Despite proven failures, many of these methods continue to be advertised and advocated by some individuals and groups as "alternate cancer therapy" (33). The American Cancer Society maintains a file of all such therapies; among these, dietary and nutritional practices play a major role (64). Shils (33) discussed the circumstances that help to explain the widespread and persistent appeal of unproven or disproven health claims of cancer patients and their families. Not mentioned by Shils is that some cancer patients inappropriately treated by physicians continue to have severe pain and eventually seek out special "quack" methods in an attempt to obtain relief.

Shils (33) emphasized why it is important for physicians, dieticians, and nurses involved with cancer patients to be aware of this problem and to know the details of some of the more common components of unproven diets, nutrients, and other questionable methods of treatment. An important issue brought up by Shils (33) is that physicians often comply with patients' requests for an unproven therapy such as metabolic "megavitamin" treatment. Most of these patients, however, receive their prescription from unorthodox practitioners, most of whom have had no medical education.

Perhaps the most famous and widely used cancer "cures" are Laetrile and vitamin B_{17} which are the twentieth century trademark names given by Krebs to amygdalin, a cyanogenetic glucoside isolated from almonds in 1830 in France. In over a century of study Laetrile has never been objectively demonstrated to be as effective or safe for cancer treatment as doing nothing. In fact, patients treated with Laetrile deteriorate and die faster than those who receive no treatment, and some evidence has shown that Laetrile might actually promote cancer (33). Although a major 1982 multiinstitution study reconfirmed the worthlessness of Laetrile as an anticancer therapy, the lucrative Laetrile industry continues. Shils (33) noted that the legislatures and governors of 21 states have actually approved the decriminalization of Laetrile, and these laws are still on the books.

C. NUTRITION AND CHRONIC NONMALIGNANT PAIN

In this section I first review some chronic painful disorders in which diet and nutritional factors can play a role in inducing the mechanism of pain and mention diets that might help to relieve it. Among these disorders are headache, arthritis, certain neuropathies, myofascial syndromes and other musculoskeletal disorders, and chronic gastrointestinal disease.

Headache

Certain foods can precipitate or contribute to the onset of headache (Chapter 39). In a significant percentage of patients who have migraine attacks, the attacks are induced by starvation, food allergy, and certain foods, especially those rich in tyramine (e.g., strong aged cheese, pickled herring, canned figs, chicken livers, and chocolate) or those that contain nitrite, nitrate, or monosodium glutamate. Beverages, particularly red wine, can also trigger an attack of migraine. Obviously, once the relationship between these foods and migraine has been established, patients should be instructed to avoid such food as a most important prophylactic measure.

Other headaches related to intake of food or alcohol include hangover, ice cream, hot dog, and Chinese restaurant syndrome headaches (page 724). Hangover headache is presumably a result of the vasodilating effect of alcohol; it lasts 5 to 10 hours, long after the alcohol has been metabolized. Ice cream headache is not caused by the ingestion of the food but by the effect of the cold substance in contact with the roof of the oropharynx. Current evidence implicates the nitrate content of foodstuffs as the cause of hot dog headache, although some claim that these headaches are provoked by the amount of pork in these products rather than by the preservatives. It has been suggested that monosodium glutamate causes headache in 30% of people who eat Chinese food. Again, prophylaxis involves avoidance of the offending food or drink.

Musculoskeletal Disorders

Arthritis

The idea that some foods might provoke and others might ameliorate arthritis has been around since ancient times. Even today literature abounds with suggestions of diets that can "cure" arthritis (65). Often reaching the best seller lists, these "nonfiction" books should be classified as fiction—for example, they purport to cure arthritis without even distinguishing among the different types of arthritis. Physicians in general, and rheumatologists in particular, consider diet therapy to be quackery; nonetheless, over 90% of arthritis patients spend nearly 1 billion dollars annually (65). As Panush (65) noted, it is surprising that despite the skepticism of rheumatologists and the enthusiasm of its advocates, little objective information exists about nutritional therapy for rheumatic disease. Klinenburg (66) stated that he believes this to be an important issue in regard to future clinical advances anticipated in the field of rheumatology.

Panush (65) stated that nutrition and rheumatic disease could be related through two possible mechanisms, which are not mutually exclusive. First, nutritional factors might alter immune and inflammatory responses and thus modify the manifestation of rheumatic disease, particularly pain. Second, food-related antigens might provoke a hypersensitivity response—that is, food allergies might produce rheumatic symptoms. The following summary is based on Panush's review of the subject (65).

Inflammatory Response

It is now well established that eicosanoids, which are arachidonic acid derivatives (prostaglandins and leukotrienes), are important mediators of the inflammatory response (Chapter 4). Qualitative and quantitative alterations of polyunsaturated fatty acids in the diet affect endogenous cellular synthesis of eicosanoids, leading to the hypothesis that modulation of dietary fatty acids can alter the host response in those with rheumatic disease. Panush (65) summarized the observations in support of this hypothesis as follows. Cold water fish contain ω-3-polyunsaturated fatty acids, such as eicosapentanoic dihydrate acid (EPA) and decosahexanoic acid (DHA). These are incorporated by cells and suppress leukotriene and prostaglandin synthesis from arachidonic acid.

Panush (65) cited experimental studies in mice in which EPA suppressed the inflammatory responses to systemic lupus erythematosus and to other collagen-induced arthritides. Although admitting that it is difficult to determine whether fish oil containing EPA and DHA is useful in the treatment of patients with rheumatic disease, Panush cited three studies that suggested beneficial effects of fish oil in patients with rheumatoid arthritis (RA). In one controlled trial, patients receiving fish oil showed a significant decrease in the number of painful and tender joints, but this number reverted toward baseline during follow-up (67). These findings are consistent with the thesis that the intake and composition of dietary fats are relevant to disease activity in patients with RA. A subsequent trial by the same group showed improvement in pain and other arthritis symptoms, a longer time to fatigue, and a decreased number of tender joints in patients taking fish oil (68). They also noted a decrease in neutrophil leukotriene B4 that correlated with improvements in joint tenderness. The third study also showed that fish oil has a beneficial effect on RA symptoms. Maggio (personal communication, 1988), as part of his integrated chronic pain management program, found that foods containing N-3 fatty acids, which include cold water fish oil, corn oil, and other vegetable oils can be helpful in the treatment of RA.

Food Allergy and Rheumatic Diseases

Immunologic mechanisms of tissue injury are important in the pathogenesis of many rheumatic diseases, but the antigens triggering these mechanisms are unknown (65, 69). Many anecdotal reports have suggested some association of RA, systemic lupus erythematosus, and other rheumatic disorders with the ingestion of certain foods or substances, such as sodium nitrate, dairy products, and alfalfa. Some reports have indicated that fasting has antirheumatic effects (see 65 for references).

Panush and associates (70) carried out a prospective, blinded, controlled trial to determine whether pain and other joint symptoms could be associated with food sensitivity in selected patients. One patient with RA noted symptomatic exacerbation associated with eating dairy products and other foods. An objective improvement during fasting was sustained with elemental nutrition. Their study showed that this patient was immunologically hypersensitive to milk. In additional studies they noted that 30% of their RA patients had alleged food-related ("allergic") arthritis. Of 15 patients who completed 19 double-blind controlled food challenge studies, 10 were negative, 2 were equivocal, and 3 clearly demonstrated subjective and objective rheumatic symptoms after the double-blind encapsulated food challenge and were asymptomatic when on elemental nutrition or when not taking the offending food. All were seronegative with palindromic symptoms and nonerosive disease. Fasting or elemental nutrition also benefited several other of these patients. On the basis of these results, Panush (65) estimated that 5% of rheumatic disease patients have an immunologic sensitivity to food(s) and can only be identified by control challenge studies. These observations suggest a possible role for food allergies, at least in some patients with rheumatoid arthritis and other types of rheumatic disease.

Vitamins, Minerals, and Rheumatic Diseases

After reviewing the literature, Panush (65) found no convincing evidence that vitamin C has clinically evident therapeutic effects in RA patients. The wearing of copper bracelets by the ancient Greeks and Romans to relieve aches and pains have prompted the recent use of copper salts concurrent with the development of gold therapy for RA. Rheumatic disease patients treated in open trials with copper compounds showed generally favorable results, but experienced many adverse effects. Panush (65) offered the comment that, although of theoretic value, copper salts are unlikely to achieve an important role in the therapy of rheumatoid arthritis or other rheumatic diseases.

Based on the observations that serum zinc levels are low in some RA patients, that zinc shows anti-inflammatory action in vitro, and that significant improvement in cellular immune response has occurred when elderly patients were given zinc sulfate, studies of zinc treatment of RA patients were instituted. Although the initial study showed that the zinc-treated RA patients fared better than the placebo-treated patients (71), the improvement was slight, and even this was not confirmed in subsequent studies (72). Finally, L-histidine (available in health food stores) has been used to treat RA patients, with possible benefit only in a small subgroup of patients. A prospective, randomized, placebo-controlled trial has suggested possible beneficial effects in patients older than 45 years with more active and prolonged RA (73).

Conclusion

These various studies relating diet to arthritis appear to be useful in the development of new therapeutic approaches for selected patients and in providing new insight into the pathogenesis of rheumatoid arthritis and other types of rheumatic disease. The hypothesis that nutrition modification (immunologically mediated) might relieve pain and other symptoms in RA patients and in those with other rheumatic diseases is of great interest but should be regarded as still in the experimental stages. More well-designed and well-controlled clinical trials are needed to define the clinical efficacy of various dietary and nutritional manipulations (65, 69).

Osteoarthritis and Obesity

Some clinicians believe that the incidence of osteoarthritis at the weight-bearing joints is higher in obese than in lean persons and that this condition tends to worsen with greater weight because it is a wear-and-tear process characterized by breakdown of cartilage and bone, with secondary proliferative changes (69). Mechanical factors that put an extra strain on joint tissues can accelerate the development or rate of progression of the disease. Studies relating dietary intake, body weight, and osteoarthritis, however, have not clearly established obesity as a factor in the pathogenesis of osteoarthritis (74). In one population survey the weight-to-height ratio correlated with the incidence of osteoarthritis (75). Because the hip joint is a common site affected by osteoarthritis, studies of the influence of body weight on the progression of the disease in the hip have been carried out. In a group of 89 patients who required total hip replacement for osteoarthritis or rheumatoid arthritis, a striking correlation was found between body weight and degree of loss of the substance of the femoral head (76).

Obviously, nutrition is an important issue in patients who are obese and have osteoarthritis. Muncie (77) reported on the results of a study involving multidisciplinary assessment and management of 77 patients with osteoarthritis over a 12-week period. In addition to receiving an anti-inflammatory analgesic, patients were evaluated and followed by health professionals in various disciplines (medicine, physical therapy, occupational therapy, nutrition, social work, and psychology). An initial assessment of the degree of pain, swelling, tenderness, stiffness, and ability to carry out activities of daily living was made; this represented the entry status of patients. Two-thirds of patients had pain, tenderness, or swelling affecting the hip, knee, or hand. Subsequent assessments were made by the multidisciplinary team every 2 weeks for 12 weeks. All 77 patients underwent at least 10 of the 12 weeks of treatment. At the end of the treatment period, 80% of patients had relief of their pain and other symptoms of osteoarthritis, and 71 patients (92%) improved in their ability to carry out activities of daily living. These results strongly support the view that a comprehensive approach to osteoarthritis can significantly reduce pain and disability and that nutrition and decrease of weight are important factors.

Gout

Gout is the most common metabolic disorder associated with arthritis. It is characterized by elevated serum urate levels, recurrent attacks of acute arthritis involving a single joint (or a few joints) over a given time, and monosodium urate dihydrate deposits (tophi) in and around the joint. Gout is one of the most painful forms of acute and chronic arthritis (Chapter 20). Studies of patients with gout have not revealed any significant differences between diet and control groups, except that patients with gout were found to consume greater amounts of beer.

Various drugs used to manage gout are discussed in Chapter 20. Dietary therapy can also be part of the management of patients with this condition. Because about 50% of the urate formed each day comes from dietary sources, a diet restricted in purine content can reduce urinary excretion of uric acid by 200 to 400 mg/day, and lowers the serum uric acid level by about 1 mg/dl (78). Although severe dietary restriction is usually not necessary, reduction in alcohol intake and, when necessary, control of hypertriglyceridemia are more important aspects of the nutritional management of gout. It is advisable for patients with gout to avoid foods high in purine, such as sweetbreads, fish roe, anchovies, sardines, liver, and kidney, and to restrict intake of foods containing moderate concentrations of purine, such as meat, seafood, beans, lentils, spinach, and peas.

Gout patients should be educated about the disease and drugs used for therapy. Weight control should be strongly recommended for obese patients, and attention should be given to blood pressure control. A 24-hour urinary uric acid measurement helps to determine the cause of the hyperuricemia in selecting appropriate urate-lowering drugs (Chapter 20).

Paget's Disease

A few reports have indicated that some bone pains can be helped by ingestion of large doses of vitamin C. In one study, 16 patients with painful Paget's disease were treated with high doses of ascorbic acid and within 5 to 7 days 8 patients had less pain and 3 had complete relief of the pain (79). Subsequent treatment with calcitonin relieved pain in most patients (79). In another report, patients with painful Paget's disease were treated for 2 weeks with combined ascorbic acid and calcitonin or with calcitonin alone (80). Of 11 patients on the combined therapy, 73% experienced pain relief; of 13 patients treated with calcitonin alone, 85% had relief of pain. In the group treated with ascorbic acid and calcitonin, however, marked pain relief was experienced, compared to only 36% of the patients who responded to calcitonin alone (80).

Myofascial Pain Syndromes

Travell and Simons (81) have emphasized that nutritional inadequacies, particularly of the water-soluble vitamins B_1, B_6, B_{12}, folic acid, and vitamin C, and certain elements, especially calcium, iron, and potassium, constitute perpetuating factors in patients with myofascial pain syndromes. They stated that almost 50% of their patients with chronic myofascial pain required resolution of vitamin inadequacies for prolonged relief. On the basis of this they have provided an extensive review (81), but only the most salient points are considered here.

According to Travell and Simons (81) vitamin inadequacies apparently increase the irritability of myofascial trigger points (TPs) by several mechanisms: impairment of the energy metabolism needed for the contraction of muscles and increased irritability of the nervous system. The affected muscles behave as though neurofeedback mechanisms are perpetually sensitizing TPs and the TP-referred phenomena are intensified. Vitamin inadequacies become a deficiency when the effects of impaired function of essential enzymes are grossly apparent, and these can be established by laboratory evidence.

Travell and Simons (81) devoted 30 pages to a detailed and elegant discussion of the history, biochemistry, function, and effects of vitamin deficiencies, and cited several hundred articles in support of their hypothesis. I could find no data from controlled clinical trials in those pages, however, to support their statement that "the patients with chronic myofascial syndrome in our experience have a remarkably high prevalence of vitamin inadequacies and deficiencies" (81). Sola, Fischer, Bonica, and others who have treated many such patients have not encountered this high prevalence of vitamin deficiencies. Although vitamin deficiencies might be a contributing factor in perpetuating myofascial syndromes, it is not as important as that suggested by Travell and Simons. I agree with them that "a full evaluation of the total vitamin status of the patient is prohibitive and difficult because of many overlapping and nonspecific findings symptomatic of vitamin deficiency." (81).

When a full battery of vitamin tests is not available, Travell and Simons (81) recommended that a complete balanced supplement is a safe and usually effective alternative. They cautioned that the body should not be overloaded with fat-soluble vitamins, particularly vitamin A. The supplement should include close to the recommended daily allowance of essential minerals. They emphasized that the cost is nominal and the amount is harmless if it is only a supplemental source and ensures a margin of safety against inadequate levels of essential nutrients. They further recommended that, when the clinical picture indicates a vitamin deficiency or inadequacy, and after blood has been withdrawn for vitamin assessment, intramuscular injection can be given in addition to oral supplementation. The injection should contain 100 mg each of vitamins B_1 amd B_6, 5 mg of folic acid, 1 mg of vitamin B_{12}, and 2 mg of protein, and should be given intramuscularly. Four or five injections might be required to bring the severely depleted reservoir of these vitamins to a functionally adequate level quickly. A balanced mixture of B-complex vitamins is preferred to supplementation of only one or two vitamins, and they suggested a mixed B complex, such as Plebex, be added to the regimen for intramuscular injection (81). I believe, however, this type of multiple "shotgun" therapy, although effective and certainly safe, is not necessary for the vast majority of patients with myofascial pain syndromes.

Chronic Visceral Disease

Painful visceral diseases are discussed in various chapters of Part IV. Those conditions in which nutritional support can be helpful in prevention or treatment are mentioned here.

Diseases of the Esophagus

Painful diseases of the esophagus include cancer, esophageal reflux, chemical injuries, and laceration and perforation of the esophagus (Chapter 56). Cancer of the esophagus has been discussed above. Esophageal reflux is a common cause of chest pain. Fatty meals, alcohol, obesity, cigarette smoking, coffee, and chocolate have been shown to reduce the tone or pressure exerted by the lower esophageal sphincter (LES) (Chapter 56). Prophylactic measures (page 1070) include strict avoidance of alcohol and smoking, reduction of fat in the diet, avoidance of citrus fruit juices (because they aggravate the pain), and a program of weight loss, because the loss of as little as 4.5 kg can relieve all symptoms in many patients.

Injury of the esophageal mucosa by infection and systemic disease causes dysphagia and odynophagia; unless promptly treated this can interfere with nutritional intake (page 1071). Injuries caused by swallowing of lye or other chemicals are usually treated by the introduction of a nasogastric tube or some larger plastic tube to provide enteral nutrition and prevent stricture formation. If stricture is severe or multiple strictures are present, esophageal interposition of the colon is performed. The nutritional status should be monitored. The same comment applies to the management of patients with laceration or perforation of the esophagus that occurred in the course of esophagoscopy.

Diseases of the Stomach and Duodenum

Gastric ulcer and gastritis cause pain and can cause undernutrition, but diet therapy is of little value because more effective therapies are available (Chapter 60). Gastric cancer often results in malnutrition that requires nutritional support (see above).

Little scientifically sound information supports the idea that diet contributes to peptic ulcer disease (82). The role of "peptic ulcer diets" in the treatment of peptic ulcer disease has been proposed, but diet has no role to play when the disease is uncomplicated. As discussed by Kimmey and Silverstein, treatment of peptic ulcer with H2 blockers can be helpful for those who can eat and tolerate food without discomfort (Chapter 60). Avoidance of cigarettes, coffee, and caffeinated drinks, which induce acid secretion, can prevent heartburn and the discomfort caused by reflux.

Idiopathic Chronic Inflammatory Bowel Disease

Idiopathic chronic inflammatory bowel disease (IBD) consists principally of ulcerative colitis and Crohn's disease. Because of their direct involvement with the gastrointestinal tract and their effects on food intake, they are commonly associated with nutritional depletion. Most patients, especially those with Crohn's disease, suffer from some degree of calorie or protein depletion. Weight loss occurs in most patients with Crohn's disease and in many with ulcerative colitis. Although micronutrient depletion occurs less often, deficiency of fat-soluble vitamins, folate, minerals, and trace minerals (especially iron and zinc) is possible (83).

Kimmey and Silverstein have emphasized that proper management of IBD requires a multidisciplinary team consisting of the physician, psychologist, surgeon, and nutritionist, who closely monitors the nutritional status of the patient to ensure compliance with dietary restrictions designed to "rest" the inflamed bowel and allow healing to proceed (Chapter 60). Significant obstructive symptoms can be relieved by eating low residue foods. Because many patients with Crohn's disease are lactose-intolerant, a trial of eliminating dairy products from the diet can decrease pain and diarrhea.

ENTERAL NUTRITION. In general, the diet should be liberal in protein and contain sufficient calories to maintain or restore weight or to support growth in children and adolescents. The diet should usually be supplemented by a multivitamin preparation containing one to five times the normal recommended dietary allowances (83). The higher therapeutic dose is indicated if clinical or laboratory evidence shows deficiency of any of several nutrients that might be poorly absorbed or whose requirements might be increased. Dietary manipulation is effective for most individuals with moderate to mild symptoms of IBD.

For patients with more severe symptoms, unresponsive to medical therapy, more intensive nutritional support might be mandatory. This can be in the form of enteral liquid formula or, for some patients, parenteral nutrition. Enteral formulas have been successful in the management of patients with ulcerative colitis or Crohn's disease, even with fistulas, growth retardation, or short bowel. Enteral formulas for the treatment of Crohn's disease patients with fistulas have resulted in a decrease in fistula drainage and healing in some individuals. Enteral formula supplements have been effective in meeting calorie requirements and restoring growth in children with growth retardation complicating Crohn's disease (84).

PARENTERAL NUTRITION. In the management of many hospitalized patients with severely active ulcerative colitis or Crohn's disease, physicians tend to place patients on a regimen of nothing by mouth and medication, including corticosteroids, in an effort to control symptoms of pain, diarrhea, and sometimes fever. Such patients can be managed by total parenteral nutrition provided through a central line for nutritional repletion and maintenance.

Combined reports of uncontrolled studies of ulcerative colitis have indicated clinical remission in about one-third of severely symptomatic patients managed with TPN, with the remainder eventually requiring surgery (85). In a controlled study of patients with colitis that compared TPN with hospitalization and drug therapy alone, however, no greater incidence of remission was observed in those on TPN (86). In Crohn's disease the experience with the use of TPN is more extensive and more positive (83). About 70% of patients in one reported series experienced clinical remission in the hospital and reversal of malnutrition deficits, but the duration of symptomatic remission was highly variable (85). Takagi and associates (87) studied the effects of TPN on IBD in 27 patients who received 32 courses of TPN. Definite

improvement of the nutritional status and a decrease or elimination of abdominal pain, diarrhea, and vomiting occurred. On short-term follow-up clinical remission was noted in 26 of 32 courses of TNP (81%), but on long-term follow-up, ranging from 6 months to 11 years, 11 of 20 patients (55%) were symptom-free without any other medical treatment. Clinical relapse occurred in 6 patients and another course of TPN was required. It was concluded that TPN was useful as an adjunctive therapy for IBD requiring bowel rest and nutritional repletion. Two patients requiring prolonged TPN returned to work with home parenteral nutrition for 2.5 and 5 years, respectively.

Chronic Pancreatitis

Chronic pancreatitis differs from acute pancreatitis in its pathogenesis, sequelae, and response to treatment (Chapter 61). Almost 100% of these patients suffer from chronic abdominal pain, which is a central feature of chronic pancreatitis. In the United States alcohol causes this condition in 80 to 90% of patients. Obstruction of the primary and secondary pancreatic ducts causes inflammation, fibrosis, loss of pancreatic exocrine tissue, and consequent exocrine insufficiency, which results in reduction of the secretion of amylase, lipase, and proteolytic enzymes. Steatorrhea and malabsorption result and contribute to progressive weight loss. These patients therefore require nutritional support in the form of a diet with a high caloric intake (2000 to 5000 kcal/day), consisting principally of carbohydrates and protein (88). Supplements of fat-soluble vitamins, such as vitamins A, B, and K, might also be required. In addition, vitamin B_{12} supplementation might be necessary. In severe cases of nutritional deficiency, a full enteral nutrition regimen administered through a nasogastric tube is indicated. Elemental diet improves nutritional status without requiring exocrine pancreatic function. Parenteral nutrition is rarely necessary but is effective if used.

Carcinoma of the Pancreas

Most patients with advanced pancreatic tumors experience severe pain and have demonstrable abnormalities in carbohydrate, fat, and protein metabolism and have vitamin and mineral deficiencies (88). The combination of these metabolic abnormalities is an important factor in causing cancer cachexia, which is associated with a hypercatabolic state and anorexia and results in malnutrition, weight loss, or wasting of lean body mass. Cancer cachexia is frequently worsened by the therapeutic modalities employed in treatment—surgery, radiotherapy, and cytotoxic chemotherapy (88). In patients with carcinoma of the pancreas, weight loss is almost invariably of dramatic onset and progressive and can precede other symptoms (88). Pain, aversion to food, diabetes mellitus, maldigestion, and malabsorption all contribute to the nutritional deficiencies. Because severe pain contributes to the anorexia and malnutrition and produces great suffering, prompt relief should be achieved with celiac plexus block with 50% alcohol (Chapter 96). If an exploratory operation is contemplated the block should be done intraoperatively under direct vision.

Because untreated tumors of the pancreas are almost invariably progressive, nutritional support of these patients has concentrated on its application as an adjunct of cancer therapy (88). The goals of nutritional support are reduction of the complications of nutritional insufficiency, possible improvement in the therapeutic response of the malnourished patient, and reduction of the morbidity caused by treatment. When surgery is performed, further catabolic effects influence the nutritional status of the patient. The degree of catabolism can be reduced significantly with continuous segmental epidural analgesia for the surgery, which is continued postoperatively for 2 to 3 days. This should be done even if patients have had a celiac plexus block prior to surgery because it decreases the massive nociceptive input consequent to the abdominal wall incision and manipulation. Good general oral nutritional support is important, together with correction of any deficiencies of vitamins, minerals, or trace elements, but unfortunately many patients have anorexia and aversion to food.

Enteral nutrition might have less of a part to play in the management of patients with pancreatic tumors than in the management of those with other malignant tumors. In patients with pancreatic tumors in whom rapid nutritional improvements are required, TPN therapy is necessary.

Neurologic Disorders

Nutritional disorders of the nervous system are most commonly seen as a consequence of chronic alcoholism, debilitating diseases that affect the gastrointestinal tract, starvation as a result of unavailable nutrients, and malnutrition caused by an individual's ignorance of proper diet and nutrition (89).

Nutritional Neuropathies

Nutritional neuropathies are probably the nutritional disorder of the peripheral nervous system that is most frequently encountered in practice, and they occur in various clinical settings (89). The characteristic clinical features of nutritional polyneuropathy in the early stages consist of symmetric impairment of sensory and motor function accompanied by reduced or absent reflex activity, affecting the legs to a greater degree than the arms. They are usually characterized by pain and other sensory changes such as paresthesia, dysesthesia, and burning. In advanced cases marked motor involvement is present. One type, beriberi neuropathy, develops from a primary deficiency of thiamine. Alcoholic polyneuropathy is caused by deficiencies of thiamine, pyridoxine, niacin, pantothenic acid, biotin, and vitamin B_{12}. The treatment of nutritional neuropathies with pain is straightforward: provision of improved nutrition, supplemental vitamins, and removal of noxious substances (89).

Neuralgia and Neuropathy

Nutritional therapy consisting of vitamins and other nutrients continues to be used in neurologic disorders of unknown cause despite a total lack of scientific rationale (89). The popularity and widespread use of large doses of vitamins as treatment for neuralgias and peripheral neuropathies of uncertain cause is said to be a result of the misinterpretation of data derived from animal studies.

Huge doses of thiamine have been and continue to be used to treat peripheral neuropathy of undetermined cause. To date no scientific evidence has shown that vitamins protect peripheral nerve fibers from further damage or enhance regeneration or remyelination, except when severe thiamine deficiency has been demonstrated by appropriate laboratory tests (89). In the first edition of this book, I cited reports of the use of large doses of vitamin B_{12} for the treatment of trigeminal neuralgia and of postherpetic neuralgia (14), but again no definitive scientific evidence has shown that these therapies are effective.

D. NUTRITIONAL MANIPULATION OF BRAIN NEUROREGULATORS FOR TREATING CHRONIC PAIN

This section discusses nutritional manipulation of neurotransmitters and neuromodulators as part of an integrated program for the management of chronic pain. I give a brief historical review, summarize the most important animal and human experimental reports, as well as reports of their clinical efficacy in patients with chronic pain, and then present my opinion about the current status and possible future role of this method.

Historical Perspective

Some remarkable advances have been made during the past 20 years in understanding the transmission and modulation of nociceptive information from the body to the brain (Chapter 4). In recent years there has been an explosion of information about how neurons in the peripheral and central nervous systems communicate with each other and how this communication is translated into sensation, perception, and behavior. This is achieved through "neuroregulators," a term proposed by Barchas and associates (90) that refers to the full panoply of interneuronal communication. Neuro-regulators are of two types, neurotransmitters and neuromodulators. Neurotransmitters are substances that carry signals from one neuron to the other unidirectionally within an identified synaptic structure. Neuromodulators are substances that alter (increase or decrease) signal transmission between neurons or neuronal activity through mechanisms other than neurotransmission.

Important advances have been made in defining the effects of various neuroregulators such as acetylcholine, dopamine, norepinephrine, serotonin, enkephalin, and other endorphins on such physiologic functions as mood, emotion, sleep, temperature regulation, appetite, motor activity, pain, and behavior. Behavioral neurochemistry has enhanced our knowledge of the function of these neuroregulators in psychologic and psychiatric disorders (91). Serotonin, catecholamines, endogenous opioids, and other neuropeptides, which have been shown to play an important role in modulating transmission of nociceptive information, have been implicated as having important causative effects on some mental illnesses, including some types of depression, some psychoses such as schizophrenia and mania and certain forms of anxiety and panic disorders (91).

Manipulation of brain neurotransmitters for the relief of pain has been achieved by the use of drugs (e.g., antidepressants), electric stimulation (e.g., TENS and PAG stimulation), autonomic nervous system conditioning (e.g., biofeedback), acupuncture, physical therapy, and other methods discussed elsewhere in this book. Another area of research carried out in the past 10 or 15 years has suggested the possibility that brain neurotransmitters can be manipulated through diet. Research that began during the period when stimulation-produced analgesia (SPA) (Chapter 4) was being intensively studied suggests that nutrients, which are precursors of neurotransmitters concerned with modulation of pain, can be manipulated through diet. In the first half of the 1970s Wurtman and colleagues (92, 93) reported that synthesis and increase in brain concentration of serotonin and catecholamines could be controlled by administration of the amino acids tryptophan and tyrosine, respectively, and that synthesis and brain concentration of acetylcholine could be controlled by the administration of choline, a component of lecithin found in egg yolk, liver, and soybeans. The results of these studies in turn provoked research on the synthesis of serotonin, catecholamine, and acetylcholine to determine their role in the hypothalamic mechanism that regulates micronutrient intake. They also led to animal and human experimental studies and clinical trials of the effects of these nutrients in patients with chronic pain (94).

Synthesis of Tryptophan

Tryptophan (TRP), an essential amino acid, appears in the blood as a result of protein ingestion and protein breakdown. It is difficult for water-soluble molecules to diffuse out of the capillaries and into the brain (blood-brain barrier) and gain access to neurons and other brain cells. Passage is facilitated by carrier molecules present in the endothelial cells that line the brain capillaries (92–95). These carrier mechanisms are charge- and size-specific for the large neutral amino acids (NAAs), which include not only TRP but also tyrosine, phenylalanine, valine, leucine, isoleucine, and methionine. The amino acids compete with one another for attachment to the carrier and uptake from the bloodstream into the brain. Because tryptophan is present in protein in relatively small amounts, a high-protein meal causes a greater increase in the amount or concentration of the large neutral amino acid relative to TRP, decreasing the ratio of plasma TRP:NAA and therefore decreasing brain TRP uptake.

A high-carbohydrate meal has the opposite effect, because the insulin secreted in response to carbohydrate intake reduces the plasma level of the competing amino acids more than it does that of the TRP (92, 93). Whereas the other amino acids circulate as free molecules, most of the tryptophan (90%) is bound to plasma albumin. TRP and fatty acids have the same binding site on albumin, so TRP binding increases after a carbohydrate meal and TRP tends to be retained in the plasma. Because binding at the blood-brain barrier is stronger than binding to albumin, tryptophan is released into the brain, thus increasing its concentration relative to that of the other large NAAs. Whereas ingestion of a protein-rich meal decreases the level of serotonin in the brain by limiting uptake of tryptophan, TRP administration and ingestion of a carbohydrate-rich diet increases the concentrations of tryptophan and serotonin in the brain.

The brain and spinal cord serotonergic cells appear to contain all the precursor compounds, enzymes, and cofactors necessary for the synthesis and catabolism of serotonin. Figure 91-9 depicts the synthesis of serotonin. Only about 1% of ingested tryptophan is metabolized to serotonin (96). Stimuli coming from certain parts of the brain cause the release of serotonin at serotonergic nerve endings into brain synapses, some of which are deaminated and oxidized by the enzyme monoamino-oxidase to form the biologically inactive metabolite 5-hydroxyindoleacetic acid. Other molecules of released serotonin interact with receptors in the postsynap-

L-Tryptophan

↓ Tryptophan hydroxylase

5-Hydroxytryptophan (5-HTP)

↓ Aromatic L-amino acid decarboxylase

Serotonin (5-hydroxytryptamine, 5-HT)

↓ Monoamine oxides and aldehyde dehydrogenase

5-Hydroxyindoleacetic acid (5-HIAA)

FIG. 91-9. Steps in the synthesis of serotonin.

tic cells to complete the process of communication (inhibition of nociceptive neurons).

Because most mammals cannot synthesize tryptophan de novo, TRP molecules available for brain serotonin biosynthesis are ultimately derived only from the lysis of protein or from circulating tryptophan obtained directly from food or small tissue storage pools (96). Because the enzyme tryptophan hydroxylase does not normally appear to be saturated with its substrates, serotonin concentration in the brain and spinal cord can be increased by injection of tryptophan or 5-hydroxytryptophan, or by feeding diets that contain higher than normal concentrations of tryptophan to animals. Injection of tryptophan produces relatively discrete increases in neurotransmitter synthesis, only in serotonergic neurons, because of the relatively specific localization of the enzyme tryptophan hydroxylase to these cells. In contrast, injection of 5-hydroxytryptophan can increase the concentration of serotonin in cells that do *not* contain the neurotransmitters, because many cells have the ability to take up amino acid and also contain the aromatic enzyme L-amino acid decarboxylase (96). Messing and Lytle (96) have presented a comprehensive review of early animal studies of the pharmacology of serotonin.

Serotonin-Induced Analgesia

Animal Studies

Animal experiments have shown that serotonin (5-HT) potentiates morphine-induced analgesia (97). Morphine increases turnover of brain serotonin, as revealed by the presence of brain serotonin breakdown products such as 5-hydroxyindoleacetic acid (98). Conversely, 5-HT depletion decreases the effectiveness of morphine (99). Electric or pharmacologic manipulation that increases brain serotonergic transmission can produce analgesia (97). Serotonin antagonists such as methysergide can modulate the pain of migraine (100). On the other hand, administration of serotonin neurotoxins, such as p-chlorophenylalanine (PCPA) or induction of medial forebrain lesions in rats depletes the CNS of 5-HT, with a consequent decrease in pain threshold (97, 101). These effects of some of the neurotoxins can be reversed by injection of 5-HTP, the precursor of 5-HT (102). Sufficient evidence has been provided by animal studies to show that the consumption of a tryptophan-poor corn diet decreases brain serotonergic neurotransmission and decreases pain threshold, whereas a single injection of L-tryptophan can reverse the increased pain sensitivity by restoring brain 5-HT concentration to normal levels (102).

Human Studies

The first report of the use of serotonin in humans to treat chronic pain was published by Sicuteri (103) in 1960. Sicuteri manipulated tryptophan in serotonin to support the thesis that migraine headache is caused by a deficiency of brain serotonin, and suggested that the administration of these substances would relieve patients with this type of headache. Fourteen years later Sicuteri and colleagues published data (100) on 27 hospitalized patients who were given L-tryptophan by intravenous infusion of doses of 2 g/day, for about 2 weeks, followed by oral administration of tryptophan, 3 to 4 g/day, continued for 2 to 6 months. A large percentage of patients had marked improvement of headaches; in some patients this was paralleled by improvement in mood, but in other the migraine improved but the mood remained depressed. Parachlorophenylalanine (PCPA), a serotonin-depleting agent, was also administered to 18 volunteer patients who had intractable migraine. It was given in daily doses of 600 to 800 mg for 1 to 3 months. After 20 to 40 days of treatment patients experienced deep and superficial hyperalgesia, spontaneous pain, and hyperpathia in the limbs, trunk, neck, and scalp. Within 5 to 10 days after discontinuation of the drug the pain gradually disappeared. Others subsequently reported the use of L-tryptophan for the successful treatment of migraine (104, 105).

The next report on the use of serotonin to treat human chronic pain was published by Sternbach and associates in 1976 (106). In a study of organic pain of long duration, usually of musculoskeletal origin, five patients received between 1.5 and 3 g/day of 5-HT in three divided doses given in capsule form for 14 days, preceded or followed by 14 days of matched placebo. Three of these patients and 2 others received L-tryptophan that was gradually increased over a 4- to 6-day period to maximum levels. Between 7 and 10 g/day was given in grapefruit juice in three divided doses for 10 days and was followed or preceded by grapefruit juice alone for 10 days. Both 5-HT and L-tryptophan were administered on a double-blind basis and the placebo-active drug sequence was counterbalanced. The results suggested that both preparations produced a trend toward decreased levels of clinical pain matched by a trend toward increased pain tolerance. It was concluded that increased brain serotonin activity decreases pain levels and seems to do so by increasing pain tolerance.

In 1978 Hosobuchi (107) reported that tryptophan reverses the tolerance induced by endogenous opioid analgesia provoked by central gray stimulation. Two years later King (108) gave tryptophan to 5 patients, each of whom demonstrated a regression of sensory deficit and progressive recurrence of pain following rhizotomy or cordotomy. He gave each patient 4 daily doses of 500 mg each. Approximately 1 month after taking tryptophan, 2 g/day, the analgesic and anesthetic areas began to spread or reappear. In about 3 to 4 months the maximum sensory deficit imposed by the operative procedure was re-established and the patients were essentially free of pain. All patients had a remarkable increase in their daily activities and all but one patient discontinued analgesic medication. Six other patients with recurrent or persistent face pain after denervation procedures had a similar beneficial course while taking the tryptophan. It was also mentioned that 8 patients with pain related to peripheral nerve injuries showed no change in sensory deficit or pain relief while taking tryptophan.

De Benedittis and associates (109) administered 5-hydroxytryptophan (5-HTP), the immediate precursor of serotonin, to 5 patients with chronic deafferentation pain or central pain that had been experienced for a mean period of 7 ± 3.7 years. The clinical pain syndromes included deafferentation pain, phantom limb pain, thalamic pain, and post-traumatic spinal pain. Prior to therapy patients underwent general medical, neurologic, and psychologic evaluation. Pain and distress levels were noted by a visual analog scale. The researchers also measured CSF 5-hydroxyindoleacetic acid, plasma 5-HT, CSF and plasma beta-endorphin, and CSF and plasma beta-lipotropin (beta-LPH). Treatment consisted of giving patients 50-mg tablets of L-5-HTP tid (150 mg total) for the first 3 days that was increased to one or two 100-mg tablets tid or qid (range, 300 to 800 mg/day; mean dose, $\pm$ SE 542 ± 78). Outcome was measured at 1- and 3-month intervals. The patients were readmitted to the hospital for evaluation of the response to treatment. Outcome parameters included self-ratings of pain and distress, sensory charts, and 5-HT and endogenous opiate assays. Figure 91-10 shows the changes in pain and distress estimates for the five patients (mean values). Pain scores were significantly lower compared to pretreatment levels ($p < 0.001$), as were the distress levels. A remarkable regression of sensory deficits was observed in all patients, especially the shrinking or diminution of the hyperpathia.

Moldofsky and Warsh (110) used tryptophan therapy in 8 patients with fibromyalgia, all of whom complained of widespread musculoskeletal pain and stiffness that were worse on awakening, weakness, easy fatigability, emotional distress, and poor work tolerance for at least 3 months. All were found to have an alpha-non-REM sleep disturbance. Patients were studied over a 3-day period, during which time no

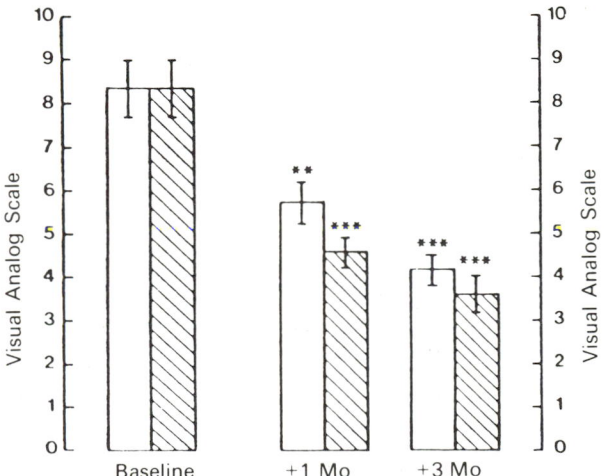

FIG. 91-10. Changes in pain and distress estimates (mean values) following 5-HTP administration at designated monthly intervals. Pain estimate, *open bar*; distress estimate, *vertical bar*; **$p < 0.01$; ***$p < 0.001$. From De Benedittis, G., et al.: Effects of 5-hydroxytryptophan on central and deafferentation chronic pain: A preliminary clinical trial. *In* Advances in Pain Research and Therapy, Vol. 5. Edited by J.J. Bonica, et al. New York, Raven Press, 1983.

medication was permitted. During this period all patients consumed a controlled diet of 2120 calories comprised of 289 g carbohydrate, 92.6 g protein, 949.5 mg tryptophan, 22.2 g saturated fat, and 35.4 g unsaturated fat. One observer measured pain with a 9 kg pressure algesiometer uniformly applied to 13 pairs of bilateral symmetric tender points in the musculoskeletal system that were commonly affected by fibromyalgia. The values were added to yield a total algesiometer score. Patients were also asked to estimate pain intensity by a visual analog scale, and mood was rated by the observer using a 27-item scale. It was found that the intensity of pain in patients with fibromyalgia was inversely related to the level of the plasma-free tryptophan, suggesting a relationship between brain serotonin metabolism and pain reactivity. When patients with this syndrome were treated with 5 g of tryptophan at bedtime for 3 weeks, however, slow-wave sleep was not increased nor were pain or mood symptoms altered (111).

Seltzer (112, 113), an authority on nutritional therapy for pain, has reported the results of 2 studies on patients with chronic pain and one double-blind study on human subjects. The randomized double-blind experimental study involved 30 normal human volunteer subjects in whom pain perception and pain tolerance thresholds were measured by an electric tooth pulp stimulation technique. Each subject was given 6 capsules, each containing 500 mg of tryptophan or placebo, to be taken 6 times a day together with the ingestion of a high-carbohydrate, low-protein, and low-fat diet for 8 days (112). The perception and tolerance threshold scores were computed for tryptophan and placebo subjects for both pretreatment and posttreatment sessions. The study revealed that the pain perception threshold did not change but that the pain tolerance threshold was significantly increased. About one-third of those in the tryptophan-treated group had itching, nausea, diarrhea, urinary changes, and weight loss; and 65% had mood elevation and 33% had rested feelings. Among those in the placebo group 2 had weight loss and 7 had mood elevation and a rested feeling.

In a noncontrolled trial of patients with chronic head and neck pain, Seltzer (113) prescribed a rigid diet consisting of approximately 80% complex carbohydrate, 10% protein, and 10% fat, to which was added 3 g of tryptophan given in 6 daily divided doses of 500 mg each. A significant reduction in pain was noted. In a randomized, double-blind, controlled study, 30 patients with chronic maxillofacial pain, including trigeminal neuralgia, atypical facial neuralgia, and myofascial pain syndromes, were treated by a similar dietary regimen (114). Of the 30 patients, 15 were allocated to a study group and 15 to a placebo group. Prior to entering the study the patients were examined clinically, tooth stimulation was used to determine pain perception and reaction thresholds, and they were subjected to a battery of psychologic tests. The patients were then given dietary instructions and placebo or tryptophan capsules, with instructions to take one 500 mg capsule 6 times daily with a carbohydrate drink such as orange juice. At the end of 1 week and 1 month the tests were readministered and pain rating scales and side effects were recorded. A significant reduction in clinical pain ratings was found, from 58 to 26 for the tryptophan subjects and from 50 to 39 in the placebo subjects (on a scale of 0 to 100) (Fig. 91-11). In addition, in those in the tryptophan group, a significant increase in pain tolerance was noted in the study group, but only a slight increase in the placebo group. All patients manifested less depression and anxiety. It was also found that the tryptophan-treated patients had a higher incidence of skin itching, nausea, diarrhea, urination, weight loss, and mood elevation than the corresponding controls.

Heinze and Lehman (115) reported that they have integrated a high-carbohydrate, low-protein, low-fat pain diet into the regimen of all patients admitted to their pain management program. Their dietary guidelines for pain management are as follows:

High complex carbohydrate (60% of total calories)
Restricted protein (15% of total calories)
Moderate fat (25% of total calories)
Diet exchanges used as a reference base and to provide options for food selections
Emphasis on fiber-rich fruits, vegetables, whole-grain breads and cereals
Increased fluid consumption to 8 to 10 cups/day
High-carbohydrate bedtime snack
Controlled calories to achieve ideal body weight
Limited caffeine
Multivitamin and mineral supplementation
L-tryptophan supplement (1 g at bedtime)

A dietician is part of their pain management team, with the responsibility of assessing the patient's nutritional and caloric needs, explaining the biochemistry of tryptophan and its conversion to serotonin to help decrease pain and the importance of diet in improving health and decreasing pain, and emphasizing that

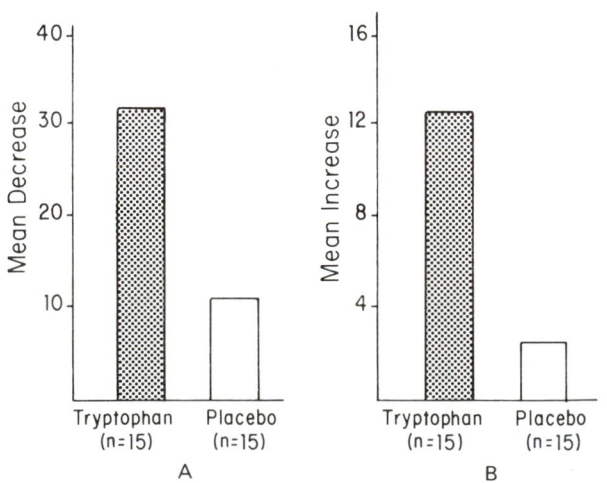

FIG. 91-11. Influence of tryptophan and placebo on patients with chronic maxillofacial pain. *A.* Pain ratings (on scale of 0–100). *B.* Pain tolerance threshold (pain became intolerable on electrical stimulation of tooth pulp using pulp tester scale of 0 to 80) (see text for details). From Seltzer, S. et al.: The effects of dietary tryptophan on chronic maxillofacial pain and experimental pain tolerance. J. Psychiatr. Res., *17*:181, 1982–1983.

tryptophan reduces the craving for sweets. Patients also received instruction about exercise. A complete laboratory examination (SMA-12) and lipoprotein electrophoresis blood tests were done on admission and during the third week of the in-hospital program. A 1-year follow-up survey of all the patients managed the preceding year revealed that 70 to 80% of patients felt immediate and long-term benefits from the diet and that they were still on the diet 6 weeks to 1 year after discharge. It was also noted that 75% of patients who wanted to lose weight lost more than 2.2 kg and 55% lost 4.5 kg or more during the 3-week hospitalization for the program. No chemical profile abnormalities were developed on the diet and lipid values frequently improved. The pain diet seemed to decrease pain and the pain became worse in patients who deviated from the diet.

Summary and Conclusion

Nutritional support for patients who have undergone major surgery for serious trauma has been one of the major advances of the past 25 years. This, together with better anesthesiologic management, intensive care, the advent of more specific antibiotics, and the widespread use of blood and blood substrates, has had a major beneficial impact in the reduction of morbidity and mortality rates among surgical and trauma patients. The use of regional anesthesia for the surgery and continuous regional analgesia for 1 to 3 days following surgery has been shown to blunt the neuroendocrine "stress" response and the hypermetabolism significantly, thus providing much appreciated pain relief, to help reduce morbidity, and to accelerate convalescence and reduce the period of hospitalization.

The use of nutritional support in the relief of pain for cancer patients has become a well-recognized advance in the management of these patients. Controversy remains regarding the use of enteral and total parenteral nutritional support in patients with advanced carcinoma, but well-controlled clinical trials are helping to resolve this. In reviewing the literature it appears that most believe that nutritional support is useful in selected patients who are to undergo intensive antineoplastic therapy. Although recent clinical trials suggest nutritional therapy in advanced cancer has no impact on tumor response to cancer therapy or survival, it might improve the quality of life and help to restore weight and strength, decrease nausea, improve performance status, and improve the psychologic and emotional status of the patient—an aspect of cancer research that needs to be explored.

The use of nutritional support in patients with various painful chronic disorders such as inflammatory bowel disease has also been established, and it is being used widely to improve the well-being of these patients.

In regard to dietary therapy in managing patients with nonmalignant chronic pain, controlled trials are critically needed. The meager available evidence suggests that it might be beneficial in patients with certain musculoskeletal disorders. Maggio, who has had extensive clinical experience that spans 25 years, is firmly convinced that patients with musculoskeletal disorders, such as certain types of arthritis, and patients with ischemic pain caused by peripheral vascular disease would benefit from specific diet as an important part of their therapeutic regimen, which should include exercise, selective nerve blocks for pain relief, neurostimulation techniques, patient education, and other multimodal therapies.

Finally, in regard to manipulation of the various neurotransmitters, especially tryptophan, review of the literature suggests that, although it might possibly prove helpful, the few clinical trials carried out to date have failed to provide convincing evidence that TRP is effective in significantly decreasing pain. Obviously, dietary control to help patients lose weight can prove beneficial for patients who have chronic pain caused by musculoskeletal disorders or other conditions. Tryptophan, like many other analgesic therapies, however, produces adverse side effects that apparently discourage patients from following the diet, and consequently no long-term benefits are produced. Moreover, the demonstration that tryptophan might contribute to the basic pathophysiology of rheumatoid arthritis suggests that patients should be carefully selected for this purpose. More well-controlled trials should be carried out, not only of tryptophan, but of other neurotransmitters that can be manipulated to enhance the various endogenous pain inhibitory systems.

REFERENCES

1. Shils, M.E., and Young, V.R. (eds): Modern Nutrition in Health and Disease. 7th Ed. Philadelphia, Lea & Febiger, 1988.
2. Hippocratis medicorum omnium facile principis opera omnia quae extant. Geneva, Chouet, 1657.
3. Wilmore, D.W., et al.: Stress in surgical patients as a neurophysiologic reflex response. Surg. Gynecol. Obstet., 142:257, 1976.
4. Souba, W.W., and Wilmore, D.W.: Diet and nutrition in the care of the patient with surgery, trauma and sepsis. In Modern Nutrition in Health and Disease. 7th Ed. Edited by M.E. Shils and V.R. Young. Philadelphia, Lea & Febiger, 1988, pp. 1306–1336.
5. Kehlet, H.: The modifying effect of general and regional anesthesia on the endocrine-metabolic response to surgery. Reg. Anaesth., 7:S38, 1982.
6. Kehlet, H.: Pain relief and modification of the stress response. In Acute Pain Management. Edited by M.J. Cousins and G.D. Phillips. London, Churchill Livingstone, 1986, pp. 49–75.
7. Bessman, F.P., and Renner, V.J.: The biphasic hormonal nature of stress. In Pathophysiology of Shock, Anoxia and Ischemia. Edited by R.A. Cowley and B.F. Trump. Baltimore, Williams & Wilkins, 1982, pp. 60–65.
8. Moore, F.D.: Metabolic Care of the Surgical Patient. Philadelphia, W.B. Saunders, 1959.
9. Holden, W.D. et al.: The effect of nutrition on nitrogen metabolism in the surgical patient. Ann. Surg., 146:563, 1957.
10. Kehlet, H: Modification of responses to surgical and neural blockade: Clinical implications. In Neural Blockade in Clinical Anesthesia and Management of Pain. 2nd Ed. Edited by M.J. Cousins and P.O. Bridenbaugh. Philadelphia, J.B. Lippincott, 1988, pp. 145–188.
11. Crile, G.W.: Phylogenetic association in relation to certain medical problems. Boston Med. Surg. J., 163:893, 1910.
12. Cannon, W.B.: The Wisdom of the Body. New York, Norton, 1939.

13. O'Shaughnessey, L., and Slome, D.: Etiology of traumatic shock. Br. J. Surg., *22*:589, 1934.
14. Bonica, J.J.: The Management of Pain. Philadelphia, Lea & Febiger, 1953.
15. Tsuji, H., et al.: Influences of splanchnic nerve blockade on endocrine-metabolic responses to upper abdominal surgery. Br. J. Surg., *70*:437, 1983.
16. Brandt, M.R., et al.: Epidural analgesia improves postoperative nitrogen balance. Br. Med. J., *1*:1106, 1978.
17. Teasdale, C., et al.: A randomized controlled trial to compare local with general anaesthesia for short-stay inguinal hernia repair. Ann. R. Coll. Surg. Engl., *64*:238, 1982.
18. Cuschieri, R.J., et al.: Postoperative pain and pulmonary complications: Comparison of three analgesic regimens. Br. J. Surg., *72*:495, 1985.
19. Yeager, M.P., et al.: Epidural anesthesia and analgesia in high-risk surgical patients. Anesthesiology, *66*:729, 1987.
20. Modig, J., et al.: Role of extradural and of general anesthesia in fibrinolysis and coagulation after total hip replacement. Br. J. Anaesth., *55*:625, 1983.
21. Pflug, A.E., et al.: The effects of postoperative peridural analgesia on pulmonary therapy and pulmonary complications. Anesthesiology, *41*:8, 1974.
22. Moss, G., et al.: Postoperative metabolic patterns following immediate total nutritional support: Hormone levels, DNA synthesis, nitrogen balance, and accelerated wound healing. J. Surg. Res., *21*:383, 1976.
23. Moss, G., et al.: Maintenance of GI function after bowel surgery and immediate enteral full nutrition. I. Doubling of canine colorectal anastomotic bursting pressure and intestinal wound mature collagen content. J. Parenter. Enteral Nutr., *4*:535, 1980.
24. Moss, G., Regal, M.E., and Lichtig, L.: Reducing postoperative pain, narcotics, and length of hospitalization. Surgery, *99*:206, 1986.
25. Moss, G.: Discharge within 24 hours of elective cholecystectomy. The first 100 patients. Arch. Surg., *121*:1159, 1986.
26. Bures-Forsthoefel, J., et al.: Feeding by tube immediately after hysterectomy. Contemp. Obstet. Gynecol., *27*:51, 1986.
27. Seidmon, E.J., et al.: Immediate postoperative feeding in urological surgery. J. Urol., *131*:1113, 1984.
28. Cuthbertson, D.P.: Further observation on disturbances of metabolism caused by injury with particular references to dietary requirements of fracture cases. Br. J. Surg., *23*:505, 1936.
29. Wilmore, D.W.: The Metabolic Management of the Critically Ill. New York, Plenum Medical Books, 1977.
30. Grant, A.: Nutritional Assessment: Guidelines for Dieticians. 2nd Ed. Seattle, Anne Grant, 1979.
31. Russell, R.I.: Nutritional support of patients with pancreatic diseases. *In* Modern Nutrition in Health and Disease. 7th Ed. Edited by M.E. Shils and V.R. Young. Philadelphia, Lea & Febiger, 1988, pp. 1114–1123.
32. Tassonyi, E., et al.: Epidural block in the treatment of acute pancreatitis. Reg. Anaesth., *6*:8, 1981.
33. Shils, M.E.: Nutrition and diet in cancer. *In* Modern Nutrition in Health and Disease. 7th Ed. Edited by M.E. Shils and V.R. Young. Philadelphia, Lea & Febiger, 1988, pp. 1380–1422.
34. Brennan, M.F.: Supportive care of the cancer patient: Nutritional support. *In* Cancer: Principles and Practice of Oncology. 2nd Ed. Edited by V.T. DeVita, Jr., S. Hellman, and S.A. Rosenberg. Philadelphia, J.B. Lippincott, 1985, pp. 1907–1919.
35. Minna, J.D., and Bunn, P.A., Jr.: Paraneoplastic syndromes: Anorexia, cachexia and intestinal abnormalities as paraneoplastic manifestations. *In* Cancer: Principles and Practice of Oncology. 2nd Ed. Edited by V.T. DeVita, Jr., S. Hellman, and S.A. Rosenberg. Philadelphia, J.B. Lippincott, 1985, pp. 1798–1842.
36. DeWys, W.D. et al.: Prognostic effect of weight loss prior to chemotherapy in cancer patients. Am. J. Med., *69*:491, 1980.
37. Baines, M.: Nausea and vomiting in patients with advanced cancer. J. Pain Symptom Management, *3*:81, 1988.
38. Theologides, A.: The anorexia-cachexia syndrome: A new hypothesis. Ann. N.Y. Acad. Sci., *230*:14, 1974.
39. Bernstein, I.: Learned taste aversions in children receiving chemotherapy. Science, *200*:1302, 1978.
40. Bernstein, I.: Etiology of anorexia in cancer. Cancer, *58*:1881, 1986.
41. Norton, J., Burt, M., and Brennan, M.: In vivo utilization of substrate by sarcoma-bearing limbs. Cancer, *45*:2934, 1980.
42. Bruera, E., and MacDonald, R.N.: Nutrition in cancer patients: An update and review of our experience. J. Pain Symptom Management, *3*:133, 1988.
43. Holroyde, C., and Reichard, G.: Carbohydrate metabolism in cancer cachexia. Cancer Treat. Rep., *65*:55, 1981.
44. Torti, F., et al.: A macrophage factor inhibits adipocyte gene expression: An in vitro model of cachexia. Science, *229*:867, 1985.
45. Theologides, A.: Anorexins, asthenins and cachectins in cancer. Am. J. Med., *81*:296, 1986.
46. Bistrian, B.: Some practical and theoretical concepts in the nutritional assessment of cancer patients. Cancer, *58*:1863, 1986.
47. Nixon, D., et al.: Protein-calorie undernutrition in hospitalized cancer patients. Am. J. Med., *68*:683, 1980.
48. DeWys, W.D.: Anorexia as a general effect of cancer. Cancer, *43*:2013, 1979.
49. Woodford, J.M., and Fielding, J.R.: Pain and cancer. *In* Pain, Clinical and Experimental Perspectives. Edited by M. Wisenberg. St. Louis, C.V. Mosby, 1975, pp. 326–332.
50. Bonica, J.J.: Principles and Practice of Obstetric Analgesia and Anesthesia. Philadelphia, F.A. Davis, 1967, pp. 675–676.
51. Nimmo, W.S.: Gastrointestinal function following surgery. Reg. Anaesth., 7:S105, 1982.
52. Jaffe, J.H., and Martin, W.R.: Opioid analgesics and antagonists. *In* Goodman and Gilman's. The Pharmacological Basis of Therapeutics. 7th Ed. Edited by A.G. Gilman, et al. New York, Macmillan, 1985, pp. 491–531.
53. Blackburn, G., Miller, M., and Bothe, A.: Nutritional factors in cancer in medical oncology. *In* Oncology. Edited by P. Calabresi and P. Schein. New York, Macmillan, 1985, pp. 1406–1432.
54. Smale, B., et al.: The efficacy of nutritional assessment and support in cancer surgery. Cancer, *47*:2375, 1981.
55. Blackburn, G., and Thornton, P.: Nutritional assessment of the hospitalized patient. Med. Clin. North Am., *63*:1103, 1979.
56. Schulze-Delrieu, K.: Metoclopramide. N. Engl. J. Med., *305*:28, 1981.
57. Cavalli, F., et al.: Randomized trial of low- versus high-dose medroxyprogesterone acetate in the treatment of postmenopausal patients with advanced breast cancer. *In* Role of Medroxyprogesterone in Endocrine-Related Tumors. Edited by A. Pellegrini and G. Robustelli. New York, Raven Press, 1984, pp. 79–90.
58. Shils, M.E., Bloch, A.S., and Chernoff, P.: Liquid Formulas for Oral and Tube Feeding. 2nd Ed. New York, Memorial Cancer Center, 1979.
59. Holter, A.R., Rosen, H.M., and Fischer, J.E.: The effects of hyperalimentation on major surgery in patients with malignant disease: A prospective study. Acta Chir. Scand. (Suppl.), *466*:86, 1976.
60. Holter, A.R., and Fischer, J.E.: The effects of perioperative hyperalimentation on complications in patients with carcinoma and weight loss. J. Surg. Res., *23*:31, 1977.
61. Koretz, R.: Parenteral nutrition: Is it oncologically logical? J. Clin. Oncol., *2*:534, 1984.
62. Evans, W., Nixon, D., and Daly, J.: A randomized study of standard or augmented oral nutritional support versus ad lib nutrition intake in patients with advanced cancer. Clin. Invest. Med., *9*:A-127, 1986.
63. Heber, D., Byerley, L., and Chi, J.: Pathophysiology of malnutrition in the adult cancer patient. Cancer, *58*:1867, 1986.
64. American Cancer Society: Unproven Methods of Cancer Management. New York, American Cancer Society, 1979.
65. Panush, R.S.: Arthritis, food, diets and nutrition. *In* Arthritis and Allied Conditions. Edited by D.J. McCarty. Philadelphia, Lea & Febiger, 1989, pp. 1010–1014.
66. Klinenberg, J.R.: ARA Presidential Address: 1984-2034: The next half-century for American rheumatology. Arthritis Rheum., *28*:1, 1985.
67. Kremer, J.M., et al.: Effects of manipulation of dietary fatty acids on clinical manifestations of rheumatoid arthritis. Lancet, *1*:184, 1985.
68. Kremer, J.M., et al.: Fish-oil fatty acid supplementation in patients with active rheumatoid arthritis, a double-blind controlled crossover study. Ann. Intern. Med., *106*:497, 1987.
69. Bollet, A.J.: Nutrition and diet in rheumatic disorders. *In* Modern Nutrition in Health and Disease, 7th Ed. Edited by M.E. Shils and V.R. Young. Philadelphia, Lea & Febiger, 1988. pp. 1471–1481.

70. Panush, R.S., Stroud, R.M., and Webster, E.: Food-induced (allergic) arthritis. Inflammatory arthritis exacerbated by milk. Arthritis Rheum., *29*:220, 1986.
71. Simkin, P.A.: Oral zinc sulfate in rheumatoid arthritis. Lancet, *2*:539, 1976.
72. Rasker, J.J., and Kardaun, S.H.: Lack of beneficial effect of zinc sulphate in rheumatoid arthritis. Scand. J. Rheumatol., *11*:168, 1982.
73. Pinals, R.S., et al.: Treatment of rheumatoid arthritis with L-histidine: A randomized, placebo-controlled, double-blind trial. J. Rheumatol., *4*:414, 1977.
74. Eising, L.: Dietary intake in patients with arthritis and other chronic disorders. J. Bone Joint Surg. [Am.], *45*:69, 1963.
75. Acheson, R.M., and Collart, A.B.: New Haven survey of joint diseases. Ann. Rheum. Dis., *34*:379, 1975.
76. Watson, M.: Femoral-head height loss: A study of the relative significance of some of its determinants in hip degeneration. Rheumatol. Rehabil. *15*:264, 1976.
77. Muncie, H.L.: Medical aspects of the multidisciplinary assessment in management of osteoarthritis. Clin. Ther. *9*(Suppl. B):4, 1986.
78. Kelley, W.N.: Gout and related disorders of purine metabolism. *In* Textbook of Rheumatology. Edited by W.N. Kelley et al. Philadelphia, W.B. Saunders, 1981, pp. 1397–1437.
79. Basu, T.K., et al.: Ascorbic acid therapy for the relief of bone pain in Paget's disease. Acta Vitaminol. Enzymol., *32*:45, 1978.
80. Smethurst, M., et al.: Combined therapy with ascorbic acid and calcitonin for the relief of bone pain in Paget's disease. Acta Vitaminol. Enzymol., *3*:8, 1981.
81. Travell, J.G., and Simons, D.G.: Myofascial Pain and Dysfunction. The Trigger Point Manual. Baltimore, Williams & Wilkins, 1983, pp. 114–144.
82. Wolman, S.L.: Nutritional effects of diseases of the stomach and duodenum. *In* Modern Nutrition in Health and Disease. 7th Ed. Edited by M.E. Shils and V.R. Young. Philadelphia, Lea & Febiger, 1988, pp. 1094–1098.
83. Rosenberg, I.H.: Nutritional support in inflammatory bowel disease. *In* Modern Nutrition in Health and Disease. 7th Ed. Edited by M.E. Shils and V.R. Young. Philadelphia, Lea & Febiger, 1988, pp. 1138–1143.
84. Kirschner, B.S., et al.: Reversal of growth retardation in Crohn's disease with therapy emphasizing oral nutritional restitution. Gastroenterology, *80*:10, 1981.
85. Bengoa, J.M., and Rosenberg, I.H.: Parenteral nutrition therapy in gastrointestinal disease. *In* Yearbook of Medicine. Edited by D.E. Rogers et al. Chicago, Yearbook Medical Publishers, 1983, pp. 363–385.
86. Dickinson, R.J., et al.: Controlled trial of intravenous hyperalimentation and total bowel rest as an adjunct to the routine therapy of acute colitis. Gastroenterology, *79*:1199, 1980.
87. Takagi, Y., et al.: Total parenteral nutrition in inflammatory bowel disease. An evaluation of its clinical response. Nippon Geka Gakkai Zasshi, *85*:1006, 1984.
88. Russell, R.I.: Nutritional support of patients with pancreatic disease. *In* Modern Nutrition in Health and Disease. 7th Ed. Edited by M.E. Shils and V.R. Young. Philadelphia, Lea & Febiger, 1988, pp. 1114–1123.
89. Dreyfus, P.M.: Diet and nutrition in neurologic disorders. *In* Modern Nutrition in Health and Disease. 7th Ed. Edited by M.E. Shils and V.R. Young. Philadelphia, Lea & Febiger, 1988, pp. 1458–1470.
90. Barchas, J.D., et al.: Behavioral neurochemistry: Neuroregulators and behavioral states. Science, *200*:964, 1978.
91. Barchas, J.D., and Elliott, G.R.: Behavioral neurochemistry, neuroregulators and behavioral states. *In* American Handbook of Psychiatry, Vol. 8. 2nd Ed. Edited by P.A. Berger and H.K.H. Brodie. New York, Basic Books, 1986, pp. 33–51.
92. Fernstrom, J.D., and Wurtman, R.J.: Brain serotonin content: Physiological dependence on plasma tryptophan levels. Science, *173*:149, 1971.
93. Fernstrom, J.D., Larin, F., and Wurtman, F.J.: Correlations between brain tryptophan and plasma neutral amino acid levels following food consumption in the rat. Life Sci., *13*:517, 1973.
94. Wurtman, R.J.: Nutrients that modify brain function. Sci. Am., *246*:42, 1982.
95. Pardridge, W.M.: Regulation of amino acid availability in the brain. *In* Nutrition and the Brain, Vol. 1. Edited by R.J. Wurtman and J.J. Wurtman. New York, Raven Press, 1977, pp. 141–204.
96. Messing, R.B., and Lytle, L.D.: Serotonin-containing neurons: Their possible role in pain and analgesia. Pain, *4*:1, 1977.
97. Akil, H., and Liebeskind, J.C.: Monoaminergic mechanisms of stimulation-produced analgesia. Brain Res., *94*:279, 1975.
98. Sparkes, C.G., and Spencer, P.S.J.: Antinociceptive activity of morphine after injection of biogenic amines in cerebral ventricle of rat. Br. J. Pharmacol., *42*:230, 1971.
99. Ogren, S.O., and Holm, A.C.: Test-specific effects of the 5-HT reuptake inhibitors alaproclate and zimelidine on pain sensitivity and morphine analgesia. J. Neurol. Transm., *47*:253, 1980.
100. Sicuteri, F., Anselmi, B., and Fanciullacci, M.: The serotonin (5-HT) theory of migraine. Adv. Neurol., *4*:383, 1974.
101. Proudfit, H.K., and Anderson, E.G.: Morphine analgesia: Blockade by raphe magnus lesions. Brain Res., *98*:612, 1975.
102. Fernstrom, J.D., and Hirsch, M.J.: Rapid repletion of brain serotonin in malnourished, corn-fed rats following L-tryptophan injection. Life Sci., *17*:455, 1975.
103. Sicuteri, F.: Emicrania e mediatori chimici. [Migraine and chemical mediators.] Presented at the International Symposium on Mediatori chimici, funzione nervosa e circolo cerebrale. Florence, Italy, 1960. Firenze, Mattioli, 1960.
104. Kangasniemi, P., et al.: Levotryptophan treatment in migraine. Headache, *18*:161, 1978.
105. Boiardi, A., et al.: 5-OH-tryptophan in migraine: Clinical and neurophysiological considerations. J. Neurol., *225*:41, 1981.
106. Sternbach, R.A. et al.: Effects of altering brain serotonin activity on human chronic pain. *In* Advances in Pain Research and Therapy, Vol. 1. Edited by J.J. Bonica and D. Albe-Fessard. New York, Raven Press, 1976, pp. 601–606.
107. Hosobuchi, Y.: Tryptophan reversal of tolerance to analgesia induced by central grey stimulation. Lancet *2*:47, 1978.
108. King, R.B.: Pain and tryptophan. J. Neurosurg., *53*:44, 1980.
109. De Benedittis, G., et al.: Effects of 5-hydroxytryptophan on central and deafferentation chronic pain: A preliminary clinical trial. *In* Advances in Pain Research and Therapy, Vol. 5. Edited by J.J. Bonica, U. Lindblom, and A. Iggo. New York, Raven Press, 1983, pp. 295–304.
110. Moldofsky, H., and Warsh, J.J.: Plasma tryptophan and musculoskeletal pain in non-articular rheumatism ("fibrositis syndrome"). Pain, *5*:65, 1978.
111. Moldofsky, H., and Lue, F.A.: The relationship of alpha- and delta-EEG frequencies to pain and mood in "fibrositis" patients treated with chlorpromazine and L-tryptophan. Electroencephalogr. Clin. Neurophysiol., *50*:71, 1980.
112. Seltzer, S., et al.: Alteration of human pain thresholds by nutritional manipulation and L-tryptophan supplementation. Pain, *13*:385, 1982.
113. Seltzer, S.: Perspectives in the control of chronic pain by nutritional manipulation. Pain, *11*:141, 1981.
114. Seltzer, S., et al.: The effects of dietary tryptophan on chronic maxillofacial pain and experimental pain tolerance. J. Psychiatr. Res., *17*:181, 1982–1983.
115. Heinze, E.G., Jr., and Lehman, K.S.: Nutritional aspects of chronic pain management. Pain (Suppl.), *4*:S299, 1987.

INTRODUCTION

JOHN J. BONICA

This section includes two chapters devoted to the use of electric stimulation for the control of acute or chronic pain. In Chapter 92, Sjölund and Eriksson discuss transcutaneous electric stimulation and Loeser presents a brief overview of the use of peripheral nerve stimulation by the application of an electrode around major peripheral nerves. In Chapter 93, Meyerson discusses spinal cord stimulation and deep-brain stimulation.

The resurgence of the use of electricity to treat pain was provoked by publication of the Melzack-Wall theory of pain (1). Indeed, the first modern application of this modality, reported by Wall and Sweet (2) in 1967, provided support for the Melzack-Wall hypothesis, which emphasized the important role of the dorsal horn of the spinal cord in modulating sensory transmission. The subsequent discovery and eventual detailed description of the anatomic, physiologic, and pharmacologic aspects of the periaqueductal gray and other brain stem sites and the descending inhibitory systems led to the use of deep-brain stimulation. To date, an unknown number of patients, probably exceeding several million, have been subjected to the techniques described in these two chapters.

Although these techniques have been considered an important recent advance in pain therapy, the practice of applying electricity to relieve pain is as old as recorded history (3–5). Egyptian tombs of the Vth Dynasty (2750 B.C.) displayed the Nile (electric) catfish (Malopterurus electricus), and the ancient Greeks, including Aristotle, described the numbness caused by the torpedo ray (Torpedo marmorata). Among the Romans, Pliny in *Natural History* and Plutarch in *Morales* referred to the numbing effect of the ray (6), and Scribonius (circa 46 A.D.) advocated electrotherapy specifically for the relief of "chronic and unbearable headache," gout, and other conditions (7). At the same time Dioscorides, a Greek army surgeon in the service of Nero, also advocated electrotherapy for a variety of painful and nonpainful disorders (8). A century later Galen, after studying live and dead electric fish, concluded that the latter had no effect; however, he wrote the following about application of a live torpedo ray to a patient suffering from headache: "It could be that this remedy is anodyne and could free the patient from pain as do other remedies which numb the senses: this I found to be so" (9). These and other Roman physicians indicated that in order to be effective, the torpedo fish should be placed on the spot where the pain was felt.

Kane and Taub (3) suggested that the characteristics of the stimuli produced by electric fish are similar to those produced artificially for local electric analgesia: The voltage ranges from 1 to 350 V (40 to 50 V for the torpedo fish). The stimulus frequency is either "fast" (maximum of 1000 impulses/s) or "slow" (generally about 200 impulses/s). The number of impulses in a train varies from 100 to several thousand (10).

The clinical application of the torpedo fish as a therapeutic modality for pain and other conditions continued throughout the Middle Ages, the Renaissance, and well into the nineteenth century; in non-Western cultures, electric fish are still used for this purpose (6). During the eighteenth century, many improvements were made in electrostatic apparatus constructed earlier by Von Guericke, including the development of the Leyden jar (5). Consequently, electrotherapy was applied even more widely despite the skepticism and opposition of a number of authorities.

During the nineteenth century, development of the electric "pile" and the subsequent development of the induction apparatus provided further impetus for electromedical application (11). Voltaic (galvanic) and faradic currents were stronger and/or more easily modulated than was static electricity, and ever-increasing, and indeed frenetic efforts were made to use electricity as a surgical anesthetic especially for tooth extraction and other dental therapies (5). In the years just before and after 1860, numerous reports were published on the use of electric anesthesia for dental surgery and subsequently for surgery on the limbs. In the United States, the most widely known exponents were Francis (12) of Philadelphia, Garratt (13) of Boston, and Oliver (14) of Buffalo. These three individuals became involved in a bitter controversy as to who was the first "discoverer" of electric anesthesia. Interestingly, this controversy occurred at about the same time as the intense controversy in regard to the discoverer of general anesthesia by demonstrating the anesthetic properties of ether and nitrous oxide.

In England, Althaus (15), a prominent electrotherapist, was the first to adopt and use the new electroanesthesia. In 1859 he applied "interrupted current" transcutaneously to peripheral nerves and eventually convinced his most prominent critic, Benjamin Richardson (who was a friend of John Snow, the patriarch of anesthesiology), of its efficacy to diminish sensation and produce analgesia by stepwise increase of the electric stimulus to Dr. Richardson's ulnar nerve. Althaus applied these techniques for the relief of neuralgia and found that analgesia was more effective and more readily attained in pathologic conditions than in normal situations (15). Unfortunately, the controversy remained and prompted the appointment of a commission headed by Richardson. After studying the efficacy of electric anesthesia in patients undergoing tooth extraction, the commission concluded that the technique produced no local anesthetic effect (16).

The use of electroanesthesia in dentistry was introduced to France in 1858, and subsequently reports also were published in Germany and Italy (3). The results obtained in these countries were variable, and toward the end of the century, this modality was virtually abandoned for surgical anesthesia, although a number of workers continued to use if for the treatment of neuralgia and other pain syndromes.

During the first six decades of this century, a number of clinicians attempted to resurrect electroanesthesia for surgical operations, but because it was much less predictable than pharmacologic anesthesia, it never became widely used. In 1928 Thompson et al. (17) of the University of California at Berkeley noted that "the cutaneous areas supplied by a nerve may be rendered insensible to light touch by subjecting the nerve trunk to the influence of an alternating current." Increasing the current produced analgesia. With this technique they determined the distribution of all the cutaneous nerves in the forearm of one individual (17). Fourteen years later Paraf (18), using the same technique, reported the successful treatment of 127 patients with sciatic pain, lumbago, postherpetic neuralgia, and tic douloureux.

In 1953 Guenot (19) wrote a thesis on local electric analgesia in which he described the work of Perrin, Bernard, LeGo, Presle, Wild, and Prolest, all of whom used local and regional electroanesthesia. Prolest (20) experimented with 50- to 100-Hz monophasic and diphasic waves, which caused initial excitation and paresthesia but soon caused "inhibition" and raised the sensory threshold to the current. During the 1950s and early 1960s, reports on the use of electric stimulation of the spinothalamic tract, the thalamus, and other parts of the brain stem for the relief of pain, with varying degrees of success, were published by Mazars et al. (21) and others (see 4 for references).

In addition to providing a scientifically plausible explanation of the mechanism of pain, the Melzack-Wall theory of pain provided the much needed impetus that, together with other factors, stimulated the revolution in pain research and therapy of the past two decades. As discussed in Chapter 4, among the most important and exciting studies were those that defined the neuroanatomic and biochemical substrates of segmental analgesia produced by transcutaneous electric nerve stimulation, spinal cord stimulation, and deep-brain stimulation. These techniques are discussed in detail in the following two chapters.

REFERENCES

1. Melzack, R., and Wall, P.D.: Pain mechanisms: A new theory. Science, 150:971, 1965.
2. Wall, P.D., and Sweet, W.H.: Temporary abolition of pain in man. Science, 155:108, 1967.
3. Kane, K., and Taub, A.: History of local electrical analgesia. Pain, 1:125, 1975.
4. Siegfried, J.: Introduction—historique. In La Neurostimulation Eléctrique Thérapeutique. Edited by R. Sedan and Y. Lazorthes. Paris, Masson, 1978, pp. 5–10.
5. Colwell, H.A.: An Essay on the History of Electrotherapy and Diagnosis. London, Heinemann, 1922.
6. Kellaway, P.: The part played by electric fish in the early history of bioelectricity and electrotherapy. Bull. Hist. Med., 20:112, 1946.
7. Scribonius, L.: Compositiones Medicae. Padua, Frambottus, 1655.
8. Dioscorides, T.: The Greek Herbal of Dioscorides. Translated by J. Goodyear. London, Oxford University Press, 1934.
9. Galen, C.: De Usu Partium. English translation by M. Tallmadge. Ithaca, NY, Cornell University Press, 1968.
10. Grundfest, H.: The mechanism of discharge of the electrical organs in relation to general and comparative electrophysiology. Prog. Biophys., 7:1, 1957.
11. Faraday, M.: On volta-electric induction, and the evolution of electricity from magnetism. Lancet, 2:246, 1831–1832.
12. Francis, J.B.: Extracting teeth by galvanism. Dent. Rep., 1:65, 1858.
13. Garratt, A.C.: Electrophysiology and Electrotherapeutics. Boston, Tricknor and Fields, 1861.
14. Oliver, W.G.: Electrical Anesthesia: Comprising a Brief History of its Discovery, a Synopsis of Experiments, also Full Directions for its Application in Surgical and Dental Operations. Buffalo, NY, Murray, Rockwell and Co., 1858.
15. Althaus, J.: A treatise on medical electricity theoretical and practical and its use in the treatment of paralysis, neuralgia and other diseases. London, Trubner, 1859.
16. Electricity as an anaesthetic agent in dental surgery. Lancet, 1:594, 1859.
17. Thompson, I.M., Inman, V.T., and Brownfield, B.: Cutaneous nerve areas of the forearm and hand. Univ. of California Publication in Anatomy. Los Angeles, Univ. of California, 1934, pp. 195–236.
18. Paraf, P.: Traitement des algies par les courants diadynamiques. Bull. Soc. Med. Paris, 64:114, 1948.
19. Guenot, J.: Contribution à l'etude de l'anesthésie locale par les impulsions rectangulaires de Basse frequence. Thesis, Paris, Universite de Paris, 1953.
20. Prolest, J.Y.: L'emploi therapeutique de certains courants electriques a bases frequences dits courants diadynamiques. Rev. Med. Suisse Romande, 70:257, 1950.
21. Mazars, G., Roge, R., and Mazars, Y.: Rèsultats de la stimulation du faisceau spino-thalamique et leur incidence sur la physiolopathologie de la douleur. Rev. Neurol., 103:136, 1960.

92 · TRANSCUTANEOUS AND IMPLANTED ELECTRIC STIMULATION OF PERIPHERAL NERVES

Bengt H. Sjölund, Margareta Eriksson, *and* John D. Loeser

THIS chapter contains discussion of the techniques for stimulation of peripheral nerves for the relief of acute and chronic pain. The material is presented in two major sections: A, Transcutaneous Electric Nerve Stimulation, written by Bengt H. Sjölund and Margareta Eriksson and B, Implanted Electric Nerve Stimulation, written by John D. Loeser. Each section includes discussion of the physiologic basis of the technique, indications for and results of its use, technical considerations including description of the equipment and technique of application, and contraindications and side effects.

A. TRANSCUTANEOUS ELECTRIC NERVE STIMULATION

Initially used largely as a screening method in selecting patients for implantable neurostimulators, transcutaneous electric nerve stimulation (TENS) has developed into a successful technique for pain relief in its own right. Technical advances and miniaturization in electronic design have contributed to the rapid and extensive adoption of TENS for clinical use, mainly for relief of chronic pain of nonmalignant origin.

Sensory stimulation (counterirritation) has a long history as a method of pain relief (1). Rubbing and massaging probably have been used to relieve pain since the dawn of time. Similarly, mildly painful stimuli, whether mechanical or thermal (e.g., cupping, acupuncture, moxa burning), and an ancient technique of electroanalgesia performed with electric fish (2) have been used to alleviate pain and suffering from disease.

With the publication of the gate theory of pain by Melzack and Wall (3) and the pioneering report by Wall and Sweet (4) on temporary abolition of pain by electric nerve stimulation, sensory stimulation was rediscovered in the 1960s as a treatment modality for pain. Today, the stimulation pulses are produced by a battery-powered, miniaturized current generator. They are delivered to nerve fibers transcutaneously via two or more epicutaneous (surface) conductive rubber electrodes, connected to the current generator by cables (Fig. 92-1). When properly applied, the stimulation gives rise to nonpainful electric paresthesia in the area of pain, called *conventional TENS*, or to muscle contractions in myotomes segmentally related to that area, labeled *acupuncture-like TENS*. Because the pain relief is temporary, stimulation has to be repeated regularly. After a period of instruction, most patients treat themselves at home several times daily, each time for 20 to 60 min. In this section, we present an overview of possible mechanisms behind the analgesia from TENS, its present indications and probable future applications, a description of the technique and mode of application, and contraindications and side effects. A note on preferred technical standards of the equipment is also given. Comprehensive reviews on the use of TENS have been published by Cotter (5) for relief of postoperative pain and by Sjölund and Eriksson (6) and Meyerson (7) for chronic pain therapy.

Physiologic Basis

All afferent nerve fibers seem to have the capacity to influence the activity of other afferent nerve fibers, mainly through mutual presynaptic inhibition (8). Based on results from animal experimentation as well as on clinical observations, Melzack and Wall (3) in 1965 postulated that a "gate" to sensory input is present in the spinal cord, which is opened by activity in small-diameter (i.e., nociceptive) afferent fibers and closed by activity in large-diameter (i.e., mainly mechanoceptive) afferent fibers. This would explain the hyperpathia of certain pain states as well as the everyday observation that rubbing a painful area often relieves pain. Although the experimental basis for the "opening part" of the gate theory has been subjected to much criticism (see Chapter 4), a temporary inhibition of transmission from small-diameter afferent nerve fibers to second-order neurons in the spinal cord by non-noxious and noxious stimuli has been amply verified experimentally (8).

If graded electric stimuli are applied to a mixed nerve, whether buried in tissue or not, the first fibers to become activated are the large-diameter ones (9). It is thus possible to induce a substantial but nonpainful barrage of impulses selectively in large afferent fibers with a small, relatively uncomplicated current generator. The first clinical report (4) on use of such a technique to relieve chronic pain in man followed soon after publication of the gate theory, but there is still no direct evidence that the analgesia from TENS in man comes from pre- or postsynaptic inhibition in the spinal cord. Although a peripheral mechanism entailing fatigue of nociceptive fibers was postulated (10), this hypothesis was shown to be highly unlikely (11). It is noteworthy, however, that the often longstanding pain relief of several hours duration after a short (20-min)

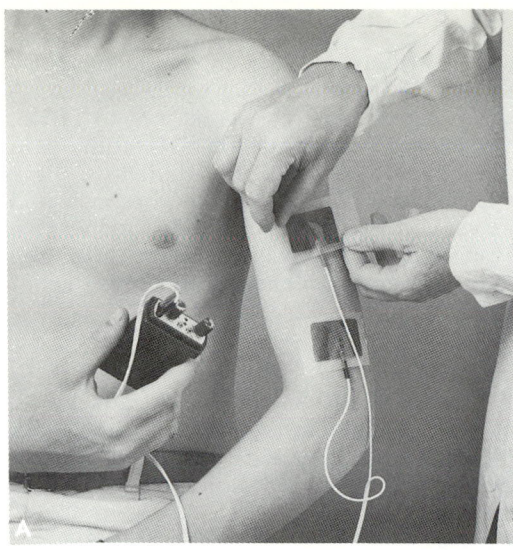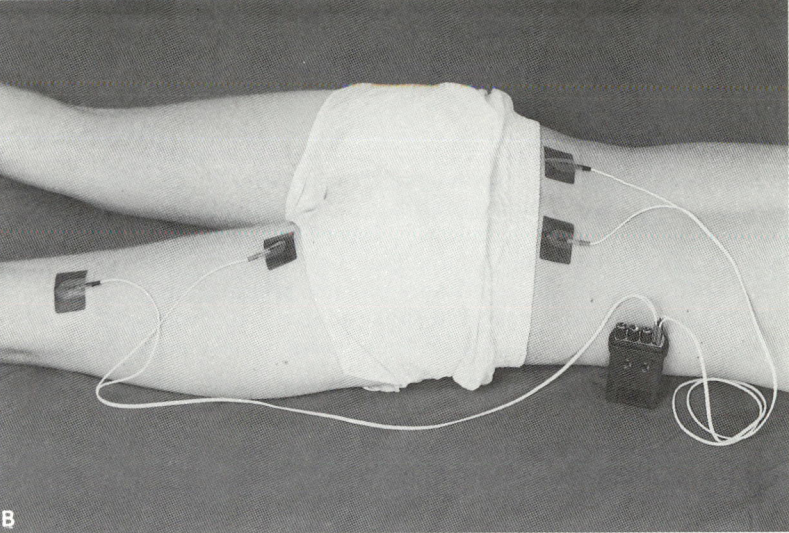

Fig. 92-1. *A.* TENS stimulator is held by the patient while carbon rubber electrodes are applied over the left radial nerve to alleviate pain from C7 rhizopathy. *B.* Dual-channel stimulation in lumbago-sciatica with irradiating pain down the right leg. Conventional TENS is given over the painful area in the lumbar region and acupuncture-like TENS is given over the right sciatic nerve, inducing twitches in L5 and S1 myotomes.

treatment period is not readily explained by ordinary inhibitory phenomena between nerve cells.

The increasing use of the TENS technique in the early 1970s soon showed that long-term treatment results were not very encouraging (12). At about the same time, several groups of investigators demonstrated a rise in experimental pain thresholds after low-frequency (0.5 to 4 Hz) electric stimulation of tissues via needle electrodes. Interestingly, Andersson et al. (13) did not find it necessary to deliver the stimuli via needles provided that the stimuli were strong enough to elicit muscle contractions when given via epicutaneous (surface) electrodes. This observation was in agreement with those of others indicating the importance of a deep afferent input for acupuncture analgesia (14).

In patients with chronic pain, eliciting strong muscle contractions via surface electrodes without discomfort was possible only when short pulse trains or tetani were used (15). The pulse trains used had an internal frequency of 100 Hz, which is well above that needed for mammalian muscle fusion (16), and were delivered at a low repetition rate (1 to 2 Hz). This technique, denoted acupuncture-like TENS (lo TENS) and utilized whenever conventional TENS (hi TENS) (4) did not give pain relief, significantly improved overall TENS treatment results (15, 17, 18).

Evidence of an endorphinergic link in the mechanism of acupuncture-like TENS has been provided by two studies. One is a double-blind study of the effect of the opiate antagonist naloxone on relief of chronic pain with this technique. The results indicate that lo-TENs analgesia is reversed by naloxone and therefore acts through links utilizing endorphins (19). The other study involved measurements of endorphin activity in the cerebrospinal fluid of patients before and after treatment (21, 22). In contrast, the analgesia from conventional (hi) TENS is not affected by naloxone (19),

even in doses up to 10 mg to an adult (20), indicating that opioids utilizing mu receptors are not involved.

Indications and Efficacy

Acute Pain

Postoperative Pain

The most common indication for TENS has been for the relief of postoperative pain. Conventional TENS has been reported effective after laparotomy, thoracotomy, laminectomy, and hernioplasty (5, 7). In patients who had pulmonary or upper abdominal operations, respiratory function was found to improve more rapidly among TENS-treated patients than in control groups (23, 24). One possible explanation for this finding is that the TENS patients received less systemic medication and thus experienced less suppression of autonomic function postoperatively. Although other workers have confirmed the pain-relieving effect of TENS, they have not found improvement of pulmonary function (25, 26).

Conventional TENS has also been shown to be of value in pain after reconstructive orthopedic surgery of the hip and knee, reducing the need for narcotic analgesics (27, 28) and enhancing the rehabilitation of the patients (29). Pain after low back surgery has also been reported to be alleviated by conventional TENS as evidenced by the reduction of narcotic intake (30).

Labor Pain

Bundsen et al. (31) in controlled studies found that parturients with labor pain experienced moderate to good pain relief from TENS. No adverse effects on the fetus or newborn were detected using the Apgar score. The analgesic effect was most pronounced on the back pain component related to cervical dilatation. The suprapubic pain during the late stages of labor responded less well, even though a special electrode for the lower abdomen, designed to reduce the risk of influencing the fetal heart rate, was used (32).

Chronic Pain

As summarized in Table 92-1, chronic neuralgic pain conditions generally respond well to TENS (17, 18, 33–38). Few, if any, studies, however, are controlled in the sense that placebo stimulation has been added in a double-blind, cross-over design. This is mainly due to the difficulty of finding a suitable placebo stimulation. Several authors have reported that relief of pain from TENS is significantly greater than pain relief from placebo stimulation without batteries (37, 38).

The clinical efficacy of TENS techniques for chronic pain has to be judged from prospective or retrospective follow-up studies. From our experience, it is vital to know the length of follow-up, since many patients drop out within the first 3 months of treatment. Patients who respond to treatment for more than 3 months, however, usually continue the treatment (17, 18).

Neuralgia

Neuralgic pain of various types has become a prime target for TENS, probably because no other effective long-term treatments exist. Acupuncture-like TENS has to be employed in many cases, typically in rhizalgia and in conditions with hyperesthesia. Pain caused by lesions in the central nervous system, such as infarction in the brain stem (facial pain), and in the somesthetic pathways (e.g., thalamic syndrome) also has been relieved by TENS. Successful outcome of TENS therapy probably depends on a sufficient sensory impulse barrage being elicited from peripheral nerves in spite of the injury sustained.

Musculoskeletal Pain

Chronic pain characterized by a continuous impulse flow from nociceptive afferents due to chronic tissue damage (somatic pain) tends to respond well to TENS. This holds for musculoskeletal pain (17), joint pain from rheumatoid arthritis (39), and arthrosis. Pain from the skeleton, such as that from osteoporosis and cancer metastases to vertebral bodies or to ribs, also may be relieved with TENS. Local visceral pain, on the other hand, such as that from abdominal cancer, is not usually susceptible to TENS treatment (17).

Peripheral Vascular Disease

Kaada (40) studied the effects of TENS on ischemic chronic pain states. He found that not only did the pain diminish in TENS-treated patients with ischemic leg ulcers but the ulcers also decreased in size and, in some patients, even healed.

Cardiac Pain

In an uncontrolled but well-quantified study, Mannheimer et al. (41) found that ischemic pain from severe angina pectoris was relieved by conventional TENS given over the chest on the site of the most intense referred pain. During TENS, patients showed an increased working capacity on a maximal bicycle ergometer test as well as reduced recovery time after the test. Interestingly, the ischemia-induced ECG changes (ST depression) were also less pronounced during TENS than before or after stimulation.

Psychogenic Pain

Pain states with heavy functional components or of probable psychogenic origin do not respond well to

TABLE 92-1. Summary of Studies on Efficacy of TENS for Chronic Pain

Source	Mode*	Type of Pain	No. of Patients	% of Patients with Pain Relief at Follow-Up (months)				
				≤1	2–6	7–12	13–24	25–36
Wynn Parry (33)	Conv.	Brachial plexus avulsion	98	30	20			
Bates and Nathan (34)	Conv.	Low back; peripheral nerve lesions; central pain	161	48		27	16	
		Postherpetic	74	35		20	15	
Sindou and Keravel (35)	Conv.	Radicular syndromes	28	60				
		Peripheral nerve lesions	55	87				80
		Postherpetic neuralgia	34	67		25		
		Brachial plexus lesions	28	25–30				
		Central pain	22	0–11				
Bohm (36)	Conv. + Acup.	Peripheral nerve injury with sympathetic hyperactivity	24			42		
Eriksson et al. (17)	Conv. + Acup.	Facial neuralgia	11		82	45		
		Neuralgia (other locations)	32		56	34		
		Rhizalgia	22		64	60	34	
		Central pain	18		67	50		
		Other organic etiology	23		52	39		
		Psychogenic pain	17		18	18		
Eriksson et al. (18)	Conv. + Acup.	Facial pain	50		58	51	45	

*Conv. = conventional TENS; Acup. = acupuncture-like TENS.

TENS (42, 43). These patients may be overenthusiastic initially but soon report no analgesia or even transient aggravation of their pain from the stimulation.

Technical Considerations

Training of Staff and Patients

The use of TENS for acute pain conditions usually takes place in a hospital setting on inpatients (postoperative pain, labor pain). In this setting, staff training is most important, because the patient does not use TENS enough to master the technique. Procedures, electrode application, and criteria for choosing stimulus parameters must be taught to physicians and nurses working in postoperative wards, recovery rooms, intensive care units, and delivery suites. Furthermore, staff members closest to patients on the ward need to understand the TENS technique and know how to detect malfunction, recharge the units, apply the electrodes, and so forth.

For chronic pain syndromes, *patients* themselves should learn to master the TENS technique. Proper selection of patients for whom TENS treatment is indicated is best done in a multidisciplinary setting. In such settings, TENS can be prescribed in conjunction with rehabilitative measures, including physical therapy and return-to-work programs. Combining TENS with oral and injectable analgesics sometimes is done if the latter contribute significantly to the relief of pain in a particular patient (18).

The usual procedure in an outpatient facility involves a trial and evaluation period before home-based TENS treatment is prescribed. The patient should be told to omit taking analgesics 6 to 12 hours before the initial appointment, so that he or she is in pain. The pain history and a standard neurologic examination provide the basis for selecting the mode of TENS and electrode positions before TENS trials are started. It is often helpful to mark the positions of electrodes including polarity with a pen on the skin. The patient is then left alone for 20 to 30 min to evaluate the ongoing stimulation. If this does not appear effective, different electrode positions and/or TENS mode are selected, followed by a new trial period. When some analgesia is reported, the patient is carefully instructed on how the stimulator functions, how to use it, and how to attach and remove the electrodes before trying the treatment at home for 1 to 2 weeks.

The patient is then seen again, preferably by the same physician, who carries out an evelution, repeats the instructions to the patient, and possibly modifies the site of electrode placement. Before the patient has his or her own stimulator prescribed, a re-evaluation is carried out after 3 months of treatment. Thereafter, the patient may require only one or two consultations per year. Of course, he or she should be informed where to get supplies for the stimulator and accessories. As an alternative, especially for weak or disabled patients or when a more intensive treatment program is preferred, the patient may be evaluated in an inpatient setting.

The Stimulator and its Accessories

The technical goal of TENS is to activate large myelinated nerve fibers buried at varying depths in the tissue. This holds both for conventional TENS, in which electric paresthesiae are produced, presumably through activation of A-beta afferents, and for acupuncture-like TENS, in which muscle contractions are produced, presumably through stimulation of alpha motoneurons, in turn evoking a deep afferent input. At the same time, activation of thin nerve fibers or endings mediating pain should be avoided.

Pulse Characteristics

For any type of nerve fiber, a strength vs. duration curve can be plotted indicating which current intensity is needed to activate the fiber at a given stimulus duration. To elicit electric paresthesiae for the relief of pain, most patients prefer a pulse duration of 0.05 to 0.15 ms (44), which is in the same range as that considered optimal for activation of large myelinated fibers in experimental situations (9). These and other experimental data strongly suggest that a monophasic square wave of 0.05 to 0.2 ms is sufficient (and optimal) for both conventional and acupuncture-like TENS.

Biphasic pulses are not necessary to avoid polarizing phenomena due to the capacitive components of the skin. The current generator should preferably be calibrated and be of the constant-current type, which compensates for the large variations occurring in the electrode–skin–electrode impedance. A current output of 50 mA per channel into a 2000-ohm external load is necessary to activate deeply situated nerve bundles (e.g., the sciatic nerve), whereas superficially situated nerves in the facial region or distally in the extremities require less energy (45). Constant-voltage generators are less suitable, because the stimulation may be rendered ineffective if the impedance is unexpectedly high for a given output setting (46).

Stimulation Frequency

Most patients seem to prefer a stimulation frequency of 30 to 100 Hz with conventional TENS and 1 to 2 Hz with acupuncture-like TENS. To avoid unpleasant sensations from too high a stimulus intensity, stimulators with a burst mode should be used for acupuncture-like TENS to elicit muscle contractions. This burst may be a short impulse train of 7 to 10 pulses at a 100-Hz internal frequency applied at a 1- to 2-Hz repetition rate (15).

Size of Stimulator

Currently available stimulators are miniaturized current generators, usually powered by rechargeable batteries. The optimum size (about $10 \times 6 \times 3$ cm) has been reached with present equipment. Further miniaturization would probably make the units, especially the dials, difficult for patients to handle. Stimulators have one or two separate output channels, the latter type being more versatile but also more expensive. The stimulation intensity and frequency are set by external dials, separate for each channel, and preferably linear with respect to output.

Available stimulation modes should include single pulses between 30 and 100 Hz (variable) for conventional TENS and short trains of pulses that can be delivered at a 1- to 2-Hz repetition rate for acupuncture-like TENS. In two-channel units, it is an advantage if the mode can be independently varied for each channel. Most patients prefer units with rechargeable batteries. For safety reasons, patients should not be able to treat themselves while a unit is being recharged.

The electrodes are usually made of conductive rubber containing carbon and have a life span of 4 to 6 months in normal use. This material has a suitable inner resistance that produces an even current distribution over the electrode surface. The size of the electrodes—a compromise between the demand for current density and the risk of skin irritation—is usually 10 to 15 cm². Larger electrodes may be advantageous when distinct nerve bundles cannot be stimulated (e.g., with pain in the back or abdomen).

A thin layer of conductive gel is put between the electrode and the skin to facilitate contact. The electrodes are attached to the skin with hypoallergenic tape (Fig. 92-1). A more expensive and short-lived alternative is self-adhesive electrodes made from conductive karaya rubber or synthetic substitutes, which eliminate the need for conductive gel and tape.

Mode of Choice, Frequency, and Intensity of Stimulation

Conventional TENS is the mode of choice in neuralgia, in causalgia, and in dull, continuous pain referred to the skeleton (spine, joints, ribs), whether from arthrosis, cancer, or muscular origin. It should also be tried in central pain states. This mode of stimulation should always evoke electric paraesthesiae in the painful area. To activate most of the large afferent fibers requires use of an intensity two to three times that at the threshold for sensation, usually 10 to 30 mA with standard-size electrodes. Stimulus frequency should be kept constant initially at 80 to 100 Hz. Later it can be varied according to the need and preference of the patient.

In some patients, the pathologic condition or previous treatment has destroyed the peripheral or central afferent pathways to the extent that a marked hypesthesia is present and electric paresthesia cannot be elicited by conventional TENS. Acupuncture-like TENS should be tried whenever conventional TENS does not give satisfactory pain relief. In addition, it is the primary choice in projected pain such as radiculopathy (sciatica) and in deep pain such as in myalgia. A positive effect with this mode requires elicitation of forceful muscle contractions in the myotomes segmentally related to the painful area. Often, a stimulus strength three to five times that at the sensory threshold, commonly 15 to 30 mA, is required to produce muscle contractions. Stimulation must produce *visible* muscle contractions to be effective. The stimulation should be started with a set repetition rate (e.g., 1.5 Hz), and the patient allowed only to modify it later after increased experience. If the stimulation causes discomfort before muscle contractions, the electrode positions should be adjusted slightly. The patient may feel muscle stiffness after the first few treatments, but this vanishes within a few days.

Electrode Placement

Electrode positions must be chosen carefully in each patient. The factors determining where to place the electrodes are the location of pain and the mode of stimulation employed. In conventional TENS, the electrodes are usually placed in or around the painful area, or mainly in the extremities, over nerves innervating the painful area (Fig. 92-2). The minimum effective requirement is that activation occurs within the same dermatome as the pain. Stimulation in the contralateral dermatome at the same level may enhance the beneficial effect. The active electrode (the cathode), from which the stimulation actually occurs, should normally be proximal. With pain in extensive areas, two electrode pairs, driven by a dual-channel unit, are suitable. Large electrodes can also be used.

In acupuncture-like TENS, the electrodes should be placed over mixed nerves supplying muscles innervated by the same segment as the site of pain or over the muscle itself (motor point maps or myotome tables may be helpful) (Fig. 90-4 p. 1817). The cathode should be distal, aiming at activating alpha motoneurons, thereby eliciting muscle contractions and a powerful, indirect, deep afferent inflow.

Contraindications and Side Effects

Transcutaneous electric nerve stimulation should *never* be used by patients carrying heart pacemakers of the "on-demand" type (47) because they may interpret the TENS pulses as electric activity from heart beats and thus become inhibited or driven. Fixed-rate pacemakers present no problems with respect to TENS, but because these are rare, it is safest not to treat any pacemaker patient with TENS. Exceptions should only be made after consulting with the physician directly responsible for the patient's pacemaker treatment.

Manufacturers of stimulators recommend that electrodes should not be placed on the anterior aspect of the neck to avoid stimulation of the carotid nerves and possible hypotension. To our knowledge, only one such case of hypotension has been reported (J. Mannheimer, personal communication). Pulses from currently available stimulators, which are 0.05 to 0.5 ms in duration and up to 100 mA in amplitude, do not carry any risk of cardiac stimulation or fibrillation when applied to the skin surface of any part of the body. This is true because these pulses carry a very low current density at the heart muscle cells, which demand a much higher energy than myelinated nerve fibers to become activated.

Only mild side effects occur with TENS. As previously mentioned, some patients report an aggravation of pain with TENS. This is, however, always transient and is most common in patients with marked functional components in their pain syndrome (42). The only significant side effect for patients who continue to use the stimulation is skin irritation. This may be due either to allergic reactions or to a minor burn (48). Care should be taken to use hypoallergenic tape, to use contact gel liberally, and to clean the skin area and the electrodes regularly with mild soap and water. If allergic reactions are suspected, the tape, gel, or electrode material should be changed. A final possibility is to use inert

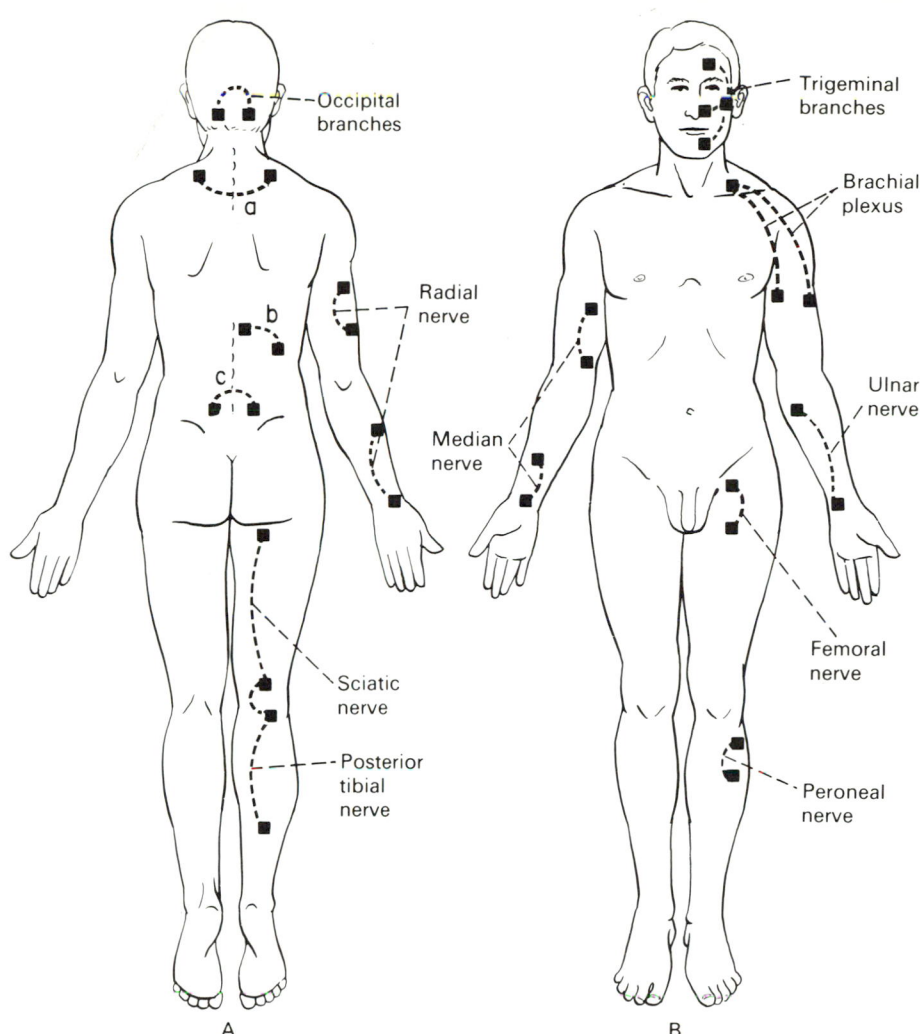

Fig. 92-2. Posterior (**A**) and anterior (**B**) electrode placement points to activate various nerves. Shown in posterior view is placement for myalgic shoulder pain (a), for intercostal postherpetic neuralgia (b), and for lumbago (c).

metal electrodes separated from the skin by moistened foam rubber in a small plastic case, marketed by some manufacturers. An additional side effect, rarely seen, is accentuation of lymphedema when lymph flow is already partly compromised.

Summary

Transcutaneous electric stimulation is a method for electric stimulation of nerves through electrodes applied to the skin. This technique produces no serious side effects or complications, is cheap, and is easy to handle. The pain-relieving effect of TENS is well documented for symptomatic treatment of acute and chronic pain. At present, TENS is commonly used and achieves good results in both acute and chronic painful conditions caused by pathology in nervous structures, in the skeleton, and in muscles. Furthermore, good results have been reported in patients with pain of ischemic origin in the extremities and angina pectoris. Best

TABLE 92-2. Summary of TENS for Various Types of Pain

Type of Pain	Mode of Choice	Impulse Pattern	Intensity	Biologic Effect
Skeletal, paravertebral, and joint pain; neuropathic (peripheral & central) pain; visceral referred pain	Conventional	Continuous at 80–100 Hz	Low (10–30 mA)	Electric paraesthesia in painful area
Muscular (deep) rhizogenic and (irradiating) pain; states with hypesthesia or dysesthesia (e.g., postherpetic pain)	Acupuncture-like	Bursts at 1–2 Hz	High but nonpainful (15–50 mA)	Twitches in related myotomes

results are obtained when TENS is used as part of a multimodal therapy.

Table 92-2 summarizes the characteristics of TENS treatment for various types of pain. In conventional TENS, paresthesiae should be evoked in the painful area by electric stimulation via surface electrodes of large cutaneous afferent nerve fibers at 30 to 100 Hz. In acupuncture-like TENS, utilized whenever the former type fails to give relief of pain, muscles segmentally related to the area of pain are stimulated with short bursts of stimuli, given at a low repetition rate (1 to 2 Hz), to evoke muscle contractions. For both modes, the stimulation is carried out with a miniaturized, battery-powered current generator connected via cables to conductive rubber electrodes placed on the skin. Individual adjustment of the technique and careful instruction to the patient are essential. The results of this therapy should be evaluated after 3 months of stimulation.

B. IMPLANTED ELECTRIC NERVE STIMULATION

Stimulation of the peripheral nerves for pain relief, using implanted devices, has been performed for over 20 years. This technique has never been extensively used, and the number of published papers is limited. Appropriate patient selection has never been adequately evaluated, and long-term follow-up of treatment outcome has been rare.

Wall and Sweet (4) demonstrated that stimulation of peripheral nerves in man was capable of blocking pain and altered the perception of a noxious stimulus. The clinical utility of this finding was not the subject of this report, and the authors saw it primarily as a corroboration of the Melzack-Wall gate hypothesis (3). Sweet and Wepsic (49) then described the use of implanted electrodes to stimulate peripheral nerve in two patients, one of whom had an implanted radiofrequency receiver to activate the electrodes.

Shelden and Pudenz (50) described stimulation of the trigeminal nerve based on the premise that electricity applied to a nerve should alter its function. The three patients in their series all had more than 2 years of pain relief, even though two of them never had any current applied to the electrodes. The third patient was stimulated for only a few weeks, but her facial pain did not recur during the 3 years of follow-up. Surgical trauma to the trigeminal ganglion was the most likely cause of pain relief for these patients, but these authors should be recognized for exploring the concept of implanting a device to chronically stimulate a peripheral nerve.

By 1970 commercial manufacturers were producing implantable electrodes and radiofrequency-coupled receivers, which could be used to stimulate peripheral nerves and the spinal cord in humans. The tremendous publicity concerning dorsal column stimulation seems to have impeded the development of peripheral nerve stimulation (PNS). Furthermore, the development of a percutaneous method of inserting electrodes for spinal cord stimulation seems to have further curtailed interest in PNS. Finally, the limited availability of suitable electrodes was also a factor in the limited usage of PNS, as reports of complications from the electrode were not uncommon.

Physiologic Basis

The physiologic basis for the efficacy of PNS has not been elucidated. Initially, some thought that inhibition of small-fiber activity by larger fibers, as proposed in the Melzack-Wall gate hypothesis, was the explanation (3). More recent evidence has shown that stimulation of A fibers selectively inhibits C-fiber and noxious evoked activity in dorsal horn neurons (51). Others have hypothesized that the applied current directly blocked axonal conduction at the electrode site (10, 52). Later, activation of the downstream modulation by enkephalins or serotonin was proposed as the mechanism of action (53). Peripheral nerve stimulation fits the general observation that anything that leads to non-noxious sensory input will alter the perception of a noxious stimulus.

Technique

The peripheral nerve to be stimulated is surgically exposed in an area that does not undergo movement (Fig. 92-3). The electrode is placed either around

TABLE 92-3. Summary of Studies on Efficacy of PNS for Chronic Pain

Source	No. of Patients	Type of Pain*	Success Rate (%)†	Follow-up	Complication Rate (%)
Long (56)	10	PNI	80	1–3 yr	10
Long and Hagfors (57)	27‡	PNI	63	?	
Cauthen and Renner (58)	3	PNI	100	4–8 mo	
Picaza et al. (46)	23	PNI, RI, SCI	87	6–20 mo	43
Campbell and Long (59)	23	PNI, RI, Ca	39	3–17 mo	13
Kirsch et al. (60)	32	PNI	53	>1 yr	13
Miles and Lipton (61)	2	PNI	50	?	
Law et al. (62)	22	PNI	71	9–88 mo	5
Nashold et al. (63)	38	PNI	40	3–10 yr	9
Waisbrod et al. (64)	19	PNI	79	4–29 mo	21

*PNI = peripheral nerve injury; RI = radicular injuries; SCI = spinal cord injuries; Ca = cancer.
†Refers to percentage of patients experiencing pain relief.
‡Includes patients in Long (55).

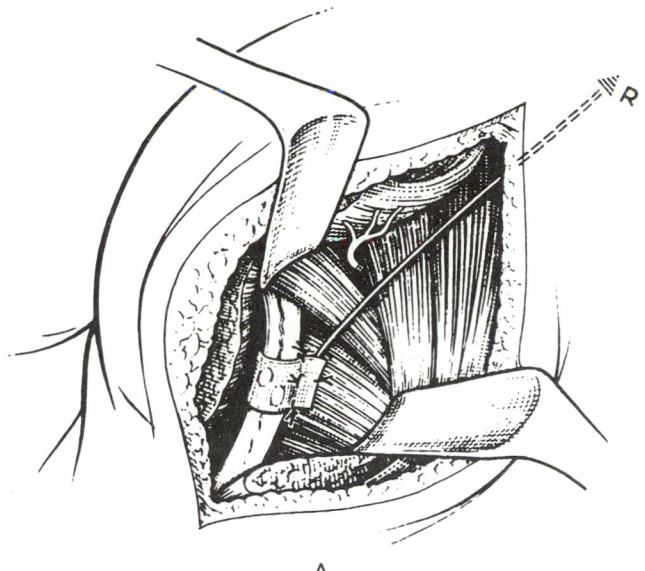

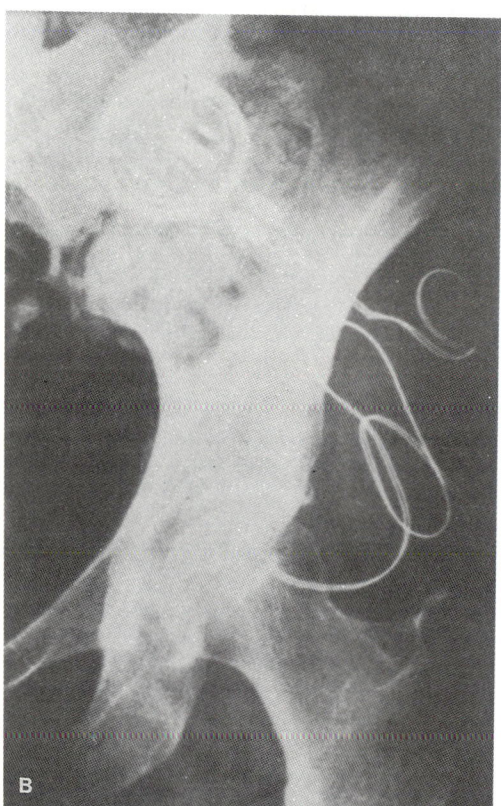

receiver to activate the device. A fully implanted stimulator, which is similar to a cardiac pacemaker, is now available, so that no external transmitter is required. This device is programmable via a radiofrequency transmitter.

Indications and Contraindications

Patient selection is obviously critical if PNS is going to be successful. First, one must be certain that the patient's pain behavior is due to an injury to the nervous system or to tissue damage in the painful area. Stimulators are not effective when pain behaviors are predominantly generated by suffering or environmental cues. Second, the patient should have some relief from TENS in the painful area or from transcutaneous stimulation of the underlying peripheral nerve, if it is superficial.

The following are possible indications for peripheral nerve implant: (a) a wider area of stimulation than can be obtained with TENS is required; (b) the patient cannot utilize skin electrodes in the painful area; or (c) a more circumscribed region of stimulation is required than spinal cord stimulation would provide. Obviously, the patient must be a suitable candidate for a surgical operation on an extremity. Specific diagnoses do not seem to correlate with long-term efficacy, but the nerve must be capable of conducting impulses to the spinal cord. Most of the reported cases are chronic pain due to injury to a peripheral nerve or nerve roots. Few cancer pain patients have been treated by PNS. Although some authors have advocated that a favorable response to a block of the involved peripheral nerve should be an indication for PNS, very little data have been reported upon which to base this conclusion.

Failure to obtain any pain relief with TENS or with temporary stimulation of the nerve with either high-intensity current passed through the skin or with temporary transdermal electrodes usually indicates a poor response to an implanted stimulator. Active infection anywhere in the body should preclude the implantation of any foreign body.

Efficacy

Table 92-3 summarizes the published results of studies on peripheral nerve stimulation using implanted devices. Most of the patients had chronic pain due to a peripheral nerve or nerve root injury. The numbers in each series are so small that meaningful generalizations are probably not warranted. There was a significant infection rate, probably related to the implantation of a large foreign body, in most studies. The cuffed electrodes, which totally surround a nerve, have been found to cause a compression neuropathy in some patients (55). Adjustments of the implanted devices may be required, particularly if the patient uses the stimulator for several months or more. Pain relief was obtained in over half of the patients in these studies. This success rate seems to be higher than that reported for spinal cord stimulation. Peripheral nerve stimulation of nerves in the upper extremity seems to be more successful than stimulation of nerves in the lower extremity.

FIG. 92-3. *A.* Illustration of the operative technique for implanting an electrode on the sciatic nerve for chronic electric stimulation. *B.* Control radiograph of the electrode on the sciatic nerve showing extension to the receiver. Reproduced with permission from R. Sedan and Y. Lazorthes.: La neurostimulation électrique thérapeutique. Neurochirurgie, *24*:1, 1978.

the nerve (cuffed electrode) or in apposition to the nerve (multicontact electrode), and the lead wires are brought to a region where the receiver can conveniently be implanted—usually the infraclavicular or subcostal area (54). The patient places an antenna connected to a small radiofrequency transmitter over the

Conclusions

Implanted peripheral nerve stimulators can alleviate the chronic pain associated with injury to the peripheral nerves or nerve roots. Some favorable results have also been reported with spinal cord lesions. Inadequate numbers of reported cases with long-term follow-up make definitive statements about efficacy and proper patient selection dubious.

REFERENCES

1. Gammon, G.D., and Starr, I.: Studies on the relief of pain by counterirritation. J. Clin. Invest., 20:13, 1941.
2. Kane, K., and Taub, A.: A history of local electrical analgesia. Pain, 1:125, 1975.
3. Melzack, R., and Wall, P.D.: Pain mechanisms: A new theory. Science, 150:971, 1965.
4. Wall, P.D., and Sweet, W.H.: Temporary abolition of pain in man. Science, 155:108, 1967.
5. Cotter, D.J.: Overview of transcutaneous electrical nerve stimulation for treatment of acute postoperative pain. Med. Instrum., 17:289, 1983.
6. Sjölund, B.H., and Eriksson, M.B.E.: Stimulation techniques in the management of pain. In Pain and Society. Edited by H. Kosterlitz and L. Terenius. Weinheim, Verlag Chemie, 1980, p. 415–430.
7. Meyerson, B.A.: Electrostimulation procedures: Effects, presumed rationale, and possible mechanisms. In Advances in Pain Research and Therapy. Vol. 5. Edited by J.J. Bonica, U. Lindblom, and A. Iggo. New York, Raven Press, 1983, pp. 495–534.
8. Schmidt, R.F.: Presynaptic inhibition in the vertebrate central nervous system. Ergeb. Physiol., 63:20, 1971.
9. Koester, J.: Functional consequences of passive electrical properties of the neuron. In Principles of Neural Science. Edited by E.R. Kandel and J.H. Schwartz. London, Edvard Arnold, 1981, p. 44.
10. Campbell, J.N., and Taub, A.: Local analgesia from percutaneous electrical stimulation. Arch. Neurol., 28:347, 1973.
11. Swett, J.E., and Law, J.D.: Analgesia with peripheral nerve stimulation: Absence of a peripheral mechanism. Pain, 15:55, 1983.
12. Loeser, J.D., Black, R.G., and Christman, A.: Relief of pain by transcutaneous stimulation. J. Neurosurg., 42:308, 1975.
13. Andersson, S.A., et al.: Electro-acupuncture: Effect on pain threshold measures with electrical stimulation of teeth. Brain Res., 63:393, 1973.
14. Chiang, C.Y., et al.: Peripheral afferent pathway for acupuncture analgesia. Sci. Sin. (B), 16:210, 1973.
15. Eriksson, M.B.E., and Sjölund, B.H.: Acupuncture-like electroanalgesia in TNS-persistent chronic pain. In Sensory Function of the Skin. Edited by Y. Zotterman. Oxford and New York, Pergamon Press, 1976, p. 575.
16. Cooper, S., and Eccles, J.C.: The isometric responses of mammalian muscles. J. Physiol. (London), 69:377, 1930.
17. Eriksson, M.B.E., Sjölund, B.H., and Nielzén, S.: Long-term results of peripheral conditioning stimulation as an analgesic measure in chronic pain. Pain, 6:335, 1979.
18. Eriksson, M.B.E., Sjölund, B.H., and Sundbärg, G.: Pain relief from peripheral conditioning stimulation in patients with chronic facial pain. J. Neurosurg., 61:149, 1984.
19. Sjölund, B.H., and Eriksson, M.B.E.: The influence of naloxone on analgesia produced by peripheral conditioning stimulation. Brain Res., 173:295, 1979.
20. Sjölund, B.H., Terenius, L., and Eriksson, M.B.E.: Increased cerebrospinal fluid levels of endorphins after electroacupuncture. Acta Physiol. Scand., 100:382, 1977.
21. Sjölund, B.H., and Eriksson, M.B.E.: Endorphins and analgesia produced by peripheral conditioning stimulation. In Advances in Pain Research and Therapy. Vol. 3. Edited by J.J. Bonica, J.C. Liebeskind, and D.G. Albe-Fessard. New York, Raven Press, 1979, pp. 587–592.
22. Freeman, T.B., Campbell, J.N., and Long, D.M.: Naloxone does not affect pain relief induced by electrical stimulation in man. Pain, 17:189, 1983.
23. Hymes, A.C., et al.: Electrical surface stimulation for control of acute postoperative pain and prevention of ileus. Surg. Forum, 24:447, 1975.
24. Ali, J., Jaffe, C.S., and Serrette, C.: The effect of transcutaneous electric nerve stimulation on postoperative pain and pulmonary function. Surgery, 89:507, 1981.
25. Cooperman, A., et al.: Use of transcutaneous electrical stimulation in the control of postoperative pain. Am. J. Surg., 133:185, 1977.
26. Rosenberg, M., Curtis, L., and Bourke, D.L.: Transcutaneous electrical stimulation for the relief of postoperative pain. Pain, 5:129, 1978.
27. Stabile, M., and Mallory, T.: The management of postoperative pain in total joint replacement: Transcutaneous electrical nerve stimulation is evaluated in total hip and knee patients. Orthop. Rev., 7:121, 1978.
28. Pike, P.M.V.: Transcutaneous electrical stimulation: Its use in the management of postoperative pain. Anaesthesia, 33:165, 1978.
29. Harvie, K.W.: A major advance in the control of postoperative knee pain. Orthopaedics, 2:26, 1979.
30. Schuster, G., and Infante, M.: Pain relief after low back surgery: The efficacy of transcutaneous electrical nerve stimulation. Pain, 8:299, 1980.
31. Bundsen, P., Ericson, K., Peterson, L.E., and Thiringer, K.: Pain relief in labor by transcutaneous electrical nerve stimulation. Acta Obstet. Gynecol. Scand., 61:129, 1982.
32. Bundsen, P., and Ericson, K.: Pain relief in labor by transcutaneous electrical nerve stimulation. Safety aspects. Acta Obstet. Gynecol. Scand., 61:1, 1982.
33. Wynn Parry, C.B.: Pain in avulsion lesions of the brachial plexus. Pain, 9:41, 1980.
34. Bates, J.A.V., and Nathan, P.W.: Transcutaneous electrical nerve stimulation for chronic pain. Anaesthesia, 35:817, 1980.
35. Sindou, M., and Keravel, Y.: Analgésie par la méthode d'électrostimulation transcutanée. Resultats dans les douleurs d'origine neurologique. A propos de 180 cas. Neurochirurgie, 26:153, 1980.
36. Bohm, E.: Transcutaneous electric nerve stimulation in the chronic pain patient after peripheral nerve injury. Acta Neurochir., 40:277, 1978.
37. Thorsteinsson, G., et al.: The placebo effect of transcutaneous electrical stimulation. Pain, 5:31, 1978.
38. Hansson, P., and Ekblom, A.: Transcutaneous electrical nerve stimulation (TENS) as compared to placebo TENS for the relief of acute orofacial pain. Pain, 15:157, 1983.
39. Kumar, V.N., and Redford, J.B.: Transcutaneous nerve stimulation in rheumatoid arthritis. Arch. Phys., 63:595, 1982.
40. Kaada, B.: Promoted healing of chronic ulceration by transcutaneous nerve stimulation (TNS). Vasa, 12:262, 1983.
41. Mannheimer, C., et al.: Transcutaneous electrical nerve stimulation in severe angina pectoris. Eur. Heart J., 3:297, 1982.
42. Richardson, R.R., et al.: Transcutaneous electrical neurostimulation in functional pain. Spine, 6:185, 1981.
43. Nielzén, S., Sjölund, B.H., and Eriksson, M.B.E.: Psychiatric factors influencing the treatment of pain with peripheral conditioning stimulation. Pain, 13:365, 1982.
44. Linzer, M., and Long, D.M.: Transcutaneous neural stimulation for relief of pain. IEEE Trans. Biomed. Eng., 23:341, 1976.
45. Mason, C.P.: Testing of electrical transcutaneous stimulators for suppressing pain. Bull. Prosth. Res., (Spring):38, 1976.
46. Picaza, J.A., et al.: Pain suppression by peripheral nerve stimulation. Surg. Neurol., 4:105, 1975.
47. Eriksson, M.B.E., Schuller, H., and Sjölund, B.H.: Hazard from transcutaneous nerve stimulation in patients with pacemakers. Lancet, 1:1319, 1978.
48. Zugerman, C.: Dermatitis from transcutaneous electric nerve stimulation. J. Am. Acad. Dermatol., 6:936, 1982.
49. Sweet, W.H., and Wepsic, J.G.: Treatment of chronic pain by stimulation of fibers of primary afferent neuron. Trans. Am. Neurol. Assoc., 93:103, 1968.
50. Shelden, C.H., Pudenz, R.H., and Doyle, J.: Electrical control of facial pain. Am. J. Surg., 114:209, 1967.
51. Chung, J.M., et al.: Factors influencing nerve stimulation produced inhibition of primate spinothalamic tract cells. Pain, 19:277, 1984.
52. Ignelzi, R.J., and Nyquist, J.V.: Direct effect of electrical stimulation on peripheral nerve evoked activity: Implication in pain relief. J. Neurosurg., 45:159, 1976.
53. Fields, H.L., et al.: Multiple opiate receptor sites on primary afferent fibers. Nature, 184:351, 1980.

54. Nashold, B.S., Jr., Miller, J.B., and Avery, R.: Peripheral nerve stimulation for pain relief using a multicontact electrode system. J. Neurosurg., *51*:872, 1979.
55. Nielson, D., Watts, C., and Clark, W.K.: Peripheral nerve injury from implantation of chronic stimulating electrodes for pain control. Surg. Neurol., *5*:51, 1976.
56. Long, D.M.: Electrical stimulation for relief of pain from chronic nerve injury. J. Neurosurg., *39*:718, 1973.
57. Long, D.M., and Hagfors, N.: Electrical stimulation of the nervous system: The current status of electrical stimulation of the nervous system for relief of pain. Pain, *1*:109, 1975.
58. Cauthen, J.C., and Renner, E.J.: Transcutaneous and peripheral nerve stimulation for chronic pain states. Surg. Neurol., *4*:102, 1975.
59. Campbell, J.N., and Long, D.M.: Peripheral nerve stimula-

tion in the treatment of intractable pain. J. Neurosurg., *45*:692, 1976.
60. Kirsch, W.M., Lewis, J.A., and Simon, R.H.: Experiences with electrical stimulation devices for the control of chronic pain. Med. Instrum., *9*:217, 1975.
61. Miles, J., and Lipton, S.: Phantom limb pain treated by electrical stimulation. Pain, *5*:373, 1978.
62. Law, J.D., Swett, J., and Kirsch, W.M.: Retrospective analysis of 22 patients with chronic pain treated by peripheral nerve stimulation. J. Neurosurg., *52*:482, 1980.
63. Nashold, B.S., Jr., Goldner, J.L., Mullen, J.B., and Bright, D.S.: Long-term pain control by direct peripheral-nerve stimulation. J. Bone Joint Surg., *64A*:1, 1982.
64. Waisbrod, H., Panhans, C., Hansen, D., and Gerbershagen, H.U.: Direct nerve stimulation for painful peripheral neuropathies. J. Bone Joint Surg. [Br.], *67*:470, 1985.

93 · ELECTRIC STIMULATION OF THE SPINAL CORD AND BRAIN

Björn A. Meyerson

In this chapter I discuss techniques for electric stimulation of various sites of the neuraxis that are currently being used for the relief of severe chronic pain. The material is presented in two major sections: A, Spinal Cord Stimulation and B, Intracerebral Stimulation. Spinal cord stimulation to relieve pain was first attempted in 1966 (1) at the same time that stimulation of peripheral nerves was being tested. A year later, Reynolds made his observation of profound analgesia during stimulation of the periaqueductal gray. As emphasized in Chapter 4, this observation provoked an unprecedented degree of research among neuroscientists, which in the course of the ensuing five years led to the definition of the descending antinociceptive system. In the early 1970s, intracerebral stimulation for the relief of severe diffuse pain was given trial. Both techniques are discussed in detail in this chapter.

A. SPINAL CORD STIMULATION

Spinal cord stimulation was the first clinical application of electric stimulation of the nervous system as a method of treating pain, and it thus signifies the introduction of nondestructive procedures as an alternative to ablative pain surgery. The publication of the first clinical trials appeared in 1967 (1). In the same year, Wall and Sweet (2) reported that electric stimulation applied via intracutaneous needles could produce local analgesia, and one year later a similar form of peripheral stimulation was documented (3). During these early years, transcutaneous nerve stimulation (TENS) was used merely to screen candidates for implantation of spinal cord electrodes, and only after several years did it become a method of treatment by itself.

Spinal cord stimulation evolved as a direct consequence of the introduction of the gate-control theory of pain (see Chapter 4), which had an enormous impact on pain research. The method of implanting electrodes onto the dorsal aspect of the spinal cord was developed with the aim of activating spinal pain-inhibiting (gating) mechanisms via the dorsal columns. For this reason the method is usually referred to as dorsal column stimulation (DCS).

Like most new methods of treating chronic pain, DCS was adopted with enthusiasm and often uncritically applied. As a consequence, the often surprisingly high incidence of favorable results obtained during the initial phase was considerably decreased at later follow-ups. Improvement of implantation techniques and a more careful selection of patients have increased the rate of long-term successful results, but there is still some divergence of opinion regarding the clinical usefulness of DCS (4, 5).

Physiologic Mechanisms

The gate-control theory has been challenged in many of its details, but the basic idea, that the interplay between noxious and non-noxious input to the spinal cord may profoundly influence the ascending activity signaling pain, still provides the conceptual framework for DCS as well as for TENS. Although several elaborate schemes based on modified versions of the original Melzack-Wall model have been proposed, many features of therapeutic electric stimulation remain poorly understood. In basic pain research, spinal inhibitory mechanisms have been studied extensively, but the relevance of the experimental findings for afferent stimulation utilized for chronic pain is difficult to evaluate. In several experimental studies, stimulation applied to the dorsal columns has been shown to effectively reduce or block activity in nociceptive neurons in the dorsal horn in response to noxious input such as heat and mechanical stimuli (6). Such inhibitory effects are generally brief, however, persisting at most for only a few seconds after cessation of the stimulation, and are not comparable to the long-lasting suppression of pain that spinal cord stimulation produces in humans. Another example of seemingly contradictory experimental findings and clinical observations is that DCS in humans does not interfere with the normal perception of acute pain, whereas in experimental animals the inhibitory effects of spinal cord stimulation may cause a marked analgesia to noxious stimuli.

Of crucial importance for understanding the mode of action of DCS is identification of the fibers or tracts in the spinal cord that are involved in activation of pain-suppressive mechanisms. As DCS is performed with an intensity just sufficient to produce paresthesia, the presence of which is usually a prerequisite for obtaining pain relief, the activation of low-threshold large fibers contained in the dorsal colunms may be critical. This does not exclude the possibility that other types of fibers, or fibers located outside the dorsal columns, also are activated, since autonomic responses (vascular, bladder tonus, etc.) are sometimes observed (7). Such effects are inconsistent, however, and therefore unlikely to be of significance for the pain-relieving effect. Some have hypothesized that the suppression of pain with DCS is brought about by a direct block of the transmission of nociceptive impulses. This would imply an excitatory effect of stimulation in the spinothalamic tract, with the conduction block occurring as a result of competition or collision with stimulation-induced spinothalamic tract activity (8). This explanation does not seem likely because pain relief persists after cessation of stimulation, and, furthermore, acute and induced pain are not influenced by DCS.

The pain-inhibitory effects of DCS may be exerted at two alternative or complementary levels, segmentally or supraspinally. The perception of stimulation-induced paresthesia necessarily involves supraspinal centers, but the often long-lasting poststimulatory relief excludes the possibility that pain is suppressed only by way of a masking effect or distraction. However, nothing contradicts the possibility of inhibition taking place also in supraspinal relays, for example the thalamus (9). Another possibility is that DCS operates via a supraspinal loop with an efferent link acting on a segmental spinal "gate."

Despite considerable research, the physiologic basis of the clinical effects of DCS, with regard to its site of action, pathways involved, and synaptic relays, is still poorly understood. As a matter of fact, no available evidence invalidates the original notion that DCS predominantly acts via antidromic activation of dorsal column collaterals, which may influence segmental inhibitory mechanisms. This idea is substantiated, for example, by the experimental finding that section of the dorsal columns caudal to the site of stimulation abolished the inhibition (10). In addition, little evidence is available on the neurochemical background of the pain-relieving effect of DCS. No data support involvement of endogenous opioids, and the effect cannot be reversed by naloxone. Circumstantial observations suggest that serotonin may be important (11), but few experimental and clinical studies have focused on this question. A more detailed discussion on physiologic mechanisms is available in an earlier publication of mine (12).

Indications and Efficacy

General Comments

The majority of pain conditions reported to be relieved by DCS can be classified as neurogenic or neuropathic (i.e., pain that chiefly originates from injury to the nervous system itself). Such painful conditions are often associated with disturbance of peripheral sensibility, either because of altered functional properties of injured afferent neurons or secondary central changes. The significance of sensibility disturbances for neuropathic pain was analyzed in detail by Lindblom (13). Some painful neuropathic conditions are characterized by a severe loss of afferent nerve fibers; these are often referred to as deafferentation conditions.

Pain that stems from pathologic processes in non-nervous tissue is less likely to respond to DCS than is neuropathic pain. Such pain can be referred to as nociceptive, implying that it originates from the activation of specific nociceptors. Therefore, pain that has a myofascial, skeletal, or inflammatory origin generally is not responsive to DCS. Pain of supraspinal origin, although neuropathic and perceived in the limbs or trunk (e.g., thalamic pain), also is not influenced by DCS.

Patients who benefit from DCS generally also show some response to TENS. This implies that the prime indications are essentially the same for both techniques, although TENS sometimes also is effective for musculoskeletal and other types of acute pain. One reason for considering DCS as an alternative treatment is insufficient pain relief with TENS because, for example, of difficulties in producing paresthesia that covers the entire painful area. There are also some patients whose pain is unaffected or even worsened by TENS but who nevertheless gain a definite and functionally useful relief with DCS.

As with many other methods of treating chronic pain, evaluating and comparing clinical reports on DCS treatment is difficult because the criteria used for defining a satisfactory outcome are not uniform. This particularly applies to long-term results, because the number of patients who initially report complete or excellent relief of pain tends to decrease with time. That many patients with perhaps less than 50% pain reduction nevertheless consider stimulation useful is often disregarded. Since no alternative treatment is available for the vast majority of these patients, however, even moderate suppression of pain is of value. Thus, patients who experience only partial pain relief commonly maintain that the treatment was worthwhile, even though they may have been subjected to one or several reimplantation procedures (14).

Following the first published reports on DCS (15, 16), large patient trials were documented in several surveys (17). Sedan and Lazorthes (18) reviewed all publications up to 1978 and presented data on some 500 patients. The long-term outcome was judged to be satisfactory in 30 to 40% of patients. In a cooperative European study comprising 281 patients (18), successful results were recorded in 62% of patients after 1 month but only in 26% after 4 years. After the technique of percutaneous trial stimulation came into use, the short-term success rate generally increased to 80% and the long-term rate to about 50% or more (19). During trial stimulation, more than half of the patients often were found to be nonresponders (see 4).

The majority of the late failures in DCS trials seem to occur within the first year; thereafter, the results seem to be more stable. Currently, there is no explanation for the occurrence of late failures, and one can only speculate that a possible reorganization of the pain-transmitting systems removes them from the modulatory influences activated by stimulation.

Unfortunately, several of the major studies on DCS only give results for the entire group of patients representing many different diagnoses. Therefore it is not possible to evaluate the clinical efficacy of DCS for each type of pain. In other studies, the numbers of patients in specific diagnostic groups are often too small to provide reliable estimates of success rates. Despite the inadequacies of published studies, I propose a tentative list of pain syndromes for which DCS is indicated (Table 93-1) based on personal experience and review of the literature. The efficacy of DCS for these conditions is discussed in the following sections.

Post-Traumatic Neuropathy

Peripheral Lesions

Results obtained with DCS applied for pain due to lesions of peripheral nerves are generally not reported with detailed information on the cause (trauma, surgery, etc.) of the lesions. However, there is no reason to assume that the cause of a nerve lesion in any way influences the responses to DCS treatment. The results obtained in patients with this type of pain were reviewed by Sedan and Lazorthes (18), who found that of 32 patients only 12 (38%) could be classified as successful. Siegfried (20) reported the effects of DSC with 84 patients with "peripheral deafferentation pain"; many of these patients likely had pain due to lesions of peripheral nerves. Good to excellent results were recorded in 54% of the patients with a 4-year follow-up, and Siegfried (20) concluded that DSC treatment could be recommended for deafferentation pain of peripheral origin. Nielson et al. (16) reported that 5 of 7 patients with post-traumatic neuropathy obtained satisfactory pain relief from DSC, but the follow-up periods were comparatively short.

Reflex Sympathetic Dystrophy

Reflex sympathetic dystrophy, or algodystrophy, as an indication for DCS has been the subject of only one study (21). Favorable results were obtained in 8 of 11 (73%) patients with follow-ups from 3 to 20 months. In most of these patients the pain was in the upper extremities; hence the electrode tip was placed in the middle cervical segments.

Postamputation Pain

Postamputation pain appears to be one of the principal indications for DCS. The largest series has been reported by Krainick et al. (22), who found that at 18-month follow-up, 36 of 64 patients treated (56%) enjoyed more than 50% pain relief. With a longer follow-up (2.5 to 5.5 years), the number of successful cases had decreased to 26 (41%). In a major cooperative European study comprising 140 amputees, satisfactory pain relief during the early phase was obtained in 67% of the patients, but after 5 years a mere 25% had retained beneficial effects (cited in 23). Burning sharp pain in the stump and in the phantom have been reported to be effectively relieved by DSC, whereas the throbbing type of pain in the stump and the lancinating, shooting pains in the phantom are generally more resistant. Nielson et al. (16) reported excellent to good results in 4 out of 5 amputees but the mean follow-up was only $1\frac{1}{2}$ years. Even though the efficacy of DCS tends to decrease with time, Krainick and Thoden (23) stated that DCS should be applied as the first surgical procedure for postamputation pain when noninvasive treatments have failed.

Coccygodynia

Coccygodynia as an indication for DCS has been occasionally reported, but the numbers of cases are too small to justify an evaluation of the efficacy of DSC for this condition. The same applies to pain associated with diabetic neuropathy.

TABLE 93-1. Neurogenic, Neuropathic, Deafferentation, and Other Pain Syndromes Likely to Respond to DCS

I. Peripheral nerve and root lesions
  Post-traumatic neuropathy
    Trauma due to injuries, surgery, entrapment, or incisional scar
    Causalgia and reflex sympathetic dystrophy
    Postamputation pain (stump and phantom)
    Coccygodynia
  Diabetic neuropathy
  Plexus lesions induced by trauma, malignancy, and radiation*
  Rhizopathy
    Postherpetic neuralgia
    Cervical syndrome
    Low back pain (particularly radicular pain due to arachnoiditis and epidural fibrosis)

II. Spinal cord lesions
  Postcordotomy dysesthesia
  Multiple sclerosis
  Paraplegia (radicular pain at level of lesion and pain below level of lesion with preservation of sensibility)

III. Peripheral vascular disease

*Plexus avulsion pain is not likely to respond to DCS.

Plexus Lesions

A few cases in which DCS was used to treat pain due to plexus lesions have been documented in the literature, but the cause of the lesion (trauma, malignancy, radiation therapy) generally has not been stated. Hood and Siegfried (24) described 8 patients with brachial plexus pain secondary to malignancy or radiation plexopathy. At 1-year follow-up, 2 (25%) patients reported good pain relief; 3 (38%), fair; and another 3, no relief. The authors concluded that DCS is indicated for this type of pain. Of 9 additional patients reported in the literature (see 18), 5 (56%) were judged to have had a satisfactory result.

In cases of pain due to lesion of the brachial plexus, it is important to determine whether avulsion of cervical roots is present or whether the lesion is confined to the plexus, distal to the spinal ganglia. Hood and Siegfried (24) convincingly demonstrated that DCS is ineffective for pain associated with root avulsion; they reported that of 12 such patients, DCS provided pain relief classified as fair only in 1 (9%), the remaining being resistant to the treatment. The reason for the lack of response of plexus avulsion pain to DCS probably is that the proximal portions of the large afferent fibers contained in the dorsal columns have degenerated, leaving no neural "substrate" for the stimulation.

Rhizopathy

Postherpetic Neuralgia

Application of DCS for postherpetic neuralgia has been reported occasionally, but the results have been inconsistent. Nonetheless, considering that this painful condition is often resistant to other forms of treatment, DCS may be worth trying. For the same reason, severe cases of cervical syndrome may be justified as an indication for DCS.

Low Back Pain

The most common condition for which DCS has been applied is low back pain, often following multiple lumbar operations and with a radiographic diagnosis of arachnoiditis or epidural fibrositis. These conditions involve several different types of pain, both neurogenic and nociceptive, which makes a thorough analysis of the pain mandatory. As a rule, radiating pain, as a symptom of rhizopathy, is more likely to respond to DCS than deep, diffuse pain confined to the lower part of the back, which is often referred to as lumbago.

In one study attempting to analyze the pain components constituting low back pain, DCS effectively reduced radicular pain, whereas a predominant lumbar pain in the same patients did not respond (25). The results of major studies on DCS of patients with low back pain and arachnoiditis are summarized in Table 93-2. On average, about half of the patients obtained 50% or more pain relief; in these studies, follow-up ranged from 6 months to 4 years. North et al. (27) and Winkelmüller (25) reported considerably higher success rates (75 and 69%, respectively).

Spinal Cord Lesions

Postcordotomy Dysesthesia

The largest series of patients treated with DCS for postcordotomy dysesthesia was reported by Nielson et al. (16), who noted that 8 of 12 patients (66%) derived excellent or good pain relief with a mean follow-up of about 1½ years. In some other studies, however, only about 25% of patients enjoyed satisfactory relief (see 18).

Multiple Sclerosis

Because the use of DCS for pain in multiple sclerosis has been reported in only a few cases, no conclusion as to its efficacy can be drawn.

Paraplegia

Pain associated with spinal cord injury and paraplegia sometimes responds to DCS if at least some sensibility is preserved in the painful area. Pain confined to a completely denervated part of the body, well below the level of the spinal injury, is not likely to benefit, because in such a case no remaining fibers are available for stimulation of the spinal cord. However, some patients present with radicular pain confined to the level of the lesion; for such pain DCS may be useful.

Several studies have included patients referred to as "spinal cord injury" or "paraplegia" with no further information on the functional severity of the injury or the degree and extent of the sensory loss. In general, the results have been unsatisfactory; for example Winkelmüller (25) reported that only 2 of 10 (20%) patients with this diagnosis benefited from DCS. Sweet and Wepsic (30) reported that among 14 patients treated with DCS, 11 (79%) experienced failure and 3 (21%) moderate or good results. Nashold and Friedman (15) treated 7 spinal cord injury patients; only 2 (29%) obtained satisfactory pain relief. It should be noted that few of these patients had been subjected to trial stimulation before permanent implantation.

TABLE 93-2. Summary of Results of Long-Term Studies on Dorsal Column Stimulation for Low Back Pain (Arachnoiditis)

Source	No. Patients	Mean Follow-up (years)	Patients with Satisfactory Relief*	
			(no.)	(%)
Ray (26)	95	1.5	46	48
North et al. (27)	24	0.5	18	75
Young (28)	25	3	10	40
Winkelmüller (25)	56	3.5	38	69
Long (14)	24	3	12	50
Ray et al. (29)	50	1.5	27	54
Siegfried & Lazorthes (4)	89	4	51	57
Siegfried (20)	67	4	29	43
All	430	—	231	54

*Classified as excellent or good, or as more than 50% relief.

Peripheral Vascular Disease

In recent years, several reports have been published on the beneficial effect of DCS for pain associated with disturbed peripheral circulation, or peripheral vasculopathy (31). In a cooperative study of 41 cases, 37 patients were permanently implanted after trial stimulation; at a mean follow-up of 25 months, substantial pain relief was experienced by 29 (78%) of the patients (32). The main reason for applying DCS in these patients was pain, but some evidence suggested that the stimulation might have favorable long-term effects on the peripheral circulation as well. For example, walking distance significantly increased in about half the patients, and small trophic ulcers healed in some. In view of these promising results, pain of vascular origin is likely to be an important indication for DCS treatment in the future, but no definitive criteria have been proposed for selection of patients.

Clinical Considerations

Surgical Technique

Stimulation applied to the dorsal aspect of the spinal cord produces paresthesia, which must be felt in the entire painful region in order to obtain relief (Fig. 93-1). The distribution of these sensations is very much dependent upon the placement of the electrode. Producing paresthesiae in the legs and arms and segmentally in the lateral aspect of the trunk generally presents no problems, whereas covering regions close to the midline, the ventral part of the trunk, and the low sacral segments often is difficult. Perianal pain, pain in the perineum, and pain in the inguinal region are examples of pain that may be difficult to treat because of location.

Presently, electrodes for stimulating the spinal cord are always placed in the epidural space, either with a percutaneous technique or a small laminectomy. The percutaneous technique is the most commonly used. The procedure is done under local anesthesia and with the patient in a sitting or prone position. The epidural space is punctured with a Touhy needle, and a lead

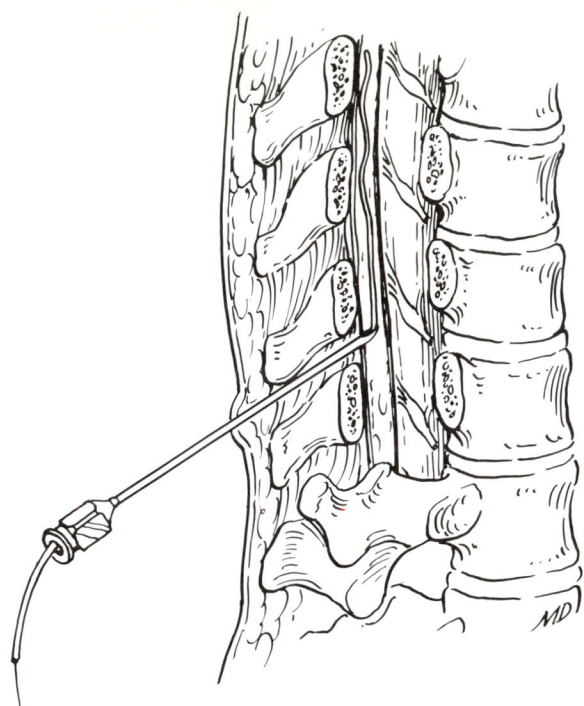

FIG. 93-1. Technique of percutaneous epidural spinal cord stimulation. The epidural puncture is achieved with a Tuohy needle inserted in the midline as described in detail in Figure 94-55. Under fluoroscopic control, a lead electrode is advanced several cm cephalad in the posterior epidural space until it is considered to be in the optimal position. Test stimulation is performed by using a surface electrode as a reference to confirm that the paresthesia covers the painful area. The electrode can be advanced if necessary, but it should not be withdrawn lest the bevel of the needle damage the lead. Once test stimulation is achieved, the interspinous ligament is exposed with a small incision, the needle is withdrawn, and the electrode is fixed to the ligament (see text for details).

electrode is advanced upward in the dorsal epidural space under fluoroscopic controls (Figs. 93-2 and 93-3). The stimulating tip of the electrode is generally placed at a mid- or lower thoracic level for pain in the legs, and in the midcervical region for pain in the arms. Test stimulation is performed by using a surface electrode as a reference to confirm that the paresthesiae cover the painful area. The interspinous ligament is exposed with a small incision, and the needle is withdrawn. The electrode is fixed to the ligament and connected to a thin lead, which is tunneled under the skin and led out some distance away from the incision (Fig. 93-26). This temporary percutaneous coupling permits trial stimulation until the clinical effect can be fully evaluated.

When it is difficult to place the electrode tip so that paresthesiae are produced in the painful area, bipolar stimulation may be helpful. This involves percutaneously implanting two electrodes with the tips separated by one or two spinal segments. An alternative method is to use a multipolar electrode implanted via a small laminectomy. Such electrodes contain four stimulating poles mounted on a thin silicon plate, which is slipped epidurally under the adjacent lamina. Using temporary percutaneous extension leads, trial stimulation can be performed. Trials with different

bipolar couplings generally will identify a combination of stimulating poles that can produce paresthesiae over the entire painful area.

Assessment of pain relief during trial stimulations is extremely important. Generally, such an evaluation is made on the basis of visual analog scales, specifically designed questionnaires, consumption of analgesics, changes in ambulation, etc. Percutaneous trial stimulation should be performed for at least 1 week, and sometimes is continued while the patient is sent home for a short period. The duration of poststimulatory pain relief appears to be at least as important as the amount of pain reduction for predicting long-term outcome. Stimulation periods of 20 to 30 min are generally sufficient to obtain a maximal effect. During the trial period, patients are encouraged to use the stimulator only when the pain is severe. The poststimulatory relief generally lasts 2 to 4 hours.

When the clinical effect is satisfactory during the trial stimulation period, permanent internalization of the system is performed. A receiver measuring 3 cm in diameter is placed in a subcutaneous pocket, generally in the infraclavicular region or onto the lower ventral part of the thoracic wall. A lead from the receiver is tunneled subcutaneously to the incision in the back and connected to the proximal part of the electrode after disconnecting the temporary percutaneous lead. Because the tunneling procedure is painful, it is usually performed under a short-acting barbiturate anesthesia. The receiver is passively activated by a disk-shaped antenna taped to the skin overlying the receiver. Fully implantable stimulators, whose on-off function is controlled by an external magnet, are now available. They also can be programmed for a cycling function, which has proven to be particularly useful for patients with pain associated with vascular disease. Lazorthes and Verdie (33) have published a detailed survey of electronic devices and techniques for neurostimulation.

Side Effects and Complications

A relatively common complaint among DCS patients is tenderness at the receiver or the stimulator site and along the subcutaneous lead; occasionally this persists for several months. Erosion of the skin at the receiver site is a rare complication, but if it occurs, the receiver and interconnecting lead must be removed and later reimplanted.

Equipment failures unfortunately are quite frequent and in some long-term studies have occurred in virtually all patients (34). Dislocation of the electrode, leading to a change in distribution of paresthesiae, is a troublesome problem and is presumably the most common cause of failure in obtaining a beneficial effect. This requires repositioning or reimplantation of the electrode. If the electrode becomes dislocated several times, switching from a percutaneously implanted electrode to a multipolar electrode positioned via a laminectomy is recommended, because these electrodes generally retain their original location. Cracks in the insulation of the lead interconnecting the receiver and the electrode causing leakage of current is another common problem that requires equipment replacement (35).

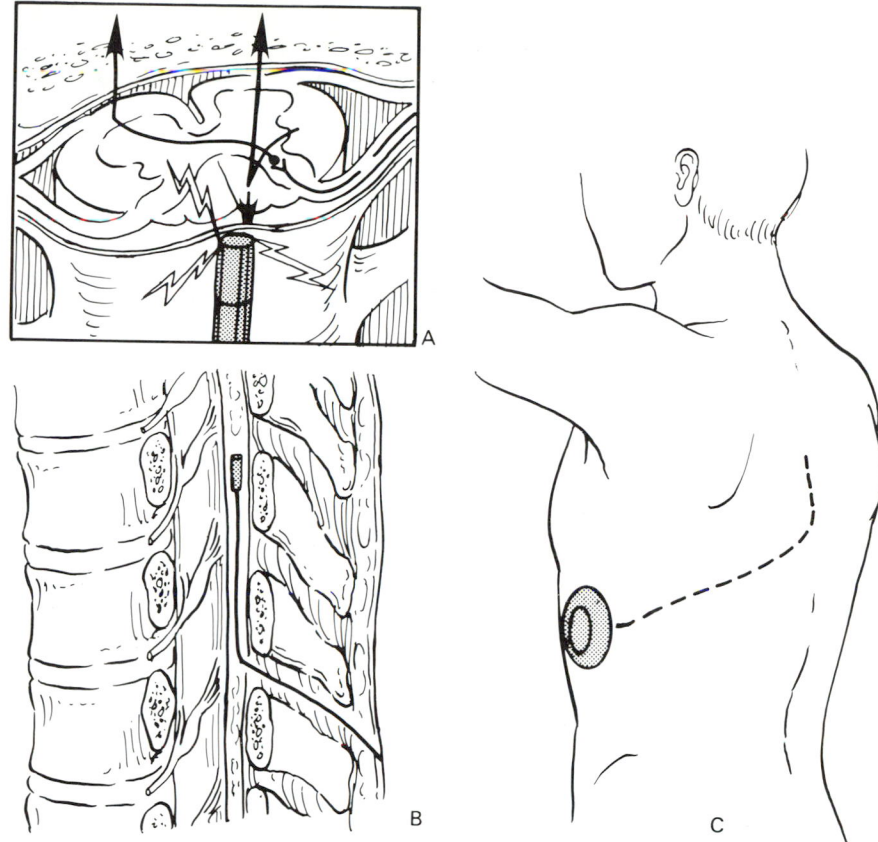

Fig. 93-2. Spinal cord stimulation. *A.* Schematic depiction of the possible mechanism of the pain-relieving effect of this procedure. Stimulation probably excites dorsal column fibers, which may activate inhibitory mechanisms in the dorsal horn of the spinal cord. *B.* The electrode and the lead in the epidural space at the midthoracic level used for achieving pain relief in the pelvis and lower limbs. Stimulation periods of 20 to 30 minutes are generally sufficient to obtain the maximal effect. *C.* When the clinical effect is satisfactory during the test stimulation period, permanent internalization of the system is performed by placing a receiver measuring 3 cm in diameter in a subcutaneous pocket in the lower anterior part of the thoracic wall. A lead from the receiver is tunneled subcutaneous to the incision in the back and connected to the proximal part of the electrode after disconnecting the temporary percutaneous lead.

The implantation techniques presently in use carry little risk of serious complications. Bleeding and infection in the epidural space can occur but appear to be exceedingly rare. The incidence of infection at the site of the receiver or along the subcutaneous lead has been reported to be about 5%, but the risk is minimized by the use of prophylactic antibiotics.

Selection of Patients

The long-term outcome of DCS is very dependent on careful patient selection. Positive though perhaps insufficient relief with TENS is a favorable predictor but cannot be relied on as a sole way of selecting patients for DCS. A somatic pain diagnosis is essential. Because poorly defined, diffuse, and multifocal pain is unlikely to respond (30), analysis of the pain—its cause and origin, character, temporal pattern, dependence on external factors, etc.—should be pushed as far as possible. Careful psychologic evaluation of the patient is particularly important, and the possible relationship between the psychologic makeup of the patient, the social situation, and the pain condition should be analyzed before the patient is accepted for trial stimulation. It has been well documented that patients with emotional disturbance or with marked psychogenic pain components (5, 14) should not be considered for implantation.

All narcotic medication should be gradually withdrawn and replaced with nonopioid analgesics before implantation and trial stimulation is performed; (in any case, narcotic analgesics are rarely effective for neuropathic pain conditions). For obvious reasons, patients must be able to learn how to operate the stimulator; they should be properly informed that DCS is not a curative treatment but a method of alleviating a symptom (pain) and that the stimulation by itself cannot be expected to improve the underlying pathologic condition. In other words, patients have to realize and accept that they will be dependent on daily usage of the stimulator for many years. Moreover, it is desirable that patients have some understanding of the mechanisms by which their pain may be suppressed by the stimulation. Finally, clinical experience has shown that many patients older than 70 to 75 years find it difficult to operate the stimulator properly. As with other pain treatments that have to be continued for years, patients considering DCS should be guaranteed that continuing contact with the implanting surgeon will be available. Any clinician who institutes this type of treatment must be prepared to take on such responsibility.

Conclusions

The clinical value of DCS for relief of chronic pain has been much disputed, and initial enthusiasm for the method faded with the realization that the long-term results were less favorable than expected. As a consequence, the method was entirely abandoned in some clinics as readily as it had once been adopted. However, since the late 1970s the use of DCS has again increased and has spread to many countries where it has previously not been practiced. Compared with its initial period of popularity, DCS is now applied more critically and more attention is given to careful

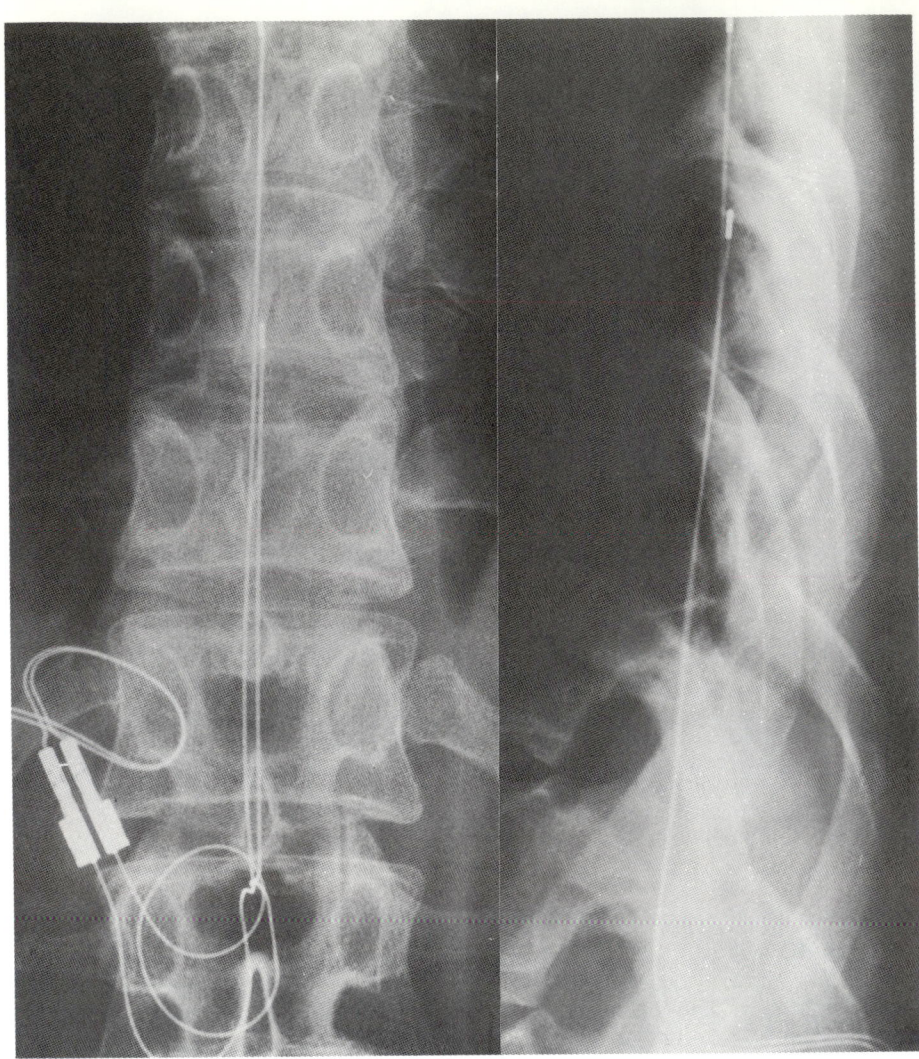

Fig. 93-3. Radiographs of the stimulating electrode for spinal cord stimulation implanted in the dorsal epidural space. *A.* Anteroposterior view showing the electrodes at the level of the lower part of the 8th and 10th thoracic vertebrae. *B.* Lateral view showing the electrodes in the posterior part of the epidural space.

A

B

selection of patients. This together with improvement of the equipment and of the implantation technique, has resulted in better long-term results. Consequently, in most clinics providing multimodal pain therapy, DCS has become a significant part of the therapeutic program and is now recognized as a routine method.

I believe that DCS is of considerable value for many painful conditions that are otherwise notoriously difficult to deal with; these include postamputation pain, painful peripheral neuropathies, and chronic sciatic pain. For such pain, effective alternative treatment often is not available, and the nondestructive nature of DCS makes it attractive in view of the well-known long-term inefficacy of ablative surgery. Moreover, patients suffering from such conditions are often severely incapacitated, and many are of a productive age and require much health care. These factors compensate for the relatively high cost of DCS equipment and its implantation.

B. INTRACEREBRAL STIMULATION

Electric stimulation applied via electrodes implanted in discrete deep-seated regions of the brain has been employed as a method of alleviating chronic pain since the mid 1970s. This technique of intracerebral stimulation (ICS), also known as deep-brain stimulation (DBS), however, is practiced in only a few neurosurgical centers. It is not established as a routine method because it requires expertise in the use of stereotaxic neurosurgical techniques, thorough knowledge of the hypothetical mechanisms behind stimulation-produced pain relief, and a good deal of experience in dealing with difficult pain conditions. When first introduced, ICS appeared to be a very promising, physiologic approach to pain treatment, because it seemed to act by employing endogenous pain-controlling mechanisms. Subsequent studies substantiated the clinical usefulness of the method for a number of pain diagnoses. Some reports during later years raised doubt about the general efficacy of ICS, and valid predictive criteria have not yet been established. Nonetheless, ICS sometimes is beneficial in pain conditions for which no alternative treatment is available.

Clinical application of ICS has evolved along two lines corresponding to two separate target regions for stimulation: the specific sensory thalamic nuclei (VPM, VPL) and the periaqueductal–periventricular gray (PAG-PVG) region (see 12, 36–38 for references). Conceivably, stimulation in these two regions influences pain by activation of different mechanisms and/or systems. Stimulation in the sensory thalamus appears to be selectively effective for relieving neuropathic pain, whereas PAG-PVG stimulation (here referred to as PVG stimulation) preferentially relieves nociceptive pain.

Physiologic Mechanisms

Sensory Thalamic Stimulation

The first trials to relieve chronic pain by stimulation of the sensory thalamus were conducted in France during the early 1960s, although clinical reports were not published until several years later (39). The conceptual basis for this approach to pain treatment was the classic theory introduced in 1911 by Head and Holmes (cited in 39), who postulated that pain can occur as a result of insufficient activity in the epicritic (non-nociceptive) sensory system. It was reasoned that artificial activation of this system in the sensory thalamic nuclei by way of electric stimulation might block or reduce transmission of the pain message. As discussed previously, publication of the gate-control theory of pain in 1965 triggered the development of TENS, DCS, and peripheral nerve stimulation. These methods appear to be effective only when the large-diameter afferent fibers in the periphery or in the spinal cord are preserved and accessible. In patients with chronic pain syndromes who lack primary afferent neurons rostral to the spinal ganglia, stimulation of the supraspinal portion of the lemniscal system seemed like a logical alternative treatment.

Only a few experimental studies have sought to elucidate the mechanisms by which pain is influenced by sensory thalamic stimulation. Some have assumed that gating mechanisms, similar to those postulated to account for pain inhibition at a segmental spinal level, are present in supraspinal relays (40). Stimulation of the ventrobasal thalamic complex in experimental animals has been shown to inhibit activity in second-order spinal dorsal horn neurons in response to peripheral noxious stimuli (see 41 for references). Moreover, such thalamic stimulation can effectively suppress responses evoked by peripheral noxious stimulation in the medial part of the thalamus (the parafascicular nucleus) (42). The relevance of all these experiments to therapeutic sensory thalamic stimulation in humans is unclear, because the animal experiments were designed to study possible suppression of responses to acute noxious stimuli, whereas in humans this type of thalamic stimulation is preferentially effective for chronic neuropathic pain. Furthermore, the clinical pain relief may last for many hours, whereas in the reported animal experiments the suppression of "thalamic pain responses" outlasts the stimulation by less than a second. The transmitter physiology involved in pain suppression with sensory thalamic stimulation is entirely unknown, and nothing suggests that endogenous opioids are of importance.

PVG Stimulation

Stimulation of the PAG-PVG region has evolved from animal experiments and from observations made during the course of stereotaxic thalamic operations. In 1969, Reynolds (43) reported that stimulation of the periaqueductal gray matter in rats could produce a powerful analgesia (see Chapter 4). This observation was a major breakthrough in modern pain research, because it demonstrated the existence of an endogenous pain-controlling system. Further studies showed that activation of this system in the core of the brain stem can inhibit pain transmission at the first synaptic relay in the dorsal horn of the spinal cord. The later demonstration of a close relationship between analgesia produced by PVG stimulation and the antinociceptive mode of action of opioids stimulated intensive research. A host of data has accumulated on the neuroanatomic, biochemical, and electrophysiologic bases for this type of stimulation-produced analgesia in animals. Much research has been addressed to the role played by novel neurotransmitters and neuromodulators with morphine-like properties as well as by serotonin and noradrenalin.

Circumstantial evidence suggests that pain relief in man and analgesia in animals as a result of periventricular-periaqueductal stimulation depend on similar mechanisms. For example, Hosobuchi et al. (44) have shown that such stimulation can cause an increase of beta-endorphin in ventricular cerebrospinal fluid, but no clear evidence shows that the activation of endorphinergic systems is a prerequisite for the alleviation of pain (45). In animals, naloxone has been extensively used to demonstrate that analgesia produced by PVG stimulation depends on opioid mechanisms. Although naloxone can reverse the effect of PVG stimulation in man, this reversal does not always occur (see 46 for discussion).

Much of the experimental data in the literature may not be relevant for understanding the physiology of pain suppression by PVG stimulation in humans. One problem is that many animal experiments with this type of stimulation are designed for the study of acute nociceptive events, and in order to quantitatively assess the analgesic effects of experimental stimulation, well-defined and reproducible pain-evoked reflexes are utilized. Moreover, it is known that the effects of antinociceptive measures are dependent upon the pain-test used (tail-flick, formalin test, etc.) (47). The relevance of nociceptive reflexes is debatable, because the mechanisms underlying chronic pain may be different from those involved in acute nociception (see Chapter 4).

Different physiologic mechanisms for the antinociceptive effects of PVG stimulation in animals and its pain-relieving effect in humans is strongly suggested by the finding that in humans the normal perception of acutely induced painful stimuli, with regard to both thresholds and tolerance, is preserved after stimulation, whereas animals may become profoundly insensitive to noxious stimuli. In addition stimulation does not seem to protect humans from new pains despite excellent relief from chronic pain (12).

Indications and Efficacy

Sensory Thalamic Stimulation

Substantial evidence indicates that stimulation applied to the sensory thalamus is effective only for pain classified as neuropathic (i.e., pain that originates from trauma or injury to the nervous system itself, including the peripheral nerves, spinal roots, spinal cord, and supraspinal structures). In cases of extensive damage, a considerable degree of deafferentation often occurs (e.g., paraplegic pain perceived below the level of the spinal injury, phantom limb pain, and anesthesia dolorosa of the face). Common pain conditions classified as neuropathic are peripheral neuralgia as a result of trauma or surgery, postherpetic pain, sciatic pain, and lesions of the brachial plexus. As described in the first part of this chapter, dorsal column stimulation is also indicated for several of these conditions.

When there is extensive damage to the spinal ganglia, the roots, or the spinal cord itself, a large number of the afferent nerve fibers in the dorsal columns may degenerate and are thus not available for spinal cord stimulation. This is most obvious in extensive spinal cord lesions and in recurrent pain after dorsal root sections. Among peripheral neuralgias that may respond favorably to sensory thalamic stimulation, postherpetic neuralgia, particularly in the face, should be mentioned. The sciatic neuropathic component of what is commonly referred to as low back pain also may benefit, but sensory thalamic stimulation for this condition has been used to a limited extent only.

Finally, central pain due to vascular or other lesions affecting the sensory pathways caudal to the thalamic relay nuclei may be considered for sensory thalamic stimulation provided the pain is confined to the face, arm and hand, or leg. For such central pain conditions caused by a lesion in the thalamus itself, stimulation of the sensory limb of the internal capsule instead may be beneficial (36).

PVG Stimulation

As noted already, PVG stimulation is chiefly effective for pain characterized as nociceptive (i.e., pain that occurs as a result of activation of specific peripheral nociceptors in musculofibrous tissue, in supportive bony-cartilaginous tissue, in the viscera, etc). In clinical practice differentiating nociceptive and neuropathic pain often is difficult, particularly in pain conditions associated with malignancy, which often represent a mixture of pains of different origins and mechanisms. Stimulation in the PAG-PVG region has been pioneered by Hosobuchi (36) and Richardson and Akil (48). The most common indication has been low back pain. In view of the preferential effect of PVG stimulation on a nociceptive type of pain, it could be expected to be more suitable for the discogenic and arthrogenic pain components, presenting as "lumbago," rather than for radicular (sciatic) pain. The differential effects of PVG stimulation on the various components constituting the syndrome of low back pain have been recognized only recently (49).

A few reports of PVG stimulation applied in patients with pancreatitis, chronic osteitis, osteoporosis, etc., have been published, but the total number of cases in each diagnostic group is too small to evaluate the validity of these indications.

Pain due to malignancy sometimes is an indication for ICS provided there is a slow progression of the underlying disease and a life expectancy of at least 6 months. The main reasons for using ICS are intolerable side effects or insufficient relief from opioids and a pain location unsuitable for destructive procedures. The selection of stimulation target—sensory thalamus or PAG-PVG region—is based on whether the dominating pain is likely to be neuropathic or nociceptive (50, 51).

Results of Clinical Studies

Cooperative studies of the clinical efficacy of intracerebral stimulation have been performed both in the United States and in Europe. The North American study comprised 339 patients treated by 7 different neurosurgeons up to 1982 (52). Patients with neuropathic and nociceptive pain conditions were included. About 75% of the patients experienced sufficient pain control by percutaneous trial stimulation to warrant permanent electrode implantation. With a mean follow-up of 16.7 months, about 75% of these patients enjoyed satisfactory relief of pain. To maintain continued control, 34 of the 173 successful patients (20%) had to undergo additional procedures involving either repair or replacement of the stimulation system. The results obtained in 304 patients with pain involving the major diagnostic groups are listed in Table 93-3.

The European cooperative study (which also included data from one North American and one South African center) was completed in 1979 and comprised 324 patients managed by 14 neurosurgical groups (53). There were 182 patients diagnosed as having neuropathic-deafferentation pain including anesthesia dolorosa, phantom limb, brachial plexus lesion, thalamic spinal cord injury, postherpetic peripheral nerve injury, and postcordotomy dysesthesia. Of these patients, 106 responded favorably to stimulation in the sensory thalamus. The largest series of patients was that of Mazars et al. (54), who reported that 83 out of 99 patients (84%) were relieved by sensory thalamic stimulation. These results, however, were much more favorable than those reported by the other groups, who had an average success rate of only 26% (23 out of 87 patients) with this type of stimulation. Of the remaining patients with the same type of pain, 76 were subjected to PVG stimulation, and 19 of these were reported to have benefited.

A large series of patients treated with ICS between 1972 and 1984 and with a mean follow-up of 5 years was reported by Levy et al. (55). In this series, 84 patients had pain classified as deafferentation (neuropathic) and 57 had nociceptive pain, in most cases referred to as low back pain. The overall results, including both types of pain and stimulation in either the sensory thalamus or PVG or in both, indicated that 60% of patients benefited from treatment in the short term, but only 30% could be judged to have benefited in the long term. Of the patients with PVG electrodes, 24 out of 47 patients (51%) had initially satisfactory results, but at long follow-up a mere 15 patients (32%) retained the effect. The authors concluded that thalamic pain and

TABLE 93-3. Summary of Results of Cooperative North American Study on Intracerebral Stimulation

Pain Syndrome	No. Patients Implanted	No. Patients Internalized	Most Common Target	Pain Relief Success* (No.)	Success* (%)	Failure (No.)	Failure (%)
Central pain	54	42	Internal capsule	30	71	12	29
Spinal cord injury	24	14	Internal capsule	11	79	3	21
Facial pain	34	19	Sensory thalamus	11	58	8	42
Peripheral nerve injury	47	38	Internal capsule or PVG	29	76	9	24
Low back pain	112	89	PVG	70	79	17	21
Cancer	33	26	PVG	22	85	4	15
All	304	228		173	76	53	24

*Percentage of success is based on the number of patients implanted for trial stimulation (second column).
From Groth, K., et al.: Deep brain stimulation for chronic intractable pain. Minneapolis, Medtronic Inc., 1982.

peripheral neuralgia were good indications for stimulation in the sensory limb of the internal capsule and in the sensory thalamus, respectively (55).

Recently Young (38) summarized the results obtained in 15 reports, including 96 patients of his own and 122 patients reported by Hosobuchi (49), for a total of 916 patients, of whom 142 (59%) experienced satisfactory long-term pain relief from ICS. In Hosobuchi's series, in which patients were followed for 2 to 14 years, 72% derived good pain relief; among Young's 96 patients, who were followed for 1 to 9 years (mean 3 years), pain relief occurred in 66.7%. Young (38) further stated that most authors reported that ICB was effective in 70 to 80% of patients with pain of peripheral origin, whereas only 50% of the patients with central (deafferentation) pain derived relief.

PVG Stimulation

The results of the major studies of PVG stimulation, summarized in Table 93-4, show that low back pain has been the main indication. The literature contains conflicting reports about the efficacy of PVG stimulation for neuropathic pain conditions. Although the two studies involving patients with neuropathic pain referred to in Table 93-4 (36, 60) found no benefit from

PVG stimulation, occasional patients diagnosed as having neuropathic pain have obtained satisfactory relief with this form of stimulation (48, 52, 53, 57). These data may perhaps invalidate the notion that PVG stimulation exclusively influences nociceptive pain (12, 49).

Sensory Thalamic Stimulation

Results of the major studies on the efficacy of stimulation in the sensory thalamic nuclei or in the internal capsule are listed in Table 93-5. Note that in two studies (49, 62), sensory thalamus stimulation was used for low back pain, albeit the authors of these studies referred to the condition as "lumbosacral radiculopathy" and "arachnoiditis," respectively.

Specific Pain Conditions

Anesthesia Dolorosa

Although anesthesia dolorosa (dysesthetic facial pain) was one of the conditions for which sensory thalamus stimulation was first tried, only small series of patients have been reported. Results published by six different groups (49, 58, 60, 61, 66, 67) and comprising 49 patients showed that 18 (37%) attained satisfactory relief. In the European cooperative study (53), only 7 of 23

TABLE 93-4. Summary of Results of Studies on PVG Stimulation

Source	No. Patients Implanted	Principal Pain Diagnosis	Follow-up (Years)	Pain Relief Success (No.)	Success (%)	Failure (No.)	Failure (%)
Richardson (56)	57	Low back	1–9	34	60	23	40
Hosobuchi (49)	22	Low back and leg	2–14	39	80	10	20
	16	Cancer and other chronic pain	2–14	11	69	5	31
Ray et al. (57)	16	Low back	2 (mean)	11	69	5	31
Plotkin (58)	48	Low back	0.5–3.5	38	79	10	21
Young et al. (45, 59)	29	Low back	2 (mean)	17	59	12	41
Siegfried (60)	13	Neuropathic	0.5–2.5	0	0	13	100
Meyerson (12)	18	Cancer	0.2–5	9	50	9	50
All	220	—	—	125	57	95	43

TABLE 93-5. Summary of Results of Studies on Stimulation in Sensory Thalamic Nuclei and Internal Capsule

Source	No. Patients Implanted	Principal Pain Diagnosis	Follow-up (Years)	Pain Relief					
				Good		Moderate		None	
				(No.)	(%)	(No.)	(%)	(No.)	(%)
Adams (61)	17	Anesthesia dolorosa	2 (mean)	3	18	11	65	3	17
Hosobuchi (49)	32	Neuropathic	2–14	25	78	—	—	7	22
	20	Lumbosacral radiculopathy	2–14	19	95	—	—	1	5
Turnbull et al. (62)	14	Arachnoiditis neuropathic	1 (mean)	8	57	5	36	1	7
Dieckmann and Witzmann (63)	32	Neuropathic	2–5	9	28	—	—	23	72
Mundinger and Neumuller (64)	18	Neuropathic	1–6	7	39	3	17	8	44
Siegfried (60)	41	Neuropathic	0.5–2.5	16	39	18	44	7	17
Namba et al. (65)	11	Thalamic	?	3	27	3	27	5	46
All	209	—	—	90	43	40	19	79	38

patients (30%) with this condition obtained relief from ICS. In the U.S. cooperative study (52), 9 patients with facial pain underwent PVG stimulation and 6 of them benefited.

Postherpetic Neuralgia

A group of 13 patients suffering from postherpetic facial pain treated with sensory thalamic stimulation was reported by Demierre and Siegfried (68). With a follow-up of 1 to 3 years, the outcome was judged to be excellent in 5 patients and good in another 5, giving a success rate of 77%. Hosobuchi (49) reported that of 5 patients with postherpetic neuralgia, 3 had initial pain relief and were implanted permanently; of these, 66% derived long-term relief.

Central Pain

Pain due to spinal cord injury has been the indication for ICS in a few studies only. Generally no information is available about the extent of the injury, but many of the patients probably were paraplegic. Four studies described sensory thalamus stimulation in 18 patients with such pain (49, 56, 57, 63); the outcome was successful in 6 patients (30%) only. In addition, in the cooperative U.S. study (52), PVG stimulation was used with 8 patients, all of whom were judged to have benefited from the treatment.

For central pain of thalamic origin, stimulation of the sensory limb of the internal capsule may be useful. In five major studies (49, 60, 63–65) comprising 28 patients, successful results were obtained in 10 patients (38%). The U.S. cooperative study (52) found that stimulation in this same target region provided satisfactory relief to 15 of 26 patients (58%).

Brachial Plexus Lesions

Treatment of patients with brachial plexus lesions, including both injury of the plexus itself and avulsion of the cervical nerve roots, with sensory thalamic stimulation has been reported in three studies (36, 63, 69). In these studies, 11 of 21 patients (52%) experienced satisfactory pain relief.

Phantom Limb Pain

Phantom limb pain has been treated with sensory thalamic stimulation in three major studies (60, 63, 64) including 21 patients; of these, 13 (62%) obtained satisfactory pain control. Mazars et al. (54) reported exceptionally favorable results, claiming that in a group of 23 patients with phantom limb pain, only 1 failed to obtain relief from thalamic stimulation.

Peripheral Nerve Injury

The U.S. cooperative study (52) suggests that pain due to peripheral nerve injury can be effectively controlled with stimulation in either the sensory limb of the internal capsule or in the PVG. Thus, 10 out of 13 patients (77%) benefited from internal capsule stimulation and 15 of 21 (71%) from PVG stimulation. No patient with stimulation in the sensory thalamus for this indication was reported in that study, whereas Mazars et al. (54) reported that such stimulation is particularly effective for pain due to peripheral nerve injury.

Cancer Pain

For pain associated with malignant disease, ICS has been performed mostly in the PVG region. Of 39 patients included in five studies (12, 49, 50, 59, 61), 27 (68%) had useful relief. In the cooperative European (53) and U.S. (52) studies, the success rates were 43% (40 patients) and 85% (26 patients), respectively. Tsubokawa et al. (51) used sensory thalamic stimulation for cancer pain and reported that 4 of 7 (57%) obtained satisfactory relief.

Low Back Pain

Low back pain is the most common indication for PVG stimulation (see Table 93-4). The long-term outcome is relatively favorable, with 60 to 70% success rates reported in most studies. Not all reports, however, give the number of patients who failed to respond to the initial phase of trial stimulation and in whom an electrode was never permanently internalized. Recently, Hosobuchi (49) reported an extended series of 49 patients treated for low back pain. With a follow-up of 2 to 14 years, 39 (80%) were classified as successful. Of these patients, 19 had electrodes implanted in both the PVG and the sensory thalamus; in the remaining 20, electrodes were implanted only in the PVG.

Clinical Considerations

Selection of Patients

In order to ensure favorable long-term results with intracerebral stimulation, patients must provide a reliable evaluation of the trial percutaneous stimulation. This procedure may be quite time-consuming and stressful for patients, as stimulation with some couplings of the stimulation poles may fail to provide pain relief. In order to assess the effect properly, patients should abstain from taking analgesics. This particular treatment requires that patients be cooperative and psychologically stable. In addition, it is desirable for patients to understand the general principles of the treatment. Therefore, patients with subnormal intelligence, those who are heavily dependent on narcotics or who may have a secondary gain of their pain condition, and those who exhibit manipulatory and hysteroid personality traits should be selected with extreme care, and generally are not good candidates for ICS.

Because much evidence indicates that the two stimulation targets are predominantly, perhaps even exclusively, effective for different types of pain, an adequate pain analysis is indispensable in order to sort out different pain components and their genesis (nociceptive or neuropathic). This is particularly important for pain in malignant disease and such complex conditions as low back pain. In these cases, testing the response to drugs may be helpful. Neuropathic pain is generally resistant to both peripherally and centrally acting analgesics, whereas the nociceptive type of pain is likely to respond. Sometimes neuropathic pain is alleviated by a test infusion of a short-acting barbiturate (70), but in practice the hypnotic effect is difficult to differentiate from a true suppression of pain. Finally, a poor effect from opioids and a beneficial effect from membrane-stabilizing drugs such as carbamazepin may suggest that the pain has a major neurogenic component.

Some have claimed that a positive response to morphine is a prerequisite for considering PVG stimulation (49). If endorphinergic mechanisms, or rather pain-controlling systems excitable by morphine, are necessarily involved in PVG stimulation, a true suppression of pain by this drug would be a reliable predictor for a positive outcome of stimulation. A morphine test is preferably performed in a double-blind fashion: four 100-ml saline infusions are prepared and coded, with two of them each containing 10 to 15 mg of morphine. The patient should not have any analgesics when tested. An infusion is given when the patient reports having pain, and he or she is asked to assess the amount of pain with the aid of a visual analog scale at 15-min intervals. If the patient reports pain relief, naloxone in a dose of 0.4 to 0.8 mg is given. If no pain relief is reported, the next infusion can be given after 2 to 3 hours. This "morphine test" has proven to be very informative and may also be used with other drugs with a possible pain-relieving effect (71, 72). A negative outcome of the morphine test, however, does not always mean a patient will not obtain effective pain relief with PVG stimulation; for example, several cases are reported in the literature about patients who did not respond to morphine or who had become tolerant to the drug and who nevertheless responded favorably to PVG stimulation (12). On the other hand, some reports indicate that cross-tolerance between opiates and PVG stimulation can occur. This seemingly contradictory evidence suggests that both opioid and nonopioid mechanisms may be involved in PVC stimulation.

Surgical Technique

Implantation of electrodes in the brain, an established technique, has been done for many years and was originally developed for depth recording in patients with epilepsy. Generally, the operation is performed with local anesthesia only and is well tolerated by most patients (Fig. 93-4). The stereotaxic technique employed requires ventriculography in order to visualize the third ventricle. Target localization is presently performed with the aid of CT. Comerically available electrodes are either monopolar or multipolar. The latter type consists of four platinum wires twisted together and has stimulating poles, 1 mm in length and placed 2 mm apart, in its distal end. The diameter of the electrode is about 1 mm. This multipolar arrangement makes it possible to explore the region along the electrode and to choose the most effective combination of stimulation poles.

The electrode is hooked onto a thin stereotaxic probe by which it is introduced to the target site (Figs. 93-5 and 93-6). It is then fixed by a plastic button in the burr hole. Percutaneous leads are tunneled under the scalp and led out through the skin a short distance away. This technique permits trial stimulation for several days, or weeks, in order to assess the effect of stimulation and to find the optimal combination of stimulation poles. If sufficient pain relief is obtained, the electrode is permanently connected to a receiver placed subcutaneously in the infraclavicular region. Since the subcutaneous tunneling of the interconnecting lead is relatively painful, this procedure is often performed with general anesthesia. The receiver is activated passively via a flat antenna taped to the skin and connected to a transmitter-stimulator of the same type as that used for spinal cord stimulation. It is also possible to perform stimulation with the aid of a fully implantable and programmable stimulator.

Sensory Thalamic Nuclei

To obtain pain relief by stimulation of the sensory thalamic nuclei, the electrode must be placed in the part of these nuclei that represents the painful region of the body, since the elicitation of paresthesiae in this area is a prerequisite for obtaining pain relief. Occasionally, a better effect is obtained with a stimulation intensity that is just subthreshold to subjective sensations. In order to obtain pain relief, stimulation must be continued for 15 to 30 min. In general, the poststimulatory effect lasts for 2 to 5 hours, but in exceptional cases the pain relief persists for a considerably longer period of time (1 to 3 days).

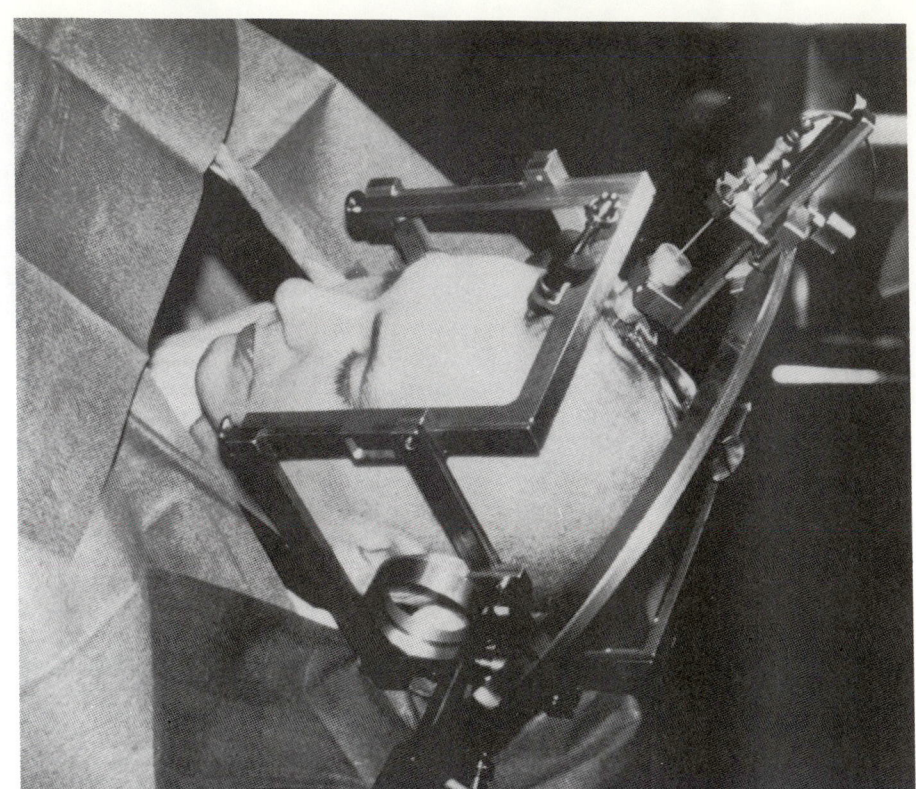

FIG. 93-4. Stereotaxic apparatus is used for the implantation of intracerebral electrodes. As a rule, the target region is explored with electric stimulation before implantation in order to ensure a proper placement (shown in the photograph).

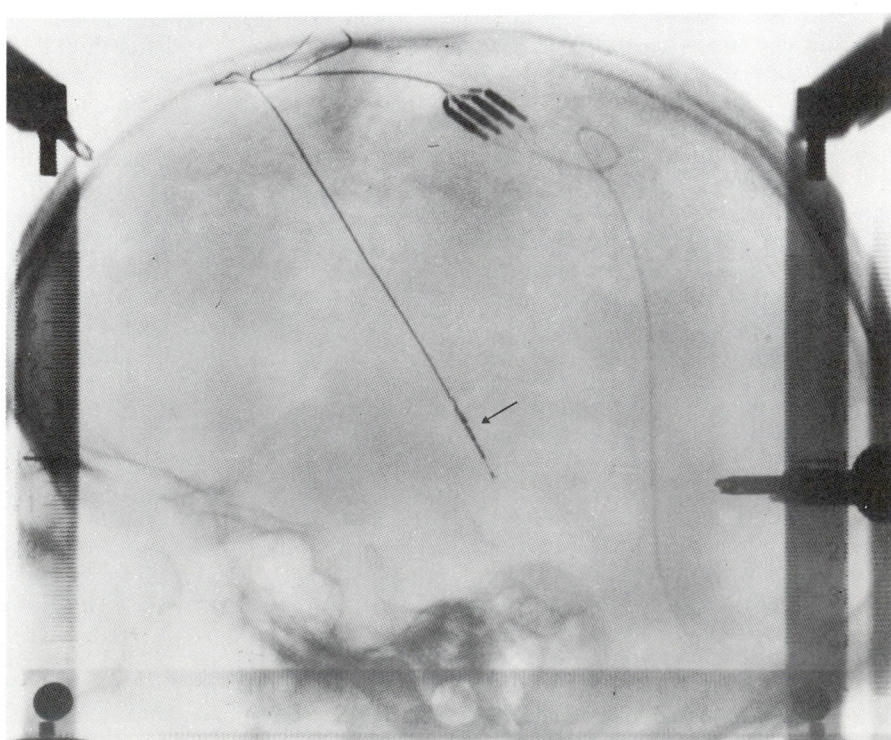

FIG. 93-5. Perioperative radiograph showing a stimulating electrode (arrow) implanted in a region where stimulation may produce pain relief. In this patient, who suffered from central pain, the electrode was implanted in the sensory thalamic nuclei. Also shown is the stereotaxic frame, which is used to determine the location of the stimulation target.

PVG Region

The sensory thalamic nuclei are comparatively large, whereas the PVG region in the medial diencephalic-mesencephalic junction zone, from where stimulation-produced pain relief is obtainable, is very small. In particular, the mediolateral extension of the susceptible region, which does not exceed 2 to 3 mm, makes the electrode placement very critical (73). The extreme precision that is required for implantation of electrodes in the PVG region presumably accounts for some of the variability in the clinical results reported in the literature.

In contrast to stimulation of sensory thalamic nuclei, PVG stimulation generally is performed at an intensity subthreshold to subjective sensations. At the onset of stimulation, however, patients generally report a pleasant feeling of warmth invading the trunk or the face, but this sensation does not necessarily imply that pain relief can be achieved. Even though stimulation is performed unilaterally, the evoked sensations have a symmetrical distribution. Increased stimulation may produce ocular oscillation, and some have claimed that this phenomenon indicates proper placement of the electrode. At excessive stimulus currents, unpleasant sensations of fear or anxiety may occur. The usual stimulation frequency is 30 Hz and the pulse duration 0.2 msec. To avoid causing fatigue of the system or inducing tolerance to stimulation, patients are instructed not to stimulate themselves for longer than 20 to 25 min at one time and, if possible, not more than three or four times per 24 hours.

Complications and Side Effects

Serious surgical complications rarely occur with intracerebral implantation of electrodes. In seven studies (36, 50, 58, 59, 61, 63, 66) comprising 310 patients, 8 patients incurred hemorrhages (3%), but no fatal outcome was reported. Introduction of an electrode into the sensory thalamus may produce mild dysesthesia, but this appears to be a rare and generally transitory complication. Electrode implantation in the PVG region may cause a slight diplopia, but in the vast majority of patients this sign subsides in 1 to 2 weeks.

Infection at the receiver site or along the subcutaneous lead has been reported in some cases (generally about 3%); this risk is minimized by the use of a prophylactic antibiotic. Even though the trial stimulation period via percutaneous extension cables is often prolonged for several weeks or even months, only a few cases of intracranial infections have been reported.

In a few patients the implanted material may give rise to local tissue reaction causing tenderness along the lead or at the site of the receiver, and sometimes serous fluid accumulates around the receiver. These problems usually subside after a few months. Malfunction of the implanted device is relatively common, occurring in 10 to 15% of the patients (59), and is corrected by reimplantation or exchange of the electrode or receiver. In a few cases, the effect may be lost due to displacement of the electrode, but this complication rarely occurs with the presently available electrodes, which are less springy than those previously used. Another cause of equipment failure is breakage of the insulation of the subcutaneous lead between the electrode contact and the receiver.

Erroneous handling of the stimulator can lead to an inadvertently high stimulation intensity, which may produce unpleasant sensations: with sensory thalamic stimulation, strong and almost painful paresthesiae

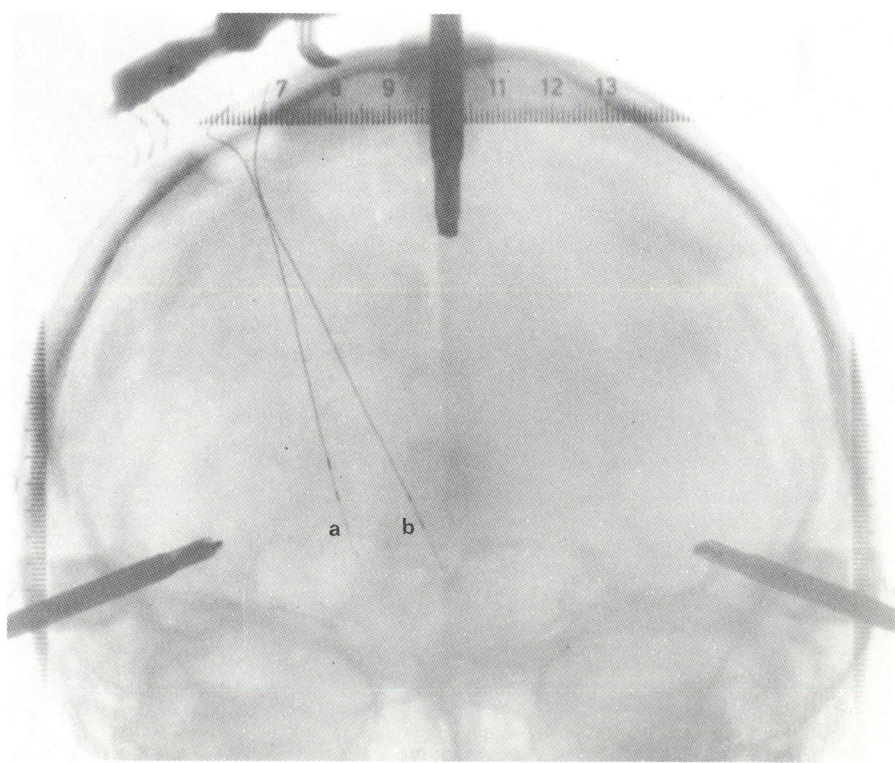

FIG. 93-6. Perioperative radiograph showing two electrodes temporarily implanted for trial stimulation. The electrodes, which contain four stimulating poles, are located in the lateral sensory thalamic nucleus (**a**) and in the PVG (**b**). The patient suffered from sciatic and low back pain presumably due to epidural fibrosis, and he later enjoyed perfect pain relief with stimulation via the sensory thalamic electrode.

can be produced and with PVG stimulation, nausea, diplopia, and anxiety. Such high-intensity stimulation has not been reported to cause any permanent sequelae, and the patients soon learn to handle the stimulator correctly.

Problems With Long-Term Treatment

Much attention has been paid to the problem of "tolerance" to ICS, which is believed to be the main reason for long-term failures. In particular, this phenomenon appears to be relatively common with PVG stimulation. Several measures have been advocated to counteract the development or the presence of tolerance to such stimulation. Some evidence suggests that a link in the descending bulbospinal pain control system, which presumably is activated by PVG stimulation, is serotonergic, and experimentally the administration of serotonin has been shown to reverse tolerance to PVG stimulation. Therefore, oral L-tryptophan, which is the precursor to serotonin, has been tried to avoid tolerance to PVG stimulation, and there is evidence that this tactic has sometimes been rewarding (36). Another way to enhance serotonergic mechanisms in PVG stimulation is the use of drugs that interfere with the reuptake of serotonin (clomipramine, amitriptyline, etc.)

Long-term failures also occur with sensory thalamic stimulation, but no evidence indicates that this phenomenon is due to the development of tolerance in the true sense of the word. Although some have claimed (51) that regular medication with L-dopa may improve the efficacy of sensory thalamic stimulation, this observation remains to be confirmed.

Conclusions

The clinical outcome of ICS is still somewhat unpredictable and the knowledge of its mode of action is fragmentary. Nonetheless, this treatment has been effective for many patients suffering from severe pain that has failed to respond to other measures. Examples of such pain conditions are postherpetic pain, anesthesia dolorosa, thalamic pain, pain due to peripheral nerve injury, and sometimes low back pain and nociceptive pain in malignancy. The two most effective and commonly used targets for stimulation are the sensory thalamic nuclei (or the sensory limb of the internal capsule) for neuropathic pain and the periventricular gray region for nociceptive pain. Consequently, it is essential to thoroughly analyze the pain with regard to its nature and origin. Intracerebral stimulation should not be applied as a routine method, and the selection of patients should be done with utmost care. On the other hand, the procedure is reversible and carries little risk of serious complications; thus, for patients with nonmalignant disease it should be considered before destructive procedures are resorted to.

REFERENCES

1. Shealy, C.N., Mortimer, J.T., and Reswick, J.: Electrical inhibition of pain by stimulation of the dorsal column: Preliminary clinical reports. Anesth. Analg., 46:489, 1967.
2. Wall, P.D., and Sweet, W.H.: Temporary abolition of pain in man. Science, 155:108, 1967.
3. Sweet, W.H., and Wepsic, J.G.: Treatment of chronic pain by stimulation of fibers of primary afferent neurons. Trans. Am. Neurol. Assoc., 93:103, 1968.
4. Siegfried, J., and Lazorthes, Y.: Long-term follow-up of dorsal column stimulation for chronic pain syndrome after multiple lumbar operations. Appl. Neurophysiol., 45:201, 1982.
5. Erickson, D.L., and Long, D.M.: Ten-year follow-up of dorsal column stimulation. In Advances in Pain Research and Therapy. Vol. 5. Edited by J.J. Bonica, U. Lindblom, and A. Iggo. New York, Raven Press, 1983, pp. 583–589.
6. Handwerker, H.O., Iggo, A., and Zimmerman, M.: Segmental and supraspinal actions on dorsal horn neurons responding to noxious and non-noxious skin stimuli. Pain, 1:147, 1975.
7. Augustinsson, L.E., Carlsson, C.A., and Fall, M.: Autonomic effects of electrostimulation. Appl. Neurophysiol., 45:185, 1982.
8. Campbell, J.N.: Examination of possible mechanisms by which stimulation of the spinal cord in man relieves pain. Appl. Neurophysiol., 44:181, 1982.
9. Nyquist, J.K., and Greenhoot, J.H.: Responses evoked from the thalamic centrum medianum by painful input: Suppression by dorsal funiculus conditioning. Exp. Neurol., 9:215, 1973.
10. Foreman, R.D., et al.: Effects of dorsal column stimulation on primate spinothalamic tract neurons. J. Neurophysiol., 39:534, 1976.
11. Richardson, D.E., and Dempsey, C.W.: Monoamine turnover in CSF of patients during dorsal column stimulation for pain control (Abstr.). Pain (Suppl.), 2:S224, 1984.
12. Meyerson, B.A.: Electrostimulation procedures: Effects, presumed rationale, and possible mechanisms. In Advances in Pain Research and Therapy. Vol. 5. Edited by J.J. Bonica, U. Lindblom, and A. Iggo. New York, Raven Press, 1983, pp. 495–534.
13. Lindblom, U.: Assessment of abnormal evoked pain in neurological pain patients and its relation to spontaneous pain. A descriptive and conceptual model with some analytical results. In Advances in Pain Research and Therapy. Vol. 9. Edited by H. Fields, R. Dubner, and F. Cervero. New York, Raven Press, 1985, pp. 409–423.
14. Long, D.M.: Patient selection and the results of spinal cord stimulation for chronic pain. In Indications for Spinal Cord Stimulation: Proceedings of a Symposium. Edited by Y. Hosobuchi and T. Corbin. Amsterdam, Excerpta Medica, 1981, pp. 1–12.
15. Nashold, B.S., and Friedman, H.: Dorsal column stimulation for control of pain: Preliminary report on 30 patients. J. Neurosurg., 36:590, 1972.
16. Nielson, K.A., Adams, J.E., and Hosobuchi, Y.: Experience with dorsal column stimulation for relief of chronic intractable pain: 1968–1973. Surg. Neurol., 4:148, 1975.
17. Long, M.D.: Current status of neuroaugmentation procedures for chronic pain. In Mechanisms of Pain and Analgesic Compounds. Edited by R.F. Beers, Jr., and E.G. Basset. New York, Raven Press, 1979, pp. 51–69.
18. Sedan, R., and Lazorthes, Y.: La neurostimulation electrique therapeutique. Neurochirurgia (Paris), 24(Suppl. 1):1, 1978.
19. Urban, B.J., and Nashold, B.S.: Percutaneous epidural stimulation of the spinal cord for relief of pain. J. Neurosurg., 48:323, 1978.
20. Siegfried, J.: Long-term results of electrical stimulation in the treatment of pain by means of implanted electrodes (epidural spinal cord and deep brain stimulation). In Pain Therapy. Edited by R. Rizzi and M. Visentin. Amsterdam, Elsevier Biomedical Press, 1983, pp. 463–475.
21. Broseta, J., et al.: Chronic epidural dorsal column stimulation in the treatment of causalgic pain. Appl. Neurophysiol., 45:190, 1982.
22. Krainick, J.U., Thoden, U., and Riechert, T.: Pain reduction in amputees by long-term spinal cord stimulation. J. Neurosurg., 52:346, 1980.
23. Krainick, J.U., and Thoden, U.: Experience with spinal cord stimulation for the control of postamputation pain. In Indications for Spinal Cord Stimulation: Proceedings of a Symposium. Edited by Y. Hosobuchi and T. Corbin. Amsterdam, Excerpta Medica, 1981, pp. 42–47.
24. Hood, T.W., and Siegfried, J.: Epidural versus thalamic stimulation for the management of brachial plexus lesion pain. Acta Neurochir. (Suppl.), 33:451, 1984.

25. Winkelmüller, W.: Experience with the control of low back pain by the dorsal column stimulation (DCS) system and by the peridural electode system (Pisces). *In* Indications for Spinal Cord Stimulation: Proceedings of a Symposium. Edited by Y. Hosobuchi and T. Corbin. Amsterdam, Excerpta Medica, 1981, pp. 34–41.

26. Ray, C.D.: Control of pain by electrical stimulation: A clinical follow-up review. *In* Advances in Neurosurgery. Vol. 3. Edited by H. Penzholz et al. Heidelberg, Springer Verlag, 1975, pp. 216–224.

27. North, R.B., Fischell, T.A., and Long, D.M.: Chronic dorsal column stimulation via percutaneously inserted epidural electrodes. Appl. Neurophysiol., *40*:184, 1977.

28. Young, R.F.: Evaluation of dorsal column stimulation in the treatment of chronic pain. Neurosurgery, *3*:373, 1978.

29. Ray, C.D., Burton, C.V., and Lifson, A.: Neurostimulation as used in a large clinical practice. Appl. Neurophysiol., *45*:160, 1982.

30. Sweet, W.H., and Wepsic, J.G.: Stimulation of the posterior columns of the spinal cord for pain control: Indications, technics and results. Clin. Neurosurg., *21*:278, 1975.

31. Tallis, R.C., et al.: Spinal cord stimulation in peripheral vascular disease. J. Neurol. Neurosurg. Psychiatr., *46*:478, 1983.

32. Broseta, J., et al.: Spinal cord stimulation in peripheral arterial disease. A cooperative study. J. Neurosurg., *64*:71, 1986.

33. Lazorthes, Y., and Verdie, J.C.: Les neurostimulateurs electriques therapeutiques. Rev. Eur. Biotech. Med., *2*:425, 1980.

34. Pineda, A.: Complications of dorsal column stimulation. J. Neurosurg., *48*:64, 1978.

35. Richardson, D.E.: Trouble-shooting in spinal stimulation. *In* Indications for Spinal Cord Stimulation: Proceedings of a Symposium. Edited by Y. Hosobuchi and T. Corbin. Amsterdam, Excerpta Medica, 1981, pp. 77–84.

36. Hosobuchi, Y.: The current status of analgesic brain stimulation. Acta Neurochir. (Suppl.), *30*:219, 1980.

37. Gybels, J.: Analgesic brain stimulation in chronic pain in man and rat. *In* Current Topics in Pain Research and Therapy. Edited by T. Yokota and R. Dubner. Amsterdam, Excerpta Medica, 1983, pp. 137–144.

38. Young, R.F.: Brain stimulation. *In* Textbook of Pain. 2nd ed. Edited by P.D. Wall and R. Melzack. Edinburgh, Churchill Livingstone, 1989, pp. 925–929.

39. Mazars, G., Merienne, S., and Cioloca, C.: Stimulations thalamiques intermittentes antalgiques. Rev. Neurol., *128*:273, 1973.

40. Nyquist, J.K., and Greenhoot, J.H.: Responses evoked from the thalamic centrum medianum by painful input: Suppression by dorsal funiculus conditioning. Exp. Neurol., *9*:215, 1973.

41. Willis, W.D.: Modulation of primate spinothalamic tract discharges. *In* Advances in Pain Research and Therapy. Vol. 6. Edited by L. Kruger and J.C. Liebeskind. New York, Raven Press, 1984, pp. 217–240.

42. Benabid, A.L., Henriksen, S.J., McGinty, J.F., and Bloom, F.E.: Thalamic nucleus ventro-postero-lateralis inhibits nucleus parafascicularis response to noxious stimuli through a non-opioid pathway. Brain Res., *280*:217, 1983.

43. Reynolds, D.V.: Surgery in the rat during electrical analgesia induced by focal brain stimulation. Science, *164*:444, 1969.

44. Hosobuchi, Y., Rossier, J., Bloom, F.E., and Guillemin, R.: Stimulation of human periaqueductal gray for pain relief increases immunoreactive beta-endorphin in ventricular fluid. Science, *203*:279, 1979.

45. Young, R.F., et al.: Electrical stimulation of the brain in the treatment of chronic pain in man. *In* Advances in Pain Research and Therapy. Vol. 6. Edited by L. Kruger and J.C. Liebeskind. New York, Raven Press, 1984, pp. 289–303.

46. Meyerson, B.A.: Biochemistry of pain relief with intracerebral stimulation: Few facts and many hypotheses. Acta Neurochir. (Suppl.), *30*:229, 1980.

47. Dennis, S.G., Choiniere, M., and Melzack, R.: Stimulation-produced analgesia in rats: Assessment by two pain tests and correlation with self-stimulation. Exp. Neurol., *68*:295, 1980.

48. Richardson, D.E., and Akil, H.: Pain reduction by electrical brain stimulation in man. Part II: Chronic self-administration in the periventricular gray matter. J. Neurosurg., *47*:184, 1977.

49. Hosobuchi, Y.: Electrical stimulation of subcortical gray matter for the control of intractable pain in humans. Report of 122 cases (1970–1984). J. Neurosurg., *64*:543, 1986.

50. Meyerson, B.A.: Central nervous stimulation for cancer pain: Possible methods of manipulating the physiology of pain modulation. *In* Management of Superior Pulmonary Sulcus Syndrome. Edited by J.J. Bonica and V. Ventrafridda. New York, Raven Press, 1982, pp. 149–164.

51. Tsubokawa, T., et al.: Thalamic relay nucleus stimulation for relief of intractable pain. Clinical results and β-endorphin immunoreactivity in the cerebrospinal fluid. Pain, *18*:115, 1984.

52. Groth, K., et al.: Deep brain stimulation for chronic intractable pain. Minneapolis, Medtronic Inc., 1982.

53. Lazorthes, Y.: European study on deep brain stimulation (Mimeo.). Resume of the 3rd European Workshop on Electrical Neurostimulation. Paris, Medtronic Europe, 1979.

54. Mazars, G.J., Merienne, L., and Cioloca, D.: Comparative study of electrical stimulation of posterior thalamic nuclei, periaqueductal gray, and other midline mesencephalic structures in man. *In* Advances in Pain Research and Therapy. Vol. 3. Edited by J.J. Bonica, J.C. Liebeskind, and D.G. Albe-Fessard. New York, Raven Press, 1979, pp. 541–546.

55. Levy, R.M., Lamb, S., and Adams, J.E.: Deep brain stimulation for chronic pain: Long-term follow-up in 145 patients from 1972–1984 (Abstr.). Pain (Suppl.), *2*:S115, 1984.

56. Richardson, D.E.: Long-term follow-up of deep brain stimulation for relief of chronic pain in the human. *In* Modern Neurosurgery 1. Edited by M. Brock. Berlin–Heidelberg, Springer Verlag, 1982, pp. 449–453.

57. Ray, C.D., Burton, C.V., and Lifson, A.: Neurostimulation as used in a large clinical practice. Appl. Neurophysiol., *45*:160, 1982.

58. Plotkin, R.: Results in 60 cases of deep brain stimulation for chronic intractable pain. *In* Modern Neurosurgery 1. Edited by M. Brock. Berlin–Heidelberg, Springer Verlag, 1982, pp. 454–459.

59. Young, R.F., et al.: Electrical stimulation of the brain in treatment of chronic pain. J. Neurosurg., *62*:389, 1985.

60. Siegfried, J.: Long-term results of electrical stimulation in the treatment of pain by means of implanted electrodes (epidural spinal cord and deep brain stimulation). *In* Pain Therapy. Edited by R. Rizzi and M. Visentin. Amsterdam, Elsevier Biomedical Press, 1983, pp. 463–475.

61. Adams, J.E.: Technique and technical problems associated with implantation of neuroaugumentive devices. Appl. Neurophysiol., *40*:111, 1977/78.

62. Turnbull, I.M., et al.: Thalamic stimulation for neuropathic pain. J. Neurosurg., *52*:486, 1980.

63. Dieckmann, G., and Witzmann, A.: Initial and long-term results of deep brain stimulation for chronic intractable pain. Appl. Neurophysiol., *45*:167, 1982.

64. Mundinger, F., and Neumuller, H.: Programmed stimulation for control of chronic pain and motor diseases. Appl. Neurophysiol., *45*:102, 1982.

65. Namba, S., et al.: Sensory and motor responses to deep brain stimulation. J. Neurosurg., *63*:224, 1985.

66. Mundinger, F., and Salomao, J.F.: Deep brain stimulation in mesencephalic lemniscus medialis for chronic pain. Acta Neurochir. (Suppl.), *30*:245, 1980.

67. Broseta, J., Roldan, P., Masbout, G., and Barcia-Salorio, J.L.: Chronic VPM thalamic stimulation in facial anaesthesia dolorosa following trigeminal surgery. Acta Neurochir. (Suppl.), *33*:505, 1984.

68. Demierre, B., and Siegfried, J.: Traitement neurochirurgical de la nevralgie postherpetiforme. Med. Hyg., *41*:1960, 1983.

69. Hood, T.W., and Siegfried, J.: Epidural versus thalamic stimulation for the management of brachial plexus lesion pain. Acta Neurochir. (Suppl.), *33*:451, 1984.

70. Tasker, R.R., Tsuda, T., and Hawrylyshyn, P.: Clinical neurophysiological investigation of deafferentation pain. *In* Advances in Pain Research and Therapy. Vol. 5. Edited by J.J. Bonica, U. Lindblom, and A. Iggo. New York, Raven Press, 1983, pp. 713–738.

71. Arner, S., Lindblom, U., and Meyerson, B.A.: Letter to the editor. Pain, *24*:117, 1986.

72. Arner, S., and Meyerson. B.A.: Lack of analgesic effect of opioids on neuropathic and idiopathic forms of pain. Pain, *33*:11, 1988.

73. Boivie, J., and Meyerson, B.A.: A correlative anatomical and clinical study of pain suppression by deep brain stimulation. Pain, *13*:113, 1982.

INTRODUCTION

JOHN J. BONICA

This section discusses regional analgesia (also called conduction analgesia and neural blockade) in the management of patients with acute pain, cancer pain, and nonmalignant chronic pain. Chapter 94 discusses various techniques of blocking peripheral somatic and sympathetic nerves with local anesthetics, and their use as diagnostic, prognostic, prophylactic, and therapeutic tools. Chapter 95 presents a comprehensive overview of the use of intraspinal opioids, which I consider to be a form of regional analgesia, and of intracerebral opioid injections for the control of acute pain and cancer pain. In Chapter 96 the use of neural blockade with neurolytic agents intended to destroy the axons or cell bodies of peripheral nerves to produce prolonged blockade is considered. Chapter 96 also reviews the role of chemical hypophysectomy in the management of cancer pain. These three chapters, as other chapters of Part V, discuss these techniques in regard to such fundamental issues as the bases for clinical application, the indications for use for the relief of various pain syndromes, the efficacy and limitations of these techniques, and brief descriptions, for those who are not acquainted with these methods. In this section the term regional *analgesia* is sometimes used intherchangeably with regional *anesthesia*. In other instances the term anesthesia has a more restrictive meaning, i.e., that all sensory modalities are eliminated by the local anesthetic or neurolytic agent. The term analgesia is used to indicate either that the primary aim of the procedure is to relieve pain or that other nerve functions are not completely eliminated. With local anesthetics, this is achieved by using dilute solutions, which block small fibers and usually do not completely interrupt other sensations. With intraspinal opioids, analgesia (pain relief) is achieved without any evidence of alteration of other sensory, somatomotor, or sympathetic functions. I generally prefer the term regional analgesia because this emphasizes the primary objective of the procedure.

Historical Perspectives

In introducing this section I present a brief historical overview of the development and use of regional anesthesia with local anesthetics as a method of pain management. Chapter 1 mentions that use of this method was really initiated by Koller's demonstration of the local anesthetic properties of cocaine (1). This, together with the pre-eminence of the specificity theory of pain, led to the development and widespread use of this method during the first 60 years of this century. The concept of injection therapy for pain relief dates back to antiquity—the Chinese used acupuncture more than 5000 years ago (2). About 2000 years ago the use of this procedure spread to Japan and other Asian countries and, in the sixteenth century, to Europe. As Mann (3) has pointed out, puncture of the skin with sharp stones, the needles of certain plants, and other instruments was practiced in ancient Egypt and Greece and, more recently, by some African and Eskimo tribes. The injection of various potions in paste or liquid form, some of which contained systemic analgesics and hypnotics, was widely practiced in ancient times and the Middle Ages (4).

The modern era of nerve blocks for pain control really began with the invention of the hollow needle by Rynd (5) in 1845 and the syringe by Pravaz (6) and Wood (7) during the 1850s. This prompted many efforts to treat painful disorders, such as trigeminal neuralgia, by injecting solutions of opiates, chloroform, bromides, tannin, alcohol, and other compounds near nerve trunks. Most of these procedures failed because all the agents (except alcohol) lacked local anesthetic action. About the time that syringes and needles were being developed, Gaedecke isolated cocaine from the juice of coca leaves, in 1855; 5 years later Niemann (8) named it cocaine and reported its tongue-numbing effect for the first time. It was then studied extensively by many pharmacologists, including Bennett (9) and Von Anrep (10), who reported its anesthetic effects and suggested its use as a surgical anesthetic. As early as 1875 Collins, Fauvel, Saglia, and other French clinicians applied an extract of cocaine leaves topically to the pharynx and larynx to control the severe pain of tuberculosis and cancer (11). These were probably the first clinical applications of local anesthesia for pain control.

Unfortunately, all these suggestions regarding its use as an anesthetic were ignored until Koller's report to the Opthalmologic Congress in Heidelberg on September 15, 1884, on the anesthetic efficacy of cocaine (1). The report was received with enthusiasm. It prompted intense laboratory research and the extensive clinical use of cocaine as a topical anesthetic for surgery in various parts of the body, and soon thereafter it was used widely to produce local infiltration analgesia. A week after the news of Koller's report was received in the United States, Halstead, who later became one of America's greatest surgeons, and his colleague, Hall, began to devise techniques for injection of various nerve trunks, including the brachial plexus and cranial nerves, to produce anesthesia for dental procedures and surgery (12). By the end of the century field block was used widely, and subarachnoid block was introduced by Bier.

Although these procedures were developed primarily for use in surgical anesthesia, it was not long before some physicians began to realize their value for the control of nonsurgical pain and other medical disorders. In 1885 Corning reported the injection of cocaine into the spinal canal of dogs to produce anesthesia of the hind legs and subsequently used the method in a man who had been suffering from "spinal weakness and seminal incontinence" (13). Corning was probably the first to produce both subarachnoid and extradural block. In 1886 Corning wrote *Local Anesthesia*, in which he described the history, effects, toxicology, and clinical application of cocaine (14). Two years later Corning (15) published *Headache and Neuralgias*, in which he described the local injection of cocaine for treatment of trigeminal neuralgia, sciatica, femoral neuralgia, and other forms of nerve pain. In 1894 Corning (16) published a book, probably the first on the subject, in which he clearly described the technique and clinical application of local anesthetics for the relief of pain of neurologic disorders, including subarachnoid injection of cocaine for the relief of severe pain. The popularity of regional anesthesia for surgery and, to a lesser extent, for pain therapy is shown by the fact that in 1899, Matas, another American surgeon, reported that 800 publications on local and regional anesthesia appeared in the literature during the period 1884 to 1898 (17).

The Golden Age of Nerve Blocks: 1900–1940

I consider the first 40 years of this century to be the golden age of regional anesthesia, particularly in regard to its use in the diagnosis and therapy of pain, because new and safer local anesthetics were developed during this period and most techniques of regional anesthesia in current use were developed and refined at that time. Efforts to apply all these techniques for the control of nonsurgical pain and other disorders were unparalleled.

In 1900 Schlösser (18) began experimenting with alcoholization of a branch of the trigeminal nerve for the treatment of tic douloureux. He noted that injection of sensory nerves with 2 ml of 80% alcohol produced transient burning pain, followed a few minutes later by numbness and anesthesia. These disappeared after a week but the analgesia persisted. Following these experiments he used this method in many patients and subsequently published several reports, the first in 1907 (18) 2 years after Ostwald made a report (19). This method was developed further by many others, particularly by Levy and Boudouin (20) and by Härtel (21). Reports on the use of alcohol for the effective relief of trigeminal neuralgia prompted others to employ alcohol nerve block for the treatment of other conditions. Levy (22) in 1911 and Fetterolf (23) in 1912 reported the injection of the superior laryngeal nerve with alcohol and obtained beneficial results in patients with intractable pain caused by advanced tuberculosis. This technique subsequently was employed by Lukens (24), Swetlow (25), and others as a means of effectively relieving intractable pain of the larynx of various causes, including cancer.

Another important development occurred in 1906 when Sellheim (26), a German surgeon, began to imploy paravertebral somatic nerve block to produce surgical anesthesia of the lower abdomen. This was followed by extensive experimentation, clinical research, and refinement of the technique for surgical anesthesia in the sacral, upper thoracic, and cervical regions by many other German and Austrian surgeons.

Paravertebral Block for Pain Research and Treatment

One of the most brilliant chapters in the history of diagnostic and therapeutic blocks involved the use of paravertebral somatic and paravertebral sympathetic nerve blocks by Austrian and German physicians for research and for the diagnosis and therapy of various pain syndromes. These procedures were used to confirm the results of animal experiments carried out during the latter part of the nineteenth century by Sherrington (27) and others, and of human studies carried out by Head (28). Head's studies helped to suggest the spinal cord segments that provide sensory (including "pain") nerves to various visceral and somatic structures. These animal and human reports prompted many, particularly the Germans, Lawen (29), Freude and Kanellis (30), Kappis (31), and Von Gaza (32), and the Austrians, Brunn and Mandl (33), to use paravertebral block to delineate the pain pathways supplying the heart, stomach, various parts of the intestine, liver, gallbladder, spleen, kidneys, ureters, and uterus. Subsequently, paravertebral block was used widely as a diagnostic tool in painful visceral disease to help differentiate, for example, epigastric pain caused by cholecystitis or gastric lesions from that caused by disease of thoracic viscera. Moreover, these physicians (29–33) and others used this procedure therapeutically in certain cases of visceral disease associated with severe pain.

In 1926 Mandl (34) published a monograph that contained a detailed account of the application of paravertebral block for the diagnosis and treatment of various visceral diseases, with emphasis on the treatment of angina pectoris. Swetlow (35), also in 1926, described alcohol block of the upper thoracic sympathetic chain to secure a lasting interruption of sensory nerves of the heart in patients with severe angina pectoris. Swetlow's report prompted White and White (36, 37), and others, to use this technique for the relief of severe angina pectoris. The use of paravertebral block was extended by Swetlow (35) and others to many other conditions associated with severe intractable pain, particularly cancer. In 1925 Leriche and Fontaine first used paravertebral sympathetic block with procaine for the relief of the intense pain associated with angina pectoris, causalgia, and other post-traumatic reflex sympathetic dystrophies, and in 1934 they reported the use of the technique of stellate ganglion block (38). This technique was also used for the diagnosis and therapy of peripheral vascular disease and reflex sympathetic dystrophies by White (39) and later by Livingston (40), and by many others in the United States, Europe, and elsewhere.

Epidural and Subarachnoid Block

In the late 1920s Dogliotti (41) began to develop two techniques that were to prove valuable as diagnostic and therapeutic tools in patients with acute and chronic pain. One was spinal epidural block, a procedure that had been proposed 10 years earlier by Pages (42), a Spanish military surgeon, but that did not gain widespread recognition until Dogliotti's publication (41). The other was the description of the technique and clinical use of injecting absolute alcohol into the subarachnoid space to achieve a chemical rhizotomy for the treatment of severe intractable pain (43). Subsequently many clinicians used the latter method for the relief of cancer pain and other chronic pain syndromes. During the 1920s Doppler (44) carried out experiments in rabbits and then in humans using phenol in the treatment of peripheral vascular disease; it was noted that phenol produced marked vasodilation when placed around blood vessels. In 1929 Woodbridge (45) injected 8 ml of 80% alcohol into the sacral canal to relieve pain caused by cancer of the bladder, a technique that had been used for a number of years by Labat (46).

Local Anesthesia in Pain Research

During the 1920s cocaine, and later procaine, tetracaine, and various nerve block procedures, were used as research tools. Following the early work of Goldscheider (47), who used cocaine to study the functional disappearance of various nerve fibers, other workers used varying concentrations of local anesthetics around different nerve trunks and noted the disappearance of different functions in a consistent sequence. These studies led to the postulate that the differential blockade was related to differences in the size and anatomic makeup of different fibers, and that different fibers had specific neurophysiologic functions. The year after Bier (48) introduced spinal anesthesia, he used this technique to study the functional disappearance of various sensory, somatomotor, and autonomic efferent fibers, and noted a similar consistent sequence. The findings of these earlier studies were confirmed by Gasser and Erlanger (49) and Heinbecker and associates (50) (and later by Sarnoff and Arrowood) (51), who used sophisticated techniques to confirm the relationship among fiber size, conduction time, difference in the time of appearance of the block, and function of the different-sized fibers. Another important and far-reaching application of paravertebral block as a research tool was found by Cleland (52), who defined the nerve pathways involved in labor pain.

Widespread Application of Diagnostic and Therapeutic Nerve Blocks

In the 1930s comprehensive reviews on the use of diagnostic, prognostic, and therapeutic nerve blocks to relieve acute and chronic pain, and other disease states, were published by Woodbridge (44), Ruth (53), and Rovenstine and Wertheim (54). These and other reports (see above) prompted many surgeons and a few anesthesiologists to use nerve blocks for the diagnosis, prognosis, and treatment of pain during the 1930s and World War II. This widespread use was related to the information contained in many reports, as well as to the pre-eminent concept of pain as a specific sensation. In addition to systemic analgesics, neural blockade represented the only nonsurgical treatment modality for pain control. Before, during, and after World War II this trend was further encouraged by the development of nerve block clinics in many parts of the United States, Great Britain, Australia, and continental Europe. In Chapter 9 I cite my own experience of the use of these procedures as diagnostic, prognostic, and therapeutic tools, the chronology that led to the publication of the first edition of this book (55), and the development and application of the multidisciplinary concept of pain research and treatment.

New Anesthetics and Refinement of Techniques

During the 1950s the publication of several books, and other events, helped to usher in a resurgence of interest in the use of regional anesthesia for surgery, obstetrics, and the diagnosis and therapy of pain. A development that had a major impact on regional analgesia and nerve blocks was the introduction of lidocaine in the early 1950s and the use of intrathecal phenol, especially by Maher (56). A decade later, mepivacaine and prilocaine were introduced, followed by the longer acting local anesthetics bupivacaine and etidocaine. A large number of studies on the pharmacokinetics and pharmacodynamics of various local anesthetics and on their local and systemic toxicity were carried out. Using the basic principles of the clinical evaluation of local anesthetics as set down by Bonica (57), Löfström (58), and Nolte et al. (59), among others, evaluated newer anesthetics in humans by employing refined neurophysiologic techniques and reassessed the sequence of blockade of various nerve fibers in different peripheral nerves.

A large series of comprehensive studies clarified the effects of different levels of sympathetic blockade and analgesia achieved with continuous epidural, subarachnoid, and brachial plexus block on circulatory, respiratory, hepatic, renal, and other functions in normal humans and in patients (60). Others used discrete somatic nerve blocks to assess extrinsic neurogenic influences on myocardial functions and respiration (61). Sympathetic blocks were also used as research tools in determining the influence of sympathetic activity on the cutaneous pain threshold (62).

During the 1950s and 1960s block of the brachial plexus, cervical plexus, and lumbar plexus, differential spinal block, percutaneous lumbar sympathectomy, and other refinements of older techniques of blocking cranial and spinal nerves were studied. A further milestone in the application of therapeutic blocks was the use of hyperbaric phenol to produce chemical rhizotomy as reported by Maher (56, 63). Initial reports prompted widespread trials, several meticulous histopathologic studies (64), and determination of its efficacy for the relief of cancer pain and other pain syndromes. Subsequently, in the 1970s, reports of results in a large number of patients were published (65). At about the same time, Moricca began to use the technique of chemical hypophysectomy or, as he later called it, "neuroadenolysis of the pituitary" (66).

Current Status of Regional Analgesia/Anesthesia

New information about pain and pain syndromes and the consequent development of new therapeutic modalities, particularly psychologic methods, neurostimulation techniques, and neurosurgical procedures, have altered the role of regional analgesia in the management of pain. Knowledge of the deleterious effects of deafferentation suggested that neurolytic blocks (as well as neuroablative surgery) not be used in patients with nonmalignant chronic pain who have a long life expectancy. The advent of intraspinal narcotics has also decreased the use of neural blockade with local anesthetics in the treatment of patients with postoperative pain, post-traumatic pain, and cancer pain.

Nevertheless, regional anesthesia and neural blockade are still important in the management of patients with acute postoperative and post-traumatic pain, cancer pain, and nonmalignant chronic pain. These procedures are essential for physicians working in small or medium-sized pain clinics to which chronic pain patients are referred, and in which the services of psychologists and of neurosurgeons skilled in neurostimulating and refined percutaneous neurosurgical procedures are not available. Also, even in large hospitals in third-world countries, anesthesiologists with the necessary skill and experience can use these procedures effectively. I believe that, although neural blockade no longer has the pre-eminent role it enjoyed 30 years ago, it remains useful to members of a multidisciplinary pain management pain program if applied correctly. Proper application requires skillful execution and careful selection of patients, taking into consideration the basis for its use and strict adherence to certain principles (Chapter 94).

REFERENCES

1. Koller, C.: On the use of cocaine for producing anaesthesia on the eye. Lancet, 2:990, 1884.
2. Bonica, J.J.: Therapeutic acupuncture in the People's Republic of China: Implications for American medicine. JAMA, 228:1544, 1974.
3. Mann, F.L.: The Treatment of Disease by Acupuncture. London, Heinemann, 1967.
4. Macht, D.I.: The history of opium and some of its preparations and alkaloids. JAMA, 64:477, 1915.
5. Rynd, F.: Treatment of neuralgia—introduction of fluid to the nerve. Dublin Med. Press, 13:167, 1845.
6. Pravaz, C.G.: Sur un nouveau moyen d'operer la coagulation du sang dans les artères, applicable à la guérison des anéyrismes. C.R. Acad. Sci. (Paris), 36:88, 1853.
7. Wood, A.: New method of treating neuralgia by the direct application of opiates to the painful points. Edinburgh Med. Surg. J., 82:265, 1855.
8. Niemann, A.: Über eine organische Base in der Coca. Annal. Chemie, 114:213, 1860.
9. Bennett, A.: An experimental inquiry into the physiological actions of theine, caffeine, guaranine, cocaine, and theobromine. Edinburgh Med. J., 19:323, 1873.
10. Von Anrep, V.: Über die physiologische Wirkung des cocaine. Arch. Ges. Physiol., 21:38, 1880.
11. Fauvel, H.: De l'anesthesie produite par le chlorhydrate de cocaine sur la muqueuse pharyngienne et laryngienne. Gas. Hôp. Nr., 134S:1067, 1884.
12. Halstead, W.S.: Practical comments on the use and abuse of cocaine, suggested by its invariably successful employment in more than a thousand minor surgical operations. N. Y. State J. Med., 42:294, 1885.
13. Corning, J.L.: Spinal anesthesia and local medication of the cord. N. Y. State J. Med., 42:483, 1885.
14. Corning, J.L.: Local Anesthesia in General Medicine and Surgery. New York, Appleton, 1886.
15. Corning, J.L.: Headache and Neuralgias. Philadelphia, J.B. Lippincott, 1888.
16. Corning, J.L.: Pain and its Neuropathologic, Diagnostic and Neurotherapeutic Relations. Philadelphia, J.B. Lippincott, 1894.
17. Matas, R.: Local and regional anesthesia with cocaine and other analgesic drugs, including the subarachnoid method, as applied in general surgical practice. Phil. Med. J., 6:820, 1900.
18. Schlösser, H.: Erfahrungen in der Neuralgiebehandlung mit Akloholeinspritzungen. Verh. Cong. Innere Med., 24:49, 1907.
19. Ostwald, F.: Traitment des neuralgies rebelles par les injections profondes d'alcohol. Presse Med., 12:812, 1905.
20. Levy, F., and Boudouin, A.: Les injections profondes dans le traitment de la neuralgie facile rebelles. Presse Med., 13:108, 1906.
21. Härtel, F.: Über die intracranielle injections behandlung der trigeminus neuralgie mit intrakraniellen alkoholeinspritzungen. Dtsch. Ztschr. f. Chir., 126:429, 1914.
22. Levy, A.P.: Analgesia of the larynx by alcohol injection of the internal branch of the superior laryngeal nerve. Laryngoscope, 21:9, 1911.
23. Fetterolf, G.: Relief of pain in advanced tuberculosis of larynx by means of alcohol injected into internal laryngeal nerve. Ann. Otol. Rhinol. Laryngol., 21:128, 1912.
24. Lukens, R.: Dysphagia in tuberculous laryngitis. N. Y. State J. Med., 107:353, 1918.
25. Swetlow, G.I.: Injection of the superior laryngeal nerve with alcohol for the relief of pain in laryngeal tuberculosis. Am. Rev. Tuberc., 12:189, 1925.
26. Selheim, H.: Cited by Matas, R.: Local and regional anesthesia. A retrospect and prospect. Am. J. Surg., 25:189, 1934.
27. Sherrington, C.S.: The integrative action of the nervous system. London, Constable, Ltd., 1906.
28. Head, H.: On disturbances of sensation with a special reference to the pain of visceral disease. Brain, 16:1, 1893.
29. Lawen, A.: Über segmentare Schmerzaufhebung durch paravertebrale Novokaininjektion zur Differential diagnose intra-abdominaler Erkrakungen. Munchen Med. Wochnschr., 69:1423, 1922.
30. Freude, E., and Kanellis, E.S.: Über die Wirkung der segmentaren paravertebral Novokainininjektion bei intraabdominallen Erkrankungen. Munchen Med. Wochnschr., 69:1432, 1922.
31. Kappis, M.: Weitere Erfahrungen mit der Sympathektomie. Klin. Wochnschr., 2:1441, 1923.
32. Von Gaza, W.: Über die physiologische Wirkung des cocaine. Arch. Ges. Physiol., 21:38, 1924.
33. Brunn, F., and Mandl, F.: Die paravertebral Injektion zur Bekampfung visceraler Schmerzen. Wien. Klin. Wochnschr., 37:511, 1924.
34. Mandl, F.: Die Paravertebral Injection. Vienna, J. Springer, 1926.
35. Swetlow, G.: Paravertebral alcohol block in cardiac pain. Am. Heart J., 1:393, 1926.
36. White, J.C.: Diagnostic novocaine block of the sensory and sympathetic nerves. Am. J. Surg., 9:264, 1930.
37. White, T.C., and White, P.D.: Angina pectoris: Treatment with paravertebral alcohol injections. JAMA, 90:1099, 1926.
38. Leriche, R., and Fontaine, R.: L'anesthesie isole du ganglion étoile. Presse Med., 41:386, 1934.
39. White, J.C.: Paravertebral alcohol block for cardiac pain. Am. Heart J. 1:393, 1926.
40. Livingston, W.K.: Pain Mechanisms: Physiologic Interpretation of Causalgia and Its Related States. New York, MacMillan, 1943.
41. Dogliotti, A.M.: Eine neue Methode der regionaren Anasthesie: "Die peridurale segmentare Anasthesie." Zentralbl. Chir., 58:3141, 1931.
42. Pages, F.: Anestesia metamerica. Rev. Sanid. Milit. Argent., 11:351, 1921.
43. Dogliotti, A.M.: Proposta di un nuovo metodo di cura delle algie periferiche. L'alcoolizzazione sottomeningea delle radici posteriori. Considerazioni sulle prime 30 osservazione cliniche. Minerva Med., 1:536, 1931.
44. Doppler, K.: Sympathikodiaphtherese (chemische Sympathikusausschalgung) an der arteria femoralis. Med. Klin., 22:1954, 1926.
45. Woodbridge, P.D.: Therapeutic nerve block with procaine and alcohol. Am. J. Surg., 9:278, 1930.
46. Labat, G.: Discussion of paper by White, J.C.: Paravertebral alcohol block for cardiac pain. Am. Heart J., 1:399, 1926.

47. Goldscheider, A.: Zur Qualität des Temperaturisians Pflüger's arch., *39*:115, 1886.
48. Bier, A.: Versuche über Cocainisirung des Rückenmarkes. Dsch. Z. Chir., *51*:361, 1899.
49. Gasser, H.S., and Erlanger, J.: Role of fiber size in establishment of nerve block by pressure or cocaine. Am. J. Physiol., *88*:581, 1929.
50. Heinbecker, P., Bishop, G.H., and O'Leary, J.: Analysis of sensation in terms of the nub of the nerve impulse. Arch. Neurol. Psychiatry, *31*:34, 1934.
51. Sarnoff, S.J., and Arrowood, J.G.: Differential spinal block. Surgery, *20*:150, 1946.
52. Cleland, J.G.P.: Paravertebral anesthesia in obstetrics. Surg. Gynecol. Obstet., *57*:51, 1933.
53. Ruth, H.: Diagnostic, prognostic and therapeutic nerve blocks. JAMA, *102*:419, 1934.
54. Rovenstine, E.A., and Wertheim, H.M.: Therapeutic nerve blocks. JAMA, *117*:1599, 1941.
55. Bonica, J.J.: The management of Pain. Philadelphia, Lea & Febiger, 1953.
56. Maher, R.M.: Relief of pain in incurable cancer. Lancet, *1*:18, 1955.
57. Bonica, J.J.: Clinical investigation of local anesthetics. Anesthesiology, *18*:110, 1957.
58. Löfström, J.B.: Ulnar blockade for the evaluation of local anaesthetic agents. Br. J. Anaesth., *47* (Suppl.):297, 1975.
59. Nolte, H., et al.: Dissociation of cold, warm, and hot sensibility during ulnar nerve block and surface anesthesia (Abstr.). *In* Advances in Pain Research and Therapy. Vol. 1. Edited by J.J. Bonica and D.G. Albe-Fessard. New York, Raven Press, 1976, pp. 673–678.
60. Bonica, J.J.: Hemodynamic changes of local and regional anesthesia. *In* Haemodynamic Changes in Anaesthesia, Vol. 3. Proceedings of the Fifth European Congress of Anaesthesiology, Paris, Sept. 4–9, 1978. Edited by J.P. Bourdarias, et al. Paris, SNPM, 1979, pp. 1137–1187.
61. Guz, A., et al.: The role of the vagus and glossopharyngeal afferent nerves in respiratory sensation, control of breathing and arterial pressure regulation in conscious man. Clin. Sci., *30*:161, 1966.
62. Porcacci, P.: The cutaneous pain threshold changes after sympathetic block in reflex sympathetic dystrophy. Pain, *1*:167, 1975.
63. Maher, R.M.: Further experiences with intrathecal and subdural phenol: Observations on two forms of pain. Lancet, *1*:895, 1960.
64. Smith, M.C.: Histological findings following intrathecal injections of phenol solutions for relief of pain. Br. J. Anaesth., *36*:387, 1964.
65. Wood, K.M.: The use of phenol as a neurolytic agent: A review. Pain, *5*:205, 1978.
66. Moricca, G.: Neuroadenolysis for diffuse unbearable cancer pain. *In* Advances in Pain Research and Therapy, Vol. 1. Edited by J.J. Bonica and D.G. Albe-Fassard. New York, Raven Press, 1976, pp. 863–866.

94 · REGIONAL ANALGESIA WITH LOCAL ANESTHETICS

JOHN J. BONICA *and* F. PETER BUCKLEY

THIS chapter discusses techniques for blocking the nerve endings, axons, or cell bodies of peripheral, somatic, and sympathetic nerves with local anesthetic in the treatment of patients with various types of acute pain, cancer pain, and nonmalignant chronic pain. In this chapter, and throughout the book, "regional analgesia" and "regional anesthesia" are terms used interchangeably with nerve block, local anesthetic block, neural blockade, and conduction block. Afferent and efferent neural impulses can be interrupted by agents other than local anesthetics, such as curare and other muscle relaxants (block of somatic motor impulses at the myoneural junction), opioids (block of nociceptive impulses in the spinal cord or other parts of the neuraxis), antagonists of neurotransmitters (e.g., alpha-2-adrenergic antagonists), or other drugs. Thus, we believe it is more precise to use the term "regional analgesia/anesthesia" or "regional neural blockade" to differentiate this method from other techniques of blocking neural impulses. As mentioned in the introduction to this section, although these procedures frequently produce blockade of nerve fibers other than those that transmit nociceptive information and consequently should properly be called regional *anesthesia*, in this and other chapters we use *analgesia* to emphasize that the application of these procedures is for the relief of pain.

In conformance with the organization of other chapters, this chapter presents the bases, indications, efficacy, side effects, and complications of local analgesia and regional nerve blocks, and provides a brief description of the techniques. The conditions for which these procedures are used are described in detail elsewhere in this book, so they are only mentioned briefly here. The information is presented in six major sections: A, Basic Considerations, including the rationale for use, indications, basic principles of application, and pharmacologic basis of regional analgesia;

B, Local Applications of Regional Analgesia; C, Block of Spinal Nerves; D, Block of the Sympathetic Nervous System; E, Intravenous Regional Blockade; and F, Neuraxial Blockade, including subarachnoid and extradural neural blockade. Because blocks of the cranial nerves and parts of the sympathetic nervous system are done predominantly with neurolytic agents, they are considered in Chapter 96.

In contrast to the detailed description of various techniques of regional anesthesia found in the first edition (1), each technique in this chapter is illustrated and described in the legend. This is not intended to be used as the sole basis for learning and applying these techniques, however, because the acquisition of proficiency in any method requires apprenticeship under the supervision of an experienced regional anesthesiologist who can teach the basic aspects of the technique and then supervise the student in carrying out the procedure so as to gain experience and skill. Rather, the primary objective of presenting the techniques in this chapter is to provide readers who do *not* practice regional anesthesia with some idea of what the procedure entails, as well as a discussion of its indications, advantages, disadvantages, and complications. This agrees with Bonica's long-held conviction that anyone managing patients with pain should be acquainted with *all* currently available therapeutic procedures. Only with such knowledge and a broad perspective can the physician inform and guide the patient as to what therapy (or combination of therapies) is suitable for a particular pain problem. A secondary reason for illustrating the techniques is to give physicians training in the field an opportunity to visualize some of the finer points, based on Bonica's 45 years of experience. The material in this chapter is a concise and updated version of material presented by Bonica (1–4); detailed descriptions of these techniques can be found elsewhere (5–7).

A. BASIC CONSIDERATIONS

Rationale for Use

Local and regional analgesia is effective in managing patients with acute or chronic pain because of the interruption of nociceptive input at its source or the blocking of nociceptive fibers that course in peripheral spinal or cranial nerves or of afferent nerve fibers that accompany autonomic nerves. Blockade also interrupts the afferent limb of the abnormal reflex mechanisms that contribute to the pathogenesis of some chronic pain syndromes. Sympathetic blockade can be used to eliminate sympathetic hyperactivity that con-

tributes to the pathophysiology of postoperative and post-traumatic pain, and is important in managing some chronic pain syndromes, such as causalgia, reflex sympathetic dystrophy, and some types of postamputation or cancer-related pain. In addition, by increasing peripheral blood flow, sympathetic block can decrease tissue damage and re-establish tissue homeostasis. Blockade of the unmyelinated C and B preganglionic fibers and small myelinated A-delta nociceptive fibers can be achieved with low concentration of the local anesthetic, with less effect on somatomotor function. Conversely, in certain conditions, it can be useful to block somatomotor nerves to relieve severe skeletal muscle spasm.

Because of the production of one or more of these effects, prompt relief of pain is often obtained. This can last for varying periods, depending on the characteristics of the local anesthetic used. Moreover, the relief of certain types of pain outlasts the transient pharmacologic action of the local anesthetic by hours or occasionally by days or even weeks. Melzack (8) has suggested that blocking sensory input for several hours stops the self-sustaining activity of the neuron pools in the neuraxis that might be responsible for some chronic pain states. Based on the concept of "hyperstimulation analgesia" first described by Fox and Melzack (9) and by Brena (10), it has been suggested that neural blockade can alter or "jam" a pattern of central neural activities.

Evidence has shown that block of afferent (nociceptive) or efferent (sympathetic) nerves produces transient relief of central pain (11, 12). This "central effect" can be a result of altering neural traffic or the disturbed neural activity ("turbulence") in the neuraxis. Central pain can also be relieved by intravenous administration of local anesthetics (13); this might be a result of selective depression of C-afferent fiber-evoked activity in the spinal cord (14).

Finally, the use of regional analgesic techniques can be important in a patient with multiple physical and psychologic impairments. Because such a patient usually has difficulty in accepting the idea that the discomfort is related to psychologic or emotional factors, a medical intervention that is aimed at the pain location can facilitate the patient's willingness to undertake psychophysiologic rehabilitation. Moreover, when structured as part of a behavioral modification program, nerve blocking enhances the patient-physician relationship and strengthens the physician's role as an educator who reinforces the global roles of rehabilitation (10).

Indications

Neural blockade can be used as a diagnostic, prognostic, prophylactic, or therapeutic tool, or as a combination of these, in managing patients with acute pain, or can be used as part of an integrated multimodal program in patients with chronic pain.

Diagnostic blocks can help the physician to do the following:

a. Determine the anatomic source of pain
b. Ascertain specific nociceptive pathways
c. Differentiate local from referred somatic pain
d. Differentiate visceral from somatic origin of thoracic or abdominal pain
e. Determine the role of the sympathetic nervous system in causing pain and associated pathophysiology
f. Differentiate local pathology from reflex muscle spasm in such disorders as torticollis, scalenus anticus syndrome, and pyriformis syndrome
g. Determine by the use of somatic block whether a painful deformity (e.g., in the limb or spine) is caused by pain and muscle spasm or by pathologic changes in a joint, tendon, capsule, or bone

h. Differentiate peripheral from central pain
i. Determine the role of nociception in patients with complex chronic pain syndromes who have major psychologic, emotional, or behavioral problems
j. Determine the reaction of patients to the elimination of the pain

Prognostic blocks can help in the following ways:

a. Provide patients with opportunities to experience sensory changes and other effects of neuroablative procedures
b. Predict the effects of neurolytic block or neurosurgery in cancer patients

Prophylactic blocks can help the physician do the following:

a. Delay the onset of postoperative pain and reduce its incidence significantly
b. Decrease incidence and prevent complications of postoperative, post-traumatic, or visceral pain
c. Decrease duration of hospitalization and convalescence
d. Prevent development of certain chronic pain syndromes such as reflex sympathetic dystrophy and phantom limb pain

Therapeutic blocks can help the physician to do the following:

a. Provide optimal relief of pain in self-limiting disorders (postoperative, post-traumatic or acute visceral disease)
b. Provide specific therapy in causalgia, reflex sympathetic dystrophy, and other disorders perpetuated by a "vicious circle" or an abnormal pattern in the CNS
c. Provide pain relief to permit more effective application of definitive therapy (e.g., traction, manipulation)
d. Improve appetite, nutrition, and physical condition of cancer patients in poor condition prior to major surgery
e. Improve peripheral blood flow through sympathetic blockade
f. Gain patient's cooperation and enhance acceptance of psychologic therapies by paying attention to the physical aspects of pain
g. Improve the patient-physician relationship and contribute to global rehabilitation program

Most of the techniques described in this chapter can be used for one or more of these indications. These are mentioned in the discussion of local blockade and other regional analgesic techniques. Here we provide an overview of these four major indications for these procedures.

Diagnostic Blocks

Neural blockade can be used as part of an integrated diagnostic process and specific nerve block procedures can be useful in helping the physician to obtain information and attain the goals listed above and presented here.

Determination of Source of Pain and Nociceptive Pathways

Local infiltration and block of small or large nerves or plexuses can provide information about the source of the pain and the pathways that mediate the nociceptive impulses. Thus, prompt and complete relief of pain following two or three direct injections of a dilute solution of local anesthetic into a trigger point, painful scar, neuroma, joint (e.g., a facet, or temporomandibular joint) or spasmodic muscle helps to determine the source of pain and helps in making the diagnosis. Similarly, prompt relief of pain following injection of 2 to 3 ml of a local anesthetic on a spinal nerve as it exits from its intervertebral foramen provides information about the nociceptive pathway(s) involved in the projected pain caused by a herniated intervertebral disk, osteophytes, fracture of the vertebra, or other vertebral pathology. Block of the appropriate nerve(s) helps to differentiate trigeminal neuralgia from atypical facial neuralgia, neuralgia of the mandibular nerve from glossopharyngeal neuralgia, and pain caused by visceral disease from pain of somatic origin.

Visceral Versus Somatic Pain

In most patients a complete history and physical examination are sufficient to differentiate pain in the chest, abdomen, or pelvis caused by visceral disease from pain in the chest wall, abdominal wall, or somatic structures of the pelvis caused by pathology. In patients who present confusing symptoms and signs, however, block of the thoracic intercostal nerves at the posterior axillary line relieves pain caused by pathologic processes in the ribs or anterior chest wall but does not relieve pain caused by disease of the thoracic viscera, the nociceptive pathways of which pass through the sympathetic nerves close to the vertebral column. Because pain in the epigastrium can be caused by disease of the thoracic viscera or of the upper abdominal viscera or by pathology in the ribs, cartilages, or soft tissue or nerves that supply the abdominal wall, blocks can be used to differentiate among these three sources of pain. Thus, block of the T6 to T9 nerves at the posterior axillary line relieves pain arising in the abdominal wall but does not relieve pain caused by visceral disease. If such a procedure does not relieve the pain the visceral source of the pain can be ascertained by blocking the upper thoracic sympathetic chain (T1 to T5 or T6), a technique that relieves pain arising from the thoracic viscera. This procedure, however, does not relieve pain arising from the abdominal viscera because these are supplied by afferent fibers contained in the thoracic splanchnic nerves (T6 to T12), which can be interrupted by a celiac plexus or splanchnic nerve block. The various pathophysiologic conditions for which these procedures can be used as diagnostic tools are discussed in more detail below.

Local Versus Referred Somatic Pain

In addition to differentiating referred pain arising from visceral disease from pain caused by somatic pathology, nerve blocks can also be used to differentiate referred pain in somatic structures that is caused by a distant somatic pathologic process from pain arising locally. Thus, pain referred to the knee is frequently caused by a pathologic process in the head and neck of the femur. Such pain can be relieved by injection of a local anesthetic into the hip joint or by block of the nerves that supply the joint. Similarly, pathology in a facet joint in the lumbar region can cause pain referred to the low back, thigh, or even the leg, and this can be relieved by injection of the facet joint or of the medial branches of the posterior primary division that supply the joint. This procedure does not relieve pain caused by pathology at the site of referred pain, but it can be relieved by infiltration into the area of the pain.

Sympathetic Versus Somatic Origin of Peripheral Pain

Sympathetic hyperactivity can cause or contribute to pain by the following mechanisms: (a) sensitization of peripheral nociceptors; (b) production of vasoconstriction with subsequent local ischemia, which causes direct nociceptor stimulation; (c) reflex changes involving afferent and efferent fibers; (d) coupling between noradrenergic postganglionic fibers and afferent fibers at the site of the lesion in tissue or a nerve trunk; (e) liberation of norepinephrine by postganglionic axon terminals, possibly leading to the release of prostaglandins that in turn decrease the threshold of nociceptive afferents (15); (g) sensitization of wide dynamic range neurons in the dorsal horn and other parts of the neuraxis; and (h) other mechanisms (Chapter 11). Recent evidence (16) also indicates that sympathetic hyperactivity contributes to the development and maintenance of trigger points of myofascial pain syndromes. Moreover, sympathetic hyperactivity can cause inhibition of the gastrointestinal and genitourinary tracts with consequent ileus and a decrease in urinary output, both of which can be a source of abdominal or suprapubic pain.

The role of sympathetic hyperactivity in causing these changes can be ascertained by blocking the regional sympathetic supply to various structures at anatomic sites that are separate from somatic nerve fibers. Thus, paravertebral block of the T2 and T3 sympathetic ganglia relieves pain in the upper limb as a result of reflex sympathetic dystrophy without involving roots of the brachial plexus. Similarly, block of the lumbar sympathetic chain relieves sympathetically maintained pain in the foot or leg without involving the roots of somatic nerves. Injection of neuromata, painful scars, trigger points, or other sites of localized disease usually results in a pure somatic block. Block of the lateral femoral cutaneous nerve to help establish the diagnosis of meralgia paresthetica or block of the saphenous nerve at the ankle also results in a purely somatic block.

Peripheral Versus Central Pain

Various techniques can be used to differentiate peripheral pain from central pain that is caused by pathology in the neuraxis. As already mentioned, evidence now shows that block of afferent and efferent nerves or intravenous injection of local anesthetics can be helpful in providing transient partial relief of central pain (13). Another technique is the use of "differential" subarachnoid or epidural block extended to the T1 thoracic spinal segment, which should eliminate pain of peripheral origin. This procedure is unlikely to eliminate pain caused by disease of the spinal cord or brain stem completely, however, and the efficacy of such methods has been questioned (see Section F). A recently introduced technique is a diagnostic epidural opioid block that might prove useful in differentiating peripheral from central pain and pain primarily of psychologic origin from pain arising from other sources. This technique is discussed in the section on extradural block (Section F).

Reaction to Pain Relief

Most patients, especially those with severe pain, are grateful when pain is relieved following neural blockade. Some patients with mild or moderate pain that is being used for secondary or tertiary gains, however, might become alarmed by the realization that the pain could be permanently eliminated. Although such instances are rare they do occur and require that the physician, with the help of nurses and others, evaluate the effects of the pain relief on patients' behavior and attitudes. At the other end of the spectrum are patients whose severe pain is caused by a musculoskeletal injury and who, on relief of pain, might disregard the physician's advice and resume strenuous activity prematurely before healing at the injury site has occurred.

Prognostic Blocks

The primary purpose of prognostic nerve blocks is to afford patients an opportunity to experience the sensory changes and other effects that follow neuroablative surgical procedures or neurolytic blocks, thus helping patients to decide whether to undergo such a procedure. It was previously believed that a single block with a local anesthetic could predict the pain-relieving effects of a neurosurgical section or neurolytic block. Ample clinical evidence now shows, however, that one such block does not predict the long-term effects of neurosurgical section, such as spinal posterior rhizotomy (17). Loeser (17) noted that, whereas the pain relief obtained immediately after a spinal posterior rhizotomy was similar to that obtained after a prior prognostic paravertebral block of certain spinal segments, many of the patients had a return of their pain in the months following the operation. It is not known if the return of pain was the result of an incomplete operation (i.e., the nociceptive fibers in the anterior root were not divided), regeneration of the nerve, or the development of other new nociceptive pathways or other mechanisms. In many patients the decision to carry out the surgical rhizotomy was done on the basis of the results of one prognostic block, an error that Bonica considers to be a "cardinal" sin in this field. In any case, we believe that prognostic blocks continued for 2 to 3 days (by continuous techniques) are still useful, not only in providing patients with the experience of sensory changes but also in predicting the effects of neurolytic blockade in patients with cancer pain whose life expectancy is limited.

Prophylactic Blocks

Various nerve blocks are used to prevent pain and thus prevent or miminize the delay of return to normal functional activity that often follows trauma, infections, or operations. In some centers nerve block procedures are considered to be one of the most efficient methods for controlling postoperative or post-traumatic pain and result in earlier functional rehabilitation, prevention of complications, and shorter hospitalization (18). Block of nociceptive afferent and efferent pathways in patients with acute pancreatitis, ileus, or other visceral disorders relieves pain, decreases morbidity, and possibly decreases mortality (see subsections on acute pancreatitis in Sections E and F). Also, evidence has shown that analgesia achieved with regional block for several days can decrease the incidence of phantom limb pain, reflex sympathetic dystrophy, and other chronic pain syndromes (19). These are discussed below in connection with various continuous techniques of neural blockade.

Therapeutic Blocks

Regional analgesia with local anesthetics is effective in treating self-limiting disease accompanied by severe pain and in breaking up the so-called "vicious circle" in patients with causalgia or other reflex sympathetic dystrophies, myofascial pain syndromes, and reflex muscle spasm. Moreover, by providing symptomatic relief, this method permits other therapeutic measures to be carried out and can be used as an adjunct to permit the more effective application of definitive therapies. For example, in patients with severe pain and severe reflex muscle spasm caused by a herniated intervertebral disk, continuous segmental epidural block not only provides prompt and complete relief of the pain but also eliminates the reflex spasm, thus permitting the more effective application of traction and other conservative measures.

In extremely sick patients with cancer pain or other chronic pain problems who are scheduled for surgical intervention, relief of pain for a week or so prior to the surgery helps to improve appetite and nutritional status and permits other therapeutic measures to be carried out. During the past decade, studies of patients with severe chronic pain have shown such pain to be associated with poor overall health, including decreased activity, impaired appetite, weight loss, and sleep disturbances. Until recently, however, no studies indicated that the pain itself contributed to the morbidity. Levine and colleagues, in a 1988 report (20), noted the contribution of pain to morbidity in a disease model of experimental arthritis in rats, who typically lost weight and were considerably less active than normal rats. To test the hypothesis that pain contributed to the general morbidity of the rats with experimental arthritis, the major ascending nociceptive transmission pathways in the ventrolateral funiculus of the spinal cord were interrupted and the effects on weight loss and decrease in activity were noted. It was found that, following the relief of pain, the treated rats had significantly less weight loss and decrease in activity as compared to those in the control group (20). These data provide strong evidence that the pain that accompanies various disease states makes an important contribution to morbidity and should therefore be eliminated promptly.

Therapeutic blocks with neurolytic agents are usually limited to patients with cancer pain, although they can be indicated in selected patients with trigeminal neuralgia, causalgia, chronic pancreatitis, severe angina pectoris, or other chronic disorders who cannot tolerate a neurosurgical operation. Neurolytic blocks are especially useful in patients with chronic peripheral vascular disease (Chapter 96).

Principles of Application

For many years neural blockade was used empirically and often haphazardly, often resulting in failure and sometimes in complications. These in turn resulted from various problems in the application of this method by anesthesiologists or other physicians, including the following: (a) inadequate knowledge of pain syndromes; (b) inadequate evaluation of patients; (c) lack of knowledge of other therapeutic measures that could be used in conjunction with nerve block as a multimodal form of therapy; (d) improper management of patients before, during, and after the procedure; and (e) lack of appreciation of the specific indications, limitations, and possible complications of the procedure.

Requisites for Optimal Results

The realization and appreciation of these problems prompted Bonica, soon after he began to use these tools, to develop certain basic principles, which were first stated in 1953 (1) and have been repeatedly reaffirmed with greater conviction as a result of increasing experience (2, 21–24). These principles are outlined here and are then discussed in greater detail.

Basic Principles of Application of Neural Blockade

I. **Requisites of the physician**
   A. The physician using neural blockade must have a thorough knowledge of pain syndromes and their pathophysiology, symptoms, and signs, and of all the diagnostic and therapeutic measures that can be used for each patient.
   B. Knowledge of the advantages, disadvantages, limitations, and complications of each procedure provides the broad perspective essential for deciding on the best therapy or combination of therapies.
   C. The physician must be highly skilled in technique and have a thorough knowledge of the following:
      1. Anatomic basis of procedure
      2. Pharmacology of local anesthetics
      3. Expected effects of procedure
      4. Side effects and possible complications of each procedure, and their prevention and *prompt* treatment

II. **Assessment of the patient**
   A. The physician must be willing and *able* to devote the necessary time and effort to evaluate the patient through a history, general physical and neurologic examination, and other studies, even when the patient has been referred by respected colleagues.
   B. The patient with a complex chronic pain problem is best managed in a multidisciplinary pain program, in which neural blockade is one of many diagnostic or therapeutic procedures available.
   C. Prior to admission for block, the physician should request the following:
      1. Comprehensive summary of previous diagnostic and therapeutic procedures and results obtained

      2. Two-week diary kept by patient regarding physical activities, characteristics of the pain, and pain medication taken, and also complete questionnaire containing demographic data of past medical and family history and other information
   D. At the time of evaluation the physician should have a comprehensive assessment of the characteristics of the pain and the results of the physical and neurologic examination and any special studies required.
   E. The physician should obtain psychologic and psychosocial assessments from clinical psychologists.
   F. On the basis of the information obtained the physician must decide whether neural blockade is indicated and for what purpose.

III. **Communication with the patient**
   A. Before neural blockade is initiated patients must be fully informed (i.e., in regard to technique, indications, and type of block). Unless patients realize the procedure is being done only to obtain information rather than to cure, they could be disappointed prematurely and might return for further care.
   B. Patients must be reassured that all is being done to minimize discomfort inherent in the procedure.

IV. **Requirements for use of diagnostic or prognostic blocks**
   A. The nerve(s) should be localized precisely by radiography or image intensifier, with or without prior injection of contrast medium.
   B. Small volumes (2 to 3 ml) of local anesthetic should be injected to avoid spillage to adjacent nerves, which could yield misleading information.
   C. No decisions should be made about the course, mechanism, or response to blockade until three blocks produce consistent results.
   D. Local anesthetics of different duration should be used, and the duration of block correlated with duration of subjective pain relief.

V. **Assessment of results of blockade by physician, nurses, and others**
   A. Note reaction of the patient to needle insertion and other manipulations to help determine "pain threshold."
   B. Ascertain if the intended nerves have been blocked with a neurologic examination and measurement of sympathetic function.
   C. Evaluate efficacy of blockade in relieving pain and pathophysiology.
   D. Correlate duration of pain relief with duration of neural blockade.
   E. Record results in detail on patient's chart.
   F. For prognostic purposes continue block for 3 to 5 days to improve predictability of neuroablative procedure.

VI. **Limitations of neural blockade**
   A. The physician, patient, and others should recognize that neural blockade is not a panacea.
   B. The results of the diagnostic or prognostic block should be considered within the framework of all other information acquired. To make a final decision according to the results of only one or two blocks is conducive to error and to the performance of useless destructive procedures.
   C. Therapeutic blocks can be supplemented by other measures in patients with acute pain.
   D. Block can be used as part of a multimodal rehabilitation program in patients with chronic pain.

Role of the Physician

The first principle, and one of the foremost, is that the anesthesiologist or any other physician who carries out these procedures must assume the responsibility of the physician and not act as a mere technician, expert only at inserting needles and injecting local anesthetic solutions. Even when acting as a consultant skilled in neural blockade, it is essential that the anesthesiologist have a thorough insight into the patient and the pain problem.

The second requisite is that the physician using this method have ample knowledge of chronic pain syndromes, including possible mechanisms and nociceptive pathways involved, pathophysiology, and symptoms and signs. It is also essential to know the advantages, disadvantages, limitations, and complications of other diagnostic and therapeutic measures that might be relevant for each pain syndrome. Only with this broad perspective can the best approach to diagnosis and the optimal therapeutic strategy be chosen for the patient with a specific pain problem.

Another important requirement is that the physician be highly skilled in carrying out the appropriate neural blockade technique and be thoroughly aware of the immediate and long-term effects of the agents used. Patients with pain are not good subjects on whom to practice nerve blocks. Skill should be acquired by first observing experts doing the blocks and then performing them repeatedly under their supervision. In patients with severe pain, especially those with complex chronic pain syndromes, neural blockade must be performed carefully with meticulous attention to anatomic detail, utmost gentleness, and the use of high-quality equipment (see below, subsection on equipment).

Assessment of the Patient and the Pain

The physician must be *willing and able to devote the time and effort* to evaluate the patient and the pain thoroughly to make or confirm the diagnosis. This is essential even if the patient has been referred by a highly competent colleague who has already made the diagnosis. A detailed history and thorough physical examination (see Chapter 31) not only provide additional information but afford an opportunity to become acquainted with the patient, to investigate his or her personality and, equally important, to establish rapport and win the patient's confidence.

In patients with complex chronic pain problems who are referred to a multidisciplinary/interdisciplinary pain management program it is essential to request that the referring physician provide a comprehensive summary of previous diagnostic and therapeutic procedures and the results obtained. Patients referred to our program at the University of Washington are required to keep a 2-week diary that contains such items as an accurate record of physical activity during each of the 14 days, "up time," "down time," and social activities, as well as a record at hourly intervals of the intensity, duration, and other characteristics of the pain and the medication taken during the waking hours. This information is supplemented by an elicitation of the history of the pain (Chapter 31).

The history begins with an assessment of the characteristics of the pain. The patient should be asked to provide details on the following: when and how the pain began; any precipitating factors; rate of onset (sudden or in minutes or hours); site(s) and radiation of the pain; intensity, quality, duration, and temporal aspects (constant, intermittent, episodic); associated symptoms or signs (e.g., muscle weakness, subjective numbness); circumstances that increase the pain and those that decrease or eliminate the pain; medication(s) prescribed and taken; and other therapeutic measures and their effects; and effect of the pain on physical activity, work, social life, sexual activity, behavior, interaction with others, and the impact on the family.

Psychologic and psychosocial assessments (see Chapter 33) should be made in the patient with a complex chronic pain problem, preferably by a clinical psychologist who has an interest and experience in pain management. In addition to the interview with the patient and spouse (or with the significant other), well-established psychologic tests such as the Minnesota Multiphasic Personality Inventory (MMPI) should be administered. The intensity and duration of the pain, factors that cause the pain, and psychosocial data provide information critical to the proper selection of a patient for therapeutic nerve block. Bonica's personal experience and that of others (25) suggest that, in a patient with severe pain of long duration, previous surgery for back pain, pain caused by injury at work, and unemployment are predictive factors suggesting less than optimal results with nerve block therapy.

PHYSICAL EXAMINATION. The physical examination should begin with a thorough and precise examination of the painful region, followed by a general physical examination. A careful neurologic and orthopedic assessment, including tests for sensory, motor, and sympathetic function, is necessary to obtain additional information on any abnormality associated with pain, and represents an essential baseline for evaluating the effects of the block. It might also be necessary to perform a radiographic examination, special laboratory tests, electromyography, myelography, and CT scan.

MEASUREMENT OF PAIN. Following completion of the patient's evaluation it is essential to assess the pain by means of the Visual Analog Scale (VAS), the McGill Pain Questionnaire (MPQ), or some other reliable method of pain measurement. It is absolutely essential that when the block is done the patient be experiencing a significant level of pain: carrying out the block in the absence of pain is less than useless.

PURPOSE OF THE BLOCK. Once the assessment is complete the physician must decide whether neural blockade is indicated; if it is, is it to be done to obtain information or predict the effect of prolonged neural interruption, or for therapeutic purposes? The empiric and haphazard use of neural blockade must be avoided, because this can do more harm than good.

Communication with the Patient

Before a neural blockade is initiated it is important to inform the patient of what is to be done, and how, and what is likely to be accomplished. The patient who does not realize that the procedure is being done only to gain information, and that it might provide only temporary relief, or none at all, might be disappointed and not return for further care. In addition to informing the patient of this during the initial visit, such information should be repeated just prior to each block. Moreover, the patient should be reassured that everything is being done to minimize discomfort from insertion of the needles, that warning is given before each step of the procedure, and that a brief rest can be requested whenever the patient thinks that it is necessary. If a series of therapeutic blocks is to be done, appropriate sedatives or narcotics can be used prior to and during the block.

Diagnostic and Prognostic Blocks

If the procedure is to be done for diagnostic or prognostic purposes, depressant drugs should not be given because the patient must be alert to answer questions and to inform the physician promptly of any unusual sensation experienced during the procedure. It is essential to locate the involved nerve(s) exactly. This can be done by using a peripheral nerve stimulator for locating somatic nerves, by checking the position of the needle by radiography or an image intensifier, with injection of the contrast medium just prior to or during the injection of the local anesthetic, or by a combination of these methods. In addition to helping ensure that the point of the needle is on (not into) the target, radiographs serve as a permanent record of the procedure.

For diagnostic or prognostic blocks, three requisites must be followed: (a) only a small volume (2 to 3 ml) of local anesthetic solution for each nerve or each sympathetic segment (ganglion) should be injected to avoid diffusion to adjacent segments, thus avoiding misleading results; (b) no decision should be made until three or more nerve blocks produce consistent responses; and (c) it is best to use local anesthetics of different duration and to correlate the duration of the block with the duration of pain relief. For prognostic purposes the block should be continuous for at least 3 to 5 days to improve the prediction of the therapeutic efficacy and side effects of destructive procedures and to provide the patient with ample time to experience prolonged sensory changes.

Assessment of Results

During and following the block the therapeutic effects must be carefully assessed. The patient's reaction to the insertion of a thin (27- to 30-gauge) needle for the formation of an intracutaneous analgesic wheal (to produce analgesia for the insertion of the larger needle) and to the advancement of the needle through fascia should be noted to help evaluate the patient's response to noxious stimuli. Similarly, noting the patient's reaction to eliciting paresthesia with the point of the needle or nerve stimulator is also useful.

After an appropriate interval subsequent to the block the patient should be examined to ascertain whether the neural pathways have been completely interrupted by repeating the neurologic examination (Chapter 31). This includes the use of pinprick, pinscratch, and hard pinch to determine changes in sensory function, muscle strength to assess motor function, and deep tendon reflexes to assess block of somatic nerves. If changes are rather vague, the abolition of twitch responses to nerve stimulation is also helpful.

If a pure sympathetic block to one of the limbs has been carried out, assessment of the completeness of the interruption is best done by determining loss of sweating or by measuring the skin conductance response (SCR), also known as the psychogalvanic reflex. The presence of Horner's syndrome alone does not ensure complete sympathetic interruption of the upper limb (see below).

Once it has been established that the block of the intended nerve(s) is complete, its effects on the pain and on the pathophysiology must be carefully assessed. This could require a few hours or several days of observation. The amount, type, and duration of pain relief should be carefully noted and recorded on the chart. In addition to observation by the physician, the results should be evaluated by patients and their family (if available) and, most importantly, by the nursing staff.

It is especially important to correlate the duration of pain relief with the duration of the neural blockade. If subjective relief is significantly shorter than the duration of the block, a nonspecific effect ("placebo") might have been achieved or the period of relief might represent a false positive result. If the duration of pain relief is similar to the duration of the block, the effect is specific and suggests the presence of an underlying pathophysiologic process. Generally, if the duration of pain relief lasts longer than the duration of the block, it suggests that the pain has an element of abnormal reflex response or the block has interrupted a "vicious circle." If the patient derives only partial or no relief, interruption of the involved nociceptive pathways might either be incomplete or the nociceptive pathway might have been entirely missed—that is, the wrong nerves have been blocked. An alternate explanation is that the patient has "central pain" and has obtained relief that is short-lasting, partial, or both. Because these possibilities exist, *it is essential for diagnostic purposes to do at least three blocks with local anesthetics of different duration before a decision is made about the results.*

Limitations of Neural Blockade

All concerned personnel must realize and appreciate that nerve blocks are not a panacea and have limitations in helping to make a diagnosis; in addition, they are even more limited in predicting the effects of prolonged interruption. Although they are effective and advantageous in a significant percentage of properly selected patients, it is essential to use the results of blockade within the framework of all other information obtained. To make the final diagnosis solely according to the results of one or even several blocks is hazardous and can subject patients to a useless destructive operation.

Nerve blocks are highly effective in treating certain types of acute pain and can be used as the primary or even the sole form of treatment, but sometimes the patient also needs an anxiolytic or sedative agent to relieve anxiety and apprehension. Moreover, some regional techniques do not completely relieve acute pain and need to be supplemented by doses of narcotics that should be significantly smaller than those that would have been required without the regional analgesia.

The role of neural blockade in managing patients with complex chronic pain problems is more limited, and should be used as part of a multimodal rehabilitation program. This applies even to some clear-cut conditions such as causalgia, reflex sympathetic dystrophy, or other chronic pain problems, in which nerve block might be considered to be the primary therapy. Because many chronic pain patients develop feelings of anxiety, depression, and other psychologic reactions, treatment of these aspects of the problem must be addressed. Moreover, because patients with prolonged chronic pain develop disuse atrophy of various muscle groups, appropriate exercises and other physical therapeutic measures must be incorporated into the treatment program. For those patients that develop deafferentation pain, nerve blocks, if included, should be supplemented with transcutaneous nerve stimulation (TENS) or other neuromodulating procedures (Chapter 92) and with tricyclic antidepressants for their analgesic effects (Chapter 79). For patients with chronic pain caused by operant or other psychologic mechanisms, blocks have a minor but important role in helping patients accept the primary psychologic therapies more readily, and they also help to strengthen the physician's role in a multimodal rehabilitation program (Chapter 100).

Pharmacology of Local Anesthetics

The effective and safe use of regional analgesic techniques with local anesthetics (LAs) requires a thorough knowledge of the pharmacology of LAs, including their pharmacokinetic and pharmacodynamic properties. Table 94-1 lists clinical characteristics, optimal concentrations, and maximal therapeutic doses of commonly used local anesthetics.

The concentration of the drug used depends on the purpose for which it is used. Local infiltration can be accomplished with a dilute concentration of a drug because the drug promptly contacts small nerve endings and readily penetrates the various tissues around the nerve endings. Consequently, it reaches the membrane of the axons quickly, where it interferes with sodium conductance (26, 27). With block of major nerves the LA must penetrate the epineurium, perineurium, endoneurium, fat, blood vessels, and lymphatics, which comprise as much as 40% of the diameter of nerve trunks. Thus, the amount of drug reaching the core of the nerve and affecting an individual axon is much smaller, because much of the drug is absorbed into the bloodstream during its diffusion from outside the nerve to the core of the nerve.

By using the low concentrations shown in Table 94-1, it is possible to achieve a block of C, A-delta, and probably B-preganglionic sympathetic fibers, with significantly less effect on the large A-beta and A-alpha fibers that are concerned with motor and tactile function and proprioception, respectively.

The degree of neural blockade depends on the potency of the drug and on the amount that reaches the target (various nerve fibers). This, in turn, depends on the amount of drug injected, its physiocochemical characteristics, and the rate of absorption into the circulation (27). The greater the amount absorbed, the less that is available to block nerve axons. The rate of absorption also influences the toxicity

TABLE 94-1. Pharmacologic and Clinical Characteristics of Local Anesthetics

Characteristic	Procaine (Novocaine)	Chloroprocaine (Nesacaine)	Lidocaine (Xylocaine)	Prilocaine (Citanest)	Mepivacaine (Carbocaine)	Bupivacaine (Marcaine)	Tetracaine (Pontocaine)	Etidocaine (Duracaine)
Physicochemical								
Potency ratio*	1	2	3	3	3	15	15	15
Toxicity ratio*	1	0.75	1.5	1.5	2.0	10	12	10
Anesthetic index (1)	1	3	3	2	1.5	1.5	1.25	1.5
pH of plain solution	5–6.5	2.7–4	6.5	4.5	4.5	4.5–6	4.5–6.5	4.5
pKa	8.9	8.7	7.9	7.7	7.6	8.1	8.6	7.7
Clinical								
Latency	Moderate	Fast	Fast	Fast	Fast	Moderate	Very slow	Fast
Penetrance	Moderate	Marked	Marked	Marked	Moderate	Moderate	Poor	Moderate
Duration	Short	Very short	Intermediate	Intermediate	Intermediate	Long	Long	Long
Duration ratio*	1	0.75	1.5–2	1.75–2	2–2.5	6–8	6–8	5–8
Concentration of Solution (%)								
Local infiltration	0.5	0.5	0.25–0.5	0.25–0.5	0.25–0.5	0.125–0.25	0.1–0.15	0.5–0.2
Regional IV	1	1	0.5	0.5	0.5	0.125–0.25	0.1–0.15	0.15–0.2
Small nerve sympathetic block	1	1	0.5	0.5	0.5	0.25	0.25	0.25
Block of large nerve or plexus	2	2	1–1.5	1–2	1–1.5	0.375–0.5	0.15–0.3	0.5–1
Extradural block								
Analgesia	1.5	1.5	1	1	1	0.25–0.375	0.2–0.4	0.5–1.0
Motor block	3	3	2	2	2	0.5–0.75	0.3–0.5	1–1.5
Maximum single dose (mg/kg)	15	15	7	8	7	3	2.5	4

*Procaine used as standard of reference = 1; ratios vary according to techniques of regional anesthesia used. Anesthetic index = potency ratio/toxicity ratio.

of local anesthetics. Absorption (uptake) depends on the vascularity of the injection site and on the drug's solubility in tissues at this site, its breakdown rate, its concentration, and its penetrance. Because local anesthetics (except cocaine) cause local vasomotor paralysis and thus increase local blood flow, this property enhances absorption (26, 27). The higher the concentration of the drug, the greater the local vasomotor action. Decreased vascularity caused by simultaneous injection of epinephrine with the LA solution retards its absorption.

Distribution of the LA depends on regional blood flow, the pH and pKa of the drug, penetrance, fat and water solubility, and protein-binding rate. The more penetrant the local anesthetic, the more readily it passes fibrous barriers and the greater the amount of drug that reaches nerve elements. The greater the fat solubility of the drug, the more drug is distributed to fat tissue (including nerves). Because LAs diffuse from tissues of high pH to those of low pH, acidosis enhances absorption into the blood. Protein binding and uptake by blood plasma and erythrocytes significantly influence the distribution of local anesthetics.

Clinical Characteristics

To select the optimal local anesthetic and concentration used, it is necessary to consider the clinical characteristics of LAs (Table 94-1). In addition to protein binding, pKa, and percentage of unionized drug at pH 7.4, it is also necessary to consider its anesthetic potency, latency or time to produce blockade, penetrance, duration of action, and local and general toxicity.

LATENCY. The latency or time required for onset of anesthesia is an important clinical property of local anesthetics. This depends on the following: (a) anesthetic activity; (b) concentrations and total dose; (c) distance between the site of injection and the site of action; and (d) penetrance of the compound.

PENETRANCE. The penetrance is the inherent ability of the drug to penetrate fibrous tissue and other structures between the site of injection and the individual nerve fibers. It is a clinically important property: the more penetrant the agent, the quicker and more intense the anesthesia.

DURATION. The duration of anesthesia depends primarily on the activity of the drug, its concentration, total dose, and vascularity of the affected region.

TOXICITY. The toxicity of LAs depends on some of the same factors as duration, as well as on the total amount of drug used, rate of absorption, distribution, and biotransformation.

Agents that Prolong or Modify the Action of Local Anesthetics

EPINEPHRINE. Inclusion of epinephrine in the LA solution causes local vasoconstriction, thus retarding the absorption of the drug from the site of injection and reducing the peak blood level. This prolongs the action of the LA and reduces the risk of systemic toxicity. Inclusion of epinephrine in solutions of local anesthetics with a short or moderate duration of action, such as procaine, chloroprocaine, or lidocaine, significantly prolongs the neural blockade. Inclusion of epinephrine with longer-acting agents, such as bupivacaine or etidocaine, however, does not prolong the duration of action as much as with the above mentioned LAs. The optimal concentration of epinephrine

to be used in adults is 1:200,000 (5 ug/ml of solution) (28) but, in children and the elderly, the use of a lower concentration, 1:300,000 (3.27 ug/ml) or even 1:400,000 (2.5 ug/ml) should be considered. (To obtain aforementioned concentrations of epinephrine in the LA solution, 0.1 ml epinephrine 1:1,000 is added to 20 ml, 30 ml, and 40 ml of LA solution respectively.)

ALKALINIZING AGENTS. Most commercially available local anesthetic agents have a pH much lower than the pKa of the drug (Table 94-1). It has been surmised that raising the pH of the LA solution increases the amount of base available, thus resulting in a faster onset of action and longer duration of blockade. Initial investigations in humans (29) indicated that lidocaine carbonate solutions produce a more rapid onset of brachial plexus block and epidural block than lidocaine hydrochloride solutions. Subsequent animal studies (30), however, as well as more recent double-blind human studies (31), have failed to substantiate the hypothesis regarding a faster action of lidocaine carbonate solutions. Conversely, the addition of sodium bicarbonate to bupivacaine solutions just prior to injection appears to produce a faster epidural block (32, 33) and increases the duration of the block (33).

DEXTRANS. Some human (34, 35) and animal studies (36) using dextrans of relatively low molecular weight (MW; mean MW less than 70,000) have shown a distinct prolongation of the duration of the action of local anesthetics, whereas other human (37, 38) and animal studies (39, 40) have not. It has been suggested that the discrepancy is caused by the difference in pH of the dextran solutions—those with a pH of 8.0 significantly increased the duration of action of the dextran-LA solution, whereas solutions with a pH of 4.5 to 5.5 did not (41). The use of dextrans of higher molecular weight (mean MW 110,000 to 150,000), with their increased viscosity, might prolong the duration of the block (42).

CORTICOSTEROIDS. A recent animal study (43) has shown that the local application of corticosteroids around or into a freshly cut nerve end prevents the development of an ectopic impulse discharge and also produces a rapid and prolonged suppression of an ongoing spontaneous ectopic discharge generated in an experimental nerve end neuroma (43). After reviewing the kinetics, Devor and colleagues (43) concluded that the suppression is brought about by a membrane-stabilizing action on nerve fiber endings, which reduces the rhythmic firing of spinal motoneurons by increasing the resting membrane polarization (hyperpolarization). Because local anesthetics also act through stabilizing the nerve membrane, it is possible that the addition of steroids to local solutions enhances and prolongs the analgesic action of local anesthetics when injected into a neuroma or trigger point. Clinical indications for the use of steroids are discussed below (B. Local Applications of Regional Analgesia).

Preliminary Considerations

Before carrying out any regional analgesic procedure, other than a minor infiltration or the use of a small volume of solution for a single nerve block, these guidelines should be followed. The patient should be told that no food or fluid is to be taken by mouth for 6 hours preceding the procedure. Suitable arrangements for care for the patient during recovery from the block, or on discharge to home, should be made, and suitable transport should be available. It should be confirmed that the patient actually does have pain, because performing a diagnostic or prognostic block in the absence of pain is fruitless. The site and side of pain should be confirmed with the patient. Other preliminary steps include discussion with and examination of the patient prior to the procedure, preparation of the site, positioning the patient correctly for the block, proper use of preblock medication, and ensuring that an assistant is present during the block.

Discussion with the Patient

It is essential to inform the patient of the details of the block technique, of the beneficial effects, and of any side effects that might occur. The importance of avoiding sudden movements should be stressed. Reassurance should be given that everything is being done to minimize discomfort, that warning will be given before each step of the procedure, and that the patient can ask for a brief rest whenever necessary. If these suggestions are followed assiduously, the confidence that can be invoked in the patient outweighs any advantages of administering sedatives, and makes their routine use unnecessary.

This briefing should be carried out at the end of the initial visit and repeated again each time the block procedure is to be executed. Failure to do so is a major reason for poor results and confusion. The patient should be given the opportunity to ask questions and to be satisfied as much as possible about the details of the procedure.

It is also advisable to obtain written consent for performance of the procedure. This is particularly important when serious potential hazards are inherent in the technique, and in all cases in which a neurolytic agent such as alcohol must be used. Obviously, it is important to present this matter to the patient so as to minimize any feelings of apprehension.

Examination of the Patient Just Prior to the Block

A preliminary examination should be done prior to every block procedure, in addition to the examination that is done to establish the diagnosis. Blood pressure, pulse, and respiration should be noted and recorded. It is also essential to determine whether the patient has hypalgesia, hyperalgesia, or any other sensory changes, motor dysfunction, or reflex abnormalities. Failure to carry out these procedures, especially when the block is being done for diagnostic or prognostic purposes, might not only preclude a precise diagnosis but could also cause the physician to be misled and commit a serious error. This type of information is also important from a medicolegal standpoint and should be recorded in detail.

Place Where the Block is Performed

Because most nerve block procedures have the potential of causing complications, it is necessary to carry out the block in a room in which *resuscitative equipment is available for immediate use for the treatment of complications.* In addition to the resuscitative equipment, it is advisable to have access to drugs for treating hypotension or other untoward reactions, including vasopressor drugs, such as ephedrine or phenylephrine in dilute solution, an ultrafast-acting barbiturate, such as thiopental, and a rapidly acting muscle relaxant, such as succinylcholine. Furthermore, it is advisable to carry out procedures that are to be of diagnostic or prognos-

tic value in patients with peripheral vascular disease in a room with constant temperature and humidity.

Positioning of the Patient

The patient should be placed in a position that best facilitates execution of the block, with the patient as comfortable as possible. Soft cushions should be placed wherever needed to avoid the discomfort caused by the pressure of bony prominences on the table and to permit the patient to be as relaxed as possible. If feasible, the recumbent position should be used, not only because it is most comfortable for the patient but because it minimizes the occurrence of syncope caused by psychogenic reactions during the procedure.

Medication Before and During the Block

Patients who are to undergo a diagnostic or prognostic block should be given reassurance and psychologic support but no depressant drugs, because they must be alert, without any mental impairment, to answer questions during and after the procedure. If a patient is still apprehensive and anxious, following the preliminary discussion it might be necessary to administer a small dose of a sedative, such as 50 to 75 mg of thiopental or 5 mg of diazepam IV. This usually produces a peak effect that lasts 3 to 5 minutes, during which time the block is performed. In patients who are to have a series of therapeutic blocks, however, an appropriate dose of narcotic should be used, such as 3 to 5 mg of morphine plus 5 to 10 mg of diazepam IV about 10 minutes before the block is to be done. This combination not only produces analgesia and sedation but also causes amnesia, so that patients do not become "needle shy."

Monitoring of the Patient

Monitoring of the patient for vital signs and for expected effects of the block, such as a rise in skin temperature or a change in the sympathogalvanic reflex, should be initiated and recorded before the block is done. For a major nerve block procedure, monitoring should include electrocardiography, blood pressure recordings, and constant verbal contact with the patient. Unless the amount of drug injected is extremely small, it is essential for the patient to have a patent IV cannula in place, with fluids running, to permit prompt injection of any appropriate resuscitative drug. Resuscitative drugs should be drawn up and readily available, along with appropriate airway management equipment (Fig. 94-1).

Personnel and Equipment for the Block

In performing local and nerve blocks it is essential to have an assistant present and to use high-quality equipment and drugs, including preservative-free fresh local anesthetic solutions in appropriate concentrations for neuraxial blocks (Fig. 94-2). Preservative-containing solutions are acceptable for peripheral nerve blocks. If epinephrine is to be used it is best to draw it up into a 0.25-ml tuberculin syringe from an ampule rather than using a stock local anesthetic solution that already contains epinephrine, because such a stock solution is less effective and more irritating. The needles used should be of appropriate length and diameter and should have short rather than long bevels, because a short-beveled needle is less likely to produce nerve damage. If a nerve stimulator is to be used to identify the nerves, appropriately insulated

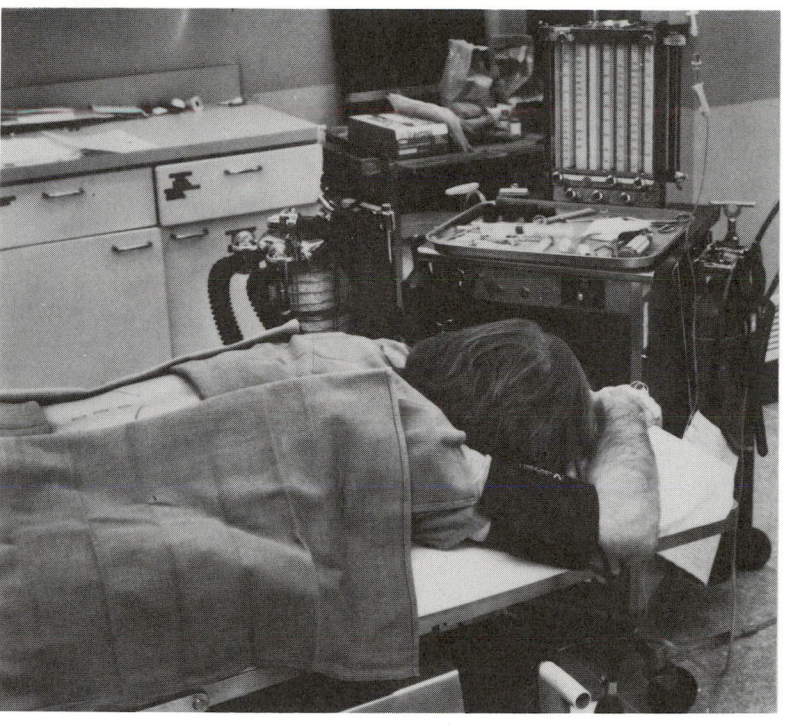

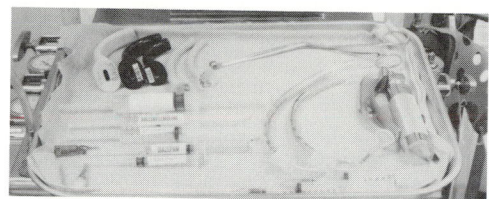

FIG. 94-1. Position of patient for bilateral celiac plexus block. An anesthesia machine, resuscitation equipment, and drugs are next to the patient, ready for immediate use. *Inset.* Close-up of the tray on top of the machine. The tray contains ampules and syringes for administering epinephrine, ephedrine, diazepam (Valium), thiopental (Pentothal), and succinylcholine; behind these are different sizes of otopharyngeal and nasopharyngeal airways (*left side*). The tray also contains a Macintosh laryngoscope, two endotracheal tubes, a Magill forceps for guiding tubes into the trachea, and a syringe for inflating the cuff of the endotracheal tube (*right side*). The anesthesia machine is not necessary as long as equipment is available for immediate administration of oxygen and for carrying out assisted or artificial ventilation. Note the patient has an intravenous catheter in a vein of the right hand and a continuous infusion of fluid for the prompt injection of resussitative drugs if reaction occurs.

needles should be available. Drugs and equipment necessary for the treatment of side effects and complications *should be available within reach of the physician for immediate use*, and an assistant should be present during the procedure to help expedite prompt treatment of any complications as well as to provide the patient with psychologic support.

Principles of Technique

The use of invasive procedures requires that sterile technique be observed, that the skin area through which injections are to be made be coated with an antiseptic, and that the area be suitably draped to maintain a sterile environment. The skin site and relevant subcutaneous tissue through which the needle(s) is to be passed should be anesthetized by injection of a dilute local anesthetic solution using a thin needle (25- to 30-gauge) of proper length.

Injection of the anesthetic solution into deeper tissue must *always* be preceded by an attempt to aspirate in two planes to avoid accidental intravascular or subarachnoid injection. The patient should be warned immediately prior to carrying out each step of the block procedure, such as the application of cold antiseptic solution to the skin or the formation of an intracutaneous wheal. Such warnings, together with constant encouragement, help the patient to tolerate these procedures better.

Again, it is important to have an assistant present to attend to the patient and to continue to give encouragement. This, along with the encouragement of the physician, has a synergistic effect and helps to minimize discomfort, anxiety, and apprehension. Having an assistant present also greatly facilitates prompt treatment of complications (see above).

The use of radiography or an image intensifier for certain diagnostic or prognostic procedures facilitates proper placement of the needle. This is especially useful in sympathetic blocks in which elicitation of paresthesia or the use of a nerve stimulator (e.g., as frequently done with a somatic block) cannot be done to aid in placing the needle accurately. In addition to being a valuable adjunct to proper needle placement, the radiograph serves as an objective record. Preliminary injection of contrast medium with radiographic visualization prior to injection of the local anesthetic solution can also be used to predict the subsequent diffusion of solution to the target.

Contraindications

Absolute contraindications to nerve blocks include the following:

(a) The patient is unwilling to undergo a nerve block.

(b) The patient has a true allergy to the drug(s) to be used. Inquire carefully about the patient's stated allergy. "Allergy" is often a label used for tachycardia in response to an epinephrine-containing solution. This is not a true allergy but is the effect of rapid systemic absorption of epinephrine. Some patients are told by their dentist that they have an "allergy" while they actually are having a psychogenic reaction to the procedure (see below).

(c) The patient has an infection at the site of injection.

(d) The blood-clotting status of the patient is in doubt.

Relative contraindications include the following:

(a) In some cases the performance of a nerve block might conceal the development of an untoward complication (e.g., a prolonged extremity block in a limb with a recent fracture might produce a compartment syndrome).

(b) If a patient is ill and debilitated the sympathetic interruption resulting from a spinal or epidural block might produce an unacceptable degree of cardiovascular compromise.

Side Effects and Complications

The regional analgesia procedures to be described are associated with various side effects, and some entail the risk of complications of varying severity. Side effects include vasomotor blockade, analgesia, anesthesia, and paresthesia, all of which disappear when the block dissipates. Complications that may occur can be of three primary types: (a) those that occur after many major nerve block procedures and consist of systemic toxicity and other systemic reactions, hematoma, and neurologic damage; (b) those that occur after high or total spinal or epidural blockade and consist of serious respiratory and cardiovascular problems; and (c) pneumothorax consequent to blocks around the chest. In addition, complications specific to each technique can occur. The three major types are briefly discussed here, and the others are discussed below in connection with individual technique. A more detailed discussion of this subject has been presented by Bonica (1), Moore (44), and Cousins and Bridenbaugh (7).

Systemic Toxic Reactions

Systemic toxic reactions to local anesthetic result from high blood levels of the drug after the following: (a) injection of an excessive dose; (b) accidental intravenous injection of all or part of a therapeutic dose; and (c) abnormal rates of absorption and biotransformation of the drug. These reactions manifest combinations of cardiovascular, respiratory, and central nervous system effects that can be arbitrarily classified as mild, moderate, or severe systemic reactions.

Symptoms and Signs

MILD REACTIONS. Mild reactions occur when the blood level of drug is just above physiologic limits. The patient experiences dysarthria, light-headedness, vertigo, tinnitus, headache, apprehension, excitement, tachycardia, slight hypertension, tachypnea, a metallic taste and dryness of the mouth and throat, occasionally nausea, and sometimes slight twitching of muscle groups.

MODERATE REACTIONS. Moderate reactions are caused by greater concentrations of local anesthetic drugs in the systemic circulation and are characterized by a progressive aggravation of the above signs and symptoms. The patient typically becomes confused or sleepy, sometimes loses consciousness, rapidly develops muscular twitching that usually progresses to convulsions, and the blood pressure and pulse

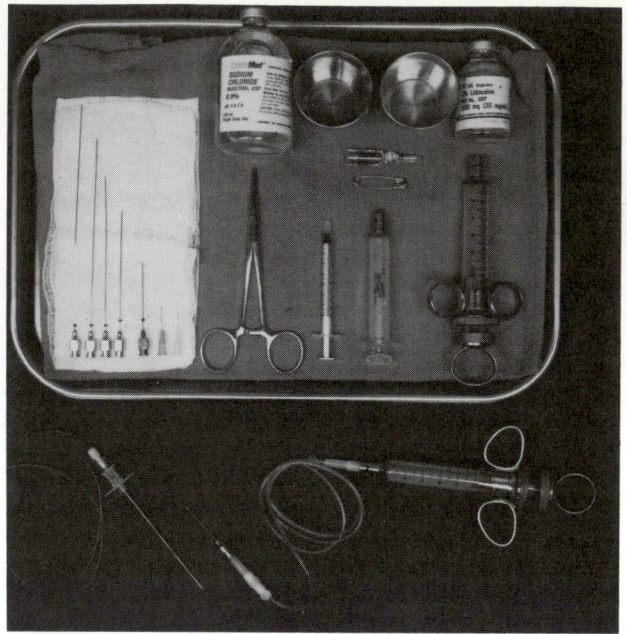

FIG. 94-2. Equipment for regional analgesia and anesthesia. On the sponge are 5 22-gauge security needles of different lengths: from the left to right, 15 cm, 12 cm, 10 cm, 8 cm, and 5 cm. On the far right is a 25-gauge 1.5-cm disposable needle. To the right of the sponge are a hemostatic forceps for grasping sponges when applying antiseptic solution to the skin, a 1-ml tuberculin syringe for measuring epinephrine solution, a 2-ml Luer-Lok syringe for syringe for injection of small volumes of local anesthetics and for aspiration tests, and a 10-ml Luer-Lok control syringe used for most regional anesthetic blocks because it facilitates aspiration and other maneuvers that are done with one hand. Above the syringes: a safety pin for skin testing and a 1-ml ampule containing 1 mg of epinephrine (1:1,000 concentration). In the back of the tray are shown a bottle of saline solution, a container for mixing the saline with local anesthetic solution to any desired concentration, a container for the antiseptic solution, and a bottle of local anesthetic. Below the tray are a Tuohy needle with a catheter threaded through it and a syringe for local anesthetic. The injecting needle is attached to the syringe by a flexible extension tube, which prevents the transference of aberrant movements of the syringe to the needle, thereby reducing the chance of the needle moving away from the target. The tubing set is used for relatively superficial blocks in which the depth of the needle insertion is so shallow that it does not afford any stability (e.g., interscalene and axillary blocks) and for femoral sheath block.

rise rapidly. Because convulsions interfere with proper ventilation, unless they are *promptly* stopped with succinylcholine the patient develops cyanosis and other signs of anoxia.

SEVERE TOXIC REACTIONS. Severe toxic reactions are usually caused by massive overdosage of the local anesthetic drug. They are manifested by loss of consciousness, coma, severe hypotension and bradycardia, respiratory depression that can end in paralysis, and other signs of severe central nervous system and cardiovascular depression. If immediate treatment is not instituted the condition can become grave, resulting in complete respiratory and cardiovascular failure and death.

Prevention

To prevent or decrease the incidence of systemic toxic reactions, the following guidelines should be followed: (a) the patient should be instructed to inform the physician performing the procedure immediately if any of the aforementioned effects occur; (b) the physician should keep in verbal contact with the patient by asking questions that require the patient to respond—among the earliest signs of a systemic toxic reaction is dysarthria and other signs of clouding of the sensorium; (c) the lowest concentration and volume of local anesthetic that ensures good results should be used; (d) epinephrine 1:200,000 should be included in the solution to retard the absorption of LA and reduce the peak plasma drug level; (e) repeated attempts to aspirate the syringe during injection should be made to ascertain that the bevel of the needle is not in a blood vessel; (f) prior to injection of a large volume of local anesthetic, 3 ml of local anesthetic containing epinephrine 1:200,000 (i.e., 15 μg of epinephrine) should be injected as a test dose—if this injection is intravenous it causes a rapid (within 20 to 30 seconds) and transient tachycardia and hypertension, which can be detected by ECG or blood pressure monitoring; and (g) if it is suspected that a toxic reaction is developing, the injection of the local anesthetic should be discontinued and the physician should monitor the patient carefully and prepare to treat any reaction.

Treatment

Oxygen should be administered whenever a systemic toxic reaction is suspected to be incipient so that if the reaction becomes more severe the patient has a store of oxygen in the lungs to decrease the incidence of hypoxia. If the reaction is mild, administration of oxygen and having the patient hyperventilate to decrease the Pa_{CO_2} (and thus decrease the convulsion threshold) might be sufficient. If the reaction progresses to convulsions, and possibly to loss of consciousness, the patient must be treated immediately to prevent hypoxia and hypercapnea (convulsions prevent adequate ventilation). Oxygen should be administered by positive pressure ventilation and a prompt IV injection of 40 to 80 mg of succinylcholine given to stop the convulsions and permit adequate ventilation. If any difficulty is encountered in maintaining a patent airway or in performing artificial ventilation, tracheal intubation should be carried out immediately. Small doses of anticonvulsant agents (5 to 10 mg of diazepam—Valium—or 50 to 100 mg of thiopental) should also be given to control the seizure activity of the cerebral cortex. Additional increments of succinylcholine and anticonvulsant should be given as necessary. The cardiovascular system must be monitored during these circumstances and any manifestation of a severe reaction, such as bradycardia and hypotension, should be promptly treated with IV fluids and vasopressors (ephedrine), as appropriate. In the case of a severe convulsions it might be appropriate to administer small quantities (0.5 mEq/kg body weight) of sodium bicarbonate to treat metabolic acidosis.

Other Systemic Reactions

Undesirable systemic reactions to local and regional analgesia frequently occur from causes other than systemic toxicity produced by the local anesthetic. These include psychogenic reactions, epinephrine reactions, allergic reactions, and idiosyncratic reactions.

PSYCHOGENIC REACTIONS. Psychogenic reactions constitute the most frequent undesirable response to local and regional analgesia. Such reactions are usually caused by fear and apprehension regarding the block procedure and frequently occur in the dentist's office, especially in a patient who is in a sitting position. They usually are manifested by dizziness, faintness, occasionally ringing in the ears, marked perspiration, tachycardia, paleness of the skin, and marked arterial hypotension, which can cause loss of consciousness. A characteristic of this type of reaction is that it occurs as soon as the procedure is initiated, even before any needle is inserted into the skin or any solution is injected, sometimes causing the reaction to be labeled by the misinformed as a sensitivity or "allergic" reaction. Treatment consists of placing the patient in the recumbent position, administering oxygen, and, if the hypotension is moderate to severe, giving small IV increments of ephedrine.

EPINEPHRINE REACTIONS. Another common cause of reactions, especially those that occur in the dentist's chair, is overdosage of epinephrine or of some other vasoconstrictor. The patient can experience an extreme degree of palpitation, tachycardia, dizziness, perspiration, and paleness of the skin. Treatment consists of the administration of a small dose of a fast-acting barbiturate to allay apprehension and to reduce the blood pressure to normal limits. If the hypertension is severe it might be necessary to administer a vasodilator such as nitroglycerine, amyl nitrite, or sodium nitrate, or to use a more potent ganglionic blocking agent.

ALLERGIC REACTIONS. Allergic reactions to local anesthetics occur rarely following repeated exposure as occurs in dentistry, and with the use of procaine or other para-aminobenzoic acid esters. They rarely, if ever, are caused by amide compounds, such as lidocaine. The patient can experience generalized urticaria, joint pains, and edema, particularly of the eyelids, hands, joints, and larynx. Treatment consists of administration of antihistamines or epinephrine. The patient should then be observed closely for severe laryngeal edema; if this occurs it might be necessary to carry out a tracheostomy.

IDIOSYNCRATIC (ANAPHYLAXIS HYPERSENSITIVITY) REACTIONS. On extremely rare occasions the administration of small amounts of a local anesthetic properly given can result in sudden cardiovascular and respiratory collapse, possibly followed rapidly by death. Although such a phenomenon could presumably occur with the use of local anesthetics the incidence must be extremely rare; Bonica, with 45 years of experience, has never seen or heard of one. Such a reaction must be classified as idiosyncratic because it occurs rarely and bears no relation to dosage. Treatment is the same as that described for severe toxic reactions and includes prompt artificial ventilation with oxygen, administration of vasopressors and, if necessary, cardiac massage.

Neurologic Complications

Most neurologic complications have occurred after the use of regional anesthesia for surgery. When and if such complications are seen, the contributions of various events during the patient's surgical experience (e.g., surgical retraction, inappropriate positioning) that might be involved with the injury should be evaluated (44, 45).

Injuries to peripheral nerves can result from direct trauma to the nerve, compression by a tourniquet or hematoma, unintentional surgical traction or compression, or the injection of an excessively high concentration of local anesthetic into the nerve. The most frequent causes of neuraxial complications following subarachnoid or extradural block are direct trauma, cord compression by hematoma, spinal cord ischemia, and lack of skill.

Most reports concerning neuropathy have involved brachial plexus block, with an overall incidence of approximately 0.4% (46). A 2.8% incidence of postblock dysesthesia has been reported with brachial plexus blocks when paresthesiae were elicited versus a 0.8% incidence of postblock dysesthesia when paresthesiae were not elicited (47, 48). Intraneural injections, which can be detected by increased resistance to the injection, have been reported to cause a higher incidence of neuropathy (49, 50) than when the injection was made around the nerve. Moreover, the use of needles with 45° bevels is associated with a lower incidence of nerve damage than the use of long-beveled needles (51). For peripheral blocks recommendations include the use of short-beveled needles, locating the nerve by a gentle technique that produces only mild paresthesia, or the use of a peripheral nerve stimulator, using the lowest appropriate concentration of local anesthetic and using epinephrine cautiously. Signs of postblock neuropathy can occur immediately after the block or within the first 7 days. These usually diminish in intensity, with recovery over a 2- to 3-month period (49).

Accidental Subarachnoid Block

The accidental injection of a local anesthetic drug into the subarachnoid space is a complication that can occur during paravertebral block of somatic or sympathetic nerves, and even with a stellate ganglion block. It can be caused by accidental invasion of the spinal canal by a needle advanced through an intervertebral foramen or by the unintentional injection of solution into an abnormal prolongation of the dura-arachnoid cuff around a formed spinal nerve projecting beyond the intervertebral foramen. Accidental injection of a dose of LA intended for epidural block into the subarachnoid space will result in total spinal anesthesia.

Prevention of this complication requires the following: (a) frequent aspiration before and after injection of a small amount of drug, (b) observation of the hub of the needle for 15 to 30 seconds for the appearance of cerebrospinal fluid, and (c) the administration of a small test dose (see above).

Treatment of this complication consists of the following: (a) immediate artificial ventilation; (b) simultaneous withdrawal of 10 to 15 ml spinal fluid to remove as much of the local anesthetic as possible, thus effecting a much earlier reversal of the subarachnoid block; and (c) support of the circulation by intravascular fluids and vasopressors.

Pneumothorax

Pneumothorax can develop after thoracic paravertebral block, supraclavicular brachial plexus block, intercostal block, or block of the celiac plexus or splanchnic nerves. In such cases the needle is misdirected and enters the lung to produce a bronchopleural fistula. Air is subsequently aspirated from the alveoli through the fistula into the pleural space with its negative pressure and can produce a progressively larger degree of lung collapse. If the pneumothorax is less than 15 to 20%, few or no symptoms or signs are likely to be present, whereas a greater collapse can produce chest pain or dyspnea or both. Symptoms can develop within minutes or, more frequently, several hours after the accident.

Diagnosis is by percussion and roentgenography. Treatment of mild cases consists of reassuring the patient and avoiding deep breathing by bed rest. Mild analgesics (e.g., codeine and non-narcotic analgesics such as aspirin) are occasionally necessary for pain relief. If pneumothorax causes moderate to severe pain, respiratory dysfunction, or both, it is necessary to aspirate the air from the pleural space continuously, preferably by a tube with one end into the pleural space and the other attached to a negative pressure pump. Oxygen and analgesics might also be necessary.

Other Complications

Hypotension

Hypotension is a frequent side effect of unintentional extensive subarachnoid or epidural blockade or extensive paravertebral sympathetic block. Each of these produces extensive vasomotor blockade, resulting in marked reduction of vascular resistance in the blocked region of the body. Celiac plexus block can also cause hypotension by the same mechanism. Prophylaxis involves an infusion of 1 L of fluids prior to carrying out these procedures. Treatment of hypotension consists of IV infusion of fluids and the IV injection of a small dose of a vasopressor, such as 15 to 25 mg of ephedrine, promptly followed by 50 mg of ephedrine IM to sustain a normal blood pressure.

Hematoma

Bleeding into the site of injection is a mild complication of nerve blocks done with large needles having a dull bevel or a hook on a long-bevel needle. Although the bleeding is often minimal, it can become serious in patients who have blood dyscrasia or who have been on anticoagulant therapy. Therefore, it is best to avoid subarachnoid or epidural block in patients on anticoagulant therapy. Treatment of hematoma consists of cold packs and pressure over the site of bleeding, transfusion if patients have lost large amounts of blood, and coagulant therapy, as appropriate.

B. LOCAL APPLICATIONS OF REGIONAL ANALGESIA

The infiltration of local anesthetics into various body structures and their topical application onto mucous membranes are simple, and frequently used techniques in the management of pain by physicians in their office. By interrupting nociceptive input at its source, pain and other symptoms and signs of various disorders can be relieved. For convenience, the use of these techniques is first considered for acute painful problems and then for chronic pain syndromes.

Local Infiltration

Acute Pain

POSTOPERATIVE PAIN. Local infiltration of a dilute solution of a long-acting local anesthetic (e.g., 0.125 to 0.25% bupivacaine) for orthopedic procedures (52) and superficial operations such as excision of breast lumps (53) and inguinal hernia (54) produces effective postoperative pain relief for 12 to 16 hours, with a consequent significant decrease in the total amount of systemic analgesic required. Injection of LA through catheters with multiple openings, placed in the wound at operation, can provide even longer pain relief (55, 56) (Fig. 94-3). Although such a procedure relieves the somatic pain caused by the incision in the abdominal or chest wall, it usually needs to be supplemented by appropriate doses of nonsteroidal anti-inflammatory drugs and opioids to relieve the visceral pain.

ACUTE BURSITIS. Acute subacromial, subcapsular, prepatellar, and trochanteric bursitis are among the most common causes of severe disabling pain that can be promptly relieved with local infiltration analgesia. The bursa should be infiltrated with 8 to 10 ml of dilute solution (e.g., 0.25%) of bupivacaine with epinephrine, 5 mg/ml solution, with the addition of 40 mg of methylprednisolone (Depo-Medrol). Pain relief occurs in 10 to 15 minutes and can last 8 hours, and not infrequently 12 hours, after which pain returns and is often intense. The patient should therefore be given systemic nonopioid or opioid analgesics to manage the postblock pain. The application

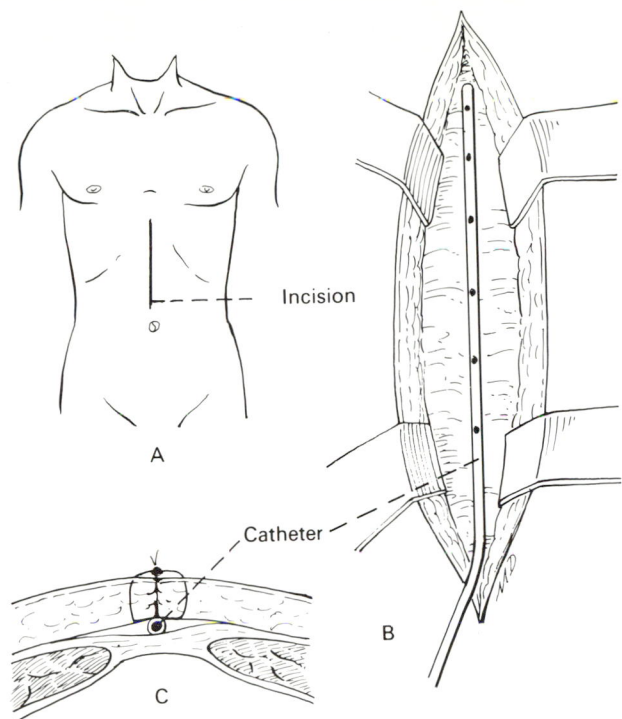

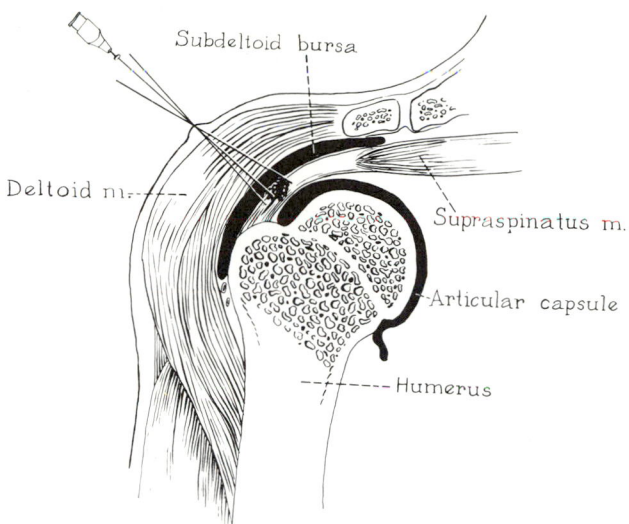

FIG. 94-4. Frontal section of the shoulder region showing injection technique for treatment of supraspinatus tendinitis and subacromial bursitis. Note the calcium deposit in the supraspinatus tendon.

FIG. 94-3. Technique for producing postoperative analgesia following a midline incision (**A**) in the upper abdomen. **B.** Just before closing the wound a catheter with multiple holes (*black*) is placed with its proximal end connected to the hub of a needle that fits into the catheter. The hub is kept sterile between injections of boluses of local anesthetic. **C.** Cross section of the abdominal wall showing the position of the catheter. Injection of a bolus of 10 to 15 ml of 0.25% bupivacaine with epinephrine results in diffusion of the drug to the surrounding structures, thus producing analgesia of the anterior abdominal wall adjacent to the incision.

of ice to the region can also relieve the pain by reducing edema and pressure within the bursa or joint. Several injections are frequently necessary. If the effusion of a joint is pronounced, frequent aspiration of the bursa is indicated.

TENDINITIS. Tendinitis is another common cause of moderate to severe and often disabling pain. The most frequent types include bicipital tendinitis, lateral epicondylitis (tennis elbow), medial epicondylitis (golfer's elbow), and supraspinatus (rotator cuff) tendinitis, often associated with subacromial bursitis (Chapter 50). Infiltration of these structures with 0.25% bupivacaine provides prompt relief of pain for 8 to 12 hours (Fig. 94-4). A long-acting steroid compound can be included in the solution for the first injection, but most orthopedic surgeons avoid repeated use because of the possible myotoxic effects and delayed sequelae (e.g., Cushing's syndrome) from the use of steroids. The inclusion of steroid in the local anesthetic for the first injection unquestionably produces prolonged pain relief for 1 to 3 or 4 weeks. Local anesthetic infiltration can be repeated several times until permanent relief is achieved.

In some patients the steroid causes a burning pain in the site of injection 24 to 48 hours after the procedure. Moreover, as with other local injections into bursa or tendon, patients might experience postblock

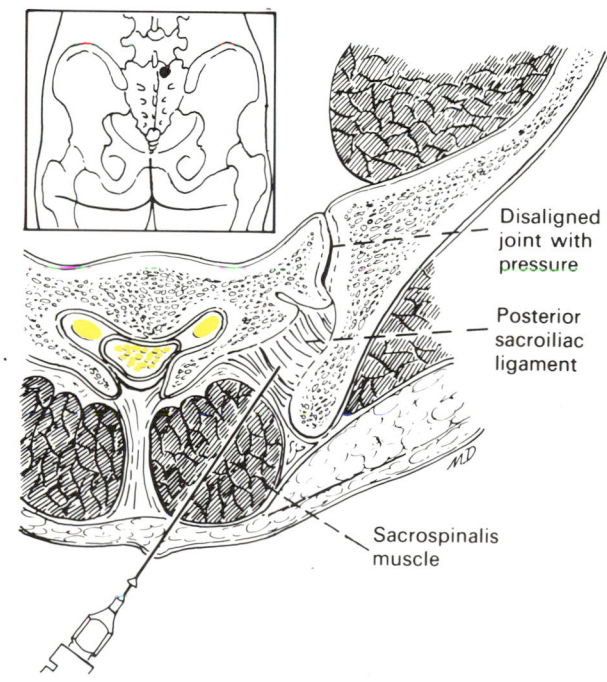

FIG. 94-5. Technique of injecting the ligaments of the right sacroiliac joint, which is shown subluxated. *Inset.* The skin wheal (*black dot*) used to anesthetize the skin for insertion of a larger needle is made in the midline at the level of the posterior superior spines of the ilium. The needle is inserted toward the affected side to make an angle of 45° with the midsagittal section. Once the point is in the ligament the LA is injected. Then an attempt is made to advance the needle into the subluxated joint, where 3 to 5 ml of solution is injected.

pain. Both types of pain should be managed with systemic analgesics.

MUSCLE SPASM. Muscle spasm with consequent severe pain can develop after injury in various locations, particularly in the low back. Muscle spasm can also be caused by poor posture or deformity of the spine (1). In all such cases LA infiltration with a dilute solution (e.g., 0.125% bupivacaine) into the entire muscle causes prompt relief of the pain and muscle spasm that can last for 8 to 12 hours. The injection should be followed by the application of heat, massage, and corrective exercises, as indicated.

Infiltration of a local anesthetic into a muscle can also be used as a diagnostic and therapeutic procedure in the rare cases of pyriformis or scalenus anticus syndrome.

Chronic Pain

PAINFUL SCARS. It is unusual for a whole scar to be painful, but frequently "trigger points" can be found in a scar. These can be associated with hyperesthesia and radiation of the pain along dermatomes from the scar. Infiltration of the scar with a dilute solution of bupivacaine (e.g., 0.25%) on about six occasions at 3- to 5-day intervals occasionally produces persistent relief. If pain relief does not persist following a series of injections of local anesthetic, transcutaneous electrical stimulation (TENS) should be tried. If this fails consideration should be given to injection of 1 ml of alcohol into the specific trigger point, which is said to produce a high incidence of success (57).

Defalque (57) reported on 69 patients who experienced persistent severe gnawing and burning pain associated with hyperesthesia, originating in postoperative scars following surgery in the inguinal, abdominal, or lumbar areas, or on an extremity. These patients were first given diagnostic local anesthetic block followed by injection of alcohol. After carefully localizing the trigger point Defalque injected 1 to 3 ml of bupivacaine with epinephrine into the scar. The injection reproduced the pain and paresthesia but within 5 to 10 mintues patients experienced complete pain relief and a small area of anesthesia that lasted from 6 to 10 hours. A second bupivacaine block was repeated a few days later with similar results. Defalque then injected 1 ml of alcohol 1 or 2 days later over a 10-minute period. Because the injection of the alcohol produced excruciating burning pain and paresthesia for up to 5 minutes, he subsequently minimized this discomfort by injection of small IV doses of fentanyl before and during the block. At the 12-month follow-up, 47 of the patients (68%) had experienced complete pain relief; in another 16 patients (23%) the severe pain and paresthesia had disappeared but some discomfort or ache persisted, especially with movement or a posture that strained the incision.

Because most other therapeutic procedures, including TENS and repeated blocks, do not relieve pain in all patients, the injection of neurolytic agents should be considered in those who have moderate to severe persistent pain from trigger points in scars.

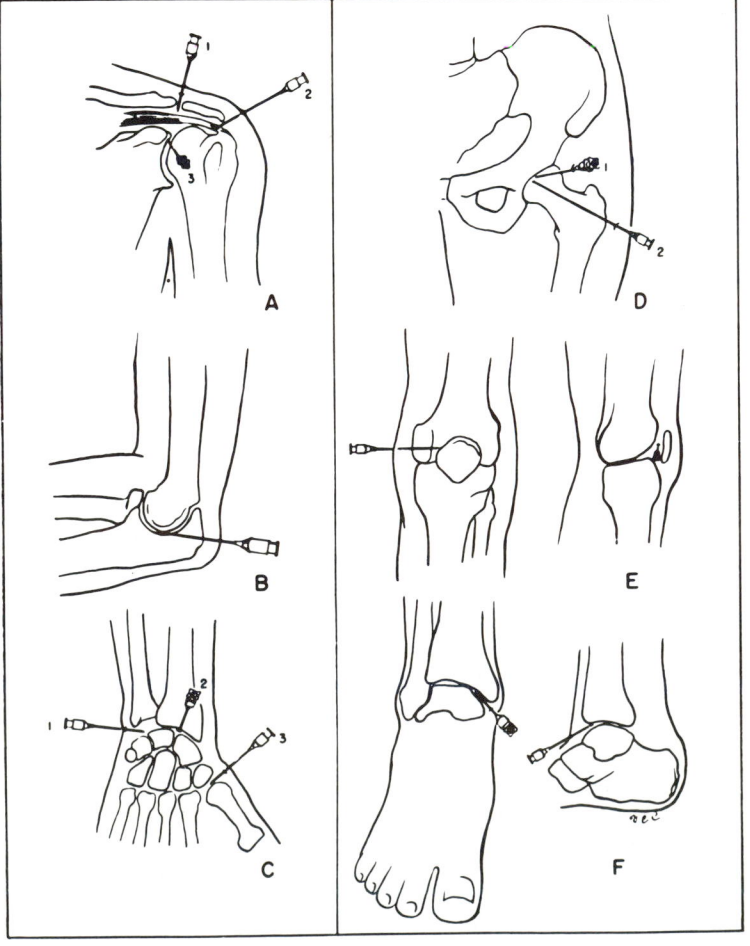

FIG. 94-6. Intra-articular injection of various joints. *A.* Techniques of injecting part of the shoulder using a 22-gauge or 25-gauge 5-cm needle: the acromioclavicular joint (1); the supraspinatus tendon for treatment of tendinitis (2); the scapulo-humeral joint (3). *B.* Technique of injecting the elbow (humeroulnar) joint. *C.* Techniques of intra-articular injection of the wrist: ulnar approach (1); dorsal approach (2); injection into the carpometacarpal joint of the thumb (3). *D.* Techniques of injection of the left hip joint by the anterior (1) and lateral approaches (2). Note the direction of the shaft of the needle to the bone. By being inserted just anterior to the greater trochanter in a sagittal direction and pointed toward the middle of Poupart's ligament, the needle point slides anterior to the periosteum and enters the joint space anteriorly near the upper reflection of the synovial sac. *E.* Technique of injecting the knee joint: anterior and lateral views. After a skin wheal is made on the anteromedial surface of the knee, about 1 to 2 cm from the medial border of the patella, a needle is inserted in a lateral and slightly posterior direction in a line aiming to slide it between the posterior surface of the patella and the patellar groove of the femur. Synovial fluid can be aspirated as soon as the joint cavity is entered. *F.* Technique of injecting the ankle joint: anterior and lateral views. From Bonica, J.J.: Clinical Applications of Diagnostic and Therapeutic Nerve Blocks. Springfield, IL, Charles C Thomas, 1959.

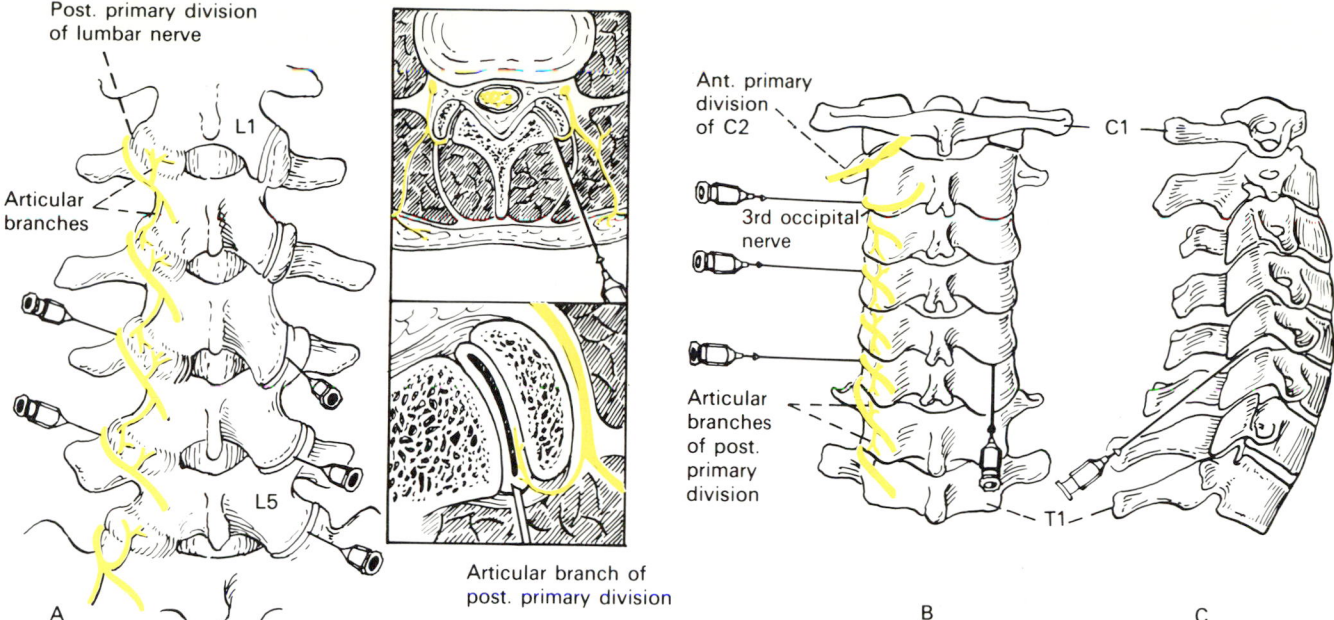

FIG. 94-7. Techniques of local injection to relieve pain resulting from pathology of a facet joint in the lumbar region (**A**) and in the cervical spine (**B** and **C**). **A.** Posterior view of the lumbar spine depicting the approach for blocking the medial branch of the posterior primary division of the lumbar spinal nerves (*left*) and the intra-articular zygapophyseal joint (*right*). Each medial branch sends articular filaments to adjacent facet joints so that each joint is supplied by two (and sometimes three) adjacent nerves, which must be blocked to interrupt sensory fibers to the particular joint. *Inset:* Cross section of lumbar spine indicating the direction of the needle (*top*); insertion of the bevel of the needle into the joint (*bottom*) **B.** Posterior view of the cervical spine depicting the approach for blocking the medial branches of the posterior primary divisions of the cervical nerves (*left*) and the direction of the needle for penetrating the zygapophyseal joint on the right. **C.** Lateral view of the cervical spine showing the course of a needle into the cavity of the right C5–C6 zygapophyseal joint. Modified from Bogduk, N.: Back pain: Zygapophyseal blocks and epidural steroids. *In* Neural Blockade in Clinical Anesthesia and Management of Pain. 2nd Ed. Edited by M.J. Cousins and P.O. Bridenbaugh. Philadelphia, J.B. Lippincott, 1988.

NEUROMATA. Neuromata can develop in nerves that are entrapped subsequent to traumatic nerve section or after surgery or amputation. Infiltration of the neuroma with a local anesthetic is a useful diagnostic procedure for determining whether the pain is arising from the neuroma. Moreover, injection of a solution containing a local anesthetic (without adrenalin) and a depot corticosteroid such as methylprednisolone (Depo-Medrol) into the neuroma can suppress the spontaneous ectopic discharges that are probably producing pain and paresthesia. Experimental studies (43) have shown that the steroid stabilizes the nerve membrane for 2 weeks or longer. Therefore, patients with painful neuromata should be given a trial with this combination at 1- to 2-week intervals for the first month and at 2- to 3-month intervals thereafter. The management of patients with this type of pain is discussed in detail in Chapter 12.

MYOFASCIAL SYNDROMES WITH TRIGGER POINTS. One of the most effective clinical applications of infiltration of local anesthetics and corticosteroids is in the management of myofascial pain syndromes with trigger points. Trigger points can develop in almost every muscle in the body, as well as in tendons and ligaments, and invariably produce local and referred pain, tenderness, reflex muscle spasm, and other signs and symptoms. In some patients such trigger points can be in the vicinity of classic acupuncture points (58). Repeated injections of trigger points with a local anesthetic alone or combined with steroid or with saline solution usually produce permanent relief of pain and eliminate the other signs and symptoms (59). (See Chapters 21, 40, 52, 58, and 77 for further discussion of myofascial pain syndromes, and Chapter 90 for a discussion of acupuncture.)

ARTHRITIS. An intra-articular injection of a dilute solution of local anesthetic alone or in combination with steroids is also indicated as a diagnostic and therapeutic procedure in patients with severe pain of chronic arthritis involving major joints in the limbs or spine (Figs. 94-5 and 94-6). It has been suggested (60, 61) that injection of corticosteroids into tender spots along the nerves supplying an osteoarthritic joint produces much better relief of pain than intrasynovial injection of steroids. The inclusion of 0.125% bupivacaine with the steroid eliminates the postinjection burning pain.

FACET SYNDROME. Intra-articular injection of local anesthetics into the facet joint in the lumbar, thoracic, and cervical regions (Fig. 94-7) has been used as an important diagnostic procedure. Although "facet syndrome" (a term first used in 1933 for diseases of the zygapophyseal joints) (62) as a cause of back pain remains controversial, it is believed that precise injection of the joint can be a valuable diagnostic tool in indicating whether pathophysiologic changes in the joint are a source of pain (63). The value of steroid injection into the facet joint as a therapeutic measure is also controversial: some clinicians have reported persistent relief of pain for at least 6 months in two-thirds of the patients, while others have reported relief in only 25% of patients. Moreover, a number of studies have suggested that this procedure or block of the medial branch of the posterior primary divisions that provide articular branches to the zygapophyseal joints above and below the nerve can be used diagnostically. (See pages 1505–1508 for detailed discussion of the subject and references). Figure 94-7 depicts both the intra-articular injection technique and block of the medial branch of the posterior primary division in the lumbar and cervical regions.

Topical Application

Topical application of a local anesthetic either in solution or in paste form is used to provide temporary relief of severe excruciating pain of the mucous membranes in the mouth, throat, and often the bladder. The most frequently used agents are 2 to 4% lidocaine, 4 to 6% cocaine, 1 to 2% tetracaine, or 0.25% dibucaine solution to produce topical analgesia for 30 to 60 minutes, or 0.5% tetracaine, 0.5% dibucaine, 2.5 to 5% lidocaine, or 30% benzocaine as constituents of an ointment, jelly, or cream to produce longer topical analgesia, with benzocaine having the longest effect. Because topical anesthetic solutions are absorbed rapidly from the vascular mucous membranes, the amount applied must be carefully measured and limited to a total dose of one-third to one-half of the total dose shown in Table 94-1. Ointments are used to relieve the excruciating pain of mucositis in cancer patients receiving chemotherapy, rectal suppositories are used for anal or rectal pain, and jellies or creams are used for pain in the urethra or urinary bladder.

C. BLOCK OF SPINAL NERVES

Outside the spinal canal the spinal nerves can be blocked in the paravertebral region or at certain points along their course (Fig. 94-8). Such procedures are usually done primarily to interrupt nociceptive pathways in the management of severe acute or chronic pain. Some of these blocks can be used to block somatomotor nerves to relieve pain of muscle spasm, however, or to block sympathetic fibers to the limbs. Blocks of the cranial nerves are used for the relief of cancer pain and chronic pain.

Cervical Spinal Nerves

The origin, course, and distribution of the cervical spinal nerves are described in Chapter 46 and depicted in Figure 94-9. As will be noted, these nerves are frequently involved in transmitting nociceptive information from the neck and upper limb and consequently are candidates for diagnostic/prognostic and therapeutic nerve blocks. The nerves can be blocked as they exit from the intervertebral foramina or they can be injected distal to the vertebral column.

Paravertebral Block

Indications

Paravertebral block of one or more of the cervical nerves is used to identify the specific nerve segment(s) in patients with segmental neuralgia caused by herniated intervertebral disk, osteophytes, root sleeve fibrosis, or paravertebral lesions, such as tumor or aneurysm. The procedure can also be used as a prognostic measure in patients with cancer pain who are scheduled to have neurolytic or neuroablative interruption of the pathways. The technique is useful for the temporary relief of severe pain resulting from musculoskeletal pathology or for the manipulation of a painful or frozen shoulder joint.

Technique

The cervical nerves exit from the spinal canal by passing laterally, lying within the sulcus of each transverse process. The tip of each transverse process consists of a smaller anterior tubercle and a larger and more superficial posterior tubercle, which is easily palpable in the average individual (Fig. 94-9). Each cervical nerve can be blocked paravertebrally by approaching the nerve as it lies in the transverse process, either from the side (lateral route) or from the back (posterior route). The lateral approach (Fig. 94-10) is the most frequently used technique for blocking these nerves. This procedure can be used to block all the cervical nerves except the C8 nerve. To block

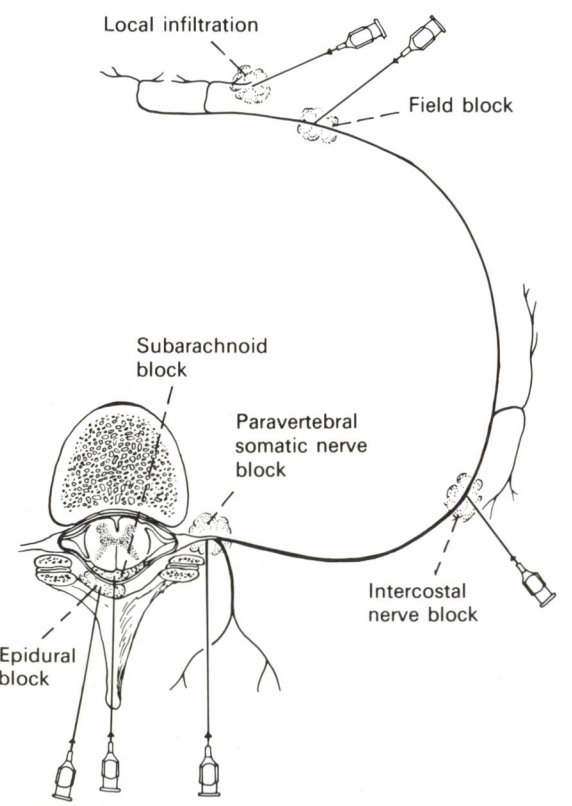

FIG. 94-8. Various sites at which a typical (thoracic) spinal nerve can be blocked.

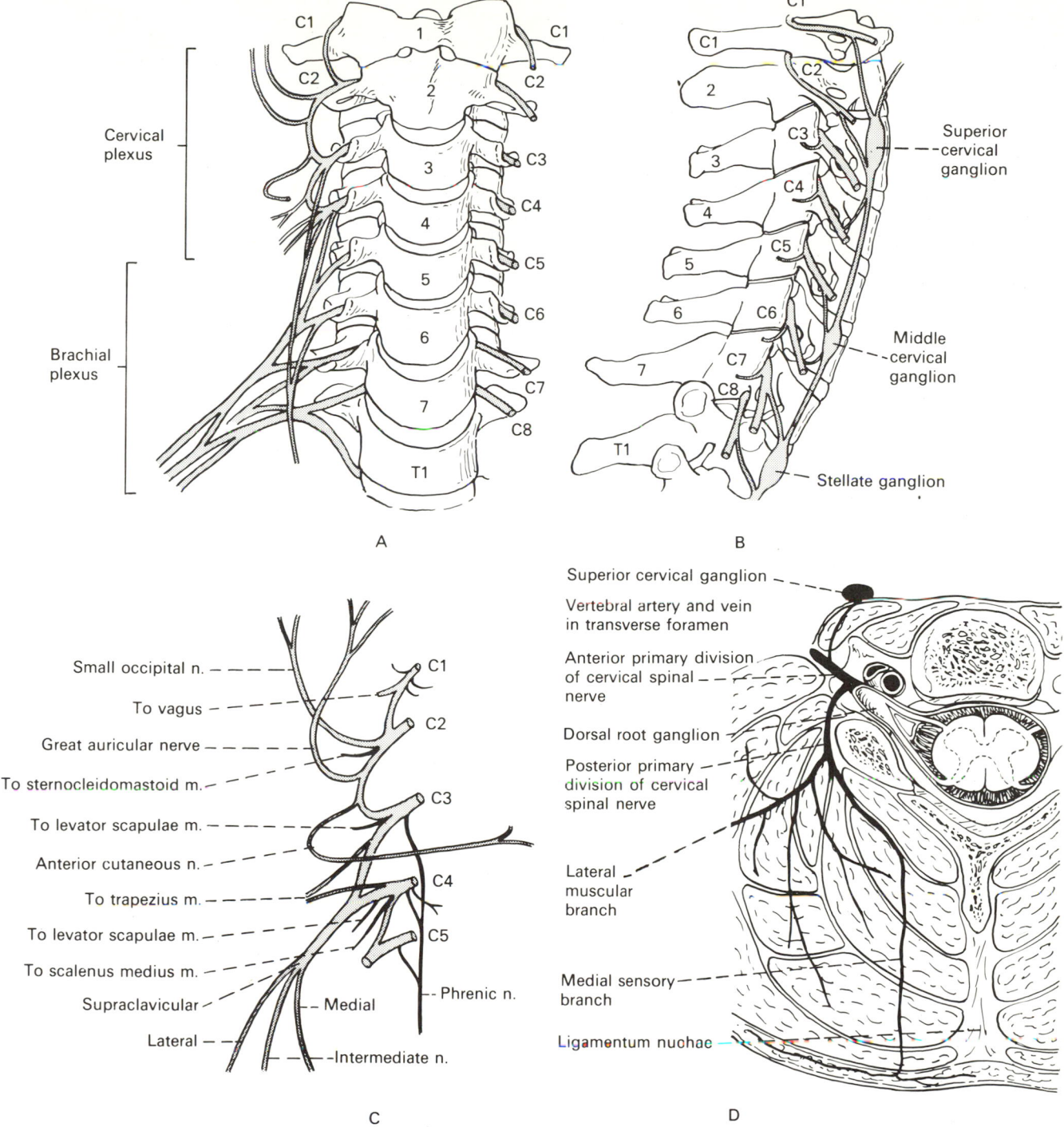

FIG. 94-9. Anatomy of the cervical nerves. *A.* Anterior view. *B.* Side view. *C.* Plan of the cervical plexus showing its origin from the anterior primary division of the upper four cervical spinal nerves and its main branches. *D.* Schematic representation of a transverse section in the neck showing the relationship of the formed nerve to various structures. Each nerve passes distally within the sulcus of each transverse process. The posterior tubercle of the transverse process is larger and more superficial, and therefore is more easily palpable than the anterior tubercle. The vertebral artery is just anterior to the formed nerve.

the C8 nerve an intracutaneous wheal of local anesthetic is made in the skin overlying the transverse process of the C7 vertebra. The needle is directed caudad and slightly mesiad and advanced slowly until contact with the nerve is made, indicated by eliciting paresthesia in its distribution.

The posterior approach, a more difficult technique,

is used in patients in whom the lateral approach is contraindicated because of skin infection, carcinoma, or other pathologic processes present in the lateral structures of the neck (Fig. 94-11).

Because some patients already have a mechanical neuropathy, extreme care must be exercised to avoid further damage to the nerve with the needle point.

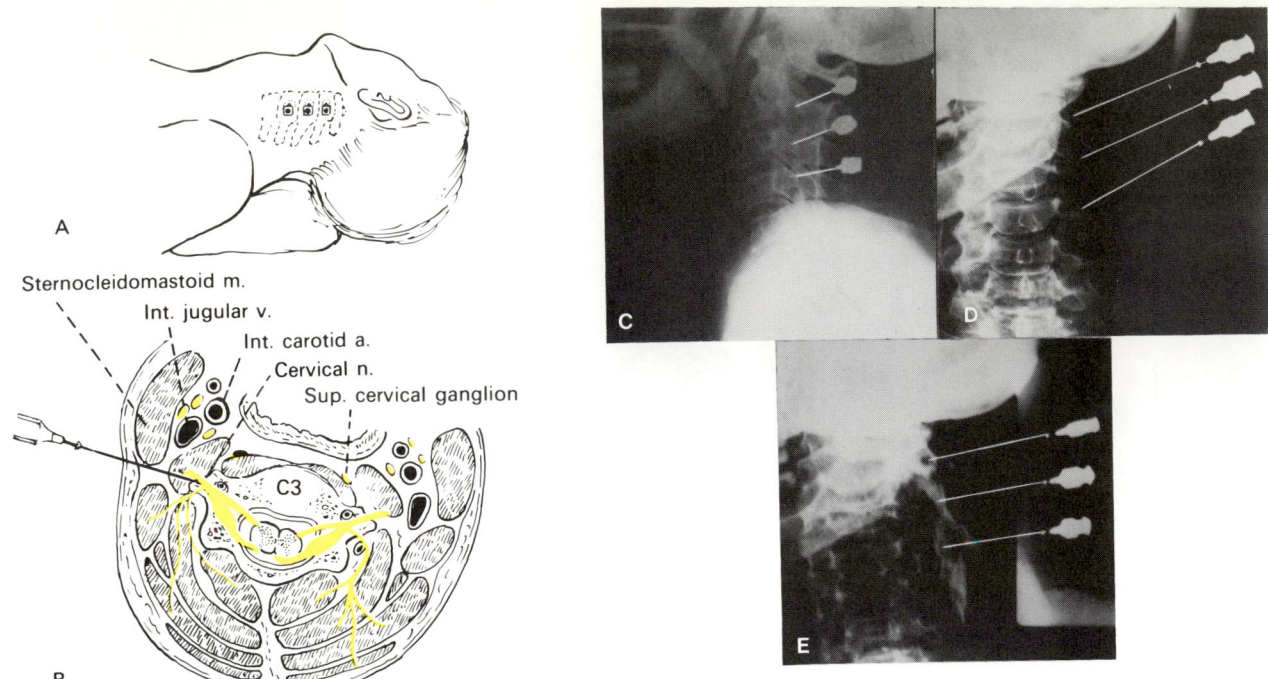

FIG. 94-10. Technique of lateral paravertebral block of the cervical nerves. **A.** Position of the patient. **B.** Cross section of the C3 vertebra with the needle in place. The patient's head is turned to the opposite side and a small pillow is placed under the upper portion of the thoracic spine and neck to make the transverse processes of the cervical vertebrae more prominent. The posterior tubercles of the transverse processes of the C3 to C7 vertebrae usually can be easily palpated, but this can be difficult in an obese patient. A line is drawn between the tip of the mastoid process and Chassaignac's (C6 posterior) tubercle, which is the most superficial and most easily felt. The second line is drawn 0.5 cm posterior to the first. Because the transverse process of the second is difficult to palpate it is usually located 1.5 cm caudad to the tip of the mastoid process on the second line. The tip of the transverse process of each subsequent vertebra is generally 1.5 cm caudad to the tip of the preceding transverse process. In a very tall or long-necked (or both) patient, the distance between adjacent transverse processes can be 1.7 and even as much as 2 cm.

After identifying the tip of the transverse process of the nerve or nerves that are to be blocked, the skin is prepared with an antiseptic solution. After 1 minute the excess is removed and an intracutaneous wheal is produced over the transverse process containing the nerve to be injected. With the fingers of the left hand immobilizing the skin a 5-cm 22-gauge needle is inserted medially and slightly caudad and advanced until the nerve or the transverse process is contacted, usually at a depth of about 2.5 to 3 cm (but possibly as deep as 4 or 5 cm in an obese patient). For diagnostic purposes the nerve can be identified by eliciting gentle paresthesia or by using a nerve stimulator. If doubt exists the nerve can be identified by lateral (**C**) and anteroposterior (**D**) radiographs. If the point of the needle is on the nerve (not *inside*), 2 ml of local anesthetic is sufficient to produce block without involving adjacent segments. If the procedure is done for therapeutic purposes, which require block of several nerves, a needle can be inserted for each segment to be blocked and 2 to 3 ml of solution injected. Alternatively, one needle can be inserted into the middle of the various segments to be blocked and 5 to 8 ml of solution injected. **E.** Anteroposterior radiograph taken 5 seconds after injecting 5 ml of 35% Diodrast solution through the middle needle. Note the wide diffusion of fluid.

Moreover, because nerve blocks are primarily used for diagnostic purposes and because of the close proximity to other nerves, the use of small quantities of local anesthetic is desirable. To identify a specific nerve either paresthesia can be elicited *gently* or a peripheral nerve stimulator and insulated needles can be used.

Complications

Paravertebral block in any segment is associated with the risk of accidental injection into the subarachnoid, subdural, or epidural space. In the cervical region this results in prompt involvement of the roots of the phrenic nerve and, with subarachnoid block, the drug rapidly diffuses to the respiratory center, with consequent respiratory paralysis. Another serious complication is the accidental injection of the drug into the vertebral artery, which promptly delivers a bolus of drug to the brain stem and brain and produces consequent transient paralysis of vital centers and often unconsciousness and seizures. Both these complications must be treated *promptly* with artificial ventilation and support of circulation until the local anesthetic drug is redistributed and biotransformed. Possible side effects include concomitant block of the cervical sympathetic chain, with development of Horner's syndrome or involvement of the superior or recurrent laryngeal nerve, or both, and perhaps even of the trunk of the vagus. These can all be avoided by using proper techniques and a small volume of solution. Because of the risk of recurrent laryngeal and phrenic nerve block, it is advisable to limit the procedure to a unilateral injection at any one time.

Occipital Nerve Block

Indications

Block of the greater and third occipital nerve can be used as a diagnostic, prognostic, or therapeutic

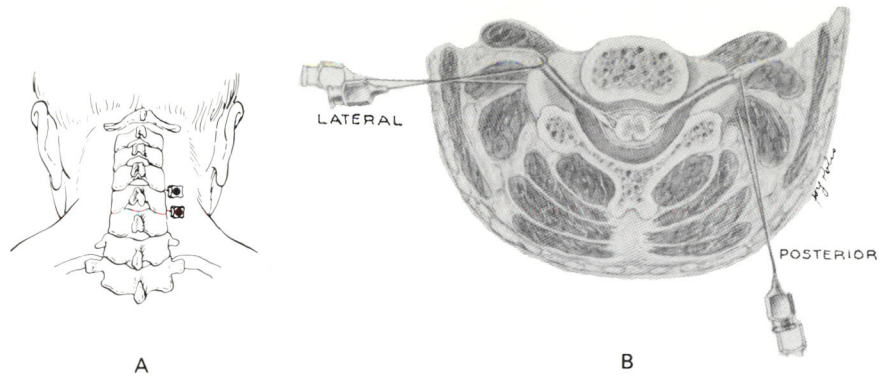

FIG. 94-11. Paravertebral block of one or more cervical nerves by the posterior approach. Following identification of the transverse process or of the processes that contain the nerves to be blocked, a line is drawn posterior to the midline with an indelible pen or marker. The patient is placed prone with a pillow under the chest, and the neck is flexed. After preparing the field an intracutaneous wheal is made 3 cm from the midline on the marked line that is at the same cross-sectional level as the transverse process of the vertebra. An 8-cm 22-gauge needle is inserted perpendicular to the skin and advanced anteriorly and slightly medially until the articular pillar is contacted, whereupon the needle marker previously threaded on the needle is placed flush with the skin. The needle is withdrawn until its point is in the subcutaneous tissue and redirected slightly more laterally so that its point is 1 cm lateral to the point of the first contact, as indicated by the needle marker. The marker is placed 1 cm from the skin and the needle is slowly advanced until contact with the nerve is made, as indicated by paresthesia. For diagnostic purposes it is essential to elicit paresthesia; it might be necessary to make several insertions, directing the needle slightly more cephalad or caudad. It is also advisable to take radiographs. Paresthesia is not necessary for therapeutic purposes but the point of the needle must be in the paravertebral space, which communicates freely in the cervical region and permits the anesthetic solution to diffuse easily to adjacent levels. The volume of local anesthetic is 2 to 3 ml for each segment or 8 to 10 ml for three or four segments.

measure in managing patients with occipital headache, neuralgia, and other painful conditions in the posterior portion of the head.

Technique

The greater occipital nerve is usually blocked just above the superior nuchal line, about 2.5 to 3 cm lateral to the external occipital protuberance (Fig. 94-12). If it is difficult to contact the nerve and elicit paresthesia, 5 ml of local anesthetic can be injected on the medial side of the artery, 2 mm superficial to the skull.

Side Effects

No side effects have been noted with the use of occipital nerve block other than accidental intraarterial injection, which is usually inconsequential because of the small volume of drug used.

Phrenic Nerve Block

Indications

Phrenic nerve block is a useful diagnostic procedure in patients who complain of pain in the shoulder caused by irritation of the central portion of the

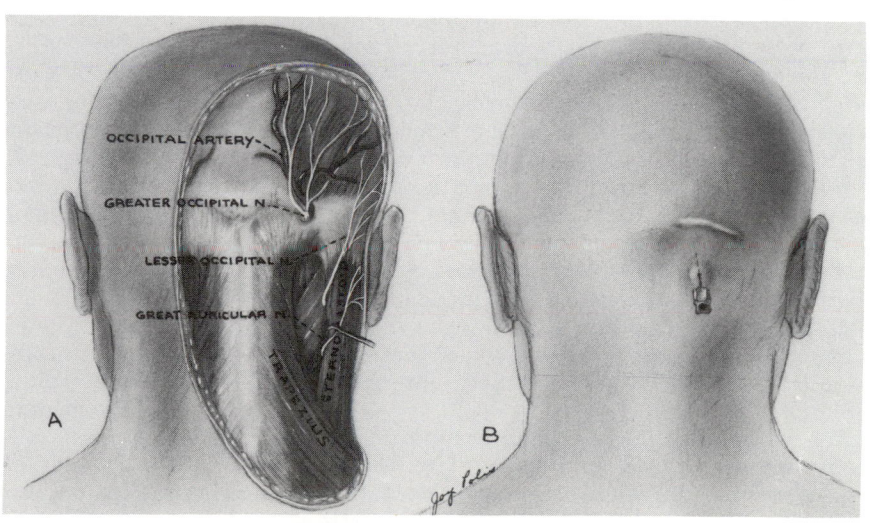

FIG. 94-12. Technique of occipital nerve block. A. Anatomy of the greater and lesser occipital nerves. The greater occipital nerve is 2.5 to 3 cm lateral to the external occipital protuberance and just medial to the occipital artery, which serves as the most reliable landmark for blocking of this nerve. The 3rd occipital nerve, which is not shown, is usually located medial to the greater occipital nerve, while the lesser occipital nerve is located about 2.5 cm lateral to the artery. B. Occipital nerve block. The greater and 3rd occipital nerves are usually blocked just above the superior nuchal line at a point medial to the occipital artery, which is easily palpated. After a thorough cleansing of the hair and scalp with an antiseptic solution, a 5-cm 25-gauge needle attached to a 5-ml syringe filled with local anesthetic is introduced about 1 cm below the level of the target and directed anteriorly and slightly superiorly, directing its point just medial to the artery. Contact with the nerve elicits paresthesia along its course, whereupon 1 ml of local anesthetic is injected if the procedure is being done for diagnostic purposes or 2 to 3 ml of solution is injected for therapeutic purposes. Anesthesia of the scalp in the distribution of the greater and 3rd occipital nerves develops within 5 to 10 minutes. If the procedure is repeated for therapeutic purposes and it is difficult to elicit paresthesia, 5 ml of local anesthetic is injected on the medial side of the artery 2 mm superficial to the skull. The lesser occipital nerve can be blocked about 2.5 cm lateral to the site of the greater occipital nerve block. If all three nerves need to be blocked with a single injection for therapeutic purposes, a simple technique involves subcutaneous injection of local anesthetic along the elevation of skin across the scalp above the needle shown in B.

diaphragm. It can also be useful in patients with intractable singultus (hiccups), in whom unilateral block is done to determine whether the condition involves one or both halves of the diaphragm.

Technique

The phrenic nerve arises from the anterior primary divisions of the C4 nerve but also receives fibers from the C3 and C5 cervical nerves. All of these join together at the lateral border of the anterior scalenus muscles; the nerve then courses caudad on the anterior surface of the muscle and enters the chest. (The course and distribution of the phrenic nerve are summarized in Chapter 53 and depicted in Fig. 53-14.) Block of the phrenic nerve is best achieved by depositing 5 to 10 ml of solution onto the anterior surface of the scalenus anticus muscle, about 3 cm above the clavicle (Fig. 94-13).

Complications

Possible complications include accidental intra-arterial injection with rapid diffusion of the local anesthetic to the brain stem, with consequent respiratory and cardiovascular depression or both, or accidental IV injection with rapid diffusion to the heart, with consequent cardiotoxic effects. Another side effect that can also cause respiratory difficulties, especially in patients with pulmonary disease, is ipsilateral hemidiaphragmatic paralysis.

Brachial Plexus Block

Indications

DIAGNOSTIC BLOCK. Block of the brachial plexus can be used as a diagnostic procedure in patients with causalgia or other reflex sympathetic dystrophies, phantom limb pain, and other types of postamputation pain. It can also be used to differentiate pain of peripheral neuralgia from that caused by disorders of the central nervous system (e.g., brachial plexus avulsion). Because all sympathetic fibers destined for the hand, forearm, and lower two-thirds of the arm are carried by nerves derived from the brachial plexus, block of the plexus is highly effective for confirming the results of cervicothoracic sympathetic block or surgical sympathectomy. For example, in patients with causalgia or reflex sympathetic dystrophy, or in painful peripheral vascular disorders in whom sympathetic block is suspected to be incomplete, as assessed by limb blood flow or SCR, block of the brachial plexus and subsequent measurement of these parameters indicate whether the sympathetic interruption is complete.

Brachial plexus block is useful diagnostically in a patient with pain and limitation of movements of joints of a limb, or with deformity associated with injury or consequent to reflex sympathetic dystrophy. Following complete block of the brachial plexus with 0.5% bupivacaine with epinephrine, pain and muscle spasm are eliminated, and passive movement can reveal a full range of motion. If little or no change in movement is noted during the block, however, the patient probably has tendon sheath fibrosis, muscle shortening consequent to chronic muscle spasm, fixed

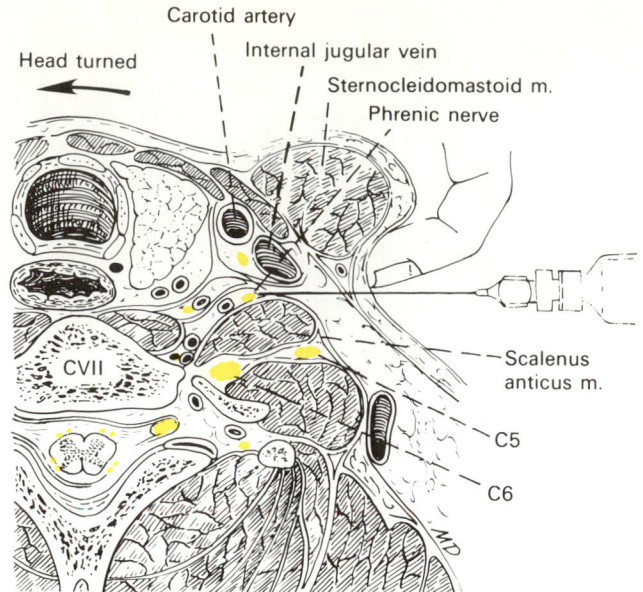

FIG. 94-13. Technique of blocking the phrenic nerve. The cross section at the level of the C7 vertebra shows the position of the phrenic nerve anterior to the fascia of the scalenus anticus muscle, with the point of the needle just touching the nerve. This procedure is best accomplished by having the patient in the supine position with the head turned to the opposite side. The posterior border of the sternocleidomastoid is identified 3 cm above the clavicle by having the patient lift the head while it is turned to the opposite side and by hooking the physician's index finger around the posterior border of the muscle. A wheal is made at this point; a short-beveled 5-cm 22-gauge needle is introduced through the wheal in a medial direction and guided with the finger of the left hand so that it passes posterior to the border of the sternocleidomastoid muscle. If the short-beveled needle is advanced slowly and carefully, one can better appreciate piercing the superficial fasica. Injection of 3 to 5 ml of solution is usually sufficient for complete block.

bony deformity, or a combination of these. Brachial plexus block can be used in a patient with muscle shortening to facilitate the task of the physical therapist in carrying out gentle and gradual stretching of the muscles to regain normal length, sometimes during several plexus blocks.

PROPHYLACTIC BLOCK. Brachial plexus block administered for surgery of the upper limb delays the onset of postoperative pain and significantly reduces its incidence. In a study by McQuay and associates (64) on patients undergoing orthopedic operations, those managed with brachial plexus block or other regional anesthesia (spinal, femoral nerve block and ankle block), the median time to first request for postoperative analgesia (TFA) was 8 hours, whereas among patients managed with general anesthesia it was 1.8 hours (64). Moreover, among the regional group, 4% required analgesia within the first 2 hours and 15% required no postoperative analgesia at all, whereas for those managed with general anesthesia, the figures were 56% and 5% respectively. Studies that will be cited in Section F in connection with epidural analgesia provide reason to believe that continuous brachial plexus block given to patients with severe pain due to occlusive arterial disease (or other causes) for 3

FIG. 94-14. *A.* Schematic depiction of the make-up of the brachial plexus. *B.* Anatomy of the brachial plexus. The brachial plexus extends from the interval between the anterior and medial scalenus muscles to the lateral border of the pectoralis muscle. The three trunks emerge from the interscalenus space at the lower border of these muscles and continue anterolaterally and inferiorly to converge toward the upper surface of the 1st rib, where they are closely grouped and thus accessible to injection of local anesthetic. In the posterior triangle of the neck the plexus is located superficially and is covered by the superficial fascia, platysma, and deep fascia. At the lateral edge of the rib each trunk divides into an anterior posterior division, which passes beneath the midportion of the clavicle to enter the axilla through its apex. Over the 1st rib the subclavian artery, lying immediately anteromedial to the plexus, is also superficial, thus affording a palpable landmark to the plexus. Throughout its course the brachial plexus and the subclavian artery are enclosed in a fascial sheath that extends from the anterior and middle scaleni muscles as far as the lower part of the axilla and the upper part of the arm (see Fig. 94-15). This sheath forms a relatively avascular enclosed space into which a local anesthetic solution can be injected thus resulting in prolonged neural blockade. (Fig. 94-15.) *C.* Superior view of first rib showing the subclavian groove, on which the brachial plexus and subclavian artery rest. *D.* Semidiagrammatic cross section to show relationships of the plexus, muscles, blood vessels, and apex of lung.

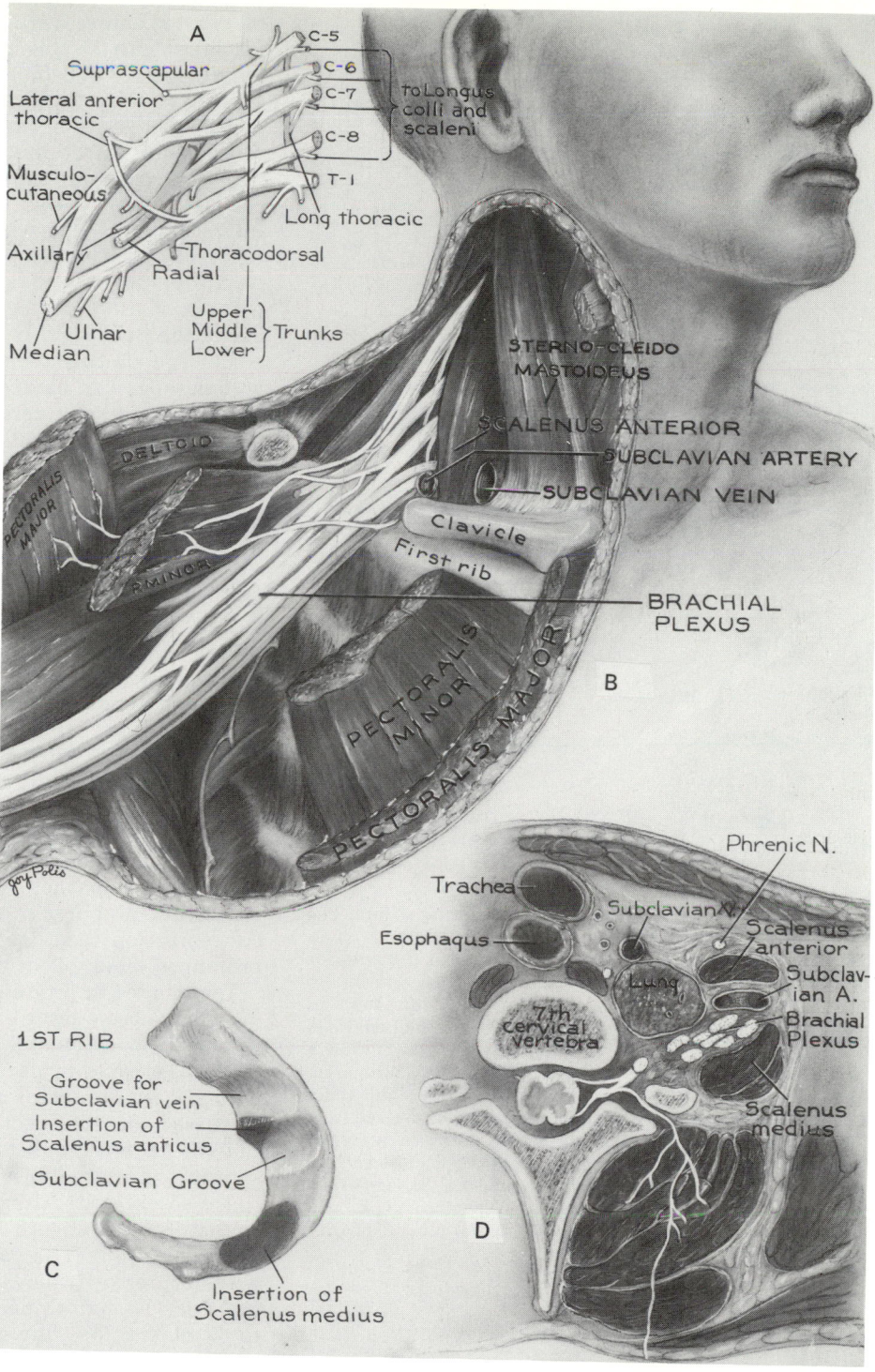

days prior to the amputation is likely to prevent or markedly reduce the incidence of postamputation phantom limb pain.

THERAPEUTIC BLOCK. Brachial plexus block is also useful in providing temporary relief in patients with severe acute pain that follows trauma or surgery, in patients with severe arteriolar spasm caused by accidental intra-arterial injection of such agents as thiopental, and in patients with severe pain consequent to an embolus. Continuous brachial plexus block is especially useful in patients who have undergone reimplantation of a severed portion of an upper limb or digit(s) and in those with other problems, in whom the blood supply to the extremities is compromised. In such circumstances prolonged sympathetic block and analgesia are useful in increasing the chance of survival of the limb and also in providing pain relief.

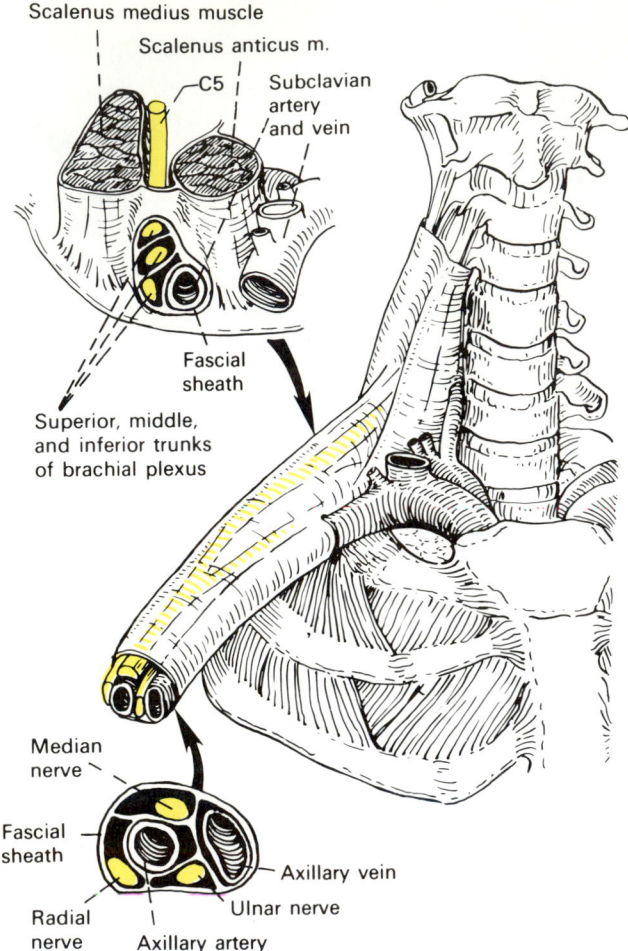

Scalenus medius muscle
Scalenus anticus m.
C5
Subclavian artery and vein
Fascial sheath
Superior, middle, and inferior trunks of brachial plexus
Median nerve
Fascial sheath
Radial nerve
Axillary vein
Ulnar nerve
Axillary artery

FIG. 94-15. The brachial and axillary neurovascular sheath. The sheath is a lateral prolongation of the prevertebral fascial layer that encloses the roots of the brachial plexus and the anterior and middle scalene muscles to form a vertical tube, continuing laterally to enclose the brachial plexus and subclavian artery. In its position above the 1st rib the subclavian vein is not enclosed in this sheath (*upper inset*) but, more distally, it is covered by a thin fascial sheath that tends to fuse with the larger neurovascular sheath. (*Lower inset*). Cross section in lower part of the axilla showing the relationships of the three major nerves derived from the brachial plexus to the axillary artery and axillary vein. Small fascial septa subdivide the main sheath to enclose each of these structures, which might constitute a fascial barrier to the diffusion of local anesthetic. Modified from Thompson, G.E., and Rorie, D.K.: Functional anatomy of the brachial plexus sheaths. Anesthesiology, *59*:117, 1983.

Technique

The anatomy of the brachial plexus is summarized in Chapter 46 and depicted in Figures 94-14 and 94-15.

Although many techniques for block of the brachial plexus have been described, the most commonly used are the supraclavicular (65) (Fig. 94-16), interscalene (66) (Fig. 94-17), and axillary approaches (67) (Fig. 94-18). During the first five decades of the century, the supraclavicular approach was the most commonly used technique, not only because it was the first of the various techniques described, but also because the site of injection is over the first rib, where all of the trunks

and cords group together and gentle paresthesia can be elicited. Moreover, when it is injected within the fascial sheath at this point, the solution will spread longitudinally and block all of the branches that are given off above the first rib. This technique requires expert knowledge of the anatomy of the plexus and its relationship to the first rib and the apex of the lung, which is medial to it. If the needle is directed medial to the rib there is a risk of puncturing the lung. In the interscalene block, which was reintroduced in the 1950s to obviate the problem of pneumothorax, the needle is introduced at the level of the transverse process of the sixth cervical vertebra, which is well above the upper end of the lung (Fig. 94-17). Another advantage of this technique is that by using large volumes, one can have diffusion of the solution cephalad to include the cervical plexus and thus provide anesthesia of the shoulder and side of the neck. The axillary block poses the least risk of serious neurologic or pulmonary complication, but unless large volumes are used, the branches of the plexus given off above the first rib are not included.

Regardless of which of the three techniques is used, a common feature is that the solution is deposited within the fascial sheath surrounding the brachial plexus (Fig. 94-15). Provided that an adequate volume of drug (30 to 40 ml in an adult) is injected into the sheath, it tends to spread longitudinally within the sheath to affect all components of the brachial plexus. Circumferential spread might not be as reliable, particularly with a small volume of solution (68).

For diagnostic purposes 1% lidocaine produces a 2- to 4-hour block. For therapeutic purposes 0.25 to 0.375% bupivacaine with epinephrine produces analgesia and sympathetic block for 8 to 12 hours. In a significant proportion of patients the use of a higher concentration (e.g., 0.5%) of bupivacaine produces a prolonged block of up to 16 to 24 hours' duration.

Techniques to produce a *continuous brachial plexus block* have been described for the supraclavicular (69), interscalene (70), and axillary routes (71–72). The plexus is located by paresthesia or loss of resistance or with the assistance of a nerve stimulator. A catheter is passed either directly into the fascial sheath or the sheath is first distended with a small volume of solution; the catheter is then passed into the distended space so created. Alternatively, a guide wire can be passed into the sheath and a catheter passed over the guide wire (73). The catheter is fixed in place either with sutures or transparent adherent dressings. Analgesia can be maintained with periodic injections of 20 to 30 ml of 0.25% bupivacaine every 6 hours, or by a continuous infusion with an infusion pump, of 0.25% bupivacaine at a rate of 6 to 12 ml/hour. With the use of these techniques the resulting blood levels of drug have been reported to be near toxic limits (74, 75). Such catheters have been left in for considerable periods of time, up to a week, with few or no complications (73).

Complications

Complications of the use of interscalene block include epidural, subdural, or subarachnoid block

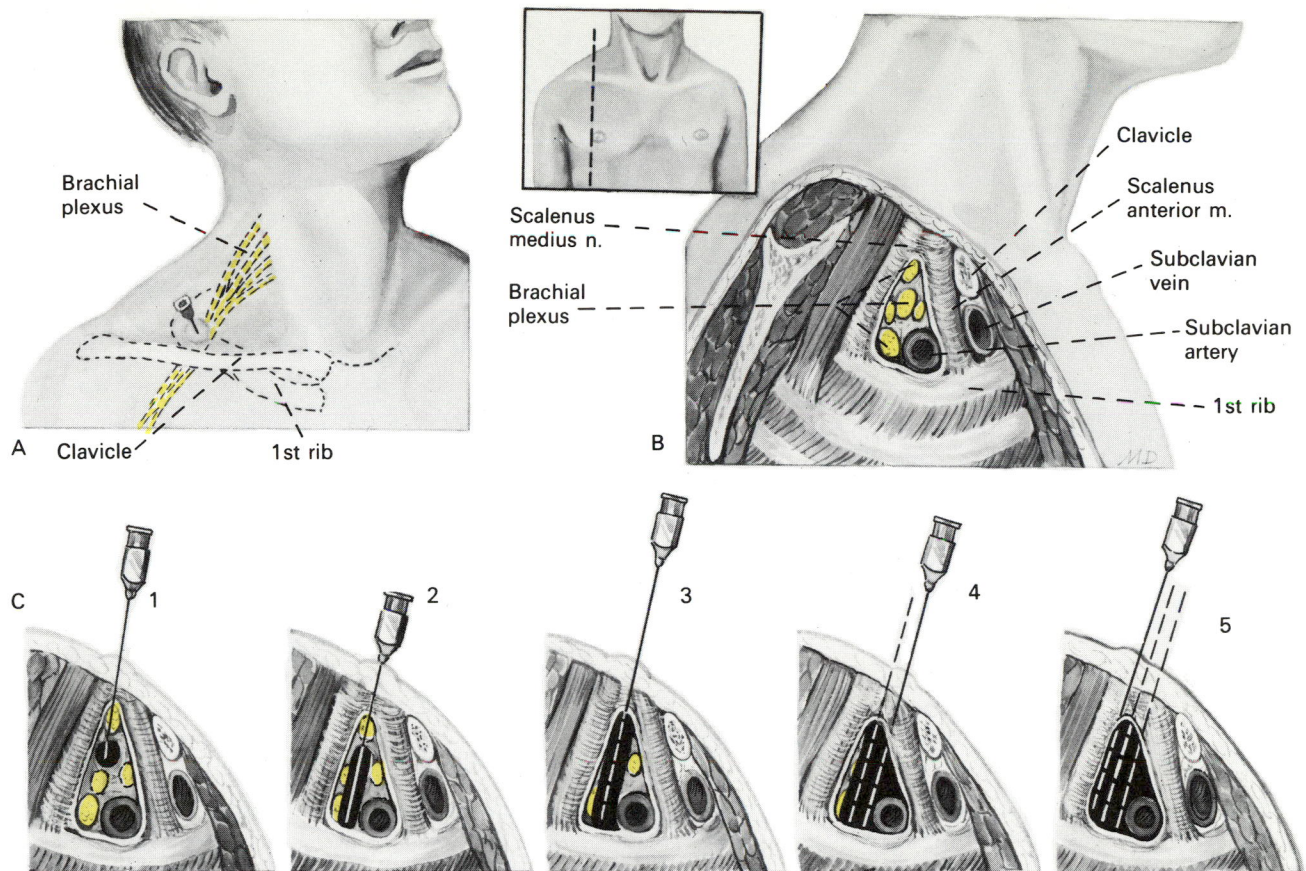

FIG. 94-16. Brachial plexus block by the supraclavicular approach using the Bonica three needle insertion technique. **A.** Anterior schematic view showing the position of the plexus and direction of the needle. **B.** Parasagittal section (inset: *dashed line*) showing the subclavian artery and brachial plexus surrounded by a sheath derived from the fascia of the scalenus anticus and scalenus medius muscles. **C.** Injection of local anesthetic solution (*black*) for each of three insertions. After informing the patient about the procedure and requesting that the patient promptly signal any feeling of paresthesia, the two ends of the clavicle are identified and the subclavian artery is palpated. The field is prepared and a skin wheal is formed about 1 cm above the midpoint of the clavicle, just posterior to the palpable subclavian artery. A 5- or 8-cm (depending on the size of the patient) 22-gauge needle attached to a 10-ml Luer-Lok control syringe filled with local anesthetic solution is inserted in a caudad and slightly dorsad and mesial direction (**A**) until paresthesia is elicited, whereupon the needle is arrested and aspiration is carried out in two places; if negative, 3 to 4 ml of local anesthetic solution is injected. The needle is then carefully advanced until the upper surface of the 1st rib is contacted (1) After injecting 2 to 3 ml on the rib, the remainder of the 10 ml of solution is injected as the needle is withdrawn between the 1st rib and the superficial fascia (2). To avoid accidental intravenous injection the needle should be withdrawn in a stepwise fashion and aspiration done prior to the injection of 1 to 2 ml of solution (3). When the point of the needle is in the subcutaneous tissue the skin is moved 1 cm anteriorly and then advanced so that the shaft of the needle is parallel to the first insertion, and the same procedure is repeated (4). Following the second step, with the needle point again subcutaneous, the skin is moved 2 cm posteriorly (i.e., 1 cm posterior to the first insertion) the needle is advanced with its shaft parallel to that in the first two steps, and the procedure is repeated (5). By injecting 10 ml of solution through each of these three insertions a wall of anesthesia is created within the entire fascial sheath containing the neuromuscular bundle (shown in black) through which the plexus passes.

(resulting from accidental injection into the sheath of dura around the nerve) or block of the sympathetic, recurrent laryngeal, and phrenic nerves. Complications of the use of the supraclavicular route include phrenic nerve block, cervical sympathetic block, and, perhaps the most serious, pneumothorax. The incidence of pneumothorax has been reported to be between 0.5 and 6.0% (44) but, in the hands of the skilled practitioner, it is lower than 1% (65). Complications of the use of the axillary route include intravascular injection, with a seizure incidence of 1.5% reported in some series (48). Minor dysesthesia can occur in approximately 3% of patients (47, 48) but, in skilled hands, the incidence is much lower, about 0.5% (46).

Suprascapular Nerve Block

Indications

The suprascapular nerve is a branch of the brachial plexus and is the major sensory nerve supply to the shoulder joint. Suprascapular nerve block is useful for the management of severe pain caused by bursitis, periarthritis, or arthritis if these conditions are not amenable to intra-articular and periarticular injection of local anesthetic and steroids.

Technique

The anatomy of the suprascapular nerve is described in Chapter 46. The nerve is composed of fibers derived

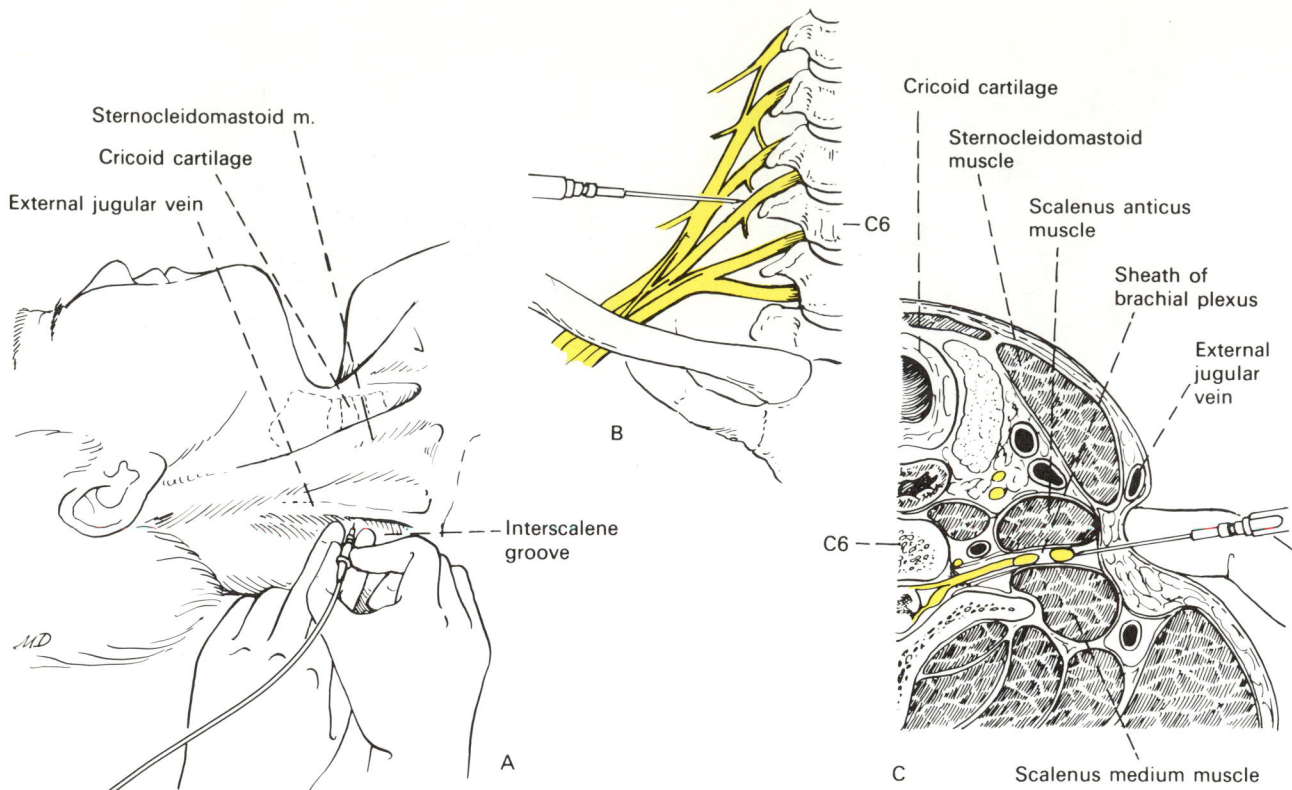

FIG. 94-17. Technique of interscalene block of the brachial plexus. **A.** The patient lies supine with the head on a pillow and rotated to the opposite side. The interscalene groove is identified by asking the patient to lift the head, which places the scaleni muscles in tension. The insertion point is determined by drawing a line that extends laterally from the cricoid cartilage to intersect the interscalene groove at the level of the transverse process of C6. After formation of a skin wheal, and with the second and third fingers of the left hand palpating the interscalene groove, a 3- or 5-cm 23- or 25-gauge short-beveled needle is inserted in a medial and slightly caudad direction toward the sulcus of the C6 transverse process. **B.** The needle is advanced slowly for 1.5 to 2 cm until paresthesia is elicited; this indicates contact with a nerve, which is usually the C7 root of the plexus. **C.** Cross section at level of C6 vertebra showing the bevel of the needle approaching the nerve, which is located between the anterior and middle scalenus muscles. The 30 to 40 ml of local anesthetic solution injected diffuses cephalad, caudad, and laterally to block the roots, trunks, and divisions of the brachial plexus and often the roots of the cervical plexus. Although this volume of solution can be injected by adapting a 10-ml Luer-Lok syringe directly to the hub of the needle, it is best to attach a length of tubing to the needle hub with its proximal end adapted to a 50-ml syringe containing the local anesthetic (as shown in **A**). To avoid unintentional intravenous or subarachnoid injection, attempts at aspiration are made before and after injection of 1 to 2 ml of solution and repeated frequently as the entire volume of the solution is injected. For a continuous technique, an 18- or 20-gauge intravenous catheter is similarly introduced, the stylet removed, and the catheter taped into place with its hub connected to a 10- to 15-cm length of tubing attached to the syringe containing the local anesthetic. Repeated injections of 20 to 30 ml of 0.25 to 0.375% bupivacaine every 6 hours, or an infusion of 0.25% bupivacaine at a rate of 6 to 12 ml/hour, produces continuous blockade.

from the C4, C5, and C6 cervical segments, which pass through the anterior primary divisions and reach the upper trunk of the brachial plexus from which the formed suprascapular nerve emerges. It then proceeds laterally, posteriorly, and inferiorly beneath the omohyoideus and trapezius muscles, but superficial to the plexus, to reach the superior border of the scapula, where it passes through the suprascapular notch beneath the superior transverse scapular ligament to enter the supraspinatus fossa (Fig. 94-19A).

The technique of suprascapular nerve block is described in Figure 94-19B–D. Although usually this block is relatively simple, it is sometimes difficult to contact the nerve and the solution is unintentionally injected within the muscle mass, resulting in failure. Radiography or a peripheral nerve stimulator can be used to aid in placement of the needle.

Complications

Side effects include paralysis of the supraspinatus and infraspinatus muscles, producing transient disability. The most serious complication is pneumothorax, which occurs if the needle is passed above the upper border of the scapula and advanced too far anteriorly into the lungs.

Block of Median, Ulnar, and Radial Nerves

Block of the median, ulnar, or radial nerves at the elbow is useful as a diagnostic or prognostic tool in patients with pain in the distribution of each specific nerve. This procedure can also be used to effect sympathetic block in the region supplied by each nerve. Block of the median or ulnar nerve, or both, at

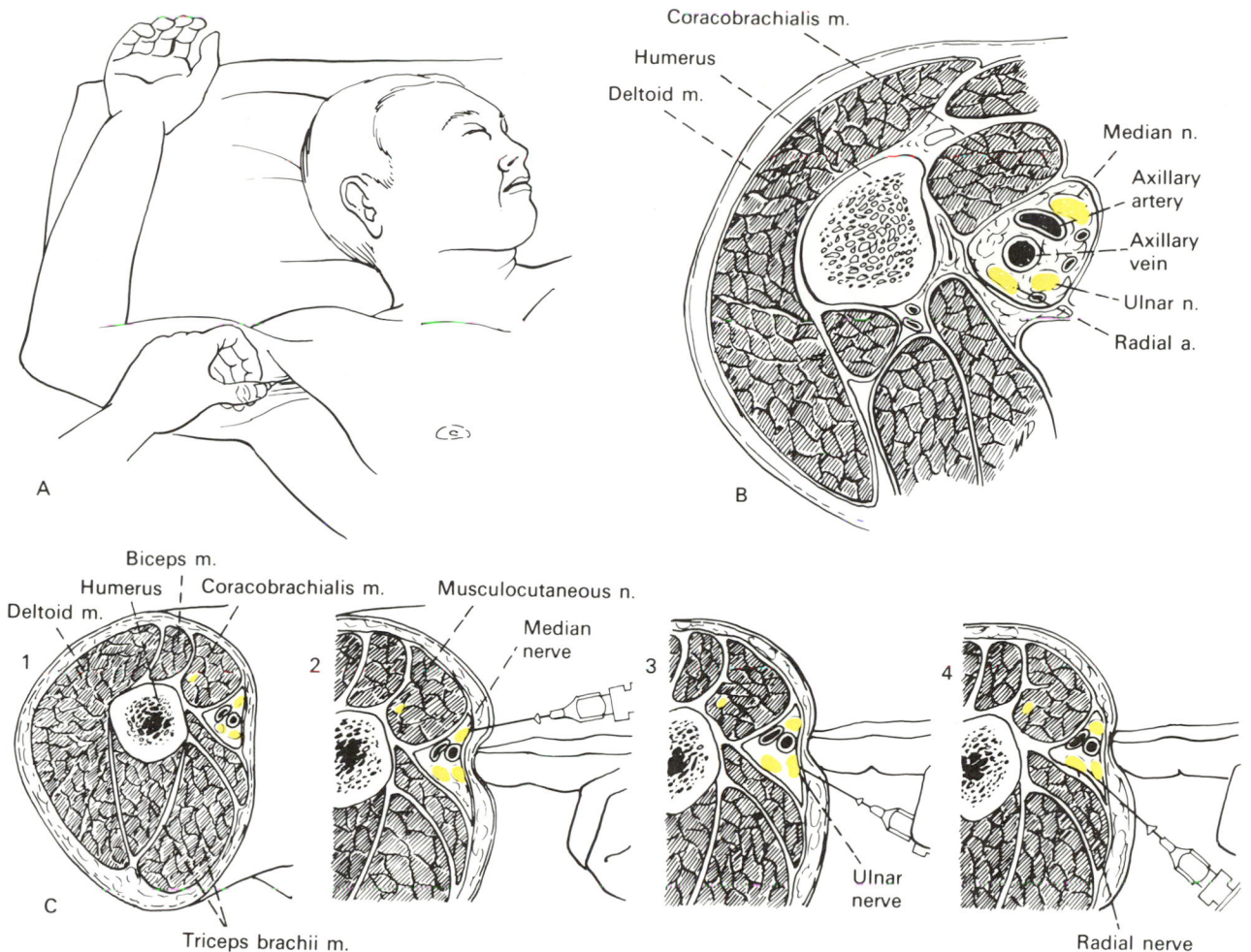

Fig. 94-18. Technique of axillary block of the brachial plexus. **A.** The patient is supine with the arm abducted to 90° and rotated externally. **B.** Cross section of the upper part of the axilla showing the relation of the nerves to the axillary arteries. The axillary artery is palpated and traced as far as possible proximally within the axilla, ideally to the pectoralis major muscle. After appropriate preparation of the skin a skin wheal is formed over the artery and a 3- or 5-cm 23- or 25-gauge short-beveled needle (attached to tubing connected to an anesthetic-filled syringe; not shown) is inserted through the wheal. The shaft of the needle should be at a 45° angle with the medial aspect of the arm (**A**), directing its point cephalad toward the apex of the axilla and advancing it slowly. A short-beveled needle can be felt to penetrate the sheath, within which lie the lower portion of the axillary artery and the four major nerves of the plexus. Penetration of the fascial sheath is felt as a "click," after which the needle is advanced 1 to 2 mm to ensure that the bevel is within the fascial sheath. Elicitation of paresthesia obviously indicates contact with one of the major nerves. Injection of 30 to 40 ml of solution while pressure is placed firmly on the neurovascular bundle and its surrounding sheath below the needle enhances diffusion of the solution proximally so as to involve all the branches of the brachial plexus, except those that leave it above the 1st rib. **C.** Some physicians prefer to elicit paresthesia and inject each of the three major nerves at the uppermost part of the arm at the beginning of the brachial artery (*1*). After identifying the artery, an intracutaneous wheal is formed just medial to the artery. A 5-cm 25-gauge short-beveled needle attached to a 10-ml Luer-Lok control syringe containing the local anesthetic solution is inserted through the wheal, and the skin is moved anteriorly about 0.5 cm. While palpating the artery with the second and third fingers of one hand, with the other hand the needle is advanced laterally through the fascial sheath, which can be felt. The needle is advanced another 2 or 3 mm until contact with the median nerve produces paresthesia in its distribution (*2*). Injection of 2 to 3 ml of solution is sufficient to anesthetize the nerve. For block of the ulnar nerve, the maneuver is repeated except, after inserting the needle through the wheal, the skin is moved posteriorly 0.5 cm and advanced until contact with the ulnar nerve elicits paresthesia in its distribution (*3*). To reach the radial nerve, which is posterolateral to the artery, the needle must be inserted 0.5 cm posterior to the point of injection of the ulnar nerve, with the needle passing posterior to the ulnar nerve in a lateral and slightly anterior direction (*4*). At this level the musculocutaneous nerve has passed laterally and is in the substance of the coracobrachialis muscle. To block this nerve it is necessary to insert the needle 0.5 cm anteriorly to where the median nerve is located and to advance the needle laterally into the substance of the muscle, in which 5 ml of solution is usually sufficient to diffuse and block the nerve. For a continuous technique, a 5-cm 18-gauge intravenous catheter is introduced through an opening in the anesthetized skin that has been made with a larger sharp needle. The catheter is directed at an angle of 30° with the skin in a central direction toward the apex of the axilla. Once the tip of the catheter pierces the sheath containing the neurovascular bundle, it is advanced about 2 cm along the side of the artery, the stylet is removed, the solution is injected, and the catheter is fixed firmly in place. Subsequent injections are repeated as necessary.

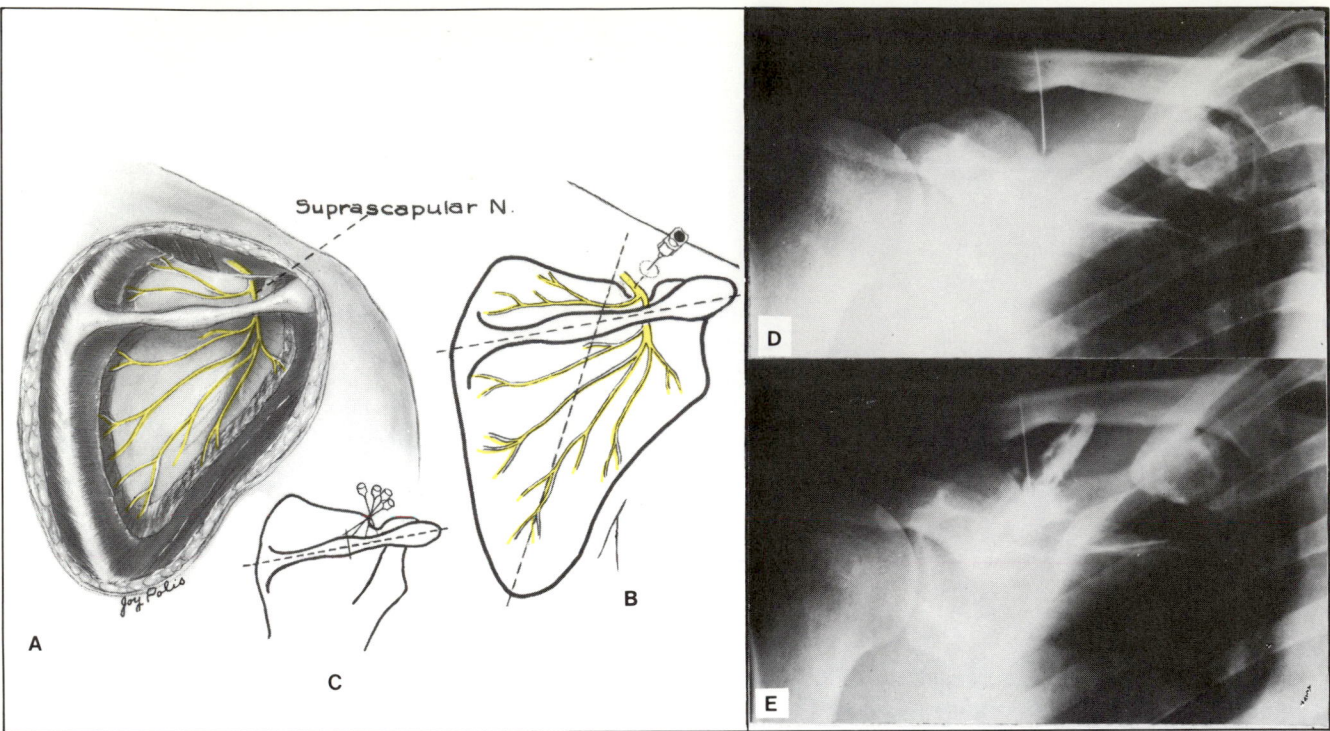

FIG. 94-19. Technique of suprascapular nerve block. **A.** Anatomy of the suprascapular nerve. **B.** Needle placement. After identifying the spine of the scapula a line is drawn on the skin overlying it, with another line bisecting the inferior angle of the scapula (*dashed lines*). The outer triangle formed by the two intersecting lines is bisected and a wheal is formed on this line, about 1.5 cm from the angle. An 8-cm 22-gauge needle is introduced through this wheal so that its shaft is directed anteriorly and slightly caudad and mesiad to make contact with the supraspinatus fossa just lateral to the suprascapular notch. The needle is withdrawn until its point is in the subcutaneous tissue and reintroduced so that its point is directed 5 mm medial to the point of first contact. Advancing the needle in this direction usually causes its point to enter the notch, make contact with the nerve, and elicit paresthesia. **C.** If the second insertion fails to produce paresthesia a third or fourth insertion is made in search of the notch. Usually 3 to 5 ml of a local anesthetic solution produces block of the nerve. The radiographs show the point of the needle in the suprascapular notch before (**D**) and after (**E**) injection of 3 ml of 30% Diodrast. Note the diffusion of the dye.

the level of the wrist can also be used for the same purpose.

The technique of blocking these nerves is described in Figure 94-20. Because the procedure entails approaching the nerve with the shaft of the needle at an angle that is perpendicular to the nerve, it is possible that the nerve could be impaled, with the needle against the underlying bone. It is essential to avoid nerve damage by using a fine (25-gauge) short-beveled needle and to elicit paresthesia gently or use a nerve stimulator. Usually 5 ml of 1% lidocaine or 0.25% bupivacaine is sufficient to block each nerve.

In addition to possible nerve damage, other preventable complications include accidental IV injection but, because the total amount of drug administered with each injection is 50 mg of lidocaine or 12.5 mg of bupivacaine, this should not cause any systemic toxicity.

Thoracic Spinal Nerves

The thoracic spinal nerves transmit nociceptive information from the chest and abdomen and therefore are good sites for diagnostic, prognostic, prophylactic, or therapeutic procedures for various painful disorders involving these structures. Paravertebral block entails injection of the nerves as they exit from the

intevertebral foramen and consequently interrupts both the anterior primary and posterior primary divisions of the nerves as well as the rami communicantes, which contain afferent fibers from the thoracic and abdominal viscera. In addition, the anterior primary division, referred to as the intercostal nerves, can be blocked at various sites along its course.

Paravertebral Block

Indications

Paravertebral block of the thoracic spinal nerves is useful in managing patients with painful disorders involving the thoracic spine, thoracic cage, and abdominal wall. Because this procedure includes the recurrent nerve that supplies the vertebrae and meninges, it is helpful to determine the nociceptive pathways in patients with segmental neuralgia caused by vertebral pathology such as osteoporosis, metastatic fracture, narrowing of the intervertebral foramen because of osteophytes, scoliosis, or herniated intervertebral disk. Unless a prolonged block (3 to 5 days) can be achieved, its value in predicting the effects of neurolytic block of thoracic nerves or surgical rhizotomy is questionable.

Paravertebral block can be used therapeutically to treat acute herpes zoster (76, 77) and fractures of

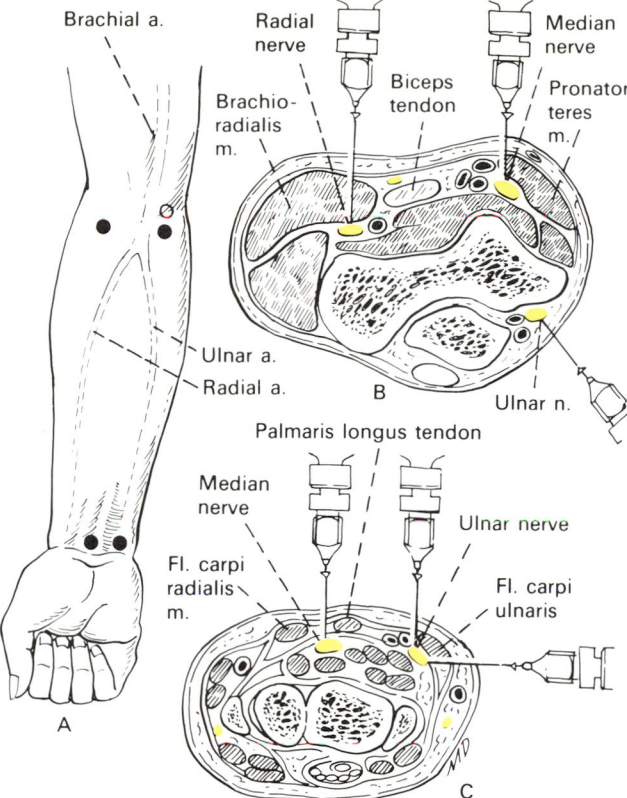

FIG. 94-20. *A.* Sites of blocking of the major nerves at the elbow and wrist. *B.* Cross section of the arm at the elbow. The median nerve is medial to the brachial artery and is at a point midway between the medial epicondyle and the medial edge of the biceps tendon. To block the radial nerve the needle is introduced 1 cm lateral to the lateral edge of the biceps tendon and advanced posteriorly. The ulnar nerve can usually be palpated just medial to the ulnar artery. Care must be exercised to use a fine needle with a short bevel to avoid damage to the nerve or eliciting paresthesia. *C.* Cross section of the arm at the wrist with needles in place to block the median and ulnar nerves. For median nerve block a skin wheal is made between the tendons of the palmaris longus and the flexor carpi radialis. A 3-cm 25-gauge needle is introduced perpendicular to the skin and advanced posteriorly until the nerve is contacted and paresthesia is elicited. For ulnar nerve block the wheal is made just lateral (radial) to the tendon of the flexor carpi ulnaris and medial to the palpable ulnar artery. A 3-cm 25-gauge needle is introduced perpendicular to the skin and directed posteriorly until the nerve is contacted. The ulnar nerve can also be blocked by a median approach, but care must be taken so that the needle is inserted just posterior to the posterior edge of the flexor carpi ulnaris tendon and advanced laterally until paresthesia is elicited.

the head or neck of the rib. Thoracic paravertebral block with local anesthetic can also be used to control severe acute post-thoracotomy pain if the chest incision extends to the paravertebral region. This procedure is also being used to manage patients with chronic post-thoracotomy and post-traumatic pain characterized by dull aching pain accompanied by occasional bouts of severe lancinating segmental pain. In a small percentage of patients, a series of paravertebral blocks with local anesthetics produced lasting benefit (1). In over a dozen patients with segmental neuralgia caused by osteoporosis Bonica noted that a series of paravertebral blocks, and on two occa-

sions a single block, produced prolonged pain relief (1). A possible explanation of the prolonged pain relief is that the block interrupted the skeletal muscle spasm that increased nociceptive input, thus interrupting a vicious circle.

Repeated injections can be used for surgical or traumatic injuries to the chest wall or upper abdomen, or a catheter can be placed in the paravertebral space. The injection of an appropriate volume of local anesthetic through the catheter produces a block of two or three segments.

Technique

The anatomy of the thoracic spinal nerve is described in detail in Chapter 53 and is shown in Figures 53-8 and 94-21. The classic technique of paravertebral block of the thoracic spinal nerves entails insertion of the needle 4 to 5 cm lateral to the spinous process. The needle is advanced anteriorly and medially, with the shaft of the needle making a 45° angle with the midsagittal plane. The needle is advanced until it strikes the appropriate transverse process and then withdrawn until it is subcutaneous. Its direction is changed and the needle readvanced in a direction that causes it to pass inferior to the transverse process until its tip reaches the nerve. Inherent in this approach is the high risk of passing the needle into the deep concavity on either side of the vertebral column that contains the posterior border of the lung, thus risking pneumothorax. Moreover, if the needle is passed further, the intervertebral foramen might be entered, with consequent puncture of the dura and even of the spinal cord.

To circumvent these problems, Bonica (2) developed the paralaminar technique described in Figure 94-22. For diagnostic purposes, 3 ml of 1% lidocaine or 0.25% bupivacaine is used. For treatment of severe acute pain, 5 ml of 0.375 to 0.5% bupivacaine with epinephrine is appropriate. Production of prolonged continuous block of multiple levels involves the injection of 10 to 15 ml of 0.375 to 0.5% bupivacaine with epinephrine through a catheter fixed in place.

Complications

Possible complications include accidental subarachnoid or epidural injection, intravascular injection, and pneumothorax. However, with the paralaminar technique correctly carried out the risk of these complications is virtually eliminated. If a number of segments are blocked, either by individual injections or by the injection of a large volume of solution, extensive sympathetic block might be produced that could result in orthostatic hypotension.

Intercostal Nerve Block

Indications

Block of specific intercostal nerves is a useful diagnostic procedure for defining nociceptive pathways of segmental pain in the chest and in the abdominal wall. Block of the intercostal nerve at the posterior axillary line is particularly useful in differentiating thoracic or abdominal visceral pain from somatic pain caused by disorders of the chest or abdominal wall. For example,

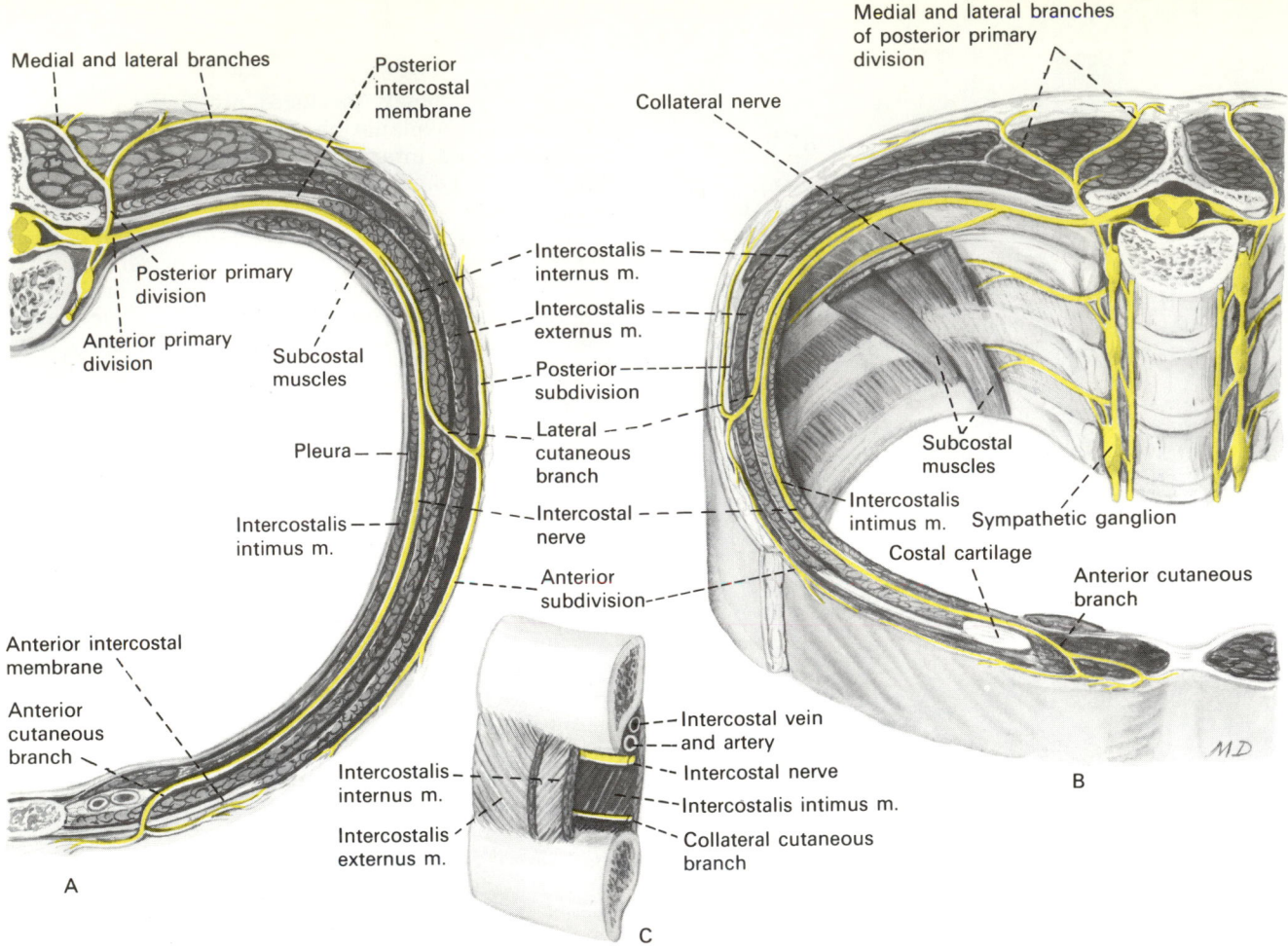

FIG. 94-21. Anatomy of the thoracic spinal nerve. *A.* Superior view of the intercostal space. *B.* Anterior view of the chest. *C.* Cut section of two adjacent ribs. Note that the nerve exits through the intervertebral foramen to reach the paravertebral region, where it promptly divides into the posterior and anterior primary divisions. The anterior primary division, which becomes an intercostal nerve, proceeds between the posterior intercostal membrane and the endothoracic fascia and adjacent pleura. At the angle of the rib it is located between the subcostal muscles and the internal intercostal muscle, and just distal to that it is situated between the intercostal intercostalis intimus and the internal intercostal muscles. The lateral cutaneous branch leaves the parent nerve near the angle of the rib. Note in *B* the relation of the intercostal nerves and their branches and these structures and the thoracic sympathetic chain; *C* shows the direction of fibers of the intercostal muscles and the position of the intercostal vessels and nerves. Modified from Netter, F.H.: The CIBA Collection of Medical Illustrations. Vol. 7. Respiratory System. West Caldwell, NJ, Ciba Pharmaceutical, 1979, p. 11.

in patients complaining of anterior chest pain, the use of intercostal nerve block at the posterior axillary line of the appropriate segments relieves pain of somatic origin but does not relieve pain arising in the thoracic viscera, which are supplied by nociceptive fibers that follow sympathetic pathways located near the vertebral column. Similarly, intercostal block relieves abdominal wall pain but does not relieve pain arising in the abdominal viscera. For most patients it is sufficient to exclude the body wall with intercostal block to implicate a visceral source of the pain, especially if visceral disease is suspected. On the other hand, if any doubt is present, it is best to carry out subsequent block of the visceral nociceptive pathways—an extensive cervicothoracic nerve block relieves the pain arising in the thoracic viscera, while a splanchnic or celiac plexus block relieves pain arising from disease of an upper abdominal viscus.

For therapeutic purposes intercostal nerve block is one of the most useful procedures for the relief of severe acute post-traumatic, postoperative, or postinfection pain in the thoracic or abdominal wall (1, 19,

78–86). It is highly effective in relieving severe pain caused by fractures of one or more ribs (81, 82) or of the sternum, dislocation of the costochondral joint (1, 16), slipped rib cartilage, chest pain associated with pleurisy, and acute herpes zoster (76, 77). It is also a useful diagnostic and therapeutic procedure in cases of entrapment of the intercostal nerve in the rectus sheath, which is said to be a common cause of abdominal pain and occasionally of chest pain (83), although rectus block might be preferable.

The widest use of intercostal block is for the treatment of severe pain after thoracotomy and sternotomy (78, 81) and after renal surgery through flank incisions (87, 88). For chest pain following thoracic surgery, for unilateral abdominal incisions (e.g., Kocher's incision), and for flank incisions for renal surgery unilateral blocks are highly effective, but bilateral intercostal blocks are necessary for sternotomy and midline upper abdominal incisions. The nerve supplying all the spinal segments through which the incision passes should be blocked and it is also necessary to block the segments above and below because of the

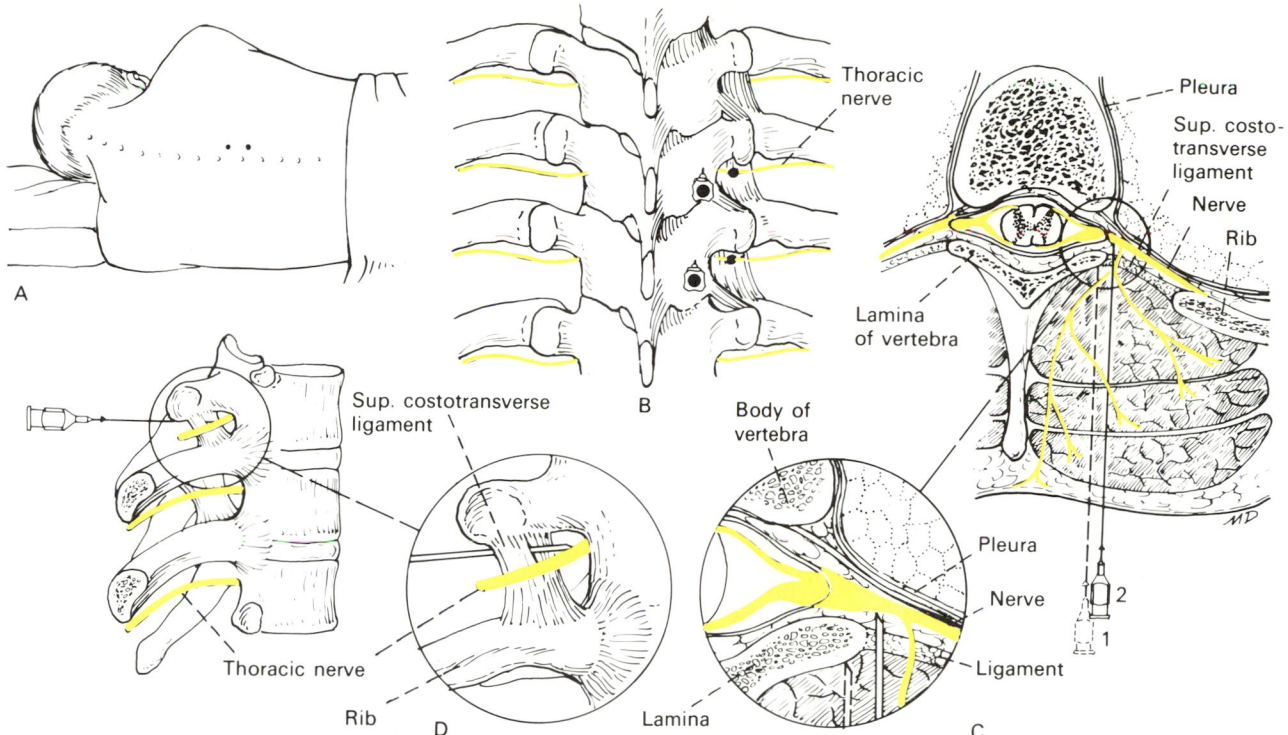

FIG. 94-22. Technique of thoracic paravertebral somatic nerve block. **A.** Position of the patient for block on the right side. Because placement of the needle depends on the relationship between the tips of the spinous processes and the laminae, it is essential to identify each spinous process and to mark it with an indelible pen or marker. After sterilizing the skin, a skin wheal is formed 1.5 cm lateral to the tip of the spinous process of the vertebra above. For block of the somatic nerve, it is best to make contact with the upper portion of the lateral aspect of the lamina. **B.** A 5- or 8-cm 22-gauge short-beveled needle is inserted through the skin wheal perpendicular to the skin. **C.** The needle is advanced until the lateral edge of the lamina is contacted (position 1). The needle is then withdrawn until its point is in the subcutaneous tissue, the skin is moved laterally about 0.5 cm, and the needle is readvanced until its point slips just lateral to the upper part of the lateral edge of the lamina and its point engages the uppermost part of the superior costotransverse ligament just below the proximal portion of the transverse process (position 2). Once the point of the needle is in the ligament, a 2-ml glass syringe filled with saline solution is attached to the needle and an attempt is made to inject the saline. It is important to test the syringe prior to its adaption to the needle to ensure that its plunger slides easily. As long as the tip of the needle is within the ligament, some resistance to the injection can be felt. By exerting constant pressure on the plunger of the syringe with the right hand and advancing the needle *slowly* with the left hand a lack of resistance is felt as soon as the bevel of the needle passes through the upper part of the superior costotransverse ligament and is in the paravertebral region in the immediate vicinity of the nerve. If paresthesia is not elicited, a nerve stimulator is used to ascertain that the bevel of the needle is on the nerve (*C*). The needle is directed in a true sagittal plane rather than at an angle, as is the case with the classical approach (see text). **D.** Lateral view showing the penetration of the superior part of the superior costotranverse ligament and the advancement of the needle until it comes in contact with the nerve.

overlap of these nerves. The intercostal nerve(s) supplying the dermatomes through which surgical drains pass must also be blocked. In patients with severe postoperative pain, the procedure not only relieves the pain but reduces or eliminates reflex muscle spasm and interrupts other reflex phenomena that are initiated by the nociceptive input (Chapters 7 and 25).

Many reports have documented that the analgesia produced by intercostal nerve block is superior to that produced by conventional narcotic analgesia. Post-thoracotomy patients managed with intercostal nerve blocks (Table 94-2) showed less impairment of effort-dependent measures of respiratory function (forced vital capacity, FVC, and peak expiratory flow, PEF, (35, 86, 89–93) and of arterial oxygenation (35, 86) than patients receiving narcotic analgesia. When compared to those receiving postsurgical narcotic analgesia for abdominal operations, patients receiving intercostal

blocks were found to have a better and earlier global recovery and an earlier discharge from hospital (79), better results on tests of respiratory function (e.g., FVC, PEF), less impairment of arterial oxygenation and a reduced incidence of respiratory complications (80) (Table 94-3). Enberg's (80, 86) detailed studies revealed that single unilateral posterior intercostal blocks in patients with subcostal incisions produce appreciable respiratory benefits. Bilateral blocks in patients with midline incisions, however, were less beneficial.

Most studies mentioned above were conducted on fit patients in whom posterior intercostal block was used. It might be expected that maximum benefits from the use of techniques would accrue in patients most likely to have postoperative respiratory difficulties—that is, those with pre-existing respiratory disease—but no studies of controlled clinical trials on the use of

TABLE 94-2. Respiratory Outcome in Post-Thoracotomy Patients Given Single-Dose Intercostal Blocks With Bupivacaine

Source	No. of Patients Studied		Time of Testing*	Parameter Measured†		
	Blocks	Control		Volume Flows‡	Pa_{O_2}	Pa_{CO_2}
Bergh et al. (89)	15	15	24 hours po	+	0	0
Galway et al. (90)	46	46	24 hours po	0	0	0
Kaplan et al. (35)	12	6	24 hours po	+ +	+	0
Delilkan et al. (91)	20	20	4 hours po	+ +	+ +	+ +
Toledo-Peraya and DeMeester (93)	10	10	1–5 days po	+ +	−	−

From Buckley, F.P.: Somatic nerve block for postoperative analgesia. *In* Acute Pain. Edited by G. Smith and B.A. Covino. London, Butterworths, 1985, pp. 205–227.
*po, postoperative.
†0, no difference between patients with nerve blocks and patients receiving opioids; +, some difference between patients with nerve blocks and patients receiving opioids; + +, marked difference between patients with nerve blocks and patients receiving opioids; −, not studied.
‡Peak flow, forced vital capacity, or both.

intercostal blocks in such patients have been reported. Anecdotal reports (94, 95) suggested that bilateral posterior intercostal blocks in patients with respiratory compromise could precipitate respiratory failure, possibly as a consequence of changes in abdominal and chest wall mechanics and in functional residual capacity (FRC) (96) produced by intercostal blocks (96–98).

Bilateral intercostal block in all of these studies was done at the angle of the rib, with consequent motor blockade and weakness or paralysis of all the intercostal and abdominal muscles supplied by the blocked segments. Obviously, unilateral block produces paresis or paralysis of the muscles on one side, which is probably compensated for by the muscles on the contralateral side. Moreover, when the block involves the thoracic intercostal nerves and is done along the posterior axillary or midclavicular line, even bilateral block does not produce ventilatory changes of the same magnitude as bilateral paravertebral or bilateral posterior intercostal block. In patients with pre-existing respiratory disease it is best to use unilateral intercostal block at the posterior axillary or midclavicular line to relieve pain on one side of the abdomen, and to use bilateral rectus block for patients with midline pain (see below). Patients with analgesia limited to the thoracic or abdominal wall require supplementation with modest doses of narcotics to relieve pain arising from the viscera and from a drain or nasogastric tube.

Although segmental epidural block is commonly used for postoperative or post-traumatic pain relief,

intercostal block has the significant advantage of producing analgesia that lasts two to four times longer than that achieved with the same dose injected into the epidural space. Moore (99) reported that, following intercostal block with 4 ml of 0.25% bupivacine with epinephrine, analgesia lasted 10 to 12 hours. This makes it practical to induce intercostal block in the morning and have the patient ambulate, cough, and be as active as possible during the analgesic stage for the remainder of the day. If necessary the block can be repeated in the evening or at least can be repeated each morning. Disadvantages of the use of intercostal block compared with epidural block include the need to make multiple injections once or twice a day and the risk of pneumothorax. The former disadvantage can be obviated by using a continuous intercostal nerve block technique (see below).

Technique

To carry out intercostal block properly, it is necessary to know the anatomy, course, and distribution of the thoracic intercostal nerves to achieve analgesia in the chest and of the thoracoabdominal intercostal nerves to achieve analgesia of the lower chest and the abdominal wall. These aspects are discussed in Chapter 53 and shown in Figures 53-8 and 94-21. Although the intercostal nerves can be blocked at any point along their course, they are usually blocked at the four sites depicted in Figure 94-23.

POSTERIOR INTERCOSTAL BLOCK. Posterior intercostal block is most easily carried out at the angle of the rib because this is the most superficial part of the

TABLE 94-3. Respiratory Outcome in Post-Abdominal Surgery Patients: Narcotics Versus Intercostal Blocks

Source	No. of Patients Studied		Incision	Time of Testing	Parameter Measured*		
	Blocks	Narcotics			Volume Flows†	Pa_{O_2}	Respiratory Complications
Bridenbaugh et al. (79)	17	15	Not stated	Days 1, 2, 3, 4	−	+	0
Engberg (80)	76	85	Unilateral	Days 1 and 2	+	+	+
	36	33	Midline	Days 1 and 2	0	0	+
Engberg (86)	41	20	Unilateral	Days 1 and 2	+	+ +	−
	16	17	Midline	Days 1 and 2	0	0	−

*+, moderate difference between patients with nerve blocks and patients receiving opioids; + +, marked difference between patients with nerve blocks and patients receiving opioids; 0, no difference between patients with nerve blocks and patients receiving opioids; −, not studied.
†Peak flow, forced vital capacity, or both.

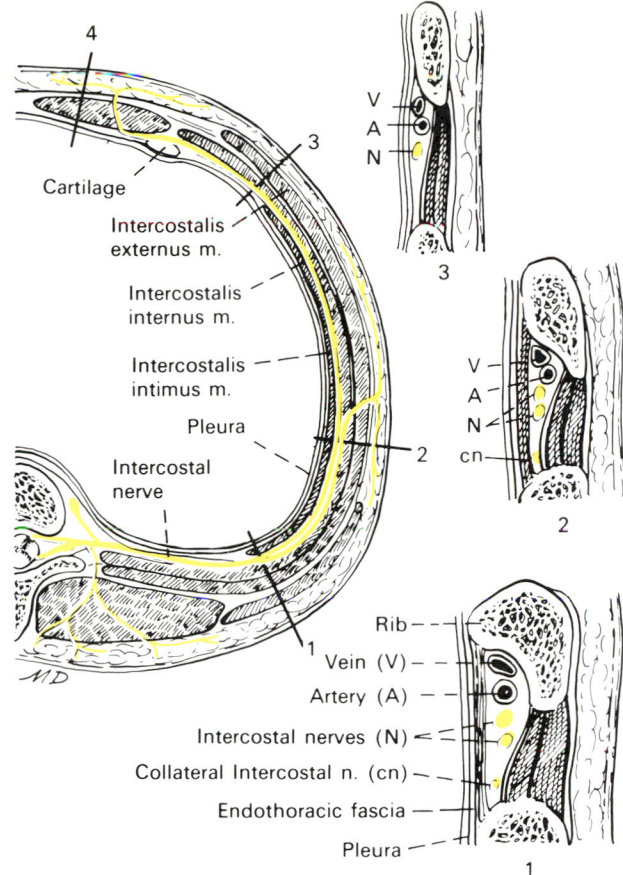

FIG. 94-23. Typical intercostal nerve and the optimal sites for intercostal block. *Left.* Cross section showing the course of the nerve *Right.* Cross sections showing the relationship of the intercostal nerves to the vessels and the muscles. 1. Angle of rib where the intercostal space is a triangular-shaped structure that contains the vein, artery, principal nerve and its lateral cutaneous branch, and collateral branch. The space is bounded medially by the pleura and the endothoracic fascia and the beginning of the intercostalis intimus muscle and laterally by the intercostal groove and the internal and external intercostal muscles. 2. Cross section along the posterior axillary line. Note the difference in shape of the space and of the cross section of the rib. 3. Cross section at the anterior axillary line.

rib and therefore the most easily palpable. Moreover, the rib is thickest and the intercostal groove is broadest and deepest at this site. Here the intercostal space is triangular, has an area of about 0.75 cm², and is filled with fat, through which the intercostal vessels and nerves course (1, 85, 100). At the angle of the rib, the intercostal nerve, its lateral cutaneous branch, and the collateral branch are located relatively close together and are therefore accessible to administration of the local anesthetic solution (1, 85, 100). As noted in Figures 94-21 and 94-23, the space is bounded externally by the intercostal groove, posterior intercostal membrane, and internal and external intercostal muscles and internally by the thin intercostalis intimus muscle and the pleura. The internal and external intercostal muscles are substantial structures bounded on their internal aspects by the posterior intercostal membrane and on their external aspects by the fascia and cutaneous structures.

The technique of posterior intercostal nerve block is described in Fig 94-24. The injection of 3 to 4 ml of local anesthetic solution at the angle of the rib spreads for several centimeters distally and proximally to involve the sympathetic chain (98). This has the advantage of also blocking visceral nociceptive pathways, thus helping to relieve pain arising from the diseased viscus. Injection of larger amounts results in both paravertebral and epidural spread of the drug (101) and, if many segments are involved, arterial hypotension can develop. Although evidence has shown that injection of the drug at one intercostal site causes its subpleural spread to adjacent intercostal nerves (85), this has been contested by Moore and associates (100). Nevertheless, several reports have indicated that a single injection of 20 ml of bupivacaine produces analgesia that involves multiple intercostal nerves (102–104). In one report it was claimed that injection of 20 ml of 0.5% bupivacaine at the T9 interspace produced good analgesia in 87.5% of patients undergoing cholecystectomy (103).

LATERAL INTERCOSTAL BLOCK. Lateral intercostal block is best achieved at the posterior axillary line, 3 to 4 cm posterior to the midaxillary line (Fig. 94-25). At the latter point the lateral cutaneous nerve pierces the intercostal muscles and divides into the anterior and posterior branches (Fig. 94-21). The anterior branch supplies the skin and subcutaneous tissues of the anterolateral chest and abdominal wall as far as 7 cm from the midline, while the posterior branch supplies these tissues as far as 7 to 10 cm from the spine. Although it has been suggested that this technique might produce inadequate analgesia (100), Bonica (1, 2) and Scott (104), among others, believe that it is a highly effective procedure for producing anesthesia during surgery, for producing postoperative analgesia, and for relieving other types of pain.

Block at this site has advantages and disadvantages when compared with posterior intercostal block. Because injection of 3 to 4 ml of solution is unlikely to diffuse to the paravertebral region, its use as a diagnostic procedure is preferable to the use of posterior intercostal block. Block at this site is particularly helpful in differentiating thoracic and abdominal visceral pain from somatic pain caused by disorders of the chest or abdominal wall. For example, in patients with anterior chest pain, the use of an intercostal nerve block of the appropriate segments relieves pain of somatic origin but does not relieve pain arising from thoracic or abdominal viscera, which are supplied by nociceptive fibers associated with sympathetic pathways located in the paravertebral region. Similarly, lateral intercostal block relieves abdominal wall pain but does not relieve pain arising from abdominal visceral disease. Moreover, intercostal block at this site produces less ventilatory impairment and might be preferable in patients with pulmonary disorders (see above). Conversely, because block at this site does not relieve postoperative pain arising from the viscera, supplementary pharmacologic analgesia in the form of nonsteroidal anti-inflammatory drugs and modest doses of opioids should also be given.

CONTINUOUS INTERCOSTAL BLOCK. A number of reports have noted the use of continuous or inter-

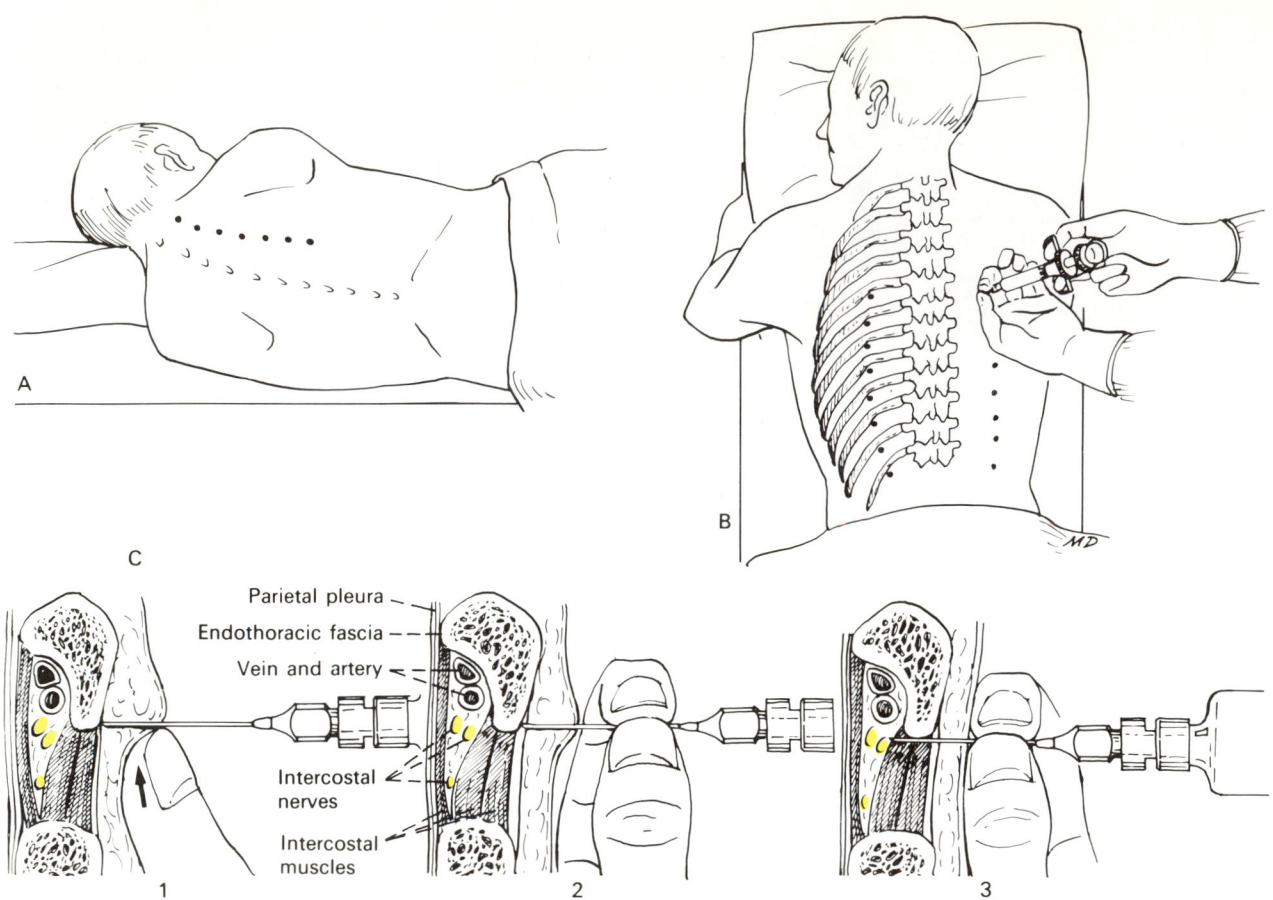

FIG. 94-24. Technique of posterior intercostal block. The injections are done at the angles of the ribs. **A.** The patient lies on the side comfortable for a unilateral block. **B.** The patient is in a prone position to facilitate bilateral block. The dots indicate the sites of injection. **C.** Details of injection. After identifying the space and sterilizing the skin over it an intracutaneous wheal is made just below the lower edge of the rib (**B**). A 3-cm 25-gauge short-beveled needle is inserted through the wheal, after which the second finger of the left hand is placed over the intercostal space and the skin is pushed slightly cephalad so that the lower edge of the rib above can be palpated at the same time the skin over lower edge of the rib is immobilized (1). This finger also protects the intercostal space, thus decreasing the risk of passing the needle too far into the lung. The needle is advanced until the lowermost part of the lateral aspect of the rib is contacted. After the rib is impinged on, the needle is grasped between the thumb and index finger of the left hand, about 3 to 5 mm from the skin (2). The skin is moved caudad with the left index finger to allow the needle to slip just below the lower border of the rib. The needle is advanced until the fingertips grasping the needle are flush with the skin (3). This simple maneuver minimizes the possibility of advancing the needle too deeply and entering the lung. With the needle held steady between the second and third fingers of the left hand, aspiration is attempted; if negative, 3 to 4 ml of solution is injected.

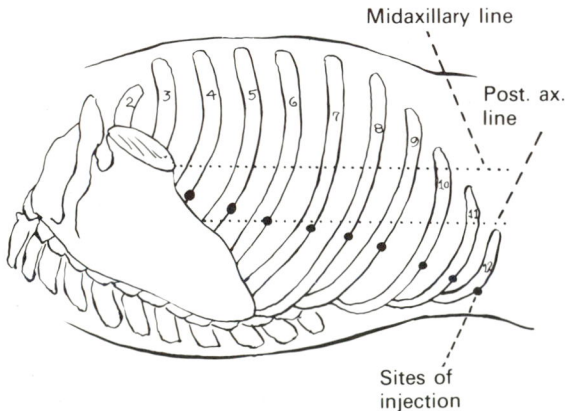

FIG. 94-25. Lateral intercostal block along the posterior axillary line. The black dots indicate the sites of injection posterior to the exit of the lateral cutaneous branches. The technique of introducing the needle is similar to that shown in Figure 94-24.

mittent intercostal nerve block for providing prolonged pain relief after surgery or for relieving post-traumatic conditions. Among the first attempts were those by Ablondi and associates (105), who inserted a Rochester plastic needle along the midaxillary or posterior axillary line into the 5th or 6th intercostal space (depending on the area required for postoperative analgesia) and injected 4 ml of 1% bupivacaine tid or qid for several days. This technique is effective in relieving pain following thoracotomy, an operation in the upper abdomen, lower abdomen, or kidneys (101, 106). Alternative techniques involve the placement of epidural catheters along the intercostal nerves at the end of an intrathoracic or renal operation, with the distal ends protruding through the closed incision (106). A similar technique was used by Blades and Ford (107) in 1950 with good results, and described by Bonica (1).

More recently, it was realized that the injection of a large volume of local anesthetic through a single intercostal injection produces multiple intercostal nerve blocks. This prompted the insertion of epidural catheters into a single space, with the injection of 20 ml of 0.5% bupivacaine at intervals of 6 to 12 hours as needed or a continuous infusion to sustain the analgesia after the initial injection proved effective. Murphy (82) reported the use of continuous intercostal block in 16 patients with multiple fractured ribs, in 33 patients who had had a cholecystectomy, and in 8 patients who had undergone renal surgery, and noted effective pain relief in 52 (91%) of the 57 patients treated. Others have reported similar results (78, 106). The technique produces good unilateral analgesia but, if the block extends posteriorly to the paravertebral region, extensive paravertebral or epidural block is possible (101).

INTRAPLEURAL BLOCK. Intrapleural block, first described by Reiestad and Stromskag (108), is another recent technique that provides unilateral analgesia involving multiple intercostal nerves and shows promise for the relief of postoperative pain and other

acute and chronic painful conditions. The technique (Fig. 94-26) entails the insertion of a standard epidural Tuohy needle and catheter into the pleural space and injection of 0.5% bupivacaine (average adult dose). Although Reiestad prefers to insert the needle and catheter at about 8 to 10 cm from the posterior midline, others have inserted it more laterally at the posterior axillary line. After the needle is removed the catheter is fixed and, after a negative aspiration, 0.5% bupivacaine with epinephrine is injected in amounts varying from 1 to 3 mg/kg body weight (i.e., 7 to 21 ml of 0.5% bupivacaine): In a more recent report, Reiestad (109) stated that more than 750 patients had been managed with this technique and, with 2 exceptions, no other form of analgesia had been necessary. On average, postoperative patients treated intermittently needed "top-up" doses every 9 hours (range, 5 to 26 hours). In patients undergoing thoracotomy, the surgeon introduces the epidural catheter through a Tuohy needle into the pleural space, one or two intercostal spaces above the incision, the internal end of

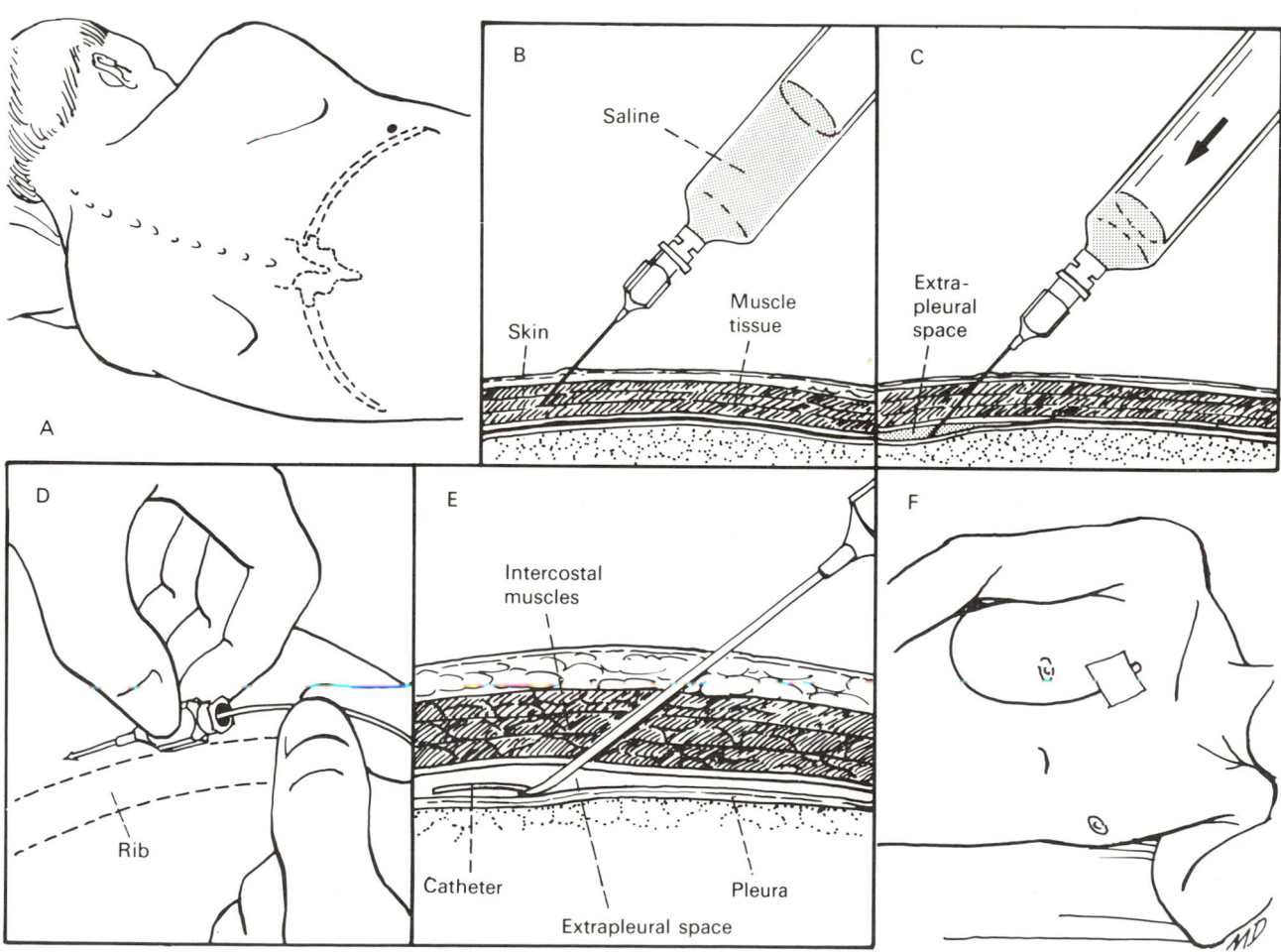

FIG. 94-26. Technique of intrapleural block. **A.** The patient lies on the unaffected side, resting comfortably on a pillow. The dot over the rib outline (*dashed lines*) shows the site of injection of a local anesthetic with a 25-gauge needle prior to insertion of the large Tuohy needle. **B.** A 17-gauge Tuohy needle attached to a syringe containing saline solution is introduced through the wheal with the bevel facing superficially as shown in **E.** The needle is directed so that its shaft makes a 60° angle with the skin. The needle is advanced slowly and carefully through the intercostal muscles and endothoracic fascia into the pleural space. **C.** The entrance of the bevel into the pleural space is indicated by the fact that the saline is sucked into the space by negative intrapleural pressure. **D.** Once the needle is in place a catheter is introduced. **E.** The catheter is advanced 4 or 5 cm, the needle is removed, and the catheter is taped in place. **F.** The patient remains with the painful side uppermost and 20 ml of 0.5% bupivacaine with epinephrine (average adult dose) is injected.

the catheter is loosely sutured next to the vertebra, and the incision is then closed. Some have indicated that, in patients with thoracotomy, this form of analgesia is inadequate because the continuous underwater suction necessary with these patients removes the local anesthetic promptly after injection. Reiestad (109), however, obviated this problem by clamping the drainage tube for about 10–15 minutes during and after injection of the local anesthetic. He has used the procedure for various operations on the chest, upper abdomen, and breast, and for herniorrhaphies. Sihota and associates (110) have reported the efficacy of this procedure in relieving pain of acute herpes zoster, chronic pancreatitis, and postherpetic neuralgia.

The underlying mechanism of intrapleural catheter analgesia is probably a combination of diffusion of local anesthetic through the pleura to block the intercostal nerves and posterior diffusion to block the somatic and sympathetic nerves near the vertebral column.

ANTEROLATERAL AND ANTERIOR INTERCOSTAL BLOCK. Anterolateral intercostal block (Fig. 94-27) is done along the anterior axillary line proximal to the takeoff of the anterior cutaneous branches of the thoracic intercostal nerves. It is useful in relieving the pain of sternotomy and fracture of the sternum or of the costal cartilages. The technique can also be used to block the upper three or four thoracoabdominal intercostal nerves (T7 to T10) just proximal to the costochondral articulation to provide analgesia in the upper abdominal wall. Figure 94-27 also depicts parasternal injection, which is done bilaterally to relieve pain caused by fractures or other pathologic processes of the sternum. This technique, like lateral intercostal block, does not interrupt visceral nociceptive pathways. Therefore, patients undergoing the procedure for postoperative pain following intrathoracic or intra-abdominal surgery, should be supplemented with nonopioid or opioid analgesics or a combination of both. On the other hand, the technique usually produces complete relief of pain arising from the anterior thoracic or abdominal wall.

RECTUS BLOCK. Bilateral rectus block (Fig. 94-28) can be used to relieve severe pain produced by a midline abdominal incision. As noted in Figures 94-21 and 94-28, the anterior branch of the thoracoabdominal intercostal nerve enters the abdominal wall by passing behind the costal cartilages and entering the space between the transversus abdominis and internal oblique muscles. These anterior cutaneous nerves then pass medially within this space as far as the semilunar line, where they perforate the posterior sheath of the rectus abdominis muscle near its lateral margin. Within the sheath they course between the posterior aspect of the muscle and the posterior sheath as far as the middle of the muscle, where they turn anteriorly and pass through the substance of the muscle and perforate its anterior sheath to become the anterior cutaneous nerves of the abdominal wall. While within the rectus sheath they give off branches to the rectus abdominis muscles. Below the arcuate line the rectus abdominis muscle lacks the posterior sheath, and is separated from the peritoneum only by the transversalis fascia and extraperitoneal fat.

Another example of the efficacy of regional anesthesia for surgery in delaying the onset of postoperative pain and reducing its incidence has been demonstrated for rectus block. Smith and associates (111) studied 24 patients who were to undergo diagnostic laparoscopy with light balanced general anesthesia alone (group A) and compared these with 22 patients who received bilateral rectus block in addition to the general anesthesia (group B). The mean pain scores at 3 postoperative assessment intervals were as follows: Group A, 7.1 at 1 hour, 4.3 at 6 hours, and 3.2 at 10 hours; Group B, 0.7 at 1 hour, 0.4 at 6 hours, and 1.6 at 10 hours. The differences were highly significant. The percentages of patients who were *pain-free* at each of the 3 postoperative assessment intervals were as follows: Group A, 0, 0, and 8; Group B, 86, 91, and 68. These differences were highly significant statistically.

Complications

The most serious complication of percutaneous intercostal block is pneumothorax, with a quoted incidence ranging from about 0.13 to 4% (44, 100). When carried out by an expert regional anesthetist who has a thorough knowledge of the anatomy and experience with the procedure, the incidence of pneumothorax should be lower than 1%.

A systemic toxic reaction can also occur. Because absorption of local anesthetic from the intercostal space occurs at a faster rate and to a greater extent

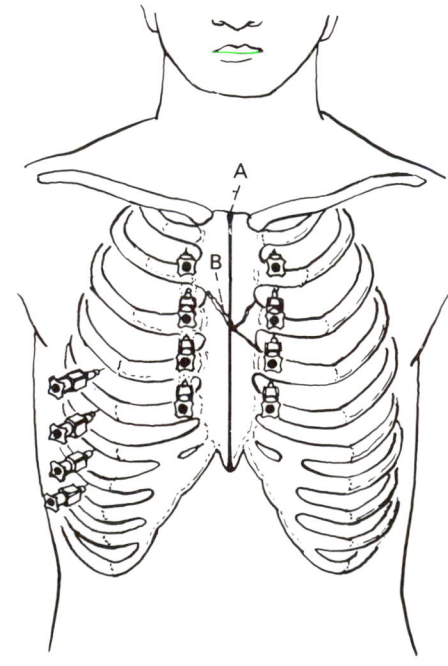

FIG. 94-27. Technique of anterolateral intercostal nerve block at the anterior axillary line (on the right side of the figure). At this point the intercostal nerve and vessels lie between the internal intercostal muscle and the endothoracic fascia and pleura (see Fig. 94-24C). To relieve the pain of sternotomy (A) or fracture of the sternum (B), an anterior intercostal block is done 2 cm lateral to the lateral edge of the sternum; the block is supplemented with subcutaneous infiltration above the sternum and medial part of the clavicle to block the branches of the cervical plexus. The technique of introducing the needle is similar to that shown in Figure 94-25.

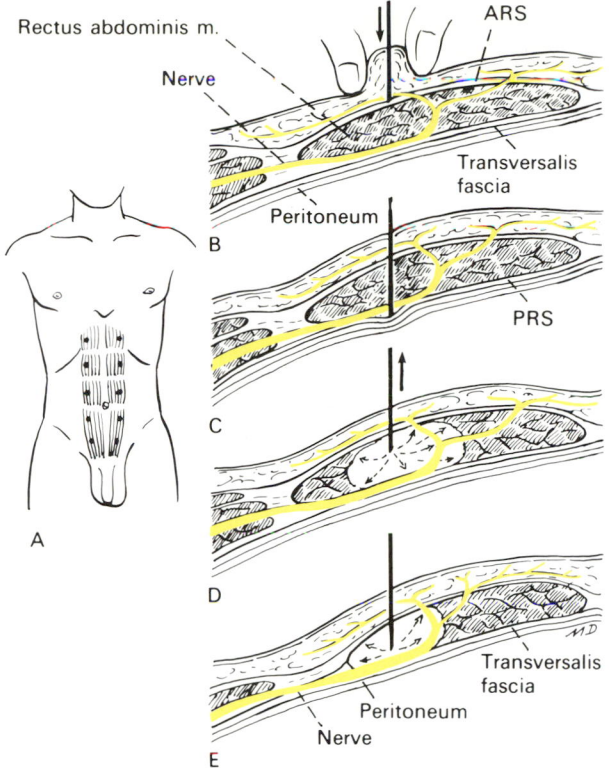

FIG. 94-28. Technique of rectus block (left side). *A.* Sites of insertion of the needle in the middle and slightly lateral part of each segment of the rectus muscle body, which can be palpated between the tendinous insertions. For an upper abdominal midline incision the upper three sites are injected bilaterally, whereas the lower two or three sites are injected bilaterally for a lower midline incision. Skin wheals and injections of the superficial subcutaneous tissue are produced at the appropriate sites for the introduction of a 5-cm 22- or 23-gauge short-beveled needle attached to a Luer-Lok control syringe filled with a local anesthetic. The needle is then passed through the skin and subcutaneous tissue. *B.* Technique for facilitating penetration of the skin by the short-beveled needle. The skin around the wheal is grasped between the thumb and second finger as the needle is passed through the skin and subcutaneous tissue and advanced until it meets the firm resistance of the anterior rectus sheath (ARS). The needle is advanced with steady pressure to penetrate the sheath. This is felt as a definite "snap." *C.* The needle is advanced slowly through the softer belly of the muscle until it meets a second site of resistance as it contacts the posterior rectus sheath (PRS). (The distance between the ARS and PRS should be noted to estimate the thickness of the muscle accurately.) *D.* As the needle rests on the PRS against which the nerve lies, 3 to 4 ml of local anesthetic solution is injected and the needle is withdrawn slowly. At the same time another 2 to 3 ml of solution is discharged within the belly of the muscle. *E.* Below the semicircular line of Douglas the PRS is lacking and the nerve is against the transversalis fascia, which provides no resistance to the needle. Therefore, after pentetration of the ARS, the needle is cautiously advanced for the same distance as noted for the upper levels of the muscle before injection of the anesthetic solution.

than after injection at most other sites (112, 113), the potential for systemic toxic reaction with intercostal block is high, especially after injection of large therapeutic doses. This problem can be obviated or at least minimized by the addition of epinephrine to the local anesthetic solution and by the use of an optimal concentration and reasonable volume of the drug, so that the total dose does not exceed the amount listed in Table 94-1.

Despite the fact that the drug can spread to involve a paravertebral nerve following percutaneous block, cardiovascular homeostasis is usually undisturbed. Following intrathoracic block (i.e., block done by the surgeon while within the thoracic cavity), hypotension or cardiovascular collapse has been reported to have been caused by subarachnoid block (114, 115) or by widespread paravertebral block (116, 117).

Lumbar and Sacral Spinal Nerves

The lumbar and sacral nerves are considered here together because they both supply the pelvis and lower extremities, and consequently are frequently involved together in conditions that indicate analgesic block. Because these nerves, like those of the upper extremities, contain somatosensory, somatomotor, and sympathetic fibers, blockade can be used to manage the same disorders as those discussed in connection with block of the brachial plexus (see above).

Paravertebral Lumbar Somatic Nerve Block

Indications

Paravertebral block of one or more of the lumbar nerves is a useful diagnostic procedure for determining the specific nociceptive pathway(s) associated with herniated intervertebral disk, vertebral pathology, or peripheral nerve pathology. It is also useful for predicting the effects of blocking the nerves involved in massive reflex spasm of the adductors in patients with such neurologic problems as multiple sclerosis or paraplegia. For these purposes the nerve must be identified precisely by carrying out radiographic verification of the level of insertion and by eliciting paresthesia or using a nerve stimulator. Lumbar paravertebral block is also useful in providing relief of severe postnephrectomy pain and severe pain caused by fracture of a lumbar vertebra.

Technique

The anatomy of the lumbar and sacral nerves and the nerves derived from the lumbar and lumbosacral plexuses is described in Chapter 70. Figure 94-29 illustrates the anatomy of the lumbar and sacral nerves and plexuses and the major nerves derived from the lumbar plexus. As they exit from the intervertebral foramina, the lumbar nerves and plexuses are located in the psoas compartment formed by the posterior fascia of the psoas muscle anteriorly, the anterior fascia of the quadratus lumborum together with the transverse processes and intertransverse ligaments posteriorly, and the bodies of the vertebrae medially. This has an important clinical application.

The technique of paravertebral block of one or more of the lumbar nerves is similar to that of blocking the thoracic spinal nerves (Fig. 94-30). For diagnostic or prognostic purposes only 2 ml of a potent local anesthetic solution (e.g., 0.5% bupivacaine with

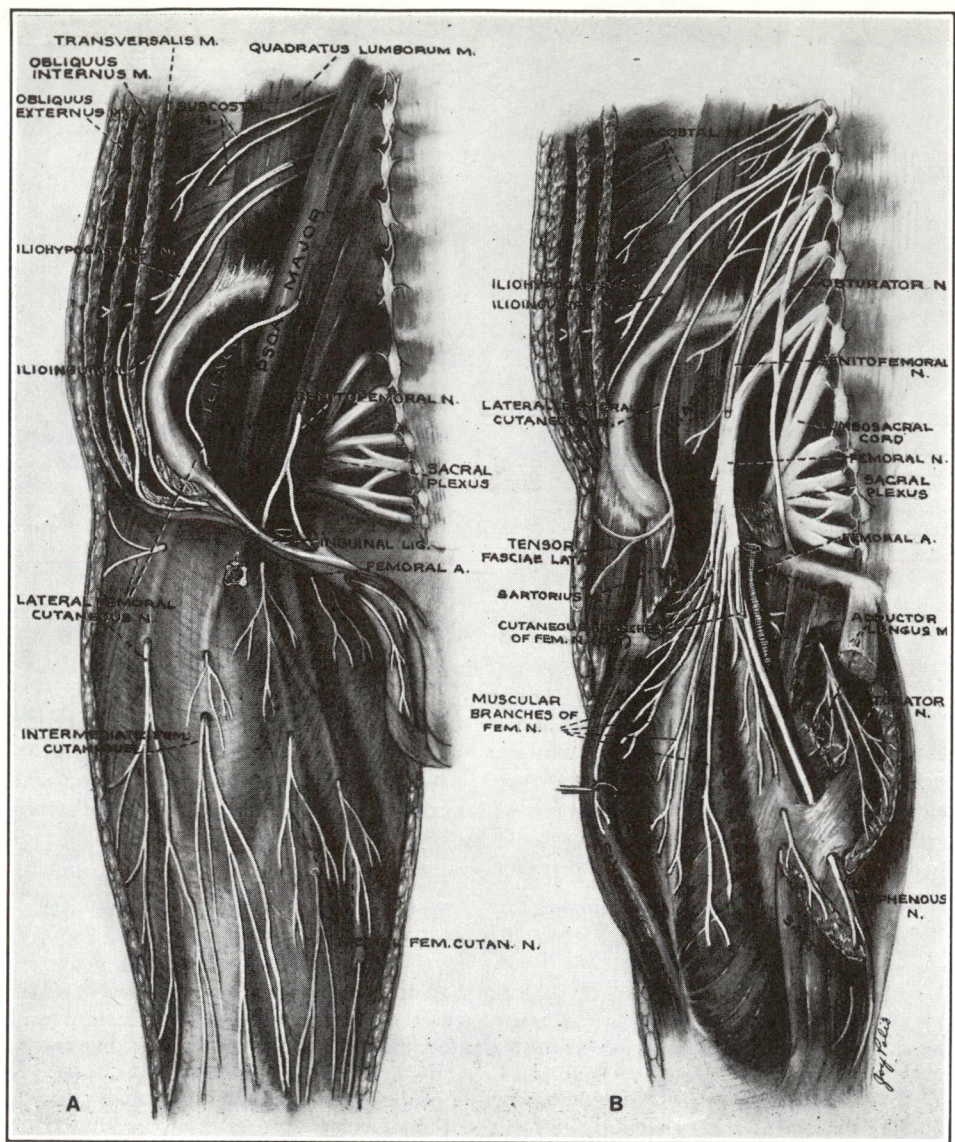

FIG. 94-29. Anatomy of the lumbar and sacral nerves, lumbar and sacral plexus, and the nerves derived from these. **A.** Course of the iliohypogastric, ilioinguinal, lateral femoral cutaneous, and genitofemoral nerves. **B.** The iliopsoas, inguinal ligament, and deep fascia of the thigh have been removed to show the formation of the lumbar and sacral plexuses and the nerves derived from the lumbar plexus. The ilioinguinal and iliohypogastric nerves are derived from the anterior primary division of the L1 nerve while the lateral femoral cutaneous nerve is derived from the L2 and L3 nerves. The femoral nerve, which is derived from the L2, L3, and L4 nerves, begins to divide into its muscular and cutaneous branches just behind (posterior to) the inguinal ligament and lateral to the femoral artery. The obturator nerve is formed within the substance of the psoas muscle by the union of the ventral branches of the anterior primary divisions of the L2, L3, and L4 lumbar nerves. It emerges from the muscle and descends, accompanied by the obturator vessels, passes through the oburator foramen, and enters the upper thigh, where it breaks up into branches.

epinephrine) should be injected after radiographic verification of the position of the bevel of the needle in the correct segment. Provided the bevel of the needle is within 1 to 2 mm of the nerve, this volume is sufficient to block the formed nerve as it exits from the intervertebral foramen. For therapeutic purposes 5 ml of solution can be used to achieve longer analgesia, but this is likely to spread to one or more adjacent segments. Indeed, because the lumbar nerves and plexus are located in the psoas compartment (Fig. 70-25), injection of 25 to 30 ml of local

anesthetic solution through one needle placed at L3 or L4 and advanced 1 cm anterior to the transverse process to place it in the compartment will cause the solution to diffuse cephalad and caudad sufficiently to block all the sympathetic nerves, the lumbar plexus, and even the lumbosacral trunk. A special technique of "psoas compartment block" has been described (118), but it is more complicated and is associated with a higher incidence of failure to block the lumbar plexus completely than the technique described here.

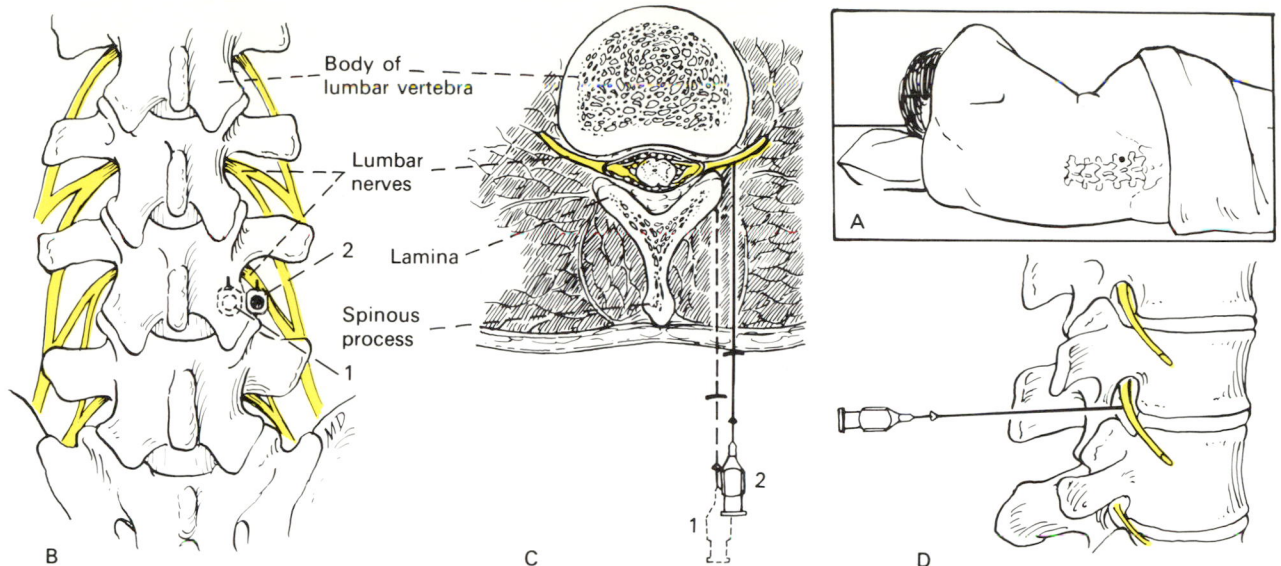

FIG. 94-30. Technique of lumbar paravertebral somatic block. **A.** Position of the patient (sterile drapes omitted for clarity). After identifying the spinous process of the appropriate vertebra (or vertebrae) and marking it with an indelible pen or marker, the skin is prepared with an antiseptic solution and a skin wheal is raised 1.5 cm lateral to the upper portion of the quadrilaterally shaped spinous process. Using a 5-cm 25-gauge needle, the subcutaneous and deeper structures are infiltrated with 5 to 7 ml of a dilute solution of local anesthetic (e.g., 0.5% lidocaine or 0.125% bupivacaine) until contact with the lamina of the vertebra is made. This infiltration should produce a region of analgesia about 2 cm in diameter for the painless introduction and advancement of an 8-cm 22-gauge short-beveled needle. The 22-gauge needle is inserted perpendicular to the skin in a parasagittal plane and advanced until it makes contact with the upper lateral part of the ipsilateral lamina of the vertebra (dashed line of hub of needle; step 1 in **B** and **C**). Care should be taken so that the point of the needle contacts the uppermost part of the lateral edge of the lamina, because this is at the same cross-section level as the nerve as it exits from the intervertebral foramen. Once the lamina is contacted a rubber marker is placed on the needle shaft 1.5 cm from the skin, the needle is withdrawn until its point is subcutaneous and the needle is then moved laterally about 0.5 cm. The needle is advanced until either the lateral edge of the lamina is contacted or the needle passes so that the marker is flush with the skin and its point makes contact with the nerve, eliciting paresthesia. It might be necessary to carry out a second or third insertion before the needle passes just lateral to the edge of the lamina. Because of the large size of the lumbar nerves, contact usually is easily made and paresthesia elicited. If difficulty is encountered, a nerve stimulator is helpful. **D.** Lateral view to show position of needle.

Complications

Complications of lumbar paravertebral block are similar to those of thoracic paravertebral block, except pneumothorax does not occur.

Trans-Sacral Block

Indications

Block of one or more of the sacral nerves by the trans-sacral technique is used for diagnostic or prognostic purposes. Block of the S1 nerve is useful for determining specific nociceptive pathways in patients with herniated intervertebral disk of this nerve root. Block of the S2, S3, and S4 nerves is also useful as a diagnostic or prognostic procedure in patients with perineal pain and can help to define specific nociceptive pathways in patients with pain in pelvic structures, such as the bladder or prostate, especially if neurolytic or ablative procedures for the relief of severe intractable pain are being considered. Because perineal pain relief can be achieved with pudendal block, a procedure that does not involve the nerves to the lower limb, it is preferable to trans-sacral block for relief of severe acute pain in the perineum.

Technique

The technique of trans-sacral nerve blocks is illustrated in Figure 94-31. For diagnostic or prognostic purposes a small volume of drug (e.g., 2 ml) should be used. For therapeutic purposes a larger volume (e.g., 3 to 5 ml) can be used.

Complications

Accidental IV injection can occur but, with the amount of local anesthetic injected, few or no systemic effects are likely to develop. Another complication is unintentional damage to the nerve caused by its penetration with a large needle. This can be prevented by using a short-beveled needle and eliciting paresthesia gently or using a peripheral nerve stimulator.

Femoral Nerve Block

Indications

Block of the femoral nerve just below the inguinal ligament can be used as a diagnostic procedure in patients with severe anterior thigh pain, or it can be used along with sciatic nerve block to produce sympathetic interruption of the lower limb. The most common use for this procedure has been for the control of severe post-traumatic or postoperative pain in the region of the distribution of the femoral nerve. It is also useful to relieve severe pain caused by fracture of the neck of the femur (119, 120).

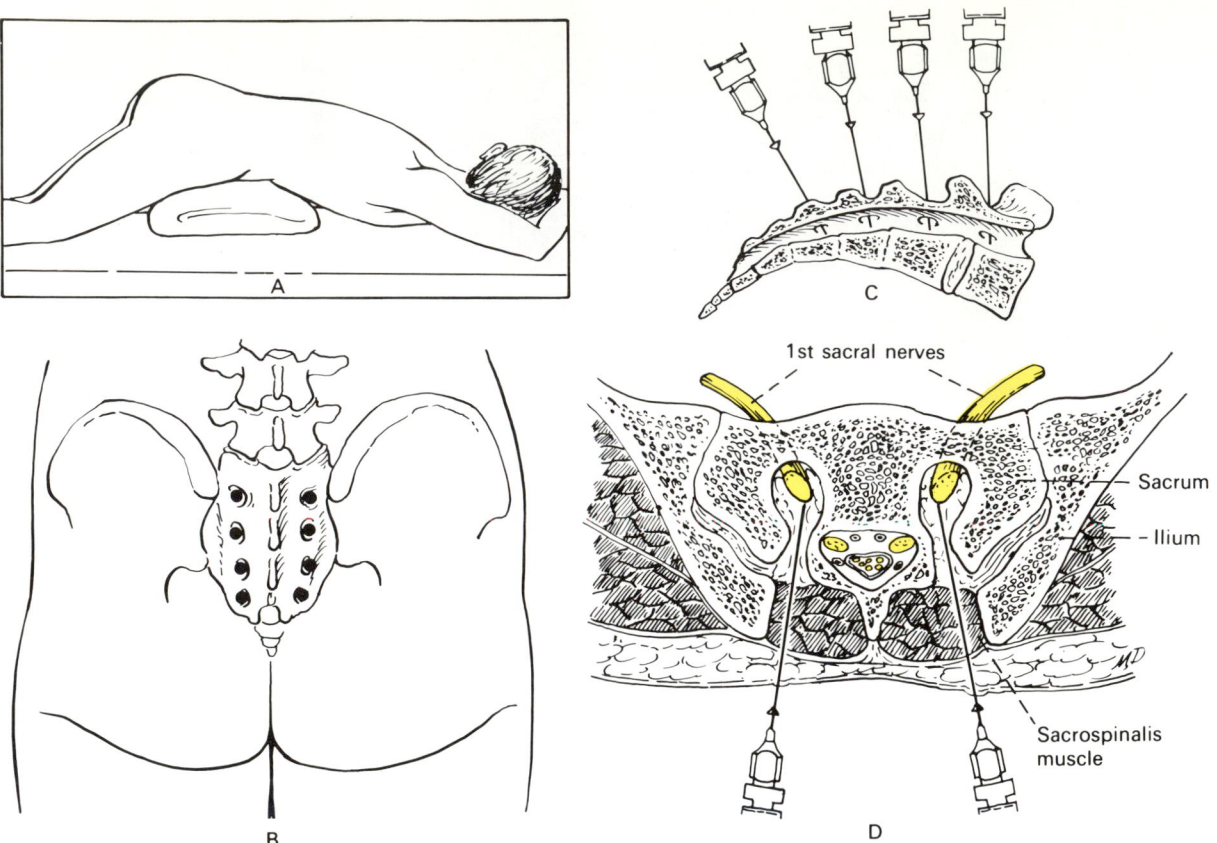

FIG. 94-31. Technique of trans-sacral nerve block. *A.* Position of the patient. *B.* Posterior view of the sacrum showing location of points of insertion. *C.* Sagittal view showing directions of needles. *D.* Cross section showing needles in position for block of the 1st sacral nerves. After identifying the posterior superior iliac spine and the sacral cornu on the ipsilateral side, a line is drawn between a point 1.5 cm medial to the spine and a point 1.5 cm lateral and cephalad to the ipsilateral cornu. For block of the S1 nerve a wheal is made on the drawn line, 1.5 cm cephalad to the level of the iliac spine. For block of the S2 nerve the wheal is made 1.5 cm below the level of the iliac spine. Because some variation exists in the location of the foramina, it is necessary to make a systematic search until the needle is felt to go through the posterior foramen to the trans-sacral canal. Contact with the nerve produces paresthesia.

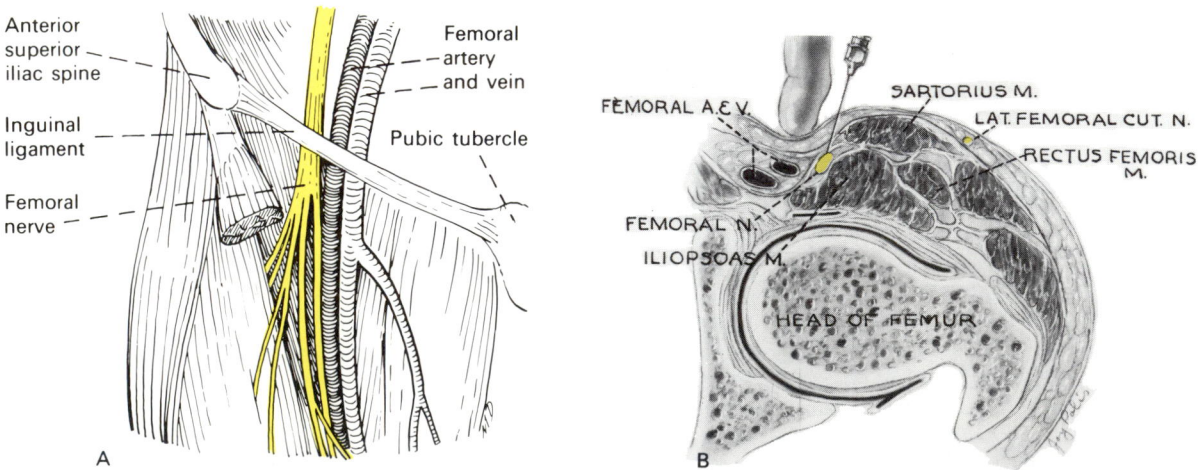

FIG. 94-32. Technique of blocking the femoral nerve. *A.* Anterior view of the region showing the relation of the femoral nerve to the artery and vein. *B.* Cross-section of the femoral nerve just below the inguinal ligament. With the patient lying supine a line is drawn joining the anterior superior iliac spine and the pubic tubercle. The midpoint of this line usually overlies the femoral artery, which is easily palpated. After preparation of the skin a skin wheal is raised 1 cm lateral to the junction of the femoral artery and inguinal ligament. With the second finger of the left hand palpating the artery, a 5-cm 22- or 25-gauge short-beveled needle is introduced through the wheal perpendicular to the skin and advanced until paresthesia is elicited in the distribution of the femoral nerve. If paresthesia is not elicited a nerve stimulator can be used. If a continuous block of this nerve is needed, a 5-cm 20-gauge intravenous catheter can be introduced so that its shaft makes an angle of 60° with the skin distal to the point of insertion. This aids in threading the catheter into the femoral sheath (see Fig. 96-35 for details of insertion).

Technique

The anatomy of the femoral nerve is described in Chapter 70 and in Figure 70-27. Figure 94-32 describes the technique of femoral nerve block. In most people the nerve does not give off its many branches until it passes below the inguinal ligament, and therefore the nerve trunk can easily be located and paresthesia elicited. In some individuals, however, the nerve breaks up into its several branches above the inguinal ligament, and it is more difficult to contact these small nerves and elicit paresthesia. Usually 8 to 10 ml of 1% lidocaine with epinephrine produces analgesia for 3 to 4 hours, whereas the same volume of 0.25% bupivacaine with epinephrine produces analgesia for 6 to 8 hours. If longer analgesia is required the concentration of the bupivacaine can be increased to 0.5% with epinephrine or a continuous block can be used by placing a catheter as described in Figure 94-35.

Complications

The only possible complication of femoral nerve block involves accidental intra-arterial or IV injection if the needle is misplaced more medially than it should be. Unintentional penetration of the nerve produces transient dysesthesia or even neurologic sequela, especially if a large long-beveled needle is used.

Obturator Nerve Block

Obturator nerve block can be used as a diagnostic or prognostic procedure in patients with adductor muscle spasm and pain caused by neurologic injury. Because the obturator nerve contributes a major portion of the nerve supply to the hip joint, it was formerly used as a diagnostic or prognostic procedure prior to obturator neurectomy in patients with severe intractable pain in the hips caused by osteoarthritis; however, the advent of arthroplasty has almost eliminated this application. In the rare patient in whom the technique might be indicated, it needs to be combined with block of the nerve to the quadratus femoris and of the articular branch of the nerve to the rectus femoris (a branch of the femoral nerve), because both also contribute to the innervation of the hip joint.

Technique

The technique of obturator nerve block is described in Figure 94-33 and is included for the sake of completeness. Because the nerve is not close to bony landmarks but is located in the center of the obturator canal, it is desirable to use a peripheral nerve stimulator to ensure accurate placement of the bevel of the needle near the target. Usually injection of 10 to 15 ml of 1% lidocaine with epinephrine produces analgesia for 3 to 4 hours. With injection of 0.25% bupivacaine with epinephrine the duration of analgesia is increased to 6 to 8 hours, and with 0.5% bupivacaine it can be as long as 8 to 12 hours.

Complications

Accidental injection into the obturator vein is likely to produce a mild systemic reaction. Accidental injection into the obturator artery is of no consequence because the drug is diluted by the time it is circulated through the limb and returned to the heart.

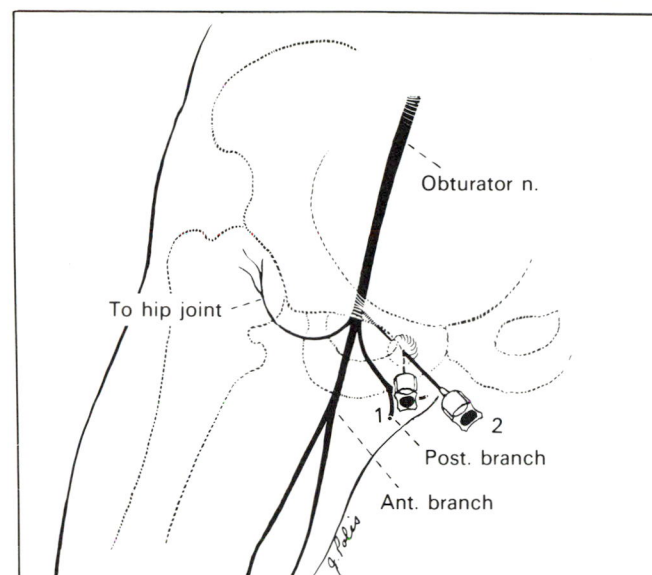

FIG. 94-33. Technique of obturator nerve block. The pubic tubercle is located and marked with the patient lying supine. After preparation of the skin, a wheal is raised 1.5 cm lateral and inferior to the tubercle. An 8-cm 22-gauge needle is introduced through the wheal perpendicular to the skin and advanced posteriorly until contact is made with the inferior ramus of the pubis (position 1). A needle marker is placed 2.5 cm from the skin and the needle withdrawn until its point is in the subcutaneous tissue. The point of the needle is redirected in a lateral and slightly superior direction so that the shaft of the needle is parallel to the superior ramus of the pubis. The needle is slowly advanced while its point is kept in contact with the inferomedial surface of the superior ramus of the pubis, until the marker is flush with the skin or contact with the bone is lost (position 2). Because paresthesia is often difficult to elicit, a nerve stimulator is used to position the point of the needle on the nerve. A volume of 10 to 15 ml of local anesthetic is injected.

Lateral Femoral Cutaneous Nerve Block

Indications

Lateral femoral cutaneous nerve block is done primarily as a diagnostic procedure in patients with pain in the anterolateral thigh, especially those who have a presumptive diagnosis of meralgia paresthetica. The latter condition has various causes, most of which can be eliminated by conservative treatment. Block is only used to confirm the diagnosis.

Technique

The technique of lateral femoral cutaneous nerve block is described in Figure 94-34. Injection of 5 to 8 ml of lidocaine with epinephrine produces analgesia for 3 to 4 hours. With 5 to 8 ml of 0.25% bupivacaine with epinephrine analgesia lasts for 6 to 8 hours, and with 0.5% bupivacaine with epinephrine it lasts for 8 to 12 hours.

Complications

Complications are rare and consist of transient neuropathy in cases of accidental damage to the nerve.

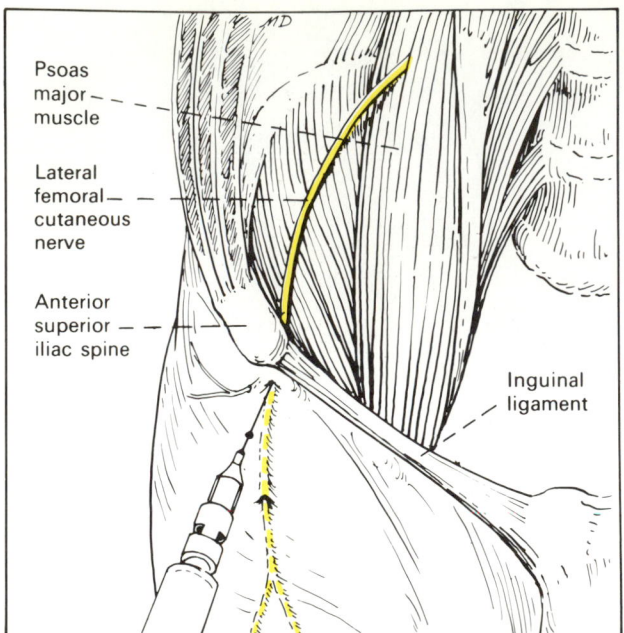

FIG. 94-34. Technique of lateral femoral cutaneous nerve block. After preparation of the skin, a wheal is produced 1.5 cm caudad to the anterior superior iliac spine just below the inguinal ligament. A 5-cm 22- or 25-gauge short-beveled needle is introduced through the skin wheal with its shaft at an angle of about 60° degrees with the skin. The needle is advanced until paresthesia is elicited or the bone is contacted. In the latter case the needle should be withdrawn until its point is subcutaneous and the skin wheal moved 0.5 cm lateral and superior; the needle is then reinserted and advanced until paresthesia is elicited. The nerve is usually located by making several insertions through the same wheal in a line parallel to the inguinal ligament. A volume of 5 to 8 ml of local anesthetic is injected.

Inguinal Perivascular (Three-In-One) Block

The nerves that make up the lumbar plexus, like those of the brachial plexus, are invested in a fascial sheath that originates from the transverse processes of the lumbar vertebrae and continues distally to enclose the plexus, forming a cone whose apex is at the femoral canal. By introducing a large volume (30 ml) of solution into the sheath of the femoral nerve at the femoral canal, and obstructing the sheath distal to the point of injection, the local anesthetic is forced to flow proximally within the sheath and diffuse toward the paravertebral region, thus producing block of the femoral, lateral femoral cutaneous, and obturator nerves in a high percentage of cases (121).

Indications

Block of these three nerves can be used for the relief of severe postoperative or post-traumatic pain located in the area supplied by these nerves, which are derived from the lumbar plexus. This technique, combined with block of the sciatic nerve, produces analgesia of the entire lower limb and sympathetic block of the foot, leg, and lower two-thirds of the thigh. It can therefore be used to confirm the effects of lumbar sympathetic block when the results of the latter technique are in doubt. By using a combination

of 0.5% bupivacaine and 1% etidocaine, the three nerves can be blocked to produce complete paralysis of the muscles of the lower limb. This procedure can then be used to differentiate limitation of motion and deformity caused by reflex muscle spasm from that produced by irreversible changes in muscles and tendons, as discussed in connection with brachial plexus block (see above).

Technique

The technique of the inguinal perivascular or three-in-one block is similar to that described for

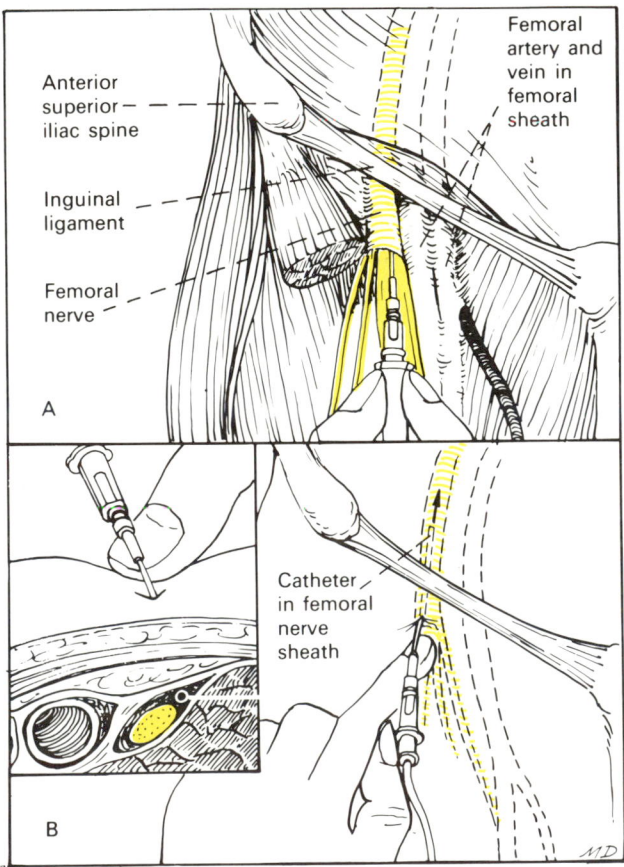

FIG. 94-35. Technique of continuous inguinal perivascular block. **A.** Following preparation of the skin with an antiseptic, an intracutaneous wheal is formed 1 cm lateral to the palpable femoral artery and 1 cm below the inguinal ligament. A 5-cm 18-gauge Teflon-coated intravenous catheter threaded over a 9-cm 22-gauge spinal needle is used. It might be necessary to make a small skin incision to facilitate introduction of the intravenous catheter through the skin. The needle is introduced through the skin wheal and advanced cephalad parallel to the artery, with its shaft making a 30° angle with the skin distal to it. This angle permits the catheter to be advanced within the sheath cephalad and minimizes damage to the nerve. **B.** Entrance into the tough sheath that surrounds the femoral nerve can be felt as a click or snap. The catheter is advanced about 3 cm within the sheath, the needle is removed, and the catheter is fixed in place. Once the catheter is in place aspiration is carried out; if negative, 30 ml of solution is injected while the second finger of the left hand presses forcefully on the artery just distal to the entrance of the catheter (*inset*), thus forcing the fluid to flow proximally. With this volume of solution, block of the femoral, lateral femoral cutaneous, and obturator nerves is achieved.

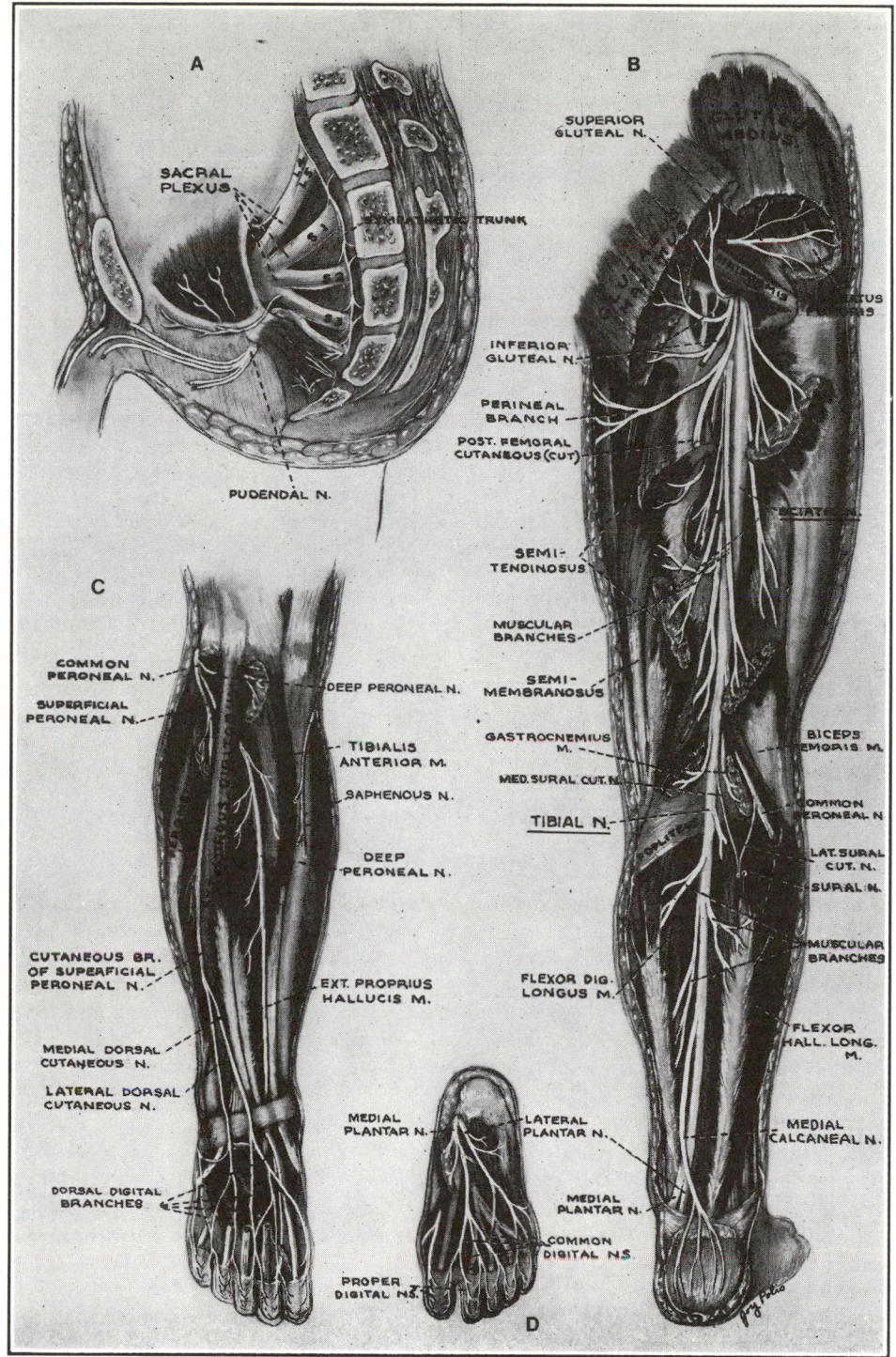

FIG. 94-36. Anatomy of the sacral plexus (*A*) and of the sciatic, tibial, and peroneal nerves and their branches (*B, C*). *D.* Plantar surface of the foot. Block of the sciatic nerve is usually performed just below the piriformis muscle. See Chapter 70 for a detailed description of these nerves.

femoral nerve block, with slight modifications (Fig. 94-35). Injection of 30 ml of 0.25 or 0.5% bupivacaine with epinephrine produces analgesia of the three nerves for 6 to 8 hours. To produce prolonged analgesia, a catheter is inserted into the femoral sheath and the local anesthetic solution is infused at a rate of 5 ml of 0.5% or 10 ml of 0.25% bupivacaine/hour (122).

Complications

Complications can include accidental IV or intra-arterial injection, with possible systemic reaction or damage to the femoral nerve and consequent dysesthesia. These can and must be prevented by the use of correct technique.

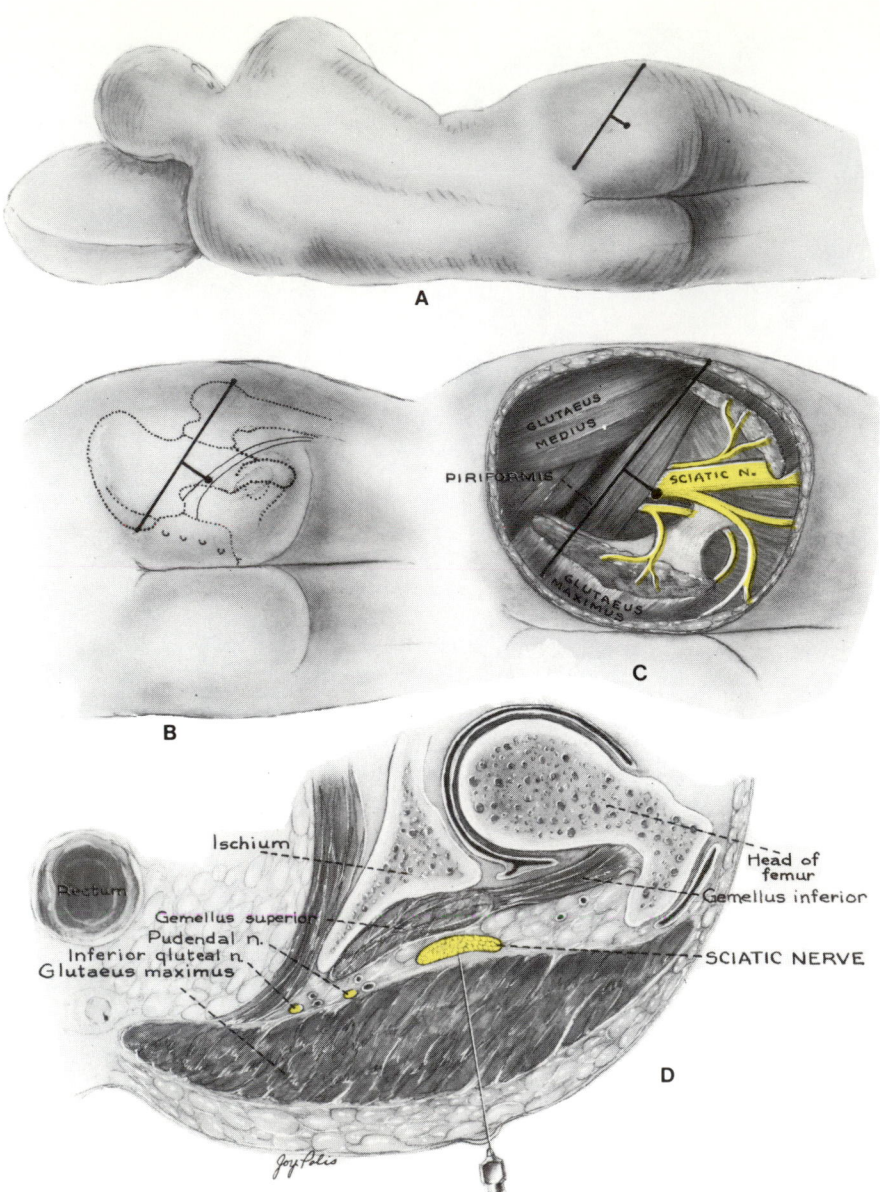

FIG. 94-37. Labat's technique of sciatic nerve block. **A.** The patient lies in a modified Sims position. A line is drawn between the posterior superior iliac spine and the superior border of the greater trochanter of the femur. The line is bisected at its midpoint and a perpendicular line 3 cm long passes caudad to it, with a solid dot indicating the site of the skin wheal and site of subsequent insertion of the block needle. **B.** Relation of the line to the bone and nerve. **C.** Relation of the nerve to muscles, with the lines superimposed. Following the creation of a skin wheal and infiltration of subcutaneous tissue, a 10-cm 22-gauge security needle is introduced in a direction perpendicular to the skin and advanced until paresthesia is obtained or bone is contacted. In the latter case, the needle is withdrawn until its point is subcutaneous and is directed a little more obliquely, either cephalad or caudad. Several such explorations should be sufficient to locate the nerve. If difficulty is encountered a nerve stimulator can be used to locate the nerve. **D.** Bevel of the needle on the nerve to elicit paresthesia, which radiates to the leg and foot. Bone depth varies from 5 cm in thin individuals to 8 cm in obese or muscular patients. If the landmark has not been determined accurately or if the needle has been improperly inserted, its point can miss the nerve and bone completely; if advanced too far, and the needle can enter the pelvis.

Sciatic Nerve Block

Indications

Because the sciatic nerve contains most of the sensory and sympathetic fibers for the lower extremity, sciatic nerve block can be used to control severe acute post-traumatic or postoperative pain in its distribution or to produce complete sympathetic interruption of interruption of the foot, leg, and posterior thigh. By combining sciatic nerve block with a three-in-one block, analgesia and sympathetic interruption of the entire lower limb can be achieved. The indications for these procedures are similar to those described for brachial plexus block for the upper limb (see above).

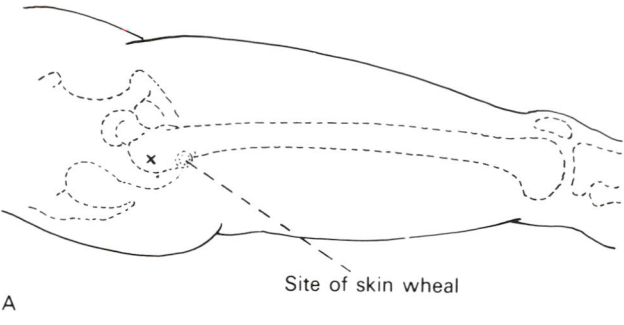

Site of skin wheal

A

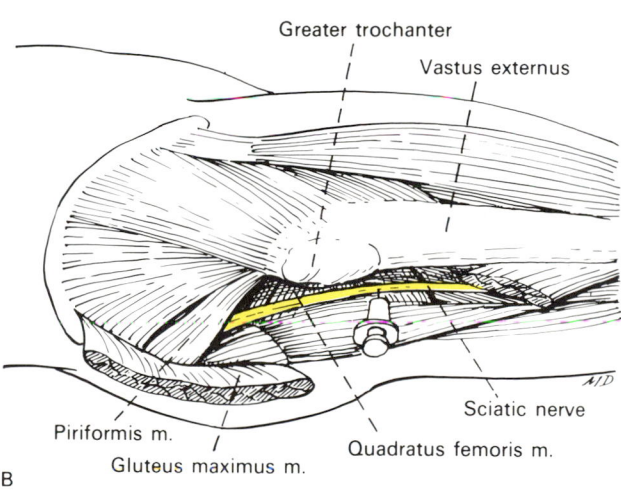

Greater trochanter

Vastus externus

Piriformis m.

Gluteus maximus m.

Sciatic nerve

Quadratus femoris m.

B

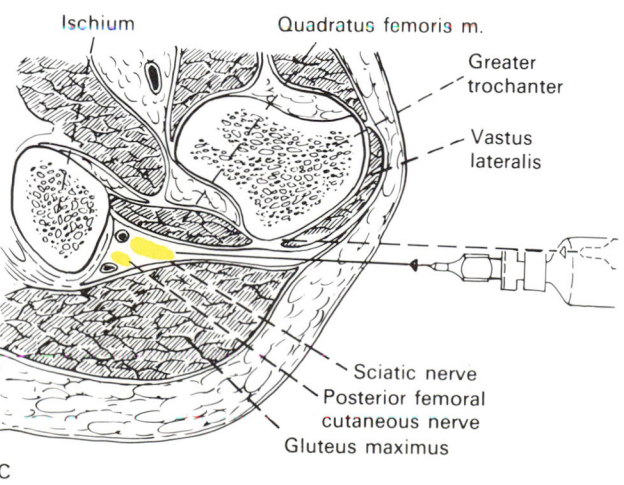

Ischium

Quadratus femoris m.

Greater trochanter

Vastus lateralis

Sciatic nerve

Posterior femoral cutaneous nerve

Gluteus maximus

C

FIG. 94-38. Technique of sciatic nerve block by the lateral approach. *A.* With the patient supine the outline of the femur (dashed lines) is drawn. An X indicates the most prominent part of the greater trochanter. The skin wheal indicates the point of penetration of the skin. *B.* View of the right thigh with the skin and subcutaneous tissue removed to show the relationship of the sciatic nerve to muscles. The sciatic nerve is anterior to the gluteus maximus and posterior to the quadratus femoris, which has been cut. The syringe is positioned so that the point is on the nerve. *C.* Cross-sectional view illustrating the technique. Following preparation of the skin and creation of a skin wheal a dilute solution of local anesthetic (e.g., 0.125% bupivacaine) is introduced through the skin wheal using a 5-cm 25-gauge needle attached to a 10-ml Luer-Lok syringe containing the anesthetic solution. The needle is advanced slowly through the skin, subcutaneous tissue, and vastus lateralis until it contacts the posterior surface of the greater trochanter. While the needle is steadily advanced the local anesthetic solution is injected into the subcutaneous tissue and the fascia of the muscle, with about 1 or 2 ml injected onto the periosteum. The depth of contact should be noted. The needle is then withdrawn until its point is in the subcutaneous tissue, the skin is moved 1 cm posteriorly, and advanced in a trajectory parallel to the first injection, and dilute solutions of the local anesthetic are injected. These leave a track of anesthesia for the subsequent painless introduction of the larger needle. A 12- or 15-cm 22-gauge needle is adapted to a 10-ml Luer-Lok control syringe containing a solution of greater strength of the local anesthetic (e.g., 0.5% bupivacaine with epinephrine) and these two steps are repeated. When the point of the larger needle contacts the periosteum or the posterior surface of the greater trochanter, the depth is noted and the needle is withdrawn until its point is in the subcutaneous tissue, and the skin is moved 1 cm posteriorly in the same fashion as earlier. The shaft of the needle should be parallel to the floor of the room. The needle is then slowly advanced. Normally, when the needle has advanced twice the distance of that in the first step, it should come in contact with the sciatic nerve and elicit paresthesia. If paresthesia is not elicited and the needle encounters bone (representing the ischial tuberosity), it is withdrawn and reinserted 2 or 3 mm anterior to its position in the second step and advanced. It might be necessary to make several penetrations before the nerve is contacted. If further difficulty is encountered in eliciting paresthesia, a nerve stimulator should be used. Special caution should be exercised in advancing the needle slowly and stopping as soon as the patient experiences paresthesia, because if the needle penetrates the nerve some axons could be damaged. It is important to inject the solution around rather than inside the nerve, because rapid expansion could also cause axonal damage. With experience and care it becomes easier to determine when the injection is extraneural because of lack of resistance. If the point of the needle is in the nerve, however, resistance can be felt and the patient experiences paresthesia during the injection.

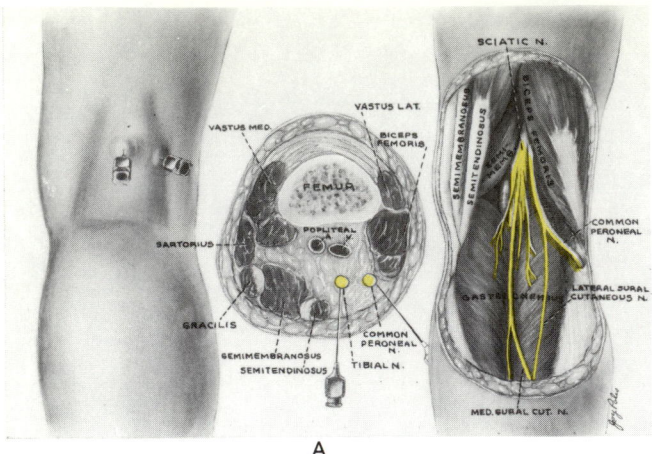

A

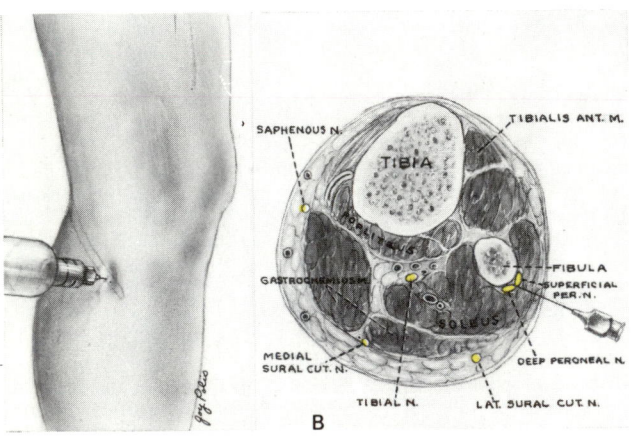

B

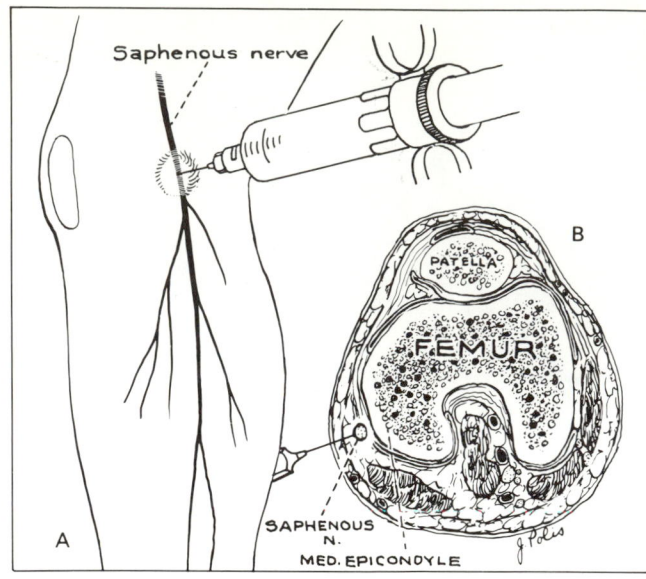

FIG. 94-40. Technique of blocking the saphenous nerve at the knee. After preparation of the skin with the patient in the supine or lateral position, a wheal is raised on the skin (*A*) over the medial surface of the medial condyle of the femur at the cross-sectional level of the apex of the patella (*B*). A 5-cm 25-gauge needle is inserted through the wheal in a direction perpendicular to the skin and advanced slowly until paresthesia along the saphenous nerve is elicited or until the bone is contacted. Several exploratory fanwise insertions are usually sufficient to locate the nerve, which is usually blocked with 3 to 5 ml of local anesthetic solution.

FIG. 94-39. Block of the three major nerves at the level of the knee. *A*. Block of the tibial and peroneal nerves in the popliteal fossa. With the patient in the prone position the bend of the knee is determined by having the patient flex the leg 90° on the thigh and the junction of the two cutaneous surfaces is traced on the skin. After skin preparation the popliteal artery is palpated 2 cm above the bend of the knee and a skin wheal is raised 1 cm lateral to this point. A 5-cm 22- or 25-gauge needle is introduced through the wheal in a direction perpendicular to the skin and advanced slowly until paresthesia radiating to the back of the leg and sole of the foot is elicited, whereupon 5 ml of local anesthetic solution is injected without moving the knee. If paresthesia is not obtained the nerve can be found by systematic exploratory fanwise insertions made in the mediolateral plane. To block the peroneal nerve the posteromedial margin of the bicep femoris is palpated at about the same level as that for tibial block. A skin wheal is raised just medial to the edge of the bicep femoris muscle and a 5-cm 22- or 25-gauge needle is introduced through it. The needle is made to pass just medial to the inner margin of the biceps and is slowly advanced until paresthesia radiating to the anterolateral aspect of the leg and dorsolateral aspect of the foot is elicited, whereupon 5 ml of solution is injected. Analgesia occurs within 5 to 8 minutes. An alternate method of blocking both nerves with one needle involves injection of 10 to 15 ml of solution when the tibial nerve is blocked. Because the two nerves are located in loose areolar tissue, the drug easily diffuses to block both nerves. *B*. Block of the peroneal nerve at the neck of the fibula. With the patient in the supine or lateral position the head of the fibula and the depression just below it, which is the neck of the fibula, are palpated. By moving the finger up and down the cord-like common peroneal nerve can be palpated. It is not necessary to make a skin wheal if a 25-gauge 2.5-cm needle is used. With the nerve held stationary by the index finger of the left hand the needle, attached to a 10 ml Luer-Lok syringe, is introduced through the skin in a direction perpendicular to it and slowly advanced until the nerve is gently contacted, as indicated by paresthesia. A volume of 3 to 4 ml of solution is sufficient to block the nerve.

Technique

The anatomy of the sciatic nerve, the peripheral nerve supply to the skin, muscles, and bones of the lower limb, and the sympathetic nerve supply to the vessels of the lower limb are described in Chapter 70 and illustrated in Figures 70-30, 70-31, and 70-32. Figure 94-36, the anatomy of the sciatic nerve and its major branches, is reproduced here for the convenience of the reader.

To block the sciatic nerve, the classic approach of Labat (123) (Fig. 94-37) or the lateral approach (Fig. 94-38) (124) is used. The lateral approach is somewhat more difficult to perform but is useful in patients who cannot move from a supine or prone position to the position required by Labat's technique because of fracture or other painful condition in the lower limb.

For over 30 years sporadic reports have appeared in regard to achieving continuous sciatic nerve block by introducing a catheter through a large needle and having its tip on the sciatic nerve (1). Because movement of the leg can displace the tip of the catheter from the nerve it has not proven consistently successful. Smith (125), however, described the use of continuous sciatic nerve block for relieving pain from ischemic gangrene of the foot for 2 days before below-the-knee amputation was carried out. It was combined with continuous inguinal paravascular block prior to surgery to provide anesthesia for the operation and to relieve postoperative pain for 2 days after surgery.

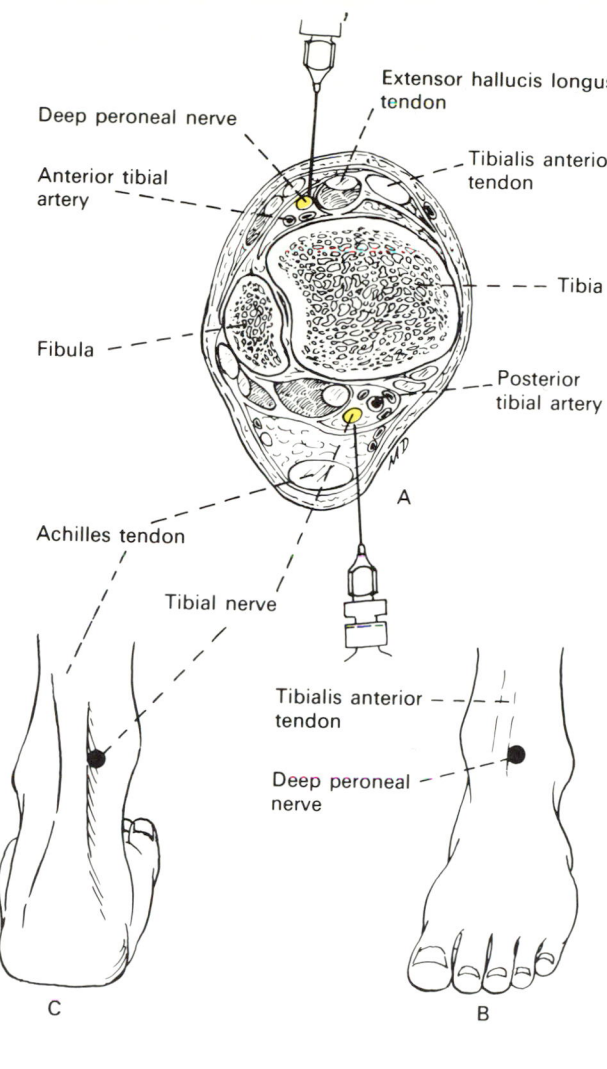

Deep peroneal nerve

Extensor hallucis longus tendon

Anterior tibial artery

Tibialis anterior tendon

Fibula

Tibia

Posterior tibial artery

Achilles tendon

Tibial nerve

Tibialis anterior tendon

Deep peroneal nerve

A

C

B

FIG. 94-41. Technique of blocking the tibial and deep peroneal nerves at the ankle. *A.* Cross section of the ankle just above the level of the malleoli. *B, C.* Anterior and posterior views showing sites of injection. The deep peroneal nerve is blocked by palpating and identifying the tendon of the extensor hallucis proprius and the anterior tibial artery. The nerve is situated between these two structures. With the patient in the supine position and the tendon and artery identified, a 5-cm 25-gauge needle is introduced through the skin (*B*), without making a preliminary skin wheal, and slowly advanced until paresthesia is elicited. If the nerve is not contacted before the needle point impinges on the anterior surface of the tibia, the needle is withdrawn until its level is subcutaneous and then reinserted so that its point is directed a little more laterally. The nerve is usually located with several fanwise insertions made along a transverse line across the ankle. Injection of 3 to 5 ml of local anesthetic solution is sufficient to produce a complete block. *A, C.* The posterior tibial nerve is blocked at the level of the malleoli. *C.* A skin wheal is raised at this level just medial to the medial border of the Achilles tendon and just lateral to the palpable posterior tibial artery (*A*). A 5-cm 25-gauge needle is introduced in an anterior direction and advanced until paresthesia is elicited or until the posterior aspect of the tibia is contacted without paresthesia. In the latter case, the needle is withdrawn and reinserted so that its point is directed a little more medially. With several fanwise insertions in the cross-sectional plane the nerve can usually be located. Injection of 3 to 5 ml of local anesthetic solution is sufficient to effect a complete block. Block of these two nerves, together with a subcutaneous infiltration around the ankle to block the subcutaneous, sural, saphenous, and superficial peroneal nerves, produces complete anesthesia of the foot.

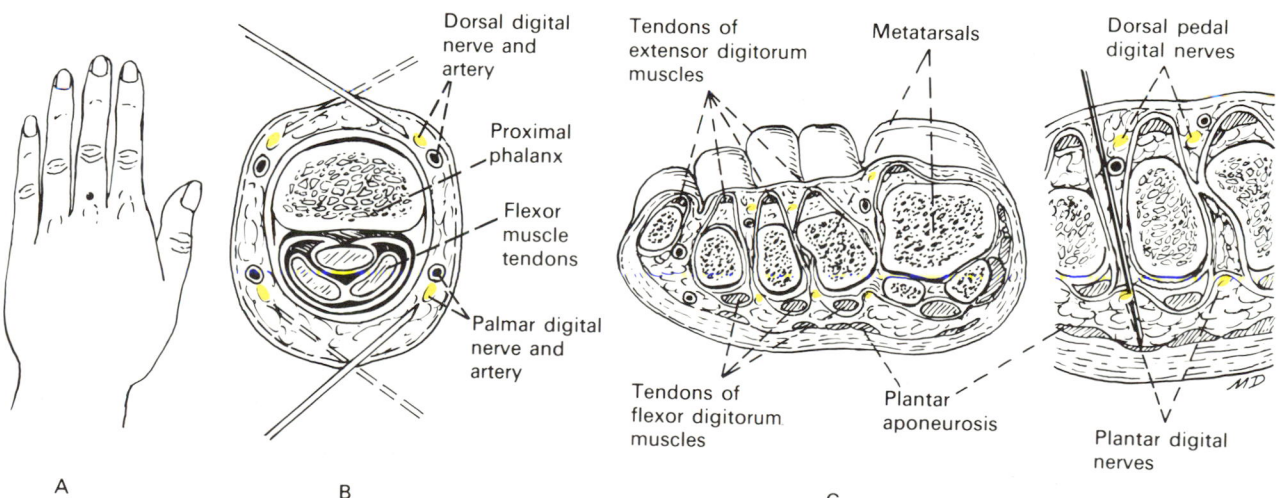

Dorsal digital nerve and artery

Proximal phalanx

Flexor muscle tendons

Palmar digital nerve and artery

Tendons of extensor digitorum muscles

Metatarsals

Dorsal pedal digital nerves

Tendons of flexor digitorum muscles

Plantar aponeurosis

Plantar digital nerves

A   B   C   D

FIG. 94-42. Techniques of blocking digital nerves. *A, B.* Block of the digital nerves in the fingers. *A.* An intracutaneous wheal is created on the dorsal and volar surfaces of the finger and a 2-cm 25-gauge needle is introduced. *B.* The needle is directed first to one side and then the other; 1.5 to 2 ml of 0.25% bupivacaine *without* epinephrine is injected at each site. Because the four digital nerves are in the same fascial space the solution diffuses to produce complete anesthesia of the finger distal to the site of injection. *C.* Cross-sectional view of the foot at the metatarsal level. *D.* Relationship of the dorsal and plantar digital nerves. Skin wheals are raised on the dorsal pedal surface of the foot over each metatarsal space that bounds the toe (or toes) to be anesthetized. A 5-cm 25-gauge needle is inserted and advanced toward the plantar surface until its point meets the resistance of the plantar aponeurosis. The needle is withdrawn 5 mm and 2 to 3 ml of local anesthetic solution is injected to block the plantar digital nerves. The needle is then withdrawn, slowly injecting 1 or 2 ml of solution between the plantar and dorsal surfaces. When the point of the needle is at the dorsal subcutaneous space 2 to 3 ml is injected, for a total of 5 ml of anesthetic solution for each metatarsal interspace.

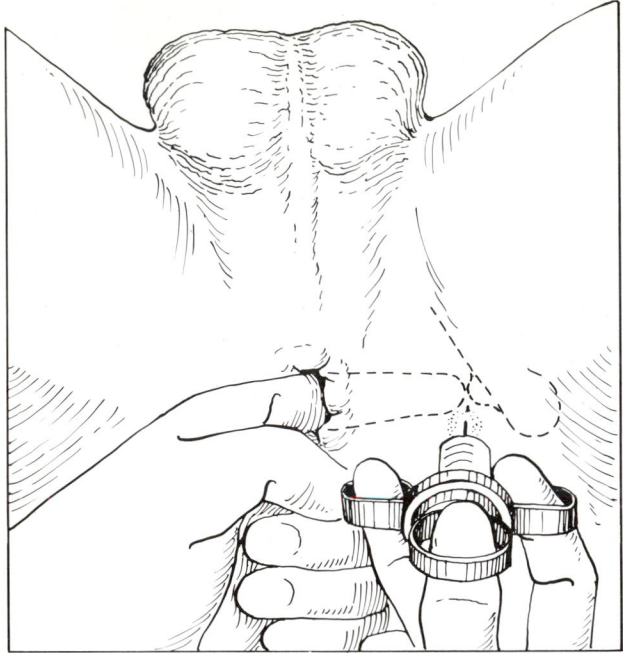

FIG. 94-43. Technique of pudendal nerve block by the transperineal approach. With the patient in the lithotomy position, the perineum is prepared and a skin wheal is made about 2.5 cm posteromedial to the tuberosity of the ischium and the subcutaneous tissue is infiltrated with a dilute solution of LA, e.g., 0.25% lidocaine. The small needle is then exchanged for a 12-cm 22-gauge needle with a security bead, which is inserted perpendicular to the skin. The index finger of the left hand (*dashed lines*) is inserted into the rectum, first to palpate the spine of the ischium and the sacrospinous ligament and then to guide the needle just posterior to the junction of these two structures, which is the optimal site for injection of the nerve. The needle is slowly advanced through the ischiorectal fossa toward the ischial spine by having it pass behind to the urogenital diaphragm and levator ani muscle. As the needle approaches the ischial spine, it is pushed posterior to it by the guiding finger. After attempting to aspirate in two planes to ensure that the point of the needle is not in a blood vessel, 5 to 7 ml of local anesthetic solution (e.g., 0.25% bupivacaine) is injected just posterior to the tip of the spine.

For single-dose techniques, injection of 10 to 15 ml of 0.25 to 0.5% bupivacaine provides analgesia for 8 to 12 hours. For the continuous technique, hourly infusions of 5 to 8 ml of 0.25 bupivacaine are used (125).

Complications

Complications associated with sciatic nerve block are rare. Obviously, if the physician penetrates the nerve and injects the solution within the nerve trunk, neurologic sequelae can occur, but these should be prevented with proper technique.

Nerve Block at the Knee, Ankle, and Foot

The nerves to the leg and foot can be blocked at the level of the knee to produce analgesia, sympathetic blockade, or both (Fig. 94-39). The tibial and common peroneal (lateral popliteal) nerves can be blocked in the popliteal fossa. The common peroneal nerve can

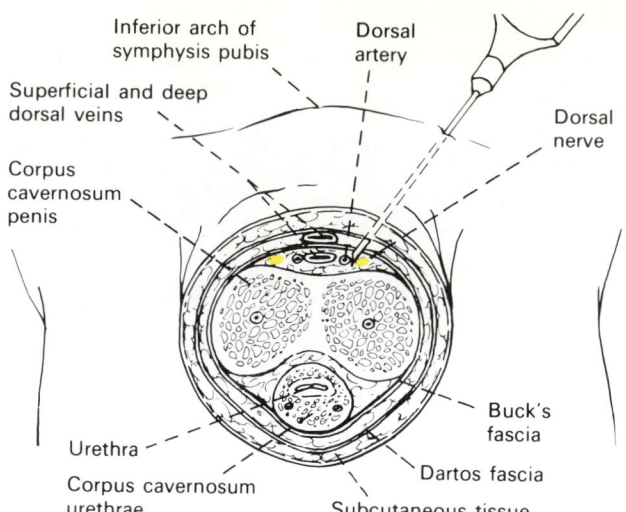

FIG. 94-44. Technique of penile nerve block. The dorsal nerves of the penis can be blocked as they pass from the pelvis to the penis. With the patient in the supine position the skin over the symphysis pubis and the base of the penis is cleansed with antiseptic solution. The inferior border of the symphysis pubis is identified and a mark is made at a level 1 cm from the midline. In an adult a 3-cm 25-gauge needle is used, but in infants a 1-cm 30-gauge needle is adapted to a Luer-Lok control syringe containing the local anesthetic solution is introduced through the mark and directed toward the midline at an angle of 30° to the skin. As the needle advances, it pierces the skin, subcutaneous tissue, dartos fascia, and Buck's fascia, which can be felt as a click. Once the needle has pierced the fascia, which is about 4 to 6 mm deep, an attempt at aspiration of blood is made and, if negative, 0.25% plain bupivacaine solution is injected. (The volumes to be injected, according to the age of the patient, are listed in the text.)

also be blocked as it winds around the neck of the tibia, while the saphenous nerve can be blocked as it lies on the medial condyle of the tibia, at the cross-sectional level of the apex of the patella. The saphenous nerve is best blocked in the medial aspect of the knee (Fig. 94-40).

Analgesia and sympathetic blockade of the foot can be achieved by blocking the deep peroneal and tibial nerves about 2 cm above the level of the malleoli (Fig. 94-41). Block of these two nerves, plus a subcutaneous infiltration around the ankle, produces analgesia of the entire foot.

Block of the digital nerves is indicated for severe pain involving one or more fingers or toes, the distal portion of the metatarsal bones, or the bones of one or more toes (Fig. 94-42). Epinephrine should *not* be used lest necrosis of the digit occur.

Pudendal Nerve Block

Indications

Block of one or both pudendal nerves is a useful diagnostic procedure in patients with severe perineal pain. It can also be used to relieve severe acute postoperative or post-traumatic pain in the perineum by carrying out the block with 0.25% bupivacaine with epinephrine. If the pain is on one side of the perineum a unilateral block is sufficient, but often it is necessary to carry out a bilateral pudendal nerve block.

Technique

The optimal site for injecting the pudendal nerve is in its position just posterior to the attachment of the sacrospinous ligament to the ischial spine. In the female this can be done transvaginally (see Fig. 66-31), and in the male a transperineal approach can be used (Fig. 94-43). Usually 5 to 7 ml of 0.25% bupivacaine is sufficient to produce block of the nerve on one side.

Complications

Unintentional involvement of the sciatic nerve and accidental IV injection are possible complications. The former can be obviated by identifying the target carefully and by limiting the volume of local anesthetic solution to 5 ml. Accidental IV injection should be avoided by aspirating before injection of the local anesthetic.

Penile Nerve Block

Indications

Penile nerve block can be used as a diagnostic procedure, but its most important application is providing postoperative analgesia subsequent to penile operations, particularly circumcision in infants and children. In these circumstances it produces prolonged analgesia and thus reduces manipulation of the dressing by the child.

Technique

The anatomy of the dorsal nerve to the penis is described in Chapter 65 and depicted in Figures 65-12 and 68-2. The technique of blocking the dorsal nerve of the penis is described in Figure 94-44. The recommended dose of 0.25% plain bupivacaine (epinephrine strictly contraindicated) is 1 ml for infants up to 1 year of age, 3 ml for children 1 to 5 years of age, 4 to 5 ml for those 6 to 12 years of age, and 5 to 7 ml for those 13 years of age or older (126–128).

Complications

Complications include puncture of the corpus cavernosum or the dorsal vessels of the penis, but if a thin (27- or 30-gauge) needle is used and intravascular injection is avoided, no serious complications develop.

D. BLOCK OF THE SYMPATHETIC NERVOUS SYSTEM

The functional relationship between the sympathetic nervous system and many disease syndromes has long been recognized. Moreover, a vast amount of experimental and clinical evidence has accumulated to indicate that interruption of certain portions of the sympathetic nervous system has beneficial effects in many of these disorders (1–3, 129). Block of the regional sympathetic pathways by injection of a local anesthetic or neurolytic agent is one of the most effective and clinically practical of the methods that have been devised to achieve interruption. Figure 94-45 depicts the entire sympathetic chain.

It is well known that clinical interruption of peripheral sympathetic pathways can be done in the following: (a) the subarachnoid space; (b) the epidural space; (c) the paravertebral and prevertebral regions; (d) the peripheral nerves; and (e) the endings of postganglionic axons (Fig. 94-46). Because subarachnoid, epidural, and peripheral nerve blocks are discussed elsewhere in this chapter, this section is limited to paravertebral and prevertebral sympathetic blockade. Segmental paravertebral injections are preferable for diagnostic and prognostic blocks because specific sympathetic pathways can be blocked by using a small volume of local anesthetic. Obviously, this is also true when alcohol or phenol is to be used for therapeutic block and the volume must be limited to 2 to 3 ml of solution. Conversely, if a large volume of local anesthetic is being used, it is not necessary to block all the involved ganglia separately because the peripheral sympathetic pathways are so arranged anatomically that they can be interrupted at certain "key" regions. Studies with contrast media have demonstrated the feasibility of blocking the entire peripheral sympathetic outflow to various body areas by placing a needle in each of three critical sites (Fig. 94-47).

With paravertebral or prevertebral techniques the local anesthetic (or neurolytic) solution interrupts all efferent (sympathetic motor) and afferent fibers, some of which are concerned with nociception. In contrast, the more recently developed technique of blocking sympathetic function to a limb by IV injection of guanethidine or some other adrenolytic agent by the Bier technique (see below) blocks only efferent impulses.

This section first presents the indications for interrupting the sympathetic efferent and afferent fibers, discusses tests for assessing the completeness of the sympathetic interruption, and then considers techniques for blocking the cervicothoracic sympathetic chain, the thoracic sympathetic ganglia, the celiac plexus, the thoracic splanchnic nerves, and the lumbar sympathetic chain. Discussion of the indications is intended to provide an overview of the efficacy of these procedures for relieving the pain of various conditions discussed elsewhere in this book. Discussion of the techniques is preceded by an overview of the regional anatomy of the sympathetic nerves; a more comprehensive discussion of the general anatomy of the sympathetic nervous system is presented in Chapter 6.

Indications

Causalgia and Other Reflex Sympathetic Dystrophies

Block of the sympathetic pathways to the limbs is the primary form of treatment for patients with causalgia and other reflex sympathetic dystrophies, conditions that Roberts (130) called sympathetically maintained pain (SMP) (Chapter 11). It is essential to properly select patients for sympathetic blockade on the basis of whether the sympathetic nervous system is involved (see below).

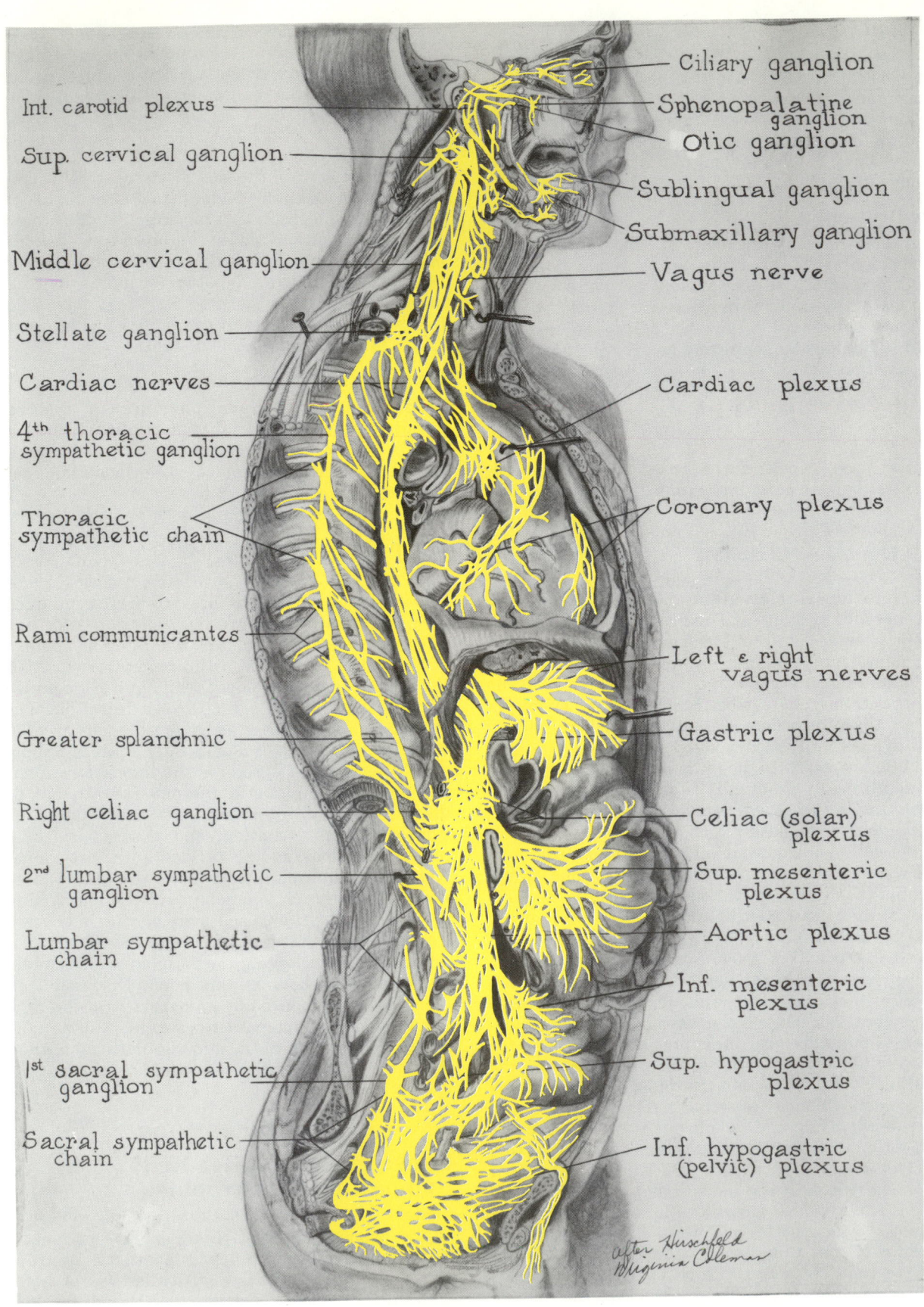

Int. carotid plexus

Sup. cervical ganglion

Middle cervical ganglion

Stellate ganglion

Cardiac nerves

4th thoracic
sympathetic ganglion

Thoracic
sympathetic chain

Rami communicantes

Greater splanchnic

Right celiac ganglion

2nd lumbar sympathetic
ganglion

Lumbar sympathetic
chain

1st sacral sympathetic
ganglion

Sacral sympathetic
chain

Ciliary ganglion

Sphenopalatine
ganglion

Otic ganglion

Sublingual ganglion

Submaxillary ganglion

Vagus nerve

Cardiac plexus

Coronary plexus

Left & right
vagus nerves

Gastric plexus

Celiac (solar)
plexus

Sup. mesenteric
plexus

Aortic plexus

Inf. mesenteric
plexus

Sup. hypogastric
plexus

Inf. hypogastric
(pelvic) plexus

after Hirschfeld
Virginia Coleman

FIG. 94-45. Anatomy of the autonomic nervous system depicting the position of the right sympathetic trunk, its branches, and the prevertebral ganglia.

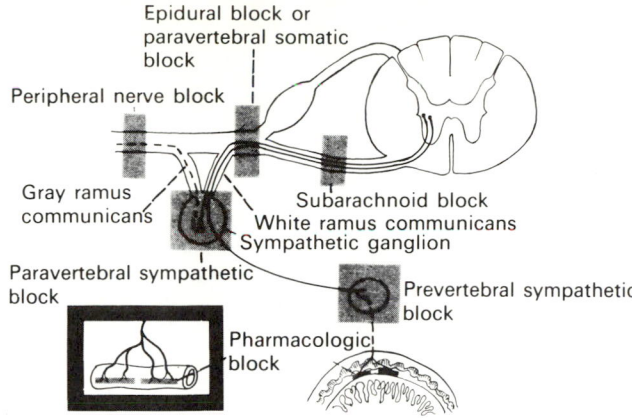

FIG. 94-46. The course of preganglionic and postganglionic sympathetic fibers and techniques that can be used to interrupt them. Modified from J.J. Bonica: Clinical Applications of Diagnostic and Therapeutic Nerve Blocks. Springfield, IL, Charles C Thomas, 1959.

Causalgia

Causalgia is a condition associated with incomplete severance of a major peripheral nerve, such as a median or sciatic nerve, and is usually caused by the effects of high-velocity missiles during wartime, although it also can occur in civilian life. The condition is characterized by severe burning pain, hyperalgesia, hyperpathia, allodynia and, not infrequently, by vasomotor and sudomotor disturbances caused by sympathetic hyperactivity.

Recent studies by Campbell and associates (131, 132) have shown that patients with nerve injuries can be of two types: those with sympathetically maintained pain (SMP) and those whose pain is independent of sympathetic hyperactivity, sympathetically independent pain (SIP). They found that in patients with SMP the pain and hyperalgesia were eliminated with sympathetic blockade, whereas in patients with SIP sympathetic blockade was ineffective. In the latter group a diagnostic block of the somatic nerve relieved the pain, and many of these patients were subsequently cured of their pain by proper peripheral nerve surgery. It was also noted that all the patients with mechanical hyperalgesia and SMP had increased pain with mild cooling (1.5 to 2° C) of the skin, effected by applying a drop of acetone, or ice water, or alcohol. In contrast, only 5 of 14 SIP patients tested reported pain response to cold, but even the 5 patients failed to obtain pain relief during sympathetic blockade. It is therefore obvious that regional sympathetic block and the response to cold stimulus can be used to differentiate patients with SMP from those with SIP.

In patients with causalgia or SMP, selective block of the regional sympathetics with a local anesthetic is an extremely useful procedure for making a definitive diagnosis. Campbell and associates (131) noted that selective blocks are not obtained by epidural analgesia or Bier blocks, because in each case other effects of the block complicate interpretation of the block. Somewhat similar issues were raised regarding the use of guanethidine blocks. To achieve specificity the sympathetic chain must be blocked by injecting a local anesthetic as close to the chain as possible, using fluoroscopic visualization if necessary. Moreover, to be a useful diagnostic procedure, it is essential that all the sympathetic nerves to the limb be interrupted, as demonstrated by various methods of monitoring sympathetic function (see below). Incomplete sympathetic interruption produces a false negative result whereas a false positive diagnostic block results if the injection also involves the somatic nerves. This is particularly relevant for knee pain because block of the L3 and L4 nerve roots can occur with lumbar sympathetic block if the correct technique is not used. Therefore, sensory testing to verify that the affected area is not hypesthetic should be performed.

When instituted early in the condition, a series of sympathetic blocks can produce prolonged and often curative effects (Chapter 11). To obtain optimal results, it is essential that the procedure produce complete sympathetic denervation of the entire limb. The mere execution of the block does not always ensure this result because, in addition to technical errors, anomalies of fascial planes and other structures can prevent the local anesthetic from diffusing sufficiently to involve the entire portion of the sympathetic chain that supplies the extremity.

For those who have not had sufficient experience with regional sympathetic blocks, the IV injection of guanethidine by the Bier block technique is the procedure of choice. Guanethidine block lasts 24 to 72 hours (see below). In Chapter 11 it is noted that phenoxybenzamine, an alpha-adrenoreceptor blocker (AAB), has also proven to be highly effective in patients with causalgia.

Following sympathetic interruption patients derive complete relief of burning pain, hyperpathia, allodynia, and other symptoms of causalgia. If sympathetic blockade with local anesthetics or with drugs produces complete but only temporary relief sympathectomy is indicated which produces complete and prolonged relief of symptoms and signs in most patients.

Reflex Sympathetic Dystrophy

Reflex sympathetic dystrophy is an all-inclusive term applied to many seemingly unrelated disorders that were formerly described separately under various other names, including minor causalgia, post-traumatic spreading neuralgia, Sudeck's atrophy, and shoulder-hand syndrome (Chapter 11). All these conditions have similar pathophysiology, symptoms and signs, and response to therapy. They are usually characterized by excessive and unduly prolonged pain, vasomotor and sudomotor disturbances, delayed functional recovery and, unless the condition is treated properly, the development of trophic changes. These disorders are much more important and serious than major causalgia because they occur more frequently and because they are often misdiagnosed, with a consequently delay in instituting therapy. Early treatment with repeated or continuous sympathetic block for 7 to 10 days produces complete and permanent relief of pain and eliminates other symptoms and signs.

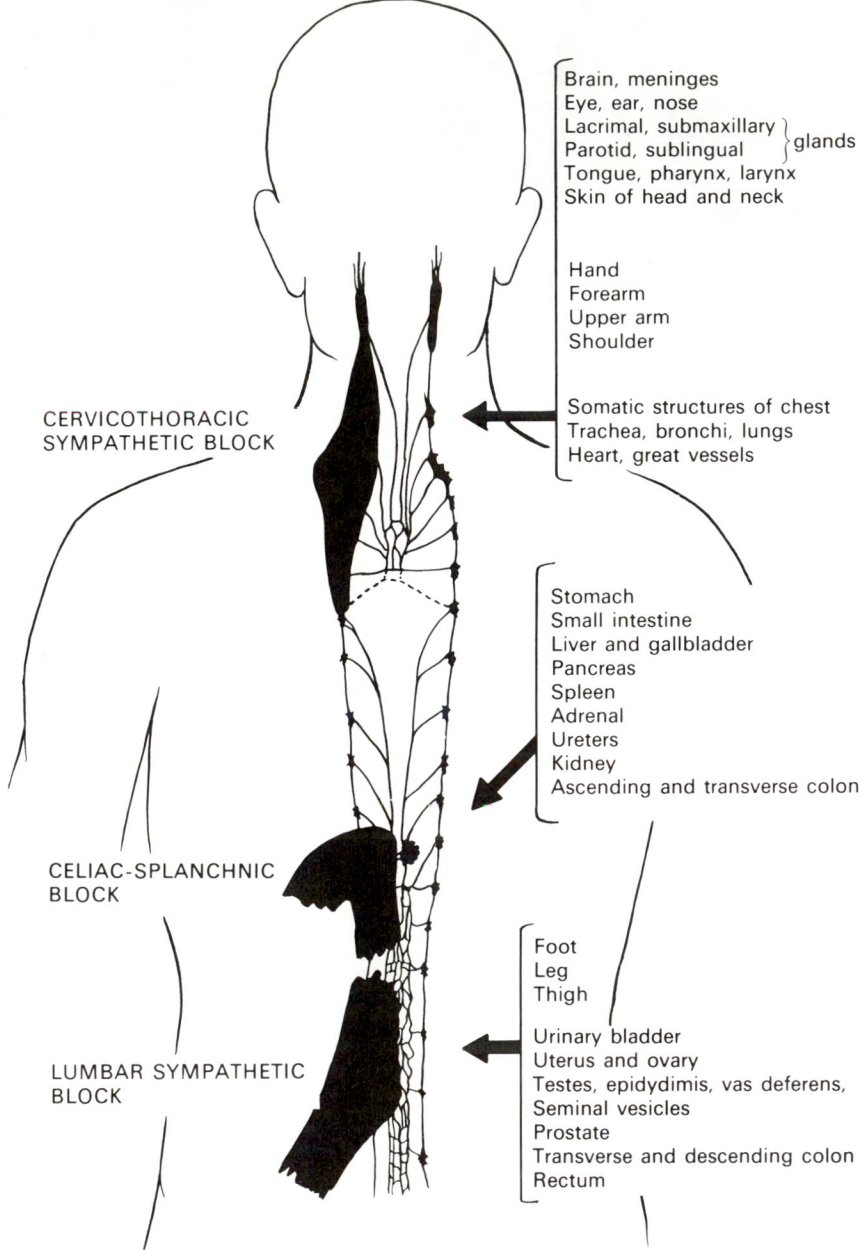

Fig. 94-47. Three "critical sites" that can be used to interrupt the peripheral sympathetic nervous system. *Left.* Pattern of diffusion (*black*) of local anesthetic solutions injected in the vicinity of the cervicothoracic (stellate) ganglion, celiac plexus, and lumbar sympathetic ganglia. Injection of 15 to 20 ml of local anesthetic solution into the proper fascial plane near the stellate ganglion spreads sufficiently to involve the sympathetic chain from the lower portion of the superior cervical ganglion to the T5 ganglion, so that all the sympathetic fibers to the head and neck, upper extremities, and the heart, and most of the fibers to the esophagus and lungs, are interrupted. Injection of 15 to 25 ml of solution bilaterally near the celiac plexus spreads sufficiently to interrupt all the sympathetic (and vagal) efferent fibers to and afferent fibers from the viscera in the upper abdomen. Injection of 15 to 20 ml of solution through a needle with its tip at the anterolateral surface of the L2 or L3 vertebra interrupts all the sympathetic fibers to the ipsilateral lower extremity and pelvis. These sympathetic nerve structures are apparently contained within fascial planes that can be considered as relatively closed spaces (or even "pouches") that facilitate the spread of the local anesthetic solution, so that an extensive sympathetic block is produced. *Right.* Names of the structures that are denervated with each block. Modified from Bonica, J.J.: Clinical Applications of Diagnostic and Therapeutic Nerve Blocks. Springfield, IL, Charles C Thomas, 1959.

Labels in figure:
Brain, meninges / Eye, ear, nose / Lacrimal, submaxillary / Parotid, sublingual } glands / Tongue, pharynx, larynx / Skin of head and neck

Hand / Forearm / Upper arm / Shoulder

Somatic structures of chest / Trachea, bronchi, lungs / Heart, great vessels

CERVICOTHORACIC SYMPATHETIC BLOCK

Stomach / Small intestine / Liver and gallbladder / Pancreas / Spleen / Adrenal / Ureters / Kidney / Ascending and transverse colon

CELIAC-SPLANCHNIC BLOCK

Foot / Leg / Thigh

Urinary bladder / Uterus and ovary / Testes, epididimis, vas deferens, / Seminal vesicles / Prostate / Transverse and descending colon / Rectum

LUMBAR SYMPATHETIC BLOCK

Postamputation Pain Syndromes

In Chapter 12, Loeser describes the various pain patterns that follow amputation of a limb or other appendage, such as the nose or breast. Following amputation of an extremity almost every patient experiences the feeling of a phantom limb (or part), but only a small percentage develop persistent severe pain in the phantom limb, stump, or both. The pain of phantom limb varies, but is usually one of three main types: (a) a burning, throbbing, aching pain not unlike that of causalgia and other reflex sympathetic dystrophies, which is described by the patient as if the hand or foot were held too close to a fire; (b) pain caused by an extremely abnormal position of the phantom limb, in which the hand or foot can be held in a painful, twisted, cramped, rigid, or flexed posture that cannot be released by the patient; or (c) a combination of these two general patterns of pain. Pain in the stump is of three predominant types: (a) a constant, diffuse, burning, throbbing pain similar to that of reflex sympathetic dystrophies; (b) a paroxysm of lancinating shooting discomfort that has a segmental or peripheral nerve distribution; or (c) a combination of these. Stump pain is usually associated with vasomotor and sudomotor disturbances and is manifested by coldness, cyanosis, edema, signs of vasocontriction, and excessive sweating.

In patients who have predominantly burning aching pain associated with vasomotor and sudomotor changes in the stump, sympathetic interruption achieved by regional sympathetic or Bier block is effective in relieving the symptoms and signs, temporarily and at times permanently. Promptly after the onset of block patients feel partial or complete relief of pain and a warming of the stump, and occasionally feel that the cramped or twisted extremity is beginning to relax and assume a normal position. If the block affords complete or good relief of pain it should be repeated on several occasions to confirm the results and also to ascertain the duration of pain relief. If relief is of progressively longer duration and significantly outlasts the duration of the block, surgical sympathectomy should be seriously considered.

Bach and associates (133) recently evaluated the efficacy of preoperative analgesia on the incidence of postamputation phantom limb pain. They studied 25 patients with preoperative limb pain that had persisted from 1 to 6 months in 23 patients and over 6 months in 2, and who were scheduled to undergo amputation. One group of 11 patients received lumbar epidural blockade with bupivacaine or morphine, or a combination of these, to achieve complete pain relief for 72 hours prior to amputation. A second control group of 14 patients who also had persistent constant limb pain were treated with nonopioid and opioid analgesics for the same period. All 25 patients received epidural or spinal anesthesia for the amputation procedure. Seven days after the surgery 3 patients (27%) in the blockade group and 9 patients (64%) in the control group had phantom limb pain ($p < 0.10$). Six months after the surgery all 11 patients in the blockade group were pain-free while 5 patients (38%) in the control group had phantom limb pain ($p < 0.05$). One year after surgery all patients in the blockade group were still pain-free but 3 patients (27%) in the control group had phantom limb pain. This study demonstrates the usefulness of regional analgesia prophylactically prior to amputation and has important clinical implications.

Other Neuropathic Painful Disorders

Regional sympathetic blockade and guanethidine blocks have also been found to be effective in relieving burning pain associated with hyperesthesia, hyperpathia, allodynia, and sensitivity to cold. Patients with painful neuromata and a number of patients with so-called "thalamic syndrome" and other central pain syndromes caused by multiple sclerosis and trauma of the spinal cord or brain stem have been relieved of their burning pain and other symptoms by sympathetic blockade (134–136). Hannington-Kiff (134) reported on six patients who had pain, hyperpathia, paresthesia, and dysesthesia in a limb following brain stem lesions who were relieved of their pain with IV guanethidine blocks. In addition, the guanethidine blocks also relieved muscle spasticity and permitted an increase in the purposeful movements of the limb. Loh and associates (135) have also noted that regional sympathetic blocks with local anesthetics or guanethidine relieved the severe pain, hyperpathia, paresthesia, and other symptoms and signs caused by lesions of the central nervous system. Schott (136) cited a number of other reports on the successful use of sympathetic interruption for the relief of central pain problems, and also presented an excellent review of the mechanisms of causalgia and related clinical conditions. It has also been suggested that sympathetic blockade be used to prevent causalgia in patients in whom exploratory surgery is being carried out to determine damage to large nerves in one of the limbs (137).

Comments

In Chapter 11 several points were made about the use of sympathetic block for causalgia, reflex sympathetic dystrophy, and postamputation pain. First, the earlier the treatment, the better the prognosis for prolonged relief of the pain. Second, if patients experience relief, even if only partial, the sympathetic interruption should be repeated because occasionally, when the first two or three blocks produce partial or no relief, subsequent blocks relieve the pain. A series of blocks can be done at 2- to 4-day intervals or weekly, depending on the response. Third, when sympathectomy is indicated, this can be done either chemically or surgically, depending on the patient's physical condition, the severity of the disease, and the patient's attitude toward the use of both techniques. Chemical sympathectomy with 7% phenol in Conray-420 or 50% alcohol produces sympathetic interruption for several weeks to several months (mean 6 months) and is especially useful in children or high-risk patients. Surgical sympathectomy is preferable in patients who are younger and in good physical condition. Finally, it is essential to ascertain that sympathetic interruption is complete. This is especially important in patients who derived complete relief of the burning pain with a local anesthetic sympathetic block but who experienced only partial or no relief of the burning pain after sympathectomy. In such cases it is likely that, although the local anesthetic diffused widely enough to involve the sympathetic chain and anomalous sympathetic pathways (which are often present in the lower cervical and upper thoracic chain and in the lower thoracic and upper lumbar region), the operation was not extensive enough, did not include the anomalous pathways, or both. In such cases, two or three sympathetic blocks should be repeated. Relief of the residual burning pain confirms that the operation did not interrupt all the sympathetic pathways to the limb.

Peripheral Vascular Disease

For nearly 50 years, sympathetic interruption achieved either by regional sympathetic block or by chemical or surgical sympathectomy was considered to be one of the most important methods of managing patients with certain peripheral vascular diseases. This was based on the fact that, in many of these conditions, an increased sympathetically induced vasoconstriction, with consequent ischemia, tissue damage, pain, and trophic changes could be partially or totally reversed by early sympathetic interruption. The advent of effective surgical therapy using bypass grafts and other procedures and the widespread use of anticoagulant therapy, however, have decreased the importance of sympathetic block in treating this group of disorders. Nevertheless, temporary or prolonged sympathetic interruption can still be a useful adjunct for a number of conditions and, in some cases, can even be one of the primary forms of treatment (Chapter 28).

Acute Vascular Disease

Acute vascular disorders for which sympathetic interruption might be indicated include post-traumatic segmentary vasospasm, generalized vasoconstriction caused by intra-arterial injection of thiopental or some other irritating agent, acute arterial occlusion caused by thrombosis, embolism or direct injury, acute venous thrombosis, and peripheral vascular disorders resulting from cold injuries (Chapter 28). In all these conditions the local lesion initiates reflex spasm of the collateral vessels, which aggravates the circulatory insufficiency, becoming more severe than if the collateral vessels had not been so affected. Sympathetic block initiated promptly, before the development of changes that favor thrombosis in the endothelium of the vasospastic collateral vessels, produces partial or complete re-establishment of normal blood flow through the collaterals and thus can decrease or prevent tissue damage that might otherwise progress to gangrene.

Sympathetic interruption can be used in these cases to determine whether severe ischemia is a result of organic obstruction, actual division of the blood vessel, or merely severe vasospasm. If anticoagulants are not being used, sympathetic interruption can be done by cervicothoracic sympathetic block for the upper limb and lumbar sympathetic block or continuous epidural analgesia for the lower limb. If anticoagulants are being used, sympathetic interruption is best achieved by the use of IV regional sympathetic block (IRSB) with guanethidine. The concomitant use of anticoagulants and regional anesthetic techniques that involve injection into a closed spaced, such as the spinal canal, is contraindicated. In cases of excruciating pain, as well as vasospasm associated with embolism of the upper limb, continuous brachial plexus block with bupivacaine can be used to provide preoperative pain relief and sympathetic blockade, anesthesia for the operation, and pain relief after surgery. The risk of serious sequelae from hemorrhage consequent to anticoagulant therapy is significantly less in the posterior triangle of the neck than in the epidural space.

Chronic Vasospastic Disorders

Chronic vasospastic disorders for which sympathetic interruption is indicated include Raynaud's disease, Raynaud's phenomenon, cold injuries, acrocyanosis, and livedo reticularis. In these and other chronic vasospastic disorders involving the small arteries and arterioles of the microcirculation, sympathetic block can be used as a diagnostic and prognostic procedure in patients in whom sympathectomy is being considered. Hannington-Kiff (137) has also suggested that sympathetic interruption achieved with a series of guanethidine blocks can be used to tide over patients with Raynaud's disease or other vasospastic syndromes aggravated by cold during the winter months. Because many of these patients are in the younger age group, surgical sympathectomy should be considered if repeated sympathetic blocks produce complete but only temporary relief of the pain and of other symptoms associated with the condition. (Chapter 28 presents a detailed discussion of all aspects of these and other peripheral vascular diseases.)

Chronic Occlusive Arterial Disease

Chronic occlusive arterial disease for which sympathetic interruption is indicated includes thromboangiitis obliterans (Buerger's disease) and arteriosclerosis obliterans. In the former condition, a nonarteriosclerotic lesion involves medium-sized arteries, veins, and nerves of the distal leg or arm. The most bothersome and most common pain problems that develop are instep claudication and ischemic rest pain (or both), which have a burning quality. Although sympathetic block can provide temporary relief of vasospasm and pain it is of minimal value as a therapeutic measure in relieving claudication; chemical or surgical sympathectomy, however, might be effective in relieving the ischemic rest pain (138, 139) (Chapter 96).

The same comments apply to patients with occlusive arteriosclerotic disease (ASO) of the lower (or upper) limb that usually produces a progressive decrease in tissue blood flow with consequent claudication, rest pain, incipient gangrene, or ulceration. In general, this condition is best treated by medical and surgical therapy with bypass grafts. In patients in whom a bypass graft cannot be used because the obliterating vascular disorder is too extensive, however, sympathectomy is effective in relieving rest pain, enhancing the healing of ischemic lesions, and postponing amputation. If and when amputation becomes necessary, it can be performed at a more distal level of the limb (132) (Chapter 28). Moreover, there is evidence that chemical sympathectomy done 1 month before an amputation to relieve severe pain is likely to reduce the incidence of postamputation phantom limb pain (see page 514 for details). The value of chemical sympathectomy for these patients is discussed in detail in Chapter 96.

Visceral Pain

Block of the sympathetic nerves to thoracic or abdominal viscera is useful in relieving severe visceral pain that is not amenable to other therapies, or it can be an important adjunct. This is based on the fact that afferent nerves that convey nociceptive impulses from the viscera accompany the efferent sympathetic nerves. Block with a local anesthetic not only relieves pain but also interrupts the afferent and efferent limbs of abnormal viscerovisceral and viscerosomatic reflexes that often develop and contribute to the pathophysiology. Segmental reflexes produce skeletal muscle spasm and sympathetic hyperactivity, which are further aggravated by suprasegmental reflexes that stimulate hypothalamic autonomic centers and invariably produce a further increase in general sympathetic tone and catecholamine release. All these responses increase cardiac output and blood pressure, the workload of the heart, and metabolism and oxygen consumption. Unless the severe pain and associated reflex responses are promptly eliminated, they can become abnormal and greatly aggravate the pathophysiology. Although potent narcotics administered in appropriate doses and by the appropriate route produce adequate pain relief, they do not eliminate the abnormal reflex responses. In contrast, block of the sympathetic nociceptive pathways achieved with local anesthetic blocks the afferent and efferent limbs of these reflexes and thus prevents or at least minimizes the reflex responses. These comments are especially relevant to certain acute thoracic and abdominal visceral painful conditions.

Thoracic Visceral Pain

ACUTE MYOCARDIAL INFARCTION. Acute myocardial infarction (AMI) often produces severe excruciating pain and associated reflex responses that, unless promptly relieved, can aggravate the myocardial pathophysiology. Segmentally induced sympathetic stimulation produces reflex coronary vasoconstriction that further impairs the delivery of oxygen to the myocardium. Moreover, the suprasegmental reflex responses are markedly enhanced by severe anxiety, which invariably develops in patients with AMI. In addition, emotional stress can cause a cortically mediated increase in blood viscosity and clotting, fibrinolysis, and platelet aggregation. All these factors greatly increase the workload of the heart and its oxygen consumption, further decrease the already compromised arteriosclerotic coronary circulation, and thus markedly increase the discrepancy between oxygen supply and oxygen demand, possibly causing extension of the infarction. It is therefore essential to relieve the pain, anxiety, and mental stress promptly and effectively and to decrease these reflex responses (Chapter 54).

Effective pain relief can be achieved with the use of potent narcotics given IV in appropriate doses. Unfortunately, even when properly administered, narcotics rarely produce complete relief in all patients, do not eliminate abnormal reflex responses, and can be associated with well-known adverse side effects. In patients with severe excruciating pain that does not respond to narcotics, cervicothoracic (stellate) sympathetic block with 20 ml of 0.25% bupivacaine provides effective analgesia for 8 to 10 hours or more. In patients with pain predominantly on one side a unilateral block suffices but, if the pain is bilateral, the block is done on the side with the most severe pain first and, after an interval of 30 minutes, is repeated on the opposite side. Unfortunately, most cardiologists are unaware of this therapeutic adjunct for the management of AMI patients.

The value of sympathetic interruption in such cases is strongly suggested by the results of animal studies done about 50 years ago (140–142). These impressively demonstrated that sympathetic denervation of the heart significantly reduced the size of an experimentally induced myocardial infarction and decreased the mortality rate of the animals in the study group as compared to results in a control group. More recent laboratory studies have confirmed these early results. In animal studies, Schwartz and Stone (143) showed that surgical sympathectomy increases the endocardial:epicardial blood flow ratio, thus improving perfusion to the myocardium and endocardium. Even more impressive beneficial effects were noted by Klassen and colleagues (144), who experimentally induced AMI in dogs: subsequent sympathetic denervation was achieved with epidural blockade. Other animal studies have shown that sympathetic denervation has a protective effect against the cardiac arrhythmias of myocardial infarction (145, 146). The protective role of beta-blocking drugs against arrhythmias has been established clinically for AMI (147) (Chapter 54).

ANGINA PECTORIS. Angina pectoris, when severe and intractable to medical therapy, was formerly managed with block of the upper four or five thoracic sympathetic ganglia with local anesthetics and subsequently with alcohol. The advent of the highly successful aortocoronary bypass graft procedure and percutaneous coronary angioplasty, however, have rendered chemical and surgical sympathectomy unnecessary. The only possible indications for these procedures are in patients with extensive coronary disease that is not amenable to surgical or other therapies and in whom the anginal pain is disabling. In such individuals, prognostic cervicothoracic sympathetic blocks with 0.25% bupivacaine effectively predict results obtained by chemical or surgical sympathectomy (1). The technique of neurolytic block of the upper thoracic sympathetic chain for the relief of angina pectoris and of the pain caused by aortic aneurysm is discussed in Chapter 96.

Abdominal Visceral Pain

Patients with severe intractable abdominal pain caused by pathology, for whom surgery is contraindicated or must be postponed, can obtain effective relief with various types of nerve blocks that interrupt pain and sympathetic pathways. If the disease is a self-limiting condition that requires block for only several days, a repeated or continuous technique with local anesthetic drugs is advisable. On the other hand, if the condition is chronic or intractable, it is necessary to administer either a neurolytic injection or to perform surgical excision of the sensory and sympathetic nerves to the viscera. If the pain is entirely a result of visceral disorders, without involvement of the abdominal wall, interruption of the splanchnic nerves or celiac plexus should provide complete relief.

ACUTE PANCREATITIS. Acute pancreatitis is frequently a cause of severe or excruciating continuous pain, severe abdominal muscle spasm and rigidity, marked abdominal tenderness, nausea and vomiting, and moderate ileus, with consequent abdominal distension (Chapter 61). In most patients the pain and associated reflex responses impair pulmonary ventilation, and some patients develop progressive hypoxia and hypercapnea that can end in death. Although potent narcotics given intravenously can be effective, this condition is more effectively managed by regional block of the nociceptive afferents achieved by splanchnic nerve block, celiac plexus block (148), or continuous segmental (T5–T10) epidural block (149). Some have suggested that, in addition to providing pain relief, interruption of nociceptive impulses decreases the severity and duration of the disease by combating reflex spasm of the duodenum, the sphincter of Oddi, and the entire ductal system (148). (See page 1960 for more details on the treatment of pancreatitis.)

BILIARY AND URETERAL COLIC. Biliary and ureteral colic are among the most excruciatingly painful conditions experienced by many patients. Although potent narcotics administered intravenously produce adequate pain relief, they do not decrease but actually increase spasm of the smooth muscle. On the other hand, paravertebral block of the splanchnic nerves and of the L1 and L2 ganglia are highly effective in providing complete pain relief. Moreover, in a number of patients, the block also relaxes the ureter sufficiently to permit a stone to move down to a point where it can be removed through a cystoscope, thus obviating an open operation (1). An alternative technique is continuous segmental (T10–L2) epidural block, which has the advantage of involving one puncture and of permitting continuous blockade for several days (see Fig. 62-7).

ADYNAMIC ILEUS. Adynamic ileus frequently follows intra-abdominal surgery but can also be caused by fracture of the thoracic vertebra or by other severe painful conditions with various causes (Chapter 64). It is now clear that the ileus is a result of sympathetic hyperactivity, which can be eliminated by sympathetic blockade that is best achieved by continuous segmental epidural blockade. The efficacy of this procedure in the treatment of adynamic ileus is discussed in detail in Chapter 64.

Other Indications

Acute Herpes Zoster and Postherpetic Neuralgia

For over 50 years block of the sympathetic nerves to the affected part has been used with variable success in the treatment of herpes zoster. Bonica has cited the relevant literature between 1938, when Rosenak (150) published the first report on the subject, and studies up to 1953, and also mentioned his personal experience in treating 43 patients during a 10-year period (1). Since then Bonica has treated 121 additional patients (see below). Our experiences, and a recent review of the literature, lead us to believe that the use of sympathetic block, alone or combined with somatic nerve blocks, if begun early after the onset of pain or the eruption of acute herpes zoster, results in a high incidence of prompt pain relief, appears to decrease the severity and duration of the eruption, and accelerates healing. The longer the interval between the onset of disease and the initiation of blocks, the lower the incidence of a satisfactory result. We recommend a regime of blocks to be done at daily intervals for 5 to 7 days and then three blocks per week until the pain relief persists. The desired effect is often obtained with three to five blocks, but it might be necessary to proceed to eight to fifteen or more blocks before obtaining prolonged pain relief. The results obtained in various studies are summarized in Table 94-4 (150–157). The following details of two studies are relevant to our thesis.

The value of sympathetic blockade in relieving the acute pain of herpes zoster has been confirmed in a double-blind crossover study (156). Tenicela and associates (156) used sympathetic blocks with 0.25% bupivacaine performed daily for 4 days and compared the results with those of placebo injections in 20 patients who were over 50 years of age (mean age, 65 years). Of the 10 patients managed with sympathetic blocks, 90% were relieved within 1 to 4 days, while only 2 of the 10 patients in the placebo group (20%) were pain-free at the end of therapy. Of the 8 patients in whom pain persisted

following placebo therapy, 7 patients were given a series of four daily blocks with bupivacaine, and 4 of these (55%) derived immediate and long-term relief. In contrast, in a study of 72 patients with acute herpes zoster who were managed with various techniques of regional analgesia or by infiltration of local anesthetics and steroids, the results were negative in regard to prevention of postherpetic neuralgia (157). Whereas regional analgesia or infiltration produced prompt pain relief in nearly all the patients, 9 of 66 patients (14%) who they were able to follow for 6 months developed postherpetic neuralgia that lasted 6 months or more. On comparing these results with other reports of the incidence of postherpetic neuralgia among patients treated with steroids or with usual medical therapy, it was concluded that blocks did not prevent postherpetic neuralgia.

During the period from 1943 to 1976, Bonica treated 164 patients with acute herpes zoster with regional sympathetic blocks alone or combined with somatic nerve blocks achieved with 0.15% tetracaine or 0.25 to 0.5% bupivacaine (unpublished data). The following results were obtained: (a) 46 patients (28%) derived persistent pain relief after 1 to 4 blocks; (b) 61 (37%) derived persistent relief with 5 to 10 blocks; (c) 44 (27%) derived good but incomplete pain relief with 10 to 15 blocks; and (d) the remaining 13 (8%) derived little or no relief with 10 blocks, and therapy was discontinued. Analysis of the data indicated that all the patients in category a were treated within 4 days of eruption, those within category b were treated within 5 to 12 days (mean, 8 days), those in category c were treated within 15 to 45 days (mean, 23 days), and those in category d were not seen and treated until 2 months after eruption.

Based on the above data and on personal experience with his own family (Chapter 58), Bonica believes that sympathetic nerve blocks, alone or combined with somatic nerve blocks, achieved with a local anesthetic and done within the first 5 to 7 days of eruption, produce prompt relief of pain, decrease the severity and duration of eruption, seem to prevent the spread of the disease, and decrease the incidence of postherpetic neuralgia by at least 30%.

Studies during the past 12 years have shown that such antiviral drugs as vidarabine and acyclovir given within 72 hours of onset of eruption reduce its spread, accelerate healing, and prevent both cutaneous dissemination and visceral complication, as compared with results obtained with placebo (158). These drugs should be combined with nerve blocks to achieve a synergistic effect and to provide patients with *prompt* relief of pain that is not obtained with the use of antiviral agents alone. Therefore, despite the lack of extensive controlled data and a negative report (157), because postherpetic neuralgia is one of the most difficult problems to treat and because promptly performed neural blockade is simple to carry out and entails little risk, such procedures should be used early in the course of acute herpes zoster.

Once postherpetic neuralgia (PHN) is established, usually by 3 months after eruption, sympathetic or other neural blockade with local anesthetic results in a 20 to 40% incidence of initial pain relief, but this falls to 10% on long-term follow-up (151, 155, 159, 160) (Table 94-5). It has been implied, however, that such blocks performed within 1 year of eruption produce an appreciably greater incidence of pain relief than if patients are managed only with the usual medical therapy (159).

TABLE 94-4. Effects of Sympathetic, Somatic, or Epidural Blocks for Acute Herpes Zoster

Source	Total No. of Patients Treated	Interval Between Eruption to Blocks‡	Protocol Used	Results (Pain Relief)†		No. of Patients who Developed PHN
				Initial Period	Long Term	
Rosenak (150)	22	<4 W	Various single blocks	90%	NS	NS
Colding (151)	205	<2 W	Daily blocks	61% CR 29% PR		7% of 71 patients developed PHN on follow-up
	38	12–20 W	Daily blocks	29% CR 26% PR		
Perkins and Hanlon (153)	7	<12 W	3 daily blocks	100% CR	All 7 CR	NS
	5	>12 W	Epidural	100% CR	Mean 25% improved	NS
Bauman (152)	28	<3 W	1–3 sympathetic blocks or epidural blocks	100% CR		No PHN developed
Dan et al. (154, 155)	(a) 529	<2 W	Regional sympathetic block or epidural block or local conduction block		88% CR	No PHN
	(b) 96	<2–4 W			86% CR	No PHN
	(c) 69	1–3 M			52% CR	?
	(d) 33	3–12 M			30% CR	?
	(e) 22	>1 year			14% CR	?
All:	749					
Tenicela et al. (156)	10	<6 W	4 stellate blocks daily	90% CR	Pain relief maintained	
	10	<6 W	Daily block in 7 placebo w failure	6% CR	4% CR	
Bonica‡	(a) 54	<4 D	1–5 daily blocks	100% CR	100% CR	0
	(b) 72	4–15 D	2–5 blocks daily, then 1–9 blocks every 3 D	100% CR	100% CR	0
	(c) 52	2–8 W	5 daily blocks, then, 5–14 blocks every 3 D	73% CR 27% PR	60% CR 32% PR	(2%)
	(d) 14	8–20 W	Same as above	6% PR 8% NR	6% PR 8% NR	8
Riopelle et al. (157)	72	30 D	Stellate, epidural peripheral block, plus local infiltration	100% CR		14% with PHN, all of whom had severe pain with with initial lesions

*D, day; W, week; M, month.
†NS, not studied; CR, complete relief; PR, partial relief; NR, no relief; PHN, postherpetic neuralgia.
‡Unpublished data.

TABLE 94-5. Results of Nerve Blocks for Pain Relief in Postherpetic Neuralgia

Source	No. of Patients	Eruption to Blocks	Protocol	Results	
				Initial Success	Long-Term Success
Colding (151)	34	3 months to 10 years	3–4 blocks	40%	10%
Forrest (159)	14	6 months to 8 years	3 epidural LA plus steroid blocks at weekly intervals	Mean pain score decreased from 84 to 8 (0–100 VAS) at 3 months' follow-up	
Dan et al. (155)	69	1–3 months	Various blocks	52% good	
	33	3–12 months		30% good	
	22	>12 months		13% good	
Milligan and Nash (160)	34	<1 year	Single stellate block	50% good, 26% improved	
	8	>1 year		25% good, 25% improved	

LA, local anesthetic; VAS, visual analog scale.

Lilley and colleagues (161) compared a control group of 28 patients (mean age 70 years) who were managed with various therapies, including a 3-week oral regimen of prednisone, with 23 patients (mean age also 70 years) who had had postherpetic neuralgia for between 2 and 12 months, and who were treated with sympathetic and somatic nerve blocks achieved with 0.25% bupivacaine. The block therapy entailed daily blocks for 5 days followed by observation for 3 days; if the pain recurred a second 5-day course was repeated. On evaluation 2 years after therapy, it was found that only 5 patients in the control group (18%) had returned to a normal life-style and 15 patients (54%) were totally disabled and did not respond to any therapeutic measures. Of those in the treated group, 11 patients (48%) had a normal life-style and only 4 patients (17%) were totally disabled.

These are surprisingly good results and far better than those we have obtained with nerve blocks. Nevertheless, given the miserable nature of postherpetic neuralgia, the relatively benign nature of the procedure, and the fact that this condition is resistant to alternative therapies, we believe it is worthwhile to give neural blockade a trial in patients with postherpetic neuralgia. We recommend a series of blocks done every other day, for a total of 7 to 10 blocks. If these do not produce lasting benefit, it is likely that the patients are not going to benefit from any additional block therapy. One report suggested that the use of epidural steroids plus local anesthetics is fairly successful in the treatment of postherpetic neuralgia in the thoracic region (159).

Cancer Pain

Sympathetic blocks can also be effective in relieving the burning aching discomfort that is experienced by some patients with cancer of the face and head. Moreover, sympathetic blocks of the upper or lower limb are indicated in patients in whom cancer infiltration or compression of the brachial or lumbosacral plexus produces the symptoms and signs characteristic of reflex sympathetic dystrophy, which responds to sympathetic blocks (Chapter 11).

Musculoskeletal Disorders

In some patients with acute bursitis, tendinitis, tenosynovitis, and other acute traumatic and infectious musculoskeletal disorders, a significant degree of reflex vasospasm, edema, and hyperhidrosis tends to aggravate the pathophysiology. Sympathetic blocks, used in combination with local infiltration of trigger areas or other therapeutic measures, are frequently helpful in relieving the pain, decreasing the pathophysiology, and shortening the disability. A recent controlled study by Bengtsson and Bengtsson (16) showed that cervicothoracic ("stellate") sympathetic block with bupivacaine that produced complete sympathetic interruption and was administered to patients with myofascial pain syndromes (which they called primary fibromyalgia) reduced the number of trigger points (TPs) and produced a marked decrease of rest pain. They administered IRSB with guanethidine 14 days later to the same patients and noted a reduction of TPs but no effect on pain. The two control groups (one group received saline injection of the stellate ganglion and the other IM bupivacaine) derived no benefit at all (no decrease in TPs or the pain). They concluded that regional sympathetic block is more effective than IRSB with guanethidine and that increased sympathetic activity contributes to the pathophysiology of these syndromes (Chapter 21).

Technical Considerations

Monitoring the Effects of Sympathetic Nerve Blocks

When performed correctly, sympathetic nerve blocks produce only minimal effects on pain threshold and cause no change in somatic sensation. To assess the completeness of sympathetic interruption in the absence of change in somatic sensation, it is necessary to measure the effects of sympathetic function. The method chosen depends on the location of the blockade and on the effects desired. Methods include the following: (a) the skin conductance response (SCR), formerly known as the sympathogalvanic reflex (Fig. 94-48); (b) sweat tests, including the Ninhydrin, cobalt

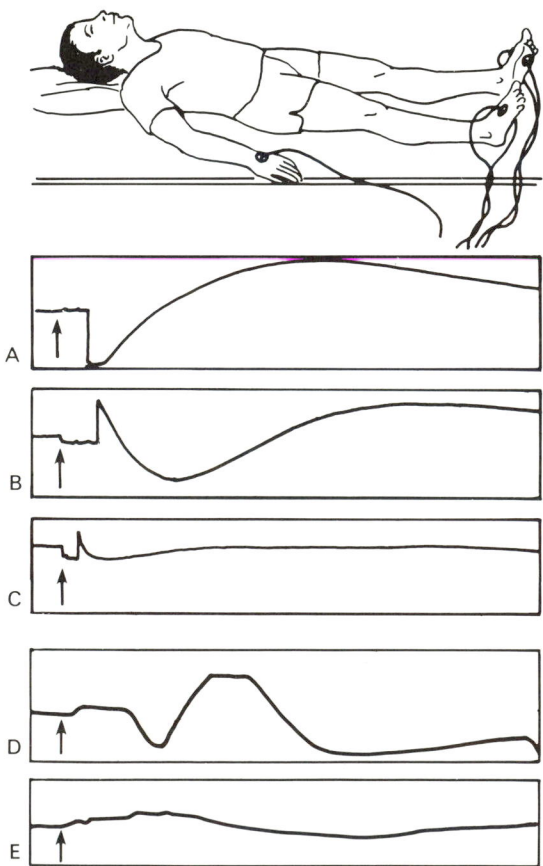

FIG. 94-48. Technique of monitoring sympathetic function by the skin conductance response (SCR). Electrodes are placed on the front and back of the hands or feet and a ground electrode is placed elsewhere on the body. *A, B.* Any unpleasant stimulus, such as a pinch or taking a deep breath, produces a typical curve. The arrow indicates the point where the pinch was applied. *C.* Flattening of the curve indicates absence of the reflex on the left leg after a left lumbar sympathetic block. *D.* Normal curve in the hand before the T2 and T3 sympathetic ganglia were blocked with 6% phenol. *E.* Tracing taken of the same hand as in *D* 2 months after the block.

blue, and starch IV tests; and (c) skin plethysmography and the "ice response test." Blood flow in the skin can be measured by change in skin temperature, a laser doppler, healing of ulcers, or tissue Pa_{O_2}. Blood flow in muscle can be monitored by plethysmography, radioisotope clearance tests, and electromagnetic measurements. Thermography has proven to be effective for measuring the effects of vasoconstriction and the changes in blood flow following sympathetic interruption.

Cervicothoracic Sympathetic Block

Block of the lower cervical and upper thoracic sympathetic chain is one of the most widely used and highly effective diagnostic and therapeutic procedures for management of certain acute and chronic pain syndromes or other disorders of the upper limb, thoracic viscera, and head and neck. Although the procedure is usually referred to as "stellate ganglion block" it is unusual for diffusion of the local anesthetic or neurolytic agent to be limited only to this structure. Studies with contrast media have shown that 5 ml of solution injected into the proper fascial plane spreads to involve the T2 thoracic and intermediate cervical ganglia as well. Injection of 10 to 12 ml of solution spreads from the level of the upper part of the C5 vertebra down to the T3 or T4 vertebra. Injection of 20 ml of solution blocks the chain from the level of the C3 vertebra to the T5 vertebra, thus interrupting all sympathetic pathways to the head and neck, upper limb, and thoracic viscera, and also interrupting the afferent (sensory or nociceptive) fibers supplying these viscera.

Anatomic Basis

The neuroanatomic basis for the clinical application of cervicothoracic sympathetic blocks is shown in Figures 94-49 and 94-50. The sympathetic nerve supply to the head and neck is discussed in Chapter 37, that to the upper limb is described in Chapter 46, and that to the thoracic viscera is described in Chapter 53. Figure 94-49 depicts the four cervical and upper three thoracic ganglia and their relationship to the brachial plexus and thoracic spinal nerves. To obtain optimal results with cervicothoracic sympathetic block, it is necessary to have a precise knowledge of the exact location of the stellage ganglion and its relationship to the upper thoracic and lower cervical ganglia (Fig. 94-50).

The stellate ganglion is an oval-shaped mass, 2.5 cm long, 1 cm wide, and 0.5 cm thick. It is located just behind the subclavian artery at the point of origin of the vertebral artery and in front of the neck of the 1st rib near the costovertebral articulation. The ganglion is situated within a concavity that is limited inferiorly by the posterior aspect of the pleura, medially by the portion of the vertebral column covered by the longus colli muscle, laterally by the scalenus muscle mass, anteriorly by the subclavian and vertebral arteries, and posteriorly by the neck of the 1st rib, the transverse process of the C7 vertebra, and the interspace between these two structures. In most instances, the ganglion extends above the 1st rib so that its upper half is in front of the interspace (Fig. 94-50). The ganglion is 5 mm anterolateral to the bony structures, being separated from them by loose areolar and adipose tissue and the longus colli muscle. The loose areolar and adipose tissue facilitate diffusion of anesthetic solutions de-

posited near the ganglion. The branches of the stellate ganglion include the communicating, anastomotic, vascular, and muscular branches, the inferior cervical cardiac and vertebral nerves, and the ansa subclavia. The gray rami communicantes that are given to the C7 and C8, T1, and sometimes the C5 and C6 spinal nerves constitute the major part of the sympathetic nerve supply to the upper limb (Fig. 94-49).

The other cervical sympathetic ganglia consist of the intermediate, the middle, and the superior cervical ganglia (Fig. 94-49). The superior ganglion is the largest, the middle is the smallest, and the intermediate ganglion is intermediate in size. These ganglia lie on the longus colli muscles and are thus in the same fascial plane as the stellate ganglion. The lower part of the stellate ganglion connects with the T2 sympathetic ganglion, which contains the largest number of synaptic connections between the preganglionic and postganglionic sympathetic fibers that supply the upper limb.

Usually all the sympathetic nerves that supply the head and neck, and most of those that supply the upper limb, traverse the stellate ganglion. Thus, blocking this structure effects a temporary sympathetic denervation of these areas. In a significant number of individuals, however, an intrathoracic somatic branch arising from the T2 spinal nerve joins the T1 spinal nerve, which of course takes part in the formation of the brachial plexus (Figs. 94-49 and 94-50) (129). This intrathoracic branch is almost always joined by gray rami communicantes carrying postganglionic fibers that arise from cell bodies in the T2 sympathetic ganglion and possibly in lower ganglia. In a smaller percentage of individuals an intrathoracic somatic branch is also present, which arises from the T3 spinal nerve and passes to the T2 spinal nerve. This second intrathoracic nerve, which also contains postganglionic sympathetic fibers that arise from the T3 ganglion, joins the T2 spinal nerve near the branch that the latter sends to the T1 nerve. These anomalous pathways, known as Kuntz's nerves, bypass the stellate ganglion so that blocks limited to the stellate ganglion or a pure stellectomy do not produce complete sympathetic denervation of the upper limb. In such cases it is also essential to block the T2 and T3 ganglia to denervate the limb completely. Moreover, because all the fibers to the upper limb pass through the T2 and occasionally the T3 ganglia, they are "key" relay stations that can be blocked with a small volume of neurolytic agent.

Technique

Various techniques for blocking the cervicothoracic (stellate ganglion) sympathetic nerves have been described, including the anterior paratracheal and the lateral, anterolateral, superior, and posterior approaches. Here only the paratracheal approach entailing the injection of the chain with local anesthetic is described. The posterior approaches to the thoracic sympathetic chain, including those that supply the upper limb, are described in Chapter 96.

The paratracheal technique (Fig. 94-51) is the simplest and most frequently used approach for blocking the cervicothoracic sympathetic chain. Because the point of the needle is near the origin of the vertebral artery and might be near a prolonged dural cuff of the C8 nerve, it is especially important to attempt aspiration in two planes before the local anesthetic is injected slowly. Another precaution against accidental intravascular or subarachnoid injection of a large volume of drug is to inject 1 ml of solution, wait about 1 minute, and repeat the aspiration test. If the test is still negative and the patient has not developed any signs of cerebral dysfunction or subarachnoid block, the remainder of the solution can be injected slowly.

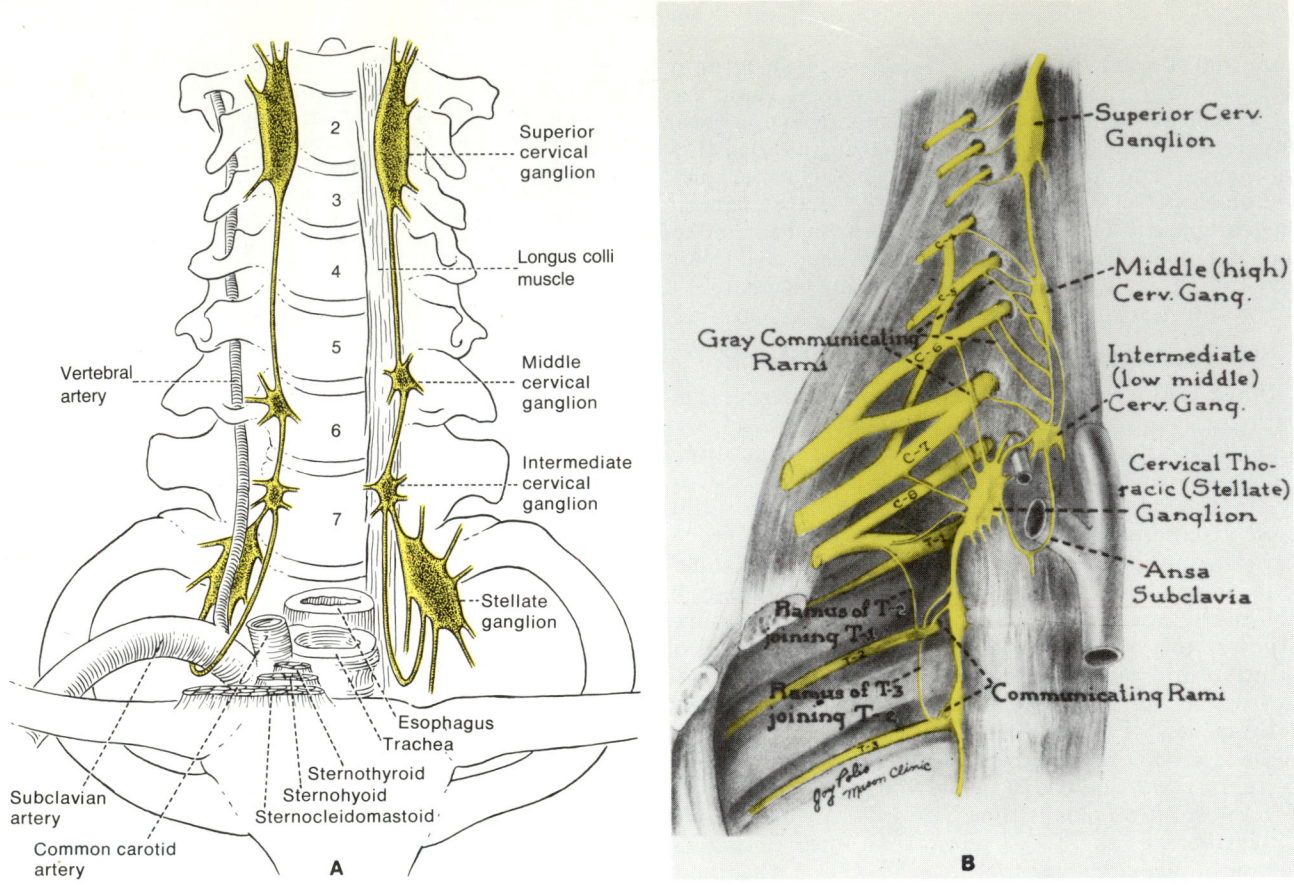

FIG. 94-49. Anatomy of the cervical sympathetic chain. **A.** Anterior view of the deep region of the lower portion of the neck showing the relationship of the sympathetic ganglia to the cervical and upper thoracic vertebrae, the longus colli muscle, and the vertebral artery. **B.** Relationship of the cervical and upper thoracic sympathetic chains and the gray rami communicantes, which connect the chain to the brachial plexus and other spinal nerves. Note the inconstant intrathoracic ramus from the T2 nerve to the T1 nerve and from the T3 nerve to the T2 nerve. Also note the beginning of the lower branches of the stellate ganglion, which include the ansa subclavia, the inferior cardiac nerve, and the nerve to the internal mammary artery. From the upper pole of the ganglion arises the vertebral nerve, which passes to the vertebral artery where it breaks up into the vertebral plexus (not shown). *A* from Bonica, J.J.: Blocks of the Sympathetic Nervous System. Vol. 2. Chicago, Frank J. Corbett, 1981, p. 64. *B* from Moore, D.C.: Stellate Ganglion Block. Springfield, IL, Charles C Thomas, 1954.

FIG. 94-50. Sagittal section of the lower portion of the neck and upper part of the thorax (*inset*) showing the relationship of the stellate ganglion and other parts of the sympathetic chain to bones, blood vessels, and apex of the lung. The longus colli muscle separates the ganglia from the bones and the stellate ganglion is immediately posterior to the beginning of the vertebral artery. Injection of a local anesthetic solution within the fascial plane containing the sympathetic chain causes the solution to diffuse cephalad and caudad to block various parts of the chain (see Fig. 94-52).

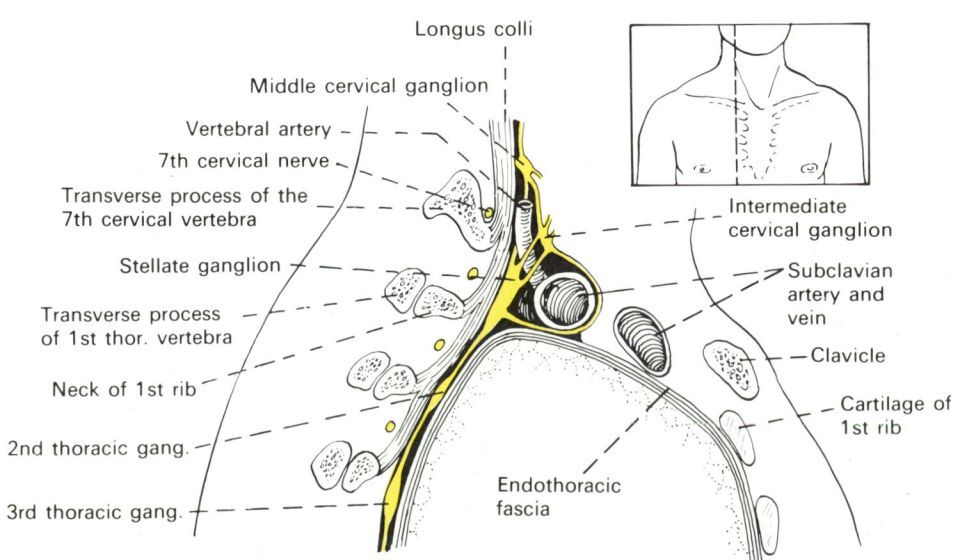

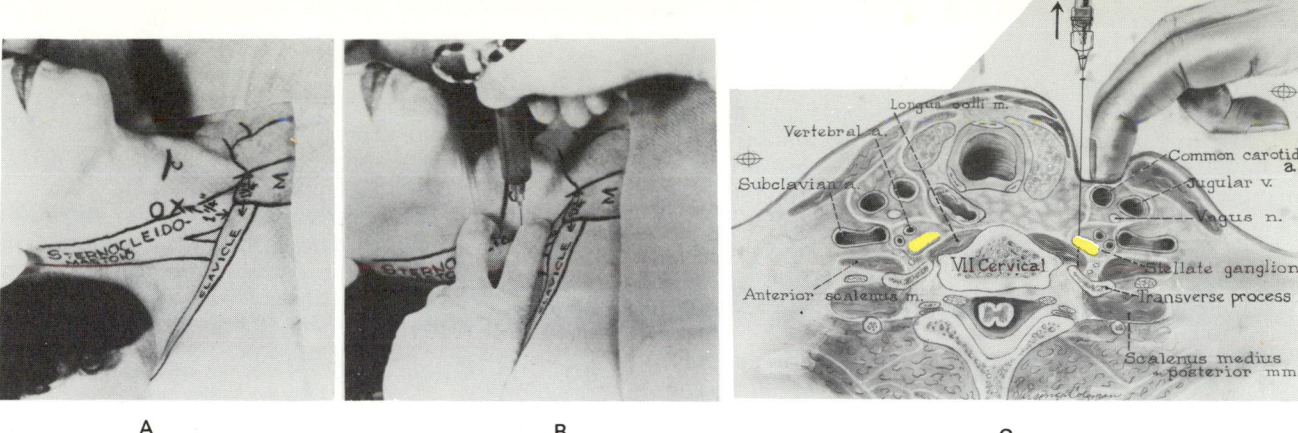

A   B   C

FIG. 94-51. Landmarks and techniques of stellate block by the anterior paratracheal approach. **A.** Outline of the clavicle and sternocleidomastoid. The level of the cricoid cartilage (c) is at the same cross-sectional level as the transverse process of the C6 vertebra (o). X lies anterior to the transverse process of the C7 vertebra and is the point on the skin where an intracutaneous wheal is formed. **B.** With the second and third fingers of the nondominant hand hooked around the medial edge of the sternocleidomastoid and the underlying carotid sheath, with its vessels and nerves retracted laterally, the needle is inserted through a wheal, directed posteriorly in the parasagittal plane, and advanced to the base of the transverse process of the C7 vertebra. **C.** Cross section of the neck at the level of the C7 vertebra depicting the placement of the needle for anterior paratracheal stellate ganglion block. The second and third fingers of the hand are retracting the medial aspect of the sternocleidomastoid muscle and the underlying vessels and the needle is advanced to the base of the transverse process of the C7 vertebra. After bone is contacted the needle is withdrawn about 0.5 cm to place its bevel anterior to the fascia of the longus colli muscle. Injection of a local anesthetic solution anterior to the fascia permits it to diffuse cephalad, caudad, and slightly laterally to block the chain. **A** and **B** from Moore, D.C.: Stellate Ganglion Block. Springfield, IL, Charles C Thomas, 1954.

If the block is intended to interrupt all sympathetic fibers to the ipsilateral upper extremity, 12 to 15 ml of solution is injected. This is sufficient to spread to and block all the sympathetic nerves that supply the upper limb, even in a patient with the anomalous Kuntz's nerves. If the block is intended to interrupt the afferents and efferents to the heart 20 ml of solution is injected, with the patient in a semirecumbent or sitting position. This volume diffuses to and interrupts all the nociceptive afferents from and the efferents (motor) to the heart and most of those to the lung and esophagus (Fig. 94-52).

It has been shown that this procedure successfully interrupts the sympathetic fibers of the head because of the appearance of Horner's syndrome (ptosis, miosis, enophthalmos, anhidrosis of the neck and face) within a few minutes of injection. Evidence that the sympathetic fibers to the upper limb have also been completely interrupted includes engorgement of the veins in the back of the hand, a rise in skin temperature, absence of an SCR, plethysmography, thermography, a sweat test, or a combination of these. Occasionally, maximal vasodilation does not develop until 10 to 20 minutes after injection.

Complications

Complications that can occur during or following cervicothoracic block by the anterior paratracheal

FIG. 94-52. Roentgenograms showing the characteristic pattern of diffusion (arrows) of 10 ml of contrast medium (Diodrast) injected in the same fascial plane as the cervicothoracic sympathetic chain. **A.** Anterorposterior view showing the spread from the top of the C5 vertebra (which includes the middle cervical ganglion) to the T4 vertebra at the level of the T4 or T5 sympathetic ganglion. **B.** Lateral view. From Moore, D.C.: Stellate Ganglion Block. Springfield, IL, Charles C Thomas, 1954.

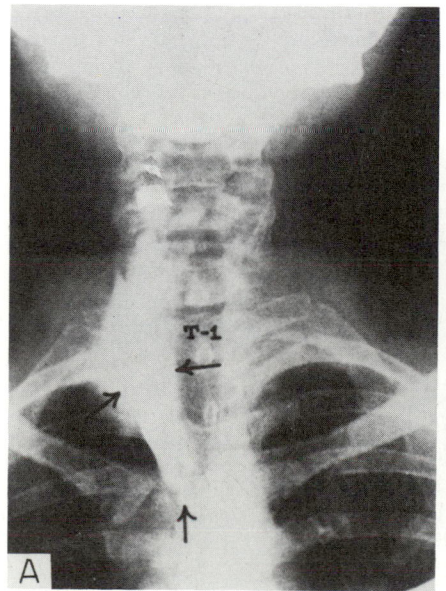 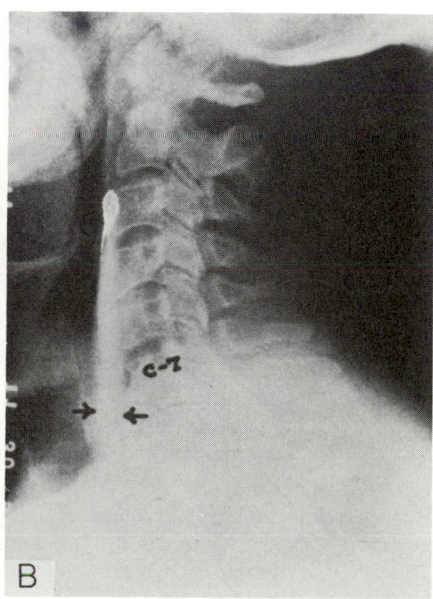

technique include accidental injection of local anesthetic drug into a vein or artery, damage to the pleura, unintentional block of the brachial plexus block, block of the recurrent laryngeal nerve, or accidental subarachnoid injection. The symptoms and signs of these various complications, their prophylaxis, and treatment have been discussed above (A. Basic Considerations). One complication of note is the accidental injection of a small amount (2 to 3 ml) of local anesthetic into the vertebral artery. This results in immediate perfusion of the brain stem and thus is likely to produce transient respiratory paralysis and unconsciousness, possibly associated with severe arterial hypotension. Treatment consists of *immediate* artificial ventilation and maintenance of arterial blood pressure.

Block of the Thoracic Sympathetic Chain

Block of one (or more) of the thoracic sympathetic ganglia and the intervening interganglionic chain is indicated as a diagnostic procedure for identifying specific nociceptive pathways or as a therapeutic measure for treating herpes zoster or some other painful disorder that might involve only a few segments. Because of its complex nature, however, most clinicians use segmental epidural block and resort to paravertebral block of the thoracic sympathetic chain with neurolytic agents in managing patients with chronic intractable pain (Chapter 96).

Block of the Celiac Plexus

Block of the celiac plexus is useful for relieving severe pain caused by acute visceral disease, hepatic embolization for the treatment of carcinoma, cancer, and other chronic visceral disorders. In addition to blocking all the nociceptive (pain) pathways that supply most of the abdominal viscera, this procedure also interrupts the efferent pathways so often involved in the reflex visceral vasospasm and other pathophysiologic processes caused by abnormal reflexes and by the persistent noxious stimulation of disease (162, 163). Because the celiac plexus contains vagal afferent and efferent fibers, block of this structure interrupts sensory fibers that transmit non-nociceptive information and the parasympathetic outflow to the abdominal viscera (164).

Celiac plexus block is also useful in treating adynamic ileus. Celiac plexus block with local anesthetic should be done to predict the effects of neurolytic blockade in patients in whom this procedure is to be used to relieve the severe pain of cancer or to treat other chronic conditions. The most frequent use of this technique is for the relief of severe chronic pain, so it is discussed in detail in Chapter 96.

Splanchnic Nerve Block

The indications for splanchnic nerve block are similar to those of celiac plexus block, except that this procedure probably does *not* involve the lumbar sympathetic chain, which is likely also to be blocked by celiac plexus block. The technique is therefore more specific and requires smaller quantities of agent with a lesser likelihood of complications. Because splanchnic nerves are usually blocked with neurolytic agents to control chronic pain, the technique is discussed in Chapter 96.

Lumbar Sympathetic Block

Indications

Block of the lumbar portion of the sympathetic chain is a useful diagnostic, prognostic, or therapeutic procedure for various painful syndromes involving the pelvis or lower limbs and for peripheral vascular disorders (see above, Cervicothoracic Sympathetic Block). The block is also important for predicting the effects of neurolytic blockade in patients with peripheral vascular disorders of the lower limbs.

Neuroanatomic Basis

The anatomy of the lumbar sympathetic chain is discussed in detail in Chapters 65 and 70. The lumbar sympathetic trunks consist of two ganglionated cords that extend from the L1 to the L5 vertebrae and are continuous above with the thoracic portion and below with the pelvic portion of the sympathetic trunk (see Fig. 94-53). Each chain lies on the anterolateral surface of the vertebral column, being more medial and anterior than the thoracic chain. Both lumbar chains are situated anteriorly and slightly medially to the aponeurotic arcades giving rise to the psoas muscle and the psoas fascia, which is also attached medially by a series of arched processes to the intervertebral disks and by the prominent upper and lower margins of adjacent vertebrae. The intervals between the arched processes of the psoas muscle and fascia and the constricted part of the vertebrae transmit the lumbar arteries and veins and sympathetic nerves that connect the lumbar sympathetic chain with the somatic lumbar nerves. The relation of the sympathetic trunks to the great vessels differs on each side. On the right side, the trunk lies posterior to the lateral edge of the vena cava, which in most cases completely covers the trunk. On the left side, the chain is rarely covered by the aorta, being from 4 to 10 mm lateral to the lateral edge of the vessel; on this side it is usually covered by the lumbar lymph glands and peritoneum. Inferiorly the cords pass posterior to the iliac vessels to become continuous with the sacral sympathetic trunks.

The lumbar sympathetic chains are the most variable portion of the sympathetic system, particularly in regard to the number of ganglia and to the general forms of the two chains; they are extremely inconstant, not only among different patients, but on each side of the same patient. It is almost exceptional to find five ganglia—it is more usual to find only four, with a fusion of the L1 and T12 ganglia; some people only have three on one side. Moreover, only rarely does one find a chain on one side that is the same shape, size, and in a similar position to the chain on the opposite side (1, 129, 162). The location of the ganglia is also inconstant: in some individuals they are segmentally located while in others they are closely grouped and lie over a particular segment. The most common location is between the L2 and the inferior border of the L4 vertebrae (129, 164). The ganglia can be situated on the body of the vertebra or anterior to the aponeurotic arcades, giving rise to the psoas muscle. In most people, they lie anterolateral to an intervertebral disk with one portion of the ganglion in front of the lower part of the vertebra above and the other portion of the ganglion in front of the upper part of the vertebra below. The same degree of variability exists in regard to the size of the ganglia and the interganglionic cord and the number of branches extending from them. Ganglia range in size from 3 to 5 mm wide and 10 to 15 mm long.

The lumbar sympathetic chain contains both the preganglionic and postganglionic neurons that supply the pelvic viscera and vessels of the lower limbs and afferent (sensory) fibers, some of which transmit nociceptive information. The cell bodies of the sympathetic preganglionic neurons that supply the lower limbs are located in the T11 and T12, L1, L2, and sometimes the T10 and L3 spinal cord segments. Their axons pass through anterior roots of the corresponding spinal nerves and through the lower four, five, or six white rami communicantes to the sympathetic trunk (Figs. 6-15 and 70-32). They descend to end in the lower three lumbar and upper three sacral ganglia, wherein they synapse with cell bodies of postganglionic neurons.

Some axons of postganglionic neurons pass directly to the iliac and femoral arteries, around which they form a plexus that passes as far as the junction of the upper and middle thirds of the thigh. Most of the postganglionic axons pass as the gray rami communicates, however, which join the spinal nerves that form the lumbar plexus and the lumbosacral plexus. These sympathetic fibers pass distally as components of the femoral, sciatic, and obturator nerves and their branches and are given off segmentally to the vessels of the lower limb (Fig. 70-33). Thus, by blocking the L2 and L3 ganglia, through which most of the fibers going to the lower limb pass, almost complete sympathetic denervation of the limb can be effected. In some subjects, however, some of the sympathetic pathways to the lower limb and pelvis bypass the sympathetic chain and make their synaptic connections in somatic spinal nerves. In these individuals, surgical sympathectomy limited to excision of the sympathetic chain fails to denervate the sympathetic supply to the limb completely.

Other branches given off by the lumbar sympathetic chain include the osseous branches, which supply the vertebrae, muscular branches, which supply the psoas muscles, and

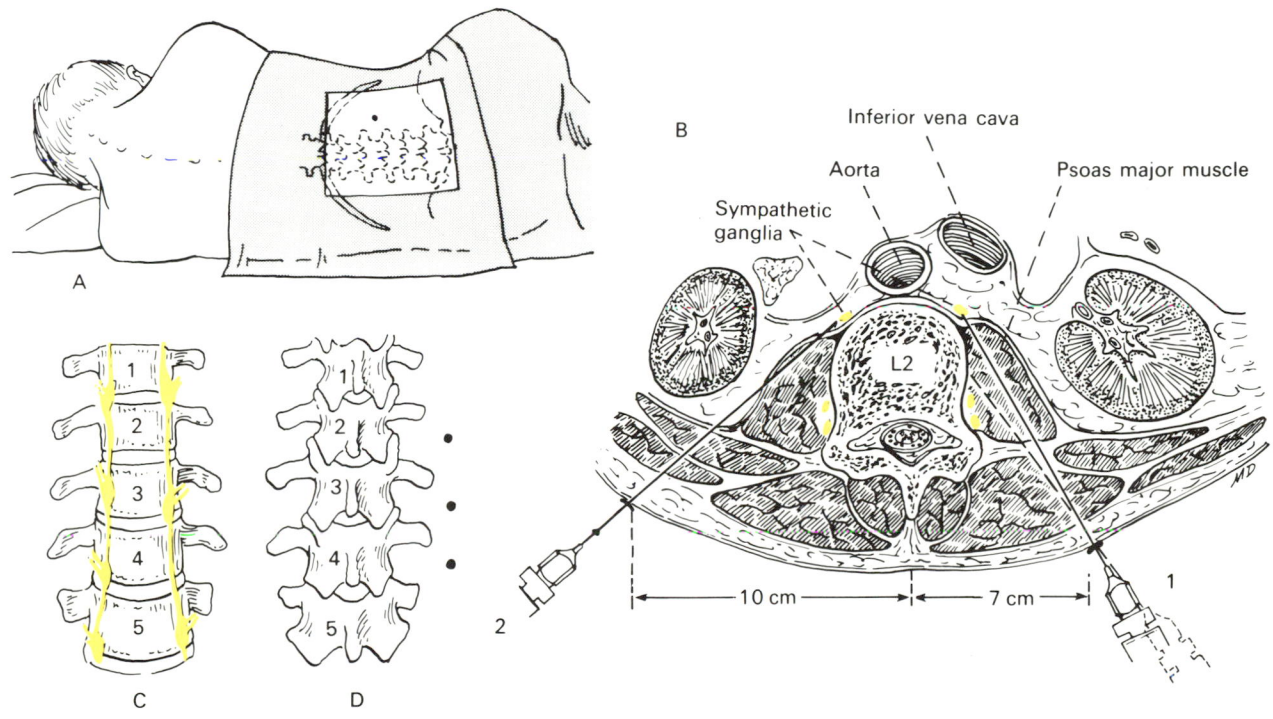

FIG. 94-53. Technique of lumbar sympathetic block. A. The patient lies on the side with the affected side uppermost. B. Cross section at L2 to show the two techniques that can be used, a so-called classic technique (using 3 or 4 needles) or a lateral technique. For the classic technique (needle #1), a skin wheal is raised 6 to 7 cm lateral to the midline at the midpoint of the quadrilaterally spaced spinous process of the lumbar vertebrae. In many patients 22-gauge 8-cm security needles with rubber depth markers are used. For patients who are obese or muscular it is best to use 10- or 12-cm 22-gauge needles. For diagnostic purposes it is best to inject through two or three needles at the levels of the L2 and L4 or L2, L3, and L4 vertebrae. Each needle is inserted through the skin wheal and advanced anteriorly and medially. The shaft of the needle should make an angle of about 75 to 80° with the skin lateral to it. The needle is advanced until the lateral aspect of the lumbar vertebra is contacted, usually at a depth of 6 to 8 cm from the skin in thin or normal individuals but possibly as deep as 10 cm from the skin in obese individuals. The skin marker is placed 2 cm from the skin and the needle is withdrawn until its point is subcutaneous and then redirected more laterally so it passes through the psoas major muscle. It might be useful to adapt a Luer-Lok control needle to a 2- or 5-ml syringe filled with air or saline solution. As the needle traverses the psoas muscle, some resistance to injection is encountered. The needle is further advanced slowly while gentle pressure is applied to the plunger of the syringe. As the point of the needle passes through the thick medial junction of the psoas fascia, significant resistance is encountered but, as soon as the bevel pierces the fascia, a sudden lack of resistance can be felt and the air or saline can be injected easily, indicating that the needle point is in the retroperitoneal space and is near the sympathetic chain. The local anesthetic solution is injected after a negative aspiration test in four quadrants. If a diagnostic procedure is being done with three needles, 3 ml of solution injected through each of the needles is sufficient. If two needles are used, 5 ml of solution is injected at L2 and L4. One needle at L2 or L3 can be used for therapeutic purposes and 15 to 20 ml of local anesthetic solution injected. If the needle is in the proper fascial plane (anterior to the vertebral insertion of the psoas fascia) the solution spreads cephalad and caudad to involve the entire lumbar sympathetic chain. The lateral technique (needle #2) entails the insertion of the needle through wheals made 10 cm lateral to the midline. With this technique no attempt is made to contact the lateral aspect of the vertebra but the needle is advanced through the psoas muscle mass for about 6 or 7 cm, after which the same test volume of air or saline solution is used as for the classic technique. As soon as the needle passes through this psoas fascia a sudden lack of resistance indicates the proper position. The rest of the technique is similar to that already described. C. Anterior view of lumbar vertebrae showing position of sympathetic chain. D. Posterior view showing sites of wheals for the lateral technique.

vascular branches, some of which accompany the lumbar arteries. They also give off four lumbar splanchnic nerves that pass anterior to the lower part of the celiac plexus to the aortic plexus and to the superior hypogastric plexuses and the plexuses that accompany the iliac vessels (Chapter 59).

Technique

Two techniques of lumbar sympathetic block are described in Figure 94-53. The classic technique, which entails insertion of four needles at the L1, L2, L3, and L4 vertebral levels, was formerly used, but this has now been simplified to a two-needle technique at L2 and L4. Boas (165) has effectively used a single needle placed at L2 or L3 and found it to be as satisfactory, even for injection of neurolytic agents. Although we believe that a one-needle technique can be effective for injection of a local anesthetic, two or even three needles should be used for neurolytic blocks (Chapter 96). Because the sympathetic trunk crosses the lumbar arteries at the constricted part (midpoint) of the vertebral body, it is best to avoid placing the point of the needle at this level. Instead, the point of the needle should be placed anterior to the attachment of the aponeurotic arcades of the psoas muscle and its fascia. This not only permits the fascia to be used for the lack of resistance test (Fig. 94-53), but also decreases the risk of damaging

the vessels and of local anesthetic solution flowing back to involve somatic nerves. To achieve the placement of the needle so that its point is in front of the aponeurotic arcades, the needle should be inserted at the same cross-sectional level as the upper part of the spinous process of the vertebra. The insertion is made a variable distance from the midline so that the needle passes either just above the tip of the transverse process or more laterally (Fig. 94-53B, left side).

If block is achieved with a fairly large volume of solution (8 to 10 ml for each needle) for therapeutic purposes, radiologic visualization is not necessary. If a block is being done for diagnostic purposes using a small volume (2 ml), however, radiographic visualization is as essential as when carrying out a neurolytic block.

Complications

In the hands of skilled anesthesiologists, complications should be extremely rare. Those that can occur include accidental injection of the drug into the inferior vena cava (on the right) or into the aorta (on the left), damage to the lumbar vessels, unintentional contact and consequent paresthesia of somatic nerves, or diffusion of the drug to block the somatic nerves, with consequent hypesthesia and even weakness of the quadriceps.

E. INTRAVENOUS REGIONAL BLOCKADE

In this section we consider two techniques of intravenous regional blockade that can be used to provide relief of a number of painful conditions. The primary method is intravenous regional sympathetic blockade, which involves the injection of guanethidine into the venous system of the limb after the circulation has been temporarily occluded with a tourniquet. The second technique is intravenous regional neural blockade, which involves the injection of a local anesthetic under the same conditions. Both techniques are used for painful conditions of the limbs and use a Bier block, proposed by August Bier, the famous German surgeon who was the first to use spinal anesthesia for surgery (166). We also discuss the use of continuous infusion of local anesthetics for pain management.

Intravenous Regional Sympathetic Blockade

For many years systemic drugs that interrupt sympathetic (efferent) function either at the pre- and postganglionic synapses or at the endings of postganglionic fibers have been used to treat various painful and nonpainful disorders. The advantages of systemic therapy over regional sympathetic block include its simplicity of administration and the avoidance of some of the complications that can follow the use of various regional sympathetic block techniques. On the other hand, systemic administration of sympatholytic drugs has the serious disadvantage of producing a sympathetic denervation that involves the entire body and is frequently incomplete.

In 1974, Hannington-Kiff (167) proposed a brilliant technique to produce prolonged sympathetic interruption in a limb without the disadvantages of systemic

drugs or regional sympathetic blocks. This procedure entails the injection of the antiadrenergic agent guanethidine into the venous system of the limb after the circulation has been temporarily occluded with a tourniquet. The technique, which has become known as intravenous regional sympathetic blockade (IRSB), has become widely used for the relief of various painful conditions in which sympathetic dysfunction is present. We present here the basis for use of the procedure, practical details, indications, advantages, disadvantages, and possible complications.

Basic Considerations

Guanethidine produces a prolonged unselective sympathetic blockade by displacing norepinephrine (NE) from presynaptic vesicles and preventing a re-uptake of NE. When guanethidine first enters the endings of the postganglionic neurons, it releases NE from its storage sites (137). The concentration of guanethidine builds up at these sites and its continued presence prevents the reuptake of NE from the synaptic cleft. Another effect of intravenous guanethidine is to inhibit the release of any remaining NE. Consequently, the adrenergic neurotransmitter is rapidly depleted, resulting in the impairment and eventual loss of sympathetic adrenergic nerve function, which has the effect of sympathetic blockade. The blockade lasts for many hours, often days, and sometimes weeks because of the strong binding and because guanethidine is eliminated slowly.

The effect of guanethidine is biphasic, first releasing NE and then causing noradrenergic block (137). Moreover, the clinical results of a guanethidine block can take time to develop and are dose-dependent. In sufficient concentration, guanethidine can cause permanent damage to the NE reuptake pump. This concentration can be reached progressively with repeated blocks because guanethidine accumulates in the nerves for a prolonged period (137).

Controlled studies have now documented the efficacy of IRSB with guanethidine in increasing blood flow (168–171) and skin temperature (168, 170) while decreasing the vasoconstrictor ice response (169) and relieving pain in vascular disease (168–170) and reflex sympathetic dystrophy (168, 172). Sweating is not reduced because this function is mediated by cholinergic postganglionic sympathetic fibers, which are unaffected by guanethidine. Bonelli and associates (168) compared the duration of effect and efficacy of guanethidine with those of stellate ganglion block in a randomized trial in patients with reflex sympathetic dystrophy (Chapter 11). They found that stellate ganglion blocks done every other day (up to a total of eight blocks) produced similar clinical effects to those of IRSB with guanethidine given every 4 days (up to a total of four blocks) in terms of pain scores and clinical signs when assessed at 1-month and 3-month follow-up.

Clinical Evaluations

ADVANTAGES. It is obvious that the IRSB technique using guanethidine has certain advantages over the regional sympathetic blocks described above. For one thing, IRSB is less "invasive" and more comfortable for patients. For another, it is simple to carry out and does not require the thorough anatomic knowledge and the technical skills necessary for performing regional sympathetic block so it can be done by physicians who are not experienced with the use of regional anesthesia. The technique is especially useful for patients who are receiving anticoagulants and for whom sympathetic interruption is indicated. Regional blocks in such patients carry the risk of hemorrhage into deeper tissues (see above). The possibility of systemic toxic reaction to local anesthetics, accidental subarachnoid injections, and other such complications are obviated with IRSB. In addition, the annoying onset of Horner's syndrome, which develops following cervicothoracic sympathetic block by the anterior paratracheal technique, is avoided. Finally, because the guanethidine technique produces blockade for several days or weeks, repeated injections are unnecessary.

DISADVANTAGES. The following are the disadvantages of the use of the IRSB technique (in comparison with regional sympathetic block): (a) the drug initially causes a transient release of noradrenalin with consequent cutaneous vasoconstriction and piloerection, and not infrequently a burning pain, especially in patients who have painful limbs; (b) unless all the guanethidine is taken up by the tissues during the occlusion of circulation by the tourniquet, some of the drug enters the systemic circulation and produces hypotension, with compensatory tachycardia, dizziness, and other symptoms and signs of systemic sympathetic blockade; and (c) the procedure can only be used to achieve sympathetic interruption in the limb. It cannot be used in patients with burning pain in the head and neck or trunk, and is of no value in relieving visceral pain. As previously mentioned, Campbell and associ-

ates (131) indicated that IRSB with guanethidine is not as specific as regional sympathetic blockade in differentiating SMP from SIP in patients with neurologic disorders. Moreover, Bengtsson and Bengtsson (16) found that, whereas normal sympathetic block eliminates trigger points and significantly reduces pain in patients with myofascial pain syndromes, IRSB with guanethidine has no effect on the pain. These differences might be related to the fact that guanethidine does not block cholinergic fibers.

Technical Considerations

The procedure should be carried out in an environment in which all appropriate resuscitative measures and equipment are available for immediate use (see pp. 1892–1895: A. Basic Considerations) and where blood pressure and other vital signs can be closely monitored. An infusion of fluid should be started in a free limb (preferably an arm) that is not the site of the block. In most patients premedication is unnecessary, but if inflation of the tourniquet causes undue anxiety and apprehension patients should be given 100 mg of thiopental or 5 to 10 mg of diazepam IV. Moreover, it might be desirable to give 3 to 5 mg of morphine IV to prevent or minimize the pain and discomfort inherent in the inflation of the tourniquet. An alternate method of minimizing the discomfort of the tourniquet is through the use of a double-cuff tourniquet applied to the upper arm or thigh and mixing the guanethidine sulfate solution with 25 to 35 mg of bupivacaine (without epinephrine).

To produce sympathetic block in the upper extremity, Hannington-Kiff (167) formerly suggested 10 to 20 mg (1 to 2 ml) of guanethidine sulfate diluted in 25 ml of saline solution and for the lower limb he recommended 15 to 20 mg guanethidine sulfate diluted in 50 ml of saline solution. Although these doses are ample for diagnostic tests and should not be exceeded when early vasodilation is required, especially in vasospastic disease, he subsequently proposed using a larger dose of 30 mg of guanethidine sulfate for repeated therapeutic blockade (137). With such doses vasodilation can be delayed for several hours, especially in sensitive patients with a history of Raynaud's phenomenon caused by the initial NE release. Hannington-Kiff suggested that this can be prevented by adding an alpha-adrenergic blocker such as thymoxamine 15 to 20 mg, which is sufficient to prevent this effect of the NE release and allows an early vasodilation. A similar but less specific method of allowing early vasodilation when using the high-dose regime of guanethidine involves the addition of 25 mg of bupivacaine (5 ml of 0.5%) to the guanethidine solution (137).

Technique

After the patient is prepared psychologically and pharmacologically and the IV infusion has been started, a thin layer of padding is wrapped around the limb and the correct size of tourniquet cuff is carefully applied and secured. The limb is raised well above the heart level for about 60 seconds to drain the venous blood and the tourniquet is inflated up to at least 50 mm Hg above systolic for an infusion in the upper limb and to 100 mm Hg above systolic for the procedure in the lower limb. Higher pressures can be used in the tourniquet for sedated patients. The limb is returned to the horizontal and the guanethidine solution is injected at a rate that conveniently passes from the 50-ml syringe through a 20-gauge butterfly needle. The treated limb soon shows patchy areas of pallor caused by the arteriolar vasoconstriction resulting from the release of NE. In his early experience, Hannington-Kiff (167) kept the tourniquet in place for 10 minutes to allow the drug to become firmly fixed to tissues. Moreover, he noted that on deflation of the tourniquet at 10 minutes it was not unusual for patients to report an evanescent slight burning sensation of the throat. Later the conjunctivae might be pink, with slight drooping of the eyelids for about an hour. These effects are uncommon with a tourniquet time of 20 minutes. On the other hand, if the condition of the limb is poor, the time can be reduced to 7 or 8 minutes, after which the tourniquet is deflated for 30 seconds and is then reinflated while the blood pressure is measured.

Following the procedure, patients are confined to bed for 2 hours and can lie horizontally on their side for the first half hour, especially if they have had any form of anesthesia. Most patients are treated on an outpatient basis. Blocks might need to be repeated, at first at 3-day intervals in severe cases and then less often. In some cases only one block, or at most two about 3 weeks apart, can suffice. The most common requirement is for two or three blocks (137).

Intravenous Regional Neural Blockade

In the introduction to this section it was noted that in 1908 Bier (166) first used intravenous regional blockade to alleviate pain. He effected localized analgesia of only one extremity by expressing the blood from the part with an Esmarch bandage and by applying a tourniquet proximal to the point of injection. This prevented the expressed blood from re-entering the extremity and the local anesthetic from leaving the extremity, thus excluding it from the general circulation. Diffusion of the local anesthetic into the tissue and block of the nerve trunks passing through the area caused analgesia of the extremity distal to the tourniquet for $1\frac{1}{2}$ to $2\frac{1}{2}$ hours. Following Bier's report, many others were published (cited in the first edition of this book) (1). In the same year intra-arterial injection of local anesthetic was used for surgical anesthesia and also for the relief of pain. Despite a number of reports this procedure did not become popular until 1935, when Leriche and Fontaine (173) reported the use of intra-arterial injection of procaine to afford relief in cases of painful arteritis obliterans. Later they advocated both IV and intra-arterial injection of procaine for other painful conditions, including Raynaud's disease, causalgia, traumatic arthritis, painful phantom limb, and leg ulcers.

Although intravenous regional blockade has become a popular method of producing surgical anesthesia of the limb, it has only been used to a limited degree in the management of acute and chronic pain. Intravenous regional blockade with local anesthetic is a convenient method for determining whether the pain arises from a peripheral source in the upper or lower limb, and can be used as a temporary measure to relieve pain. Boas and Cousins (174) suggested that pain relief can be assessed only while the cuff is inflated because generalized effects would be produced as soon as the local anesthetic is released into the circulation. Moreover, local anesthetic can escape under the cuff and by intraosseus blood flow, even when the cuff is inflated. Nevertheless, this procedure can be used to help in differential diagnosis and also as a temporary measure to relieve severe pain.

Technique

The technique is similar to that described for IRSB with guanethidine. After the patient is prepared with an IV infusion, the limb is elevated and snugly wrapped with an Esmarch bandage, beginning just proximal to the site of the needle in the hand. The tourniquet is inflated to a pressure above the patient's systolic pressure, as with the IRSB technique. Using a 50-ml disposable syringe, 30 to 40 ml of 0.5% lidocaine or procaine without epinephrine or other vasoconstrictors is injected slowly. As the drug is injected the skin usually becomes mottled, and analgesia develops rapidly. Usually sufficient analgesia and frequently muscle relaxation develop within 5 to 10 minutes. Unfortunately, the tourniquet does produce significant discomfort that might require IV injection of sedatives and a small dose of narcotics. If the technique is being used for diagnostic purposes, however, use of an opioid can confuse the issue. For this and other reasons, intravenous neural blockade has limited application in the management of pain.

Continuous Infusion of Local Anesthetics

Following the report by Leriche and Fontaine (173), single-dose and subsequently continuous infusion of intravenous local anesthetics were used to relieve various painful and nonpainful conditions. During the 1940s and early 1950s, continuous infusion of local anesthetic drugs was used so widely as to prompt Bonica (1) to devote an entire chapter to a description of the techniques and the results obtained. Because many of the reports were subsequently unsubstantiated, however, use of the technique was practically abandoned.

During the past 15 years interest has been rekindled in the use of IV lidocaine and procaine for treating central pain states. Boas and colleagues (13) have used IV lidocaine in patients with neuralgia and deafferentation syndrome, with good results. Atkinson (175) reported the efficacy of IV lidocaine for relief of the severe intractable pain of adiposis dolorosa. He administered a 0.1% lidocaine solution IV until 200 mg had been given over a 35-minute period. The pain relief lasted for 2 to over 12 months. Hatangdi and associates (176) reported on the use of a combination of antiepileptic and tricyclic drugs with IV lidocaine. They found that IV lidocaine in doses of 1 to 1.5 mg/kg body weight during a paroxysmal attack usually produced complete relief of lancinating pain within seconds of injection and provided an indication of the likely response to antiepileptic drugs taken orally. Tocainide, a primary amine congener of lidocaine with a longer duration of action, has been found to be effective for the relief of tic douloureux and causalgia (177).

The efficacy of IV local anesthetics in relieving neuralgia, deafferentation pain, and other central pain problems has been supported by experimental studies. Woolf and Wiesenfeld-Hallin (14) and Wiesenfeld-Hallin and Lindblom (177) demonstrated that IV administration of lidocaine or tocainide produced a selective depression of C-afferent fiber-evoked activity in the spinal cord by increasing the inactivation of sodium channels. It has also been shown that lidocaine can depress synaptic transmission; this is thought to be the likely mechanism involved in the central antinociceptive action of these drugs. In this regard, tocainide has an advantage over lidocaine in that it can be administered orally and produces a longer antinociceptive action. Wiesenfeld-Hallin and Lindblom (177) reported that, given in doses of 4 to 8 mg/kg body weight, oral tocainide is effective in producing the same degree of pain relief in patients with trigemimal neuralgia as carbamazepine.

Technique

The local anesthetics were formerly given IV as a bolus, but more recently continuous infusion of lidocaine or chloroprocaine has been used. Boas and co-workers (13) administered lidocaine at a rate of 4 mg/minute using a Harvard pump for 1 hour in patients with deafferentation syndrome, and pain relief was achieved with serum lidocaine levels of 1.5 to 2 μg/ml. Raj (178) recommended the use of 1% chloroprocaine administered by volumetric infusion to control the incidence of side effects. The drug is administered at a rate of 1 to 1.5 mg/kg/minute until a total dose of 10 to 20 mg/kg is delivered.

It is essential that the infusion be done in a controlled environment that permits continuous ECG monitoring and frequent measurement of blood pressure, heart rate, and mental function. Moreover, resuscitative equipment and drugs must be immediately available to treat any systemic local anesthetic toxicity. Following completion of therapy patients are required to rest for 1 to 2 hours; if in satisfactory condition they can then be discharged home accompanied by an escort.

The efficacy of an IV infusion of local anesthetics in relieving chronic pain must be evaluated, particularly with conditions that do not respond to usual therapy (e.g., postherpetic neuralgia and deafferentation syndrome). Pain relief scores should be elicited from patients before, during, and after infusion. For the period between treatments, which is usually a 1-week interval, patients should be requested to assess and record their degree of pain relief and psychologic scores on a visual analog scale at least four times daily (i.e., morning, afternoon, evening, and night) (176). Sufficient evidence now suggests that IV local anesthetics given at regular intervals do provide partial pain relief. Bonica (1) has noted that Livingston and Haugen (personal communication, 1952) reported favorable results with weekly IV infusions of procaine in patients with postherpetic neuralgia and other types of deafferentation pain. They emphasized that, to be effective, this method must be employed with persistence because a number of treatments are often required before patients experience consistent pain relief. More recent reports suggest that 50% require four to six treatments, while the remainder require additional therapeutic measures at intervals of 2 to 3 weeks (174, 178). Obviously, the decision to continue is based on the fact that the initial series produces some degree of relief.

F. NEURAXIAL BLOCKADE

Subarachnoid Block

Subarachnoid block, also known as spinal anesthesia, is achieved by introducing a small amount of local anesthetic (e.g., 100 to 150 mg procaine, or 50 to 100 mg lidocaine, or 5 to 15 mg bupivacaine) into the subarachnoid space, where it mixes readily with the cerebrospinal fluid (CSF). Because the drug comes into contact with nerve axons without the necessity of traversing the epineurium and perineurium, as with other analgesic techniques, it produces a rapid onset of analgesia. Moreover, subarachnoid injection is the simplest regional anesthetic technique to administer and, in experienced hands, permits better control of the degree, extent, and duration of blockade than can be obtained with other regional techniques. Thus, by making the local anesthetic solution hyperbaric (i.e., its specific gravity is greater than that of the CSF), the spread of block can be controlled by changing the position of the patient.

Notwithstanding these advantages, subarachnoid block with local anesthetic has a limited place in managing patients with acute pain and even less of a role in managing patients with chronic pain, except as

a prognostic block prior to subarachnoid injection of a neurolytic agent. This technique, which entails injection of 1 mg of tetracaine or bupivacaine at a vertebral level at which the subarachnoid space contains the rootlets of the midportion of all the spinal segments to be blocked, is described in detail in Chapter 96. Here we limit our comments to "differential" or graduated subarachnoid block.

Differential Subarachnoid Block

Indications

Differential subarachnoid block was introduced as an effective method for differentiating pain caused primarily by sympathetic hyperactivity from pain caused by nociceptive input along sensory nerves. The technique was also intended to differentiate peripheral nociception from central pain. This procedure was based on the long-held assumption that fibers of different sizes are blocked by different concentrations of local anesthetics. It was believed that the small sympathetic preganglionic axons in the subarachnoid space, being the smallest diameter fibers, were susceptible to a concentration of local anesthetic that did not block somatic nociceptive impulses, and that the A-delta and C fibers in somatic nerves could be blocked by concentrations that would not block the large A-beta and A-alpha fibers that carry tactile and motor functions, respectively. Differential or graduated subarachnoid block (179, 180) has been used to permit differentiation of the source of pain. The technique was considered to be most suitable for investigating patients with lower extremity, pelvic, lower abdominal, and lumbar spine pain. It was considered to be less suitable for investigating patients with pain from the upper abdomen, thorax, or cervical spine, because high blocks in these regions inevitably entail an extensive autonomic block, along with its cardiovascular sequelae.

This classic concept of differential blockade has recently come into question. It is now clear that no sure way exists for producing a "pure" block of sympathetic, sensory, or motor fibers. A number of studies have drawn attention to other factors, such as frequency-dependent conduction block and spinal cord long tract block (174). Moreover, it has been shown that the preganglionic fibers in the subarachnoid space, though smaller than A-delta fibers, are more resistant to a low concentration of local anesthetic than are the nociceptive fibers (181). These findings make the concept of the "differential" neural blockade increasingly contentious, and cast considerable doubt on the interpretation of such block. On the other hand, graduated spinal block can be used to determine the segmental level from which pain is derived or transmitted. This is accomplished by producing ascending spinal blockade with dose increments that produce rising segmental anesthesia (174). Subarachnoid injection is the procedure of choice here because smaller doses of local anesthetic can be used, so that much less drug is absorbed into the vasculature, and the direct effect of absorbed local anesthetic on spinal neurons is avoided.

Technique

A differential or graduated subarachnoid block is best achieved by inserting a microcatheter into the

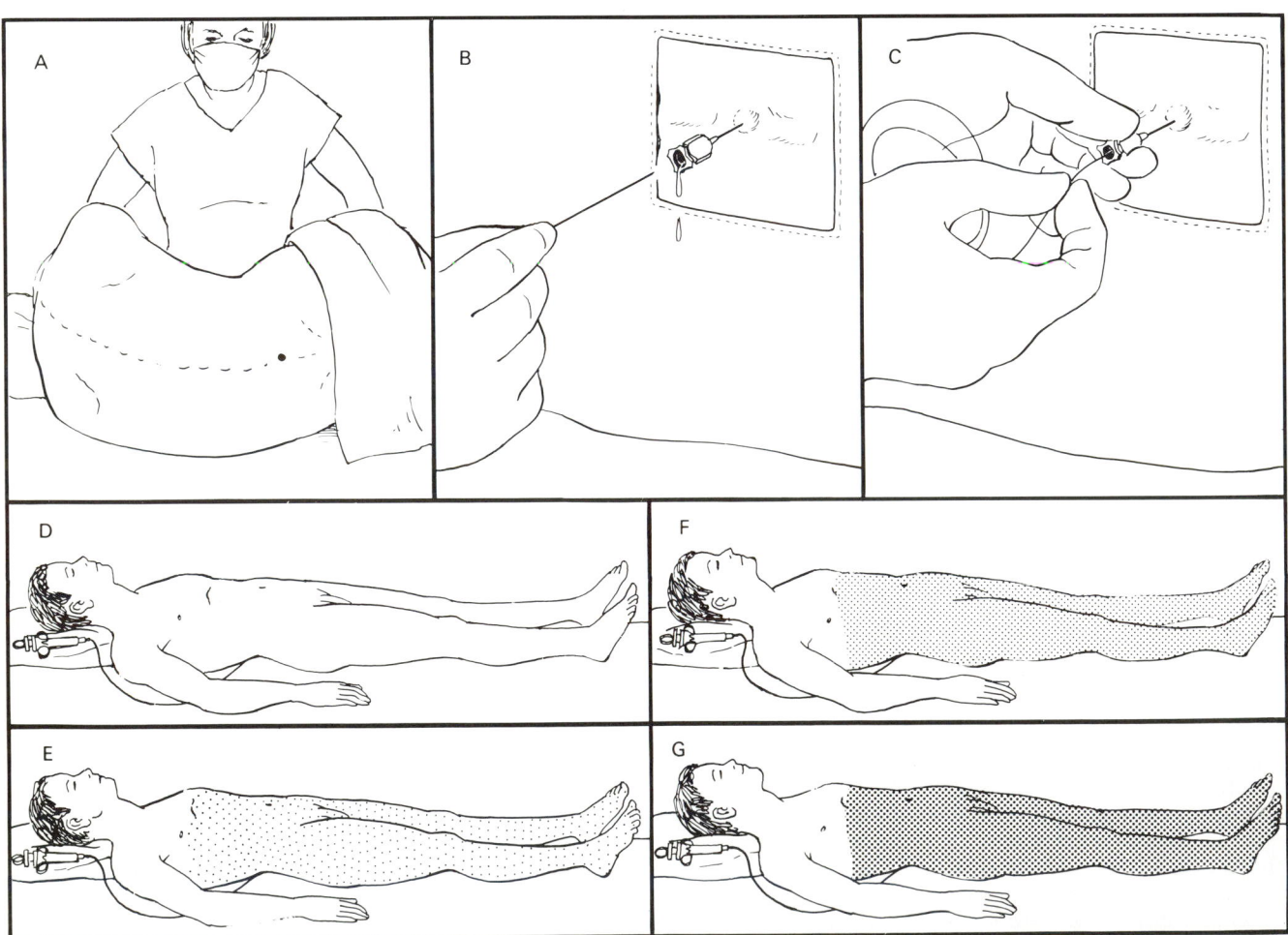

FIG. 94-54. Technique of graduated subarachnoid (spinal) block. *A.* Technique of lumbar puncture and insertion of the catheter: lateral position for the puncture. *B.* After formation of the skin wheal a special 25-gauge needle is advanced toward the subarachnoid space. The point of the needle is in the subarachnoid space, as shown by the emergence of cerebrospinal fluid. *C.* Introduction of the thin catheter through the needle into the subarachnoid space. *D.* The patient is supine. After injection of 8 ml of saline solution no change is noted in sensation. *E.* Injection of 8 ml of 0.25% procaine produces a sympathetic nerve block (*light stippling*). *F.* Injection of 8 ml of 0.5% procaine produces analgesia to pinprick, pin scratch, and pinch (*heavy stippling*). *G.* Injection of 8 ml of 1% procaine produces motor block, as indicated by the inability of the patient to move the limbs; also, the abdominal wall is relaxed.

subarachnoid space. A 32-gauge polyimide micro-catheter 91 cm long has been developed that can be inserted through a 25- or 26-gauge spinal needle.* Prior to insertion of the catheter the patient should be properly prepared and the sympathetic, sensory, and motor functions assessed and vital signs continuously monitored. After insertion of the catheter, the classic technique entails injection of different solutions at 10-minute intervals in the following sequence (Fig. 94-54):

a. 8 to 10 ml of saline solution is injected. Because controversy remains regarding whether normal saline solution produces a change in sensation (182, 183), some have advocated the aspiration of 8 ml of CSF and its reinjection.
b. 8 to 10 ml of 0.25% procaine is injected, which should produce a sympathetic nerve block as indicated by measuring sympathetic function.
c. 8 to 10 ml of 0.5% procaine is injected, which should produce a sensory block as assessed by pinprick, pin scratch, and pinch.
d. 8 to 10 ml of 1% procaine is injected, which should produce a motor block.

The amount of pain the patient has, the sensory level of block, the neurophysiologic and behavioral changes in response to the block, and the analgesia produced should be established and noted between each injection. Interpreted simplistically, pain that responds to "placebo" is presumed to have a non-nociceptive origin and has been classified as psychogenic. Pain reliability removed by a sympathetic blockade and accompanied by objective evidence of sympathetic interruption has been interpreted to imply a sympathetic hyperactivity component to the pain. Recent evidence, however, casts doubt on this assumption (174, 184). Elimination of the pain by 0.5 or 1% procaine solution indicates a somatic origin of the pain. Failure of any solution or block to relieve pain implies a central pain.

The distinctions between the various causes and responses are by no means as concrete as that implied by the simplistic interpretations given above. It is almost impossible to produce a pure sympathetic block or a pure block of A-delta fibers. Another problem is the method by which the patient is questioned and how the technique is presented, which can contribute to difficulties in interpretation. It is important that the technique be used according to a strict protocol that minimizes bias in both the patient's report and the observer's interpretation, and that the results of such a diagnostic block are interpreted within the context of the other clinical, investigative, and behavioral information that has been obtained about the patient and the pain problem (184). Finally, the graduated procedure can be used to determine the uppermost segment of nociceptive input into the neuraxis.

Extradural Neural Blockade

Extradural neural blockade for the management of pain involves the injection of a local anesthetic or

*Manufactured by TFX Medical, Duluth, Ga.

neurolytic agent into the epidural (extradural, peridural) space. The site of injection can be the sacral canal, the so-called "caudal block," or in the lumbar, thoracic, or cervical epidural space. The blockade can be achieved with a single injection of local anesthetic through a needle placed at the appropriate level or, more preferably, by the introduction of a catheter through a thin-walled 18- or 17-gauge needle, advancing its tip to any vertebral level that is considered to be the optimal site for injection. In this section we first mention the indications for extradural analgesia with local anesthetics, which are applicable to any of the techniques, and briefly describe the anatomic bases and techniques of caudal and spinal epidural block. We then consider the indications and efficacy of various extradural techniques in managing acute and chronic pain, and finally discuss the adverse effects and possible complications of extradural analgesia.

Basic Considerations

General Indications

Continuous epidural block is one of the most practical techniques for managing patients with acute and chronic pain because, by placing the catheter at different levels of the extradural space, analgesia of one or more spinal segments can be produced in almost any part of the body below the head. Continuous segmental epidural analgesia is a most effective and practical procedure for relieving the severe pain of acute pancreatitis, biliary colic, renal or ureteral colic, multiple fractures of ribs, and other severe post-traumatic pain, for controlling postoperative pain in the thorax, abdomen, pelvis, and lower limbs. It is also useful for providing temporary relief of severe local and segmental pain caused by herniated intervertebral disk or severe pain caused by fractures of the vertebrae. In all these acute conditions the blockade provides not only *complete* relief by interrupting nociceptive pathways from somatic structures and viscera but, through its block of efferent somatic and efferent sympathetic nerves, decreases or eliminates the reflex muscle spasm, sympathetically induced ileus, and neuroendocrine response that usually develop with such injuries or acute diseases. In some of these conditions, such as intervertebral disk, epidural analgesia facilitates the administration of conservative therapy. Continuous segmental epidural block extended for 5 to 8 days or longer is also useful as a therapeutic measure for providing pain relief in patients with severe cancer pain while they are being prepared for more definitive pain-relieving procedure. In such patients the pain relief and elimination of the sympathetically-induced gastrointestinal atony improve appetite and nutrition and permit more physical activity to improve the condition of the patient further. Finally, continuous epidural blockade is useful as a therapeutic measure in causalgia and other reflex sympathetic dystrophies in patients in whom other procedures cannot provide the continuous sympathetic interruption possible with the use of epidural analgesia.

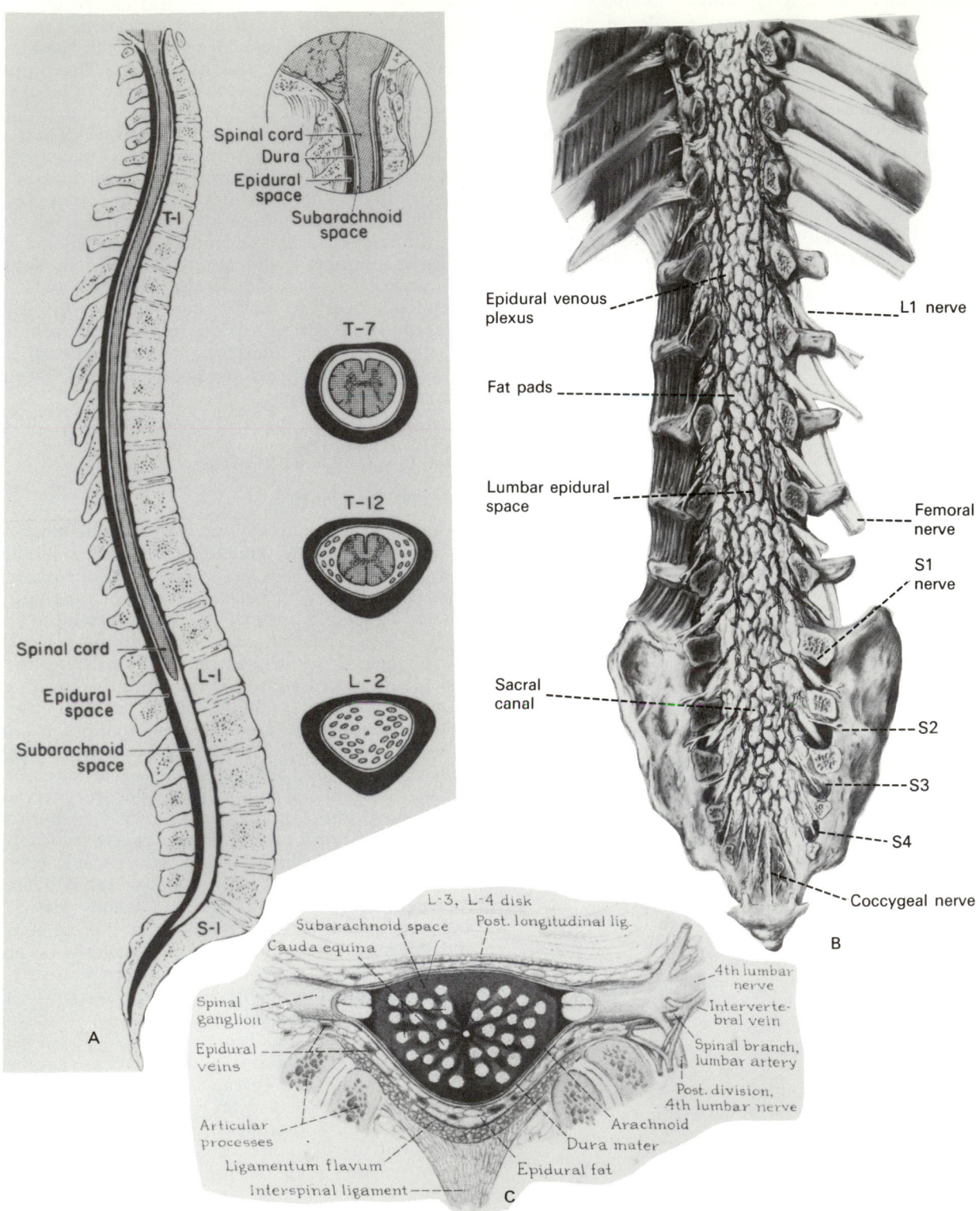

FIG. 94-55. Anatomy of the epidural space. *A.* Sagittal section of the spinal column. *Inset.* Enlarged view of the upper cervical region indicating that the epidural space does not extend beyond the foramen magnum, where the dura attaches to the entire circumference of the foramen. Below the inset are three cross-sectional views of various levels of the vertebral column. The epidural space has a different shape in the midthoracic and midlumbar regions. *B.* Posterioranterior view of the epidural space after the spinous processes and lamina have been removed, showing that its contents consist of an internal vertebral venous plexus accompanied by loose areolar tissue and fat. *C.* Schematic cross section of the spinal canal at the level of the intervertebral disk between the L3 and L4 vertebrae showing the shape and size of the epidural space and its contents and the position of the rootlets that make up the cauda equina. From Bonica, J.J.: Principles and Practice of Obstetric Analgesia and Anesthesia, Vol. 1. Philadelphia, F.A. Davis, 1967.

Anatomic Basis

The epidural space is the interval between the periosteum that lines the vertebral canal and the various ligaments that connect the vertebrae and the pachymeninges (dura-arachnoid) surrounding the spinal cord and roots in all of their extension from the foramen magnum to the conus terminalis, which in the adult extends to the S2 vertebra. The epidural space continues inferiorly as the sacral canal and laterally it communicates with the paravertebral tissues and spaces by the 48 intervertebral foramina through which the spinal nerves make their exit (Fig. 94-55).

The width of the epidural space varies greatly, with the anterior portion being narrow and almost theoretic because of the close contact of the dura with the posterior longitudinal ligament (see Fig. 53-7). The posterolateral portion of the epidural space is found between the dura and the ligamenta flava and laminae. Because of the shape of the spinal canal, the epidural space in the posterolateral region is somewhat triangular, being widest in the midline between the dura and the junction of the two laminae. This triangular space varies in its anteroposterior diameter as follows: 1.5 to 2.0 mm at C7; 3.0 to 4.0 mm at T2; 3.0 to 5.0 mm in the midthoracic region; 5.0 to 6.0 mm at L2; and only 2 mm at the lumbosacral junction (185, 186).

The contents of the epidural space include solid and liquid fat and loose areolar tissue, through which run the internal vertebral venous plexus, lymphatics, and the dural projections that surround the spinal nerve roots (Fig. 94-55). Fat is abundant in the posterolateral space, where it forms pads that intervene between the dura and the laminae and ligamentum flava. Although this tissue is loosely adherent to the vertebral canal and dura it is easily stripped from the dura by fluids that disperse from the point of injection.

Because the spinal cord ends at the level of the lower part of the L1 or the middle part of the L2 vertebra in 90% of adults, the dura arachnoid below the L2 vertebra contains only the cauda equina. This obviates the risk of injuring the conus medullaris with the epidural needle or catheter if the puncture is done below L2. Experienced anesthesiologists, however, can safely perform epidural punctures and introduce catheters at any level, including the lower cervical, thoracic, or lumbar region, as well as the sacral canal to produce caudal analgesia.

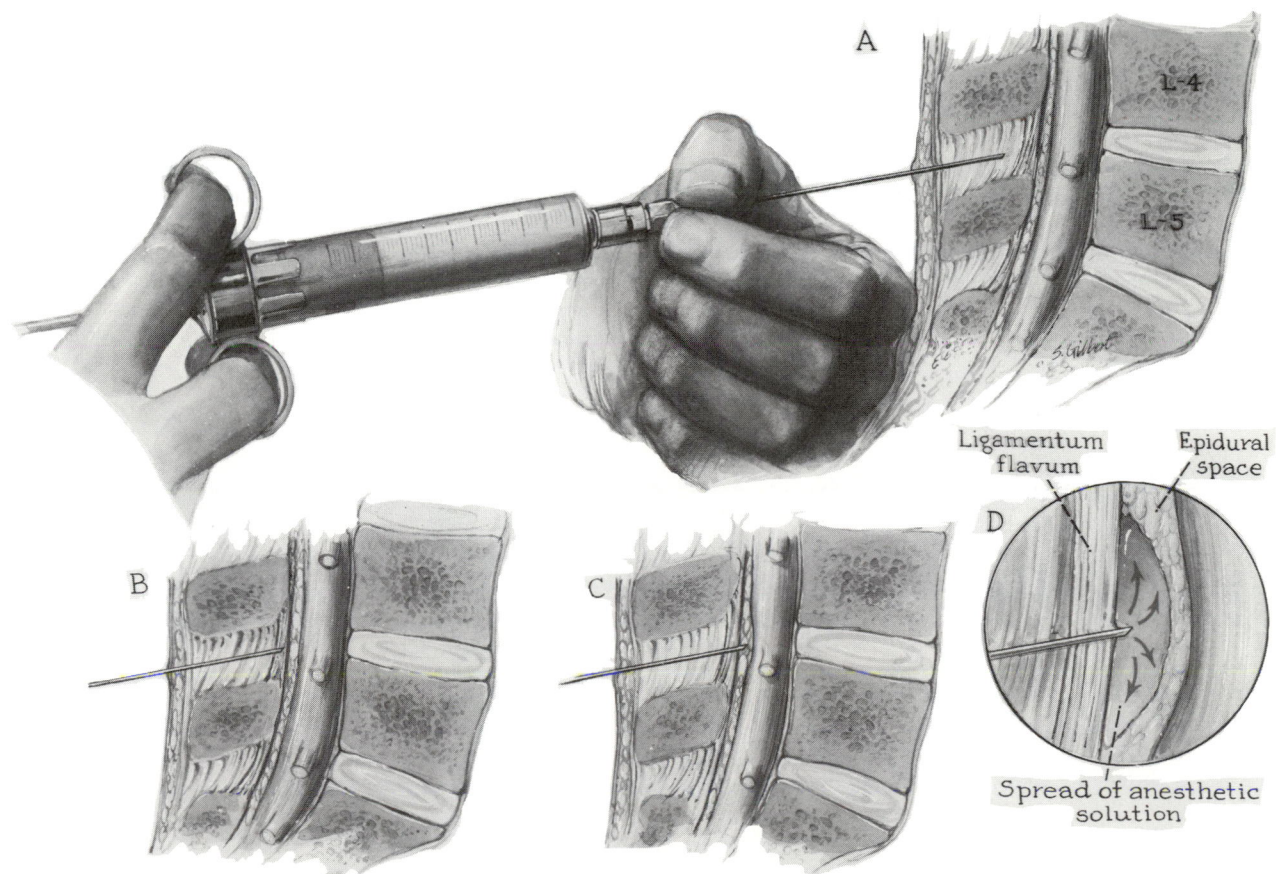

FIG. 94-56. Technique of epidural puncture into the lumbar region using the midline approach. *A.* After producing an intracutaneous wheal in the midline between the tips of adjacent spinous processes, a 20-gauge short beveled needle attached to a syringe filled with saline solution is introduced into the interspinous ligament. The back of the left hand is held against the patient's back, with the thumb and index finger grasping the hub of the needle; these act as a fine control of the advance of the needle while it is being pushed anteriorly with the right hand. An attempt to inject the saline solution while the point of the needle is in the interspinous ligament meets with some resistance. *B.* The point of the needle is in the ligamentum flavum, which offers marked resistance and makes it impossible to inject the solution. *C.* Entrance of the point of the needle into the epidural space is discerned by the sudden lack of resistance to the injection of the saline solution. *D.* The force of injection of 8 to 10 ml of saline solution pushes the dura-arachnoid away from the point of the needle. From Bonica, J.J.: Principles and Practice of Obstetric Analgesia and Anesthesia, Vol. 1. Philadelphia, F.A. Davis, 1967.

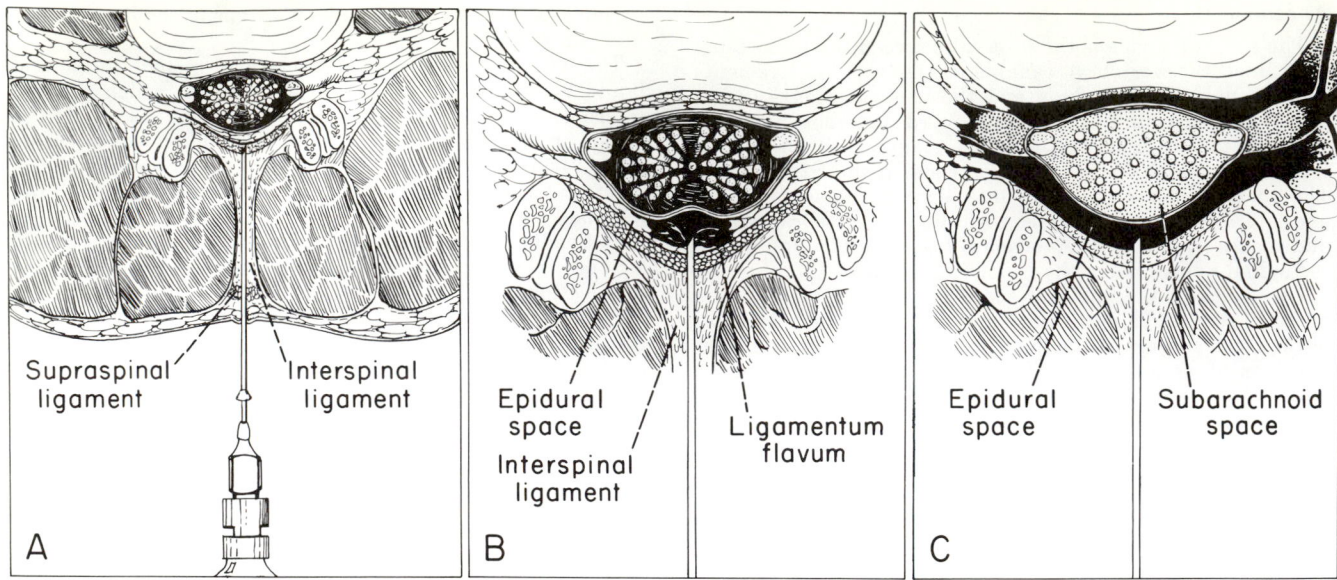

FIG. 94-57. Cross section at the midlumbar region to show the technique of epidural puncture using the midline. ***A.*** The point of the needle is in the ligamentum flavum, which offers marked resistance to the injection of saline solution. ***B.*** Injection of saline pushes the dura slightly anteriorly, thus decreasing the risk of puncture of the dura by the bevel of the needle. ***C.*** Injection of the local anesthetic solution causes diffusion throughout the epidural space and penetrates the dura-arachnoid to involve the rootlets. From Bonica, J.J.: Principles and Practice of Obstetric Analgesia and Anesthesia, Vol. 1. Philadelphia, F.A. Davis, 1967.

Technical Considerations

Spinal Epidural Block

The single-injection technique for block of the epidural space in the lumbar, thoracic, or cervical region is best carried out with a 20-gauge short-beveled spinal needle. For the continuous technique a special 18-gauge thin-walled needle that allows passage of a catheter is used. Bonica prefers the Tuohy needle for reasons given below. The most important part of the procedure is to advance the point of the needle through the thick ligamentum flavum *slowly* using the lack of resistance test and *promptly* arresting the advance of the needle once its bevel has passed into the epidural space. Unless this step is done slowly and cautiously, with full control of the advance of the

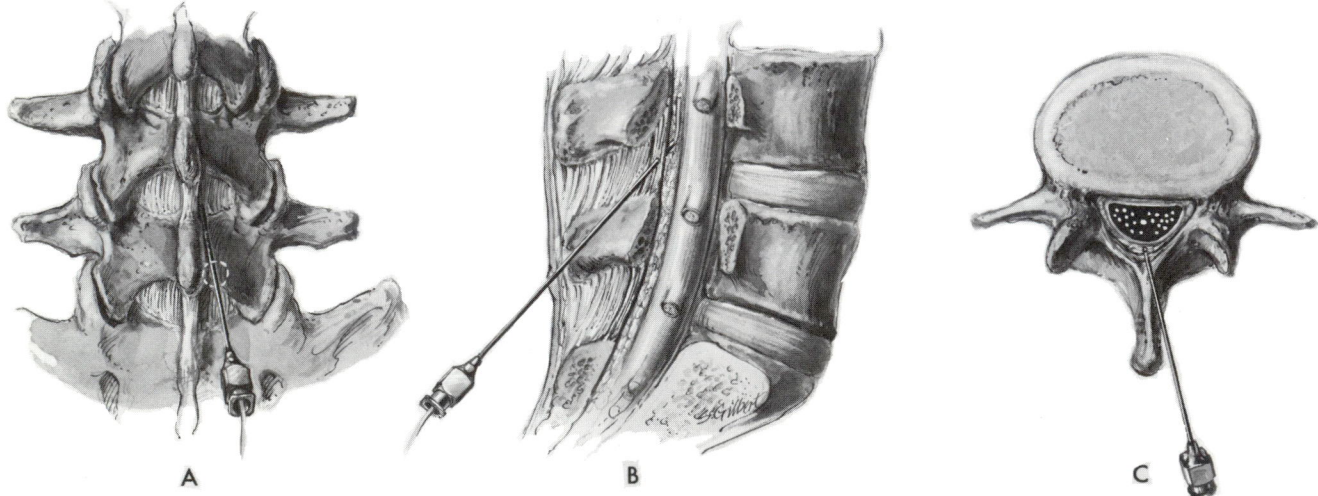

FIG. 94-58. Technique of continuous epidural block in the lumbar region using the paramedian approach. ***A.*** Posterior view showing the relationship of site of puncture, direction of needle, and spinous process. The anesthetic wheal is made 1.5 cm from the midline at the same cross-sectional level as the lower tip of the spinous process. Following formation of the wheal a 22-gauge needle is used to infiltrate the subcutaneous tissue, muscle, and upper medial part of the lamina with about 10 ml of a dilute local anesthetic solution (0.5% lidocaine). A special 18-gauge thin-walled Tuohy needle is introduced so that its axis makes an angle of approximately 15° with the midsagittal plane. ***B.*** Side view showing the same relationship and position of tubing in the epidural space as in ***A.*** The laminae and pedicles of the vertebrae have been removed. The needle makes a 35° angle with the skin inferior to the point of insertion. ***C.*** Superior view showing the relationship of the needle to the midsagittal plane and the position of the needle point in the epidural space, with the bevel of the needle facing cephalad. From Bonica, J.J.: Principles and Practice of Obstetric Analgesia and Anesthesia, Vol. 1. Philadelphia, F.A. Davis, 1967.

FIG. 94-59. Technique of continuous epidural block in the midthoracic region using the paramedian approach. **A.** The obliquity of the spinous processes is extreme and bony spurs are usually on the surface of the adjacent spinous processes, making introduction of the needle through the supraspinous and intraspinous ligaments difficult, so the paramedian approach facilitates the puncture and the introduction of a catheter. The skin wheal is made 1.5 cm lateral to the tip of the spinous process of the vertebra above the interspace to be penetrated. The first step is to contact the medial upper part of the lamina. (The syringe, which is usually attached to the needle throughout its advancement, is not shown for the sake of clarity.) **B.** The bevel of the needle is in the ligamentum flavum in the midline. At this point injection of saline solution creates resistance until the ligament is traversed, after which a sudden lack of resistance can be felt. **C.** Cross-sectional depiction of the relationship of the needle to the soft tissue, spinous process, lamina, and ligaments. The bevel of the needle is near the midline of the epidural space and is facing cephalad. **D.** Sagittal section with the lamina and pedicles removed showing the relationship of the needle to the surrounding structures and to the catheter in the epidural space. From Bonica, J.J.: Continuous peridural block. Anesthesiology, *17*:626, 1956.

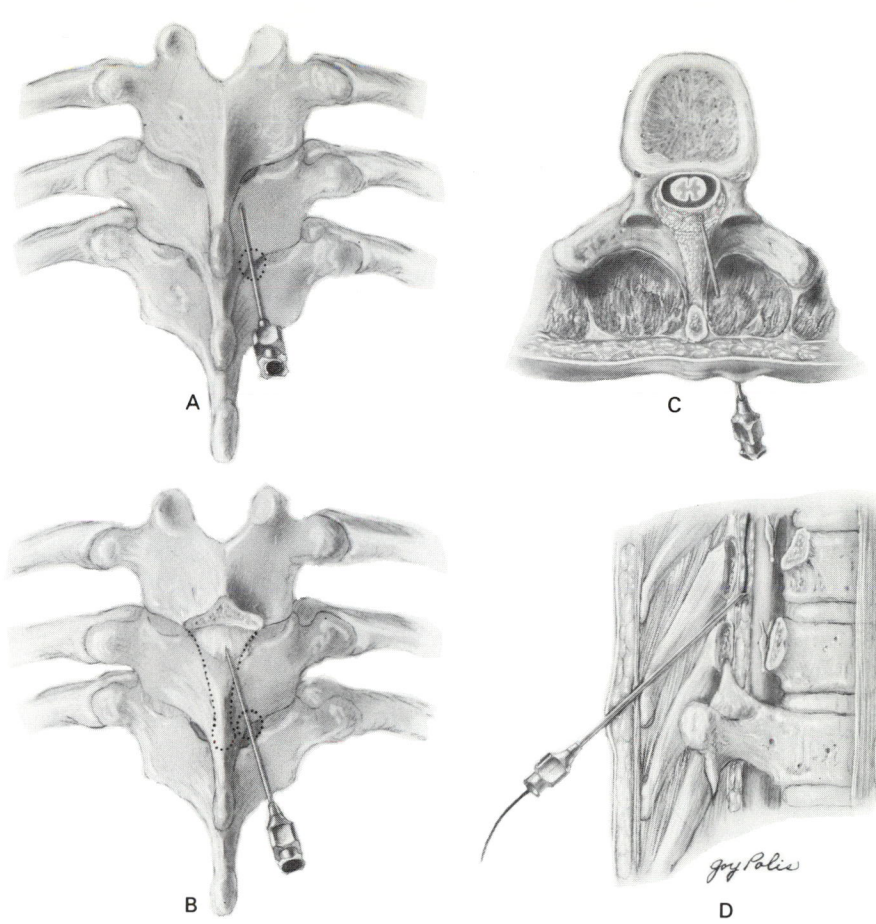

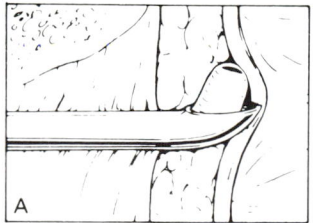 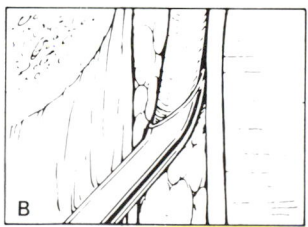

FIG. 94-60. Schematic depiction of the advantage of introducing the Tuohy needle by a paramedian approach in the lumbar region at an angle that facilitates advancement of the catheter through the needle as compared to use of the midline approach. **A.** A Tuohy needle is introduced through the midline and advanced sufficiently so that its entire bevel is within the epidural space. If the space is narrow the dura might be partially punctured. Also, because of the direction of the bevel of the Tuohy needle, the tip of the catheter is directed anterosuperiorly against the dura in an attempt to make a 90° turn cephalad; not infrequently it is prevented from advancing by a fat pad or a vein lying on the dura. **B.** A paramedian approach with the Tuohy needle causes the catheter to be directed more cephalad, thus facilitating its advance within the epidural space. Moreover, because the point of the needle is directed cephalad, the possibility of puncturing the dura is small. From Bonica, J.J.: Obstetric Analgesia and Anesthesia. Seattle, University of Washington Press, 1980.

needle, the needle point could be accidentally advanced too far into the subarachnoid space. For a single injection the midline approach can be used (Figs. 94-56 and 94-57). To introduce a catheter, Bonica prefers the paramedian approach, which he described in 1956 (187) (Figs. 94-58 and 94-59). Figure 94-60 illustrates the paramedian approach which facilitates the advance of the catheter in the epidural space. The technique of inserting a needle and catheter into the sacral canal is shown in Figure 66-65.

Once the bevel of the needle is actually within the epidural space, an injection can be made. Alternately a catheter is passed through the needle and the needle is subsequently withdrawn. Using currently available catheters, only 4 to 5 cm should be inserted into the epidural space beyond the bevel of the needle. Attempts to introduce a greater length of catheter, or to thread the catheter to points remote from the site of puncture, lead to an unpredictable position of the catheter tip (188, 189).

When segmental epidural analgesia is being used the site of injection or catheter placement should be close to the center of the spinal segments that the physician wishes to block with the local anesthetic. This ensures that drug placement is accurate and that the dose of drug necessary to produce the desired effect is relatively small when compared to that of an injection at a remote site (190).

Indications

DIAGNOSTIC BLOCK. Segmental epidural blockade can be used as a diagnostic aid in determining the levels of nociceptive input in patients with visceral or somatic disorders. Because the technique invariably produces block of sympathetic and sensory fibers, which supply both somatic structures and viscera, this procedure is not as useful as selective sympathetic or somatic nerve block. Winnie and Collins (180) advocated the use of differential epidural block to overcome some of the limitations of differential spinal subarachnoid block. They contended that the use of an epidural catheter allows better patient movement and associated testing for pain, while providing for repeated tests if some responses are equivocal. Avoidance of headache, especially in young patients, was a further advantage. Despite these considerations, diagnostic differential epidural local anesthetic block carries the same limitation of interpretation as subarachnoid differential block (174). On the other hand, by using a volume of anesthetic at various intervals the segmental level(s) of nociceptive input can be established and, if pain persists in or below a fully blocked area, it can be presumed that the pain is of a higher central focus (e.g., central pain or psychologic pain).

In this regard we should mention the use of what might be considered as "differential" epidural opioid blockade combined with epidural lidocaine as a diagnostic adjunctive tool in patients with chronic pain. This procedure is based on the assumption that epidural opioids block nociceptive input at the level of the dorsal horn, leaving sensory, sympathetic, and motor functions unchanged without giving patients "cues" that blockade has occurred. Cherry and associates (191) studied eight patients in whom both physical and psychosocial assessment in a pain management unit left doubt as to their diagnosis. They were subjected to a sequence of the following solutions injected into the epidural space at 20-minute intervals: two injections of normal saline (placebo), one injection of 1 μg/kg fentanyl, 0.4 mg IV naloxone and, depending on the results obtained, 15 to 20 ml of 2% lidocaine injected through the epidural catheter. If the visual analog pain score decreased following epidural fentanyl and subsequently increased following naloxone, then a predominantly physical basis for the pain was considered to be likely. In contrast, little change in the visual analog score following the administration of fentanyl and naloxone suggested a predominantly emotional basis for the pain. The diagnosis was substantiated by subsequent follow-up and treatment.

Boas and Cousins (174) pointed out two problems with this technique: (a) some types of pain might not be abolished by spinal opioids (e.g., intermittent deep somatic and visceral pain) (192); and (b) opioids migrate in the CSF to the brain and are absorbed into the vasculature, which might provide "cues" to the patient and possibly also exert a significant analgesic effect on the brain. To resolve these problems, they

TABLE 94-6. Diagnostic Epidural Opioid Blockade*

Step	Amount/Agent Used	Site of Injection
1	10 ml of 0.9% saline without preservative	Epidural; placebo
2	10 ml of 0.9% saline without preservative	Epidural; placebo
3	10 ml solution of fentanyl, 100 μg	Epidural
4	Naloxone 0.4 mg	IV
5	Lidocaine 2% 20 ml	Epidural

From Boas, R.A., and Cousins, M.J.: Diagnostic neural blockade. *In* Neural Blockade. 2nd Ed. Edited by M.J. Cousins and P.O. Bridenbaugh. Philadelphia, J.B. Lippincott, 1988, p. 893.
*A visual analog scale is used to record pain relief. The pattern on response is suggested as being useful.

suggested that the following steps be done: (a) use of blood and CSF pharmacokinetic studies after epidural and intrathecal opioids for diagnostic purposes; (b) simultaneous documentation of pharmacodynamic effects; and (c) statistical analysis of the reliability of diagnostic opioid blockade in predicting the cause of pain syndromes that are precisely documented. They recommend a modification of the original technique (174) (Table 94-6).

PROGNOSTIC BLOCK. Epidural blocks with local anesthetic can be used as prognostic procedures as an alternative to individual nerve blocks, but suffer the same limitations as noted above in regard to diagnostic blocks. A more recent indication is the use of epidural blocks as prognostic indicators for the possible efficacy of epidural narcotics for patients with cancer pain. Most physicians who use epidural opioids for pain therapy determine the placement of the catheter and the efficacy of the technique in relieving pain by injecting a local anesthetic into the epidural space and noting its analgesic spread (Chapter 95).

PROPHYLACTIC BLOCK. In earlier parts of this chapter mention has been made that continuous relief of severe pain due to occlusive arterial disease can prevent or at least reduce the incidence of phantom limb pain. Bach and associates (19) demonstrated this beneficial effect in a prospective study of 25 patients scheduled to undergo lower limb amputation for occlusive arterial disease, 11 (44%) of whom also had diabetes mellitus. Two of the patients had had pain for more than 6 months, and the other 23 reported having had pain for less than 6 months but more than 1 month. All of the patients were in constant pain and regularly received analgesia, including intramuscular opioids.

Eleven patients received a continuous lumbar epidural block that provided complete pain relief for 3 days postoperatively while a control group of 14 patients, also with preoperative pain, were treated with various analgesic drugs such as opioids alone or in combination with nonopioid analgesics. The continuous epidural block consisted of epidural morphine hydrochloride or 0.25% bupivacaine or a combination of the two with the overall aim of complete relief of pain. All 25 patients received epidural or spinal anesthesia for the operation; postoperatively they were managed with meperidine, paracetamol (acetaminophen), or aspirin.

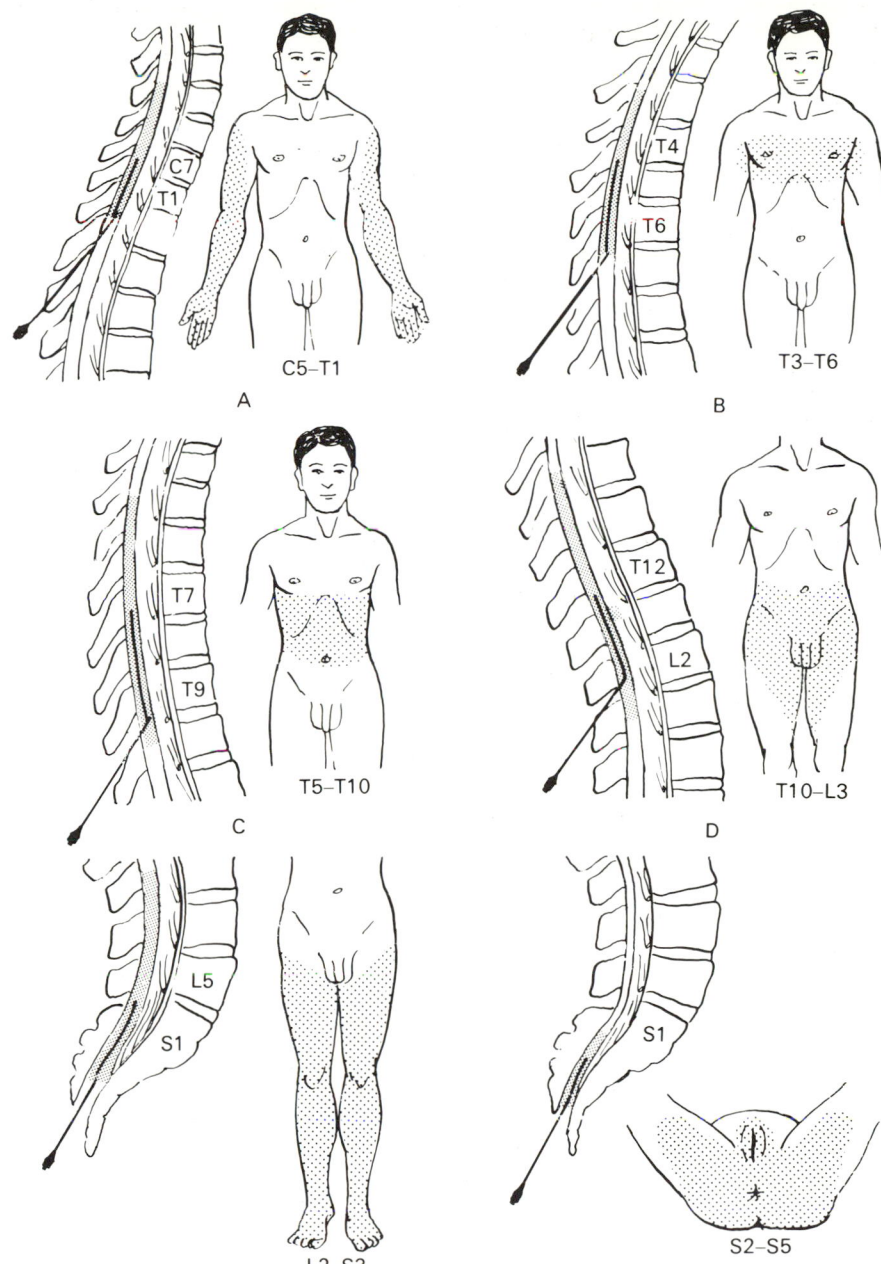

FIG. 94-61. Patterns of segmental epidural analgesia, achieved with injection of a local anesthetic for the relief of pain in various regions of the body. On the left of each part of the figure is a sagittal section showing the site or level of the epidural puncture for placement of the Tuohy needle and subsequent insertion of the catheter (*black*), which is advanced 4 to 5 cm in the epidural space so that its tip is in the center of the band of analgesia desired. The right part depicts the region of the body in which pain is relieved (*stippled area*). *A.* Analgesia for pain in the upper limbs bilaterally. *B.* Analgesia to control pain in the upper part of the chest. *C.* Analgesia to control pain following upper abdominal surgery. *D.* Segmental analgesia following lower abdominal surgery to control pain and to produce continuous lumbar epidural block. *E.* Analgesia to relieve pain in the deep pelvis and the lower limbs. *F.* Continuous low caudal analgesia (S2–S5) to relieve pain after hemorrhoidectomy or after other operations involving the perineum.

The patients were interviewed by means of a standard questionnaire 5 days before operation and at 7 days, 6 months, and 1 year after surgery. Figure 77-11 depicts the results obtained. At 7 days, 3 patients (27%) in the group who received the epidural block and 9 patients (64%) in the control group had phantom limb pain (p<0.10). At 6 months and thereafter, all patients in the blockade group were pain-free, whereas 5 patients (38%) in the control group had phantom limb pain. After 1 year, all of the patients in the blockade group were still pain-free and 3 patients (27%) in the control group had phantom limb pain (p<0.20). One patient in each of the groups complained of stump pain promptly after the operation, but at 6 months and 1 year all the patients were free of stump pain. None of the patients in the block group experienced nonpainful phantom limb sensations, whereas among the control group 1 patient experienced phantom limb sensation at 7 days and 6 months, and 2 had phantom limb sensation after 1 year. If these results are replicated, continuous regional analgesia for several days should be considered in patients who have severe preamputation pain. The possibile mechanisms of this phenomenon are discussed in Chapter 77.

THERAPEUTIC BLOCKS. Continuous segmental epidural or caudal analgesia with local anesthetics can be used for the relief of acute postoperative or post-traumatic pain that occurs below the clavicle

(Fig. 94-61). The introduction of continuous epidural narcotics for the relief of acute postoperative or post-traumatic pain has markedly decreased the indications for which local anesthetics are used. Little doubt remains that epidural analgesia with local anesthetics is much more effective in blocking nociceptive input as well as efferent pathways, thus providing a superior quality of analgesia and decreasing reflex responses (see Fig. 25-9). Therefore, it can be used to provide pain relief in patients in whom epidural narcotics have not provided sufficient pain relief, as might occur in patients with pain who require respiratory therapy maneuvers or have pain on movement.

More recently the use of a combination of continuous epidural block with boluses or continuous infusion of solution containing both opioids and local anesthetics has been increasing. This technique permits the use of smaller amounts of local anesthetic, with less risk of systemic effects, while at the same time providing the advantages of local anesthetics as well as the relief of pain. This technique probably evolved from the observation that, in patients receiving continuous epidural block with local anesthetic who developed tachyphylaxis, IV administration of opioids halted and indeed reversed the regression of the analgesia. In a double-blind study comparing the epidural infusion of bupivacaine (0.1% at 3 to 4 ml/hour), morphine (0.3 to 0.4 mg/hour), or both (with a saline control group and a nonepidural group), it was found that the combination was statistically superior to the other groups (193). Better results could probably have been obtained with higher doses of bupivacaine.

Epidural Blockade for Acute Pain

CHEST INJURIES. Patients with chest injuries present a spectrum of severity of trauma, ranging from severe chest wall instability with pulmonary contusion and pulmonary failure as a consequence, to chest wall injury with or without instability but with little or no pulmonary contusion and little or no evidence of respiratory failure. Formerly, great importance was placed on the necessity of providing mechanical chest wall stability by "internal pneumatic stabilization" using tracheal intubation and positive pressure ventilation. Consequently, many patients with extensive chest injuries were managed with this regime. It is now recognized, however, almost irrespective of the degree of chest wall instability, and provided that there is little or no pulmonary contusion or respiratory failure once hemothorax and pneumothorax have been drained, that patients with chest injuries can be safely managed with supplemental oxygen and respiratory therapy maneuvers (194, 195), especially when effective epidural analgesia with local anesthetic is provided (196, 197). Moreover, trials of such a conservative technique in comparison to tracheal intubation and positive pressure ventilation in patients with similar degrees of chest and lung injuries have had lower morbidity and mortality rates and a shorter duration of intensive care unit stay (195).

Prospective trials of treatment in which the management protocol was individualized, as based on

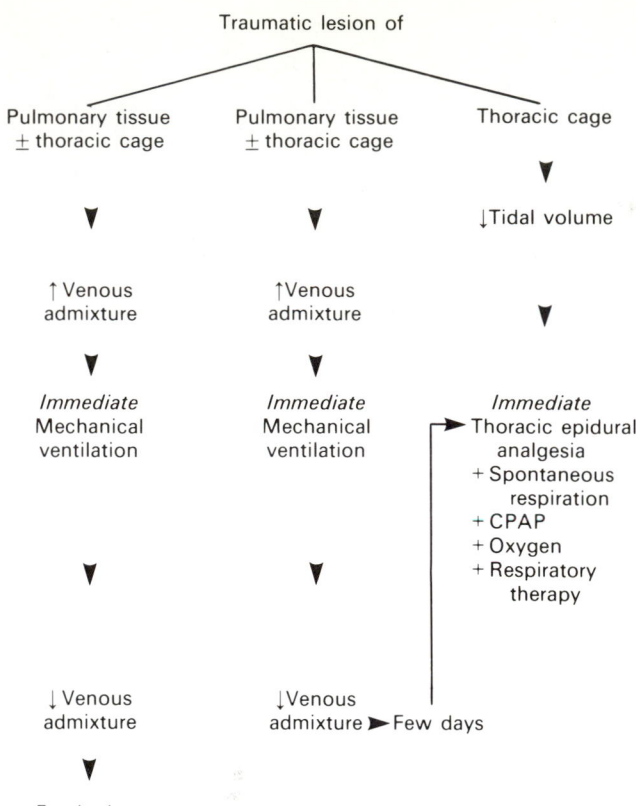

FIG. 94-62. Management protocol for patients with chest injury. Modified from Dittmann, M., et al.: A rationale for epidural analgesia in the treatment of rib fractures. Intensive Care Med., 8:89, 1982.

patients' respiratory status (198–200), have tended to confirm the value of the conservative management protocol (Fig. 94-62). Patients with severe pulmonary contusions and respiratory failure (manifested by tachypnea, dyspnea, Pa_{O_2} of less than 60 mm Hg, Pa_{CO_2} greater than 50 mm Hg) are in need of respiratory support and should be treated with tracheal intubation and positive pressure ventilation (Table 94-7, group 1). Patients with major pulmonary injury, or those who might need artificial ventilation for other reasons, should initially be treated with artificial ventilation but, as the pulmonary lesion and pulmonary status improve, they can be weaned from such support, have the endotracheal tube removed, and be managed with spontaneous ventilation and epidural analgesia (Table 94-7, group 2). Patients with chest wall instability but little or no discernible pulmonary injury and respiratory failure, once hemothorax and pneumothorax are drained, can be managed with epidural analgesia, oxygen, and respiratory therapy (Table 94-7, group 3). If patients are managed by the conservative protocol, as in group 3, it is important to monitor the pulmonary status closely and to treat any incipient or declared respiratory failure by positive pressure ventilation. This was necessary in 5 of 112 patients managed by Dittmann et al. (200) (Table 94-7B, group 3).

TABLE 94-7. Results of Management of Chest Injuries*

Parameter	A. Shackford et al. (195) Group			B. Dittmann et al. (200) Group		
	1	2	3	1	2	3
No. of patients	13	7	16	155	21†	112
Mean no. of rib fractures	5.7	4.7	5.5	6.6		6.8
No. of patients with hemothorax or pneumothorax	9	3	8	91		40
No. of patients with pulmonary contusion	13	2	4	50		1
Mean duration of hospitalization (days)	27	11	18	26		17
Deaths	2	0	1	38	0	5

*Endotracheal intubation and positive pressure ventilation (group 1); endotracheal intubation and positive pressure ventilation followed by early extubation and pain management with epidural LA (group 2); or epidural LA plus supportive oxygen and respiratory therapy only (group 3). See text for more detailed definitions of groups.

†This group, which was part of Group 1 that was primarily ventilated, could be extubated early under thoracic epidural analgesia without fatal course.

Although the patients managed by the conservative protocols (Table 94-7, groups 2 and 3) had a lower mortality rate they had a lower incidence of associated injuries, such as head, abdominal, or long bone injuries, which might have contributed to the lower morbidity and mortality rates. Nonetheless, it appears that the conservative management protocol has a definite place in the management of chest injuries and is associated with a more benign intrahospital course.

If epidural analgesia is to be used in patients with chest injuries it is critical that the technique not be started until the patient has been adequately resuscitated with blood or crystalloid solutions, as needed. The adequacy of resuscitation should be ascertained by the measurement of central venous pressure and other parameters. The technique should also be used with caution in patients with central nervous system injuries or extensive injuries elsewhere.

When epidural analgesia is used for chest injuries the catheter should be placed close to the middle of the segment(s) in which the analgesia is desired. If it is anticipated that the catheter might have to be in place and in use for a long period of time, consideration should be given to tunneling the catheter subcutaneously to minimize the risks of catheter displacement and infection (Fig. 24-11). The doses of local anesthetic necessary for providing epidural analgesia are 5 to 10 ml of 0.5% bupivacaine with epinephrine or an infusion of 0.25% bupivacaine at a rate of 8 to 10 ml/hour (201, 202). Rankin and Comber (203) have used epidural opioids as a baseline analgesic technique, supplemented with epidural injection of local anesthetics for painful maneuvers such as coughing, deep breathing, or other respiratory therapy techniques for which epidural narcotics did not provide effective analgesia.

POSTOPERATIVE PAIN. Epidural analgesia with local anesthetic provides excellent analgesia after thoracic or abdominal surgery, and most of the experience gained with prolonged epidural neural blockage has been for this indication. For pain consequent to upper abdominal operations, the catheter should be placed with its tip at the T8 interspace whereas for post-thoracotomy pain the tip is placed at T4 (Fig. 94-61). Although satisfactory analgesia can be obtained with catheters placed at lower levels, this requires an increase in the volume of drug used and results in a high incidence of lower extremity paresis and urinary retention. For the relief of pain that follows lower abdominal operations the catheter is inserted into the T12 or L1 interspace, while for lower limb surgery the tip of the catheter should not be higher than the L4 interspace, which would require puncture at L5. An alternative technique is to insert the catheter into the sacral canal and advance it 7 to 8 cm so that its tip is at the lower part of the S1 vertebral level. Advancing the catheter with the stylet in place, and kept in the midline of the sacral canal, entails little risk of deviation of the catheter as it proceeds cephalad.

To relieve pain following abdominal operations, intermittent top-up doses of 4 to 6 ml of 0.25 to 0.5% bupivacaine with epinephrine produce analgesia for 2 to $2\frac{1}{2}$ hours. To relieve pain following lower abdominal surgery, 6 to 10 ml of 0.25 to 0.5% bupivacaine with epinephrine produces analgesia for 2 to $3\frac{1}{2}$ hours. To relieve pain following pelvic or lower limb surgery, the same volumes can be used provided that the tip of the catheter is at the S1 level. After the initial dose is injected, persistent analgesia can be achieved either with top-up doses of similar or greater amounts if the patient develops tachyphylaxis. Better still, an infusion of bupivacaine 0.25% at a rate of 6 to 10 ml/hour or 0.125% at a rate of 15 ml/hour can be initiated (104, 201). A roller infusion pump is ideal because it is unaffected by the resistance of the catheter. Once good sustained analgesia has been achieved it is essential to prepare a reservoir of drugs sufficient to last 24 hours and to use a pediatric drip set to avoid accidental overdose. A set with a 30-ml measuring chamber is ideal and, although it must be refilled every 2 to 3 hours from the reservoir, allows accurate monitoring of the infusion rate (104). Obviously, the patient should be monitored closely for hypotension or other adverse affects, which should be promptly treated.

The quality of postoperative analgesia produced by epidural neural blockade with local anesthetic is superior to that produced by parenteral narcotics (204). Abdominal surgery, particularly that involving viscera in the upper abdomen, is attended by significant changes in indexes of respiratory function and oxygenation and by a substantially higher incidence of chest infection (Chapter 25). When compared to patients receiving conventional narcotic analgesia, patients receiving epidural analgesia with local anesthetics have a better forced vital capacity (FVC) and peak expiratory flow rate (PERF) (18, 205, 206), but most studies have shown no difference in functional residual capacity (FRC) (207–209). On the other hand, Bromage (185), one of the foremost authorities on epidural neural blockade, reported a lesser decrease in FRC with epidural analgesia than with narcotics (see Table 25-3). Most, but not all patients, tend to maintain a more normal Pa_{O_2} (204–206) and to have a lower incidence of chest infection (204, 205).

Although these beneficial effects of epidural analgesia compared to narcotics have not been observed by some investigators, Bonica's personal experience with epidural anesthesia used for cholecystectomy and for the postoperative period, as well as a combined observation of patients and the favorable reports noted above, suggest that epidural analgesia expertly executed on a cooperative patient results in better pulmonary function than that seen when narcotic analgesia is used. Pflug and associates (18) studied 40 patients who had undergone upper abdominal surgery or hip operations and were managed with epidural analgesia; they left the hospital 3 days earlier than the control group managed with narcotics (Table 25-4). In morbidly obese patients with a high risk of pulmonary complications, the use of continuous epidural local analgesia for brief periods of time postoperatively is associated with a decrease in incidence of respiratory complications (210, 211).

Continuous epidural block that extends from T5 to the sacral segments during and following lower abdominal operations markedly reduces the postoperative metabolic and neuroendocrine response to surgery and the postoperative tissue damage. Marked increases in levels of the catabolically acting pituitary hormones (e.g., growth hormones, prolactin, ACTH, ADH), adrenal hormones (e.g., cortisol, aldosterone, catecholamines) normally seen in patients given general anesthesia during surgery and managed with postoperative narcotics are minimized, and the incidence of postoperative hyperglycemia is greatly attenuated (212, 213). Patients receiving epidural analgesia show fewer changes in hepatic enzymes (214). The significance of the reduction of these metabolic and neuroendocrine responses to trauma is certain and clinically important.

Segmental epidural anesthesia for upper abdominal surgery and epidural analgesia during the postoperative period have fewer effects on these responses to tissue damage than are seen after lower abdominal and leg operations (212, 213), but this is because not all afferent and efferent neural pathways are interrupted. Because the phrenic nerves provide significant supply to some of the viscera in the upper abdomen and to the diaphragmatic peritoneum, they constitute important pathways for afferent input, together with the vagus nerves. To achieve total blockade it is essential to combine epidural anesthesia with extensive celiac plexus block using large volumes of local anesthetic to cause diffusion of the drug on the inferior surface of the diaphragm. Epidural analgesia with local anesthetic is much more effective in attenuating the metabolic and neuroendocrine response during and after upper abdominal surgery than epidural opioids (Fig. 25-9).

Postoperative pain following back, hip, and lower extremity surgery managed with epidural analgesia is associated with a much better respiratory function (18) and with a lower incidence of deep vein thrombosis and pulmonary embolus (215) than in patients receiving opioid analgesia. Based on his own personal experience with 11 hip operations, of which 8 were done with regional anesthesia for the surgery followed by epidural analgesia during the postoperative period and 3 were done with general anesthesia and postoperative pain managed with modest doses of meperidine, Bonica is firmly convinced of the immense superiority of the use of epidural neural blockade over opioids. Moreover, based on experience with postoperative pain that followed 3 laminectomies, epidural analgesia with local anesthetic is more effective in relieving pain caused by reflex muscle spasm or movement than epidural opioids and far better than patient-controlled analgesia. Finally, evidence is accumulating that the use of regional anesthesia during surgery and regional analgesia with local anesthetics during the postoperative period, compared with general anesthesia and narcotic analgesia, suggests a decrease in mortality rate following hip operations with the former method compared with the latter (216, 217). In the elderly, the use of epidural analgesia rather than general anesthesia can result in a lesser decrement in mental function subsequent to operations (218).

ACUTE VISCERAL PAIN. In Section E of this chapter (see above) the efficacy of regional analgesia with local anesthetics for relieving severe pain associated with acute pancreatitis, ureteral colic, and biliary colic was noted. Although celiac plexus block or splanchnic nerve block relieves the pain arising from the viscera, segmental epidural block has the following advantages: (a) the block is easier to carry out; (b) it is more effective in relieving pain, not only that coming from the viscera but also that caused by irritation of the peritoneum (which is supplied by somatic nerves); (c) by blocking motor fibers it eliminates the reflex muscle spasm and the decrease in chest wall compliance consequent to it; and (d) it is much easier to produce sustained analgesia for a number of days than with other techniques.

For acute pancreatitis the catheter is best placed with its tip at the T7 or T8 spinal cord segmental level with 5 to 8 ml of 0.5% bupivacaine with epinephrine injected as the initial dose. Once adequate analgesia has been established the patient should be placed on an infusion pump that delivers 5 to 8 ml of 0.5% bupivacaine with epinephrine every 2 to 3 hours, as required, and continued for 5 to 12 days, as necessary. A number of older reports cited by Bonica (1) and a more recent report (219) provide impressive evidence that continuous epidural analgesia not only relieves pain but also eliminates the reflex muscle spasm and decreased chest wall compliance consequent to it. It also decreases or eliminates ileus within 12 to 24 hours, improves renal blood flow, and combats reflex spasm of the duodenum, the sphincter of Oddi, and the entire ductal system, so that extraductal pressure is rapidly released. In addition, it helps to empty toxic fluids from the extrabiliary and pancreatic ductal systems, relieves the visceral vasospasm that contributes to the pathophysiology, and improves pulmonary function. Through these and other beneficial effects, epidural analgesia helps to lower morbidity and mortality rates, which in most cases are caused by respiratory insufficiency and anuria.

Tassonyi and associates (219) reported their results in 83 patients with acute pancreatitis managed with epidural analgesia over a 6-year period. By early institution of the procedure they observed all of its beneficial effects, reduced the incidence of early surgery, and reduced the mortality rate from the 28% that was seen prior to the start of this therapy to lower than 11% in those treated with epidural analgesia. They also noted that, during the first $4\frac{1}{2}$ years of their study, surgical intervention was undertaken early in the course of disease in 45% of the 58 patients managed during this period and, of these, 14% died, whereas of 25 patients managed during the last 18 months of the study period, only 4% underwent surgery, with a mortality rate of 4%.

For the relief of biliary colic a segmental analgesia of the same type is used, whereas for the relief of ureteral colic the segments to be blocked are lower and depend on the site of the impacted stone. For pain caused by obstruction in the pelvis of the kidney or ureter, block of T10 to L2 provides pain relief.

Epidural Analgesia for Chronic Pain

Epidural neural blockade with local anesthetics combined with steroids has been given clinical trials in patients with postherpetic neuralgia, post-traumatic pain, and low back pain.

POSTHERPETIC NEURALGIA. One report (220) on the use of a series of two or three epidural blocks with local anesthetic combined with steroids injected at the segments affected at intervals of 1 to 2 weeks produced a 60% improvement rate. The best results were obtained with treatment within 3 months of onset of the neuralgia. In view of the lack of controls, and because this is a difficult problem, however, epidural analgesia can be tried to provide temporary relief, but it is unlikely to produce prolonged pain relief.

CHRONIC LOW BACK PAIN. Epidural injection of varying volumes of steroids with or without local anesthetics has been widely used for low back pain with varying degrees of success (221). Some reports claimed an immediate success rate ranging from 25 to 89% (221). In other reports success rates were between 35 and 85% at follow-up which was 6 weeks to 5 years after treatment (222). The average success rate was about 60% at 3 to 6 months follow-up. A decline in success rate over time has been noted. One longitudinal study revealed a drop from 68 to 42% by 2 years and another from 90 to 70% at 6 months (221).

Analysis of the factors that contribute to success shows that the inclusion of steroids (80 mg of methylprednisolone) is the most important, whereas the volume of the solution and the presence of local anesthetic and its concentration are relatively unimportant (223). One report suggested that factors in patients that predict a good result include a relatively acute low back pain condition or an acute episode of chronic back pain in patients not having had surgery for back problems and patients being employed, not taking sedatives, and not receiving compensation (224). Disease diagnoses predicting a good success rate are spinal stenosis and irritative radiculopathy. Patients with a proven herniated disk or postsurgical pain derive little benefit.

The overall assessment of the efficacy of the technique is difficult and complex. In a comprehensive review, Kepes and Duncalf (223) concluded that the rationale for the use of spinal injection of local anesthetics with steroids or the use of IM steroids for low back pain or sciatica has not been scientifically proven. Moreover, because complications with the use of subarachnoid steroids are sufficiently serious, this form of therapy should be abandoned. In another review article published in the same journal, however, Benzon (225) had a more favorable conclusion: relief is usually effective in patients with signs and symptoms of acute nerve root irritation caused by intervertebral disk. Patients with acute radiculopathy have a better response compared to patients with chronic symptoms, and improvement might not be noted until 6 days after injection.

The recommended procedure for performing such blocks is to place small quantities of dilute local anesthetic (5 to 8 ml of 1% lidocaine or 0.25% bupivacaine) containing steroid (methylprednisolone, 40 to 80 mg) into the epidural space as close as possible to the pain site. Benefits from such an injection can take up to a week to appear, and the injections can be repeated at 2- to 3-week intervals. This interval is chosen because, with the recommended doses of steroid, adrenal suppression can occur for about 2 weeks (225).

CHRONIC NECK PAIN. Reports of the use of cervical epidural injections for various pain problems in the neck and upper limb have recently begun to appear in the literature. As with lumbar epidural injections, the procedure can be done with local anesthetics alone or with local anesthetics combined with corticosteroids (226, 227). Injections are usually done at the C7 to T1 interspace but can be done at other interspaces. The volume of the local anesthetic should be small—for example, 1 to 3 ml of dilute solution (e.g., 0.25% bupivacaine so as not to produce extensive motor block of cervical nerves). Injections usually consist of a series of three or four blocks performed at intervals of 2 to 3 weeks. Obviously, particular caution is necessary in performing these blocks because the epidural space is narrow and damage to the spinal cord can occur.

In one report, 16% of patients who received steroid injection in the cervical epidural space for acute cervical radicular pain with sensory deficit had a good to excellent response (227). The authors of this study attempted to correlate success rate with other objective findings, such as motor weakness, plain radiographs, CT scan, and EMG, but found no specific correlation. Similar rates of success have been reported with degenerative cervical disease and chronic neck strain, but the response of postherpetic and occipital neuralgia was not as encouraging (228).

REFERENCES

1. Bonica, J.J.: The Management of Pain. Philadelphia, Lea & Febiger, 1953.
2. Bonica, J.J.: Clinical Applications of Diagnostic and Therapeutic Nerve Blocks. Springfield, IL, Charles C Thomas, 1959.
3. Bonica, J.J.: Blocks of the Sympathetic Nervous System, Vol. 1, 2. Chicago, Frank J. Corbet, 1981.
4. Bonica, J.J.: Local anaesthesia and regional blocks, In Textbook of Pain. 2nd Ed. Edited by P.S. Wall and R. Melzack. Edinburgh, Churchill Livingstone, 1989, pp. 724–743.
5. Moore, D.C.: Regional Blockade. 4th Ed. Springfield, IL, Charles C Thomas, 1963.
6. Katz, J.: Atlas of Regional Anesthesia. Norwalk, CT, Appleton-Century-Crofts, 1985.
7. Cousins, M.J., and Bridenbaugh, P.O.: Neural Blockade in Clinical Anesthesia and Management of Pain. 2nd Ed. Philadelphia, J.B. Lippincott, 1988.
8. Melzack, R.: The Puzzle of Pain. New York, Basic Books, 1973.
9. Fox. A.J., and Melzack, R.: Transcutaneous electrical stimulation in acupuncture: Comparison of treatment of low back pain. Pain, 2:141, 1976.
10. Brena, S.F.: Nerve blocks and chronic pain states—an update. Postgrad. Med., 78:62, 1985.
11. Kibler, R.F., and Nathan, P.W.: Relief of pain and paresthesiae by nerve blocks distal to a lesion. J. Neurol. Neurosurg. Psychiatry, 23:91, 1960.
12. Loh, L., Nathan, P.W., and Schott, G.: Pain due to lesions of the central nervous system removed by sympathetic block. Br. Med. J., 282:1026, 1981.
13. Boas, R.A., Covino, B.G., and Shahwarian, A.: Analgesic response to IV lignocaine. Br. J. Anaesth., 54:501, 1982.
14. Woolf, C., and Wiesenfeld-Hallin, Z.: The systemic administration of local anesthetics produces a selective depression of C-afferent fiber evoked activity in the spinal cord. Pain, 23:361, 1985.
15. Jänig, W.: The pathophysiology of nerve following mechanical injury. In Pain Research and Clinical Management, Vol. 3. Proceedings of the Fifth World Congress on Pain. Edited by R. Dubner, G.F. Gebhart, and M.R. Bond. Amsterdam, Elsevier, 1988, pp. 87–108.
16. Bengtsson, A., and Bengtsson, M.: Regional sympathetic blockade in primary fibromyalgia. Pain, 33:161, 1988.
17. Loeser, J.D.: Dorsal rhizotomy for the relief of chronic pain. J. Neurosurg., 36:745, 1972.
18. Pflug, E.A., et al.: The effects of postoperative peridural analgesia on pulmonary therapy and pulmonary complications. Anesthesiology, 41:8, 1974.
19. Bach, S., Noreng, M.F., and Tjellden, N.U.: Phantom limb pain in amputees during the first 12 months following limb amputation, after preoperative lumbar epidural blockade Pain, 33:297, 1988.
20. Levine, J.D., Coderre, T.J., and Basbaum, A.I.: The peripheral nervous system and the inflammatory process. In Pain Research and Clinical Management, Vol. 3. Proceedings of the Fifth World Congress on Pain. Edited by R. Dubner, G.F. Gebhart, and M.R. Bond. Amsterdam, Elsevier, 1988, pp. 33–43.
21. Bonica, J.J.: Diagnostic and therapeutic blocks. A reappraisal based on 15 years' experience. Anesth. Analg., 37:58, 1958.
22. Bonica, J.J.: Current role of nerve blocks in the diagnosis and therapy of pain. In Advances in Neurology, Vol. 4. Edited by J.J. Bonica. New York, Raven Press, 1974, p. 445.
23. Bonica, J.J.: Management of pain with conduction analgesia. Bull. Reg. Anesth., 3:42, 1983.
24. Bonica, J.J.: Management of pain with regional analgesia. Postgrad. Med., 60:897, 1984.
25. Abram, S.E., Anderson, R.A., and Maitra-D'Cruze, A.M.: Factors predicting short-term outcome of nerve blocks in the management of chronic pain. Pain, 10:232, 1981.
26. Covino, B.G.: Clinical pharmacology of local anesthetic agents. In Neural Blockade in Clinical Anesthesia and Management of Pain. 2nd Ed. Edited by M.J. Cousins and P.O. Bridenbaugh. Philadelphia, J.B. Lippincott, 1988, pp. 111–144.
27. Tucker, G.T., and Mather, L.E.: Properties, absorption, and disposition of local anesthetic agents. In Neural Blockade in Clinical Anesthesia and Management of Pain. 2nd Ed. Edited by M.J. Cousins and P.O. Bridenbaugh. Philadelphia, J.B. Lippincott, 1988, pp. 47–110.
28. Bieter, R.N.: Applied pharmacology of local anesthetics. Am. J. Surg., 35:500, 1936.
29. Bromage, P.R.: A comparison of the hydrochloride and carbon dioxide salts of lidocaine and prilocaine in epidural analgesia. Acta Anaesthesiol. Scand. [Suppl.], 16:55, 1965.
30. Buckley, F.P., Duval-Neto, G., and Fink, B.R.: Acid and alkaline solutions of local anesthetics. Duration of nerve block and tissue pH. Anesth. Analg., 64:477, 1985.
31. Morrison, D.H.: A double-blind comparison of carbonated lidocaine and lidocaine hydrochloride in epidural anaesthesia. Can. Anaesth. Soc. J., 28:387, 1981.
32. Galindo, A.: pH-adjusted local anesthetics: Clinical experience. Reg. Anesth., 8:35, 1983.
33. Hilger, M.: Alkalinization of bupivacaine for brachial plexus block. Reg. Anesth., 10:59, 1983.
34. Loder, R.E.: A long-acting local anesthetic solution for the relief of pain after thoracotomy. Thorax, 17:375, 1962.
35. Kaplan, J.A., Miller, E.D., and Gallagher, E.C. Postoperative analgesia for thoracotomy patients. Anesth. Analg., 54:773, 1975.
36. Rosenblatt, R.M., and Fung, R.L.: Optimal ratio of bupivacaine and dextran for regional anesthesia. Reg. Anesth., 4:2, 1979.
37. Bridenbaugh, L.D.: Does the addition of low molecular weight dextran prolong the duration of action of bupivacaine? Reg. Anesth., 3:6, 1978.
38. Kingsnorth, A.N., Wijesinha, S.S., and Grixti, C.S.: Evaluation of dextran with local anesthetic for short-stay inguinal herniorraphy. Ann. R. Coll. Surg. Engl., 61:456, 1979.
39. Scurlock, J.E., and Curtis, B.M.: Dextran-local anesthetic interactions. Anesthesiology, 54:265, 1980.
40. Buckley, F.P., and Fink, B.R.: Duration of action of nerve blocks produced by mixtures of local anesthetic and low molecular weight dextran: Studies in rat infraorbital nerve blocks. Anesth. Analg., 60:142, 1981.
41. Rosenbladt, L.D., and Fung, R.L.: Mechanisms of action of dextran prolonging regional anesthesia. Reg. Anesth., 5:3, 1980.
42. Navaratnarajah, R.M., and Davenport, H.T.: The prolongation of local anesthetic with dextran. Anaesthesia, 40:259, 1985.
43. Devor, M., Govrin-Lippmann, R., and Raber, P.: Corticosteroids suppress ectopic neural discharge originating in experimental neuromas. Pain, 22:127, 1985.
44. Moore, D.C.: Complications of Regional Anesthesia. Springfield, IL, Charles C Thomas, 1955.
45. Thompson, G.E.: The role of regional analgesia in peri-operative nerve injuries. Reg. Anesth., 10:48:, 1985.
46. Winchell, S.W., and Wolfe, R.: The incidence of neuropathy following upper extremity blocks. Reg. Anesth., 10:12, 1985.
47. Selander, D., Edshage, S., and Wolff, T.: Paresthesia or no paresthesia. Nerve lesions after axillary blocks. Acta Anaesthesiol. Scand., 23:27, 1979.
48. Plevak, D.J., Linstromberg, J.W., and Danielson, D.R.: Paresthesia vs. nonparesthesia. The axillary block. Anesthesiology, 59:A216, 1983.
49. Löfström, B., Wennberg, A., and Widen, I.: Late disturbances in nerve function after block with local anesthetic agents. Acta Anaesthesiol. Scand., 10:111, 1966.
50. Selander, D., Brattsand, R., and Lundborg, G.: Local anesthetics: Importance of mode of application, concentration, and adrenaline for the appearance of nerve lesions. Acta Anaesthesiol. Scand., 23:127, 1979.
51. Selander, K.D., Dhuner, K.G., and Lundborg, G.: Peripheral nerve injury due to injection needles used for regional anesthesia. Acta Anaesthesiol. Scand., 21:182, 1977.
52. Porter, K.M., and Davies, J.: The control of pain after Keller's procedure—a controlled, double-blind prospective trial with local anesthetic and placebo. Ann. R. Coll. Surg. Engl., 67:293, 1985.
53. Owen, M., Galloway, D.J., and Mitchell, K.G.: Analgesia by wound infiltration after surgical excision of benign breast lumps. Ann. R. Coll. Surg. Engl., 67:130, 1985.
54. Hashimi, K., and Middleton, M.D.: Subcutaneous bupivacaine for postoperative analgesia after herniorraphy. Ann. R. Coll. Surg. Engl., 65:38, 1983.
55. Thomas, D.F.M., Lambert, W.S., and Lloyd, W.K.: The direct perfusion of surgical wounds with local anesthetic solution: An approach to postoperative pain. Ann. R. Coll. Surg. Engl., 65: 226, 1983.

56. Levack, S.P., Holmes, J.D., and Robertson, J.S.: Abdominal wound perfusion for the relief of postoperative pain. Br. J. Anaesth., 58:615, 1986.

57. Defalque, R.J.: Painful trigger points in surgical scars. Anesth. Analg., 61:518, 1982.

58. Melzack, R.: Myofascial trigger points: Relation to acupuncture and mechanisms of pain. Arch. Phys. Med. Rehabil., 62:114, 1981.

59. Simons, D.G.: Myofascial pain syndromes of head, neck and low back. In Pain Research and Clinical Management, Vol. 3. Proceedings of the Fifth World Congress on Pain. Edited by R. Dubner, G.F. Gebhart, and M.R. Bond. New York, Elsevier, 1988, pp. 186–200.

60. Pybus, P.K.: Osteoarthrosis of the knee. Practitioner, 224:928, 1980.

61. Pybus, P.K.: The control of pain and stiffness in osteoarthritis of the hand. S. Afr. Med. J., 59:514, 1981.

62. Ghormley, R.K.: Low back pain with special reference to the articular facets with presentation of an operative procedure. JAMA, 10:1773, 1933.

63. Bogduk, N.: Back pain: Zygapophyseal blocks and epidural steroids. In Neural Blockade in Clinical Anesthesia and Management of Pain. 2nd Ed. Edited by M.J. Cousins and P.O. Bridenbaugh. Philadelphia, J.B. Lippincott, 1988, pp. 935–954.

64. McQuay, H.J., Carroll, D., and Moore, R.A.: Postoperative paediatric pain—the effects of opiate premedication and local anaesthetic blocks. Pain, 33:291, 1988.

65. Bonica, J.J., Moore, D.C., and Orlov, M.: Brachial plexus block anesthesia. Am. J. Surg., 78:65, 1949.

66. Winnie, A.P.: Interscalene brachial plexus. Anesth. Analg., 49:455, 1970.

67. Eather, K.F.: Axillary brachial plexus block. Anesthesiology, 19:683, 1958.

68. Thompson, G.E., and Rorie, D.K.: Functional anatomy of the brachial plexus sheath. Anesthesiology, 59:117, 1983.

69. Dekrey, J.A., Schroeder, C.F., and Buechel, D.R.: Continuous brachial plexus block. Anesthesiology, 30:332, 1969.

70. Tash, E., and Aaronson, M.B.: Continuous interscalene block for surgical operations on the hand. Anesthesiology, 53:356, 1980.

71. Selander, D.: Catheter technique in axillary brachial plexus block. Acta Anaesthesiol. Scand., 21:324, 1977.

72. Rosenblatt, R., Pepitone-Rockwell, R., and McKillop, R.J.: Continuous axillary analgesia for traumatic hand injury. Anesthesiology, 51:565, 1979.

73. Ang, E.T., Lassale, B., and Goldfarb, G.: Continuous axillary brachial plexus block—a clinical and anatomical study. Anesth. Analg., 63:680, 1984.

74. Tuominen, M., Rosenberg, P.M., and Kalso, E.: Blood levels of bupivacaine after single dose, supplementary dose and during continuous infusion in axillary brachial plexus blockade. Acta Anaesthesiol. Scand., 27:303, 1983.

75. Kirkpatrick, A.F., and Bednarczyk, L.R.: Bupivacaine blood levels during continuous interscalene block. Anesthesiology, 62:65, 1985.

76. Colding, A.: The effect of regional sympathetic blocks in the treatment of herpes zoster. Acta Anaesthesiol. Scand., 13:133, 1969.

77. Dan, K., Higa, K., and Tanaka, K.: Herpetic pain and cellular immunity. In Current Topics in Pain Research and Therapy. Edited by Y.O. Yokota and R. Dubner. Amsterdam, Excerpta Medicus International Congress Series, 1983, pp. 293–305.

78. Restelli, L., Movilia, P., and Bossi, L.: Management of pain after thoracotomy and technique of multiple intercostal blocks. Anesthesiology, 61:353, 1984.

79. Bridenbaugh, P.O., Du Pen, S.L., and Moore, D.C.: Postoperative intercostal nerve block analgesia vs. narcotic analgesia. Anesth. Analg., 52:81, 1973.

80. Engberg, G.: Single-dose intercostal blocks with etidocaine for pain relief after upper abdominal surgery. Acta Anaesthesiol. Scand. [Suppl.], 60:43, 1975.

81. O'Kelly, E., and Garry, B. Continuous pain relief for multiple fractured ribs. Br. J. Anaesth., 53:989, 1981.

82. Murphy, D.F.: Intercostal nerve blockade for fractured ribs and postoperative analgesia. Description of a new technique. Reg. Anesth., 8:151, 1983.

83. Applegate, W.V.: Abdominal cutaneous nerve entrapment syndrome. Surgery, 71:118, 1972.

84. Cronin, K.D., and Davis, M.J.: Intercostal block for postoperative pain relief. Anaesth. Intensive Care, 4:259, 1976.

85. Nunn, J.F., and Slavin, A.: Posterior intercostal nerve block for pain relief after cholecystectomy. Anatomic basis and efficacy. Br. J. Anaesth., 53:253, 1980.

86. Engberg, G.: Respiratory performance after upper abdominal surgery. A comparison of pain relief with intercostal blocks and centrally acting analgesics. Acta Anaesthesiol. Scand., 29:427, 1985.

87. Humphreys, C.F., and Kay, M.: The control of postoperative pain with the use of bupivacaine injections. J. Urol., 122:506, 1976.

88. Crawford, E.D., and Skinner, D.B.: Intercostal nerve block with thoracoabdominal and flank incisions. Urology, 19:25, 1982.

89. Bergh, N.P., et al.: Effect of intercostal block on lung function after thoracotomy. Acta Anaesthesiol. Scand. [Suppl.], 24:85, 1966.

90. Galway, J.E., Caves, P.K., and Dundee, J.W.: Effect of intercostal nerve block during operation on lung function and the relief of pain following thoracotomy. Br. J. Anaesth., 47:730, 1975.

91. Delilkan, A.E., et al.: Postoperative local analgesia for thoracotomy with direct bupivacaine blocks. Anesthesiology, 28:561, 1973.

92. Faust, R.J., and Nauss, L.A.: Post-thoracotomy intercostal block: Comparison of its effects on pulmonary function with those of intramuscular meperidine. Anesth. Analg., 55:542, 1976.

93. Toledo-Peraya, L.M., and DeMeester, T.R.: Prospective randomized evaluation of intrathoracic block with bupivacaine in postoperative ventilatory function. Ann. Thorac. Surg., 19:355, 1978.

94. Cory, P.C., and Mulroy, M.F.: Postoperative respiratory failure following intercostal block. Anesthesiology, 59:418, 1981.

95. Casey, W.F.: Respiratory failure following intercostal nerve blockade. Anaesthesia, 39:351, 1984.

96. Cory, P.C., and Horton, W.G.: Lung volume changes produced by intercostal block with 0.5% bupivacaine. Anesthesiology, 55:A144, 1981.

97. Jakobson, S., and Ivarson, F.: Effects of intercostal nerve block (bupivacaine 0.25% and etidocaine 0.5%) on chest wall mechanics in healthy men. Acta Anaesthesiol. Scand., 21:489, 1977.

98. Jakobson, S., et al.: Effects of intercostal nerve blocks on pulmonary mechanics in healthy men. Acta Anaesthesiol. Scand., 24:482, 1980.

99. Moore, D.C.: Intercostal nerve block for postoperative somatic pain following surgery of the thorax and upper abdomen. Br. J. Anaesth., 47:284, 1975.

100. Moore, D.C., Bush, W.K., and Scurlock, J.E.: Intercostal nerve block: A roentgenographic study of technique and absorption in humans. Anesth. Analg., 59:815, 1980.

101. Middaugh, R.E., Menk, E.J., and Reynolds, W.J.: Epidural block using large volumes of local anesthetic solution for intercostal block. Anesthesiology, 63:214, 1985.

102. Ishizuku, I., et al.: Continuous block for pain relief after lumbar incisions. J. Urol., 122:506, 1979.

103. Kirno, K., and Lindell, K.: Intercostal nerve blockade. Br. J. Anaesth., 58:246, 1986.

104. Scott, D.B.: Acute pain management. In Neural Blockade in Clinical Anesthesia and Management of Pain. 2nd Ed. Edited by M.J. Cousins and P.O. Bridenbaugh. Philadelphia, J.B. Lippincott, 1988, pp. 861–883.

105. Ablondi, M.A., et al.: Continuous intercostal blocks for postoperative pain relief. Anesth. Analg., 45:185, 1966.

106. Lyles, R., et al.: Continuous intercostal catheter techniques for treatment of post-traumatic thoracic pain. Anesthesiology, 65:A205, 1986.

107. Blades, B., and Ford, W.: A method for control of postoperative pain. Surg. Gynecol. Obstet., 91:524, 1950.

108. Reiestad, F., and Stromskag, K.E.: Intrapleural catheter in the management of postoperative pain—a preliminary report. Reg. Anesth., 11:89, 1986.

109. Reiestad, F.: Intrapleural regional analgesia. Presented at the Second International Symposium on Regional Anesthesia. Williamsburg, VA, May, 1988.

110. Sihota, M.K., et al.: Successful management of chronic pancreatitis and postherpetic neuralgia with intrapleural technique. Reg. Anesth., 13:40, 1988.

111. Smith, B.E., et al.: Rectus sheath block for diagnostic laparoscopy. Anaesthesia, 43:947, 1988.

112. Braid, D.P., and Scott, D.B.: The systemic absorption of local anaesthetic agents. Br. J. Anaesth., 37:394, 1965.
113. Tucker, G.T., et al.: Systemic absorption of mepivacaine in commonly used regional block procedures. Anesthesiology, 37:277, 1972.
114. Benumof, J.L., and Semenza, J.: Total spinal anesthesia following intrathoracic intercostal blocks. Anesthesiology, 43:124, 1975.
115. Moore, M.C., and Reitan, J.D.: Sudden total spinal block after intraoperative intercostal injections. Anesth. Rev., 5:36, 1978.
116. Brodsky, J.B., and Mark, J.B.D.: Hypotension from intra-operative intercostal blocks. Reg. Anesth., 4:17, 1979.
117. Skretting, P.: Hypotension after intercostal block during thoracotomy under general anesthesia. Br. J. Anaesth., 53:527, 1984.
118. Chayen, D., Nathan, M., and Chayen, M.: The psoas compartment block. Anesthesiology, 45:95, 1976.
119. Brands, E., and Callahan, V.L.: Continuous lumbar plexus block. Analgesia for femoral neck fractures. Anesth. Intensive Care, 6:265, 1978.
120. Berry, F.R. Analgesia in patients with fractured neck of femur. Anaesthesia, 37:577, 1977.
121. Winnie, A.P., Ramamarthy, S., and Durranii, A.: The inguinal perivascular technique of lumbar plexus anesthesia: the 3-in-1 block. Anesth. Analg., 52:989, 1973.
122. Rosenblatt, R.M.: Continuous femoral anesthesia for lower extremity surgery. Reg. Anesth., 4:2, 1980.
123. Labat, G.: Regional Anesthesia. 2nd Ed. Philadelphia, W.B. Saunders, 1930, pp. 330–337.
124. Guardini, R., Waldron, B.A., and Wallace, W.A.: Sciatic nerve block: A new lateral approach. Acta Anaesthesiol. Scand., 29:515, 1985.
125. Smith, B.D.: Continuous sciatic nerve block. Anaesthesia, 39:155, 1984.
126. Soliman, M.A., and Tremblay, N.A.: Nerve block of the penis for postoperative pain relief in children. Anesth. Analg., 57:495, 1977.
127. Goulding, F.J.: Penile block for postoperative pain relief in penile surgery. J. Urol., 126:337, 1981.
128. Carlsson, P., and Svensson, J.: The duration of pain relief after penile nerve block in boys undergoing circumcision. Acta Anaesthesiol. Scand., 28:432, 1984.
129. Kuntz, A.: Autonomic Nervous System. 4th Ed. Philadelphia, Lea & Febiger, 1953.
130. Roberts, W.J.: A hypothesis on the physiologic basis for causalgia related pain. Pain, 24:297, 1986.
131. Campbell, J.N., Raja, S.N., and Meyer, R.A.: Painful sequelae of nerve injury. In Pain Research and Clinical Management, Vol. 3. Proceedings of the Fifth World Congress on Pain. Edited by R. Dubner, G.F. Gebhart, and M.R. Bond. New York, Elsevier, 1988, pp. 135–143.
132. Frost, S.A., et al.: Does hyperalgesia to cooling stimuli characterize patients with sympathetically maintained pain (reflex sympathetic dystrophy)? In Pain Research and Clinical Management, Vol. 3. Proceedings of the Fifth World Congress on Pain. Edited by R. Dubner, G.F. Gebhart, and M.R. Bond. Amsterdam, Elsevier, 1988, pp. 151–156.
133. Bach, S., Noreng, M.F., and Tjellden, N.U.: Phantom limb pain in amputees during the first 12 months following limb amputation after preoperative lumbar epidural blockade. Pain, 33:297, 1988.
134. Hannington-Kiff, J.B.: In Limbo. Jacksonian Prize Dissertation In Libres. Edinburgh, Royal College of Surgeons, 1980.
135. Loh, L., Nathan, P.W., and Schott, G.: Pain due to lesions of the central nervous systems removed by sympathetic block. Br. Med. J., 282:1026, 1981.
136. Schott, G.D.: Mechanisms of causalgia and related clinical conditions. The role of the central and of the sympathetic nervous system. Brain, 109:717, 1986.
137. Hannington-Kiff, J.B.: Antisympathetic drugs in limbs. In Textbook of Pain. Edited by P.D. Wall and R. Melzack. London, Churchill Livingstone, 1984, pp. 566–573.
138. Cousins, M.J., et al.: Neurolytic lumbar sympathetic blockade: Duration of denervation and relief of rest pain. Anesth. Intensive Care, 7:2, 1979.
139. Reid, W., Watt, J.K. and Gray, G.: Phenol injection of the sympathetic chain. Br. J. Surg., 57:45, 1970.
140. Cox, W.V., et al.: The effect of stellate ganglionectomy on the cardiac function of intact dogs and its effect on the extent of myocardial infarction and on cardial function following coronary artery occlusion. Am. Heart J., 12:285, 1936.
141. McEachern, C.G., et al.: Sudden occlusion of coronary arteries following removal of cardiosensory pathways. Arch. Intern. Med., 65:661, 1940.
142. Schauer, G., et al.: Hemodynamic studies in experimental coronary occlusion. IV. Stellate ganglionectomy experiments. Am. Heart J., 14:669, 1937.
143. Schwartz, P.J., and Stone, H.L.: Tonic influence of the sympathetic nervous system on myocardial reactive hyperemia and on coronary blood flow distribution in dogs. Circ. Res., 41:51, 1977.
144. Klassen, G.A., et al.: Effect of acute sympathectomy by epidural anesthesia on the canine coronary circulation. Anesthesiology, 52:8, 1980.
145. Schaal, S.F., et al.: Protective effect of cardiac denervation against arrhythmias of myocardial infarction. Cardiovasc. Res., 3:241, 1969.
146. Vik-Mo, H., Ottesen, S., and Renck, H.: Cardiac effects of thoracic epidural analgesia before and during acute coronary artery occlusion in open chest dogs. Scand. J. Clin. Lab. Ivest., 38:737, 1978.
147. Jewitt, D.E., et al.: Practolol in the treatment of cardiac arrhythmias due to acute myocardial infarction. Lancet, 2:227, 1969.
148. Gage, I.M.: Treatment of acute pancreatitis. Surgery, 23:723, 1948.
149. Walker, T., and Pembleton, W.E.: Continuous epidural block in the treatment of pancreatitis. Anesthesiology, 14:33, 1953.
150. Rosenak, S.: Procaine injection treatment of herpes zoster. Lancet, 2:1056, 1938.
151. Colding, A.: The effect of regional sympathetic blocks in the treatment of herpes zoster. Acta Anaesthesiol. Scand., 13:133, 1969.
152. Bauman, J.: Treatment of acute herpes zoster neuralgia by epidural injection or stellate ganglion block. Anesthesiology, 51:523, 1979.
153. Perkins, H.M., and Hanlon, P.R.: Epidural injection of local anesthetic and steroids for relief of pain secondary to herpes zoster. Arch. Surg., 113:253, 1978.
154. Dan, K., Higa, K., and Tanaka, K.: Herpetic pain and cellular immunity. In Current Topics in Pain Research and Therapy. Edited by Y.O. Yokoda and R.T. Dubner. Amsterdam, Excerpta Medicus International Congress Series, 1983.
155. Dan, K., Higa, K., and Noda, B.: Nerve block for herpetic pain. In Advances in Pain Research and Therapy, Vol. 9. Edited by H.L. Fields, R.W. Dubner, and F. Cervero. New York, Raven Press, 1985, pp. 831–838.
156. Tenicela, R., Lovasik, D., and Eaglstein, W.: Treatment of herpes zoster with sympathetic blocks. Clin. J. Pain, 1:64, 1985.
157. Riopelle, J.M., Naraghi, M., and Grush, K.P.: Chronic neuralgia incidence following local anesthetic therapy for herpes zoster. Arch. Dermatol., 120:747, 1984.
158. Price, R.W.: Herpes zoster: An approach to systemic therapy. Med. Clin. North Am., 66:1105, 1982.
159. Forrest, J.B.: The response to epidural steroid injections in chronic dorsal root pain. Can. Anaesth. Soc. J., 27:40, 1980.
160. Milligan, N.S., and Nash, T.P: Treatment of post-herpetic neuralgia: A review of 77 consecutive cases. Pain, 23:381, 1985.
161. Lilley, J.P., Su, D., and Wang, J.K.: Sensory and sympathetic nerve blocks for postherpetic neuralgia. Reg. Anesth., 11:165, 1986.
162. Ward, E.M., et al.: The celiac ganglia in man. Normal anatomic variation. Anesth. Analg., 56:461, 1979.
163. Moore, D.C., Bush, W.K., and Burnett, L.L.: Celiac plexus block: A roentgenographic anatomic study of technique and spread of solution in patients and corpses. Anesth. Analg., 60:369, 1981.
164. Hovelacque, A.: Anatomie des Nerfs Craniens et Rachidiens et du Systéme Grand Sympathique chez l'Homme. Paris, G. Doin & Cie, 1927.
165. Boas, R.A.: The sympathetic nervous system and pain relief. In Relief of Intractable Pain. Edited by M. Swerdlow. Amsterdam, Elsevier, 1983.
166. Bier, A.: Über einen neuen weg Lokalanesthesie an den Gliedmassen zu erqueugen. Arch. Klin. Chir., 86:1007, 1908.

167. Hannington-Kiff, J.C.: Intravenous sympathetic blockade with guanethidine. Lancet, 1:1019, 1974.
168. Bonelli, S., et al.: Regional intravenous guanethidine vs. stellate ganglion block in reflex sympathetic dystrophies: A randomized trial. Pain, 16:297, 1983.
169. Glynn, C.J., Basedow, R.W., and Walsh, J.A.: Pain relief following postganglionic sympathetic blockade with IV guanethidine. Br. J. Anaesth., 53:1297, 1981.
170. McKain, C.W., Bruno, J.U., and Goldner J.L.: The effects of intravenous regional guanethidine and reserpine. J. Bone Joint Surg., 6:808, 1983.
171. Vaughan, R.S., Lawrie, B.W., and Sykes, P.J.: Use of intravenous regional sympathetic block in upper limb angiography. Ann. R. Coll. Surg. Engl., 67:309, 1985.
172. Driessen, J.J., et al.: Clinical effects of regional intravenous guanethidine (Ismelin) in reflex sympathetic dystrophy. Acta Anesthesiol. Scand., 27:505, 1983.
173. Leriche, R., and Fontaine, R.: On the use of intra-arterial injections of novocaine for painful forms of arteritis obliterans. Bull. Mem. Soc. Nat. Chir., 61:244, 1935.
174. Boas, R.A., and Cousins, M.J.: Diagnostic neural blockade. In Neural Blockade in Clinical Anesthesia and Management of Pain. 2nd Ed. Edited by M.J. Cousins and P.O. Bridenbaugh. Philadelphia, J.B. Lippincott, 1988, pp. 885–898.
175. Atkinson, R.L.: Intravenous lidocaine for the treatment of intractable pain of adiposis dolorosa. Int. J. Obesity, 6:351, 1982.
176. Hatangdi, V.S., Boas, R.A., and Richards, E.G.: Management with antiepileptic and tricyclic drugs. In Advances in Pain Research and Therapy. Vol. 1. Edited by J.J. Bonica and D. Albe-Fessard. New York, Raven Press, 1976, pp. 583–587.
177. Wiesenfeld-Hallin, Z., and Lindblom, U.: The effect of systemic tocainide, lidocaine and bupivacaine on nociception in the rat. Pain, 23:357, 1985.
178. Raj, P.P.: Prognostic and therapeutic local anesthetic blockade. In Neural Blockade in Clinical Anesthesia and Management of Pain. 2nd Edition. Edited by M.J. Cousins and P.O. Bridenbaugh. Philadelphia, J.B., Lippincott, 1988, pp. 899–933.
179. Ahlgren, E.W.: Diagnosis of pain with a graduated spinal block technique. JAMA, 193:813, 1966.
180. Winnie, A.P., and Collins, V.S.: Differential neural blockade in pain syndrome of questionable etiology. Med. Clin. North Am., 52:123, 1968.
181. Bengstsson, M., Löfström, J.B., and Malmquist, L.A.: Skin conductance responses during spinal analgesia. Acta Anaesthesiol. Scand., 29:67, 1985.
182. Urban, B.J., and McKain, C.W.: Local anesthetic effect of intrathecal normal saline. Pain, 5:43, 1978.
183. Teeple, E., Scott, D.L., and Ghia, J.N.: Intrathecal saline without preservative does not have a local anesthetic effect. Pain, 14:3, 1982.
184. Ghia, J.N., et al.: Toward an understanding of chronic pain mechanisms. The use of psychological tests and a refined differential spinal block. Anesthesiology, 50:20, 1979.
185. Bromage, P.R.: Epidural Analgesia. Philadelphia, W.B. Saunders, 1980.
186. Cheng, P.A.: The anatomical and clinical aspects of epidural anesthesia. Curr. Res. Anesth. Analg., 42:398, 1963.
187. Bonica, J.J.: Continuous peridural block. Anesthesiology, 17:626, 1956.
188. Sancha, R., Aman, L., and Rocha, F.: An analysis of radiological visualization of catheters placed in the extradural space. Br. J. Anaesth., 39:485, 1967.
189. Bridenbaugh, L.D., et al.: The position of plastic tubing in continuous block techniques. An X-ray study of 552 patients. Anesthesiology, 29:1047, 1968.
190. Sjögren, S., and Wright, B.: Circulation, respiration and lidocaine concentration during continuous epidural blockade. Acta Anaesthesiol. Scand. [Suppl.], 46:5, 1972.
191. Cherry, D.A., et al.: Diagnostic epidural opioid blockade and chronic pain. Pain, 21:143, 1985.
192. Arner, S., and Arner, B.: Differential effects of epidural morphine in the treatment of cancer-related pain. Acta Anaesthesiol. Scand., 29:32, 1985.
193. Cullen, M.L., et al.: Continuous epidural infusion for analgesia after major abdominal operations: A randomized, prospective double-blind study. Surgery, 98:718, 1985.
194. Trinkle, J.K., et al.: Management of flail chests without mechanical ventilation. Ann. Thorac. Surg., 19:355, 1975.
195. Shackford, S.R., Virgilio, R.W., and Peters, R.M.: Selective use of ventilator therapy in flail chest injury. J. Thorac. Cardiovasc. Surg., 31:194, 1981.
196. Gibbon, J., James, O., and Quail, A.: Management of 130 cases of chest injury with respiratory failure. Br. J. Anaesth., 45:1130, 1973.
197. Gibbon, J., James, O., and Quail, A.: Relief of pain in chest injuries. Br. J. Anaesth., 45:36, 1973.
198. Conacher, J.D., et al.: Epidural analgesia following thoracic surgery. A review of two years experience. Anaesthesia, 38:546, 1983.
199. Dittmann, M. Keller, R., and Wolff, G.: A rationale for epidural analgesia in the treatment of multiple rib fractures. Intensive Care Med., 4:193, 1978.
200. Dittman, M., et al.: Epidural analgesia or mechanical ventilation for multiple rib fractures? Intensive Care Med., 8:89, 1982.
201. Griffiths, D.R.G., Diamond, A.W., and Cameron, J.D.: Postoperative extradural analgesia following thoracic surgery. A feasibility study. Br. J. Anaesth., 47:48, 1975.
202. Shuman, R.L., and Peters, R.M.: Epidural analgesia following thoracotomy in patients with chronic obstructive airway disease. J. Thorac. Cardiovasc. Surg., 71:82, 1976.
203. Rankin, A.P.N., and Comber, R.M.: Management of fifty cases of chest injury with a regimen of epidural bupivacaine and morphine. Anesth. Intensive Care, 12:311, 1984.
204. Addison, N.V., et al.: Epidural analgesia following cholecystectomy. Br. J. Surg., 161:850, 1974.
205. Spence, A.A., and Smith, G.: Postoperative analgesia and lung function. A comparison of morphine with extradural block. Br. J. Anaesth., 43:144, 1971.
206. Miller, J.L., et al.: A comparison of the effects of narcotic and epidural analgesia on postoperative respiratory function. Am. J. Surg. 131:291, 1976.
207. Wahba, W.M., Don, M.F., and Craig, D.B.: Postoperative epidural analgesia: Effects on lung volume. Can. Anaesth. Soc. J., 22:519, 1975.
208. Spence, A.A., and Logan, D.A.: Respiratory effects of extradural nerve block in the postoperative period. Br. J. Anaesth., 47:281, 1975.
209. Drummond, G.B., and Littlewood, D.G.: Respiratory effects of extradural analgesia after lower abdominal surgery. Br. J. Anaesth., 49:999, 1977.
210. Fox, G.S, Whalley, D.G., and Bevan, P.R.: Anaesthesia for the morbidly obese. Experience with 110 patients. Br. J. Anaesth., 53:811, 1981.
211. Buckley, F.P., et al.: Anaesthesia in the morbidly obese: A comparison of anesthetic and analgesic regimes for upper abdominal surgery. Anaesthesia, 38:840, 1983.
212. Kehlet, H.: The modifying effect of general vs. regional anaesthesia on the endocrine metabolic response to surgery. Reg. Anesth., 7:538, 1982.
213. Kehlet, H.: Epidural analgesia and the endocrine-metabolic response to surgery. Acta Anaesthesiol. Scand., 28:125, 1984.
214. Rem, J., et al.: Influence of epidural analgesia on postoperative changes in various serum enzymes and serum bilirubin. Acta Anaesthesiol. Scand., 25:142, 1981.
215. Modig, J., Borg, T., and Karlstrom, G., et al.: Thromboembolism after total hip replacement: Role of epidural and regional anaesthesia. Acta Anaesthesiol. Scand., 62:174, 1983.
216. McClaren, A.D., Stockwell, M.C., and Reid, V.T.: Anesthetic techniques for surgical correction of fractured neck of femur. A comparison of spinal vs. general anesthesia in the elderly. Anaesthesia, 33:10, 1978.
217. Davis, F.M., and Laurenson, V.C.: Spinal anaesthesia or general anesthesia for emergency hip surgery in elderly patients. Anesth. Intensive Care, 9:352, 1981.
218. Hole, A., Terjeson, T., and Breivik, M.: Epidural versus general anaesthesia for total hip arthroplasty in elderly patients. Acta Anaesthesiol. Scand., 24:279, 1980.
219. Tassonyi, E., et al.: Epidural block in the treatment of acute pancreatitis. Reg. Anesth., 6:8, 1981.
220. Forrest, J.B.: The response to epidural steroid injections in chronic dorsal root pain. Can. Anaesth. Soc. J., 27:40, 1980.
221. Cappio, M.: Il trattanmento idrocortisonico per via epidurale sacrale delle lombosciatalgie. Reumatismo, 9:60, 1957.

222. Lindholm, R., and Salenius, P.: Caudal epidural administration of anesthetics and corticoids in the treatment of low back pain. Acta Orthop. Scand., *1*:114, 1964.

223. Kepes, E.R., and Duncalf, D.: Treatment of backache with spinal injections of local anesthetics, spinal and systemic steroids. A review. Pain, *22*:33, 1985.

224. Abram, J.A., and Anderson, R.A.: Using a pain questionnaire to predict response to steroid epidural. Reg. Anesth., *5*:11, 1980.

225. Benzon, H.T.: Epidural steroid injections for low back pain and lumbosacral radiculopathy. Pain, *24*:277, 1986.

226. Catchlove, R., and Braha, A.: The use of cervical epidural blocks in the management of chronic head and neck pain. Can. Anaesth. Soc. J., *31*:188, 1985.

227. Rowlingson, J.C., and Kirschnenbaum, L.P.: Epidural analgesic techniques in the management of cervical pain. Anaesth. Analg., *65*:938, 1986.

228. Purkis, L.E.: Cervical epidural steroids. Pain Clinic, *1*:3, 1986.

95 • REGIONAL ANALGESIA WITH INTRASPINAL OPIOIDS

L. BRIAN READY

OPIATE receptors were identified in the central nervous system in 1973 (1), and in 1977 large populations of these receptors were localized in the dorsal horn of the spinal cord (2). These observations, coupled with the discovery of endogenous opioids (3, 4), led to animal studies that demonstrated that intrathecal administration of opioids produces analgesia (5). Detailed reviews on the physiology and pharmacology of the analgesic effects produced by the action of opioids in the spinal cord have been presented by Benedetti and Bonica (6) and by Yaksh (7).

In 1979, Wang (8) and associates reported pain relief using intrathecal morphine in cancer patients; in the same year Behar and colleagues achieved the same result by injecting the drug into the epidural space (9). Subsequent authors have confirmed that selective long-duration analgesia was possible using these techniques in various clinical settings. As more studies were done it became clear that a number of side effects might be expected, ranging from annoying (e.g., sedation, pruritus, nausea, vomiting, urinary retention) to life-threatening (e.g., early and delayed respiratory depression). It is now apparent, however, that with attention to patient selection, appropriate choice of drugs, dosage, route of administration, and adequate patient monitoring, the benefits of intraspinal opioid analgesia can be obtained with a high degree of safety.

This chapter contains a discussion of the basis and clinical application of intraspinal opioids for the management of pain. The material is presented in three major sections: A, Basic Considerations, including discussion of the physiology of opiate receptors, the mechanism of action of intraspinal opioids, and their pharmacokinetics and pharmacology; B, Clinical Applications, including the management of acute pain, cancer pain, and nonmalignant chronic pain; C, Technical Considerations, including selection of patients, procedural techniques, selection of opioids, patient monitoring, contraindications to these procedures, and complications and their treatment. The term "intraspinal" has been used to include both the intrathecal (subarachnoid) and extradural (epidural) routes when considering them together. Because of long usage, in this chapter the terms "opiates" and "narcotics" are used interchangeably with the term "opioids," which is currently the preferred name for these drugs.

A. BASIC CONSIDERATIONS

Physiology

Physiologic and Anatomic Substrates and Spinal Opiate Receptors

Nerve impulses resulting from noxious stimuli and transmitted predominantly by slow-conducting A-delta and C fibers are modulated in the spinal cord before ascending to higher nerve centers in the brain. This modulation occurs through interactions at sensitive interneurons and associated receptors found in high concentrations in the substantia gelatinosa of the dorsal horn (2). It is mediated by endorphins, naturally occurring peptides that impair the transmission of nociceptive impulses and consequently diminish or eliminate the perception of pain without affecting somatic, autonomic, or motor functions.

Since the initial discovery of central nervous system opiate receptors, five types have been demonstrated—mu, kappa, delta, sigma, and epsilon (10). Narcotics administered by the intrathecal or epidural route can act on these receptors, like endorphins, to produce profound selective analgesia. It is likely that the specificity, affinity, and intrinsic activity of each agent reaching the various receptors determine its pharmacologic effects. The mu receptor is probably the dominant site in mediating analgesia, although delta and kappa receptors are also believed to play a role (Chapter 78). The receptors most important in mediating somatic pain can differ from those mediating visceral pain (11), which could explain the clinical observation that, although intraspinal narcotics might completely relieve incisional pain, the bowel distension accompanying ileus can still be distressing.

Mechanisms of Action

Intrathecal Injection

With the injection of an opioid the cerebrospinal fluid (CSF), a reservoir of drug is created that diffuses passively into the dorsal horn of the spinal cord. There it binds to opiate receptors, where it is presumed to inhibit the release of substance P, a neurotransmitter believed to be responsible for relaying nociceptive information across synapses. This inhibition is reversible with a narcotic antagonist such as naloxone.

Extradural Injection

A narcotic injected into the epidural space produces analgesia by two mechanisms. First, a portion of the drug crosses the dura mater to enter the CSF. From there it penetrates into the dorsal horn of the spinal cord, as after direct intrathecal injection. In addition, systemic absorption of the extradural bolus occurs to produce a plasma profile that resembles that of intramuscular injection (12). The systemic levels of opioid aid in producing analgesia as the drug is distributed to both the brain and spinal cord.

Comparison of Intrathecal and Extradural Injection

When a narcotic is injected into the CSF directly, only small doses are required because no anatomic barriers have to be crossed and removal by vasular absorption is slow. Administration by this route creates a reservoir of concentrated drug close to its site of action, where its effects should be limited to the spinal cord.

If the epidural route is chosen, the narcotic dose must be higher than that used with the intrathecal route to produce comparable analgesia. In the case of morphine a tenfold increase is needed (12). The CSF uptake of morphine administered epidurally is only about 2% but, because of the small volume of distribution within the spinal CSF (approximately 70 ml), morphine concentrations achieved in CSF are more than 100 times higher than those found after intramuscular injection (12). The highly vascular epidural space clears drug more rapidly than the relatively avascular subarachnoid space. Even so, the epidural opioid dose is only a fraction of that required to produce analgesia by intramuscular or intravenous administration.

After initial human experience with both intrathecal and epidural narcotics, the epidural route has achieved much greater popularity. This is partly because of the ease with which indwelling catheters can be placed in the epidural space for use over extended periods. In addition, it has become clear that certain complications, including the most serious (e.g., delayed respiratory depression), are more common after intrathecal than after epidural administration (13).

Comparison with Regional Analgesia with Local Anesthetics

It is useful for the clinician familiar with offering pain relief using local anesthetic neuraxis blocks (e.g., spinal, epidural) to compare and contrast these with intraspinal narcotics. Table 95-1 provides this information in a manner used previously by Cousins and Mather in a comprehensive review (14). A major difference between these techniques relates to the highly specific "block" of nociceptive pathways with intraspinal narcotics and the implications that this selectivity has for patient mobility while obtaining analgesia.

Pharmacokinetics and Pharmacology

Uptake and Distribution

The efficacy of intraspinal opioids is dependent on their availability from the site of injection to the spinal cord receptors in the dorsal horn. After intrathecal injection the rate at which a drug penetrates the tissue of the spinal cord is closely related to its lipid solubility. More rapid uptake and more rapid onset of action are seen with highly lipid-soluble drugs such as meperidine and fentanyl than with a less lipid-soluble agent such as morphine. Table 95-2 contrasts a drug of low lipid solubility (morphine) with one of high lipid solubility (fentanyl) with regard to clinically observable analgesic effects.

After epidural injection, a narcotic must also penetrate the dura, a relatively thick membrane that significantly slows its rate of diffusion. Arachnoid protrusions have been identified in the spinal root sleeves. These structures represent a possible route for passage of epidurally injected drugs into CSF (15). The possible role of uptake and delivery to the dorsal horn by the posterior radicular arteries has also been described (14).

The rate of dural penetration of epidural opiates is influenced by lipid solubility (16), molecular weight (17), and dissociation constant (pKa). Fentanyl, meperidine, and methadone all have a relatively high pKa. Because this favors high concentrations of freely diffusible nonionized molecules, these drugs exhibit

TABLE 95-1. Comparison of the Use of Intraspinal Narcotics and Local Anesthetic Block

Characteristic	Narcotics	Local Anesthetics
Action		
Site	Opiate receptors in dorsal horn of spinal cord (substantia gelatinosa)	Nerve roots and rootlets
Inhibition	Neural cell excitation	Axonal membrane impulse conduction
Pathways blocked	Pain	Pain, sympathetic, sensory, motor
Side effects		
Cardiovascular		Hypotension
Respiratory	Early depression—systemic absorption; late depression—rostral spread in CSF	
CNS		
Sedation	Variable, less than with parenteral narcotics	
Nausea and vomiting	Yes	Occasional
Urinary retention	Yes	Yes
Pruritus	Yes	
Convulsions		With high systemic drug level

TABLE 95-2. Effects of Narcotic Lipid Solubility on Analgesia

Effect	Lipid Solubility of Drug	
	Low (e.g., Morphine)	High (e.g., Fentanyl)
Spinal cord receptor uptake (onset of analgesia)	Slow	Rapid
Duration of action	Long	Short
CSF concentration	High	Low
Rostral spread of narcotic	Extensive	Limited

rapid onset and limited duration of spinal analgesia. Morphine, with a lower pKa, has a lower concentration of nonionized molecules following injection. This factor further contributes to its slow onset and long duration of action.

After epidural injection, vascular absorption decreases the concentration gradient across the dura, thus reducing the rate of transfer. The addition of epinephrine to epidural morphine has been reported to increase the speed of onset, quality, and duration of analgesia and intensity of side effects by reducing systemic absorption (18). In another study, however, only an increased frequency of side effects was found (19). Most clinicians do not use solutions that contain epinephrine.

Some portion of an opioid injected epidurally diffuses into extradural fat and thus does not cross the dura. The more lipophilic drugs show the fastest and greatest uptake by fat.

Highly lipophilic agents such as meperidine and fentanyl move rapidly from CSF into the lipid-rich tissues of the spinal cord. With such agents, onset of analgesia is rapid and the effect is relatively segmental near the injection site. Low lipid solubility, as in the case of morphine, leads to prolonged high CSF drug concentration, low tissue fixation, and the possibility of rostral spread in CSF. The drug continues to be available to receptors, resulting in a long duration of action.

Metabolism and Clearance

The role of metabolism in the termination of the spinal action of narcotics following intrathecal or extradural injection has not yet been established but, considering the high concentrations of drug present, it is unlikely that it is a major factor.

Loss of analgesia following intraspinal injection results from drug clearance from the site of action. The strong receptor binding seen with polar agents such as morphine retards clearance as compared with that of more lipophilic agents.

Intrathecal opioids are removed by two routes, diffusion along the neuraxis and vascular absorption. Rostral spread of CSF from the spinal subarachnoid space to the supraspinal cisternae has been demonstrated (20), making clearance through intracranial arachnoid granulations a likely mechanism.

Vascular absorption of intraspinally administered opiates can occur as a result of movement into spinal cord blood vessels or, following epidural injection, into the venous plexus found in the epidural space. High lipid solubility favors passage of drug into blood vessels at either site.

Tolerance

Tolerance, the decrease in effect over time with a given dose of narcotic, has been demonstrated in animals with both the intrathecal and epidural routes (21, 22), as has cross tolerance between intrathecal and systemically administered morphine (23).

In humans, conflicting information has been found. Rapid development of tolerance similar to that seen in animals has been reported in cancer patients who received 1 mg/day of intrathecal morphine (24). In contrast, cancer patients receiving epidural morphine in divided doses by intermittent injection showed little or no need for increased dose for as long as 280 days (25).

The mechanism leading to the development of tolerance is not known. A number of observations, however, might be of practical clinical importance. First, consumption of parenteral narcotics prior to commencing epidural treatment can increase the required dose (7). Second, the rate of onset of tolerance seems to be proportional to the concentration of the narcotic at the receptor—that is, the degree of receptor activation. Therefore the rate of development of tolerance might be minimized by the following factors: (a) selection of the lowest effective narcotic dose; (b) precise placement of narcotic for optimal segmental effect; (c) administration of small divided doses rather than large single daily doses into intraspinal catheters; and (d) possibly the use of low-dose continuous infusion systems when extended periods of analgesia are needed.

Toxicology

The toxicology of intraspinal opioids has been examined in various animal and clinical studies. Repeated intrathecal and extradural injections of analgesic doses of opioids lead to no neurologic symptoms or observable adverse effects on spinal cord cells or fibers. No turbidity is seen when morphine, meperidine, or methadone is added to CSF, but it is present after the addition of heroin, suggesting the precipitation of CSF protein (26).

Vast worldwide human experience indicates that intraspinal opioids, even when administered in high doses for long periods, do not cause neural injury. A number of opioids are supplied by their manufacturers in additive-free forms. Others contain preservatives, antioxidants, and buffering agents. It is not known whether any of these additives can be damaging following intraspinal or epidural injection. Sodium bisulfite, an antioxidant present in some local anesthetic and narcotic solutions, does appear to be a dose-related neurotoxin (27).

Preservative-free preparations of morphine (e.g., Duramorph, Astramorph) are marketed specifically for intraspinal use. They are considerably more expensive, however, than preservative-containing morphin preparations, a significant consideration in cancer patients who might require large doses over extended periods. A method has been described for preparing a preservative-free morphine solution from oral tablets (28).

B. CLINICAL APPLICATIONS

Acute Pain

Since 1979, following the initial reports of the clinical efficacy of intraspinal narcotics by Wang and colleagues (8) and by Behar and associates (9), investigators have reported their application in a wide variety of clinical settings. Claims of efficacy vary, but profound analgesia has generally been noted. Many of these reports, however, represent uncontrolled observations, and the possibility of bias cannot be eliminated. A number of randomized blind studies have been carried out, such as the one by Rawal and co-workers (29), which showed superior postoperative analgesia with opioids in obese patients following gastroplasty, and by Writer and colleagues (30) in patients undergoing various surgical procedures.

Experience with intraspinal opioids for the control of severe postoperative pain, post-traumatic pain, and other severe pain associated with acute disorders is summarized in this section.

Postoperative Pain

Intraspinal narcotics have been reported to control pain effectively following various surgical procedures, as shown in Table 95-3. Because authors varied widely in their choice of opioids, dose, site of injection, and characteristics of surgical population, these are not listed.

Intrathecal opioids have the appeal of ease of administration, either at the time of spinal local anesthetic injection for surgical anesthesia or as a separate technique when general anesthesia is administered. Because most clinicians give a single injection, this technique can be used most effectively when surgical pain is expected to be of relatively short duration. Many patients remain comfortable for 24 hours or more after a single injection of intrathecal morphine; some require no additional pain relief during their postoperative course, or find that their remaining pain is easily managed by oral analgesics.

The epidural route has been used much more extensively than the subarachnoid route for postoperative pain control. Reasons include popularity of the technique alone or in combination with light general anesthesia during surgery, willingness to leave an epidural catheter in place for extended periods to maintain analgesia, familiarity with postoperative analgesia using local anesthetics, and freedom from the risk of postlumbar puncture headache. Narcotics have been effective when injected by the caudal route into the epidural space of children following genital surgery (42).

A number of studies have been done regarding the use of epidural narcotics for postoperative pain control. Stenseth and Breivik reported a prospective study of the efficacy and side effects of epidural morphine in 1085 patients after thoracic, abdominal, urologic, or orthopedic surgery (32). This large experience from a single institution provides a wealth of observations that are instructive for those contemplating the use of epidural narcotics.

Rawal and colleagues (29), in a randomized double-blind study of 30 obese patients undergoing gastro-plasty for weight reduction, compared the effects of intramuscular and epidural morphine with respect to analgesia, time to ambulation, gastrointestinal motility, early and late pulmonary function, duration of hospitalization, and occurrence of deep vein thrombosis in the postoperative period (Table 95-4). The protocol allowed morphine to be given by the assigned route until pain was adequately controlled.

Yeager and associates (52) compared the outcomes of high-risk surgical patients randomized to receive either general anesthesia and conventional postoperative analgesia or epidural anesthesia and epidural morphine analgesia. The epidural group had a significantly lower mortality rate and lower incidence of major complications, shorter intensive care unit and hospital stays, and lower hospital and physician costs.

The use of intraspinal narcotics for control of pain following cesarean section is widespread. These can be offered when spinal or epidural anesthesia is provided for surgery (43), although most reports have focused on the latter application. Pain after vaginal delivery originating from a large episiotomy repair or perineal repair can also be managed with intraspinal narcotics.

Post-Traumatic Pain

A small dose of epidural morphine (2 mg) has been reported to be effective in controlling the pain that accompanies rib fractures (45, 46). Its advantages over epidural bupivacaine for the same purpose were longer duration of action and absence of hypotension. Pain resulting from lower extremity fractures has also been relieved by epidural morphine (46) (Table 95-3).

Morphine by both the spinal and epidural routes has been used to treat pain after multiple trauma in patients on mechanical ventilator support in an intensive care unit (41). Because communication was difficult or impossible, the adequacy of analgesia was documented by noting the marked reduction in doses of parenteral narcotics and sedatives needed to eliminate objective signs of pain (e.g., restlessness, sweating, tachycardia, lacrimation, pupil dilation, hypertension) after beginning intraspinal narcotics. Another group of patients who could communicate clearly after multiple trauma also experienced good analgesia with epidural narcotics (47).

Other Acute Painful Conditions

The pain of acute myocardial infarction has been treated effectively with 0.5 mg of intrathecal morphine (48). The analgesia it produced was more rapid in onset, more intense, and of longer duration during the first 24 hours than that obtained in a control group with total doses of morphine 40 times larger administered by the intravenous or intramuscular route. In another report, 1.2 to 3.6 mg of epidural morphine was effective in relieving postmyocardial infarction pain in six patients after conventional intravenous analgesic agents had failed (49). Epidural meperidine has been used successfully to control the ischemic pain that follows renal infarction or ablation in patients with renal adenocarcinoma (50) (Table 95-3).

TABLE 95-3. Applications of Intraspinal Narcotics for Relief of Acute Pain

Source	Route	Procedure	Total No. of Patients	Pain Relief Efficacy (%)
		POSTOPERATIVE		
Gjessing and Tomlin (31)	S	General Surgery	13	100
Bromage et al. (16); Rawal et al. (29); Writer et al. (30); Stenseth and Breivik (32)	E		571	90
Takasaki and Asno (33)	S	Gynecology	92	100
Writer et al. (30); Ready et al. (34); Chambers et al. (35)	E		99	85
Stenseth and Breivik (32)	E	Urology	139	91
Gjessing and Tomlin (31); Kalso (36)	S	Orthopedics	49	100
Writer et al. (30); Stenseth and Breivik (32)	E		351	90
Mathews and Abrams (37)	S	Cardiac	40	100
El-Baz and Goldin (38)	E		30	80
Samii and Viars (39)	S	Thoracic	13	100
Stenseth and Breivik (32); El-Baz et al. (40)	E		111	95
Rawal and Tandon (41)	E	Peripheral vascular	1	100
Jensen (42)	C	Pediatric (genital)	13	100
Chadwick and Ready (43)	S	Cesarean section	195	85
Writer et al. (30); Chadwick and Ready (43); Kotelko et al. (44)	E		492	85
		POST-TRAUMATIC		
Johnson and McCaughey (45); Magora et al. (46)	E	Rib fracture	9	100
Magora et al. (46)	E	Lower extremity fracture	2	75
Rawal and Tandon (41)	S	Multiple trauma	5	100
Rawal and Tandon (41); Torda and Pybus (47)	E		13	100
		OTHER ACUTE PAIN		
Pasqualucci (48)	S	Myocardial infarction	108	100
Skoeld et al. (49)	E		6	100
Jordan et al. (50)	E	Renal infarction	8	100
Magora et al. (46)	E	Thrombophlebitis	2	75
Magora et al. (46); Torda and Pybus (47)	E	Lumbar disk prolapse	4	50
Magora et al. (46); Torda and Pybus (47)	E	Acute herpes zoster	3	100
Magora et al. (46)	E	Nephrolithiasis	1	100
Rawal and Tandon (41)	S	Pancreatitis	1	100
Rawal and Tandon (41)	E		2	100
Erickson et al. (51)	S	Pain or spasm after spinal cord injury	4	100
Magora et al. (46); Torda and Pybus (47)	E	Ischemic leg pain	15	85

*S, spinal; E, epidural; C, caudal.

Patients suffering from various other acute painful conditions have experienced relief with intraspinal opioids. These conditions include acute lumbar disk prolapse, thrombophlebitis, acute herpes zoster, nephrolithiasis, and ischemic pain (41, 46, 47). Patients in an intensive care unit suffering severe pain as a result of pancreatitis improved with either spinal or epidural narcotics (41). Although the results of these reports are promising, the numbers of patients receiving treatment have been small (Table 95-3).

An interesting and useful application of spinal narcotics is the reduction of muscle spasm and the pain that can accompany it in patients with spinal cord lesions (51). Implanted infusion devices were used in some of these patients, permitting treatment to continue for extended periods.

Cancer Pain

Consistently good pain relief has been obtained in patients with cancer using either spinal or epidural opioids (Table 95-5). Results differed in regard to effective doses and the need for supplemental analgesics, probably reflecting differences in the magnitude of the pain problems in the populations studied. Patients with the most severe pain are typically on large narcotic doses before intraspinal narcotics are used. Effective intraspinal doses in these groups are

TABLE 95-4. Comparison of Effects of Intramuscular and Epidural Morphine in 30 Gastroplasty Patients

Parameter	Route	
	IM	Epidural
Mean morphine use over 36 hours (mg)	66	9
Patients with adequate pain relief (%)	93	100
Patients ambulating at 24 hours (%)	13	93
Mean time to passage of flatus (hr)	75	57
Patients with pulmonary complications (%)	40	13
Evidence of deep vein thrombosis (%)	20	0
Mean postoperative hospitalization (days)	9.0	7.1

Data from Rawal, N., et al.: Comparison of intramuscular and epidural morphine for postoperative analgesia in the grossly obese: Influence on postoperative ambulation and pulmonary function. Anesth. Analg., *63*:583, 1984.

higher than those in narcotic-naive patients. With advancing disease and increasing pain, intraspinal narcotics combined with local anesthetics or supplemental analgesics by another route might be required for satisfactory analgesia.

Intraspinal Injection

Both the spinal and epidural routes are effective for the relief of cancer pain. Intermittent injections through conventional catheters, catheters tunneled subcutaneously, subcutaneously implanted reservoirs, and infusion pumps all have their advocates.

The benefits of intraspinal narcotics to control cancer pain are largely related to the lower doses required compared to those needed when administered by other routes. Patients are more alert, ambulation is easier when less sedation and freedom from pain are combined, and increased appetite and weight gain are frequently noted. All these advantages facilitate patient care at home, leading to a higher quality of life and to substantial economic savings as compared with hospital care. Unlike local anesthetic or lytic blocks, sympathetic tone, motor power, and sphincter function are preserved. No irreversible changes are produced as compared with neurosurgical procedures.

Reports of narcotic tolerance, with the need for escalating doses and frequency of injection, vary among investigators (see Table 95-5). This appears to be an uncommon problem during the first several weeks or even months of therapy, but becomes progressively more likely the longer therapy is continued. Tolerance can be difficult to distinguish from rapid malignant tumor progression. A sudden increase in pain should prompt a thorough re-evaluation for a new cause for the pain—for example, tumor extension into the neuraxis.

It is well known that nonorganic factors such as anxiety or depression can lead to reporting of increased pain. Effective treatment of these factors should not be overlooked.

Technical problems with spinal or epidural catheters are not uncommon. These include obstruction, leaking, and dislodgment. Such problems result in failure of the injected narcotic to reach its site of spinal action, with an accompanying increase in previously well-controlled pain. Periodic catheter replacement might be necessary in some patients.

Radicular pain in some patients during epidural catheter injection has been noted in several reports. Caputi and colleagues (57) have stated that this is a result of the narcotic fluid bolus causing distension of the dural sleeve of a spinal nerve root near the tip of the catheter. They found that this could be resolved by the injection of triamcinolone through the catheter several times at intervals of 3 or 4 days. Others have found that catheter replacement solves the problem.

Except for superficial skin inflammation, infection has not been a problem with the use of indwelling intraspinal catheters. This is remarkable, because many of these catheters have been in place for many months in patients receiving steroids, immunosuppressants, and chemotherapy.

No serious respiratory depression has been reported in cancer patients treated with intraspinal narcotics even when high doses have been administered. It is believed that exposure to narcotics by other routes prior to starting intraspinal injections confers tolerance to the respiratory depressant effects sometimes seen in other populations with the use of these agents.

TABLE 95-5. Applications of Intraspinal Narcotics for Cancer Pain

Source	Route*	No. of Patients	Morphine (mg/day)	Duration of Treatment (months)	Onset of Tolerance
Coombs et al. (53)	S	6	0.5–75	1.5–13	6 months
Coombs et al. (53)	E	8	2–50	NR	NR
Malone et al. (25)	E	15	4–45	0.2–9	Gradual
Zenz et al. (54)	E	40	4–80	0.1–4	25 days
Findler et al. (55)	E	6	4–8	4–5	NR
Penn et al. (56)	S	11	0.2–8	1–13	6 weeks (1 patient)
Penn et al. (56)	E	3	6–10	NR	NR
Caputi et al. (57)	E	43	1–5	0.1–8.5	NR

*S, spinal; E, epidural; NR, not reported.

Intraventricular Injection

A new approach that appears to be promising is the injection of morphine into the lateral ventricles of selected patients suffering from the uncontrolled pain of advanced cancer. In 1982 Leavens and co-workers (28) described their early clinical experience with a technique of ventricular catheter insertion and attachment to a subcutaneously implanted Ommaya reservoir. Lobato and colleagues (58) reported experience with the technique and analyzed the results of 7 other authors. They showed that, among 197 patients treated, 95% obtained excellent pain relief with initial morphine doses of 0.25 to 4.0 mg. Dose requirements increased to as high as 36 mg with continued use. Obbens and associates (59) found that patients who had used large doses of oral and parenteral narcotics required higher intraventricular doses. With the development of tolerance, as much as 15 mg of morphine every 6 hours was needed by some patients.

Complications of intraventricular morphine administration included reservoir malfunction and contamination, resulting in meningitis. The most common side effects were nausea and somnolence.

Nonmalignant Chronic Pain

A few reports have documented experience with intraspinal narcotics in patients with various chronic nonmalignant pain syndromes (Table 95-6).

Cohn and colleagues (60) reported that a single epidural administration of morphine and methylprednisolone acetate produced pain relief lasting from 6 to 12 months in 100% of patients with chronic postlaminectomy low back pain. Other investigators, however, were unable to duplicate this result. Magora and associates (46) found that about 50% of their patients with chronic low back pain reported good relief over

TABLE 95-6. Applications of Intraspinal Narcotics for Chronic Non-Neoplastic Pain

Source	Condition	No. of Patients
Cohn et al. (60)	Low back pain	16
Magora et al. (46)		19
Torda and Pybus (47)		4
Coombs et al. (61)		5
Coombs et al. (62)		2
Magora et al. (46)	Ischemic pain	5
Torda and Pybus (47)		10
Magora et al. (46)	Causalgia	4
Magora et al. (46)	Cervical spine syndrome	2
Magora et al. (46)	Old vertebal fracture	1

an observation period of a few days. Coombs and co-workers (61) found that, compared with cancer patients with similar levels of reported pain, chronic low back pain patients showed no sustained improvement.

Magora and colleagues (46) used epidural narcotics in small numbers of patients with various chronic pain syndromes that included ischemic pain caused by peripheral vascular disease, causalgia, cervical spine syndrome, and an old vertebral fracture. They found that the results obtained in this group were comparable to those of other, more standard methods of treatment (e.g., physical therapy, extradural block, and nerve block with local anesthetics and steroids).

It appears that currently used techniques of intraspinal narcotic analgesia do not have widespread application for treating nonmalignant chronic pain. They might have occasional short-term use for managing intermittent episodes of severe pain in this population. Regular use with currently available opioids would be expected to lead to tolerance, as is the case with cancer patients.

C. TECHNICAL CONSIDERATIONS

Patient Selection

Patients suffering from painful medical conditions, cancer, or trauma, or undergoing various surgical procedures can benefit from the superior analgesia possible with intraspinal opioids. This is particularly true in patients in whom uncontrolled pain can compromise pulmonary function, leading to atelectasis and pneumonia. Examples include patients with rib fractures and those with pain resulting from abdominal and thoracic incisions. Patients with underlying medical conditions such as respiratory insufficiency or obesity might derive particular benefit.

In patients receiving regional anesthesia for surgery, it is particularly easy to offer intraspinal narcotics for postoperative pain. For example, a single dose of morphine can be added to the local anesthetic solution chosen for subarachnoid injection prior to transurethral prostatectomy. Similarly, a narcotic can be injected repeatedly or infused continuously into a catheter placed in the epidural space to provide

anesthesia for surgical patients (e.g., for cholecystectomy, hip surgery, thoracotomy).

If general anesthesia is used for the surgery, an epidural catheter can be placed at any time in the postoperative period if pain control by conventional methods proves inadequate. It appears to be easier to establish good pain control immediately after surgery with these methods than to treat severe pain once it is established (35).

Intraspinal narcotics should be considered for patients with cancer pain when control by moderate doses of oral or parenteral narcotics is ineffective or when the side effects from large doses of narcotics interfere with the quality of life and the wish to be cared for at home. Although elimination or a marked reduction in the dose of systemic narcotics might be possible, this should be done gradually to avoid opiate withdrawal syndrome.

Although not as effective as regional analgesia with local anesthetics for controlling the pain associated with vaginal delivery, epidural or spinal narcotics produce excellent analgesia for postoperative pain following cesarean section (43).

Needle and Cathether Placement

Subarachnoid Needle or Catheter

Lumbar puncture is usually performed at the second or third lumbar interspace, as described in Chapter 94, but it can be done at other levels by those experienced with the technique. For a single injection of narcotic, a small needle (25- or 26-gauge) minimizes the risk of postlumbar puncture headache. When it is necessary to provide analgesia for extended periods, an epidural cathether can be threaded into the subarachnoid space through an 18-gauge needle. The catheter is then secured to the skin at its exit site and used for bolus injections or for continuous infusion of narcotic. Alternately, it can be tunneled subcutaneously to exit anteriorly, where it is less likely to become dislodged and is more accessible to the patient. There it can be injected intermittently or attached subcutaneously to one of a number of reservoirs or infusion devices that can be refilled as necessary with transdermal injections.

Epidural Needle or Catheter

Opioids can be introduced into the epidural space through the sacral hiatus (caudal approach) or in the lumbar, thoracic, or cervical regions, as described in Chapter 94. When the site of injection is close to the desired site of action, satisfactory analgesia might be obtained with lower doses of narcotic. As with intrathecal narcotics, a single injection can be given with a needle placed in the epidural space. If analgesia is necessary for a few days (e.g., following surgery), an epidural catheter is advanced through the needle and secured to the skin at its point of exit. For extended analgesia over several weeks or months, an epidural or special Silastic catheter can be tunneled subcutaneously to a convenient location on the anterior abdominal wall. There, as with spinal catheters, it can be injected intermittently or attached subcutaneously to a reservoir or infusion pump that is refilled transdermally using a syringe and small-gauge needle (62).

In the cervical, thoracic, or high lumbar regions the spinal cord is near the tip of a correctly placed spinal or epidural needle. To minimize the risk of spinal cord injury, needle and catheter placement in these areas is most safely accomplished in patients who are awake and who can report any paresthesias or severe pain that would be indicative of impending spinal cord damage. These sites should only be used by experts in regional anesthetic techniques.

Some use micropore filters on intrathecal and epidural catheters. These can reduce the risk of contamination by pathogenic organisms and prevent injection of foreign material, such as glass particles. When filters were not used, however, infections were not found to be a problem. Aspiration of epidural catheters to check for intravenous or subarachnoid migration is made difficult when some of these devices are used. Needles with filters in their hubs can be used to remove particulate matter while drawing up narcotic solutions for injection or infusion.

Patients receiving intraspinal narcotics in a hospital setting require an indwelling intravenous cannula to facilitate immediate treatment of complications.

Choice of Opioids

Table 95-7 lists the suggested dose ranges, expected latency, and duration of analgesia with various opioids. Doses necessary to produce analgesia and their duration of effect vary considerably from one patient to another depending on age, medical condition, site of injection, type of pain, and other factors. The recommended doses are therefore given only as rough guidelines. A dynamic ongoing assessment of adequacy of pain relief for a particular patient with changes in dose or frequency of injection as necessary is therefore the logical approach. Elderly patients in particular might need remarkably small doses. In reviewing our experience treating women after abdominal hysterectomy, we found a significant negative correlation between age and effective dose of epidural morphine needed every 24 hours to achieve analgesia (34). The relationship can be expressed by the following equation:

$$\text{Effective 24-hour dose (mg)} = 18 - (\text{age} \times 0.15)$$

Suggested initial doses of epidural morphine for the relief of incisional pain in various clinical situations are listed in Table 95-8.

Morphine is by far the most widely used narcotic for both spinal and epidural injection. It is manufactured specifically for intraspinal analgesia as a preservative-free isobaric solution (1 mg/ml) in a single-use ampule. Standard preparations have been used in a wide range of concentrations, however, with no apparent difference in efficacy. Delayed and profound respiratory depression rarely occur, particularly with the spinal route. The use of a hyperbaric morphine solution (10% dextrose), along with the patient's head tilted up 30 to 45°, has been recommended during and after subarachnoid injection to limit rostral spread (63). This measure has not proved effective in eliminating respiratory depression with the epidural route (64).

Although most experience with morphine has involved intermittent injection, it has been used successfully as a continuous infusion with various external pumps or implanted devices (40, 51, 53, 65, 66).

TABLE 95-7. Suggested Dose Ranges, Latency, and Duration of Analgesia with Intraspinal Opioids

Route; Drug	Dose (mg)*	Onset (min)	Duration (hours)†
Epidural			
Morphine	1–10	30	6–24
Meperidine	20–200	5	6–8
Methadone	1–10	10	6–10
Hydromorphone	1–2	15	10–16
Diamorphine	4–6	5	12
Fentanyl	0.025–0.15	5	4–6
Subarachnoid			
Morphine	0.1–0.5	15	8–24
Merperidine	10–30	?	10–30
Diamorphine	1–2	?	20

*Low doses can be effective when administered to the elderly or when injected in the cervical or thoracic region.

†Duration of analgesia varies widely; higher doses produce longer duration of action.

TABLE 95-8. Epidural Morphine for the Relief of Incisional Pain*

Patient Age (years)	Starting Dose (mg)†		
	Nonthoracic Surgery With Lumbar or Caudal Catheter	Thoracic Surgery	
		Thoracic Catheter	Lumbar Catheter
15–44	5	4	6
45–65	4	3	5
66–75	3	2	4
Over 75	2	1	2

*These doses should only be considered as guidelines. Safe and effective doses for individual patients can vary considerably.
†These doses are based on the use of undiluted 0.1% preservative-free morphine.

A lipophilic agent such as fentanyl is useful when rapid onset of epidural analgesia is important. Its short duration, a drawback for most applications, can be offset by the use of a 50 to 100 μg epidural bolus followed by a continuous infusion (25 to 150 μg/h) with an accurately calibrated pump. Severe delayed respiratory depression using these doses has not been reported to date with fentanyl.

Regional Analgesia with Mixtures of Opioids and Local Anesthetics

Although continuous infusion of local anesthetics in the usual clinical concentrations produces effective analgesia, it can also produce undesirable side effects, including hypotension, sensory and motor block, nausea, and urinary retention. In an attempt to achieve postoperative analgesia free of side effects, combinations of dilute local anesthetics and opioids infused continuously through an epidural catheter have been advocated. This is done with the assumption that nociceptive pathways are interrupted at different sites with the two drugs—namely, the nerve axon with the local anesthetic and the spinal opiate receptor with the narcotic. Bupivacaine appears to be well suited to this application because dilute solutions produce minimal motor block.

Cullen and colleagues (66) used a mixture of bupivacaine 0.1% plus morphine 0.01% infused at a rate of 3 to 4 ml/h and compared it to the same concentrations of bupivacaine or morphine infused alone. Pain scores among those in the morphine and combination groups were superior to those in the bupivacaine group. The only significant difference in side effects was a higher incidence of pruritus in those who had received morphine. Hypotension or difficulty with ambulation were not apparent in those who received bupivacaine.

It remains unclear whether the combination of epidural opioids and local anesthetics is superior for certain patients. I have used a combination of fentanyl 0.00025 to 0.0005% (2 to 5 μg/ml) plus 0.0625% bupivacaine infused at a rate of 10 ml/h with good effect in patients with a known tolerance to narcotics and in patients whose pain was not adequately controlled with epidural narcotics alone. In addition to the monitoring recommended for patients receiving only epidural narcotics, frequent measurement of blood pressure and sensory and motor examination should be added. With further experience it might be determined that these measures are not necessary.

Monitoring

Until it is possible to identify and eliminate the factors that occasionally lead to severe respiratory depression in patients receiving intraspinal opioid analgesia, it must be assumed that all patients offered these techniques are at risk. The subarachnoid route appears to carry a higher risk than the epidural route. Because severe respiratory depression can occur with either route of administration, however, and because a catheter in the epidural space can migrate through the dura at any time, equal vigilance must be exercised with the use of both techniques. Patients are at greater risk during the immediate postoperative period. The times of peak risk using morphine are the first 2 hours after injection and between the sixth and twelfth hours.

Nothing can replace a high level of vigilance to prevent serious injury or death. This can be provided by a nurse who checks the rate and depth of respiration as well as the general status of the patient at frequent intervals. A respiratory monitor that sounds an alarm if ventilation is not detected can aid in this process but should not be viewed as a substitute for alert, well-trained human observers. The following criteria can be used to identify patients at extra risk of respiratory depression:*

a. Age > 50
b. ASA physical status: III, IV, or V
c. Surgical site: thorax or upper abdomen
d. Duration of surgery > 4 hours
e. General anesthetic, narcotics, or other long-acting CNS depressants used before or during surgery
f. Epidural morphine dose: 6 mg or more; subarachnoid morphine dose: 0.5 mg or more

Intensive care facilities are well suited to the monitoring needs of higher risk patients (e.g., advanced age, poor underlying condition, extensive surgery), but the expense and limited availability of these facilities render them impractical for routine use. A "step-down unit," intermediate between an intensive care unit and regular ward with regard to the level of monitoring and nursing care available, is an appealing alternative. Many practitioners believe that, with extensive nursing education, careful patient selection, frequent monitoring of ventilation, protocols for immediate treatment of complications, and immediate availability of medical personnel, this care can safely be offered on conventional hospital wards (67). A set of "standard orders" used throughout an institution can facilitate a uniform high standard of care. A sample of such orders is presented in Figure 95-1. They must be individualized to meet the unique needs of each institution. Delegation of all responsibility for

*These are only suspected risk factors. Others can apply to individual patients.

1. Operating room dose: drug ____ mg ____ Time____
2. Drug for continuing analgesia:
   a. PF Morphine (1 mg/ml): ____ mg q6–12 h.
   b. Fentanyl (5 μg/ml): Infuse ____ μg (____ ml) per hour
   c. Other drug: ____ Concentration ____ Dose ____
      Interval ____
3. For inadequate analgesia with prescribed dose of epidural narcotic, give Fentanyl 50 μg (1.0 ml) into epidural catheter q3h prn
4. Maintain IV access (drip, heparin lock) for 24 hours after last dose of epidural narcotic
5. Naloxone, 0.4 mg at bedside
6. *No narcotics or other CNS depressants* to be given except as ordered by the Acute Pain Service
7. Monitoring of respiration (MR):
   a. Respiratory rate and sedation scale q1h for first 24 hours
   b. Respiratory monitor for first 24 hours: Yes ____ No ____
8. Nausea and vomiting prophylaxis: Metoclopramide, 10 mg IV slowly q8h × 3; then q8h prn for nausea and vomiting
9. Treatment of side effects:
   a. RR < 10/min: Call Acute Pain Service
      RR < 8/min: Naloxone 0.4 mg *IV stat.* MR prn. Call Acute Pain Service
   b. Naloxone 0.1 mg IV for severe itching. MR q10 min × 5
   c. Transdermal scopolamine patch to either mastoid area if metoclopramide ineffective for nausea and vomiting. Change patch q72h prn
   d. Naloxone 0.1 mg IV for urinary retention. MR q10 min × 5. If ineffective, "in-and-out" bladder catheter
10. For inadequate analgesia or other problems related to epidural, call Acute Pain Service

Date _____   _____ M.D.

FIG. 95-1. Sample epidural narcotic standard orders.

pain control to one group of physicians within an institution can minimize errors of conflicting or duplicated orders and of inadvertent administration of parenteral narcotics to patients receiving intraspinal narcotics.

Contraindications

Intraspinal narcotic analgesia is best avoided under some circumstances. These include the following: (a) inexperience in performing lumbar puncture or epidural block, particularly in the cervical or thoracic regions; (b) inadequate nursing education or monitoring capabilities; (c) known narcotic allergies; and (d) infection at the site of needle insertion. It remains controversial whether these techniques should be used in patients with coagulopathies or who are receiving anticoagulant therapy. Decisions should be based on the relative risks and benefits for individual patients.

Complications and Their Treatment

Complications have been reported with the use of intraspinal narcotics (Table 95-9). The range in incidence reflects differences in type of pain treated, technique used, drug and dose, age and status of population, concomitant use of other drugs, and criteria for defining a complication.

Respiratory Depression

Early respiratory depression occurring in the first 2 hours following injection is a feature only of epidural

TABLE 95-9. Complications of the Use of Intraspinal Narcotics

Complication	Reported Incidence (%)*		Treatment
	Spinal	Epidural	
Respiratory depression	5–7	0.1–2	Support ventilation; naloxone
Pruritus	60	1–100	Antihistamine; naloxone
Nausea and vomiting	20–50	20–30	Antiemetic; transdermal scopolamine; naloxone
Urinary retention	50	15–25	Catheterize; naloxone

*Reported incidences vary widely, appear to be related to dose, and are higher with spinal than with epidural administration.

opioid administration and is a result of vascular uptake and redistribution (i.e., the same mechanism that follows intramuscular injection). Delayed respiratory depression occurring between 6 and 12 hours following subarachnoid or epidural injection is probably the consequence of rostral spread of narcotic in CSF. The target site is thought to be the respiratory center, located superficially in the floor of the fourth ventricle. The actual incidence of respiratory depression is not known and depends on a number of factors, including the population studied, how it is monitored, and the definition of respiratory depression. In a large multi-institutional Swedish survey the incidence of "depression requiring naloxone" was 0.25 to 0.40% (68). In a survey of 74 American institutions the incidence of "respiratory insufficiency" was 1.9 to 2.3% (69). In a prospective study of 1085 patients in a single institution, the incidence of "respiratory depression" was 0.9% (32).

It is not known whether the risk of severe respiratory depression is greater after intraspinal narcotics than that following narcotic administration by more conventional routes. It has been reported that 860 hospitalized patients receiving morphine orally or parenterally (IV, IM, SC) for pain showed a 0.9% incidence of "life-threatening respiratory depression" (70).

The risk of severe delayed respiratory depression after intraspinal narcotics appears to be greatest early in the course of therapy. This complication has not been reported to occur later than 24 hours after administration of the initial dose of drug. The clinical features of reported cases were tabulated in a recent review (13). From this report, and also from a large prospective study (32) and a large Swedish retrospective study (68), a number of possible predisposing risk factors have been identified. Consistently impressive among these are large intraspinal narcotic doses, advanced age, concomitant use of systemic narcotics or other CNS depressants, high-risk surgical patients, and extensive surgery.

Respiratory rate alone is not an adequate indicator of ventilatory status in volunteers (71) or in postoperative patients (72) receiving epidural narcotics. A more global assessment is necessary, particularly during the first 24 hours of treatment. This should include assessment of level of consciousness because increasing sedation (presumably as a result of CO_2 narcosis) has

TABLE 95-10. Sedation Scale

Level of Sedation	Feature
0: None	Patient alert
1: Mild	Occasionally drowsy; easily aroused
2: Moderate	Frequently drowsy; easily aroused
3: Severe	Somnolent; difficult to arouse
S: None	Normal sleep; easily aroused

commonly been noted with advanced respiratory depression (32, 65). Table 95-10 is a sedation scale that ward nurses can use to classify deterioration in level of consciousness in patients receiving intraspinal narcotics. Healthy volunteers breathing CO_2 mixtures have been noted to lose consciousness at Pa_{CO_2} levels of about 80 mm Hg (73). Thus, every patient receiving intraspinal narcotics whose level of consciousness deteriorates unexpectedly should be assumed to have respiratory depression until disproved by the results of arterial blood gas analysis.

The immediate treatment of severe respiratory depression is support of ventilation. Equipment to deliver oxygen with positive pressure must be readily available, and personnel in the area must be familiar with its use. Naloxone 0.4 mg IV usually restores adequate spontaneous ventilation promptly, but repeated doses are sometimes necessary.

Pruritus

Pruritus is common but seldom bothersome. The incidence is particularly high in obstetric patients. The itching can be generalized or localized, the face being the most common site. Pruritus is seen both with narcotics containing preservatives and with preservative-free preparations. Although it is probably not due to histamine release, antihistamines often provide symptomatic relief. Naloxone is consistently effective but might need to be administered frequently. The mechanism of action of this side effect is not known.

Urinary Retention

The incidence of urinary retention has been found to be higher in volunteers than in patients, and higher in males. Naloxone can help to prevent or reverse urinary retention, but doses approaching those that antagonize analgesia might be needed. Some patients require bladder catheterization.

Nausea and Vomiting

Nausea and vomiting are distressing symptoms that are believed to be the result of rostral spread of the opioid in CSF to the vomiting center and to the chemoreceptor trigger zone located superficially in the floor of the fourth ventricle. The symptoms usually subside with repeated injections, so they are rarely a problem in cancer patients receiving long-term therapy. Relief is frequently possible with antiemetics, but these can also produce unwanted sedation or can even increase the risk of respiratory depression (74).

Preliminary experience (74) suggests that preoperative application of transdermal scopolamine patches to the mastoid area designed to deliver 0.5 mg/day is remarkably effective in reducing the incidence and severity of nausea and vomiting in patients receiving epidural morphine.

Sedation

When any patient receiving intraspinal narcotics appears to be excessively sedated, hypercarbia should be suspected and, if present, treated. The possible contributing role of other drugs such as antiemetics should also be considered (75).

Sedation produced by intraspinal narcotics, rarely a significant problem with moderate drug doses, can be the result of spread of the drug in CSF to receptors in the thalamus, limbic system, or cortex. Pharmacologic treatment is seldom indicated, but physostigmine 1 mg IV can be effective (76).

Summary

Intraspinal opioids represent a powerful tool for the control of severe pain. The selective manner with which they block transmission of nociceptive impulses gives them unique advantages over the use of other methods for producing analgesia. Because the potential exists for life-threatening complications, however, a high level of vigilance must accompany their use. Although it is not known whether the risks accompanying these techniques exceed those associated with more traditional methods of controlling severe pain, concern about possible complications has been the major factor limiting widespread acceptance of intraspinal opioid analgesia in clinical practice. As new information becomes available, intraspinal opioid techniques can be further refined to reduce or eliminate the risk of serious complications.

REFERENCES

1. Pert, C.B., and Synder, S.H.: Opiate receptor: Demonstration in nervous tissue. Science, 179:1011, 1973.
2. Atweh, S.F., and Kuhar, M.J.: Autoradiographic localization of opiate receptors in rat brain. I. Spinal cord and lower medulla. Brain Res., 124:53, 1977.
3. Hughes, J., et al.: Identification of two related pentapeptides from the brain with potent opiate agonist activity. Nature, 285:577, 1975.
4. Tseng, L.F., Loh, H.N., and Li, C.H.: β-Endorphin as a potent analgesic by intravenous injection. Nature, 263:239, 1976.
5. Yaksh, T.L., and Rudy, T.A.: Analgesia mediated by a direct spinal action of narcotics. Science, 192:1357, 1976.
6. Benedetti, C., and Bonica, J.J.: Symposium on recent advances in intraspinal pain therapy. Acta Anaesthesiol. Scand., 31:S85, 1987.
7. Yaksh, T.L.: Spinal opiate analgesia: Characteristics and principles of action. Pain, 11:293, 1981.
8. Wang, J.K., Nauss, L.A., and Thomas, J.E.: Pain relief by intrathecally applied morphine in man. Anesthesiology, 50:149, 1979.
9. Behar, M., et al.: Epidural morphine in treatment of pain. Lancet, 1:527, 1979.
10. Rance, M.J.: Multiple opiate receptors—their occurrence and significance. In Clinics in Anaesthesiology, Vol. 1. Edited by R.E.S. Bullingham. Philadelphia, W.B. Saunders, 1983, pp. 183–199.

11. Schmauss, C., and Yaksh, T.L.: In vivo studies on spinal opiate receptor systems mediating antinociception. II. Pharmacological profiles suggesting a differential association of mu, delta, and kappa receptors with visceral chemical and cutaneous thermal stimuli in the rat. J. Pharmacol. Exp. Ther., 228:1, 1984.

12. Nordberg, G.: Pharmacokinetic aspects of spinal morphine analgesia. Acta Anaesthesiol. Scand. [Suppl. 79], 28:1, 1984.

13. Jacobson, L.: Intrathecal and extradural narcotics. In Advances in Pain Research and Therapy, Vol. 7. Edited by C. Benedetti, et al. New York, Raven Press, 1984, pp. 199–236.

14. Cousins, M.J., and Mather, L.E.: Intrathecal and epidural administration of opiates. Anesthesiology, 61:276, 1984.

15. Bromage, P.R.: Epidural Analgesia. Philadelphia, W.B. Saunders, 1978, pp. 23–26.

16. Bromage, P.R., Camporesi, E., and Chestnut, D.: Epidural narcotics for postoperative analgesia. Anesth. Analg., 59:473, 1980.

17. Moore, R.A., et al.: Dural permeability to narcotics: In vitro determination and application to extradural administration. Br. J. Anaesth., 54:1117, 1982.

18. Bromage, P.R., et al.: Influence of epinephrine as an adjuvant to epidural narcotics. Anesthesiology, 58:257, 1983.

19. Fasano, M., and Waldvogel, H.H.: Peridural administration of morphine, with or without adrenalin, for postoperative analgesia. Acta Anaesthesiol. Belg., 33:195, 1982.

20. Dichiro, G.: Observations on the circulation of the cerebrospinal fluid. Acta Radiol. [Diagn.] (Stockh.), 5:988, 1966.

21. Tung, A.S., Yaksh, T.L., and Wang, J.Y.: Tolerance to intrathecal opiates in the rat. Anesthesiology, 55:A171, 1981.

22. Yaksh, T.L., and Reddy, S.V.R.: Studies on the analgesic effects of intrathecal opiates, alpha-adrenergic agonists and baclofen: Their pharmacology in the primate. Anesthesiology, 54:451, 1981.

23. Yaksh, T.L., Kohl, R.L., and Rudy, T.A.: Induction of tolerance and withdrawal in rats receiving morphine in the spinal subarachnoid space. Eur. J. Pharmacol., 42:275, 1977.

24. Ventafridda, V., et al.: Clinical observations on analgesia elicited by intrathecal morphine in cancer patients. In Advances in Pain Research and Therapy, Vol. 3. Edited by J.J. Bonica, et al. New York, Raven Press, 1979, pp. 559–565.

25. Malone, B.T., Beye, R., and Walker, J.: Management of cancer pain in the terminally ill by administration of epidural narcotics. Cancer, 55:438, 1985.

26. Borner, U., et al.: Epidurale opiatanalgesie. Gewebe- und liquorvertraglichkeit der opiate. Anaesthesist, 29:570, 1980.

27. Ready, L.B., et al.: Neurotoxicity of intrathecal local anesthetics in rabbits. Anesthesiology, 63:364, 1985.

28. Leavens, M.E., et al.: Intrathecal and intraventricular morphine for pain in cancer patients: Initial study. J. Neurosurg., 56:241, 1982.

29. Rawal, N., et al.: Comparison of intramuscular and epidural morphine for analgesia in the grossly obese: Influence on postoperative ambulation and pulmonary function. Anesth. Analg., 63:583, 1984.

30. Writer, W.D.R., et al.: Epidural morphine prophylaxis of postoperative pain: Report of a double-blind multicentre study. Can. Anaesth. Soc. J., 32:330, 1985.

31. Gjessing, J., and Tomlin, P.J.: Postoperative pain control with intrathecal morphine. Anaesthesia, 36:268, 1981.

32. Stenseth, O.S., and Breivik, H.: Epidural morphine for postoperative pain: Experience with 1085 patients. Acta Anaesthesiol. Scand., 29:148, 1985.

33. Takasaki, M., and Asno, M.: Intrathecal morphine combined with hyperbaric tetracaine. Anaesthesia, 38:76, 1983.

34. Ready, L.B., Chadwick, H.S., and Ross, B.: Age predicts effective epidural morphine dose after abdominal hysterectomy. Anesth. Analg., 66:1215, 1987.

35. Chambers, W.A., Sinclair, C.J., and Scott, D.B.: Extradural morphine for pain after surgery. Br. J. Anaesth., 53:921, 1981.

36. Kalso, E.: Effects of intrathecal morphine injected with bupivacaine, on pain after orthopedic surgery. Br. J. Anaesth., 55:415, 1983.

37. Mathews, E.T., and Abrams, L.D.: Intrathecal morphine in open heart surgery. Lancet, 1:543, 1980.

38. El-Baz, N., and Goldin, M.: Continuous epidural infusion of morphine for pain relief after cardiac operations. J. Thorac. Cardiovasc. Surg., 93:878, 1987.

39. Samii, K., and Viars, P.: Postoperative spinal analgesia with morphine. Br. J. Anaesth., 53:817, 1981.

40. El-Baz, N., Faber, L.P., and Jensik, R.J.: Continuous epidural infusion of morphine for treatment of pain after thoracic surgery. A new technique. Anesth. Analg., 63:757, 1984.

41. Rawal, N., and Tandon, B.: Epidural and intrathecal morphine in intensive care units. Intensive Care Med., 11:129, 1985.

42. Jensen, B.H.: Caudal block for post-operative pain relief in children after genital surgery. A comparison between bupivacaine and morphine. Acta Anaesth. Scand., 25:373, 1981.

43. Chadwick, H.S., and Ready, L.B.: Comparison of intrathecal and epidural morphine sulfate for post-cesarean section analgesia. Anesthesiology, 68:925, 1988.

44. Kotelko, D.M., et al.: Epidural morphine analgesia after cesarean delivery. Obstet. Gynecol., 63:409, 1984.

45. Johnston, J.R., and McCaughey, W.: Epidural morphine. A method of management of multiple fractured ribs. Anaesthesia, 35:155, 1980.

46. Magora, F., et al.: Observations on extradural morphine analgesia in various pain conditions. Br. J. Anaesth., 52:247, 1980.

47. Torda, T.A., and Pybus, D.A.: Clinical experience with epidural morphine. Anaesth. Intensive Care, 9:129, 1981.

48. Pasqualucci, V.: Advances in the management of cardiac pain. In Advances in Pain Research and Therapy, Vol. 7. Edited by C. Benedetti, C.R. Chapman, and G. Moricca. New York, Raven Press, 1984, pp. 511–513.

49. Skoeld, M., Gillberg, L., and Ohlsson, O.: Pain relief in myocardial infarction after continuous epidural morphine analgesia. N. Engl. J. Med., 312:650, 1985.

50. Jordan, G.H., et al.: Pain control following renal infarction/ablation using continuous epidural combined anesthesia/analgesia. J. Urol., 130:861, 1983.

51. Erickson, D.L., et al.: Control of spasticity by implantable continuous flow morphine pump. Neurosurgery, 16:215, 1985.

52. Yeager, M.P., et al.: Epidural anesthesia and analgesia in high-risk surgical patients. Anesthesiology, 66:729, 1987.

53. Coombs, D.W., et al.: Outcomes and complications of continuous intraspinal narcotic analgesia for cancer pain control. J. Clin. Oncol., 2:1414, 1984.

54. Zenz, M., et al.: Long-term peridural morphine analgesia in cancer pain. Lancet, 1:91, 1981.

55. Findler, G., Olshwang, D., and Hadani, M.: Continuous epidural morphine treatment for intractable pain in terminal cancer patients. Pain, 14:311, 1982.

56. Penn, R.D., et al.: Cancer pain relief using chronic morphine infusion. Early experience with a programmable implanted drug pump. J. Neurosurg., 61:302, 1984.

57. Caputi, C.A., et al.: Evaluation of tolerance in long-term treatment of cancer pain with epidural morphine. Int. J. Clin. Pharmacol. Ther. Toxicol., 21:587, 1983.

58. Lobato, R.D, et al.: Intraventricular morphine for intractable cancer pain: Rationale, methods, clinical results. Acta Anaesthesiol. Scand., 85:68, 1987.

59. Obbens, E.A.M.T., et al.: Intraventricular morphine administration for control of chronic cancer pain. Pain, 28:61, 1987.

60. Cohn, M.L., et al.: Computed tomographic and electromyographic evaluation of epidural treatment for chronic low back pain. Anesthesiology, 59:A194, 1983.

61. Coombs, D.W., et al.: Relief of continuous chronic pain by intraspinal narcotic infusion via an implanted reservoir. JAMA, 250:2336, 1983.

62. Coombs, D.W., et al.: Epidural narcotic infusion reservoir: Implantation technique and efficacy. Anesthesiology, 56:469, 1982.

63. Samii, K., et al.: Selective epidural analgesia. Lancet, 1:1142, 1979.

64. Jensen, F.M., et al.: Respiratory depression after epidural morphine in the postoperative period. Influence of posture. Acta Anaesthesiol. Scand., 28:600, 1984.

65. Chrubasik, J., and Wiemers, K.: Continuous-plus-on-demand epidural infusion of morphine for postoperative pain relief by means of a small, externally worn infusion device. Anesthesiology, 62:263, 1985.

66. Cullen, M.L., et al.: Continuous epidural infusion for analgesia after major abdominal operations: A randomized, prospective, double-blind study. Surgery, 98:718, 1985.

67. Ready, L.B., et al.: Development of an anesthesiology-based postoperative pain management service. Anesthesiology, 68:100, 1988.

68. Gustafsson, L.L., Schildt, B., and Jacobsen, K.J.: Adverse effects of extradural and intrathecal opiates: Reports of a nationwide survey in Sweden. Br. J. Anaesth., *54*:479, 1982.
69. Mott, J.M., and Eisele, J.H.: A survey of monitoring practices following spinal opiate administration. Anesth. Analg., *65*:S1, 1986.
70. Miller, R.R., and Greenblatt, D.J. (eds.): Drug Effects in Hospitalized Patients. New York, John Wiley & Sons, 1976, pp. 151–152.
71. Camporesi, E.M., et al.: Ventilatory CO_2 sensitivity after intravenous and epidural morphine in volunteers. Anesth. Analg., *62*:633, 1983.
72. Rawal, N., and Wattwil, M.: Respiratory depression after epidural morphine—an experimental and clinical study. Anesth. Analg., *63*:8, 1984.
73. Sechzer, P.H., et al.: Effect of CO_2 inhalation on arterial pressure, ECG and plasma catecholamines and 17-OH corticosteriods in normal man. J. Appl. Physiol., *15*:454, 1960.
74. Loper, K.A., Ready, L.B., and Dorman, B.H.: Prophylactic transdermal scopolamine patches reduce nausea in postoperative patients receiving epidural morphine. Anesth. Analg., *68*:144, 1989.
75. Cohen, S.E., Rothblatt, A.J., and Albright, G.A.: Early respiratory depression with epidural narcotic and intravenous droperidol. Anesthesiology, *59*:559, 1983.
76. Shulman, M.S., Sandler, A., and Brebner, J.: The reversal of epidural morphine-induced somnolence with physotigmine. Can. Anaesth. Soc. J., *31*:678, 1984.

96 · NEUROLYTIC BLOCKADE AND HYPOPHYSECTOMY*

John J. Bonica
with contributions by
F. Peter Buckley, Guido Moricca, *and* Terence M. Murphy

THIS chapter contains an overview of the clinical application of neurolytic blockade in the management of chronic cancer pain and of a few other specific nonmalignant chronic pain syndromes. As the term implies, a chemical agent is injected into the subarachnoid, subdural, or epidural space or into some other appropriate site to produce prolonged destruction of axons or prolonged and at times permanent destruction of the cell bodies of peripheral somatic, or sympathetic nerves or a combination. These agents include ethyl alcohol, phenol, chlorocresol, glycerol, and ammonium sulfate. The application of extreme cold with a cryoprobe or of heat with a laser produces similar effects, and these are reviewed. Alcohol is also used to destroy the pituitary gland in patients with severe diffuse cancer pain. We discuss the indications, techniques, and results, including the efficacy, limitations, side effects, and complications of each technique. Because many of these techniques are described in Chapter 94 they are not repeated here, but

we emphasize the important technical differences that apply to the use of neurolytic blocks.

The material in the chapter is presented in seven sections: A, Basic Considerations, including re-emphasis of some basic principles discussed in Chapter 94 and a concise description of the pathophysiologic changes in the target nerve produced by the neurolytic agents; B, Block of Cranial Nerves; C, Neuraxial Neurolytic Blocks, including the subarachnoid, epidural, and subdural techniques; D, Neurolytic Sympathetic Blockade; E, Neurolytic Block of Somatic Spinal Nerves, including cryoanalgesia and laser therapy; F, Neuroadenolysis of the Pituitary, primarily achieved with alcohol, but other techniques entailing surgery are also presented; and G, Neurolytic Blocks for Control of Spasticity. Buckley contributed some information relevant to Sections B and C, Moricca contributed up-to-date information relevant to Section F, and Murphy contributed Section G.

A. BASIC CONSIDERATIONS

The introduction to this section of the book notes that neurolytic blocks were widely used during the first six decades of this century (1) for several reasons: (a) the specificity theory of pain was pre-eminent, and it was mistakenly believed that destruction of peripheral "pain" pathways would result in prolonged and even permanent relief of severe intractable pain; (b) other than pharmacologic drugs, neural blockade was the only nonsurgical method available that produced effective pain relief in patients who could not tolerate major neuroablative operations; and (c) the efficacy, side effects, and complications of the use of opioids were not precisely understood, particularly in regard to tolerance and addiction, resulting in improper use of these drugs in the management of patients with cancer pain. This was in contrast to the effective pain relief produced by neurolytic blockade when it was skillfully carried out in properly selected patients.

The acquisition of more information about pain and pain syndromes and the consequent development of new therapeutic modalities (particularly psychologic methods, opioid preparations, neurostimulation techniques, intraspinal narcotics, and neurosurgical procedures), together with information about the deleterious effects of deafferentation, have significantly decreased the indications for the use of neurolytic blocks. The more effective use of opioids and of "coanalgesics" has made it possible to treat 70% of cancer pain patients with these measures alone. In one study by Ventafridda and co-workers (2), who managed 1249 cancer patients with moderate to severe pain, neurolytic blocks were required in less than 30% of patients and a significant percentage of these patients still needed to continue with a reduced dose of oral opioids. Many of these patients had advanced or terminal cancer and were managed at home.

Nevertheless, neurolytic blockade remains an important tool that offers significant pain relief to patients with severe pain caused by advanced cancer, certain types of neuralgias, and incurable conditions, such as occlusive vascular disease (3). This is particularly true in situations in which neurosurgeons skilled in neuroablative procedures are not available, and especially in developing countries, in which anesthesiologists with the necessary skill and experience can perform neurolytic blocks effectively.

The techniques of neurolytic cranial nerve block, subarachnoid block, celiac plexus block, and lumbar sympathetic block, when properly executed, result in a high degree of success with an acceptable incidence of side effects in patients who have not obtained satisfactory pain relief by other methods (1, 3). To obtain such desirable results it is essential that the basic

*This chapter is dedicated to my dear friend Prof. Guido Moricca (who died August 4, 1989) in appreciation of the very significant contributions he made to pain management worldwide.

principles of application discussed in detail in Chapter 94 be strictly followed. Neurolytic blockade, however, represents only one of many therapeutic measures that should be used in the overall management of patients with severe intractable pain.

Principles of Application

As with other therapeutic modalities used for the relief of chronic cancer or nonmalignant persistent pain, proper application of neurolytic blocks requires a thorough understanding of the mechanisms of action of the various agents used and of the pathophysiologic effects that produce not only pain relief but that also can result in undesirable side effects and complications.

Because of the potential harm that can follow neurolytic blocks, the following requisites are especially important:

a. Only physicians with extensive experience, skill, and knowledge of these procedures, and who have managed patients with chronic pain, should consider using neurolytic blocks.

b. As discussed in Chapter 24, neurolytic blocks should be used as one therapeutic measure in a multimodal therapy program for patients with severe cancer pain. Even when a neurolytic block has been a technical success, supplementary analgesics and adjuvants might be required because the disease might have spread beyond the anatomic limits of the block.

c. Careful selection of patients and of the optimal procedures that provide them with maximum pain relief, with the least risk of adverse side effects or complications, should be done. Obviously, this requires a thorough assessment of patients (Chapters 31 and 94). It is especially important to consider neurolytic blockade for the relief of severe persistent pain. At the time of the "workup," in addition, it is necessary to determine the degree of pain using a visual analog scale or other more sophisticated measures that can be repeated after the procedure to assess the degree of pain relief achieved. Moreover, it is essential that the physician be aware of other therapeutic modalities that might be useful, including their advantages, disadvantages, limitations, and complications. Only with this broad perspective can the optimal therapeutic strategy be chosen for all patients with specific chronic pain syndromes. Other than hypophysectomy, neurolytic blocks for the management of severe cancer pain are indicated in patients who have relatively localized pain.

d. It is essential to thoroughly inform the patient and the family of the details of the procedure, to state what is likely to be accomplished and, especially, to discuss possible adverse side effects and complications. These should be discussed before the procedure is carried out so that the patient and the family have sufficient time to consider the risk-to-benefit ratio and make the proper decision about whether to accept this therapy.

e. All patients who are to have neurolytic blocks should have at least two or three diagnostic or prognostic blocks with a local anesthetic (Chapter 94).

Although temporary blocks do not necessarily predict the long-term effects of surgical section, they do allow patients to experience any side effects inherent in interruption of sensory and motor pathways and, if properly carried out, to provide the physician with the opportunity to predict the analgesic efficacy of the neurolytic block in patients with cancer pain whose life expectancy is limited.

f. It is essential to assess the results of the block, including determination of whether the procedure has completely interrupted the nociceptive pathways and the degree and duration of pain relief. This requires several days of observation, not only by the physician but also by the house staff, nurses, and family. In addition to patients' verbal reports, the results of the block should be determined objectively by noting any reduction in drug requirements and improvements in sleep pattern, appetite, general activity, and mood. If patients state that no significant relief of pain is felt one should consider the fact that the block might have been successful but could have unmasked other pain, or patients are preoccupied with side effects of the block, are depressed, or have developed narcotic dependence. In patients who have become physically dependent on strong opioid analgesics, it might be difficult to assess the efficacy of a neurolytic block or to plan a satisfactory sequential analgesic regimen. In any case, it is essential to follow patients and to record the degree and duration of pain relief and side effects on the chart.

g. Sudden cessation of pain consequent to a neurolytic block in patients who have been on large doses of opioids might also eliminate the respiratory stimulating effect of the pain, and patients could develop respiratory depression. Obviously this requires close monitoring of patients and appropriate treatment if such depression occurs. On the other hand, too rapid cessation of analgesic therapy can produce withdrawal symptoms that could further complicate determination of the efficacy of the block. Therefore, strong opioids should be reduced gradually.

Other important basic principles are not repeated in considering the techniques described in this chapter, but it is assumed that patients have been properly prepared and that the physician carrying out the blockade has adhered to these basic principles, as well as to those mentioned in Chapter 94. Moreover, to conserve space, discussion of the immediate preparation of patients is omitted, including monitoring of vital signs and the aseptic preparation and draping of the field.

Mechanisms of Action and Pathophysiology

Alcohol

Alcohol is the classic neurolytic agent, and has been used extensively in concentrations from 3 to 100% (1). Its effects are brought about by a destruction of nerve fibers, resulting in wallerian degeneration that is similar to that which results from nerve section, except that usually the basal lamina around the Schwann cell tube is spared and the axon can regenerate without the formation of a neuroma. If the cell bodies of the nerve are completely destroyed no regeneration takes place, whereas if they are only partially destroyed regeneration does occur.

Effects on Somatic Nerves

The effects of alcohol on somatic nerves were studied by Schlosser (4) soon after he began to use alcohol block of branches of the trigeminal nerves for the treatment of tic douloureux in 1900. He noted and recorded that injection of alcohol into nerves was followed by a degeneration and absorption of all the components of the nerve, except the neurolemma. A few years later Finkelburg (5) studied this problem by injecting 0.5 to 1.5 ml of 60 to 80% alcohol into the exposed sciatic nerve of dogs and rabbits and found that persistent paralysis resulted with these concentrations. In the ensuing two decades the effects of alcohol on somatic nerves were studied by May, Gordon, Nasaroff, and Labat, all of whom used different concentrations of alcohol in an attempt to produce a selective block of small-diameter nerves, thus resulting in analgesia without motor paralysis or paresis (see 1 for references). The conclusions reached were that a concentration of at least 50 to 70% alcohol was needed to produce nerve damage to achieve good pain relief; in lower concentrations than 50% less nerve damage resulted. In later clinical studies Labat and Greene (6) reported satisfactory results in the management of painful disorders by employing 33% alcohol in peripheral nerves, with little or no muscular paralysis.

More recent studies have shown that alcohol acts on nervous tissue by extraction of cholesterol, phospholipids, and cerebrosides and also causes precipitation of lipoproteins and mucoproteins (7). Alcohol applied topically to peripheral nerves damages both the axon and the Schwann cell, which develops swollen mitochondria, and the myelin sheath is disrupted (8). Dilated vesicles can be seen in the dystrophic axons and wallerian degeneration is a prominent feature. In vivo electrophysiologic investigation of peripheral nerves of cats revealed significant depression of compound action potentials (CAPs) when tested 8 weeks after injection of alcohol close to the nerve (9). A slight increase in the effect on CAPs was noted as the alcohol concentration increased from 50 to 100%.

Effects on Sympathetic Neurons and Ganglia

Merrick (10) was the first to study the changes that occur after injection of alcohol into a sympathetic ganglion and the rami communicantes, and noted differences between the two structures. Injection of the ganglion resulted in a permanent block to all effector organs innervated by the postganglionic fibers that originated from the injected ganglion because the alcohol destroyed the ganglion cells, whereas injection of the rami alone resulted in temporary block only. Blocking of preganglionic fibers paravertebrally did not directly affect their cells of origin, because the latter are located in the spinal cord. Block of postganglionic fibers was also accomplished without affecting the ganglion cell bodies, especially because the ganglia were more resistant to alcohol than the rami. Merrick (10) also found that the alcohol affects the axons at the site of infiltration by partially dissolving the myelin (if the fibers are myelinated) and by interrupting the continuity of the axons so that the distant segment underwent typical wallerian degeneration. Retrograde changes also occurred in nearby cell bodies, which caused some neurons to undergo complete degeneration while others suffered to a lesser degree and eventually recovered. Merrick (10) noted that, following block of the rami, regeneration was apparent in 90 days and complete at 170 days. The effects of alcohol on sympathetic afferents are similar to that of its effects on somatic nerves as described in the preceding section.

Effects on Rootlets with Subarachnoid Injection

Following subarachnoid injection of 100% alcohol, the initial histologic appearances are of myelin sheath disruption and beading of the axon cylinder within the rootlets, with subsequent development of an inflammatory response (11). Damage to the spinal cord is usually limited to the dorsal rootlets and roots, Lissauer's tract, and posterior columns, which show spotty areas of demyelination and mild focal inflammatory changes in the meninges (11). In some cases, however, the whole superficial surface of the spinal cord at the site of injection can reveal damage. Later histologic findings consist of wallerian degeneration at the site of the initial insult, particularly in the dorsal horns. Extensive lesions of the rootlets, remote demyelination and degeneration of the spinal cord, arachnoidal lesions with cyst formation, and lesions of the pial vessels have been reported, but these were probably a result of the injection of a large volume of alcohol at one time. When alcohol is introduced into the cerebrospinal fluid (CSF) it is removed relatively rapidly, with only 10% of the initial dose remaining in the CSF 10 minutes after injection (12).

Phenol

The history of the introduction and subsequent use of phenol to produce prolonged sympathetic block, somatic nerve block, and subarachnoid and epidural blocks, has been summarized in the introduction to this section. Stimulated by reports of studies carried out in the preceding two decades and prompted by a desire to establish prolonged sympathetic block without the undesirable reaction of alcohol, Mandl (13) in 1945 investigated the sympathetic neurolytic effects of phenol in animals. After injecting 0.2 ml of 6% phenol into the cervical ganglia, he observed that complete necrosis occurred within 24 hours, which progressed to complete degeneration in 45 days and regeneration in 75 days. These studies indicated that phenol injection of sympathetic nerves is followed by more rapid recovery of function than that following alcohol injection—a fact that correlates well with the observed duration of chemical sympathectomy in patients. The injection of phenol into the subarachnoid space or intraneurolytic administration produces pathophysiologic effects similar to those of alcohol.

Effects of Subarachnoid Phenol

The introduction of hyperbaric phenol solution for subarachnoid neurolysis in 1955 by Maher (14), and his subsequent claim that it produced a selective block of small fibers without affecting large fibers (15), prompted a number of experimental studies. Iggo and Walsh (16) and Nathan and Sears (17) carried out animal studies of CAPs in the cat spinal root and their results led them to conclude that 5% phenol produced selective block of small fibers, but subsequent studies by Stewart and Lourie (18), Nathan and colleagues (19), Smith (20), and Shaumburg and associates (21) disputed these findings. They noted that, in low concentrations, phenol exhibited a transient local anesthetic effect but, if a concentration high enough to produce long-lasting pain relief was used, the block was not at all selective but was similar to that produced by alcohol. It was also found that phenol damaged all neural elements to a similar extent as alcohol and, indeed, Shaumburg and co-workers (21) found that phenol produced more damage of large-diameter fibers than small-diameter fibers.

The primary effect of phenol is to coagulate protein, and it is similar to alcohol in regard to potency and nonselective damage to nervous system tissue. Subarachnoid injection of 5 to 8% phenol produces a mild meningeal reaction but a higher concentration causes extensive fibrosis and thickening of the arachnoid. Histologic studies after subarachnoid injection of phenol were done by Smith (20) in cats and in 18 patients. It was found that phenol destroyed axons regardless of their size and that the lesions occurred along the length of the rootlets between the posterior dorsal ganglion and spinal cord, without distortion of the rootlets. Destruction of axons in the anterior roots adjacent to the affected posterior rootlets occurred but was of a lesser degree, and no destruction of cell bodies in the posterior root ganglion was seen. All the patients showed degeneration of the posterior columns. It is obvious that the damage to the posterior rootlets is similar to that produced by ethyl alcohol, causing segmental demyelination and wallerian degeneration characteristic of intrathecal phenol. The degree and extent of the lesions are related to the volume and concentration used, and axonal abnormalities and wallerian degeneration are apparent only with concentrations high enough to produce effective pain relief (21).

Like alcohol, phenol injected into the subarachnoid space decreases rapidly in concentration. In a study of patients with cancer, Ichiyanagi and colleagues (22) injected 7% phenol in glycerin and subsequently measured its concentration in CSF at frequent intervals. They noted a rapid decrease to 30% of the original concentration by 1 minute and, by 15 minutes, the concentration was 0.1%, thus reaching an isobaric concentration. Based on these data they suggested that it is probably safe for patients to change position 15 minutes after injection (see below, C. Neuraxial Neurolytic Block).

Effects on Peripheral Nerves

Studies of 3% phenol injected into rat sciatic nerves showed consistent acute and chronic damage to both axonal and myelin elements; at 6 weeks postlesion regeneration of axons began to appear (23). When applied to peripheral nerves in concentrations above 5%, phenol causes protein coagulation and necrosis, with axonal degeneration and subsequent wallerian degeneration.

Electrophysiologic and histopathologic studies by Gregg and associates (23), who injected phenol and Renografin close to the peripheral nerves of cats in vivo, revealed a highly significant concentration-related depression of CAPs 1 and 2 weeks after injection. The maximum effect required 12% phenol. By 8 weeks postinjection remyelination was clearly evident and the CAPs had returned to normal.

The excellent comprehensive review by Wood (24) summarized the most important laboratory and clinical studies published prior to 1978. It was concluded that the overall destructive effect of phenol contributed to the neurolytic (pain-relieving) effects of the agent. One in vitro study cited by Wood (24) indicated that the affinity of phenol was greater for vascular tissue than for brain neurophospholipid, and it was suggested that injury to blood vessels might be an important pathophysiologic factor contributing to the observed neuropathology. Smith (20), however, in both animal and human studies, did not see much damage to blood vessels following subarachnoid injection of phenol. Wood's suggestion raises concern about the use of large volumes of phenol near major blood vessels, and might be the basis for some physicians preferring the use of alcohol over phenol for celiac plexus block.

Glycerol

Häkanson's report (25) of the efficacy of glycerol injected into the trigeminal ganglion for the treatment of trigeminal neuralgia without producing significant sensory deficits led to its widespread use in the treatment of this condition (26, 27) and to further histologic and electrophysiologic studies. Topical application of 50% glycerol solution onto the nerve produces localized subperineurial damage but, following intraneural injection, glycerol is more damaging than topical application (28). Histologic changes include the presence of numerous inflammatory cells, extensive myelin swelling, and axonolysis (29).

Myelin disintegration occurs weeks after the injection along with concomitant axonolysis during periods of myelin restitution, indicating an ongoing nerve fiber injury possibly caused by secondary events such as compression of transperineurial vessels and ischemia. Electron microscopic studies have revealed evidence of wallerian degeneration and, with intraneural injection, almost all nerve fibers are destroyed (29). Lipid droplets are seen in Schwann and phagocytic cells, and mast cell degranulation occurs. Burchiel and Russell (30) carried out studies on rat saphenous nerve and found differential effects of glycerol on the electrophysiologic function of the nerve. At this time, however, histologic data to support these observations are lacking.

Ammonium Compounds

In 1931 Judovich (see 31) prepared an aqueous solution derived from a pitcher plant distillate (Sarracenia purpurea) and found it to relieve the pain of neuralgia without producing changes in skin sensation and deleterious effects on motor nerves. This selective action on the pain was of much longer duration than with procaine. Subsequent laboratory investigations revealed that the ammonium ion, in the form of ammonium chloride or ammonium hydroxide (depending on the pH of the distillate) was the active component. Using the unsophisticated technology available at that time, Judovich and associates found that ammonium salts eliminated C-fiber potential, with only a small effect on A fibers. In 1942 Bates and Judovich (32) reported 5000 administrations of ammonium salts (in a 6% concentration) by paravertebral injection or local infiltration, with highly favorable results. I have reported (1) on extensive clinical trials that yielded disappointing results: the drug was found to lack uniformity of action and produced pain relief in a small percentage of cases and in an unpredictable manner. Similar results were reported to me by F. A. D. Alexander (personal communication, 1951), one of the foremost authorities on neural blockade of the past 50 years. Subsequent reports on the use of 10% concentrations, predominantly for intercostal nerve block or other peripheral nerve blocks, suggested that good analgesia without loss of motor function can be achieved (33, 34). Limited pathologic studies, however, indicated that injections of ammonium salts around a peripheral nerve cause an acute degenerative neuropathy affecting all fibers (29).

Cryotherapy

It has long been known that cooling causes a reversible conduction block in nerves. In 1945, Denney-Brown and colleagues (35) reported on the pathology of nerves subjected to cold and noted the sensitivity of A-delta and C fibers to damage. Subsequent studies have revealed that a prolonged axonal potential results when nerve fibers are cooled to 5° C (29). It has also been found that unmyelinated axons are blocked at a lower temperature than myelinated axons (36) and that conduction is blocked in all myelinated fibers at about the same temperature (37). Early cytopathologic studies revealed abnormalities of Schwann cells and endoneurial capillaries that were attributed to accelerated enzyme production, which affected Schwann cell metabolism (29). More recent studies have shown that freezing results in the formation of ice crystals and causes necrosis of all tissue elements, including nerves (38). Freezing produces a longer lasting clinical deficit and has become a method of neurolysis of intercostal nerves following thoracotomy for relief of post-thoracotomy pain.

The technique is based on the freezing of a small nerve segment with a 2-mm diameter cryoprobe cooled to about $-60°$ C by the rapid expansion of pressurized nitrous oxide from its tip. When the cryoprobe is left in contact with the nerve for 60 seconds, a 2 to 4-mm diameter ice ball is formed that freezes the nerve and completely damages the nerve fibers (39). This initially produces severe vascular injury and edema, with diapedesis of polymorphonuclear cells through vessel walls (29, 38). The endoneurial fluid pressure (EFP) is elevated within 90 minutes of the lesion and rises to a level of about 20 cm H_2O, or twice that observed in edematous neuropathies developing more slowly. In the ensuing 24 hours the EFP is reduced, presumably because of the changes in the elastic characteristics of the perineurium (29). The EFP then increases again to reach a plateau at 6 days that is associated with wallerian degeneration of the distal fibers, a prominent pathologic feature that affects the entire nerve. Although freezing causes complete damage to the nerve, the basal lamina is fortunately spared and provides a conduit for nerve fiber regeneration. Thus, freezing causes an acute and severe injury to all nerve fibers that persists for about 1 month, after which regeneration occurs; this is aided by the presence of Schwann cell basal lamina, which makes the complete and appropriate reinnervation of distal structures possible (29).

Laser and Radiofrequency Lesions

Heating of peripheral nerves with ultrasonic energy produces three levels of nerve conduction effects: enhancement, reversible depression, and irreversible depression, with the latter characterized by a functional deficit that lasts longer than 18 hours (40). With such lesions the axis cylinder is fragmented but the perineurium is unaffected. Recently lasers have been used to heat peripheral nerves more precisely—the energy produced by the laser heats the nerve directly without affecting the surrounding tissue, and the output of the laser can be controlled in regard to both magnitude and duration. Laser irradiation of peripheral nerves produces localized lesions characterized histologically

by a concentric zone of coagulation necrosis surrounded by persistent nerve edema (41). The perineurium is not damaged but the resulting edema increases the EFP. Sections of laser-injured nerves show discrete endoneurial lesions characterized by greatly swollen axons packed with organelles; these changes are characteristic of the axonal dystrophy that occurs during acute wallerian degeneration (29). Because laser injury produces wallerian degeneration and can be finely controlled and focused, it should prove to be useful as a neurolytic technique, provided that direct visual access to the nerve is possible. Radiofrequency lesions also produce coagulation of the nerve (see Chapter 97).

Conclusion

Neurolytic agents in the form of alcohol, phenol, and glycerol injected around or into a nerve produce pathophysiologic changes of varying degree, depending on the concentration of the agent that comes in direct contact with the nerve tissue. These agents, applied onto the surface of the nerve or nerve rootlets (in the subarachnoid space), alter perineurial permeability and provide access to axons or occasionally to nerve cells. Intraneural injection of these agents produces severe nerve damage, consisting of significant axonal abnormality and wallerian degeneration. Techniques that physically damage the nerve with cold by means of the cryoprobe or with heat by means of a laser or radiofrequency produce similar results. It has now been impressively shown that a differential block of only A-delta and C fibers, without affecting larger fibers and with good pain relief still being obtained, is usually not possible. Although variations in concentration produce different clinical findings, suggesting a dose-related response, the nerve needs to be damaged sufficiently to produce wallerian degeneration to achieve desirable long-lasting pain relief. The persistence of basal lamina around the Schwann cell tube allows the successful and appropriate degeneration of nerve fibers, thus eliminating the formation of painful neuroma. This is in contrast to surgical section of a nerve, which invariably results in neuroma formation. This difference justifies the use of neurolytic agents over surgical interruption of peripheral nerve fibers for the treatment of chronic pain.

B. BLOCK OF CRANIAL NERVES

From 1900 to 1960, block of the gasserian ganglion or of branches of the trigeminal nerve with alcohol or other neurolytic agents was widely used for the treatment of trigeminal neuralgia, severe intractable cancer pain, and a few other chronic pain syndromes. Block of the facial nerve with a local anesthetic or alcohol has been used for the treatment of facial spasm, while block of the glossopharyngeal and vagus nerve with a local anesthetic has been used as a diagnostic or prognostic procedure in patients with neuralgia or cancer pain in the distribution of these nerves. Even block of the spinal accessory nerve has been used to treat spasm of the trapezius muscle.

The advent of the use of Tegretol and other anticonvulsant drugs, of the highly successful microvascular decompression operation, and of controlled thermo-

gangliolysis has superseded the use of neurolytic blocks for the relief of the pain of trigeminal neuralgia. Moreover, the use of thermogangliolysis and other more sophisticated neurosurgical procedures has also reduced the use of neurolytic block in the treatment of cancer pain.

Nevertheless, neurolytic block of the gasserian ganglion or of one of the major branches of the trigeminal nerve remains an important tool for the treatment of severe intractable facial pain caused by cancer or neuralgia and of other types of severe chronic pain in those situations in which sophisticated neurosurgical techniques are unavailable. A few other painful conditions in the head have also been and continue to be managed with neurolytic blockade. One of these is the injection of 50% alcohol to relieve persistent eye pain in patients with glaucoma but who retain good vision. Moreover, the injection of 70 to 100% alcohol is used to relieve severe intractable eye pain in patients who have lost their vision (Chapter 42).

Although block of branches of the trigeminal nerve or of the glossopharyngeal and vagus nerves with local anesthetic is not used widely, such a procedure can be highly effective in patients who have severe excruciating acute postoperative or post-traumatic pain or pain caused by other self-limiting conditions. As mentioned below, block of the nerve as well as of the gasserian ganglion with local anesthetic should be done prior to the injection of a neurolytic agent or destruction of the nerve.

Basic Considerations

Optimal results with these procedures require adherence to the requirements and preliminary considerations discussed in Chapter 94. One of the most important is a thorough knowledge of the anatomy of the target nerve, of adjacent structures with which the solution might come in contact, and also of structures that are traversed by the needle. The anatomy of the cranial nerves is discussed in detail in Chapter 37 and shown in Figures 37-1 to 37-8.

The physician must also follow the principles of the technique noted in Chapter 94, and should be aware of contraindications. When carrying out these procedures it is essential to have fluoroscopic control of needle placement and to determine the pattern of diffusion of the contrast medium that might be injected prior to injection of the neurolytic agent.

Based on my extensive experience in carrying out these procedures, I believe that it is essential to carry out two or three diagnostic or prognostic blocks with a long-lasting local anesthetic to determine whether the neurolytic blockade can provide complete pain relief. Moreover, as stressed in Chapter 94, a local anesthetic block provides the patient with an opportunity to evaluate the degree of pain relief as well as to experience the sensory anesthesia that follows alcohol or phenol injection.

Because neurolytic agents diffuse to a much lesser extent than local anesthetics, prognostic blocks require that the volume of local anesthetic be the same as or less than the volume of neurolytic agent to be used. For example, neurolytic block of the gasserian ganglion with 1 ml of alcohol should be preceded by two prognostic blocks with 0.75 to 1.0 ml of bupivacaine, each done at intervals of 1 day or longer between the blocks and before the neurolytic block.

Because the face and head have special meaning for most people, and because having a needle inserted into these structures invariably causes a great degree of anxiety, apprehension, and even fear, and because the procedures do produce moderate discomfort, it is best to administer a sedative or anxiolytic drug such as 2.5 mg droperidol 30 minutes before and a small dose (2 to 3 mg) of morphine IV about 5 to 10 minutes before the procedure.

The patient should be positioned appropriately according to the specific gravity of the injected solution.

Technical Considerations

Gasserian Ganglion Block

The anatomy of the trigeminal nerve is depicted in Figure 96-1 and that of the gasserian ganglion is shown in Figure 96-2. Figure 96-3 depicts the common sites of blocking the trigeminal nerve and its branches. Block of the gasserian ganglion is achieved by various intraoral, oral, or extraoral routes, but the best and most commonly used technique is that originally described by Härtel (42, 43) (Fig. 96-4).

FIG. 96-1. Anatomy of the trigeminal nerve. The root of the trigeminal is short, extending from the ventrolateral surface of the pons to the apex of the petrous portion of the temporal bone, where it expands into the gasserian ganglion. The cresent-shaped gasserian ganglion lies lateral to the internal carotid artery and cavernous sinus and occupies Meckel's cave, located just posteromedial to the foramen ovale. The ophthalmic nerve passes through the superior orbital fissure to reach the orbit. The maxillary nerve passes through the foramen rotundum and leaves the cranial cavity to reach the pterygopalatine fossa, where this nerve can be blocked. The mandibular nerve is formed by the union of a large sensory root and a smaller motor root that arises from the pons and passes beneath the gasserian ganglion to reach the foramen ovale, through which, together with the sensory root, it leaves the cranial cavity.

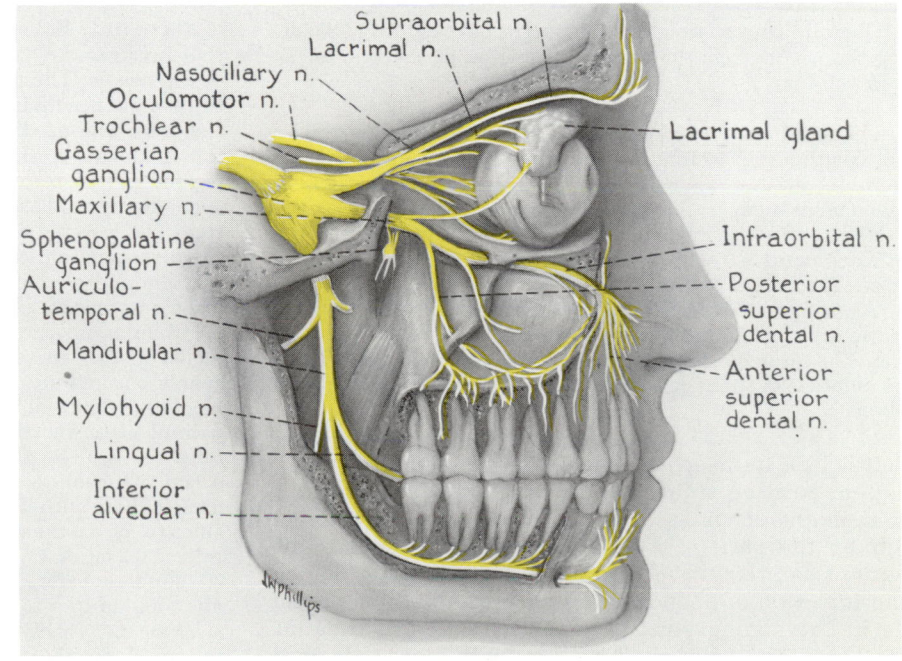

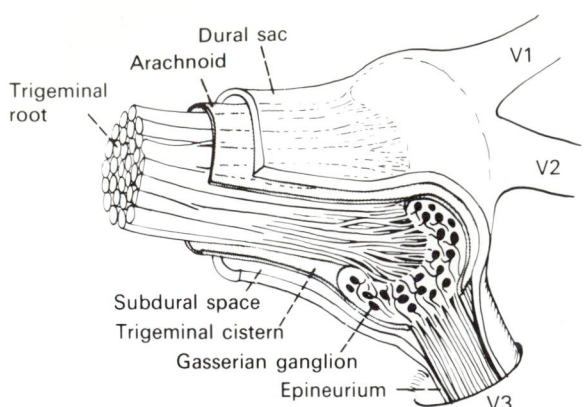

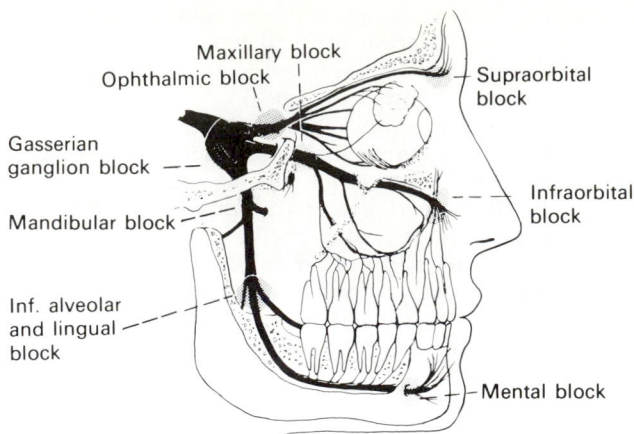

FIG. 96-2. Gasserian ganglion, which contains cell bodies that have pseudounipolar axons. These break up into central branches that constitute the sensory root of the trigeminal nerve and into peripheral branches that comprise the three major nerves. The ganglion is canoe-shaped, with the three peripheral branches of the nerve attached to its anterior convex aspect. The roots emerge from the concave side of the ganglion to comprise the triangular portion of the root. A variable number of anastomoses exists between the group bundle in this triangular portion, which is just behind the ganglion. The dural-arachnoidal envelope surrounding the ganglion is an evagination of the dura from the posterior cranial fossa to a position under the dura mater of the middle fossa. The dural-arachnoid pouch behind the ganglion constitutes the trigeminal cistern, which normally contains cerebrospinal fluid that communicates with the infratentorial bases of the cisterns through the trigeminal porus. The anterior convex surface of the ganglion is adherent to the dural-arachnoidal covering and, as the latter passes distally, it becomes the epineurium of the mandibular, maxillary, and ophthalmic nerves. Also note the relationship of the subdural and arachnoid spaces. Modified from Ferner, H.: The anatomy of the trigeminal root and the gasserian ganglion and their relations to the cerebral meninges. In Trigeminal Neuralgia. Edited by R. Hassler and A.E. Walker. Stuttgart, Georg Thieme Verlag, 1970.

FIG. 96-3. Various sites (stippled areas) at which the gasserian ganglion, the three major nerves, and their most important branches can be blocked.

The following anatomic points might be useful in introducing the needle from the point of insertion in the skin to the foramen (1):

a. The foramen is an oval or elliptic canal 5 mm long, with an axis that has an inferior and slightly anterolateral direction. Its greater diameter averages 8 mm and its smaller diameter is 4 mm.

b. It is situated immediately posterior to the smooth hard infratemporal surface of the greater wing of the sphenoid bone. The center of this plate, which serves as an important landmark, is about 4 cm medial to the midpoint of the zygomatic arch in the same frontal plane.

c. The foramen is approximately 4 cm medial to the articular tubercle of the zygomatic arch in exactly the same frontal plane.

It is best to insert the needle with the patient in the supine position to avoid any orthostatic hypotension that might occur as a result of severe apprehension felt by the patient. For the injection of alcohol the patient can remain in this supine position but, during the injection of phenol or glycerol, the patient should be in the sitting position. Usually a 10-cm 22-gauge security needle threaded with a depth marker is used

for this procedure. Aspiration should be attempted with a 2-ml Luer-Lok syringe to ensure that the needle point is not in a blood vessel or in the subarachnoid space. It is best to guide the placement of the needle by radiographic control (Fig. 96-5). Aliquots of 0.1 ml of alcohol or of 5% phenol or glycerol should be injected. After each injection detailed sensory testing is done and the patient questioned about the extent of analgesia and numbness to determine the effects of each aliquot. A total of 0.5 to 0.75 ml is injected, depending on the needs and responses of the patient.

During the 1960s and 1970s several refinements of blocking the gasserian ganglion or the sensory root were done to decrease the risk of serious complications. These included modifications of blocking with alcohol and the introduction of phenol in glycerin and of glycerol for gasserian ganglion block. The most important of these are briefly described.

ALCOHOL. Ecker and Perl (44) developed a technique that involves the use of radiographic control of the position of the needle. The patient is supine with the head extended so that the needle is inserted in a direction perpendicular to the floor. The needle is advanced through the center of the foramen ovale so that its tip lies on the target exactly 4 mm beyond the posteromedial border of the foramen ovale and 2 mm above the base of the skull, at the petrosphenoid junction. The injected alcohol enters the ganglionic sinus where the juxtaganglionic rootlets are arrayed as in the peripheral division and also are the thinnest, most widely spread, and least interwined. With the patient in this position the mandibular fibers are the highest so that the alcohol, injected in tiny increments, rises to affect them and usually spares corneal sensation. Ecker and Perl (44) injected the alcohol in 0.05-ml aliquots, after which sensation in the painful area was tested. Additional aliquots were injected until the desired affects were obtained, usually with 0.2 to 0.3 ml of absolute alcohol. More recently Delfino (45) reported that, with Ecker's technique using an image intensifier to locate the exact center of the foramen ovale, he first injects 0.2 ml of 2% lidocaine solution as a prognostic block 30 minutes before injecting the ethyl alcohol in 0.05-ml aliquots, up to a total of no more than 0.2 ml.

PHENOL. In 1936 Putnam and Hampton (46) were the first to report on the use of the injection of phenol into the

Fig. 96-4. Technique of injection of the gasserian ganglion or of the mandibular nerve by the anterolateral (Härtel) approach. *A.* A skin wheal is made 3 cm lateral to the angle of the mouth at the level of the upper second molar. A 10-cm 22-gauge needle threaded with a depth marker is introduced through the wheal and advanced posteromedially and superiorly so that, when viewed from the side, its axis points to the midpoint of the zygomatic arch (χ). *B.* When viewed from the front the axis of the needle points to the pupil. A guiding finger of the other hand is placed in the oral cavity to ensure that the needle does not enter the mouth, which could introduce contaminating bacteria into deeper structures. As the needle advances it passes through the buccinator muscle, beneath the mucous membrane between the mandibular ramus and tuberosity of the maxilla, and finally through the external pterygoid muscle before it contacts the infratemporal plate lateral to the base of the pterygoid process and just anterior to the foramen ovale, at a depth of 6 to 7.5 cm. The depth marker is placed 1.25 cm from the skin surface and the needle is withdrawn until its point is subcutaneous. The needle is then reinserted so that the axis of the needle, when viewed from the side, points to the articular tubercle (●) and, when viewed from the front, it still points to the pupil. When the needle has been advanced to a depth just 1 cm short of the rubber marker its point usually contacts the mandibular nerve, causing paresthesia along its course. The needle is further advanced until the marker is flush with the skin.

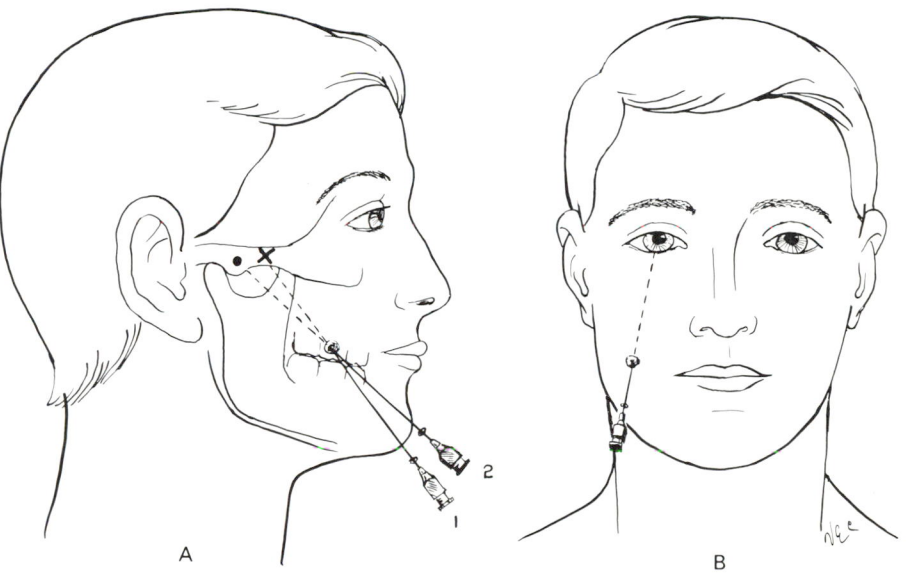

Fig. 96-5. Radiographic visualization of gasserian ganglion block. *A.* The point of the needle is entering the foramen ovale. *B.* The needle has passed through the foramen and rests over the trigeminal depression of the petrous portion of the temporal bone. After *B* was taken absolute alcohol, in 0.1-ml aliquots, for a total of 0.5 ml, produced analgesia of the 2nd and 3rd divisions.

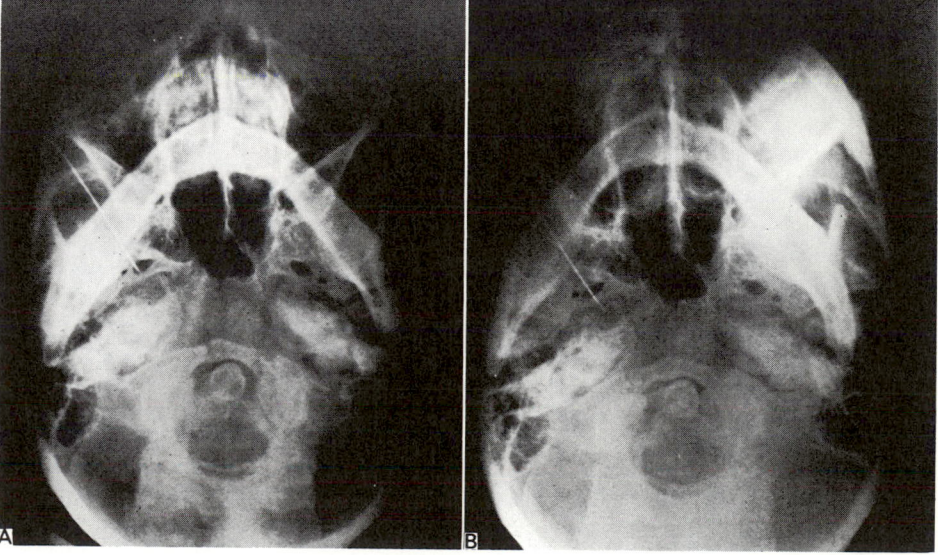

gasserian ganglion under roentgenographic control for the treatment of trigeminal neuralgia, but published no follow-up of their preliminary report. In 1963 Jefferson (47) reported on the use of 5% phenol in glycerin for the treatment of trigeminal neuralgia as well as for postherpetic pain and cancer pain. The technique entailed inserting the needle into the foramen ovale under radiographic control, getting spinal fluid about half the time, and sitting the patient up with the head flexed forward on the chest so that the needle points vertically upward. Jefferson (47) then injected increments of 0.05 to 0.1 ml of phenol in glycerin until the desired results were achieved and then kept the patient upright for 20 to 30 minutes. The technique was subsequently used by Mousel (48) and by Frothingham and associates (49).

GLYCEROL. The technique of placing the needle for injecting glycerol into the trigeminal cistern, as advocated by Häkanson (25), is similar to that shown in Figures 96-4 and 96-5, with the notable difference that the needle is inserted while the patient is in the sitting position and the dura arachnoid is purposely penetrated so that there is spontaneous flow of CSF. Häkanson (25) has emphasized that, if spontaneous CSF drainage through the needle does not occur, the needle is not in the proper position and it is necessary to reposition it or to use the first needle as a guide and insert a second needle into its proper place. Once the needle is considered to be in the correct place and the CSF fluid has drained, 1 ml of metrizamide is injected slowly in 0.2-ml increments using a 1-ml tuberculin syringe and its diffusion is visualized by fluoroscopy. To fill the cistern completely, 2 ml of metrizamide is injected with the patient's chin against the chest. If the point of the needle is in the proper position the contrast medium is seen to fill the cistern, escaping into the posterior fossa through the trigeminal porus.

Lateral and anteroposterior radiographs are then taken to show the pattern of diffusion of the contrast medium and to define the outline of the cistern. After the correct position of the needle tip has been verified, the metrizamide is evacuated from the trigeminal cistern by removing the syringe from the needle and placing the patient in a recumbent position for about 5 minutes. A total of 0.2 to 0.4 ml of pure sterile glycerol is then injected slowly. Because the size and shape of the trigeminal cistern are highly variable, it is necessary to vary the total volume of glycerol injected. To affect all three divisions one must fill the cistern entirely, using 0.3 to 0.4 ml of glycerol with the patient's head in a ventrally flexed position (Fig. 96-6). For the relief of neuralgia in the 3rd division or in the 2nd and 3rd divisions, 0.2 to 0.35 ml of glycerol is injected. Because the specific gravity of glycerol is 1.242 (compared to that of CSF, which is 1.0065 to 1.007), with the patient's head in the flexed position the glycerol remains in the inferolateral portion of the trigeminal cistern, which contains the rootlets of the mandibular and maxillary nerves (Fig. 96-6A). Because the specific gravity of metrizamide is even heavier than that of glycerol (1.329 versus 1.242), leaving a small amount of metrizamide in the bottom of the cistern protects the rootlets of the 3rd branch in patients who have trigeminal neuralgia in the 1st and 2nd divisions (Fig. 96-6B).

Results

TRIGEMINAL NEURALGIA. Gasserian ganglion block with 90 to 100% ethyl alcohol, 5% phenol in glycerin, or glycerol should only be done in high-risk patients who have severe pain in all three divisions of the nerve and in whom drugs are no longer effective and neurosurgical procedures are not available. Because of the significant incidence of paralytic keratitis it might be better, even in such patients, to block the

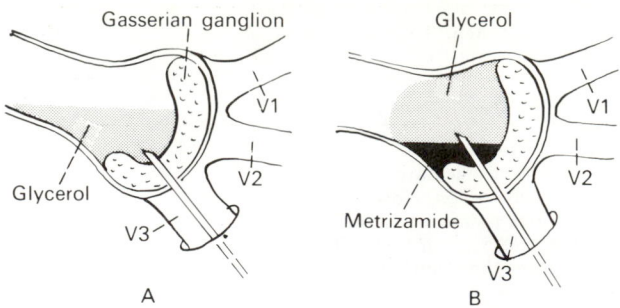

FIG. 96-6. Häkanson's technique of injecting the sensory root of the trigeminal nerve with glycerol. **A.** After drainage of the cerebrospinal fluid, and subsequent injection of metrizamide (see text), pure sterile glycerol is injected in 0.1-ml aliquots for a total of 0.4 ml if all three divisions are to be affected. By adjusting the volume of injected glycerol, it is possible to affect the different trigeminal divisions selectively. Because of the density of glycerol it remains in the bottom of the cistern and a smaller volume (0.2 ml) therefore affects only the 3rd division, while a larger volume also involves the 2nd division (**A**). **B.** For the treatment of 1st- and 2nd-division neuralgia the rootlets of the 3rd division can be spared by leaving a small amount of metrizamide, which is heavier then glycerol, in the bottom of the cistern. The amount of metrizamide left in the cistern is controlled before the glycerol is injected. Modified from Häkanson, S.: Trigeminal neuralgia treated by the injection of glycerol into the trigeminal cistern. Neurosurgery, 9:638, 1981.

2nd and 3rd divisions and the branches of the ophthalmic nerve that are involved in the neuralgia (usually the supraorbital and supratrochlear as they curve over the supraorbital ridge), thus sparing the nerve supply to the cornea.

ETHYL ALCOHOL. In one of the largest series on the use of ethyl alcohol for trigeminal neuralgia, Harris (50) treated a total of 2500 patients. Of 457 patients followed 3 years or longer, 360 (70%) had no recurrence of pain but, unfortunately, the incidence of keratitis or of anesthesia dolorosa was not reported. The results obtained by others using ethyl alcohol, phenol, and glycerol are shown in Table 96-1. Most of these reports, however, lack specific data on the incidence of complications.

I have described (1) the use of the Härtel technique of gasserian alcohol block with ethyl alcohol in 28 patients, and reported on a technique of blocking only the 2nd and 3rd divisions within the ganglion in 4 other patients who had had injections of the nerves outside of the skull and had recurrence of pain. The 32 patients received 39 injections. Of those in this group, 28 patients (88%) had good relief following the injection, but the pain recurred in 17 patients (53%) during the follow-up period, which ranged from 14 months to 8 years or until the death of the patient. Of the 28 patients who had complete trigeminal analgesia, 4 (14%) developed keratitis (despite meticulous ophthalmologic care), 1 developed anesthesia dolorosa, and 1 sustained paresis of other cranial nerves from an accidental subarachnoid injection of the alcohol. This was the most serious complication I encountered during my extensive experience with neurolytic blocks (1). These complications and less serious but annoying side effects such as numbness, paresthesia, and herpetic eruptions in patients with a fairly long life expectancy,

TABLE 96-1. Results of Therapy of the Pain of Trigeminal Neuralgia With Neurolytic Gasserian Ganglion Block

Source	No. of Patients	Results (Pain Relief)* (% of Patients Treated)		Permanent or Serious Complications (% of Patients Treated)
		Immediate	Long-Term (years)	
Alcohol				
Harris (50)	457	95	70 (7+)	NSD
Kulenkampff (51)	800	90	80 (NSD)†	NSD
Thurel (52, 53)	3,000	85	?	NSD
Henderson (54)	196	81	33 (1+)	6, NU
Ecker and Perl (44)	133	97	97 (7+)	10, CU
Ecker (55)	312	90	77 (7+)	None
Miles (56)	130	90(?)	59	3, NU, CU
Delfino (45)	741	98	91	NSD
Phenol				
Jefferson (57)	50	96+	96 ($2\frac{1}{2}$)	2
Mousel (48)	34	90	87 (1)	3
Frothingham (49)	12	92	75 (NS)	15
Glycerol				
Häkanson (25)	75	98	81 (0.2–4)	None
Häkanson (58)	100	96	96 (2.5)	None
Sweet el al. (27)	27	89	89 (NSD)	33, MD
Lumsford and (26)	112	?	67, CR	6.6
All/Mean:	6,179	86	75	

*Results with one or more blocks.
†NSD, no specific data available; CR, complete relief; CU, corneal ulcer; NU, nasal ulceration; MD, mild dysesthesia.

together with the advent of more refined and specific neurosurgical operations, caused me to discontinue the use of gasserian ganglion block with alcohol for the treatment of trigeminal neuralgia in the late 1950s.

Modern radiologic technology, which has permitted the use of the image intensifier, the widespread use of the nerve stimulator, the advent of newer and safer

TABLE 96-2. Comparison of Results of Treatment of the Pain of Trigeminal Neuralgia

Parameter	Radiofrequency Coagulation	Surgical Root Section	Neurolytic Ganglion Block
Number or patients	36	33	130
Recurrence of pain (in 1% of procedures done)	14	21	32
Complications (% of total)			
Loss of corneal reflex	8	36	15
Corneal ulceration	0	6	1
Trigeminal motor weakness	11	12	1
Oculomotor weakness	0	6	1
Facial weakness	0	0	0
Facial ulceration	0	12	1
Anesthesia dolorosa	3	0	0
Mean, complications (%):	22	67	22

From Miles, J.: Trigeminal neuralgia. *In* Persistent Pain: Modern Methods of Treatment, Vol. 2. Edited by S. Lipton. New York, Grune & Stratton, 1980.

contrast media, and the use of glycerol, together with skillful administration, make gasserian ganglion block easier and safer than it was two decades ago (Tables 96-1 and 96-2). Notwithstanding the better results obtained with neurolytic blocks, patients with the pain of trigeminal neuralgia who are not relieved with drug therapy should be managed with microvascular decompression, which is successful in about 80 to 90% of patients; the remainder can be managed with retrogasserian rhizotomy and neurogangliolysis (Chapters 38, 97, and 99).

CANCER PAIN. In contrast to its use in a trigeminal neuralgia patient with a long life expectancy, alcohol block remains a useful procedure for those with severe intractable pain in the anterior two-thirds of the face caused by advanced or terminal cancer. Prior to selection of the optimal method it is essential to determine the type of cancer, the predicted rate and direction of spread, the condition of the patient, and the availability of a physician skilled in block techniques (Chapter 24). If the neoplasm is slow-growing and involves structures in the 2nd or 3rd division, or in both, block of the nerves is preferable to avoid keratitis. If it is possible that the neoplasm could spread to affect the 1st division, however, or if it is difficult to block the 2nd division because the tumor occupies the pterygopalatine fossa, it is better to carry out gasserian ganglion block at the outset to produce a widespread field of analgesia into which the cancer can spread without producing subsequent pain. Although this technique carries the risk of corneal anesthesia and possibly keratitis, the problem is different than when dealing with a patient with trigeminal neuralgia in whom life expectancy is long and in whom corneal ulcer would be a serious complication. In a patient with advanced or terminal cancer, effective relief of severe excruciating pain is considered to be worth the risk of these complications.

Obtaining radiographs prior to block is useful and necessary to ascertain that the foramen ovale has not been invaded, which could impair the proper positioning of the needle. In patients with carcinoma of the nasopharynx and floor of the mouth, the tumor can destroy bone structures of the base of the skull and make it impossible to identify the foramen ovale. In such cases a different approach for the block must be adopted or a different procedure must be used. Because alcohol diffuses poorly in tissues the point of the needle must be in the precise position. Another important step is to carry out block with a local anesthetic to predict the efficacy of the neurolytic agent before it is injected.

Between 1945 and 1977 I used gasserian ganglion block with absolute alcohol in 107 patients. Of these, 79 patients (74%) obtained effective pain relief and, together with small or moderate doses of sedatives, codeine, or adjuvant drugs, they were made comfortable until their death, 2 weeks to 7 months later. Another 16 patients (15%) obtained only partial relief with the first injection and required either a second injection of the ganglion (9 patients) or a supplementary injection of one of the major nerves (7 patients), together with modest doses of drugs. The procedure produced little or no relief in the remaining 12 patients, and they were managed with opioids. Similar results were reported by my former colleague, Dr. Jose Madrid, at the First International Symposium on Cancer Pain in 1979 (59). Madrid reported that he had done 371 blocks of the gasserian ganglion—72% were done with absolute alcohol, 22% were done with phenol in glycerin, and the remainder (6%) were done with hypertonic saline solution, which he gave up because of poor results. Good pain relief was obtained in over 80% of these patients, and an additional 10% obtained partial relief of pain. Complications in 12 to 15% of those in each group included keratitis, weakness of the ipsilateral muscles of mastication because of block of the motor root of the mandibular nerve, and annoying paresthesia and dysesthesia (59). No cases of paralysis of other cranial nerves and no deaths were attributable to the use of neurolytic block in either group. (See Figs. 45-1 to 45-4, pp. 807, 808).

These results compare favorably with those achieved with the use of major neuroablative techniques, and are actually better in regard to mortality rate in such patients. This does not suggest that neurolytic block of the gasserian ganglion should be used instead of neurosurgery in patients who can tolerate the stress of a surgical procedure. Rather, in patients with advanced or terminal cancer, serious consideration should be given to the use of this technique *provided* that personnel with the necessary experience and skill are available if neuroablative procedures are not feasible for some reason. This also applies to patients who require large doses of oral or parenteral opioids to obtain adequate relief.

Complications

Most of the complications that occur with neurolytic block of the gasserian ganglion block have been mentioned; some complications and unwanted side effects are avoidable, and some are not. Unavoidable side effects that are usually transient, and that are not serious, include Horner's syndrome from block of the paratrigeminal sympathetic fibers and involvement of the motor root, with transient weakness of the muscles of mastication. If the entire ganglion is affected by the neurolytic agent, corneal anesthesia, with consequent loss of corneal reflex and possibly paralytic keratitis, loss of sensation on the ipsilateral side of the face and half of the tongue, paresthesia, herpetic eruptions, trophic ulcerations, and anesthesia dolorosa can and do develop. The incidence, degree, and duration of these complications from neurolytic blockade varies, however, depending on the completeness of the destruction of nerve cells.

Following injection of a small amount of neurolytic agent (less than 0.5 ml of alcohol, phenol, or glycerol) many of these pathologic processes have been found to be transient and some do not occur at all but, after injection of a larger amount (more than 1 ml) they are likely to occur more frequently and to last longer. That such is the case has been confirmed by Miles (56), who compared the effects of neurolytic ganglion injection with those of surgical root section and radiofrequency coagulation in one center in which each of these procedures was carried out by highly experienced and skilled personnel (Table 96-2). The data suggest that the use of neurolytic ganglion block results in fewer complications than surgical root section, but also show that the incidence of the recurrence of the neuralgia is greater with neurolytic ganglion block than with surgical root section (32 versus 21%). Techniques of gasserian ganglion block that spare the cell bodies or rootlets of the 1st division, such as those used by Håkanson (25), Ecker and Perl (44, 55), and Jefferson (57), are not followed by corneal ulceration or anesthesia dolorosa. Accidental subarachnoid injection of alcohol is likely to involve other cranial nerves and is probably the most serious complication of this technique. Its incidence can be minimized by repeated attempts at aspiration prior to injection of each aliquot.

Block of the Ophthalmic, Maxillary, and Mandibular Nerves

Indications

Block of the maxillary or mandibular nerve, or of both, remains useful for the relief of severe tic douloureux or of cancer-related pain affecting one or both of these nerves if neuroablative procedures cannot be carried out. For patients with trigeminal neuralgia it is essential to use prognostic blocks with local anesthetics to determine which branch needs to be blocked, especially those who have trigger areas in one branch and pain distribution in another branch. If touching the upper lip causes pain in the lower jaw, for example, it is likely that the 2nd division needs to be blocked instead of the 3rd division. Occasionally, however, both nerves need to be blocked.

NEURALGIA. White and Sweet, in their classic textbook (60), listed six indications for injection of the major branches of the trigeminal nerve in patients with trigeminal neuralgia: (a) to provide prompt pain relief so that patients weakened by poor fluid intake might be strengthened preparatory to an operation for permanent relief; (b) to enable those likely to die soon to live out their lives pain-free and without major surgery; (c) to aid in the differential diagnosis of patients whose pain has characteristics transitional between those of trigeminal neuralgia and other forms of facial neuralgia; (d) to relieve pain on the second side of the face when bilateral neuralgia has developed so as to avoid complete, lasting anesthesia on both sides of the face; (e) to relieve pain by the use of alcohol block in the distribution of branches of the 1st division, but without involving the eye to avoid the corneal anesthesia produced by rhizotomy of the ophthalmic nerve; and (f) to help patients adjust to the dysesthesia that might follow posterior rhizotomy.

Obviously, the advent of anticonvulsant drugs has virtually eliminated the first two indications. Block with a local anesthetic remains useful to help in the diagnosis of patients with neuralgia with confusing symptoms and to obviate the need of bilateral rhizotomy in patients with bilateral neuralgia. White and Sweet (60) were of the opinion that neurolytic block should be used prior to trigeminal rhizotomy to give a clear-cut and sustained (but reversible) indication of

the sensory changes that accompany denervation to help patients decide whether they prefer temporizing drugs or surgery to produce lasting anesthesia and consequently permanent relief. A large number of internationally known neurosurgeons concurred, and data were presented that showed that patients who had had alcohol injection prior to rhizotomy (as a criterion of selection for surgery) had an incidence of postoperative paresthesia or dysesthesia that was 10% of the incidence among those patients who had not had alcohol injection (60). This is now a moot point because neurosurgeons with expertise in microvascular decompression, surgical rhizotomy, and neuroganglioysis are available in many medical centers.

CANCER PAIN. Block of the maxillary or mandibular nerve, or of both, with neurolytic agents remains useful in managing patients with severe and intractable cancer-related pain, especially if experienced neurosurgeons are not available and if life expectancy is shorter than 3 months. Cancer of the nasal cavity and paranasal structures is predominantly adenocarcinoma, which unfortunately is highly malignant and all too often is inoperable when first seen. Eventually this cancer produces severe symptoms, including nasal obstruction, nasal discharge,

FIG. 96-7. Block of the branches of the ophthalmic nerve. *A, B.* Anterior views showing, from left to right, lateral orbital block, supraorbital block, and medial orbital block. *C.* Schematic cross section of the orbit with the nerves left intact to show the techniques of lateral and medial orbital block. To block all the branches within the orbit the lateral superior route is used. A 5-cm 25-gauge needle is introduced through a wheal made just above the lateral canthus and advanced posterolaterally until contact is made with the bone of the lateral wall of the orbit. With its bevel flush with the bone the needle is then advanced posteromedially toward the apex of the orbit, keeping constant contact with the bone. At a depth of 3.5 cm the point of the needle usually loses contact with the bone, being situated at the lateral portion of the superior orbital fissure. It is then advanced another 3 to 5 mm, aspiration is attempted and, if no blood or cerebrospinal fluid is obtained, 2 to 3 ml of local anesthetic are slowly injected. To block the supraorbital nerve as it curves around the supraorbital ridge a 1.5-cm 30-gauge needle adapted to a 2-ml syringe, which contains a local

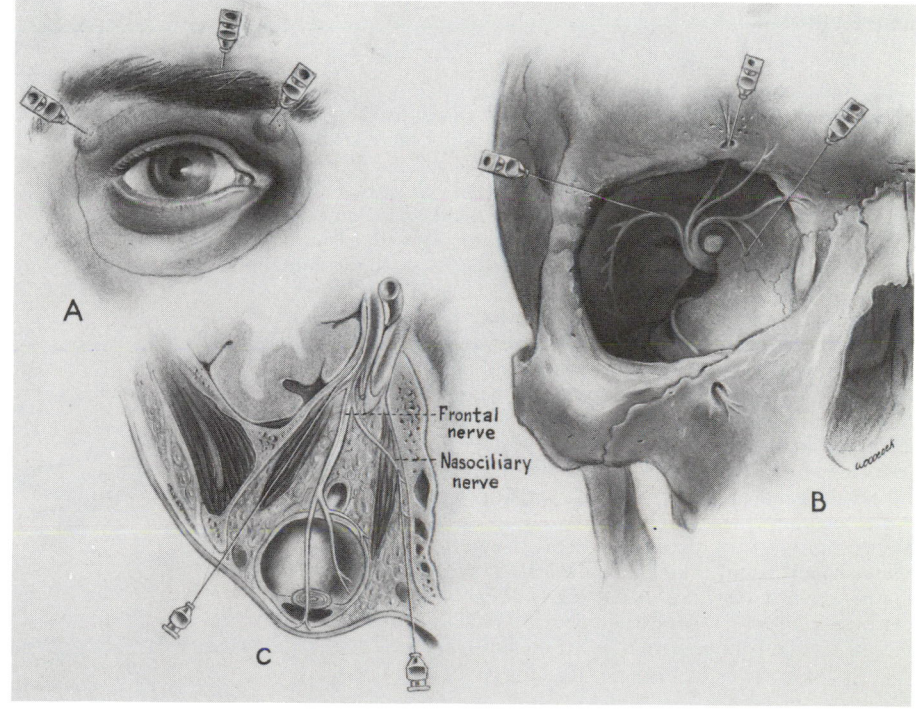

anesthetic, or a 1-ml tuberculin syringe which contains alcohol, is held like a dart and thrust through the skin of the upper lid in a direction perpendicular to it. The supraorbital foramen or notch through which the nerve passes is easily palpable through the skin of the upper lid by retracting the eyebrow upward at a point 2.5 cm from the midline. The needle is advanced slowly until paresthesia is elicited or until bone is contacted. For neurolytic block it is essential to contact the nerve, and several reinsertions might be necessary to locate it so that the neurolytic agent can be deposited intraneurally. To block the nasociliary nerve or its branches a 5-cm 25-gauge needle is inserted through a wheal 1 cm above the inner canthus and directed posterolaterally, always keeping contact with bone. At a depth of 2 cm the point of the needle should be at the anterior ethmoidal foramen, and 1.5 to 2 ml of local anesthetic solution is then injected. This blocks the anterior ethmoidal nerve, which eventually becomes the internal and external nasal branches. The needle is then advanced 1 cm further to reach the posterior ethmoidal foramen, where 1.5 to 2 ml of solution are injected to block the posterior ethmoidal nerve that supplies the ethmoidal cells and the sphenoid cavity. These two injections are also likely to block the infratrochlear nerve, which supplies the conjunctiva, lacrimal sac, inner canthus, and root of the nose.

epistaxis, and intractable pain, which is usually diffuse, dull, and aching and is frequently referred to the face. The pain can be satisfactorily relieved by blocking the maxillary nerve with alcohol. If the pterygopalatine fossa is invaded and block of the 2nd division is impossible, gasserian ganglion block must be carried out.

Cancer of the lower jaw, particularly Ewing's sarcoma and osteogenic sarcoma, two common tumors originating in the mandible, often produces severe intractable pain. The ulcerating type of carcinoma of the lower gingiva and floor of the mouth, which has resulted in extensive invasion of the mandible or overlying skin, or both, also produces intense pain. In many of these cases the pain becomes progressively more intense and is often accompanied by trismus and otalgia, all of which prevent patients from eating and sleeping, thus enhancing cachexia. Because many of these patients are in poor physical condition, alcohol block of the mandibular nerve alone or in combination with block of C2 and C3 is indicated. Alcohol block of the lingual nerve should be considered in patients with severe pain caused by cancer of the tongue, especially if the pain involves both sides, thus obviating bilateral masticatory paralysis, which usually follows bilateral mandibular nerve block. Inferior alveolar nerve block should also be considered for patients with severe pain caused by cancer of the mandible.

In 1951 I analyzed the results of neurolytic blocks (61). These were included, with subsequent cases, in the first edition of this book (1). A total of 76 patients were studied; they had undergone 102 neurolytic blocks of the maxillary or mandibular nerve, or a combination of these or one of their branches. Of these, 69% had complete or almost complete relief of pain, 19% had partial relief of pain, and the remainder (12%) had no relief; there were no deaths in this group. Subsequently I managed 61 additional patients with these techniques and obtained similar results. Murphy has also used these techniques in patients with cancer pain, but progressively fewer of these procedures have been done at the UW Pain Center, for two major reasons: (a) many of these patients are managed by former trainees of the Pain Training Program and by other anesthesiologists practicing in other hospitals; and (b) the Pain Center has become involved predominantly in the management of patients with complex, nonmalignant, chronic pain problems. These techniques remain important tools, however, especially in those hospitals in which sophisticated neurosurgical techniques are not available and in medical centers in developing countries. Properly done they provide much-needed relief to patients with cancer pain.

OTHER INDICATIONS. Block of the mandibular or maxillary nerve, or of both, with long-lasting local anesthetic (e.g., 0.5% bupivacaine with epinephrine 1:200,000) can be used in patients who experience excruciating pain postoperatively or post-injury. The block usually lasts 8 to 12 hours and can be repeated one, two, or even three times to tide patients over. Obviously, patients with post-traumatic pain can have distortion of the bones of the face, making the classic lateral extraoral route difficult or impossible. In such cases the orbital (Matas) route is used.

RETROBULBAR BLOCK. Retrobulbar block, with varying concentrations of alcohol for the relief of severe persistent eye pain, has been used for the past seven decades. Grüter (62) in 1918 reported the injection of 3 ml of 80 to 90% ethyl alcohol as an alternative to the enucleation of blind painful eyes. Weekers (63) in 1930 first described the use of a dilute solution of alcohol in patients with "seeing eyes" (i.e., patients who had vision) to relieve severe persistent eye pain consequent to corneal ulcers, keratitis, uveitis, and glaucoma. Since then many ophthalmologists have used alcohol block for the relief of pain in both types of patients, as well as for the control of photophobia and blepharospasm following corneal surgery and after penetrating keratoplasty. The duration of pain relief varies but usually is 3 to 6 months and even longer, although pain can return sooner if the underlying pathologic process remains uncontrolled.

In 1949, Maumenee (64) published a comprehensive report summarizing the development of this technique, the results

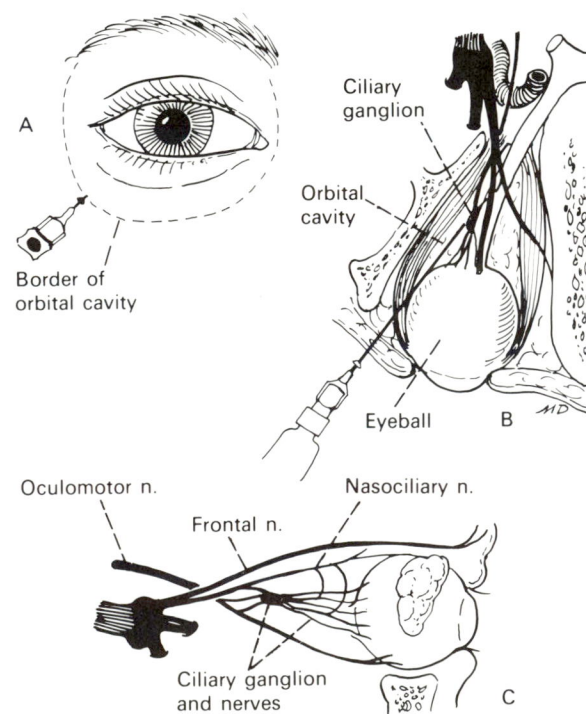

FIG. 96-8. Technique of retrobulbar alcohol block. Following appropriate preparation of the field, the needle, adapted to a 5-ml syringe containing 1 or 2% lidocaine, is inserted into the lateral third of the lower eyelid just above the rim of the orbit. The needle is advanced and made to pass through Tenon's capsule (the thin membrane that envelops the eyeball) between the lateral rectus and inferior rectus muscles into the muscle cone. The needle should be advanced until its tip is just behind the globe. Aspiration is attempted to ensure that the bevel of the needle is not in a blood vessel; if negative, 2 ml of lidocaine are injected. The syringe is then removed, leaving the needle in place. After 15 to 20 minutes a 2-ml Luer-Lok syringe containing either 50% alcohol (for patients with vision) or absolute alcohol (for patients with no vision) is adapted. An attempt at aspiration is again made to ensure that the needle has not entered a blood vessel and the alcohol is injected slowly.

obtained by Grüter from the time he first described the technique to 1943, and those of others up to 1949. Maumenee also described the technique and analyzed the results of injection of 95% alcohol in 41 eyes with less than 10/200 vision ("blind eyes") and in 15 patients whose visual acuity ranged from 10/200 to 20/20 ("seeing eyes"). Of the patients with "blind eyes" 68% had glaucoma and the remainder (32%) had corneal ulcers, keratitis, uveitis, and keratoplasty. Those with "seeing eyes" had various forms of infectious keratitis, including herpes zoster, uveitis, glaucoma secondary to uveitis, and epidemic keratoconjunctivitis. No patients in the latter group had reduction of visual acuity after the injection of alcohol and, in all of these patients, vision improved with therapy of the underlying condition. Histologic studies of the optic nerves of 15 eyes that had been removed after alcohol injection showed no evidence of damage to the nerve from the alcohol (64). It was concluded that the optic nerve is apparently protected from the effects of alcohol by the thick sheath that surrounds it.

FIG. 96-9. Technique of maxillary nerve block. A. Needles in place for the lateral and anterolateral routes. For the lateral route a wheal is raised below the sigmoid notch of the zygomatic arch and an 8-cm 22-gauge needle threaded with a depth marker is introduced through it perpendicular to the skin and slowly advanced until the point strikes the lateral pterygoid plate at a depth of about 4 cm (B, step 1). The marker is then set 1 cm from the skin, the needle is withdrawn until its point is subcutaneous, and it is readvanced in a slightly anterior and superior direction so that its point is 1 cm anterior and 1 cm superior to the point of bone contact made on the first insertion. The needle is carefully advanced in this direction until the marker is flush with the skin and the point of the needle is within the pterygopalatine fossa (step 2 in B and C). For local anesthesia 2 ml are injected slowly. If a neurolytic block is required it is essential that the bevel of the needle be on or in the nerve. The nerve is located by eliciting paresthesia or by using a nerve stimulator. If the point of the needle is on the nerve 1 ml of alcohol is injected, but, if the needle bevel is within the nerve, 0.4 ml is sufficient to destroy the nerve. D. Inferior view of the skull showing needle 1 with its bevel against the lateral pterygoid plate and needle 2 with its distal centimeter in the pterygopalatine fossa and its bevel in front of the foramen rotundum. E. Radiograph showing the needle in place and its bevel in front of the foramen rotundum. For the anterolateral route a skin wheal is raised at the angle formed by the coronoid process of the mandible and the inferior border of the zygomatic arch and an 8-cm 22-gauge needle is introduced and advanced medially, superiorly, and slightly posteriorly (A, C). At a depth of 4 cm the upper part of the posterior surface of the maxilla is contacted and the needle is advanced further with its bevel facing the bone to a depth of 4 to 5 cm, where contact with the bone is lost and paresthesia in the upper jaw is elicited. If difficulties are encountered a nerve stimulator and radiographic control can be used. Once contact is made the same volumes of local anesthetic or neurolytic agent, as mentioned for the lateral route, are injected.

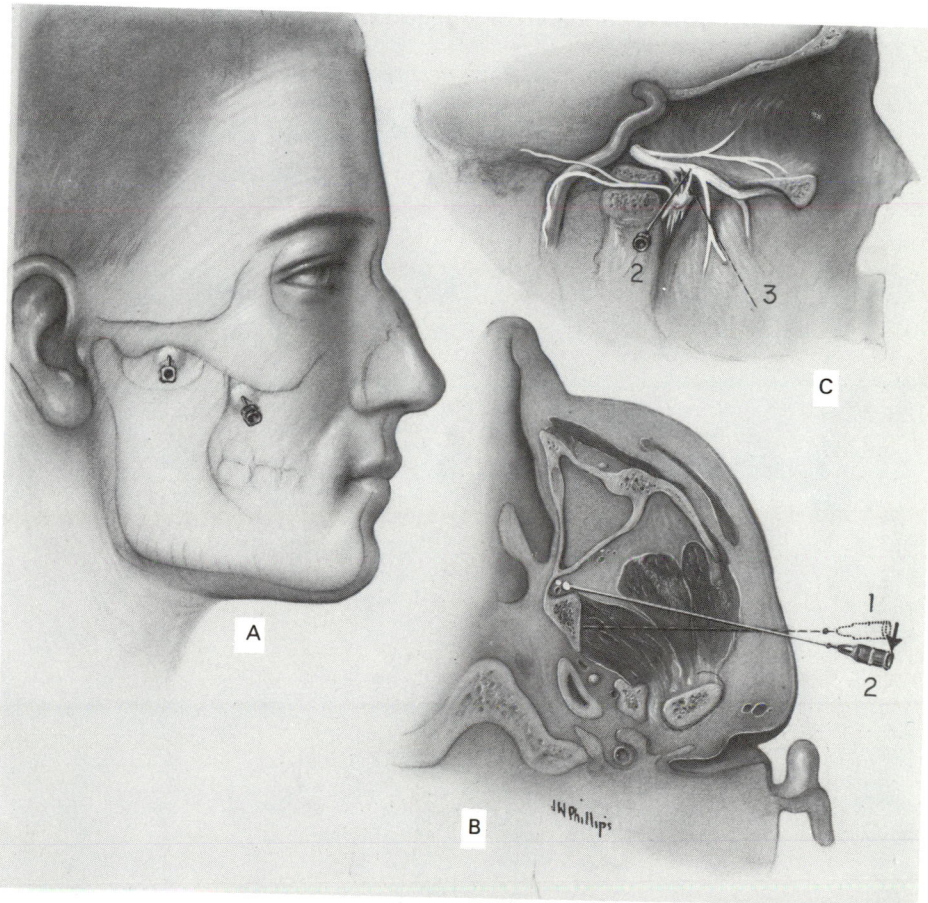

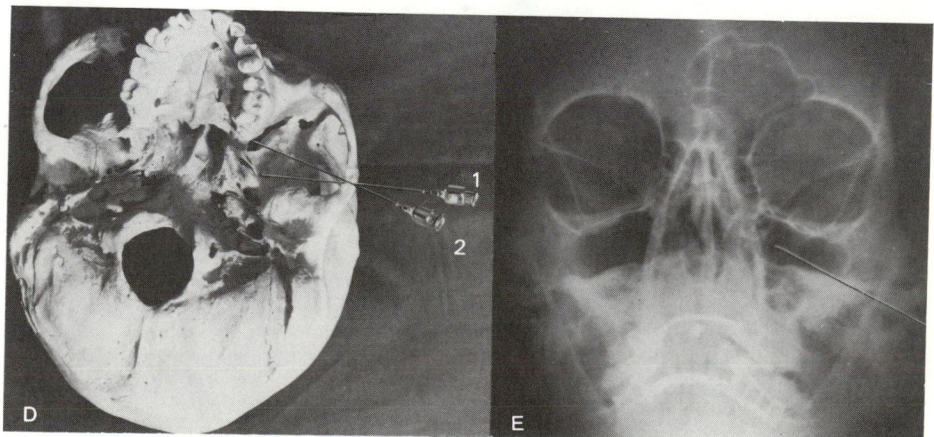

Techniques of Block

The anatomy of the ophthalmic, maxillary, and mandibular nerves is described in detail in Chapter 37 and depicted in Figures 37-4, 37-5, 37-6, and 37-8. Figure 96-7 illustrates various techniques of blocking the branches of the ophthalmic nerve, and Figure 96-8 shows the technique of retrobulbar alcohol block. Figure 96-9 depicts procedures for blocking the maxillary nerve by the lateral and anterolateral extraoral routes. Figure 96-10 shows the technique of maxillary nerve block by the orbital (Matas) route, which is used if the lateral technique cannot be carried out because of a tumor in the path of the needle. Figure 96-11 shows mandibular nerve block by the lateral extraoral route, which is the most frequently used technique for injection of this nerve.

The neurolytic block should always be preceded by a block with a long-lasting local anesthetic, such as bupivacaine. As noted above, the volume of local anesthetic should be the same or smaller than the volume of neurolytic agent to be used. I prefer alcohol injected intraneurally to obtain a longer-lasting neural blockade. This is best done with the mandibular nerve because of its size and position below the foramen ovale, whereas the maxillary nerve in the pterygopalatine fossa is smaller and it is more difficult to place the point of the needle into the nerve. In any case, good results require that the point of the needle be in or very near the nerve as indicated by eliciting paresthesia; if difficulty is encountered a nerve stimulator should be used.

With absolute alcohol the average duration of blockade, as reported by many workers, has been 12 to 14 months for the maxillary nerve and 16 to 18 months for the mandibular nerve (60, 65). In my series maxillary nerve block afforded relief for an average of 14.6 months, with a range of 8 to 27 months, and mandibular nerve block provided relief for an average of 18.4 months, with a range of 7 to 29 months.

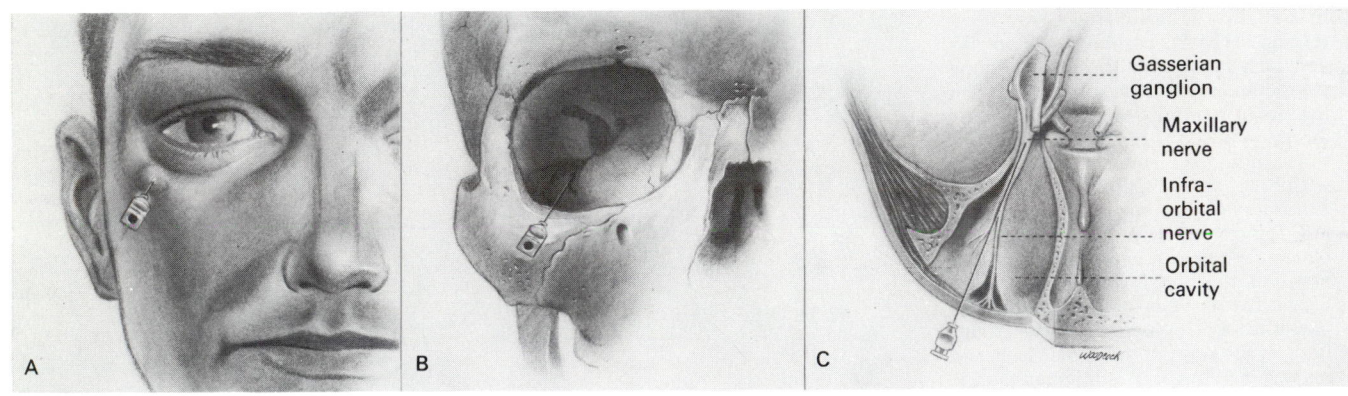

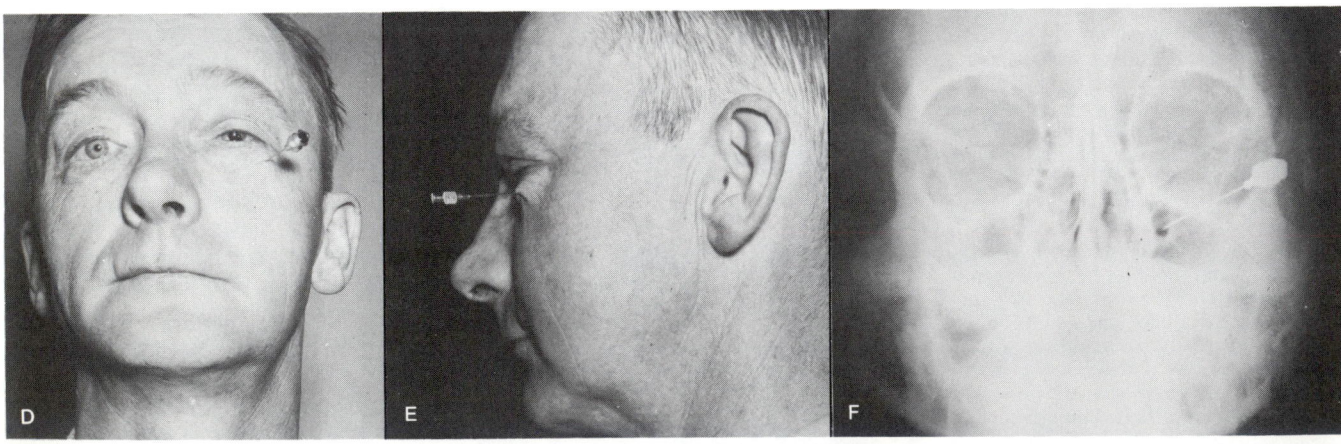

FIG. 96-10. Maxillary nerve block by the orbital (Matas) route. **A.** An 8-cm 22-gauge needle is introduced through a wheal made just above the inferior orbital margin, 1 cm medial to the inferior lateral angle of the orbital rim. Contact with the floor of the orbit is made and the needle is advanced posteriorly and slightly medially, keeping constant contact with the bone. **B.** At a depth of about 3.5 cm the point of the needle enters the inferior orbital fissure and loses its contact with bone. **C.** The needle is then slowly advanced so that its point passes through the pterygopalatine fossa and it finally enters the foramen rotundum at a depth of about 5 cm. Paresthesia can be elicited while the needle is advancing through the pterygopalatine fossa and should always be elicited when the needle enters the foramen rotundum containing the nerve. **D,** and **E.** Patient with the needle in place. **F.** Radiograph showing the bevel of the needle within the foramen rotundum. Injection of 0.5 ml of alcohol is sufficient to destroy the nerve.

FIG. 96-11. Mandibular nerve block by the lateral extraoral route. *A.* A skin wheal is raised just below the midpoint of the zygomatic arch and an 8-cm 22-gauge needle threaded with a rubber marker is inserted through it perpendicular to the skin. *B.* The needle is advanced until its point strikes the lateral pterygoid plate at a depth of about 4 cm from the skin (needle position 1). The marker is set 5 mm from the skin surface and the needle is withdrawn until its point is subcutaneous and reinserted so that its point is 1 cm posterior to its previous position (needle position 2). The needle is gently advanced until the marker is flush with the skin, at which depth the bevel of the needle usually contacts the nerve just inferior to the foramen ovale and elicits paresthesia. For a diagnostic block, 2 to 3 ml of local anesthetic can be injected on the nerve but, for a neurolytic block, it is best to inject 1 ml of alcohol intraneurally. Because intraneural injection of alcohol is painful it is essential either to give the patient a short-acting opioid, such as fentanyl, before injecting the alcohol or to inject 0.5 ml of 2% lidocaine, wait about 30 minutes, and then inject the alcohol. *C.* Inferior part of the skull showing two needles in place. Needle 1 has it bevel against the lateral pterygoid plate while needle 2 has its bevel in the center of the foramen ovale. *D.* Radiograph showing the needle below the foramen ovale.

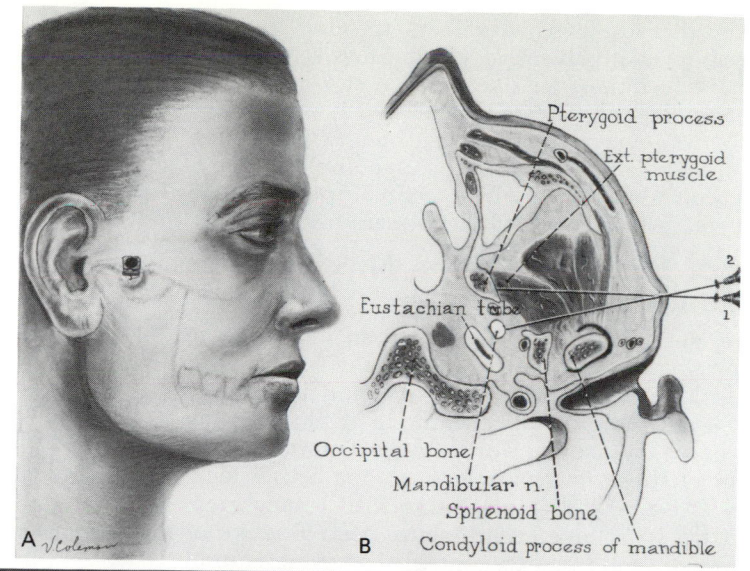

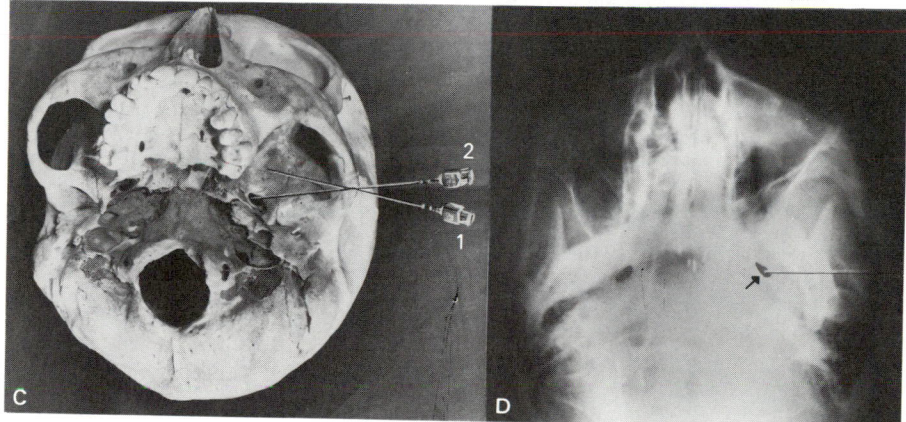

The technique of injecting alcohol to relieve persistent eye pain (Fig. 96-8) is somewhat different from that described for ophthalmic nerve block. Most ophthalmologists use a 3.5-cm 22-gauge needle, but a 25-gauge needle produces less tissue damage. As part of the psychologic preparation patients should be reassured about the procedure and instructed to alert the physician promptly if a flash of bright light is experienced, which indicates that the needle has penetrated the optic nerve. In some patients the injection is done during the course of surgery with general anesthesia.

Complications

RETROBULBAR BLOCK. Following retrobulbar alcohol injection patients have routinely developed some degree of ptosis, proptosis, chemosis, and extraocular muscle palsy within hours of injection, but all these are resolved in 2 days to several weeks (64). Temporary muscle paralysis is commonly seen if injection is done too far posteriorly in the muscle cone, instead of using the technique described above. Properly done, little or no risk of optic nerve damage is involved, because the nerve is protected by the thick sheath that surrounds it. Moreover, no permanent muscle palsy or other serious complications have been noted. Several cases of optic nerve damage, however, have been reported following accidental injection of alcohol into the optic nerve (64).

MAXILLARY NERVE BLOCK. Because of the highly vascular nature of the contents of the pterygopalatine fossa, bleeding often occurs with maxillary nerve block but is usually not serious. Injection of neurolytic agents in excess of 1 ml increases the risk of having the drug pass through the inferior orbital fissure into the orbit and of damage to the oculomotor and abducens nerves, producing visual difficulties; for reasons noted above this does not damage the optic nerve. Moore (66) reported a case of necrosis of the mucosa and cartilage of the palate, with a consequent large defect in half of the roof of the mouth on the ipsilateral side following alcohol injection of the maxillary nerve. In view of the numerous patients who have received maxillary nerve blocks with alcohol, these are rare complications that can be minimized and even eliminated by using a small volume of alcohol and precise technique.

MANDIBULAR NERVE BLOCK. Other than postinjection pain and the infrequent incidence of hemorrhage in the cheek that occur during and following mandibular block by the anterolateral extraorbital route, and that are transient effects, the most frequent complication is involvement of the motor root with consequent weakness or paralysis of the muscles of mastication of the affected side, which causes the mandible to deviate from the midline. If more than 1 ml of alcohol is injected into the mandibular nerve it is likely that some of the solution can diffuse cephalad and affect the lower part of the gasserian ganglion.

Block of Branches of the Maxillary and Mandibular Nerves

Figure 96-12 depicts the technique of blocking the infraorbital nerve, Figure 96-13 shows the technique of blocking the lingual and inferior alveolar nerves, and Figure 96-14 illustrates the technique of blocking the mental nerve by the intraoral and extraoral routes. Injection of these branches with a long-acting local anesthetic (e.g., 0.25% bupivacaine with epinephrine) can be used to relieve severe acute postoperative or post-traumatic pain and to control the severe pain of herpes zoster in the distribution of each of these branches. Because of their simplicity, and with the use of 25-gauge needles, injections can be repeated twice daily until the pain subsides.

Alcohol block of these nerves is used as a prognostic and therapeutic procedure in patients with tic douloureux, postherpetic neuralgia, and severe cancer pain limited to their distribution. For optimal results it is best to inject the drug intraneurally to destroy these nerves, thus producing a prolonged effect. Some patients develop postinjection neuropathy with neuralgia, with degeneration of the nerve. Swerdlow (65) reported a patient with a small area of ulceration on the cheek following infraorbital nerve block with 10%

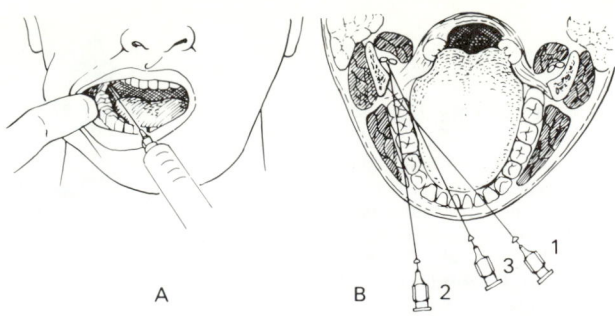

FIG. 96-13. Technique of blocking the inferior alveolar and lingual nerves by the oral route. **A.** After the mucous membrane of the retromolar trigone is topically anesthetized and prepared with an antiseptic solution, a 10-cm 22-gauge needle attached to a 5-ml syringe containing local anesthetic, or a 1-ml tuberculin syringe containing alcohol, is introduced 1 cm above the triturating surface of the last molar tooth. **B.** The angle is such that the shaft of the needle rests 1 cm above the dental arch between the canine and first premolar tooth of the opposite side (position 1). After contact is made with the trigone at its medial side, the needle is swung horizontally so that its shaft rests parallel to the teeth of the same side and it is gently and slowly advanced so that its point slips to the medial border of the trigone (position 2). The needle is swung back so that its shaft finally rests above the first incisor of the same side and it is advanced about 1.5 cm to bring the point midway between the anterior and posterior margins of the ascending ramus (position 3). At this juncture the bevel of the needle is just medial to the mandibular foramen, where 2 to 3 ml of local anesthetic solution (or 1 ml of alcohol) are injected. For neurolytic block it is essential to contact the inferior alveolar and lingual nerves separately and to elicit paresthesia before injecting alcohol.

aqueous phenol and cited Churcher, who reported a similar complication. Churcher had another patient in whom injection of 0.2 ml of absolute alcohol caused rapid ischemic necrosis of the mucosa and cartilage of the palate and produced a defect in the roof of the mouth, which was attributed to intense spasm of the maxillary artery.

Block of the Glossopharyngeal and Vagus Nerves

Indications

Block of the glossopharyngeal or vagus nerve, or both, is indicated for patients with severe intractable pain caused by tic-like neuralgia or with cancer-related pain in the distribution of these nerves. Block of these nerves with a long-lasting local anesthetic is used to help in the differential diagnosis of tic-like pain in the angle of the jaw, which can be caused either by glossopharyngeal or mandibular neuralgia. Glossopharyngeal block is used in differentiating glossopharyngeal neuralgia from the geniculate ganglion neuralgia that causes pain deep in the ear and has some of the features of glossopharyngeal neuralgia. Because geniculate neuralgia involves the sensory root of the facial nerve (nervus intermedius), glossopharyngeal nerve block at the jugular foramen or below the styloid process does not relieve it. In such cases the initial step involves provoking glossopharyngeal neuralgia by applying a cotton applicator to the

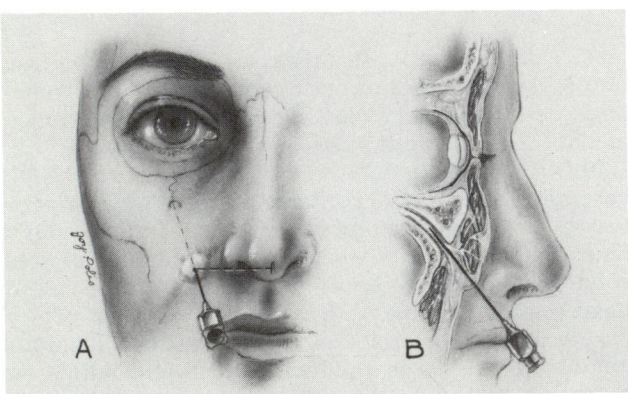

FIG. 96-12. Technique of infraorbital nerve block. **A.** A 5-cm 25-gauge needle attached to a 2-ml Luer-Lok syringe and containing a local anesthetic, or a 1-ml tuberculin syringe containing alcohol, is introduced through a skin wheal made 1 cm lateral to the middle part of the ala nasa, or 2.5 cm from the midline, and advanced superiorly, posteriorly, and slightly laterally. The bone just inferior to the foramen is contacted at a depth of 1 to 1.5 cm and paresthesia is elicited, usually radiating to the upper lip. To block the branch that supplies the lip the injection is made at this point but, to block the nerve supply to the front teeth, it is necessary to pass the needle into the canal 7 to 10 mm (**B**). Paresthesia is usually elicited during the advance. After negative aspiration tests 1 ml of local anesthetic or 0.3 to 0.5 ml of alcohol is sufficient to destroy the nerve.

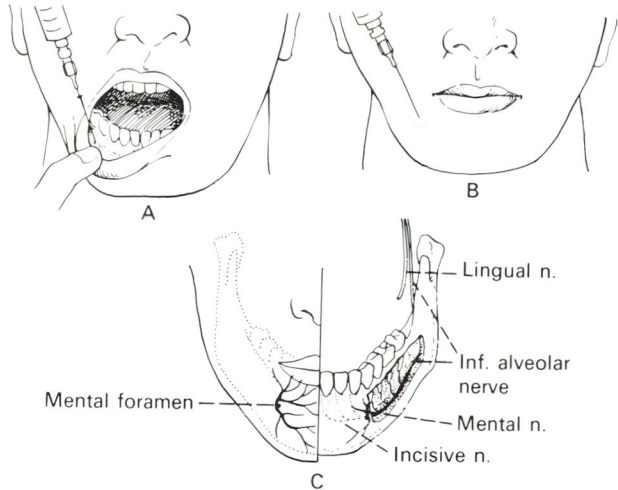

FIG. 96-14. Technique of mental nerve block by the oral and extraoral routes. **A.** Oral route. A 5-cm 25-gauge needle is introduced through the gingivobuccal reflection on a line drawn between the premolar teeth. After contacting the upper margin of the mandible the needle is advanced inferiorly on the same line to a point midway between the upper and lower margins, where the nerve is usually contacted and paresthesia is elicited. **B.** Extraoral route. A 5-cm 25-gauge needle is introduced through a wheal raised on the skin of the lower lip inferior and anterior to the root of the second premolar tooth. On making a contact with the bone the needle is advanced anteriorly, inferiorly, and medially until it passes into the foramen, which faces posteriorly, superiorly, and laterally, and paresthesia is elicited. Usually 2 ml of local anesthetic are used for prognostic block but, for neurolytic block, 0.3 ml of absolute alcohol is injected intraneurally or into the mental canal. **C.** View of the mandible to show the emergence of the mental nerve through the mental foramen (left) and dissection of the inferior alveolar canal to show the distribution of the inferior alveolar nerve to the teeth.

tonsils, posterior pharynx, or back of the tongue and then applying a topical anesthetic such as 4% cocaine or 2% tetracaine, which produces analgesia of the trigger points within 10 to 15 minutes.

A small percentage of patients develops a variant of glossopharyngeal neuralgia, in which the vagus nerve is also involved. Robson and Bonica (67) reported a method of aiding the diagnosis of this type of neuralgia. In two patients who presented with typical clinical pictures of glossopharyngeal neuralgia, complete topical anesthetization of the entire pharynx, which completely relieves the pain of neuralgia limited to the glossopharyngeal nerve, failed to do so. Block of the glossopharyngeal and vagus nerves below the jugular foramen, however, afforded complete relief. In these patients resection of the sensory root of the glossopharyngeal nerve, as well as of the anterior half of the sensory root of the vagus nerve, produced permanent and complete relief of the neuralgia.

Block of the vagus nerve with a local anesthetic is also useful as a diagnostic or prognostic procedure in patients with cancer pain in the tracheobronchial tree. This type of pain is effectively treated with section of the vagus nerve below the recurrent laryngeal nerve (Chapter 57). Because block of each of these two nerves is best done at the base of the skull motor

nerves are also interrupted, and therefore neurolytic blocks are contraindicated because they produce prolonged paralysis of the pharyngeal and laryngeal muscles and the consequent loss of the ability to swallow and phonate.

In earlier years I advocated the cautious use of unilateral glossopharyngeal block with neurolytic agents for the relief of severe cancer pain in patients who could tolerate intracranial rhizotomy. As noted in Chapters 24 and 45, however, the recent development and clinical application of percutaneous thermocoagulation of the glossopharyngeal nerve, described by Broggi and Siegfried (68) and used by other workers for the treatment of glossopharyngeal neuralgia and cancer pain, have decreased the need for unilateral neurolytic blockade of this nerve. Using the thermocoagulation procedure (see Fig. 97-5), several workers have reported good pain relief in about half of patients with glossopharyngeal neuralgia and in about two-thirds of patients with cancer pain. The procedure produces transient vagal dysfunction and occasionally causes dysarthria and dysphagia. This procedure is done only in a few medical centers worldwide,

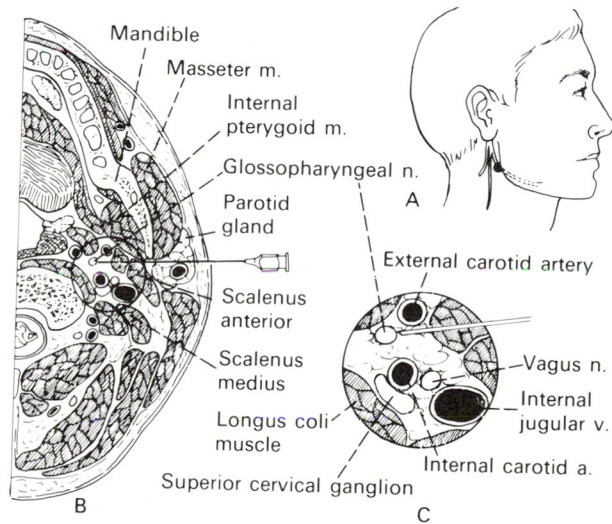

FIG. 96-15. Technique of glossopharyngeal nerve block. **A.** A skin wheal is made just posterior to the angle of the mandible and a 5-cm 22-gauge Teflon-coated needle attached to a stimulator is passed through the wheal. At this level the glossopharyngeal nerve is about 1.5 to 2 cm anterior to the vagus nerve and can be blocked exclusively with small volumes of solutions without involving the vagus nerve. **B.** The needle is advanced medially and just posterior to the mandible until its bevel is 4 cm deep and the stimulator is used to help locate the nerve. Once the nerve has been found 2 to 2.5 ml of the local anesthetic or 1.5 to 2 ml of alcohol are injected. **C.** Enlargement of the circled area in **B** to show the point of the needle on the nerve. Because the section is below the tip of the styloid process this is not seen as it is in Fig. 96-16C. If the nerve cannot be located with the stimulator at this level, the classic approach is used. This involves the passage of the needle through a wheal raised at the point of bisection of a line drawn between the mastoid process and the angle of the mandible. The needle is advanced perpendicular to the skin until the styloid process is contacted, the rubber marker is placed 5 mm from the skin, and the needle is withdrawn and reintroduced to pass anterior to the styloid process and advanced until the marker is flush with the skin, at which point paresthesia should be elicited.

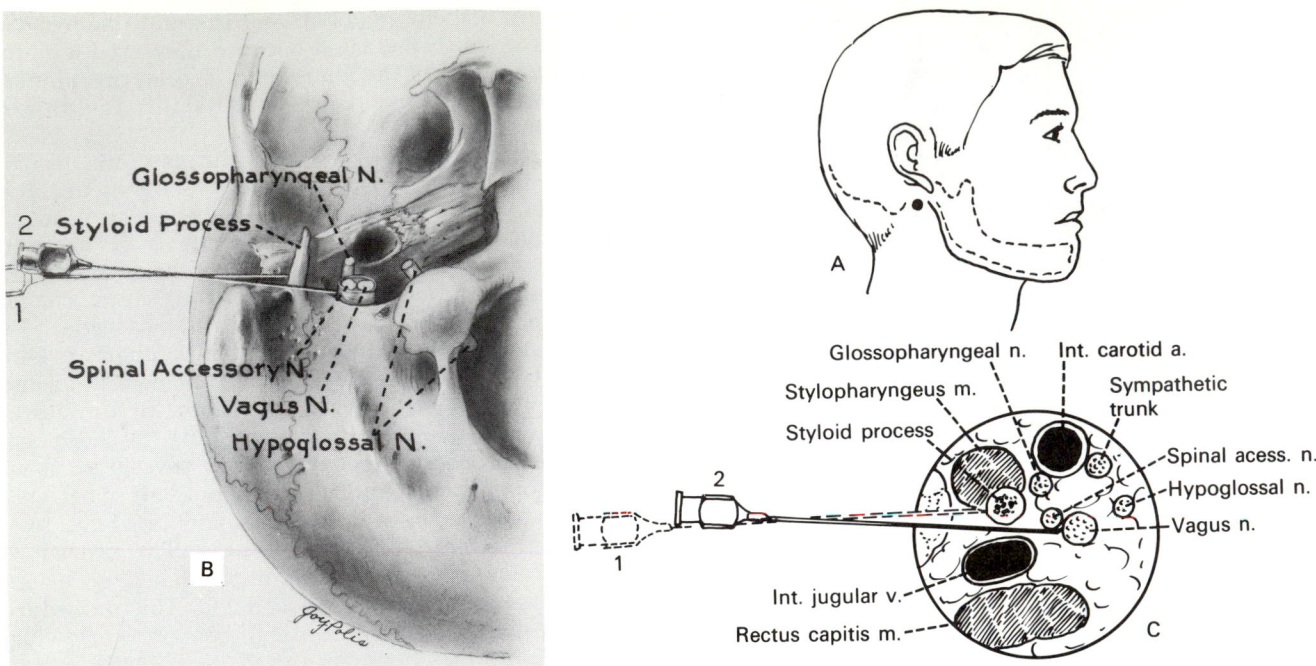

FIG. 96-16. Technique of vagus nerve block. *A.* A skin wheal is raised just anterior to the mastoid process and immediately below the external auditory meatus. *B.* The relations of the styloid process and cranial nerves 9, 10, 11, and 12. *C.* Cross section enlargement of the area just below the jugular foramen. Note the close proximity of the various nerves, vessels, and the styloid process. A 5-cm 25-gauge needle is introduced through the wheal and advanced until the styloid process is contacted (needle position 1 in *B* and *C*), whereupon the needle marker is placed 1 cm from the skin. The needle is withdrawn until its bevel is subcutaneous and reintroduced so that it passes posterior to the styloid process until it is flush with the skin (needle position 2 in *C*). A volume of 2 to 4 ml of local anesthetic solution is injected, which is likely to block not only the vagus but also the 9th, 11th, and 12th cranial nerves because of their close proximity. Neurolytic block of the vagus nerve is not done at this level.

however, and is not available to most patients with severe cancer pain in the throat. If patients can tolerate it intracranial section of the sensory root of the glossopharyngeal nerve should be done, but if patients are in poor physical condition and the pain cannot be controlled with opioids, a unilateral neurolytic block should be done.

Block of the internal laryngeal branch of the superior laryngeal nerve with local anesthetic and subsequently with alcohol or phenol can be used to control severe neuralgia, cancer pain, or other chronic painful conditions in the larynx. In patients who have cancer pain involving branches of the glossopharyngeal or mandibular nerves, block of the internal laryngeal

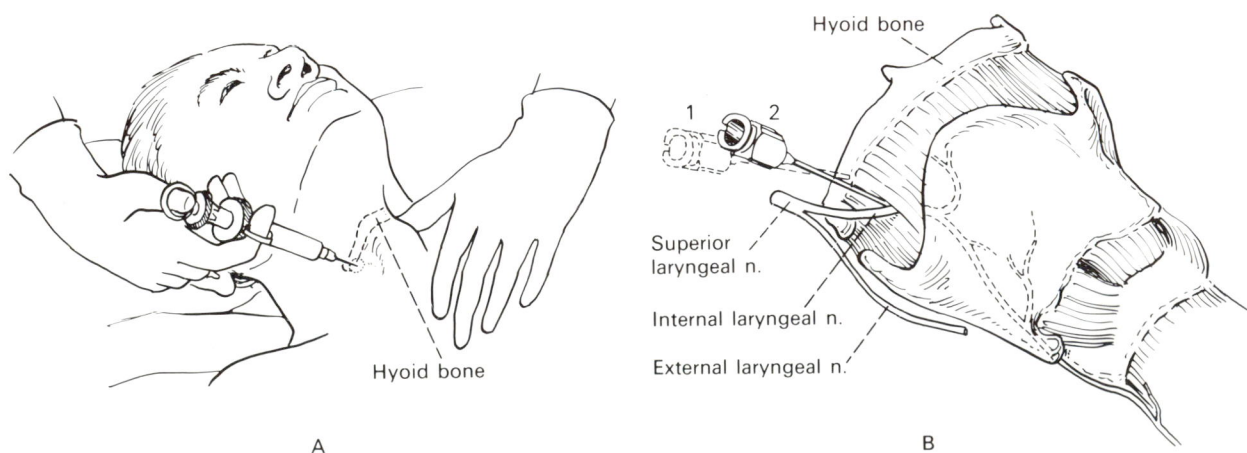

FIG. 96-17. Technique of blocking the internal branch of the superior laryngeal nerve. *A.* After identifying the great cornu of the hyoid bone on the side to be blocked (facilitated by exerting pressure on the oppostie side of the bone to render the great cornu more prominent), a wheal is raised in the skin overlying the tip of the cornu. A 5-cm 25-gauge needle is inserted through the wheal and advanced perpendicularly to the skin until the hyoid bone is contacted. *B.* The needle is withdrawn and redirected inferiorly and slightly medially until its bevel lies midway between the inferior border of the hyoid bone and the superior border of the thyroid cartilage, about 1 cm anterior to the lateral thyrohyoid ligament, where the nerve is usually contacted. Injection of 2 ml of local anesthetic produces analgesia of the laryngeal inlet down to the level of the vocal cords. Injection of a neurolytic agent (e.g., 0.5 ml of alcohol) should be done only when the nerve is contacted.

nerve must be supplemented with block of these nerves.

Techniques

The anatomy of the glossopharyngeal and vagus nerves is described in detail in Chapter 37 and shown in Figure 37-9. The technique of blocking the glossopharyngeal nerve is depicted in Figure 96-15, and block of the vagus nerve is shown in Figure 96-16. Because of the proximity of both nerves just below the jugular foramen, selective block of the glossopharyngeal nerve is possible (but difficult). Inserting the needle just posterior to the angle of the mandible, which is about 5 cm below the level of the jugular foramen, the glossopharyngeal nerve is 1.5 to 2 cm anterior to the vagus nerve (Fig. 96-15C). By using a nerve stimulator and a Teflon-coated needle, the nerve is contacted about 2 or 3 cm below and anterior to the tip of the styloid process. Once the nerve has been contacted, 1 to 1.5 ml of 0.5% bupivacaine with epinephrine is injected. If the block produces analgesia limited to the distribution of the glossopharyngeal nerve, one can consider following it up with the injection of 5% aqueous phenol to obtain a block of several months. Figure 96-17 shows the technique of blocking the internal branch of the superior laryngeal nerve.

Complications

Glossopharyngeal block causes dysphagia from paralysis of the pharyngeal muscle, whereas block of the vagus causes paralysis of the ipsilateral vocal cord with impairment of phonation, and block of vagal fibers to the heart produces tachycardia. If the block is done below the jugular foramen it is likely to involve the spinal accessory and hypoglossal nerves, so that the patient develops paralysis of the trapezius muscles and of half of the tongue on the same side as the block. Furthermore, use of excessive amounts of neurolytic solution can cause sloughing and fibrosis in surrounding tissues, particularly the carotid artery and internal jugular vein, but this is usually a result of improper technique (65).

C. NEURAXIAL NEUROLYTIC BLOCKS

Injection of a neurolytic agent into the subarachnoid, extradural, or subdural space is one of the most effective methods of relieving severe intractable pain caused primarily by advanced or terminal cancer. The use of these techniques for chronic nonmalignant pain is to be discouraged, however, except in special circumstances that are considered in this section.

Agents that have been used for this purpose include ethyl alcohol, phenol in glycerin, chlorocresol in glycerin, aqueous phenol, hypertonic saline solution, and ammonium compounds. Most of this section discusses basic considerations, including indications, techniques, results, and complications of the use of subarachnoid alcohol and subarachnoid phenol in glycerin. Extradural neural blockade and subdural neural blockade are also considered briefly.

Subarachnoid Neurolytic Block

Basis for Application

The bases for the injection of a neurolytic agent into the subarachnoid space to relieve severe pain include the following:

a. Most nociceptive impulses from the skin, subcutaneous tissue, deep somatic structures, and viscera pass to the spinal cord through the posterior roots and their rootlets.

b. By proper positioning of the patient, hypobaric alcohol or hyperbaric phenol in glycerin can be made to diffuse predominantly to the posterior rootlets involved in the transmission of nociceptive information.

c. On contact with the rootlets, neurolytic agents destroy axons (wallerian degeneration) of the rootlets, extending from the dorsal root ganglion to their attachments to the spinal cord.

d. By using appropriate technique, the solution can be made to block as many segments as are involved in the transmission of pain information. Thus, with this method, it is possible to produce a predominantly posterior chemical rhizotomy to relieve pain for weeks, months, and even for a year or more.

e. Because cell bodies are not affected, regeneration occurs over varying periods of time, depending on the degree of destruction caused by the neurolytic agent.

Indications and Advantages

In properly selected patients subarachnoid rhizotomy is an effective method for controlling severe intractable pain located below the head. Dogliotti (69), when first describing the technique, advocated the use of subarachnoid alcohol not only for the relief of cancer pain but also for nonmalignant severe pain caused by other pathologic processes. The procedure has been used mostly for the management of cancer pain; best results are obtained in patients with pain in the trunk. Because of involvement of the anterior root and weakness of the intercostal muscle, dysfunction occurs only in patients with severe respiratory disease. The technique has also been used for the relief of pain in the neck, upper limbs, pelvis, and lower limbs, but in such patients it is associated with varying degrees of complications (see below). Subarachnoid neurolysis is also effective for managing patients with spasticity.

Intrathecal neurolysis is relatively simple to carry out. It is not associated with much pain and causes few serious complications. It can be carried out in patients in poor physical condition and in the elderly. Because it involves only a brief stay in the hospital, it can be made available to a relatively large number of patients and requires no special, costly, or highly sophisticated equipment or facilities. Subarachnoid neurolytic injection can be repeated or extended if the pain spreads or persists. It is useful for patients in poor physical condition, who can be made to improve so that a neurosurgical procedure can be performed at a later time. In patients with terminal cancer the duration of pain relief is usually sufficient to afford a relatively comfortable end.

It is generally agreed that, in patients who are in fairly good physical condition and who have an anticipated survival of longer than 4 to 6 months, a surgical or percutaneous cordotomy can provide a longer and more certain period of pain relief. In patients with a shorter life expectancy and in those who are unable, unfit, or unwilling to undergo surgery, however, intrathecal neurolytic injection offers a good prospect of worthwhile pain relief so that patients can remain ambulatory and on minimal oral analgesic medication. Subarachnoid neurolytic blockade is also valuable for patients with extensive bilateral cancer pain, because the risk of performing bilateral cordotomy is great. This risk can be minimized by performing cordotomy on the side with the most intense and extensive pain and the subarachnoid neurolytic block can be done on the other side.

Some authorities (3) have stated that, in patients with bilateral pain, subarachnoid neurolysis should be used with great caution, if at all, but at the UW Pain Center this procedure has been used in patients with bilateral pain in the trunk with good results. Some clinicians (70) have advocated treating bilateral pain by placing patients prone but, to obtain effective relief, it is necessary to use large volumes of neurolytic agents, which consequently increases the risk of complications. It is extremely important to avoid increasing disability through motor weakness, sphincteric incompetence, and loss of positional sense, unless it can be justified by the degree of pain relief achieved. Usually ambulatory patients choose not to lose control of bladder function, even if pain relief with the use of an alternative method is inferior. On the other hand, for a patient whose bladder is already involved with a tumor and who has a bladder catheter in place, bladder paresis is not an unacceptable price to pay.

Disadvantages and Contraindications

The most significant disadvantages of intrathecal neurolysis (or of any other neurolytic procedure) in managing patients with cancer pain are that some patients obtain inadequate pain relief and some incur complications. Inadequate pain relief results either from failure of the original injection to interrupt all the nociceptive pathways completely or from spread of the pain beyond the anesthetized region. The fact that pain of malignant disease has a tendency to spread in time and space is well known and accounts for some failures: the block might initially interrupt the nerves to the painful region and afford complete relief of pain but, in a few days, weeks, or months, the neoplasm can spread beyond the confines of the analgesia and cause additional pain.

Occasionally chemical interruption might not last long enough to afford the patient relief of pain until death. This can be the result of failure of the block to last as long as anticipated, or because the patient has lived longer than expected. Fortunately, the block can be repeated several times without further taxing the patient's already overburdened physiologic status, so not all these disadvantages are as significant as they might seem.

A more important disadvantage includes complications that can occur during or following the procedure. Muscle weakness in the limbs and involvement of the rectal and vesicular sphincters are the most serious of these. Relative contraindications to the use of subarachnoid neurolysis include the following: (a) pain that is diffuse or is extensive and poorly localized; (b) intraspinal tumor infiltration, with involvement of the cord or the spinal column at the level of injection; (c) two diagnostic or prognostic procedures with a local anesthetic that provide no relief of pain.

Principles of Application

Subarachnoid neurolytic block should be used as part of a multimodal program, which can include sedatives, antidepressants, anxiolytic drugs and moderate doses of opioids and, most importantly, psychologic care for the patient's anxiety, depression, and other serious emotional reactions (Chapter 24). I have stressed (1) that optimal results require adherence to the following steps and principles:

a. If subarachnoid neurolytic blockade is considered as the method of choice for controlling severe pain, it should be carried out at the earliest possible time.

b. Patients should be admitted to the hospital 1 or 2 days before the procedure to allow proper preinjection assessment and management, including carrying out one or more diagnostic or prognostic blocks at intervals of 8 to 10 hours between each injection.

c. Assuming that a detailed history already has been taken and a comprehensive physical and neurologic examination has been carried out at the previous outpatient consultation, it is still necessary to reassess and record the site, quality, intensity, and other characteristics of the pain using the visual analog scale, descriptors, or other measures discussed in Chapters 24 and 32. It is also important to repeat a neurologic examination even if one has been done because it is important to determine whether any changes have occurred during the interval between the preceding and the present examinations.

d. The patients, family, and referring physician should be thoroughly informed about the incidence and degree of pain relief expected and about any complications associated with the procedure. It is important to inform patients that the procedure might not relieve all the pain, and that it is frequently necessary to repeat the injection once or twice to achieve optimal pain relief. Patients must also be told that the procedure is intended to relieve the pain and *not* to cure the disease, so that they do not develop a false hope of cure when the pain is eliminated.

e. The diagnostic or prognostic blocks should be carried out at least 12 hours prior to the intrathecal neurolysis. If alcohol is to be used for the neurolysis, hypobaric tetracaine is used, whereas if phenol in glycerin is to be employed hyperbaric tetracaine or bupivacaine is used.* The slow injection of a 0.2-ml volume containing 1 mg of either drug and using a tuberculin syringe for precise measurement usually blocks the rootlets of one or two segments.

f. Generally, premedication should be avoided because the full cooperation of patients is necessary to decide on immediate localization of the neurolytic solution after it is injected. If patients are unduly apprehensive, an anxiolytic, sedative,

---

*Hypobaric tetracaine is made by dissolving niphanoid crystals containing 20 mg of the drug in 4 ml of sterile distilled water to produce a mixture with a specific gravity of 1.003. Hyperbaric solutions are made by adding glucose to the local anesthetic solution to produce a mixture with a specific gravity of 1.24.

or combination should be given in moderate doses that do not impair mentation. Although some authorities (71) have suggested that no opioid analgesic be given after 4 hours of the block to assess the degree of pain and pain relief with the procedure properly, circumstances do exist in which the position required for the injection is so painful that modest doses of opioids should be given IV. This not only helps patients but permits dural puncture during the peak effects of the analgesic and thus decreases any associated discomfort. It is important to wait long enough so that the drug concentration has decreased below the minimum effective analgesic concentration.

Little difference has been noted between the use of hypobaric alcohol or hyperbaric phenol in glycerin in regard to the degree and extent of nerve damage. Thus, it is reasonable to expect that the incidence of pain relief and complications would be similar with both techniques. Different results occur primarily because of the knowledge, skill, and experience of the administrator with a particular agent and the technique used. On the other hand, the comparison between the two agents given below does suggest differences in the hands of some who have had extensive experience with both techniques.

Techniques

SUBARACHNOID ALCOHOL. The technique of subarachnoid alcohol block is based on the fact that ethyl alcohol is a neurolytic agent that destroys nerve fibers and is hypobaric, with a specific gravity of 0.789. Therefore, when it is slowly injected into the cerebrospinal fluid (CSF), which has a specific gravity of 1.0065 to 1.007, the alcohol diffuses upward and forms

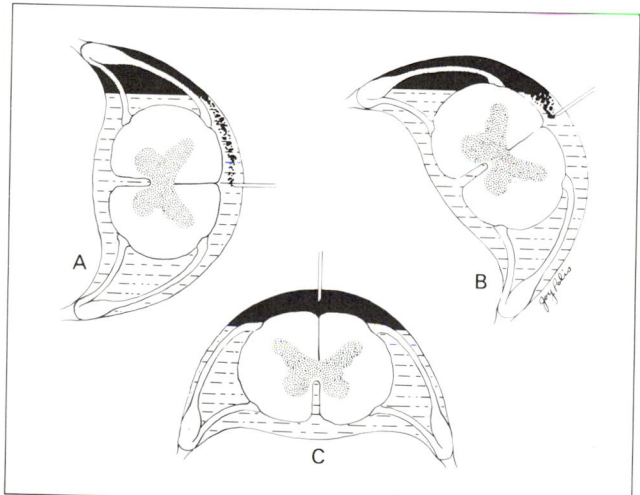

FIG. 96-18. Diffusion of alcohol into the subarachnoid space. **A.** With the patient in the lateral position both the anterior and posterior roots are affected. **B.** The patient is in the lateral-prone position, with the posterior rootlets uppermost. The bevel of the needle is just anterior to the dura-arachnoid. The alcohol, which is hypobaric, is injected in small aliquots so that it diffuses along the surface of the arachnoid membrane and comes in contact predominantly with the posterior rootlets. **C.** With the patient in the prone position small amounts of alcohol are insufficient to affect the posterior rootlets. The use of larger volumes increases the risk of damaging the posterior columns of the spinal cord and other complications.

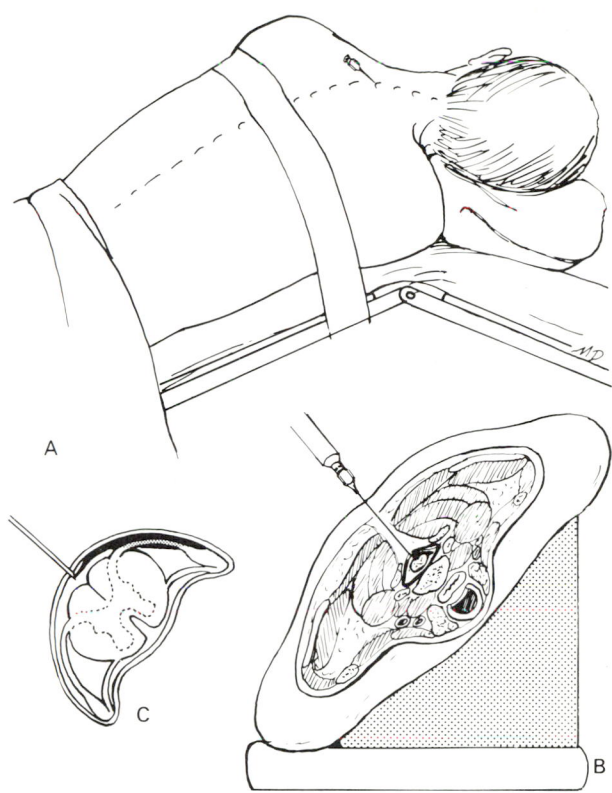

FIG. 96-19. Subarachnoid alcohol block for pain in the lower cervical and upper thoracic regions. **A.** Position of the patient, showing the angle the body with the surface of the table. **B.** Cross-sectional representation of the body showing the angle it makes with the table. **C.** Enlargement of the intrathecal structure showing diffusion of the alcohol to bathe the posterior rootlets and root.

somewhat of a layer on top of the spinal fluid (Fig. 96-18). To achieve the best results it is therefore necessary to have the patient placed on an operating table that can be moved to various positions (Fig. 96-19 through 96-22). Once the patient is in position and the area has been properly prepared, puncture is carried out with an 8- or 10-cm 22-gauge short-beveled needle using the technique depicted in Figure 96-23.

The patient is placed in the lateral position on the side opposite the one to be blocked, with one or two pillows under the region to produce a scoliosis with a maximum curve corresponding to that of the nerve rootlets conveying the nociceptive impulses (Figs. 96-19 and 96-20). The convexity of the curve, which is upward, can be accentuated by "breaking" the table or by employing the gallbladder or kidney lifts (Figs. 96-21, 96-22). This places the involved posterior nerve rootlets uppermost, with the head and lower part of the body below the puncture site. In addition, the patient is turned forward 45° so that the posterior rootlets of the nerves of the upper side are horizontal (Fig. 96-18) and they become bathed with the injected solution, while the anterior roots are (theoretically) less affected. The patient is made as comfortable as possible and is loosely strapped in place with adhesive tape to prevent movement from the desired position.

The site of puncture also depends on the segments involved. It is best to deposit the alcohol at the level where the involved rootlets originate from the spinal cord and not at the point of exit of the roots through the intervertebral

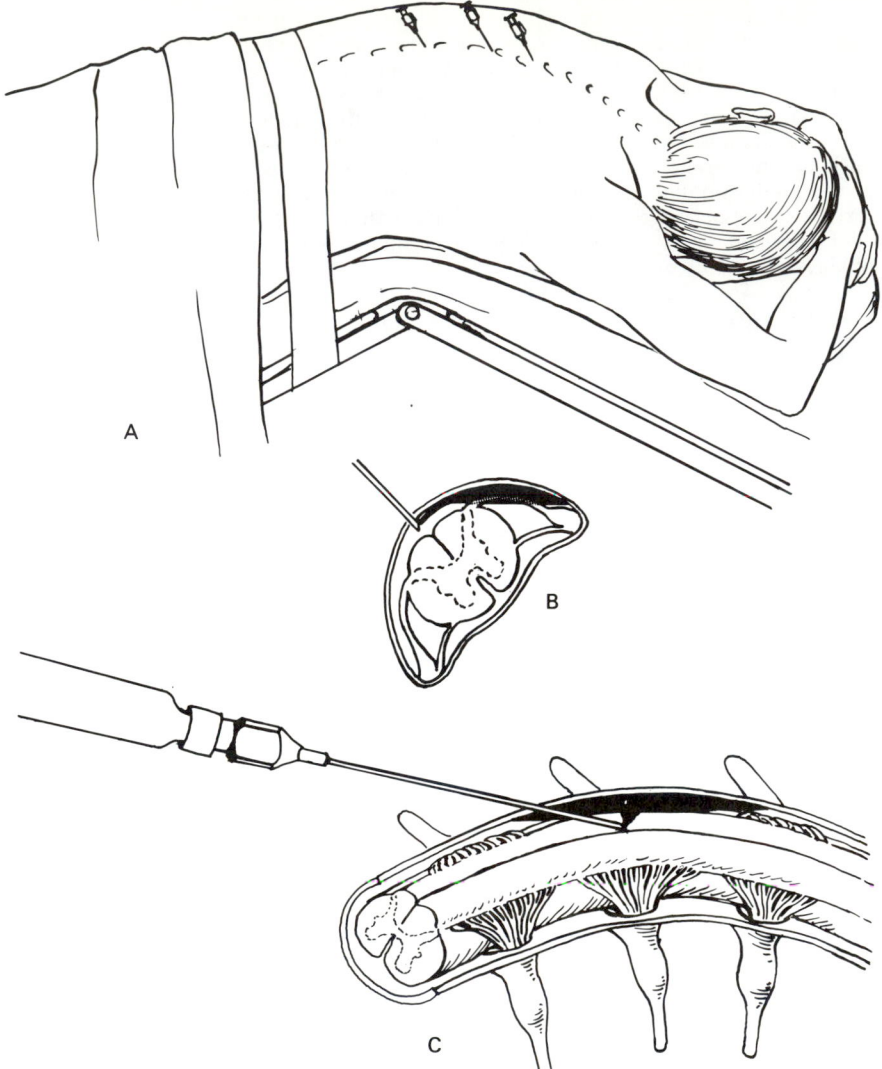

FIG. 96-20. Position of a patient for subarachnoid alcohol block in the thoracic region. *A.* One or two pillows are placed under the region to be blocked and the table is flexed to produce a scoliosis of the spine, with a maximum curve corresponding to that of the nerve rootlets conveying the nociceptive impulses. This places the posterior (sensory) nerve rootlets and roots uppermost, with the head and extremities lower than the point of injection. *B.* Cross section of the thoracic subarachnoid space, showing diffusion of the alcohol uppermost to involve the posterior rootlets. *C.* Schematic representation of the spinal cord (posterolateral view). The alcohol diffuses to affect the rootlets of two segments by injection of 0.1-ml aliquots over 90 seconds, repeated at 3-minute intervals until 0.4 to 0.5 ml of alcohol has been injected through each needle. *D, E.* Patient in position for block of the left side to relieve chest pain caused by metastasis to and multiple fractures of the ribs. These produced pain during normal respiration and severe pain during deep respiration, causing the patient to hypoventilate markedly. Three needles were used to permit injection of small volumes of solution and thus minimize complications. The first injection on the left side produced good relief from pain, extending from T4 to T10. The procedure was repeated 10 days later on the right side and the patient derived sufficient pain relief to permit adequate ventilation for 4 weeks. A second series of blocks produced relief until death, 7 weeks after the second series of subarachnoid alcohol therapy, for a total of 11 weeks of pain relief.

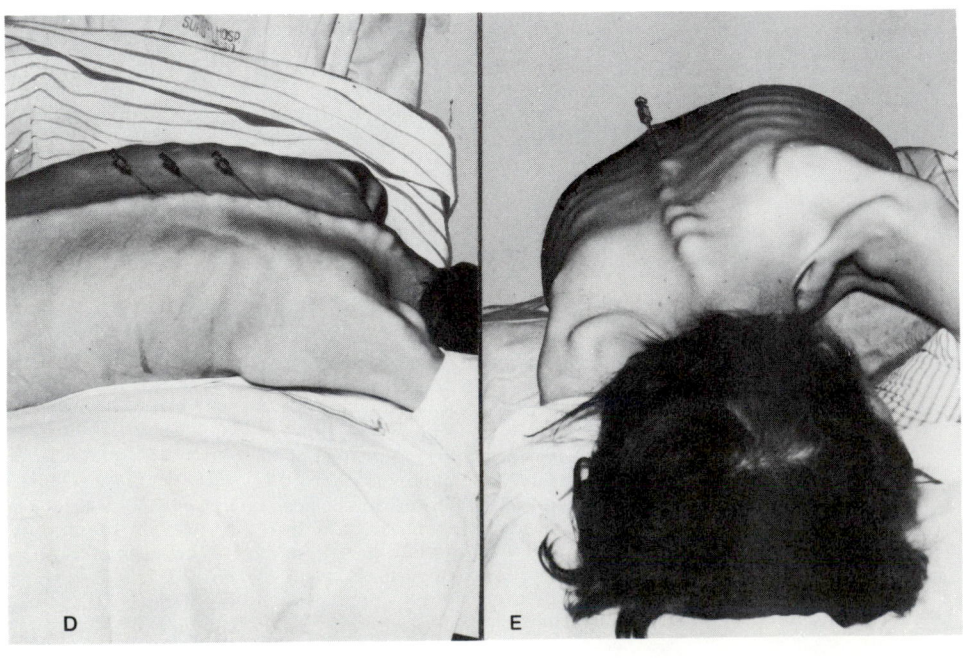

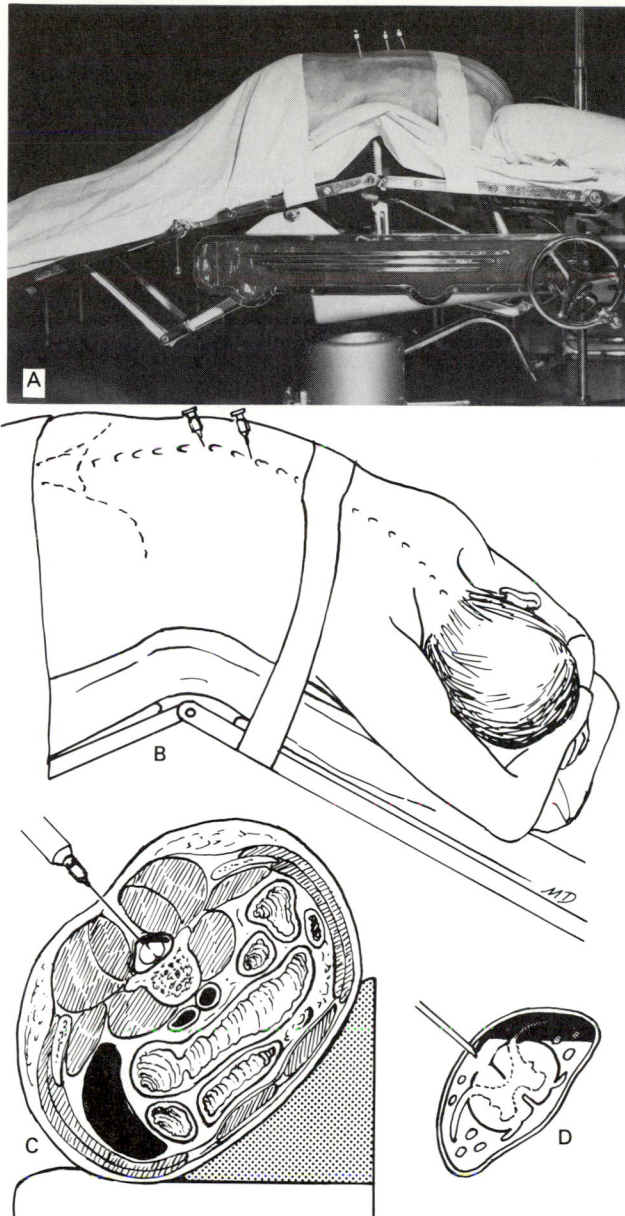

FIG. 96-21. **A, B.** Position of the patient for subarachnoid alcohol block of the lower thoracic vertebral levels for the relief of cancer pain in the pelvis and thigh. The gallbladder lift and the pillow over it are used to obviate lumbar lordosis. The table was then moved so that the upper part of the body was lower than the lower trunk. Three needles are in place for the injection of 0.05-ml aliquots of alcohol. **C.** Cross-sectional representation of the body showing the angle it makes with the table. **D.** Diffusion of the alcohol to bathe the posterior rootlets and roots.

foramen, as suggested by some (3). At their attachment to the cord are 8 to 12 fila radicularia, which provide a greater surface area and are thus much more susceptible to the action of the neurolytic agent than the root or the dorsal root ganglion. To place the bevel of the needle precisely at the desired segment(s), it is necessary to recall that below the 3rd cervical spinal segment the spinal cord levels from which the rootlets of a spinal nerve originate are not at the same levels of the corresponding vertebrae (Fig. 96-23). This is particularly true for the thoracic, lumbar, and sacral segments. Although a patient might not have the exact correlation between spinal cord segments and vertebrae as that shown, it is sufficiently accurate so that it can be followed

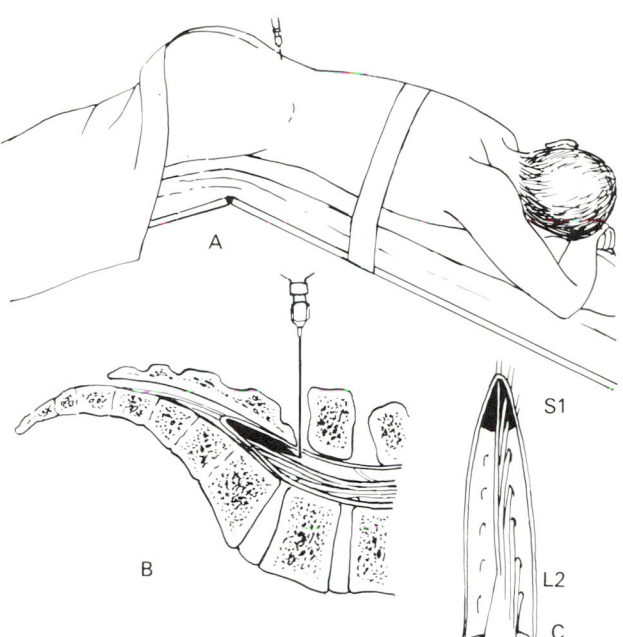

FIG. 96-22. **A.** Patient in steep Kraske's position for injection of alcohol to destroy the rootlets of S4, S5, and the coccygeal nerve to relieve severe perineal pain. The needle puncture is made at the L5–S1 interspace, with the bevel of the needle just anterior to the dura arachnoid. **B.** Injection of hypobaric alcohol drop by drop causes the alcohol to rise to above the cerebrospinal fluid level and eventually to settle in the lowest part of the sac. **C.** Diffusion of the alcohol is limited to S4, S5, and the coccygeal nerves. Properly done, this produces analgesia in the perianal region and posterior part of the perineum. The procedure is especially indicated for patients with severe pain after abdomino-perineal resection and subsequent metastasis to the region.

with a certain degree of assurance. Once the interspaces are decided on, the spinous processes of the vertebrae must be counted carefully, beginning with C7 downward, and the findings confirmed by counting from the L5 interspace upward.

Puncture in the lumbar region is usually simple because the interspaces are wide and almost perpendicular to the skin and the subarachnoid space contains the cauda equina, but puncture is much more difficult above the T11 or T12 interspace because of two anatomic facts: (a) between the T2 and T8 or T9 vertebrae the laminae and spinous processes of the vertebrae are imbricated, making the interspaces narrow (moreover, elderly people can have bony spurs on the tips of the adjacent spinous processes and, in some cases, the supraspinous ligament is ossified, making a midline approach impossible); and (b) the subarachnoid space in this region is much narrower. Thus, the greatest of care must be exercised in placing the short bevel of the needle in the posterior part of the subarachnoid space just anterior to the dura-arachnoid. Equally important is the fact that the injection must be made in the most posterior part of the subarachnoid space so that the alcohol, as it is injected drop by drop, rises along the curvature of the arachnoid to the top of the CSF as a layer and thus bathes only the desired posterior rootlets. By using the technique illustrated in Figure 96-24 it is possible to puncture the dura-arachnoid safely and obtain CSF and to inject the neurolytic agent without difficulty.

Once the bevel of the needle is in the subarachnoid space, the alcohol is slowly injected in 0.1-ml aliquots with 60 to 90 seconds between each injection. Before and during injection the patient should be told to

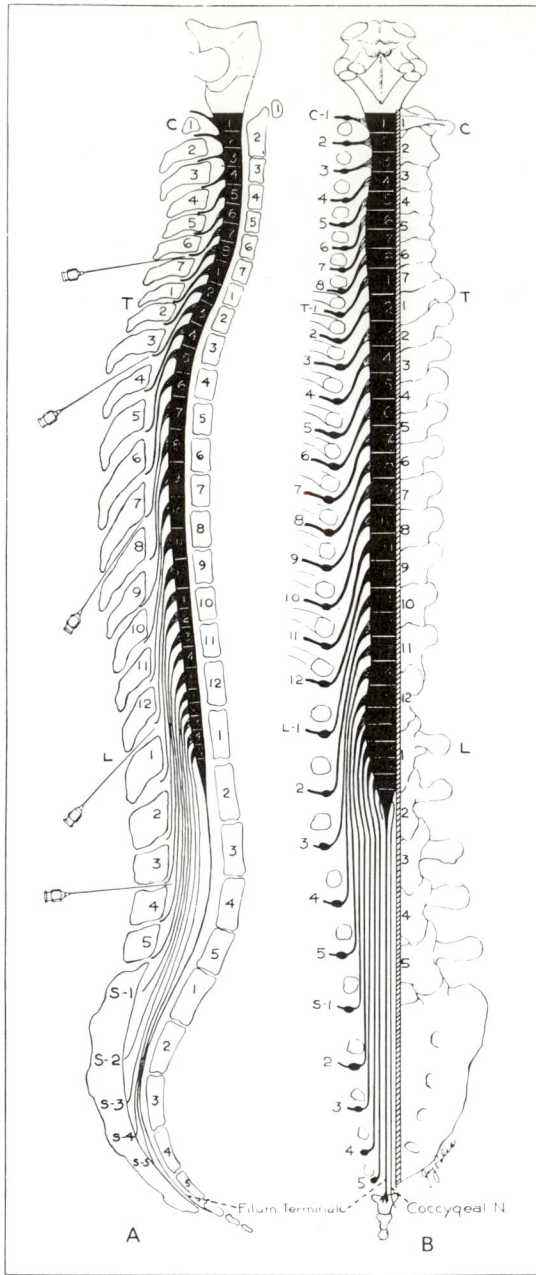

Fig. 96-23. Schematic representation of relationships of the spinal column, the spinal cord, the spinal nerves, and the sites of attachment of their rootlets. **A.** Lateral view. Also shown are the angles of the shafts of needles inserted for dural puncture at different vertebral levels. **B.** Posterior view showing relationships of the vertebrae to the spinal cord segments and to the rootlets of various spinal nerves.

expect a feeling of warmth, burning pain, and tingling that lasts a few seconds and then fades. In addition, the skin of the segments involved manifests hyperemia. After injection of each aliquot the effect of alcohol in producing hypalgesia should be assessed by the pin scratch technique (Chapter 31).

Based on extensive experience I firmly believe that, if more than two segments of the spinal cord are involved in transmitting nociceptive impulses, it is preferable to insert multiple needles and inject small amounts through each needle rather than to inject a large amount of alcohol through one needle to obtain a widespread effect. If, for example, the pain involves the T5 to T10 segments, a needle is placed in the T3, T5, and T7 interspaces and 0.2 ml of alcohol is injected through each needle in 0.1-ml aliquots. This drop-by-drop injection technique prevents widespread diffusion of the alcohol and thus increases its concentration to the target rootlets and decreases the risk of complications. This is especially important in blocks to provide relief of pain in the upper limb, where it is essential to minimize the diffusion of the alcohol to the anterior roots.

During and following the injection the blood pressure, pulse, respiration, and color are noted and recorded. The patient should remain in the same position for 25 to 30 minutes to ensure that the alcohol is completely "fixed" to the nerve tissue and that none is left in the CSF to diffuse to undesired rootlets. Following this period the patient is placed in a supine position with the head slightly lower than the rest of the body, remaining in this position for the next 24 hours to decrease the risk of loss of spinal fluid and encouraged to drink as much fluid as possible to minimize the incidence of postpuncture headache.

SUBARACHNOID PHENOL OR CHLOROCRESOL. The technique of injecting phenol or chlorocresol in glycerin is different from that for subarachnoid alcohol for several reasons: (a) because the solution is hyperbaric, the patient needs to be placed on the table with the affected rootlets lowermost; (b) because the solution is viscid, a 20-gauge short-beveled needle is required, and the injection with the tuberculin syringe requires considerable force; and (c) the onset of definitive blockade can be evaluated within a day of the injection, whereas it requires a longer period with alcohol. The procedure is carried out with the affected side down and the back turned, so that its surface makes a 45° angle with the surface of the table (Figs. 96-25 and 96-26). Swerdlow (71) has used a total dose of phenol or chlorocresol in glycerin ranging from 0.5 to 1.0 ml, depending chiefly on the number of segments being blocked, the length of the spine, and the part of the spine being injected, with a smaller volume injected in the sacral segments and a larger one in the thoracic region. Whereas phenol invariably produces sensory changes, chlorocresol frequently does not cause any sensory changes. Thus, Mehta (72) has used a mixture of equal parts of phenol and chlorocresol in glycerin in the hope of obtaining the benefits of localization by the phenol along with the longer duration of action of chlorocresol.

Evaluation of Results and Reinjection

When the block is effective and is localized to the involved segments, the relief of pain is remarkable. Such relief can occur within a few hours or a day after injection of phenol or chlorocresol, or it might not be complete until several days after injection of alcohol. Following injection, zones of hypalgesia, analgesia, and hypesthesia occur, frequently with diminution or complete loss of pinprick and temperature sensation. The stretch afferents are usually also blocked and

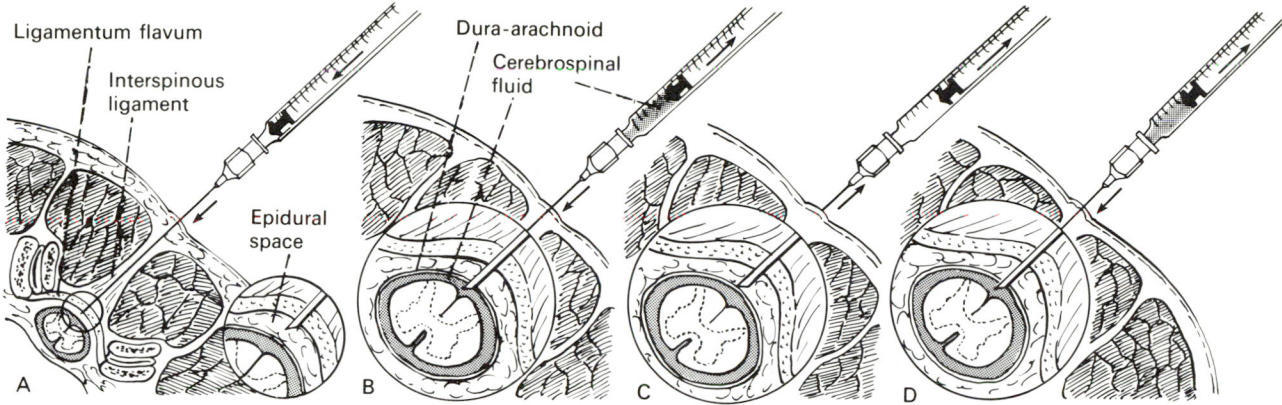

Ligamentum flavum
Interspinous ligament
Epidural space
Dura-arachnoid
Cerebrospinal fluid

FIG. 96-24. Technique of puncture of the dura arachnoid for subarachnoid injection of neurolytic agents. It is *essential* to have the bevel of the needle just anterior to the anterior surface of the arachnoid membrane to limit diffusion of the neurolytic agent to the posteromedial part of the subarachnoid space. *A.* The needle is inserted in the usual manner except that, when the needle is felt to pass through the tough ligamentum flavum and into the epidural space (using the lack of resistance test described in Chapter 94), the needle is attached to the 2-ml Luer-Lok syringe and advanced about 3 to 4 mm within the lumbar epidural space or 2 to 3 mm in the thoracic epidural space and 1 to 2 mm in the cervical epidural space. To detect penetration of the dura-arachnoid promptly, the plunger of the syringe is withdrawn while aspirating to cause a negative pressure at the bevel of the needle. *B.* The needle is advanced *slowly* until its passage through the dura-arachnoid and its entrance into the arachnoid space is indicated by the usual snap and the almost simultaneous appearance of cerebrospinal fluid (CSF) in the syringe. *C.* The proper position of the bevel of the needle is further ascertained by first reinjecting the CSF into the subarachnoid space and then attempting to aspirate fluid with the empty syringe while the needle is slowly withdrawn, until the free flow of fluid stops. If the needle point has been properly placed it need only be withdrawn 1 or 2 mm before its point leaves the subarachnoid space. *D.* The needle is advanced again until CSF can be aspirated once more. Because aspiration of fluid is frequently impeded by a veil of arachnoid, and in the lumbar region by nerve rootlets, the injection of 0.3 to 0.5 ml of air or saline solution causes the obstructing structure to move away from the bevel. Once the bevel of the needle is just anterior to the anterior surface of the arachnoid the neurolytic agent can be slowly injected. (Insets represent an enlargement of the region to show details of the structures.)

certain reflexes are diminished or absent. Sometimes a zone of hyperesthesia extends beyond the zone of analgesia, possibly also with fibrillary muscle twitching and muscle jerking; all of these effects disappear within a few days. Because the maximum effects of alcohol block might not be obvious for several days, assessment must be postponed until 3 to 5 days after injection. If the patient is still having pain after this period it is advisable to reinject the various segments that remain painful. It has been our experience that the initial injection provides adequate relief in about 60% of patients, so that about 40% require a second injection and 50% of these require a third injection (73).

If a patient has been on a strong opioid for over 2 weeks and derives good pain relief with one or more subarachnoid neurolytic injections, special care should be exercised in continuing the opioid analgesic; it should not be stopped suddenly, because withdrawal symptoms could develop. Such symptoms might cause patients to complain and confuse the issue of whether the subarachnoid neurolytic blockade is completely effective. It is therefore important in such instances to taper the dose of opioid given over a period of 7 to 10 days. Often it is necessary to continue to give patients small or moderate doses of opioids to relieve "other pain" that might be present outside of the area of the neurolytic blockade.

In patients who have bilateral pain, it is preferable not to attempt to block both sides with one injection because this would require a large volume of solution and consequently increase the risk of complications.

Usually the side that has the most intense pain is blocked and the injection is repeated until good relief is achieved. After an interval of several days blocks are carried out for the other side.

It has been claimed that subarachnoid alcohol or phenol does not produce the same beneficial effect in the upper thoracic and cervical segments (71, 74, 75) because of several factors: (a) the dural sheath in which the neurolytic agent "settles" in the cervical segments is relatively short; (b) the cervical nerve roots and rootlets have a short intrathecal course and therefore have less exposure to the neurolytic agent; and (c) the spinal canal is narrow, with a stronger current of CSF that tends to carry the neurolytic agent away from the target nerve rootlets. We have obtained good results, however, by inserting a needle through each of the interspinous spaces involved and injecting 0.2 ml of absolute alcohol in 0.05-ml aliquots through each of two or three needles (Fig. 96-20). Others have used extradural or subdural injection of phenol for this purpose (74–77).

Results

Various reports on the results of therapy using subarachnoid neurolytic blockade are difficult to compare because of differences in the assessment of pain and of pain relief, the types and sites of tumor for which the procedure was done, and the sites and doses of alcohol injection. Moreover, many of the reports lack specific data on the incidence, severity, and duration of side effects and complications.

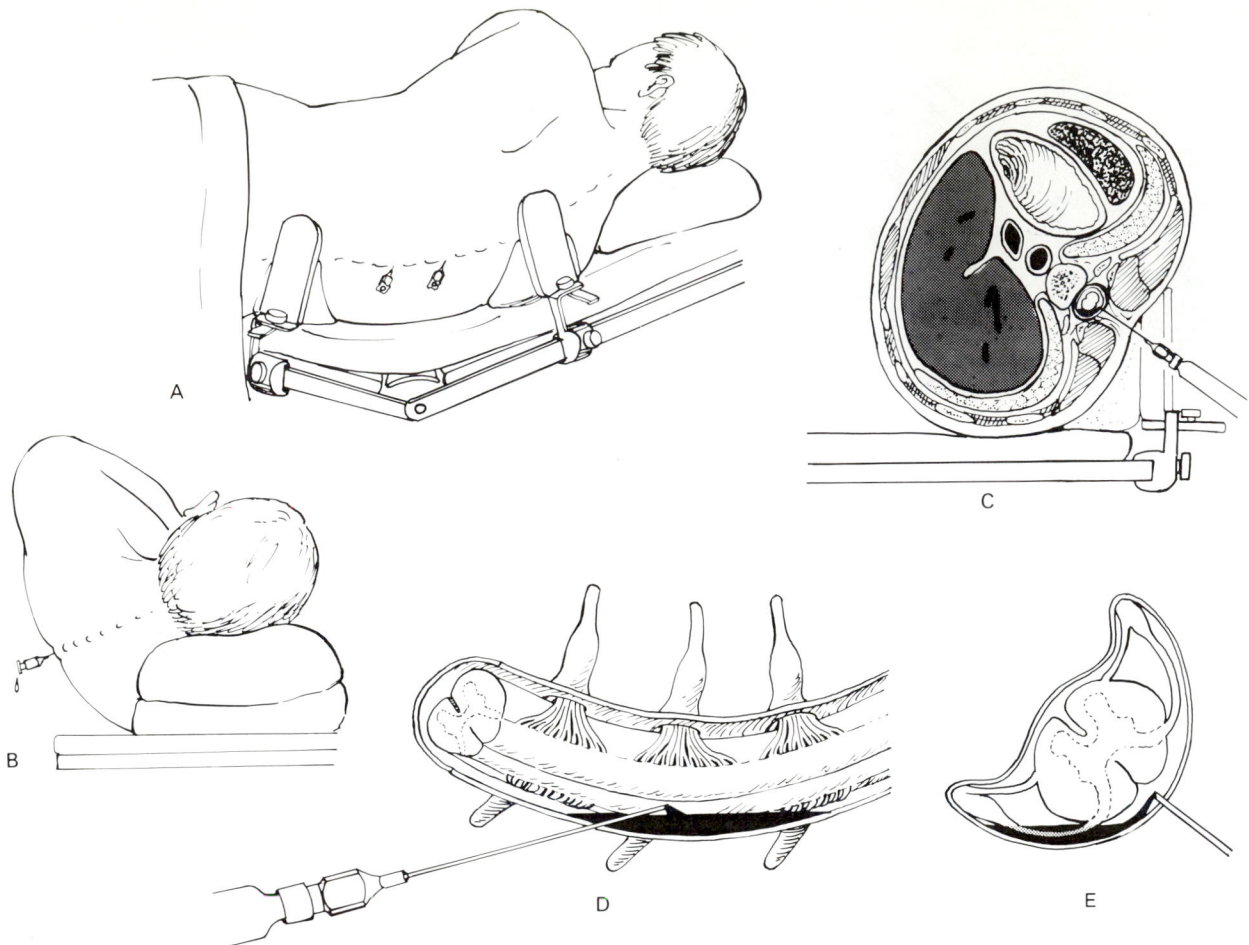

FIG. 96-25. Technique of subarachnoid injection of hyperbaric phenol in glycerin. **A.** The dural-arachnoid puncture is made with the patient on the side, with the affected side underneath. **B.** Once CSF emerges from the hub of the needle the upper part of the body is displaced posteriorly so that the posterior surface of the back makes an angle of 45° with the superior surface of the table. **C.** Cross-sectional representation of the body in the same position as **B.** This position is maintained with kidney rests or with wide adhesive tape across the patient's body attached to the lateral edges of the table. Schematic longitudinal section (**D**) and cross section (**E**) to show diffusion of hyperbaric phenol to the posterior (sensory) rootlets that transmit nociceptive information, which are lowermost.

Table 96-3 summarizes some of the most important reports of results with subarachnoid alcohol, and Table 96-4 summarizes some reports of results obtained with phenol in glycerin. "Good" pain relief indicates that the patient obtained complete or almost complete relief of pain for which the procedure(s) was done until the death of the patient. "Fair" relief means complete relief of pain for less than 1 month or pain relief of 50% or more until the patient's death, and "poor" relief indicates that the patient experienced partial relief for a few days or no relief at all. In many cases more than one block was done to achieve the reported results. Based on personal experience I believe that in those reports in which the incidence of combined good and fair relief was lower than 60%, an improper technique was used. For example, the neurolytic agent was injected into the lumbar region and then change in posture was used in an attempt to direct the neurolytic agent to the affected segments in the mid-thoracic or high thoracic area. As I have emphasized (1), such a technique not only produces

inadequate pain relief but results in an unacceptably high complication rate because the drug diffuses sufficiently caudad to cause urinary and bowel dysfunction, as well as weakness in the lower limbs.

In 1951 I presented the first report (later published) (61) containing an analysis of the results obtained in 194 patients with cancer pain who were treated with various neurolytic techniques, including 68 patients who received 107 subarachnoid blocks with alcohol. As noted in Table 96-3 (61), 37 patients (54%) obtained complete or almost complete relief of pain, which permitted the gradual reduction in dosage of strong opioids in those who had received them. Another 22 patients (32%) had partial relief and were made comfortable with moderate doses of opioids and adjuvants (usually less than half the amount they had been receiving at the time of the block). Despite one or even two reinjections, 9 patients (14%) derived only transient relief of pain and required strong opioids.

In 1958, 7 years later, I published a summary of the results obtained in an additional 114 patients, which was added to the results of the first group and shown as a second series in

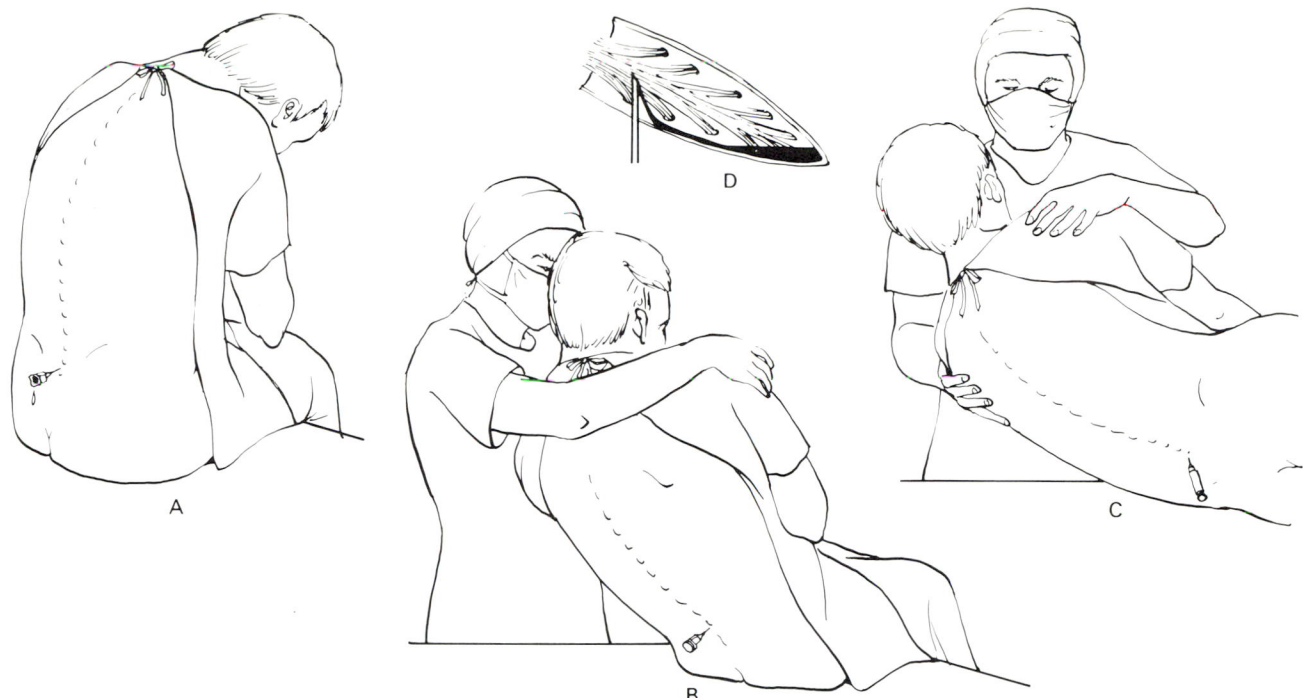

Fig. 96-26. Technique of injecting hyperbaric phenol in glycerin to block the rootlets of the lower sacral and coccygeal nerves. **A.** Position of the patient for puncture at the L5–S1 interspace. **B.** Position of the patient for injection of phenol to achieve bilateral block. **C.** Position of the patient for unilateral block of the lower lumbar and sacral roots. **D.** Diffusion of phenol along the left side of the subarachnoid space to contact the rootlets of the S4, S5, and coccygeal nerves.

Table 96-3 (84). Although the results regarding pain relief were similar, those in the second group experienced a lower incidence of complications (see Table 96-5). This was because the earlier experience (when one needle was used to inject 1 to 1.5 ml of alcohol to block several segments) prompted me to adopt the multiple-needle technique and to inject small volumes of alcohol (see above: Techniques, Subarachnoid Alcohol). All these patients were managed in a community hospital in a medium-sized city, which facilitated careful follow-up (61). In the ensuing 19 years I carried out subarachnoid block with alcohol in an additional 167 patients, who received a total of 228 blocks (Table 96-3) (unpublished data). As noted in Tables 96-3 and 96-5, the analgesia improved slightly, with a further decrease in complications, reflecting a more conservative attitude and a more careful selection of patients.

TABLE 96-3. Comparison of Results with Subarachnoid Alcohol Block for the Relief of Cancer Pain

Source	No. of Patients	Results (% of Patients Treated)		
		Good	Fair	Little or None
Dogliotti (69)	150	59	25	16
Stern (78)	50	63	25	10
Abbott (79)	25	84	18	8
Poppen (80)	57	72	18	10
Peyton et al. (81)	27	59	23	18
Truelsen (82)	69	59	23	18
Greenhill and Schmitz (83)	100	60	10	30
Bonica (61)	68	54	32	14
Bonica (84)	182	55	29	16
Parese (85)	95	57	32	11
Hay (86)	322	46	32	22
Kuzucu et al. (87)	322	58	26	16
Bonica (unpublished data)	167	62	23	14
All/Mean:	1,634	61 85*	24	15
Gerbershagen (73)	1,478	60 81	21	19
Papke (88)	1,908	60 81	21	19

*The combined good and fair percentages.

TABLE 96-4. Comparison of Results with Intrathecal Phenol in Glycerin or Iophendylate for the Relief of Cancer Pain

Source	No. of Patients	Results (% of Patients Treated)			
		Good	Fair	Good-Fair*	Poor
Brown (89)	38			79	21
Mark et al. (90)	66			55	45
Tank et al. (91)	23	48	18		34
Wilkinson et al. (92)	27			67	23
Ball et al. (93)	51	41	33		36
Maher (74)	352	66	2		32
Stovner and Enderson (76)	151			77	23
Maher (75)	433	62	6		32
Brown (77)	114	68	5		27
Lifshitz (94)	117			77	23
Papo and Visca (95)	290	40	35		25
Swerdlow (71)	320	57	19		24
All/Mean:	1982	58	16	73	28

*Reports that combined good and fair results in one number.

It is generally acknowledged that, in the hands of those who have experience extensive enough with one or the other agent to be considered as an "expert," the results of therapy with subarachnoid alcohol are similar to those obtained with phenol in glycerin. Pain relief appears to be better and to last longer with alcohol, however, than with phenol. On the other hand, Maher (14, 74) stated that phenol is easier to handle, spares "non-pain-conducting fibers," and yields better results than alcohol. The latter two advantages are disputed by the histologic evidence cited above (A. Basic Considerations) and also by the clinical experience of those who have used both agents. Brown (96) stated that "alcohol has proved to be easier to control and to achieve better results than when phenol solutions are employed." Gerbershagen (73), who has used both agents, also prefers alcohol. Tank and colleagues (91) studied a number of patients who had been treated either with alcohol or phenol in glycerin, and found that the risk of sphincter paralysis with phenol was lower, but that otherwise alcohol was superior. Our own experience suggests that sphincter control can be minimized, but not eliminated, by giving a small volume through multiple needles in properly positioned patients (Figs. 96-20 and 96-25).

Important causes of failure with the use of subarachnoid neurolytic agents include intraspinal tumor infiltration, as frequently occurs in those with Pancoast's tumor, which prevents the neurolytic agent from coming into contact with the rootlets. Therefore, prior to carrying out the procedure, it is essential to rule out this possibility by appropriate radiographic tests, such as CT scanning, especially in patients who have tumors that are likely to spread or metastasize to the intraspinal canal. If such screening has not been done and the first injection, which should otherwise produce analgesia, has no effect, it is advisable for the physician to consider such a possibility. Prior radiation therapy to the spinal canal can also interfere with the pathophysiologic effects of neurolytic agents. It is also important to consider assessing patients for other sites or causes of pain, such as physical disabilities. A frequent cause of "failure" is the development of extension of the lesion, with consequent pain beyond the area in which block for the previous pain remains effective. Obviously in such a case it would be necessary either to carry out an additional subarachnoid block or some other neurolytic technique or, possibly, to consider percutaneous cordotomy, if available.

Complications

Complications can occur even when a flawless technique is employed, but the incidence of serious complications can be minimized by proper selection, preparation, and positioning of patients and by the use of precise technique. Some complications are not serious and are transient; others occur rarely and only with a break in aseptic technique, whereas still others can occur as a result of diffusion of the neurolytic agent to the anterior roots in the lower cervical and T1 regions or to the lumbosacral region. Headache can occur following the block, but this is transitory and responds well to conservative therapy. Aseptic meningitis, caused by irritation by the neurolytic agent, occurs but is rare. Septic meningitis can also occur but only a few cases have been reported (65).

Paresis or paralysis of the muscles occurs if the anterior rootlets are sufficiently involved in the pathophysiologic process to interrupt motor function. Involvement of the anterior roots by the neurolytic agent in the three middle sacral segments interrupts the parasympathetic fibers to the bladder and the rectum and lower colon, which could cause loss of sphincteric function, urinary retention, and bowel incontinence. Annoying and sometimes distressing side effects of block of the posterior rootlets include loss of proprioception and touch and troublesome dysesthesias. Complication rates reported by various authors are presented in Table 96-5. Fortunately, most of these complications are transient. A case of fatal meningitis was believed to have been caused by meningeal irritation by silver nitrate incorporated into the phenol solution (65). Few patients with postblock paraplegia were subsequently found to have vertebral metastasis (65).

TABLE 96-5. Complications with the Use of Subarachnoid Neurolytic Block for the Relief of Cancer Pain

Source	No. of Patients	Complications (% of Patients Treated)			
		Bladder Paresis	Bowel Paresis	Muscle Weakness	Other
Alcohol					
Peyton et al. (81)	27	20 (4)*		15 (6)	6 (6)
Bonica (61)	68	7 (1)	6 (1)	9 (2)	3 (1)
Bonica (84)	162	4 (1)	5 (2)	8 (1)	6 (1.5)
Hay (86)	252	0.7	1	1	3.4
Kuzucu et al. (87)	322	0.6 (0.1)	0.6 (0.1)	1.5 (0.1)	1.5
Bonica (unpublished data)	167	3 (1)	4 (1)	7 (1)	
Phenol or chlorocresol					
Papo and Visca (95)	290	4.7 (1.7)		6.8 (3.8)	
Stover and Enderson (76)	151	4 (1)	1.5 (1.5)	7 (2)	2
Lifshitz et al. (94)	133	22	2.2	23	
Swerdlow (71)	300	12	1.5	3.5	4

*Percentage in parenthesis represents prolonged complications.

Muscle weakness in the upper or lower limbs occurs as a result of involvement of the anterior roots, with the risk being much higher in the lower limbs because of the proximity of the anterior and posterior roots in the lumbosacral enlargement of the cord (at the T10 and L1 vertebral levels). Below the L1 level injection is made into the cauda equina, where the anterior and posterior rootlets are not as well separated as above these levels. Except in patients who have severe respiratory disease, paresis of the intercostal muscles, of segments of the abdominal muscles on one side, or even of a few segments bilaterally, does not significantly affect ventilation.

Bladder dysfunction occurs most frequently with injection below the T10 interspace. Although some have reported that injection to relieve perineal pain at the L5 interspace is associated with an incidence of bladder paresis ranging from 25 to 60% (97), use of the technique shown in Figure 96-22 is associated with an incidence lower than this.

Gerbershagen (73) reviewed reports that provided data on the duration of 303 complications (Table 96-6) and obtained the following results: 28% disappeared within 3 days; 23% disappeared within 1 week; 21% disappeared within 1 month; 9% disappeared within 4

TABLE 96-6. Complications of 2125 Alcohol Subarachnoid Blocks

Complication	Duration of Complication					
	Transient		Permanent		Total	
	No.	(%)	No.	(%)	No.	(%)
Paresis or paralysis	92	(4.3)	18	(0.8)	110	(5.2)
Bladder dysfunction	137	(6.4)	16	(0.8)	153	(7.2)
Bowel disorder	8	(0.4)	3	(0.1)	11	(0.5)
Other	19	(0.9)	10	(0.5)	29	(1.4)
All	256	(12)	47	(2.0)	303	(14.0)

From Gerbershagen, H.Y.: Neurolysis: Subarachnoid neurolytic blockade. Acta Anaesthesiol. Belg., 1:45, 1981.

months; and 18% lasted longer than 4 months. Table 96-7 presents an analysis by Swerdlow (71) of the incidence of complications in 300 patients managed with 5 or 7% phenol in glycerin, 2 or 2.5% chlorocresol in glycerin, or a combination of these.

Epidural Neurolytic Blockade

The theoretic advantages of the use of epidural injection over intrathecal neurolysis include less risk of meningeal irritation, less spread of the solution to cranial nerves, and supposedly less risk of bladder and rectal involvement. Swerdlow (71) has employed epidural neurolytics in patients suffering from extensive nonterminal intractable pain, and a fair degree of success was achieved with the injection of phenol in glycerin. Madrid (98) used 7.5% phenol in glycerin and noted good pain relief in a high percentage of patients. Others have used aqueous phenol injected through an epidural catheter. Rafferty (99) reported employing an epidural catheter and used intermittent doses of 0.5 to 1 ml of 6% aqueous phenol, which produced good pain relief in 65% of 27 patients. My former colleagues, Colpitts and associates (100), while staff members of the Clinical Pain Service at the University of Washington, used epidural phenol on patients with cancer-related pain and obtained prolonged pain relief in slightly more than 80% of patients. Racz and co-workers (101) have used phenol in saline for the same purpose. More recently Korevaar (102) reported favorable results using transcatheter thoracic epidural neurolysis achieved with ethyl alcohol.

Technique

Most authors use phenol in glycerin, but some use an aqueous solution of phenol. The technique of epidural puncture is described in detail in Chapter 94. A 22-gauge needle can be used for a single injection of aqueous phenol, but it is necessary to use a 20-gauge spinal needle for injection of phenol in glycerin. Once the bevel of the needle is in the epidural space the patient is tilted backward into a 45° angle (as for subarachnoid phenol injection) and a test dose of 0.2 ml of phenol is injected. After ascertaining that the

TABLE 96-7. Complications Lasting Longer Than 7 Days in 300 Patients

Drug(s)	No. of Patients	Complication						
		Bladder Paresis	Bowel Paresis	Muscle Paresis	Headache	Paresthesia	Numbness	Total
		No. (%)	No. (%)	No. (%)	No. (%)	No. (%)	No. (%)	No. (%)
Phenol	145	7 (5)	1 (0.7)	4 (3)		1 (0.7)	4 (3)	17 (12)
Chlorocresol	138	10 (7)	1 (0.7)	7 (5)	1 (0.7)	1 (0.7)	4 (4)	25 (1)
Phenol and chlorocresol	17	3 (18)	1 (6)		1 (6)		1 (6)	6 (35)
All/Mean:	300	20 (7)	3 (1)	11 (4)	2 (1)	2 (0.7)	9 (3)	47 (16)

From Swerdlow, M.: Intrathecal and extradural block and pain relief. *In* Relief of Intractable Pain. Edited by M. Swerdlow. Amsterdam, Elsevier, 1983.

solution has not been deposited into the subarachnoid space, about 2 ml of 7% phenol in glycerin or of 8 to 10% aqueous phenol is injected for each nerve root to be blocked. Swerdlow (71) has recommended that in the cervical region the dose should be 1.5 ml/dermatome. After injection the patient remains in the tilted position for about 40 minutes. With successful blocks pain disappears in about 10 to 15 minutes.

Some authors have reported relief of pain for as long as 9 months (71) but Madrid (98), using 7.5% phenol in glycerin for pain in the neck, noted that pain relief lasted only a few days. Some clinicians have used an epidural catheter to allow repeated injections of phenol in glycerin into the cervical region. The epidural puncture is made at the C7–T1 interspace and the catheter is advanced about 4 to 5 cm.

Placement of the catheter can be checked by injection of a small amount of metrizamide, which should produce a rather diffuse outline immediately anterior to the posterior wall of the pierced canal. Catheter placement can also be checked by injection of small doses of a local anesthetic, such as 2 ml of 1% lidocaine at 15- to 20-minute intervals, and this should produce a narrow band of segmental sensory loss. If a local anesthetic is used for this purpose it is essential to allow the anesthetic to dissipate and to wait 2 hours more after its disappearance before the neurolytic agent is injected.

Racz and co-workers (101) have reported on the use of the Racz catheter for multiple epidural injections of 5.5% phenol in saline. After confirmation of the position of the catheter in the cervical region by radiographic control and by the injection of 3 ml of 0.5% bupivacaine and the aspiration test, injection of aliquots of phenol 24 hours after the prognostic block can be initiated using a total of 2.5 to 5 ml for the cervical region. This technique has been used to treat not only cancer pain but also radiculopathy, reflex sympathetic dystrophy, and chronic pain syndromes in patients with spasticity.

In a series of 18 patients with cancer pain treated with this technique (101), 6 of 11 patients (54%) with metastatic cancer and 6 of 7 patients (86%) with primary cancer derived good relief. In patients with primary cancer, pain relief lasted less than a month in 1 patient (17%), 1 to 3 months in 3 patients (50%), 3 to 6 months in 1 patient (17%), and longer than 6 months in 1 patient (17%); in those with metastatic cancer the figures were 3 (49%), 2 (33%), 0 (0%), and 1 (15%), respectively. Among those patients whose pain returned within 1 month a second series of injections increased the duration of relief by 1 to 3 months.

In treating patients with cancer-related pain, Colpitts and associates (100) first stabilized them on a narcotic-containing "pain cocktail." Once patients were stabilized, the amount of narcotics was gradually reduced until patients began to experience moderate pain. The pain cocktail, given in a time-contingent manner (Chapter 81), was intended to eliminate the psychologic factors that were contributing to the pain. The epidural catheter was inserted and placed with its tip in the center of the band of pain and 3 to 4 ml of 1 to 2% lidocaine was injected to ascertain the proper position of the catheter and the volume of phenol required to relieve the pain. Colpitts and colleagues then injected the same volume of phenol, and patients were observed for 24 hours. Patients were followed in a VA hospital, where they were either inpatients or outpatients who returned for follow-up every 2 weeks. Pain relief lasted until all the patients who had initial relief died, which varied from 3 weeks to $4\frac{1}{2}$ months.

Korevaar (102) has recently reported on the use of a technique similar to that reported by Rafferty (99) for phenol. He used "transcatheter" thoracic epidural neurolysis with alcohol in 36 consecutive inpatients with intractable somatic or visceral pain of malignant and nonmalignant origin that was referable to the cervical or thoracic nerve roots. These included 14 patients with cancer of the pancreas, 13 with metastatic cancer in the abdominal or thoracic region, 4 with chronic pancreatitis, 2 with postherpetic neuralgia (in the T4 and T5 regions), and 3 with diffuse abdominal pain of unknown origin.

The epidural catheter was introduced so that its tip was in the center of the dermatomal pain distribution. Five to 7 ml of 0.25% bupivacaine was injected in 2-ml increments to determine correct catheter placement. Patients were in a 30° head-up supine position for bilateral visceral or somatic pain or were positioned with the affected side up in a lateral position for unilateral somatic pain. Once the efficacy of the local anesthetic block had been ascertained, Korevaar (102) injected increments of 0.2 ml of absolute alcohol until 3 to 5 ml of neurolytic agent had been injected over a 20- to 30-minute period.

After completion of the alcohol injections the catheter was flushed with 0.25 ml of the 0.25% bupivacaine solution and capped. Patients were returned to their hospital rooms 30 minutes after completion of the injections and followed for pain relief. The second and third alcohol injections were done on a daily basis unless patients experienced 100% pain relief that persisted over a 24-hour period and decreased their narcotic use by at least 25%. On the second and third days 3 to 5 ml of ethyl alcohol was slowly injected 10 minutes after the catheter was tested using 2 ml of 0.5% bupivacaine.

Patients were monitored closely; 89% of patients were judged to have been successfully treated because they reported 70% pain relief or greater, supported by a decrease in narcotic dose of 25% or more. All 27 patients who had pancreatic and metastatic cancer had immediate pain relief that continued for the first week, as compared to pain relief in 55% of patients with nonmalignant chronic pain. The overall duration of pain relief for patients who had been successfully treated ranged from 2 weeks to 7 months (mean 3.3 months), reflecting the large number of patients who died of their underlying illness during the period of study. Twelve patients with cancer died within 4 months after treatment. Twenty patients who died during the study reported continued relief of pain until death, and 12 patients survived long enough to have recurrence of pain. The duration of pain relief in these patients extended from 3 weeks to 7.25 months, (mean 4.4 months). Although a few complications such as hypotension, vomiting, pain on injection, and pain at the site of the catheter during the first 3 days were noted, no long-term serious complications occurred. Korevaar's (102) results are impressive and suggest that the technique should be given more extensive trial.

Subdural Neurolysis

In 1960 Maher (66) introduced the use of the subdural injection of phenol in glycerin for the cervical and upper thoracic regions as an alternative to subarachnoid neurolysis because of difficulty in achieving good results with the latter method. Since then the technique has been used only by a few others, whose results have not been impressive.

Anatomic Basis

The subdural space is a potential space between the dura and arachnoid, separated by a thin film of fluid. This space is separated from the subarachnoid space by the arachnoid mater and extends laterally for a short distance, where it widens into the region of the nerve roots. Injection of any fluid creates a potential space that extends cephalad to the foramen magnum and caudally to the level of the termination of the dura at the level of the S2 vertebra. The subdural space is wider in the cervical region and thus is easier to enter here than at other levels of the spine. Trabeculae of connective tissue throughout the subdural space course between the dura and arachnoid, similar to those seen between the arachnoid and pia mater except that the subdural space is much narrower. These trabeculae account for the "honeycomb" appearance in radiographs taken after subdural injection of contrast media.

Technique

The procedure is best done with the patient's affected side down and a pillow under the head, and the cervical spine is flexed as much as possible. Following appropriate preparation of the skin and the production of analgesia of the skin and subcutaneous tissue with a 25-gauge needle, a short-beveled 5- or 8-cm 20-gauge spinal needle is inserted into the exact midline and advanced until the epidural space is entered, using the lack of resistance test described in Chapter 94. Image intensification is used to check that the needle is properly placed: in the lateral view the needle should be in line with the posterior wall of the cervical canal, while in the anteroposterior view the needle tip should lie precisely in the midline, aligned with spinous processes. Once the bevel of the needle has entered the epidural space, a 0.5- or 1-ml tuberculin syringe filled with saline is connected to the needle, which is advanced slowly while continuous pressure is exerted on the plunger of the syringe. As soon as the bevel of the needle contacts the dura the patient might experience a transient bout of pain that promptly ceases. Entrance of the bevel of the needle into the subdural space is indicated when *increased* resistance to the injection is felt. This is followed by injection of 0.1 to 0.2 ml of contrast medium to ascertain that the bevel is in the correct space (103). The radiograph taken following injection usually reveals a classic fine line that is a few millimeters anterior to the plane of the posterior wall of the spinal canal; a second line is produced anteriorly, where the contrast medium tends to arrange itself like beads on a necklace in the dural root sleeves (103, 104). An anteroposterior radiograph shows that the bilateral spread is confined to the interior of the canal in what Ischia and colleagues (104) have called the "nail scratch shape" confined to the interior of the canal and extending three or four segments. Once it has been ascertained that the needle is in the subdural space, 5 to 10% phenol in glycerin is injected in doses ranging from 0.5 to 2.5 ml. Cousins and collaborators (3) have suggested that 10% phenol in metrizamide has the advantage of direct visualization during injection.

Results

I could not find specific data on the results achieved by Maher with this technique. Ischia and associates (104) used the procedure in a group of 47 patients, of whom 25 had severe cancer pain and 22 had pain caused by nonmalignant pathologic processes. The results were evaluated as "good" if patients were free of pain until death or until the end of follow-up at 3 months, as "fair" if the analgesic dosage was decreased or if the pain disappeared completely for at least 20 days, and as "poor" or "failure" if patients had lesser degrees of pain relief. Of the 25 cancer patients, 9 patients (36%) had good relief, 7 patients (28%) had fair relief, and 9 patients (36%) were considered to be failures. Results in the 22 patients with nonmalignant pain were 36.5, 9, and 54%, respectively. No complications were reported in any of the patients.

D. NEUROLYTIC SYMPATHETIC BLOCKADE

In Chapter 94 Bonica and Buckley review indications for sympathetic blocks with local anesthetics for various painful conditions in the upper limb, visceral pain, severe pain caused by disease of the thoracic or abdominal viscera, and other painful conditions in the lower limbs (refer to Chapter 94 for details). This section describes the injection of neurolytic agents to cause destruction and consequent prolonged interruption of sympathetic pathways in various parts of the body, including indications, techniques, results, and complications of neurolytic block of the thoracic chain, celiac plexus, splanchnic nerves, and lumbar sympathetic chain.

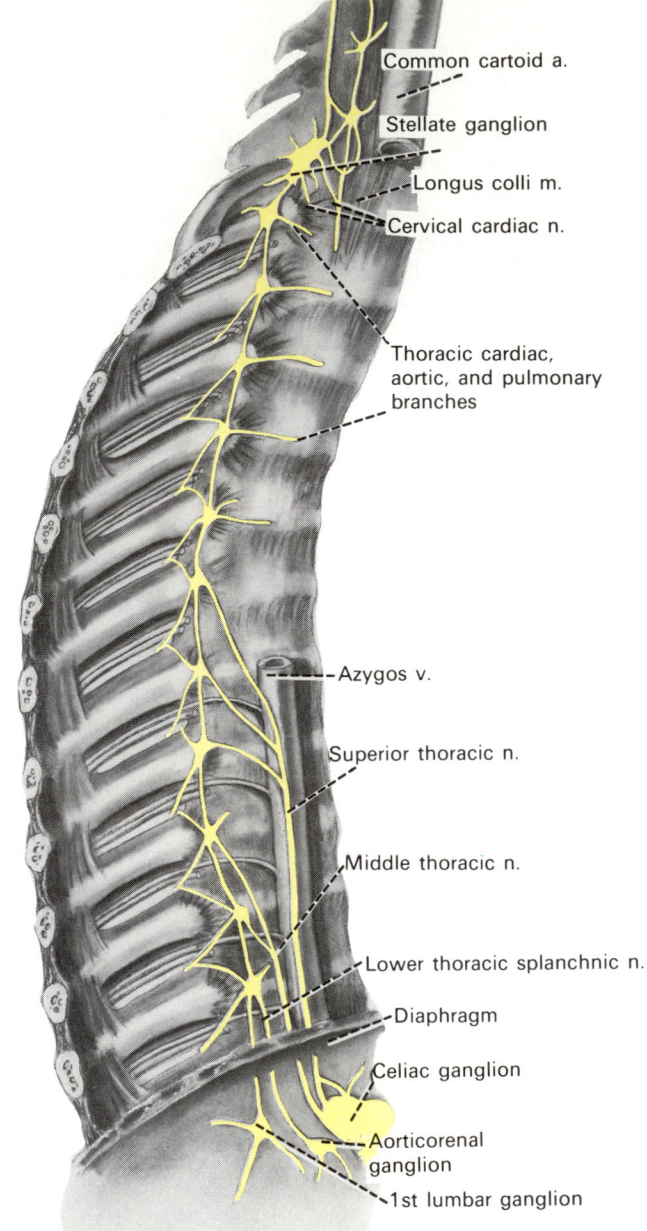

Common cartoid a.

Stellate ganglion

Longus colli m.

Cervical cardiac n.

Thoracic cardiac, aortic, and pulmonary branches

Azygos v.

Superior thoracic n.

Middle thoracic n.

Lower thoracic splanchnic n.

Diaphragm

Celiac ganglion

Aorticorenal ganglion

1st lumbar ganglion

FIG. 96-27. Anatomy of the right thoracic sympathetic chain showing the precise relation of the ganglia to the vertebrae and ribs at various levels, as well as the major branches given off by the chain. The T2 sympathetic ganglion is located anterior to the medial portion of the neck of the ribs, the T3 to T6 ganglia are located in front of the head of the corresponding ribs, the T7 to T10 ganglia are located anterior to the radiate ligaments of the costovertebral joints, and the T11 and T12 ganglia are more anteriorly placed than the rest and are on the lateral surface of the vertebral bodies. In the upper three or four segments the lower half of each ganglion is located in front of the upper portion of the neck or head of the rib. In the lower thoracic segments the ganglia are located in front of the head of the ribs, extending their total length. This is clinically significant because the point of the needle cannot be placed in contact with the lower ganglia. In the upper three segments the intercostal vessels are immediately posterior to part of the ganglia, whereas in the lower segments, where the ganglia rest wholly on the periosteum of the neck or head of the ribs, these vessels are superior to the ganglia. The somatic spinal nerves pass posterior and cephalad to the interganglionic chain. Moreover, the pleura is immediately in front of and closely related to the ganglia, being separated from the ganglia by the thin endothoracic fascia.

To obtain optimal results with these procedures it is essential to adhere to the basic principles of application, including preliminary preparation and various other considerations (Chapter 94). Because the use of neurolytic agents can be associated with serious and unwanted side effects and complications, it is especially important to prepare the patient psychologically and physiologically, to discuss the procedure, anticipated results, and possible complications with the patient and family, to monitor the patient continuously, including monitoring of sympathetic function (Chapter 94), and to adhere to the principles of technique. Neurolytic blocks of this part of the nervous system must be preceded by two or more diagnostic or prognostic blocks (Chapter 94) using local anesthetics with different durations of action to confirm the diagnosis, to determine the pathophysiologic mechanism(s) underlying the condition, and to ascertain whether prolonged interruption is going to be beneficial.

Block of Thoracic Sympathetic Chain

Indications

BLOCK OF SYMPATHETICS TO THE UPPER LIMB. Block of the sympathetics to the upper limb achieved by the neurolytic blockade of T2 and T3 and the interganglionic part of the chain fibers is indicated in the management of causalgia and other reflex sympathetic dystrophies, postamputation pain syndromes, and other painful neuropathic conditions mentioned in Chapter 94 and discussed in detail elsewhere in this book (Part IV: Regional Pains). Block of the same structures is indicated for certain chronic occlusive vascular diseases affecting the upper limb in patients in whom preliminary blocks with local anesthetic have indicated that prolonged interruption would prove beneficial.

The anatomic and physiologic bases of limiting neurolytic block to the T2 and T3 ganglia and the interganglionic chain to produce prolonged interruption of the sympathetics of the upper limb is discussed in detail in Chapter 46 and shown in Figures 46-20 and 46-21. The peripheral portion of the sympathetic supply to the upper limb is composed of preganglionic neurons whose cell bodies are in the intermediolateral horn of the spinal cord at the T2 to T8 or T9 levels, while their axons pass along the anterior root of the spinal nerves, the white rami communicantes, and pass to the lateral sympathetic chain. Here they ascend cephalad and synapse with the postganglionic fibers, primarily in T2 but also in T3 and in the stellate and middle cervical ganglia. By blocking T2 and T3, which are considered to be "key" synaptic stations, all the sympathetic nerves destined for the upper limb can be interrupted.

Sympathetic block of the upper limb is usually achieved by anterior paratracheal block of the cervicothoracic sympathetic chain (see Chapter 94 and Fig. 94-51). With this technique, however, injection of a neurolytic agent carries a high risk of producing a prolonged Horner's syndrome, prolonged block of the recurrent laryngeal nerve with impairment of phonation, unintentional block of the brachial plexus, or accidental injection of the neurolytic agent into the vertebral artery. Moreover, a small number of patients apparently have fascial barriers that prevent the caudad diffusion of the neurolytic agent to involve the T3 and sometimes even the T2 ganglia. In the latter case, this would result in an incomplete sympathetic denervation of the upper limb in those patients who have the anomalous sympathetic pathway known as Kuntz's nerve, which bypasses the stellate ganglion (Chapter 46 and Figs. 94-49 and 94-50). The posterior approach to the T2 and T3 sympathetic ganglia and the interganglionic chain obviates this problem and is less likely to produce the other complications of paratracheal block.

BLOCK OF SYMPATHETICS TO THE CHEST. Neurolytic block of the sympathetic chain at the levels of the T1 to T5 ganglia is used for the relief of pain in the rare patient with severe intractable cardiac pain that is not relieved by medical therapy and is not amenable to aortocoronary bypass surgery or to percutaneous intramural angioplasty (Chapter 54). Neurolytic block of the sympathetic chain from T2 to T8 using multiple needles can be used in patients with severe intractable pain caused by carcinoma of the esophagus or by some other chronic pathologic process of the upper two-thirds of the esophagus. If the lesion is in the lower part of the esophagus it is necessary to block the splanchnic nerves, which contribute an important sensory nerve supply to the lower third of the intrathoracic part and to the abdominal portion of the esophagus (Chapter 56 and Fig. 56-1 and 56-2).

In all these cases neurolytic block is intended to destroy the sensory fibers that convey nociceptive impulses from the thoracic viscera. Interruption of sympathetic efferent fibers can also help to relieve pain by eliminating any arterial vasospasm that might exist, which could contribute to the pathophysiology of these conditions. Finally, neurolytic block of the sympathetic chain extending from T2 to T6 is indicated in patients who have chronic intractable pain caused by aortic aneurysm and who are not suitable

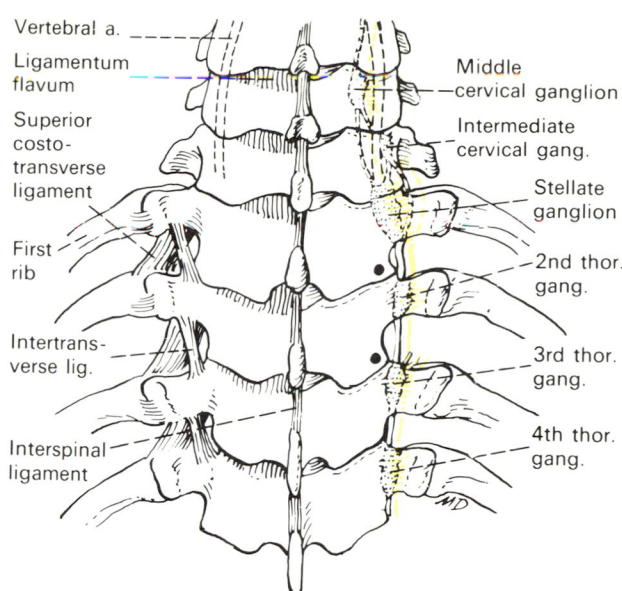

FIG. 96-28. Posterior view of the lower cervical and upper thoracic vertebrae showing the relationships of the sympathetic chain to the vertebra and vertebral artery. The supraspinous ligament has been removed to more easily identify the posterior tips of the spinal processes. The sympathetic ganglia (on the right) are depicted by stippled areas surrounded by dashed lines and are lying in front of the necks of the ribs. The black solid circles indicate the site of contacting the lower and lateral part of the lamina with the bevel of needles inserted by the paralaminar technique (see Fig. 96-29). Injection at the level of the T2 and T3 ganglia causes block of this portion of the chain and consequently completes interruption of the sympathetic supply to the upper limbs, while block of T1 to T5 denervates the heart. Modified from Bonica, J.J.: Sympathetic Nerve Blocks for Pain Diagnosis and Therapy. New York, Breon Laboratories, 1981.

for neuroablative surgery. White and Sweet (60) used this technique in a number of patients with large and intensely painful aneurysms of the aortic arch after a preliminary block with procaine produced complete pain relief. In the first edition of this book (p. 1342) I described White's experience, that of two other neurosurgeons, and my own experience with three patients who were relieved with paravertebral alcohol block. Subsequently I used the technique in three other patients, with similar results.

BLOCK OF SYMPATHETICS TO THE ABDOMINAL VISCERA. Neurolytic block of the lower two-thirds of the thoracic sympathetic chain is indicated in patients with severe intractable pain produced by cancer of one or more of the viscera, by chronic pancreatitis, or by some other chronic disease of one or more of the abdominal viscera that is not amenable to other therapy. Whereas block of individual segments that supply each of the various viscera with a local anesthetic is often used as a diagnostic procedure, in most patients with severe intractable persistent pain it is preferable to carry out a neurolytic block of the celiac plexus or of the three thoracic splanchnic nerves (see below).

Technical Considerations

The anatomy of the thoracic sympathetic trunk is discussed in detail in Chapter 53 and depicted in

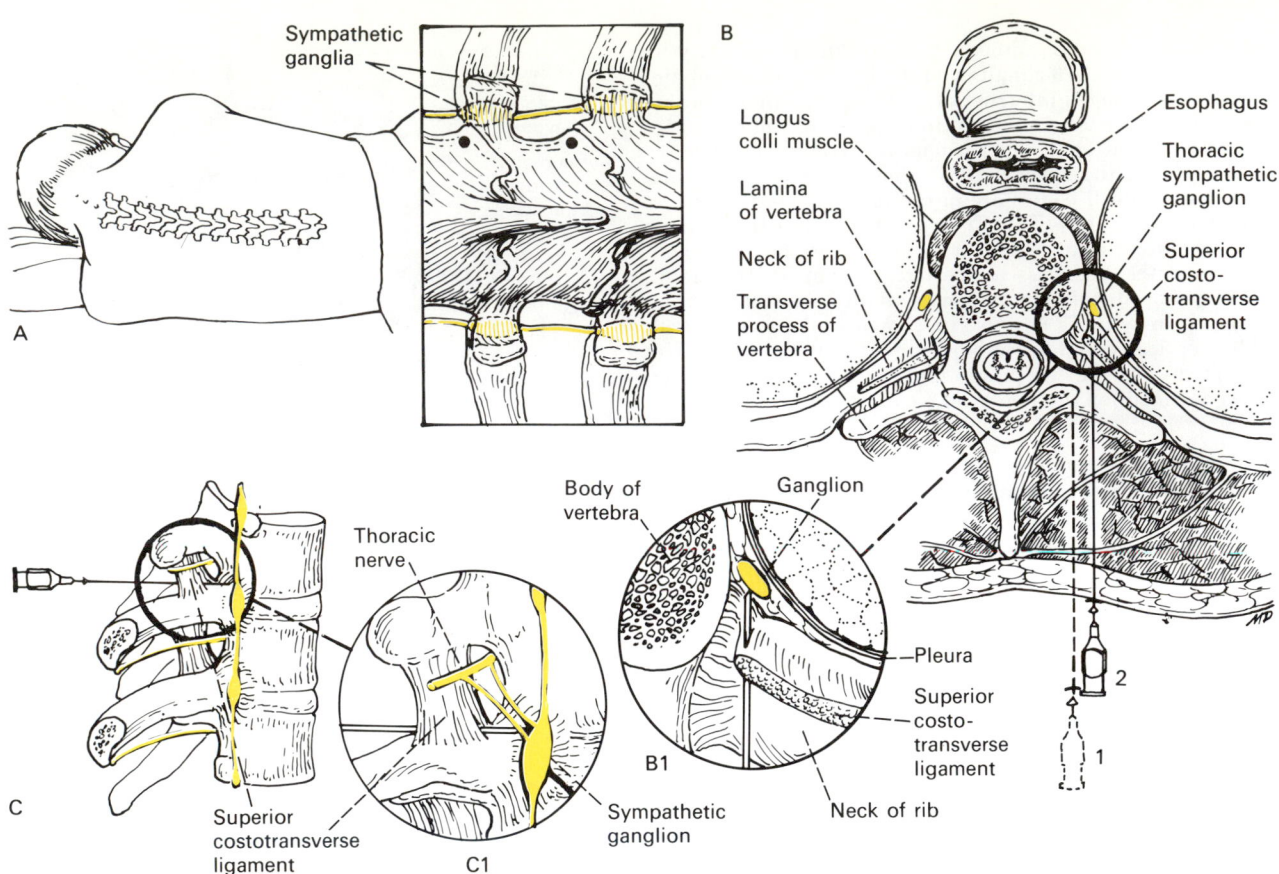

FIG. 96-29. Paralaminar technique of blocking the thoracic sympathetic ganglia and interganglionic part of the chain. **A.** Position of the patient on the side, with the spine flexed. *Inset.* Close-up of the T5 and T6 vertebrae to show the relation of the sympathetic ganglia anterior to the necks of the ribs and the sites of contact of the bevel of the needles with the laminae of the vertebrae. At this level the site of puncture is at the same cross-sectional plane as the posterior end of the spinous processes of one vertebra above (T4 and T5). Skin wheals are made 2 cm lateral to the midline of the back with a 5-cm 25-gauge needle, which is then inserted and directed anteriorly. The dilute local anesthetic solution is liberally injected into the subcutaneous tissue and muscle and onto the periosteum of the ipsilateral laminae to produce a tract of analgesia. **B.** Cross sectional view at the level of the T5 vertebra showing the two steps in placing the point of the needle. After a few minutes, an 8- or 10-cm 22-gauge short-beveled needle adapted to a 2-ml glass syringe with a Luer-Lok and containing saline is inserted and advanced until the lamina is again identified (needle 1). At this point a depth marker is placed 1.5 cm from the skin, the needle is withdrawn until its point is in the subcutaneous tissue, and the skin is moved 0.5 cm laterally. The needle is then advanced in the same sagittal plane parallel to the first insertion (needle 2 in **B**). When advanced to the same depth as the lamina its point either contacts the lateral edge of the lamina or the superior costotransverse ligament, which is lateral to the lateral edge of the lamina and just above the transverse process of the vertebra below. Here the needle encounters a structure that is much less resistant than bone but more resistant than muscle—the superior costotransverse ligament—as shown in **C**, which is a schematic lateromedial view of the vertebrae, the proximal parts of the ribs, and the superior costotransverse ligament. Once the point of the needle has engaged the ligament, the needle is advanced *slowly* (2 mm at a time) while simultaneously exerting continuous *unremitting* pressure on the plunger of the syringe. A sudden loss of resistance indicates that the bevel of the needle has traversed the ligament and is wholly anterior to the anterior surface of the ligament. The needle is then advanced another 7 to 10 mm so that its bevel is in the same coronal plane as the anterior surface of the neck or head of the rib, as shown in position 2 in **B** and in inset B1, which is an enlargement of the circled area in **B** and shows the point of the needle in contact with the upper pole of the sympathetic ganglion. Inset C1 is an enlargement of the circled area in **C** showing the needle through the ligament. Its point is in contact with the upper pole of the ganglion. Once the needle is considered to be in a proper position, 1 ml of saline solution is injected to dislodge any tissue in the needle. Aspiration is then attempted in two planes to ensure that the point of the needle is not in a vessel or within a prolonged dural-arachnoid cuff. After a negative aspiration a test dose of 1 ml of 0.5% bupivacaine anesthetic solution is injected. If no sign of subarachnoid block or other complications is evident, 2 to 3 ml of 0.25% bupivacaine or 2 to 3 ml of a neurolytic agent are injected. This volume is usually sufficient to block one segment (a ganglion and its upper interganglionic fibers). The procedure is repeated at subsequent lower levels.

Figure 96-27. The classic technique of blocking the thoracic sympathetic chain involves creation of an anesthetic wheal through which the needle is inserted 5 to 6 cm lateral to the spinous process. The needle is directed anteromedially toward the lateral aspect of the body of the vertebra, based on the misconception that this is where the chain is located. Such an approach requires that the needle make an angle of 45° with the sagittal plane, which causes the needle to pass through the posterior trough of the thoracic cage created by the angles of the rib. Because the parietal and visceral pleurae "hug" the trough closely,

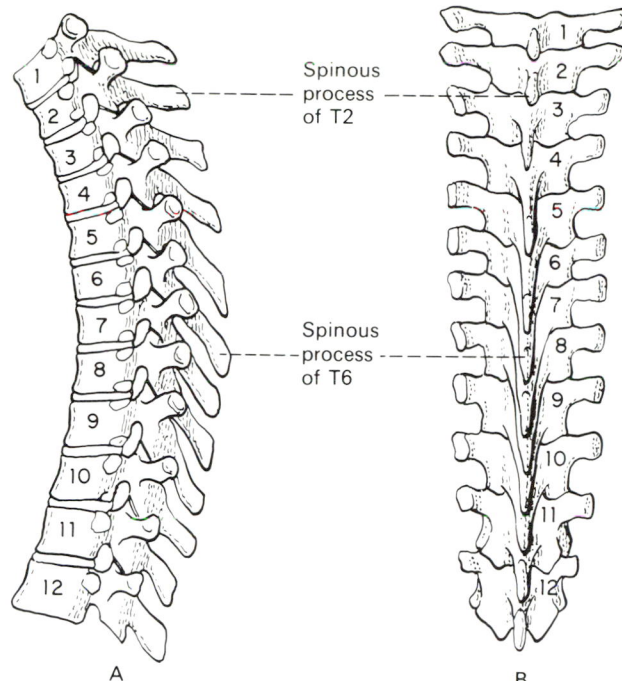

Spinous process of T2

Spinous process of T6

A   B

FIG. 96-30. Posterior view (*A*) and lateral view (*B*) to show relationship at the cross-sectional level of the spinous processes and laminae. The spinous process of the T1 vertebra is at the same cross-sectional level as the lamina of the T2 vertebra. Because of the greater imbrication of the spinous processes in the middle thoracic region, the spinous process of the T6 vertebra is at the same cross-sectional level as the upper portion of the lamina of T8 (i.e., two segments below). In the lower portion of the thoracic vertebra there is much less imbrication, and consequently the spinous process of T11 is at the same cross-sectional level as the lamina of T11, and the spinous process of T12 is at the same cross-sectional level as the middle of the lamina of T12.

the needle is likely to puncture these structures and create a bronchopleural fistula that could cause pneumothorax.

To obviate this problem, I developed the paralaminar technique (Figs. 96-28 and 96-29). For injection of the neurolytic solution an 8- or 10-cm 22-gauge short-beveled needle is used with a 2-ml glass syringe that has been tested to ensure that its wet plunger fits properly so that it can be advanced and withdrawn without any resistance. This is crucial to the second step of determining passage of the bevel of the needle through the superior costotransverse ligament. For verification of the level of the injection it is highly desirable to use an image intensifier and to know the relationship between the spinous process of one vertebra and the lamina to be contacted at the cross-sectional plane (Fig. 96-30).

The needle is inserted only 2 cm lateral to the spinous process and its contact is made in the *lower portion of the lateral part of the lamina*. The second insertion places the bevel of the needle just above the upper surface of the rib below and at some distance below and anterior to the thoracic somatic nerve (Fig. 96-29C and C1). This decreases the risk of involving the somatic nerve with the neurolytic agent. Compare

Figure 96-30 with Figure 94-22 (p. 1913), which shows the technique of blocking the thoracic somatic nerve. As can be noted, for somatic nerve block the needle is inserted more cephalad to contact the upper portion of the lateral part of the lamina and then is made to pass through the upper portion of the superior costotransverse ligament below the transverse process of the vertebra above.

If the technique is carried out by someone who has a thorough knowledge of the anatomy, is skilled in regional analgesia, and proceeds slowly and cautiously, less risk of contacting the somatic spinal nerve and of puncturing the dura is involved than with the use of the classic posterior approach. Even the approach described here, however, requires patience and skill to avoid advancing the needle too far anteriorly, which could pierce the lung.

Complications

Complications with the use of the paralaminar technique for blocking the thoracic sympathetic chain include the following: (a) puncture of the lung from placing the needle too far anteriorly, producing pneumothorax; and (b) puncture of the intercostal vein or artery or contact with the thoracic somatic nerve if the bevel of the needle is placed higher than recommended. If aspiration is not carried out in two planes the neurolytic agent might be injected into the vessel, with consequent necrosis, or into the subarachnoid space of a prolonged dural cuff, with consequent diffusion to the subarachnoid space, prolonged block of the somatic nerve, or both. All these complications can be prevented with proper technique. In the past 30 years I have carried out more than 125 of these procedures without causing any of these problems.

Neurolytic Block of the Celiac Plexus

Indications

ACUTE PAIN. Celiac plexus block with a local anesthetic is now being used to obviate or reduce drastically the excruciating epigastric and generalized abdominal pain caused by arterial embolization of the liver for the treatment of carcinoma. Until very recently the procedure was carried out with relatively high intravenous doses of morphine given just prior to the embolization. It had little pain-relieving effect. My colleagues K.A. Loper and D.C. Moore, in collabora-

TABLE 96-8. Comparison of Intravenous Morphine (in mg) & Celiac Plexus Block for Control of Pain Caused by Hepatic Arterial Embolization (HAE)

Method of Pain Control	Prior to and During Embolization	Postembolization	
		6–8 hrs	8–24 hrs
A. Morphine (in mg) —mean (range)	5.5 (2.5–12.5)	22 (16–46)	37 (24–68)
Pain score 0–10	6.5 (2–8)	8.0 (4–10)	5.4 (3–8)
B. Celiac plexus block Pain scores	0	0	1.2 (0–2)
Morphine given in mg —mean (range)	0	0	3.4 (1–5.6)

tion with members of the Department of Radiology (personal communication, 1989), carried out a comparative study of the efficacy of morphine and celiac plexus block in five patients who required hepatic arterial embolization (HAE). For the first HAE, patients were managed with morphine, given for the procedure and for postoperative pain during the first 24 hours after the procedure was completed. Pain was evaluated by patient report using a 0–10 verbal scale, 0 being "no pain" and 10 being "extreme pain." For the subsequent HAE procedure, they were given celiac plexus block performed under radiographic guidance for proper placement of the needle. There was a marked difference in pain scores between the two procedures. The data from this study provide impressive evidence of the superiority of celiac plexus block over systemic analgesics in controlling the pain caused by hepatic arterial embolization (Table 96-8).

CHRONIC PAIN. Neurolytic block of the celiac plexus is useful in relieving severe intractable pain caused by cancer or chronic visceral disease. In addition to blocking all the nociceptive (pain) pathways that supply the viscera in the upper abdomen, the procedure relieves visceral vasospasm and other pathophysiologic processes caused by abnormal reflexes consequent to persistent noxious stimulation by the disease process. Because the celiac plexus contains vagal afferents and efferents, block of this structure interrupts the sensory fibers that transmit non-nociceptive information and the parasympathetic outflow to the abdominal viscera. In considering the use of neurolytic block of the celiac plexus, it is essential to carry out at least one and preferably two diagnostic or prognostic blocks with a local anesthetic to predict the effects of the neurolytic blockade in patients in whom this procedure is to be used to relieve the severe pain of cancer or of some other chronic condition. The neurolytic agent diffuses to a lesser extent than the local anesthetic, so it is essential to carry out the preliminary block with a volume of local anesthetic that is about two-thirds the volume of neurolytic agent to be injected.

Anatomic Basis

The neuroanatomic basis for block of the celiac plexus is summarized in Chapters 53 and 59 and illustrated in Fig. 96-31. Hovelacque (105), more than 60 years ago, emphasized that, contrary to the classic textbook description, the celiac ganglia vary in number, size, and location, and this point was also made in the first edition of this book (1); more recently, Ward and associates (106) "rediscovered" this fact. The number of ganglia varies from 1 to 4 or 5 and the size of each ranges from 0.5 to nearly 5 cm in diameter (Chapter 59). Moreover, they are located at a variable distance in the anteroposterior plane from the anterior surface of the L1 vertebra, which is used as a landmark in blocking the plexus. In addition to understanding the anatomy of the celiac plexus itself, it is also essential to understand the anatomy of the surrounding structures, which might be subjected to potential trauma by needles, drugs, or both. On the right side, and anterior to the plexus, is the inferior

vena cava, and on the left side is the aorta, with the kidneys posterolateral to these vessels. Anteriorly the plexus is near the posterior surface of the pancreas.

Technique

The technique of neurolytic celiac plexus block (NCPB) is illustrated in Figure 96-32. Preparation of patients should include discontinuing antihypertensive agents, which could enhance the hypotensive effect of the block, and anticoagulants, which could produce excessive bleeding. No sedatives or narcotics should be given for the prognostic block, which, if done correctly, should be rather painless. Because the injection of alcohol causes severe pain, however, sedatives and opioid analgesics can be given IV 15 minutes before the block and should not interfere with the results. All patients should have supplemental IV fluids (crystalloid form) in doses of 10 to 15 ml/kg as a bolus at the time of the alcohol block.

It is important to use a needle that is of sufficient length—10 cm for thin individuals, 12 cm for average patients, and 15 cm for obese or muscular persons. Thompson and Moore (107) have suggested that a 20-gauge needle is far better than a 22-gauge needle because it is easier to insert without buckling and, more important, offers much less resistance than the 22-gauge needle, which they claimed requires a firm pressure during injection and therefore makes it difficult to feel any difference in resistance in different tissues. A study by Brown and associates (108), however, Thompson's co-workers, showed no significant difference in the quality of block between the two sizes. Except in muscular individuals, I prefer to use a 22-gauge needle because it is less traumatic.

The neurolytic solution consists of equal parts of absolute alcohol and saline solution or, preferably, 0.75% bupivacaine or 2% lidocaine to lessen the severe alcohol-induced pain. If radiographic control of the spread of the solution is to be done, a mixture containing 25 ml absolute alcohol, 18 ml local anesthetic, and 7 ml of contrast medium (e.g., Conray-420) is used.

The needle should pass through the crura of the diaphragm and have its bevel lateral to both sides of the aorta, just below the level of the celiac plexus (Fig. 96-32). Although the plexus is presumably in loose areolar tissue behind the pancreas, which enhances the diffusion of local anesthetic drugs, Moore (109) verified needle placement and spread of injected solution by conventional radiography and by CT scan, and showed that spread of the solution tends to be confined to the side of the injection. Therefore, it is essential to do a bilateral block to obtain maximum pain relief.

Recently several modifications of the classic technique have been described. Some authors insist that radiographic control is absolutely essential for proper placement of the needle and for visualization of the neurolytic agent. In a critical analysis of results in 136 patients who underwent NCPB for the relief of pancreatic cancer pain, however, Brown and associates (108) found that radiographic verification of needle position does not influence the quality of the block. Neverthe-

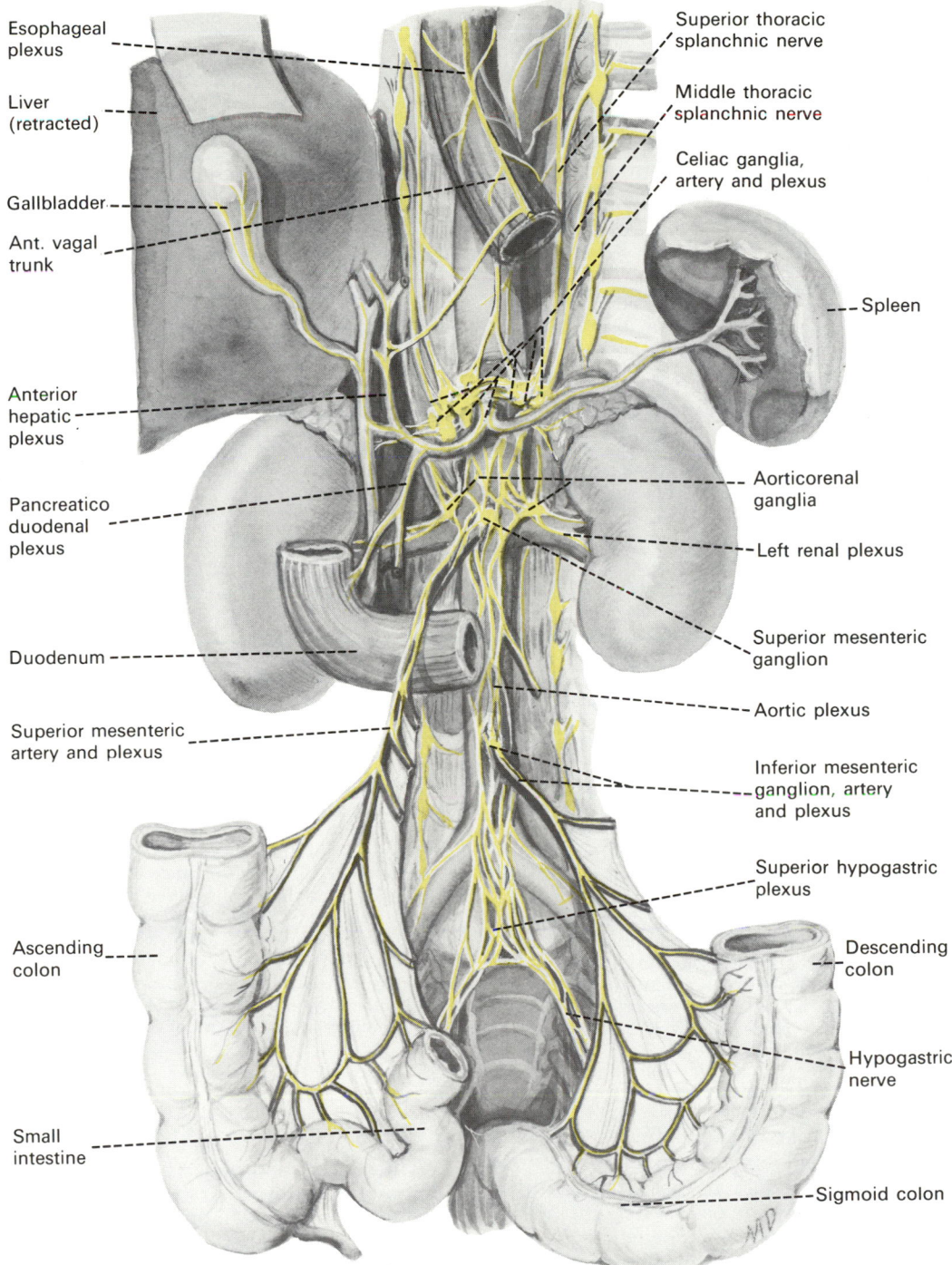

Esophageal plexus

Liver (retracted)

Gallbladder

Ant. vagal trunk

Anterior hepatic plexus

Pancreatico duodenal plexus

Duodenum

Superior mesenteric artery and plexus

Ascending colon

Small intestine

Superior thoracic splanchnic nerve

Middle thoracic splanchnic nerve

Celiac ganglia, artery and plexus

Spleen

Aorticorenal ganglia

Left renal plexus

Superior mesenteric ganglion

Aortic plexus

Inferior mesenteric ganglion, artery and plexus

Superior hypogastric plexus

Descending colon

Hypogastric nerve

Sigmoid colon

FIG. 96-31. Anatomy of the celiac plexus and subsidiary plexuses. The celiac plexus occupies an area 3 cm long and 4 cm wide between the two adrenal glands. It is located in the epigastrium just anterior to the crura of the diaphragm around and below the celiac axis, and on either side of the midline. It is often subdivided into right and left portions and consists of a number of prevertebral ganglia and a dense network of autonomic fibers that unite and enmesh these ganglia. The autonomic fibers include sympathetic preganglionic fibers contributed by the thoracic splanchnic nerves, sympathetic postganglionic fibers provided by the lumbar splanchnic nerves (contributed by the lumbar sympathetic chain), and parasympathetic preganglionic fibers contributed by both vagus nerves. Sensory fibers are contributed by the phrenic nerves, the vagus nerves, and the splanchnic nerves, which provide sympathetic afferents. Only the phrenic and sympathetic afferents transmit nociceptive information from the upper abdominal viscera. Although the celiac ganglia are usually depicted as two large masses, semilunar in shape and located on each side of the origin of the celiac axis, their shapes and sizes are actually variable. Note the location of the superior and inferior mesenteric ganglia and plexuses. (See Chapter 59 for a detailed description of these plexuses.)

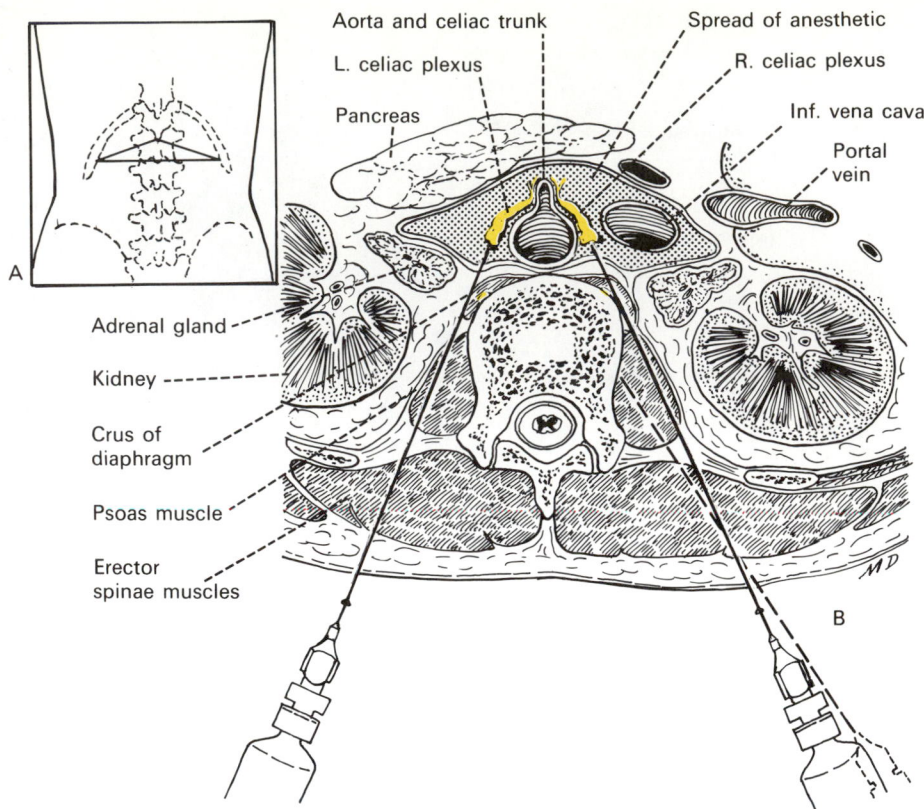

FIG. 96-32. Technique of blocking the celiac plexus. The patient is placed prone with a pillow under the abdomen after an IV infusion has been started. **A.** The spinous processes of T12 and L1 are marked, as are the lower borders of both 12th ribs, and these are connected to make a flattened isosceles triangle. Skin wheals are raised 6 to 7 cm lateral to the inferior part of the quadrilaterally shaped spinous process of L1. **B.** Using a 25-gauge disposable spinal needle, the subcutaneous fascia and muscles are infiltrated with a dilute solution of local anesthetic. Security needles of proper length are selected for injection of the local anesthetic or of a neurolytic agent. Each needle, with a depth marker attached, is inserted through the skin wheal with its bevel facing medially and directed so that its shaft makes an angle of 40° with the midsaggital plane. The first needle should be inserted on the left side so that contact with the lateral aspect of the aorta can be ascertained by feeling the transmitted pulsation up the shaft of the needle, which is held firmly. This provides an approximation of how far the right needle needs to be advanced. The needle is then advanced slowly until contact with the lateral surface of L1 is made, usually at a depth of 8 to 9 cm. If bony contact is made more superficially it is likely that the needle has contacted the transverse process; if this occurs the needle must be withdrawn and redirected to advance below the transverse process. Once the needle impinges on the lateral side of the body of the L1 vertebra, the rubber marker is placed 4 cm from the skin. The needle is withdrawn until its point is in the subcutaneous tissue, the angle is decreased by 30° on the left side, and it is readvanced slowly until the marker is flush with the skin. At this point the pulsation of the aorta should be felt, indicating that the needle is lateral to the vessel. If bone is encountered before the marker is flush with the skin, the needle is withdrawn and readvanced so that its shaft makes an angle of 25° with the sagittal plane. This permits passage of the needle without further bony contact; it is then advanced until the marker is flushed with the skin. The depth is noted and the right needle is similarly inserted and advanced, except that, on the second insertion, the needle is directed so that its shaft makes an angle of 35°. If bone is contacted the needle is withdrawn and the angle is decreased to 30° because the aorta is to the left of the midline. Once the needles have been positioned, aspiration is attempted in four quadrants to rule out accidental intravascular or subarachnoid injection. For diagnostic purposes with local anesthetics, 15 ml of 0.5% bupivacaine with epinephrine is injected through each needle. This is usually sufficient to spread and involve the celiac and subsidiary plexuses laterally as far as the adrenal glands. The injection of solution should offer no resistance because it is made into the loose areolar tissue of the retroperitoneal space. An effective block generally relieves abdominal pain within 15 minutes and the patient manifests orthostatic hypotension. If difficulty is encountered it is advisable to use an image intensifier or CT scanning to place the bevels of the needles correctly. A volume of 15 to 20 ml of 50% alcohol is injected through each needle for a neurolytic block.

less, radiographic control can be helpful, especially to those who have not had extensive experience with celiac plexus block. It should be used if the initial block fails to produce complete pain relief (Fig. 96-33).

Ischia and colleagues (104) have developed a technique that uses a combination of fluoroscopy and fingertip feel to penetrate the aorta with a 20-gauge needle intentionally. The needle is advanced until its bevel penetrates the anterior wall and no blood can be withdrawn. Theoretically, this places the bevel of the needle directly in the middle of the preaortic network of the celiac plexus and should guarantee correct placement, but it entails the risk of producing postblock hemorrhage: in this series six patients (104) developed retroperitoneal hematoma, as shown by CT scan.

Results

The results obtained by some who used the "classic" technique and by others who used modifications of the technique are shown in Table 96-9. With use of the classic technique between 70 and 85% of patients with severe upper abdominal cancer pain obtained pain relief lasting from 1 month up to 1 year. Best results were obtained in patients with severe pain caused by cancer of the pancreas.

Brown and colleagues (108), in their comprehensive analysis of 166 patients with cancer of the pancreas whose ages ranged from 29 to 87 years, found that 141 patients (85%) obtained good pain relief, which lasted until death in 75% and for longer than 50% of the survival time in an additional 12.5%. Analysis of patient variables revealed that the quality

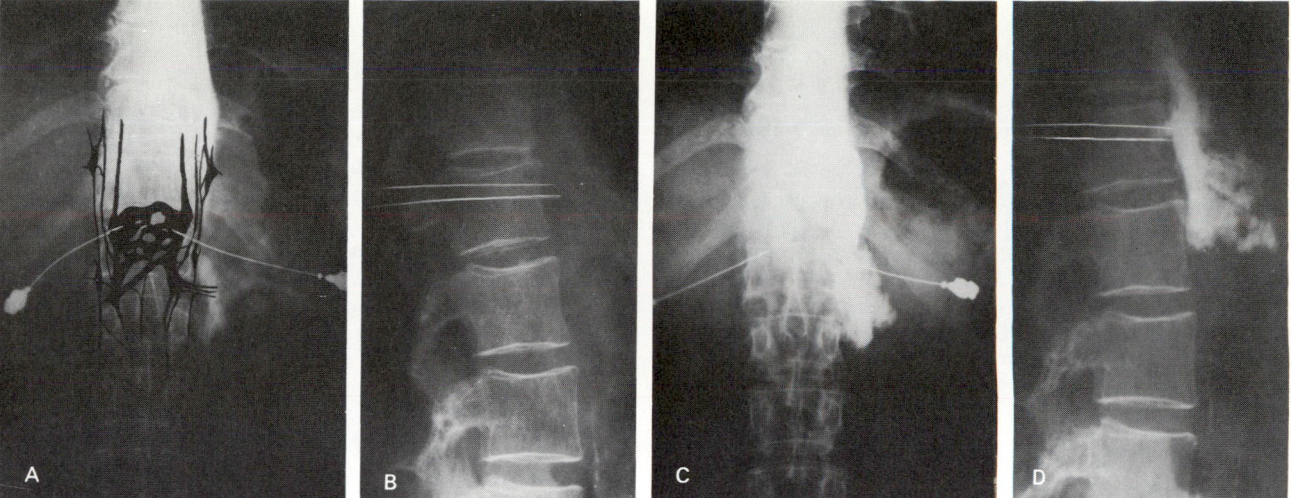

FIG. 96-33. Radiographs showing needles in place for injection of the celiac plexus. **A.** Anteroposterior view with drawing of the plexus superimposed in front of the body of the L1 vertebra in the upper part of the L2 vertebra. **B.** Lateral view with both needles in place. The distal 3 cm of the needle are anterior to the anterolateral surface of the vertebral body. **C, D.** Diffusion of 10 ml of 35% Diodrast injected through the right needle, with most of the spread being anterior to the anterior surface of the L1 and upper part of the L2 vertebrae.

of the block was not affected by age or sex, by whether or not they had metastasis, or by anticancer therapy such as surgery, chemotherapy, radiation therapy, or a combination of these. When block was repeated for recurrence of pain after a successful first block, 81% of patients again obtained beneficial pain relief. Moreover, repetition of the block did not increase the incidence of complications which was limited to pneumothorax in 2 patients, without neurologic sequelae. In patients in whom an initial poor result was obtained, a second NCPB was performed with CT scanning

to verify the spread of injected solution. In a subsequent report by Brown (110) on another 66 patients who had other types of abdominal cancer pain and who underwent 75 NCPBs, 48 patients (73%) had good pain relief until their death, which occurred at a mean of 17.4 weeks and a median of 8 weeks. Moreover, NCPB provided pain relief for the remainder of these patients' lives in 59% and for more than half of their remaining lives in an additional 15%. Four reports from the Virginia Mason Medical Center, Seattle (108, 110, 111, 115) indicated that those in the group led by

TABLE 96-9. Comparison of Results with Neurolytic Celiac Plexus Block

Source	Indications	No. of Patients	Pain Relief (% of Patients Treated)		
			Good	Fair	Poor
Bridenbaugh et al. (111)	Pancreatic cancer	25	88	8	4
	Other abdominal cancer	16	94	6	0
Gorbitz and Leavin (112)	Pancreatic cancer	5	80	20	0
	Other abdominal cancer	3	100	0	0
Black and Dwyer (113)	Pancreatic cancer	15	73	27	0
	Other abdominal cancer	35	71	17	12
	Chronic pancreatitis	15	67	5	28
Jones and Gough (114)	Abdominal cancer	100	48	43	0
Thompson et al. (115)	Abdominal cancer	97	62	35	3
Flanigan and Kraft (116)*	Pancreatic cancer (NCPB)	32	78	9	13
	Pancreatic cancer (surg.)	19	0	21	79
	Pancreatitis (NCPB)	1	100	0	0
Hegedus (117)	Pancreatic cancer	36	44	44	12
	Pancreatitis	9	33	22	45
Bonica et al. (unpublished data)	Pancreatic cancer	84	79	13	8
	Other abdominal cancer	72	68	17	15
	Pancreatitis	12	43	21	36
Brown (110)	Pancreatic cancer	136	85	12.5	2.5
	Other abdominal cancer	66	74	15	11
All/Mean:	Pancreatic cancer	333	78	16	6
	Other abdominal cancer	389	64	28	8
	Pancreatitis†	37	51	16	33

*Comparison of surgery alone (surg.) with surgery plus open splanchnicectomy (NCPB).
†Good pain relief only transient.

Moore carried out a total of 370 NCPBs over a 25-year period, with an impressively high success rate. Many of these were done without radiographic control. An important factor for the high success rate is that Moore and associates routinely used celiac plexus block combined with intercostal nerve block for most patients undergoing upper abdominal surgery.

I began to report on the results of the celiac plexus block for cancer pain of the abdomen in 1951 (1), and was one of the first to suggest the use of radiographic control by injecting contrast medium with a local anesthetic. Extensive experience with celiac plexus–intercostal block for surgery, however, prompted my group to carry out most NCPBs successfully without radiographic control. In the ensuing 20 years I and my colleagues have carried out 168 NCPBs with results similar to those reported by Moore and associates (unpublished data).

The value of neurolytic celiac plexus block for the management of severe pain caused by unresectable cancer of the pancreas has been impressively demonstrated by Flanigan and Kraft (116). They compared the results of relief of pain with palliative surgery alone, including biliary and duodenal bypasses, with those obtained with the operation and also injected the celiac plexus and splanchnic nerves with 15 to 20 ml of 6% phenol at the time of operation. All patients had severe preoperative pain. Of the 19 patients who had conventional operations alone only 4 patients (21%) experienced partial relief of pain postoperatively, whereas, of the 32 patients who had the operation and NCPB, 28 patients (88%) experienced excellent pain relief postoperatively for a mean duration of 4.3 months. The mean postoperative survival time was 5 months, and 84% of patients experienced no recurrence of their pain prior to death. In commenting on the report of Flanigan and Kraft (116), White, one of our colleagues, reported similar highly successful results with the injection of 25 ml of 50% alcohol in each side of the celiac plexus at the time of operation. In view of these and other results (Table 96-8) it is surprising that most surgeons do not use neurolysis of the celiac plexus and of the splanchnic nerves during the course of surgery.

In the treatment of chronic pancreatitis and other nonmalignant chronic pain syndromes, the initial results were almost as good as those in patients with cancer pain, but the pain recurs with time, so that long-term results can be considered to be only fair. Flanigan and Kraft (116) had one patient who remained pain-free for 3 years postoperatively. In most patients, however, the technique should be viewed as a temporary measure to aid in the management of these patients. The same comment could apply to other nonmalignant abdominal chronic pain syndromes.

Complications

A frequent adverse side effect of celiac plexus block with a local anesthetic is extensive vasomotor block, because the drug diffuses to involve not only the plexus but also the upper part of the lumbar sympathetic chain, and subsequently hypotension develops. The degree of hypotension in normovolemic patients in the supine position is mild, but elderly patients, or those who are hypovolemic, are likely to develop moderate to severe orthostatic arterial hypotension, especially if they attempt to assume the upright position too quickly. The treatment of hypotension is discussed in Chapter 94, p. 1896 (A. Basic Considerations).

Possible complications include accidental injection of the entire volume of local anesthetic into the inferior vena cava, which causes a systemic toxic reaction because the drug promptly reaches the heart and brain. Accidental injection of the drug into the aorta is less likely to cause a reaction because it is diluted as it passes with the blood to the lower part of the body before it is returned to the heart. Accidental intravascular injection of alcohol or phenol can produce necrosis of the vessels. In patients with coagulation defects, puncture of the inferior vena cava with a large needle, which has a hook created on contacting the vertebra, can result in retroperitoneal hematoma. Pneumothorax can develop if the pleura extends below its normal caudad border of the 12th rib.

Other more serious complications of NCPB that have been reported include postinjection neuropathy with neuralgia that persisted for several months, paraplegia consequent to thrombosis of a major feeder artery to the spinal cord, accidental neurolytic injection into the kidney with consequent necrosis or hemorrhage, and failure of ejaculation, presumably because of involvement of the hypogastric plexus (65).

Neurolytic Block of Splanchnic Nerves

Indications for blocking the splanchnic nerves with neurolytic agents are similar to those for celiac plexus block except that the procedure is less likely to involve the lumbar sympathetic chain than is celiac plexus block. The technique is therefore more discrete, requires a smaller volume of neurolytic agent, and entails a lower risk of complications. Boas (118, 119) has indicated a preference for block of thoracic splanchnic nerves rather than celiac plexus block because it has the advantage of a true compartmental block, thus being safer for the patient.

Technique

The anatomy of the thoracic splanchnic nerves is discussed in detail in Chapter 53 and depicted in Figure 96-34. My technique of blocking these nerves is shown in Figure 96-35.

Complications

Hypotension consequent to vasomotor block is of a lesser degree with splanchnic block than with celiac plexus block because the lumbar sympathetics are usually not interrupted. Pneumothorax occurs if the needle is not kept in contact with the lateral surface of the vertebra. Accidental injection of the neurolytic agent into the azygous vein on the right side or into the hemiazygous vein on the left side results in necrosis of these vessels. The thoracic duct might be damaged, leading to a chylothorax, or it might become obstructed, leading to lymphedema. All these complications can and must be prevented by correct technique.

Neurolytic Lumbar Sympathetic Block

Chapter 94 presents the indications for lumbar sympathetic block with a local anesthetic. The

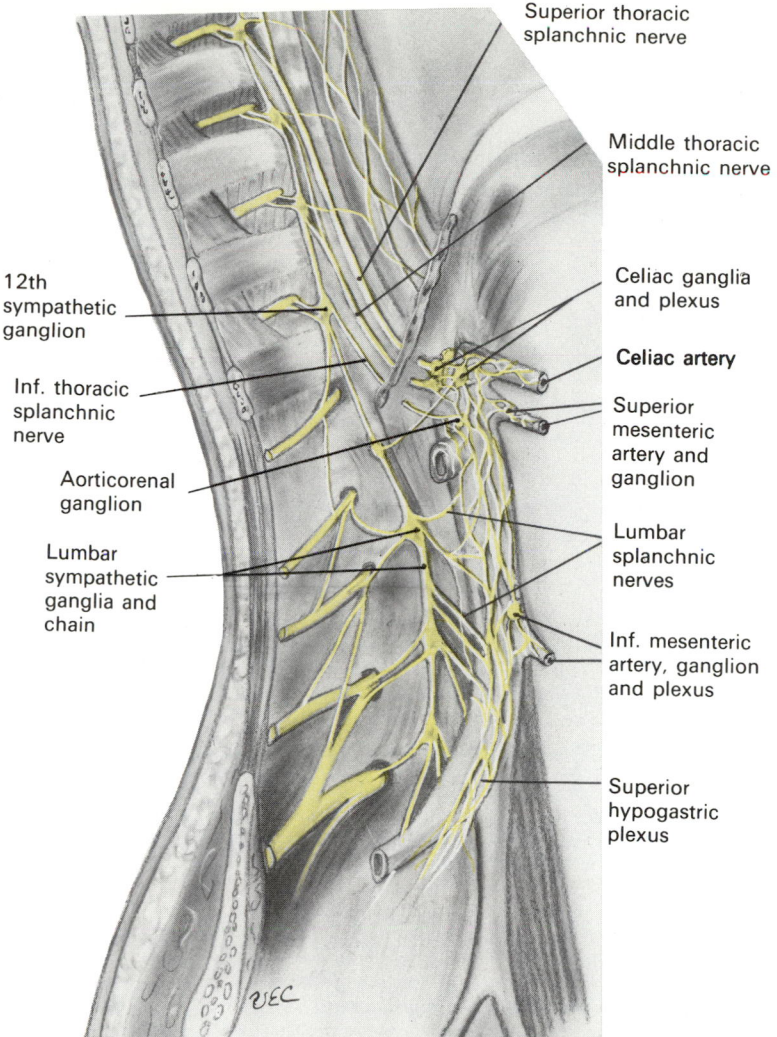

Superior thoracic
splanchnic nerve

Middle thoracic
splanchnic nerve

Celiac ganglia
and plexus

Celiac artery

Superior
mesenteric
artery and
ganglion

Lumbar
splanchnic
nerves

Inf. mesenteric
artery, ganglion
and plexus

Superior
hypogastric
plexus

12th
sympathetic
ganglion

Inf. thoracic
splanchnic
nerve

Aorticorenal
ganglion

Lumbar
sympathetic
ganglia and
chain

FIG. 96-34. Relationship of the lower thoracic and lumbar sympathetic chains, splanchnic nerves, celiac ganglia and plexuses, and their branches (lateral view). These relationships serve as a basis for block of the splanchnic nerves and block of the lumbar sympathetic chain.

neuroanatomy and technique are also described in Chapter 94 (Fig. 94-53 p. 1946). Here the indications for neurolytic blockade of the lumbar sympathetic chain are discussed.

Indications

Neurolytic block is indicated for the relief of various chronic painful conditions in the lower limbs in patients who achieve good but transient results from local anesthetic block but are elderly and not suitable for surgical sympathectomy. These conditions include causalgia and other reflex sympathetic dystrophies, phantom limb and other postamputation pain, other neuropathic conditions that are temporarily relieved with local anesthetics, various chronic peripheral vascular disorders, pain caused by cancer of the pelvic viscera, and severe persistent tenesmus. Duthie and Ingham (120) reported on patients with persistent lower abdominal pain that had not been relieved by surgical excision of various organs but that was completely relieved by several lumbar sympathetic blocks with local anesthetic. These results prompted them to carry out lumbar sympathectomy with 7.5% aqueous phenol. Because all nociceptive pathways from the uterus and cervix pass through the lumbar sympathetic chain (Chapter 66), persistent pain caused by cancer limited to the uterus or nonmalignant chronic painful conditions not amenable to other forms of treatment should be given several bilateral diagnostic or prognostic lumbar sympathetic blocks with local anesthetic. If good relief is obtained, bilateral sympathectomy can be considered. Obviously these procedures are ineffective when cancer begins to infiltrate the lumbosacral plexus.

The largest experience to date with neurolytic lumbar sympathetic block, which is often referred to as lumbar chemical sympathectomy, is in the treatment of occlusive vascular disease of the lower limbs. Based on my own experiences, as well on those of Löfstrom and Zetterquist (112), Reid and colleagues (122), Boas and associates (119, 123), and Cousins and co-workers (124), it is clear that chemical sympathectomy is highly effective in relieving rest pain and in helping to heal ischemic lesion. It can even relieve the pain of intermittent claudication in a smaller percentage of patients. The procedure is indicated in patients for whom bypass

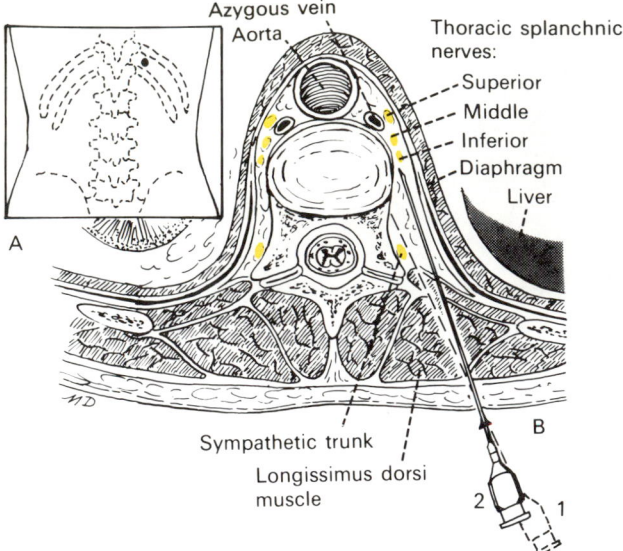

Azygous vein
Aorta
Thoracic splanchnic
nerves:
- Superior
- Middle
- Inferior
- Diaphragm
Liver

A

Sympathetic trunk
Longissimus dorsi
muscle

B

2   1

FIG. 96-35. Technique of blocking the thoracic splanchnic nerves. *A.* Following identification and marking of the lower tip of the spinous process of the T11 vertebra, the area is prepared and an intracutaneous wheal is produced about 6 to 7 cm lateral to the lower tip of the spinous process of the T11 vertebra (black dot). This is at the same cross-sectional level as the upper part of the body of the T12 vertebra. A 10- or 12-cm 22-gauge needle is adequate for the thin or average individual, whereas a 15-cm 22-gauge needle is necessary for an obese or muscular person. *B.* The needle is introduced through the skin wheal and directed anteriorly and medially so that its shaft makes an angle of 45° with the midsagittal plane. The needle is advanced until the posterolateral surface of the upper part of the body of the T12 vertebra is contacted (position 1). A marker is then placed about 2 cm from the skin. The needle is withdrawn until its point is in the subcutaneous tissue and reinserted in a slightly more lateral direction, which places the bevel of the needle just lateral to the anterolateral surface of the body of the vertebra where the three thoracic splanchnic nerves are located near each other (position 2). To avoid damage to the pleura it is essential that the bevel of the needle be maintained in contact with the vertebra during its anterior advance. Injection of 10 ml of 0.25 to 0.5% bupivacaine with epinephrine solution diffuses throughout the region to involve all three nerves on one side. A bilateral block is often essential for the relief of upper abdominal pain.

graft surgery cannot be used because the obliterating disorder is too extensive.

For many years consensus favored subjecting patients with lower limb disease to surgical sympathectomy, especially of the lumbar region, because in skilled hands it was considered to be a simple procedure, with low morbidity and mortality rates. Chemical sympathectomy with alcohol or phenol was considered only in patients in poor physical condition. Moreover, sympathetic block with a local anesthetic was thought to be of little value in predicting the effects of sympathectomy, presumably because the duration of such a block was too short. With the widespread use of continuous epidural analgesia and the advent of long-acting local anesthetics such as bupivacaine, however, diagnostic and prognostic sympathetic blocks have resumed an important role in the management of these

patients. With recent improvements in fluoroscopic control of needle placement and spread of the solution, the use of chemical sympathectomy has come to be preferred over surgical section, especially in debilitated patients. Reid and colleagues (122) found a mortality rate of 1/1666 injections (0.06%) and, in the series of 386 blocks reported by Cousins only one death (0.26%) occurred, within 1 week of blockade, and this was in a patient who had severe ischemic heart disease with congestive cardiac failure prior to the procedure. These data compare favorably with those for surgical sympathectomy, which has a mortality rate ranging from 6 to as high as 20% in patients with severe vascular disease (122).

Because the duration of sympathetic interruption is similar for surgical and chemical sympathectomy (mean of 6 months), neurolytic blockade is preferred even in patients in good physical condition because it offers significant advantages over surgery. The procedure can be done on an outpatient basis, allowing patients a rapid return to their home environment. This reduces postoperative morbidity, especially the risk of thrombosis associated with surgery and bed rest, and drastically decreases the duration and cost of hospitalization. Moreover, in a busy service, use of the procedure permits a large turnover: as many as eight to ten can be done in a single day (123). If a bilateral procedure is required it can be performed with the second side blocked 1 week later, also on an outpatient basis.

Technique

The neuroanatomic basis for block of the lumbar sympathetic chain is described in Chapter 94. (Consult that chapter for more information on the anatomy of the lumbar sympathetic chain, which is not described in most surgery textbooks or in those dealing with nerve blocks.)

The lumbar sympathetic chain is the most variable portion of the sympathetic system, particularly in regard to the number of ganglia and to the general form of the two chains; these differ greatly, not only among different patients but on each side of the same patient. In most individuals they lie anterolateral to the intervertebral disk, with one portion of the ganglion being in front of the lower part of the vertebra above and the other portion of the ganglia being in front of the upper part of the vertebra below. In addition, the size of the ganglia and the interganglionic cord and the number of branches extending from them show great variation. The lumbar sympathetic chain contains both preganglionic and postganglionic neurons that supply the pelvic viscera and vessels of the lower limbs and have afferent (sensory) fibers, some of which transmit nociceptive information.

Boas (118, 119) has effectively used a single needle placed at L2 or L3 and has found it to be satisfactory for injection of the neurolytic agent. It is best, however, to use two needles at L2 and L4 or even three needles at L2, L3, and L4, placed in the center of the vertebral body. Insertion of the needle is the same as that illustrated in Figure 94-53 (p. 1946). For placement of the block needle it is essential not only to anesthetize the skin but also the subcutaneous tissue and fascia of muscles, using the lack of resistance test to determine passage of the point of the needle through the psoas fascia.

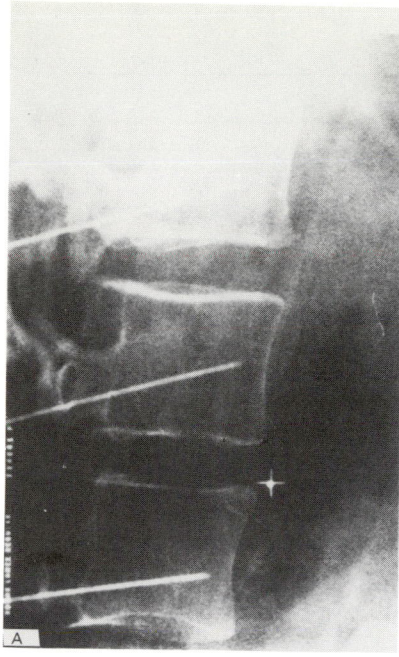
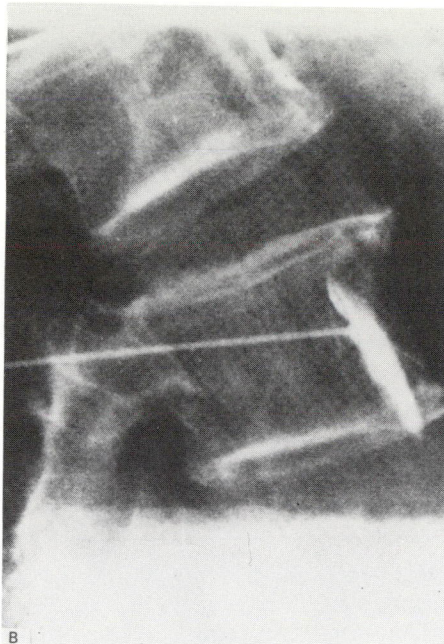
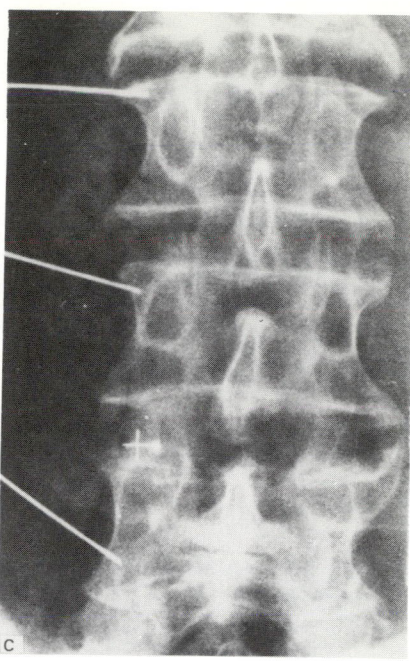

Fig. 96-36. **A.** Radiographs showing lateral views of lumbar vertebrae with needles in place to carry out lumbar chemical sympathectomy. **B.** Injection of 1 ml of 10% phenol in Conray-420 at each level causes spread of the solution from L2 to L4. **C.** Posteroanterior view. From Cousins, M.J., et al.: Neurolytic lumbar sympathetic blockade: Duration of denervation and relief of rest pain. Anaesth. Intensive Care, 7:121, 1979.

Although some clinicians have the patient in the prone position during the procedure, the lateral position is preferable because it facilitates monitoring of diffusion of the solution in the lateral view, probably diminishes its retroperitoneal spread, and enhances its cephalad-caudad spread. Once the needles are in place the positions of the bevels are checked with fluoroscopy or, better, with a bi-planar image intensifier, which permits obtaining both lateral and anteroposterior views. The lateral view should show the bevel of the needle near the anterior of the bodies of the vertebrae, the anterolateral view should show the bevels of the needles to be 1 cm medial to the lateral edges of the vertebrae and the anteroposterior view should show the needles close to the lateral aspects of the vertebral bodies. When this has been accomplished a 2-ml syringe containing a solution of Conray-420 dye or Angiographin is adapted, and aspiration is attempted in two planes to ascertain that the bevel is not in a blood vessel or in a dural cuff. If the aspiration is negative, 0.5 ml of contrast solution is injected under image intensifier monitoring using the lateral view. If each needle is in the correct position, the contrast medium spreads in a thin linear fashion that conforms to the anterior edge of the vertebra (Fig. 96-36). The appearance of a "blob" or fuzzy patch of the contrast medium indicates that the injection was made into the psoas muscle or fascia, both of which offer resistance to injection. Occasionally a small vessel is entered without backflow of blood during aspiration, but on injection of the contrast medium it is promptly whisked away along the path of the vessel. In either case the needle should be readjusted and the preliminary injection of contrast medium should be repeated.

Once it has been confirmed that the bevels of all the needles are correctly positioned, 3 to 4 ml of 10% phenol in Conray-420 (or in some other water-based iodinated contrast medium) is injected through the needles at L2 and L4. If three needles are used 2 ml of solution is injected at L2 and L3 and 3 ml of the solution is injected at L4. With one needle at L2 or L3 10 ml of phenol-contrast medium is injected. The image intensifier is used to monitor the spread of the solution. Using these volumes the phenol-containing solu-

tion spreads in the same linear fashion as above, extending from the upper level of L2 or the lower level of L1 to the level of L5. With such a spread the phenol can destroy the entire sympathetic nerve supply to the limb below the knee.

Permanent roentgenograms of needle placement and solution spread are taken in two planes, and 0.5 ml of air or saline is then injected through each needle before it is removed. This is done to prevent spilling of the small amount of neurolytic agent in the needle onto a somatic nerve during needle withdrawal, thus minimizing the risk of postinjection neuralgia.

Patients are kept on their side for 10 to 15 minutes to prevent the spread of the solution laterally toward the genitofemoral nerve or posteriorly through the aponeurotic arcades or spaces in the origin of the psoas muscle and its fascia along the fibrous tunnel occupied by the rami communicantes. The latter, of course, connect the sympathetic chain with the lumbar spinal (somatic) nerves.

Because this entire procedure requires that the patient stay in the same position for about 90 to 120 minutes it is essential to give moral support, encouragement, and reassurance frequently during the entire procedure. Moreover, if the patient manifests apprehension or anxiety or complains of discomfort, it might be necessary to give an additional dose of a sedative, an IV injection of 4 to 5 mg of morphine, or both—especially if the discomfort develops early in the procedure and is likely to persist. If additional medication is not necessary during the procedure the patient should be given a "reward" in the form of a sedative as soon as the procedure is completed. Properly administered, this supplementary medication should not interfere with evaluation of the block.

After the 10-minute waiting period the patient is turned supine but is instructed not to raise the head for 1 hour, during which time observations of skin temperature, blood pressure, and pulse are made at frequent intervals. If blood pressure remains stable after this period the patient is allowed to sit for 45 minutes and resume oral intake. Blood pressure and pulse are checked 1 hour later with the patient sitting and standing and, if unchanged, the infusion is

TABLE 96-10. Comparison of Results of Lumbar Chemical Sympathectomy for the Relief of Pain of Occlusive Peripheral Vascular Disease (relief in Percent of Patients Treated)

Parameter	Source				
	Löfstrom et al. (121)	Cousins et al. (124)	Boas et al. (123)	Other Studies*	
				No. of Reports	Mean (Range)
Total number of patients	72	246	250	?	
Rest pain					
Number of patients	18	194	175	?	
Good relief	100	49	75	8	48 (48–50)
Partial relief	0	31			
None	0	20	25		
Gangrene					
Number of patients	42	40			
Good relief	52	50		9	49 (33–64)
Partial relief	30				
None	18	50			
Intermittent claudication					
Number of patients	12	12	63	?	?
Relief	58	50	30	3	25 (13–41)
No relief	42	50	70		75
Healing of ulcer					
Number of patients			75		
Good healing			60		

*Cited in Cousins, M.J., Dwyer, B., and Gibb, D.: Chronic pain and neurolytic neural blockade. In Neural Blockade in Clinical Anesthesia and Management of Pain. 2nd Ed. Edited by M.J. Cousins and P.O. Bridenbaugh. Philadelphia, J.B. Lippincott Company. 1988. pp. 1053–1084.

removed and the patient is allowed to ambulate. The patient with unstable cardiovascular disease should be observed and vital signs monitored for at least 24 hours after the block.

In patients in whom the chemical sympathectomy is being done for relief of burning pain of causalgia in the thigh associated with major nerve injury or with reflex sympathetic dystrophy or following an above-the-knee amputation, it might be necessary to block the uppermost lumbar and lowermost thoracic portions of the sympathetic chain to eliminate all sympathetic function to the entire limb and provide complete relief. During World War II I saw a number of patients with causalgia or reflex sympathetic dystrophies who derived complete relief of pain from prognostic blocks with local anesthetic but who obtained only partial relief from a subsequent lumbar sympathectomy, limited to the L2, L3, and L4 ganglia. A second series of prognostic blocks done after the sympathectomy, which included L1 and T12, produced complete relief from pain, suggesting that the surgical sympathectomy was incomplete. A second operation, in which the chain between T10 and L1 was removed, resulted in complete and permanent relief. Because such extensive sympathectomy can produce sexual impotence, especially if done bilaterally, it should be considered only when severe pain is present and patients are informed about the complications and agree to proceed.

Results

Three sets of results on the use of lumbar chemical sympathectomy are summarized in Table 96-10.

Löfstrom and associates (121, 125) treated patients with occlusive peripheral arterial disease by continuous lumbar sympathetic block with a local anesthetic. They then proceeded to carry out the block with phenol for those who were only temporarily relieved of their symptoms. The local anesthetic block produced prolonged pain relief in 28 of 55 patients (51%) with arteriosclerotic gangrene, in 14 of 28 patients (50%) with pain caused by diabetes, in 5 of 23 patients (22%) with severe rest pain, and in 1 of 16 patients (6%) with intermittent claudication.

In a series of 250 percutaneous chemical sympathectomies done by Boas and colleagues (123), 70% of patients had rest pain, 30% had trophic changes with ulcerations, gangrenous changes, or both, and 25% had intermittent claudication. Long-term results included relief of rest pain in 75% of patients (better than that achieved with surgical sympathectomy), healing of the ischemic lesions in 60%, and improvement of claudication in only 30% of patients with this complaint. Subsequently, Boas (119) mentioned that his group had done phenol block on over 500 patients with arteriosclerotic symptoms and signs, with similar results.

In the series reported by Cousins and associates (124), relief from rest pain was complete in 49% of patients and partial in 31%. In those without pre-existing gangrenous changes 84% of patients derived partial or complete relief as compared to 56% of those with gangrenous lesion. The onset of pain relief coincided with the onset of sympathetic block and with increases in skin blood flow and temperature. The mean duration of pain relief was 5.9 ± 0.6 months, which was similar to the mean duration of sweat modification (6.0 ± 0 months). Two years after the blockade 35% of patients were alive and the skin was intact, without evidence of ulcer or gangrene, 15% had undergone reconstructive surgery, and 25% required either local debridement or major amputation within an average of 10 months after the block. Only 10% of patients required a repeat block on the same side within a period of 3 to 12 months. Pain relief after the second block was always at least equal to that obtained with the first block. Cousins and colleagues (124) also noted that another, often neglected, benefit of sympathectomy is that it shortens the time to a clear demarcation area of the amputation level and improves the vascular supply to the stump. Moreover, because early sympathectomy is beneficial in treating some types of phantom limb pain, sympathectomy for pain relief performed 1 month before amputation can prevent postamputation pain. This is suggested by the fact that none of their patients who underwent amputation developed severe phantom limb pain.

Cousins and associates (124) used prognostic block of the lumbar sympathetic chain with 0.5% bupivacaine in most of their patients. They believed that, unless this is carried out, some patients manifest the "stealing" phenomenon because of the response of healthy vessels and the lack of response of diseased vessels. Moreover, Cousins and co-workers (124), as well as Boas and associates (123), excluded patients whose primary complaint was intermittent claudication on the premise that they are best treated with reconstructive surgery. Löfstrom and Cousins (125), in a review of 14 studies, cited the percentage of patients with occlusive vascular disease who responded to lumbar sympathetic block in regard to such parameters as rest pain, skin lesion, and intermittent claudication. Rest pain was relieved in a mean of 48% of patients, with a range of 48 to 80%.

Over a 30-year period, my associates and I carried out chemical sympathectomy in more than 200 patients, with good relief of rest pain being obtained in about 50% and partial relief in another 25% (unpublished data). About 50% of patients had healing of their skin ulcers and derived relief from pain caused by gangrene. As others have demonstrated, the poorest results were obtained in regard to intermittent claudication, with only 30% of patients deriving good or partial relief. My results with chemical sympathectomy for the production of prolonged sympathetic interruption in patients with causalgia and reflex sympathetic dystrophy are presented in Chapter 11.

Complications

In addition to the complications mentioned in Chapter 94 associated with the use of lumbar sympathetic block with local anesthetics, the most serious complication with chemical sympathectomy is genitofemoral neuralgia, which occurs in 5 to 7% of patients. It is presumably caused by the diffusion of the alcohol to the genitofemoral nerve as it lies on the anterior surface of the psoas major muscle, not too far from the lumbar sympathetic chain. This same complication follows surgical sympathectomy, suggesting that the nerve is damaged during the course of the operation. The condition is characterized by the usual burning and aching pain and can be relieved by transcutaneous electric nerve stimulation. Although some authors have claimed that the incidence of this complication is much higher with alcohol, this has not been my experience in the more than 50 patients in whom chemical sympathectomy was done with 50% alcohol.

E. NEUROLYTIC BLOCK OF SOMATIC SPINAL NERVES

Based on early experience with neurolytic block of somatic spinal nerves I have continued to insist that, except in patients with severe terminal cancer pain not amenable to any other procedure, neurolytic block of somatic nerves should not be used. The primary rationale for this is that, during nerve regeneration, patients experience severe neuralgia in the nerves supplying the limb, invariably producing a weak and often useless limb. Although some authorities (3) have suggested that the neuralgia is related to the fact that the nerve damage is caused by imprecise needle placement and incomplete neurolysis, I have had this condition occur in patients in whom the neurolytic agent was injected intraneurally, with complete destruction of the nerve. For some unknown reason neurolytic block of the branches of the trigeminal nerve does not usually produce neuralgia during regeneration. *In any case I feel that, with a few special exceptions, neurolytic block of somatic spinal nerves should not be done in patients with nonmalignant chronic pain.*

On the other hand I do believe that, in patients with severe intractable pain caused by advanced or terminal cancer in whom other therapeutic measures are not effective, it is appropriate to inject somatic nerves with absolute alcohol or with aqueous phenol. I have reported (1) on patients with terminal Pancoast's tumor who could not be relieved with large doses of morphine IM given every 3 hours in whom the roots of the brachial plexus were blocked with alcohol (Fig. 96-37). I have also done paravertebral block using 1 ml of alcohol injected into each of the several nerves involved in patients with severe pain in the chest or abdomen caused by vertebral or paravertebral neoplasms (as well as visceral neoplasms), in whom the tumor invaded the parietal peritoneum and celiac plexus block, as expected, did not relieve the somatic pain. In all these patients two or three blocks with a long-lasting local anesthetic indicated that interruption of the nerve would provide good pain relief.

In several patients with severe pain and edema, which made the limb useless, I have injected the brachial plexus with 20 ml of 95% alcohol after two prognostic blocks with 0.15% tetracaine produced good pain relief but also paralysis of the limb; patients chose neurolytic block after being informed of its prolonged effects. Pain relief in the limb lasted until the death of these patients. I have also used 5% aqueous phenol for block of the brachial plexus, with consequent analgesia that lasted from 3 weeks to $3\frac{1}{2}$ months. Mullin (126) has reported on the injection of 10 ml of 3% aqueous phenol following diagnostic or prognostic blocks with a local anesthetic to ensure good pain relief. The phenol block provided good pain relief for 2 to 5 weeks and was repeated as often as five times, until death ensued. Others have reported on the use of neurolytic block of the brachial plexus with either alcohol or phenol, with effective pain relief being produced in patients with terminal cancer.

Feldman and Yeung (127) cited the use of lumbar somatic nerve block with 5 to 10 ml of 7.5% phenol in myodil under radiographic control in 26 patients with severe intermittent claudication not amenable to bypass surgery. Of those in this group, 24 patients (93%) showed improvement, as reflected by an increase of 1.5 to 9 times the original claudication walking distance. Follow-up at 3 months showed improvement in 19 of 22 patients (86%), at 6 months in 10 of 14 patients (71%), and at 1 year in 6 of 7 patients (88%). They

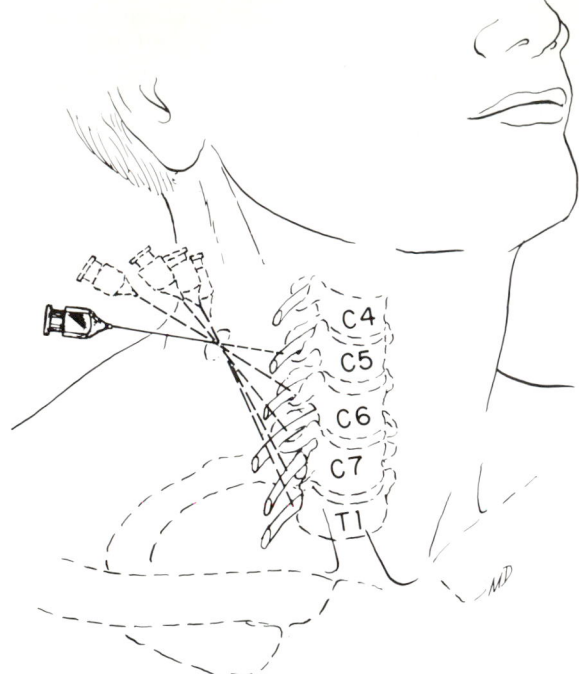

Fig. 96-37. Technique of injecting the roots of the brachial plexus with a neurolytic agent using one needle inserted through a skin wheal made just lateral to the transverse process of the C5 vertebra. The first insertion is directed medially to contact the C5 spinal nerve as it lies in the sulcus of the transverse process. The needle penetrates the nerve and 0.5 ml of alcohol is injected. The second and subsequent needles are passed through the same skin wheal, but directed progressively more caudad.

attributed these benefits to the fact that, with pain relief, patients walked more freely, promoting the development of collateral vessels. Other than transient back pain and hypesthesia, only 2 of 24 patients (7%) had troublesome burning over the distribution of their lower lumbar segment which lasted for some months.

Trans-sacral nerve block with a neurolytic agent is useful in patients with severe unremitting perineal pain caused by inoperable cancer of the rectum or by that which occurs after abdominoperineal resection not relieved by subarachnoid neurolysis. Because the S4 segment provides predominant sensory innervation to the perineum, trans-sacral block of this segment with 2 ml of 6% aqueous phenol has been used to provide prolonged pain relief. Robertson (128) reported the use of this technique in 9 patients with cancer of the rectum: 8 had undergone abdominoperineal resection and 1 had an inoperable lesion and a defunctioning colostomy. The pain was asymmetric in all 9 patients, being more pronounced on one side of the perineum than the other, and was of such severity to be considered an indication for intrathecal neurolysis. All patients received a prognostic block with 2.5 ml of 0.5% bupivacaine and an equal volume of 6% aqueous phenol was injected 24 hours later. The first injection provided pain relief of less than 1 week's duration in 6 patients, of 10 days duration in 1 patient, and of 202 and 414 days duration in the other 2 patients, respectively. A second injection produced pain relief lasting from 18 to 122 days, and 3 patients received a third block. Treatment was carried out on an outpatient basis, with no disturbances of bladder or motor function and with sensory changes limited to the perineum.

Neurolytic Somatic Block for the Relief of Chronic Nonmalignant Pain

Brief mention is made here of several indications for the use of neurolytic block in patients with nonmalignant chronic pain. These include trans-sacral block for severe bladder pain and spasticity, the abdominal nerve entrapment syndrome, coccyodynia, and the injection of small neuromas consequent to surgery.

CYSTITIS. Simon and associates (129) reported on a prospective study to evaluate the results of the injection of 2 ml of 6% aqueous phenol at S3 in 15 patients with severe pain caused by interstitial or hemorrhagic cystitis and in 1 patient who had a neurogenic spastic bladder. Following a diagnostic block with 0.5% bupivacaine, 2 ml of 6% aqueous phenol was injected through the right S3 foramen (Chapter 94). Of these patients 10 who received bupivacaine subsequently received phenol and, of these, 7 reported significant long-lasting pain relief, 1 had pain relief for 1 week, and 2 received no benefit. The average follow-up period was 24 months and the duration of response in patients with persistent pain was at least as long. No patients suffered urinary or rectal incontinence.

ABDOMINAL NERVE ENTRAPMENT SYNDROME. The abdominal nerve entrapment syndrome (Chapter 63) is a source of significant discomfort that can be disabling. The condition is usually treated with repeated injections of a long-lasting local anesthetic. Recently McGrady and Marks (130) reported on a series of 76 patients treated with 1 ml of 6% aqueous phenol using a nerve stimulator to locate the optimal point of injection. Of those in the group of 44 patients whose diagnosis had been definitively made, 95% derived complete or partial relief of symptoms at follow-up lasting from 6 months to 4 years, while in a group of 32 patients who had other symptoms that made the diagnosis less certain 48% gained partial relief and 8% obtained complete relief.

COCCYODYNIA. Coccyodynia is often a difficult pain problem to manage (Chapter 69). If the pain is severe a series of local anesthetic blocks using 1 to 2 ml of 0.25% bupivacaine with epinephrine injected into the S5 and coccygeal nerves should be tried. If a series of at least four blocks produces complete but transient pain relief, the injection of either 6% phenol or 10% ammonium sulfate should be considered.

Cryoanalgesia

The term "cryoanalgesia" was coined by Lloyd and colleagues (131) to describe the destruction of peripheral nerves by extreme cold to achieve pain relief. The histologic effects of cryoanalgesia on nerves has been summarized above (A. Basic Considerations). The procedure produces a small ice crystal that causes a second-degree nerve injury that consists of wallerian degeneration with axonal disintegration and break-up of the myelin sheath but with minimal disruption of the endoneurium and the basal lamina. It is claimed that cryolesions produce less fibrous tissue reaction than other forms of destruction (132). Since its introduction in 1976 this method has had limited clinical application and the number of published reports is small (133–136).

Indications

Cryoanalgesia has been used for local destruction of brain tissue and to block cranial and spinal nerves to relieve such problems as intractable facial pain, post-thoracotomy pain, post-traumatic chest pain, and cancer pain. Because the duration of pain relief averages about 2 weeks (range, 2 days to 7 months), however, the most fruitful use is to relieve postoperative and post-traumatic chest pain and to provide medium duration of relief in patients with various chronic pain syndromes.

Technique

Cryoanalgesia is done with a 15-gauge cryoneedle. Blockade is based on the principle of the Joule-Thompson effect, with nitrous oxide being used as the refrigerant gas (137). The Joule-Thompson effect occurs when gas at about 700 psi pressure is injected through a nozzle; as it expands it cools to about $-75°C$. The cooled gas impinges on the inner surface of the needle tip and absorbs heat from the surrounding tissue, and the warm gas is exhausted back up the needle and vented through the scavenger system. The Spembley-Lloyd cryoneedle uses a thermocouple to confirm the temperature achieved at the tip and an electric connection at the tip of the probe is connected to a peripheral nerve stimulator for precise location of the nerve. The probe is connected by a 6-foot piece of flexible tubing (Fig. 96-38) to a console that has a gas pressure regulator switch, a nerve stimulator socket, and dials for displaying gas pressure and probe tip temperature.

The probe can be introduced percutaneously or under direct vision by the surgeon at the end of the thoracotomy. For percutaneous application the skin is anesthetized with a local anesthetic and a Sise introducor is used to create a tract through the tissue through which the probe is inserted. Using the stimulator, maximum response with minimum current indicates that the tip is lying adjacent to the target nerve. A cryolesion is then produced and is confirmed by the temperature. Because the small ice ball cannot be visualized, temperature monitoring is the only check on probe function. It has been shown that repeated freeze-thaw cycles are likely to increase the destructive effect, so Lloyd and associates (131) have recommended two freeze-thaw cycles each time for 2 minutes from when a steady low temperature of about $-60°C$ is established. After each freeze the temperature returns to about $0°C$ before refreezing or withdrawal of the probe.

Cousins and co-workers (3) have made three important points about the procedure: (a) the cryoprobe should not be withdrawn until it has fully thawed because otherwise the surrounding tissue might adhere to the probe, which could tear blood vessels, neural structures, or both; (b) great care should be exercised with cryoprobe blockade in the paravertebral region where the dural cuff might be extended because the cold lesion could extend to the spinal cord or cause thrombosis of a major "feeder" artery by the marked local reduction of temperature—thus, somatic block should be carried out away from the paravertebral space unless it is necessary to block the posterior primary division of the spinal nerve; and (c) a major disadvantage of percutaneous use is that the freezing that occurs along the needle can result in full-thickness destruction of the skin, which leaves a depigmented scar after healing. This problem can be minimized by heating the skin with an ordinary infrared lamp or by using a large IV cannula to provide a sheath for insertion of the cryoprobe. Cryoanalgesia should not be used on a mixed spinal nerve that supplies the limb because this results in complete loss of function in the nerve, including paralysis of the muscles supplied by that nerve.

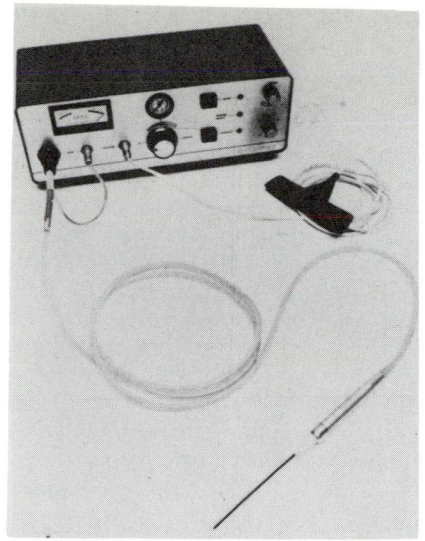

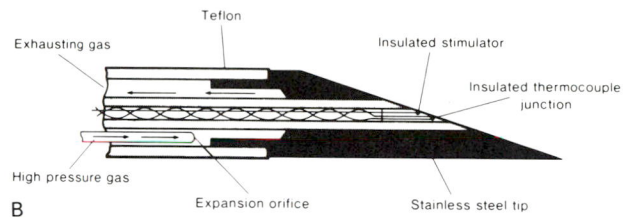

FIG. 96-38. A. Spembley-Lloyd cryoanalgesia apparatus. The unit incorporates a cryosurgical system that is coupled to a nerve stimulator for accurate positioning of the probe. The probe is connected by 6 feet of flexible tubing to a console that has a gas pressure regulator switch, a nerve stimulator socket, and dials to display gas pressure and probe tip temperature. **B.** Details of the cryoprobe tip. A chrome-constantan thermocouple is fitted to the tip of the probe to monitor the temperature. The probe is 10 cm long and is constructed from a 15-gauge stainless steel hypodermic tube with an 18° short-beveled point. An electrical connection is made to the tip of the probe from the nerve stimulator and all parts of the probe are insulated from the patient and operator by a Teflon coating. From Lloyd, G.W., Bernard, J.D., and Glynn, C.J.: Cryoanalgesia: A new approach to pain relief. Lancet, 2:933, 1976.

Results

Lloyd and colleagues (131) reported on the use of cryoanalgesia in 64 patients, of whom 52 obtained good relief of pain that lasted for a median period of 11 days, up to 7 months. Best results were obtained in providing pain relief to 88% of 17 patients with intercostal nerve pain, to all of 6 patients with facial neuralgia who were subjected to infraorbital or mental nerve block, and to 8 of 9 patients (89%) who had cancer (4 of these had intercostal blocks and 5 had the cryoprobe introduced through the sacral hiatus to produce caudal analgesia). Subsequently the same group reported on 29 patients who received intercostal block with cryoprobe under direct vision prior to closure of the thoracotomy. They compared postoperative opioid requirements with those of a control group of 29 patients who were matched for sex, age, and diagnosis and managed with intramuscular opioids (133). Those patients in the cryoanalgesia group derived more effective relief and required significantly fewer opioid injections for less time as compared to those in the control group. Barnard and colleagues (134) used cryoanalgesia in the management of chronic facial pain in 43 patients who received 85 cryogenic blocks of branches of the trigeminal nerve for the relief of the pain of tic douloureux, postoperative neuralgia, postherpetic neuralgia, and other types of facial pain. In 67% of patients with nonherpetic neuralgia the pain relief persisted for a median of 93 days. Of 26 patients with postherpetic neuralgia only 42% derived relief, which lasted 6 weeks. None of those in the three groups of patients treated by Lloyd and co-workers (131, 133, 134) developed neuralgia subsequent to treatment and no other serious complications have been reported.

Katz and associates (135) reported good relief of post-thoracotomy pain following intercostal cryoanalgesia carried out under direct vision. Katz also stated (personal communication, 1988) that he and co-workers have used cryoanalgesia in nearly 150 patients, with good pain relief being produced in over 85% of patients. Jones and Murrin (136) reported results with the use of percutaneous cryotherapy of intercostal nerves in patients with various chronic chest pain syndromes who had had pain for 6 months to 2 years. Of 32 patients with post-thoracotomy scar pain, 13 (40%) derived good relief, 30% had partial relief, and 30% had little or no relief. Among 15 patients with postherpetic neuralgia 74% derived good relief, 13% had partial relief, and 13% had little or no relief. The duration of pain relief for those in the latter group was less than 7 days in 79% of patients, while for those in the former group relief lasted considerably longer (136).

F. NEUROADENOLYSIS OF THE PITUITARY

Neuroadenolysis of the pituitary (NALP) has purposely not been discussed in this chapter until all other neurolytic blocks for pain control had been described. I consider it to be the most useful neurolytic procedure for patients with diffuse advanced cancer pain for whom all other neurolytic blocks are impractical or produce inadequate pain relief, or both. Based on personal observations, review of the literature, and discussion with clinicians who have had extensive experience with the use of NALP, I am convinced that this procedure should be learned by anesthesiologists and neurosurgeons involved in the management of cancer pain. Properly carried out, NALP produces a remarkable and, at times, almost incredible degree of relief of diffuse pain.

This section first presents the technique developed by Moricca (138, 139) because it can be done in any hospital in which skilled personnel and the usual radiographic equipment are available. Thus, it could also be carried out in hospitals in third-world countries. The evolution of the NALP procedure is mentioned and, after Moricca's technique is described, some modifications and results obtained are discussed, including the degree of pain relief and complications reported by a number of clinicians. The stereotaxic techique developed by Levin, Katz, and associates is also summarized (140, 141).

General Considerations

Perspective

The history of the destruction of the pituitary for pain relief began with the early work of Huggins (142), who showed that hormonal manipulation through gonadectomy, adrenalectomy, or both to produce regression of cancer of the breast and prostate was often followed by relief of pain.*

---

*For a comprehensive review of the history, evolution, and other aspects of the destruction of the pituitary, see the article by Gianasi (139).

In the early 1950s several workers, including Scott (143) and Luft and Olivecrona (144), reported on the use of transcranial hypophysectomy for the treatment of breast or prostate cancer, or both. This procedure represents the practical application of the then well-known fact that the hypothalamic-pituitary axis constitutes the integrating and coordinating center for the entire endocrine system. Although these workers carried out surgical hypophysectomy primarily to produce objective regression of metastatic breast or prostatic carcinoma, they noted that reduction or elimination of pain was a more consistent effect than tumor regression.

These preliminary reports apparently did not arouse as much interest as might be expected, partly because such major surgery in patients with advanced metastatic cancer had certain limitations. Among the most important of these limitations is that such procedures cannot be performed on high-risk patients, for whom any major operation might be contraindicated. Consequently, less stressful methods of pituitary inactivation were devised. In 1955 Forrest and Brown (145) published a report on their experience with the insertion of radon into the pituitary by a rhinotranssphenoidal approach. Later, Lewis and Baxton (146) studied the results of treating hormone-dependent tumors by inserting radioisotopes or injecting alcohol into the gland or by ligating peduncle of the pituitary.

During the 1950s Moricca, working at the Cancer Institute Regina Elena in Rome, was evaluating surgical adrenalectomy, oophorectomy, and hypophysectomy for the therapy of advanced breast cancer with diffuse metastasis. He soon realized that surgical procedures, especially hypophysectomy, presented serious problems in patients in poor physical condition. Because of his extensive experience with neurolytic blocks achieved by "blindly" injecting alcohol through percutaneously placed needles, Moricca began to consider the injection of alcohol into the pituitary through a needle passed into the gland through the nose and ethmoid and sphenoid bones. He first carried out studies on cadavers to determine the best approach for insertion of the needle by this route and observed the diffusion of 2 to 3 ml of methylene blue stain, noting the spread into the gland and also into suprasellar spaces. In 1958 Moricca performed the procedure in 7 patients, with encouraging results (see 139 for a list of all Moricca's publications). At the same time Greco and associates (147), independent of Moricca but following the suggestions of Lewis and Baxton (146), injected alcohol into the pituitary of 5 patients with cancer, with good results. In a series of papers published in 1965 Greco reported on 150 patients; by 1973 other reports were published. Recently Carbonin (148) summarized all the reports published by Greco.

Moricca continued to use and improve the technique. In the 1960s he performed several studies indicating the procedure to be highly effective in eliminating the pain of hormone-dependent tumors, such as those of the breast, prostate, thyroid, and uterus, which had progressed to an advanced phase of visceral and bony metastasis (see 139 for references). In many of these patients the severe intractable pain could only be partially or transiently relieved by more aggressive and stressful neurosurgical ablative procedures, and could not be controlled by large doses of morphine or other potent narcotics. In 1974 Moricca published his experiences with the use of NALP for the treatment of cancer pain caused by advanced nonhormone-dependent tumors (138).

The use of the procedure initiated a controversy among those oncologists and neurosurgeons who preferred other measures for removing or inactivating the pituitary gland. The advent of stereotaxic surgery and microsurgery caused some clinicians to replace the classic method of hypophysectomy through craniotomy with the use of the rhino-transsphenoidal route. Others used such procedures as stereotaxic cryohypophysectomy, open microsurgical hypophysectomy, and thermal coagulation of the pituitary by the transsphenoidal route—techniques that made pituitary ablation presumably safer than the classic surgical procedure. Some advocated pituitary inactivation through conventional radiotherapy, external irradiation with heavy particles (especially alpha rays and protons), and ultrasonic destruction of the pituitary. Still others used direct implantation of radioactive substances, such as seeds or pellets of ^{90}Y, ^{198}Au, and ^{32}P, into the sella turcica (see 139 for review and references). Moricca long maintained that these interventions compare unfavorably with NALP because they have the same limitations as surgical hypophysectomy or require sophisticated or expensive equipment or materials.

NALP does not require expensive equipment and can be practiced in any hospital in which skilled and experienced physicians can carry it out, even on patients in poor physical condition. Moreover, the procedure has the advantage that it can be repeated freely whenever the need arises, either for recurrence of the pain or for manifestations of new signs of tumor growth without impairing patients' mental faculties, which can occur with the administration of large doses of opioids or neuroleptic agents. During the past 15 years NALP has been used by many clinicians throughout the world. Most reports indicate that the procedure completely or partly relieves cancer pain in 65 to 90% of patients, and that the onset of pain relief is rapid and usually complete within hours of the procedure in those who respond (149, 150). In some patients pain relief is present by the time they wake up from the anesthesia, while in others it can take 24 to 48 hours (150). The degree and duration of relief are not strictly related to tumor regression because in about 50% of the patients with long-lasting pain relief no evidence of tumor regression is found, while in others it is (150). Finally, and most impressively, the procedure does not produce changes in skin sensation and does not seem to affect the functioning of the ascending nociceptive systems.

Mechanisms of Action

Many investigators have attempted to explain the pain relief produced by the use of NALP by hypothesizing a single mechanism. Some have suggested that the procedure eliminates the hormones produced by the pituitary that are responsible for enhancement of nociceptive transmission, while others have hypothesized that it disturbs hormonal balance through effects on certain parts of the central nervous system, so that it directly or indirectly influences the ubiquitous dopaminergic and endorphinergic receptors in the structures affected by alcohol. Still others have implicated certain structures in the hypothalamus and third ventricle (139, 141).

Clinical observations and experimental work have suggested that the pain relief might be a result of activation of a hypothalamus-suppressing response, a hypothesis that was first suggested by Moricca in the early 1970s when he began to insist that the procedure acts on the hypothalamus and other suprastructures rather than on the pituitary (138, 139). Evidence supporting the stimulation of hypothalamic function includes the fact that oophorectomy, adrenalectomy, or orchidectomy produces pain relief within hours of operation in patients with metastatic breast or prostate cancer. This pain relief occurs well before any evidence of tumor regression and the timing of its onset is similar to that of NALP, suggesting a hypothalamic pain-suppressing response activated by the elimination of hormonal feedback (149). Moreover, following the procedure, retrograde cell loss occurs in the hypothalamus in the region of the paraventricular and supraoptic nuclei, and this appears to be quite adequate to initiate pain relief. Pituitary stalk section also produces retrograde cell loss in the hypothalamus and associated pain relief.

On the other hand, apart from these effects, overt hypothalamic damage is not required to obtain prompt pain relief, even when anatomic or endocrinologic destruction of the pituitary is incomplete (149). Although many animal experimental studies have implicated endogenous opioid systems as a mechanism for pain relief following NALP, the evidence to support this hypothesis in humans with cancer pain is weak. Finally, Levin and Ramirez (141) suggested that analgesia following NALP can result from similar pain-suppressing hypothalamic mechanisms that produce stress-induced analgesia (Chapter 4).

Although no data available at present have defined the precise mechanisms of NALP, clinicians should not be deterred from using this procedure. After all, general anesthesia has been used for 150 years and we still do not know the precise mechanism of its action. In addition, the lack of information on the mechanism of action of the procedure should spur researchers to exert even greater efforts.

Clinical Considerations

Indications

NALP is indicated for patients with severe cancer pain that is widespread because of multiple metastases. It is useful, and indeed indispensable, for relieving such pain, especially that resulting from hormone-dependent tumors. Thus, when all anticancer procedures have been exhausted and diffuse pain persists or has recurred after other pain-relieving methods have failed, NALP should be considered if appropriate resources are available. Some authorities (3) have proposed that intraspinal opioids can be used, and do produce good pain relief, but NALP has the advantage of relieving pain in patients who have become tolerant to intraspinal opioids; in addition, it might have neoplasm-arresting action. Properly carried out it can be used in patients who are in poor physical condition, and it can always be repeated when the pain recurs or if the progression of the tumor is not arrested.

It has been impressively shown that NALP produces highly effective and long-lasting relief in a substantial proportion of patients, with a significant reduction in dosage or total gradual elimination of opioids. Obviously, ethical and humane limits are inherent in any technique used to treat cancer patients in the terminal phase of the disease when death is likely to occur in a few days. Such patients are best managed with opioids.

Techniques

When a decision that the patient can benefit from NALP is made, an explicit and formal consent must be obtained from the patient and family and the algologist should carry out a preoperative physiologic and psychologic evaluation and preparation of the patient (Chapters 31 and 94). It is important to obtain radiographs of the cranium in the anteroposterior and lateral projections to estimate the size and position of the pituitary fossa and sphenoid sinus, and to detect the presence of any nasal spurs or deviation of the septum. Bony abnormalities of the cranium do not contraindicate the technique but can create difficulties in positioning the needle in the sella turcica.

MORICCA'S TECHNIQUE. The Moricca technique for NALP has been described in detail elsewhere (138, 139). The equipment necessary is as follows:

For needle placement:

> Two Moricca needles
> Two bayonet forceps
> One small metal hammer
> One 2-ml insulin syringe
> One long Killian forceps
> One long Klemmer forceps
> One spinal needle
> One 10-ml syringe

Auxiliary equipment:

> Disinfection equipment for nasal cavity
> Disposable suction catheter for nasal cavity
> Antiseptic solution
> Gauze—sponges, strips
> Steroids—hydrocortisone, methylprednisolone
> Absolute alcohol
> Coagulants

The Moricca needle is made of stainless steel and has a stylet to prevent obstruction by blood clots. Its surface is smooth except for six notches in the proximal quarter of its length, which serve as reference points if

readjustment of the needle is necessary. It is strong enough to penetrate the bone without difficulty. Accurate positioning of the patient is essential for the correct and rapid execution of the procedure. The patient is placed supine on the operating table with the head semiflexed on a radiotransparent head rest that allows the patient to be comfortable and, at the same time, holds the head steady in the required position (Fig. 96-39). The image intensifier is arranged to swing around the head through 90° to obtain lateral and anteroposterior skull films. Some units have a television monitor attached to the image intensifier so that the needle placement can be seen instantly. Light general endotracheal anesthesia that preserves pupillary responses is used by Moricca and most other clinicians. Usually the thiopental, nitrous oxide–oxygen, and muscle relaxant technique is used and the endotracheal tube is inserted after topical anesthesia of the larynx and trachea has been achieved. When the patient has been anesthetized and is in the proper position, the following steps for the procedure are carried out:

a. The catheter is introduced into the nasal cavity and pharynx to aspirate secretions.

b. The antiseptic solution is applied to the skin around the nasal cavity.

c. The needle is introduced through the disinfected nasal cavity and directed posteriorly, superiorly, and slightly medially toward the glabella when viewed from the frontal plane and toward the midpoint of the zygomatic arch when viewed from the side (Fig. 96-40).

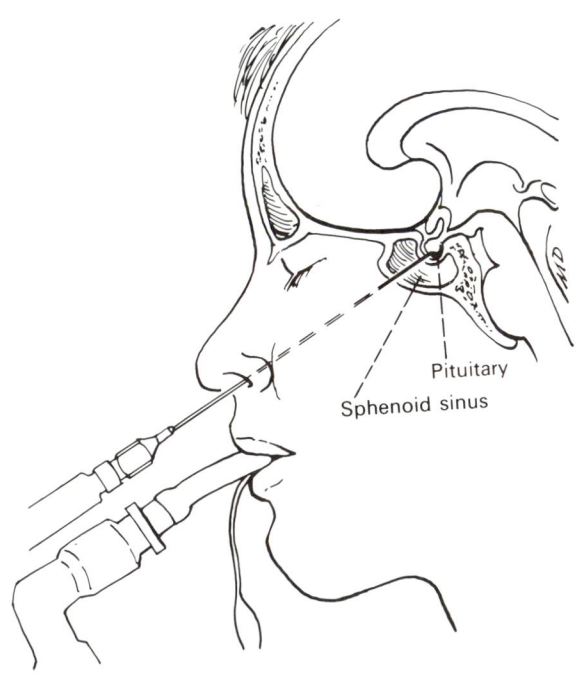

FIG. 96-39. Technique of injection of alcohol into the pituitary gland showing a lateral view of the head with some of the important bony landmarks. Although the patient is supine with the head flexed on a pillow, here it is shown upright for easier visualization. The Moricca needle or some other apparatus is passed transnasally and directed superiorly and medially to penetrate through the sphenoid sinus until its point is in the posterior part of the sella turcica.

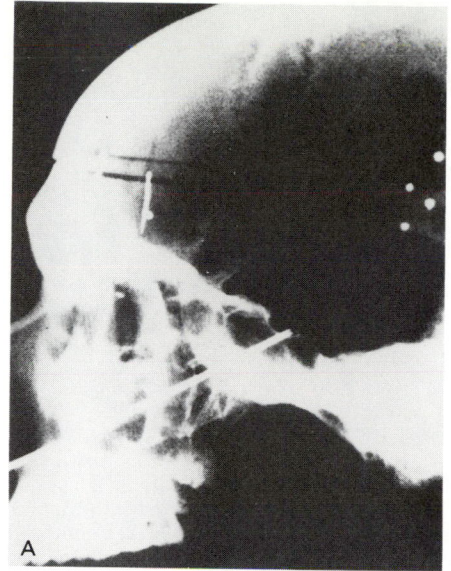 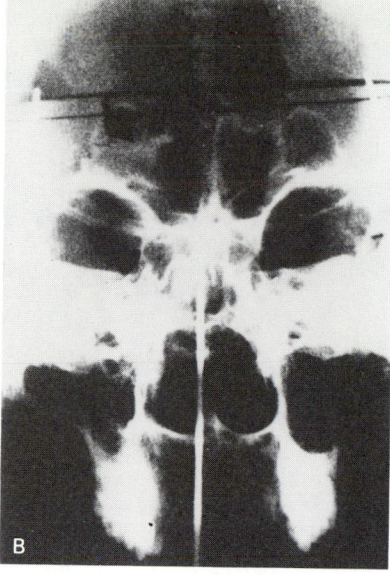 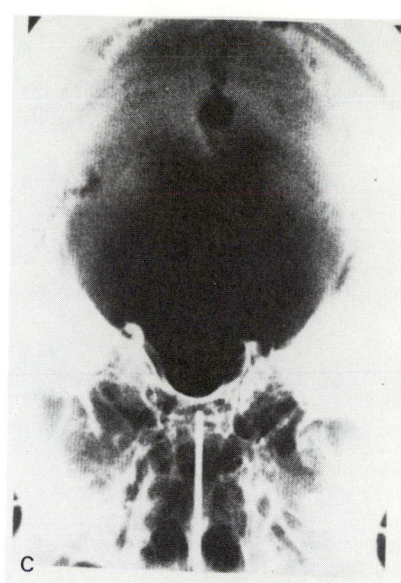

Fig. 96-40. Radiographs showing Moricca's technique of placing the Moricca needle in the sella turcica. *A.* Lateral view. The tip of the needle is close to the posterior wall of the sella turcica to favor the diffusion of alcohol along the pituitary stalk and involve the pituitary-hypothalamic structures. *B.* Anteroposterior view of the same needle. The point of the needle is in the exact midline. *C.* Radiograph taken with the patient in Fowler's position shows the correct position of the needle point in the sella turcica prior to the injection of alcohol.

d. The needle is inserted through the mucous membrane of the posterior nasal cavity toward the sphenoid bone and advanced through the base of the cranium with light strokes of the hammer. Passage through the various structures can be ascertained by noting variation in resistance and in the tone of the percussion.

e. Once the base of the sella has been perforated the stylet is retracted slightly and the needle is advanced by slight percussion of the hammer. Once the dorsum sella has been reached the stylet is advanced, but not as far as the entire length of the needle.

f. Radiographs of the position of the needle are taken in anteroposterior and lateral views.

g. The Queckenstedt maneuver is performed to detect any CSF or blood flow from the needle hub. If negative, proceed to injection of the alcohol.

Once proper positioning of the needle has been ascertained (Fig. 96-40), the patient is awakened sufficiently to be able to cooperate and collaborate with the operator. At this point the alcohol is injected in fractional doses of approximately 0.25 ml at intervals of 15 to 20 seconds. During this time the diameter of the pupil and the pupillary reflex response to light continue to be monitored in a darkened room. If pupillary dilatation occurs the injection of alcohol is discontinued and the patient is given 200 to 500 mg of hydrocortisone IV immediately. If things otherwise proceed satisfactorily, the injection is carried out gently and slowly to avoid a transient headache referred to the glabella. After 2 ml of alcohol has been injected the needle is withdrawn slightly and another series of injections is carried out, if deemed necessary. Indeed, a third series of injections, up to a total of 6 ml of alcohol, can be used during the first treatment.

After injection of alcohol is complete the stylet is reintroduced into the needle and the needle is withdrawn gently in a rotating fashion. After the needle has been withdrawn nasal tamponade is done with sterile gauze soaked in antiseptic.

OTHER TECHNIQUES. Some clinicians have modified the Moricca technique slightly as follows. The nose is packed with a varying concentration (7.5 to 20%) of cocaine solution with or without epinephrine 1:200,000 (140, 141, 150, 151). After 10 minutes the packs are removed and the anterior nasal mucosa is prepared with antiseptic solution and draped. The anterior nasal mucosa and deep tissues are infiltrated with a solution of 1% lidocaine containing 1:200,000 epinephrine. Some clinicians use a 15-gauge trocar to introduce a 15-cm 15-gauge needle (150), while others use a 8.5-cm 17-gauge styleted spinal needle to introduce a 15-cm 20-gauge needle (151). The cannula or introducer is advanced under biplanar fluoroscopic guidance until its tip rests against the anterior wall of the sella turcica, at which point plain radiographs are taken to confirm its position. Once this is done the injection needle is introduced into the pituitary gland, as for the Moricca technique. If pupillary dilatation occurs during injection of the alcohol, some clinicians discontinue the injection and turn the patient on the side, make a cisternal puncture, and inject 50 mg of hydrocortisone, 25 mg of prednisone and hydrocortisone, or 25 mg of prednisone (149, 150). After the injection of alcohol is complete the needle is withdrawn until its tip reaches the anterior wall of the sella, at which point 0.5 ml of cyanomethacrylate resin is injected through the 20-gauge needle to seal the hole in the sella and to prevent CSF leakage (140, 141, 151). Both needles are then removed and the mucosa is observed for bleeding or CSF leakage. Levin and

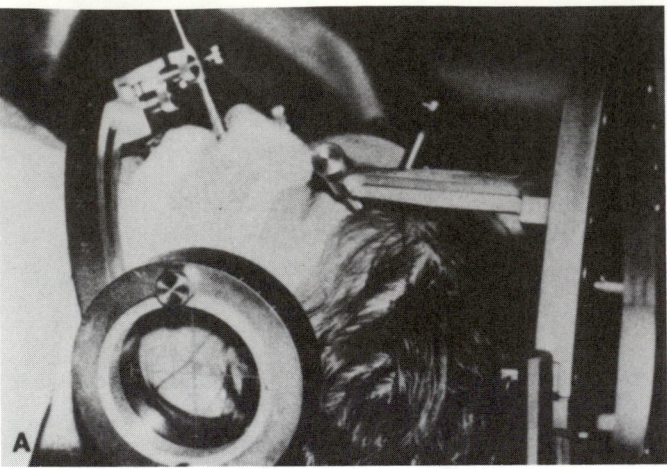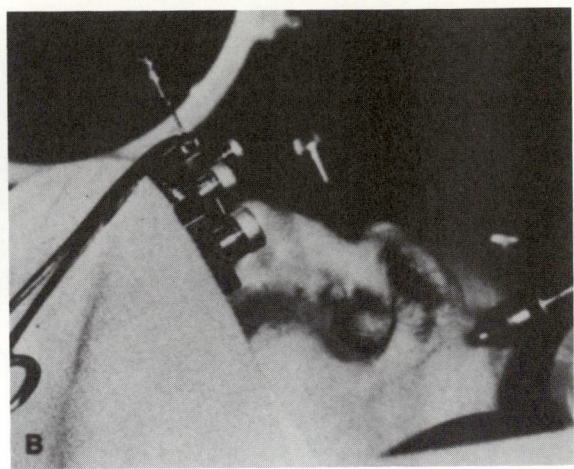

FIG. 96-41. Technique of neuroadenolysis of the pituitary using a stereotaxic apparatus. **A.** Lateral view. The patient is positioned in a Todd-Wells Stereotaxic head holder using a transverse quadrant assembly. The needle guide has been inserted into the nostril and is passed as far back toward the superior aspect of the nasal passage as possible. Under fluoroscopic lateral control and radiographic anteroposterior control following anesthesia of the mucosa, a 16-inch 18-gauge spinal needle is passed through the needle guide and advanced to the floor of the sphenoid sinus. **B.** The 18-gauge needle is then removed and a 6-inch 20-gauge spinal needle is passed through the guide and gently inserted through the floor of the sella turcica. From Levin, A.B., and Ramirez, L.L.: Treatment of cancer pain with hypophysectomy: Surgical and chemical. *In* Advances in Pain Research and Therapy, Vol. 7. Edited by C. Benedetti et al. New York, Raven Press, 1984.

co-workers (141) and Waldman and colleagues (151) have reported that nasal packing has not been required if the resin is used.

STEREOTAXIC NEUROADENOLYSIS OF THE PITUITARY. Levin and associates (140, 141) have developed a stereotaxic technique to produce NALP to permit the use of a fine needle to prevent large holes in the floor of the sella turcica and thus decrease the chance of CSF leakage, and to permit the use of a large volume of alcohol with one needle. The technique is similar to the "free-hand" procedure used by Moricca and others except that the patient is placed in a Todd-Wells stereotaxic head holder using a transverse quadrant assembly (Fig. 96-41). A 4% cocaine paste is applied to the nasal mucosa of the nostril with the least septal deviation and the angle of the transverse quadrant is adjusted so that the needle has the greatest possible penetration of the tubular glands on its way to the target. The mucosa is infiltrated with the lidocaine epinephrine solution (see above). The 18-gauge needle is removed and a 15-cm 20-gauge spinal needle is passed through the guide and gently inserted into the floor of the sella turcica (Fig. 96-42B). After the image intensifier ascertains that the needle has followed its intended path to the floor of the sella turcica, it is advanced to its target just below the posterior clinoid processes in the midline (Fig. 96-42). Once correct placement is confirmed, 1 to 2 ml of absolute alcohol is slowly injected while the patient's pupils are monitored. If pupillary dilatation occurs injection is suspended; if not, the needle is withdrawn to halfway between the target and the floor of the sella turcica and a second injection of 1 to 2 ml of alcohol is made. The needle is further withdrawn to a point halfway between that of the second injection and the floor of the sella turcica, and a third dose of 1 to 2 ml of alcohol is injected. The needle is then withdrawn, and cyanoethoacrylate resin (see above) is used to seal the hole of the sella and to prevent CSF leakage. As the needle is withdrawn the needle guide is withdrawn from the nostril, which is then observed. If bleeding occurs the nostril is packed with gauze impregnated with petroleum jelly.

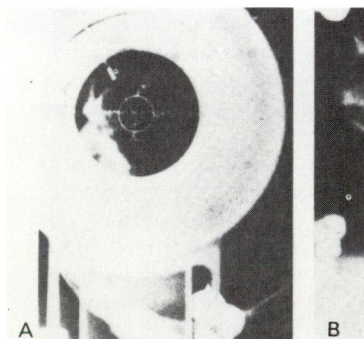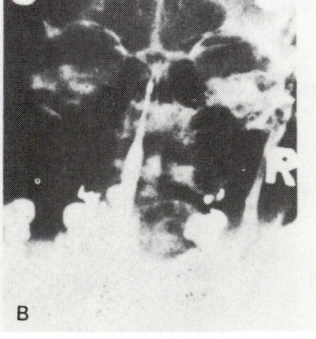

FIG. 96-42. **A.** Lateral view radiograph showing needle at target of stereotaxic apparatus. **B.** Anteroposterior view showing needle in midline of target. From Levin, A.B., and Ramirez, L.L.: Treatment of cancer pain with hypophysectomy: Surgical and chemical. *In* Advances in Pain Research and Therapy, Vol. 7. Edited by C. Benedetti et al. New York, Raven Press, 1984.

Postoperative Care

During the immediate postoperative period it is essential to monitor intake and output and vital signs carefully and to carry out laboratory studies, includ-

TABLE 96-11. Moricca's Results with NALP*

Parameter	Results (% of Patients Treated)
Complete pain relief	
After first NALP	59
After second NALP	9
After third NALP	28
All:	96
Incomplete pain relief after third NALP	4

*These unpublished data were compiled by Moricca from 1963 to 1987. A total of 2887 patients were treated; of these, 91% had hormone-dependent cancer and 9% had nonhormone-dependent cancer. During each session 3 to 6 ml of alcohol were injected.

TABLE 96-12. Gianasi's Results with NALP

Parameter	Results
Patients treated	109
With hormone-dependent tumors	73 (67%)
High-risk patients	83 (76%)
Age (years)	66 (52–78)*
Procedures performed	
Total	248†
Average/patient	2.27
Alcohol injected (ml)	
Each procedure	3 (0.5–7)*
Total/patient	5 (0.5–11)*
Procedures not completed‡	16
Follow-up to 3 months or death	93
Total pain relief	82 (88%)
Partial pain relief	11 (12%)
Total pain relief in hormone-dependent cancer	60 of 64 (94%)
Total pain relief in hormone-autonomous cancer	22 of 29 (76%)

Data from Gianasi, G.: Neuroadenolysis of the pituitary of Moricca: An overview of development, mechanisms, technique, and results. In Advances in Pain Research and Therapy, Vol. 7. Edited by C. Benedetti, C.R. Chapman, and G. Moricca. New York, Raven Press, 1984, pp. 647-678.

*Average values with range in parentheses.

†This total includes 17 NALPs that were repeated to control the pain, which had returned after the first set of NALPs had controlled it for a significant period of time.

‡Cases in which it was not possible to perform enough NALPs to introduce a total of 6 ml of alcohol.

ing determination of blood glucose, blood and urinary electrolyte, and creatinine levels. Many workers continue antibiotics for 24 hours and give endocrine replacement each morning, consisting of 15 mg hydrocortisone or prednisone and 0.5 mg Synthoid (138–141, 149–151). It is also important to watch for the metabolic alterations that frequently occur in patients with disorders of certain organs, either caused by cancer by chemotherapeutic procedures. The patient is allowed oral intake, first clear liquids and later food, 3 to 6 hours after the procedure. That afternoon or the next day the patient is allowed to ambulate if able to do so preoperatively. If the patient was taking opioids before the procedure, these are continued for 24 hours and then tapered. Assessment of results should be made over a period of several days.

Results

Incidence of Pain Relief

The incidence of pain relief recently reported by Moricca (152) and by Gianasi (139), a former colleague of Moricca, is presented in Tables 96-11 and 96-12; Table 96-13 contains the results of Levin and associates (140, 141) and of others who have reported the use of the procedure in more than 20 patients. The discrepancies among the various results are seen because of several factors: (a) differences in criteria for patient selection; (b) variations in type of tumor causing the pain; (c) differences in criteria for evaluation of analgesic efficacy; (d) varying lengths of follow-up; and (e) differences in technique. In regard to the selection of patients, it is generally agreed that NALP should be used exclusively in patients with widespread malignant disease who are suffering severe pain. Most patients treated by Moricca (138, 152) and by Gianasi (139, 153) had hormone-dependent tumors, and others have obtained better analgesic results with NALP for relieving the pain of hormone-dependent than that of nonhormone-dependent tumors (150, 155, 162). On the other hand, the results obtained by others who

TABLE 96-13. Comparison of Results with NALP for the Relief of Cancer Pain

Source (Country)	No. of Patients Treated	No. of NALPs Performed	Total Alcohol Injected (ml)	Pain Relief (% of Patients Treated)		
				Complete or Good	Fair	Poor or None
Katz and Levin (140) (USA)	22	24	5–6	87		13
Levin and Ramirez (141) (USA)	85	85	4–6	84		16
Gianasi (139) (Italy)	109	248	3–5	82	12	6
Lloyd et al. (155) (UK)	25	25	1–2	71		29
Lipton (150) (UK)	187	292	1–2	40	32	28
Farcot et al. (154) (France)	21	27	1–1.3	39	33	28
Corssen et al. (156) (USA)	32	34	1–2	69	28	3
Grunwald (157) (Uruguay)	60	?	0.5–2	65	25	10
Ischia et al. (158) (Italy)	83	100	2–3	57	32	11
Madrid (159) (Spain)	516	650	2–3	57	29	14
Cook et al. (160) (UK)	26	43	1–2	27	38	35
Romoli (161) (Italy)	148	188	1.5–2	75	17	8
Takeda (162) (Japan)	90	122	2–2.5	81	11	8
Waldman et al. (151) (USA)	55	55	4–6	75	17	8
Lahuerta et al. (163) (UK)	28	54	1–2	39	36	25
All/Mean:	1,471	2,024		63 86*	23	14

*Mean percent for all reports combining good and fair pain relief.

used NALP for patients with nonhormone-dependent tumors have been comparable to those for hormone-dependent cancers (140, 141, 150, 156, 158, 160, 163).

Moricca and Gianasi (138, 139, 152, 153) claimed that those whose results of complete and partial relief were lower than 80 to 85% used an insufficient volume of alcohol, usually 0.5 to 1 ml. This position is supported by Katz (personal communication 1988), who firmly believes that at least 4 to 6 ml of alcohol must be injected to obtain maximum results. The same position has been expressed by Waldman and colleagues (151) and, as noted, Levin (141), Katz's former collaborator, has also used large volumes of alcohol. On the other hand, Lipton (150) stated that in the series of patients treated by his group the volume of alcohol injected was not found to be critical in regard to the incidence of pain relief reported by the patient.

Moricca also noted that the differences in the results reported might be a result of insufficient experience with the technique. Thus, the results obtained by those who reported on a limited number of patients could reflect the results of the initial phase of the application of the technique, before it was mastered and perfected. Another factor might be that some of the reports contain data on the use of only one injection, and that the procedure was not repeated when it became necessary because of pain recurrence. In Moricca's own series (Table 96-11) good pain relief was obtained by 59% of patients after the first injection, by 9% of patients after the second injection, and by 28% of patients after the third procedure. Regardless of the effect on the pain, Moricca repeated the procedure until a total volume of at least 5 ml of alcohol was injected. This constitutes one cycle of therapy, and about 90% of patients obtained good pain relief from the first cycle of NALP. In a significant percentage of these patients, however, pain recurred several months later, at which point another cycle of NALP was repeated.

In assessing pain relief, some authors have considered pain relief to be "complete" if the patient required no opioids after they were gradually reduced following the procedure, and to be "good" or "partial" if pain was controlled by the procedure and by reduced doses of opioids and nonopioid analgesics. Other clinicians have reported "good" pain relief for patients who derived sufficient relief to reduce significantly but not eliminate the daily intake of opioids. As noted in Table 96-13, the means of 15 reports indicate that 86% of patients treated with NALP obtained complete (63%) or partial (fair) (23%) relief. The duration of pain relief varied from 3 weeks to several months, with more that 50% of patients having pain relief lasting 3 to 5 months, and for more than 1 year in a few patients (138–141, 149–151, 156–163).

Side Effects and Complications

Postinjection headache and rhinorrhea occur in 40 to 60% of patients. Diabetes insipidus, which occurs in 15 to 60% (mean, 40%) (138–142, 149–162), is not so much a complication as a natural concomitant of destruction of the pituitary gland. It is only dangerous if dehydration or abnormality of electrolyte balance occurs (150). In almost all patients it responds satisfactorily to desmopressin in daily dosages of 10 to 40 mg. Rhinorrhea occurs in 1 to 17% (161, 162) but is always transient. Diarrhea occurs in a few patients and usually lasts a few hours, but in a small percentage of patients it can last as long as 4 days. Other complications include drowsiness, slow mentation, and even coma for a few days postoperatively.

Theoretically, visual defects could be profound, but they actually occur infrequently and are transient, although some authors have reported permanent defects in about 5% of their patients (150, 158). Other complications that could occur as a consequence of destruction of the pituitary include hyperthermia, hyperphagia, hypopituitarism, and steroid deficiency. The latter two need temporary hormonal replacement but, as in diabetes insipidus, they usually resolve spontaneously within 1 or 2 weeks. Death caused directly by NALP is either absent or has a low incidence and, when it occurs several days after the procedure, it is related to infection (meningitis), hypothalamic damage, or acute pituitary insufficiency. Most of these can be prevented by the use of aseptic technique, antibiotics, and hormone replacement therapy.

Conclusion

After reviewing the available data, I concur with Miles (149), Lipton (150), Levin and associates (140, 141) and many others who have used this procedure extensively (151, 155–159, 160, 162, 163) that it is useful in patients with severe diffuse cancer pain. Indeed, destruction of the pituitary gland and probably hypothalamic mechanisms with alcohol results in complete or partial pain relief in some 70 to 85% or more of these patients. Pain relief can occur immediately on pituitary destruction or can occur within 1 or 2 days after the procedure. The duration of pain relief varies: whereas the pain usually returns in 3 to 5 months, in some patients it is possible for relief to last longer than 1 year (150, 151), and in patients with cancer of the breast or prostate pain relief can be associated with evidence of regression of the tumor. These data suggest that NALP is one of the most, if not the most, effective ablative procedure for the relief of severe diffuse cancer pain in patients who are in poor physical condition.

Some authorities (3) have suggested that the results obtained by Levin and colleagues (140, 141) using stereotaxic equipment are much better than those reported by authors using the "free-hand" technique (i.e., introduction of the needle without the stereotaxic apparatus). As noted in Table 96-13, however, Waldman and associates (151) reported the use of NALP in 55 patients using the technique of Levin and Ramirez (141), but without the advantage of the stereotaxic apparatus, and obtained similar results. This is not mentioned to detract from the use of the stereotaxic apparatus, which does provide some advantages, but rather to re-emphasize that, if such apparatus is not available, NALP can be carried out with less sophisticated radiographic equipment, which is generally available. A high success rate for pain relief can still be achieved provided, of course, that the operator is skilled in the technique.

G. NEUROLYTIC BLOCKS FOR CONTROL OF SPASTICITY

Indications

Although neurolytic nerve blocks are usually used for the control of chronic pain, they are also important for the treatment of spasticity consequent to injuries to the central nervous system (e.g., stroke and spinal cord damage secondary to trauma or disease, such as multiple sclerosis). Such patients often develop spasticity that results in profound spasms of various muscle groups, which can be painful. These spasms are usually uncontrolled and often produce sporadic spontaneous and uncontrolled flexor or extensor movements that can severely compromise the patients' ability to sit in a wheelchair. Sometimes such spasms can be so violent as to catapult patients out of their wheelchairs. Many patients with spinal cord injury develop spasms of the adductor muscles of the thigh, which in addition to the painful spasm affects the ability to perform perineal toilet hygiene and to carry out other aspects of nursing care.

Reduction of such profound skeletal muscle spasm by neurolytic block has been helpful in these patients (164–170). Less commonly, such blocks can be used to treat muscle spasms in the trunk or in the upper extremity that are associated with quadriplegia (164).

Some special indications for producing reversible spasms in such individuals also exist. Many use the muscle spasms as an integral part of their support for sitting and functioning both during recreation and at work. It is sometimes necessary, however, to reduce such spasms temporarily. For example, a patient might need to be nursed in the prone position for some length of time (e.g., during and after placement of a skin graft for a gluteal bed sore). Therefore, prolonged and complete elimination of flexion spasms would not be indicated because such spasms are useful to the individual during normal activities. In such a case prolonged reversible therapy for the spasms is needed.

The novel use of epidural or intrathecal opioids seems to be effective for producing this reversible relief of spasm. This can be accomplished by the use of an externalized epidural catheter for short-term needs. Longer control of spasticity has been accomplished by the implantation of subcutaneous morphine pumps and reservoirs (171–173).

Most interventions for the control of spasm are usually done to relieve adductor and flexor spasm in the thigh. Discrete paravertebral somatic nerve block of the L2 and L3 levels, which control motor function to the adductor muscles of the thigh (adductor magnus, adductor longus, and gracilis), can be done. These same spinal roots also control flexion of the thigh. Extension of the thigh is controlled by the more caudad segments of L4 and L5. Selective block of these different roots can diminish motor activity in these myotomes and thereby relieve excessive spasm and pain, if present.

Block of specific peripheral nerves is indicated for certain conditions. For example, block of the musculocutaneous nerve with phenol is effective in relieving excessive elbow flexion (167) and block of the posterior tibial nerve is effective in relieving excessive plantar flexion (164). Block of the sciatic and femoral nerves with alcohol has also been used to relieve spasticity in the lower limbs (170).

Another approach to spasticity resulting from head injuries is injection of small volumes of neurolytic agent into motor end points in specific muscles (167). Another technique is the injection of the neurolytic agents into the epidural space for the control of spasticity (168). I am of the opinion that greater specificity and accuracy can be achieved with the use of the subarachnoid and paravertebral techniques.

Technical Considerations

Block with Local Anesthetics

Prior to carrying out a neurolytic block it is preferable to perform diagnostic-prognostic blocks with a long-acting local anesthetic (e.g., 0.5% bupivacaine with epinephrine) to ascertain the segments that need to be interrupted. Local anesthetic blocks repeated daily can also be used by therapists in carrying out rehabilitation measures. In some patients these temporary blocks are sufficient for a successful rehabilitation program.

Agents for Neurolytic Blocks

The neurolytic agents used for spasticity are the same as those used for pain control—alcohol and phenol. Although nerve impairment could occur with a weaker solution, it is usually necessary to use absolute alcohol and at least 5% or preferably 10% phenol to produce predictable motor blockade. As emphasized above (Subarachnoid Alcohol Block), alcohol, when injected into the subarachnoid space, is administered in a hypobaric solution and phenol is usually mixed with glycerin to make it hyperbaric. When phenol is used for peripheral nerve block it is in an aqueous solution.

Alcohol is usually supplied in small 2-ml ampules of "absolute" alcohol. It is used in small volumes when injected into the subarachnoid space, usually in 0.25- to 0.5-ml aliquots for each spinal segmental neurolysis required. Phenol is usually "custom-prepared" in the hospital pharmacy but it is preferable to obtain the phenol in crystal form, usually 1 g of phenol crystal in an ampule. The solvent of choice, either glycerin or water, can then be added. Dissolving the phenol crystals in the glycerin is a slow process that can be hastened by adding sufficient glycerin to the ampule containing the phenol crystals to produce the desired concentration (5 to 10%) and then standing the ampule in a basin of warm water. Agitation of the vial also speeds up the process.

Glycerin is viscid and consequently difficult to inject through narrow-bore needles. It is therefore necessary to use at least a 22-gauge, preferably a 20-gauge, needle for administering the phenol mixed in the glycerin base.

Techniques

The technique of subarachnoid injection of alcohol or phenol for the relief of pain is described above (Section C). The injection of hypobaric alcohol requires that the rootlets and roots of the nerves to be interrupted are uppermost. In contrast to the use of subarachnoid alcohol for pain control, which requires that the posterior rootlets and roots be uppermost, for the relief of spasticity the patient must be positioned so that the anterior rootlets and roots are uppermost. The surface of the patient's back should make an angle of 45° with the surface of the table. The middle of the table is raised just below the segments to be blocked.

For injection of the hypobaric phenol in glycerin the patient needs to be positioned so that the anterior rootlets and roots are lowermost. The table must be flexed and the patient placed with the side to be blocked lowermost, with the body positioned so that the anterior surface of the abdomen makes a 45° angle with the surface of the table. For the lower limb interruption it is necessary to have the patient positioned with the segments to be interrupted lowermost. Meticulous attention to position technique is required for subarachnoid neurolytic block, to prevent unintentional spread to other spinal segments, especially to those sacral segments involved in sphincter control.

The techniques of paravertebral somatic nerve block and block of various peripheral nerves to the upper or lower limbs are described in detail in Chapter 94. It is helpful to use an electrical nerve stimulator to locate the target nerve because hemiplegic and paraplegic patients usually cannot report paresthesia.

It is preferable to use an initial conservative approach with neurolytic blocks and to return at a later date to extend it, if necessary, rather than to risk production of a too-extensive block during the initial attempt.

Results

Garland and associates (166) reported that neurolytic block produced a high success rate in terms of restoration of normal functional position in the limb. The duration of block was usually 4 to 6 months, but after this period normal function of the limb was not maintained. During the period of blockade, however, considerable progress was achieved and more definitive treatment (e.g., lengthening of the Achilles tendon) was planned. Our group and others who have reported on the use of neurolytic block also noted significant success with the use of these procedures.

Few blocks are truly "permanent," and the return of spasticity occurs over time. Paravertebral and peripheral nerve blocks usually last 3 to 6 months and subarachnoid neurolytic blocks generally last 4 to 6 months. In certain patients, however, for reasons not understood, they can last a year or more. If unintentional spread to segments involved in sphincter control occurs, resulting in incontinence, pre-existing bladder and bowel reflex function usually returns in 1 to 2 months in most patients (65).

REFERENCES

1. Bonica, J.J.: The Management of Pain. Philadelphia, Lea & Febiger, 1953.
2. Ventafridda, V., et al.: A validation study of the WHO method for cancer pain relief. Cancer, *59*:850, 1987.
3. Cousins, M.J., Dwyer, B., and Gibb, D.: Chronic pain and neurolytic neural blockade. *In* Neural Blockade in Clinical Anesthesia and Management of Pain. 2nd Ed. Edited by M.J. Cousins and P.O. Bridenbaugh. Philadelphia, J.B. Lippincott, 1988, pp. 1053–1084.
4. Schlosser, H.: Erfahrungen in der Neuralgiebehandlung mit Alkoholeinspritzungen. Verh. Cong. Innere Med., *24*:49, 1907.
5. Finkelburg, R.: Experimentelle Untersuchungen über den Einfluss von Alkoholinjektionen und periferische Nerven. Verh. Cong. Innere Med., *24*:75, 1907.
6. Labat, G., and Greeme, M.B.: Contribution to modern method of diagnosis and treatment of so-called sciatic neuralgias. Am. J. Surg., *11*:435, 1931.
7. Rumsby, M.G., and Finean, J.B.: The action of organic solvents on the myelin sheath of peripheral nerve tissue—II (short-chain aliphatic alcohols). J. Neurochem., *13*:1509, 1966.
8. Woolsey, R.M., Taylor, J.J., and Nagel, H.H.: Acute effects of topical ethyl alcohol on the sciatic nerve of the mouse. Arch. Phys. Med. Rehabil., *53*:410, 1972.
9. Gregg, R.V., et al.: Electrophysiologic investigation of alcohol as a neurolytic agent. Anesthesiology, *63*:A250, 1985.
10. Merrick, R.L.: Degeneration and recovery of autonomic neurones following alcoholic block. Ann. Surg., *113*:298, 1941.
11. Gallagher, H.S., et al.: Subarachnoid alcohol block. II. Histologic changes in the central nervous system. Am. J. Pathol., *35*:679, 1961.
12. Matsuki, M., Kato, Y., and Ichiyanagi, K.: Progressive changes in the concentration of ethyl alcohol in the human and canine subarachnoid spaces. Anesthesiology, *36*:617, 1972.
13. Mandl, F.: Aqueous solution of phenol as a substitute for alcohol in sympathetic block. J. Int. Coll. Surg., *13*:566, 1950.
14. Maher, R.M.: Relief of pain in incurable cancer. Lancet, *1*:18, 1955.
15. Maher, R.M.: Neurone selection in relief of pain. Lancet, *1*:16, 1957.
16. Iggo, A., and Walsh, E.G.: Selective block of small fibres in the spinal roots by phenol. Brain, *83*:701, 1960.
17. Nathan, P.W., and Sears, T.A.: Effects of phenol in nervous conduction. J. Physiol. (Lond.), *150*:565, 1960.
18. Stewart, W.A., and Lourie, H.: An experimental evaluation of the effects of subarachnoid injection of phenol-Pantopaque in cats. J. Neurosurg., *20*:64, 1963.
19. Natan, P.W., Sears, T.A., and Smith, M.C.: Effects of phenol solutions on the nerve roots of the cat: An electrophysiological and histological study. J. Neurol. Sci., *2*:7, 1965.
20. Smith, M.C.: Histological findings following intrathecal injections of phenol solutions for the relief of pain. Anaesthesia, *36*:387, 1964.
21. Schaumburg, H.N., Byck, R., and Weller, R.O.: The effect of phenol on peripheral nerves. A histological and electrophysiological study. J. Neuropathol. Exp. Neurol., *29*:615, 1970.
22. Ichiyanagi, K., et al.: Progressive changes in the concentrations of phenol and glycerin in the human subarachnoid space. Anesthesiology, *42*:622, 1975.
23. Gregg, R.V., et al.: Electrophysiologic and histopathologic investigation of phenol in Renografin as a neurolytic agent. Anesthesiolology, *63*:A239, 1985.
24. Wood, K.M.: The use of phenol as a neurolytic agent: A review. Pain, *5*:205, 1978.
25. Håkanson, S.: Trigeminal neuralgia treated by the injection of glycerol into the trigeminal cistern. Neurosurgery, *9*:638, 1981.
26. Lunsford, L.D., and Bennett, M.H.: Percutaneous retrogasserian glycerol rhizotomy for tic douloureux: Part I. Technique and results in 112 patients. Neurosurgery, *14*:424, 1984.

27. Sweet, W.H., Poletti, C.E., and Macon, J.B.: Treatment of trigeminal neuralgia and other facial pain by retrogasserian injection of glycerol. Neurosurgery, 9:647, 1981.
28. Rengachary, S.S., et al.: Effect of glycerol on peripheral nerve: An experimental study. Neurosurgery, 13:681, 1983.
29. Myers, R.R., and Katz, J.: Neural pathology of neurolytic and semidestructive agents. In Neural Blockade in Clinical Anesthesia and Management of Pain. 2nd Ed. Edited by M.J. Cousins and P.O. Bridenbaugh. Philadelphia, J.B. Lippincott, 1988, pp. 1031–1051.
30. Burchiel, K.J., and Russell, L.C.: Glycerol neurolysis: Neurophysiologic effects of topical glycerol application on rat saphenous nerve. J. Neurosurg., 63:784, 1985.
31. Judovich, B., and Bates, W.: Pain Syndromes: Treatment by Paravertebral Nerve Block. Philadelphia, F.A. Davis, 1950, pp. 242–249.
32. Bates, W., and Judovich, B.D.: Intractable pain. Anesthesiology, 3:663, 1942.
33. Miller, R.D., Johnston, R.R., and Hosbuchi, Y.: Treatment of intercostal neuralgia with 10% ammonium sulfate. J. Thorac. Cardiovasc. Surg., 69:476, 1975.
34. Davies, J.J., Stewart, P.B., and Fink, A.P.: Prolonged sensory block using ammonium salts. Anesthesiology, 28:244, 1967.
35. Denney-Brown, D., et al.: The pathology of injury to nerve induced by cold. J. Neuropathol. Exp. Neurol., 4:305, 1945.
36. Douglas, W.S., and Malcolm, J.L.: Effect of localized cooling on conduction in cat nerves. J. Physiol. (Lond.), 130:63, 1955.
37. Paintal, A.S.: Block of conduction in mammalian myelinated nerve fibers by low temperatures. J. Physiol., 180:1, 1965.
38. Thomas, P.K., and Holdroff, B.: Neuropathy due to physical agents. In Peripheral Neuropathy. Edited by P.J. Dyck, et al. Philadelphia, W.B. Saunders, 1984, p. 1479.
39. Myers, R.R., et al.: Endoneurial fluid pressure: Direct measurement with micropipettes. Brain Res., 148:510, 1978.
40. Lele, P.P.: Effects of focused ultrasound radiation on peripheral nerves, with observations on local heating. Exp. Neurol., 8:47, 1963.
41. Myers, R.R., James, H.E., and Powell, H.C.: Laser injury of peripheral nerve: A model for focal endoneurial damage. J. Neurol. Neurosurg. Psychiatry, 48:1265, 1985.
42. Härtel, F.: Über die Intrakranielle Injections Behandlung der Trigeminus Neuralgie. Med. Klin., 1:582, 1914.
43. Härtel, F.: Die Behandlung der Trigeminus Neuralgie mit Intrakraniellen Alkohol einspritzungen. Dtsch. Z. Chir., 126:429, 1914.
44. Ecker, A., and Perl, T.: Alcoholic gasserian injection for the relief of tic douloureux. Preliminary report of a modification of Penman's method. Neurology, 8:461, 1958.
45. Delfino, U.: An advance in trigeminal therapy. In Persistent Pain, Vol. 4. Edited by S. Lipton and J. Miles. New York, Grune & Stratton, 1983, pp. 145–157.
46. Putnam, T.J., and Hampton, A.O.: A technique of injection into the gasserian ganglion under roentgenographic control. Arch. Neurol. Psychiatry, 35:92, 1936.
47. Jefferson, A.: Trigeminal root and ganglion injections using phenol in glycerin for the relief of trigeminal neuralgia, J. Neurol. Neurosurg. Psychiatry, 26:345, 1963.
48. Mousel, L.H.: Treatment of intractable pain of the head and neck. Anesth. Analg., 46:705, 1967.
49. Frothingham, R.E., Atchison, J.W.D., and Bailey, C.C.: Treatment of facial pain by percutaneous injection of the gasserian ganglion. J.S.C. Med. Assoc., 70:160, 1974.
50. Harris, W.: An analysis of 1,433 cases of paroxysmal trigeminal neuralgia (trigeminal tic) and the end results of gasserian alcohol injection. Brain, 63:209, 1940.
51. Kulenkampff, D.: Die Behandlung der Trigeminusneuralgie Muenchen. Med. Wachenscht., 89:670, 1942.
52. Thurel, R.: Nevralgie faciale et alcoolisation du ganglion de Gasser. A. Rev. Neurol. (Paris), 104:75, 534, 1961.
53. Thurel, R.: Nevralgie faciale et alcoolisation du ganglion de Gasser. B. Rev. Neurol. (Paris), 105:62, 346, 1961.
54. Henderson, W.R.: Trigeminal neuralgia: The pain and its treatment. Br. Med. J., 1:7, 1967.
55. Ecker, A.: Sensory loss and prolonged remission of tic douloureux after selective alcoholic gasserian injection. In Advances in Pain Research and Therapy, Vol. 1. Edited by J.J. Bonica and D. Albe-Fessard. New York, Raven Press, 1976, pp. 895–900.
56. Miles, J.: Trigeminal neuralgia. In Persistent Pain: Modern Methods of Treatment, Vol. 2. Edited by S. Lipton. New York, Grune & Stratton, 1980, pp. 223–248.
57. Jefferson, A.: Trigeminal neuralgia: Trigeminal root and ganglion injection used in phenol and glycerin. In Pain. Edited by R.S. Knighton and P.R. Dumke. Boston, Little, Brown & Company, 1966, pp. 365–372.
58. Häkanson, S.: Retrogasserian glycerol injection as treatment of tic douloureux. In Advances in Pain Research and Therapy, Vol. 5. Edited by J.J. Bonica, U. Lindblom, and A. Iggo. New York, Raven Press, 1983, pp. 927–933.
59. Madrid, J.L., and Bonica, J.J.: Cranial nerve blocks. In International Symposium on Pain of Advanced Cancer. Advances in Pain Research and Therapy, Vol. 2. Edited by J.J. Bonica and V. Ventafridda. New York, Raven Press, 1979, pp. 347–355.
60. White, J.C., and Sweet, W.H.: Pain and the Neurosurgeon. A Forty-Year Experience. Springfield, IL, Charles C Thomas. 1969.
61. Bonica, J.J.: The management of pain of malignant disease with nerve blocks. Anesthesiology, 15:134, 1954.
62. Grüter, W.: Orbital injection of alcohol for relief of pain in blind eyes. Berl. Versammlung Ophthalmol. 3:85, 1918.
63. Weekers, L.: Treatment of painful diseases with persistent vision by orbital injection of weak solutions of alcohol. Arch. Ophthalmol., 47:299, 1930.
64. Maumenee, A.E.: Retrobulbar alcohol injections. Relief of ocular pain in eyes with and without vision. Am. J. Ophthalmol., 32:1502, 1949.
65. Swerdlow, M.: Complications of neurolytic neural blockade. In Neural Blockade in Clinical Anesthesia and Management of Pain. 2nd Ed. Edited by M.J. Cousins and P.O. Bridenbaugh. Philadelphia, J.B. Lippincott, 1988, pp. 719–735.
66. Moore, D.C.: Complications of Regional Anesthesia. Springfield, IL, Charles C Thomas, 1965, pp. 119–140.
67. Robson, J.T., and Bonica, J.J.: The vagus nerve in surgical consideration of glossopharyngeal neuralgia. J. Neurosurg., 7:482, 1950.
68. Broggi, G., and Siegfried, J.: Percutaneous differential radiofrequency rhizotomy of the glossopharyngeal nerve in facial pain due to cancer. In Advances in Pain Research and Therapy, Vol. 2. Edited by J.J. Bonica and V. Ventafridda. New York, Raven Press, 1979, pp. 469–473.
69. Dogliotti, A.M.: Traitment des Syndromes Douloureux de la Peripherie par l'Alcoolisation Sub-arachnoidienne des Racines Posterieures à leur emergence de la Moelle Épinière. Presse Med., 39:1249, 1931.
70. Derrick, W.S.: Subarachnoid alcohol block for the control of intractable pain. Acta Anesthesiol. Scand. [Suppl.], 24:167, 1966.
71. Swerdlow, M.: Intrathecal and extradural block and pain relief. In Relief of Intractable Pain. Edited by M. Swerdlow. Amsterdam, Elsevier, 1983, pp. 175–214.
72. Mehta, M.: Intractable Pain. London, W.B. Saunders, 1973.
73. Gerbershagen, H.U.: Neurolysis: Subarachnoid neurolytic blockade. Acta Anaesthesiol. Belg., 1:45, 1981.
74. Maher, R.M.: Phenol for pain and spasticity. In Pain: Henry Ford Hospital International Symposium. Edited by R.S. Knighton and P.R. Dumpke. New York, Little, Brown & Company, 1966, pp. 335–341.
75. Maher R.M.: Results of subarachnoid phenol block. In Relief of Intractable Pain. Edited by M. Swerdlow. Amsterdam, Elsevier, 1983, p. 192.
76. Stovner, J., and Endresen, R.: Intrathecal phenol for cancer pain. Acta Anaesth. Scand., 16:17, 1972.
77. Brown, A.S.: Pain relief in malignant disease. Symposium on malignant disease. R. Coll. Phys. Edin., 47:86, 1976.
78. Stern, E.L.: Relief of intractable pain by intraspinal (subarachnoid) injection of alcohol. Am. J. Surg., 25:217, 1937.
79. Abbott, W.D.: Intraspinal injection of absolute alcohol for intractable pain. Am. J. Surg., 31:351, 1936.
80. Poppen, J.L.: Relief of pain by use of subarachnoid alcohol injection; Indications, contraindications, technic, and results in 82 patients. Med. Clin. North Am., 16:1663, 1936.
81. Peyton, W.T., Semansky, E.J., and Baker, A.B.: Subarachnoid injection of alcohol for relief of intractable pain with discussion of cord changes found at autopsy. Am. J. Cancer, 30:709, 1937.
82. Truelsen, F.: Subarachnoid alcohol injection for relief of intractable pain. Acta Chir. Scand., 88:17, 1943.
83. Greenhill, J.P., and Schmitz, H.E.: Intraspinal (subarachnoid) injection of alcohol for pain associated with malignant conditions of female genitalia. JAMA, 105:406, 1935.

84. Bonica, J.J.: Diagnostic and therapeutic blocks: A reappraisal based on 15 years' experience. Anesth. Analg. Curr. Res., *37*:58, 1958.
85. Perese, D.M.: Subarachnoid alcohol block in management of pain of malignant disease. Arch. Surg., *76*:347, 1958.
86. Hay, R.C.: Subarachnoid alcohol block in the control of intractable pain. Anesth. Analg. Curr. Res., *41*:12, 1962.
87. Kuzucu, E.Y., Derrick, W.S., and Wilber, S.A.: Control of intractable pain with subarachnoid alcohol block. JAMA, *195*:133, 1966.
88. Papke, H.: Indikationen Möglichkeiten und Grenzen der subarachnoidalen alkoholinjektionen. M.D. thesis, University of Mainz, Germany, 1974.
89. Brown, A.S.: Treatment of Intractable Pain by Nerve Block with Phenol. Amsterdam, Excerpta Medica, International Congress Series 36, E59, 1961.
90. Mark, V.H., et al.: Intrathecal use of phenol for the relief of chronic severe pain. N. Engl. J. Med., *267*:589, 1962.
91. Tank, T.M., Dohn, D.F., and Gardner, W.J.: Intrathecal injection of alcohol and phenol for the relief of intractable pain. Cleve. Clin. Q., *30*:11, 1963.
92. Wilkinson, H.A., Mark, V.H., and White, J.C.: Further experiences with intrathecal phenol for the relief of pain. J. Chron. Dis., *17*:1055, 1964.
93. Ball, H.J.C., Pearce, D.J., and Davies, J.A.H.: Experiences with therapeutic nerve blocks. Anaesthesia, *19*:250, 1964.
94. Lifshitz, S., Debacker, L.J., and Buchsbaum, H.J.: Subarachnoid phenol block for pain relief in gynecologic malignancy. Obstet. Gynecol., *48*:316, 1976.
95. Papo, I., and Visca, A.: Phenol subarachnoid rhizotomy for the treatment of cancer pain: A personal account on 290 cases. *In* Advances in Pain Research and Therapy. Vol. 2. Edited by J.J. Bonica and V. Ventafridda. New York, Raven Press, 1979, pp. 339–346.
96. Brown, A.S.: Current views on the use of nerve blocking in the relief of chronic pain. *In* The Therapy of Pain. Edited by M. Swerdlow. Lancaster, England, M.T. Press Ltd., 1981, pp. 111–134.
97. Drechsel, U.: Treatment of cancer pain with neurolytic agents. Recent Results Cancer Res., *89*:137, 1984.
98. Madrid, J.L.: Experience de 363 cas d'analgesie par alcool et phenol. Cah. Anesthesiol., *23*:825, 1975.
99. Rafferty, H.: Extradural injection of 5% aqueous solution of phenol for cervical pain. Presented at the Annual Meeting of the Intractable Pain Society of Great Britain. London, March 1977.
100. Colpitts, M.R., Levy, D.A., and Lawrence, M.: Treatment of cancer-related pain with phenol epidural block (Abstr.) Presented at the Second World Congress on Pain. Montreal, August 27–September 1, 1978.
101. Racz, G.B., Heavner, J., and Haynsworth, P.: Repeat epidural phenol injections in chronic pain and spasticity. *In* Persistent Pain: Modern Methods of Treatment, Vol. 5. Edited by S. Lipton. New York, Grune & Stratton, 1985, pp. 157–180.
102. Korevaar, W.C.: Transcatheter thoracic epidural neurolysis using ethyl alcohol. Anesthesiology, *69*:989, 1988.
103. Maher, R.M., and Mehta, M.: Spinal (intrathecal) and extradural analgesia. *In* Persistent Pain: Modern Methods of treatment. Edited by S. Lipton. New York, Grune & Stratton, 1977, pp. 61–99.
104. Ischia, S., et al.: Subdural extra-arachnoid neurolytic block in cervical pain. Pain, *14*:347, 1982.
105. Hovelacque, A.: Anatomie des Nerfs Craniens et Rachidiens et du système Grand Sympathique chez l'Homme. Paris, G. Doin & Cie, 1927, pp. 375–397.
106. Ward, E.M., Rorie, D.K., and Nauss, L.A.: The celiac ganglia in men: normal anatomic variations. Anesth. Analg., *58*:461, 1979.
107. Thompson, G.E., and Moore, D.C.: Celiac plexus, intercostal, and minor peripheral blockade. *In* Neural Blockade in Clinical Anesthesia and Management of Pain. 2nd Ed. Edited by M.J. Cousins and P.O. Bridenbaugh. Philadelphia, J.B. Lippincott, 1988, pp. 503–530.
108. Brown, D.L., Bulley, S.K., and Quiel, E.L.: Neurolytic celiac plexus block of pancreatic cancer pain. Anesth. Analg., *66*:869, 1987.
109. Moore, D.C.: Intercostal nerve block and celiac plexus block for pain therapy. *In* Advances in Pain Research and Therapy, Vol. 7. Edited by C. Benedetti, C.R. Chapman, and G. Moricca. New York, Raven Press, 1984, pp. 309–329
110. Brown, D.L.: A retrospective analysis of neurolytic celiac plexus block for nonpancreatic intra-abdominal cancer pain. Reg. Anaesth., *14*:63, 1989.
111. Bridenbaugh, L.D., Moore, D.C., and Campbell, D.D.: Management of upper abdominal cancer pain. Treatment with celiac plexus block with alcohol. JAMA, *190*:877, 1964.
112. Gorbitz, C., and Leavens, M.E.: Alchohol block of the celiac plexus for control of the upper abdominal pain caused by cancer and pancreatitis. J. Neurosurg., *34*:575, 1971.
113. Black, A., and Dwyer, B.: Coeliac plexus block. Anaesth. Intensive Care, *1*:15, 1973.
114. Jones, J., and Gough, D.: Coeliac plexus block with alcohol for relief of upper abdominal pain due to cancer. Ann. R. Coll. Surg. Engl., *59*:46, 1977.
115. Thompson, G.E., et al.: Abdominal pain and alcohol celiac plexus nerve block. Anesth. Analg., *56*:1, 1977.
116. Flanigan, D.P., and Kraft, R.O.: Continuing experience with palliative chemical splanchnicectomy. Arch. Surg., *113*:509, 1978.
117. Hegedus, V.: Relief of pancreatic pain by radiography-guided block. Am. J. Radiol., *133*:1101, 1979.
118. Boas, R.A.: Sympathetic blocks in clinical practice. Int. Anesthesiol. Clin., *16*:149, 1978.
119. Boas, R.A.: The sympathetic nervous system and pain relief. *In* Relief of Intractable Pain. Edited by M. Swerdlow. Amsterdam, Elsevier, 1983, pp. 215–237.
120. Duthie, A.M., and Ingham, V.: Persistent abdominal pain. Treatment by lumbar sympathetic lysis. Anaesthesia, *36*:289, 1981.
121. Löfstrom, B., and Zetterquist, S.: Lumbar sympathetic blocks in the treatment of patients with obliterative arterial disease of the lower limb. Int. Anesthesiol. Clin., *7*:423, 1969.
122. Reid, W., Watt, J.K., and Gray, T.G.: Phenol injection of the sympathetic chain. Br. J. Surg., *57*:45, 1970.
123. Boas, R.A., Hatangdi, V.S., and Richards, E.G.: Lumbar sympathectomy—a percutaneous chemical technique. *In* Advances in Pain Research and Therapy, Vol. 1. Edited by J.J. Bonica and D. Albe-Fessard. New York, Raven Press, 1976, pp. 685–689.
124. Cousins, M.J., et al.: Neurolytic lumbar sympathetic blockade: Duration of denervation and relief of rest pain. Anaesth. Intensive Care, 7:121, 1979.
125. Löfstrom, J.B., and Cousins, M.J.: Sympathetic neural blockade of upper and lower extremity. *In* Neural Blockade in Clinical Anesthesia and Management of Pain. 2nd Ed. Edited by M.J. Cousins and P.O. Bridenbaugh. Philadelphia, J.B. Lippincott, 1988, pp. 641–500.
126. Mullin, V.: Brachial plexus block with phenol for painful arm associated with Pancoast's syndrome. Anesthesiology, *53*:431, 1980.
127. Feldman, S.A., and Yeung, M.L.: Treatment of intermittent claudication: Lumbar paravertebral block with phenol. Anaesthesia, *30*:174, 1975.
128. Robertson, D.H.: Trans-sacral neurolytic nerve block. An alternative approach to intractable perineal pain. Br. J. Anaesth., *55*:873, 1983.
129. Simon, D.L., Carron, H., and Rowlinson, J.C.: Treatment of bladder pain with trans-sacral nerve block. Anesth. Analg., *61*:46, 1982.
130. McGrady, E.M., and Marks, R.L.: Treatment of abdominal nerve entrapment syndrome using a nerve stimulator. Ann. R. Coll. Surg. Engl., *70*:120, 1988.
131. Lloyd, J.W., Barnard, J.D.W., and Glynn, C.J.: Cryoanalgesia: A new approach to pain relief. Lancet, *2*:932, 1976.
132. Barnard, J.D.W.: The effects of extreme cold on sensory nerves. Ann. R. Coll. Surg. Engl., *62*:180, 1980.
133. Glynn, C.J., Lloyd, J.W., and Barnard, J.D.W.: Cryoanalgesia in the management of post-thoracotomy pain. Thorax, *35*:325, 1980.
134. Barnard, J.D.W., Lloyd, J., and Evans, J.: Cryoanalgesia in the management of chronic facial pain. J. Maxillofac. Surg., *9*:101, 1981.
135. Katz, J., et al.: Cryoanalgesia for post-thoracotomy pain. Lancet, *8*:512, 1980.
136. Jones, M.J.T., and Murrin, K.R.: Intercostal block with cryotherapy. Ann. R. Coll. Surg. Engl., *69*:261, 1987.
137. Amoils, S.P.: The Joule-Thompson cryoprobe. Arch. Ophthalmol., *78*:201, 1967.
138. Morrica, G.: Neuroadenolysis for the antalgic treatment of advanced cancer patients. *In* Recent Advances in Pain. Edited by J.J. Bonica, P. Procacci, and C. Pagni. Springfield, IL, Charles C Thomas, 1974, pp. 313–328.

139. Gianasi, G.: Neuroadenolysis of the pituitary of Moricca: An overview of development, mechanisms, technique, and results. *In* Advances in Pain Research and Therapy, Vol. 7. Edited by C. Benedetti, C.R. Chapman, and G. Moricca. New York, Raven Press, 1984, pp. 647–678.

140. Katz, J., and Levin, A.B.: Long-term follow-up study of chemical hypophysectomy and additional cases. Anesthesiology, *51*:167, 1979.

141. Levin, A.B., and Ramirez, L.F.: Treatment of cancer pain with hypophysectomy: Surgical and chemical. *In* Advances in Pain Research and Therapy, Vol. 7. Edited by C. Benedetti, C.R. Chapman, and G. Morrica. New York, Raven Press, 1984, pp. 631–645.

142. Huggins, C.: Endocrine-induced regression of cancer: Nobel Prize lecture 1966. Cancer Res., *27*:1925, 1966.

143. Scott, W.W.: Endocrine management of disseminated prostate cancer including bilateral adrenalectomy and hypophysectomy. Trans. Am. Assoc. Genito-urinary Surg., *44*:101, 1952.

144. Luft, R., and Olivecrona, H.: Hypophysectomy in man. Experiences in metastatic cancer of the breast. Cancer, *8*:261, 1955.

145. Forrest, A.P.M., and Brown, D.A.: Pituitary radon implant for breast cancer. Lancet, *1*:1054, 1955.

146. Lewis, J.L., and Baxton, L.: Discussione dell' Adunanza Scientifica del 21 dicembre 1957. Boll. Mem. Soc. Tosco-Umbra Chir., *19*:78, 1958.

147. Greco, T., Sbaragli, F., and Cammilli, L.: L'alcolizzazione della ipofisi per via transfenoidale nella terapia di particolari tumori maligni. Settim. Med., *45*:355, 1957.

148. Carbonin, G.: Hypophysectomy in pain relief in cancer. J. Neurosurg., *48*:666, 1978.

149. Miles, J.: Pituitary destruction. *In* Textbook of Pain. 2nd Ed. Edited by P.D. Wall and R. Melzack. New York, Churchill Livingstone, 1989, pp. 856–867.

150. Lipton, S.: Percutaneous cervical cordotomy and pituitary injection of alcohol. *In* Relief of Intractable Pain. 3rd Ed. Edited by M. Swerdlow. Amsterdam, Elsevier, 1983, pp. 269–304.

151. Waldman, S.D., Feldstein, G.S., and Allen, M.L.: Neuroadenolysis of the pituitary: Description of a modified technique. J. Pain Symptom Management, *2*:45, 1987.

152. Moricca, G., and Moricca, P.: Updated statistics on neuroadenolysis of the pituitary (NALP) for the treatment of severe diffuse cancer pain. Unpublished communication, 1988.

153. Moricca, G., and Gianasi, G.C.: Neuroadenolysis of the pituitary in the treatment of cancer pain and hormone-dependent tumours. *In* Pain Treatment. Pituitary Neuroadenolysis in the Treatment of Cancer Pain and Hormone-Dependent Tumours. Edited by S. Ischia, S. Lipton, and G.F. Maffezzoli. Verona, Corina International, 1983, pp. 71–78.

154. Farcot, J.M., et al.: L'hypophysiolyse et l'alcool. Indications, techniques et résultats. Observations sur le mécanisme d'action. Anésthsie, Analgésie Réanim., *38*:361, 1981.

155. Lloyd, J.W., Rawlinson, W.A.L., and Evans, P.J.D.: Selective hypophysectomy for metastatic pain. A review of ethyl alcohol ablation of the anterior pituitary in a Regional Pain Relief Unit. Br. J. Anaesth., *53*:1129, 1981.

156. Corssen, G., Edwards, T.W., and Ford, A.: Control of intractable cancer pain in man: Further experimental and clinical experience with pituitary neuroadenolysis (NALP). *In* Pain Treatment. Pituitary Neuroadenolysis in the Treatment of Cancer Pain and Hormone-Dependent Tumors.

Edited by S. Ischia, S. Lipton, and G.F. Maffezzoli. Verona, Corina International, 1983, pp. 55–58.

157. Grunwald, I.: Pituitary neuroadenolysis: Two years' experience of treating cancer pain and hormone-dependent tumours. *In* Pain treatment. Pituitary Neuroadenolysis in the Treatment of Cancer Pain and Hormone-Dependent Tumours. Edited by S. Ischia, S. Lipton, and G.F. Maffezzoli. Verona, Cortina International, 1983, pp. 79–83.

158. Ischia, S., et al.: NALP: Personal experience and results. *In* Pain Treatment. Pituitary Neuroadenolysis in the Treatment of Cancer Pain and Hormone-Dependent Tumors. Edited by S. Ischia, S. Lipton, and G.F. Maffezzoli. Verona, Cortina International, 1983, pp. 65–70.

159. Madrid, J.L.: Pituitary neuroadenolysis (NALP): Immediate and long-term results. *In* Pain Treatment. Pituitary Neuroadenolysis in the Treatment of Cancer Pain and Hormone-Dependent Tumours. Edited by S. Ischia, S. Lipton, and G.F. Maffezzoli. Verona, Cortina International, 1983, pp. 59–64.

160. Cook, P.R., Campbell, F.N., and Puddy, B.R.: Pituitary alcohol injection for cancer pain use in a district general hospital. Anaesthesia, *39*:540, 1984.

161. Romoli, R.: Our experience with pituitary neuroadenolysis in the treatment of various neoplastic forms. *In* Pain Treatment. Pituitary Neuroadenolysis in the Treatment of Cancer Pain and Hormone-Dependent Tumours. Edited by S. Ischia, S. Lipton, and G.F. Maffezzoli. Verona, Cortina International, 1983, pp. 97–102.

162. Takeda, F.: Results of cancer pain relief and tumor regression by pituitary neuroadenolysis and surgical hypophysectomy. *In* Pain Treatment. Pituitary Neuroadenolysis in the Treatment of Cancer Pain and Hormone-Dependent Tumours. Verona, Cortina International, 1983, pp. 103–114.

163. Lahuerta, J., et al.: Update on percutaneous cordotomy and pituitary alcohol neuroadenolysis: An audit of recent results and complications. *In* Persistent Pain, Vol. 5. Edited by S. Lipton and J. Miles. London, Grune & Stratton, 1985, pp. 197–223.

164. Wainapel, S.F., Haigney, D., and Labib, K.: Spastic hemiplegia in a quadriplegic patient. Treatments with phenol nerve block. Arch. Phys. Med. Rehabil., *65*:786, 1984.

165. Essam, A.A.: Phenol block for control of hip flexor and adductor spasticity. Arch. Phys. Med. Rehabil., *53*:554, 1972.

166. Garland, D.E., Lucie, R.S., and Waters, R.L.: Current uses of open phenol nerve block for adult acquired spasticity. Clin. Orthoped Rel. Res., *165*:217, 1982.

167. Garland, D.E., Lilling, M., and Keenan, M.A.: Percutaneous phenol blocks to motor points of spastic forearm muscles in head-injured adults. Arch. Phys. Med. Rehabil., *65*:243, 1984.

168. Tardieu, G., et al.: Developmental treatment of spasticity by injection of dilute alcohol at motor point or by epidural route. Dev. Med. Child Neurol., *10*:564, 1968.

169. Carpenter, E.B.: Role of nerve blocks in the foot and ankle in cerebral palsy. Therapeutic and diagnostic. Foot Ankle *4*:164, 1983.

170. Singler, R.C.: Alcohol neurolysis of sciatic and femoral nerves. Anesth. Analg., *60*:532, 1981.

171. Erickson, D.L., et al.: Control of spasticity by implantable continuous flow morphine pump. Neurosurgery, *16*:215, 1985.

172. Loubser, P.G., Sharkey, P., and Dimitri-Jevic, N.: Control of chronic spasticity following spinal cord injury using intrathecal morphine. Anesth. Analg. *67*:S266, 1988.

173. Gall, D.H., et al.: Intrathecal morphine for treatment of spasticity. Anesthesiology, *69*:A353, 1988.

INTRODUCTION
JOHN D. LOESER

This section, composed of three chapters, presents a concise discussion of the neurosurgical procedures used for the management of chronic pain. Each chapter contains sections devoted to specific operations, which have been arbitrarily divided into three groups. Thus, Chapter 97 discusses operations on the peripheral nerves, Chapter 98 discusses operations on the spinal cord, and Chapter 99 discusses operations on the brain and brain stem. Like other chapters in this part of the book, each chapter contains sections with an up-to-date summary of the fundamental basis of the procedure, indications for its use, the clinical results obtained by the author and others who have had extensive experience with the procedure, a brief description of the operation, and a summary of the possible complications. The material is intended to provide an overview to physicians (and other health professionals) who might not be pain specialists. As emphasized elsewhere in this book, it is essential for physicians to be knowledgeable about various therapeutic procedures so that they can discuss them objectively with their patients.

This introductory section commences with a brief historical perspective on surgery performed to relieve pain and then analyzes the requirements and guidelines for applications of the various operative procedures used to obtain relief of nonmalignant chronic pain and pain caused by cancer. The importance of patient selection is emphasized, and criteria for choosing a particular operation are identified. More detailed discussions of the indications, techniques, and results of neurosurgical procedures for pain relief have been superbly presented by White and Sweet (1) and by Wilkins and Rengachary (2). The neuroanatomy, physiology, and biochemistry of the pain system are discussed in more detail in Chapters 3 and 4.

Historical Considerations of Surgical Procedures

In Chapter 1, Bonica mentions the concepts and surgical procedures used by the ancients in their attempts to understand and relieve pain. Ambroise Paré recognized in the late sixteenth century that cutting a nerve in the arm could relieve chronic pain secondary to a penetrating wound of the extremity. By the end of the seventeenth century, Maréchal, the surgeon to the court of Louis XIV, was performing peripheral neurotomies for tic douloureux. Modern neurosurgery began in the latter part of the nineteenth century after the advent of anesthesia and Lister's concepts of asepsis. Probably the first procedure to be used was peripheral neurotomy, described in a book published in 1873 by Letievant (3), in which he discussed sectioning of cranial nerves and of nerves supplying the extremities. One of the greatest neurosurgical pioneers was Horsley, who inaugurated surgery on the gasserian ganglion for tic douloureux in 1891. His work was continued by Krause and perfected by Frazier. The first spinal dorsal rhizotomies are accredited to Abbé and to Bennett in 1889. Spiller and Martin performed the first cordotomy in 1912. Förster continued the clinical studies of cordotomy and made many contributions to the surgery of pain (4).

The development of sympathectomy was mainly the work of Leriche, with major contributions by Jonnesco and Gomoiu. Many other great men of early twentieth century neurosurgery played important roles in the development of neurosurgical procedures for pain relief: Chippault, Jaubolay, Sicard, Van Gehuchten, de Beule, Thiersch, Sjöqvist, Cushing, Dandy, and White all made significant contributions. Horsley and Clark's apparatus for producing lesions in animal brains was brilliantly adapted by Spiegel and Wycis in their pioneering work on human stereotaxis. Certainly, the major neurosurgical treatise on pain relief of the twentieth century was the text by White and Sweet (1), which introduced the modern era of surgical pain relief.

There is little doubt that developments in our understanding of the anatomy, physiology, and psychology of chronic pain will spur the advance of surgical procedures directed at new targets. Events of the past decade have already shown the inventiveness of surgeons in applying both new information and new technologic methods to the problems of chronic pain.

Some of the most dramatic changes in the domain of neurologic surgery have occurred in regard to procedures designed to relieve pain. Early neurosurgical operations, in the late nineteenth and early twentieth centuries, involved section of nerves, roots, spinal cord, and then brain stem. The development of frontal lobotomy permitted a new approach—alteration of the suffering component of the patient's complaints rather than interruption of the pain pathways. Surgeons added new stereotaxic procedures for interruption of both specific and diffuse pain pathways at specific sites for the alleviation of suffering. Finally, the development of new theories of the nature of pain and of technologic refinements in the electronic industry has led to the use of both surface and implanted electrical stimulators to augment rather than reduce sensory input in attempts to relieve pain (Chapters 92 and 93).

Another important technical development has been the use of controlled radiofrequency current or cold probes to generate a thermally destructive lesion; this has enabled surgeons to make discrete lesions through a needle rather than by a surgical incision. Patients who could not withstand the physical and psychologic stress of a surgical operation can now be offered a percutaneous procedure that does not entail significant risk of infection, hemorrhage, or problems with wound healing. Technologic developments of the twentieth century continue to add to the surgeon's repertoire for alleviating pain and suffering, and new operations are described regularly. Long-term results are often not included in the initial optimistic appraisal of the value of each procedure, and some caution seems warranted before new procedures are widely used.

Guidelines for Optimizing Surgical Results

The role played by the neurosurgeon in the treatment of chronic pain is a function of local patterns of medical care and the success of the patient's interactions with the health care delivery system. The development of multidisciplinary groups and pain clinics has altered the conceptual approach to the patient with chronic pain and, hopefully, can lead to more sophisticated approaches for using surgical methods to deal with the patient with chronic pain. Ablative procedures, whether by knife, alcohol, or thermal coagulation, are often not the primary choice for the management of the patient with chronic pain caused by nonmalignant diseases; they are more useful for cancer pain. Unfortunately, far too many have been subjected to destructive surgical procedures that have not provided long-term relief of symptoms.

The neurosurgeon usually is well advised to avoid destructive operations for chronic pain unless the patient is known to have a life-shortening malignancy or has been thoroughly studied, and all other feasible treatments attempted. Of course, the patient with classic tic douloureux who has not responded to intensive medical therapy is an exception, because the response of this disease to various surgical procedures is likely to be favorable. A few other diseases respond well to surgery—causalgia and compression neuropathy stand out. I suspect that, for every patient who achieves long-term benefit from a destructive operation, two are unimproved or made worse because of increased pain or neurologic deficit. This can be a function of the personality of a particular chronic pain patient, as well as of the nature of the operation performed. Technical success is not always mirrored by patient improvement; reciprocally, the good results ascribed to an operation can be related to events other than the destruction of a portion of the nervous system.

The Role of Technical Skill and Experience

Undoubtedly the results of an operation are directly related to the surgeon's knowledge and skill. Appropriate training and experience should be prerequisites for performing operative procedures of any type, especially those affecting the nervous system. Most neurosurgeons have the necessary skills, but few have had adequate experience dealing with the many facets of many chronic pain patients. Most errors in the management of these patients do not occur in the operating room, but are made during the preoperative and postoperative evaluation of the patients by the surgeon. The

operation is often technically adequate, but patients might have been unwisely selected for the procedure.

Experience in Managing Chronic Pain Patients

Few neurosurgery training programs currently offer adequate exposure to the multiple problems of patients with chronic pain; the overall poor therapeutic results are often not known, and short-term successes are considered adequate reasons for major surgery. For example, it is well known that the "success rate" for initial lumbar diskectomy varies from 60 to 85% as a function of the patient population, but long-term follow-up in a 20-year multicenter Veterans Hospital study did not show an advantage for surgical therapy over conservative treatment (4).

Such data should make the neurosurgeon consider the indications for diskectomy carefully. Other studies have indicated that the natural history of patients who have a ruptured disk is not altered by surgery when the patients are followed for 5 years (5). Furthermore, the long-term results after second or third lumbar disk operations have long been known to be dismal, yet surgeons still use this approach to chronic low back pain, often before other less hazardous avenues are explored.

This situation can be ascribed to various aspects of the systems of medical care: I choose to identify inadequate long-term follow-up and feedback to the surgeon as the primary reasons for its continuation, although economics can be a factor. Careful long-term follow-up and increased participation by the neurosurgeon in the overall management of the patient with chronic pain are needed. Major neurosurgical textbooks often describe operative procedures with little or no discussion of long-term success rates. Many operations can be done to alleviate pain and suffering; the tough decision is not which one, however, but whether any destructive procedure is warranted at a specific time in the patient's course.

In contrast to the circumspect attitude that a neurosurgeon should exhibit toward destructive operative procedures for most nonmalignant diseases, certain types of patients should be promptly offered appropriate surgical relief of their pain or suffering. Two common examples of specific diseases are causalgia that has not been cured by a series of sympathetic blocks and tic douloureux that has not responded to anticonvulsants. The pain resulting from uncontrolled cancer is also an appropriate indication for a surgical procedure.

Some guidelines for the management of cancer pain are important for the surgeon. If the patient has a short life expectancy (less than 60 to 90 days), it is unwise to consider a major surgical procedure; narcotics or a percutaneous neurolytic procedure is usually more appropriate. The patient who is this close to death rarely has adequate infection resistance, wound healing, or blood coagulation, and is a high surgical risk. For the patient who is going to survive more than 6 months, it is unlikely that oral narcotics or percutaneous procedures are optimal, and a surgical procedure is often indicated. Intermediate survival periods are often best managed by percutaneous procedures such as cordotomy, rhizotomy, epidural narcotics, or intrathecal injections of phenol or alcohol.

The patient with cancer is more likely to have a good result from a surgical procedure because the pain most likely is a result of nociception, which is eliminated by ablative procedures, and the patient is not likely to survive long enough for the beneficial effects of the surgical procedure to disappear. Furthermore, I suspect (but cannot prove) that those personality factors that play such a large role in the pain behavior of some patients with chronic pain secondary to a nonmalignant disease process are not usually found in the patient with a malignancy. These factors can predispose a patient with chronic pain of nonmalignant origin to operative failure. It is the younger patient with a vague pain syndrome related to a nonmalignant disease who so often fails to obtain pain relief from an operative procedure that seemed so promising.

Prediction of Long-Term Results

The major problem for the neurosurgeon is the prediction of long-term operative results for individual patients. A few studies of adequate numbers of patients followed for more than 3 months are available, but how can particular patients be related to a larger group? Are any reliable predictors of operative outcome available? For patients with low back pain, several studies now indicate that return to work 1 year after surgery is not related to the preoperative examination or the findings at surgery, but is predictable from preoperative psychologic testing results (6). Few, if any, studies for such procedures as cordotomy, myelotomy, and rhizotomy have been done. The latter operation has been the subject of several reviews, which clearly show that spinal rhizotomy does not provide long-term relief for most patients (7, 8).

Role of Psychologic and Psychiatric Evaluation

A patient with chronic pain not caused by a malignancy is frequently referred to a psychiatrist or psychologist for evaluation. Unfortunately, few of these patients have been evaluated prior to embarking on a career of chronic pain, so we do not know if the psychologic evaluation describes the type of patient who suffers from chronic pain or describes the effects of chronic pain on the patient. It is clearly unwise to perform a major surgical procedure on a psychotic or severely depressed patient, not so much because of the risk of technical failure but because of the patient's inability to handle the stresses of hospitalization and surgery.

Hysterical or highly suggestible patients are likely to respond favorably on a short-term basis to any procedure, but little is known about its long-term efficacy in hysterical patients versus patients with a better integrated ego. The indications for surgery in hysterical patients must be thoroughly scrutinized; these patients seem all too likely to receive more therapies for body ailments than is required. A significant proportion of patients with chronic pain are labeled as having psychologic needs for their pain behavior. With the exception of the malingerer or the overtly emotionally ill,

this type of diagnostic evaluation does not seem to influence the therapeutic results. Therapy should be based on the identification of specific factors that indicate the need for operative intervention.

Many surgeons have relied on the Minnesota Multiphasic Personality Inventory (MMPI) as an indicator of the suitability of patients for surgical therapy. No controlled studies have been done to validate this use of the MMPI, but the test does eliminate the problem of observer bias and seems to predict the types of behavior patterns patients manifest and their responses to illness and stress. The MMPI can effectively identify people who have great readiness to convey to others that something is wrong with their body; to the extent that such tendencies are present (hypochondriasis), surgery or any other therapy is unlikely to reduce health care seeking behavior. The MMPI can be used to identify those individuals whose characteristic modes of responding to environmental stresses make it unlikely that any surgical procedure can restore them to a productive life-style.

Influence of Compensation and Litigation

Neurosurgeons have long been aware of the roles of compensation and litigation as factors in the determination of therapeutic outcome. I am not sure that these are particularly valid, because their effects have never been separated from such factors as the passage of time and intervening therapies. It is now quite obvious that environmental factors can and do influence pain behavior regardless of the cause of the pain. Compensation and litigation are only two of the many environmental influences impinging on our patients. Family interactions can perpetuate pain behavior long after healing has occurred. Health care and insurance programs should be designed to offer rewards for recovery, not prolonged illness; some clearly have the opposite effect and lead to unnecessary surgical procedures.

The lack of motivation to "get well" can influence the search for continued medical assistance. Several studies of specific operations, however, failed to show a poorer prognosis for patients receiving compensation for their illness (8). It is too simplistic to consider only economic compensation when psychologic and environmental factors can play such large roles in the genesis of pain behavior (9). Issues such as these have made it difficult to assess the results of surgical procedures.

The influences of duration of pain and prior attempts to alleviate pain have not been ascertained. Santayana's statement that "He who is ignorant of the lessons of history must be prepared to repeat them" is probably relevant to patients with chronic pain who fail to respond to many other well-chosen treatment regimens.

Role of Prognostic Nerve Blocks

The role of nerve blocks in the selection of patients for surgical procedures must be scrutinized. The proper use of diagnostic blocks is discussed in Chapter 94 and other sections of this book; certain points need to be emphasized for the neurosurgeon. A single nerve block cannot be relied on to provide meaningful information—too many extraneous factors can influence the patient's response. A carefully planned series of blocks is often helpful but does not, as far as I can tell, predict long-term outcome of an ablative procedure except for sympathectomy for causalgia, or trigeminal neurectomy for tic douloureux. Nerve blocks can identify the source of pain and the nerves or roots that must be cut to isolate that region of the body from the spinal cord or brain stem. They can also determine if the patient's responses seem to be related to the duration of the anesthetic agents used and the nerve structure injected; these seem to be important measures of patient reliability. This issue is difficult to clarify, because no results have been reported in regard to operations performed on the patient who does not respond to nerve blocks in the region of the proposed surgery. Another indication for preoperative nerve block involves allowing the patient to experience the expected numbness on a short-term basis. Some prefer their pain to this numbness.

Managing Narcotics in the Preoperative and Postoperative Periods

The neurosurgeon must have a strategy for dealing with patients who are taking significant amounts of narcotics and are being considered for an operative procedure. If the genesis of the pain has been clearly established as nociception, as in many patients with cancer-related pain, it is reasonable to relieve the pain with an operation and then taper the medications. Patients with an unclear cause of their pain behavior (e.g., associated with nonmalignant diseases) should be converted from short-duration narcotics to a long-acting drug such as methadone, and the dosage gradually tapered (10). In many of these patients the pain behavior diminishes as the narcotic level falls, and no operation is required. In others a more accurate diagnosis can be made as the narcotic-induced mental impairment clears; surgical indications might then be more clear-cut (10).

Pain relief obtained with a surgical procedure is likely to reduce the patient's tolerance for narcotics dramatically, and consequently respiratory depression and even apnea can develop (Chapter 78). The dosage should be sharply curtailed in the immediate postoperative period while the patient is under close observation and, if respiratory depression becomes evident, incremental doses of naloxone are used. Patient-controlled analgesia is an excellent method for controlling postoperative pain (Chapters 25, 78, and 95).

Informed Consent

Another issue that must be considered concerns informed consent. The patient and family should be thoroughly informed about the therapeutic options and the risks and benefits of alternative treatment strategies. Not only the neurosurgeon but also the patient's primary care physician(s) must be knowledgeable about the likely outcomes from alternative treatments. As emphasized in Chapter 31, the patient's physician should have a clear idea of what a proposed neurosurgical procedure entails so that this can be discussed with the patient. The options currently available do not allow traditional biases to determine health care.

The neurosurgeon who deals with patients with chronic pain must recognize that the greatest problems lie in the selection of therapeutic methods rather than in the application of the techniques themselves. Every operation and every other form of therapy has its advantages and disadvantages (9). What is appropriate at one point in time for a patient might not be optimal during any other phase of treatment. Not infrequently, surgical procedures must be performed in conjunction with other modes of therapy if the patient as a total human being is to be rehabilitated. In general, destructive procedures should not be considered until other modes of therapy have been thoroughly evaluated. When indicated, surgical intervention should not be delayed. That decision reflects the art of neurosurgery.

REFERENCES

1. White, J.C., and Sweet, W.H.: Pain and the Neurosurgeon. Springfield, IL, Charles C Thomas, 1969.
2. Wilkins, R.H., and Rengachary, S.S.: Neurosurgery. New York, McGraw-Hill, 1985.
3. Letievant, E.: Traité des sections nerveuses. Paris, J.B. Balliere et Fils, 1873.
4. Nashold, B.S., Jr., and Hrubec, Z.: Lumbar Disc Disease. St. Louis, C.V. Mosby, 1971.
5. Nachemson, A.L.: The natural course of low back pain. In Symposium on Idiopathic Low Back Pain. Edited by A.A. White III and S.L. Gordon. St. Louis, C.V. Mosby, 1982, pp. 46–51.
6. Pondaag, W., and Oostdam, E.M.M.: Predicting the outcome of lumbar disc surgery by means of preoperative psychological testing. In Advances in Pain Research and Therapy, Vol. 3. Edited by J.J. Bonica, J.C. Liebeskind, and D. Albe-Fessard. New York, Raven Press, 1979, pp. 713–717.
7. Onofrio, B.M., and Campo, H.K.: Evaluation of rhizotomy. Review of 12 year's experience. J. Neurosurg., 36:751, 1972.
8. Loeser, J.D.: Dorsal rhizotomy for the relief of chronic pain. J. Neurosurg., 36:745, 1972.
9. Loeser, J.D., and Fordyce, W.L.: Chronic pain. In Behavioral Sciences in the Practice of Medicine. Edited by J.E. Carr and H.A. Dengerink. New York, Elsevier, 1983, pp. 331–345.
10. Halpern, L.: Substitution-detoxification and its role in the management of chronic benign pain. J. Clin. Psychiatry, 43:10, 1982.

97 • NEUROSURGICAL OPERATIONS INVOLVING PERIPHERAL NERVES

JOHN D. LOESER, WILLIAM H. SWEET, JOHN M. TEW, JR., *and* HARRY VAN LOVEREN
with contributions by
JOHN J. BONICA

THIS chapter discusses neurosurgical techniques involving peripheral spinal, cranial and sympathetic nerves used for relief of chronic pain, and is presented in five sections: A, Peripheral Neurectomy; B, Spinal Dorsal Rhizotomy; C, Sympa-

thectomy; D, Trigeminal Gangliolysis; and E, Cranial Rhizotomy. Loeser wrote Sections A, B, and E, Sweet wrote Section C, Tew and van Loveren wrote Section D, and Bonica contributed to Sections C, D, and E.

A. PERIPHERAL NEURECTOMY

Neurectomy, which entails resection of a part of one or more peripheral branches of the cranial or spinal nerves, was the first neurosurgical procedure to be used for chronic pain. Today, however, it has only a small role in managing patients with chronic pain. This section discusses the advantages and disadvantages of neurectomy in different parts of the body, followed by a brief consideration of the indications, techniques, and results for cranial neurectomy, extremity neurectomy, and neurectomy in the trunk.

Basic Considerations

Advantages

The foremost advantages of resection of a peripheral nerve are the ease of the operation and the predictable loss of function. If the two ends of the nerve are widely separated functional regeneration does not occur, except in the trigeminal nerve. Exposing the peripheral nerve and dividing it should be a quick and safe operative procedure that can be done under local or regional anesthesia. Neurectomy can be expected to produce complete anesthesia in the territory of the sectioned nerve.

Disadvantages

The disadvantages of this technique outweigh all the supposed advantages. With the exception of the trigeminal and a few minor cutaneous nerves of the extremities, most peripheral nerves are mixed; motor loss occurs and persists even longer than the sensory changes following peripheral neurectomy. Another disadvantage can be the loss of all sensory modalities and the complications of anesthesia in skin or joints. This is in contrast with cordotomy, in which only pain and temperature sensation are lost.

In addition to these immediate complications several long-term problems often arise. Adjacent intact sensory nerves sprout into the denervated area, producing a general circumferential decrease in the

region of anesthesia. If the original anesthetic area is small, the sensory loss can completely vanish in several months. Associated with the decreasing anesthesia is the return of the original painful sensation. In addition, changes in the spinal cord or perhaps in more rostral neural structures can lead to decreased anesthesia or to a new pain syndrome, called denervation hypersensitivity or anesthesia dolorosa. Although this is most common after cranial neurectomy, it can occur in an extremity and is a most distressing complication, because no reliable therapy is currently available. Finally, whenever a peripheral nerve is transected, a neuroma is formed. Not all neuromata are painful, but those that occur in pressure areas frequently cause pain. This new iatrogenic disorder can be worse than the original pain.

Clinical Considerations

Cranial Neurectomy

The most frequently performed neurectomies involving the trigeminal nerve have been resection of the supraorbital, infraorbital, and mandibular nerves in patients with intractable trigeminal neuralgia. Beneficial results have been obtained by denervation either of the region of pain or of trigger areas (1, 2). Peripheral neurectomy, however, is no longer a primary surgical procedure in the management of tic douloureux. Percutaneous gangliolysis produces longer pain relief with less sensory loss, and has just as low a morbidity rate. Only when gangliolysis has failed and the patient is not a candidate for an intracranial procedure should peripheral neurectomy be undertaken (see Cranial Neuralgias, Chapter 38). Sections of sensory branches more proximal to this involve intracranial surgical procedures (see below, Section 97E). Cranial peripheral neurectomies have been used for all types of headaches and atypical facial pains. They are rarely successful and have little place in the current management of these pain syndromes (3, 4).

2044

Properly controlled studies of the efficacy of peripheral neurectomy are rare, in spite of many claims for the value of this type of surgery.

Techniques

The supraorbital nerve is approached through a skin incision paralleling and within the eyebrow. This nerve enters the scalp through a foramen or notch in the supraorbital rim directly above the pupil when the eye is in midposition. The nerve is grasped with two hemostats and sectioned between them; the proximal and distal stumps are avulsed.

The infraorbital nerve is approached through a sublabial incision, as for a Caldwell-Luc procedure. The cheek is elevated by blunt dissection and the nerve is identified as it exits the infraorbital foramen. Two hemostats are applied, the nerve is cut between them, and both are avulsed proximally and distally.

The mandibular nerve is approached transorally by most dentists and oral surgeons and by a submandibular lateral approach by most neurosurgeons. For the latter approach, a 3-cm curved incision is made to conform to the skin lines at the angle of the jaw. The skin is reflected superiorly and the masseter fibers are spread to expose the angle of the ramus overlying the mandibular nerve canal. A high-speed drill is then used to expose the nerve, which is divided and avulsed; the accompanying blood vessels must be coagulated.

Results

The results of trigeminal neurectomies have rarely been reported in a useful format. Rasmussen's study (3) is a good source of long-term follow-up data (Table 97-1). In general, prior to gangliolysis with modern equipment, trigeminal neurectomies were a reasonable first surgical step. Today they are indicated only when gangliolysis is not available.

Neurectomy in the Extremities

The disadvantages of neurectomy, as mentioned above, are especially relevant to neurectomy involving nerves to the extremities. With the exception of the lateral femoral cutaneous and saphenous nerves in the lower limbs and the cutaneous nerves in the forearm, most nerves of the extremities are mixed and resection results in motor loss that persists longer than the sensory changes. Of course, all sensory modalities are lost. The amount of motor loss is so great that any neurectomy of major nerves to the intact extremity is rarely justified. In addition, the anesthesia produced can result in repeated trauma to the numb area and in the development of decubiti and Charcot joints. Without proprioception an extremity is useless. If the patient has useful function in the distal musculature, nerves such as the ulnar, medial, or sciatic should almost never be sectioned.

Indications

Few indications for peripheral neurectomy are seen today. This procedure can occasionally be helpful in the amputee who has a neuroma in a weight-bearing area. Resecting the nerve so that its end lies in a more protected region can provide relief of a distressing stump pain syndrome if the pain is clearly caused by pressure on the neuroma. In the absence of local pressure, resection of a neuroma in a stump is usually futile (5, 6) (Chapter 12).

Extremity nerves that have been traumatized or entrapped can develop a neuroma in continuity that is a source of pain. Resection of the neuroma and neurorrhaphy can provide the patient with pain relief and with the opportunity for restoration of function. Selected severe cases of meralgia paresthetica can benefit from lateral femoral cutaneous nerve section but, in almost all cases, the pain can be managed without this operation. Crush or destruction of a peripheral nerve to alleviate the pain of gangrene or a terminal neoplasm is a theoretic possibility, and in earlier years was probably a satisfactory use of peripheral neurectomy. Phantom limb pain cannot be relieved by neuroma resection.

Pain in the distribution of the radial nerve is notoriously refractory to section of the sensory branch in the forearm. I have seen four patients who had this minor branch sectioned an average of three times each in the hopes of relieving post-traumatic wrist pain. These twelve operations were all failures.

Technique

If a peripheral neurectomy is to be undertaken, it is imperative that the proximal nerve stump be treated so as to minimize the risk of postoperative neuroma pain. The level of the neurectomy should be carefully planned to avoid placing the proximal end in a weight-bearing or pressure area. The literature is replete with nostrums to prevent the formation of a neuroma. Clearly, if regeneration is not desired, the proximal and distal stumps should be widely separated and the ends either capped with some inert material or buried in the bone. Little evidence has been found, however, to indicate that such measures or the injection of sclerosing substances are truly effective in eliminating painful neuromata (7). It does seem to be helpful to bury the proximal stump of the nerve so that it is not distorted by scarring during activity in adjacent muscles. Strategies to cap the proximal stump or to seal axons within the epineurium have no proven efficacy.

TABLE 97-1. Avulsions of Branches of the Trigeminal Nerve

Nerve	No. of Operations	Results (% of Patients)		
		Initial Success*	2-Year Success	Pain Still Relieved at Time of Death
Supraorbital				
Tic douloureux	59	79	14	12
Non-neuralgic pain	37	54	16	
Infraorbital				
Tic douloureux	82	74	23	2
Non-neuralgic pain	11	55	27	

*Success = good pain relief.
From Rasmussen, P.P.: Facial Pain. Copenhagen, Ejnar Munksgaards Forlag, 1965, p. 211.

Summary

Many reasons for avoiding peripheral neurectomy in the extremity are apparent, so it would be advisable to reconsider any patient who seems to be a candidate for such an operation carefully. Few long-term successes can be anticipated.

Neurectomy Involving Nerves of the Trunk

Intercostal neurectomy has far fewer theoretic disadvantages than neurectomy in the extremity; unfortunately, it too is often a practical failure. Although the intercostal nerves are mixed, the motor loss that follows their transection is usually not significant to the patient. In addition, the loss of all sensation over a segment of the body wall is generally not a major problem, unlike anesthesia in an extremity. The chest and abdomen are usually covered and are protected from environmental trauma. Similar problems with sensory overlap, sprouting, and anesthesia dolorosa can occur after intercostal or upper lumbar neurectomy.

Indications

Intercostal neurectomy has been used in the attempt to alleviate the pain of chest wall invasion by malignancy or by painful costochondral junctions. Painful scars in the upper abdomen have also been treated by appropriate neurectomy. Long-term results have not been satisfactory. None of the neuralgias following thoracotomy or herpes zoster, or caused by other unknown factors, is likely to respond to intercostal neurectomy; this operation should not be contemplated for patients with such diagnoses.

Technique

Intercostal nerves can be most readily transected at the anterior or posterior axillary line. Care must be taken to control bleeding from the accompanying artery and vein and to divide the nerve, and not just one of the vascular structures. Facilities should be available to treat a pneumothorax in case this complication occurs. A series of intercostal nerve blocks should be used preoperatively to identify those nerves that must be divided to denervate the painful area fully. Because overlap from adjacent nerves is common, it is wisest to divide an additional nerve above and below the apparently involved segments.

Techniques to perform the neurectomy with a cryoprobe or radiofrequency lesion are available and can obviate the need for an open surgical procedure (8, 9). Whether such new methods of destroying nerves yield better long-term results is unclear at present. Such percutaneous techniques to reduce operative risks can result in increased numbers of patients having neurolytic procedures without any increase in the percentage of those who obtain long-term symptomatic relief. Multiple sequential neurectomies can render a segment of the abdominal wall flaccid and can lead to abdominal asymmetry and cosmetic complaints.

Summary

In summary, few if any indications for intercostal or lumbar neurectomy exist. Damaging the nerves further is not a likely remedy, especially for those patients whose pain is associated with a nerve injury. Although painful body wall invasion by a neoplasm can be treated by neurectomy, dorsal rhizotomy or cordotomy is usually a better choice.

B. SPINAL DORSAL RHIZOTOMY

The deliberate section of a spinal dorsal root in the attempt to alleviate pain was first described in the American literature in 1889 by Abbé; the operation was apparently first performed in England shortly thereafter by Bennett (10, 11). Since then innumerable neurosurgeons have performed this operation, and thousands of patients have obtained pain relief from this procedure.

It is somewhat startling to realize that so few reports have been published on patients who have undergone dorsal rhizotomy; equally troubling, many of those reported series did not describe particularly satisfactory long-term results. Dorsal rhizotomies are less commonly performed today as the knowledge of the discrepancy between short-term and long-term results has become disseminated throughout the neurosurgical community. Newer techniques, such as percutaneous neurolysis with radiofrequency current or a cryoprobe, or modification of the surgery by the addition of ganglionectomy, might alter the long-term outcome. No one has yet identified the criteria for optimal patient selection, and this probably is a factor in the less than desired long-term successes (12).

Cervicothoracic dorsal rhizotomy was once used to treat angina pectoris, because it is possible to eliminate afferent input from the heart and coronary blood vessels with this operation (13, 14). Little, if any, use of dorsal rhizotomy is now made for cardiac pain, as pharmacologic and surgical approaches to the coronary arteries have become the accepted standards of care.

At various times there has been enthusiasm for the use of upper cervical dorsal rhizotomy for the relief of intractable headaches (15). The role of afferent fibers from the upper cervical roots in specific types of headache has not been adequately evaluated, and the proper indications for the use of dorsal rhizotomy to relieve different types of headache remains unclear. On the other hand, a definite place exists for upper cervical rhizotomy in conjunction with section of the 5th and 9th cranial nerves in patients with face and neck cancer.

Basic Considerations

Advantages

Theoretic advantages of spinal dorsal rhizotomy make this operation superior to peripheral neurectomy. White (16) has expressed the belief that it is also more effective than cordotomy. The primary advantage is the sparing of motor fibers and the absence, therefore, of muscle paralysis. The complete sectioning of all the dorsal roots to an extremity, however, renders that limb anesthetic, paralyzed, and functionally useless because of the loss of gamma and proprioceptive afferent fibers. Total dorsal rhizotomy to a functional limb should therefore not be performed. This is clearly not a problem in the uppermost four cervical, the thoracic, or the uppermost two lumbar nerves, in which motor loss is usually not a clinically significant deficit.

Six or more consecutive roots can be sectioned without damaging cord function if the radicular vessels are spared (17). Partial selective rhizidiotomy, achieved by sectioning the lateral rootlets, is thought by some to be a useful strategy when cervical or lumbar rhizotomy is required to eliminate pain in an extremity with preserved function (17–19). Data on long-term results for such operations are sparse.

Another theoretic advantage of spinal dorsal rhizotomy is the ability to render a definite region of the body totally anesthetic. The area of anesthesia can be determined in advance by prognostic paravertebral somatic nerve blocks with a local anesthetic (Chapter 94), or intraoperatively by applying local anesthetic to the rootlets intradurally. Although individual variations in segmental cutaneous innervation can be present, certain generally applicable patterns can help in the planning of which dorsal roots to cut to alleviate pain in a specific area. The region of sensory change is restricted to the side of the body in which the dorsal roots are sectioned, and sensory loss only occurs in those regions whose segmental innervation has been cut (see Chapter 6 for dermatomal patterns).

The studies of Coggeshall (20) and others have suggested that some unmyelinated afferent fibers have their cell bodies in the dorsal root ganglia, appear to enter the ventral roots, and synapse in the dorsal horns in a pattern identical to that of dorsal root unmyelinated afferents. If such fibers exist, their persistence can be a factor in the failure of dorsal rhizotomy to relieve pain (21). Many neurosurgeons now perform spinal ganglionectomy, therefore, whenever dorsal rhizotomy is undertaken (22).

Smith (23) described dorsal rhizotomy and ganglionectomy long before the presence of ventral root afferent fibers was recognized. No reports have been published to allow standard dorsal rhizotomy to be compared to ganglionectomy and rhizotomy. Hence, it is unclear if the addition of ganglionectomy improves the long-term efficacy of dorsal rhizotomy. Sindou and colleagues (19) have described selective rhizidiotomy of the intraspinal dorsal root fibers. Although they reported favorable results, little confirmation from other surgeons has been received in regard to the value of this modification of dorsal rhizotomy.

Intradural dorsal rhizotomy requires a laminectomy over each root to be sectioned except over the conus or cauda equina, where many roots can be visualized in a restricted area (24). Although laminectomy and durotomy is a major operative procedure, it should not carry a significant complication rate if the operation is well planned and executed. It is not a particularly difficult operation and can be carried out successfully by any skilled neurosurgeon. An operating microscope

and microtools are essential to ensure visualization of all rootlets and preservation of the radicular blood supply.

Extradural dorsal rhizotomy does not require a laminectomy but does require a small laminotomy and medial facetectomy to expose the root sleeve. The extradural approach is particularly useful in the lumbar region. If a ganglionectomy is to be performed the exposure must unroof the facet completely to follow the root into the lateral foramen. The operating microscope is particularly helpful in performing a ganglionectomy.

Disadvantages

Spinal dorsal rhizotomy has certain theoretic and practical disadvantages. It cannot be used to relieve extremity pain when complete denervation is required, as has been discussed. Only when the causative lesion, such as cancer, has already rendered extremity function useless can all the dorsal roots from a limb be sectioned. Sparing portions of several roots can obviate this problem but, particularly in the upper limb, the loss of function can be as devastating as the pain itself. Midline or bilateral pain, either dorsal or ventral, requires bilateral dorsal rhizotomies for relief. In the sacral region this can lead to loss of anal and bladder sphincter control and render pain relief by this technique impractical. On the other hand, when the sphincters are already inoperative, sacral rhizotomy can be effective in the management of perineal or perianal pain (24, 25). Coccygodynia can be treated by S4 to Co1 rhizotomy without endangering sphincters (25). It must also be ascertained that the patient's pain is not a result of visceral afferent activity entering the spinal cord, with the sympathetic afferents rostral to the somatic segments. Careful use of selective nerve blocks can demonstrate the neuronal circuits involved in nociceptive input and allow the surgeon to plan the appropriate operation.

Another disadvantage is the initial loss of all sensory modalities in the dermatomes that have undergone dorsal rhizotomy. Sensations of light touch and joint position are lost, along with those of pain and temperature. Decubiti and Charcot joints can occur in traumatized and denervated regions of the body. The anesthetic area usually diminishes in size over time and, if initially less than three segments wide, can eventually disappear completely. When this occurs the pain usually recurs.

Causes of Failures

Several theories have been proposed to explain the high failure rate of dorsal rhizotomy for pain relief. One involves the concept of sprouting from intact nerves in adjacent skin into the denervated regions. This phenomenon has been histologically demonstrated and is confirmed by the common observation that the return of sensation usually starts at the interface with normally innervated skin, and proceeds circumferentially into the anesthetic area. This type of cutaneous sprouting rarely extends beyond one dermatome.

Another theory invokes the concept of sprouting within the spinal cord so as to alter the receptive fields of existing neurons (26). Although histologic evidence for sprouting within the spinal cord is available, the new connections have never been shown to be functional. Also, "latent" synapses are electrically silent until adjacent dorsal roots are cut, thereby establishing new sensory fields for dorsal horn neurons immediately after rhizotomy. The time course for this phenomenon is too rapid to be explained by sprouting within the spinal cord. Finally, the receptive fields of dorsal horn neurons are not fixed but can be modified pharmacologically, as shown by Hodge and King (27). Others have proposed that return of sensation could be attributed to anastomoses between roots or to incomplete root section, with return of conduction in fibers that were only traumatized but not transected (16).

Although laminectomy and dorsal rhizotomy are well tolerated by a healthy patient, it certainly can be a hazardous operation in the cachectic patient with a preterminal malignancy. The proper biologic substrate for wound healing must be present if this operation is to be undertaken. If the region of pain input is extensive, the multilevel laminectomy required can become prohibitive. Although 6- to 12-level rhizotomies have been undertaken, although rarely with long-term success, they certainly are a far more formidable procedure than the more common 2- to 4-level operation.

Strategies for dorsal rhizotomy without laminectomy and open operation have evolved in the past decade or so. Lazorthes and associates (8) and Uematsu and co-workers (28) have described percutaneous radiofrequency lesioning of the dorsal roots just lateral to the spinal foramina. Others have used a cryoprobe to produce a freezing lesion. Nash (29) used percutaneous radiofrequency lesions of dorsal root ganglia in 26 patients with severe neuralgia or other intractable chronic pain problems in the cervical, thoracic, lumbar, or sacral region with excellent to good results in 15 (58%) and this persisted in 13 (50%) until death of the patients or follow-up that ranged from 6 to 72 months. Similar results have been reported by others (see p. 2028). Percutaneous rhizotomy and/or ganglionectomy can be offered to a patient who might not withstand the stress of an open operation.

Complications

Operative complications of open dorsal rhizotomy should be minimal but are by no means unknown. Among the problems described are wound infection, meningitis, postoperative intradural or extradural hemorrhage, infarction of the spinal cord, mechanical trauma to the cord with ensuing paralysis, and cerebrospinal fluid fistula. Almost all of these catastrophes are preventable by strict adherence to the principles of neurologic surgery and to the realization that major vessels in the dorsal roots must be preserved; the operating microscope or a loupe is a valuable aid in the latter task.

A final and devastating complication is the development of anesthesia dolorosa, pain in an anesthetic area. Cutting additional dorsal roots does not solve this problem. In contrast, patients who have had extensive dorsal rhizotomies might complain of continued pain in the apparently denervated area. Careful examination can reveal that total anesthesia has not actually been

obtained—poorly localized pain perception can still be present. I have found in several such patients that ganglionectomy or ventral rhizotomy (in the thoracic area) can alleviate the persisting pain. These results suggest corroboration of the existence of ventral root afferent fibers (21).

Clinical Considerations
Criteria for Patient Selection

The selection of a patient for spinal dorsal rhizotomy requires knowledge of the pathology leading to the chronic pain, the patient's overall health status and prognosis, and the availability of alternative modes of therapy. As is true for most major operative procedures for pain relief, it is imperative to ascertain that therapy directed at the cause of pain is unlikely to succeed before selecting a destructive operative procedure. Spinal dorsal rhizotomy is not the procedure of choice if the patient's life expectancy is less than 30 to 60 days. Problems with wound healing are common in the preterminal patient; it is unwise to keep a patient in the hospital for postoperative recuperation that occupies more than 25% of the remaining lifetime. Pharmacologic methods or percutaneous procedures should be used in the patient who has such a short life expectancy.

The existence of drug dependence because of chronic pain need not be a contraindication to dorsal rhizotomy; a successful operative result makes it all the easier to gradually taper the dosage of narcotics in the postoperative period. The presence of significant systemic infection or even a minor infection adjacent to the operative area is an absolute contraindication to dorsal rhizotomy.

Technique

The technical aspects of dorsal rhizotomy are well known among neurosurgeons. The operation is greatly facilitated by the use of the operating microscope and of microdissection tools but does not require any other specialized equipment. Most surgeons prefer an intradural approach in the cervical, thoracic, and lumbar areas; in the sacral region extradural rhizotomies are more common. Scoville (23), Smith (30), and Dubuisson (31) have described extradural approaches in the thoracic region, and Crue and Todd (24) have described the extradural sacral rhizotomy.

Dorsal rhizotomy can be performed under local, regional, or general anesthesia; the choice of type of anesthetic is a function of the level of surgery, preoperative evaluation, patient personality, and surgeon's preference. The patient can be in the prone, lateral decubitus, oblique, or seated position during surgery. Several factors influence this choice. It is unwise to perform a dorsal rhizotomy under local or segmental anesthesia in the seated position because of the inevitable loss of cerebrospinal fluid and the ensuing headache, nausea, and vomiting during the time when the patient's cooperation is required. Segmental epidural anesthesia is quite effective but should only be undertaken by anesthesiologists highly skilled in the technique, because errors can occur that result in a high spinal anesthetic.

Operation under local anesthesia allows the surgeon to evaluate the effects of blocking each root by the application of pledgets soaked with lidocaine (Xylocaine) prior to cutting the root. Roots or rootlets can be serially sectioned and the effects on the patient's pain and the area of sensory loss can be ascertained. In this fashion a technically adequate initial operative result can be guaranteed and the hazards of sectioning the wrong dorsal root(s) are reduced. The patient often rejects a major operation under local anesthesia, however, and good physician-patient rapport is required to convince the patient of the wisdom of local anesthesia when the neurosurgeon feels that it is warranted. Techniques of general anesthesia that permit the patient to be awakened during the operation to assess the effects of blocking individual roots have also been described (12).

Preoperative evaluation by radiographically controlled paravertebral nerve blocks with local anesthetics can often obviate the need for an operation under local anesthesia. One block is *never* an adequate evaluation for surgery; it is essential to carry out a carefully planned sequence if meaningful information is to be obtained (Chapter 94). Preoperative localization should be undertaken with appropriate roentgenography and a skin marker; intraoperative ambiguities about the operative level can be answered by a roentgenogram during surgery. Various strategies for localizing the operative level have been described, but none is foolproof. The surgeon is well advised to take special precautions to operate at the correct level by using intraoperative roentgenography (17).

Unilateral Rhizotomy

I prefer to perform unilateral intradural dorsal rhizotomies in the lateral decubitus position with the side of the rhizotomies superior. After a midline incision of the skin, the paraspinal musculature is dissected from the spinous processes and laminae unilaterally and a hemilaminectomy is performed (Fig. 97-1). The dura is opened in the middle of the bony defect and the roots and rootlets can be readily identified as they travel from the inferiorly lying spinal cord to their superior dural sheaths. The arachnoid is opened to gain access to the roots and rootlets. It is rarely necessary to touch the spinal cord as the roots and rootlets are identified and the major vessels are dissected free. The surgical microscope is a valuable adjunct.

I use a bipolar coagulator on each root before applying a single silver clip to mark the rootlets of each transected root at its dural investment, and then section the root (Fig. 97-1). Because this step of the operation is extremely painful, either the root must be blocked with a local anesthetic or the general anesthesia must be quite deep to prevent profound cardiovascular responses. Watertight closure of the dura and fascial planes is essential to minimize the risk of cerebrospinal fistula. It is usually necessary to remove one more lamina than the number of roots to be sectioned to ensure adequate exposure. It is prudent to plan to section two roots above and two roots below the segments shown by nerve blocks to be responsible for the pain.

Extradural rhizotomies or rhizotomy and ganglionectomy can also be performed through a midline skin incision and unilateral muscle dissection to expose the lateral facet joints and origins of the transverse process. The high-speed drill is the tool of choice for unroofing the neural foramen and exposing the dural root sleeve and dorsal root ganglion. The dura is incised and the dorsal root transected just proximal to the ganglion. The root is reflected laterally and the ganglion is separated from the ventral root. The dorsal root is transected just lateral to the ganglion and the surgical specimen removed. Because this approach is lateral to the arachnoid cuff on the dorsal root, it entails little risk of cerebrospinal fluid leakage.

Bilateral Rhizotomy

I perform bilateral dorsal rhizotomies with the patient prone or occasionally seated if the operation is to

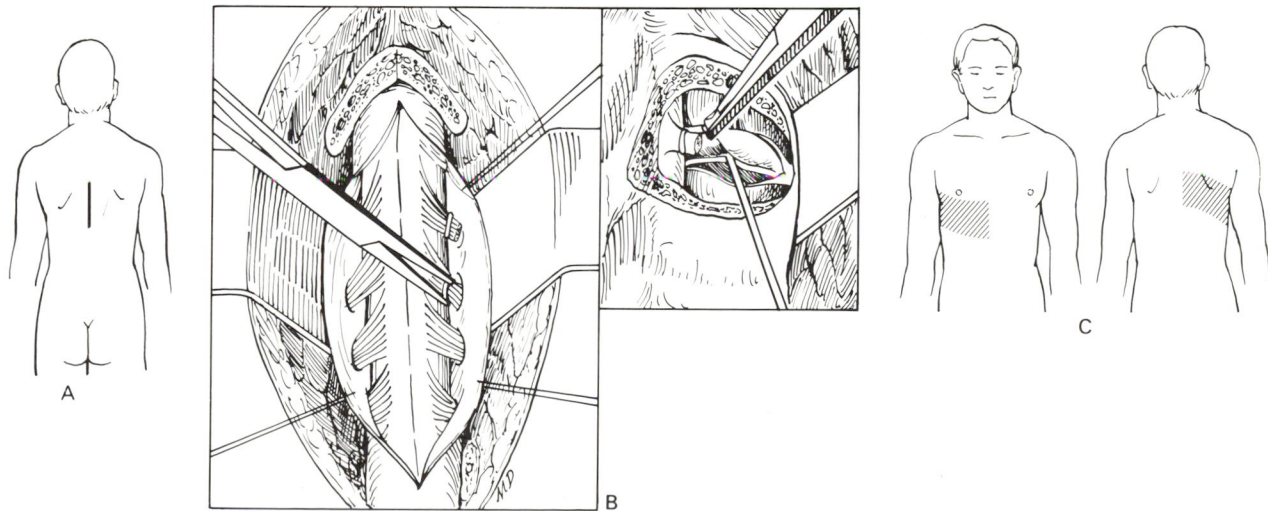

FIG. 97-1. Dorsal rhizotomy. *A.* Location of midline dorsal incision for T4–T7 dorsal rhizotomy. *B.* Intradural dorsal rhizotomy with application of metal clip on the rootlets of a root already transected above and being applied to the rootlets of a root below just prior to sectioning them. Inset on the right depicts extradural dorsal rhizotomy showing division of the dorsal root central to the ganglion prior to extirpation of the ganglion by a lesion which will be made just distal to the ganglion. *C.* Expected area of sensory loss following right T4 to T7 dorsal rhizotomy.

TABLE 97-2. Results with Dorsal Rhizotomy

Disease	Approximate No. of Reported Cases	Approximate Long-term Relief (% of Total Cases)
Occipital neuralgia	60	50
Cervicothoracic lumbar neuralgias	120	60
Postherpetic neuralgia	20	25
Failed lumbar disk	200	33*
Coccygodynia	70	60
Cancer	600	50

*Range of 10 to 86%

be in the cervical or upper thoracic region. Bilateral muscle dissection and laminectomy are required, and a midline dural incision is used. Postoperative local wound pain is a much more common problem than after the unilateral approach. In the upper thoracic region wound dehiscences caused by pulling with the arms in the immediate postoperative period are also a hazard. Patients should not be allowed to use their arms to pull themselves up for 2 weeks after upper thoracic laminectomy.

Postoperative Care

The typical patient is kept at bed rest until the postoperative headache abates, usually for 2 to 3 days. Activities are then progressively augmented until discharge, 5 to 7 days after surgery. Strenuous activity is interdicted for the first postoperative month, by which time tissue healing should be essentially complete. Failure to achieve anesthesia in the desired area is a complication that should be dealt with by prompt reoperation and sectioning of the correct roots. Lack of pain relief in spite of adequate anesthesia in the region of the pain is not an indication for further dorsal rhizotomies. Return of pain a few weeks after dorsal rhizotomy usually indicates that the original good result was either a placebo response or that central reorganization has occurred in the spinal cord. Cutting additional roots at a second operation a few weeks later is almost certain to be a failure.

Indications

As is true for almost every operation or other form of treatment, it is useful to consider the indications for dorsal rhizotomy in the two major groups of chronic pain patients: those with pain secondary to cancer, and those with pain ascribed to a nonmalignant disease process. In my experience the best results are

obtained in cancer patients, although the published reports often suggest equally good results with non-malignant diseases (Table 97-2). Better results with cancer pain are obtained because the diagnosis is clear-cut and the pain is likely to be a result of tissue damage and not other factors, and the patient is not likely to survive long enough for the late loss of efficacy that characterizes almost all ablative surgical procedures. Moreover, it is not likely that prior neuro-destructive procedures can have given the patient a denervation pain syndrome. Cancer pain in any region of the body can be treated by dorsal rhizotomy although the most common area for this operation is the thoracoabdominal region (see above). In association with lower cranial rhizotomies, upper cervical rhizotomies have a place in the management of head and neck cancer pain. When the anal and vesicular sphincters are not functional or are bypassed by surgical diversions, sacral rhizotomies can be effective in managing perineal and perianal pain.

Although chronic pain caused by cancer is one of the better indications for dorsal rhizotomy, some problems must be considered by the surgeon. First, the tumor is likely to grow and the noxious stimulation arises from outside the denervated area. Second, the tumor can grow to involve visceral afferents that enter the spinal cord at levels outside of the rhizotomy, thereby gaining access to the central nervous system even though the somatic afferents have been sectioned.

Chronic pain caused by a nonmalignant disease is, in my experience, much less likely to respond to dorsal rhizotomy. The results of reported series vary widely for reasons that are not clear. Some have reported good results from single- or double-level dorsal rhizotomies in the management of the failed lumbar disk patient (17, 32, 33). Others have reported consistent failures. Dorsal rhizotomy is not useful in the management of post-thoracotomy pain, postherpetic neuralgia, or postparaplegic pain (19, 34, 35). When nerve roots are trapped in a spinal fracture site, however, rhizotomy can be beneficial.

Whether the addition of ganglionectomy to dorsal rhizotomy can alter the long-term outcome in patients with pain caused by benign diseases is presently unknown, although some suggestions of its additional efficacy have been noted (8, 9, 23, 29). Perfecting percutaneous techniques with a low morbidity rate might expand the indications for dorsal rhizotomy and/or ganglionectomy to patients too ill for major surgery. The vagaries of the patient's response to this operation, however, prevent its widespread use. Dorsal rhizotomy should become a popular surgical procedure only when we learn the factors that predict outcome.

C. SYMPATHECTOMY*

Surgical sympathectomy for painful states presently involves three main sites of denervation: the limbs, the heart, and the abdominal viscera. The probability that operative denervation will stop the pain can be

*I wish to express my gratitude to the Neuro-Research Foundation for its support in the preparation of this section on sympathectomy and to John J. Bonica for his contributions.—William H. Sweet.

assessed in all these areas by temporary pharmacologic sympathetic blockade interspersed with placebo blocks (Chapter 94E). These have the advantage not only of establishing the crucial role of the sympathetic activity in causing the pain, but the repetition of effective blocks might stop the pain and eliminate the need for any surgical treatment. Indeed, increasing information regarding specific sympathetic blocking agents and new methods of administration have reduced the need for operative sympathectomy. Thus, Hannington-Kiff (36) has introduced the tactic of regional sympathetic block, which by use of a proximal tourniquet on a limb largely confines the agent injected into a distal vein to that limb. The best-studied agent, guanethidine, displaces norepinephrine, the neurotransmitter at the sympathetic nerve endings, occupying the storage sites to which it binds so strongly that complete elimination of the drug requires days. Repeated injections of guanethidine sulfate can achieve a "chemical sympathectomy." Details of the method and the extended indications for its use have been given in Chapter 94E.

An intelligent exploration of nonoperative sympatholytic treatments is a prerequisite to consideration of surgery. When a surgical procedure is required, sympathectomy appears to have a much lower rate of recurrence of pain than any other ablative operation.

Pains originating from the thoracic or abdominal viscera are alleviated by sympathectomy because the afferent fibers from the viscera travel in the sympathetic nerves, trunks, ganglia, and rami. Sympathectomy for visceral pain is therefore analogous to peripheral neurectomy or dorsal rhizotomy for somatic pain.

When causalgia, reflex sympathetic dystrophy, or Raynaud's phenomenon is alleviated by sympathectomy, the explanation for pain relief is not as obvious. Some have argued that afferent fibers are present in the sympathetic nerves to the extremities. Others believe that abnormal efferent activity in the sympathetic nerves is alleviated by sympathectomy. Another explanation is the abolition of ephaptic connections. The observation that dorsal rhizotomy does not stop causalgia suggests both afferent and efferent roles for the sympathetic nervous system in this syndrome. White and Sweet (5) and Sweet (37) have discussed sympathectomy further.

Sympathectomy of Limbs

Indications

The most common disorders for which such operations are indicated involve the limbs, and are classified as causalgia, (reflex) sympathetic dystrophy, Sudeck's atrophy (38), and painful ischemic states, including Raynaud's phenomenon.

Causalgia

From 2 to 5% of peripheral nerve injuries in the limbs caused by gunshot and war wounds and a smaller percentage of nerve injuries from other causes produce spontaneous disabling pain within a few days that is usually most intense distally in the hand or foot. The causative injury is commonly much more proximal in the limb. The greater the severity and duration of the pain, the less likely is sustained relief from temporary diagnostic or therapeutic nerve blocks. Accordingly, it is not advisable to defer the active low-risk sympatholytic medical and, if necessary, surgical treatments in the hope of spontaneous disappearance of the pain.

The results of operations at the site of injury are grossly inferior to those of sympathectomy. This latter operation stops the burning pain in over 90% of patients, with low morbidity and mortality rates and with the persistence of slight and various forms of residual discomfort in only about one-third of patients. Chapter 11 analyzes the results of sympathectomy as reported by about 25 authors. I have also studied data derived from long-term extensive follow-up of causalgia veterans of World War II (37). Postganglionic sympathectomy for the upper limb by removal of the stellate ganglion, as insisted on by de Takats (39), has been proven to be actually less effective than the preganglionic section, which spares that ganglion and does not lead to a Horner's syndrome (37).

More recent experience in 40 consecutive cases of soldiers who developed causalgia after wounds sustained in the wars in Lebanon revealed remarkable results by the simple oral use of phenoxybenzamine (40). This agent is about 100 times as potent a blocker of postsynaptic (alpha-1) receptors as of presynaptic (alpha-2) receptors, producing "an irreversible and insurmountable type of blockade." When given tid in doses gradually increased from 30 mg/day to a maximum of 120 mg/day, it stopped the pain in every case, requiring only 6 to 13 weeks of full administration followed by slow tapering and discontinuation. Two cases involved the greater occipital nerve and 5 involved the cauda equina; peripheral nerves to the limbs comprised the rest. Complications were minor; orthostatic hypotension in 17 patients was successfully treated by stockinettes or abdominal girdle or both, in only 8; 3 men described reduction of seminal fluid, which returned to normal after the medication was discontinued. As yet no confirmation has been received from other sources in regard to these results.

Reflex Sympathetic Dystrophy

The painful disorders subsumed under the terms minor causalgia, (reflex) sympathetic dystrophy (RSD), and Sudeck's atrophy have been given 52 other English, German, and French names, as listed by Ascherl and Blümel (41). They are characterized by burning pain in the extremity, often with a major component of joint and muscle throbbing, cramping, or aching. Osteoporosis and trophic changes in skin and deeper tissues develop if treatment is not prompt and effective. The patient usually dates the onset of pain to relatively minor trauma that clearly did not involve injury to a major nerve, thus distinguishing reflex sympathetic dystrophy from causalgia.

Early use of sympathetic blocks for the dystrophies carries an even better chance of achieving cure without any surgery than in major causalgia. On the basis of his own experience and analysis of data in several reports, Bonica (42) estimated 80% cure by this approach. The use of intra-arterial reserpine as a predictor of the results of sympathectomy also has its adherents (43). The same positive recommendation for sympathectomy applicable for major causalgia is also appropriate here, once the benefit of temporary blocks has proven to be consistent and repeated blocks do not permanently eliminate the pain. Wirth and Rutherford (44) summarized the results in 5 papers: 95 of 108 patients were either totally relieved or significantly improved. In the personal series of Thompson (45), 46% of his 120 cases required sympathectomy (T2–T3 ganglia for the upper limb, L2–L3 for the lower limb). Sympathetic blocks proved to be a definitive treatment in 49%; the remainder required only medical measures. "Excellent" results were achieved in 81% of patients, and "good" results in 13%. Noteworthy is the delay between trauma and diagnosis of 5 months, but good results often ensued once effective treatment had begun.

Pain persisting after digital amputations can respond to sympathetic block and sympathectomy. Thus, White (5) had seven cases, with five excellent and two good results—the longest follow-up was 20 years. We have never found sympathetic denervation to be of value for stump pain, however, in amputations at or above the wrist or ankle.

Peripheral Vascular Disease

In cases of occlusive disease angiography can be required to demonstrate proximal focal lesions susceptible to direct vascular attack in contrast to distal arterial occlusion. The painful structural occlusive lesions of the small distal vessels of the limbs are likely to benefit temporarily from sympathetic blockade and, if more lasting types of chemical sympathectomy fail, surgical sympathectomy is advisable. The correlation between the results of sympathetic block and sympathectomy is, of course, not perfect. Thus, Berguer and Smit (43) had two of nine patients whose symptoms did not subside after stellate block but who were relieved by sympathectomy. Dale and Lewis (46) reported twelve patients whose arterial occlusions in the wrist, hand, or fingers were successfully treated in every instance by excision of the sympathetic trunk from the caudal part of T1 through T3 ganglia. The only complications were a Horner's syndrome in three patients and one patient with intercostal pain of several months' duration. Berguer and Smit (43) reported three of four good results from a T2 to T4 ganglionectomy in such patients (Chapter 28 presents a detailed discussion of peripheral vascular disease and treatment with sympathectomy).

Primary and Secondary Raynaud's Disease

RAYNAUD'S DISEASE.   A thorough study on sympathectomy for Raynaud's disease was undertaken by Baddeley (47) in Great Britain, where the low temperatures at which houses are maintained in the winter can contribute to the large numbers of patients with distal vasospasm. Table 97-3 includes his discouraging long-term follow-up after 104 upper dorsal sympathectomies of varying extent for primary Raynaud's disease done between 1950 and 1957. In 24 patients the disease involved the feet as well, but in only 7 did its severity warrant lumbar sympathectomy. The results of the more extensive denervations were not better. Baddeley concluded that, in primary Raynaud's disease, sympathectomy should be restricted to patients with severe painful progressive lesions in whom trophic changes threaten the integrity of a digit. Baddeley (47) cited his own studies and those of several others, which indicated that sympathetic neural activity invariably returns over months or years and is associated with symptomatic relapse.

The comprehensive report by Mattassi and colleagues (48) agreed with Baddeley that it is the presence of trophic lesions rather than persistent pain that constitutes the indication for sympathectomy in the group with primary Raynaud's disease. More optimistic results have been obtained by Fontaine who, in collaboration with Leonard (48), treated 65 patients with Raynaud's disease by sympathectomy. On follow-up, which extended from 5 to 20 years, they noted "success" in 60% of patients. Even when the disorder was accompanied by scleroderma or some other collagen disease 30% of patients had successful results. (Chapter 28 presents a detailed discussion of Raynaud's disease and Raynaud's phenomenon and their treatment with sympathectomy.)

RAYNAUD'S PHENOMENON.   The use of sympathectomy for secondary Raynaud's phenomenon has been reported by numerous workers. Mattassi and associates (49) have records of follow-ups ranging from 2 to 11 years after T2 to T3 thoracic sympathectomy on 16 patients whose Raynaud's phenomenon was secondary to arteriosclerosis obliterans. The operation produced good results; recurrence was noted in only 1 patient. They (49), as well as Touati and co-workers (50), also reported good results from sympathectomy in workers with Raynaud's phenomenon who developed the condition from prolonged use of vibrating tools. In contrast, both groups reported poor results in cases of Raynaud's phenomenon associated with scleroderma, as have many other clinicians who used sympathectomy for this condition. Arnulf (51) emphasized the particular efficacy of the operation for frostbite injuries with ulceration.

Other Indications

The uncertain causes of many chronic pain states has made it worthwhile to try sympathetic blockade by injection of local anesthetics, regional blocking agents, or oral blocking agents. When the pain is described as burning or is associated with trophic vasomotor or sudomotor changes, a trial of sympathetic blockade is particularly warranted. When a series of blocks provides only temporary relief surgical sympathectomy should be considered, even if the diagnosis is unclear. Table 97-3 presents the results of some reported series concerning the use of sympathectomy for pain.

Operative Techniques

Uncertainty as to the extent of denervation required to relieve pain in either the upper or lower limb has been at least partially resolved by the use of careful preoperative studies. Perhaps the most critical of these is the tactic proposed by Erdemir and colleagues (52) of determining the level of sympathectomy required for the lower limb by slowly injecting 1% lidocaine into the midlumbar posterior epidural space and ascertaining the upper level of the somatosensory block required to provide complete relief of pain. They cited two patients in whom a sensory level of T10 was

TABLE 97-3. Sympathectomy for Painful Disorders

Source	Year(s) of Report	Indication	No. of Cases (No. of Operations)	Results (% of Total Cases)			
				Success*	Complications	Mortality Rate	Comments
Dorsal and lumbar sympathectomy for lymph disorders							
Various authors (Chapter 11)	1940–1969	Causalgia	518	95			One-third had minor residual discomfort
Wirth and Rutherford (44)	1970	Reflex sympathetic dystrophy (RSD)	108	88			
Thompson (45)	1979	RSD	55	81 excellent, 13 fair			
White and Sweet (5)	1969	RSD	7	71 excellent, 29 fair			
Baddeley (47)	1965	Raynaud's disease	59 (104)	0			Only useful for trophic changes and ulceration
Mattassi et al. (48)	1981	Raynaud's disease	87 (125)	0			
		Raynaud's phenomenon	16	100			Recurrence in one case*
Fontaine and Leonard (49)	1979	Raynaud's disease	65	60			
Touati et al. (50)	1982	Raynaud's disease	67 (84)	0			
		Raynaud's phenomenon		Good			See text
Cardiac sympathectomy (T1–T4)							
Raney (77)	1939	Angina pectoris	11	100		0	Preganglionic operation
Lindgren and Olivecrona (74)	1947	Angina pectoris	71	93		7	
Lindgren (75)	1950	Angina pectoris	105	71		8.5	27% pain remission in control group
Burnett and Evans (73)	1956	Angina pectoris plus hypertension	33	86		5	
Palumbo and Lulu (76)	1963	Angina pectoris	20	100		10	
		Assorted arm pain	23	79	7	0	
Birkett et al. (72)	1965	Angina pectoris	52	80	21	7.5	
White and Sweet (5)	1969	Angina pectoris	19	89		16	Three failures when T3 not cut
		Nerve trauma	8	88		0	
		Brachial neuralgia	1	100	0	0	
Dorsal and lumbar sympathectomy for cancer pain							
Heisey and Dohn (89)	1967	Neoplasm	10	100	0	0	Less than 4 mo. survival*
		Neoplasm	12	33	3+	0	More than 4 mo.
		Postoperative intercostal pain	17	82	4+	0	
Presacral sympathectomy (superhypogastric plexus) for pelvic pain							
Fontaine and Hermann (84)	1932	Severe dysmenorrhea	22	86	0	5	15 of 20 long-term Follow-up (3 mo.)
		Pelvic malignancy	6	100	0	0	
Counseller and Craig (85)	1934	Severe dysmenorrhea	14	100	0	0	
Meigs (86)	1939	Severe dysmenorrhea	20	75	0	0	
Phaneuf (87)	1947	Severe dysmenorrhea	76	88	0		
Frier (88)	1965	Nonmalignant pelvic pain	20	10		0	
White and Sweet (5)	1969	Postamputation	7	86		0	

*Success = pain relief at time of follow-up at least 3 months after surgery.

needed for temporary pain relief, and who then maintained relief of their post-traumatic sympathetic dystrophic pain for many years after thoracolumbar sympathectomies to the T10 level.

In general, a cause of failure has been an inadequate level of denervation, especially in the lower limbs. Thus, in seven of Mayfield's (53) patients, his standard L2 to L3 or L2 to L4 ganglionectomy still permitted sweating in the foot. In three of these patients removal of the L1 ganglion completed the denervation and stopped the pain, but in the other four patients removal of the T11 and T12 ganglia was required to achieve relief.

Regeneration of the sympathetic nerves can cause recurrences, and it can even be remarkably complete. An especially convincing case is that of Mattassi and associates (48), whose patient with recurrent pain after the first histologically proven sympathectomy had re-operation. The specimen, removed again from the lower T1 through T3 ganglia, was confirmed histologically to be another completely normal sympathetic chain. Such counter-regeneration tactics as encasement of the disconnected ganglia in a nylon sleeve, which is sutured to muscles to guide the regenerating fibers into fruitless areas, have become common practice (Fig. 97-2). The actual extent of a surgical sympathectomy should be checked about 1 month after operation by sweating tests, cutaneous thermometry, or skin resistance measurements (54, 55). If pain recurs the possibility of regeneration to account for a recurrence can be studied in the same fashion and confirmed with sympathetic block, which should produce positive results (Chapter 94). In the lower limbs, recurrence of pain is less of a problem and special operative measures are thus not required to preclude it (56).

The usual open thoracic operations through supraclavicular, transaxillary, or posterior costotransversectomy approaches all have low rates of complications—for example severe branchial plexus injuries occurred in only 3 of Adar's (57) 456 thoracic sympathectomies by the supraclavicular approach, and even these 3 recovered after 3 to 6 months. All are performed under general endotracheal anesthesia; all have some risk of pneumothorax. The transaxillary approach of Atkins (58), although it provides the best view of the long length of the upper thoracic trunk, is also fraught with the most minor complications such as pneumothorax, pain, and dysesthesias somewhere in the chest or medial arm (43). The choice of surgical approach is based on the surgeon's preference because no data are available to favor one over another. The positioning of the patient is determined by the planned approach.

The open lumbar operations, now customarily performed by an anterior extraperitoneal approach, have been re-evaluated extensively in the last decade. Two major collections of articles involving many centers have been published (59, 60). Regeneration is "much less likely" if the L2 through L4 ganglia are removed (56). This extent of removal usually suffices to control the pain although, as already noted above (Causalgia), a more rostral ganglionic excision might be needed. Ray and Console (61) have shown that, on occasion, combining ventral rhizotomy of T12, L1, and L2, along with lumbar ganglionectomy, might even be required to produce complete sympathetic denervation.

On the basis of their 1344 lumbar sympathectomies, Goldstein and co-workers (62) described the complications as almost always transient, with a mortality rate of 0.6% that was largely confined to elderly arteriosclerotics with advanced disease. Prolonged paralytic ileus lasted 5, 6, and 12 days in only 3 patients; paradoxic transitory partial ischemia of a sympathectomized lower limb occurred in 2 patients, both of whom were effectively treated medically.

The most frequent complication, specifically related to the sympathectomy and apparently unrelated to any particular operative technique, is a "postsympathectomy neuralgia." This puzzling, severe, deep aching or burning pain, usually worse at night, is referred to the proximal part of the limb only—the shoulder and upper arm after upper thoracic surgery, and the groin and anterior thigh after lumbar operations. Patients begin to experience the aching burning pain about the second week after operation, often after they have left the hospital. As pointed out by Tracy and Cockett (63) for the leg, sympathetic activity at the site of the pain in the anterior thigh increases, as shown by greatly lowered skin resistance that denotes increased sudomotor activity. The increased sweating over the anterior thigh did not occur in their patients, who did not develop this peculiar neuralgia. In over 20 publications on the problem, most found that this type of neuralgia appears in less than 20% of patients, with about equal frequency in upper and lower limbs. Happily, unlike many syndromes of deafferentation pain, this neuralgia subsides spontaneously in nearly all patients in from 12 days to 6 months (64, 65).

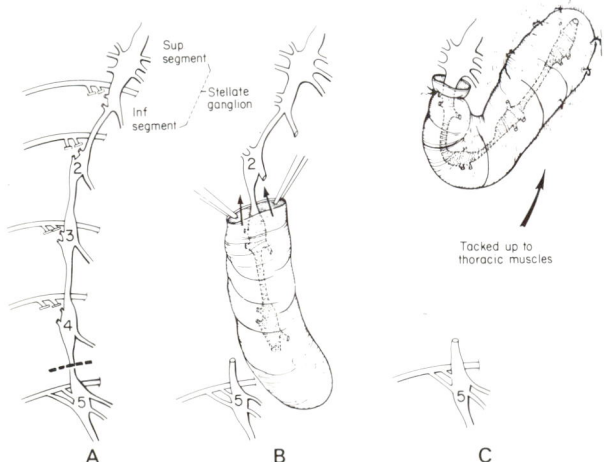

FIG. 97-2. Technique of upper thoracic sympathectomy for retarding regeneration. *A.* Note the division of pairs of rami communicantes at the T1 through T4 levels and the application of metal clips near their junctions with the somatic thoracic nerves. *B.* The sympathetic trunk is divided above the T5 ganglion and is then enclosed in a nylon "sack" tied rostrally above the lower pole of the stellate ganglion. *C.* The sack containing the four ganglia is then brought outside the thoracic cage and sewn to the muscles external to it. This procedure does not produce a Horner's syndrome.

Sexual dysfunction in men can occur after bilateral removal of the 1st or 2nd lumbar ganglia or of the presacral plexus. The most comprehensive report is that of Whitelaw and Smithwick (66), which was based on a massive series of predominantly bilateral sympathectomies, including the upper lumbar ganglia for hypertension. Even in the 8 patients with the most extensive bilateral removals, including a portion of the thoracic chain, the splanchnic nerves, and the L1 and L2 ganglia, only three patients had a significant disturbance of erection or permanent loss of ejaculation. In similar operations, except that L1 ganglia only were removed, such loss of sexual function occurred in only 20% (13) of 66 patients. Bilateral removals confined to L2 plus various combinations of L1 and L3 ganglia in 11 patients disturbed erection in 63% and eliminated ejaculation permanently in 54%. Such unilateral removals in 12 men produced only disturbances of erection confined to two patients.

Percutaneous Sympathectomy

Thermocoagulation of Upper Thoracic Sympathetic Trunk.

Radiographically guided percutaneous introduction of electrodes against the bodies of the upper thoracic vertebrae at the expected site of the sympathetic chain has been pioneered by Wilkinson (67). Only local anesthesia is required, and a trial of stimulation and heating ensures that the electrode is not so close to an intercostal nerve as to provide pain and not so close to the stellate ganglion as to cause a Horner's syndrome. "Good sympathetic" interruption ensued in 24 of 27 procedures. Two or three ganglia—if appropriate—can be destroyed bilaterally at the same session. The only complications in the pain patients were minor—one small pneumothorax and medial brachial pain lasting 2 to 3 months in three patients. The patient can usually be discharged from the hospital on the day of the procedure.

Thoracic Endoscopic Sympathectomy

This slightly more complex procedure, introduced by E. Kux in Vienna in 1954, had been performed by M. Kux (68) 166 times by 1977. The procedure entails initially collapsing the lung with 1000 ml of room air through a pneumothorax needle in the midaxillary line; then, through a 1.5-cm incision just caudal to the inferior angle of the scapula, a special endoscope is introduced and the sympathetic ganglia can be dissected free, from T2 as far down as T6, if desired. The lung is reinflated and the patient can often be discharged within 48 hours. Rösner and Goldberg (69) followed 23 patients for a minimum of 6 years after such an operation for Raynaud's syndrome. No significant complications were found but no lasting cures were obtained; this contrasts with a 35% cure rate after open sympathectomy. The procedure has been modified by using electrocoagulation under direct vision to destroy the sympathetic trunk by Weale (70) in England (10 cases) and Malone and colleagues (71) in Ireland (30 cases).

Cardiac Sympathectomy

Medically intractable angina pectoris was effectively treated in many hospitals by some form of upper thoracic sympathectomy, usually stellate ganglion through T4, (5, 72–77). Birkett and associates (72) and White and Sweet (5) have reviewed the surgical anatomy and carefully described the long-term results. In spite of the high likelihood of success and reasonably low complication rate, this indication for sympathectomy has been virtually eliminated by better pharmacologic management of angina pectoris and by the development of coronary artery bypass graft surgery, which restores blood supply to the ischemic myocardium directly (extensive studies done on this topic are discussed in Chapter 54).

Sympathectomy for Abdominal Visceral Pain

Technique of Open Operation

Although all the upper abdominal viscera send their nociceptive afferents through the greater, lesser, and least splanchnic nerves, the pancreas is the organ most likely to be the site of chronic pain that can be effectively treated by sympathectomy. Painful chronic relapsing pancreatitis, often with calculi obstructing the ducts, has long been treated by splanchnicectomy. By 1950 Mallet-Guy and de Beaujeu (78) could already report on 70 cases treated by a left-sided operation, with 31 of 37 satisfactory results in patients followed 1 to 6 years. American surgeons improved on these figures by the bilateral removal of all 3 splanchnic nerves and the lower 4 thoracic ganglia by a simple 1-hour extrapleural procedure, originated by Peet for the treatment of essential hypertension. White and Sweet (5) summarized their own results and those of 7 other groups in a total of 26 cases. The documentation was brought up to date by Vosschulte and Wagner (79) in 1970. Their own preference was for bilateral splanchnicectomy with resection of the upper pole of the celiac ganglion. They collected data from 25 publications reporting 141 cases with 94 (67%) satisfactory results. When the 84 cases followed from 1 to several years were considered separately, 64% were still satisfactory. In a smaller group of 39 cases followed 5 or more years, 69% remained in this same category. Recently, a group of French surgeons have used the transhiatal approach of Dubois to perform bilateral splanchnicectomy at the esophageal hiatus (80). They described achievement of relief in all of their 12 patients with chronic pancreatitis. Many surgeons in the United States do not agree that chronic pancreatitis can be successfully treated by splanchnicectomy, and I can find no articles in the English language on the subject in the past 15 years.

The early reports on low thoracic sympathectomy plus splanchnicectomy for relief of pain of pancreatic carcinoma were discouraging, presumably because operation was delayed until invasion of the somatic nerves in the abdominal wall had occurred. Since 1950 Sadar and Hardy (81) have treated the pain of 56 patients with this disorder first by laparotomy, at which any feasible palliative procedure was done. This was followed at the same operation by turning the patient to a prone position and doing the above-described Peet type of bilateral extensive sympathectomy in the low thoracic extrapleural space. They usually preceded this operation by repetitive lidocaine blocks but had at times achieved relief from surgery when the lidocaine blocks were ineffective. The operation had a mortality rate of 7% but yielded good or complete relief in 70% of patients, with poor or no relief in the remainder. Pain recurred to some extent in 23% of the 70% of patients, and was noted especially in the longer term survivors (average, 11 months). The Michotey group (80) described 100% early pain relief in their 11 cases of cancer but did not indicate the later results. They had no operative mortality but had one significant complication of splenic injury, which required splenectomy during the hiatal dissection.

Chemical Sympathectomy of Celiac Plexus and Splanchnic Nerves

Chemical sympathetomy of the celiac plexus and splanchnic nerves has been carried out either by direct injection of phenol and alcohol into the junction of splanchnic nerves and celiac ganglia at the time of exploratory laparotomy or by radiographically guided percutaneous injection of alcohol. Of 2 substantial series of cancer patients treated by the first method, Flanigan and Kraft (82) reported 41 patients, with a 15% operative mortality rate. Although 88% of survivors had initial relief, this lasted only an average of 4.3 months. No complications were attributed to the injection. Of the 37 patients reported by Gardner and Solomon (83), 70% were relieved of pain until death, with a 5% operative mortality rate. They cited 3 other articles describing relief in, respectively, 70% of 10 patients, 33% of 9 patients, and 75% of 28 patients. All groups attributed the operative mortality rate to the severe primary disease. In the course of the study I carried out decades ago, I was impressed by the dispersal into many tissues planes of this enormous plexus and the many ganglia that comprise the celiac ganglion (Chapter 59). (The more favorable results reported by a number of anesthesiologists, cited on pages 2018 and 2020, are probably a result of the fact that because of their extensive experience with needle techniques they were able to place the needle more precisely and, more importantly, they used larger volumes of neurolytic agents.)

Presacral Neurectomy

In the first 50 years of this century, presacral neurectomy was a commonly undertaken surgical procedure for women who complained of severe chronic dysmenorrhea (5, 84–89). Such an operation provided varying amounts of autonomic denervation of the pelvic viscera and was reputed to have high efficacy. Presacral neurectomy has been undertaken much less commonly in the past 30 years, and in the United States it is no longer a standard method of treating dysmenorrhea.

D. TRIGEMINAL GANGLIOLYSIS*

This section describes the technique of percutaneous stereotaxic rhizotomy (PSR), which is most frequently used in the treatment of trigeminal neuralgia (tic douloureux). This procedure is commonly called gangliolysis, although the lesion is usually in the rootlets behind the ganglion. PSR is one of the truly elegant procedures in surgery. PSR involves the freehand passage of a special electrode through the cheek, into the mandibular branch of the trigeminal nerve, through the foramen ovale, and into the gasserian ganglion in an awake patient (Fig. 97-3). The specific nerve fibers coming from the region of the lancinating pains are localized and selectively destroyed by controlled heating with radiofrequency current. A specific degree and distribution of sensory loss is exchanged for relief of facial pain. We emphasize our personal experiences; alternative techniques have been described and are briefly discussed.

Historical Perspective

Although tic douloureux was well described as a clinical entity by John Fothergill in 1773, misdirected attacks on the facial nerve did not end until Charles Bell's classic dissertation in 1821 distinguished between the sensory function of the trigeminal nerve and the motor function of the facial nerve (90). The injection of chemical substances into the trigeminal nerve and gasserian ganglion became common practice during the nineteenth century. By the early twentieth century the list of injected substances included alcohol, phenol, and boiling water, all of which achieved a certain degree of success (91–93).

In 1932 Kirschner (94) introduced the use of an electrocoagulating current to produce more discrete lesions and to overcome the spreading effect observed with chemical substances. Roentgenography and stereotaxic instrumentation facilitated proper placement of the electrode through the foramen ovale into the gasserian ganglion (95). Sweet and Wepsic (96) refined the technique with the following modifications: (a) use of a short-acting anesthetic agent with rapid awakening for sensory testing during the operation; (b) reliable radiofrequency current for discrete lesion production; (c) electric stimulation for precise localization of pain-producing fibers; and (d) temperature monitoring for precise control of lesion configuration and density.

The development of an adjustable curved-tip electrode with increased maneuverability inside the ganglion has further decreased our operative complications and side effects (97). More detailed discussion of the various techniques and results can be found elsewhere (96, 98–104). Other neurosurgeons use straight electrodes of varying diameters and lengths of

*We express appreciation to Marjorie M. Carleton, Scientific Illustrator, and to Stephanie Gates for the preparation of the manuscript for this section on trigeminal gangliolysis. —John M. Tew, Jr., and Harry van Loveren

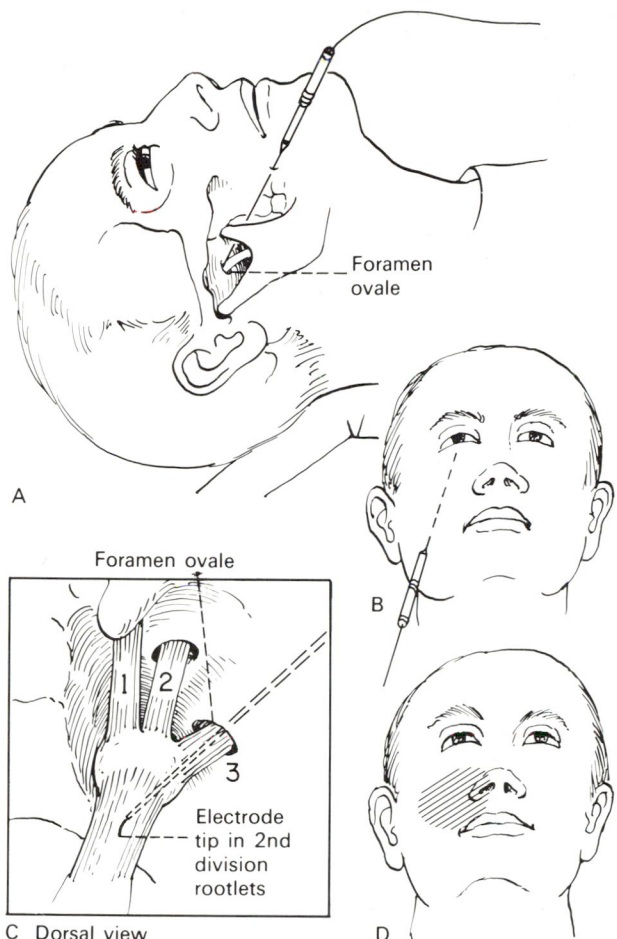

Foramen
ovale

Foramen ovale

1 2

3

Electrode
tip in 2nd
division
rootlets

A

B

C Dorsal view

D

FIG. 97-3. Technique of placing the curved electrode freehand through the cheek into the mandibular branch of the trigeminal nerve, through the foramen ovale, and into the gasserian ganglion and posterior rootlets. *A.* Lateral view to show that the needle electrode is inserted into the cheek 2.5 cm lateral to the corner of the mouth in the occlusal plane and directed so that its bevel will be 2 cm anterior to the tragus. *B.* Anterior view showing the trajectory of the needle toward the pupil. *C.* Major branches showing the tip of the electrode passed to the rootlets of the second division. *D.* Area of analgesia resulting from coagulation of some of the rootlets of the second division. *A* and *B* original by M. Domenowske; *C* and *D* modified by M. Domenowske from illustrations provided by Drs. Tew and van Loveren that had been developed by M.M. Carleton.

FIG. 97-4. Curved electrode, which is 0.5 mm in diameter, shown emerging from the 20-gauge cannula with its tip among the trigeminal rootlets inside the trigeminal cistern. The inset shows that the flexible curved electrode tip can be manipulated to produce lesions in the V1, V2, and V3 fibers, respectively. Illustration developed by M.M. Carleton for the authors.

uninsulated tips. The development of gangliolysis by glycerol injection has potential advantages as well as disadvantages when contrasted with radiofrequency gangliolysis (105–107).

Technique

Percutaneous trigeminal rhizotomy is performed in the radiography suite. Landmarks on the face and bony landmarks identified by lateral fluoroscopy are used to guide the insertion of a 20-gauge cannula and stylet through the cheek, lateral to the pterygoid plate and through the foramen ovale by a simple freehand technique (Fig. 97-3). During any parts of the procedure that might be painful the patient is sedated for several minutes with an intravenous injection of 30 to 50 mg of methohexital (Brevital).

Once the cannula is within the gasserian ganglion, the stylet is removed and the curved-tip electrode is inserted and connected to the lesion generator. Final placement of the electrode tip is determined by the patient's response to electric stimulation. A current of 0.2 to 0.3 V at 50 to 75 cycles/s reproduces the paroxysmal bouts of pain reminiscent of trigeminal neuralgia. By manipulating the electrode, including rotation of the curved tip through a 360° axis, those fibers responsible for the patients's pain are identified (Fig. 97-4).

Using radiofrequency current, graded heat lesions (60° to 100°C) are created to partially destroy the pain-generating fibers. A short-acting IV anesthetic is again used to obviate discomfort to the patient. One or several lesions in succession might be necessary to achieve the desired result. Best results are obtained when hypalgesia or analgesia is produced in the trigeminal divisions that are painful or serve as trigger zones for the development of pain. Sensory loss is not created in uninvolved divisions, nor is anesthesia produced in any involved division.

The patient remains in the hospital overnight for observation. Prior to discharge the patient is informed of the necessity for eye care, the avoidance of jaw strain, and the consequences of facial analgesia.

The pathophysiology of trigeminal neuralgia remains an issue for debate, as does the mechanism by which percutaneous rhizotomy relieves the pain. Existing laboratory data and clinical observation, however, support the contention that percutaneous rhizotomy with radiofrequency current destroys unmyelinated and thinly myelinated C and A-delta fibers that subserve nociception while preserving the larger and more heavily myelinated A-alpha and A-beta fibers responsible for touch sensation (100).

TABLE 97-4. Characteristics of 700 Patients Treated for Trigeminal Neuralgia

Characteristic	Findings
Average age (yr)	65
Gender: female (%)	62
Duration of neuralgia (yr)	8
Prior procedure (%)	42
Side with neuralgia (%)	
Right	60
Left	35
Both	5
Distribution (%)	
V1	1
V2	16
V3	15
V1, V2	15
V2, V3	40
V1–V3	13

TABLE 97-5. Results of Percutaneous Stereotaxic Rhizotomy in 750 Patients with Trigeminal Neuralgia

Results	Patients No.	%
Immediate postoperative relief	940	99
Persistent relief (no recurrence)		
Excellent (no tic pain, no D/P*)	618	65
Good (no tic pain with minor D/P)	257	27
Fair (no tic pain with moderate D/P)	49	5
Poor (no tic pain with major D/P)	9	1
Subtotal	933	99
Failure	19	2
Recurrence		
Minor (no medication required)	47	5
Moderate (medication required)	38	4
Severe (requiring surgery)	47	5
Subtotal	132	14
Mean follow-up in years (range)	8(1–18)	

*D, dysesthesia; P, paresthesia.

Criteria for Patient Selection

We have treated over 1400 patients with classic trigeminal neuralgia, and of these about 1100 have been treated surgically by percutaneous stereotaxic rhizotomy. For this report we have analyzed the data for 950 patients (Table 97-4). The diagnosis of trigeminal neuralgia was based on typical clinical features, including the following: (a) intense paroxysms of superficial pain confined to the trigeminal distribution; (b) pain confined to one side of the face; (c) pain provoked by cutaneous stimuli to trigger zones; and (d) absence of a detectable neurologic deficit or a subtle sensory deficit within the distribution of the trigeminal nerve (101). Diagnostic criteria are presented because proper diagnosis is the most important determinant of outcome for medical or surgical therapy.

All patients were initially treated with medical therapy consisting of diphenylhydantoin (Dilantin) (102) or carbamazepine (Tegretol) (103). Although 90% of patients had an initial favorable therapeutic response, 75% failed to achieve satisfactory long-term relief because of side effects or failure of the drug to control the pain adequately (104, 108). Following discussions of alternate forms of therapy, about 1100 patients chose to undergo radiofrequency neurolysis. The sensory loss inherent to the procedure is not severe and occasionally is demonstrated to patients by temporary lidocaine nerve block. The morbidity rate of the procedure is low. We have had no mortality and usually only 1 day of hospitalization is required. Neither advanced age nor medical illness, excluding irreversible intrinsic or extrinsic coagulopathy, represents an absolute contraindication to the procedure.

Results

Of the 950 patients for whom data were analyzed, in the initial 700 we used the straight electrode and in the other 250 we used the curved electrode with some modification of tactic and technique. Immediate relief of pain was obtained in 99% of patients (Table 97-5), but at the end of the follow-up period, which averaged 8 years with a range of 1 to 18 years, pain recurred in 14%. Recurrence can readily be treated with a repeat of this procedure; similar excellent results are obtained on second or third operations. In fact, our current tactic is to begin with a minimal lesion that increases the risk of recurrence but allows many patients to remain pain-free, with minor sensory loss. Those patients who had a successful procedure without recurrence rated their results as excellent in 65% and good in 27%. The results were rated as fair in 5% of patients, principally because of troublesome dysesthesias. Any return of tic-like pain, no matter how slight, was considered a recurrence, even though many of those patients still rated their results as excellent or good.

Although this procedure has been used for other types of facial pain, its primary usefulness is for tic douloureux. Patients with atypical facial pain rarely report effective pain relief and are often made worse.

Side Effects and Complications

The nature of radiofrequency trigeminal rhizotomy is such that sensory loss must be exchanged for the patient's pain. The most common complication of the procedure is the production of a degree of sensory loss that is troublesome to the patient.

The precision of the new curved electrode reduced the incidence of minor dysesthesias to 11.2% in our last

TABLE 97-6. Complications with Use of Curved and Straight Electrodes for Percutaneous Rhizotomy

Complication	Incidence (% of Total)		
	Curved Electrode*	Straight Electrode†	Combined Series
Masseter weakness	5	24	18
Paresthesias/dysesthesia			
Minor	12	22	20
Major	0	5	3
Diplopia	0	2	1.5
Keratitis	1.6	4	3.0

*250 procedures.
†700 procedures.

TABLE 97-7. Results of Percutaneous Stereotaxic Rhizotomy for Trigeminal Neuralgia

Source	No. of Cases	Initial Relief (%)	Average Follow-up	Complications (% of Total Cases)			
				Paresthesias	Anesthesia Dolorosa	Motor Root Weakness†	Recurrence
Apfelbaum (109)	48	88	1–36 mo	*	12	2	23
Burchiel et al. (110)	78	83	4.7 yr	15	4	*	64
Menzel et al. (111)	315	97	12 yr	93	2	50	80
Nugent (112)	643	*	4.7 yr	14	1	25	23
Onofrio (113)	135	98	*	*	1.4	38	12
Rhoton et al. (114)	149	98	1–53 mo	34	13	60	18.7
Siegfried (115)	416	98	15 mo	1.8	0.8	30	4.3
Sweet and Wepsic (96)	274	91	4 yr	2	1	43	22
Tew et al. (98)	950	99	8 yr	22	5	18	14

*Not reported.
†Usually transient.

250 patients (Table 97-6). The desired end point of the procedure is analgesia in the region severely affected by pain and hypalgesia in regions secondarily affected or harboring trigger zones. If a division is rendered completely anesthetic, a constant severe dysesthesia (anesthesia dolorosa) is more likely to develop. This was a rare complication using the straight electrode that has not been observed with the curved electrode.

The motor root of the trigeminal nerve travels along the medial surface of the mandibular division. Inadvertent heating of the motor root results in masseter weakness in about 5% of patients. This is an axonotmesis and therefore nearly always resolves within 6 months. Transient diplopia caused by palsy of the abducens or trochlear nerve has been eliminated as a complication with use of the curved electrode. Application of this technique by other investigators has yielded similar results (Table 97-7).

Discussion

We have presented our results in the treatment of trigeminal neuralgia using a single technique. Table 97-7 lists the results of several major series of radiofrequency lesions. Different neurosurgeons have developed their own technical strategies for this procedure; if only patients with classic tic douloureux are treated, the results are similar. Larger lesions usually produce more sensory loss and higher initial and long-term success rates, but they are accompanied by a higher incidence of disturbing sensory changes.

Percutaneous stereotaxic rhizotomy is the initial surgical procedure of choice for most patients with tic douloureux. It can be accomplished with a radiofrequency lesion or, as recently described, with the injection of glycerol (105–107). It is much safer than alcohol injections (91, 93) and produces a more selective and less dense sensory loss than peripheral neurectomy (see above, section A).

Increased recognition that neural compression by blood vessels in the posterior fossa is a significant mechanical factor in the production of most cases of trigeminal neuralgia has led to debates regarding the preferred initial surgical procedure for tic douloureux (99, 116–118). Posterior fossa exploration for possible neurovascular decompression can be considered for select patients who are without medical contraindications to a major surgical procedure.

Trigeminal neuralgia is an excruciatingly painful condition of the face but is otherwise benign. Ideal treatment requires elimination of pain without sensory loss, an extremely low morbidity rate, and no mortality. This ideal remains elusive and will continue to do so until the cause of trigeminal neuralgia is understood. Percutaneous stereotaxic rhizotomy is an established, safe, and effective technique for this condition. We reserve posterior fossa exploration for younger patients who express a desire to avoid any sensory disturbance of the face and recommend it to patients who have failed with all other forms of therapy, including repeated PSR. These patients must be informed of the minimal risk of serious side effects and of the possibility of partial sensory rhizotomy if significant neurovascular compression is not found. In our hands percutaneous stereotaxic rhizotomy remains the procedure of choice in most patients with trigeminal neuralgia.

E. CRANIAL RHIZOTOMY

The intracranial approach to the trigeminal nerve and ganglion was first popularized in the 1890s; the pioneers in this field were Hartley, Krause, Tiffany, and Horsley. They independently demonstrated that it was possible to alleviate pain in the face by extirpating the gasserian ganglion or sectioning the trigeminal root just behind it. The initial approaches were transtemporal and intradural; in 1901 Frazier performed the first procedure using the extradural approach to the trigeminal nerve root. Frazier was also the first to spare the motor root deliberately and to perform a partial rhizotomy. His contributions to this type of surgery spanned 35 years, and the transtemporal extradural approach is still known to many surgeons as "Frazier's operation" (119). In 1925 Dandy described the approach to the trigeminal root through the posterior fossa. Many other variations have been described and are of historical interest only, because the management of orofacial pain has changed significantly in the past 20 years. The large personal series amassed before the use of diphenylhydantoin and carbamazepine for the treatment of tic douloureux can never again be equaled, and the surgical skills and results of the masters might never be duplicated. Percutaneous trigeminal gangliolysis was discussed above in detail (Section D); percutaneous glossopharyngeal gangliolysis is also mentioned in this chapter.

Basic Considerations

Advantages

Trigeminal rhizotomy was once the surgical procedure of choice for all types of facial pain. Newer techniques have relegated rhizotomy to a secondary place for treatment of all pains of nonmalignant origin, but it is still useful for pain caused by orofacial cancer. Although the transtemporal approach was once the most popular, it is now obsolete and rarely used. The suboccipital route, coming through the cerebellopontine angle to the fifth cranial nerve, has also given way to the retromastoid supracerebellar approach, which allows much better visualization of the trigeminal nerve. A lateral approach is useful when sectioning of the nervus intermedius or glossopharyngeal nerve is required to denervate the pharynx completely; this is easily combined with the supracerebellar route.

The primary advantage of trigeminal rhizotomy is its ability to denervate the face totally, which is usually required for relief of cancer pain. When required, the other cranial sensory nerves can be sectioned during the same operation. The pains of tic douloureux can also be effectively managed, but gangliolysis or microvascular decompression is a wiser choice for initial surgical treatment of this disease (Chapter 38).

Disadvantages

The major disadvantages of trigeminal rhizotomy are: major surgery, potential recurrence of pain, development of unwanted neurologic deficits, production of keratitis, which can lead to loss of vision in the eye, and sensory changes ranging from paresthesias to anesthesia dolorosa (120). All of these can occur with any type of rhizotomy. The recurrence rate is a function of at least two variables, degree of sensory loss and duration of postoperative survival of the patient. The lowest recurrence rates are associated with persisting sensory loss in the region of the original pain, but some tic patients have a return of their pain in spite of complete facial anesthesia. The degree of anesthesia produced must be limited because of several other potential complications; keratitis, facial paresthesias, and anesthesia dolorosa. When the pain does not involve the first division of the trigeminal nerve, it is wisest not to produce a lesion large enough to cause corneal anesthesia. This prevents the development of keratitis, although it can lead to a higher rate of recurrence of pain. When the cornea is hypesthetic, the patient must be carefully instructed to protect the eye at all times and to examine it regularly for foreign bodies or signs of irritation. Damage to the motor branch can lead to paralysis of the muscles of mastication and secondary temporomandibular joint dysfunction.

Published reports appear to indicate that injury to other cranial nerves is much less common during the suboccipital than the subtemporal approach to the trigeminal nerve. Facial palsy is seen more commonly after use of the transtemporal route than of the suboccipital, which is probably the result of mechanical trauma to the greater superficial petrosal nerve and swelling within the bony canal. Loss of tearing can ensue from this injury and further jeopardize the eye.

The development of annoying paresthesias or even painful dysesthesias and anesthesia dolorosa is a well-recognized sequel of any procedure that destroys some of the sensory input to the brain stem. Paresthesias are almost universally noted by patients after rhizotomy and are more frequent in those patients with significant sensory loss. Anesthesia dolorosa is much less common but is a devastating complication. When it occurs, carbamazepine or other anticonvulsants should be tried. Tricyclic antidepressants are sometimes helpful. Further denervation almost never succeeds; trigeminal tractotomy or deep brain stimulation can be effective. The risk of this complication of denervation is a major deterrent to complete trigeminal rhizotomy.

Other nonspecific problems are found during and after these operative procedures, including a small risk of infection, cerebrospinal fluid fistula, or damage to other intracranial structures, such as major vessels, nerves, or the cerebellum. Some typical reports are summarized in Table 97-8; a listing of all published series would require over 50 entries.

Clinical Considerations

The development of percutaneous radiofrequency or glycerol gangliolysis has eliminated most of the indications for rhizotomy of the trigeminal nerve in the management of tic douloureux and other neuralgias. This technique, which is safe, rapid, and effective, is also superior to peripheral nerve avulsion. If percutaneous radiofrequency or glycerol gangliolysis fails to relieve the patient's pain, it is then reasonable to consider an intracranial procedure. Microvascular decompression is the best initial open surgical procedure for tic douloureux; rhizotomy is indicated only when microvascular decompression has failed to control tic pain. A percutaneous approach to the glossopharyngeal nerve has also been described and is discussed below. There is no percutaneous route to the nervus intermedius.

Chronic facial or oral pain caused by malignancy should be treated with a lesion large enough to produce total denervation of the involved structures and to allow for extension of the pain by the growth of the malignancy. Tumors in the pharynx therefore usually require sectioning of both the fifth and ninth cranial nerves, and retromastoid craniectomy is the best approach. If a component of deep ear pain is present, sectioning of the nervus intermedius should also be undertaken. Tumors that involve the jaw and upper cervical region can require dorsal rhizotomy of the C1 to C3 nerves in addition to the appropriate cranial nerves. Bilateral facial pain cannot be successfully managed by denervating the entire face and mouth; most surgeons prefer partial juxtapontine trigeminal rhizotomies or a trigeminal tractotomy contralateral

TABLE 97-8. Typical Results of Trigeminal Rhizotomy for Neuralgia

Source	Year of Report	No. of Cases	Operation Route*	Operation Type†	Success‡	Complications	Paresthesia	Anesthesia Dolorosa	Mortality	Comments
Grant (121)	1938	359	TT	T	98	24	15	?	?	Tic douloureux and other types of neuralgia
Grant (121)	1938	510	TT	P	92	10	14	?	1.3	
Peet and Schneider (122)	1952	544	TT	T	86	25	55	?	1.6	9 posterior fossa operations, complications mainly transient
Stookey and Ransohoff (90)	1959	710	TT	P	87	8	10	?	0.8	
Ruge et al. (123)	1958	627	S	T & P	99	10	20	?	0.6	65 patients with partial section
Wertheimer (124)	1960	326	TT	P	84	10	11	?	1.5	
Olivecrona (125)	1961	445	TT	P	91	12	13	3.1	0.4	
Morello (126)	1969	409	TT	P	85	5	?	1.6	0.7	
White and Sweet (5)	1969	305	TT	P	85	16	?	26	1.3	Follow-up on 238 patients

*TT = transtemporal; S = suboccipital.
†T = total; P = partial; ? = not reported.
‡Success = pain relief at least 3 months past surgery.

to a complete rhizotomy. No rhizotomy should be undertaken until patients have experienced at least one local anesthetic block that produces numbness in the same area as the planned surgery. All forms of intracranial surgery are contraindicated in patients with clinically significant coagulopathies, systemic infections, or debilitation that would interfere with wound healing.

Techniques

The standard Frazier operation is the starting point for all transtemporal variations. The patient is placed in the seated position with the zygoma horizontal and the head tilted slightly toward the operator. Most surgeons prefer general endotracheal anesthesia. A vertical 6- to 8-cm scalp incision is made extending upward from the root of the zygoma 1 to 2 cm anterior to the external auditory meatus. The temporalis muscle is incised parallel to its fibers and held with a self-retaining retractor. A burr hole is made in the squamosal portion of the temporal bone and enlarged with rongeurs until the craniectomy is carried to the floor of the middle fossa and is 6 to 8 cm in diameter. The dura is elevated from the floor of the middle fossa by blunt dissection and the foramen spinosum is identified. The middle meningeal artery is coagulated and divided and the dura is further elevated to expose the foramen ovale.

The dura propria is then separated from the dura covering the temporal lobe. The greater superficial petrosal nerve is visualized beneath the third division and is protected. When the dura propria is dissected free it is incised, and the rootlets of the trigeminal nerve are visualized posterior to the semilunar ganglion. The motor root lies beneath the sensory fascicles; it should always be spared. If the ophthalmic division is to be spared the lateral three-fourths of the rootlets are divided. After the rootlets have been sec-

tioned the dura is allowed to fall back into place and the temporalis muscle, fascia, and scalp are closed.

The posterior fossa approach can be done with the patient seated or in the lateral decubitus position with the operative side superior and the head slightly rotated. Most surgeons now use a vertical retromastoid incision, which allows exposure of the traverse sinus superiorly and the sigmoid sinus laterally. A burr hole is made and a craniectomy of the lateral occipital bone is carried out superiorly and laterally as defined by the major venous structures. The dura is opened and the fifth cranial nerve is identified by allowing the cerebellum to fall away from the petrous bone and by dividing the petrosal vein. Use of the operating microscope is essential. The nerve is coagulated and divided, either partially or totally, as desired. The dura is closed and the muscles, fascia, and skin are sutured in layers.

Results

Typical results with open trigeminal rhizotomy are listed in Table 97-8. From 85 to 95% or more of patients derived relief. All trigeminal root destructive procedures, however, have possible complications, including mortality, recurrence of pain, postoperative paresthesias, anesthesia dolorosa, other cranial nerve pareses, keratitis, sequelae of numbness such as trophic changes of skin and mucous membranes, and nonspecific problems such as infection, faulty wound healing, or cerebrospinal fluid fistula. The mortality rate is lowest with percutaneous gangliolysis, as is the incidence of damage to any other cranial nerves. The incidence of keratitis is directly related to the production of anesthesia in the first division, regardless of the operative technique used. Postoperative paresthesias and anesthesia dolorosa seem to be a function of the completeness of the sensory loss produced by any operative technique. Pain recurrence is a function of the cause of the pain and the amount of sensory loss.

Few areas of neurologic surgery have been as thoroughly discussed in the literature as the treatment of facial pain. Trigeminal rhizotomy has been a classic approach, but it is now rarely done for tic. Atypical facial pain is often made worse by rhizotomy. Pain from a malignancy, however, should be expeditiously treated by appropriate denervation procedures.

Glossopharyngeal and Nervus Intermedius Rhizotomy

Rhizotomy of the glossopharyngeal nerve and nervus intermedius can also be performed to alleviate pain that is perceived in the pharynx or ear. The efficacy of procedures directed at these two nerves seems to be a function of the type of pain and its cause and is generally similar to the results seen after trigeminal rhizotomy (Table 97-9). Extracranial destruction of either the nervus intermedius or glossopharyngeal nerves is not feasible; pain from their peripheral distribution should be alleviated only by intracranial rhizotomy or descending trigeminal tractotomy.

Sectioning the nervus intermedius produces variable anesthesia in the auditory canal and in structures within the inner ear and eustachian tube, variable loss of taste in the anterior two-thirds of the tongue, and decrease of salivation and lacrimation; none of these is significant when lost unilaterally. The glossopharyngeal nerve variably supplies taste to the posterior third of the tongue and pharynx and sensation to the pharynx. Although a unilateral lesion is usually well tolerated, bilateral sectioning is not usually performed because of the fear of loss of the protective and swallowing reflexes. Some patients have had bilateral glossopharyngeal nerve sections without detectable sensory or reflex loss, but this remains a risky approach to the treatment of bilateral pain.

Glossopharyngeal tic douloureux that has not responded to medications or microvascular decompression of that nerve can be alleviated by rhizotomy. Tic douloureux can involve both glossopharyngeal and trigeminal nerves; Brzustowicz (130) described five patients who obtained good long-term relief from sections of both nerves, as did Peet and Schneider (123). Glossopharyngeal nerve block should always be done prior to rhizotomy to localize the pain and to give patients a trial of numbness. Some patients prefer their pain to the numbness produced by rhizotomy. It is not possible to block the nervus intermedius with local anesthetics injected through a foramen, because this nerve does not have an accessible discrete exit site from the skull. The case reports of ninth cranial nerve section have failed to document a single case of anesthesia dolorosa or paresthesias in its territory—a sharp contrast with trigeminal rhizotomy. Other painful conditions involving the glossopharyngeal nerve and nervus intermedius can be alleviated by rhizotomy, but results are usually poor for atypical pains or pain of unknown cause. Pain resulting from a malignancy can be relieved if all the innervation is destroyed; thus, it is usually wisest to treat pain in the pharynx by a combined section of the trigeminal and glossopharyngeal nerves, including the nervus intermedius if any of the pain is referred to the ear.

Tew and associates (98) have described a percutaneous technique for the destruction of glossopharyngeal and vagal nerves using a needle passed through the cheek into the jugular foramen. A small number of patients have been treated and pain relief has been reported in cases of both neuralgia and cancer pain. A significant risk of vocal cord paralysis (2 of 11 patients) has been noted, and cardiovascular complications can also occur (135).

Others have reported the use of percutaneous rhizotomy of the glossopharyngeal nerve alone or in combination with CN X for therapy of neuralgia and cancer pain. Lazorthes and Verdie (134) used percutaneous rhizotomy of CN IX and X for 11 patients with cancer pain with long-term relief in 8 (73%) and rhizotomy of CN IX for 1 patient with glossopharyngeal neuralgia with complete pain relief. Isamat et al. (135) carried out a total of 5 thermocoagulation rhizotomies on 3 patients with glossopharyngeal neuralgia who remained pain free at follow-up that ranged from 5 months to 2.8 years. Giorgio and Broggi (136) reported its use in 5 patients with neuralgia and 5 patients with

TABLE 97-9. Results of Glossopharyngeal and Nervus Intermedius Rhizotomy

Source	Year of Report	Operation*	Indication	No. of Patients	Results (% of Total)			
					Success†	Complications	Paresthesia	Mortality Rate
Dandy (127)	1927	CN IX	Tic douloureux	2	100	0	0	0
Dandy (128)	1929	CN V, IX	Cancer	1	100	0	0	0
Peet (129)	1935	CN V, IX	Tic douloureux	5	100	0	0	0
Peet (129)	1935	CN IX	Tic douloureux	7	100	0	0	0
Brzustowicz (130)	1955	CN V, IX	Tic douloureux	5	100	0	0	0
Bohm and Strang (131)	1962	CN IX	Neuralgias	16	70‡	0	0	0
Sachs (132)	1966	NI	Cluster headache	4	100	0	0	10
Chawla and and Falconer (133)	1967	CN IX	Neuralgias	10	90	0	0	10
Lazorthes and Verdie (134)	1979	CN IX, X	Cancer	11	73	0	0	0
		CN IX	Neuralgia	1	100	0	0	0
Isamat et al. (135)	1980	CN IX, X	Neuralgia	3	100	0	0	0
Giorgi and Broggi (136)	1984	CN IX, X	Neuralgia	5	80	0	0	0
	1984	CN IX, X (X)	Cancer	5	100	0	0	0

*V = trigeminal rhizotomy; IX = glossopharyngeal rhizotomy; X = vagal rhizotomy; NI = nervus intermedius rhizotomy.
†Success = complete relief.
‡Two patients subsequently relieved by CN X section, long follow-up.

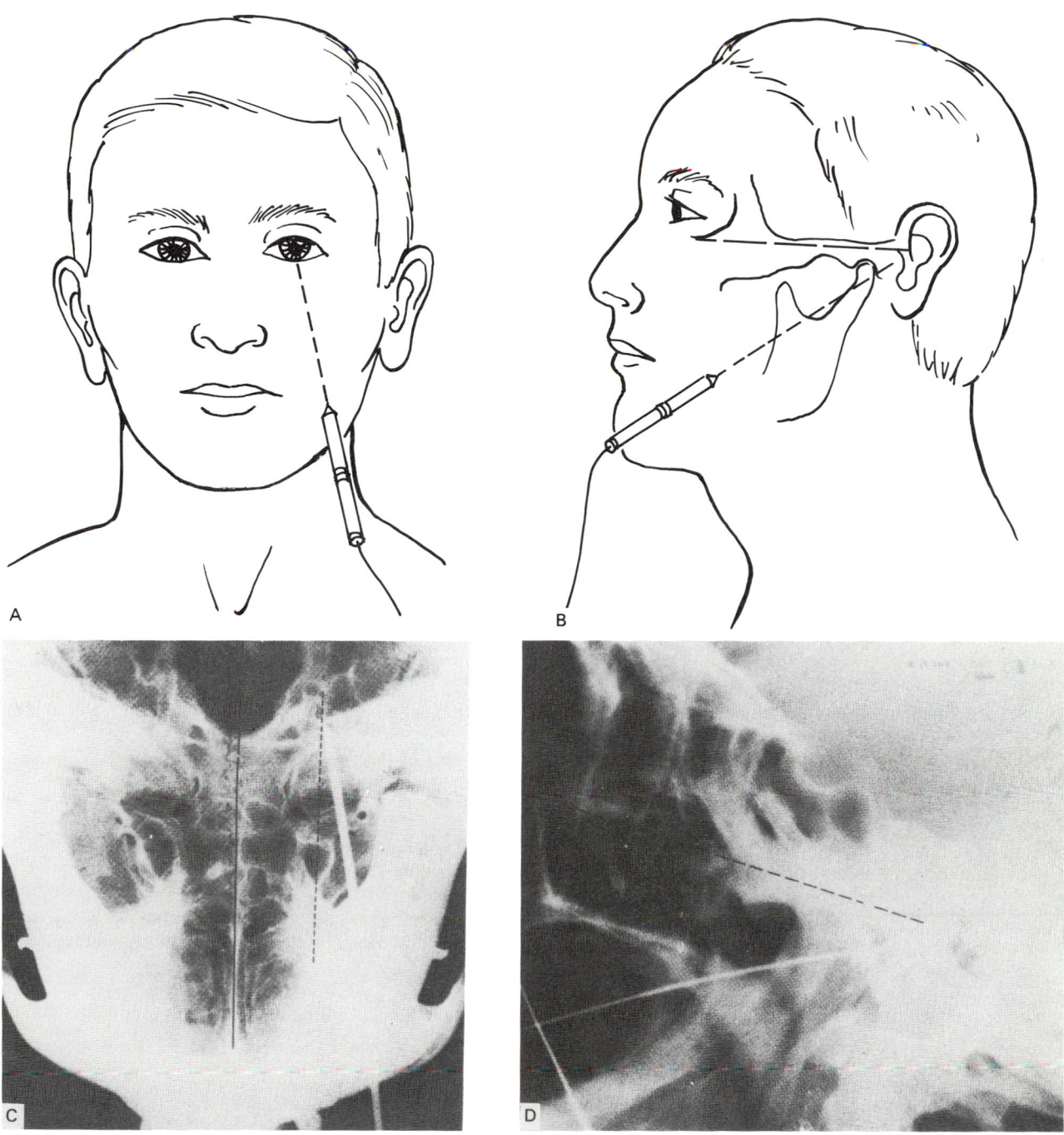

FIG. 97-5. Technique of percutaneous rhizotomy of cranial nerves IX and X. *A.* Anterior view of the face. The needle is inserted into the skin 2.5 cm lateral to the labial commissure and directed under fluoroscopic control along two planes, one at a 12° angle to the vertical plane through the pupil of the eye. *B.* Lateral view. The second plane is at a 40° angle to the plane passing through the internal auditory meatus and the inferior margin of the orbit. The needle is advanced to a point lateral to the internal carotid artery, where its tip should be in the pars nervosa of the posterior foramen lacerum. This position is checked by roentgenography; electrophysiologic control is then carried out by checking the impedance and by evoking responses from cranial nerves IX, X, and XII to confirm the exact position of the needle. ECG monitoring is recommended because of possible cardiac dysrhythmia. *C.* Anteroposterior roentgenogram of the dry skull showing the position of the needle. Note the angle to the plane parallel to the midsaggital plane. A single bolus of 100 to 150 mg of thiopental is administered before radiofrequency coagulation to produce amnesia during the period of coagulation. The temperature of the probe should be kept between 65° and 75° C. The lesion is repeated if intraoperative evaluation is necessary. *D.* Lateral roentgenogram taken with a fluoroscopic intensifier depicting the position of the needle where radiofrequency coagulation was performed after electrophysiologic control. The axis of the needle makes a 40° angle with the line passing through the internal auditory meatus and the inferior margin of the orbit. C and D from Broggi, G., and Siegfried, J.: Percutaneous differential radiofrequency rhizotomy of glossopharyngeal nerve in facial pain due to cancer. In Advances in Pain Research and Therapy, Vol. 2. Edited by J.J. Bonica and V. Ventafridda. New York, Raven Press, 1979, pp. 471, 472.

cancer pain. Of the 5 patients with neuralgia, in 1 it was limited to CN V, while the other 4 also had involvement of CN IX. Percutaneous rhizotomy produced relief of pain that persisted for periods of 3 to 5 years in 4 and in the fifth, for 3 years, after which open rhizotomy provided relief. Of the 5 patients with cancer pain, 4 also required retrogasserian trigeminal rhizotomy, which produced pain relief until death of the patients, which ranged from 4 months to 3 years.

Conclusions

Rhizotomy of the cranial sensory nerves—trigeminal, nervus intermedius, and glossopharyngeal—remains a useful primary procedure for pain secondary to cancer but is not often indicated for any form of facial neuralgia. When such patients fail medical management, gangliolysis or microvascular decompression of the cranial nerves is the initial procedure of choice. The number of rhizotomies performed in the past 20 years has decreased markedly because of the new surgical procedures available for the treatment of tic douloureux. Only when microvascular decompression has failed should rhizotomy be considered for tic douloureux. Trigeminal rhizotomy is associated with annoying paresthesias and the occasional development of anesthesia dolorosa; these complications make gangliolysis and microvascular decompression the primary procedures for tic pain. Rhizotomy is not a suitable operation for atypical facial pain.

REFERENCES

1. Penman, J., and Walsh, L.S.: Great auricular neurotomy for tic douloureux: A controlled clinical trial. B. Med. J., 1:22, 1957.
2. Marguth, F.: The surgical treatment of trigeminal neuralgia. In Pain. Edited by R. Janzen et al. Baltimore, Williams & Wilkins, 1972, pp. 213–214.
3. Rasmussen, P.P.: Facial Pain. Copenhagen, Ejnar Munksgaards Forlag, 1965, pp. 210–296.
4. Murphy, J.P.: Occipital neurectomy in the treatment of headache. Md. State Med. J., 18:62, 1969.
5. White, J.C., and Sweet, W.H.: Pain and the Neurosurgeon. Springfield, IL, Charles C Thomas, 1969.
6. Jensen, T.S., and Rasmussen, P.: Textbook of Pain. Edited by P.D. Wall and R. Melzack. Edinburgh, Churchill Livingstone, 1984, p. 409.
7. Sunderland, S.: Nerves and Nerve Injuries. Edinburgh, Churchill Livingstone, 1972, pp. 486–503.
8. Lazorthes, Y., Verdie, J.C., and Lagarrigue, J.: Thermocoagulation percutanée des nerfs rachidiens a visée analgesique. Neurochirurgie, 22:445, 1976.
9. Uematsu, S.: Percutaneous electrothermocoagulation of spinal nerve trunk, ganglion and rootlets. In Operative Neurosurgical Techniques: Indications, Methods and Results. 2nd Ed. Edited by H.H. Schmidek and W.S. Sweet. New York, Grune & Stratton, 1988, pp. 1207–1221.
10. Abbe, R.: A contribution to the surgery of the spine. Med. Rec. [NY], 35:149, 1889.
11. Bennett, W.H.: A case in which acute spasmodic pain in the left lower extremity was completely relieved by sub-dural division of the posterior roots of certain spinal nerves. Med. Chir. Trans. [Lond.], 72:329, 1889.
12. White, J.C., and Sweet, W.H.: Pain and the Neurosurgeon. Springfield, IL, Charles C Thomas, 1969, pp. 635–660.
13. Haven, H., and King, R.: Section of the posterior roots for the relief of pain in angina pectoris. Surg. Gynecol. Obstet., 75:298, 1942.
14. White, J.C., Garrey, W.E., and Atkins, J.A.: Cardiac innervation. Experimental and clinical studies. Arch. Surg., 26:765, 1933.
15. Hunter, C.R., and Mayfield, F.H.: Role of the upper cervical roots in the production of pain in the head. Am. J. Surg., 78:743, 1949.
16. White, J.C.: Posterior rhizotomy: A possible substitute for cordotomy in otherwise intractable neuralgias of the trunk and extremities of non-malignant origin. Clin. Neurosurg., 13:30, 1966.
17. White, J.C., and Kjellberg, R.N.: Posterior spinal rhizotomy: A substitute for cordotomy in the relief of localized pain in patients with normal life expectancy. Neurochirurgie, 16:141, 1973.
18. Sindou, M.: Étude de la jonction radiculo-medullaire posterieure la radicellotomie posterieure selective dans la chirurgie de la douleur. Lyon, Travail de L'Hôpital Neurologique et de L'Unite de Recherches de Physiopathologie de Systeme Nerveux, 1972, pp. 1–182.
19. Sindou, M., et al.: Posterior spinal rhizotomy and selective posterior rhizidiotomy. Prog. Neurosurg., 7:201, 1976.
20. Coggeshall, R.E.: Afferent fibers in the ventral root. Neurosurgery, 4:443, 1979.
21. Hosobuchi, Y.: The majority of unmyelinated afferent axons in human ventral roots probably conduct pain. Pain, 8:167, 180, 1980.
22. Osgood, C.P., et al.: Microsurgical ganglionectomy for chronic pain syndromes. J. Neurosurg., 45:113, 1976.
23. Smith, F.P.: Trans-spinal ganglionectomy for relief of intercostal pain. J. Neurosurg., 32:574, 1970.
24. Crue, B.L., and Todd, E.M.: A simplified technique of sacral rhizotomy for pelvic pain. J. Neurosurg., 21:835, 1964.
25. Felsoory, A., and Crue, B.L.: Results of 19 years' experience with sacral rhizotomy for perineal and perianal cancer pain. Pain, 2:431, 1976.
26. Liu, C.N., and Chambers, W.W.: Ultraspinal sprouting of dorsal root axons. Arch. Neurol., 79:46, 1958.
27. Hodge, C.J., Jr., and King, R.B.: Medical modification of sensation. J. Neurosurg., 44:21, 1976.
28. Uematsu, S., et al.: Percutaneous radiofrequency rhizotomy. Surg. Neurol., 2:319, 1974.
29. Nash, T.P.: Percutaneous radiofrequency lesioning of dorsal root ganglia for intractable pain. Pain, 24:67, 1986.
30. Scoville, W.B.: Extradural spinal sensory rhizotomy. J. Neurosurg., 25:94, 1966.
31. Dubuisson, D.: Root surgery. In Textbook of Pain. 2nd Ed. Edited by P.D. Wall and R. Melzack. Edinburgh, Churchill Livingstone, 1989, pp. 784–794.
32. Bertrand, G.: The "battered" root problem. Orthop. Clin. North Am., 6:305, 1975.
33. Strait, T.A., and Hunter, S.E.: Intraspinal extradural rhizotomy in patients with failure of lumbar disc surgery. J. Neurosurg., 54:193, 1981.
34. Loeser, J.D.: Dorsal rhizotomy for the relief of chronic pain. J. Neurosurg., 36:745, 1972.
35. Onofrio, B.M., and Campa, H.K.: Evaluation of rhizotomy. Review of 12 years' experience. J. Neurosurg., 36:751, 1972.
36. Hannington-Kiff, J.G.: Intravenous regional sympathetic block with guanethidine. Lancet, 1:1019, 1974.
37. Sweet, W.H.: Causalgia: Sympathetic dystrophy (Sudeck's atrophy). In Neurosurgery. Edited by R.H. Wilkins and S.S. Rengachary. New York, McGraw-Hill, 1985, pp. 1886–1893.
38. Sudeck, P.: Über die akute, entzundlishe Knochenatrophie. Arch. Klin. Chir., 62:147, 1900.
39. De Takats, G.: Sympathectomy revisited: Dodo or phoenix? Surgery, 78:644, 1975.
40. Ghostine, S.Y., et al.: Phenoxybenzamine in the treatment of causalgia: Report of 40 cases. J. Neurosurg., 60:1263, 1984.
41. Ascherl, R., and Blümel, G.: Zum Krankheitsbild der Sudeck'schen Dystrophie. Fortschr. Med., 99:712, 1981.
42. Bonica, J.J.: Causalgia and other reflex sympathetic dystrophies. In Advances in Pain Research and Therapy, Vol. 3. Edited by J.J. Bonica, J.C. Liebeskind, and D.G. Albe-Fessard. New York, Raven Press, 1979, pp. 141–166.
43. Berguer, R., and Smit, R.: Transaxillary sympathectomy (T2 to T4) for relief of vasospastic/sympathetic pain of upper extremities. Surgery, 89:764, 1981.
44. Wirth, F.P., and Rutherford, R.B.: A civilian experience with causalgia. Arch. Surg., 100:633, 1970.
45. Thompson, J.E.: The diagnosis and management of post-traumatic pain syndromes (causalgia). Aust. N.Z. J. Surg., 49:299, 1979.
46. Dale, W.A., and Lewis, M.R.: Management of ischemia of the hand and fingers. Surgery, 67:62, 1970.

47. Baddeley, R.M.: The place of upper dorsal sympathectomy in the treatment of primary Raynaud's disease. Br. J. Surg., 52:426, 1965.
48. Mattassi, R., Miele, F., and D'Angelo, F.: Thoracic sympathectomy. Review of indications, results and surgical techniques. J. Cardiovasc. Surg., 22:336, 1981.
49. Fontaine, J.-L., and Leonard, P.: Indikationen und Grenzen der Sympathikus-Chirurgie. Münch. Med. Wochenschr., 121:413, 1979.
50. Touati, Y., et al.: Indications actuelles de la sympathectomie dorsale supérieure. A propos de 84 cas. J. Mal. Vasc., 7:187, 1982.
51. Arnulf, G.: La chirurgie du sympathique dans la douleur de R. Leriche à nos jours. Bull. Acad. Natl. Med. (Paris), 163:928, 1979.
52. Erdemir, H., Gelman, S., and Galbraith, J.G.: Prediction of the needed level of sympathectomy for posttraumatic reflex sympathetic dystrophy. Surg. Neurol., 17:353, 1982.
53. Mayfield, F.H.: Causalgia. Springfield, IL, Charles C Thomas, 1951.
54. Benassy, J.: A propos du Procès-verbal. Au sujet de la communication de MM. Motta et Afanassieff: Traitement des moignons douloureux et causalgies. Chirurgie, 103:926, 1977.
55. Van der Stricht, J.: Signification de la thermométrie cutanée; application à l'étude circulatoire de membres. Paris, Journées Angéiologiques de Langues Francaise, Expansion Scientifique Paris, 1972, pp. 233–237.
56. Simeone, F.A.: The anatomy of the lumbar sympathetic trunks in man (with special reference to the question of regeneration after sympathectomy). J. Cardiovasc. Surg., 20:283, 1979.
57. Adar, R.: Iatrogenic brachial plexus injuries. Mayo Clin. Proc., 54:277, 1979.
58. Atkins, J.H.B.: Sympathectomy by the axillary approach. Lancet, 1:538, 1954.
59. Fontaine, R., et al.: Lumbar sympathectomy. Acta Chir. Belg., 76:1, 1977.
60. Van der Stricht, J.: 50 years of lumbar sympathectomy. J. Cardiovasc. Surg., 20:283, 1979.
61. Ray, B.S., and Console, A.D.: The relief of pain in chronic (calcareous) pancreatitis by sympathectomy. Surg. Gynecol. Obstet., 89:1, 1949.
62. Goldstein, M., et al.: Les complications de la sympathectomie lombaire. Étude rétrospective de 791 malades. Acta Chirg. Belgica, 76:73, 1977.
63. Tracy, G.D., and Cockett, F.B.: Pain in the lower limb after sympathectomy. Lancet, 1:12, 1957.
64. Litwin, M.S.: Postsympathectomy neuralgia. Arch. Surg., 84:591, 1962.
65. Longoni, F., et al.: La neuralgia postsimpatectomia lumbar. Angiologia, 33:118, 1981.
66. Whitelaw, G.P., and Smithwick, R.H.: Some secondary effects of sympathectomy with particular reference to disturbance of sexual function. N. Engl. J. Med., 245:121, 1951.
67. Wilkinson, H.: Percutaneous radiofrequency upper thoracic sympathectomy: A new technique. Neurosurgery, 15:811, 1984.
68. Kux, M.: Thoracic endoscopic sympathectomy for treatment of upper-limb hyperhidrosis. Lancet, 1:1320, 1977.
69. Rösner, K., and Goldberg, S.: Der Stellenwert der thorakoskopischen Sympathikotomie bei der Behandlung des Raynaud-Syndrom. Z. Gesamte Inn. Med., 34:127, 1979.
70. Weale, F.E.: Upper thoracic sympathectomy by transthoracic electrocoagulation. Br. J. Surg., 67:71, 1980.
71. Malone, P.S., Duignan, J.P., and Hederman, W.P.: Transthoracic electrocoagulation (T.T.E.C.)—a new and simple approach to upper limb sympathectomy. Irish Med. J., 75:20, 1982.
72. Birkett, D.A., et al.: Bilateral upper thoracic sympathectomy in angina pectoris: Results in 52 cases. Br. Med. J., 2:187, 1965.
73. Burnett, C.F., Jr., and Evans, J.: Follow-up report on resection of the anginal pathway in thirty-three patients. JAMA, 162:709, 1956.
74. Lindgren, I., and Olivecrona, H.: Surgical treatment of angina pectoris. J. Neurosurg., 4:19, 1947.
75. Lindgren, I.: Angina pectoris, clinical study with special reference to neurosurgical treatment. Acta Med. Scand., (Suppl.), 243:1, 1950.
76. Palumbo, L.T., and Lulu, D.J.: Transthoracic upper dorsal sympathectomy. Surgery, 53:563, 1963.
77. Raney, R.B.: A hitherto undescribed surgical procedure relieving attacks of angina pectoris. JAMA, 224:1619, 1939.
78. Mallet-Guy, P., and de Beaujeu, M.J.: Treatment of chronic pancreatitis by unilateral splanchnicectomy. Arch. Surg., 60:233, 1950.
79. Vosschulte, K., and Wagner, E.: Splanchnicectomy in chronic pancreatitis. Minn. Med., 53:1053, 1970.
80. Michotey, G., et al.: La splanchnicectomie par voie transhiatale de Dubois. Á propos de 25 sections. J. Chiru. (Paris), 120:487, 1983.
81. Sadar, E.S., and Hardy, R.W., Jr.: Thoracic splanchnicectomy and sympathectomy for relief of pancreatic pain. In Surgery of the Pancreas. Edited by A.M. Cooperman and S.O. Herr. St. Louis, C.V. Mosby, 1978, pp. 141–152.
82. Flanigan, D.P., and Kraft, R.O.: Continuing experience with chemical palliative splanchnicectomy. Arch. Surg., 113:509, 1978.
83. Gardner, A.M.N., and Solomon, G.: Relief of the pain of unresectable carcinoma of pancreas by chemical splanchnicectomy during laparotomy. Ann. R. Coll. Surg. Engl., 66:409, 1984.
84. Fontaine, R., and Hermann, L.G.: Clinical and experimental basis for surgery of the pelvic sympathetic nerves in gynecology. Surg. Gynecol. Obstet., 54:133, 1932.
85. Counseller, V.S., and Craig, W.: The treatment of dysmenorrhea by resection of the presacral sympathetic nerves: Evaluation of end results. Am. J. Obstet. Gynecol., 28:161, 1934.
86. Meigs, J.V.: Excision of the superior hypogastric plexus (presacral nerve) for primary dysmenorrhea. Surg. Gynecol. Obstet., 68:723, 1939.
87. Phaneuf, L.E.: Presacral neurectomy in intractable dysmenorrhea. J. Mt. Sinai Hosp., 14:553, 1947.
88. Frier, A.: Pelvic neurectomy in gynecology. Obstet. Gynecol., 25:48, 1965.
89. Heisey, W.G., and Dohn, D.F.: Splanchnicectomy for the treatment of intractable abdominal pain. Cleve. Clin. Q., 34:9, 1967.
90. Stookey, B., and Ransohoff, J.: Trigeminal Neuralgia. Its History and Treatment. Springfield, IL, Charles C Thomas, 1959, pp. 132–166.
91. Harris, W.: An analysis of 1,433 cases of paroxysmal trigeminal neuralgia (trigeminal-tic) and the end-results of gasserian alcohol injection. Brain, 63:209, 1940.
92. Jaeger, R.: The relief of tic douloureux (trigeminal tic) and other pains of fifth cranial nerve by injections of hot water into gasserian ganglion. J. Am. Geriatr. Soc., 3:416, 1955.
93. Sharr, M.M., and Garfield, J.S.: The place of ganglion or root alcohol injection in trigeminal neuralgia. J. Neurol. Neurosurg. Psychiatry, 40:286, 1977.
94. Kirschner, M.: Electrocoagulation des ganglion gasseri. Zentralbl. Chir., 59:2841, 1932.
95. Kirschner, M.: Die Behandlung der Trigeminusneuralgie (nach Erfahrungen an 1113 Kranken). Münch. Med. Wochenschr., 89:235–239, 1942.
96. Sweet, W.H., and Wepsic, J.G.: Controlled thermocoagulation of trigeminal ganglion and rootlets for differential destruction of pain fibers. Part 1. Trigeminal neuralgia. J. Neurosurg., 40:143, 1974.
97. Tew, J.M., and Keller, J.T.: The treatment of trigeminal neuralgia by percutaneous radiofrequency technique. Clin. Neurosurg., 24:557, 1977.
98. Tew, J.M., Tobler, W.D., and van Loveren, H.: Percutaneous rhizotomy in the treatment of intractable facial pain (trigeminal, glossopharyngeal, and vagal nerves). In Operative Neurosurgical Techniques. Edited by H.H. Schmidek and W.H. Sweet. New York, Grune & Stratton, 1982, pp. 1083–1106.
99. Van Loveren, H., et al.: A 10-year experience in the treatment of trigeminal neuralgia: Comparison of percutaneous stereotaxic rhizotomy and posterior fossa exploration. J. Neurosurg., 57:757, 1982.
100. Frigyese, T.L., Siegfried, J., and Broggi, G.: The selective vulnerability of evoked potentials in the trigeminal sensory root to graded thermocoagulation. Exp. Neurol., 49:11, 1975.
101. Lewy, F.H., and Grant, F.C.: Physiopathologic and pathoanatomic aspects of major trigeminal neuralgia. Arch. Neurol. Psychiatry, 40:1126, 1938.
102. Braham, J., and Saia, A.: Phenytoin in the treatment of trigeminal and other neuralgias. Lancet, 2:982, 1960.
103. Taylor, J.C.: Tegretol in the treatment of trigeminal neuralgia. J. Neurol. Neurosurg. Psychiatry, 29:478, 1966.

104. Garvan, N.J., and Siegfried, J.: Trigeminal neuralgia—earlier referral for surgery. Postgrad. Med. J., 59:435, 1983.
105. Hakanson, S.: Trigeminal neuralgia treated by the injection of glycerol into the trigeminal cistern. Neurosurgery, 9:638, 1981.
106. Sweet, W.H., Poletti, C.E., and Macon, J.B.: Treatment of trigeminal neuralgia and other facial pains by retrogasserian injection of glycerol. Neurosurgery, 9:647, 1981.
107. Lundsford, L.D., and Bennett, M.H.: Percutaneous retrogasserian glycerol rhizotomy for tic douloureux. I. Technique and results in 112 patients. Neurosurgery, 14:424, 1984.
108. Loeser, J.D.: What to do about tic douloureux. JAMA, 239:1153, 1978.
109. Apfelbaum, R.I.: A comparison of percutaneous radiofrequency trigeminal neurolysis and microvascular decompression of the trigeminal nerve for the treatment of tic douloureux. Neurosurgery, 1:16, 1977.
110. Burchiel, K.J., et al.: Comparison of percutaneous radiofrequency gangliolysis and microvascular decompression for the surgical management of tic douloureux. Neurosurgery, 9:111, 1981.
111. Menzel, J., Piotrowski, W., and Penzhole, H.: Long-term results of gasserian ganglion electrocoagulation. J. Neurosurg., 42:140, 1975.
112. Nugent, G.R.: Technique and results of 800 percutaneous radiofrequency thermocoagulations for trigeminal neuralgia. Appl. Neurophysiol., 45:504, 1982.
113. Onofrio, B.M.: Radiofrequency percutaneous gasserian ganglion lesions. J. Neurosurg., 42:132, 1975.
114. Rhoton, A.L., et al.: Percutaneous stereotaxic radiofrequency lesions for trigeminal neuralgia. J. Fla. Med. Assoc., 64:448, 1977.
115. Siegfried, J.: 500 percutaneous thermocoagulations of the gasserian ganglion for trigeminal pain. Surg. Neurol., 8:126, 1977.
116. Dandy, W.E.: Concerning the cause of trigeminal neuralgia. Am. J. Surg., 24:447, 1934.
117. Jannetta, P.J.: Microsurgical approach to the trigeminal nerve for tic douloureux. Prog. Neurol. Surg., 7:180, 1976.
118. Hardy, D.G., and Rhoton, A.L., Jr.: Microsurgical relationships of the superior cerebellar artery and the trigeminal nerve. J. Neurosurg., 49:669, 1978.
119. Frazier, C.H.: Subtotal resection of sensory root for relief of major trigeminal neuralgia. Arch. Neurol. Psychiatry, 13:378, 1925.
120. Grant, F.C.: Complications accompanying surgical relief of pain in trigeminal neuralgia. Am. J. Surg., 75:42, 1948.
121. Grant, F.C.: Results in the operative treatment of major trigeminal neuralgia. Ann. Surg., 107:14, 1938.
122. Peet, M.M., and Schneider, R.C.: Trigeminal neuralgia. A review of six hundred and eighty-nine cases with a follow-up study on sixty-five per cent of the group. J. Neurosurg., 9:367, 1952.
123. Ruge, D., Brochner, R., and Davis, L.: A study of the treatment of 637 patients with trigeminal neuralgia. J. Neurosurg., 15:528, 1958.
124. Wertheimer, P.: Neurochirurgie Fonctionelle. Paris, I. Masson, 1960, p. 177.
125. Olivecrona, H.P.: Trigeminal neuralgia. Triangle, 5:60, 1961.
126. Morello, G.: Results of trigeminal rhizotomy by intradural route in 409 personal cases of trigeminal neuralgia. Minerva Neurochir., 13:183, 1969.
127. Dandy, W.E.: Glossopharyngeal neuralgia (tic douloureux). Its diagnosis and treatment. Arch. Surg., 15:198, 1927.
128. Dandy, W.E.: Operative relief from pain in lesions of the mouth, tongue and throat. Arch. Surg., 19:143, 1929.
129. Peet, M.M.: Glossopharyngeal neuralgia. Ann. Surg., 101:256, 1935.
130. Brzustowicz, R.: Combined trigeminal and glossopharyngeal neuralgia. Neurology, 5:1, 1955.
131. Bohm, E., and Strang, R.R.: Glossopharyngeal neuralgia. Brain, 85:371, 1962.
132. Sachs, E.: The role of the nervus intermedius in facial neuralgia. Report of four cases with observations on the pathways for taste, lacrimation, and pain in the face. J. Neurosurg., 28:54, 1966.
133. Chawla, J.C., and Falconer, M.A.: Glossopharyngeal and vagal neuralgia. Br. Med. J., 2:529, 1967.
134. Lazorthes, Y., and Verdie, J.C.: Radiofrequency coagulation of the petrous ganglion in glossopharyngeal neuralgia. Neurosurgery, 4:512, 1979.
135. Isamat, F., Ferran, E., and Acebes, J.J.: Selective percutaneous thermocoagulation rhizotomy in essential glossopharyngeal neuralgia. J. Neurosurg., 55:575, 1981.
136. Giorgi, C. and Broggi, G.: Surgical treatment of glossopharyngeal neuralgia and pain from cancer of the nasopharynx: A 20 year experience. J. Neurosurg., 61:952, 1984.

98 · NEUROSURGICAL OPERATIONS ON THE SPINAL CORD

Hubert L. Rosomoff, Isacco Papo, *and* John D. Loeser
with contributions by
John J. Bonica

THIS chapter discusses various neurosurgical operations carried out on the spinal cord for the relief of chronic pain. The material is presented in three sections: A, Anterolateral Cordotomy, written by Rosomoff, B, Myelotomy, written by Papo and Loeser, and C, Dorsal Root Entry Zone Lesions, written by Loeser. Bonica collaborated with Loeser in editing and amplifying the text and in supervising the development of the illustrations by M. Domenowske from those provided by the authors and computing and rearranging the data in the tables to present them in a uniform format. A more detailed discussion of the techniques presented can be found in major textbooks of neurosurgery, as cited in the introduction to section F.

A. ANTEROLATERAL CORDOTOMY

Anterolateral cordotomy is the operative procedure by which the spinal anterolateral ascending system for the transmission of pain, also known as the spinothalamic tract, is interrupted for the relief of pain. Both percutaneous and open techniques are available; the anatomic goal is the same and results differ only with respect to the risks of each strategy and to long-term results.

The concept of relieving pain by section of the pain-conducting pathways in the anterolateral quadrant of the spinal cord was first proposed by Schuller (1) in 1910. It was not until 2 years later, however, that Martin (2), at the urging of Spiller, performed the initial thoracic cordotomy in humans. Foerster and Gagel (3) were the first to use the cervical route for access. The literature contains numerous reports concerning technique, results, and complications, which suggest that open surgical cordotomy is a useful short-term method for the alleviation of pain in patients with malignant disease, although with some risk of complications, and with questionable duration of effect in those fortunate enough to survive beyond expectations.

To avoid or minimize the risks of open surgery the concept of a percutaneous stereotaxic procedure evolved, a procedure that could be accomplished under local anesthesia simply, easily, and with a low morbidity rate in patients who otherwise might not be suitable for a major open operation. Mullan and associates (4, 5) are to be recognized for this visionary innovation. Their original technique underwent several modifications, incorporating the experiences of Rosomoff and co-workers (6), before arriving at standard methodology currently used for this procedure.

The initial method for percutaneous cordotomy used a radioisotope-tipped needle that was inserted into the spine at the C1–C2 interspace laterally and came to lie anterolaterally in the subarachnoid space adjacent to the ventral quadrant of the spinal cord. The next approach introduced a wire electrode into the parenchyma of the spinal cord, with the direct current source for lesion-making in the ventral quadrant. Rosomoff and associates proposed a technique using a radiofrequency (RF) current to produce the lesion, which allowed for rapid and solid lesion-making; the equipment was available commercially or easily built, and the intrumentation was portable. This technique became standard, although a number of modifications of access route have been used—anterior, posterior, medullary, and low cervical—as well various methods of target localization and electrode design, and modifications of RF lesion makers (Table 98-1). The operation to be presented is one that Rosomoff has used, as first described in 1965 (6), and as modified by his experiences to date. After discussing the percutaneous technique, the open operation will be considered.

Basic Considerations

The anatomy and physiology of the spinothalamic and other important ascending tracts in the anterolateral quadrant of the spinal cord that transmit nociceptive information are discussed in detail in Chapter 3 (pages 52–66) and are depicted in Figures 3-28 to 3-43.

Indications

The technique of percutaneous cordotomy can be considered for any patient with somatic pain below the level of the mandible. Percutaneous cordotomy is indicated for patients with pain from cancer, including those who previously could not be subjected to the major operation of laminectomy and spinothalamic section because of debilitation or a preterminal state. It is also indicated for some patients with painful conditions that are intractable and nonmalignant in nature. In the selection of patients, it is necessary to differentiate pain of a lancinating or toothache-like quality from distressing dysesthesias, such as burning, prickling, pressure, or crawling. The former is mediated by the lateral spinothalamic tract, and ventrolateral cordotomy alleviates pain in more than 90% of patients. The latter is not transmitted entirely

TABLE 98-1. Developments in Percutaneous Cordotomy

Source	Technique	Comments or Modifications
Mullan et al. (4)	Isotope needle; lateral cervical	Unpredictable, radiation risk, complex to prepare
Mullan et al. (5)	Unipolar electrode; lateral cervical	Erratic lesion, prolonged current time, unpredictable
Rosomoff et al. (6)	Radiofrequency current; bilateral or unilateral cervical	Rapid, solid lesion, portable, predictable
Crue et al. (7)	Radiofrequency; high cervical	Posterior approach, traverses spinal cord, higher levels (?)
Fox (8)	Radiofrequency	Current related to lesion size
Gildenberg et al. (9, 10); Lin et al. (12)	Radiofrequency; low cervical, transdiskal	Anterior approach, decreased respiratory complications (?), more difficult technically, impedance measurements, increased safety
Hitchcock (11)	Radiofrequency; high cervical	Posterior approach, traverses spinal cord, higher levels (?)
Taren et al. (13), Tasker and Organ (14)	Radiofrequency, lateral cervical	Physiologic identification of target site
Todd et al. (15)	Radiofrequency; high cervical, medulla	Posterior approach; useful for somatic and facial pain
Mullan (16)	Radiofrequency; lateral cervical	Electric stimulation to identify tract, increased safety

through the ventral quadrant and these discomforts are relieved imperfectly or not at all. In fact, in patients with a mixed pain picture (i.e., lancinating pain and dysesthesias), the initial response to a successful cordotomy might be relief of all types of discomfort. Within a few days to weeks, however, the dysesthesias return to conscious perception. Their perception sometimes appears to be heightened by the absence of the lancinating component that was formerly the overriding sensation.

It is still possible to demonstrate dense analgesia to pinprick, confirming ablation of the anterolateral ascending pain system. It therefore follows that dysesthetic "pain" is transmitted elsewhere but in closely approximate structures, in which conduction is interrupted temporarily by the trauma of surgery only to return to function with resolution of the posttraumatic operative effects. One exception to this is the relief of tabetic or pseudotabetic pain, which does have a dysesthetic quality but in which cordotomy is an effective means of producing relief. When bilateral cordotomy is required the contralateral procedure is performed as a second stage no less than 1 week after the first.

Contraindications

Severe pulmonary dysfunction is the major contraindication to either percutaneous or open surgical cordotomy. The absence of a lung per se does not interdict the procedure, however, providing that remaining pulmonary function is satisfactory. Recently incurred neurologic deficits, such as paresis or rectalbladder disturbance, can be aggravated or recovery delayed by the superimposition of cordotomy; if this is the case the effect is usually temporary.

Clinical Considerations

Technique

The patient is premedicated and is placed in the supine position with the head fixed in flexion and the neck extended at the shoulders (Fig. 98-1). A no. 18 short-beveled spinal needle is introduced into the spinal canal using local infiltration anesthesia between the 1st and 2nd cervical vertebrae. An external sighting device is used in conjunction with an image intensifier to define the point of entry anterior to the position of the spinal cord.

Once the needle has been introduced into the subarachnoid space of the spinal canal, air is injected to produce an air myelogram, which visualizes the anterior border of the spinal cord. The needle is then directed toward the ventral quadrant of the spinal cord, and an electrode is inserted through the needle into the parenchyma of the spinal cord (Fig. 98-2). Impedance measures or electrical stimulation, or both, can be used at this point to ensure spinal cord penetration and correct localization of the electrode tip.

The cables of an RF generator are attached to the electrode and a lesion is made by increasing the duration of a preselected current (Fig. 98-3). The patient is tested carefully after each increment of current, both for the level of analgesia and for the possibility of complications—in particular, ipsilateral hemiparesis.

The procedure can be accomplished using cinefluoroscopy in about 15 to 20 minutes. When Polaroid techniques are necessary (e.g., as in hospitals that do not have cinefluoroscopy), the procedure can take twice as long.

Results

In Rosomoff's series 789 patients have undergone a total of 1279 cordotomies (Table 98-2), with a slight preponderance of males. Old age and infirmity were not contraindications. An analysis of the disease states for which the procedures were done indicates a preponderance of malignant disease among the initial 300 patients but, once the value of the procedure had become established, patients with benign conditions were referred more often for pain relief. Cancer of the

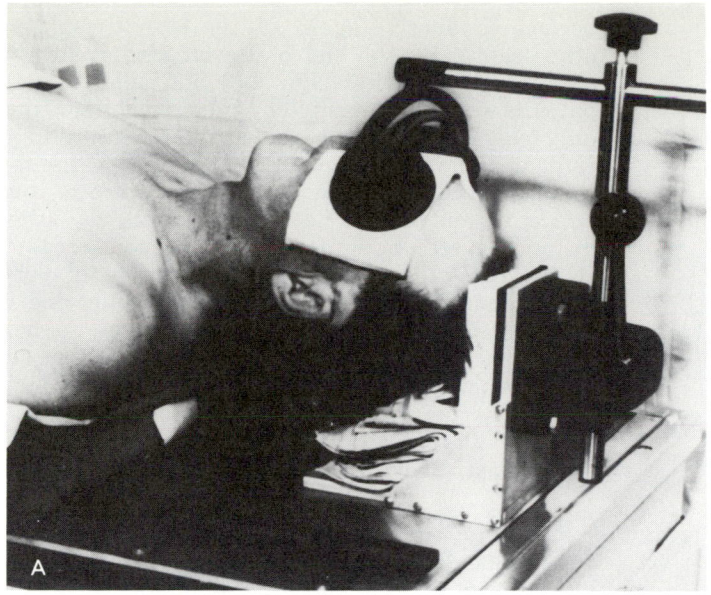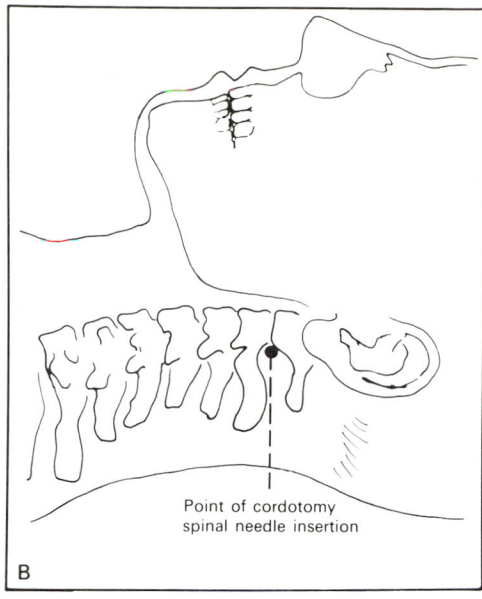

Point of cordotomy
spinal needle insertion

FIG. 98-1. *A.* Position of patient for percutaneous C1–C2 cordotomy. *B.* Site of insertion of needle for percutaneous C1–C2 cordotomy.

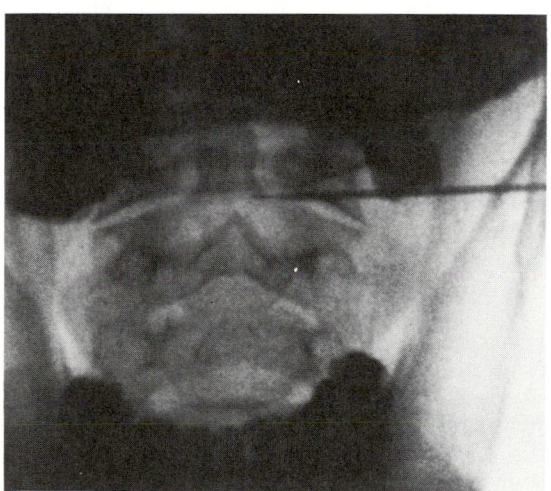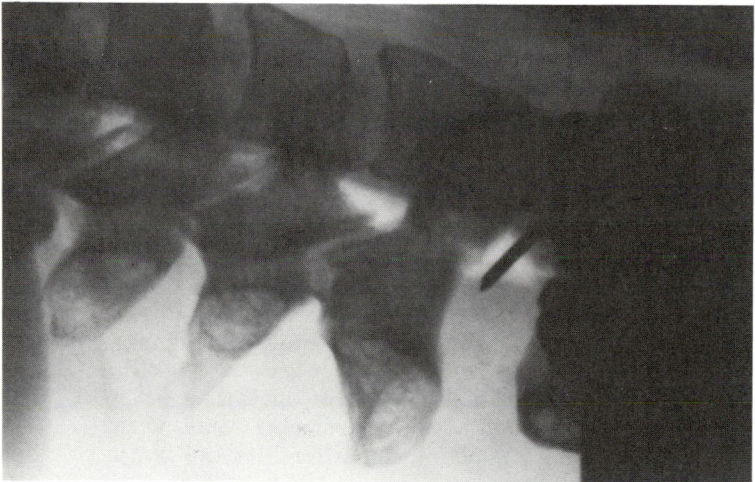

FIG. 98-2. Position of needle electrode for percutaneous C1–C2 cordotomy as seen on anteroposterior (*A*) and lateral (*B*) radiographs.

lung and gastrointestinal neoplasia were the most common diagnoses among the malignant diseases. Lumbar radiculopathy, as found in the unsuccessfully multiply operated back, and peripheral neuropathies were the most common indications for intervention in benign states.

A total of 531 patients underwent unilateral cordotomy for pain relief; 258 patients had bilateral cordotomies. These were staged operations, at least 1 week apart. Of the patients with malignant disease, 35% required bilateral intervention. Only 30% of those with benign disease required bilateral intervention. Repeat cordotomies were necessary in 18% of cordotomies—that is, in 24% of patients undergoing pain relief. In most cases this was the result of an imperfect lesion placed at the first operation because of caution

exercised by the surgeon. The less common reason for repetition was the loss of analgesia at a later date or the return of islands of pain perception.

Approximately 30% of patients had pain in the neck, upper extremities, or thorax. The remaining patients had pain in the abdomen, perineum, back, or lower extremities. Approximately 60% of those undergoing cordotomy procedures ended with analgesia at cervical or high thoracic levels.

At follow-up, analgesic levels were found to be the same or higher in 54% of those who had cordotomies, with the 19% that were higher offering additional protection; 32% were lower, usually within the accepted criterion of two to four dermatome segments; and 13% proved to be inadequate, requiring repetition if the patient was willing. Interestingly, 9% of the

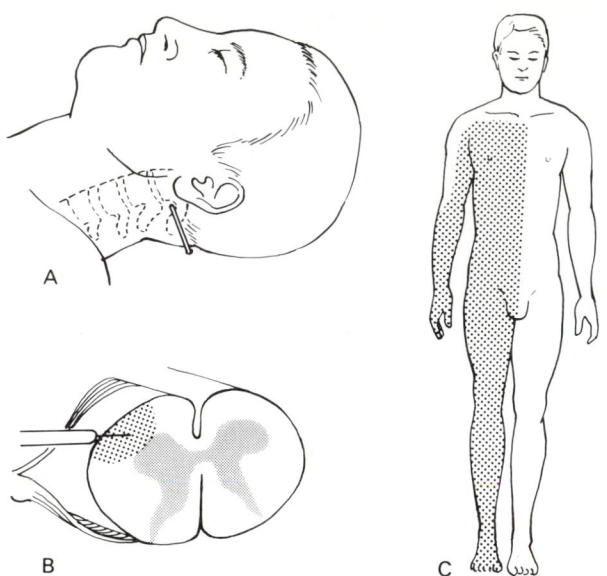

FIG. 98-3. *A.* Site of percutaneous C1–C2 cordotomy. *B.* Lesion produced by percutaneous C1–C2 cordotomy. *C.* Extent of analgesia produced by left C1–C2 percutaneous cordotomy.

analgesic levels disappeared, a still unsolved problem of cordotomy whatever type of technique is employed. Repeat of the cordotomy, however, invariably reproduced an acceptable level of analgesia. The remaining 4%, with no analgesic level or spotty analgesia, were technically inadequate and they too were repeated.

Unfortunately, follow-up data were obtained by questionnaires because many patients were referred for treatment from distant areas. The patients examined themselves and reported the historical and physical results. Because of the preponderance of malignant diseases, almost two-thirds of patients were dead or lost to follow-up within 3 months of operation. Only 25% were available for analysis after 1 year, with rapidly decreasing numbers thereafter into the tenth year.

Immediately following cordotomy, more than 90% of the patients considered themselves to be pain-free or so comfortable that no analgesics were necessary. By the end of 3 months, however, these measures of success had decreased to 84%. Dysesthesias, which had become prominent and could not be distinguished from lancinating toothache-like pain, were one reason for failure. Incomplete analgesia, originally or from fibers that were temporarily blocked by the RF current to

TABLE 98-2. Results of Percutaneous Cordotomy

Duration of Follow-Up	No. of Operations	Results (Successful)	
		No.	%
3 mo	599	495	84
3 mo–1 yr	304	185	61
1–5 yr	299	127	43
5–10 yr	86	32	37

become conductive again at this later time, was another cause. By the end of 1 year almost 40% were classified as failures. This does not mean that these patients were not benefited by the procedure; rather, it only means they did not have absolute pain relief. It is estimated that more than 50% of these patients felt they had received major help, could return to routine activities, and did not have problems of drug usage or distress severe enough to undergo repeat cordotomy. By 2 years and thereafter, an average of 60% of patients no longer had complete pain relief and were therefore classified technically as failures. As before, 50% of those in this group still considered themselves to be benefited. These data could be interpreted as being disappointing but they probably are not, because about 70% continue to have beneficial effects and are satisfied with their results.

Complications

The complication rate was low (Table 98-3). Ipsilateral hemiparesis appeared temporarily in 5% of those who had cordotomies, lasting usually only a few days to a few weeks but permanent in 3%. Ataxia, in 20%, was the most common complication, but it was sometimes present for only a few hours. Permanent ataxia, in 3%, was difficult to distinguish from a mild paresis. Catheterization was required in 10% of the procedures, usually in patients whose bladder mechanism was already disturbed by disease; 2% were left with permanent catheters, mostly for nursing convenience. Information relative to sexual function was difficult to obtain. The 4% incidence of difficulty was described usually as a decrease in voluptuous sensation about the genitals on the side rendered analgesic. Impotence was reported only occasionally, even with bilateral cordotomies. Postcordotomy dysesthetic syndromes—that is, burning distress throughout the entire area that was made analgesic, was uncommon, occurring in less than 1%. Its pathophysiologic mechanism is still unknown. Dysesthesias, in 16%, are noted separately. These sensations (e.g., tingling, burning, prickling in the area of pathologic implication) are not complications per se. They are uncomfortable feelings that were usually present preoperatively but were not conspicuous because of overriding pain. Once the pain

TABLE 98-3. Complications of 1279 Percutaneous Cordotomies

Type of Complaint	Temporary		Permanent	
	No.	%	No.	%
Paresis	63	5	34	3
Ataxia	252	20	44	3
Urinary	123	10	29	2
Sexual			54	4
Postcordotomy dysesthetic syndrome			10	1
Respiratory				
Minor	36	3		
Major	23	2	12	1*
Dysesthesias			199	16

*Includes 1 death.

had been ablated by the cordotomy, the dysesthesias became discernible and prominent.

Respiratory changes require separate discussion. An ascending system contributes to the control of ventilation mediated through the upper cervical spinal cord (17). Bilateral interruption can sometimes interfere with control so that the patient breathes normally when awake but becomes apneic when asleep. This phenomenon has been called sleep-induced apnea, or "Ondine's curse." The incidence of this major complication, the only life-threatening consequence of cordotomy, was 3%. It is delayed in onset and can be predicted by testing the patient's response to breathing carbon dioxide (18). Ablation of the response, which is normally a two- to threefold increase in minute volume, predicts the appearance of the syndrome, but not all patients go on to apnea. Such individuals, however, are candidates for apnea and must be observed carefully. They might require intubation with supportive artificial ventilation if respiration fails. The process is usually self-limiting, lasting a few days to 3 weeks. Minor changes in respiration, such as intermittent shortness of breath without compromised blood gas levels, occur in another 3%. These pass without event. The only death in this series was attributable to sleep-induced apnea that went undiscovered or was treated inadequately, especially early in my experience when little was known about the problem.

Open Surgical Cordotomy

Although percutaneous cordotomy has largely replaced the open surgical technique, circumstances still remain in which open cordotomy might be indicated. This usually pertains to facilities in which percutaneous cordotomy equipment is not available or the surgeon has not mastered the percutaneous technique or performs it so infrequently as to lose skill in the procedure. Rarely, the patient creates the indication by being unable to tolerate the procedure while awake, or by having an unusual anatomic condition that would require use of the open method. The historical development of open surgical cordotomy was outlined above; of course, it preceded the development of the percutaneous technique. The indications for both forms of the procedure are the same, as modified by the facilities available and by the training and expertise of the operating surgeon.

Technique

Although it is technically possible to perform open surgical cordotomy under local anesthesia, these procedures are usually carried out under general anesthesia with endotracheal intubation. Another option is segmental epidural blockade, which requires a skilled anesthesiologist. One of four basic surgical techniques can be used. High cervical cordotomy is done if levels of analgesia above C8 are required. It is carried out with the patient in either the sitting or prone position. If the sitting position is chosen a right atrial catheter should be placed and cardiac Doppler monitoring used to detect possible air embolism. A lower level cervical cordotomy can be carried out through an anterior approach with the patient in the supine position. Thoracic cordotomy is carried out with the patient in the prone or lateral decubitus position.

The posterior cordotomy approach in the cervical or thoracic area is essentially the same. A midline incision is made from the inion to C4 for cervical cordotomy and the thoracic cordotomy incision is centered over T2 to T4. A laminectomy is carried out, which is extended to the facet on the side of the spinal cord to be incised (Fig. 98-4). The dura is opened and sewn to the muscles laterally so as to gain maximum exposure. The arachnoid is opened and the dentate ligament is identified. The lateral attachment of the dentate to the dura can be cut or left intact, but in either case the dentate is held with a fine clamp.

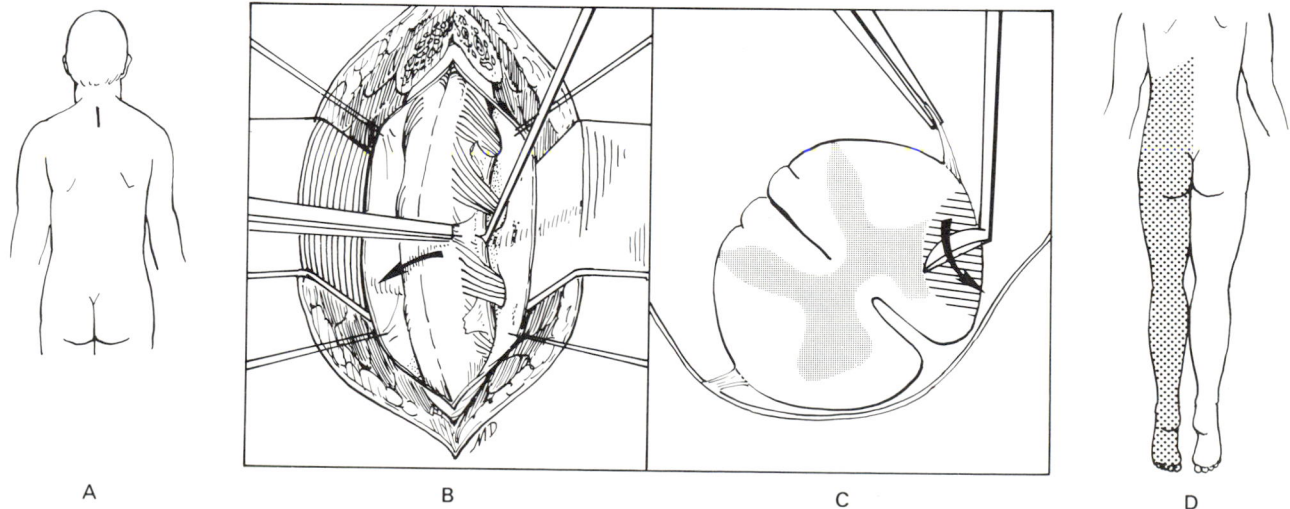

A   B   C   D

FIG. 98-4. A. Site of open thoracic cordotomy. B. and C. Method of performing open thoracic cordotomy. B. After T1–T2 laminectomy, the dura is opened and the dentate ligaments sectioned. The linea alba is grasped in a hemostat and the spinal cord is rotated 45°. C. A special cordotomy knife is used to section the anterolateral quadrant. D. Extent of analgesia on dorsal surface produced by right T1–T2 open cordotomy.

TABLE 98-4. Comparison of Results of Percutaneous and Open Cordotomy

Source	No. of Cases	Success (% of Total)		Follow-Up
		Early	Late	
Percutaneous operation				
Rosomoff (19)	1,279	93	40	10 yr
Ventafridda et al. (20)*	369	80	47	3 mo
Lipton (21)	809	84	76	1–10 yr
Tasker (22)	380	88	71	1 mo to death
Gildenberg (23)	288	90	65	6 mo
Mullan (24)	183	62		
White and Sweet (25)†	3,357	85		
Open operation				
White and Sweet (26)				
High thoracic	271 (M)	86		No late survivors
High thoracic	70 (NM)	85	62	1–30 yr
High cervical	30 (NM)	70	32	1–30 yr
French et al. (27)‡	200 (NM)	87	84	1 yr
Tasker (28)§	141 (NM)	84	69	

*Data from 18 centers.
†Data from 21 centers.
‡High thoracic.
§High cervical.
M, malignant; NM, nonmalignant.

The anterolateral surface of the spinal cord is viewed and an avascular area is found for the incision. A down-cutting cordotomy knife or a piece of angled razor blade held in a clamp is used to make the incision. The knife blade projects 6 mm in the cervical area and 4 to 5 mm in the thoracic area. The point is inserted just ventral to the dentate ligament, pulling the spinal cord onto the knife blade so as to penetrate cleanly. The blade cuts ventrally so as to transect the ventral quadrant down through the exit of the motor rootlets but to spare the medial funiculus.

In the thoracic area, if a bilateral cordotomy is required, the second side is sectioned one or two segments below the first cut. The dura is closed and the muscles and skin are approximated in layers. In the anterior approach, a collar incision at the C4 to C5 level is made from the right side. The midline muscles are retracted along with the trachea and esophagus and the C4 to C5 intervertebral disk is removed. An 18-mm hole in the opposing vertebral bodies is drilled down to the dura, which is then opened to expose the spinal cord beneath. The incision into the spinal cord is carried out in the same fashion as described for posterior cervical cordotomy. After the dura is closed a bone plug taken from a bone bank or from the patient's analgesic hip is inserted between the vertebrae, and the incision is closed in layers.

Results

After open cordotomy immediate relief was reported in 70 to 90% of patients who had undergone unilateral procedures and in 40 to 78% of those with bilateral procedures. Early failures were caused by postoperative pain, inadequate denervation, and immediate spread of pain to the opposite side. Late failures occurred from spread of the disease and from loss of analgesia. A comparison of results from a sample of the larger series is presented in Table 98-4.

Complications

Mortality rates for open cordotomy ranged from 3% for the unilateral procedure to 20% for bilateral procedures. Paresis was reported in 10 to 15% of patients after unilateral procedures and in 24 to 39% after bilateral procedures. Urinary complications were high, ranging from 14% for unilateral procedures to 92% for bilateral procedures. Major risk from hypotension was found in 22% of those who had undergone cordotomies. Respiratory complications comprised the most common cause of death, but the exact numbers were not listed. The respiratory morbidity rate was probably well in excess of 10% with a mortality rate as high as 20%. Postcordotomy dysesthetic syndromes can occur in 11% of patients. Open surgical cordotomy seems to be less effective and certainly has a higher risk of complication than the percutaneous techniques.

Conclusion

Percutaneous cordotomy is simpler and better tolerated than open surgical techniques. Because the anatomic and physiologic bases for pain relief are the same for all cordotomies, true differences in long-term results might not be discernible. However, such advantages as the ease of performance, drastic reduction of risk, and the additional advantages of and repeatability literally ad infinitum, make percutaneous cordotomy the procedure of choice.

B. MYELOTOMY

Commissural myelotomy for the treatment of pain was first described by Armour (29) in 1927. Putnam (30) was apparently unaware of this report when he claimed to have performed the first myelotomy in 1934. Since then the popularity of this operation has waxed and waned. It seems quite logical that neurosurgeons would aim at producing bilateral pain relief with a single low-risk procedure that has little risk of damage to the important spinal axonal systems. Unfortunately, this apparently attractive operation has not been as effective as predicted on theoretic grounds. After the initial attempts on a few patients, commissural myelotomy was applied on a relatively large scale by French and German neurosurgeons in the 1940s and 1950s (31–33), subsequently becoming relatively obsolete for several years. At the end of the 1960s Sourek (34–36) published encouraging results and once more aroused the interest of neurosurgeons in this technique. In the last 15 years the topic has recurred sporadically in the neurosurgical literature, with various results reported (37–51). Approximately 425 myelotomies have been reported in the neurosurgical literature.

Basic Considerations

The original aim of commissural myelotomy was the interruption of all the decussating spinothalamic fibers subserving pain perception on both sides of the body as they travel in the anterior commissure of the spinal cord. Theoretically, bilateral symmetric analgesia should have been achieved, with pain relief restricted to the segments where sensation had been altered. The length of the myelotomy incision should have been proportional to the extent of pain. What was seen, however, even after extensive longitudinal splitting of the spinal cord over several centimeters, was that a girdle of analgesia was present in the expected area but that pain relief extended caudally into regions that had no demonstrable sensory changes. Hence, the role of the spinothalamic fibers in pain relief after myelotomy is not clear. Various hypotheses have been proposed to explain this antalgic but not analgesic effect of myelotomy. Sourek (34–36) theorized that the spinal commissurotomy interrupts two systems that conduct pain information: the slow-conducting anterolateral system and the fast-conducting mediodorsal system. The latter was believed to have a somatotopic arrangement, and was contained in the medial portion of the posterior columns.

Sunder-Plassmann and Grunert (37) have reported their experiences with 56 midline myelotomies and described only bilateral segmental analgesia appropriate to the level of the myelotomy. In contrast, Hitchcock (38, 39) and Schvarcz (40, 51) carried out cervical stereotaxic myelotomies and reported extensive areas of pain relief without sensory changes. They thought that their procedure specifically interrupts an extralemniscal centrospinal multisynaptic pathway, with Schvarcz referring to "extralemniscal tractotomy."

From an anatomic standpoint, the only experimental findings have been published by Kerr and Lippman (52). They reported that the projections to the periaqueductal gray matter seen in cordotomy are topographically different from those seen in myelotomy. They also observed that in their experimental animals severe postoperative edema extended over a number of segments caudal or rostral to the end of the myelotomy incision. In patients who have had an open myelotomy, disorders attributable to damage to the posterior columns are frequently observed for several weeks after surgery. It is possible, therefore, that the region of the spinal cord that must be damaged to produce pain relief by midline myelotomy has not yet been clearly identified. It is unlikely that a specific axonal system is unrecognized in the spinal cord; more probable is the existence of a multisynaptic mesial system that surrounds the central canal and ascends to the mesial thalamus. Perhaps the interruption of a centrospinal multisynaptic system with no somatotopic arrangement provides pain relief. It is also possible that a downstream modulatory system is altered by this operation. In addition, some antalgic role could be ascribed to damage to fibers in the medial posterior columns.

Clinical Considerations

Technique

The two basic strategies for midline myelotomy are the following: open, requiring a laminectomy, opening of the dura, and making a lesion under direct vision; and closed, making a lesion through a needle that has been passed through the skin, between adjacent laminae, and into the spinal cord.

The open operation requires a midline dorsal incision that is usually performed in the low thoracic and upper lumbar area. A laminectomy is performed and the dura is opened widely. Retention sutures are used to hold the dura open and the spinal cord is visualized. The arachnoid is incised and the dorsal midline of the spinal cord is identified. The incision in the spinal cord is made in the exact midline between the two gracilis tracts and carried down ventrally until the ventral pia has been divided. The spinal cord is therefore totally transected so that the right and left sides no longer communicate. The central gray matter is of course destroyed, as are the decussating fibers that go on to form the spinothalamic tract (Fig. 98-5).

Different techniques have been described over several decades. It is obvious that spinal commissurotomy or midline myelotomy is by no means a standardized procedure. Similar results have been obtained with quite different operations: the level, length, and depth of the spinal lesions vary extensively. For example, some neurosurgeons have reported limited myelotomies or even single stereotaxic RF lesions; on the other hand, others have used complete longitudinal splitting of the spinal cord over multiple segments from 100 to 110 mm long. It appears that no reliable or widely accepted criteria exist as to how long or how deep the incision should be to interrupt all fibers subserving a given painful area. Most do agree that the depth of the incision should extend to the anterior sulcus of the spinal cord. Second, postoperative sensory changes are too variable to allow any physiologic appraisal of the effect of myelotomy; consequently, correlations between lesion size and site and outcome are impossible. Finally, the mechanism of pain relief after myelotomy is not understood.

Open myelotomy is a major surgical procedure that should be considered with caution. Patients in poor condition who have a short life expectancy are not often suitable. On the other hand, even the most extensive myelotomies have not guaranteed long-lasting pain relief. The variability of reported results indicates that at present this operation should not be considered to be a routine procedure (Table 98-5). Complications have been reported in 5 to 10% of the reported cases: postoperative dysesthesia can be distressing, and might last several weeks. Sensory disorders (mostly impairment or loss of proprioception) and motor and sphincter disturbances have not been rare.

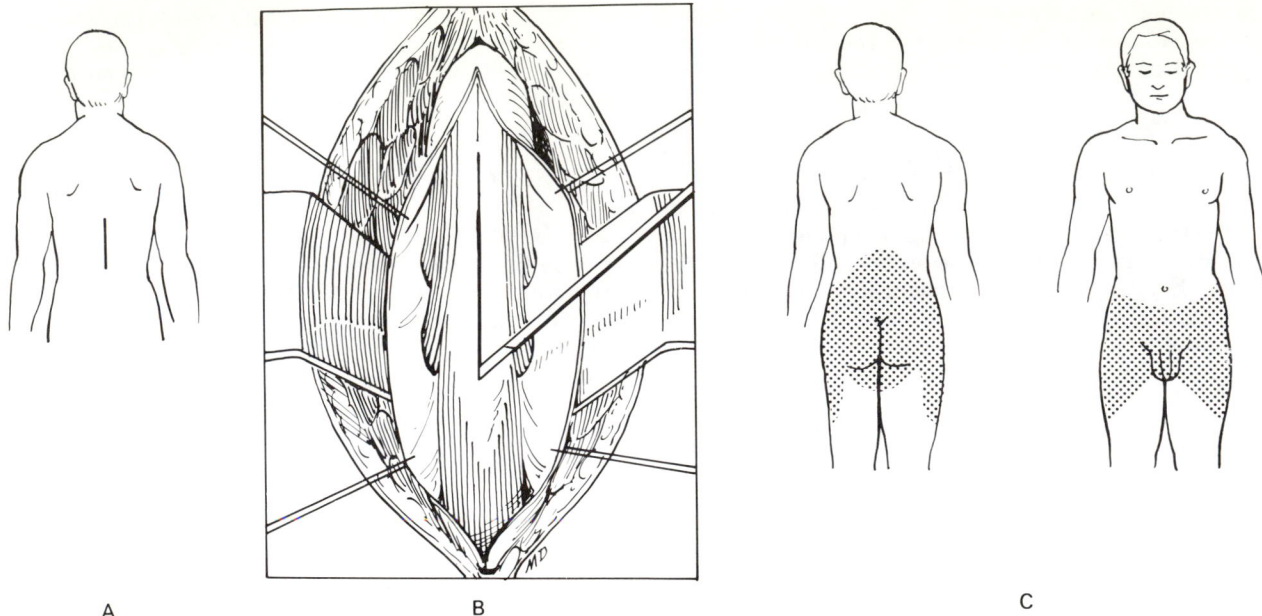

FIG. 98-5. *A.* Site of thoracolumbar midline myelotomy. *B.* Method of performing midline myelotomy in thoracolumbar region. After a laminectomy of T9–L1, the dura is opened and the dorsal midline of the spinal cord identified. A microknife is used to make a midline incision to the ventral pial surface. *C.* Extent of analgesia produced by thoracolumbar midline myelotomy.

TABLE 98-5. Results of Commissural Myelotomy

Source	Year of Report	No. of Cases	Results (% of Total)		Mortality Rate	Comments
			Success*	Complications		
Open operation						
Armour (29)	1927	1	0	0	100	Cancer
Putnam (30)	1934	3	67		33	Cancer
Wertheimer and Lecuire (31)	1953	107	65	14	7	93 cancer
Lembcke (33)	1964	12	100	0	0	
White and Sweet (26)	1969	1	100	0	0	Ultrasound lesion
Broager (42)	1974	34	82	6	3	31 cancer
Lippert et al. (44)	1974	16	94	6	0	12 cancer
Sunder-Plassmann and Grunert (37)	1976	58	26†	6	8	52 cancer
Papo and Luongo (45)	1976	10	20	20	0	9 cancer
Sourek (35)	1977	39	82	15	3	27 cancer
Cook and Kawakami (43)	1977	24	71	8	0	17 cancer
King (46)	1977	9	100	22	0	6 cancer
Gildenberg and Hirshberg (41)	1984	14	71	0	0	2 RF lesion; all cancer
Payne (47)	1984	24	75	8	0	Pelvic, lower limb cancer
Fink (48)	1984	1	100	0	0	Laser
Sweet and Poletti (49)	1984	9	67	22	0	Cancer
Adams et al. (50)	1988	24	63 CR‡ 30 PR§	17	0	21 neoplasms
All (mean):		329	65	10	4.5	
Percutaneous operation						
Hitchcock (39)	1974	26	50	0	0	Mainly cancer
Schvarcz (40)	1976	45	84	0	0	35 cancer
Gildenberg (41)	1984	2	0	0	0	Cancer
Schvarcz (51)	1984	79	78	Transient ataxia	0	Pelvic cancer
All (mean):		73	70	0	0	

*Success = pain relief for more than 3 months or until death.
†32% of patients had no follow-up.
‡CR, complete relief.
§PR, pertial relief.

Percutaneous myelotomy has been described by only four surgeons; the procedure has probably been performed in about 150 patients. Hitchcock (38, 39), Schvarcz (40), and Gildenberg and Hirshberg (41) have described making a lesion at C1, and Sourek (34–36) made lesions both at C1 and at D9–D10. The C1 lesion produced dramatic changes in sensation and pain relief over variable but widespread regions of the body. Follow-ups have been variable and the duration of pain relief is not clear.

Results

Despite the well-documented shortcomings, rewarding clinical results, mostly in cancer patients, have been reported in the literature (Table 98-5). Wertheimer and Lecuire (31), who applied myelotomy on a large scale nearly 40 years ago, initially stated that myelotomy provided satisfactory pain relief in most patients with bilateral pain in the lower half of the body. The same clinical material was subsequently reanalyzed by Dargent and colleagues (32), who concluded that myelotomy was effective only for the management of vaginal and visceral pain, whereas rectal and lower limb pain were not significantly influenced. Later, Sourek (34–36) and Broager (42) reported good results for the relief of lower limb pain, whereas Cook and Kawakami (43) and Lippert and associates (44) did not succeed in relieving lower limb or spinal pain. As for the pain located in the upper part of the body, Lembcke (33) and Cook and Kawakami (43) reported satisfactory results, whereas Sourek's (34–36) experience was disappointing. With stereotaxic cervical procedures, Hitchcock (38, 39) and Schvarcz (40) succeeded in most patients irrespective of the location of pain, whereas Papo and Luongo (45) obtained only short-lasting relief with a cervical mixed procedure (superficial splitting and deep coagulation) regardless of the type and location of pain, which always recurred in patients who survived more than 2 to 3 months. Sunder-Plassmann and Grunert (37) claimed that 91% of their patients were pain-free after midline myelotomy; 26% remained pain-free until their deaths or for the duration of follow-up, which lasted up to 4 years. Myelotomy is an uncommonly performed procedure confined to selected patients, even in the series reported by the authors who declared themselves satisfied with this procedure. All the published series have contained small numbers of patients.

Most surgeons agree that the typical open longitudinal midline myelotomy produces only a temporary loss of pain and temperature sensation in a girdle area that corresponds to the region of the cord incision. Loss of pain without sensory change caudal to the pain and temperature loss are also seen. How long this unexplained sensory loss persists is unclear, which is why myelotomy has not found widespread usage.

Conclusions

Myelotomy remains controversial; no reliable criteria are available for selecting patients suitable for this operation. In the absence of new information, caution should be exercised in regard to recommending myelotomy as the initial procedure for the relief of cancer pain. This procedure can be useful for the relief of bilateral pelvic and perineal pain because the other surgical alternative is bilateral cordotomy, which carries increased risk of bladder dysfunction (Chapter 98A). Epidural and intrathecal narcotics have unquestionably greatly reduced the numbers of patients who need ablative surgery for cancer pain. For the management of noncancer pain, open myelotomy is even more difficult to accept. So few surgeons have reported on C1 radiofrequency myelotomy that it is impossible to adequately evaluate this variant, which can have a different anatomic substrate from the low thoracic myelotomy. Certainly, the reports by Hitchcock (38, 39) and Schvarcz (40) are encouraging. At present, specific indications for myelotomy are rare. It is conceivable that increased understanding of the anatomy and physiology of mesial spinal cord systems can lead to a clearer picture of the optimal technique and indications for midline myelotomy. This might be an effective procedure, which has just not had a thorough trial.

C. DORSAL ROOT ENTRY ZONE LESIONS

The dorsal root entry zone (DREZ) operation entails making a series of lesions aimed at the substantia gelatinosa Rolandi and the surrounding fiber tracts. This operation was conceived and first used by Nashold and co-workers (53) in 1975 in a patient with severe pain secondary to brachial plexus avulsion. That patient has been reported to be free of pain ever since. By 1989 the Nashold group had done a total of 550 operations for various conditions (personal communication to Bonica 1989). Moreover, about 100 additional operations had been reported by others, and probably an equal number had been done but not reported. Although Nashold and associates have the most extensive experience with this operation, a number of other neurosurgeons are carrying it out. The data published to date permit us to make some inferences regarding its efficacy.

Basic Considerations

The premise of this operation is the destruction of dorsal horn neurons and perhaps of the axons traveling in juxtaposition to the gray matter, in those segments that correspond to the patient's reported area of pain. The detailed anatomy of the human dorsal horn is discussed in Chapter 3; this chapter contains only a superficial review relevant to this operation. The dorsal horn can be segmented on a cytoarchitectonic basis into six laminae; the five most superficial are clearly involved in the transmission of nociceptive information from the periphery and can play an essential role in some deafferentation or central pain states.

Not only are the synaptic connections from peripheral nociceptors localized in laminae I through V, but recent studies have shown major concentrations of opiate receptors, substance P, and other biologically active peptides in these regions. Indeed, many believe that the "gate," as described by Wall and Melzack (54), resides in this region of the spinal cord. The combination of classic neurophysiology and modern pharmacology points to this region as being critical in the processing of sensory information. In 1967, Loeser and Ward (55) reported that neurons in the dorsal horn become hyperactive when deafferentated. Nashold and co-workers (53) subsequently designed an operation to destroy the dorsal horn in patients with deafferentating lesions and severe pain. Initial successes have led to increasing use of this procedure; it has been almost exclusively used for pain states characterized by an injury to the nervous system referred to in this book as "deafferentation pain," and thought to have a peripheral-central pain mechanism; others have used the term "central pain."

Few, if any, traditional surgical procedures have a significant chance of alleviating the pain that follows deafferentation (56). Certainly, rhizotomy, cordotomy, myelotomy, or sympathectomy is unlikely to produce long-term pain relief. DREZ lesions appear to be remarkably effective in brachial plexus avulsion and are reasonably effective for the relief of postparaplegic pain, postamputation pain, postherpetic neuralgia, and for a small number of miscellaneous neuropathies and myelopathies.

The following chronic pain states represent diagnoses that thus far have been considered to be appropriate for treatment by DREZ lesions: brachial plexus avulsion; other brachial plexus lesions; sacral root avulsion; postparaplegic pain; phantom limb pain; stump pain; post-thoracotomy pain; postherpetic neuralgia; peripheral mononeuropathy; spinal cord tumor; multiple sclerosis; causalgia; and postrhizotomy pain.

Specific predictive factors to indicate a favorable outcome are being developed.

Indications

The indications for consideration of DREZ lesions as a treatment of chronic pain are the following: well-established diagnosis; failure of medical management; and the patient's understanding of alternative strategies, risks, and potential benefits. As already mentioned, the diagnoses listed above are those that have thus far been considered to be appropriate for DREZ lesions. The number of patients treated, however, is currently limited in some of these diagnostic groups.

Contraindications

Contraindications relate to the patient's general health and ability to withstand a major operation, including such factors as infection resistance, wound healing and coagulation of blood, and cardiopulmonary status. Patients who have significant emotional disturbances are rarely good surgical candidates, although the ravages of chronic pain can alter patients' judgment and emotions.

Clinical Considerations

Technique

Spinal Cord Lesions

DREZ lesions are performed under general anesthesia and require a laminectomy over each segment to be lesioned. For brachial plexus avulsion involving C5 to T1 dorsal roots, it is necessary to do a C4 through T1 laminectomy (Fig. 98-6). In the sacral segments the anatomy of the conus permits extensive lesioning with a more limited laminectomy. The dura is opened and

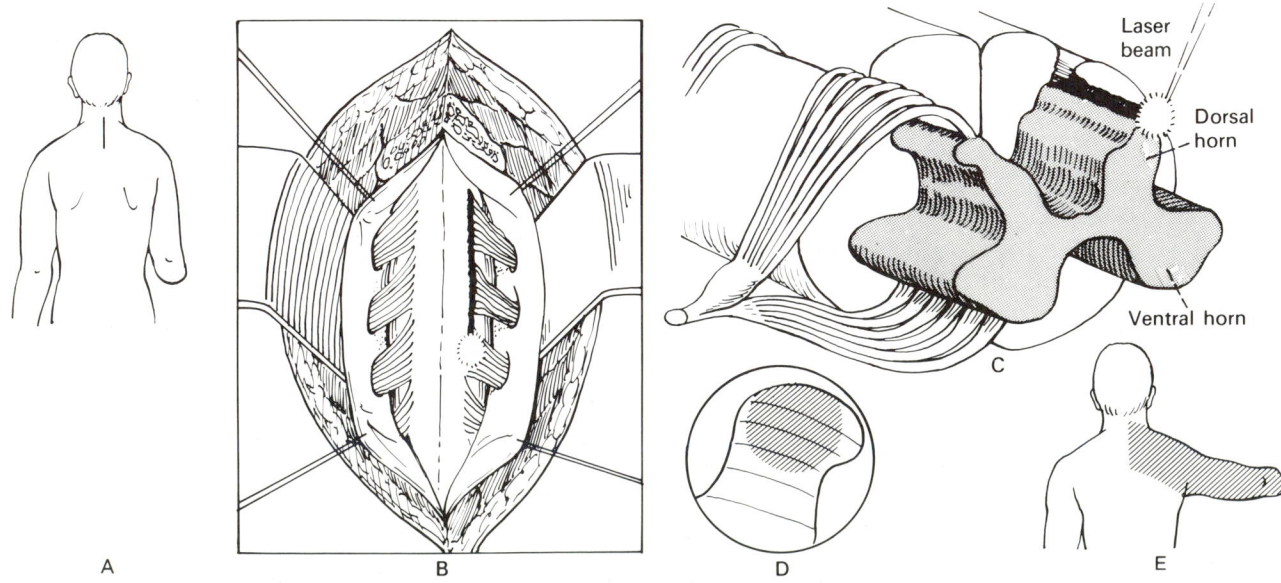

FIG. 98-6. A. Site of C5–T1 dorsal root entry zone (DREZ) lesions. B and C. Production of DREZ lesion using CO_2 laser. B. After a laminectomy of C5–T1, the dura is opened and the dorsolateral sulcus is identified. The pial vessels are coagulated and a continuous lesion made in the dorsolateral sulcus to destroy the dorsal root entry zone. C. After the laser is used, a microprobe is inserted into the dorsal horn to verify its destruction. D. Extent of lesion in dorsal horn. E. Analgesia produced by right C5–T1 DREZ lesions.

the spinal cord is visualized. The dorsolateral sulcus is identified; the operating microscope is an important adjunct. Most neurosurgeons section the dentate ligaments so that the spinal cord can be rotated to orient the dorsal horn vertically. When the dorsal roots have been avulsed the dorsolateral sulcus has a series of microcysts and gliosis. It is essential to see the intact dorsal roots rostral and caudal to the avulsion to identify the dorsolateral sulcus positively. Injury to nerves in the periphery or herpes zoster often leads to atrophic dorsal roots.

Nashold's (53, 65) careful studies of this new operative procedure should be required reading for any surgeon who wants to use DREZ lesions. His original RF electrode made too large a lesion and was apparently responsible for the high incidence of postoperative dorsal column and pyramidal tract dysfunction. The neurologic complication rate has fallen dramatically since Nashold shifted to a smaller thermistor-controlled electrode, which is 0.25 mm in diameter and 2 mm long for DREZ lesions in the spinal cord and 3 mm long for subnucleus caudalis lesions (65). Each lesion is made at 75° C for 15 seconds, and a series of lesions is done at 1-mm intervals; the longest series in one patient extending over a 5-cm length of the spinal cord. Using these parameters, each lesion in the spinal cord will measure 2×1.5 mm, which is adequate to destroy laminae I–V of the dorsal horn (65).

Sweet and Poletti (66) have described the deliberate use of a larger lesion in a small number of cases, and others have used variations of lesion making; none of the reports has been published. In the past few years the advent of the laser as a surgical tool has led to reports of the use of both CO_2 and argon lasers to lesion the DREZ (67, 68). In a recent cat study (69), the lesions in dorsal horn produced by the radiofrequency probe were compared with those produced by CO_2 laser. Histologic examination revealed that depths of the laser and RF lesions were similar but the RF lesions showed more lateral spread. Laser lesions comprised $4.4 \pm 1.6\%$ of the cross-sectional area of the spinal cord, whereas the RF lesions occupied $22.8 \pm 4\%$, demonstrating that the CO_2 laser produces smaller lesions than the RF electrode. This seems to be a promising technique that is less traumatic to the spinal cord if the parameters are carefully chosen. The dura is then closed in a watertight fashion.

The postoperative course is usually benign; many patients have transient dorsal column or pyramidal tract dysfunction, but few have permanent deficits. It is presently unclear which method of destroying the dorsal horn is safest and most effective; use of the laser is certainly faster than any other technique.

It is also unclear why lesions in the dorsal horn stop deafferentation pain states. Two or three autopsy reports published to date showed that DREZ lesions made at 40–50 nA for 5 to 15 seconds destroyed laminae I through IV of the dorsal horn and some of the white matter medial and lateral to the dorsal horn (66, 70). In the third patient, who died on the 28th postoperative day and in whom the DREZ lesions were done according to the parameters mentioned above, the lesions involving the dorsal horn extended halfway into lamina 6 but there was minimal impingement on the white matter (71). These findings suggest that the technique described above accomplishes the objective and that additional neurologic deficits in either the posterior column or pyramidal tract functions are not required for effective pain relief.

A major problem with DREZ lesions is proper localization of the lesions. The dorsolateral sulcus is varyingly discernible; when the dorsal roots have been avulsed, the dorsolateral region can be densely adherent to the arachnoid or to the dura. The dorsal horn is obliquely oriented and the electrode, knife, or laser beam must be angled or the spinal cord rotated to create the desired lesion and avoid damage to the pyramidal tract or the dorsal column. When roots have been avulsed or the spinal cord damaged, it is helpful to expose the levels rostral and, when feasible, caudal to the proposed operative area so that normal dorsal roots can be visualized and the dorsolateral sulcus can be identified. Evoked potentials can also be used to localize the superficial tracts in the spinal cord and assist in the placement of lesions (71).

Subnucleus Caudalis Lesions

More recently Nashold and associates (73, 74) reported the use of DREZ lesions on the subnucleus caudalis for the treatment of severe postherpetic neuralgia and other severe intractable facial pain. Following laminectomy of the C1–C3 vertebrae and a small suboccipital craniectomy, the lesion is made to extend from the upper dorsal rootlet of C2 to the turberculum cinereum, slightly rostral to the level of the obex and the fourth ventricle. Production of DREZ lesions in the subnucleus caudalis also entails destruction of the descending trigeminal tract; the anatomic correlate of pain relief is unclear (73, 85).

Results

Brachial Plexus Avulsion

The most common and most successful application of DREZ lesions is for the relief of the pain of brachial plexus avulsion. This traumatic disaster is most common in young men who ride motorcycles. Nashold's first patient suffered from this injury; at the time of this writing 155 patients have been reported, with an overall 83% success rate and many follow-ups of longer than 5 years (53, 57, 61, 67, 75 83). A few patients with sacral root avulsions are included in this series. No other diagnosis has as high a likelihood of success, and no other operation is as likely to relieve this type of deafferentation pain. Table 98-6 summarizes the results obtained to date.

Postparaplegic or Postquadriplegic Pain

Postparaplegic or postquadriplegic pain has also been relieved by DREZ lesions (61, 62, 67, 68, 75, 77, 83). To date 46 patients have been reported. The long-term success rate is 54%, but the duration of follow-up has been variable (Table 98-7). Some of the reported patients had drainage of post-traumatic syringomyelia at the same time; it is unclear if DREZ lesions alone are responsible for their pain relief. It is puzzling that distal spinal cordectomy does not often relieve this type of pain but that DREZ lesions are sometimes

TABLE 98-6. Results of DREZ Operation for Brachial Plexus Avulsion

Source	Year of Report	No. of Cases	Results (% of Total)		Follow-Up (Months)
			Success	Complications†	
Nashold et al. (53)*	1976	4	100	25	6–12
Nashold and Ostdahl (60)*	1979	18	72	50	6–42
Nashold et al. (61)*	1983	18	72		60
Levy et al. (67)	1983	1	100	0	12
Nashold (57)*	1984	57	80		60
Richter and Seitz (75)	1984	7	57	86	5–30
Samii and Moringlane (77)	1084	22	91	0	NR‡
Thomas and Jones (78)	1984	34	85	12	4–44
Nashold et al. (59)*	1985	37	62	33	96
Friedman and Bullitt (80)	1988	39	67	0	12–96
Campbell et al. (81)	1988	10	85	10	7–52
Ishijima et al. (82)	1988	19	82	10	21
Powers et al. (83)	1988	6	100	0	24
All (mean):		155	83	16	

†Complication defined as any permanent undesirable outcome.
*Same patients in series, so 57 is the total for the five Nashold series.
‡NR, not reported.

TABLE 98-7. Results of DREZ Operation for Paraplegic Pain

Source	Year of Report	No. of Cases	Results (% of Total)		Follow-Up (Months)
			Success	Complications†	
Nashold and Bullitt (58)*	1981	13	85	23	5–38
Levy et al. (67)	1983	2	50	0	8
Richter and Seitz (75)	1984	2	0	0	
Samii and Moringlane (77)	1984	5	80	0	
Sweet and Poletti (49)	1984	2	0	0	13
Nashold et al. (59)*	1985	28	54		60
Wiegand and Winkelmüller (84)	1985	20	50	5	5–34
Friedman and Bullitt (80)	1988	56	59	5	6–72
Powers et al. (83)	1988	9	67	22	4–40
All (mean):		96	56	5	

†Complication defined as any permanent undesirable outcome.
*Same patients in series.

TABLE 98-8. Results of DREZ Operation for Postamputation Pain

Source	Year of Report	No. of Cases	Results (% of Total)		Follow-Up (Months)
			Success	Complications†	
Nashold et al. (61)*	1983	5	100		6–12
Samii and Moringlane (77)	1984	2	50	0	NR§
Thomas and Jones (78)	1984	1	0	0	
Nashold et al. (59)*	1985	10	60		12–24
Saris et al. (85)*	1988				
Phantom		9	67		
Stump		6	0	45	6–48
Phantom and Stump		7‡	29‡		
Powers et al. (83)	1988	4	50	25	12
Ishijima et al. (82)	1988	6	50	15	21
All (mean):		35	37	6	

*Same patients in series.
†Complication defined as any permanent undesirable outcome.
‡Total number of cases in Saris et al. Series = 22, with a mean success rate of 36%.
§NR, not reported.

TABLE 98-9. Results of DREZ Operation for Postherpetic Neuralgia

Source	Year of Report	No. of Cases	Results (% of Total)		Follow-Up (Months)
			Success	Complications*	
Friedman et al. (62)†	1984	12	67	42	6–21
Friedman and Nashold (63)†	1984	17	59	35	6–25
Nashold et al. (59)†	1985	7	57	57	21
Friedman and Bullitt (80)†	1988	32	91, 53, 25‡	33	18–48
Powers et al. (83)	1988	3	67	33	24
All		35	56	38	

*Complication defined as any permanent undesirable outcome.
†Same patients in series.
‡100% immediate relief, 50% relief at 6 months, 25% relief at 18 months.

TABLE 98-10. Results of DREZ Operation for Other Neuropathies and Myelopathies

Source	Year of Report	No. of Cases	Results (% of Total)		Follow-up (Months)
			Success	Complications*	
Samii and Moringlane (77)	1984	11	73	0	NR†
Thomas and Jones (78)	1984	4	50	12	NR
Nashold et al. (59)	1985	7	86	NR	6–12
Ishijima et al. (82)	1988	6	50	33	22
Powers et al. (83)	1988	18	39	22	40
All		46	57	18	

*Complication defined as any permanent undesirable outcome.
†NR, not reported.

effective. It should be recognized that this is not radicular pain, nor is it the pain associated with osseous instability that can occur with traumatic injury to the vertebral column. Although cordotomy is sometimes effective for this type of pain, the long-term results do not approach those obtained with DREZ lesions.

Postamputation Pain

Another type of central pain that has responded to DREZ lesions is postamputation pain (59, 61, 77, 78, 82–83, 85) (Table 98-8). Hidden in this category are two different types of pain syndromes, stump pain and phantom limb pain. Until a recent paper by the Nashold group, these two types of pain that follow amputation had not been analyzed separately (64, 85). The overall results for postamputation pain are 39% success in a group of 28 patients. Phantom limb pain is highly likely to respond (6 of 9 patients), whereas stump pain was never relieved (0 of 6 patients). When phantom limb pain and stump pain were both present good results were noted in 2 of 7 patients, but only the phantom pain responded regularly. None of the other reports clearly discriminated between phantom limb pain and stump pain. Because of the aforementioned failures, Nashold no longer does DREZ lesion for stump pain (personal communication to J.J. Bonica 1989).

Postherpetic Neuralgia and Other Disorders

In the earlier reports on the use of DREZ lesion for postherpetic neuralgia, Nashold and associates (59, 62, 63) reported that 10 of 17 patients (59%) had good pain relief accompanied by a complication rate of 35%. In

the most recent report by the Nashold group (80) on 32 patients who had postherpetic pain for 6 months to 11 years and were followed 6 months to 6 years postoperatively, 29 (91%) had immediate relief, but at 6 months the figure dropped to 17 (53%) and at 18 months and thereafter only 8 (25%) had persistent relief of postherpetic neuralgia involving the spinal nerves (Table 98-9). Thirty-one patients with various myelopathies and neuropathies have also been treated with DREZ lesions (56, 65, 71, 72). Approximately two-thirds had good results, with follow-ups of 6 to 19 months and a complication rate of 10 to 20%. The results are summarized in Table 98-10.

Results with Subnucleus Caudalis DREZ Lesions

In the most recent report the Nashold group (74) had done DREZ lesions of the subnucleus caudalis in 28 patients with severe facial pain. Of these 6 of 9 patients (67%) with postherpetic neuralgia and 2 of 3 patients (67%) with anesthesia delorosa derived prolonged relief whereas only 1 of 5 patients (20%) with tic douleureux and 1 of 4 patients (25%) with cancer pain had pain relief that persisted over time. Ishijima et al. (82) also reported a 67% relief of postherpetic neuralgia and only partial relief in 8 patients with tic douleureux.

Comments and Conclusions

Until more reports are published, it is impossible to describe the optimal indications for DREZ lesions in the management of chronic pain. The DREZ lesion is the only operation that was specifically designed to treat central and deafferentation pains. It is widely recognized that all standard ablative neurosurgical procedures are much more effective against the pains associated with nociception (especially cancer pain) than they are against peripheral-central pain states. It is presently unclear whether DREZ lesions are ever to be tried in patients with cancer pain; dorsal rhizotomy seems to be a less formidable operation for denervation of the painful area. The results of rhizotomy are variable, however, and it is not known if the addition of ganglionectomy can improve them. Perhaps DREZ lesions will be effective in this type of pain. If so, this new operation might be used with greater frequency.

More than any other ablative procedure, use of DREZ lesions can achieve variable results because of differences in lesion placement. It is not known how many segments above or below the level of injury the lesions should be made. Patients who have failed to obtain good pain relief might continue to suffer because the lesions did not extend far enough rostrally or caudally, yet the failure to relieve pain is ascribed to a deficiency of the operation itself. The poor results that sometimes follow DREZ lesions could be caused by failure of the surgeon to destroy the necessary amount of tissue, or could be a result of inherent shortcomings in the operation as a concept (57).

REFERENCES

1. Schuller, A.: Über operative Durchtrennung der Reckenmarksstrange (chordotomie). Wien. Med. Wochenschra, 60:2292, 1910.
2. Spiller, W.G., and Martin, E.: The treatment of persistent pain of organic origin in the lower part of the body by division of the anterolateral column of the spinal cord. JAMA, 58:1489, 1912.
3. Foerster, O., and Gagel, O.: Die Vorderseiten strangdurchschneidung beim Menschen. Eine klinisch-pathophysiologisch-anatomische Studie. Z. Gesamte Neurol. Psychiatr., 138:1, 1932.
4. Mullan, S., et al.: Percutaneous interruption of spinal-pain tracts by means of a strontium-90 needle. J. Neurosurg., 20:931, 1963.
5. Mullan, S., et al.: Percutaneous intramedullary cordotomy utilizing the unipolar anodal electrolytic lesion. J. Neurosurg., 22:548, 1965.
6. Rosomoff, H.L., et al.: Percutaneous radiofrequency cervical cordotomy: Technique. J. Neurosurg., 23:639, 1965.
7. Crue, B.L., Todd, E.M., and Carregal, E.J.A.: Posterior approach for high cervical percutaneous radiofrequency cordotomy. Confin. Neurol., 30:11, 1968.
8. Fox, J.L.: Experimental relationship of radiofrequency electrical current and lesion size for application to percutaneous cordotomy. J. Neurosurg., 33:415, 1970.
9. Gildenberg, P.L., et al.: Anterior percutaneous cervical cordotomy. Determination of target point and calculations of angle of insertion. Technical note. J. Neurosurg., 28:173, 1968.
10. Gildenberg, P.L., et al.: Impedance measuring device for detection of penetration of the spinal cord in anterior percutaneous cervical cordotomy. Technical note. J. Neurosurg., 30:87, 1969.
11. Hitchcock, E.: Stereotaxic spinal surgery: A preliminary report. J. Neurosurg., 31:386, 1969.
12. Lin, P.M., Gildenberg, P.L., and Polakoff, P.P.: An anterior approach to percutaneous lower cervical cordotomy. J. Neurosurg., 25:553, 1966.
13. Taren, J.A., Davis, R., and Crosby, E.C.: Target physiologic correlation in stereotaxic cervical cordotomy. J. Neurosurg., 30:569, 1969.
14. Tasker, R.R., and Organ, L.W.: Percutaneous cordotomy. Physiologic identification of target site. Confin. Neurol., 35:110, 1973.
15. Todd, E.M., Crue, B.L., and Carregal, E.J.A.: Posterior percutaneous tractotomy and cordotomy. Confin. Neurol., 31:106, 1969.
16. Mullan, J.: Percutaneous cordotomy. J. Neurosurg., 35:360, 1971.
17. Krieger, A.J., et al.: Changes in ventilatory patterns after ablation of various respiratory feedback mechanisms. J. Appl. Physiol., 33:431, 1972.
18. Rosomoff, H.L., Krieger, A.J., and Kuperman, A.S.: Effects of percutaneous cervical cordotomy on pulmonary function. J. Neurosurg., 31:620, 1969.
19. Rosomoff, H.L.: Stereotaxic cordotomy. In Neurological Surgery, Vol. 6. Edited by J.R. Youmans. Philadelphia, W.B. Saunders, 1982, pp. 3672–3685.

20. Ventafridda, V., DeConno, F., and Fochi, C.: Cervical percutaneous cordotomy. In Advances in Pain Research and Therapy. Edited by J.J. Bonica, et al. New York, Raven Press, 1982, pp. 185–198.
21. Lipton, S.: Percutaneous cordotomy. In Textbook of Pain. Edited by P.D. Wall and R. Melzack. New York, Churchill Livingstone, 1984, pp. 632–638.
22. Tasker, R.R.: Percutaneous cervical cordotomy. In Operative Neurosurgical Techniques: Indications, Methods, and Results. 2nd Ed. Edited by H.H. Schmidek and W.H. Sweet. Orlando, FL, Grune & Stratton, 1988, pp. 1191–1205.
23. Gildenberg, P.L.: Percutaneous cervical cordotomy. Appl. Neurophysiol., 39:97, 1976–1977.
24. Mullan, S.: Percutaneous cordotomy for pain. In Pain. Edited by R.S. Knighton and P.R. Dumke. Boston, Little, Brown & Co., 1966, pp. 321–330.
25. White, J.C., and Sweet, W.H.: Anterolateral cordotomy: Open vs. closed comparison of end results. In Advances in Pain Research and Therapy. Vol. 3. Edited by J.J. Bonica et al. New York, Raven Press, 1979, pp. 911–919.
26. White, J.C., and Sweet, W.H.: Pain and the Neurosurgeon. A Forty-Year Experience. Springfield, IL., Charles C Thomas, 1969.
27. French, L.A., Chou, S.N., and Story, J.L.: Cervical tractotomy: Technique and clinical usefulness. In Pain. Edited by R.S. Knighton and P.R. Dumke. Boston, Little, Brown & Co., 1966.
28. Tasker, R.R.: Open cordotomy. Prog. Neurosurg., 8:1,14, 1977.
29. Armour, D.: Surgery of the spinal cord and its membranes. Lancet, 1:691, 1927.
30. Putnam, T.J.: Myelotomy of the commissure. Arch. Neurol. Psychiatry, 32:1189, 1934.
31. Wertheimer, P., and Lecuire, J.: La myélotomie commissurale postérieure. Acta Chir. Belg., 52:568, 1953.
32. Dargent, M., et al.: Les problemes posées par la douleur dans l'évolution des cancers gynécologiques. Lyon Chirurgical, 59:62, 1963.
33. Lembcke, W.: Über die mediologitudinale Chordotomie in Halsmarkbereich. Z. Chir., 89:349, 1964.
34. Sourek, K.: Commissural myelotomy. J. Neurosurg. 31:524, 1969.
35. Sourek, K.: Mediolongitudinal myelotomy. Prog. Neurosurg., 8:15, 1977.
36. Sourek, K.: Central thermocoagulation of the cord for the relief of pain. In Neurological Surgery. Proceedings of the World Federation of Neurosurgery-Society of Munich. Edited by Stuttgart, Georg. Thiem Verlag., 1981, pp. 66–72.
37. Sunder-Plassmann, M., and Grunert, V.: Commissural myelotomy for drug-resistant pain. In Clinical Microsurgery. Edited by W.T. Koos, F.W. Boeck, and R.F. Spetzler. Stuttgart, Georg. Thiem Verlag., 1976, pp. 165–170.
38. Hitchcock, E.: Stereotactic cervical myelotomy. J. Neurol. Neurosurg. Psychiatry, 33:224, 1970.
39. Hitchcock, E.: Stereotactic myelotomy. Proc. R. Soc. Med., 67:771, 1974.
40. Schvarcz, J.R.: Stereotactic extralemniscal myelotomy. J. Neurol. Neurosurg. Psychiatry, 39:53, 1976.

41. Gildenberg, P.N., and Hirshberg, R.M.: Limited myelotomy for the treatment of intractable cancer pain. J. Neurol. Neurosurg. Phychiatry, *47*:94, 1984.

42. Broager, B.: Commissural myelotomy. Surg. Neurol., *2*:71, 1974.

43. Cook, A.W., and Kawakami, Y.: Commissural myelotomy. J. Neurosurg., *47*:1, 1977.

44. Lippert, R.G., Hosobuchi, Y., and Nielsen, S.L.: Spinal commissurotomy. Surg. Neurol., *2*:373, 1974.

45. Papo, I., and Luongo, A.: High cervical commissural myelotomy in the treatment of pain. J. Neurol. Neurosurg. Psychiatry, *39*:705, 1976.

46. King, R.B.: Anterior commissurotomy for intractable pain. J. Neurosurg., *47*:7, 1977.

47. Payne, N.S.: Dorsal longitudinal myletomy for the control of perineal and lower body pain. Pain (Suppl. 2):S320, 1984.

48. Fink, R.A.: Neurosurgical treatment of non-malignant intractable rectal pain: Microsurgical commissural myelotomy with the carbon dioxide laser. Neurosurgery, *14*:64, 1984.

49. Sweet, W.H., and Poletti, C.E.: Operations in the brain stem and spinal canal, with an appendix on open cordotomy. *In* Textbook of Pain. Edited by P.D. Wall and R. Melzack. Edinburgh, Churchill Livingstone, 1984, pp. 615–631.

50. Adams, J.E., Lippert, R., and Hosobuchi, Y.: Commissural myelotomy. *In* Current Techniques in Operative Neurosurgery. 2nd Ed. Edited by W.H. Sweet and H.H. Schmidek. New York, Grune & Stratton, 1988, pp. 1185–1189.

51. Schvarcz, J.R.: Stereotactic high cervical extralemniscal myelotomy for pelvic cancer pain. Acta Neurochir. (Suppl. 33):431, 1984.

52. Kerr, F.W.L., and Lippman, H.H.: The primate spinothalamic tract as demonstrated by anterolateral cordotomy and commissural myelotomy. *In* Advances in Neurology, Vol. 4. Edited by J.J. Bonica. New York, Raven Press, 1974, pp. 147–156.

53. Nashold, B.S., Jr., Urban, B., and Zorub, D.S.: Phantom pain relief by focal destruction of the substantia gelatinosa of Rolando. *In* Advances in Pain Research and Therapy, Vol. 1. Edited by J.J. Bonica and D. Albe-Fessard. New York, Raven Press, 1976, pp. 959–963.

54. Wall, P.D., and Melzack, R.: Pain mechanisms: A new theory. Science, *150*:971, 1965.

55. Loeser, J.D., and Ward, A.A., Jr.: Some effects of deafferentation on neurons of the cat spinal cord. Arch. Neurol., *17*:629, 1967.

56. Zorub, D.S., Nashold, B.S., Jr., and Cook, W.A., Jr.: Avulsion of the brachial plexus: I. A review with implications on the therapy of intractable pain. Surg. Neurol., *2*:347, 1974.

57. Nashold, B.S., Jr.: Current status of the DREZ operation: 1984. Neurosurgery, *15*:942, 1984.

58. Nashold, B.S., Jr., and Bullitt, E.: Dorsal root entry zone lesions to control central pain in paraplegics. J. Neurosurg., *55*:414, 1981.

59. Nashold, B.S., Jr., Higgins, A.C., and Blumenkopf, B.: Dorsal root entry zone lesions for pain relief. *In* Neurosurgery. Edited by R.H. Wilkins and S.S. Rangachary. New York, McGraw-Hill, 1985, pp. 2433–2437.

60. Nashold, B.S., Jr., and Ostdahl, R.H.: Dorsal root entry zone lesions for pain relief. J. Neurosurg., *51*:59, 1979.

61. Nashold, B.S., Jr., et al.: Dorsal root entry zone lesions: A new neurosurgical therapy for deafferentation pain. Adv. Pain Res. Ther., *5*:739, 1983.

62. Friedman, A.H., and Nashold, B.S., Jr.: Dorsal root entry zone lesions for the treatment of postherpetic neuralgia. Neurosurgery, *15*:969, 1984.

63. Friedman, A.H., Nashold, B.S., Jr., and Ovelmen-Levitt, J.: Dorsal root entry zone lesions for the treatment of postherpetic neuralgia. J. Neurosurg., *60*:1258, 1984.

64. Saris, S.C., Iacono, R.P., and Nashold, B.S., Jr.: Dorsal root entry zone lesions for post-amputation pain. J. Neurosurg., *62*:72, 1985.

65. Nashold, B.S., Jr.: Neurosurgical technique of the dorsal root entry zone operation. Appl. Neurophysiol., *51*:136, 1985.

66. Sweet, W.H., and Poletti, C.E.: Operations in the brain stem and spinal canal, with an appendix on open cordotomy. *In* Textbook of Pain. 2nd Ed. Edited by P.D. Wall and R. Melzack. Edinburgh, Churchill Livingstone, 1989, pp. 811–831.

67. Levy, W.J., et al.: Laser-induced dorsal root entry zone lesions for pain control: Report of three cases. J. Neurosurg., *59*:884, 1983.

68. Powers, S.K., et al.: Pain relief from dorsal root entry zone lesions made with argon and carbon dioxide microsurgical lasers. J. Neurosurg., *61*:841, 1984.

69. Elias, Z., Powers, S.K., and Bullitt, E.: Evalutation of laser- and rediofrequency-generated dorsal root entry zone lesions in the cat. Appl. Neurophysiol., *51*:255, 1988.

70. Richter, H., and Schachenmayr, W.: Is the substantia gelatinosa the target in dorsal root entry zone lesions? An autopsy report. Neurosurgery, *15*:913, 1984.

71. Iacono, R.P., Aguirre, M.L., and Nashold, B.S., Jr.: Anatomic examination of human dorsal root entry zone lesions. Appl. Neurophysiol., *51*:225, 1988.

72. Campbell, J.A., and Miles, J.: Evoked potentials as an aid to lesion making in the dorsal root entry zone. Neurosurgery, *15*:951, 1984.

73. Nashold, B.S., Jr., and Brophy, B.P.: The neurosurgeon and chronic pain. *In* Handbook of Chronic Pain Management. Edited by G.D. Burrows, D. Elton, and G.V. Stanley. New York, Elsevier, 1987, pp. 383–440.

74. Bernard, E.J., Nashold, B.S., and Caputi, F.: Clinical review of nucleus caudalis dorsal root entry lesions for facial pain. Appl. Neurophysiol., *51*:218, 1988.

75. Richter, H., and Seitz, K.: Dorsal root entry zone lesions for the control of deafferentation pain: Experiences in ten patients. Neurosurgery, *15*:956, 1984.

76. Samii, M.: Thermocoagulation of the substantia gelatinosa for pain relief (preliminary report). *In* Phantom and Stump Pain. Edited by J. Siegfried and M. Zimmerman. Berlin, Springer-Verlag, 1981, pp. 156–159.

77. Samii, M., and Moringlane, J.R.: Thermocoagulation of the dorsal root entry zone for the treatment of intractable pain. Neurosurgery, *15*:953, 1984.

78. Thomas, D.G.T., and Jones, S.J.: Dorsal root entry zone lesions (Nashold's procedure) in brachial plexus avulsion. Neurosurgery, *15*:966, 1984.

79. Thomas, D.G.T., and Sheehy, J.P.R.: Dorsal root entry zone lesions (Nashold's procedure) for pain relief following brachial plexus avulsion. J. Neurol. Neurosurg. Psychiatry, *46*:924, 1983.

80. Friedman, A.H., and Bullitt, E.: Dorsal root entry zone lesions in the treatment of pain following brachial plexus avulsion, spinal cord injury and herpes zoster. Appl. Neurophysiol., *51*:164, 1988.

81. Campbell, J.N., Solomon, C.T., and James, C.S.: The Hopkins experience with lesions of the dorsal horn (Nashold's operation) for pain from avulsion of the brachial plexus. Appl. Neurophysiol., *51*:170, 1988.

82. Ishijima, B., et al.: Lesions of spinal and trigeminal dorsal root entry zone for deafferentation pain: Experience of 35 cases. Appl. Neurophysiol., *51*:175, 1988.

83. Powers, S.K., Barbaro, N.M., and Levy, R.M.: Pain control with laser-produced dorsal root entry zone lesions. Appl. Neurophysiol., *51*:243, 1988.

84. Wiegand, H., and Winklemüller, W.: Behandlung des Deafferentierungsschmerzes durch Hochfrequenzläsion der Hinterwurzeleintrittszone. Deutsche Med. Wochenschr., *110*:216, 1985.

85. Saris, S.C., Iacono, R.P., and Nashold, B.S.: Successful treatment of phantom pain with dorsal root entry zone coagulation. Appl. Neurophysiol., *51*:188, 1988.

99 • OPERATIONS ON THE BRAIN AND BRAIN STEM FOR CHRONIC PAIN

PETER J. JANNETTA, PHILLIP L. GILDENBERG, JOHN D. LOESER,
WILLIAM H. SWEET, *and* GEORGE A. OJEMANN

with contributions by JOHN J. BONICA

THIS chapter is the last devoted to a discussion of neuroablative and research procedures for the relief of chronic pain. It focuses on operations on the brain and brain stem, and consists of five sections: A, Microvascular Decompression for Trigeminal Neuralgia, written by Jannetta; B, Medullary and Mesencephalic Tractotomy, written by Loeser and Gildenberg; C, Thalamotomy and Hypothalamotomy, written by Gildenberg and Loeser; D, Precentral and Postcentral Gyrectomy, written by Sweet; and E, Frontal Lobe Operations for Pain, written by Ojemann. Bonica collaborated with Loeser in editing and amplifying the text and in the development of some of the illustrations and the computations and revision of all of the tables so that they are presented in the same format.

A. MICROVASCULAR DECOMPRESSION FOR TRIGEMINAL NEURALGIA

The development of microvascular decompression as a treatment for trigeminal neuralgia depended on the application of modern technology to operative neurosurgery. In the 1930s, Dandy (1, 2) made significant observations regarding compression of the trigeminal nerve in the cerebellopontine angle by blood vessels and tumors in many patients with trigeminal neuralgia. Gardner and Miklos (3), and Gardner (4), in a small series of patients operated on in the 1950s and early 1960s, observed similar abnormalities and in 1959 actually reported a case in which a blood vessel was mobilized away from the trigeminal nerve. Neither Gardner nor Miklos, both superb neurosurgeons, could formulate complete hypotheses about a vascular cause of trigeminal neuralgia, and their ideas were not accepted by others in the field.

With the advent of the surgical binocular microscope in neurosurgical procedures, and specifically for cranial nerve problems in the cerebellopontine angle, further observations on the causes of trigeminal neuralgia have been made and validated. The first microvascular decompression of the facial nerve in a patient with hemifacial spasm was performed in June 1966 (5). General acceptance of the vascular cause of trigeminal neuralgia took many years to develop.

Basic Considerations

It is now generally acknowledged that trigeminal neuralgia is a problem of the aging process that depends primarily on two degenerative conditions. The first is arterial elongation and deterioration, presumably arteriosclerotic in nature (6). This causes the blood vessels around the base of the brain to loop and compress various cranial nerves, including the trigeminal nerve, at root entry zones and the junctional area between central and peripheral myelin. The second condition is sagging of the hindbrain, which can contribute both to venous and to arterial compression of the cranial nerves. Vascular compression is the primary cause of trigeminal neuralgia even if tumors are present, because tumors almost always cause trigeminal neuralgia by dislocating blood vessels into the root entry zone of the trigeminal nerve. Blood vessels can be multiple and small, and the compression can be quite subtle. This is amply emphasized by my operative findings and those of others (Tables 99-1 and 99-2).

Configuration of Compressions

Various configurations of compressing blood vessels that have been found in patients with trigeminal neuralgia are shown in Figure 99-1. A fairly precise clinical correlation exists between the location of the blood vessel on the nerve and the distribution of the pain. An elongated superior cerebellar artery is the most common (80%) cause of trigeminal neuralgia and lower facial pain. The most common cause of pain exclusively in the distribution of the second division (V2) is a blood vessel on the lateral side of the nerve, usually an aberrant trigeminal vein bridging to the dura mater near Meckel's cave. The rare V1 pain is caused by a blood

TABLE 99-1. Results of Microvascular Decompression for Trigeminal Neuralgia

Findings	Patients	
	No.	%
Arterial compression	242	58.9
Venous compression	54	13.0
Mixed arterial-venous compression	96	23.3
Aneurysm	1	0.2
Arteriovenous malformation	1	0.2
Tumor	15	4.0
No pathologic lesion identified	1	0.2
Unrecorded	1	0.2
All:	411	100.0

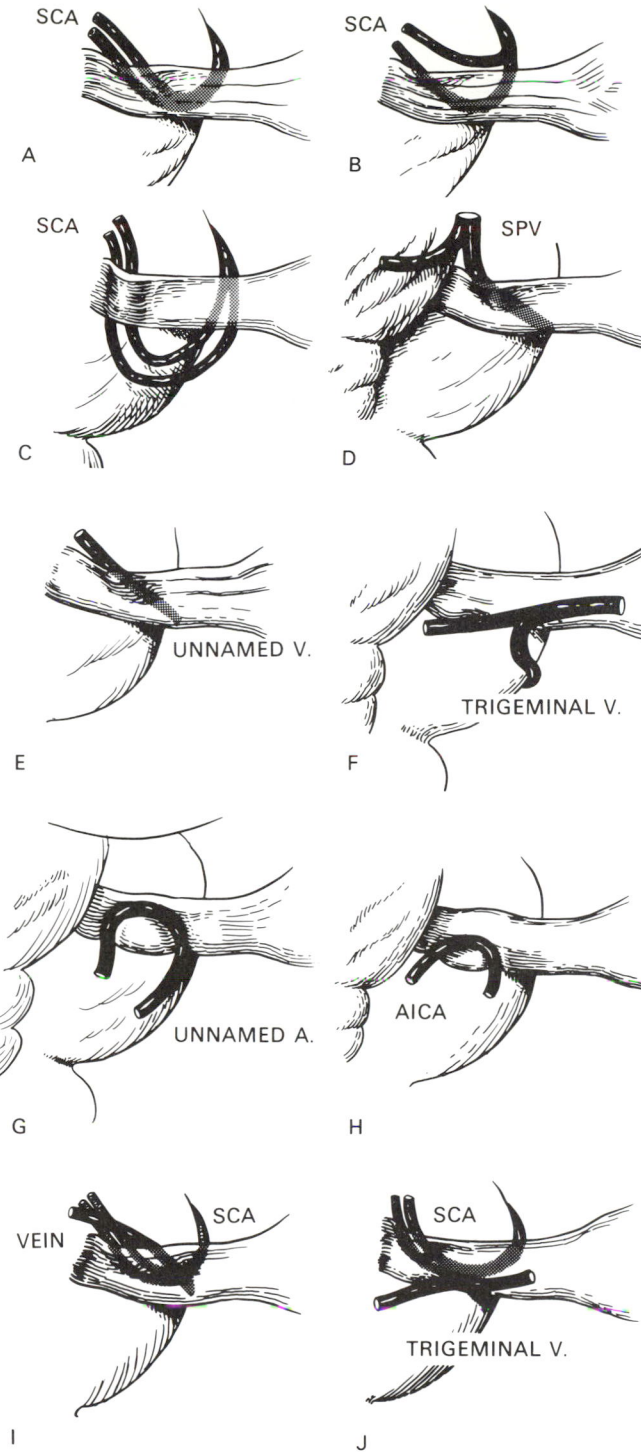

FIG. 99-1. Vascular relationships of the trigeminal nerve in patients with trigeminal neuralgia. ***A–C.*** Various configurations of the superior cerebellar artery (SCA) can be hidden by the ala of the cerebellum. ***D.*** The superior petrosal vein (SPV) can be the cause of trigeminal neuralgia. ***E–G.*** Veins or arteries on the lateral aspect of the nerve are the most common cause of neuralgia in the second division. ***H.*** A loop of the anterior inferior cerebellar artery (AICA). ***I*** and ***J.*** Multiple blood vessels on the same or all sides of the trigeminal nerve are not infrequently found in patients with trigeminal neuralgia. Modified from Jannetta, P.J.: Trigeminal neuralgia: Treatment by microvascular compression. *In* Neurosurgery. Edited by R.H. Wilkins and S.S. Rengachary. New York, McGraw-Hill, 1984, p. 2360.

vessel on the caudal side of the nerve. The junctional area of central and peripheral myelin in the trigeminal nerve is at the brain stem in the motor proprioceptive and intermediate fascicles, but extends quite distally in the portio major. Therefore, caudal and lateral blood vessels causing V1 or V2 tic can be distal on the nerve.

In the past, the best operative treatment for trigeminal neuralgia consisted of a "tradeoff" in which the surgeon traded numbness in the patient's face for the prior pain. I believe that microvascular decompression (MVD) is a definitive procedure that eliminates the cause of the pain and should be the first indicated operative treatment (7–9). Denervative procedures including alcohol injection, rhizotomy, and even a highly refined current technique such as glycerol rhizotomy (10, 11) should be used in those who fail to obtain relief with MVD or who are too frail to undergo general anesthesia and a major intracranial operation. The quality of survival is better in the patient who is not made numb prior to the operation by neurolytic or ablative procedures and who has less threat of recurrence. A fairly large number of reports have now been published by other investigators that indicate findings, complications, and operative results (7–9, 12–22). Other neurosurgeons might prefer gangliolysis as the initial surgical procedure.

Results

Table 99-3 lists my operative results for MVD and Table 99-4 presents those reported by others. It is apparent that MVD produces complete relief of pain without numbness in about 82 to 85% of patients; some patients do have late relapses. Another 10% of patients, usually those with a protracted history of tic douloureux (over 8 to 10 years), can have some intermittent residual pain that is relieved by phenytoin or for which no medication is necessary. The failure rate is about 10%, in which case exploration is indicated and a second or even third MVD done. If no lesion can be found, a denervative procedure such as glycerol or radiofrequency rhizotomy might be warranted. I have also used microvascular decompression in a much smaller number of patients with glossopharyngeal neuralgia and in whom the root of the nerve was compressed by a vessel with beneficial results similar to those for trigeminal neuralgia.

MVD can be accomplished with a mortality rate of about 0.5% and a relatively small incidence of complications (Tables 99-5 and 99-6). In regard to the rate of recurrence of pain, Barba and Alksne (23) found that the recurrence rate is 50% in those patients who have had a prior destructive procedure, versus 7% when MVD is the primary procedure. This is obviously helpful information in the surgical decision-making process.

Since these data were analyzed we have done over 600 additional operations with similar beneficial results and no deaths in the last 850 patients (personal communications to J.J. Bonica 1989).

Clinical Considerations

Technique

Microvascular decompression is performed with the patient under general anesthesia in the lateral

TABLE 99-2. Results of Microvascular Decompression for Trigeminal Neuralgia

Source	No. of Patients	Vascular Compression		Tumors		Indefinite Pathology		Other	
		No.	%	No.	%	No.	%		
Petty (12); Petty et al. (13, 14)	50	44	88	3	6	3	6		
Apfelbaum (15)	55	54	98	1	2				
Lazar (16)	15	14	93					1 (MS)*	
Rhoton (17)	10	10	100						
Weidmann (18)	10	10	100						
Voorhies and Patterson (19)	32	24	75	4	12.5			4 (1 MS)†	
Burchiel et al. (20)	42	36	86			6	14		
Rushworth and Smith (21)	17	17	100						
All/mean:	231	209	90.5	8	3.4	9	3.9	5	2.2

*MS, multiple sclerosis.
†REZ not visualized in 2, adhesions in 1, MS in 1.

TABLE 99-3. Results of Microvascular Decompression for Trigeminal Neuralgia

Results of Operation	Patients	
	No.	%
Well after one MVD*	328	79.8
Well after repeat MVD	14	83.2
Well after third MVD	1	83.5
Subtotal:	343	83.5
Well after MVD and RFL†	17	87.6
Well after MVD and medication	38	96.9
Subtotal:	398	96.9
Slight pain, no medication	2	0.5
Severe pain	5	1.2
Deceased‡	5	1
Status unknown	1	0.2
All:	411	100

*MVD, microvascular decompression.
†RFL, radiofrequency lesion.
‡Three postoperative deaths, 1 suicide, and 1 accident.

decubitus position. Brain stem auditory evoked potential (BAEP) monitoring is recommended to decrease the risk of ipsilateral hearing loss caused by inadvertent traction on or compression of the auditory nerve (24). A high lateral retromastoid craniectomy up to $3\frac{1}{2}$ cm in diameter is performed through a small retromastoid incision (Fig. 99-2). Using microsurgical techniques, the subarachnoid space is opened and a supralateral exposure of the cerebellum and of the trigeminal nerve in the cerebellopontine angle is then achieved so that the cerebellum falls away (Fig. 99-2B).

The vascular compression is noted and relieved by mobilizing arterial loops and holding them away with small implants of a soft plastic material, such as shredded Teflon felt (Fig. 99-2E, F, and G). Large bridging veins can be decompressed in this way or can be coagulated and divided. Small veins intrinsic to the nerve can be coagulated and divided. After completion of the decompression the dura is closed in a watertight fashion, and the bone chips are replaced so that no "soft spot" is left; the subcutaneous tissues and skin are then closed.

TABLE 99-4. Results of Microvascular Decompression for Trigeminal Neuralgia

Source	No. of Patients	Results						Follow-up
		Free of Pain		Improved		Recurrence		
		No.	%	No.	%	No.	%	
Petty (12); Petty et al. (13, 14)	50	46	92	2	4			4 mo–8 yrs
Apfelbaum (15)	55	42	76	8	14.5	5	9	1–14 mo
Lazar (16)	15	14	93					3–24 mo
Rhoton (17)	10	10	100					7–21 mo
Weidmann (18)	10	10	100					6–18 mo
Voorhies and Patterson (19)	32	22	69			3	9	9–40 mo
Burchiel et al. (20)	42	30	71			6	14	Mean, 25 mo
Rushworth and Smith (21)	17	16	94			1	6	5–36 mo
All/mean:	231	190	82	10	4	15	6.5	

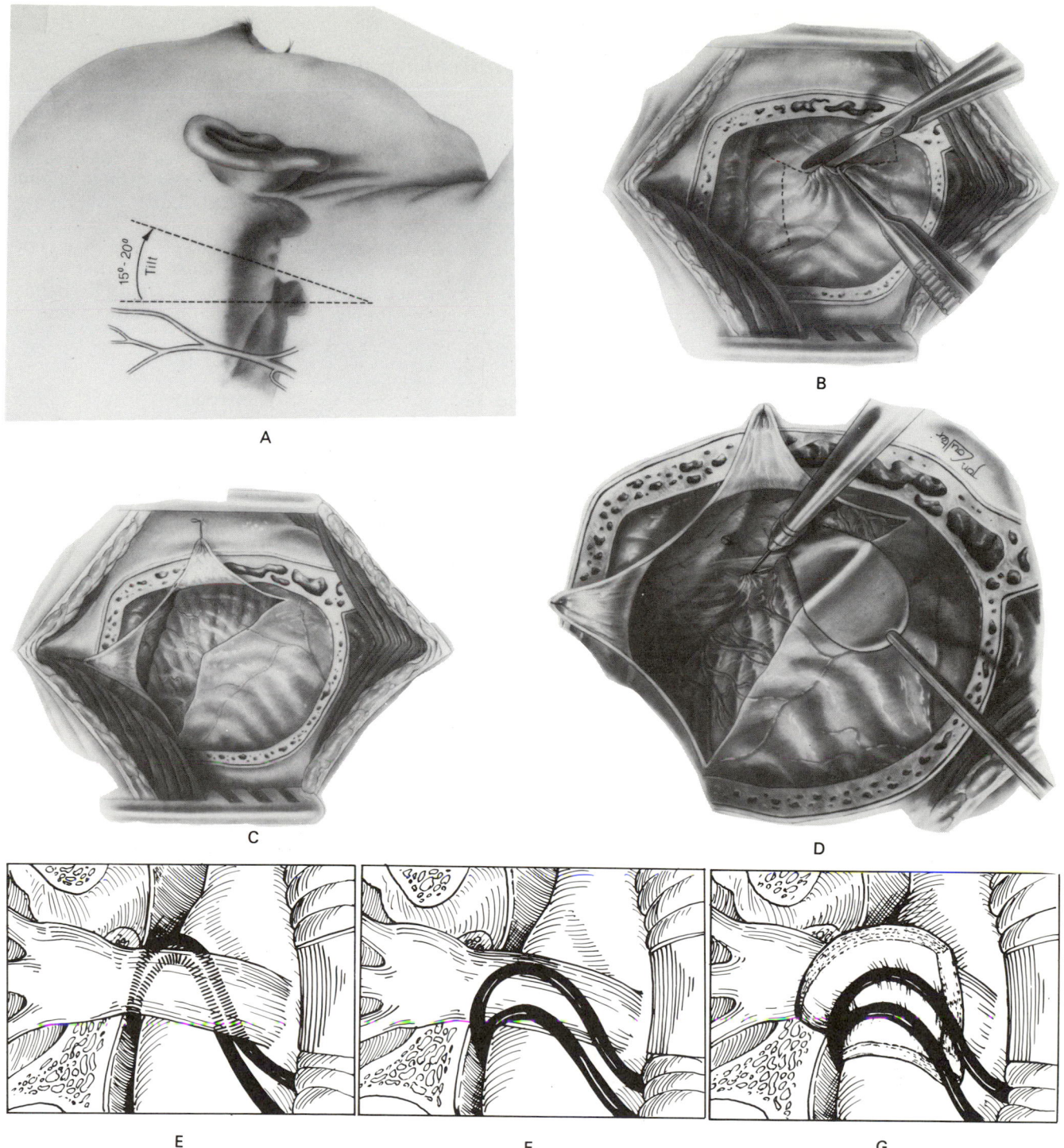

FIG. 99-2. Operative technique of microvascular decompression for treatment of trigeminal neuralgia. **A.** The patient is anesthetized and placed in the contralateral lateral decubitus position. The incision is placed one finger breadth behind the mastoid eminence following the hairline (*dotted lines*). The occipital nerve must be avoided. The craniectomy, 3 cm in diameter, is placed to expose the lateral sinus and to permit progression to the sigmoid sinus. **B.** Following the craniectomy the dura mater is opened and incised into the upper lateral corner at the junction of the lateral and sigmoid sinuses. **C.** The dura is then sewn back out of the way to expose the cerebellum. **D.** The tractor is placed superolaterally over the cerebellum to expose the superior petrosal vein. The vein might be a cause of the trigeminal neuralgia, and this relationship must be established. The vein is then coagulated and divided and the arachnoid opened using a no. 22 needle on a handle. **E.** The artery lies along the pons, extending caudally posteriorly and then rostrally, and impinges on the rostral anterior aspect of the root entry zone. **F.** The artery is mobilized into a horizontal position. **G.** It is held away from the nerve in its new position with an implant made of shredded Teflon felt. Modified from Jannetta, P.J.: Trigeminal neuralgia: Treatment by microvascular decompression. *In* Neurosurgery. Edited by R.H. Wilkins and S.S. Rengachary. New York, McGraw-Hill, 1984, pp. 2359, 2360.

TABLE 99-5. Postoperative Complications of Microvascular Decompression for Trigeminal Neuralgia

Complications	Patients	
	No.	%
Permanent cranial nerve deficit	23	5.6
Aseptic meningitis	21	5.1
Intracranial hematoma	4	1.0
Bacterial meningitis	3	0.7
Infarction	3	0.7
Pneumonia	2	0.5
Cerebrospinal fluid	2	0.5
Pulmonary embolism	2	0.5
Death	2	0.5
All/mean:	62	15.1

implication seems to be that high doses of adrenocorticosteroids should not be used. Infection is rare (26).

Clinical Application

Microvascular decompression is a useful primary operative treatment for trigeminal neuralgia in reasonably healthy patients of any age. I have discarded age as a limiting factor, but use an expected 5-year life survival as the limitation in decision-making. An excellent quality of life with "normal" patients, with no reminder of prior pain, can be expected in 80% or more of all patients and in over 90% of patients who have not had a primary destructive procedure. If patients are free of pain for a year, they have a less than 1% chance of recurrence for 5 years. Recurrent pain after a year is

TABLE 99-6. Postoperative Complications of Microvascular Decompression for Trigeminal Neuralgia

Source	No. of Patients	Complications		Type*	Mortality†	
		No.	%		No.	%
Petty (12); Petty et al. (13, 14)	50	3	6	2 AT, 1 DH	MVD*	1(?)
Apfelbaum (15)	55	9	16	2 TCNP, 1 PCNP, 2 DH, 2 AT		
Lazar (16)	15	2	13	2 CNP(?)		
Rhoton (17)	10					
Weidmann (18)	10	1	10	T AT/BP		
Voorhies and Patterson (19)	32	1	3	Wound hematoma		
Burchiel et al. (20)	42	1	2.4	Subdural hematoma	1	‡
Rushworth and Smith (21)	17	2	12	1 deafness, 1 DH		
All/mean:	231	19	8		2	0.9

*AT, ataxia; DH, decreased hearing; CNP, crania l nerve palsy; TCNP, transient cranial nerve palsy; PCNP, persistent cranial nerve palsy; BP, bulbar palsy.
†Mortality associated with tumor.
‡Mortality with microvascular decompression.

Side Effects and Complications

The impressive positive results with MVD are obtained with low mortality and morbidity rates. The operative mortality rate is generally less than 1% and approaches 0% with increased experience. Major postoperative problems include ipsilateral hearing loss, which has occurred in up to 10% of patients in various series. These statistics improve with increased experience and are substantially improved with the use of BAEP monitoring. Cerebrospinal fluid leaks are not uncommon, but are almost always treated effectively with a short period of closed system drainage (25). Preliminary data from a double-blind study have shown that the incidence of cerebrospinal fluid leaks is associated with the use of high doses of adrenocorticosteroids and that patients have no more headache, malaise, and discomfort without steroids than with steroids. The

generally a result of new vascular elongation that has produced compression of the trigeminal nerve root entry zone.

Summary

Microvascular decompression is indicated as a primary operative treatment in patients with trigeminal neuralgia that is intractable to medical therapy. Mortality and morbidity rates are low. The operation is a safe procedure with one caveat: the neurosurgeon performing this procedure should have ample experience with microsurgery in the cerebellopontine angle. I recommend that all surgeons who would perform such a procedure have some special training to learn the nuances of this operative technique so that they can operate safely, identify the pathologic blood vessel(s) present in almost all patients, and perform the decompression effectively (27).

B. MEDULLARY AND MESENCEPHALIC TRACTOTOMY

The term "medullary tractotomy" has been applied to two different and distinct procedures, section of the spinothalamic tract and section of the descending trigeminal tract at the level of the nucleus caudalis.

The division of the spinothalamic tract for the treatment of pain involving the contralateral body, especially the arm and shoulder, was first described by Schwartz and O'Leary (28) in 1941. Their publication, however, appeared after White (29) performed an almost identical procedure and reported it the same year. Section of the descending trigeminal tract and adjacent nucleus caudalis was reported by Sjöqvist (30) for the treatment of face pain in 1938. The operative techniques are quite similar because both pathways lie close to the lateral surface of the medulla at the level of the obex, the spinothalamic tract just dorsal to and the nucleus caudalis just ventral to the line dividing the dorsal and ventral halves of the spinal cord (Fig. 3-38).

Medullary and Pontine Spinothalamic Tractotomy (MSTT)

Basic Considerations

Anatomy

The lateral spinothalamic tract ascends through the medulla at the posterior portion of the anterolateral quadrant just below the pial surface immediately in front of the line of emergence of the rootlets of the spinal accessory nerve, which marks the division between the ventral and dorsal medulla (Fig. 99-3). At that site it is approximately 6 × 6 mm in cross section and is somatotopically oriented, with the sacral fibers anterolateral and the cervical fibers posteromedial (31). It lies ventral to the descending tract of the trigeminal nerve, which is also somatotopically oriented in continuity. As the fibers ascend to pontine levels they take a somewhat more medial course as they are overlain by the transverse pontine fibers and the associated corticobulbar pathways. At the level of the mesencephalon the spinothalamic tract lies just underneath the pial surface anterior to the plane of the aqueduct and posterior to the lateral edge of the peduncle (32) (Fig. 99-3B). Just medial to the spinothalamic fibers are those of the quintothalamic pathway, and

just medial to that is an area of the reticular formation that encroaches on the periaqueductal gray and appears to be a portion of the ascending extralemniscal spinoreticular system (33). Most of the spinothalamic fibers do not actually ascend to the thalamus but project medially to the reticular formation. At the upper cervical levels the spinothalamic pathway consists of approximately 15,000 fibers but, by the level of the mesencephalon, only 1,500 remain (33).

It is thought that the spinothalamic or lemniscal fibers are concerned with perception of discrete somatic pain, whereas the extralemniscal spinoreticular pathways might be more involved in patients with intractable pain caused by an injury to the nervous system. The spinoreticular formation projects to the limbic lobe by way of the posterior hypothalamus, as well as to the nonspecific thalamic nuclei such as the centrum median, parafascicular nuclei, and intralaminar area (32). (See Figs. 3-29 to 3-40 and pages 59 to 65 for detailed discussion of the spinothalamic tract and other ascending pathways that transmit nociceptive information.)

Indications

Ablative procedures such as medullary tractotomy are used primarily for the relief of cancer pain, because most patients who undergo such ablative procedures for pain of nonmalignant origin eventually have a recurrence of pain, sometimes with the addition of dysesthesias that can be more distressing than the original symptoms (34, 35).

Medullary spinothalamic tractotomy can be indicated for patients with cancer who have unilateral pain involving the entire contralateral body and limbs or who have pain of the upper extremity or shoulder. It is more effective than high cervical cordotomy in those patients whose pain is in the upper arm, shoulder, or neck. The advent of percutaneous cervical cordotomy at the C1–C2 level, however, has lessened the need for medullary tractotomy for such pain because this procedure is better tolerated, less hazardous, and easier to perform (36–38) (Chapter 98A). If a pneumonectomy has been done previously, or significant respiratory impairment exists on the side of the pain, especially from pulmonary involvement with tumor, both high cervical cordotomy and medullary tractotomy are relatively contraindicated because they could lead to further respiratory impairment or sleep-induced apnea (39); mesencephalotomy or thalamotomy, however, might be considered for such patients (Chapter 99C).

The pain associated with Pancoast's tumor responds variably to medullary or pontine ST tractotomy. Pain caused by tumor of tissues about the shoulder—sharp somatic radiating pain—is frequently relieved, but aching, dysesthetic pain can remain even after a successful tractotomy with dense analgesia. Such patients can be treated with the production of dorsal root entry zone (DREZ) lesions (Chapter 98C), intralaminar thalamotomy (Chapter 99C), or chronic deep brain stimulation (Chapter 93B) (40–43).

Results

A success rate of 80 to 90% permanent relief of cancer pain can be anticipated in contrast to a success rate

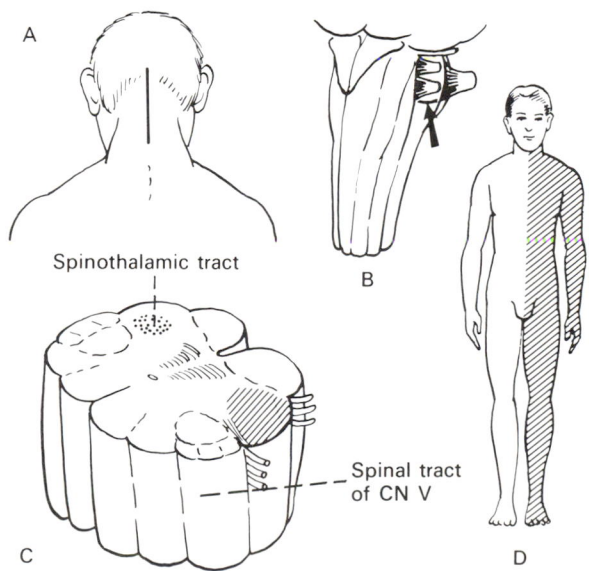

FIG. 99-3. Medullary spinothalamic tractotomy. *A.* Site of skin incision. *B.* Dorsolateral view of medulla indicating site of incision in brain stem. *C.* Cross-section of medulla indicating depth of incision into dorsolateral medulla. *D.* Extent of analgesia after right medullary spinothalamic tractotomy.

of approximately 50% and a complication rate of about 14% after long-term follow-up in cases of nonmalignant pain (31, 34, 35) (Table 99-7). Of the 50 patients having medullary tractotomy in reports reviewed by White and Sweet (31), 45 had initial relief of pain; long-term follow-up was unavailable, however, because most of the operated patients had cancer pain and survived for less than 6 months. It was indicated that medullary tractotomy is superior to high cervical cordotomy for relief of neuralgia in the upper extremity, even though a number of patients had a return of pain or lowering of their sensory levels with time. White and Sweet (31) concluded that, in patients with pain not caused by cancer, medullary tractotomy was most valuable for pain following nerve injury of the upper extremity or for postamputation pain, with an acceptable risk after unilateral operations in individuals in good physical condition with nonmalignant neuralgia. Since the introduction of DREZ lesions for that group of patients or selective posterior rhizotomy, however, the indications for open medullary spinothalamic tractotomy are even less certain (40, 44).

Hitchcock et al. (46) have used stereotaxic pontine spinothalamic tractotomy on 8 patients with severe pain due to malignancy. This technique, which Hitchcock first described in 1973, has been refined with the hope of avoiding problems of respiratory difficulty, dysesthesia, and sphincter disturbances. Of 8 patients subjected to the procedure 7 (88%) obtained good pain relief until death. Barberá et al. (48) have reported the use of this stereotaxic technique in 5 cancer patients, all of whom had pain relief without serious complications.

Clinical Considerations

Anesthesia

Open medullary spinothalamic tractotomy is usually performed through a suboccipital craniectomy; a small number of surgeons have used a percutaneous stereotaxic approach (46, 47). Because it is desirable to control the extent of the lesions by testing the patient for analgesia at the time of surgery, some have used light general anesthesia so that the patient can be awakened briefly following production of the lesion to assess whether the lesion is adequate or needs to be enlarged (31). The risk of air embolism, particularly under light anesthesia, has led most surgeons to perform the operation with the patient in the lateral position (31). Bonica has suggested (Chapter 94) that bilateral deep cervical plexus block limited to C2 and C3 nerves, achieved with a local anesthetic (e.g., 0.5% bupivacaine) and combined with mild sedation, is an excellent alternative because it provides anesthesia of the skin, deep somatic structures, vertebrae, posterior part of the skull, and dura. Pain provoked by manipulation of the rootlets of the uppermost cervical nerves can be eliminated by topical application of a local anesthetic.

Technique

A limited unilateral suboccipital craniectomy is made and the posterior arch of the atlas is removed. The dura is opened on the side of the intended lesion. The level of the obex is identified so that the lesion can be made 2 to 10 mm below that level to avoid involvement of the vestibular nuclei or restiform body, which could lead to ataxia or lateropulsion (31, 49). The line of emerging rootlets of the spinal accessory nerve marks the dorsal extent of the incision. A cordotomy knife, adjusted to make an incision 6 mm deep, is inserted, and a 4-mm transverse incision is made. The patient is awakened and tested. If the analgesia does not extend high enough, the incision should be extended dorsally until the patient notices sensation in the ipsilateral forehead and orbit from contact of the blade with the fibers of the ophthalmic division of the descending trigeminal tract (31). It might be necessary to extend the lesion 1 mm more to ensure adequate analgesia (31). This procedure has been well described by White and Sweet (31). Some surgeons perform the operation without awakening the patient and rely exclusively on anatomic landmarks.

The Hitchcock technique for pontine spinothalamic tractotomy entails radiologically demonstrating the position of the aqueduct and the floor and fastigium of the fourth ventricle (45). The target is identified by electric stimulation and the lesion carried out by an electrode that is 3 mm long and 1.1–1.8 mm in diameter to make a radiofrequency lesion at 75° C for 60 seconds.

Side Effects

The major side effect that has been reported is ipsilateral ataxia, which is usually temporary. It is caused by involvement of fibers of the restiform body. This problem can be minimized by making the transection below the level of the obex. Risk of bleeding can be minimized by observation with the operating microscope to avoid incision into local blood vessels. Side effects of pontine spinothalamatic tractotomy include transient dysesthesia, vertigo, and paresis.

Summary

Open medullary spinothalamic tractotomy can occasionally be useful for the management of cancer pain involving large areas of unilateral pain, including the shoulder or base of the neck. It has little advantage over high cervical cordotomy, however, and is used infrequently.

Medullary Trigeminal Tractotomy

Rationale and History

Treatment of pain involving the face or head, particularly cancer pain, is difficult, because the face and head are innervated by cranial nerves V, VII, IX, and X. Section of one or even several of these nerves might produce only incomplete denervation and an unsuccessful result. The pain components of all these nerves, however, converge in the nucleus caudalis of the trigeminal nerve, which uniquely serves pain and temperature sensation (Chapter 3). Consequently, destruction of that nucleus and the overlying descending tract can produce excellent loss of pain sensation to the head and pharynx but spare other sensations and protective reflexes. There is no risk of producing a motor deficit.

Medullary trigeminal tractotomy was first described by Sjöqvist (30). The procedure did not obtain widespread use because of the difficulty in interrupting all the descending fibers of the nucleus caudalis without injuring adjacent portions of the medulla and producing significant neurologic deficit. Improved techniques for localizing the descending trigeminal tract suggest that reconsideration of this procedure is in order (51, 52). A percutaneous stereotaxic approach to the descending trigeminal tract and nucleus caudalis has been described (45, 47).

Basic Considerations

Anatomy

The fibers of the trigeminal nerve concerned with pain sensation descend to medullary and uppermost cervical levels in the descending tract of the trigeminal nerve, terminating at various levels in the nucleus caudalis according to anatomic distribution. They are joined by pain fibers from cranial nerves VII, IX, and X (Figs. 3-46 and 3-47, p. 69). As the nucleus caudalis descends, it lies below the surface of the medulla at the level of the lower third of the inferior olive. It emerges from beneath the restiform body and continues as low as C4, where it becomes contiguous with the tract of Lissauer. It lies just dorsal to fibers of the lateral spinothalamic and dorsal spinocerebellar tracts; this junction can be identified on the surface by the emerging fibers of the spinal accessory nerve. Just dorsal to the nucleus caudalis is the fasciculus cuneatus, from which the descending trigeminal tract is separated on the surface by the dorsolateral sulcus. The somatic organization is inverted so that the ophthalmic division fibers descend to the C3–C4 level, the maxillary fibers descend to the C1–C2 level, and the mandibular fibers descend near the cervicomedullary junction (53–55). The fibers for pain from the territories of cranial nerves VII, IX, and X travel in the medial portion of the trigeminal tract, adjacent to the cuneate tract (Chapter 3 presents a detailed discussion of the trigeminal system).

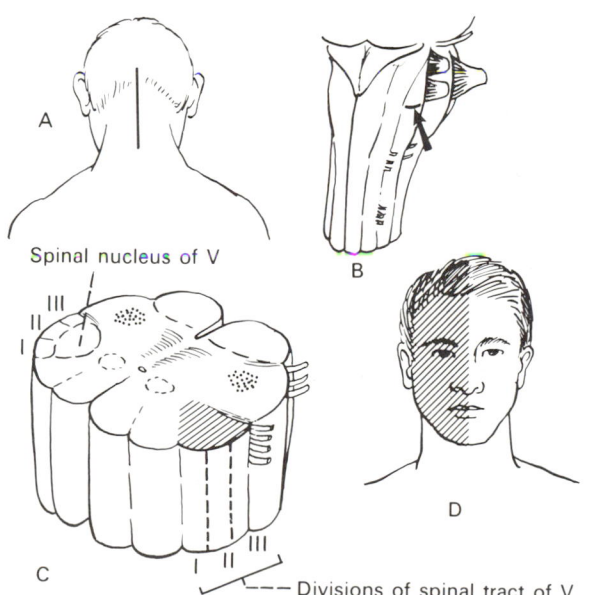

Fig. 99-4. Medullary trigeminal tractotomy. **A.** Site of skin incision. **B.** Dorsolateral view of medulla indicating site of incision into brain stem. **C.** Cross-section of medulla indicating depth of incision into dorsolateral medulla. **D.** Extent of analgesia after right medullary trigeminal tractotomy.

Some pain fibers to the base of the skull and certainly the upper portion of the neck are carried through the uppermost cervical nerve roots, which might necessitate section of the dorsal roots of C2, C3, or C4 (or a combination of these) to provide complete relief of cranial and upper neck pain (Fig. 99-4).

Indications

This procedure has been particularly helpful for relief of intractable pain caused by malignancy of the head and neck. It has been advocated for postherpetic neuralgia and anesthesia dolorosa of the face. The excellent results described by Kunc (56) have not been reported by others. It has also been recommended as a secondary procedure for the management of tic douloureux, especially when the patient has a contralateral impairment such as blindness, absent corneal reflex, facial palsy, or trigeminal motor loss, because the procedure is less likely to cause those problems than section of the peripheral nerve or ganglion (57).

Results

A success rate of 75 to 85% of substantial and sustained pain relief has been reported in patients with malignant disease (57). The mortality rate should be under 2% (58). Bricolo (51) reported complete, immediate relief of cancer pain in 10 patients, but later 2 had a partial but not distressing return of pain; these good results were possibly a result of accurate localization of the descending tract of V with intraoperative stimulation (Table 99-8).

Clinical Considerations

Open descending trigeminal tractotomy is performed under general anesthesia, although some surgeons prefer to awaken patients during the operation to ascertain the adequacy of the lesion. It is usually possible to obtain adequate exposure by performing a C1 and C2 laminectomy; in some patients the posterior rim of the foramen magnum must also be removed. The dura is opened and the obex and dorsal lateral sulcus are identified. The operating microscope is an important adjunct. An incision is made 2 mm below the obex, 3 mm deep to the pial surface, extending from the dorsolateral sulcus laterally to the accessory nerve filaments. The trigeminal tract can also be identified by the use of evoked potentials (56, 58–60).

Stereotaxic Trigeminal Tractotomy

The descending trigeminal tract in the medulla can be interrupted by a stereotaxic technique (47). The procedure is done under local anesthesia with the patient in the prone or sitting position, depending on the type of stereotaxic apparatus. One reason this procedure has not gained popularity is the difficulty in obtaining a satisfactory suboccipital approach with most types of stereotaxic apparatus, but the Hitchcock apparatus is particularly suited for this approach (45). The electrode is angulated 30° craniad and introduced 6 mm from the midline, where the trigeminal fibers lie 4 mm below the surface. A fine sharpened electrode is used because the pia is quite firm in this area. Verification of the electrode position can be obtained by electric stimulation at 50 Hz. With proper placement of the electrode, sensation is projected to the face at a low voltage. If the electrode is too deep or lateral in the spinothalamic tract, sensation can be projected elsewhere in the body. Stereotaxic trigeminal tractotomy has been used both in cancer pain and as a secondary procedure for various noncancer chronic pains (47).

Hitchcock (45) reported pain relief in 4 out of 5 patients with head and neck pain caused by malignancy, in 1 out of 2 with neuralgia-like facial pain, and in 2 out of 3 with postherpetic pain. Schvarcz (47) reported 100 patients, with an 87.5% success rate for postherpetic neuralgia, 57% for anesthesia dolorosa, 72% for dysesthesia, and 83.8% for relief of pain from malignancy (Table 99-9).

Medullary trigeminal tractotomy can be helpful in selected patients with pain secondary to malignancy of the head and neck. Its role in the relief of other pain-states has not been well established. A small number of neurosurgeons have used percutaneous tractotomy for other pain states; results have been encouraging.

Mesencephalotomy

Interruption of the spinothalamic tract by open surgery at the level of the mesencephalon was originally advocated by Walker (61) in 1942. The procedure proved to be technically hazardous, however, and postoperative neurologic complications were common, especially disagreeable dysesthesias in the early postoperative period (61, 62).

The treatment of pain by interruption of the spinothalamic tract in the mesencephalon was the first use of stereotaxic surgery by Spiegel, Wycis et al. (63) in 1947. They reported their long-range results 15 years later (64). They recognized that spinal transmission of pain was mediated by the spinoreticular pathways in the central gray as well as by the spinothalamic tract, and achieved improved results by interrupting both the spinothalamic tract and a limited adjacent portion of the spinoreticular pathway (64).

Basic Considerations

Anatomy

At mesencephalic levels the spinothalamic tract lies immediately below the pia in the region just anterior to the corpora quadrigemini, directly lateral to the aqueduct of Sylvius (Chapter 3). Just medial to it is the quintothalamic tract, which carries pain fibers from the nucleus caudalis of the trigeminal nerve to the contralateral thalamus. These two pathways are organized in somatotopic continuity to provide an integrated homunculus, with the head medial and the feet lateral. Just medial to the quintothalamic tract is the periaqueductal gray, which contains the spinoreticular fibers. The spinothalamic and quintothalamic tracts ascend to the ventroposterior nuclei of the thalamus but give off collaterals to the spinoreticular central gray area, which in turn projects to the parafascicular and intralaminar areas of the thalamus, the so-called extralemniscal pathway (43).

Indications

Some patients with central pain resulting from thalamic syndrome can respond to mesencephalotomy, as can patients with facial dysesthesia or anesthesia dolorosa following unsuccessful trigeminal surgery, postherpetic facial pain, or unilateral cancer pain (34, 35, 65, 66). Patients often considered for mesencephalotomy are those with unilateral head or neck pain of cancer, especially if combined with unilateral pain in the shoulder or body. Cancer patients with arm or shoulder pain can be considered for mesencephalotomy even if they have significant respiratory impairment or have had a pneumonectomy; perhaps this is the single most important group of patients who can be offered relief by this procedure. Because respiratory dysfunction never occurs after mesencephalotomy, it can be used in patients who could not safely undergo cervical cordotomy. Although mesencephalotomy has a slightly higher morbidity rate than medial thalamotomy, it is often preferred because it is somewhat more effective (67, 68). Those patients whose pain is bilateral or more diffuse, or who have a dysesthetic quality to their pain, such as with Pancoast's syndrome, might benefit more from basal or intralaminar thalamotomy, which can readily be combined with mesencephalotomy during the same procedure (69).

Results

For pain of central origin, such as a thalamic syndrome, a stereotaxic mesencephalotomy can provide pain relief in 50% of patients, although the pain often returns (33, 35, 65). Patients who have bilateral diffuse face or neck pain can sometimes be afforded bilateral pain relief by a unilateral lesion on the side of the greatest pain, even without bilateral analgesia, especially when the extralemniscal fibers are interrupted and if the lesion encroaches on the periaqueductal gray. If the pain persists on the other side a contralateral lesion can be made during a separate surgery (70, 71).

The mortality rate following stereotaxic mesencephalotomy averages 3 to 5% (33). In addition, 37% of patients develop temporary neurologic deficits, particularly changes in ocular motility (72). Dysesthesias have occurred in less than 5% (64, 66, 73, 74), in contrast to a 70% incidence after open surgical mesencephalotomy for pain (34, 61, 63) (Tables 99-10, 99-11).

Clinical Considerations

Because the hazards of open surgical mesencephalotomy have long been considered to be unacceptable, mesencephalotomy is always performed stereotaxically (34). A rigid frame is attached to the skull under local anesthesia and targets are selected by use of contrast radiography or CT scanning.

Technique

A small hole is made in the skull to allow the introduction of an electrode toward the target site. Stimulation should always be applied before production of a lesion. When the electrode is in the spinothalamic tract the patient reports a tingling or numb sensation over the contralateral half of the body at a relatively low voltage. The eyes should be observed for extraocular movement or myosis on stimulation, which would indicate that the electrode is too low and is encroaching on the oculomotor fibers. If low-frequency stimulation at low voltage causes movement of the contralateral extremities, the electrode might be too far anterior or lateral in the corticospinal pathway. If facilities are available to record evoked potentials during surgery, the lateral spinothalamic tract can be readily identified on stimulation of the contralateral median nerve (33, 75).

Effects of Lesion

After a lesion is made it is usually possible to demonstrate hypalgesia over wide areas of the contralateral body, face, or both, sometimes with a dense analgesia in those regions. If the sensory loss is not in the area of the body with the most pain, additional lesions should be made in adjacent areas. If the pain has a dysesthetic or chronic aching quality, involves both sides of the body at all, or has a diffuse nature, the extralemniscal

TABLE 99-7. Results of Medullary Spinothalamic Tractotomy

| Source | Year of Report | No. of Cases | Pain Relief | | | | Complications | | Deaths† | |
| | | | Initial | | Long-Term* | | | | | |
			No.	%	No.	%	No.	%	No.	%
Schwartz and O'Leary (28)	1941	1	1	100	0	0	0	0	1	100
Schwartz and O'Leary (76)	1942	1	1	100	0	0	NR		NR	
Adams and Munro (77)	1944	3	3	100	1	33	1	33	0	0
Crawford (78)	1947	11	9	82	5	45	5	45	4	36
Klemme (79)	1949	9	8	89	NR**		0	0	0	0
D'Errico (50)	1950	12	10	83	NR		3	25	1	8
Crawford and Knighton (80)	1953	8	6	75	2	25	?		1	12
Crawford (81)	1960	4	4	100	NR		1	25	NR	
Birkenfeld and Fisher (82)	1963	1	1	100	1	100	0	0	0	0
White and Sweet (31)†	1969‖	10	8	80	4	40	2	20	2	20
White and Sweet (31)†	1969#	8	6	75	0	0	2	25	1	12
White and Sweet (31)‡	1969	50	45	90	NR		NR		NR	
Barberá et al. (46)	1976	5	5	100	5	100	0	0	0	0
Hitchcock et al. (45)	1985	8	7	88	7	88	0	0	0	0
All/mean: §		131	114	87	25	45	14	23	10	13

*Long-term relief considered to be until death of cancer patients and longer than 8 mo postoperatively in cases of nonmalignant pain.
†Personal cases.
‡Review of cases in literature.
§Computed only on reports with data.
‖Knife lesions.
#Radiofrequency lesions.
**NR, not reported.

TABLE 99-8. Results of Medullary Trigeminal Tractotomy (Open)

| Source | Year of Report | No. of Cases | Indications | Results (% of Total Cases) | | | | |
				Success	Complications	Paresthesia	Anesthesia Dolorosa	Death
Grant and Weinberger (83)	1941	7	Neuralgia	67	100	50	0	0
Grant and Weinberger (83)	1941	12	Cancer	50	50	0	0	0
Hamby (84)	1948	35	Neuralgia	79	33	43	0	5.7
Hamby (84)	1948	13	Cancer					46
Falconer (85)	1949	15	Neuralgia	100	40	80	0	0
Falconer (85)	1949	5	Postherpetic neuralgia (4); lupus vulgaris (1)	0	0	0	0	20
Raney et al. (86)	1950	59	Neuralgia		2			2
Guidetti (87)	1950	124	Neuralgia	63	35	6	0	1.6
McKenzie (88)	1955	38	Neuralgia	85 ⎫				
					25	93	0	0
McKenzie (88)	1955	3	Cancer	100 ⎭				
Olivecrona (58)	1961	101	Neuralgia	70	0	0	0	2
Irsigler (89)	1963	22	Neuralgia	78	41	18	0	5
Kunc (90)	1965	6*	CN IX neuralgia	100	0	0	0	0
Kunc (56)	1966	216	Neuralgia	87				0.92
All/mean:		669		75	25	18	0	2

*Selective tractotomy for glossopharyngeal neuralgia.

TABLE 99-9. Results of Percutaneous Trigeminal Tractotomy

Source	Year of Report	No. of Cases	Indications	Results (% of Total Cases)				
				Success	Complications	Paresthesia	Anesthesia Dolorosa	Death
Hitchcock (91)	1970	5	Cancer	80	0	0	0	0
Hitchcock (91)	1970	2	Neuralgia	50	0	0	0	0
Hitchcock and Schvarcz (92)	1972	3	Postherpetic neuralgia	100	33	0	0	0
Crue et al. (93)	1972	8	Cancer	75	0	0	0	0
Crue et al. (93)	1972	4	Neuralgia	50	25	0	0	0
Fox (94)	1973	4	Chronic pain	75	39*	0	0	0
Fox (94)	1973	14	Cancer	100		0	0	0
All/mean:		40		82.5	22.5	0	0	0

*Ataxia or contralateral analgesia of leg.

TABLE 99-10. Results of Mesencephalic Tractotomy (Open)

Source	Year of Report	No. of Cases	Indications	Results (% of Total Cases)			
				Success	Complications	Paresthesia	Mortality Rate
Dogliotti (95)	1938	4	Cancer	100	0	100	25
Walker (61)	1942	2	Cancer	100	0	0	50
Walker (96)	1942	3	2 cancers, 1 amputation	100	0	100	0
Drake and McKenzie (97)	1953	6	4 cancers	100	0	100	0
White and Sweet (31)	1969	11	5 cancer (personal); 6 cancer, neuralgia reviewed	54	54	9	72
All/mean:		26		77	23	54	38

TABLE 99-11. Results of Stereotaxic Mesencephalotomy

Source	Year of Report	No. of Cases	Indications	Results (% of Total Cases)			
				Success	Complications	Dysesthesia	Mortality Rate
Mazars et al. (98)	1960	86	Varied diagnoses	90			1.2
Wycis and Speigel (63)	1962	54	12 cancers	30	35	14.8	7.4
Nashold et al. (65)	1969	15	Central pain	69	100	33	0
Zapheltal (99)	1969	14		50	75	7	0
Hageman and DeGrood (100)	1970	5	Cancer	80	0	0	20
		3	Plexus trauma	66	0	0	0
		2	Central pains	0	50	0	0
Nashold (66)	1972	8	3–22-month follow-up, all had ocular motility abnormalities	100	100	0	0
Whisler and Voris (70)	1978	38	Cancer	92	30	10	0
Frank et al. (101)	1983	14	Cancer	100	7	0	0
Amano et al. (102)	1986	6	Cancer	83	26	0	0
		23	Deaffer. pain	64			
Frank et al. (103)	1987	109	Cancer	84	13	7	0
Tasker (68)†	1989	92	Cancer / Deaffer. pain	80	15–20	5–10	0
Tasker (68)‡	1989	32	Cancer	68	9	0	10
All/mean:		501		76	22	6.5	1.3

†Data collected form published reports.
‡Personal data.

fibers should be included by extending the mesencephalic lesion more medially (33, 63, 66).

Side Effects

Side effects can include changes in ocular motility and contralateral weakness of the arm, leg, or both. Postoperative dysesthesia can occur, with or without good pain relief, and it can occur in the original painful area (72).

Summary

Stereotaxic mesencephalotomy can be effective for patients with cancer pain, especially those whose pain is unilateral or involves the shoulder, neck, or head, or those in whom respiratory function is impaired. The use of this operation is not widespread because so few neurosurgeons perform stereotaxic surgery.

Tables 99-7 through 99-10 present the operative findings of various authors for medullary spinothalamic tractotomy, open medullary trigeminal tractotomy, percutaneous trigeminal tractotomy, open mesencephalic tractotomy, and stereotaxic mesencephalotomy.

C. THALAMOTOMY AND HYPOTHALAMOTOMY

Thalamotomy

Despite both theoretic advantages and good short-term results, stereotaxic thalamotomy never achieved widespread use as a procedure for the relief of chronic pain. The first thalamotomy for pain relief was performed in 1953 by Spiegel and Wycis (104), who combined a lesion of the dorsomedian thalamus with mesencephalotomy to combat both the affective and perceptual aspects of the pain. Hecaen and colleagues (105) reported the first group of patients with lesions confined to the thalamus for the treatment of pain. These patients had lesions in the ventrobasal complex, centromedian nucleus, dorsomedial nucleus, or various combinations of these sites. These early attempts to treat pain by medial thalamic lesions were not too successful, but careful studies of target areas and lesion effects led to improved outcomes (Chapter 3 presents a detailed description of the anatomy and physiology of the thalamus, hypothalamus, and limbic system.)

Basic Considerations

Anatomy and Physiology

The thalamus receives the termination of the neospinothalamic pathway—that is, the portion of the lateral spinothalamic pathway that terminates in the ventral posterior nuclei—which is the lemniscal system. Most fibers of the lateral spinothalamic system actually end in the reticular formation and form the spinoreticular pathway, which is the diffusely projecting multisynaptic paleospinothalamic system. These axons, together with archispinothalamic fibers, ascend around the central gray from spinal cord levels and project to the medial thalamus, specifically to the intralaminar area, parafascicular nucleus, and centromedian nucleus. It is believed that these axons play a role in the suffering component of severe chronic pain (106–108). Fibers from the same central gray areas also project to the dorsomedial nucleus, from which there are connections to the frontal lobes and the limbic system that are known to be active in the emotional responses to pain. Additional fibers project from the central gray to the posterior hypothalamus, which is involved in the visceral responses to pain.

In the ventroposterior nuclei of the thalamus, the fibers of the spinothalamic system intermingle with axons that subserve all other sensory modalities. Lesions in these nuclei do not reliably lead to relief of pain and often create both numbness and a new type of dyses-thetic pain (109–110). The spinothalamic fibers can be selectively interrupted by making a lesion just below the ventroposterior nuclei, just rostral to the site of mesencephalotomy. Such a lesion can be extended into the intralaminar area of the medial thalamus if the pain is diffuse, boring, or aching (69, 111).

The most commonly selected target sites are in the medial thalamus (112–115). These nuclei receive fibers from the nonspecific systems that originate in the spinal cord and brain stem reticular formation (central gray). Their projections are to the association cortex and a wide variety of the basal nuclei. Unlike the ventroposterior nuclei, no somatotopic representation is found in these nuclei, and lesions produce the loss of pain perception over wide areas of the body.

A third general target area has been the posteromedial thalamus and pulvinar (113, 115). These regions are not known to play a major role in sensory pathways from either the specific or diffusely projecting thalamic systems. They project to the parietal cortex and receive fibers from the reticular formation; lesions in this area do not produce motor or sensory deficits.

A fourth general target area includes the dorsomedial and anterior thalamic nuclei, which project to the frontal and limbic lobes. Lesions in these nuclei produce the loss of the complaint of suffering but do not affect the detection of a noxious stimulus. The effects resemble those of cingulumotomy or frontal lobotomy: affective responses are blunted.

Spiegel and colleagues (107, 116) and White and Sweet (117) have described their successes with patients who have had lesions placed in both dorsomedial and posteromedial targets. The theoretic basis of the production of such dual lesions is the control of both the perception of the noxious stimulus and the suffering response to the pain and underlying disease (usually cancer). Orthner and Roeder (118) described the combination of mesencephalotomy with dorsomedial thalamotomy for the same reason.

Indications

The most frequent indication for thalamotomy is pain caused by cancer. Thalamotomy is particularly useful for cancer patients in whom a procedure lower in the nervous system is unlikely to succeed, such as those with widespread metastatic disease or with midline, bilateral, or head and neck pain. Basal or intralaminar thalamotomy can be especially helpful when much disagreeable sensation is felt in addition to pain, as in Pancoast's syndrome.

The initial success rate seems to be similar for that of relief of pain in any region of the body; it is the long-term failure rate that limits the usefulness of thalamotomy. Consequently, this operation should be used for noncancer pain only under the most unusual circumstances. Successful results have been recorded for pains of the thalamic syndrome, especially when CT scanning or magnetic resonance imaging reveals that the lesion is extrinsic to the thalamus (119). Coccygodynia has also been cured. Almost all forms of chronic pain have been treated unsuccessfully by thalamotomy; the general rule is that the benefits of this operation at any thalamic site do not often last more than a year or so. Hence, cancer pain is almost the only reasonable indication.

Medial or basal thalamotomy is usually performed on the side opposite the greatest pain. If necessary, a contralateral lesion can be performed several weeks after the first. Thalamotomy can also be combined with mesencephalotomy or cingulumotomy for more effective relief of pain and suffering (69, 106, 120, 121).

Results

Medial and basal thalamotomies have an initial success rate of approximately 80% (69, 122). By 1 year of postoperative survival the success rate falls to 30% (106, 110, 116). Tasker (123) attempted to summarize the results of thalamotomy as published in many series but found that incomplete case descriptions and inadequate surgical data made a comprehensive review extremely frustrating. Patients with pain caused by cancer certainly had better results than those with pain resulting from injury to the nervous system (124).

The effects of basal and medial thalamotomies are fascinating, because the patient experiences pain relief but does not have demonstrable analgesia (125). This contrasts with dorsomedial thalamotomy or cingulumotomy, after which the patient states that pain is still felt but is no longer distressing. Both contrast with a procedure such as anterolateral cordotomy, which produces pain relief only insofar as it leads to analgesia.

All surgical procedures have complications, and thalamotomy is no exception. A small risk of infection or intracerebral hemorrhage is involved (1 to 3%). It is possible to make a lesion in an unselected area and produce undesired neurologic deficits. This is certainly a procedure that should only be done in a center that frequently undertakes stereotaxic procedures.

Clinical Considerations

Thalamotomy is a stereotaxic procedure that is performed under local anesthesia. The patient's head is rigidly held in a frame that permits identification of the target site, either by CT scanning or by the injection of contrast agents into the ventricular system and the use of roentgenography for definition of the anatomic landmarks. A small hole is made in the skull and an electrode is directed toward the target site. The electrode is fixed to the frame and is guided to the target after calculating the optimal trajectory. The target is stimulated to determine the evoked responses that corroborate with the anatomic data. For example, if extraocular movements are produced, the electrode lies

below the optimal level for a thalamotomy. The report of sensory phenomena indicates that the electrode is too close to the fibers projecting to the ventroposterior complex (126). By combining the anatomic and physiologic evidence, it is possible to achieve an accuracy to the nearest 1 mm in deep brain structures. Thalamotomy is, in fact, a minor surgical procedure with a low complication rate.

Conclusions

Thalamotomy has a role in the management of cancer pain, especially when the involved areas are the head and neck or widespread metastases. Lesions in the nonspecific pain projection systems are particularly effective when undue suffering is experienced. Thalamotomy can be combined with other stereotaxic lesions for maximal efficacy. When specific therapy or segmental procedures are unavailable, thalamotomy can be a reasonable surgical choice. Unquestionably, only a limited number of neurosurgeons have extensive experience with this operation, and the published series are difficult to interpret because of different lesion sites, diagnoses, and follow-up.

The poor long-term success rate is probably related to the ability of the nonspecific projection system to reorganize itself after injury, and not to inaccurate lesion localization or size. Possibly better anatomic and physiologic data, as well as new lesions sites, might increase the efficacy of this operation in the future.

Hypothalamotomy

The procedure of making small stereotaxic lesions in the posterior hypothalamus was introduced by Sano (127) in 1962 for the treatment of violent aggressive behavior, especially in those with epilepsy and mental retardation. Because of the theoretic consideration that painful stimulation always causes signs of sympathetic discharges, Sano and associates began to perform posteromedial hypothalamotomy for intractable pain in 1971 (121, 128). It was also reported by Fairman (129) at about the same time but has not become widely used.

Basic Considerations

Anatomy and Physiology

The anatomy of the area of the hypothalamus in which a lesion is made for pain relief does not correspond to a specific nucleus as defined by anatomic studies. It corresponds, however, to the area in which microelectrode recording demonstrates evoked activity at a latency of more than 100 ms on stimulation of the contralateral superficial radial nerve, which has been shown to be a result of C-fiber stimulation transmitted along a multisynaptic pathway (128, 130).

This area of the posteromedial hypothalamus has connections with the parafascicular nucleus and probably with the primary and secondary somatosensory cortex, as well as with the ipsilateral ventrocaudalis parvocellularis but not the dorsomedial nucleus.

The physiologic basis of hypothalamotomy is the normalization of ergotropic and trophotropic balance coordinated by that area (128).

Indications

Stereotaxic posteromedial hypothalamotomy is used infrequently and is generally reserved for the patient with cancer pain, particularly if it involves the face and especially if the patient manifests a great deal of suffering, anxiety, or depression in addition to the pain. It has been used with mixed success for pain of postherpetic neuralgia involving the face (128, 129).

Results

Patients who obtain pain relief after hypothalamotomy behave differently from patients who obtain relief after frontal lobotomy. After lobotomy, cingulumotomy, or dorsomedial thalamotomy, patients might be relieved of suffering and no longer require pain medications but might indicate, when asked, that the pain is still perceived. After hypothalamotomy the response is much more like that seen after an intralaminar thalomotomy: patients report that they no longer perceive the pain. Satisfactory pain relief was obtained with hypothalamotomy for cancer pain in 70% of patients in one series (131) and in 5 of 6 patients in another series (128), but it must be recognized that this group of patients does not ordinarily require long-term follow-up. Partial relief has been reported in the use of hypothalamotomy for herpes zoster, causalgia, and thalamic pain (129). Two-thirds of patients with somatic pain, particularly after cancer, had relief from hypothalamotomy, but in general those patients with dysesthetic pain did poorly.

Clinical Considerations

Anesthesia

Hypothalamotomy is always done under local anesthesia because of the desirability of identifying electrode localization by stimulation or recording.

Sedation must be carefully selected so as not to interfere with those activities (132).

Lesion Site

An electrode is introduced stereotaxically to a target 2 mm below the midpoint of the intercommissural line and 2 mm lateral to the lateral wall of the third ventricle. The operation can be done bilaterally in cases of widespread pain, but success can result from a unilateral lesion placed contralateral to the location of pain.

Electrode Localization by Stimulation

Recording of evoked activity on painful electric stimulation of the contralateral radial or medial nerve can verify proper position of the electrode. In addition, application of pinpricks to the skin over wide areas of the body can produce evoked responses, with latencies of 300 to 2000 msec (128). Electric stimulation causes signs of sympathetic discharge such as rise in blood pressure, tachycardia, pupillary dilation, or occasionally neck movement or ocular movement. Patients report a sensation of fear or horror during stimulation, but no sensation of pain.

Conclusions

More logical and potentially more successful procedures than hypothalomotomy currently exist for the treatment of pain. Few reports have been presented in the literature, and few neurosurgeons have found the procedure to be particularly helpful.

Hypothalamotomy is a surgical procedure that does not have a rational foundation in our understanding of the anatomy and physiology of the brain. Other stereotaxic procedures have a clearer anatomic substrate and appear to have a higher likelihood of success. The indications for hypothalamotomy are not clear, nor is it clear that it offers any advantages over more commonly performed thalamotomies.

D. PRECENTRAL AND POSTCENTRAL GYRECTOMY

Excision of portions of the sensory cortex was first proposed by Leriche (133) and apparently was first performed by De Gutiérrez-Mahoney (134, 135). Although the initial short-term results of excision of the postcentral gyrus were encouraging, the vast majority of patients who have had this procedure have described recurrence of their pain.

Basic Considerations

Anatomy and Physiology

The postcentral gyrus, which includes Brodmann's areas 1 to 3 and part of area 5, is the principal cortical region for the integration and interpretation of sensory information. The precentral gyrus plays a similar role for motor activities; the precise localization of function varies from patient to patient. It has been known since the turn of the century that lesions involving the human postcentral gyrus could dramatically alter sensation and could alter chronic pain states. Precise localization could only be determined by autopsy studies, and these were infrequent. The role of the cerebral cortex in the perception and response to pain

is not clear, and major disagreements remain as to the rational basis of cortical resection for relief of pain (Chapter 3).

Indications

Certainly, gyrectomy is not a primary procedure for relief of pain. The development of stereotaxic surgery and implanted electrodes for stimulation have probably played a role in the infrequent use of this surgical procedure. The lack of data makes it difficult to determine the possible advantages of gyrectomy.

Clinical Considerations

Technique

With the technology currently available this operation is best performed under local anesthesia so that cortical mapping can be undertaken, and the resection can be based on both physiologic and anatomic data. A large craniotomy is required to expose the central and precentral regions, similar to that used for cortical resection of an epileptic focus.

TABLE 99-12. Results of Postcentral Gyrectomy

Source	Year of Report	No. of Cases	Indications	Results (% of Total Cases)			
				Success	Complications	Paresthesia	Mortality Rate
Hamby (139)	1961	1	Thalamic pain	100	0	0	0
White and Sweet (136)*	1969	38	Thalamic and phantom pains	47	10	0	3
Lende et al. (138)	1971	2	Precentral, post-central, and secondary sensory area resections	100	0	0	0
All/mean:		41		51	10	0	2.8

*Review of literature plus three personal cases.

Results

In 1969 White and Sweet (136) summarized their review of 21 publications, which included data on 38 patients (Table 99-12). Of the 18 initial successes, only 4 were said to be relieved of their pain when assessed 1 or more years later. Even the much more extensive lesion used by Pool and Bridges (137), which undercut the parietal lobe for 7.5 cm posterior to the central sulcus, provided pain relief for only a little more than a year. Lende and co-workers (138) removed both the pre- and postcentral gyri of the face projection area to the upper border of the insula. This resection included both the primary and secondary sensory areas for the face as well as all of the precentral motor-sensory cortex. Only mild contralateral facial weakness was noted, probably because of the bilateral cortical representation for the face. Data were reported on two patients. One had con-tinuous unilateral burning facial pain secondary to a pontine stroke and was rendered pain-free until he died 20 months later from heart disease. The other had continuous facial pain after a retrogasserian rhizotomy for trigeminal neuralgia and was pain-free for at least 17 years.

It is possible that removal of the entire primary and secondary sensory areas along with the corresponding motor area can succeed where less extensive operations have failed (139). I am not aware of any reports of such operative procedures.

Complications

Cortical excisions do involve some risk of focal epilepsy, especially in the region of the central sulcus. Extensive cortical lesions can also result in contralateral sensory and motor loss.

E. FRONTAL LOBE OPERATIONS FOR PAIN

Prefrontal Leukotomy

Contemporary frontal lobe operations for pain evolved from prefrontal leukotomy, an operation originally devised for the treatment of severe intractable psychiatric disorders (140). No other class of surgical procedures has been subjected to the political and scientific scrutiny that has accompanied "psycho-surgery." The abusive use of prefrontal leukotomy in the first 25 years of its widespread acceptance led to a rebound that, at least in the United States, makes it difficult to perform any psychosurgical procedure. Although prefrontal leukotomy probably has no contemporary application, its descendant, cingulumotomy, can be effective for the relief of pain in properly selected patients.

Basic Considerations

Anatomy and Physiology

The prefrontal leukotomy procedure was based on experimental observations in animals of calming effects following bilateral division of white matter fibers immediately anterior to the frontal horns of the lateral ventricles (141). These fibers project from the cingulate gyrus and dorsomedial thalamus to areas 9 through 14 of the frontal cortex. They are the rostral projection of the reticular activating system and diffuse thalamic projection pathways. Subsequent reports indicated that some patients with complaints of pain as part of their mental illness lost their pain after prefrontal leukotomy (142, 143). These reports stimulated the use of bilateral prefrontal lobotomy for the treatment of various chronic pain states (144–149). The operation, whether primarily for psychiatric disorders or chronic pain, was then refined, at first by restricting the bilateral leukotomy to medial frontal white matter (150).

Clinical Considerations

Techniques

Although prefrontal lobotomy is popularly regarded as a surgical procedure done by inserting an ice pick through the orbital roof and blindly traumatizing the frontal lobes, most neurosurgeons have used a trephine hole placed anterior to the coronal suture, either laterally or superiorly. The dura is opened in a cruciate fashion and blood vessels on the cortical surface are coagulated. A ventricular needle is passed in the plane of the proposed leukotomy to ensure that it is anterior to the frontal horn of the lateral ventricles. A leukotome is then inserted to transect the bulk of the white matter. The operation is usually performed under local anesthesia.

Variations in the surgical technique include suction-coagulation under direct vision, injection of sclerosing solutions, and use of radiofrequency current to make lesions. Limited leukotomies have been performed by manually directing the lesion to the area of interest.

Results

The effectiveness and limitations of these procedures in the treatment of various pain states were well described by Elithorn and colleagues (151). They evaluated 25 patients managed with standard bilateral prefrontal leukotomy or with the more restricted bilateral section of only the medial frontal white matter. Evaluation, at a minimum of 6 months after operation (mean 24 months), was based on patients' and relatives' opinions and on a social functioning rating scale. All patients but 1 had chronic pain; the largest groups were 5 with postherpetic neuralgia, 4 with atypical facial pain, and 3 with painful torticollis.

These operations did *not* change the perception of acute pain or responses to it except for a suggestion of a more intense but briefer response to noxious stimulus. Two-thirds of the patients were considered to be improved, however, with 6 of 25 much improved based on the social function rating scale, although only one-third of the patients or relatives thought there had been improvement. Patients with the most extensive operations had the best outcomes based on the evaluation by the patients and relatives, but not on the social function rating scale. Those with the most severe pain did least well by any measure. Older patients had better outcomes. Patients with large "standard" leukotomies all showed some personality change, which was considered severe in one-third. Eight of 13 patients with more limited medial frontal leukotomies demonstrated personality changes; these were severe in 2.

Benefit in patients with severe organic pain usually required some personality change. Elithorn and associates (151) concluded that the major beneficial effect of these operations was to reduce depression and anxiety, with a more variable effect on obsessive behavior. In pain patients the typical postleukotomy picture was one in which patients still complained of severe pain but at the same time showed an inappropriately cheerful affect and the inability to sustain an attitude or mood. Unfortunately, only 13 of 25 patients returned to their preoperative level of intellectual and physical activities. Generally similar results were reported by others (152).

Unilateral Prefrontal Leukotomy

The value of unilateral prefrontal leukotomy in chronic pain of diverse causes was evaluated by Scarff (153, 154) in 33 patients. They found that two-thirds of patients were improved without major personality changes. White and Sweet (155) disagreed with this conclusion, however, and stated that mental changes were always present when suffering had been alleviated, although unilateral prefrontal leukotomy was less likely to lead to the severe personality changes seen after bilateral lesions. White and Sweet (155) also indicated that suffering returned if patients survived more than 6 months after a unilateral prefrontal lobotomy. When psychologic functioning returned to normal, patients were likely to suffer again.

Summary

In these reports the major features of frontal lobe procedures for pain were evident: major effects on depression and anxiety, little or no effect on pain perception or on the patient's report of pain, but an apparent reduction in the impact of the pain on the patient's affect and functioning. These same features also apply to modern, more limited, frontal operations for pain, although these newer operations have no measurable effect on personality or intellectual performance. Prefrontal leukotomy is no longer considered to be a reasonable operation for pain relief because of its devastating effect on social activities and intellectual performance.

Cingulumotomy

Basic Considerations

Anatomy and Physiology

Modern frontal lobe operations for pain arose from several procedures. One was the limited resection of regions of the prefrontal cortex (rather than white matter) for pain. Topectomies of areas 9, 10, 11, and 12 in various combinations were reported by White and Sweet (155), Scoville (156), and Pool and Bridges (157). Like frontal leukotomy, these operations did not dissociate effects on suffering from effects on other emotional and intellectual functions. A more limited operation, however, topectomy of the anterior cingulate gyrus, or cingulectomy, seemed to relieve suffering sometimes without producing major personality changes (158). Several more recent reports include a few cases in which this operation was used (Tables 99-13 and 99-14).

Most modern series of frontal lobe operations for pain or psychiatric disorders include cases in which frontal lobe white matter lesions are placed with stereotaxic techniques. These evolved from the use of radiofrequency (RF) lesions for prefrontal leukotomy (159). When combined with stereotaxic techniques for placement of the RF electrode, specific frontal white matter pathways can be focally lesioned. Most current frontal lobe operations for psychiatric disorders and chronic pain are based on these technical advances and on the clinical and experimental observations that two focal areas of frontal lobe are particularly important to therapeutic benefit.

One of these areas is the inferior medial frontal lobe. Destruction of that area has been called "innominotomy" (160) or "subcaudate capsulotomy" (161). The other area is that portion of the superior posterior medial white matter deep to the cingulate gyrus, a fiber bundle known as the cingulum—hence the operation's name, "cingulumotomy." Selection of the cingulum as an area of importance in frontal lobe

TABLE 99-13. Results of Cingulumotomy for Cancer Pain

Source	Year of Report	No. of Cases	Pain "Relief" (% of Total Cases)*	
			Initial	Long-Term
Cingulumotomy alone				
Foltz and White (164)	1957	11	82	
Faillace et al. (170)	1971	7	43	
Turnbull (174)	1972	13	0	
Hurt and Ballantine (168)	1973	32	32	11 (over 3 mo)
Wilson and Chang (171) (cingulectomy)	1974	19	53	100 (in only 2 patients over 6 mo) (See text)
Voris and Whisler (172)	1975	5	100	
All/mean:		87	31	
Cingulumotomy combined with interruption of pain pathways				
Turnbull (174)	1972	10	90	50 (2 patients over 1 yr)
Voris and Whisler (172)	1975	2	100	
All/mean:		12	92	

*"Complete" and "marked," "good" and "excellent," "improved," "relieved."

operations for pain is also partly on theoretic grounds, because the cingulate gyrus represents the frontal lobe component of Papez' limbic lobe, a portion of brain thought to be important for emotion, with the cingulum one of the major frontal limbic pathways (162, 163).

An additional basis for the use of cingulumotomy in the relief of pain states was the observation that these lesions attenuated withdrawal symptoms after morphine addiction in monkeys (164). Moreover, cingulumotomy was reported to cure addiction to narcotics and alcohol in a substantial number of addicted humans, independent of any effects on pain (163, 165). Cingulum lesions in monkeys were shown to reduce hyperactive motor and autonomic (gut) responses induced by stress and to reduce conditioned responses to minor stimuli without altering acquisition of conditioned responses to intense stimuli (166).

Thus, anatomic, clinical, and experimental studies suggest that cingulumotomy might alter the response to stressful stimuli such as pain. In addition, bilateral cingulumotomy is not associated with measurable postoperative deterioration in personality or intellect, even when assessed with sensitive neuropsychologic measures (167). This altered response to pain can therefore be achieved without a deterioration in personality or intellect. As a consequence, considerable experience with cingulumotomy for the relief of both neoplastic and non-neoplastic chronic pain, alone and in combination with operations that interrupt afferent pain pathways, has been reported. By contrast, the other operation that represents a modern refinement of frontal leukotomy, subcaudate capsulotomy, or innominotomy, has been little used to relieve pain states although, like cingulumotomy, it often diminishes depression and anxiety and can be even more effective than cingulumotomy for relieving obsessive symptoms.

TABLE 99-14. Results of Cingulumotomy for Nonmalignant Chronic Pain*

Source	Year of Report	No. of Cases	Pain "Relief" (% of Total Cases)†		Comments
			Initial	Long-Term	
Foltz and White (163)	1968	24	67	42 (1 year plus)	
Faillace et al. (170)	1971	2	50	50 (2 yr)	
Turnbull (174)	1972	7	57		Alone
Turnbull (174)	1972	6	50	17	With mesencephalotomy
Hurt and Ballantine (168)	1973	36	22	22 (over 6 mo)	
Wilson and Chang‡ (171)	1974	4	50	0 (over 1 yr)	
Voris and Whisler (172)	1975	11	73	18 (over 3 yr)	Alone
Voris and Whisler (172)	1975	7	71	0 (over 3 yr)	With mesencephalotomy (5) or thalamotomy (2)
Broager and Olesen (173)‡	1972	17		82 (over 6 mo)	
Corkin et al. (167)	1979	11	82	82 (over 1 year)	
All/mean:		125	51	38	

*Alone or in combination with other procedures.
†"Complete" and "marked," "good" and "excellent," "improved," "relieved."
‡Includes cases of cingulectomy.

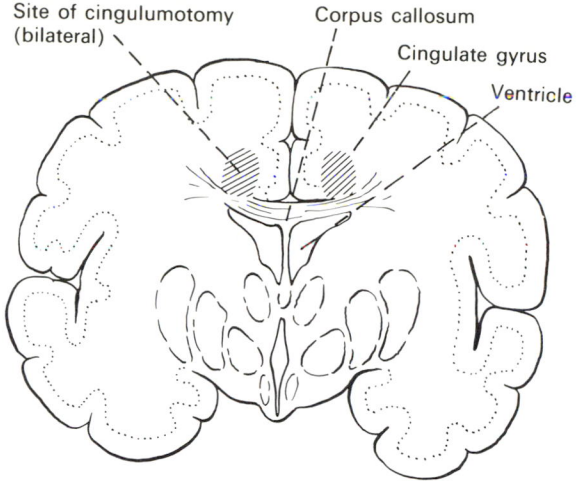

FIG. 99-5. Coronal section of brain indicating sites of lesions for cingulumotomy.

Clinical Considerations

Technique

Cingulumotomy can be performed under local or general anesthesia. A stereotaxic technique is used. The target area (Fig. 99-5) is 2 to 4 cm posterior to the tip of the frontal horns of the lateral ventricles, 1 mm above the ventricle, beginning 1.3 cm on either side of the midline (163, 168). The target is approached through bilateral frontal burr holes or twist drill holes placed 9.5 cm posterior to the nasion, centered 1.3 cm on either side of the midline. The frontal horn of the lateral ventricle is punctured by a needle inserted through one of these holes and 6 ml of air is introduced. This outlines the frontal horn of the lateral ventricle on appropriate anteroposterior and lateral roentgenograms, allowing for calculation of the target. Electrodes with 8- to 10-mm exposed tips are introduced to the target. There are no physiologic guides to target placement, although stimulation in the cingulum further posterior, more than 4 cm from the tip of the frontal horn, sometimes evokes trunk movements. Relatively large lesions are created, about 1 cm in diameter, extending 2 cm above the target point; most often these are made by a thermistor-controlled RF technique. Neuropathologic studies have shown that such lesions destroy some fibers of the corpus callosum as well as of the cingulum (169). Similar lesions placed more superiorly in frontal white matter failed to diminish symptoms of depression and anxiety.

Results

When conducted under local anesthesia, some reduction in anxiety is often noticeable after placement of a lesion on one side, but bilateral lesions have been used in most reported series. The behavioral effects on pain and anxiety are usually apparent immediately, if they are to occur. As with all stereotaxic surgery, the procedure should not be done on patients with blood clotting disorders or uncontrolled hypertension.

Application and Results

Cancer Pain

The value of cingulumotomy alone in the control of the chronic pain caused by malignant disease has been noted in a number of reports (Table 99-13). Most of this experience is with head and neck cancers, in which an element of "suffering" related to respiratory impairment, dysarthria, or choking was also thought to be present. Several reports suggested that many patients receive benefit, at least initially. Foltz and White (163) reported 9 of 11 patients with "good" or "excellent" outcomes, with unspecified follow-up. Wilson and Chang (171) reported that the operation benefited 53% of 19 patients, and Voris and Whisler (172) reported that all of 5 patients were relieved until their deaths, which occurred in less than 1 year. Hurt and Ballantine (168) reported marked or complete relief in 32% of 32 patients evaluated at 3 months postoperatively or less, but this degree of relief was present in only 11% (1 patient) of the 9 patients of this group who survived long enough to be evaluated over a longer period.

In other reports of patients with pain secondary to neoplasia, cingulumotomy has been combined with stereotaxic procedures to interrupt afferent pain pathways, most often mesencephalotomy. Good initial pain relief has been reported in most patients undergoing these combined procedures (Table 99-13), but few long-term results have been reported.

Nonmalignant Chronic Pain

Cingulumotomy has also been used in the therapy of various chronic non-neoplastic pain states (Table 99-14). The initial experience of Foltz and White (163) was quite positive, with 10 of 24 patients with psychogenic or organic chronic pain said to have "good" or "excellent" outcomes with 1 year or more follow-up; this has been replicated in some other studies (167, 174). Other reports have been less enthusiastic; Hurt and Ballantine (168), in the largest reported series, noted marked or complete pain relief in only 22% of 36 patients with chronic pain, whether evaluated acutely or with more than 6 months' follow-up. The addition of procedures to interrupt afferent pain pathways might increase the initial "success" rate in patients with chronic pain but does not seem to improve the long-term outcome (171, 173). Enlarging a cingulum lesion by repeating cingulumotomy in patients with recurrence of pain has been of value in some series (163) but not others (167). This contrasts with the generally reported value of repeating the cingulumotomy when the major goal was relief of depressive symptoms (169).

Criteria for Patient Selection

Criteria for selection of patients likely to benefit from cingulumotomy have been relatively vague, with the suggestion that a favorable outcome is more likely in patients with substantial elements of depression or "suffering." Foltz and White (163) proposed that the "augmentor-reducer" criterion of Petrie (175) derived from a kinesthetic after-image test, might be used for patient selection, with greater benefits from cingulumotomy more likely to occur in those pain patients who were "augmentors," but this proposal seems never to have been tested systematically. Patients with apparent long-term pain relief after cingulumotomy differ in a number of ways from those with long-term pain relief after frontal leukotomy. Patients benefiting from cingulumotomy do not necessarily have measurable personality changes (167), there was general agreement on outcome regardless of whether evaluation was by self-assessment, physician assessment, or level of activity (168).

Side Effects and Complications

Complications and unwanted side effects of cingulumotomy have been relatively few in most reports. A few days to a week of headache and fever, occasionally with transient incontinence, have been described in a number of reports. Postoperative intracranial hemorrhage is the most serious complication; death from that cause has been reported but is rare (173). Postoperative seizures have been reported in several series in a small proportion of patients. Extensive neuropsychologic testing of patients before and after cingulumotomy has shown few changes (167). IQ measures have tended to improve. Some older patients demonstrated subtle decrements in some visuospatial measures. Assessment with formal neuropsychologic tests has also documented the clinically evident improvement in symptoms of depression after cingulumotomy, alone or in combination with innominotomy (176).

Summary

Of all the frontal lobe operations for pain, only cingulumotomy seems to have a sufficiently low incidence of complications or undesirable side effects, with a high enough reported rate of major or complete control of pain, to be considered as an option for pain control. Cingulumotomy seems to have some value in the control of neoplastic pain, especially when associated with depression and suffering, as in some head and neck malignancies. Cingulumotomy generally does not alter the response to acute pain or patients' reports of pain. It does reduce the impact of the pain and neoplasia on behavior. The addition of procedures to interrupt afferent pain pathways might result in a more favorable outcome in these patients than either those operations alone or cingulumotomy alone. As is evident from the lack of recent reports in Table 99-13, however, cingulumotomy alone or in combination is now rarely reported in the management of pain of malignancies, having been displaced by the use of more effective and less invasive techniques such as intraventricular or intrathecal opiates (Chapter 95).

The value of cingulumotomy in chronic pain states not caused by cancer is more difficult to assess. I believe that in such cases the major effect of the operation is on intractable depression, and that a favorable long-term outcome is more likely in those patients in whom depressive symptoms, rather than pain symptoms, dominate the clinical picture. The selection criteria for cingulumotomy for pain, then, might be the same as the selection criteria for cingulumotomy in the treatment of intractable depression (167, 175).

REFERENCES

1. Dandy, W.E.: Section of the sensory root of the trigeminal nerve at the pons. Bull. Johns Hopkins Hosp., *36*:105, 1925.
2. Dandy, W.E.: Treatment of trigeminal neuralgia by the cerebellar route. Ann. Surg., *96*:787, 1932.
3. Gardner, W.J., and Miklos, M.V.: Response of trigeminal neuralgia to "decompression" of sensory root. JAMA, *170*:1773, 1959.
4. Gardner, W.J.: Concerning the mechanism of trigeminal neuralgia and hemifacial spasm. J. Neurosurg., *19*:947, 1962.
5. Jannetta, P.J.: Microsurgical exploration and decompression of the facial nerve in hemifacial spasm. Curr. Top. Surg. Res., *2*:217, 1970.
6. Sunderland, S.: The arterial relationships of the internal auditory meatus. Brain, *68*:23, 1945.
7. Jannetta, P.J.: Structural mechanisms of trigeminal neuralgia: Arterial compression of the trigeminal nerve at the pons in patients with trigeminal neuralgia. J. Neurosurg., *26*:159, 1967.
8. Jannetta, P.J.: Treatment of trigeminal neuralgia by suboccipital and transtentorial cranial operations. Clin. Neurosurg., *24*:538, 1977.
9. Jannetta, P.J.: Neurovascular compression in cranial nerve and systemic disease. Ann. Surg., *192*:518, 1980.
10. Hakanson, S.: Trigeminal neuralgia treated by the injection of glycerol into the trigeminal cistern. Neurosurgery, *9*:638, 1981.
11. Lunsford, L.D.: Treatment of tic douloureux by percutaneous retrogasserian glycerol injection. JAMA, *248*:449, 1982.
12. Petty, P.G.: Arterial compression of the trigeminal nerve at the pons as a cause of trigeminal neuralgia. Inst. Neurol. Madras, Proc., *6*:93, 1976.
13. Petty, P.G., and Southby, R.: Vascular compression of lower cranial nerves: Observations using microsurgery with particular reference to trigeminal neuralgia. Aust. N. Z. J. Surg., *47*:314, 1977.
14. Petty, P.G., Southby, R., and Siu, K.: Vascular compression. Cause of trigeminal neuralgia. Med. J. Aust., *1*:166, 1980.
15. Apfelbaum, R.I.: A comparison of percutaneous radiofrequency trigeminal neurolysis and microvascular decompression of the trigeminal nerve for the treatment of tic douloureux. Neurosurgery, *47*:16, 1977.
16. Lazar, M.L.: Management of tic douloureux. JAMA, *240*:1715, 1978.
17. Rhoton, A.L.: Microsurgical neurovascular decompression for trigeminal neuralgia and hemifacial spasm. J. Fla. Med. Assoc., *65*:425, 1978.
18. Weidmann, M.J.: Trigeminal neuralgia. Med. J. Aust., *2*:628, 630, 1979.
19. Vorrhies, R., and Patterson, R.H.: Management of trigeminal neuralgia (tic douloureux). JAMA, *245*:2521, 1981.
20. Burchiel, K.J., et al.: Comparison of percutaneous radiofrequency gangliolysis and microvascular decompression for the surgical management of tic douloureux. Neurosurgery, *9*:111, 1981.
21. Rushworth, R.G., and Smith, F.F.: Trigeminal neuralgia and hemifacial spasm. Treatment by microvascular decompression. Med. J. Aust., *1*:424, 1982.
22. Van Loveren, H., et al.: A 10-year experience in the treatment of trigeminal neuralgia. J. Neurosurg., *57*:757, 1982.
23. Barba, D., and Alksne, J.F.: Success of microvascular decompression with and without prior surgical therapy for trigeminal neuralgia. J. Neurosurg., *60*:104, 1984.
24. Grundy, B.L., et al.: BAEP monitoring during cerebellopontine angle surgery. Anesthesiology, *55*:A127, 1981.
25. McCallum, J.E., Tenicela, R., and Jannetta, P.J.: Closed external drainage of cerebrospinal fluid in treatment of postoperative CSF fistulae. Surg. Forum, *24*:465, 1973.
26. Malis, L.I.: Prevention of neurosurgical infection by intraoperative antibiotics. Neurosurgery, *5*:339, 1979.
27. Jannetta, P.J.: Trigeminal neuralgia: Treatment by microvascular decompression. *In* Neurosurgery. Edited by R.H. Wilkins and S.S. Rengachary. New York, McGraw-Hill, 1984, pp. 2357–2363.

28. Schwartz, H.G., and O'Leary, J.L.: Section of the spinothalamic tract in the medulla with observations on the pathway for pain. Surgery, *9*:183, 1941.
29. White, J.C.: Spinothalamic tractotomy in the medulla oblongata. An operation for the relief of intractable neuralgias of the occiput, neck and shoulder. Arch. Surg., *43*:113, 1941.
30. Sjöqvist, O.: Studies on pain conduction in the trigeminal nerve. A contribution to the surgical treatment of facial pain. Acta Psychiatr. Scand. (Suppl.), *17*:1, 1938.
31. White, J.C., and Sweet, W.H.: Pain and the Neurosurgeon. A Forty-Year Experience. Springfield, IL, Charles C Thomas, 1969, pp. 712–726.
32. Carpenter, M.B.: Human Neuroanatomy, 7th Ed. Baltimore, Williams & Wilkins, 1976.
33. Nashold, B.S., Jr.: Brain stem stereotaxic procedures. *In* Stereotaxy of the Human Brain. Anatomical, Physiological and Clinical Applications. Edited by G. Schaltenbrand and A.E. Walker. New York, Georg Thieme Verlag, 1982, pp. 475–483.
34. Spiegel, E.A., and Wycis, H.T.: Stereoencephalotomy. New York, Grune & Stratton, 1965, p. 504.
35. Spiegel, E.A.: Guided Brain Operations. Basel, S. Karger, 1984.
36. Gildenberg, P.L.: Percutaneous cervical cordotomy. Clin. Neurosurg., *21*:24, 1974.
37. Lin, P., Gildenberg, P.L., and Polakoff, P.P.: An anterior approach to percutaneous lower cervical cordotomy, J. Neurosurg., *25*:5553, 1966.
38. Rosomoff, H.L., Brown, C.J., and Sheptak, P.: Percutaneous radiofrequency cervical cordotomy. Technique. J. Neurosurg., *23*:639, 1965.
39. Rosomoff, H.L., Kriger, A.J., and Kupman, A.S.: Effects of percutaneous cervical cordotomy on pulmonary function. J. Neurosurg., *31*:620, 1969.
40. Nashold, B.S., Jr., and Ostdahl, P.H.: Dorsal root-entry zone lesions for pain relief. J. Neurosurg., *51*:59, 1979.
41. Spiegel, E.A., et al.: Medial and basal thalamotomy in so-called intractable pain. *In* Pain. Edited by P.R. Dumke. Boston, Little, Brown & Co., 1966, pp. 503–517.
42. Spiegel, E.A., et al.: Combined dorsomedial, intralaminar and basal thalamotomy for relief of so-called intractable pain. J. Int. Coll. Surg., *42*:160, 1964.
43. Richardson, D.E., and Akil, H.: Pain reduction by electrical brain stimulation in man. II. Chronic self-administration in the periventricular gray matter. J. Neurosurg., *47*:184, 1977.
44. Sindou, M., and Goutelle, A.: Surgical posterior rhizotomies for the treatment of pain. *In* Advances and Technical Standards in Neurosurgery, Vol. 10. Edited by H. Krayenbuhl. New York, Springer-Verlag, 1983, pp. 147–185.
45. Hitchcock, E.R.: Sterertactic cervical myelotomy. J. Neurol. Neurosurg. Psychiatry, *33*:224, 1970.
46. Hitchcock, E., Sotelo, M.G., and Kim, M.Ch.: Analgesic levels and technical method in stereotaxic pontine spinothalamic tractotomy. Acta Neurochir., *77*:29, 1985.
47. Schvarcz, J.R.: Spinal cord stereotactic techniques. Re: Trigeminal nucleotomy and extralemniscal myelotomy. Appl. Neurophysiol., *41*:99, 1978.
48. Barberá, J., Barcia-Salorio, J.L., and Broseta, J.: Stereotaxic pontine spinothalamic tractotomy. Surg. Neurol., *11*:111, 1979.
49. Grant, F.C., and Weinberger, L.M.: Experiences with intramedullary tractotomy. I. Relief of facial pain and summary of operative results. Arch Surg., *42*:681, 1941.
50. D'Errico, A.: Intramedullary spinothalamic tractotomy. J. Neurosurg., *7*:294, 1950.
51. Bricolo, A.: Medullary tractotomy for cephalic pain of malignant disease. *In* Advances in Pain Research and Therapy, Vol. 2. Edited by J.J. Bonica and V. Ventafridda. New York, Raven Press, 1979, pp. 453–462.
52. Hosobuchi, Y., and Rutkin, B.: Descending trigeminal tractotomy, neurophysiological approach. Arch. Neurol., *25*:115, 1971.
53. Taren, J.A.: The position of the cutaneous components of facial, glossopharyngeal and vagal nerves on the spinal tract of V. J. Comp. Neurol., *122*:389, 1964.
54. Dubner, R., Gobel, S., and Price, D.D.: Peripheral and central trigeminal "pain" pathways. *In* Advances in Pain Research and Therapy. Edited by J.J. Bonica and D. Albe-Fessard. New York, Raven Press, 1976, pp. 137–148.
55. Yokota, T.: Trigeminal subnucleus caudalis neurons excited by tooth pulp stimulations. *In* Advances in Pain Research and Therapy, Vol. 1. Edited by J.J. Bonica and D. Albe-Fessard. New York, Raven Press, 1976, pp. 171–176.
56. Kunc, Z.: Significance of fresh anatomic data on spinal trigeminal tract for possibility of selective tractotomies. *In* Pain. Edited by R.S. Knighton and P.R. Dumke. Boston, Little Brown, 1966, pp. 351–366.
57. King, R.B.: Medullary tractotomy for pain relief. *In* Neurosurgery. Edited by R. Wilkins and S. Rengachary. New York, McGraw-Hill, 1983, pp. 2452–2454.
58. Olivecrona, H.: Trigeminal neuralgia. Triangle, *5*:60, 1961.
59. Grant, F.C., Groff, R.A., and Levy, F.H.: Section of the descending spinal root of the fifth cranial nerve. Arch. Neurol. Psychiatry, *43*:490, 1940.
60. Olivecrona, H.: Tractotomy for the relief of trigeminal neuralgia. Arch. Neurol. Psychiatry, *47*:544, 1942.
61. Walker, A.E.: Relief of pain by mesencephalic tractotomy. Arch. Neurol. Psychiatry, *48*:865, 1942.
62. Maxwell, R.E.: Craniofacial pain syndromes: An overview. *In* Neurosurgery. Edited by R. Wilkins and S. Rengachary. New York, McGraw-Hill, 1983, pp. 2327–2336.
63. Spiegel, E.A., et al.: Stereotaxic apparatus for operation on the human brain. Science, *106*:349, 1947.
64. Wycis, H.T., and Spiegel, E.A.: Long-range results in the treatment of intractable pain by stereotaxic midbrain surgery. J. Neurosurg., *19*:101, 1962.
65. Nashold, B.S., Jr., Wilson, W.P., and Slaughter, D.G.: Stereotactic midbrain lesions for central dysesthesia and phantom pain. J. Neurosurg., *30*:116, 1969.
66. Nashold, B.S., Jr.: Extensive cephalic and oral pain relieved by midbrain tractotomy. Confin. Neurol., *34*:382, 1972.
67. Tasker, R.R.: Stereotactic surgery: Principles and techniques. *In* Neurosurgery. Edited by R. Wilkins and S. Rengachary. New York, McGraw-Hill, 1983, pp. 2465–2481.
68. Tasker, R.R.: Stereotaxic surgery. *In* Textbook of Pain. 2nd Ed. Edited by P.D. Wall and R. Melzack. Edinburgh, Churchill Livingstone, 1989, pp. 840–855.
69. Gildenberg, P.L.: Functional neurosurgery. *In* Operative Neurosurgical Techniques, Vol. II. 2nd Ed. Edited by H.H. Schmidek and W.H. Sweet. New York, Grune & Stratton, 1988, pp. 1035–1068.
70. Whisler, W.W., and Voris, H.C.: Mesencephalotomy for intractable pain due to malignant disease. Appl. Neurophysiol., *41*:52, 1978.
71. Voris, H.C., and Whisler, W.W.: Results of stereotaxic surgery for intractable pain. Confin. Neurol., *37*:86, 1975.
72. Nashold, B.S., Jr.: Defects of ocular motility after stereotactic midbrain lesions in man. Arch. Ophthalmol., *88*:245, 1972.
73. Orthner, H., and Roeder, F.: Further clinical and anatomical experience with stereotactic operations for the relief of pain. Confin. Neurol., *27*:418, 1966.
74. Roeder, F., and Orthner, H.: Erfahrungen mit stereotaktischen Eingriffen, III. Mitteilung. Über zerebrale Schmerzoperationen, insbesondere mediale Mesencephalotomie bei thalimischer Hyperpathic und bei Anesthesia dolorosa. Confin. Neurol., *21*:51, 1961.
75. Lieberson, W.T., Voris, H.C., and Uematsu, S.: Recording of somatosensory evoked potentials during mesencephalotomy for intractable pain. Confin. Neurol., *32*:185, 1970.
76. Schwartz, H.G., and O'Leary, J.: Section of the spinothalamic tract at the level of the inferior olive. Arch. Neurol. Psychiatry, *47*:293, 1942.
77. Adams, R., and Munro, D.: Surgical division of the spinothalamic tract in the medulla. Surg. Gynecol. Obstet., *78*:591, 1944.
78. Crawford, A.S.: Medullary tractotomy for relief of intractable pain in the upper levels. Arch. Surg., *55*:523, 1947.
79. Klemme, R.: Relief of pain by section of the spinothalamic tract at the level of the olivary nucleus. J. Int. Coll. Surg., *12*:754, 1949.
80. Crawford, A.S., and Knighton, R.S.: Further observations on medullary spinothalamic tractotomy. J. Neurosurg., *10*:113, 121, 1953.
81. Crawford, A.S.: Medullary spinothalamic tractotomy for high intractable pain. J. Maine Med. Assoc., *51*:233, 1960.
82. Birkenfeld, R., and Fisher, R.G.: Successful treatment of causalgia of upper extremity with medullary spinothalamic tractotomy. J. Neurosurg., *20*:303, 1963.
83. Grant, F.C., and Weinberger, L.M.: Experiences with intramedullary tractotomy. IV. Surgery of the brain stem and its operative complications. Surg. Gynecol. Obstet., *72*:747, 1941.

84. Hamby, W.B.: Trigeminal tractotomy. Observations on 48 cases. Arch. Surg., *57*:171, 1948.
85. Falconer, M.A.: Intramedullary trigeminal tractotomy and its place in the treatment of facial pain. J. Neurol. Neurosurg. Psychiatry, *12*:297, 1949.
86. Raney, R., Raney, A., and Hunter, C.R.: Treatment of major trigeminal neuralgia through section of the trigeminospinal tract in the medulla. Am. J. Surg., *80*:11, 1950.
87. Guidetti, B.: Tractotomy for the relief of trigeminal neuralgia. J. Neurosurg., *7*:499, 1950.
88. McKenzie, F.G.: Trigeminal tractotomy. Clin. Neurosurg., *2*:50, 1955.
89. Irsigler, F.J.: Sjöqvist's tractotomy: experiences in 22 cases. Neurochirurgie, *6*:136, 1963.
90. Kunc, Z.: Treatment of essential neuralgia of the 9th nerve by selective tractotomy. J. Neurosurg., *23*:494, 1965.
91. Hitchcock, E.: Stereotactic trigeminal tractotomy. Ann. Clin. Res., *2*:121, 1970.
92. Hitchcock, E.R., and Schvarcz, J.R.: Stereotaxic trigeminal tractotomy for post-herpetic facial pain. J. Neurosurg., *37*:412, 1972.
93. Crue, B.L., Carregal, E.J.A., and Felsoory, A.: Percutaneous stereotactic radiofrequency trigeminal tractotomy with neurophysiological recordings. Confin. Neurol., *34*:389, 1972.
94. Fox, J.L.: Percutaneous trigeminal tractotomy for facial pain. Acta Neurochir., *29*:83, 1973.
95. Dogliotti, M.: First surgical sections, in man, of the lemniscus lateralis (pain-temperature path at the brain stem, for the treatment of diffused rebellious pain). Curr. Res. Anesth. Analg., *17*:143, 1938.
96. Walker, A.E.: Mesencephalic tractotomy. A method for the relief of unilateral intractable pain. Arch. Surg., *44*:953, 1942.
97. Drake, C.G., and McKenzie, K.G.: Mesencephalic tractotomy for pain. Experience with six cases. J. Neurosurg., *10*:457, 1953.
98. Mazars, G., Roge, R., and Pansini, A.: Stereotactic coagulation of the spinothalamic tract for intractable trigeminal pain. J. Neurol. Neurosurg. Psychiatry, *23*:352, 1960.
99. Zapheltal, B.: Indications for the brain stem operations and the division of patients for the resultant evaluation. Acta Neurochir., *N16–18*:63, 1968–1969.
100. Hageman, R., and DeGrood, M.P.A.M.: Experience with stereotaxic treatment of intractable pain. Psychiatr. Neurol. Neurochir., *73*:113, 1970.
101. Frank, F., et al.: Stereotaxic rostral mesencephalotomy in treatment of malignant faciothoracobrachial pain syndromes. J. Neurosurg., *56*:807, 1982.
102. Amano, K., et al.: Long-term follow-up study of rostral mesencephalic reticulotomy for pain relief—report of 34 cases. Appl. Neurophysiol., *49*:105, 1986.
103. Frank, F., et al: Stereotactic mesencephalotomy versus multiple thalamotomies in the treatment of chronic cancer pain syndromes. Appl. Neurophysiol., *50*:314, 1987.
104. Spiegel, E.A., and Wycis, H.T.: Mesencephalotomy in treatment of "intractable" facial pain. Arch. Neurol. Psychiatry, *69*:1, 1953.
105. Hecaen, H., et al.: Coagulations limitées du thalamus dans les algies du syndrome thalamique. Rev. Neurol. (Paris), *81*:917, 1949.
106. Willis, W.D., Jr.: The Pain System. The Neural Basis of Nociceptive Transmission in the Mammalian Nervous System. Basel, S. Karger, 1985, pp. 241–244.
107. Spiegel, E.A., et al.: Combined dorsomedial, intralaminar and basal thalamotomy for relief of so-called intractable pain. J. Int. Coll. Surg., *42*:160, 1964.
108. Tasker, R.R.: Stereotactic surgery principles and techniques. *In* Neurosurgery. Edited by R.H. Wilkins and S.S. Rengachary. New York, McGraw-Hill, 1985, pp. 2465–2481.
109. Mark, V.H., Ervin, F.R., and Hackett, T.P.: Clinical aspects of stereotactic thalamotomy in the human. Arch. Neurol., *3*:351, 1960.
110. Spiegel, E.A., and Wycis, H.T.: Present status of stereoencephalotomies for pain relief. Confin. Neurol., *27*:7, 1966.
111. Spiegel, E.A.: Guided Brain Operations. Basel, S. Karger, 1982.
112. Fairman, D.: Evaluation of results in stereotactic thalamotomy for the treatment of intractable pain. Confin. Neurol., *27*:67, 1966.
113. Richardson, D.E.: Thalamotomy for intractable pain. Confin. Neurol., *29*:139, 1967.
114. Sano, K., et al.: Thalamolaminotomy. Confin. Neurol., *27*:63, 1966.
115. Yoshii, N., Kazuma, A., and Tatsuyuki, K.: Further studies on the stereotaxic thalamotomy for pain relief. Tohoku J. Exp. Med., *102*:225, 1970.
116. Spiegel, E.A., and Wycis, H.T.: Stereoencephalotomy. Part II. Clinical and Physiological Applications. Basel, S. Karger, 1962.
117. White, J.C., and Sweet, W.H.: Pain and the Neurosurgeon. Springfield, IL, Charles C Thomas, 1969, pp. 843–887.
118. Orthner, H., and Roeder, F.: Further clinical and anatomical experiences with stereotactic operations for relief of pain. Confin. Neurol., *27*:418, 1966.
119. White, J.C., and Sweet, W.H.: Pain and the Neurosurgeon. A Forty-Year Experience. Springfield, IL, Charles C Thomas, 1969, p. 387.
120. Sano, K.: Intralaminar thalamotomy (thalamolaminotomy) and posterior-medial hypothalamedial hypothalamotomy in the treatment of intractable pain. *In* Progress in Neurological Surgery, Vol. 8. Edited by H. Krayenbuhl, P.E. Maspes, and W.H. Sweet. Basel, S. Karger, 1977, pp. 50–103.
121. Turnbull, I.M.: Bilateral cingulumotomy combined with thalamotomy for mesencephalic tractotomy for pain. Surg. Gynecol. Obstet., *134*:958, 1972.
122. Roth, D.A., and Mark, V.H.: Thalamotomy for pain relief. *In* Neurological Surgery, Vol. 3. Edited by J.R. Youmans. Philadelphia, W.B. Saunders, 1973, pp. 1783–1789.
123. Tasker, R.R.: Thalamic stereotaxic procedures. *In* Stereotaxy of the Human Brain. Edited by G. Schaltenbrand and A.E. Walker. Stuttgart, Georg Thieme Verlag, 1982, pp. 484–497.
124. Pagni, C.A.: Central pain and painful anesthesia. *In* Progress in Neurological Surgery. Edited by H. Krayenbuhl, P.E. Maspeth, and W.H. Sweet. Basel, S. Karger, 1977, pp. 132–257.
125. Voris, H.C., and Whisler, W.W.: Results of stereotaxic surgery in intractable pain. Confin. Neurol., *37*:86, 1975.
126. Tasker, R.R., Organ, L.W., and Hawrylyshyn, P.A.: The Thalamus and Midbrain of Man. A Physiological Atlas Using Electrical Stimulation. Springfield, IL, Charles C Thomas, 1982.
127. Sano, K.: Sedative neurosurgery with special reference to posteromedial hypothalamotomy. Neurol. Med. Chir., *4*:112, 1962.
128. Sano, K., et al.: Posteromedial hypothalamotomy in the treatment of intractable pain. Confin. Neurol., *37*:285, 1975.
129. Fairman, D.: Hypothalamotomy as a new perspective for alleviation of intractable pain and regression of metastatic tumors. *In* Present Limits of Neurosurgery. Edited by I. Fusek and Z. Kunc. Prague, Avicenum, 1972, pp. 525–528.
130. Dafny, N., Bental, E., and Feldman, S.: Effect of sensory stimuli on single unit activity in the posterior hypothalamus. Electroencephalogr. Clin. Neurophysiol., *19*:256, 1965.
131. Fairman, D.: Neurophysiological basis for the hypothalamic lesion in stimulation by chronic implanted electrodes for the relief of intractable pain in cancer. *In* Advances in Pain Research and Therapy, Vol. 1. Edited by J.J. Bonica and D. Albe-Fessard. New York, Raven Press, 1976, pp. 843–847.
132. Gildenberg, P.L.: Stereotactic surgery. *In* Clinical Anesthesia in Neurosurgery. Edited by E.A.M. Frost. New York, Butterworth & Co., 1984, pp. 279–292.
133. Leriche, R.: La Chirurgie de la Douleur. Paris, Masson, 1937, p. 186.
134. De Gutiérrez-Mahoney, C.G.: The treatment of painful phantom limb by removal of postcentral cortex. J. Neurosurg., *1*:156, 1944.
135. De Gutiérrez-Mahoney, C.G.: The treatment of painful phantom limb. A follow-up study. Surg. Clin. North Am., *28*:481, 1948.
136. White, J.C., and Sweet, W.H.: Pain and the Neurosurgeon. A Forty-Year Experience. Springfield, IL, Charles C Thomas, 1969, pp. 79–83, 835–842.
137. Pool, J.L., and Bridges, T.J.: Subcortical parietal lobotomy for relief of phantom limb syndrome in the upper extremity: A case report. Bull. N. Y. Acad. Med., *30*:302, 1954.
138. Lende, R.A., Kirsch, W.M., and Druckman, R.: Relief of facial pain after combined removal of precentral and postcentral cortex. J. Neurosurg., *34*:537, 1971.
139. Hamby, W.B.G.: Reversible central pain. Arch. Neurol., *5*:528, 1961.
140. Moniz, E.: Tentatives operations dans le traitement de certaines psychoses. Paris, Masson, 1936.
141. Fulton, J., and Jacobsen, C.: The functions of the frontal lobes, a comparative study in monkeys, chimpanzees and man. Abstract. Second International Neurological Congress, London, 1935, p. 70.

142. Freeman. W., and Watts, J.: Pain mechanisms and the frontal lobes: A study of prefrontal lobotomy for intractable pain. Ann. Intern. Med., *28*:747, 1948.
143. Watts, J.W., and Freeman, W.: Psychosurgery for the relief of unbearable pain. J. Int. Coll. Surg., *9*:679, 1946.
144. Dynes, J.B., and Poppen, L.L.: Lobotomy for intractable pain. JAMA, *140*:15, 1949.
145. Falconer, M.A.: Relief of intractable pain of organic origin by frontal lobotomy. Res. Publ. Assoc. Res. Nerv. Ment. Dis. *27*:706, 1948.
146. Hamilton, F.E., and Hayes, G.J.: Prefrontal lobotomy in the management of intractable pain. Arch. Surg., *58*:731, 1949.
147. Love, J., Petersen, M.C., and Moersch, F.P.: Prefrontal lobotomy for the relief of intractable pain. Minn. Med., *32*:148, 1949.
148. Otenasek, F.J.: Prefrontal lobotomy for the relief of intractable pain. Bull. Johns Hopkins Hosp., *83*:229, 1948.
149. Poppen, J.L.: Prefrontal lobotomy for intractable pain: Case report. Lahey Clinic Boston Bull., *2*:205, 1946.
150. Greenblatt, M., and Solomon, H.: Survey of nine years of lobotomy investigations. Am. J. Psychiatry, *109*:262, 1952.
151. Elithorn, A., Glithero, E., and Slater, E.: Leucotomy for pain. J. Neurol. Neurosurg. Psychiatry, *21*:249, 1958.
152. Bertrand, C., Martinez, N., and Hardy, J.: Frontothalamic section for intractable pain. *In* Pain. Henry Ford Hospital International Symposium. Edited by R.S. Knighton and R.R. Dumke. Boston, Little, Brown & Co., 1966, pp. 531–535.
153. Scarff, J.E.: Unilateral prefrontal lobotomy with relief of ipsilateral, contralateral and bilateral pain. A preliminary report. J. Neurosurg., *5*:288, 1948.
154. Scarff, J.E.: Unilateral prefrontal lobotomy for the relief of intractable pain and termination of narcotic addiction. Surg. Gynecol. Obstet., *89*:385, 1948.
155. White, J.C., and Sweet, W.H.: Pain and the Neurosurgeon. Springfield, IL, Charles C Thomas, 1969, pp. 773–814.
156. Scoville, W.B.: Selective cortical undercutting as a means of modifying and studying frontal lobe function in man. J. Neurosurg., *6*:65, 1949.
157. Pool, J.L., and Bridges, T.J.: Subcortical parietal lobotomy for relief of phantom limb syndrome in the upper extremity. Bull. N.Y. Acad. Med., *30*:302, 1954.
158. LeBeau, J.: Anterior cingulectomy in man. J. Neurosurg., *11*:268, 1954.
159. Grantham, E.G.: Prefrontal lobotomy for relief of pain—with a report of a new operative technique. J. Neurosurg., *8*:405, 1951.
160. Knight, G.: Stereotactic tractotomy in the surgical treatment of mental illness. J. Neurol Neurosurg. Psychiatry, *28*:304, 1965.
161. Meyerson, B., Bergström, M., and Greitz, T.: Target localization in stereotactic capsulotomy with the aid of computed tomography. *In* Modern Concepts in Psychiatric Surgery. Edited by E. Hitchcock, H. Ballantine, and B. Meyerson. Amsterdam, Elsevier, 1979.
162. Papez, J.: A proposed mechanism of emotion. Arch. Neurol. Psychiatry, *38*:725, 1937.
163. Foltz, E., and White, L.: The role of rostral cingulumotomy in "pain" relief. Int. J. Neurol., *6*:353, 1968.
164. Foltz, E., and White, L.: Experimental cingulumotomy and modification of morphine withdrawal. J. Neurosurg., *14*:655, 1957.
165. Kanaka, T., and Balasubramaniam, V.: Stereotactic cingulumotomy for drug addiction. Appl. Neurophysiol., *41*:86, 1978.
166. Foltz, E., and Lockard, J.: Recovery of homeostasis by cingulumotomy in monkey. *In* Modern Concepts in Psychiatric Surgery. Edited by E. Hitchcock, H. Ballantine, and B. Meyerson. Amsterdam. Elsevier, 1979, pp. 111–130.
167. Corkin, S., Twitchell, T., and Sullivan, E.: Safety and efficacy of cingulumotomy for pain and psychiatric disorders. *In* Modern Concepts in Psychiatric Surgery. Edited by E. Hitchcock, H. Ballantine, and B. Meyerson. Amsterdam, Elsevier, 1979, pp. 253–272.
168. Hurt, R.W., and Ballantine, H.T.: Stereotactic anterior cingulate lesions for persistent pain: A report on 68 cases. Clin. Neurosurg., *21*:334, 1973.
169. Bernad, P., Ballantine, H.T., and Giriunas, I.: Neuropathological study of bilateral cingulumotomy for mood disturbance. *In* Modern Concepts in Psychiatric Surgery. Edited by E. Hitchcock, H. Ballantine, and B. Meyerson. Amsterdam, Elsevier, 1979, pp. 283–302.
170. Faillace, L., et al.: Cognitive deficits from bilateral cingulumotomy for intractable pain in man. Dis. Nerv. Syst., *32*:171, 1971.
171. Wilson, D., and Chang, E.: Bilateral anterior cingulectomy for the relief of intractable pain. Confin. Neurol., *36*:61, 1974.
172. Voris, H., and Whisler, W.: Results of stereotaxic surgery for intractable pain. Confin. Neurol., *37*:86, 1975.
173. Broager, B., and Olesen, K.: Psychosurgery in sixty-three cases of open cingulectomy and fourteen cases of bifrontal prehypothalamic cryolesion. *In* Second International Conference on Psychosurgery. Edited by E. Hitchcock and K. Vaernet. Springfield, IL, Charles C Thomas, 1972, pp. 253–257.
174. Turnbull, I.: Bilateral cingulumotomy combined with thalamotomy or mesencephalic tractotomy for pain. Surg. Gynecol. Obstet., *134*:958, 1972.
175. Mitchell-Heggs, N., et al.: Further experience in limbic leucotomy. *In* Modern Concepts in Psychiatric Surgery. Edited by E. Hitchcock, H. Ballantine, and B. Meyerson. Amsterdam, Elsevier, pp. 327–336, 1979.
176. Petrie, A.: Individuality in Pain and Suffering. Chicago, University of Chicago Press, 1967.

INTRODUCTION

JOHN J. BONICA

In contrast to most sections of this book, this last section has only one chapter. It describes the multidisciplinary/interdisciplinary team approach using multimodal therapies in the management of patients with complex chronic pain problems. Each chapter that precedes this one has been written by an authority in a specific field, and of course it is natural to emphasize the indications for and efficacy and advantages of specific therapies as well as complications and disadvantages. Although each modality used alone is effective for one or more specific types of pain, no single modality can be expected to be effective for all types of pain, especially chronic pain syndromes. This chapter is presented at this point to emphasize the critical importance of integrating various modalities by multidisciplinary/interdisciplinary teams who work in an exquisitely coordinated and collaborative fashion to make the diagnosis and develop the most effective therapeutic strategies.

In Chapter 9 I describe in some detail the evolution and current status of these types of programs. As noted there, soon after I began my assigned responsibility of attending patients with pain problems in a large military hospital during World War II, I realized that although nerve blocks and the use of narcotics—the two procedures I knew as an anesthesiologist—were effective in managing some patients with acute pain or cancer pain and a few nonmalignant chronic pain syndromes, they were ineffective in dealing with patients with complex problems. From reading the available literature and observing patients, I realized that many if not most patients with complex chronic problems had psychologic/psychiatric, neurologic, or orthopedic substrates to their problems—often a combination of all of these—and that I was wholly ignorant of these conditions. Indeed I came to the conclusion that regardless of a physician's thorough knowledge and utmost skill in his specific field, these were not enough to solve many problems. I therefore began to request consultations of colleagues in other specialties.

Initially, these consultations were done in the manner inherent in traditional medical practice of that period: The consultants would see the patient in their offices or on the ward, then write the findings in the chart. After all consultants saw the patient I read their evaluations and attempted to come to some conclusion as to the diagnosis and what treatment to recommend. This proved not only difficult and frustrating, but very time consuming. I therefore suggested to my colleagues from different specialties who had seen the patient that we meet face-to-face as a group and review each other's findings and discuss the case until we could reach consensus on the diagnosis and therapy. After several months' experience I became convinced that complex chronic pain problems could be more effectively treated by a multidisciplinary/interdisciplinary team, each member of which would contribute his or her specialized knowledge and skills to the common goal of making a correct diagnosis and developing the most effective therapeutic strategy. In addition to providing much needed service to the patient, this was a highly effective mechanism for the exchange of information that proved an excellent educational process for each member of the team.

After the war I developed a similar program in a private hospital, and in 1960 I developed the University of Washington program. I also spent much time expounding the concept in various parts of the world, but until the late 1960s it was ignored by the health professions. Fortunately, in the late 1960s and early 1970s a number of factors (see page 199) converged to cause an increasing number of clinicians to put the concept into practice. (For details of the growth of pain programs, the types of pain centers or clinics that developed, the numbers in various parts of the world, the concerns provoked by this rapid development of centers, and the evolution of the pain program at the University of Washington, see pages 200–208.)

The chapter that follows describes two interdisciplinary, multimodal pain management programs: one at the University of Washington directed by Dr. John D. Loeser and staffed by faculty and trainees of numerous disciplines in the Health Sciences Division of the University of Washington, and the other at the Northwest Pain Center in Portland, Oregon, organized and directed by Dr. Joel L. Seres and Dr. Richard I. Newman. The Portland program primarily manages patients with operant chronic pain and patients with pain of unknown origin manifesting disability out of proportion to their impairment. The University of Washington program manages patients with cancer pain and various nonmalignant chronic pain syndromes, a significant proportion of whom have developed chronic pain behavior as a result of environmental factors. The University of Washington program also has an acute pain service that provides an outstanding service to patients with acute postoperative and post-traumatic pain and with acute pain caused by visceral disease (see Chapter 25). The University Pain Center also has a very large research program that is discussed in Chapter 9.

In Chapter 100, Loeser, Seres, and Newman focus on the interdisciplinary, multimodal approach to the management of patients who have failed to respond to traditional medical modalities and discuss the organization and function of the program in much more detail than in Chapter 9. An even more detailed description of this program is given in a recently published monograph edited by Loeser and Egan that includes chapters written by virtually every member of the faculty (1).

Despite the intrinsic and extrinsic problems encountered during the early years (see page 206) and the skepticism expressed by some national authorities who apparently were medical traditionalists, most of the comprehensive pain programs of the type described in Chapter 100 have been successful in returning a significant percentage of patients to a productive life. The results reported from a number of such programs are summarized in the last section of the chapter. The usefulness and value of such programs has been emphasized by two important task groups, one in the United States and the other in Canada. In the United States the prestigious Institute of Medicine (IOM) appointed a *Committee on Pain, Disability, and Chronic Illness Behavior* to consider the various aspects of chronic pain and disability (2). In Canada the *Quebec Task Force on Spinal Disorders* focused on pain in all parts of the spine, with emphasis on the rates of such disorders among workers in Quebec (3). In their reports, both groups encouraged physicians and other health professionals to refer patients with chronic pain who have failed to respond to the usual medical therapy to a multidisciplinary pain team.

The Quebec Task Force suggested that if management by the treating physician and a consultant specialist has not been successful and the patient still has pain after 3 to 6 months, he or she should be referred to a multidisciplinary team, which should focus primarily on psychologic and psychosocial elements, on the premise that these factors are primarily responsible for the persistence of pain. Nothing is said of having the team reassess for pathologic or pathophysiologic bases for the pain. It is widely known that persistent pain due to pathologic lesions can cause serious psychologic and psychosocial disorders and that they should therefore be included in the assessment, but I believe that the team has as much responsibiltiy to evaluate the patient for physical and pathologic processes that might have been missed and which might be responsible for the persistent pain and consequent psychologic and psychosocial dysfunction. Dr. H. LaRocca, Editor-in-Chief of the journal *Spine* (in which a summary of the report is published as a supplement), expressed concern about this issue in an editorial (4) in which he stated that "many patients with symptoms of six months' duration or more can still have intractable organic disease without significant psychologic component. Every effort must be made to identify them." In Chapter 72 I cite a number of reports concerning many patients in whom the pathologic processes had not been diagnosed by the primary physician and even by consultants but were identified by the multidisciplinary team to which the patients were referred. Stoeckle and Boyd (5), members of the IOM committee, also mention the unresolved problem posed by patients with chronic pain in whom a diagnosis of an underlying physical illness was missed because of inadequate diagnostic assessment or because the assessment was carried out before identification of the disease process was possible. They cite three publications reporting morbidity rates of undiagnosed physical illness presenting as psychiatric disease. As emphasized by Loeser et al. in Chapter 100, time and effort must be expended to carry out a comprehensive evaluation to diagnose organic pathology that can be eliminated.

Although currently many if not most of the programs in the United States accept as referrals and manage patients who have developed chronic pain behavior and disability long after the healing process and have minimal or no obvious pathology, I believe that the same principles of diagnosis and rehabilitation therapy should be applied to the management of patients with obvious chronic pathology that cannot be removed such as arthritis, cancer, deafferentation pain, and other chronic pain syndromes. Because chronic persistent pain that is not adequately relieved causes the patient to develop psychologic, psychosocial, and behavioral problems as well as progressive physical deterioration, these patients should also be managed by multidisciplinary teams.

In Chapter 24 I describe the application of this concept to the management of patients with cancer-related pain. There are a number of comprehensive cancer centers that have a division or department of cancer pain therapy composed of interdisciplinary teams that are able to manage not only the physical, but also the psychologic and psychosocial aspects of the pain and frequently the cancer. Similar teams also exist in the many hospices, as described by Twycross in the last section of Chapter 24. The experience of these teams provides impressive evidence that this integrated approach is much more effective in improving the quality of life of patients with advanced or terminal cancer than can be achieved with the traditional way, in which the oncologist manages the patient with the support of nurses. Indeed, in Chapter 24 evidence is presented that many oncologists have little or no interest in the problem of pain or knowledge about it (in contrast to the problem of cancer). In very recent years the difference between the team approach and the traditional care of cancer patients has become more and more appreciated, and I predict that within the next decade every hospital or other facility that cares for cancer patients will have interdisciplinary cancer management teams. Moreover, as the benefits of the interdisciplinary, multimodal approach in treating patients with chronic pain becomes known within institutions that have them, the approach will be applied to patients with other types of chronic pain.

As emphasized by Loeser, Seres, and Newman, we must mount a multipronged program to educate physicians (particularly practicing family physicians), other health care professionals, the consumers of health care, and third-party carriers about the critical importance of the team approach in managing patients with chronic pain. We must inform and indeed encourage treating physicians and even specialists who have been unsuccessful with the first or at most the second attempt in using surgery or other medical therapies in managing complex pain problems; they should seriously consider referring the patient to a multidisciplinary/interdisciplinary pain center that can carry out an exquisitely coordinated effort in making the diagnosis and developing the most effective therapeutic strategy.

Although such comprehensive centers in the past have been viewed as "court of last appeal" for treatment of chronic pain, health professionals should refer patients with complex problems early in order to abort the development of what some improperly refer to as "chronic pain syndrome" and—most important—reduce the suffering among millions of patients with chronic pain. The success rate reported by a number of such programs suggests that increasing use of such facilities is likely to obviate the multiple, often useless, and at times mutilating operations and attendant complications. Recently Loeser and his colleagues were referred a patient who had had 46 operations for low back pain or for complications of previous surgery or other therapies. At the time of the interview the patient was taking over 60 daily medications prescribed by 14 different doctors; none of them knew that other colleagues had seen the patient. Review of the records revealed that the initial operation for back pain that led to this incredible series of misadventures was not indicated. I would think that physicians who saw the patient after the third or fourth operation would have come to the conclusion that further surgery might not be the answer to the problem and would have referred the patient to a multidisciplinary pain rehabilitation program.

REFERENCES

1. Loeser, J.D., and Egan, K.J. (eds.): Managing the Chronic Pain Patient: Theory and Practice at the University of Washington Multidisciplinary Pain Center. New York, Raven Press, 1989.
2. Osterweis, M., Kleinman, A., and Mechanic, D.: Pain and Disability. Washington DC, National Academy Press, 1987.
3. Spitzer, W.O., et al.: Scientific approach to the assessment and management of activity-related spinal disorders. Spine, 12(Suppl. 1), 1987.
4. La Rocca, H.: Editorial. Scientific approach to the assessment and management of activity-related spinal disorders. Spine, 12(Suppl. 1):S8, 1987.
5. Stoeckle, J.D., and Boyd, R.: Chronic pain in medical practice. In Pain and Disability. Edited by M. Osterweis, A. Kleinman, and D. Mechanic. Washington, DC, National Academy Press, 1987, pp. 189–210.

100 • INTERDISCIPLINARY, MULTIMODAL MANAGEMENT OF CHRONIC PAIN

JOHN D. LOESER, JOEL L. SERES, *and* RICHARD I. NEWMAN, JR.

MULTIMODAL, multidisciplinary pain diagnosis and therapy programs focusing on the needs of patients with chronic pain have developed from the increasing awareness that individual physicians often do not possess the skills, knowledge, and attitudes necessary to deal successfully with complex chronic pain problems.

We believe that a taxonomy of pain treatment is required so that the public can know what it is receiving, and so that governmental agencies and third-party payers can evaluate the services provided (see Chapter 9).

We suggest that the terminology used throughout this chapter and in Chapter 9 provides reasonable criteria for classifying pain treatment facilities. These can be evaluated on the nature of the services they provide and the types of health care providers in their employ. The term *clinic* refers to a unit that offers only outpatient services; a *center* offers both inpatient and outpatient activities. A facility that treats only one type of pain problem is best described in terms of that disease, e.g., headache clinic/center or foot pain clinic/center. The phrases *pain clinic* and *pain center* are reserved for organizations of multiple health care providers who treat a variety of chronic pain problems. A *multidisciplinary or interdisciplinary pain clinic/center* has at least three professionals from different disciplines who are available to deal with patients, and care is provided in a coordinated, integrated fashion. The designation *comprehensive multidisciplinary or interdisciplinary pain center* is used to describe a complex organization that has many different types of health care providers and engages in teaching and research. Most comprehensive pain clinics or centers have a strong component of behavioral medicine and owe their intellectual heritage to the work of Fordyce and his associates (1). In such a facility, the members of the treatment team interact with each other so as to present to the patient a single, unified approach to his or her pain problem. A properly functioning pain clinic or pain center is not only multidisciplinary but also interdisciplinary.

In this chapter we focus on the multidisciplinary pain center or clinic, which is the dominant type of facility in the United States. This is the optimal type of pain management facility when the appropriate resources and personnel are available. Our discussion is based primarily on the experiences of two pain centers, the University of Washington Multidisciplinary Pain Center founded by Bonica and White in 1960 and the Northwest Pain Center run by Seres and Newman since 1972. The former is a part of a major medical center, and its medical and psychological staff are all faculty members, whereas the latter is a free-standing pain treatment unit, whose staff are private practitioners. Additional information about the University of Washington Multidisciplinary Pain Center can be found in Chapter 9.

The integration of multiple modalities and disciplines for the treatment of pain has probably been the single most important advance in the modern care of the patient who suffers from chronic pain (1–5). Standing apart from those sufferers who respond to conventional approaches is an ever-enlarging group of people for whom individual treatment modalities have failed to provide adequate relief of pain and its life-controlling impact. They are the failures of the traditional health care delivery system, because society has defined their problem to be medical.

The interdisciplinary approach requires a different role for the patient and for the providers of care. Whereas specific-modality therapies often allow passivity of the patient who receives them, interdisciplinary treatment demands *active* participation. Whereas the physician is usually in control of the care and the outcome of medical efforts in single-modality therapy, other health care providers and the patient become *equally* important in an interdisciplinary approach. Without the integration of all the health care providers, a treatment plan disintegrates quickly into a series of isolated single-modality therapies. The physician on an interdisciplinary team must become an integrator, open to the views and the approaches of other health care providers. Heading an interdisciplinary team calls for special skills (4, 5).

CHRONIC PAIN

The differentiation of chronic pain from acute pain has been an important breakthrough in the formulation of the mechanisms involved and the treatment strategies that can be expected to work (Chapters 7, 8, 16, and 81). Several efforts have been made to define pain syndromes and it is clear that acute pain, pain due to progressive malignant disease, and pain due to long-standing nonmalignant causes each responds differently to the same treatment modalities. It is therefore important to develop some guidelines for the treatment of each of these types of pain in order to effect appropriate results. Multidisciplinary pain clinics/centers must be prepared to assess and treat appropriately all types of chronic pain patients.

Acute pain syndromes respond with predictable results to narcotics, sedatives, muscle relaxants, and other families of drugs. Acute problems usually respond to rest, initial immobilization, and a willingness of the patient to help the normal healing process, essentially a passive role (Chapter 7). With the passage of time, however, changes occur in many patients, and these same treatment approaches become less effective, then ineffective, and finally counterproductive (6–9). Interventions such as surgery, local blocks, and efforts at further diagnosis all lose their effectiveness as time passes (Chapter 8).

A different set of problems exists in the management of chronic pain due to cancer. Nociception is highly likely to play a significant role in this type of chronic pain, and physicians must be available to utilize pharmacologic, anesthesiologic, and surgical techniques to obtain pain relief. Of course, psychologic issues can be present and must also be addressed. The management of pain due to cancer and its treatments can be facilitated by multidisciplinary assessment and treatment, and pain clinics/centers associated with major hospitals should be prepared to treat cancer pain patients with multidisciplinary strategies.

It is also important to identify those patients whose chronic pain is not due to cancer and whose diagnosis and treatment can be facilitated by a multidisciplinary approach, even though they might not require the full array of services offered in a pain clinic/center. The multidisciplinary approach can lead to more accurate diagnosis, a wider array of treatment options, and prompt recognition of treatment failure. Hence, referral to a pain clinic/center can be appropriate even when the patient has a clear-cut diagnosis and medical treatments are available that have some likelihood of success. Pain clinics/centers are not just for the failures of health care delivery; appropriate care can help patients early in their chronic illness.

This chapter, however, focuses on the chronic pain patients who appear to have failed to respond to traditional medical modalities. They are a distinct subgroup of the patients seen in pain clinics/centers who can best be described as suffering from pain of unknown origin and manifesting disability out of proportion to their impairment. The Portland Pain Center does not treat patients with cancer pain or specific chronic pain syndromes; the University of Washington Multidisciplinary Pain Center does, and it also has an acute pain service that provides therapy to patients with acute pain. The topic of cancer pain management is discussed in Chapter 24; it is not discussed in this chapter.

For those who would treat them, an essential aspect of too many chronic pain patients lies in the important and often distasteful prospect of *incurability*. A physical problem, for which modern therapy has not evolved a treatment to eradicate the cause, now emerges as the therapeutic challenge. There is, therefore, a distinction between the patient with chronic pain who functions well in spite of the pain, without manifesting pain and suffering, and the individual with whatever intensity of pain who is unable to

function because of it. Wherever possible, efforts must be expended to look for a treatable cause. This does not imply, however, that every patient should have every test available repeated again and again. It certainly does not suggest that another surgical procedure should be done "as a last resort" or "to see what happens" in a blind effort to satisfy the physician's need to "try everything."

Judicious use of diagnostic procedures and interventions must be the keystone of the care plan. The complexity of the chronic pain problem does not allow the patient to decide on further surgery without the direct guidance of the physician. In the setting of chronic pain, offering a patient who is depressed and desperate another surgical procedure is an abrogation of responsibility by the physician and the exploitation of the confused, discouraged, and frustrated patient who will grasp at almost any straw offered, often without regard to the risks involved or, indeed, any chance for significant improvement.

As an important part of the picture, the roles of the participants must now change. The physician cannot cure the problem and must be willing to deal with that fact; others must be brought into the plan to work closely with the physician to help the patient develop more effective coping mechanisms, support systems, and life-planning. In short, all the players in the drama must now deal with the reality that the problem will persist unless a different approach is adopted and should help the patient integrate that fact into an effective and satisfactory life-plan. It is essential that the patient become an active and willing participant in this effort.

The patient and physician both must come to recognize that the patient is "hurting more than he needs to" because of the effects of deconditioning and social contingencies. These issues must be appropriately addressed at the same time pain management and pain reduction techniques are taught.

Chronic pain of unknown cause that has failed to respond to traditional medical therapy demands alternate goals. The purpose of therapy is to reduce irritating factors as much as possible and expanding coping ability. Reactive depression, anger, frustration, fear, anxiety, and other usually constructive emotional responses become impediments to a normal life-style. Recognition of these elements becomes an important part of diagnosis and treatment, and overlooking them can be one of the major reasons for the failure of traditional treatment approaches. Sometimes financial considerations on the part of insurance carriers limit our abilities to examine and treat emotional concomitants out of fear that these psychologic issues will become "part of the claimant's disability" and thereby significantly increase the company's financial exposure. In reality, early recognition and treatment of these behavioral and emotional factors can make the difference between success and failure of treatment (10–14).

A significant number of nonpatients, when asked, will report having chronic pain of more than trivial severity. These people might consume some health care, but the pain does not take over their lives. They might lose some time from the job or household activities, but although they say they have chronic pain they do not appear to suffer and are functional (15). These are not the people who come to pain clinics/centers in the United States. To the extent that such people seek assistance, the principles elucidated in this chapter can be applied.

Furthermore, there is a large group of individuals who function well using single-modality therapy to control their chronic pain. For example, there are many people whose pains are satisfactorily controlled with the judicious use of nerve blocks, acupuncture, the various forms of manipulative therapy, or other treatment methods. So long as objective improvement and maintenance of function can be seen, the approach used is acceptable. However, our personal observations over several years in multidisciplinary pain treatment programs have made clear that these approaches are, in all too many patients, continued without objective evidence of improvement or enhanced function. Unless judiciously used, such isolated treatment strategies can become supportive of the passivity of the patient and his disability and can perpetuate the patient's pain behaviors.

The expectations of the patient entering treatment must be understood. Often patients will report significant improvement when asked by their treating physician, but report incapacitating problems when asked by others. For many patients anything short of complete restoration is often viewed as abject failure of the therapy, even though such expectations are clearly unreasonable. Physicians and patients may not share the same goals and patients may say what they think physicians want to hear. Thorough discussion of expectations and obligations of the patient and the treatment team is essential.

Chronic pain therefore means many different things. Its treatment and the results obtained are expressed in ways carrying very different meanings for patient, family, physician, therapists, and those dealing with the emotional adaptation of the individual. For the purposes of this discussion the most refractory of those problems will be our focus.

DEVELOPMENT OF INTERDISCIPLINARY, MULTIMODAL APPROACH TO CHRONIC PAIN

As early as 1945, Bonica (16) realized that "complex pain problems required a vast amount of knowledge and experience, much more than that possessed by any individual." As a result he conceived the notion "that complex pain problems can be treated more effectively by a multidisciplinary/interdisciplinary team, each member of which contributes his/her specialized knowledge and skills to the common goal of making a correct diagnosis and developing the most effective therapeutic strategy" (3, 16) (see Chapter 9). From this emerged the importance of defining acute and chronic pain (2, 10, 17, 18). The concept of individuals from different disciplines working together led to the development of an integration of their knowledge and approaches into an *inter*disciplinary whole from *multi*disciplinary origins.

Members of the treatment team contribute not only their own knowledge and experience, but also contribute to the integration of that information into the multifaceted team approach. Of especial importance is the development of changes in the approaches of individuals involved in the team. Each individual learns from other members of the treatment team. In the interdisciplinary team the individual members become most effective as the edges of their territorial limits become less sharply defined. They then become truly specialists in pain management (algologists) in a way that supersedes the fields of their basic disciplines.

Techniques of coping with chronic pain patients evolved through deeper understanding of the mechanisms involved in the pain behaviors observed as the usual stimulus for the initiation of therapy. Fordyce (1, 19) observed that profound changes in behavior can be effected by behavioral techniques without addressing directly the alleged causes or trying to modify the intensity of nociceptive stimuli from a somatic source. In chronic pain, he pointed out, "When there are physical findings, those findings typically characterize what might have originated the pain problem. They do not necessarily establish a causal relationship between the current pain manifestations and those earlier nociceptive-producing events: the initiating trauma" (1).

The observation that all chronic pain *behaviors* are operants is an important concept that affects outcome in the interdisciplinary treatment program. These behaviors "which began in response to nociception may occur totally or in part for other reasons, namely, because of reinforcing consequences provided by the environment.... behaviors which are contingently and positively reinforced will tend to increase in frequency or probability of occurrence." Changing the reinforcers results in changes in the resultant suffering behaviors (2). It is thus clear that the complaints of pain, the physical findings, and the indications for care take on different meaning in the operant chronic pain patient.

A corollary of Fordyce's work is the way in which operants work in the usual management of the patient. The physician or therapist is rewarded by positive feedback from the patient. Thus reinforced, the physician tends to continue or to increase the therapeutic efforts. A patient who indicates that improvement is occurring and that the treatment is working can be reinforcing the escalation of treatment attempts rather than reporting objectifiable improvement. Because the problem is so refractory, the positive statements of the patient serve as reinforcers for continued treatment and an inappropriate sense of effectiveness in the provider of care. Eventually, the patient will admit the failure of the approach and move on to a new provider when the reinforcers of that behavior so dictate. Of course, unless the operant factors are observed and reinforcers changed, any new therapy will also result in failure. The new treatment approach will most always result in initial dramatic improvement until, again, the operant principles emerge. To miss the presence of operant factors in all individuals demonstrating any degree of chronic pain behavior is to miss the single most important element in providing effective care.

The goal is for the therapy to relate to the reinforcers so that the patient now receives satisfaction through new and more constructive behaviors or reengagement in activities that themselves maintain performance. For example, an individual who is not setting appropriate activity restrictions given significant physical limitations will experience progressively increasing pain. A willingness to find a way to satisfy the activity needs of patients and to help them to set reasonable limits is a prerequisite for any plan to result in continued improvement. Another example is the obese person with a knee or low back pain problem who refuses to participate on a regular basis in a weight-reduction program. In such cases the operant factors are more powerful determinants of success or failure than the organic problem being presented. The integration of operant principles forms the basis of the well-constructed interdisciplinary program.

Sternbach (14) has provided an essential insight to the problem of chronic pain. He points out that whereas the person in chronic pain due to life-threatening disease "must learn how to die," the person in chronic pain due to nonmalignant disease "must learn how to live." Interpersonal relationships play a great role in this. An understanding of the meanings of the observed behaviors in terms of relationships of the needs of various parts of the personality is a keystone in building the integrated approach to the treatment of chronic pain. Again, this is an especially severe problem in the patient with chronic pain primarily due to operant mechanisms. Personal-ity factors are more predictive of surgical outcome than the physical or organic findings on diagnostic studies (13). Yet, the complexity of the psychologic and environmental factors does not permit standard psychologic testing to predict outcome in the multidisciplinary pain center (20).

The behavioral approach to chronic pain has given us a better understanding of the reasons for failure of conventional medical therapy in patients with operant factors and reasons for relapse after initial improvement. This perspective has provided a basis for an integration of multiple modalities into a cohesive interdisciplinary approach in which the necessity of the patient's full participation both in the development of goals and in their achievement is fully recognized. Success or failure hinges on the willingness of the patient and those important others who will be reinforcing the new behaviors. Based on our experience in our pain clinics/centers, all these players must see this new approach in a positive light for any significant degree of success to persist.

Reactive depression is often a component of chronic pain behavior (Chapters 8 and 18). The diagnosis is often difficult for the physician. Missing it often results in inadvertent augmentation of its presence. Depression can be looked upon as an impediment in coping ability. Profound depression often defeats any treatment approach that might otherwise stand a good chance of success. Indeed, merely recognizing its presence can result in dramatic improvement in affect and in activity levels. Reactivation, already an integral part of effective treatment, can in itself ameliorate depression. Medications that produce or increase depression must be avoided. False expectations must be eliminated. The depressed patient might not be able to return to a former occupation even if his or her pain is eliminated.

INTERDISCIPLINARY/MULTIDISCIPLINARY THERAPY

In this section we describe in more detail the composition of multimodal therapy for chronic pain (3, 6, 7, 10–13, 21). The make-up of the multidisciplinary pain clinic is documented elsewhere (Chapter 9) (3, 16).

Specific modalities that have been used to varying degrees in pain treatment programs include:

1. Medical assessment
2. Psychologic assessment
3. Diagnostic procedures
4. Medical treatment
5. Physical therapy
6. Occupational therapy
7. Psychologic treatment
8. Vocational counseling
9. Vocational aptitude testing
10. Family therapy
11. Nerve blocks
12. Trigger point injections
13. Acupuncture
14. Biofeedback
15. Relaxation therapy
16. Autogenic training
17. Education
18. Assertiveness training
19. Communication training
20. Massage therapy
21. TENS
22. Ablative neurosurgery
23. Implanted stimulators

Obviously, not all programs utilize all these modalities. Based upon the results, not all these are indicated. Results may be based more on the personnel and their involvement with the patients than on which treatment modalities are used. Palliative treatment modalities must not be allowed to become contingent on pain behavior; their use should have a predetermined end point. Systematic fading of the frequency of their use is often indicated. As yet, testing of each of these in terms of the success generated has not been accomplished. Overall program effectiveness, however, has been evaluated (5, 12, 13, 21).

In the traditional medical model, each specialist evaluates the patient within the constraints of his or her field of interest, leaving to the attending physician the job of integrating that information into a cohesive and therapeutically sound treatment plan. The interdisciplinary approach requires intercommunication between specialists; the process integrates all those involved with the patient. The patient cannot be just sent to Physical Therapy for "treatment." PT must be part of the overall plan, and therapists must be conversant with others on the team. Only in this way will objectives not be circumvented and defeated. Frequent communication between all team members and the sharing of responsibility are important. The psychologist and physician who observe the patient during physical activity, for example, might gain insights that could not be made at any other time. A breakdown of traditional barriers between disciplines begins to occur. This may be threatening to those health care providers who are accustomed to functioning independently in their own autonomous areas, but it must occur if the team is to be effective and efficient. The staff must be educated in the modes of functioning of the interdisciplinary approach.

It is the job of the director to see not only that the necessary interaction occurs, but also that professional egos are somehow protected and maintained. There is no place for dogmatism. Empathy and understanding hold the team together and make it work. It is often the physician who has the greatest difficulty adapting to this approach. Probably the most important element in the efforts of the interdisciplinary team is the provision of a supportive milieu. Not only must the patient feel a part of the program, but the members of the treatment team must recognize that the maintenance of the milieu is more important than their usual autonomous roles. Unless all members of the treatment team work for the conjoint approach, resentments develop and the therapeutic effect disintegrates. In this approach the individual therapist is less important than his or her impact on the whole. The therapeutic milieu is greater than the sum of its parts; it is protective, supportive, directing, coaxing, educating, and criticizing, and it effects growth in both patients and staff. This interdisciplinary approach requires the integration of somatic, psychologic, social, and economic factors (10–13).

An important problem in the maintenance of an effective interdisciplinary team is staff morale. The therapy environment must have built-in reinforcers and support for the staff to maintain a high level of enthusiasm and mutual involvement in patient care. Criticism must be laced with empathy; staff communication and sharing of goals are critical parameters (7).

An example of the function of the interdisciplinary mechanism can be seen in the following anecdote. Early in the development of the Northwest Pain Center, it was noted that many patients with chronic low back pain were not performing exercises properly. The physical therapist was providing appropriate instruction, but the nurses and the biofeedback technicians were not aware of the basic principles of low back exercises. The nursing program changed to include activities in which appropriate posture mechanics could be observed, and the nurses in the program became more knowledgeable about the principles of the exercise program.

In addition, for the difficult problem patient, EMG biofeedback was combined with physical activities supervised by the biofeedback therapist as a further training tool. The biofeedback technician became, thereby, an active member of the team with a therapeutic approach that was now specific for the patient's complaints. The resultant integration of therapy functions now created better communication between professionals and a combined therapeutic regime that no single therapeutic modality could achieve on its own. An important fallout of this improved treatment process was improvement in staff morale and a reduction in staff burnout and depression. Members of the pain treatment team became enthusiastic and felt they were providing a unique and valuable service. This promoted a willingness to stay at the job, resulting in the expertise that only experience can provide.

THE UNIVERSITY OF WASHINGTON MULTIDISCIPLINARY PAIN CENTER

The general organization of the University of Washington Multidisciplinary Pain Center (UWPC) is described in Chapter 9. It is composed of three clinical divisions: the Acute Pain Service, the Inpatient Pain Service, and the Outpatient Pain Service. The Center evaluates and treats patients with all types of chronic pain, including that due to cancer and disease of the nervous and musculoskeletal systems and chronic visceral pain. Although the functions of this program are discussed in Chapters 9 and 31, the most important points are repeated here.

Initial Assessment Options

The UWPC sees patients by referral only. A letter or a phone call from the patient's treating physician is reviewed by a Pain Center physician and the initial patient assessment option is determined. These options are:

1. Further information is required before the patient's suitability for one of our treatment programs is determined. The patient and the referring physician must provide past medical records, radiographs, and so on before the Center will go any further.
2. The patient has a clear-cut, diagnosable pain problem that one UWPC physician can manage. We label this a "consult" patient. Cancer pain and pain related to nerve injury usually fall into this category.
3. The patient has a complex, long-standing pain problem that requires multidisciplinary evaluation. This patient is labeled a "screener."

4. The patient has unresolved medical issues that require further evaluation before consideration of pain management. Either the local physician or the UWPC will arrange for these.

5. The UWPC will not evaluate the patient. Usually this indicates failure of prior, similar pain treatment programs, addiction to street drugs, or coercion of the patient by a governmental or insurance agency.

Screening Evaluation

The majority of new patients at UWPC have complex pain problems of long duration. The first task is to collect the facts. Patients scheduled for screening must arrange with their physicians to have them send their complete medical records and diagnostic tests (or they can bring the records with them). Prior to the initial visit the patient is sent a demographic form and diary materials to be completed for the 2 weeks prior to screening. All patients must bring their spouse or significant other to the screening visit. The UWPC will not screen a patient without this person in attendance to participate in the evaluation and to take part in the discussion of treatment options.

The screening process takes 4 to 5 hours. The patient is seen by a physician who completes a history and physical examination. The patient is interviewed by a psychologist and completes an MMPI, which is immediately scored and interpreted. The patient's spouse or significant other is interviewed by the psychologist. The physician and the psychologist and other members of the evaluation team (nurses, residents, and fellows) then meet to discuss their findings and establish a diagnosis and treatment plan. The patient and significant other then join the group and participate in the discussion (Fig. 100-1), which leads to a mutually agreed-upon management plan. If the inpatient program is recommended and return to work is a likely treatment objective, vocational assessment is arranged prior to admission. About half of the complex pain patients screened are admitted to the inpatient program. The remainder are treated as outpatients or are returned to their referring physician for continuing treatment.

The physician and the psychologist complement each other during the assessment process. The essential role of the physician is to document the history of the patient's illness with the goals of achieving an understanding of the medical facts that led to the patient's present condition and determining the present physical status of the patient, including medication intake. The psychologist's task is to elucidate the role of affective and environmental factors in the patient's chronic pain state. The physician focuses on the contribution of nociception and pain, and the psychologist focuses on suffering and pain behavior; they jointly attempt to put the pieces together to plan a rational treatment.

The evaluation process is essential to the well-being of the UWPC pain center. The staff of the Center has learned over a 29-year span that not all patients are amenable to the UWPC treatment programs. The strategies employed, just like those used by a surgeon, have specific indications and contraindications. The patient characteristics that indicate a likelihood of success with the UWPC inpatient program are:

Physician-prescribed inappropriate medications
Physical deactivation
Depression
Superstitious behaviors and beliefs about the body
Reasonable outcome goals

The UWPC management strategies can often successfully address these issues and restore the patient to an appropriate functional level.

Inpatient Treatment Program

The UWPC standard inpatient treatment program lasts 19 days and keeps the patient busy 13 hours per day. It is very intensive, for both patients and staff. The UWPC runs a continuous 10-patient group to which five patients are admitted on week 1, five patients on week 2, and no patients on week 3. A psychologist, a physician, and a nurse are jointly responsible for each 3-week group. At present, four psychologists, six physicians, and six nurses rotate this responsibility. The daily schedule is shown in Table 100-1.

There are three group sessions each weekday: Group I, called "Pain Education Conference," takes place from 8:00 to 9:00 a.m. and is a didactic session given by one of the physicians or psychologists or by an invited speaker. Topics are listed in Table 100-2. Table 100-3 lists the issues discussed about drugs used for pain relief. The goal of this session is to provide the patient with information that will help him or her to understand how the body works and how the outside world deals with him or her as a disabled pain patient.

Patients then have a combination of physical therapy and occupational therapy from 9:00 until 11:30. The physical therapy consists of a set of exercises relevant to the individual patient's pain problem as well as aerobic exercises and stretching. The exercises are designed to gradually increase the patient's work, starting from the individual patient's entry level abilities.

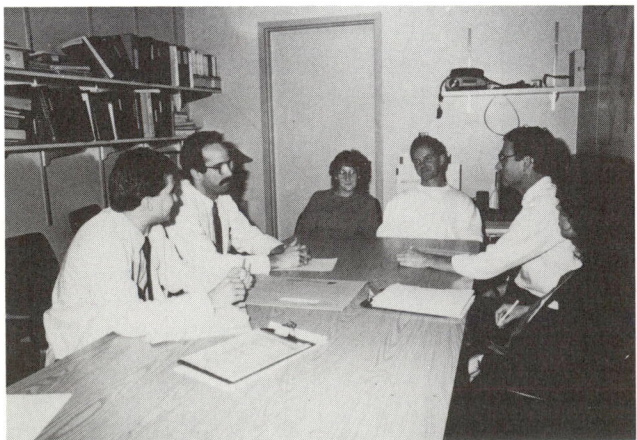

FIG. 100-1. Screening evaluation at University of Washington Multidisciplinary Pain Center. Patient and spouse meet with physician, psychologist, and other staff to discuss evaluation and options for treatment.

TABLE 100-1. Daily Schedule for Inpatients at University of Washington Multidisciplinary Pain Center

Weekdays	
7:30	Breakfast
8:00	Group I: Pain education conference
9:00	Physical therapy
	Occupational therapy
	Vocational counseling
	Individual psychotherapy
12:00	Lunch
1:00	Group II: Skills training
2:00	Physical therapy
	Occupational therapy
	Vocational counseling
	Individual psychotherapy
5:00	Free time
5:45	Dinner
7:00	Group III: Relaxation and consolidation
8:00	Free time, sleep

Tuesday 5:00–5:30 P.M.: Food and nutrition information group

Wednesday 6:00–8:00 P.M.: Swimming (optional)

Weekends	
7:30	Breakfast
8:30	Physical therapy
10:00	Planning for weekend activities
11:00	Occupational therapy
12:00	Lunch
1:00	Physical therapy
2:00	Pass or free time
8:00	Group III: Relaxation and consolidation

From Loeser, J.D., and Egan, K.J.: Inpatient pain treatment program. *In* Managing the Chronic Pain Patient: Theory and Practice at the University of Washington Multidisciplinary Pain Center. Edited by J.D. Loeser and K.J. Egan. New York, Raven Press, 1989, p. 39.

TABLE 100-3. Didactic Session: Drugs for Pain Relief

I. Classes of drugs useful for pain relief

  A. Peripherally acting
    1. Mode of action
    2. Clinical uses
    3. Potential side effects
    4. Common drugs: aspirin, Tylenol, nonsteroidal anti-inflammatories

  B. Centrally acting analgesic adjuvant drugs
    1. Narcotics
      a. Modes of action
      b. Clinical uses
      c. Potential side effects
      d. Acute vs. chronic pain
      e. Habituation, tolerance, addiction
    2. Tricyclic antidepressants
      a. Mode of action
      b. Clinical uses
      c. Potential side effects
    3. Anticonvulsants
      a. Mode of action
      b. Clinical uses
      c. Potential side effects

II. Drugs to avoid in chronic pain patients

  A. Sedative-hypnotics
  B. Benzodiazepines
  C. Muscle relaxants
  D. Alcohol
  E. Others

III. Rational use of medications

  A. Resist propaganda
  B. Ask physician, pharmacist
  C. Duration of treatment
  D. Relative costs

Occupational therapy consists of activities designed to help the patient do those things that he cannot accomplish on admission that are relevant to his or her goals. For example, if the patient has difficulty sitting, activities such as operating a keyboard or other tasks accomplished in the seated position will be employed. All such activities are started at the patient's level of ability on admission and are gradually increased. The patients keep graphs of their daily accomplishments (Fig. 100-2); these are frequently reviewed by the treatment staff.

After lunch, the second group session of the day occurs. This group session, called "Skills Training," is led by a psychologist and focuses on such topics as

TABLE 100-2. Topics in Group I: Pain Education Conference

Pain mechanisms	Depression
Gate theory	Effects of exercise and inactivity
Headaches	Low back pain
Biomechanics	Role of surgery for pain
Drugs: Use and abuse	Dealing with doctors
Workman's Compensation	Program orientation
Former patient visit	Maintenance of gains
Acute vs. chronic pain	Discharge planning
Healing and disuse	

From Loeser, J.D., and Egan, K.J.: Inpatient pain treatment program. *In* Managing the Chronic Pain Patient: Theory and Practice at the University of Washington Multidisciplinary Pain Center. Edited by J.D. Loeser and K.J. Egan. New York, Raven Press, 1989, p. 40.

stress management, control of aggression, assertiveness training, and relaxation (Table 100-4). Following this, another 3-hour segment of physical therapy and occupational therapy occurs. The patients then have 45 minutes of free time before dinner.

Following dinner, a third daily group session occurs, called "Relaxation and Consolidation." It is usually led by a nurse. This group includes both physical and psychologic programs such as speed walking,

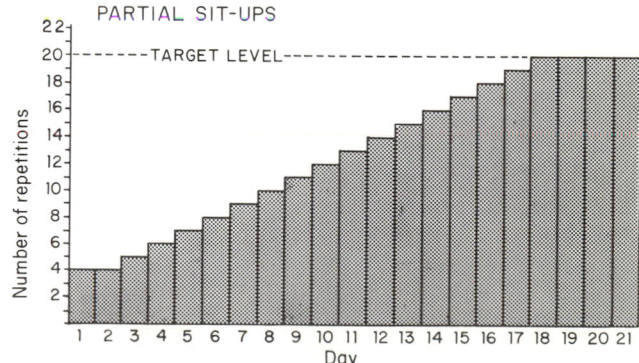

FIG. 100-2. Sample of a patient's daily activity graph (partial sit-ups) for inpatient program. First 2 days are baseline; an incremental program is established until target level is achieved. The patient maintains graphs of this type for each physical activity in the pain management program.

TABLE 100-4. Topics for Group II: Skills Training

Stress management	Assertiveness training
Relaxation training	Cognitive strategies
Coping skills	Communication skills
Anger management	Dealing with depression
Pain behaviors	Crisis management
Sleep disorders	Costs/meanings of pain
Physiology of stress	

From Loeser, J.D., and Egan, K.J.: Inpatient pain treatment program. *In* Managing the Chronic Pain Patient: Theory and Practice at the University of Washington Multidisciplinary Pain Center. Edited by J.D. Loeser and K.J. Egan. New York, Raven Press, 1989, p. 41.

TABLE 100-5. Topics for Group III: Relaxation and Consolidation

Maintenance of gains	Program orientation
Making and using a coping plan	Purposes of group sessions
	Program goals
Relaxation training	Goal setting
Physiology of stress	Focused breathing
Quieting response	Hurt vs. harm
Evaluation of use of coping plan	Identifying gains
	Review of patient education materials
Preparing for new patients	
Time planning	

From Loeser, J.D., and Egan, K.J.: Inpatient pain treatment program. *In* Managing the Chronic Pain Patient: Theory and Practice at the University of Washington Multidisciplinary Pain Center. Edited by J.D. Loeser and K.J. Egan. New York, Raven Press, 1989, p. 41.

TABLE 100-6. Points of Rehabilitation Counselor Intervention

Outpatient screening evaluation
  When physician and psychologist identify need for early intervention
    Individual assessment—is a return to work desired and realistic?
      Motivation
      Funding issues
      Litigation issues
      Other potential barriers
Inpatient treatment
  Individual assessment
    All Workman's Compensation patients with vocational potential
    Work-related issues
  Intervention when appropriate
    Vocational counseling
    Job-seeking skills training
    Placement counseling
    Job station
    Education
    Liaison services
Postdischarge follow-up
  Routine follow-up when appropriate
  Intensive follow-up when necessary
    Outpatient treatment program
    Job station/work hardening
  Other liaison, follow-up services

From Weinhouse, S.: Vocational issues in the rehabilitation of pain patients: The role of the rehabilitation counselor. *In* Managing the Chronic Pain Patient: Theory and Practice at the University of Washington Multidisciplinary Pain Center. Edited by J.D. Loeser and K.J. Egan. New York, Raven Press, 1989, p. 145.

TABLE 100-7. Rehabilitation Counselor Functions

Vocational evaluation (individual assessment)
  Interests
  Education
  Aptitude
  Physical capabilities
  Learning capabilities
  Vocational goals
  Work experience
  Transferable skills
Goal
  Identify realistic vocational options
  Identify actual or potential barriers
Vocational counseling
  Information gathering
  Evaluation
  Decision making
  Goal setting
  Goal attainment (structure)
Job-seeking skills training
  Job-seeking strategies
    Networking
    Informational interviewing
    Hidden job market
  Interviewing
  Applications
  Résumé
  Cover letters
  Time management
Placement counseling
  One-to-one active process
    Passive mode
    Active mode
Job station program
  Build physical work tolerance
  Trial work/test skills
  Evaluate work behaviors
  Identify interest
  Assess physical capabilities
  Build confidence
  Provide recent work experience
Education
  Systems
    Realistic expectations
  Self-help community resources
Liaison services
  Department of Vocational Rehabilitation, Department of Labor and Industry, Department of Social and Health Services, insurance companies

From Weinhouse, S.: Vocational issues in the rehabilitation of pain patients: The role of the rehabilitation counselor. *In* Managing the Chronic Pain Patient: Theory and Practice at the University of Washington Multidisciplinary Pain Center. Edited by J.D. Loeser and K.J. Egan. New York, Raven Press, 1989, p. 146.

relaxation training, discussion of the morning's didactic session or the content of the afternoon group, and individual problem-solving (Table 100-5).

On weekends and holidays there is only one physical therapy or occupational therapy session per day and the morning and afternoon groups are not held. The daily schedule lasts $5\frac{1}{2}$ hours; patients may go on pass from 2:00 p.m. until 8:00 p.m. This is the only time that patients are permitted to be on pass.

Vocational counseling, individual psychotherapy, and conferences with the patient and significant other are worked into the physical therapy and occupational therapy schedules.

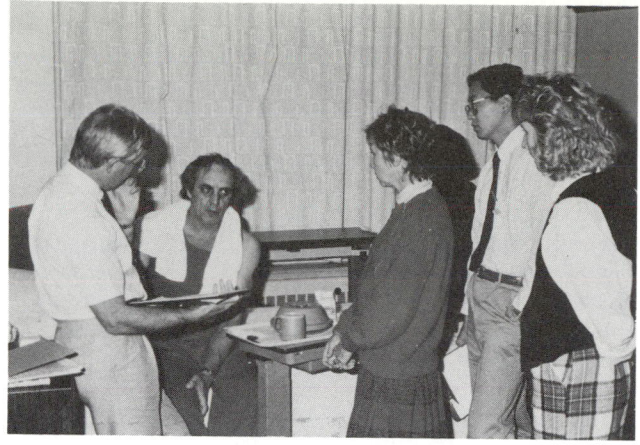

FIG. 100-3. Inpatient management team making rounds to discuss with the patient his progress at the University of Washington Multidisciplinary Pain Center. Physician, psychologist, nurse, and house staff participate in rounds twice each day.

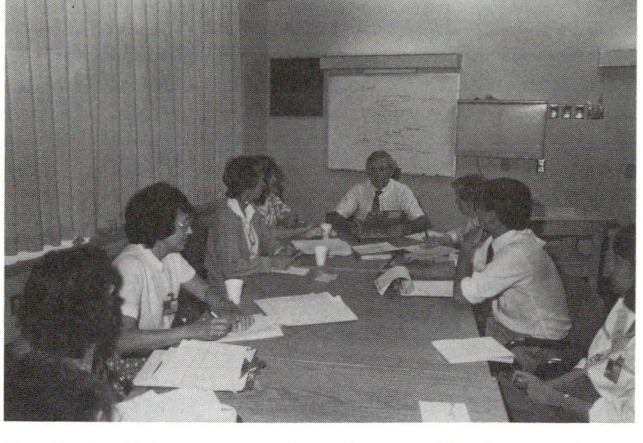

FIG. 100-4. Pain management conference. The treatment team meets Wednesday afternoon to discuss each patient's progress and problems and to plan the next segment of treatment.

The rehabilitation counselor is trained in vocational reassessment, evaluation, and counseling as well as the medical, psychologic, and social aspects of disability. The rehabilitation counselor is a more specialized professional than a vocational counselor and is specifically trained to understand and deal with the vocational need of the disabled person. He or she can assess and treat a broad range of issues as appropriate even if they are outside of the traditional vocational realm, including work-related problems stemming from injury or disability if the patient is working, job modification if appropriate to facilitate a return to work, a patient's fears regarding return to work, and counseling to help a patient accept loss and/or physical limitation. The vocational counselor is involved in all phases of patient evaluation and treatment as listed in Table 100-6. Table 100-7 summarizes the functions of the rehabilitation counselor.

The inpatient management team, consisting of the physician, psychologist, nurse, and various students and observers, makes rounds every morning and reviews each patient's progress (Fig. 100-3). Every Wednesday the entire treatment team reviews each patient in a formal conference setting; plans and goals are established for each patient at this time (Fig. 100-4).

The day prior to discharge we ask that the patient's significant other attend all of the activities to see what has been accomplished and to learn how to minimize recidivism. A formal discharge conference is held with the treatment team; the patient prepares a maintenance-of-gains worksheet that details the plans for continued physical activities, job-related activities, and strategies for avoiding the pitfalls of chronic pain behaviors.

THE NORTHWEST PAIN CENTER

The Northwest Pain Center Program (NPC) is a multidisciplinary day treatment pain program designed to treat up to 30 chronic pain patients at a time. It is a $3\frac{1}{2}$ week program operated out of a large freestanding clinic with classrooms, treatment areas, and other designated spaces. It accommodates an average census of 25 patients and has a staff of 38 full-time specially trained and coordinated personnel (10–13, 21) (Table 100-8).

The NPC program has been in existence since 1972 and has evaluated and treated over 8000 chronic pain patients. Patients with cancer pain are not treated at NPC. Staff clinicians at NPC have an average of 10 years of experience in the evaluation and treatment of chronic pain. The program is directed jointly by a neurosurgeon and a medical psychologist. Two full-time orthopedic surgeons and a part-time neurologist complete the physician staff. Four full-time and one half-time clinical psychologists constitute the psychological staff. Two full-time registered physical thera-

pists and three full-time registered occupational therapists, two full-time biofeedback technicians, two full-time registered nurses, three part-time nurses, and a licensed practical nurse round out the clinical treatment team. Clerical and clinical staff members are coordinated by a master's level administrator/licensed vocational counselor. The clinical staff is divided into two working clinical teams, each representing various appropriate treatment disciplines.

The interdisciplinary concept used at the Northwest Pain Center helps integrate the multiplicity of

TABLE 100-8. Staff at Northwest Pain Center

Neurosurgeon (FTE) (1)	Physical therapists (2)
Orthopedic surgeons (2)	Occupational therapists (3)
Neurologist ($\frac{1}{2}$)	Biofeedback technicians (2)
Clinical psychologists ($4\frac{1}{2}$)	Nurses ($4\frac{1}{2}$)
	Vocational counselor (1)

theories, strategies, and experiences into a single common approach to patient care. The nature of the clinical population demands significant crossover between disciplines, and it is common for psychologists to render instruction in anatomy and for physicians to counsel patients on the impact of pain on marriage and communication processes. Although this might seem unusual, the fact that the therapeutic team has worked together daily for years has led to a tremendous amount of cross fertilization of ideas and knowledge which makes each member familiar with the basic application of others' disciplines, a point repeatedly emphasized by Bonica (see Chapter 9).

Treatment teams meet twice each week to discuss patients' progress. Refinement of the diagnoses and therapeutic strategies occurs in an orderly fashion, taking into account multiple observers, different contexts, and different times of observation and thereby producing a more accurate and complete picture of the patient's pain behavior. Patients must complete behavioral treatment contracts and achieve reasonable goals in order to remain in the treatment program. Treatment personnel and the patients themselves are both responsible for definition and refinement of these goals.

The therapeutic modalities used in the pain program have been modified and changed over the years on the basis of experience (11–13, 21). Each therapy is designed to be active, with emphasis on patient responsibility, as opposed to palliative or passive treatments.

Because the program addresses not only the reduction of nociceptive input but also the emotional, psychologic, and environmental concomitants of the chronic pain experience, it is important to address areas of secondary gain, financial compensation, operant reinforcers, time out from work, body mechanics, muscle strengthening, and the physiologic mechanisms of pain. The team approach places heavy emphasis on patient responsibility. Patients are educated on such topics as the biomechanics of the spine, the effects of drugs on the body, various types of spinal surgery, sexual dysfunction, depression, and other problems that relate to the chronic pain experience. Analgesic and tranquilizing medications are withdrawn gradually over the first 7 to 10 days of treatment. Frequently, antidepressant medications are used to reduce pain and restore normal sleep patterns.

New patients are admitted and discharged on a weekly basis, thereby producing overlap of patients in various stages of progress through the programs. Being able to see others in various stages of pain management helps to instill feelings of hope and encouragement. The therapeutic milieu itself is a powerful source of modeling because of the development of an intense level of camaraderie that frequently goes far beyond the patient's stay in the treatment program.

Medicine

The team physicians are responsible for monitoring the medical care of patients by assessing the need for diagnostic procedures, more medical consultation, management of medication, and their physical progress through the program. The physicians must be capable of giving up the concept of complete control of all aspects of patient care and be willing to blend their talents with those of the other health care providers on the interdisciplinary team. They must also be able to accept that there is no single therapeutic modality or approach that will be completely effective in ameliorating pain in the chronic pain patient.

Medical Psychologist

A clinical psychologist in a pain center must have a working familiarity with neurology, neurosurgery, and orthopedic medicine. He or she must feel comfortable in dealing with issues that have been defined traditionally as medical areas. The psychologist does not practice medicine, but he or she must be comfortable discussing issues that involve biomedical causes of pain and instructing and educating of patients in posture and body mechanics. The psychologist must be familiar with the physical as well as the psychologic effects of the chronic use of medications on the chronic pain patient. The psychologist must recognize that most chronic pain patients reject the notion that there is anything psychologically wrong with them and fear that their problems will be defined as psychologic in origin and therefore not legitimate for Workman's Compensation benefits.

Occupational and Vocational Therapies

Most patients with chronic pain have experienced a devastating loss in regard to their ability to work. Careful evaluation and analysis of patients' work histories, physical limitations, intelligence, and emotional make-up are critical in vocational planning. Work capacity evaluation and standardized work sample assessments are important factors in planning for vocational rehabilitation of these patients. Integration of these data with objective measures of physical function, combined with both medicine and psychology in the total data base, results in a more complete picture of the impact of the pain on the patient and his or her family.

Nursing Services

Nurses with special expertise in pain management are an integral part of the one-to-one relationship that is developed with each patient. It is the nurse who is responsible for monitoring the drug withdrawal program, nutritional counseling, instruction in transcutaneous nerve stimulation, communications training, stress management skills, and relaxation training. The nurse establishes significant rapport with each patient and often provides the basic fabric of the interdisciplinary team.

Biofeedback Therapy

Neuromuscular re-education and biologic feedback modalities include electromyographic training, thermal training, and galvanic skin resistance (GSR) training. Biofeedback is used to help patients understand that they indeed have some capacity to control their own physiology. Many patients seek pain treatment with little or no understanding of the role that they can play in self control. Inappropriate muscular bracing and generalized muscular tension are characteristic of our chronic pain patients; reduction of these maladaptive neuromuscular behaviors can play a key role in relieving some of the patient's pain. Thermal mode biofeedback can promote a feeling of generalized control and help patients learn to manage their own pain problems. In addition, substantial use is made of portable EMG units. Patients are instructed in body mechanics, a work hardening program, and engage in other physical activities while being monitored and fed back information about excess activity of their paravertebral muscles or other muscles involved in their pain problem. Because of this form of objective feedback, patients learn many of the maladaptive postural behaviors that have exacerbated their underlying mechanical pain problem.

Physical Therapy

Each patient is involved in active physical therapy with emphasis on stretching of muscles, increasing range of motion, mobility, endurance, and strength.

Increasing pain tolerance, utilization of appropriate modeling, videotape feedback, and one-to-one group instruction from a registered physical therapist are critical parts of the treatment program. Extensive flexion exercises, use of the pelvic tilt, and other postural activities are taught in conjunction with aerobics, walking exercises, and gait training. Videotape and mirror feedback modalities are used in neuromuscular retraining and correction of faulty postures and gaits. The NPC does not generally use passive modalities such as massage, manipulation, or whirlpool. These modalities might temporarily make a patient feel better, but the focus of the program is on long-term gains, which are achieved through teaching patients mechanisms of self-control and responsibility for the management of their own pain problems. If a specific passive modality is used, three criteria must be met: (1) the use must be time-contingent, not pain-contingent (see Chapters 16 and 81), (2) a clearly specified end point must be established, and (3) the patient must demonstrate improved performance after the treatment.

RESULTS OF THE INTERDISCIPLINARY APPROACH

Many reports are available regarding the results of pain center care, and Fordyce et al. have reviewed and synthesized them (5, 22, 23). Until recently the lack of a standard method of reporting made it difficult to compare results or even, in some cases, to understand them. Reports have used many different parameters as measures of success. Return to work, cessation of suffering behaviors, increase in well behaviors, decrease in analgesic medication usage, improvement in affect, attitude, and communications, and reduction in physician visits are some of the elements studied. An important criticism made by Sternbach (24) is that the reports of all these groups are of outcome studies of programs using a variety of treatments (e.g., group therapy, physical therapy, operant conditioning), so that their results reflect overall program effects rather than those of behavioral treatment alone.

Efforts are being made to standardize care in patient treatment programs and to define the meaning of the interdisciplinary team approach in specific operational terms. The Commission on Accreditation of Rehabilitation Facilities (CARF) has established national standards for the specific types of programs and a means for the collection of data regarding program effectiveness. From their influence, perhaps standard result data will be available. In addition, the diagnostic system proposed by IASP (see Chapter 2) will assist in the collection of meaningful data.

Improvements in activity level, range of motion, and exercise tolerance can be seen as the result of the multidisciplinary approach. Reduction in subsequent medical contacts and drug use is well documented (25). Yet some patients remain dissatisfied with whatever level of improvement has occurred and continue to present their problems to the next physician or pain center for care. Some, for whom further surgery was not indicated, have nevertheless undergone additional surgical procedures, with disastrous results. Most of these people are now firmly entrenched in their role as disabled, and no form of available therapy can be expected to effect significant change. A very few have benefited from further attempts at surgery, but in no case has there been enough improvement to warrant the risk involved.

Because the pain team approach provides the patient the education and the tools for self-improvement, the recidivism that occurs is an interesting and educational phenomenon to study. Indeed, should not people who have suffered view their improvement as a positive achievement? Unfortunately, for some patients and their families this is not always the case. Improvement might be seen as a threat by the spouse as more independent activity occurs. Contact with the physician might be seen as a support that is removed with well behavior. Often a patient will again see the doctor in order to maintain a human contact; the patient is legitimated by the complaint of pain. The physician rushes in with a prescription, and the cycle of dependent behavior and suffering starts anew. The patient who responds to the operant approach is initially very fragile and responds dramatically to environmental cues that encourage and reinforce the previously well-practiced behaviors. It is essential that the attending physician understand the operant factors present in all relationships with the patient and be willing to be supportive without necessarily reinstating therapy for old complaints that now have a much different symbolic meaning. Family members might have been playing a key role in the reinforcement of pain behaviors prior to treatment (1, 2, 19, 21). They also can play a key role subsequent to treatment in influencing whether gains persist or fade away. These issues must be addressed in evaluation of treatment and in preparing the home environment to help maintain gains. These points are discussed in more detail in Chapter 81.

Recidivism After Initial Improvement

Fairly characteristic of the patient with chronic pain is the repetitious history of improvement after all previous treatment attempts with the rapid recurrence of symptoms. An understanding of this phenomenon can lead to a significant decrease in treatment attempts, including surgery, which often fails, even in the presence of acceptable indications. Understanding the factors leading to recidivism can effect a significant cost-saving.

The whole issue of recidivism, maintenance of gains, and outcome measurements needs to be viewed from a different perspective. Treatment must consist of teaching people to act differently, and to seek solutions to life's problems differently. Moreover, the patient can hardly ever control all of these tasks. Of necessity, they entail what others (e.g., spouse, employer) do as well. Therefore, outcomes or recidivism rates need to be understood as indexes not only of treatment effectiveness for the patient but also of the degree to which the patient's environment can be influenced to support treatment gains and promote their expansion. The patients treated at NPC and UWPC have been carefully followed after discharge. We have noted that treatment success or failure is not correlated with self-reported pain levels either at initial evaluation or at discharge from the program. The major determinants of unsuccessful long-term outcome appear to be lack of suitable employment opportunities, patient attitude about treatment, age greater than 50, and lack of incentives to improve one's status (21, 26).

Positive Results

Several outcome studies have looked at the results after discharge. Fordyce et al. (2) (Chapter 16) reported behavioral improvements after treatment. Painter et al. (11) similarly used mailed questionnaires and found that 77% of patients felt improved as a result of their pain center treatment, with an average pain reduction of 35%. Aronoff and colleagues (27, 28) reported that 57.5% of respondents no longer had significant problems with pain. They also reported improvements in social functioning and other activities important to the patient. McCann et al. (29) reported significant reductions in medication use and in utilization of medical care resources and increased meaningful activity. Anderson et al. (30), in personal interviews with a small number of patients, reported a decrease in the impact of pain as the result of participation in the pain center program.

Crue and Pinsky (17), Sternbach (24), Aronoff and Evans (28), Wang et al. (31), and Swanson and associates (32) reported similar studies, all using pretreatment measures as the comparison for success. Again, significant reduction of pain was observed in about half of the patients. Malec et al. (33) reported success as measured in the nonuse of narcotic and muscle-relaxing medications, employment status, and increased activities without an increase in pain. Vasudevan et al. (34) reported improvements in activity levels, subjective pain reports, use of analgesic drugs, rehospitalizations, and employment status. Herman and Baptiste (35) used a combined scoring method that included physical, psychologic, and behavioral factors as a measure of success. They reported that 41 of their 50 patients were successful during their stay in the program. Of these 58% improved further after discharge, 27% remained unchanged, and 15% had deteriorated one year later.

Roberts and Reinhardt (25) compared those who had been admitted to the program with those who refused treatment and those who were rejected. The results of this study demonstrated that those admitted to the program did significantly better than the others.

Chapman et al. (36) and Rosomoff et al. (37) found no significant differences in results between those involved in litigation and those who were not. The return to work issue as an index of success was used in a review of results by Addison (38). He found that close to 82% of patients had returned to work.

It is clear the dependent measures of success of pain center treatment vary greatly depending on the research data in question, but it is equally clear that positive benefits in the form of pain reduction, increased functional capacity, vocational rehabilitation, and reduction in overutilization of medical resources occur as a result of the interdisciplinary pain treatment mode.

Significant improvements in physical range of motion and activity level were documented by measurement in a study by Seres et al. (13). In this study patients reported little change in pain level. This study is of importance because it demonstrated the important lack of correlation between the "complaint of pain" and functional capacity. In practical terms, it is not the intensity of the pain experienced by the chronic pain patient that creates the disability syndrome, but rather the impact of the pain and its consequences.

Cost-Benefit Analysis of the Interdisciplinary Approach

Several efforts have been made to assess the cost-benefit ratio for pain clinic treatments (12, 39). In one study, data were obtained from a worker's compensation insurance company regarding a group of 75 injured workers (12). Seventy-one of these were admitted to an interdisciplinary treatment program and were

TABLE 100-9. Cost-Benefit Analysis for Patients Admitted to Northwest Pain Center in 1976 (Data Obtained from Insurance Carrier)

Average cost of admission	$3,413.15		
Total cases reviewed	75		
Total enrolled in program	71		

	1977	1978	1979
Open claims	34	13	12
Closed claims	27	56	58 (82%)
Continuing regular medical care	43	20	15
Vocational rehabilitation	14	11	4
Returned to work	5	15	18 (25%)

From Seres, J.L., et al.: Evaluation and management of chronic pain by nonsurgical means. In Pain Management: Symposium on the Neurosurgical Treatment of Pain. Edited by L.J. Fletcher. Baltimore, Williams & Wilkins, 1977.

followed by the insurance company for 3 years. Patients in this study had claims that had been open an average of 4½ years prior to coming into the pain center program. At the completion of the 3-year follow-up of this patient group, 82% had closed claims, demonstrating a significant cost saving to the insurance carrier. In addition, at the time of final follow-up, 30% were either working or actively involved in vocational placement (Table 100-9).

Conclusions

Chronic pain clearly is a complex network of phenomena that transcends the experience of any single profession. In order to diagnose and treat it, an array of resources is essential. Thus an interdisciplinary approach, as described here, is more than a simple sum of its parts. It is the integrated and coordinated use of multiple skills and expertise that makes the difference. We must now strive to educate health care professionals, particularly practicing physicians, and consumers of health care, be they patients or third-party carriers, about the importance of recognizing the critical distinctions between acute and chronic pain. They should support the implementation of diagnostic and treatment procedures that recognize and apply those distinctions (40).

Multidisciplinary pain centers must carefully report their results using standardized methods of describing patients and reporting outcomes. New treatment approaches must continue to evolve; the tendency to apply a biomedical model to all human suffering must be reversed.

The increasing number of citizens in the developed nations who claim disability due to pain is a major economic, political, and human disaster.

REFERENCES

1. Fordyce, W.E.: Behavioral Methods in Chronic Pain and Illness. St. Louis, C.V. Mosby, 1976.
2. Fordyce, W.E., et al.: Operant conditioning in the treatment of chronic pain. Arch. Phys. Med. Rehabil., 54:399, 1973.
3. Bonica, J.J.: Introduction to Conference on Multidisciplinary Clinics. In New Approaches to Treatment of Chronic Pain: A Review of Multidisciplinary Pain Clinician Pain Centers. Edited by L.K.Y. Ng. Rockville, MD, NIDA Research Monograph 36, 1981, pp. 3–6.
4. Melzack, R., and Wall, P.D.: The Challenge of Pain. New York, Basic Books, 1982, pp. 356–361.
5. Linton, S.: Behavioral remediation of chronic pain: A status report. Pain, 24:125, 1986.
6. Melvin, J.L.: Interdisciplinary multidisciplinary activities and ACRM. Arch. Phys. Med. Rehabil., 61:379, 1980.
7. Fordyce, W.E.: On interdisciplinary peers. Arch. Phys. Med. Rehabil., 62:51, 1981.
8. Bortz, W.M.: The disuse syndrome. West. J. Med., 141:691, 1984.
9. Berntzen, D., and Gotesstam, K.: Effects of on-demand or fixed interval schedules in the treatment of chronic pain with analgesic compounds: An experimental comparison. J. Consult. Clin. Psychol., 55:213–217, 1987.
10. Newman, R.I., Painter, J.R., and Seres, J.L.: A therapeutic milieu for chronic pain patients. J. Human Stress, 6:8, 1978.
11. Painter, J.R., Seres, J.L., and Newman, R.I.: Assessing benefits of the pain center: Why some patients regress. Pain, 8:101, 1980.
12. Seres, J.L., et al.: Evaluation and management of chronic pain by nonsurgical means. In Pain Management: Symposium on the Neurosurgical Treatment of Pain. Edited by L.J. Fletcher. Baltimore, Williams & Wilkins, 1977.
13. Seres, J.L., Painter, J.R., and Newman, R.I.: Multidisciplinary treatment of chronic pain at the Northwest Pain Center. In New Approaches to Treatment of Chronic Pain: A Review of Multidisciplinary Pain Clinics and Pain Centers. Edited by L.K.Y. Ng. Rockville, MD, NIDA Research Monograph 36, 1981, pp. 41–65.
14. Sternbach, R.A.: Pain Patients: Traits and Treatment. New York, Academic Press, 1974.
15. The Nuprin Pain Report. New York, Louis Harris & Associates, 1985, pp. 1–233.
16. Bonica, J.J.: General clinical considerations (including organization and function of a pain clinic). In Recent Advances in Pain. Edited by J.J. Bonica et al. Springfield, IL, Charles C Thomas, 1974, pp. 274–298.
17. Crue, B.L., and Pinsky, J.L.: Chronic pain syndrome: Four aspects of the problem. New Hope Pain Center and Pain Research Foundation. In New Approaches to Treatment of Chronic Pain: A Review of Multidisciplinary Pain Clinics and Pain Centers. Edited by L.K.Y. Ng. Rockville, MD, NIDA Monograph 36, 1981, pp. 137–168.
18. Steig, R.L., and Williams, R.C.: Chronic pain as a biosociocultural phenomenon: Implications for treatment. Semin. Neurol., 3:370, 1983.
19. Fordyce, W.E.: Behavioral concepts in chronic pain and illness. In Behavioral Management of Anxiety, Depression and Pain. Edited by P.W. Davidson. New York, Brunner-Mazel, 1976, pp. 147–188.
20. Cummings, C., et al.: Use of the MMPI to predict outcome of treatment for chronic pain. Adv. Pain Res. Therapy, 3:667, 1979.
21. Newman, R.I., et al.: Multidisciplinary treatment of chronic pain: Long term follow-up of low back pain patients. Pain, 4:283, 1978.
22. Fordyce, W.E.: Environmental factors in the genesis of low back pain. Adv. Pain Res. Therapy, 3:659, 1979.
23. Fordyce, W.E., Roberts, A.H., and Sternbach, R.A.: The behavioral management of chronic pain: A response to critics. Pain, 22:113, 1985.
24. Sternbach, R.A.: Clinical aspects of pain. In The Psychology of Pain. Edited by R.A. Sternbach. New York, Raven Press, 1978, pp. 241–264.
25. Roberts, A.H., and Reinhardt, L.: The behavioral management of chronic pain: Long-term follow-up with comparison groups. Pain, 8:151, 1980.
26. Crue, B.L.: Chronic Pain. New York, Spectrum, 1979.
27. Aronoff, G.M., Evans W.O., and Enders, P.L.: A review of follow-up studies of multidisciplinary pain units. Pain, 16:1, 1983.
28. Aronoff, G.M., and Evans, W.O.: The prediction of treatment outcome at a multidisciplinary pain center. Pain, 14:67, 1982.
29. McCann, V.J., Redford, J.B., and Jacobs, R.R.: Long-term effectiveness of a multidimensional treatment program for persons with low back pain (Abstr.). Pain, 1:S225, 1981.
30. Anderson, T.P., et al.: Behavioral modification of chronic pain: A treatment program by a multidisciplinary team. Clin. Orthop., 129:9, 1977.
31. Wang, J.K., et al.: Outpatient pain clinic: A long term follow-up study. Minn. Med., 63:663, 1980.
32. Swanson, S.W., Maruta, T., and Swanson, W.M.: Results of behavioral modification in the treatment of chronic pain. Psychosom. Med., 41:55, 1979.
33. Malec, J., et al.: Pain management: Long-term follow-up of an in-patient program. Arch. Phys. Med. Rehabil., 62:369, 1981.
34. Vasudevan, S.V., Lynch, N.T., and Abrams, S.: Effectiveness of an ambulatory chronic pain management program (Abstr.), Pain, 1:S294, 1981.
35. Herman, E., and Baptiste, S.: Pain control: Mastery through group experience. Pain, 10:79, 1981.
36. Chapman, S.L., Brena, S.F., and Bradford, L.A.: Treatment outcome in a chronic pain rehabilitation program, Pain, 11:255, 1981.
37. Rosomoff, H.L., et al.: Pain and low back rehabilitation program at the University of Miami School of Medicine. In New Approaches to Treatment of Chronic Pain: A Review of Multidisciplinary Pain Clinics and Pain Centers. Edited by L.K.Y. Ng. NIDA Research Monograph 36, Rockville, MD, 1981, pp. 92–111.

38. Addison, R.G.: Treatment of chronic pain. The Center for Pain Studies Rehabilitation Institute of Chicago. *In* New Approaches to Treatment of Chronic Pain: A Review of Multidisciplinary Pain Clinics and Pain Centers. Edited by L.K.Y. Ng. Rockville, MD, NIDA Research Monograph 36, 1981, pp. 12–32.

39. Podobnikar, I.G., and MacIntosh, S.: Pain center: A cost-effective approach to the treatment of chronic pain due to industrial injury (Abstr.). Pain, *1*:S295, 1981.

40. Fordyce, W.E.: Back pain, compensation and public policy. *In* Prevention in Health Psychology. Edited by J. Rosen and L. Solomon. Boston, University Press of New England, 1985, pp. 390–400.

INDEX

Page numbers in *italics* refer to illustrations, numbers followed by the letter "t" refer to tabular matter.

maxillary, mandibular, or ophthalmic nerve and, 1994-1995
pituitary adenolysis and, 280
retrobulbar, 763, *1992*
spasticity and, 2035
subarachnoid, 1106, 2001, *2002,* 2003-2004, 2007t
complications and, 2009t
Vail's syndrome and, 810
Alcohol use or abuse
cluster headache and, 718
depression and, 316
gout and, 345
headache and, 670t, 724
neuropathy and, 218
pancreatitis and, 1222-1223, 1223t, 1225, 1226
patient evaluation and, 574
psychologic evaluation and, 598
ulcers and, 1195
ALF; *see* Anterolateral fasciculus
Algesic substances, 96
Algogenic substance, 96
chronic pain and, 183
surgery and, 463, 464
Algology, 20
Algology fellowship at University of Washington Pain Center, 204
Algometer, *359*
Algorithm
epidural spinal cord compression and, 1111, *1111*
pain measurement instruments and, *592*
Alkalizing agent in anesthetic, 1891
Alkaloid
cancer and, 1798t
naturally occurring opium, 1656-1657
Alkalosis, respiratory, 177
Alkaptonuria, 335
Alkylating agent, 1797t
ALL (Anterior longitudinal ligament), 817
Allen test, 508, *508*
Raynaud's phenomenon and, 528
thromboangiitis obliterans and, 515
Allergy
Churg-Strauss granulomatosis and, 492t, 493-494
food
abdominal pain and, 1183t
migraine and, 706-707
rheumatic disease and, 1839-1840
gingival pain and, 755
heterocyclic antidepressant and, 1680
nerve block and, 1893, 1895
nonopioid analgesic and, 1661t
nonsteroidal anti-inflammatory drug, 1662
vulvovaginal irritation and, 1353
vulvulitis and, 1304t
Allodynia
brain lesion and, 278
causalgia and, 221, 224
central pain and, 271
characteristics of, 265
definition of, 20
reflex sympathetic dystrophy and, 232-233
Roberts' hypothesis and, 240
superficial pain and, 161-163
Allograft, 1761
Allopurinol, 347
Alpha-adrenergic blocker, 1055
Alphaprodine
description of, 1658

pharmacokinetics and pharmacodynamics and, 1648t
systemic effects of, 1650t
Alprazolam, 1685t
Alrheumat; *see* Ketoprofen
Alternating current, 1777
Altitude headache, 670t, 724
Alveolar bone abscess, 751-752
Alveolar nerve, posterior superior, 656-657
Alveolar nerve block, inferior, *1996*
Alzheimer's dementia, 558
Amantadine hydrochloride, 259
Ambulation
gait cycle and
foot and, 1604
hip and, 1538-1539
knee function and, 1568
pain behavior and, 586
Amebic abscess, 1176t
Amebic dysentery, 1175t
American Cancer Society, 400
American Medical Association Guides to the Evaluation of Permanent Impairments, 645
American Psychiatric Association, 324
Amine, depression and, 312
Amine antagonist for migraine, 711, 712t
Amino acid, 105t
Aminoglycan, 348
δ-Aminolevulinic acid, 1273
Amitriptyline
cancer-related pain and, 423t, 424, 433
dosages and effects of, 1678t
migraine and, 711, 712t
muscles of mastication disorder and, 733t
neuropathy and, 215t
diabetic, 217
pain reduction and, 316
primary fibromyalgia syndrome and, 389, 1499
pudendal neuralgia and, 1390
tension headache and, 716
Ammonium compounds in neurolytic blockade, 1983
Amniotic fluid, 1056
Amoxapine, 317
Amoxicillin
gonococcal arthritis and, 348
pelvic inflammatory disease versus, 1349
sinusitis and, 777
Amphetamine
cancer-related pain and, 423t, 425
postoperative pain and, 472
Amphiarthrodial joint, 329
Ampicillin
gonococcal arthritis and, 348
pelvic inflammatory disease versus, 1349
septic renal calculus and, 1242
sinusitis and, 777
tracheobronchitis and, 1050
Amplitude of response in nerve conduction study, 627, 628
Ampulla of Vater
pancreatitis and, 1223
postcholecystectomy pain and, 1221
Amputation, 244-256, 250t; *see also* Phantom limb pain; Stump pain
arteriosclerosis obliterans and, 509, 1631
cancer-related pain and, 407t, 409
digital
reflex sympathetic dystrophy and, 236
sympathectomy and, 2052
dorsal column stimulation and, 1864

dorsal root entry zone lesion and, 2078t, 2079
indications for, 1766-1767
lower extremity and, 1446t, *1629,* 1629-1630
malignancy and, 1767
neurectomy and, 2045
sympathetic nerve block and, 1934-1935
Amylase
abdominal examination and, 1166
gastric ulcer and, 1194
pancreatitis and, 1224
Amyloid, 217
Amyotrophy, 216
Anabolism in convalescence, 1823
Anal fissure, 1210-1211
differential diagnosis and, 1311t
Anal muscles and fascia, 1293-1294
Analgesia, 1640-1675
application principles and, 1667-1672, *1669, 1670,* 1670t, 1671t, 1672t
burn pain and, 484-488
cancer-related pain and, 421-422; *see also* Cancer pain
central pain and, 272
child and, 548t, 548-549
childbirth and, 1323-1326, *1324-1326,* 1332t
clinical pharmacology and, *1644,* 1644-1645
continuous; *see* Continuous analgesia
definition of, 20, 574
development of, 11
elderly patient and, 555
electrical stimulation and; *see* Electrical stimulation; Transcutaneous electrical nerve stimulation
epidural; *see* Epidural analgesia
first use of, 5
inhalation
burn patient and, 485
childbirth and, 1334
trauma and, 372
intrinsic, 117-119
measurement of, 589-591
migraine and, 711
muscle tension and, 388
muscles of mastication disorder and, 733t
narcotic; *see* Opioid analgesia
nerve block and; *see* Nerve block; Regional analgesia
nonopioid, 1660t, 1660-1667, 1661t
cancer-related pain and, 421-422
development of, 11
migraine and, 707, 710t, 712t
nonsteroidal; *see* Nonsteroidal anti-inflammatory drug
phantom limb pain and, 250
postoperative pain and, 472
stress-induced pain and, 117-118
nonulcer dyspepsia and, 1192
nutrition and, 1835
ocular pain and, 763
opioid; *see* Opioid analgesia
patient-controlled
burn pain and, 485
head and neck pain and, 804-805
intermittent porphyria and, 1294
mild to moderate pain and, 1669, *1669, 1670,* 1670t
nutrition and, 1825-1826
postoperative pain and, 471, 542
reflex spasm of quadriceps muscle and, 1574

Heparin *(Cont.)*
  intestinal ischemia and, 1260-1261
  livedoid vasculitis, 491, 492t
  pulmonary embolism and, 1058
  venous thrombosis and, 533
Hepatic artery, 1207
Hepatic disorder; *see* Liver
Hepatic flexure syndrome, 1182t
Hepatic plexus, *1158*, 1158-1159, *1159*
Hepatitis, 1214-1215
  differential diagnosis and, 1176t
Hepatization, red, 1052
Hepatobiliary disorder, 1220
Hepatocellular carcinoma, 1217
  differential diagnosis and, 1176t
Hepatoma, 1216-1217
  differential diagnosis and, 1176t
Hereditary disease; *see* Genetic disorder
Hernia
  Bochdalek, 1181t
  hiatal, 991t, 1078-1080, *1080*, 1189
    abdominal pain and, 1173t
Herniated disk, 1118-1119
  cervical, 267t
  cervicobrachial neuralgia and, 872
  low back pain and, 1469-1471
  patient history and, 1454
  postoperative muscle spasm and, 1387
Herniation
  compartment syndrome and, 381
  diaphragm and, 1265-1266
    differential diagnosis and, 1181t
  diverticulitis and, 1202-1203
  nucleus pulposus and
    cervicobrachial neuralgia and, 872, *872*
    lumbosacral neuralgia and, 1517-1518,
      1519
  phantom limb pain and, 245
Heroin
  cancer-related pain and, 426t, 428
  pharmacokinetics and
    pharmacodynamics and, 1648t
  systemic effects of, 1650t
Herpes simplex, 772
  esophageal pain and, 1070, 1072t
  genital, 1381
    differential diagnosis and, 1304t, 1308t
    treatment of, 1352
    urethritis and, 1376
    vulvovaginal infection and, 1351
  skin and, 495-496
Herpes zoster, 257-260, 258t, 260t, 772,
    1116-1118, *1117*
  abdominal pain and, 1277
  cancer and, 805
  cancer pain and, 409
  cervical neuralgia and, 853
  chest pain and, 1116-1118, *1117*
  dermatomes and, 134-135, *136*
  differential diagnosis and, 258
  ear and, 674t
  geniculate neuralgia and, 683
  incidence of, 257
  mononeuropathy and, 215
  pathology and, 257-258
  postherpetic neuralgia and; *see*
    Postherpetic neuralgia
  skin and, 495
  sympathetic nerve block and, 1938,
    1939t, 1940
  treatment of, 259-260
  trigeminal neuralgia and, 667-668t, 682
  uveitis and, 765
Hester Career Evaluation System, 646
Heterocyclic antidepressant, 317

administration techniques and, 1677-
    1679
  complex techniques and, 1684
  dosages and effects of, 1678t
  efficacy of, 1679
  indications for, 1676t
  side effects and complications and, 1679-
    1681
Hexamethylmelamine, 1798t
5-HIAA (5-Hydroxyindoleacetic acid), 312
Hiatal hernia, 1078-1080, *1080*
  differential diagnosis and, 991t
  paraesophageal, 1189
    abdominal pain and, 1173t
Hidradenitis suppurativa, 497, 1305t
  genital pain and, 1392, 1393
  perineum and external genitalia and,
    1311t
High-threshold mechanoreceptor, 33, 34
High-threshold polymodal C fiber, 95
Hill operation for sliding hiatus hernia,
    1079-1080
Hindfoot
  diagnostic tests for, 1607t
  differential diagnosis and, 1442t
  pes cavus and, 1613-1615
Hinge joint
  ankle and, 1591-1592
  elbow and, 893-894
Hip pain, 1530-1556
  anatomy and, 1530-1538, *1531-1537*
  arthrodesis and, 1764
  arthroplasty and
    muscle spasm and, 1622
    osteoarthritis and, 1551
    postoperative period and, 461, 467
  biomechanics and, 1538-1540
  classification of, 1530
  developmental disorder and, 1551
  differential diagnosis and, 1433-1435t
  epiphyseal disorder and, 1551-1552
  extra-articular disorder and, 1552-1554
  infection and inflammation and, 1548-
    1551
  metabolic and endocrine disorders and,
    1554-1555
  myofascial pain syndromes and, 357
  nerve supply of muscles to, 143t
  osteoarthritis and, 333, 1551
  patient evaluation and, 1540-1546, 1541t,
    1541-1545
  plexitis and, 215
  trauma and, 1546-1548
Hippocrates, 4
Hirschsprung's disease, 1208
Histamine, 700
Hitchcock apparatus, 2989-2090
HLA-B27
  inflammatory bowel disease and, 343
  Reiter's syndrome and, 341
Hodgkin's disease, 1795
Hollow foot, 1444t, 1613, *1613*
Home care
  nursing and, 1697
  terminal patient and, 449
Homogentisic acid oxidase deficiency, 335
Horizontal flexion test, 1127
Hormonal challenge in depression, 316
Hormonal disorder, 1183t
Hormone; *see also* Endocrine *entries*
  chronic dysmenorrhea and, 1356
  female sex, 1273
  female urethral syndrome and, 1377
  labor and, 1320-1322
  mastalgia and, 1138

stress-induced analgesia and, 118
Hormone therapy for cancer, 1800t, 1801-
    1802, 1836
  breast cancer and, 1094-1095
  palliative, 419, 420t
  prostatic cancer and, 1379
Horn
  dorsal
    anatomy and physiology and, 87-89
    causalgia and reflex sympathetic
      dystrophy and, 240
    medullary, 45-52, *45-52*, 104
    modulation and, 115, 116
    morphology of, 69-72
    peripheral neuropathies and, 213-214
    phantom limb pain and, 245, 248
    spinal, 45-52, *45-52*
    substance P and, *99*
    termination of primary afferent and,
      41-45
  ventral, 49
Horner's syndrome, 1097, 1097t
  cervicobrachial neuralgia and, 877
Horseradish peroxidase, 42
Horseshoe kidney, 1178t, 1238
Hospice, 447-448
  nursing and, 1698, 1698t
Hot dog headache, 707, 724
Hot pack, 1770-1771, *1771*
  quadratus lumborum syndrome and,
    1494
HPT (Hyperparathyroidism), 398, 1223
HRP (Horseradish peroxidase), 42
5-HT; *see* Serotonin
Huang Ti Nei Ching Su Wen, 3
Humeral head, 885
Humerus
  abduction and, 893
  elbow joint and, 894
  fracture and, 916-917
  radiography and, 920
Humoral circumflex artery, posterior, 835
Humors, 4
H-wave response, *627*, 629, 634
Hyaline cartilage, 961
Hydrocephalus, otitic, 774
Hydrocortisone
  Crohn's disease and, 1204
  esophageal chemical injury and, 1072
Hydrocortisone enema, 1205
Hydrogen peroxide, 757
Hydrolysis
  drug metabolism and, 1642t
  systemic analgesic and, 1641
Hydromorphone
  burn pain and, 484-485
  intraspinal injection and, 1974t
  pharmacokinetics and
    pharmacodynamics and, 1648t
  systemic effects of, 1650t
Hydronephrosis
  differential diagnosis and, 1179t
  intermittent, 1242
  pregnancy and, 1243
Hydrotherapy, 1771-1772
Hydroxurea, 1798t
Hydroxyapatite arthropathy, 344
Hydroxychloroquine, 339
Hydroxycortisone, 1800t
5-Hydroxyindoleacetic acid, 312
Hydroxyl radical, 612
Hydroxyprogesterone, 1800t
Hydroxyzine
  burn pain and, 487

Lateral compartmental syndrome, *380*
Lateral cord of brachial plexus, 826
Lateral costotransverse ligament, 963
Lateral cutaneous branch of intercostal
    nerve, 968-969, *969*
Lateral cutaneous nerve entrapment, 945
Lateral femoral cutaneous nerve, 1415
Lateral femoral cutaneous nerve block,
    1923, *1924*
    inguinal paravascular block and, 1924
Lateral femoral nerve entrapment, 1525,
    1525
Lateral gastrocnemius bursa, 1565
Lateral intercostal nerve block, 1915
Lateral ligament, temporomandibular joint
    and, 728
Lateral longitudinal arch of foot, 1598,
    1599
Lateral pectoral nerve, 891
Lateral plantar nerve, 1596
Lateral rotation
    arm and, 142t
    hip/thigh and, 143t
Lateral spinothalamic tract, 56
Lateral sympathetic trunk, 152
Lateral trapezoid ligament, 887
Latissimus dorsi muscle, 892
    anatomy of, 890
    bursa and, 890
Latissimus dorsi muscle syndrome, *1134*,
    1134-1135
Laxity of ankle, 1610
LCT (Liquid crystal thermography), 612,
    618
Lead poisoning, 1294
    differential diagnosis and, 1183t
Learned helplessness, 314
Learned pain, 291-299, 297t
    abdominal pain and, 1251
        differential diagnosis and, 1184t
    avoidance learning and, 296
    back pain and, 1509
    chest pain and, 999t, 1142
    chronic pain and, 189
    cognitive processing and, 294
    reinforcing consequences and, 295-296
    respondent and operant pain and, 292-
        293
    suffering and, 294-295
    superstitious learning and, 297
    treatment and, 298
Learning process, 126-127
Least thoracic splanchnic nerve, 972-973
Left gastric plexus, 1159
Left hypochondriac region pain, 1170
Left lower quadrant abscess, 1267
Left vagus nerve, 1155
Left ventricle, 1031
Leg; *see* Lower extremity
Leg brace, 1759
Leg raising, straight, 1456
Legal aspects of psychologic evaluation,
    600
Legg-Calvé-Perthes disease, 1435t, 1551-
    1552
Lemniscal trigeminothalamic pathway, *72*,
    73
Length of limb, *1542*, 1542-1543, *1544*
Leprosy
    peripheral mechanisms and, 184-185
    phantom limb pain and, 245
Leptomeningeal carcinomatosis, 406t
Leptomeningeal metastasis
    cervicobrachial neuralgia and, 870-871
    lumbosacral neuralgia and, 1516-1517

LES (Lower esophageal sphincter), 1067
Lesser cavernous nerve, 1292, 1371
Lesser occipital nerve
    cervical plexus and, 824, *824*
    ear and, 769
Lesser omentum, 1154
Lesser palatine nerve, 656
Lesser pelvis, 1283
Lesser sciatic foramen, 1286
Lesser splanchnic nerve, 972
LET (Linear energy transfer), 1791
Leukeran; *see* Chlorambucil
Leukocytoclastic vasculitis, 491-493, 492t
Leukotomy
    cancer-related pain and, 445
    prefrontal, 2096-2097
Leukotrine
    action of, 97
    pain mediation and, 96
Levator ani muscle, 1287
    coccygodynia and, 1384
Levator ani syndrome, 1498, *1498*
Levator muscle, pelvic pain and, 1359-1360
Levator scapulae muscle
    anatomy of, 889-890
    myofascial pain syndrome and, 948
    scapular movement and, 892
    trigger points of, *357*
Levator scapular syndrome, 859
Levatores costarum muscle, 964-965
Levine-Pilowsky Depression Questionnaire
    chronic pain and, 194
    psychiatric illness and, 325
Levo-Dromoran; *see* Levorphanol
Levopromazine, 710t
Levoprome; *see* Methotrimeprazine
Levorphanol
    cancer-related pain and, 426t, 427
    description of, 1657
    pharmacokinetics and
        pharmacodynamics and, 1648t
LHRH (Luteinizing hormone releasing
    hormone), 1379
Lichen planus, 755
Lidocaine
    brachial plexus block and, 1906
    chronic pancreatitis and, 1226
    continuous infusion of, 1948-1949
    hemorrhoids and, 1209
    ointment, 1202
    orchitis and, 1380
    pharmacology of, 1890t
    proctitis and, 1210
    ruptured intervertebral disk and, 1119
    septic renal calculus and, 1241
    topical application of, 1900
    trauma and, 372
    trigger point injection and, 363
        chest pain and, 1130
        head and facial pain and, 743
        neck and, 860, *860*
        upper extremity and, 948
Lifting injury, 1409, *1409*, 1502
Ligament
    accessory, of knee, *1563*, 1564
    acromioclavicular joint and, 887
    ankle and, 1592, 1593, *1594*, *1595*
    anterior longitudinal
        cervical spine and, 817
        lumbosacral spine and, 1397
        thoracic spine and, 1397
        whiplash and, 856
    back pain and, 1501-1508, *1502-1506*
    broad, 1289, *1289*, 1359
    calcaneonavicular, 1593

cervical, foot and, 1593
cervical spine and, *816*
    occipitovertebral, 816-817
    posterior longitudinal, 815-816, 817
collateral
    ankle and, 1592, 1593
    knee and, 1564, *1571*
coracoclavicular, 893
costotransverse, 963
elbow and, *895*
entrapment and, 842t
fingers and, *902*
flexor retinacula of wrist and, 899
foot and, 1598, *1599*
    biomechanics and, 1600
hip joint and, 1532-1533, *1533*
intercarpal, 898
interosseous, 1587
interspinous, 1857
    cervical spine and, 817
    dorsal column stimulation and, 1857
    lumbosacral spine and, 1400
    retraction of testicle and, 166-167
    thoracic, 176, 962
knee and, 1437t, *1563*, 1577-1578, *1578*
local anesthetic injection and, 1461
lumbar spine and
    movement and, 1407
    retraction of testicle and, 166-167
lumbosacral spine and, 1396, *1398*, 1400
nuchal, 850
palmar, 903
plantar, 1593
posterior longitudinal, 1401-1402
    cervical spine and, 815-816, 817
    meningeal nerves and, 1401-1402
    thoracic spine and, 962
pubic symphysis and, 1286
radiocarpal joint and, 897
reconstruction of, 1764, *1765*
round, 1344, 1345
sacroiliac, 1284-1285
shoulder girdle and arm and, 886t
sports injury and, 383-384
sprains and, 375-376
sternoclavicular joint and, 888
stylohyoid, 782
synovitis of hand and, 939
talocalcaneal interosseous, 1593
tarsal tunnel syndrome and, 1614-1615
tear of, 381-382
temporomandibular joint and, 728, 729
thermography and, 616
thoracic interspinous, 176
thorax and, 961-963, *963*
upper extremity and, 954
uterine
    broad, 1288-1289, *1289*, 1359
    round, 1344, 1345
vertebropelvic, 1285-1286, *1286*
wrist and, 900
Ligamenta flava
    calcification of, 864
    cervical spine and, 817
    lumbosacral spine and, 1400
    thoracic spine and, 962
Ligamentum nuchae, 817
Ligation
    hemorrhoids and, 1209
    inferior vena cava and, 1058
Light
    migraine and, 707
    ultraviolet keratitis and, 766
Limb; *see* Extremity; Lower extremity;
    Upper extremity